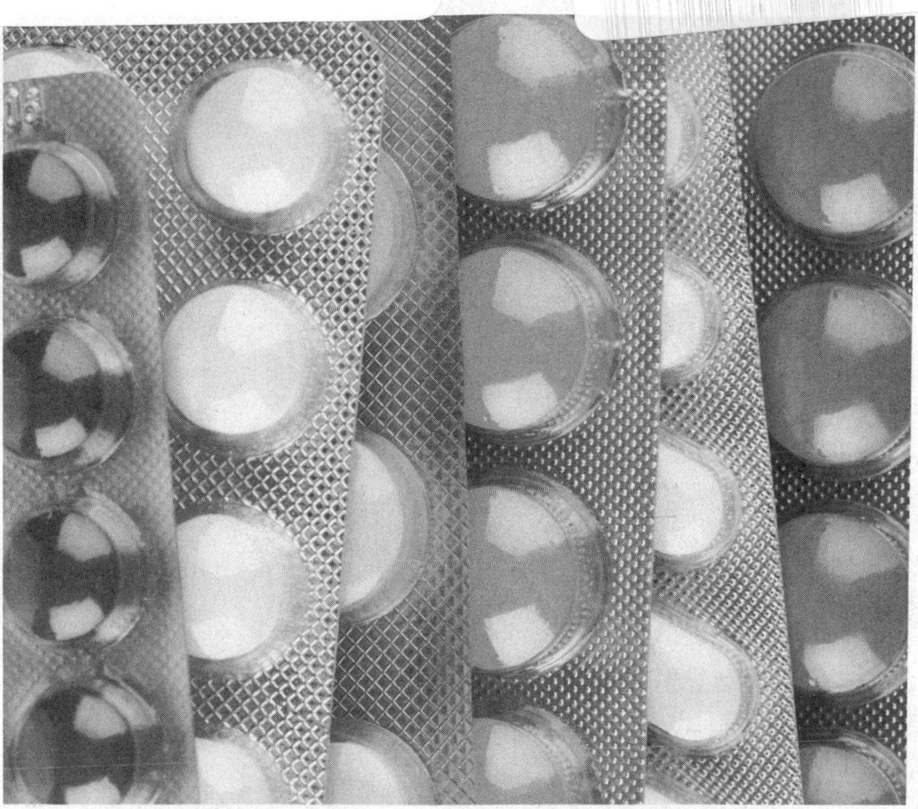

Philip D. Hansten ▪ John R. Horn

Drug Interactions
Analysis and Management
2012

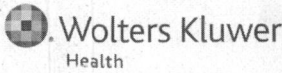 . Wolters Kluwer | Facts & Comparisons®
Health

Drug Interactions
Analysis and Management

AUTHORS

Philip D. Hansten, PharmD
University of Washington, Seattle

John R. Horn, PharmD
University of Washington, Seattle

FACTS AND COMPARISONS® PUBLISHING GROUP

Senior Director Content Development	Scot E. Walker, PharmD, MS, BCPS, BCACP
Senior Clinical Managers	Paul B. Johnson, RPh
	Cathy A. Meives, PharmD
Product Manager	Melissa Kennedy, PharmD, BCPS
President & CEO, Clinical Solutions	Arvind Subramanian, MBA
Acquisitions Manager	Angela J. Bush
Managing Editor	Sarah W. Gremillion
Senior Editors	Sharon M. McCarron
	Michelle M. Polley
	Sara L. Schwean
Associate Editor	Jennifer A. Besserman
Managing Editor, Quality Control	Susan H. Sunderman
Senior Quality Control Editor	Kirsten V. Ketner
Senior Composition Specialist	Beverly A. Donnell
Managing Technical Editor	Wendy L. Bell
Inventory Analyst	Barbara J. Hunter

Adapted from *Hansten and Horn's Drug Interactions Analysis and Management* loose-leaf information service through the January 2012 update.

ISBN 1-57439-342-1
ISBN 978-1-57439-342-2

Printed in the United States of America

Wolters Kluwer Health
77 Westport Plaza, Suite 450
St. Louis, Missouri 63146-3125
Phone 314/392-0000 • 800/223-0554
Fax 314/392-0160
www.factsandcomparisons.com

Drug Interactions
Analysis and Management

TABLE OF CONTENTS

Introduction

    Foreword   ix

    Preface   xi

    Instructions to Users   xiii

Principles and Mechanisms

    Pharmacokinetic Drug Interaction Mechanisms and Clinical Characteristics . . .   PM-1

    Mechanisms of Drug Interactions: Extrahepatic First-Pass Metabolism PM-33

    Cytochrome (CYP) P450 Isozyme Drug Interactions PM-37

Monographs   1

Index   1859

INTRODUCTION

INTRODUCTION

Drug Interactions
Analysis and Management

FOREWORD

Hansten and Horn's Drug Interaction Analysis and Management (DIAM) is researched and written by Philip D. Hansten, PharmD and John R. Horn, PharmD, both recognized as experts in the field of drug interactions. Because of their tireless pursuit, *DIAM* remains a trusted source of information. It is used in daily patient care and management of the patient's drug therapy. The drug interaction monographs are practical and concise. They are written and presented in a format allowing for in-depth evaluation as well as determining the proper course of action quickly and easily. Both of these features are important factors in today's health care environment.

Facts and Comparisons is pleased to provide health care professionals with quality publications such as *DIAM*. It is our intent to provide our subscribers with the most up-to-date information on drug interactions. However, we are constantly seeking ways to improve our publications so that Facts and Comparisons remains the most trusted source for drug information. Therefore, comments, suggestions, and criticisms are encouraged.

Drug Interactions
Analysis and Management

PREFACE

The first edition of this book went to press over 40 years ago. The first edition had but a few hundred drug-drug interactions, while this edition has expanded to include thousands. The title has also undergone inflation. The earlier edition, called simply *Drug Interactions*, has given way to *Drug Interactions Analysis and Management*. The addition of the latter words in the title reflects a change in emphasis from the earlier editions.

A critical "analysis" of drug interactions depends not only on assessment of the published drug interaction literature, but also on other factors such as the predictability of the interaction, the likelihood that the drugs will be used clinically in the same manner as they were in the published reports, and potential medicolegal considerations. We have taken these and other factors into consideration in our analysis of the clinical importance of the drug interactions described.

The "management" of drug interactions is emphasized in this book. Unlike adverse drug reactions to individual drugs, adverse drug *interactions* are almost completely preventable. Hence, we have devoted considerable effort to providing management options for each interaction. These options allow the health care provider to select one or more courses of action that are designed to reduce the likelihood that the patient will suffer an adverse consequence from the interaction.

We designed this book to be used by health care providers who prescribe, dispense, or administer medications. We have included both prescription and non-prescription medications, and increasingly, herbal remedies. Nonetheless, there are a few types of drug interactions that one is *not* likely to find in this book: drugs used primarily in the practice of anesthesiology, drugs of abuse, and some well-known and predictable pharmacodynamic interactions such as combinations of CNS depressants.

We would like to thank our students and colleagues for their many helpful suggestions on previous editions of this book. Special thanks go to Edward Hartshorn, PhD, who has shown an unflagging commitment to providing timely updates of the drug interaction literature for over a third of a century. We would also like to thank the Drug Interaction Foundation for the five-step classification system used in this book. The foundation has made this classification available to anyone who would like to use it, and many health care providers have found it to be a particularly useful system.

Philip D. Hansten, PharmD
John R. Horn, PharmD
Authors

Drug Interactions
Analysis and Management

INTRODUCTION

Instructions to Users

When first introduced in 1981, the monograph format of *Hansten and Horn's Drug Interactions Analysis and Management* was based on the author's evaluation of the interaction's clinical significance. The clinical significance was established by considering the potential harm to the patient and the degree of documentation available. Each interaction was assigned to one of three classes: Major, Moderate, or Minor. While this classification system has been adapted by many other providers of drug interaction information, the authors became increasingly dissatisfied with the utility of this system. By emphasizing the "clinical significance" of an interaction, the format did not focus on the most important aspect of drug interaction assessment: **prevention of patient harm**.

Knowing the clinical significance of an interaction provides only minimal information for selection of appropriate management strategies for a particular patient. Thus, we have revised the format of the monographs to emphasize the management options available for a patient receiving an interacting pair of drugs. This change enables the reader to quickly select one or more appropriate standardized management options. These options still are based, in part, on the severity of the potential interaction outcomes, but other factors such as the availability of alternative, noninteracting drugs also contribute. The goal of each monograph is to provide the reader with information necessary to assess the degree of risk to the patient, and to prevent an adverse outcome as a result of exposure to the interacting drugs.

Interacting drugs are assigned to one of five classes based on the intervention needed to minimize the risk of the interaction. This classification system originally was developed by the Drug Interaction Foundation. The interactions are assigned the following Significance numbers:

1 = **Avoid Combination.** Risk always outweighs benefit.

2 = **Usually Avoid Combination.** Use combination only under special circumstances.

3 = **Minimize Risk.** Take action as necessary to reduce risk.

4 = **No Action Needed.** Risk of adverse outcomes appears small.

5 = **No Interaction.** Evidence suggests no interaction.

The goal of *Hansten and Horn's Drug Interactions Analysis and Management* is not simply to provide the reader with an abstract of reported interactions, rather to provide the authors' analysis of each interaction and its implication to the patient. The purpose of each of the monograph sections is detailed below.

Summary provides a concise description of the potential outcome of the interaction and its clinical significance.

Risk Factors outlines patient or drug specific factors that have been identified as contributing to the magnitude or severity of the interaction. Obvious factors that apply universally are not listed. For example, virtually all drug interactions are dose dependent, or more precisely, dependent on the concentration of the precipitant drug at the site of the interaction. The larger dose or the higher the concentration of the precipitant drug, the greater the magnitude of the interaction and the larger the risk that an adverse outcome may result. If the literature provides specific data on dose- or concentration-effect relationships, they are included here.

Mechanism provides the mechanism currently thought to be responsible for the interaction. It includes both pharmacokinetic and pharmacodynamic mechanisms. Please refer to the *primary literature* cited within the Reference section for more detailed information than presented here.

Clinical Evaluation focuses on the authors' evaluation of the interaction. It includes specific details such as dose, route of administration, or time course of the interaction as necessary for clarity and understanding. The authors do not attempt to cite every report of an interaction: in many cases they are simply redundant. The cited reports bring new understanding of an interaction's mechanism or help explain its variable outcomes.

Related Drugs cites examples of closely related agents that would be expected to interact in a similar manner as the monograph agents. Related drugs usually are confined to the chemical class as those in the monograph that have similar pharmacokinetic or pharmacodynamic interaction potential. This listing aids in selecting alternative therapy by noting those drugs that should be eliminated from consideration as alternatives. Prediction of potential interactions that are as yet undocumented are simplified by consulting this section. When specific data are available, related drugs also appear in individual monographs.

Management Options includes different options for patient management based on the actions necessary to avoid patient harm. These management options are placed into five classifications that assist the reader in eliminating or minimizing the risk to the patient. Each drug interaction in the Index identifies the management class to which it has been assigned.

Class 1 Interactions. Avoid administration of the drug combination. The risk of adverse patient outcome precludes the concomitant administration of the drugs.

Class 2 Interactions. Should avoid administration unless it is determined that the benefit of coadministration of the drugs outweighs the risk to the patient. The use of an alternative to one of the interacting drugs is recommended when appropriate. Patients should be monitored carefully if the drugs are coadministered.

Class 3 Interactions. Several potential management options are available for class 3 interactions. When an alternative agent should be considered, examples of documented noninteracting drugs are provided. Changes in drug dosage or route of administration that can circumvent or minimize the potential interaction are suggested. Again, patient monitoring is suggested in case the interacting drugs are administered.

Class 4 Interactions. Include interactions where the potential for patient harm is low and no specific action is required other than to be aware of the possibility of the drug interaction.

Class 5 Interactions. Include combinations of drugs for which the available evidence suggests no interaction.

References will contain pertinent citations that provide meaningful insight for the interaction.

Monographs are organized alphabetically and both interacting drugs are placed in the Index. All drugs are listed by generic name and not pharmacological class except combination products like antacids that are listed under Antacids as well as brand name. The few exceptions are, from the standpoint of drug interactions, homogenous (eg, thyroid, oral contraceptives, and thiazides) where interactions apply equally to all members of the class.

The monograph profiling the drug interaction between Rifampin and Tamoxifen that follows illustrates the organization and format used throughout *Hansten and Horn's Drug Interactions Analysis and Management.* Your comments and suggestions are welcome.

Rifampin (eg, *Rifadin*)

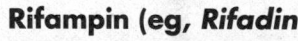

Tamoxifen

SUMMARY: Rifampin administration markedly reduces tamoxifen plasma concentrations; loss of tamoxifen's antiestrogenic effect is likely.

RISK FACTORS: No specific risk factors are known.

MECHANISM: Rifampin is known to induce the activity of CYP3A4, the isozyme that metabolizes tamoxifen. Rifampin appears to increase the first-pass and systemic clearance of tamoxifen.

CLINICAL EVALUATION: Ten healthy subjects took either rifampin 600 mg or placebo daily for 5 days.[1] On day 6, a single oral dose of tamoxifen 80 mg was administered 17 hours after the last rifampin dose. The administration of rifampin reduced the area under the plasma concentration-time curve (AUC) of tamoxifen 86% and its peak concentration 55%. The half-life of tamoxifen was reduced from 118 to 68 hours following rifampin dosing. Rifampin increased the metabolism of toremifene (*Fareston*), a derivative of tamoxifen, by a similar amount (87% reduction in AUC). The effect of long-term rifampin therapy on tamoxifen is unknown, but the magnitude of the interaction may be greater than that observed in this study.

RELATED DRUGS: Rifabutin (*Mycobutin*) is likely to affect tamoxifen and toremifene metabolism similarly.

MANAGEMENT OPTIONS:

➡ *Monitor.* Monitor patients taking tamoxifen for loss of efficacy if rifampin is coadministered. The dosage of tamoxifen may need to be increased.

REFERENCES:

1. Kivistö KT, et al. Tamoxifen and toremifene concentrations in plasma are greatly decreased by rifampin. *Clin Pharmacol Ther.* 1998;64(6):648-654.

PRINCIPLES AND MECHANISMS

Pharmacokinetic Drug Interaction Mechanisms and Clinical Characteristics

The administration of more than one drug is a frequent occurrence, and the probability of a drug interaction increases with the number of drugs a patient is taking. The same pharmacokinetic and pharmacodynamic principles that determine the behavior of drugs in the body can be applied to drug interactions. The absorption, distribution, or elimination of one drug can be altered by another. Additionally, the pharmacodynamics of an agent may be altered independently from changes in its pharmacokinetics. An understanding of these basic principles as they apply to drug interactions enhances the ability to predict possible outcomes resulting from the coadministration of two drugs known, or suspected, to interact. Likewise, knowledge of the various mechanisms of drug interactions is helpful in understanding how to avoid the adverse effects of drug interactions. This chapter reviews the basic information regarding common properties and mechanisms of drug-drug interactions.

THE TIME COURSE OF DRUG INTERACTIONS

The time course of drug interactions can vary dramatically; some interactions occur in a matter of seconds or minutes, while others develop over several weeks. When considering the time course of drug interactions, there are several time points that are of clinical interest:

- Time of onset of the interaction (when the interaction first becomes detectable).
- Time for maximal pharmacokinetic or pharmacodynamic effect of the interaction.
- Time that the patient experiences an adverse response to the interaction.
- Time required for the dissipation of the interaction.

For some drug interactions, clinical information is available on one or more of these time points, such as the time of onset, maximal pharmacokinetic or pharmacodynamic effect, and dissipation. Although the time that the patient will experience an adverse effect from an interaction is more difficult to predict, one often can estimate the time of maximal risk and take appropriate precautions.

Estimates of the time course of drug interactions in specific patients are just that—estimates. Even though the time course for an interaction may be relatively consistent in a group of similar patients, some patients, for unknown reasons, will develop the interaction much more quickly or slowly than others.

Importance of Considering Time Course

Estimating the time course of a drug interaction in a given patient can help the clinician minimize the likelihood of an adverse effect from the interaction and reduce the costs of monitoring for the interaction.

Patient Monitoring. Knowledge of the time course allows the clinician to select the most appropriate times to monitor the interaction. For example, assume a patient receiving warfarin (eg, *Coumadin*) is started on a drug that gradually increases the hypoprothrombinemic response over several weeks. It probably would be sufficient to obtain prothrombin times no more often than every 4 or 5 days to prevent excessive hypoprothrombinemia. On the other hand, if a drug rapidly increases the hypoprothrombinemic response to warfarin, the prothrombin time should be monitored more frequently.

Assessing Clinical Importance. Knowledge of the time course of an interaction may allow the clinician to estimate the clinical importance of an interaction in a given patient. For example, nonsteroidal anti-inflammatory drugs (NSAIDs) are known to gradually reduce the effect of a variety of antihypertensive drugs over a period of 1 to 2 weeks.[1] Thus, the short-term administration of an NSAID to treat dysmenorrhea or headache is unlikely to adversely affect blood pressure control in a clinically important way. Similarly, use of the enzyme inducer rifampin (eg, *Rifadin*) for 2 days (eg, prophylaxis of bacterial meningitis) is unlikely to stimulate the metabolism of other drugs sufficiently to reduce the desired therapeutic effect. This is because enzyme induction is a gradual process that generally takes several days to a week or more to maximally reduce the effect of a drug.

Discovering New Interactions. When performing clinical research, it is important to study a drug interaction over a sufficient time period to minimize the likelihood of false-negative conclusions. For example, in early studies, tricyclic antidepressants (TCAs) were not observed to alter the antihypertensive response of guanethidine (*Ismelin*). The drug interaction was not detected because these studies were performed over a period of hours. When the period of study was extended, the interaction was found to take 1 or 2 days to develop, and the TCAs were noted to substantially inhibit the antihypertensive response to guanethidine.[2]

Determinants of Time Course

Numerous factors can affect the time course of drug interactions, and it often is necessary to consider several when estimating the time course of a given interaction in a particular patient.

Half-Lives of Drugs Involved. The half-life of the *precipitant drug* (ie, drug that causes the altered action of the other drug) can be an important consideration because the half-life dictates the time course of the precipitant drug's accumulation to steady state. If it takes a long period of time for the precipitant drug to reach a plateau level, the interaction may be delayed. For example, when phenobarbital therapy is started, it generally takes approximately 1 week to reach steady-state serum phenobarbital concentrations. Thus, the maximal interactive effects of phenobarbital would not be expected during the first few days of therapy. Similarly, the discontinuation of phenobarbital tends to result in a gradual dissipation of its interactions at least in part because the serum concentrations of phenobarbital gradually decline over approximately 1 week.

The half-life of the *object drug* (ie, drug whose action is altered by the interaction) is also an important determinant. As an example, consider what happens when cimetidine (eg, *Tagamet*) is added to the chronic therapy of a patient receiving either theophylline (eg, *Theolair*) or warfarin. Since theophylline has a relatively short half-life, patients receiving theophylline will usually manifest the new increased steady-state serum theophylline concentrations a few days after starting cimetidine.[3] On the other hand, when cimetidine is added to the therapy of a patient stabilized on warfarin, serum warfarin concentrations will increase over 1 week or more.[4] When estimating how long it will take for an object drug to reach a new plateau level in these situations, remember it is the *new* half-life that has been prolonged (or reduced) by the precipitant drug that must be considered. Thus, it typically takes more time (or less time) for the new steady-state serum concentrations to be achieved than might be expected from an average half-life value in the population at large.

Drug Dosage. The dosage of the object drug can influence the time course of an interaction. For example, if a patient is receiving a large dose of an object drug and the serum concentration of that drug is at the upper end of the therapeutic range, it may take only a short time for the serum concentration to rise into the toxic range following administration of another drug that inhibits the elimination of the object drug. Conversely, when a patient is receiving a low dose of the same object drug or when this patient has a serum concentration that is in the low therapeutic or subtherapeutic range, it will take more time for the serum concentration to rise to the toxic range (if it gets there at all) following the administration of a drug that inhibits its elimination.

In general, larger doses of a precipitant drug would result in a somewhat more rapid onset of the interaction since the serum concentration necessary to produce the interaction may be achieved more rapidly. Similarly, it may take longer for the interaction to dissipate after discontinuation of large doses of the precipitant drug because it may take longer for the serum concentration of the precipitant drug to drop below the threshold level required for the interaction.

Routes of Administration. Routes of administration that rapidly achieve therapeutic serum concentrations of interacting drugs will tend to result in more rapid development of drug interactions. For example, in a patient receiving a CNS depressant, the IV administration of an additional CNS depressant is likely to more rapidly affect the patient than if the second agent is given orally.

Drug Metabolites. If it is the metabolite rather than the parent form of the precipitant drug that is involved in the interaction, it may take longer than expected for the interaction to occur. For example, there is some evidence that a metabolite of erythromycin (eg, *E-Mycin*), rather than erythromycin itself, is responsible for the inhibition of theophylline metabolism in patients taking the combination.[5] It would be expected that adding an inhibitor of hepatic metabolism such as erythromycin to theophylline therapy would significantly increase serum theophylline concentrations within 2 or 3 days of starting the erythromycin. However, in most patients, increases in serum theophylline caused by erythromycin are delayed by at least 5 days. This may reflect the time required for the erythromycin metabolite to be produced and to accumulate in the serum until there is a sufficient concentration to inhibit the hepatic metabolism of theophylline.

The metabolites of object drugs also may affect the time course of drug interactions, particularly if active metabolites are involved. For example, cimetidine inhibits the hepatic metabolism of diazepam (eg, *Valium*) and its active metabolite, desmethyldiazepam.[6] Thus, in estimating the lag time before the maximal effects of the interaction are seen, consider not only the half-life of diazepam, but also its active metabolite. Accordingly, the dissipation of this interaction following discontinuation of cimetidine is dependent upon the half-life of both the parent drug and active metabolite.

Dose-Dependent Pharmacokinetics. Consider dose-dependent pharmacokinetics when estimating the time course of drug interactions. When the elimination of an object drug is dose dependent, the addition of a drug that reduces its elimination can increase the serum concentrations of the object drug into the zero order range. As a consequence, the increased half-life of the object drug can result in serum concentrations that increase over a longer time period than would be expected on the basis of its "normal" half-life. For example, isoniazid (INH; *Nydrazid*) inhibits the hepatic metabolism of phenytoin (eg, *Dilantin*), a drug that displays dose-dependent pharmacokinetics.[7] When INH is added to phenytoin therapy, the serum phenytoin concentration can be increased into the range where its half-life is prolonged, and the serum phenytoin concentrations can increase steadily over a period of several weeks.

Effect of Drug Interaction Mechanisms on Time Course

Knowledge of the mechanism for a given drug interaction is useful in estimating the likely time course, but it is important to realize that the mechanism must be considered in concert with the other determinants discussed above.

GI Absorption Interactions. When a precipitant drug binds with or otherwise inhibits the GI absorption of an object drug, the serum concentration of the object drug usually will *begin* to decrease within hours of concurrent use of the 2 drugs. This situation is like lowering the dose of the object drug. However, the rate of decline of the serum concentration of the object drug depends upon its half-life.

Some drugs may interfere with the enterohepatic circulation of an object drug. When the object drug is excreted into the GI tract, the precipitant drug can bind to it and prevent its reabsorption back into the systemic circulation. The bound object drug then is excreted in the feces, thus effectively shortening its half-life. An example of this mechanism would be the concurrent administration of warfarin and cholestyramine (eg, *Questran*). The half-life of warfarin is shortened by oral cholestyramine even if the warfarin is given IV. Thus, a new steady-state serum concentration of warfarin will be achieved more rapidly than might be expected given the "normal" half-life of warfarin.

Plasma Protein-Binding Interactions. When one drug displaces another drug from plasma protein-binding sites, the free serum concentration of the displaced drug increases, and its pharmacologic effect tends to increase. However, the unbound fraction of the drug is not only more available to sites of action but also is more readily eliminated. Thus, protein-binding displacement interactions tend to be self-correcting with time. Typically, the pharmacologic activity of the displaced drug initially is increased for several days or more, depending upon the pharmacokinetics of the displaced drug. This period is followed by a return of the pharmacologic response back to "normal" (ie, the unbound serum concentration of the object drug returns to that seen before administration of the displacing drug) even if the patient is continued on therapy with both drugs. Thus, if the patient does not manifest an adverse response from the interaction during the first week or so of administration of the displacing drug, an adverse effect probably will not occur even if the patient chronically receives both drugs in a constant dose.

Enzyme-Induction Interactions. Enzyme inducers stimulate the metabolism of other drugs gradually, primarily because enzyme induction results in the synthesis of new drug metabolizing enzymes. Although the initial effects of an enzyme inducer may be detected within the first 2 days of concurrent therapy, it generally takes at least 1 week before the effects of maximal enzyme induction are manifested. However, the onset of enzyme induction also depends upon the half-life of the inducing agent. For example, an enzyme inducer, such as rifampin, with a relatively short half-life will reach steady-state serum concentrations rather quickly; thus, rifampin would induce drug metabolizing enzymes more rapidly than phenobarbital because more than a week would be required to reach plateau phenobarbital serum concentrations. Clinical studies substantiate that rifampin induces enzymes more rapidly than inducers with longer half-lives. The dissipation of enzyme induction after discontinuation of an enzyme inducer also occurs gradually because of dependence upon both the elimination of the inducing agent from the body and the gradual decay of the enhanced enzymatic activity in the liver. Thus, an enzyme-inducing agent with a long half-life, such as phenobarbital, probably sustains enzyme induction for several days after it is discontinued; this is followed by the gradual decay of the increased enzyme stores. For this reason, phenobarbital-induced enzyme induction may still be detectable 2 weeks or longer after the discontinuation of phenobarbital.

Enzyme-Inhibition Interactions. Inhibition of hepatic drug metabolism tends to begin as soon as sufficient concentrations of the inhibitor appear in the liver (usually within hours), and inhibition of metabolism of the object drug is usually maximal within the first 24 hours of administration of the inhibitor. Although the effect of enzyme inhibitors develops rapidly, the time required to reach a new steady-state serum concentration or toxicity of the object drug is dependent upon a variety of factors. These include the following: 1) the new (prolonged) half-life of the object drug; 2) its pre-existing serum concentration; 3) whether or not it displays concentration-dependent pharmacokinetics; and 4) the patient's susceptibility because of disease, organ malfunction, or other response modifiers. Enzyme inhibition generally dissipates more rapidly than enzyme induction.

Renal Excretion Interactions. Renal excretion interactions, like interactions involving enzyme inhibition, are generally of a competitive type. Thus, they tend to begin as soon as sufficient concentrations of the 2 drugs appear in the kidney (ie, usually within hours of administration of the second drug). These interactions tend to have a fairly rapid onset; however, the time until a new steady state is reached or until drug toxicity appears depends upon a variety of factors (see Enzyme-Inhibition Interactions). Because renal excretion interactions are generally competitive, discontinuation of one of the drugs results in fairly rapid dissipation of the interaction. After 2 or 3 half-lives of the discontinued drug have passed, the effect on the elimination of the object drug is usually minimal.

Pharmacodynamic Interactions. These interactions often involve additive or antagonistic pharmacologic effects and are usually rapid in onset. For example, when drug combinations result in additive hypotensive or sedative effects, the interaction can be detected as soon as the pharmacologic effect of the second drug is manifest. Nevertheless, some pharmacodynamic interactions take place more slowly. For example, the inhibitory effect of TCAs on the antihypertensive response to guanethidine takes place over several days; and when NSAIDs are added to patients stabilized on an antihypertensive drug regimen, the blood pressure may increase gradually over a period of weeks. Thus, simple additive or antagonistic pharmacodynamic drug interactions tend to occur rapidly, and the time course is more predictable; while the time course of at least some of the more complex pharmacodynamic interactions develops over a more prolonged period.

Summary

The time course for the onset and offset of drug interactions varies considerably from one drug interaction to another. The same drug interaction also can have a different time course depending on the way in which the drugs are used and the patient. Based upon clinical studies and theoretical principles, the likely time course of an interaction in a specific patient often can be estimated. Such estimates are important in determining the risk of the interaction in a particular patient and in the design of the safest and most cost-effective schedule for monitoring the effects of an interaction.

DRUG INTERACTIONS DURING ABSORPTION FROM THE GI TRACT

The absorption of orally administered drugs from the GI tract is a complex process and is subject to many sources of variability. One cause of the variation in response to orally administered drugs is the concomitant administration of drugs that are capable of affecting the absorption process.

GI Absorption: General Principles

Dissolution. When a solid dosage form such as a tablet is administered orally, it disintegrates into progressively smaller particles. This disintegration process is important for optimal absorption, since the smaller the particles, the more rapidly the drug goes into solution. Drugs must be in solution before they are capable of crossing the intestinal epithelium and entering the bloodstream.

Sites of Absorption. The small intestine is the primary site from which orally administered drugs are absorbed; few drugs are absorbed to any significant extent from the stomach.[26,27] There are several reasons for this finding. The intestine has an absorptive area approximately 200 times greater than that of the stomach. In addition, the intestinal epithelium is much more permeable to drugs than is the stomach. Moreover, total blood flow through the intestinal capillaries is considerably greater than the stomach. In short, the intestine is an organ designed for absorption while the stomach is not. Thus, the stomach can be considered a reservoir from which drugs are released in increments to the small intestine for absorption.

Rate vs Extent of Absorption. For most chronically administered drugs, the *rate* of absorption from the GI tract is of little clinical importance as long as there is no alteration in the *extent* of drug absorption. When the extent of absorption is unaffected, the mean steady-state plasma concentration (and the pharmacologic response) will remain the same. Accordingly, when evaluating the literature on GI absorption interactions of drugs administered chronically, it is important to determine whether the study was performed in such a way that the *extent* of absorption was assessed. Although alterations in absorption rate tend to be unimportant for chronically administered drugs, effects on absorption rate can be clinically important when a drug is being used for an acute effect (eg, analgesics or hypnotics).

Mechanisms of GI Absorption Drug Interactions

There are several mechanisms by which one drug may affect the GI absorption of another:

- Drug binding in the GI tract.
- Alterations in GI motility.
- Alterations in GI pH.
- Alterations in intestinal flora.
- Alterations in drug metabolism within the wall of the intestine.

Nevertheless, for many GI absorption interactions, the exact mechanism is not established.

Drug Binding in the GI Tract. Drug binding in the GI tract occurs through a variety of mechanisms. Some agents with a large surface area can adsorb other drugs onto their surfaces, thus preventing passage of the drug across the wall of the intestine. Examples of agents that may interfere with drug absorption by this mechanism include activated charcoal and, possibly kaolin-pectin and antacids. In the case of charcoal, this property is used to advantage in the treatment of drug overdose; when unintended, however, such binding may reduce the therapeutic response to the affected drug.

Other agents are capable of forming insoluble (and thus nonabsorbable) complexes or chelates with drugs. For example, iron salts substantially inhibit the GI absorption of several tetracyclines,[28] methyldopa (eg, *Aldomet*),[29] and levodopa (eg, *Larodopa*),[30] probably by producing such complexes. This mechanism appears to be responsible for the ability of both antacids and sucralfate (eg, *Carafate*) to reduce the GI absorption of quinolones (eg, norfloxacin [*Noroxin*] and ciprofloxacin [*Cipro*]).[31,32]

Binding resins such as cholestyramine and colestipol (*Colestid*) bind not only bile salts in the intestine, but several drugs as well. For example, the GI absorption of thyroxine, warfarin, and thiazide diuretics may be inhibited by such binding resins.[33-35]

Alterations in GI Motility. As mentioned previously, orally administered drugs are generally not well absorbed before reaching the small intestine; thus, gastric emptying is an important determinant of drug absorption rate. Acetaminophen (eg, *Tylenol*) is a good example of a drug whose absorption rate is affected by other drugs that affect GI motility. Pretreatment with the anticholinergic agent, propantheline (eg, *Pro-Banthine*), slows gastric emptying and delays the absorption of orally administered acetaminophen. Conversely, pretreatment with metoclopramide (eg, *Reglan*) speeds gastric emptying, thereby hastening the absorption of acetaminophen.[36]

Although the absorption *rate* of many drugs is likely to be affected by alterations in GI motility, there are relatively few examples of changes in extent of absorption as a result of this mechanism. One situation where changes in *extent* of absorption may occur due to effects on GI motility involves drugs that do not dissolve well in GI fluids. In this situation, slowing GI motility may allow more of the drug to dissolve before reaching the absorption sites in the small bowel, thus increasing bioavailability. Conversely, speeding GI motility would have the opposite effect on dissolution, thus reducing the extent of absorption. For example, the bioavailability of one digoxin tablet formulation (not *Lanoxin*) was enhanced by treatment with propantheline and reduced by treatment with metoclopramide.[37] Propantheline also increases the extent of absorption of nitrofurantoin (*Furadantin*), another drug that is poorly soluble in the GI tract.[38]

Another situation in which alteration of GI motility may affect the extent of absorption involves drugs that are degraded to inactive products in the stomach. Here, a slowing of gastric emptying would tend to allow more of the drug to be inactivated before reaching the absorbing areas in the small intestine, while speeding gastric emptying would deliver more intact drug to the intestine for absorption. A possible example of this phenomenon involves levodopa, where speeding gastric emptying with an antacid was associated with enhanced levodopa bioavailability.[39]

Alteration in GI pH. Many drugs are weak acids or weak bases, and it is their nonionized (more lipid-soluble) form that can traverse the intestinal membranes into the bloodstream. Thus, drugs that are weak acids theoretically would be better absorbed in an acidic medium because a greater proportion of the drug would be present in its more lipid-soluble form. The opposite would be true for weak bases. On the other hand, weak acids do not *dissolve* as well in an acidic medium, and dissolution is a prerequisite to absorption. Moreover, some drugs manifest pH-dependent degradation to inactive products in the GI tract. In addition, the pH of the GI tract may affect GI motility as well as other determinants of drug absorption. Thus, the effect of GI pH on drug absorption can be complex, and it often is difficult to predict what effect pH changes will have on the absorption of a given drug.

The importance of pH on drug dissolution can be seen with ketoconazole (eg, *Nizoral*), which requires an acidic medium in order to dissolve adequately for absorption.[40] Thus, the administration of H_2-antagonists, proton pump inhibitors, or antacids, by increasing gastric pH, may markedly reduce the bioavailability of ketoconazole.

Drugs that are degraded by gastric acid or are particularly irritating to the gastric mucosa sometimes are formulated in an enteric-coated product. Enteric-coated drugs are designed to remain intact in the stomach and release the drug from the dosage form after reaching the more alkaline small intestine. Theoretically, concurrent administration of an antacid and a drug with a pH-dependent enteric coating would result in premature release of the drug. Indeed, enteric-coated aspirin does appear to be absorbed more rapidly when combined with antacids.[41] Nevertheless, few other examples of this type of interaction have been demonstrated in humans, and their clinical importance is not established.

Effects on Intestinal Flora. Although bacterial flora are present in large numbers in the large bowel, the stomach, duodenum, jejunum, and upper ileum normally contain relatively few bacteria.[42] Thus, drugs that are well absorbed from the small bowel would have little opportunity to be affected by changes in GI tract flora. Accordingly, drugs that have been shown to be affected by the bacteria in the intestine tend to be those that are incompletely absorbed in the small intestine or those drugs that are secreted back into the intestine after absorption.

Digoxin (eg, *Lanoxin*) absorption can be affected by alterations in intestinal flora in certain patients. In most patients, degradation of digoxin by intestinal bacteria has little effect on plasma digoxin concentrations. The administration of an antibiotic such as erythromycin may substantially increase plasma digoxin concentrations due to reduced bacterial inactivation of digoxin; however, the major mechanism of the erythromycin/digoxin interaction is inhibition of P-glycoprotein by erythromycin.[43]

Alterations in bacterial flora also may be involved in the controversial interaction between oral contraceptives and oral antibiotic therapy. Numerous cases of unintended pregnancy have occurred in women on oral contraceptives who have received oral antibiotics such as ampicillin (eg, *Principen*) and tetracycline, but conclusive proof of the interaction is lacking.[44] The mechanism proposed for this interaction is as follows: Estrogens from the oral contraceptive are conjugated in the liver and are secreted into the intestine via the bile. Normally bacteria in the intestine hydrolyze the conjugated estrogen, yielding free estrogen that can be reabsorbed back into the bloodstream. Thus, the bacteria help maintain the plasma estrogen concentration at a level sufficient to prevent conception. Antibiotics can reduce the numbers of intestinal bacteria, and thereby interrupt the enterohepatic circulation of the estrogen, resulting in increased fecal excretion of estrogen and reduced plasma estrogen concentration. Menstrual irregularities and unintended pregnancies can result because of these alterations in estrogen metabolism.

Drug Metabolism within the Intestinal Wall. Most drugs have been thought to pass through the wall of the intestine with little or no metabolic alteration. Nevertheless, most research on drug metabolism is not designed to differentiate between metabolism in the GI wall vs the liver. Thus, there may be more drug metabolism within the intestinal wall than is commonly appreciated. Several types of metabolism are known to occur in the wall of the intestine (eg, sulfation, glucuronidation, cytochrome P450 oxidation, monoamine oxidation).[45]

Monoamine oxidase in the GI wall helps protect the body against tyramine in foods and against some pressor amines, such as phenylephrine.[46] Thus, monoamine oxidase inhibitors (MAOIs) may predispose patients to hypertensive reactions when the pressor substance is metabolized by intestinal wall monoamine oxidase. (Note: indirect-acting sympathomimetics, such as amphetamines and phenylpropanolamine, interact with MAOIs via a different mechanism).

Ethinyl estradiol, an estrogen found in many oral contraceptives, is sulfated in the intestinal wall. Ascorbic acid 1 g orally increases the plasma concentrations of ethinyl estradiol in women receiving low-dose oral contraceptives, possibly by interfering with the sulfation of ethinyl estradiol in the intestinal wall.[47,48] The clinical implications of this interaction are not clear, but intermittent use of ascorbic acid in women on oral contraceptives might result in fluctuating plasma concentrations of estrogen.

Cimetidine inhibits the hepatic metabolism of a variety of drugs, including alcohol. In one study, cimetidine inhibited the elimination of orally administered alcohol but did not affect the disposition of alcohol administered IV.[49] These findings were consistent with the authors' contention that cimetidine interfered with the metabolism of alcohol in the GI wall.

How to Avoid GI Absorption Drug Interactions

When a patient is receiving two drugs that potentially interact with each other in the GI tract, it may be necessary to take action to prevent the unwanted effects of the interaction. However, as seen in the following discussion, separating the doses of the interacting drugs may not always circumvent the interaction (see Table 1 for a listing of GI absorption drug interactions).

TABLE 1. GI Absorption Drug Interactions

Mechanism:	Precipitant Drug(s)[1]	Object Drug(s)[2]	Effect(s)
Adsorption	Charcoal, antacids, kaolin-pectin	Numerous drugs	↓ absorption of object drug
		Digoxin	↓ bioavailability of digoxin
		Lincomycin	↓ bioavailability of lincomycin
Complexation or chelation	Iron, antacids	Tetracyclines, methyldopa, levodopa	↓ bioavailability of object drugs
		Quinolones	↓ bioavailability of ciprofloxacin, norfloxacin
Resin binding	Cholestyramine, colestipol	Thyroxine, warfarin, thiazides	↓ bioavailability of object drugs
↓ GI motility	Anticholinergics, opiates, aluminum hydroxide	Nitrofurantoin, digoxin tablets (some)	↑ bioavailability of object drugs due to enhanced dissolution
		Levodopa, chlorpromazine	↓ bioavailability of object drug
↑ GI motility	Metoclopramide, laxatives	Digoxin tablets (some), nitrofurantoin	↓ bioavailability of object drug

TABLE 1. GI Absorption Drug Interactions

Mechanism:	Precipitant Drug(s)[1]	Object Drug(s)[2]	Effect(s)
↑ Gastric pH	H₂-antagonists, antacids	Ketoconazole	↓ bioavailability of ketoconazole due to ↓ dissolution
	Proton pump inhibitors	Enteric-coated drugs	Premature dissolution of enteric coating
↓ Intestinal flora	Antibiotics (eg, ampicillin, tetracycline)	Digoxin	↓ bacterial destruction of digoxin in GI tract; ↑ digoxin effect
		Estrogens (eg, oral contraceptives)	↓ bacterial hydrolysis of conjugated estrogen in GI tract; ↓ contraceptive efficacy
Inhibition of metabolism in GI wall	MAOIs	Tyramine, phenylephrine	↑ pressor response to tyramine or phenylephrine

[1] Precipitant Drug = Drug that causes the interaction.
[2] Object Drug = Drug affected by the interaction.

Binding Interactions. In general, these interactions can be minimized if the object drug is given at least 2 hours before the binding agent is given because the object drug can be absorbed in the absence of the binding agent. Nevertheless, the absorption of the object drug may be affected if the object drug is absorbed slowly, or the object drug undergoes enterohepatic circulation.

GI Motility Interactions. In general, separating the doses of the interacting drugs would not circumvent GI motility interactions, because the altered motility usually results from a systemic response to the precipitant drug. Nonetheless, in some situations the object drug may be administered after the effect of the precipitant drug on GI motility has dissipated.

Alterations in GI pH. In many cases, these types of interactions may be avoided by adjusting the dosing times. For example, the alkalinizing effect of antacids on the GI tract is transient; therefore, it may be possible to administer the object drug when the effect of the antacid on GI pH is minimal. Similarly, because H₂-blockers often are given in a once nightly dose, their effect on GI pH during the following day is largely dissipated. Thus, appropriate adjustment of dosing times for the object drug may minimize the likelihood of an interaction.

Effects on Intestinal Flora. Adjustment of dosing times of the precipitant and object drugs would not be expected to alter these interactions, because effects on GI flora take place gradually and dissipate gradually.

Drug Metabolism within the Intestinal Wall. Few details are known about these interactions, so the effect of separating doses of the interacting drugs is not established. However, to the extent that these interactions result from competitive inhibition of metabolism, it would be expected that the simultaneous administration of the agents would result in a greater magnitude of interaction.

MECHANISMS OF DRUG INTERACTIONS: PROTEIN-BINDING DISPLACEMENT

The binding of drugs to proteins can change as a result of disease, accumulation of endogenous compounds, or concomitant drug administration. The outcome and clinical significance of drug interactions that are mediated by displacement of drug from protein-binding sites are frequently misunderstood and often result in an overestimation of their importance.

Basics of Drug Protein Binding

Serum proteins can act as a transport medium for drugs, carrying them to their site of action or to an organ of elimination. Serum proteins also can serve as a drug reservoir, thereby limiting the drug's distribution outside of the vascular space. Albumin is negatively charged at pH 7.4, which makes it the principal plasma protein responsible for the binding of acidic drugs, such as warfarin. However, it also is capable of binding basic and neutral drugs. Albumin concentrations can be altered by several disease states, such as cirrhosis,[8] renal failure, nephrotic syndrome,[9] and burns.[10] Alpha$_1$-acid glycoprotein (AAG) is the site of plasma binding for many basic compounds, such as propranolol (eg, *Inderal*), amitriptyline (eg, *Elavil*), disopyramide (eg, *Norpace*), and lidocaine (eg, *Xylocaine*).[11] AAG, an acute phase reactant, is increased by a number of clinical conditions, including burns,[10] trauma,[12] inflammatory disease,[11] and MI.[13] The capacity of AAG to bind certain basic drugs (eg, disopyramide) is rather limited and drug binding sites on AAG can be saturated at therapeutic plasma concentrations. Other proteins that bind drugs in the plasma include the lipoproteins (which bind lipophilic basic drugs such as cyclosporine (eg, *Neoral*) and transcortin, an alpha-globulin to which corticosteroids may bind.

The tissues also bind drugs, with albumin in interstitial fluid providing many of the drug binding sites. Digoxin is bound to tissue to a significant extent. The primary tissue-binding site for digoxin is the myocardial receptor, sodium-potassium ATPase. Tissue binding of digoxin in the myocardium is so extensive that a 60:1 myocardial tissue-to-plasma concentration ratio has been reported.[14]

When one drug displaces another from its binding sites, the drug with the lower association constant or affinity for the binding site will be displaced by the drug with higher affinity. Acidic drugs, which are primarily bound to albumin, frequently are involved in displacement interactions. A less common mechanism responsible for a reduction in protein binding is a drug-induced decrease in concentration of binding protein.[3] For example, chronic phenobarbital administration reduces the concentration of AAG 10% and increases the free fraction of verapamil (eg, *Calan*) 33%.[15] Conversely, when AAG levels rise, an increase in drug binding can occur.

The expression commonly used to describe drug binding is "percent bound" and is related to the concentrations of *protein-bound* drug (C_b) and *unbound drug* (C_u). Thus:

$$\% \text{ Bound} = \left(\frac{C_b}{C_u + C_b}\right)(100)$$

The unbound concentration in the serum also is referred to as the *free concentration*. The free concentration is dependent upon the *free fraction* (f_u) and the total drug concentration. Thus:

$$C_u = (f_u)(C_u + C_b)$$

The free fraction is the free drug concentration divided by the total drug concentration and can be calculated as follows:

$$f_u = \frac{C_u}{C_u + C_b}$$

The unbound fraction of drug in the serum is determined by several interrelated factors, including the drug's affinity for the binding site on the protein, the concentration of binding proteins, the binding capacity of the proteins, and in some cases the drug concentration. The terms "free fraction" and "free concentration" should not be confused. Free fraction represents the fraction of the total drug concentration that is not bound, while free concentration is the absolute concentration of unbound drug.

Displacement of drugs that are highly protein bound tends to have a greater effect on the free drug concentration than displacement of drugs that are less highly bound. To illustrate, of the total concentration of warfarin in the blood, approximately 98% is protein bound; the remaining 2% represents the free fraction. If an additional 2% is displaced from warfarin's binding sites, the percent bound will remain high (96%), but the free fraction will double (from 2% to 4%). The net effect is a doubling of the free drug concentration. In contrast, the displacement of an additional 2% from binding sites for a drug that is 60% protein bound will result in only a 5% increase in the free drug concentration. Therefore, highly bound drugs, such as warfarin, are more likely to be affected by drug protein displacement interactions to a clinically significant degree.

Such drug protein binding is a reversible process; an equilibrium is established between bound and free drug. A similar equilibrium is maintained between free plasma concentrations and drug bound to tissue protein. Therefore, if the free drug concentration in the plasma is increased, the drug will tend to move into the tissues. Conversely, a falling plasma free drug concentration will result in a shift of drug from tissues to plasma.[16]

Results of Protein-Binding Changes

Changes in drug protein binding can alter pharmacokinetic and pharmacodynamic parameters. These changes, and the interaction between them, determine the net outcome of a drug binding interaction. It has been widely held that the biological effect of a drug correlates best to its free concentration. This is because drug bound to plasma proteins will be retained in the vascular space, and only unbound drug is capable of crossing tissue membranes to reach extravascular receptors. Some drugs, however, appear to be transported into tissues in a bound state, or their binding may be altered within an organ's microcirculation. For example, propranolol has a free fraction of only 5% to 10%, yet over 70% of this drug is extracted from the blood as it passes through the liver. Thus, one of two things happens:

- A portion of the protein bound drug also must be taken up by the liver.
- Propranolol's binding is changed within the hepatic circulation.

Nevertheless, when changes in drug binding are accompanied by altered free drug concentration, corresponding changes in the pharmacodynamic response should be expected.

Volume of Distribution. Drugs that are highly bound to plasma proteins tend to remain in the vascular space; a small percentage distributes into the tissues. The volume of distribution of highly bound drugs is usually low. Warfarin, which is extensively bound to albumin, has a volume of distribution of approximately 0.1 L/kg. Conversely, drugs such as digoxin, with a plasma protein binding of 20% to 30% can be distributed widely to body tissues and can have a large volume of distribution (6 to 7 L/kg). In general, an increase in the free fraction of drug in plasma will result in an increase in the volume of distribution.[8,16] Thus, the initial increase in plasma unbound drug concentration at the onset of an interaction involving protein-binding displacement is blunted.

For example, the effects of aspirin on the plasma binding of the NSAID tenoxicam have been reported. Subjects received chronic therapy with tenoxicam alone and following 3 weeks of aspirin 2.6 to 3.9 g/day. Similar to other NSAIDs, tenoxicam is extensively (more than 99%) bound to albumin. Its volume of distribution increased from 7.7 to 11.5 L during the aspirin therapy. In vitro binding studies demonstrated the ability of aspirin to displace tenoxicam from plasma binding sites. The free fraction of tenoxicam increased from 0.56% in the absence of aspirin to 1.24% in the presence of aspirin.[17]

Drug Clearance. Protein-binding changes have complex and variable effects on drug clearance. These changes in clearance depend upon the drug's metabolism. Generally, drugs that are metabolized by the liver are divided into 2 subgroups. The first group of drugs has an intrinsic clearance that is much less than liver blood flow; the metabolism of this group of drugs is considered restrictive because it is restricted to unbound drug. For these drugs, passive diffusion is required for the drug to enter the liver cell. Drugs in this subgroup may be thought of as having a greater affinity for their plasma protein binding sites than for the hepatic metabolizing enzymes. For this reason, they are partially protected from metabolism by protein binding.

The second group of drugs has an intrinsic clearance that may be greater than liver blood flow; their metabolism is independent of protein binding. These drugs are considered to undergo nonrestrictive metabolism because clearance is not restricted to free drug molecules. The liver enzyme affinity for these drugs is large. As unbound drug is cleared from the blood, bound drug rapidly dissociates from protein-binding sites and becomes available for metabolism.[18]

Examples of highly protein-bound drugs with relatively low clearances restricted to unbound drug include warfarin, phenytoin (eg, *Dilantin*), valproic acid (eg, *Depakene*), and diazepam (eg, *Valium*). Because the systemic clearance of these drugs is dependent upon the free concentration of drug passing through the liver and the intrinsic clearance of the drug, changes in free drug concentration will cause a nearly proportional change in systemic clearance.

The plasma concentration of total (free + bound) drug at steady state is determined by the dosage of drug administered, the free fraction of the drug, and the intrinsic ability of the liver to metabolize the drug (intrinsic clearance). As the free fraction increases, the systemic clearance increases proportionally and the total drug concentration will decrease. The plasma concentration of free drug is dependent upon dose and intrinsic clearance. As drug is released from protein-binding sites, additional free drug becomes available for metabolism; therefore, no change in steady-state free drug concentration occurs (assuming there is no change in intrinsic clearance).[19] There will be, however, a transient rise in the free drug concentration but it will quickly return to pre-interaction levels. A theoretical exception to this model involves drugs with nonlinear metabolism such as phenytoin. In this case, as the concentration of unbound drug increases, metabolic clearance may not increase proportionately and unbound drug can accumulate (see Figure 1). In the example of

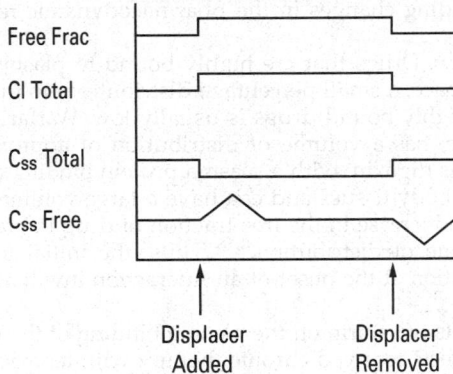

Free Frac

Cl Total

C$_{ss}$ Total

C$_{ss}$ Free

Displacer   Displacer
Added   Removed

FIGURE 1 • Restrictive Metabolism

Free Frac = Free fraction of drug in the plasma: Cl Total = systemic clearance; C$_{ss}$ Total = Steady-state concentration of bound plus free drug; C$_{ss}$ Free = Steady-state concentration of unbound drug.

the interaction between aspirin and tenoxicam cited previously, the volume of distribution was noted to increase approximately 50%.[17] This increase is likely the result of the increase in the free fraction of tenoxicam. Because tenoxicam is a highly bound drug with relatively low clearance, the clearance of tenoxicam would be expected to increase and the steady-state concentration to decrease. The authors reported that the steady-state tenoxicam concentration fell from 11.2 to 6.3 mcg/mL and clearance increased approximately 80%. No concentrations of unbound tenoxicam were reported. Thus, it is important not to be misled by measurements of total drug plasma concentrations. If a decrease in the total drug concentration is the consequence of a protein displacement drug interaction, increasing the dose may cause toxic free drug concentrations.

Examples of drugs with nonrestrictive clearances include lidocaine and propranolol. These drugs have systemic clearances that are limited only by liver blood flow because both bound and unbound drug are removed from the blood. Changes in protein binding will not alter the clearance of these drugs. Because displacement of bound drug will not increase clearance, free drug concentrations will tend to rise in the blood while total drug concentrations remain unchanged. (see Figure 2). Consequently, more free drug will distribute from the plasma to the tissues, potentially increasing drug action. Protein-displacement drug interactions with non-restrictive

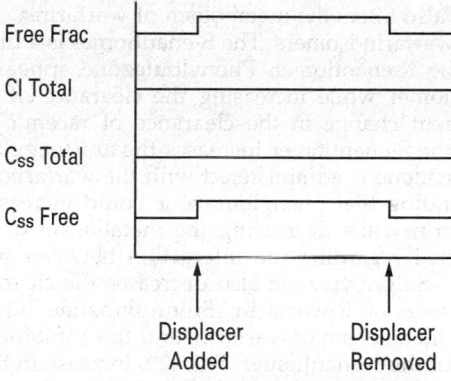

FIGURE 2 • Non-Restrictive Metabolism

Free Frac = Free fraction of drug in the plasma; Cl Total = Total systemic clearance; C_{ss} Total = Steady-state concentration of bound plus free drug; C_{ss} Free = Steady-state concentration of unbound drug.

drugs are rarely reported because most have low protein binding. Additional factors that may limit the observation of these interactions include the relatively wide therapeutic ratio of some of the drugs; the common practice of assaying and reporting only total drug concentrations; and the binding of the drugs to albumin if they are displaced from alpha$_1$-acid glycoprotein.

Bioavailability. Plasma protein-binding displacement can also alter bioavailability. The pharmacokinetics of oxazepam (eg, *Serax*) were studied before and during the administration of diflunisal (eg, *Dolobid*).[20] Both drugs are extensively protein bound and have similar metabolic pathways. Diflunisal increased the free fraction of oxazepam by up to 56% in vitro. The coadministration of the 2 drugs resulted in a reduction in oxazepam's maximum concentration (C_{max}) 38% without a change in cumulative (ie, drug and metabolites) urinary recovery. Absorption probably was not altered, but the presystemic or "first-pass" metabolism of oxazepam was increased. When the oxazepam was administered 20 minutes after the diflunisal dose, high concentrations of diflunisal in the portal blood may have displaced oxazepam from binding sites making more oxazepam available for first-pass metabolism. The reduction in peak oxazepam concentrations was accompanied by an increase in oxazepam metabolites.

Warfarin Interactions. Drug interactions with warfarin can serve as prototypes for drug interactions mediated through altered protein binding. Warfarin is a highly protein-bound drug that has a small volume of distribution; it also has a relatively low clearance which is restricted to unbound drug. Therefore, the concomitant administration of a second drug that competes with warfarin for protein-binding sites should have a transient effect on both the warfarin concentration and the pro-thrombin time, and long-term changes should not occur.

The prototypical drug that illustrates these predictions is chloral hydrate. A pri-mary metabolite of chloral hydrate, trichloroacetic acid, competes with warfarin for binding sites on albumin. Displacement of warfarin causes an increase in its hypo-prothrombinemic effect that may last for up to a week, but with continued therapy, the total plasma warfarin concentration declines and the free warfarin concentration returns to pre-interaction levels.[21-23] A hemorrhagic episode is most likely to occur if a high dose of the displacer is administered or if the patient's prothrombin time is excessive before chloral hydrate administration.

Phenylbutazone is a potent displacer of warfarin, and concomitant use prolongs prothrombin times and increases bleeding episodes. However, the prolongation of the prothrombin time resulting from this combination does not abate with time because phenylbutazone also alters the metabolism of warfarin.[24] Warfarin is a race-mic mixture of R- and S-warfarin isomers. The S-enantiomer is 4 times more active as an anticoagulant than the R-enantiomer. Phenylbutazone appears to decrease the clearance of the S-enantiomer while increasing the clearance of the R-enantiomer. This results in no apparent change in the clearance of racemic warfarin, but the diminished clearance of the S-enantiomer increases the anticoagulant effect that per-sists as long as phenylbutazone is administered with the warfarin.

The rather unusual finding that phenylbutazone could increase the clearance of one enantiomer of warfarin while decreasing the metabolism of the other may be explained by data reported regarding the interaction between sulfinpyrazone (eg, *Anturane*) and warfarin.[25] Sulfinpyrazone also decreases the clearance of S-warfarin and increases the clearance of R-warfarin. Sulfinpyrazone inhibits only 1 of 4 enzymes involved in the metabolism of warfarin, and this inhibition accounts for the reduced clearance (40%) of the S-enantiomer. The 42% increase in the clearance of the R-enantiomer was not caused by enzyme induction but was due to a greater than 40% reduction in the protein binding of the R-enantiomer following the addition of sulfinpyrazone.

Summary

The displacement of drugs with restrictive clearance from protein-bound sites will produce transient increases in unbound drug concentrations and, perhaps, pharma-codynamic effects. Pharmacodynamic changes are most likely to be clinically impor-tant for drugs with narrow therapeutic indices, particularly when large doses of the displacing drugs are administered. At steady state, total plasma drug concentrations will be decreased, but unbound concentrations will remain unaltered. It may be nec-essary to monitor unbound drug concentrations to avoid inappropriate dosage increases based upon reduced total drug concentrations. Dosage adjustments usually will be unnecessary unless the displacing drug also alters the intrinsic clearance of the displaced drug. Altered pharmacodynamic effects can occur if drugs with nonre-strictive clearance are displaced from their binding sites, but these changes may not be clinically important. At this time, little information regarding displacement inter-actions with nonrestrictive drugs is available.

INTERACTIONS ASSOCIATED WITH MODIFIED DRUG EXCRETION

Drugs are eliminated from the body unchanged, as metabolites, or both. The lipid-soluble drugs usually are metabolized to more polar compounds before elimination, while drugs that are highly polar tend to be eliminated unchanged. Generally, the liver is the organ responsible for the metabolism of drugs and the kidney is the site of drug or metabolite elimination or excretion from the body. Most interactions involving drug excretion occur in the kidney, but the liver and GI tract are occasion-ally sites of drug excretion interactions. The mechanisms responsible for these inter-actions will be reviewed and representative examples will be discussed.

Drugs excreted in breast milk are important to consider for their potential effects in the nursing infant; however, no interaction data specific to breast milk drug excretion are available at this time. Similarly, there is a lack of data providing examples of drug interactions involving drugs eliminated by pulmonary excretion.

The kidney has 3 primary methods to excrete drugs and their metabolites: 1) glomerular filtration; 2) active tubular secretion; and 3) passive tubular reabsorption. Glomerular filtration depends upon the drug's plasma protein binding and glomerular filtration rate (GFR). The proximal tubule is the site of active secretion and, in some cases (eg, uric acid), reabsorption of organic acids and bases. Nonionized forms of weak acids and bases undergo passive reabsorption in the proximal and distal tubule.

Glomerular Filtration

The glomerulus is a semipermeable membrane that filters the plasma using the hydrostatic pressure of the blood. Much of the fluid portion of the plasma as well as small molecules pass through the capillary membrane of the glomerulus. Lipids, proteins, and substances bound to proteins do not, and are retained in the blood. Thus, only nonprotein-bound drugs or metabolites are filtered into the tubular fluid. A drug-induced decrease in plasma protein binding of a drug that is eliminated by glomerular filtration would increase the excretion of the drug and would serve to offset the increased free concentration of the drug in the plasma. The net result of this type of an interaction usually would not be clinically significant.

Most changes in glomerular filtration are the result of changes in the filtration pressure. These changes typically originate with alteration in either the systemic blood pressure or the glomerular hydrostatic pressure. Drugs can alter either blood pressure or, by altering the vascular tone of the afferent and efferent renal arterioles, glomerular hydrostatic pressure. A reduction in glomerular pressure will reduce the ability of the glomerulus to excrete a drug. An absolute reduction in the number of glomeruli will also reduce the ability of the kidney to filter drugs.

Perhaps the most commonly observed drug interactions involving glomerular filtration result from the combination of a nephrotoxic drug with a second drug that is primarily eliminated from the body by glomerular filtration. This is an indirect interaction and often is not considered a drug-drug interaction because it originates with drug-induced renal toxicity. For example, a patient stabilized on digoxin is treated with an aminoglycoside antibiotic. If the patient develops an aminoglycoside-induced renal failure, digoxin toxicity may develop if the digoxin dose is not appropriately adjusted. Excess antihypertensive therapy can result in hypotension and reduced renal blood flow. Under these circumstances, drugs principally eliminated by glomerular filtration will accumulate and potentially result in drug toxicity. The clinical significance of these interactions will depend upon the degree and duration of the reduction in glomerular filtration and the characteristics of the accumulating drug. The appropriate adjustment of the dosage of drugs eliminated by glomerular filtration will avoid drug accumulation secondary to drug-induced nephrotoxicity.

Active Tubular Secretion

Many drugs, in addition to undergoing glomerular filtration, are subject to tubular secretion. Numerous acidic and basic drugs are susceptible to tubular secretion and to drug interactions resulting from altered secretion (see Table 2). Inhibition of tubular secretion can result in accumulation of the drug in the serum.

TABLE 2. Drugs Secreted by the Renal Tubules

Basic (Cationic) Agents	Acidic (Anionic) Agents
Amiodarone (eg, *Cordarone*)	Aspirin
Cimetidine (eg, *Tagamet*)	Cephalosporins

TABLE 2. Drugs Secreted by the Renal Tubules

Basic (Cationic) Agents	Acidic (Anionic) Agents
Diltiazem (eg, *Cardizem*)	Chlorpropamide (eg, *Diabinese*)
Digoxin (eg, *Lanoxin*)	Clofibrate (*Atromid-S*)
Procainamide (eg, *Pronestyl*)	Indomethacin (eg, *Indocin*)
Quinidine (eg, *Quinora*)	Methotrexate
Quinine	Penicillins
Ranitidine (eg, *Zantac*)	Probenecid
Trimethoprim (eg, *Proloprim*)	Salicylic acid
Triamterene (*Dyrenium*)	Sulfinpyrazone (eg, *Anturane*)
Verapamil (eg, *Calan*)	Thiazides

Tubular secretion occurs in the proximal portion of the renal tubule. The secretion of organic acids and bases is an active process and requires the substance to bind to a carrier at the cell membrane and to be released at the opposite side of the membrane. For a drug molecule to be secreted by the tubule, it must pass from the blood through the basolateral membrane and into the proximal tubular cell cytoplasm. After crossing the tubular cell fluid to the luminal side of the cell, the molecule must pass through the brush border membrane and into the tubular lumen where it joins the glomerular filtrate.

The transport of organic anions and cations tends to rely on distinct and unique systems. These transport systems are considered to be composed of a series of proteins located in the basolateral and brush border membranes. Each protein has a unique affinity for an anion or cation and different capacities for the transportation of an organic molecule (transport maximum [Tm]).[50,51] Usually, substances that are excreted by one system of proteins (eg, the organic anion system), do not compete for excretion with the other system. It is more common that drugs that share a similar transport system may interact by competitive inhibition of the transport proteins. When two drugs compete for the same transport proteins, saturation of the transport system may occur, reducing the Tm of one or both drugs. Since the active transport of drug molecules requires the expenditure of energy, drugs that inhibit cellular energy production also could alter the excretion of other agents.[52]

Interactions with Acidic Drugs. The interaction between probenecid and penicillins has been used to enhance the therapeutic effect of the penicillins, particularly in the treatment of sexually transmitted diseases.[53] Probenecid competes with penicillin to reduce its tubular secretion and renal clearance. Likewise, probenecid can reduce the renal excretion of cephalosporins.[54] Other acidic drugs, such as indomethacin (eg, *Indocin*), salicylates, and sulfinpyrazone, reduce the excretion of penicillin, but in general these changes are of no clinical significance.[55]

While the accumulation of penicillin or cephalosporin resulting from concomitant probenecid administration may not cause the patient harm, this is not true for all drugs. For example, probenecid significantly inhibits the tubular secretion of methotrexate, which can lead to a 2- to 3-fold increase in methotrexate concentrations and serious methotrexate toxicity.[56,57] Likewise, NSAIDs, including salicylates, have been shown to enhance methotrexate toxicity, particularly when administered to patients taking antineoplastic doses of methotrexate.[58,59]

The uricosuric activity of probenecid and sulfinpyrazone is related to their ability to block the active reabsorption of uric acid from the urine to the blood in the proximal tubule. The administration of 5 or 6 g/day of aspirin also inhibits the reabsorption of uric acid. However, doses of aspirin producing salicylate concentrations at least 5 to 10 mg/dL will reduce the uricosuric action of probenecid and sulfinpyrazone.[60] Likewise, probenecid and sulfinpyrazone inhibit the uricosuric action of high-dose aspirin.[61] Concentrations of salicylates that inhibit the uricosuric effects of probenecid do not alter probenecid's impediment of penicillin excretion.[62] The mechanism of these interactions is not certain. It may involve different affinities for the uric acid transport proteins and competitive binding with the proteins by the various uricosuric agents.

The concomitant use of acidic drugs may produce drug interactions by mechanisms in addition to inhibition of tubular secretion. For example, the hypoglycemic activity of the sulfonylureas has been reported to be enhanced when clofibrate (*Atromid-S*) is administered.[63] The mechanism of this interaction probably involves reduced tubular secretion, as with chlorpropamide (eg, *Diabinese*),[64] or plasma protein-binding displacement with tolbutamide (eg, *Orinase*).[65]

Drugs also can indirectly interact through changes in tubular secretion or reabsorption. Chronic administration of thiazide diurctics results in a compensatory increase in proximal tubule reabsorption of sodium. If a patient is also taking lithium carbonate (eg, *Eskalith*), the increase in sodium reabsorption will result in increased tubular lithium reabsorption as well. The reduction in lithium renal clearance can result in the accumulation of lithium in the serum and the development of toxicity.[66,67]

Interactions with Basic Drugs. Perhaps the best known interaction involving altered renal excretion involves quinidine (eg, *Quinora*) and digoxin. In addition to inhibition of digoxin's nonrenal clearance and tissue binding, quinidine reduces digoxin renal clearance 30% to 50% by inhibiting the tubular secretion of digoxin.[68,69] Amiodarone (*Cordarone*) inhibits the renal and nonrenal clearance of digoxin in a similar manner.[70]

Studies of the effects of verapamil on digoxin renal clearance indicate a reduction[71] or no change[72] in digoxin renal clearance following verapamil administration. These differences may be partially explained by the findings that the effects of verapamil on digoxin renal clearance may be transient. A 35% reduction in digoxin renal clearance following 1 week of verapamil administration was noted to have returned to pre-verapamil rates after 6 weeks of continuous verapamil administration.[73]

The renal tubular secretion of digoxin has been reported to be inhibited by trimethoprim (eg, *Proloprim*) and spironolactone (eg, *Aldactone*).[74,75] In one report, the combination of spironolactone and quinidine produced a larger effect on digoxin clearance than either drug administered alone.[76] Captopril (eg, *Capoten*) administration reduces digoxin renal clearance to a significantly greater degree than its effect on creatinine clearance, indicating a reduction in digoxin renal secretion.[77]

Procainamide (eg, *Pronestyl*) is a basic drug, which is metabolized *and* undergoes renal tubular secretion. Amiodarone appears to produce a significant increase in the procainamide serum concentration by inhibition of its renal and nonrenal clearance.[78] The coadministration of cimetidine with procainamide results in a reduction in the tubular secretion of procainamide.[79,80] The effect of ranitidine (eg, *Zantac*) on procainamide renal clearance has been less consistent. No significant effect was reported following ranitidine 300 mg over 12 hours while a dose of 750 mg over 12 hours produced a 35% reduction in procainamide's renal clearance.[81] The effect of ranitidine on procainamide clearance is variable and dependent upon baseline procainamide clearance and ranitidine concentrations.[82]

Passive Tubular Reabsorption

The excretion and reabsorption of most drugs from the renal tubules is by passive diffusion across the cell membranes. This diffusion is governed by the concentration and lipid solubility of the nonionic form of the drug on each side of the membrane. Nonionized drug molecules in the tubular fluid are preferentially reabsorbed over ionized molecules. The relative ratio of nonionized to ionized molecules is dependent upon urinary pH and the pKa of the drug. Strong acids and bases tend to be ionized when urine pH is approximately 5 to 8. For weak acids with pKas between 3 and 7 and weak bases with pKbs between 7 and 11, the proportion of the drug in the ionized vs nonionized states will depend upon urine pH. In an acidic urine, weakly acidic drugs tend to be reabsorbed while basic drugs will tend to be excreted in the urine. Conversely, in an alkaline urine, acidic drugs will be excreted and basic drugs will be reabsorbed.

Interactions with Basic Drugs. Quinidine is a weak base whose urinary excretion may be altered by changes in urine pH. The urinary excretion of quinidine was reduced nearly 90% when the urine pH was increased from less than 6 to over 7.5.[83] Alkalinization of the urine with systemic antacids or acetazolamide (eg, *Diamox*) can result in accumulation of other weak bases, including amphetamine.[84] Acidification of the urine would increase the excretion of weak bases.

Interactions with Acidic Drugs. Drugs that are weak acids will tend to accumulate if the urine is made more acidic. Vitamin C ingestion has been suggested as a method of urinary acidification, but its administration does not uniformly alter urine pH or salicylate concentrations.[85] However, urinary alkalinization may be useful to increase the excretion of weak acids when toxicity is present.

Interactions Involving Nonrenal Excretion

The nonrenal clearance of digoxin has consistently been reported to be reduced by quinidine administration.[86,87] Quinidine administration also resulted in a 42% reduction in the biliary clearance of digoxin.[88] Data from in vitro animal studies[89] and studies in human subjects[156] indicate that several basic drugs have the ability to inhibit the hepatic uptake of digoxin. One mechanism that may be responsible for the reduced uptake observed is the inhibition of oxidative phosphorylation, a cellular process that provides energy for active transport functions. Whether this mechanism is common to the numerous basic drugs that alter digoxin renal and nonrenal excretion remains to be determined.

Drugs excreted into the GI tract may undergo enterohepatic reabsorption. The presence of drugs in the GI tract that inhibit the reabsorption of these agents will reduce their serum concentrations and, perhaps, therapeutic effectiveness. Binding resins, such as cholestyramine and colestipol, are capable of reducing the reabsorption of several drugs, including amiodarone, digitalis glycosides, and warfarin.[34,90,91] Binding interactions involving drugs that undergo enterohepatic circulation are difficult to avoid since biliary secretion continues throughout the day.

Summary

It is difficult to predict which drugs will alter the excretion of another drug, particularly when the mechanism involves active transport processes. Acidic and basic drugs appear to be more likely to interact with drugs of similar acid-base nature. Changes in passive tubular reabsorption are most likely to be clinically significant when the urine is made more alkaline during administration of a weak base. Interference with the active uptake of drugs by the liver may explain the reduced clearance observed with several interactions involving agents not usually considered to be hepatic cytochrome P450 inhibitors. Clinically significant interactions are more likely to occur when they involve drugs excreted unchanged, having narrow therapeutic ranges, and dosed to relatively high plasma concentrations.

DRUG INTERACTION MECHANISMS: ENZYME INDUCTION

The primary function of drug-metabolizing enzymes is to transform lipid-soluble drugs into more water-soluble metabolites, thus facilitating their excretion via the urine and bile. The metabolites usually are not recognized by the drug receptor, and this results in a loss or diminution of pharmacologic activity. For this reason, the rate of metabolism often is the primary factor regulating the time course of drug activity. Oxidative metabolizing enzymes have been found in virtually all life forms and appear to enhance survival by enabling the organism to eliminate the undesirable chemicals to which it is exposed. These enzymes have low substrate specificity and thus are able to transform almost any xenobiotic into more water-soluble products.[92,93] They also are involved in the metabolism of endogenous substances such as estrogens, thyroxine, vitamin D, and bilirubin.

The liver is the most important drug metabolizing organ, although metabolism also takes place in organs such as the GI tract, lung, skin, kidney, blood, and placenta. Drug metabolism generally is divided into Phase I (oxidation, reduction, hydrolysis) and Phase II (conjugation with glucuronide, sulfate, glycine). Phase I metabolism generally involves the hepatic *cytochrome P450* system (also called "mixed function oxidases" or "monooxygenases"). Although some drugs undergo only a Phase II conjugation reaction (eg, the glucuronidation of oxazepam), most Phase II reactions are preceded by a Phase I process that prepares the drug molecule for conjugation.

Enzyme Induction: The Process

Some drugs and other xenobiotics are capable of increasing mixed function oxidase enzymes in the liver, a process called "enzyme induction." Enzyme induction can be considered an adaptive process resulting from the body's perception that there is an onslaught of lipid-soluble compounds that need to be eliminated from the body. Enzyme induction affects primarily Phase I metabolism, although some Phase II reactions also may be affected. Some enzyme inducers (eg, carbamazepine [eg, *Tegretol*]) enhance their own metabolism as well as the metabolism of other drugs. This autoinduction tends to result in pharmacokinetic changes over time.

The process of enzyme induction is more complex than originally thought. Different enzyme inducers may preferentially induce certain isozymes of cytochrome P450, resulting in greater effects on the metabolism of some drugs versus others. Thus, it cannot be certain that a given object drug will be affected by an enzyme inducer until the interaction has been specifically studied in humans. Moreover, the marked species differences in enzyme induction preclude the extrapolation of the results of animal studies to humans.

Enzyme-Inducing Drugs

A wide variety of chemically unrelated xenobiotics, including several drugs, act as enzyme inducers in humans. The only chemical characteristic common to them all is lipid solubility. Most of the enzyme-inducing drugs that have exhibited clinically important drug interactions are anticonvulsants, although one antimicrobial agent, rifampin, has proven to be a potent enzyme inducer. Cigarette smoking and chronic alcohol consumption also may induce drug metabolizing enzymes and alter drug response (see Table 3 for a listing of drugs affected by enzyme-inducing drugs).

TABLE 3. Drugs Affected by Enzyme-Inducing Drugs

Object Drug	Outcome
Anticoagulants, oral	↓ hypoprothrombinemic response; ↑ hypoprothrombinemia when barbiturate is stopped
Beta-adrenergic blockers	↓ effect of beta blockers metabolized by the liver
Chloramphenicol	↓ chloramphenicol effect; chloramphenicol may ↓ metabolism of phenytoin or barbiturates
Contraceptives, oral	↑ risk of unintended pregnancy
Corticosteroids	↓ corticosteroid response; especially a problem when barbiturates started in a patient carefully titrated on corticosteroid for chronic disease
Cyclosporine	↓ cyclosporine effect; possible rejection of transplant
Digitoxin	↓ digitoxin response; digoxin less likely to interact
Disopyramide	↓ disopyramide response with phenytoin, rifampin, and probably other enzyme inducers
Doxycycline	↓ doxycycline serum concentrations shown with several enzyme inducers; possible ↓ in antimicrobial effect

TABLE 3. Drugs Affected by Enzyme-Inducing Drugs

Object Drug	Outcome
Methadone	↓ methadone serum concentrations; ↑ likelihood of methadone withdrawal
Mexiletine	↓ mexiletine serum concentrations; possible ↓ in mexiletine response
Neuroleptics	↓ neuroleptic serum concentrations; possible ↓ in neuroleptic response
Quinidine	↓ quinidine serum concentrations shown with several enzyme inducers; ↑ quinidine dose or use alternative agent
Theophylline	↓ theophylline serum concentrations; possible ↓ in theophylline response
Thyroid	↑ metabolism of thyroxine and triiodothyronine; may result in hypothyroidism in patients without normal thyroid-pituitary-hypothalamus axis
Tricyclic Antidepressants	↓ antidepressant effect; may need substantial ↑ in tricyclic dosage
Verapamil	↓ verapamil serum concentrations; interaction minimal with IV verapamil

Barbiturates. The enzyme-inducing ability of barbiturates has been known for decades and has resulted in several clinically important drug interactions. It is likely that most barbiturates are capable of producing enzyme induction, although there may be differences in the magnitude and time course of the inducing effects. Among the barbiturates that have produced enzyme induction in humans are phenobarbital,[94,95] pentobarbital (eg, *Nembutal*),[96,97] secobarbital (*Seconal*),[98,99] amobarbital (*Amytal*),[100] butabarbital (eg, *Butisol*),[101] and heptabarbital.[102] Although the enzyme-inducing ability of other barbiturates is not well studied, it seems likely that enzyme induction also would occur with barbiturates such as aprobarbital (*Alurate*), mephobarbital (*Mebaral*), and talbutal.

Carbamazepine. Although carbamazepine (eg, *Tegretol*) is structurally related to tricyclic antidepressants, its 3-dimensional structure appears to be spatially similar to another enzyme inducer, phenytoin. Carbamazepine can induce its own metabolism as well as the metabolism of several other drugs.

Glutethimide. Glutethimide, a rarely used hypnotic agent, possesses a chemical structure that is closely related to phenobarbital. Information on the enzyme-inducing effects of glutethimide is limited, but it does appear to enhance the hepatic metabolism of warfarin. The related drug, aminoglutethimide (*Cytadren*), has been shown to stimulate the metabolism of several other drugs.

Phenytoin. Like the barbiturates, the enzyme-inducing ability of phenytoin (eg, *Dilantin*) has been repeatedly documented.[103-114] Little research has been conducted on the enzyme-inducing ability of other hydantoins (eg, ethotoin [*Peganone*], mephenytoin [*Mesantoin*]). However, due to their structural similarity to phenytoin and their high lipid solubility, they also may be capable of producing enzyme induction; it should be assumed they are enzyme inducers until proven otherwise.

Primidone. Primidone (eg, *Mysoline*) is partially metabolized to phenobarbital, and it is not unusual for primidone-treated patients to have serum concentrations of phenobarbital that are capable of producing enzyme induction. Primidone itself also may contribute to the enzyme induction observed.

Rifampin. Rifampin (eg, *Rifadin*), one of the few nonanticonvulsant enzyme inducers, is a potent inducer of the metabolism of numerous drugs (see Table 3). Other antimicrobials do not appear to result in significant enzyme induction, with the possible exception of griseofulvin (eg, *Fulvicin*).

Characteristics of Enzyme Induction

Time Course. The time course of enzyme induction as it relates to the duration of therapy with the enzyme inducer can be divided into the following categories:

- How long does it take before enzyme induction can be detected?
- How long does it take to reach maximum enzyme induction?

- When are adverse effects of the interaction likely to occur?
- How long will it take for enzyme induction to dissipate?

The onset and offset of enzyme induction from phenobarbital, for example, tends to be quite gradual; induction can be detected after approximately 1 week and takes 2 to 3 weeks to become maximal. Enzyme induction may take up to 1 month or more to dissipate after the phenobarbital is discontinued.[115,116] The dose and duration of phenobarbital treatment may affect these times. For example, dissipation of phenobarbital enzyme induction would take considerably longer in a patient receiving large doses of phenobarbital for several months than in a patient receiving small doses over 2 weeks.

Rifampin, on the other hand, tends to have a more rapid onset and offset of enzyme induction than phenobarbital. Enzyme induction following rifampin usually can be detected after 2 to 4 days and becomes maximal after approximately 6 to 10 days. Induction dissipates over 2 to 3 weeks. The onset and offset of induction for most other enzyme-inducing drugs probably falls somewhere between that of phenobarbital and rifampin; nonetheless, for most enzyme inducers, only partial information is available regarding the time course of this effect.

In general, the onset and offset of enzyme induction is a gradual process when compared with other mechanisms of drug interactions. In addition to the time required for the inducer to achieve serum concentrations sufficient to produce enzyme induction, time is also required for the concentration of the drug metabolizing enzymes to build to their maximal level and for the serum concentration of the object drug to decline. Similarly, the dissipation of enzyme induction after discontinuation of the inducer is dependent not only upon the elimination rate of the inducing agent but also upon the decay of the drug metabolizing enzymes to normal (noninduced) levels. Because dissipation of enzyme induction tends to take longer than initiation, it appears that the formation of drug-metabolizing enzymes is a more rapid process than the decay of these enzymes.

Dose of Inducer. Enzyme induction, like virtually all drug interaction mechanisms, appears to be dose related. Nevertheless, this may be more obvious for some inducers than for others, since some drugs may induce enzymes at all usual dosages. The enzyme-inducing effects of phenobarbital appear to be dose related. Eight healthy subjects took 7.5 mg/day for 4 weeks followed by 15 mg/day for 4 weeks; 5 subjects took 30 mg/day for an additional 2 weeks.[117] The clearance of antipyrine 1 g oral at the end of each dosing period increased as the dose of phenobarbital was increased. Similar results were obtained in another study of 4 healthy subjects[118] (see Figure 3). Larger phenobarbital doses (eg, 60 to 100 mg/day) appear to produce greater effects on antipyrine clearance (50% to 100% increases instead of the 10% to 30% increases noted in the studies just described).[115] The enzyme-inducing effect of other barbiturates probably also is dose dependent. In 1 patient, 100 mg/day of secobarbital had no effect on plasma warfarin concentrations while 200 mg/day had a marked effect.[119] Nonetheless, a study in 6 healthy subjects found 100 mg/day of secobarbital sufficient to enhance warfarin metabolism.[99]

As indicated previously, carbamazepine can induce its own metabolism (autoinduction); this process also may be dose related. In 13 epileptic patients receiving 800 mg/day or more of carbamazepine, a dosage increase resulted in a disproportionately small increase in plasma carbamazepine concentrations in 10 of the patients.[120] One plausible explanation for this finding would be increased carbamazepine autoinduction at the higher dosage level.

The dose dependency of enzyme induction also may vary depending upon the specific object drug involved. For example, 1,200 mg/day of rifampin may increase antipyrine clearance twice as much as 600 mg/day, but the two doses of rifampin appear to produce a similar effect on propranolol clearance.[115]

In general, enzyme induction appears to be dose related, with larger doses of the inducer tending to produce a greater degree of enzyme induction. Nevertheless, due

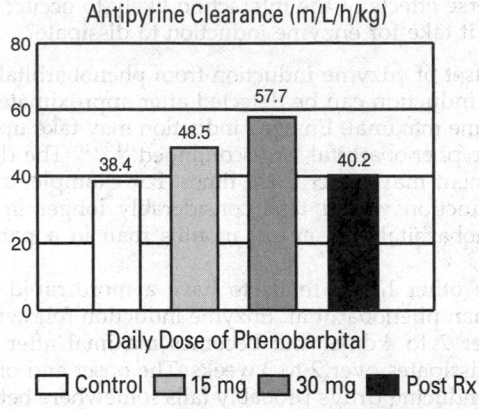

FIGURE 3 • Antipyrine/Phenobarbital Clearance
Increasing clearance of antipyrine with increasing doses of phenobarbital in 4 healthy subjects. A 2-day loading dose of phenobarbital was given at the beginning of each 4-week treatment period. The 30 mg, but not the 15 mg, dose of phenobarbital produced a statistically significant effect compared with control. The posttreatment value was approximately 6 weeks after stopping phenobarbital.

to factors such as high interpatient variability and differences in susceptibility of various object drugs, it is difficult to predict what dose of the inducer will produce what degree of enzyme induction in any given patient.

Variability. As previously mentioned, there is considerable variability in the magnitude of enzyme induction from patient to patient. For example, the ability of phenobarbital and glutethimide to inhibit the hypoprothrombinemic response in patients on chronic warfarin therapy varies from a marked response to no detectable effect.[121] Among the factors that may affect the magnitude of enzyme induction are dose of inducer (discussed previously), age, genetics, concurrent therapy with more than one enzyme inducer, concurrent therapy with an enzyme inhibitor, and the presence of hepatic disease.

Effect of Age. Some evidence suggests that the elderly do not manifest enzyme induction to the same degree as younger individuals.[122] Cigarette smoking did not affect antipyrine clearance in the elderly as much as in younger adults, and others also have found the elderly to be less likely to manifest enzyme induction.[123]

Genetic Influences. Genetics appear to play an important role in the outcome of enzyme induction. Four sets of identical twins and 4 sets of fraternal twins were given a single oral dose of antipyrine before and after phenobarbital 2 mg/kg/day for 2 weeks.[124] The shortening of antipyrine half-time due to phenobarbital showed considerably more variability in the fraternal twins than in the identical twins, suggesting genetic control over the ability of phenobarbital to induce antipyrine metabolism. In addition, phenobarbital induces the metabolism of sparteine in rapid sparteine metabolizers but not in poor sparteine metabolizers.[125]

Presence of Other Enzyme Inducers. It would be expected that initiation of therapy with an enzyme inducer in a patient already receiving another enzyme inducer would not result in the same degree of change in the metabolism of the object drug as compared to a patient not already receiving an enzyme inducer. In other words, if inducer A alone increases the clearance of the object drug 100% and inducer B alone does the same, concurrent use of inducers A and B may produce less than a 200% increase in clearance of the object drug. There is some evidence to indicate this is true. For example, in 122 patients with seizures, antipyrine clearance was about the same in those receiving monotherapy with carbamazepine, phenytoin, phenobarbital, or primidone (eg, *Mysoline*) as it was in patients receiving combinations of these drugs.[126]

Presence of Enzyme Inhibitors. Available evidence suggests that administration of a hepatic microsomal enzyme inhibitor such as cimetidine would attenuate the stimulatory effect of enzyme inducers on drug metabolism. For example, cimetidine 800 mg/day markedly attenuates the effect of rifampin 600 mg/day on antipyrine metabolism.[127]

Summary

Several commonly used drugs are capable of increasing hepatic microsomal drug metabolizing enzymes in the liver, a process called "enzyme induction." The elimination of drugs and endogenous substances metabolized by these enzymes is increased by enzyme inducers, usually resulting in a reduction in the pharmacologic response of the induced drug. Examples of enzyme-inducing drugs include barbiturates, carbamazepine, glutethimide, phenytoin, primidone, and rifampin. The time course of drug interactions involving enzyme induction tends to be gradual, and it varies depending upon factors such as the specific inducer involved, the dose and duration of therapy with the inducer, and the pharmacokinetics and pharmacodynamics of the object drug. The magnitude of the alteration in response to the object drug also is variable, depending upon factors such as age, genetics, and the presence of other enzyme inducers or inhibitors.

DRUG INTERACTION MECHANISMS: ENZYME INHIBITION

Inhibition of drug metabolism is perhaps the most commonly reported mechanism responsible for the interaction between two drugs. Most often, these interactions result in an increased plasma concentration and pharmacologic response to one of the drugs, thereby increasing the potential for adverse effects. Enzyme inhibition interactions are so common that if a new drug is known to be metabolized by the liver, often it is studied to determine if it interacts with cimetidine or other common inhibitors before being released into the market. Enzyme inhibition interactions are complex in that they involve a variety of drugs and can be modified by several factors. Furthermore, the outcomes of these interactions can vary tremendously.

Hepatic Drug Metabolism

Many drugs undergo metabolism via the smooth endoplasmic reticulum of the liver as the first step in their elimination from the body. Oxidation is involved in the metabolism of many drugs; it is dependent upon a group of enzymes called *mixed-function oxidases*, often collectively referred to as *cytochrome P450*. There are several cytochrome P450 enzymes (isozymes) that have different specificity and activity. Table 4 lists some of the common isozymes, drugs that are metabolized by the isozyme (substrates), and common drugs that inhibit or induce the isozyme. Most drugs are metabolized primarily by one enzyme while each enzyme is capable of metabolizing several different drugs. The knowledge of which drugs are metabolized by which enzyme enables one to predict interactions between substrate drugs and potential inhibitors.

TABLE 4. Drug Metabolizing Enzymes and Selected Inhibitors and Inducers

Isozyme[1]	Drugs or Substrates	Inhibitors	Inducers
CYP1A2	Caffeine, tacrine, theophylline, lidocaine, R-warfarin	Cimetidine, ciprofloxacin, erythromycin, tacrine	Omeprazole, smoking, phenobarbital
CYP2B6	Cocaine, ifosphamide, cyclophosphamide	Chloramphenicol	Phenobarbital
CYP2C9/10	S-warfarin, phenytoin, tolbutamide, diclofenac, piroxicam	Amiodarone, fluconazole, lovastatin	Rifampin, phenobarbital

TABLE 4. Drug Metabolizing Enzymes and Selected Inhibitors and Inducers

Isozyme[1]	Drugs or Substrates	Inhibitors	Inducers
CYP2C19	Diazepam, omeprazole, mephenytoin	Fluvoxamine, fluoxetine, omeprazole, felbamate	Rifampin, phenobarbital
CYP2D6	Codeine, haloperidol, dextromethorphan, tricyclic antidepressants, phenothiazines, metoprolol, propranolol (4-OH), venlafaxine, risperidone, encainide, paroxetine, sertraline, venlafaxine	Quinidine, fluoxetine, sertraline, amiodarone, propoxyphene	None known
CYP2E1	Acetaminophen, alcohol	Disulfiram	Isoniazid, alcohol
CYP3A3/4	Nifedipine, verapamil, cyclosporine, carbamazepine, terfenadine, cisapride, astemizole, tacrolimus, midazolam, alfentanil, diazepam, verapamil, loratadine, ifosphamide, cyclophosphamide	Erythromycin, cimetidine, clarithromycin, fluvoxamine, fluoxetine, ketoconazole, itraconazole, grapefruit juice, metronidazole, ritonavir, indinavir, mibefradil	Rifampin, phenytoin, phenobarbital, carbamazepine

[1] CYP = Cytochrome P450.

Drug metabolizing enzymes are grouped into families based on their genetic makeup. Enzymes that have at least 40% of their genes in common are considered to be from the same family. Family groups are labeled with Arabic numbers (eg, 1, 2, 3, etc). The cytochrome (CYP) families most important for human drug metabolism are CYP1, CYP2, and CYP3. Subfamilies of enzymes consist of enzymes having at least 55% of their genes in the same sequence. The subfamily members are designated with a capital letter (eg, CYP1A, CYP2B, or CYP2C). Individual members of an enzyme family are named with another Arabic number and have at least 97% of their genes in the same sequence. CYP1A2 and CYP3A4 represent individual drug metabolizing isozymes.

Drugs that are metabolized in the liver can be classified according to the ability of the liver to extract the drug from the blood that flows through this organ. When more than 60% to 70% of the drug in the hepatic blood is removed (extracted) by the liver, it is classified as a *high extraction* drug (eg, propranolol and lidocaine). If less than 30% of the drug is extracted, it is designated as a *low extraction* drug (eg, theophylline and phenytoin). Drugs that do not fit into either of these categories are designated as *intermediate extraction* drugs. Following oral administration, the clearance from the body of drugs in all three extraction categories depends upon the intrinsic ability of the liver to metabolize the drug (intrinsic clearance). The same is true following IV administration, except for high extraction drugs whose clearance is principally dependent upon hepatic blood flow when administered IV. Thus, enzyme inhibition will have the least effect on high extraction drugs administered IV.

Inhibition of Hepatic Metabolism

Mechanisms of Inhibition. The inhibition of hepatic enzyme activity by drugs is usually competitive. The inhibiting drug competes with the object drug for binding sites of the metabolizing enzyme and reduces the ability of the liver to metabolize the object drug. Noncompetitive inhibition occurs when the enzyme's metabolic activity is suspended even though the object drug may continue to bind normally to the enzyme. In both competitive and noncompetitive inhibition, the metabolism of the object drug is reduced. The inhibiting drug may or may not be metabolized by the enzyme it inhibits.[128] Enzyme inhibition most frequently affects Phase I metabolism; however, Phase II metabolism is also affected by some drugs. Some enzyme inhibitors (eg, verapamil) tend to inhibit their own metabolism as well as the metabolism of other drugs. Studies with animal hepatocytes have demonstrated reduced digoxin uptake in hepatocytes by several basic drugs.[89] This could represent an additional mechanism for interactions thought to be caused by enzyme inhibition. For example, inhibiting the access of a drug to the metabolizing enzyme or to biliary secretion would likely result in reduced body clearance.

Characteristics of Enzyme Inhibition

Time Course. The inhibition of drug metabolism begins as the inhibitor reaches a critical concentration. Unless the inhibitor has a very long half-life and is not administered with a loading dose, inhibition usually reaches maximal intensity within 24 hours.[116] Once the inhibition begins, the time required for the object drug to reach a new steady state will primarily depend upon the new, post-interaction half-life of the object drug. When an inhibitor is discontinued, the decreased metabolism of the object drug will reverse based upon the elimination of the inhibitor. As with the interaction onset, its offset will occur within 24 hours for most common inhibitors. The object drug concentration will decline in relationship to its half-life. When the half-life of the inhibitor is less than that of the object drug, the offset of an inhibition interaction will be quicker than its onset (see Table 5 for a listing of drugs that inhibit drug metabolism with potentially significant results).

TABLE 5. Drugs that Inhibit Drug Metabolism with Potentially Significant Results

Allopurinol (eg, *Zyloprim*)	Itraconazole (*Sporanox*)
Amiodarone (eg, *Cordarone*)	Ketoconazole (eg, *Nizoral*)
Chloramphenicol (eg, *Chloromycetin*)	Metronidazole (eg, *Flagyl*)
Cimetidine (eg, *Tagamet*)	Mibefradil
Ciprofloxacin (*Cipro*)	Miconazole
Clarithromycin (*Biaxin*)	Monoamine oxidase inhibitors
Diltiazem (eg, *Cardizem*)	Phenylbutazone
Disulfiram (eg, *Antabuse*)	Propoxyphene (eg, *Darvocet-N*)
Enoxacin (*Penetrex*)	Quinidine
Erythromycin (eg, *E-Mycin*)	Ritonavir (*Norvir*)
Ethanol (acute ingestion)	Sulfinpyrazone (eg, *Anturane*)
Fluconazole (*Diflucan*)	Trimethoprim-Sulfamethoxazole (eg, *Bactrim*)
Fluoxetine (*Prozac*)	Troleandomycin (*TAO*)
Indinavir (*Crixivan*)	Verapamil (eg, *Calan*)
Isoniazid (INH; *Nydrazid*)	

Dose of the Inhibitor. Figure 4 displays the results of increasing doses of cimetidine on antipyrine clearance.[129] Cimetidine, in a similar dose-dependent manner, inhibits the clearance of theophylline and phenytoin.[130,131] While few dose-response studies have been completed with enzyme inhibitors, it appears that enzyme inhibition is generally dose related. Higher doses of the inhibitor will result in greater inhibition, although some inhibitors may have a maximum effect within their usual dosage range.

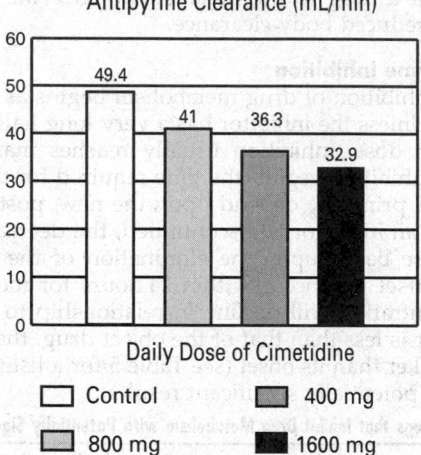

FIGURE 4 • Antipyrine/Cimetidine Clearance

Decreasing clearance of antipyrine with increasing doses of cimetidine in six subjects. Cimetidine doses were administered 4 times daily for 24 hours before and 30 hours after antipyrine dosing.

Potential Changes in Response. The major question relevant to all drug interactions relates to potential clinical significance. One of the major determinations of significance is the magnitude of change in the plasma concentration of the object drug. Drug clearance (Cl) and dosage determine a drug's steady-state plasma concentration (C_{ss}), where F is the fraction of the dose absorbed into the systemic circulation, D is the dose, and τ is the dosing interval. If an enzyme inhibition interaction alters only

$$C_{ss} = \frac{(F)(D)}{(Cl)(\tau)}$$

Cl, the change in C_{ss} will be determined by the change in Cl. The new C_{ss} can be estimated from the following equation:

$$\text{New } C_{ss} = (\text{Original } C_{ss}) \left(\frac{1}{1 - \text{fraction change in Cl}} \right)$$

Thus, a 20% reduction in clearance (0.2) would cause a 25% increase (1.25) in C_{ss}. Table 6 lists the changes in C_{ss} expected following a variety of reductions in Cl. Few drug interactions involve inhibition exceeding 50%, but a 15% to 20% change in clearance usually is necessary to produce observable effects.

TABLE 6. Percent Increase in Steady-State Plasma Concentrations Resulting from Various Percent Decreases in Clearance

Decrease in Cl	Increase in C_{ss}
10%	11%
15%	18%
20%	25%
25%	33%
30%	43%
50%	100%
75%	400%

For any change in object drug clearance, the effect observed will depend upon the object drug's concentration before the interaction. For example, if cimetidine reduces theophylline clearance 30%, a 43% increase in theophylline concentration would be expected. If a patient's theophylline concentration is 10 mcg/mL before the addition of cimetidine, the theophylline concentration probably would increase to approximately 14 mcg/mL. However, a theophylline concentration of 20 mcg/mL before cimetidine administration would be expected to increase to 29 mcg/mL. The risk of developing toxicity is greater in a patient with a theophylline concentration of 29 mcg/mL than a patient with a concentration of 14 mcg/mL.

Specificity. As previously noted, drugs that inhibit one cytochrome P450 isozyme tend to inhibit several P450 isozymes. The ability to inhibit drug metabolism may be related to specific structures common to interacting drugs. For example, it is the imidazole nucleus of cimetidine that is thought to bind to cytochrome P450.[132] Ketoconazole, itraconazole (*Sporanox*), metronidazole (eg, *Flagyl*), and miconazole all contain the imidazole ring structure and are known inhibitors of P450 metabolism.[133-136] Omeprazole (*Prilosec*) also contains the imidazole ring structure and has been shown to interact with diazepam, phenytoin, and other drugs that undergo oxidative metabolism.[137,138]

Many drugs, such as warfarin, are administered as a racemic mixture of 2 or more optical isomers. Often, these isomers have markedly different pharmacokinetic and pharmacodynamic properties, including their response to interacting drugs. For example, S-warfarin is approximately 4 times more potent in its hypoprothrombinemic activity than R-warfarin. Cimetidine significantly reduces the clearance of R-warfarin, but has little effect on S-warfarin.[139] However, cimetidine has been reported to prolong the prothrombin time and cause hemorrhagic complications in patients receiving warfarin.[140] Similarly, omeprazole only inhibits the metabolism of R-warfarin.[141] Other drugs, including metronidazole, trimethoprim-sulfamethoxazole (eg, *Bactrim*), phenylbutazone, and sulfinpyrazone, selectively inhibit the more active enantiomer S-warfarin and are probably more likely to produce significant changes in prothrombin times.[24,25,135,142,143] Sulfinpyrazone also exhibits stereoselective protein-binding displacement of R-warfarin.[25]

Variability. The large variability in response among patients following the administration of an enzyme inhibitor is due to several factors. The dose of the inhibitor and object drug are probably the most important determinants of the final result of inhibitor interactions. Other factors that can alter the incidence and magnitude of enzyme inhibition include genetic differences, age, concurrent therapy with an enzyme inducer, concurrent therapy with multiple enzyme inhibitors, and the presence of hepatic disease.

Genetic Influences. Drug metabolism may be genetically determined.[144] The most common metabolic pathways that are genetically controlled are N-acetylation, mephenytoin (CYP2C19) oxidation, and debrisoquin (CYP2D6) oxidation. Subjects are labeled as extensive or poor metabolizers based upon their inherited metabolic activity. Approximately 50% of Americans are poor N-acetylators, while 5% to 10% appear to lack the CYP2C19 or CYP2D6 enzymes. Although N-acetylation is independent of cytochrome P450, cimetidine reportedly has a greater effect on the clearance of antipyrine in slow acetylators (48% reduction) than in rapid acetylators (22% reduction).[145] Antipyrine, however, is not metabolized by acetylation, and slow acetylators had higher baseline antipyrine clearances than the fast acetylators. Quinidine, another well-known inhibitor of CYP2D6 isozyme activity, also affects rapid metabolizers to a greater extent than poor metabolizers. Drugs whose metabolism is inhibited by quinidine include codeine, sparteine, metoprolol (eg, *Lopressor*), propafenone (*Rythmol*), and encainide (*Enkaid*).[146-150]

Effect of Age. Age has not been shown to affect the magnitude of enzyme inhibition. Cimetidine inhibits the metabolism of theophylline and antipyrine to the same extent in young and elderly adults.[129,130] However, elderly patients may be at greater risk from inhibition reactions. The increased risk in the elderly is probably related to their potential for higher drug concentrations that result from age-induced reduction in drug clearance, and their reduced ability to withstand the insult of the drug interaction.

Presence of Enzyme Inducers. Smoking is a well-known inducer of hepatic drug metabolism. The inhibitory effect of cimetidine on theophylline metabolism was shown in one study to be greater in smokers than nonsmokers.[151] However, another study found no such relationship.[152] In subjects pretreated with rifampin, an inducer of cytochrome P450 enzymes, cimetidine reduced antipyrine clearance 44% compared with a 24% reduction before rifampin induction.[129]

Presence of Other Enzyme Inhibitors. Limited data indicate that combinations of enzyme inhibitors may have additive effects on the inhibition of drug clearance.[153] As with increasing cimetidine doses, however, there may be limits to the degree of inhibition that can be enhanced by combinations of inhibitors.[129] Hepatic cirrhosis can reduce drug clearance, and the combination of extrinsic inhibitors could potentiate disease-induced inhibition. For example, cimetidine can further depress drug clearance in patients with hepatic disease.[154,155]

Summary

Many commonly used drugs can inhibit the activity of hepatic drug metabolizing enzymes. Drug interactions involving enzyme inhibition tend to occur soon after the inhibiting drug is started, and disappear quickly with the elimination of the inhibitor. Inhibitors of oxidative drug metabolism are most prevalent and tend to affect many cytochrome P450 isozymes. The clinical significance of an enzyme inhibition interaction depends upon a variety of factors, including the dose of the object drug and the inhibitor and certain patient-specific characteristics.

CONCLUSION

This review of the general principles of drug interactions is intended to enable the practitioner to predict and evaluate potential drug interactions. A knowledge of the characteristics of drug interactions enables the practitioner to avoid or minimize the risk of potential drug interactions. Interactions tend to follow predictable patterns in time course and mechanism but express large interpatient variability in outcome. Each potential interaction should be evaluated using patient-specific parameters. Only then can a judgment be made regarding alternative responses designed to minimize the clinical impact of the interaction.

REFERENCES:
1. Radack KL. Ibuprofen interferes with the efficacy of anti-hypertensive drugs. A randomized, double-blind, placebo-controlled trial of ibuprofen compared with acetaminophen. *Ann Intern Med.* 1987;107:628.
2. Mitchell JR, et al. Guanethidine and related agents. III. Antagonism by drugs which inhibit the norepinephrine pump in man. *J Clin Invest.* 1970;49:1596.

3. Lalonde RL, et al. The effects of cimetidine on theophylline pharmacokinetics at steady state. *Chest.* 1983;2:221.
4. Serlin MJ, et al. Cimetidine: interactions with oral anticoagulants in man. *Lancet.* 1979;2:317.
5. Danan F, et al. Self-induction by erythromycin of its own transformation into a metabolite forming an inactive complex with reduced cytochrome P450. *J Pharmacol Exp Ther.* 1981;218:509.
6. Klotz U, et al. Elevation of steady-state diazepam levels by cimetidine. *Clin Pharmacol Ther.* 1981;30:513.
7. Miller RR, et al. Clinical importance of the interaction of phenytoin and isoniazid. *Chest.* 1979;75:356.
8. Wood AJJ, et al. The influence of cirrhosis on steady-state blood concentrations of unbound propranolol after oral administration. *Clin Pharmacokinet.* 1978;3:487.
9. Grossman SH, et al. Diazepam and lidocaine plasma protein binding in renal disease. *Clin Pharmacol Ther.* 1982;31:350.
10. Jeevendra Martyn JA, et al. Plasma protein binding of drugs after severe burn injury. *Clin Pharmacol Ther.* 1984;35:535.
11. Piafsky KM. Disease-induced changes in the plasma binding of basic drugs. *Clin Pharmacokinet.* 1980;5:246.
12. Edwards DJ, et al. Alpha-1–acid glycoprotein concentration and protein binding in trauma. *Clin Pharmacol Ther.* 1982;31:62.
13. Routledge PA, et al. Relationship between alpha-1–acid glycoprotein and lidocaine disposition in myocardial infarction. *Clin Pharmacol Ther.* 1981;30:154.
14. Jusko WJ, et al. Myocardial distribution of digoxin and renal function. *Clin Pharmacol Ther.* 1974;16:449.
15. Pieper JA, et al. Effects of phenobarbital on serum protein concentrations and verapamil binding. *Clin Pharmacol Ther.* 1987;41:165.
16. McElnay JC, et al. Protein binding displacement interactions and their clinical significance. *Drugs.* 1983;25:495.
17. Day RO, et al. The effect of concurrent aspirin upon plasma concentrations of tenoxicam. *Br J Clin Pharmacol.* 1988;26:455.
18. Rowland M. Protein binding and drug clearance. *Clin Pharmacokinet.* 1984;9(Suppl. 1):10.
19. MacKichan JJ. Pharmacokinetic consequences of drug displacement from blood and tissue proteins. *Clin Pharmacokinet.* 1984;9(Suppl. 1):32.
20. Van Hecken AM, et al. The influence of diflunisal on the pharmacokinetics of oxazepam. *Br J Clin Pharmacol.* 1985;20:225.
21. Udall JA. Warfarin-chloral hydrate interaction: pharmacological activity and clinical significance. *Ann Intern Med.* 1974;81:341.
22. Sellers EM, et al. Kinetics and clinical importance of displacement of warfarin from albumin by acidic drugs. *Ann NY Acad Sci.* 1971;179:213.
23. Griner PF, et al. Chloral hydrate and warfarin interaction: clinical significance? *Ann Intern Med.* 1971;74:540.
24. Lewis RJ, et al. Warfarin. Stereochemical aspects of its metabolism and the interaction with phenylbutazone. *J Clin Invest.* 1974;53:1607.
25. Toon S, et al. The warfarin-sulfinpyrazone interaction: stereochemical considerations. *Clin Pharmacol Ther.* 1986;39:15.
26. Rowland M, et al. Clinical Pharmacokinetics. Concepts and Applications. 2nd ed. Philadelphia: Lea & Febiger; 1988.
27. Cadwallader DE. Biopharmaceutics and Drug Interactions. 3rd ed. New York: Raven Press; 1983.
28. Neuvonen PJ, et al. Inhibitory effect of various iron salts on the absorption of tetracycline in man. *Eur J Clin Pharmacol.* 1974;7:357.
29. Campbell NRC, et al. Alteration of methyldopa absorption, metabolism and blood pressure control caused by ferrous sulfate and ferrous gluconate. *Clin Pharmacol Ther.* 1988;43:381.
30. Campbell NRC, et al. Ferrous sulfate reduces levodopa bioavailability: chelation as a possible mechanism. *Clin Pharmacol Ther.* 1989;45:220.
31. Schentag JJ, et al. Time dependent interactions between antacids and quinolone antibiotics. *Clin Pharmacol Ther.* 1988;43:135.
32. Parpia SH, et al. The effect of sucralfate on the oral bioavailability of norfloxacin. *Pharmacotherapy.* 1988;8:140. Abstract.
33. Northcutt RC, et al. The influence of cholestyramine on thyroxine absorption. *JAMA.* 1969;208:1857.
34. Jahnchen E, et al. Enhanced elimination of warfarin during treatment with cholestyramine. *Br J Clin Pharmacol.* 1978;5:437.
35. Hunninghake DB, et al. The effect of cholestyramine and colestipol on the absorption of hydrochlorothiazide. *Int J Clin Pharmacol Ther Toxicol.* 1982;20:151.
36. Nimmo J, et al. Pharmacological modification of gastric emptying: effects of propantheline and metoclopramide on paracetamol absorption. *BMJ.* 1973;1:587.
37. Manninen V, et al. Altered absorption of digoxin in patients given propantheline and metoclopramide. *Lancet.* 1973;1:398.
38. Jaffe JM. Effect of propantheline on nitrofurantoin absorption. *J Pharm Sci.* 1975;64:1729. Letter.
39. Champion MC. Domperidone. *Gen Pharmacol.* 1988;19:499.
40. Van der Meer JWM, et al. The influence of gastric acidity on the bioavailability of ketoconazole. *J Antimicrob Chemother.* 1980;6:552.
41. Feldman S, et al. Effect of antacid on absorption of enteric-coated aspirin. *JAMA.* 1974;227:660. Letter.
42. Boxenbaum HG, et al. Influence of gastrointestinal tract microflora on bioavailability. *Drug Metab Rev.* 1979;9:259.

43. Lindenbaum J, et al. Inactivation of digoxin by the gastrointestinal tract flora: reversal by antibiotic therapy. *N Engl J Med.* 1981;305:789.
44. Back DJ, et al. Evaluation of committee on safety of medicines. Yellow card reports on oral contraceptive-drug interactions with anticonvulsants and antibiotics. *Br J Clin Pharmacol.* 1988;25:527.
45. Griffin JP. Drug interactions occurring during absorption from the gastrointestinal tract. *Pharmacol Ther.* 1981;15:79.
46. Anon. Foods potentially harmful to patients taking MAO inhibitors. *The Medical Letter.* 1976;18:32.
47. Back DJ, et al. Interaction of ethinyl estradiol with ascorbic acid in man. *BMJ.* 1981;282:1516.
48. Morris JC, et al. Interaction of ethinyl estradiol with ascorbic acid in man. *BMJ.* 1981;283:503.
49. Caballeria J, et al. Effects of cimetidine on gastric alcohol dehydrogenase activity and blood ethanol levels. *Gastroenterology.* 1989;96:388.
50. Rennick BR, et al. Renal excretion of drugs: tubular transport and metabolism. *Ann Rev Pharmacol Toxicol.* 1972;12:141.
51. Rennick BR, et al. Renal tubule transport of organic cations. *Am J Physiol.* 1981;240:F83.
52. Kosoglou T, et al. Drug interactions involving renal transport mechanisms: an overview. *DICP Ann Pharmacother.* 1989;23:116.
53. Kvale PA, et al. Single oral dose ampicillin-probenecid treatment of gonorrhea in the male. *JAMA.* 1971;215:1449.
54. Griffith RS, et al. Effect of probenecid on the blood levels and urinary excretion of cefamandole. *Antimicrob Agents Chemother.* 1977;11:809.
55. Kampmann J, et al. Effect of some drugs on penicillin half-life in blood. *Clin Pharmacol Ther.* 1972;13:516.
56. Lilly MB, et al. Clinical pharmacology of oral intermediate-dose methotrexate with or without probenecid. *Cancer Chemother Pharmacol.* 1985;15:220.
57. Howell SB, et al. Effect of probenecid on cerebrospinal fluid methotrexate kinetics. *Clin Pharmacol Ther.* 1979;26:641.
58. Ellison NM, et al. Acute renal failure and death following sequential intermediate-dose methotrexate and 5-FU; a possible adverse effect due to concomitant indomethacin administration. *Cancer Treat Rep.* 1985;69:342.
59. Liegler DG, et al. The effect of organic acids on renal clearance of methotrexate in man. *Clin Pharmacol Ther.* 1969;10:849.
60. Regal RE, et al. Aspirin and uricosurics: interaction revisited. *Drug Intell Clin Pharm.* 1987;21:219.
61. Yu TF, et al. Mutual suppression of the uricosuric effects of sulfinpyrazone and salicylate: a study in interactions between drugs. *J Clin Invest.* 1963;42:1330.
62. Boger WP, et al. Probenecid and salicylates: the question of interaction in terms of penicillin excretion. *J Lab Clin Med.* 1955;45:478.
63. Daubresse JC, et al. Clofibrate and diabetes control in patients treated with oral hypoglycemic agents. *Br J Clin Pharmacol.* 1979;7:599.
64. Petitpierre B, et al. Behavior of chlorpropamide in renal insufficiency and under the effect of associated drug therapy. *Int J Clin Pharmacol Ther Toxicol.* 1972;6:120.
65. Ferrari C, et al. Potentiation of hypoglycemic response to intravenous tolbutamide by clofibrate. *N Engl J Med.* 1976;294:613.
66. Petersen V, et al. Effect of prolonged thiazide treatment on renal lithium clearance. *BMJ.* 1974;2:143.
67. Solomon K. Combined use of lithium and diuretics. *South Med J.* 1978;71:1098.
68. Leahey EB, et al. Reduced renal clearance of digoxin during chronic quinidine administration. *Circulation.* 1979;60:11.
69. Schenck-Gustafsson K, et al. Renal function and digoxin clearance during quinidine therapy. *Clin Physiol.* 1982;2:401.
70. Fenster PE, et al. Pharmacokinetic evaluation of the digoxin-amiodarone interaction. *J Am Coll Cardiol.* 1985;5:108.
71. Pedersen KE, et al. Digoxin-verapamil interaction. *Clin Pharmacol Ther.* 1981;30:311.
72. Johnson BF, et al. The comparative effects of verapamil and a new dihydropyridine calcium channel blocker on digoxin pharmacokinetics. *Clin Pharmacol Ther.* 1987;42:66.
73. Pedersen KE at el. The long-term effect of verapamil on plasma digoxin concentration and renal digoxin clearance in healthy subjects. *Eur J Clin Pharmacol.* 1982;22:123.
74. Pedersen KE, et al. Digoxin-trimethoprim interaction. *Acta Med Scand.* 1985;217:423.
75. Waldorff S, et al. Spironolactone-induced changes in digoxin kinetics. *Clin Pharmacol Ther.* 1978;24:162.
76. Fenster PE, et al. Digoxin-quinidinespironolactone interaction. *Clin Pharmacol Ther.* 1984;36:70.
77. Cleland JGF, et al. The effects of captopril on serum digoxin and urinary urea and digoxin clearances in patients with congestive heart failure. *Am Heart J.* 1986;112:130.
78. Windle J, et al. Pharmacokinetic and electrophysiologic interactions of amiodarone and procainamide. *Clin Pharmacol Ther.* 1987;41:603.
79. Somogyi A, et al. Cimetidine-procainamide pharmacokinetic interaction in man: evidence of competition for tubular secretion of basic drugs. *Eur J Clin Pharmacol.* 1983;25:339.
80. Rodvold KA, et al. Interaction of steady-state procainamide with H2- receptor antagonists cimetidine and ranitidine. *Ther Drug Monit.* 1987;9:378.
81. Rocci ML at et. Ranitidine-induced changes in the renal and hepatic clearances of procainamide are correlated. *J Parmacol Exp Ther.* 1989;248:923.
82. Somogyi A, et al. Dose and concentration dependent effect of ranitidine on procainamide disposition and renal clearance in man. *Br J Clin Pharmacol.* 1984;18:175.

83. Gerhardt RE, et al. Quinidine excretion in aciduria and alkaluria. *Ann Intern Med.* 1969;71:927.
84. Beckett AH, et al. Influence of urinary pH on excretion of amphetamines. *Lancet.* 1965;1:303.
85. Hansten PD, et al. Effect of antacids and ascorbic acid on serum salicylate concentrations. *J Clin Pharmacol.* 1980;24:326.
86. Hager WD, et al. Digoxin-quinidine interaction: pharmacokinetic evaluation. *N Engl J Med.* 1979;300:1238.
87. Schenck-Gustafsson K, et al. Pharmacokinetics of digoxin in patients subjected to the quinidine-digoxin interaction. *Br J Clin Pharmacol.* 1981;11:181.
88. Angelin B, et al. Quinidine reduces biliary clearance of digoxin in man. *Eur J Clin Invest.* 1987;17:262.
89. Okudaira K, et al. Effects of basic drugs on the hepatic transport of cardiac glycosides in rats. *Biocherm Pharmacol.* 1988;37:2949.
90. Nitsch J, et al. Enhanced elimination of amiodarone by colestyramine. *Dtsch Med Wochenschr.* 1986;111:1241.
91. Brown DD, et al. A steady-state evaluation of the effects of propantheline bromide and cholestyramine on the bioavailability of digoxin when administered as tablets or capsules. *J Clin Pharmacol.* 1985;25:360.
92. Cayen MN. Metabolism of xenobiotics. *Pharm International.* 1984;5:53.
93. Lu AYH. Multiplicity of liver drug metabolizing enzymes. *Drug Metab Rev.* 1979;10:187.
94. Orme M. Enantiomers of warfarin and phenobarbital. *N Engl J Med.* 1976;295:1482.
95. Mantyla R, et al. Pharmacokinetic interactions of timolol with vasodilating drugs, food and phenobarbitone in healthy human volunteers. *Eur J Clin Pharmacol.* 1983;24:227.
96. Gibson GA, et al. Influence of high-dose pentobarbital on theophylline pharmacokinetics: a case report. *Ther Drug Monit.* 1983;7:181.
97. Alvan G, et al. Effects of pentobarbital on the disposition of alprenolol. *Clin Pharmacol Ther.* 1977;22:316.
98. Paladino JA, et al. Effect of secobarbital on theophylline clearance. *Ther Drug Monit.* 1983;5:135.
99. O'Reilly RA, et al. Interaction of secobarbital with warfarin pseudoracemates. *Clin Pharmacol Ther.* 1980;28:187.
100. Stevenson IH, et al. Changes in human drug metabolism after long-term exposure to hypnotics. *BMJ.* 1972;4:322.
101. Antlitz AM, et al. Effect of butabarbital on orally administered anticoagulants. *Curr Ther Res* 1968;10:70.
102. Aggeler PM, et al. Effect of heptabarbital on the response to bishydroxycoumarin in man. *J Lab Clin Med.* 1969;74:229.
103. Boylan JJ, et al. Phenytoin interference with dexamethasone. *JAMA.* 1976;235:803.
104. Petereit LB, et al. Effectiveness of prednisolone during phenytoin therapy. *Clin Pharmacol Ther.* 1977;22:912.
105. Kessler JM, et al. Disopyramide and phenytoin interaction. *Clin Pharm* 1982;1:263.
106. Nightingale J, et al. Effect of phenytoin on serum disopyramide concentrations. *Clin Pharm.* 1987;6:46.
107. Morris S. Drug interaction between phenytoin and oral contraceptives. *Drug Intell Clin Pharm.* 1984;18:135.
108. Notelovitz M, et al. Interaction between estrogen and dilantin in a menopausal woman. *N Engl J Med.* 1981;304:788.
109. Tong TG, et al. Phenytoin-induced methadone withdrawal. *Ann Intern Med.* 1981;94:349.
110. Begg EJ, et al. Enhanced metabolism of mexiletine after phenytoin administration. *Br J Clin Pharmacol.* 1982;14:219.
111. Farringer JA, et al. Quinidine and 3-hydroxyquinidine levels during initiation of anticonvulsant therapy and after chronic anticonvulsant administration. *Drug Intell Clin Pharm.* 1985;19:461.
112. Urbano AM. Phenytoin-quinidine interaction in a patient with recurrent ventricular tachyarrhythmias. *N Engl J Med.* 1982;308:225.
113. Miller M, et al. Influence of phenytoin on theophylline clearance. *Clin Pharmacol Ther.* 1984;35:666.
114. Sklar SJ, et al. Enhanced theophylline clearance secondary to phenytoin therapy. *Drug Intell Clin Pharm.* 1985;19:34.
115. Powell JR, et al. Induction and inhibition of drug metabolism. In: Evans E, et al. Applied Pharmacokinetics. 2nd ed. Vancouver: Applied Therapeutics; 1986;139–186.
116. Dossing M, et al. Time course of phenobarbital and cimetidine mediated changes in hepatic drug metabolism. *Eur J Clin Pharmacol.* 1983;25:215.
117. Price DE, et al. The effect of low-dose phenobarbitone on three indices of hepatic microsomal enzyme induction. *Br J Clin Pharmacol.* 1986;22:744.
118. Perucca E, et al. Effect of low-dose phenobarbitone on five indirect indices of hepatic microsomal enzyme induction and plasma lipoproteins in normal subjects. *Br J Clin Pharmacol.* 1981;12:592.
119. Whitfield JB, et al. Changes in plasma gamma-glutamyl transpeptidase activity associated with alterations in drug metabolism in man. *BMJ.* 1973;1:316.
120. Tomson T, et al. Relationship of intraindividual dose to plasma concentration of carbamazepine: indication of dose-dependent induction of metabolism. *Ther Drug Monit.* 1989;11:533.
121. Corn M. Effect of phenobarbital and glutethimide on biological half-life of warfarin. *Thromb Diath Haemorrh.* 1966;16:606.
122. Vestal RE, et al. Antipyrine metabolism in man: influence of age, alcohol, caffeine, and smoking. *Clin Pharmacol Ther.* 1975;18:425.
123. Salem SAM, et al. Reduced induction of drug metabolism in the elderly. *Age Aging.* 1978;7:68.
124. Vesell ES, et al. Genetic control of the phenobarbital-induced shortening of plasma antipyrine half-lives in man. *J Clin Invest.* 1969;48:2202.

125. Eichelbaum M, et al. The influence of enzyme induction on polymorphic sparteine oxidation. *Br J Clin Pharmacol.* 1986;22:49.
126. Perucca E, et al. A comparative study of the relative enzyme-inducing properties of anticonvulsant drugs in epileptic patients. *Br J Clin Pharmacol.* 1984;18:401.
127. Feely J, et al. Inhibition of drug metabolism: dose response and sensitivity of elderly and induced subjects. *Br J Clin Pharmacol.* 1983;15:589P.
128. Testa B, et al. Inhibitors of cytochrome P450s and their mechanism of action. *Drug Metab Rev.* 1981;12:1.
129. Feely J, et al. Factors affecting the response to inhibition of drug metabolism by cimetidine-dose response and sensitivity of elderly and induced subjects. *Br J Clin Pharmacol.* 1984;17:77.
130. Cohen IA, et al. Cimetidine-theophylline interaction: effects of age and cimetidine dose. *Ther Drug Monit.* 1985;7:426.
131. Bartle WR, et al. Dose-dependent effect of cimetidine on phenytoin kinetics. *Clin Pharmacol Ther.* 1983;33:649.
132. Rendic S, et al. Characterization of cimetidine, ranitidine and related structures' interaction with cytochrome P450. *Drug Metab Dispos.* 1983;11:137.
133. Shepard JH, et al. Cyclosporine-ketoconazole: a potentially dangerous drug-drug interaction. *Clin Pharm.* 1986;5:648.
134. Kwan JTC, et al. Interaction of cyclosporine and itraconazole. *Lancet.* 1987;2:282.
135. O'Reilly RA. The stereoselective interaction of warfarin and metronidazole in man. *N Engl J Med.* 1976;295:354.
136. Coloquhoun MC, et al. Interaction between warfarin and miconazole oral gel. *Lancet.* 1987;1:695.
137. Gugler R, et al. Omeprazole inhibits oxidative drug metabolism: studies with diazepam and phenytoin in vivo and 7-ethoxycoumarin in vitro. *Gastroenterology.* 1985;89:1235.
138. Jensen JC, et al. Inhibition of human liver cytochrome P450 by omeprazole. *Br J Clin Pharmacol.* 1986;21:328.
139. Choonara IA, et al. Stereoselective interaction between the R enantiomer of warfarin and cimetidine. *Br J Clin Pharmacol.* 1986;21:271.
140. Kerley B, et al. Cimetidine potentiation of warfarin action. *Can Med Assoc J.* 1982;126:116.
141. Sutfin T, et al. Stereoselective interaction of omeprazole with warfarin in healthy men. *Ther Drug Monit.* 1989;11:176.
142. O'Reilly RA. Stereoselective interaction of trimethoprim-sulfamethoxazole with the separated enantiomorphs of racemic warfarin in man. *N Engl J Med.* 1980;302:33.
143. O'Reilly RA. Stereoselective interaction of sulfinpyrazone with racemic warfarin and its separated enantiomorphs in man. *Circulation.* 1982;65:202.
144. Relling MV. Polymorphic drug metabolism. *Clin Pharm.* 1989;8:852.
145. Gachalyi B, et al. Pharmacogenetic differences in the inhibitory effect of cimetidine on the metabolism of antipyrine. *Eur J Clin Pharmacol.* 1987;31:613.
146. Sindrup SH, et al. The effect of quinidine on the analgesic effect of codeine. *Eur J Clin Pharmacol.* 1992;42:587.
147. Brinn R, et al. Sparteine oxidation is practically abolished in quinidine-treated patients. *Br J Clin Pharmacol.* 1986;22:194.
148. Leemann T, et al. Single-dose quinidine treatment inhibits metoprolol oxidation in extensive metabolizers. *Eur J Clin Pharmacol.* 1986;29:739.
149. Funck-Brentano C, et al. Genetically-determined interaction between propafenone and low dose quinidine: role of active metabolites in modulating net drug effect. *Br Clin Pharmacol.* 1989;249:134.
150. Funck-Brentano C, et al. Effect of low dose quinidine on encainide pharmacokinetics and pharmacodynamics. Influence of genetic polymorphism. *J Pharmacol Exp Ther.* 1989;249:134.
151. Grygiel JJ, et al. Differential effects of cimetidine on theophylline metabolic pathways. *Eur J Clin Pharmacol.* 1984;26:335.
152. Cusack BJ, et al. Cigarette smoking and theophylline metabolism: effects of cimetidine. *Clin Pharmacol Ther.* 1985;37:330.
153. Loft S, et al. Inhibition of antipyrine elimination by disulfiram and cimetidine: the effect of concomitant administration. *Br J Clin Pharmacol.* 1986;21:75.
154. Nelson DC, et al. The effect of cimetidine on hepatic drug elimination in cirrhosis. *Hepatology.* 1985;5:305.
155. Rollinghoff W, et al. Inhibition of drug metabolism by cimetidine in man: dependence on pretreatment microsomal liver function. *Eur J Clin Invest.* 1982;12:429.
156. Hedman A. Inibition by basic drugs of digoxin secretion into human bile. *Eur J Clin Pharmacol.* 1992;42:457.

Mechanisms of Drug Interactions: Extrahepatic First-Pass Metabolism

The most common route of drug administration is oral. The passage of a drug from the GI tract to the systemic circulation requires a series of interrelated steps that begin with drug dissolution and end with the drug exiting the portal circulation. For a drug to exert its pharmacologic effect, it must survive this journey as an intact, pharmacologically active molecule. The drug initially dissolves into solution, then passes through the intestinal epithelial cells and enters the portal vein system. From the intestinal tract, the drug is carried to the liver where it must "first pass" by the hepatocytes before entering the systemic blood for transport to its site of action. A number of factors have been identified that can affect the drug absorption process including the time of day that drug administration occurs, age and gender of the patient, pathologic alterations in GI motility, pH or flora, diet, rate of hepatic blood flow, and genetically determined differences in a patient's drug metabolism.

DRUG INTERACTIONS FOLLOWING ORAL DRUG ADMINISTRATION

Drug interactions arising from changes in the absorption of an object drug have been widely reported. Common examples include reduced bioavailability of tetracycline and quinolone antibiotics by antacids and the binding of thyroxine by cholestyramine. These physical-chemical interactions are usually predictable and may be minimized by careful selection of drug administration times. Alteration in drug metabolism during the absorption process is a common occurrence and can cause large changes in the plasma concentrations of the object drug. This review will consider the mechanisms involved in this presystemic metabolism and its role in drug interactions.

A brief review of the pharmacokinetic parameters involved in determining plasma concentrations following oral drug administration is helpful to understand the clinical consequences of interactions with oral drugs. If the dose (D) and dosing interval (τ) are not changed, the mean steady-state drug concentration (C_{ss}) will be determined by the fraction of the dose absorbed (F) and the total clearance of the drug (Cl_t). Equation 1 describes this relationship:

$$C_{ss} = \frac{(F)(D)}{(Cl_t)(\tau)}$$

Effect of Changes in Bioavailability or Clearance

The fraction of the dose absorbed, or bioavailability, can be thought of as the amount of a dose actually entering the systemic circulation and is reduced from 100% absorption by anything that reduces the amount of drug leaving the GI tract (eg, cholestyramine binding). Any metabolism that occurs prior to the entry of the drug into the systemic circulation will also reduce the bioavailability of the drug. The liver has been considered the primary site of this presystemic metabolism. Since this metabolism occurs during the first pass of the drug through the liver immediately after absorption, it is referred to as "first-pass metabolism" or the "first-pass effect." As can be seen from Equation 1, a change in F causes a direct change in C_{ss} while a change in Cl_t will produce an inverse change in C_{ss}. Thus, a decrease in F decreases C_{ss} while a decrease in Cl_t will result in an increase in C_{ss}. It is important to remember that the changes in F and Cl_t produce proportionately different changes in C_{ss}. Table 1 shows how changes in a drug's F and Cl_t are reflected in its steady-state plasma concentrations.

TABLE 1. The Relationship Between Changes in Bioavailability or Total Clearance and Steady-State Plasma Concentrations

Change in F	Change in C_{ss}	Change in Cl_t	Change in C_{ss}
Increase 20%	Increase 20%	Increase 20%	Decrease 17%
Increase 50%	Increase 50%	Increase 50%	Decrease 33%
Decrease 20%	Decrease 20%	Decrease 20%	Increase 25%
Decrease 50%	Decrease 50%	Decrease 50%	Increase 100%

Several trends that are helpful in predicting the potential clinical significance of drug interactions are demonstrated by Table 1. Consider the situation where an object drug is metabolized by CYP3A4 in the intestine and liver. An equal degree (percent of baseline activity) of CYP3A4 inhibition in the liver will produce a larger increase in C_{ss} than inhibition of intestinal CYP3A4. For example, a 50% decrease in hepatic metabolic activity would produce a 100% increase in C_{ss}, while a similar decrease in intestinal metabolism would raise the bioavailability and C_{ss} only 50%. Stimulation of CYP3A4 activity by 50% would reduce bioavailability and C_{ss} 50% but a similar increase in hepatic metabolism would only reduce C_{ss} 33%. Thus, for interactions involving inhibition of enzyme activity, a larger change in C_{ss}, and clinical effect, will occur with hepatic vs intestinal enzyme inhibition. Conversely, when enzyme induction occurs, greater changes in C_{ss} will result from intestinal enzyme induction compared with hepatic induction. Of course a change in both hepatic and intestinal enzyme activity would produce greater effects on C_{ss} than a change in only one site of metabolism.

Extrahepatic First-Pass Metabolism and P-Glycoprotein
In addition to first-pass metabolism occurring in the liver, it has been known for some time that certain drugs are also metabolized in the intestine and therefore undergo extrahepatic first-pass metabolism. For example, monoamine oxidase in the intestinal wall metabolizes tyramine in foods and some amines such as phenylephrine. Inhibition of monoamine oxidase predisposes patients to hypertensive reactions when phenylephrine is taken orally. Recently, the discovery of one of the cytochrome P450 enzymes responsible for hepatic metabolism (CYP3A4) in the wall of the intestine has provided another mechanism for extrahepatic first-pass metabolism. CYP3A4 is the major cytochrome P450 enzyme in the liver and its concentration and activity vary widely between subjects.[1] This enzyme, which is found in intestinal epithelial cells, plays an important role in the metabolism of a large number of drugs including calcium antagonists, cyclosporine, benzodiazepines, and nonsedating antihistamines. Changes in the activity of this enzyme can alter the bioavailability and hepatic clearance of these drugs, producing large variations in plasma concentrations.

The discovery of a transporter protein in the intestine has added another modulator of drug bioavailability. P-glycoprotein is an efflux pump located in the brush border on the luminal surface of the enterocyte. It functions as a pump that transports drugs from the cell cytoplasm back into the intestinal lumen.[2,3] This would result in a reduction in the rate and perhaps amount of drug absorption. Drugs that are pumped out of the intestinal cell back into the intestinal lumen could be reabsorbed at a later time or may remain in the gut to be excreted. The function of P-glycoprotein may be to limit the rate of absorption of toxins, including drugs, into the body by reducing their transport through the intestinal wall and into the portal circulation. By limiting the absorption rate of a drug, P-glycoprotein increases the efficiency of enzymes located in the intestinal wall (eg, CYP3A4) to metabolize the drug. P-glycoprotein serves as a kind of valve, slowing the presentation of the drug to the intestinal enzymes. This may enable more complete drug metabolism by avoiding saturation of the enzyme by very high intracellular concentrations of the drug that would occur following oral administration or by increasing the time of drug exposure to the enzymes. Inhibition of P-glycoprotein would produce changes in bioavailability similar to those seen after inhibition of CYP3A4. The nature of the relationship between P-glycoprotein and CYP3A4 in the enterocyte awaits further study.

Drug interactions involving altered first-pass metabolism may result from changes in intestinal enzyme activity, hepatic enzyme activity, P-glycoprotein activity, or a combination of changes in these mechanisms. Many interactions that were initially considered to be due to altered hepatic first-pass metabolism may require re-evaluation to discern the role, if any, of intestinal enzyme and P-glycoprotein activity. Identifying the mechanism(s) responsible for a specific interaction can be difficult. By evaluating the pharmacokinetic changes that occur during interactions involving different object and precipitant drugs and different routes of administration, it is possible to gain some insight into the mechanisms involved.

Factors Affecting the Clinical Outcome of Oral Drug Interactions

The changes in an object drug's pharmacokinetic parameters may help establish the relative contribution of changes in bioavailability or systemic clearance produced by the precipitant drug. For example, changes in peak plasma concentrations (C_{max}) primarily reflect altered first-pass metabolism in the liver or intestine. Drug half-life changes, assuming no change in volume of distribution (V_d), will reflect changes in oral clearance. The effect of erythromycin on oral buspirone pharmacokinetics was studied in healthy subjects.[4] In this study, erythromycin administration resulted in a 5-fold increase in buspirone C_{max} but no change in its half-life. The bioavailability of buspirone is only approximately 5%, making it very susceptible to changes in first-pass metabolism. These results would suggest that erythromycin's effect was primarily limited to increasing the bioavailability of buspirone without altering its systemic clearance. Assuming no erythromycin-induced change in buspirone volume of distribution, this could represent a selective inhibition of intestinal CYP3A4, inhibition of P-glycoprotein, or both.

In another study, alprazolam was administered orally alone and following erythromycin pretreatment.[5] In this study, erythromycin increased the area under the concentration-time curve (AUC) of alprazolam 147% and increased its half-life from 16 to 40 hours. The peak concentration of alprazolam was not increased by erythromycin administration. This lack of effect on alprazolam's C_{max} is probably due to its rather high bioavailability (approximately 92%) that will be minimally affected by inhibition of first-pass metabolism. Thus, it would appear that the primary effect of erythromycin was to reduce the oral clearance of alprazolam. This reduction in hepatic metabolism was reflected by an increase in alprazolam's half-life.

Grapefruit Juice: A Selective Inhibitor of Intestinal Metabolism

As can be seen by the examples above, it is often impossible to separate the effects of an inhibitor on hepatic vs intestinal first-pass enzyme activity. In addition, the effects of erythromycin, or other inhibitors, on P-glycoprotein activity is not readily discernible from these studies. What is needed is a precipitant drug that has a limited site of action. Fortunately, such a compound exists: Grapefruit juice. Grapefruit juice is known to inhibit CYP3A4 in the intestinal cells but has minimal effect on hepatic CYP3A4 and no effect on intestinal P-glycoprotein.

The effects of grapefruit juice and erythromycin on the pharmacokinetics of felodipine illustrate the differences in intestinal vs hepatic enzyme inhibition.[6] In one investigation, subjects received 10 mg extended-release felodipine alone, following 1 day of pretreatment with erythromycin 250 mg 4 times daily, and following a single dose of grapefruit juice. Compared with administration with water, erythromycin increased the AUC and C_{max} of felodipine 294% and 243%, respectively. Felodipine half-life increased from a mean of 6.9 hours with water to 11.1 hours after erythromycin. Grapefruit juice increased felodipine's AUC and C_{max} 225% and 270%, respectively, but no change in felodipine half-life was noted after grapefruit juice. It would appear that grapefruit juice and erythromycin increase the bioavailability of felodipine from its usual 15% to 35% or 40%. Because both drugs produced a similar increase in felodipine C_{max}, most of the effect must have been due to enzyme inhibition in the intestinal wall. In addition, erythromycin-induced increase in felodipine half-life indicates that it inhibits the hepatic metabolism of felodipine.

If grapefruit juice only affects intestinal CYP3A4, its effects would be expected to be limited to object drugs that are administered orally. The effects of grapefruit juice on the pharmacokinetics of felodipine following oral and IV administration have been reported.[7] In this study, felodipine was administered as a 1-hour 1.5 mg IV infusion or orally as a 10 mg extended-release tablet. Water or grapefruit juice was given just before drug administration. Because felodipine was administered IV and orally, absolute bioavailability could be determined. Grapefruit juice did not affect the pharmacokinetics of felodipine after IV administration. Following oral administration of felodipine, grapefruit juice increased its C_{max} 173% and its AUC 72%. Felodipine half-life was not changed by preadministration of grapefruit juice. The mean bioavailability of felodipine increased from 14.2% with water to 25.3% after grapefruit juice.

CONCLUSION

A number of different mechanisms can be responsible for drug interactions involving drugs that are administered orally. During the past few years, our knowledge and understanding of the role of presystemic metabolism has expanded to include extrahepatic metabolism. The function of P-glycoprotein and its relationship to enterocyte metabolism is just beginning to be studied. Several characteristics of oral drug interactions have emerged as critical in determining the potential clinical significance of an oral drug interaction. Drugs with extensive first-pass metabolism, particularly if they are CYP3A4 substrates, are more likely to undergo large increases in plasma concentrations as a result of enzyme or P-glycoprotein inhibition. Precipitant drugs that are capable of influencing intestinal and hepatic enzymes as well as P-glycoprotein activity are likely to produce interactions of greater clinical significance. Until the potential contribution of each of these mechanisms is defined, assessment of the change, or lack of change, in object drug pharmacokinetic parameters will help identify the mechanisms responsible for specific interactions.

REFERENCES:
1. Shimada T, et al. Interindividual variations in human liver cytochrome P-450 enzymes involved in the oxidation of drugs, carcinogens and toxic chemicals: studies with liver microsomes of 30 Japanese and 30 Caucasians. *J Pharmacol Exp Ther.* 1994;270:414.
2. Saeki T, et al. Human P-glycoprotein transports cyclosporin A and FK506. *J Biol Chem.* 1993;268:6077.
3. Saitoh H, et al. Possible involvement of multiple P-glycoprotein-mediated efflux systems in the transport of verapamil and other organic cations across rat intestine. *Pharm Res.* 1995;12:1304.
4. Kivisto KT, et al. Plasma buspirone concentrations are greatly increased by erythromycin and itraconazole. *Clin Pharmacol Ther.* 1997;62:348.
5. Yasui N, et al. A kinetic and dynamic study of oral alprazolam with and without erythromycin in humans: in vivo evidence for the involvement of CYP3A4 in alprazolam metabolism. *Clin Pharmacol Ther.* 1996;59:514.
6. Bailey DG, et al. Erythromycin-felodipine interaction: magnitude, mechanism, and comparison with grapefruit juice. *Clin Pharmacol Ther.* 1996;60:25.
7. Lundahl J, et al. Effects of grapefruit juice ingestion—pharmacokinetics and haemodynamics of intravenously and orally administered felodipine in healthy men. *Eur J Clin Pharmacol.* 1997;52:139.

Cytochrome (CYP) P450 Isozyme Drug Interactions

Many commonly used drugs can inhibit the activity of hepatic drug metabolizing enzymes. Drug interactions involving enzyme inhibition tend to occur soon after the inhibiting drug is started and disappear quickly with the elimination of the inhibitor. Inhibitors of oxidative drug metabolism are most prevalent and tend to affect many cytochrome P450 isozymes. The clinical significance of an enzyme inhibition interaction depends upon a variety of factors, including the dose of the object drug and the inhibitor and certain patient-specific characteristics. For additional information on cytochrome P450 isozyme inhibitors, see Pharmacokinetic Drug Interaction Mechanisms and Clinical Characteristics. In particular, see the section on Drug Interaction Mechanisms: Enzyme Inhibition.

TABLE 1. Cytochrome (CYP) P450 Isozyme

Generic Name	1A2	2C9	2C19	2D6	2E1	3A4
Acetaminophen					Substrate	
Alcohol		Inhibitor, Inducer			Substrate	
Alfentanil						Substrate
Alfuzosin						Substrate
Almotriptan				Substrate		Substrate
Alprazolam						Substrate
Amiodarone		Inhibitor		Inhibitor		Substrate, Inhibitor
Amitriptyline	Substrate		Substrate	Substrate		Substrate
Amlodipine						Substrate
Amprenavir		Substrate		Substrate		Substrate, Inhibitor
Aprepitant	Substrate	Inducer	Substrate			Substrate, Inhibitor
Aripiprazole				Substrate		Substrate
Artemisinin	Inhibitor		Inducer			
Astemizole						Substrate
Atazanavir	Inhibitor					Substrate, Inhibitor
Atomoxetine				Substrate		
Atorvastatin						Substrate
Barbiturates	Inducer	Inducer	Inducer			Inducer
Basiliximab						Inhibitor
Bepridil						Substrate

TABLE 1. Cytochrome (CYP) P450 Isozyme

Generic Name	1A2	2C9	2C19	2D6	2E1	3A4
Bexarotene						Substrate, Inducer
Bosentan		Substrate, Inducer				Substrate, Inducer
Bromocriptine						Substrate
Budesonide						Substrate
Bupropion				Inhibitor		
Buspirone						Substrate
Caffeine	Substrate					
Capecitabine		Inhibitor				
Carbamazepine	Inducer	Inducer				Substrate, Inducer
Carvedilol				Substrate		
Chloramphenicol			Inhibitor			Inhibitor
Chloroquine				Inhibitor		
Chlorpheniramine				Substrate, Inhibitor		Substrate
Chlorpromazine				Substrate, Inhibitor		
Chlorpropamide		Substrate				
Cigarette smoking	Inducer					
Cimetidine	Inhibitor		Inhibitor	Inhibitor		
Cinacalcet	Substrate			Substrate, Inhibitor		Substrate
Ciprofloxacin	Inhibitor					
Cisapride						Substrate
Citalopram			Substrate	Substrate, Inhibitor		Substrate
Clarithromycin						Substrate, Inhibitor
Clomipramine	Substrate		Substrate	Substrate		Substrate
Clonazepam						Substrate
Clopidogrel		Inhibitor	Substrate			Substrate
Clozapine	Substrate		Substrate	Substrate		Substrate
Codeine conversion to morphine				Substrate		
Colchicine						Substrate
Conivaptan						Substrate, Inhibitor
Corticosteroids						Substrate

TABLE 1. Cytochrome (CYP) P450 Isozyme

Generic Name	1A2	2C9	2C19	2D6	2E1	3A4
Cotrimoxazole		Substrate, Inhibitor				Substrate
Cyclophosphamide (Cytoxan)						Substrate
Cyclosporine						Substrate, Inhibitor
Danazol						Inhibitor
Dapsone					Substrate	Substrate
Darifenacin				Substrate		Substrate
Darunavir						Substrate, Inhibitor
Dasatinib						Substrate, Inhibitor
Delavirdine		Inhibitor	Inhibitor			Substrate, Inhibitor
Desipramine			Substrate	Substrate		
Desvenlafaxine				Inhibitor		Substrate
Dexamethasone						Substrate, Inducer
Dextromethorphan				Substrate		Substate
Diazepam			Substrate			Substrate
Diclofenac		Substrate				Substrate
Dihydrocodeine				Substrate		
Dihydroergotamine						Substrate
Diltiazem						Substrate, Inhibitor
Diphenhydramine	Substrate		Substrate	Substrate, Inhibitor		
Disopyramide						Substrate
Disulfiram		Inhibitor			Inhibitor	
Docetaxel						Substrate
Dofetilide						Substrate
Dolasetron				Substrate		Substrate
Donepezil				Substrate		Substrate
Doxepin		Substrate	Substrate	Substrate		
Doxorubicin						Substrate
Dronedarone				Inhibitor		Substrate, Inhibitor
Droperidol						Substrate
Duloxetine	Substrate			Substrate, Inhibitor		

TABLE 1. Cytochrome (CYP) P450 Isozyme

Generic Name	1A2	2C9	2C19	2D6	2E1	3A4
Dutasteride						Substrate
Ebastine						Substrate
Efavirenz		Inhibitor	Inhibitor			Substrate, Inducer
Eletriptan						Substrate
Encainide				Substrate		
Enoxacin	Inhibitor					
Eplerenone						Substrate
Ergotamine						Substrate
Erlotinib	Substrate					Substrate
Erythromycin						Substrate, Inhibitor
Escitalopram			Substrate	Substrate, Inhibitor		Substrate
Esomeprazole			Substrate, Inhibitor			Substrate
Estazolam						Substrate
Eszopiclone						Substrate
Ethinyl estradiol	Inhibitor					Substrate, Inhibitor
Etoposide						Substrate
Etravirine		Substrate, Inhibitor	Substrate, Inhibitor			Substrate, Inducer
Everolimus						Substrate
Felbamate			Inhibitor			
Felodipine						Substrate
Fentanyl						Substrate
Fesoterodine				Substrate		Substrate
Finasteride						Substrate
Flecainide				Substrate, Inhibitor		
Fluconazole		Inhibitor	Inhibitor			Inhibitor
Fluorouracil		Inhibitor				
Fluoxetine		Substrate, Inhibitor	Substrate, Inhibitor	Substrate, Inhibitor		Inhibitor
Flurazepam						Substrate
Flurbiprofen		Substrate				
Fluvastatin		Substrate, Inhibitor				

TABLE 1. Cytochrome (CYP) P450 Isozyme

Generic Name	1A2	2C9	2C19	2D6	2E1	3A4
Fluvoxamine	Substrate, Inhibitor	Inhibitor	Inhibitor	Substrate, Inhibitor		Inhibitor
Fosamprenavir (Lexiva)						Substrate, Inhibitor
Frovatriptan	Substrate					
Galantamine				Substrate		Substrate
Gefitinib				Substrate		Substrate
Gemfibrozil		Inhibitor				
Glimepiride		Substrate				
Glipizide		Substrate				
Glyburide		Substrate				
Granisetron						Substrate
Grapefruit juice						Inhibitor
Griseofulvin		Inducer				Inducer
Haloperidol				Substrate, Inhibitor		Substrate
Hydrocodone				Substrate		
Hydroxychloroquine				Inhibitor		
Ibuprofen		Substrate				
Ifosfamide						Substrate
Imatanib		Inhibitor		Inhibitor		Substrate, Inhibitor
Imipramine	Substrate		Substrate	Substrate		Substrate
Indinavir						Substrate, Inhibitor
Indomethacin		Substrate				
Irbesartan		Substrate				
Irinotecan						Substrate
Isoniazid			Inhibitor		Substrate, Inhibitor	Inhibitor
Isradipine						Substrate
Itraconazole						Substrate, Inhibitor
Ketoconazole						Substrate, Inhibitor
Lapatinib						Substrate, Inhibitor
Lansoprazole			Substrate			Substrate
Leflunomide		Inhibitor				

TABLE 1. Cytochrome (CYP) P450 Isozyme

Generic Name	1A2	2C9	2C19	2D6	2E1	3A4
Levomethadyl						Substrate
Lidocaine	Substrate					Substrate
Loperamide						Substrate
Lopinavir						Substrate
Loratadine				Substrate		Substrate
Losartan		Substrate				Substrate
Lovastatin						Substrate
Maprotiline				Substrate		
Maraviroc						Substrate
Meloxicam		Substrate				Substrate
Mephenytoin			Substrate			
Mesoridazine				Substrate		
Methadone			Substrate	Substrate		
Methamphetamine				Substrate		
Methylprednisolone						Substrate
Metoclopramide				Substrate		
Metoprolol				Substrate		
Metronidazole		Inhibitor				
Mexiletine	Substrate, Inhibitor			Substrate		
Mianserin				Substrate		
Miconazole		Inhibitor				Inhibitor
Midazolam						Substrate
Mifepristone						Substrate, Inhibitor
Mirtazapine	Substrate			Substrate		Substrate
Moclobemide			Substrate, Inhibitor	Inhibitor		
Modafinil		Inhibitor	Inhibitor			Substrate, Inducer
Montelukast		Substrate				Substrate
Nafcillin						Inducer
Naproxen		Substrate				
Nefazodone						Substrate, Inhibitor
Nateglinide		Substrate				Substrate
Nebivolol				Substrate		
Nelfinavir			Substrate			Substrate, Inhibitor

TABLE 1. Cytochrome (CYP) P450 Isozyme

Generic Name	1A2	2C9	2C19	2D6	2E1	3A4
Nevirapine						Substrate, Inducer
Nicardipine						Substrate, Inhibitor
Nifedipine						Substrate
Nilotinib						Substrate, Inhibitor
Nimodipine						Substrate
Nisoldipine						Substrate
Nitrendipine						Substrate
Norfloxacin	Inhibitor					
Nortriptyline				Substrate		Substrate
Olanzapine	Substrate			Substrate		Substrate
Omeprazole			Substrate, Inhibitor			Substrate
Ondansetron	Substrate			Substrate		Substrate
Oxcarbazepine			Inhibitor			Inducer
Oxybutynin						Substrate
Oxycodone				Substrate		Substrate
Paclitaxel						Substrate
Palonosetron	Substrate			Substrate		Substrate
Pantoprazole			Substrate			Substrate
Paroxetine				Substrate, Inhibitor		
Parsugrel		Substrate	Substrate			Substrate
Pazopanib				Inhibitor		Substrate, Inhibitor
Perhexiline				Substrate		
Perphenazine				Substrate, Inhibitor		
Phenobarbital	Inducer	Substrate, Inducer	Substrate, Inducer			Inducer
Phenytoin	Inducer	Substrate, Inhibitor	Substrate, Inducer			Inducer
Pimozide	Substrate					Substrate
Pioglitazone						Substrate
Piroxicam		Substrate				
Posaconazole						Inhibitor
Prednisolone						Substrate

TABLE 1. Cytochrome (CYP) P450 Isozyme

Generic Name	1A2	2C9	2C19	2D6	2E1	3A4
Prednisone						Substrate
Primidone	Inducer	Inducer	Inducer			Inducer
Promethazine				Substrate, Inhibitor		
Propafenone	Substrate			Substrate, Inhibitor		Substrate
Propoxyphene				Substrate, Inhibitor		Substrate, Inhibitor
Propranolol			Substrate	Substrate		
Protriptyline				Substrate		
Quazepam						Substrate
Quetiapine						Substrate
Quinacrine				Inhibitor		Substrate
Quinidine				Inhibitor		Substrate
Quinine				Inhibitor		Substrate
Quinupristin						Inhibitor
Rabeprazole			Substrate			
Ramelteon	Substrate	Substrate				Substrate
Ranolazine				Substrate, Inhibitor		Substrate, Inhibitor
Rasagiline	Substrate					
Repaglinide						Substrate
Rifabutin						Substrate, Inducer
Rifampin	Inducer	Inducer	Inducer	Inducer		Inducer
Rifapentine		Inducer				Inducer
Risperidone				Substrate, Inhibitor		Substrate
Ritonavir				Inhibitor		Substrate, Inhibitor
Ropinirole	Substrate					
Rosiglitazone		Substrate				
Rosuvastatin		Substrate				
Saquinavir						Substrate, Inhibitor
Selegiline	Substrate					Substrate
Sertindole				Substrate		Substrate
Sertraline			Substrate	Substrate, Inhibitor		Substrate

TABLE 1. Cytochrome (CYP) P450 Isozyme

Generic Name	1A2	2C9	2C19	2D6	2E1	3A4
Sibutramine						Substrate
Sildenafil		Substrate				Substrate
Simvastatin				Substrate		Substrate
Sirolimus						Substrate
Solifenacin						Substrate
Sorafenib						Substrate
St. John's Wort			Inducer			Inducer
Sufentanil						Substrate
Sulfamethoxazole		Substrate, Inhibitor				Substrate
Sulfinpyrazone		Inhibitor				
Sunitinib						Substrate
Tacrine	Substrate, Inhibitor					
Tacrolimus						Substrate
Tadalafil						Substrate
Tamoxifen				Substrate		Substrate, Inhibitor
Tamsulosin				Substrate		Substrate
Telithromycin						Inhibitor
Teniposide						Substrate
Terbinafine				Inhibitor		
Terfenadine						Substrate
Testosterone						Substrate
Theophylline	Substrate					Substrate
Thioridazine	Substrate			Substrate, Inhibitor		Substrate
Tiagabine						Substrate
Ticlopidine			Inhibitor			
Timolol				Substrate		
Tizanidine	Substrate					
Tolbutamide		Substrate				
Tolterodine				Substrate		Substrate
Topiramate			Inhibitor			Substrate, Inducer
Torsemide		Substrate				
Tramadol				Substrate		Substrate
Trazodone				Substrate		Substrate

TABLE 1. Cytochrome (CYP) P450 Isozyme

Generic Name	1A2	2C9	2C19	2D6	2E1	3A4
Triamterene	Substrate					Substrate
Triazolam						Substrate
Valdecoxib		Substrate				Substrate
Valproic Acid		Inhibitor				
Valsartan		Substrate				
Vardenafil						Substrate
Venlafaxine				Substrate		Substrate
Verapamil						Substrate, Inhibitor
Vesnarinone						Substrate
Vinblastine						Substrate
Vincristine						Substrate
Vinorelbine						Substrate
Voriconazole		Substrate, Inhibitor	Substrate, Inhibitor			Substrate, Inhibitor
R-Warfarin	Substrate		Substrate			Substrate
S-Warfarin		Substrate				
Yohimbine				Substrate		Substrate
Zafirlukast	Substrate, Inhibitor	Inhibitor				Inhibitor
Zaleplon						Substrate
Zileuton	Substrate, Inhibitor					
Ziprasidone						Substrate
Zolmitriptan	Substrate					
Zolpidem		Substrate				Substrate
Zonisamide						Substrate
Zopiclone						Substrate

MONOGRAPHS

Acarbose (*Precose*) 4

Acetaminophen (eg, *Tylenol*)

SUMMARY: Animal studies suggest that acarbose may increase the risk of acetaminophen-alcohol hepatotoxicity, but the clinical importance of this effect is not established.

RISK FACTORS:

➡ *Other Drugs.* Patients who regularly ingest alcohol may be at greater risk for this interaction.

MECHANISM: Not established. It is proposed that acarbose increases the activity of CYP2E1, resulting in an increase in the conversion of acetaminophen to its hepatotoxic metabolite, NAPQI.

CLINICAL EVALUATION: Studies in rats suggest that acarbose increases the hepatotoxicity of acetaminophen in the presence of alcohol.[1] The extent to which acarbose increases hepatotoxicity in the absence of alcohol was not studied. Although studies in humans are not available, the potential severity of the adverse outcome prompted the authors to suggest that this interaction may be of clinical importance.

RELATED DRUGS: No information is available.

MANAGEMENT OPTIONS: No specific action is required, but be alert for evidence of the interaction.

REFERENCES:

1. Krahenbuhl S. Acarbose and acetaminophen—a dangerous combination? *Hepatology.* 1999;29:285.

Acenocoumarol (*Sintrom*) 4

Chlorpromazine (eg, *Thorazine*)

SUMMARY: Animal studies indicate that chlorpromazine enhances the effect of acenocoumarol, but clinical information concerning a similar effect in humans is lacking.

RISK FACTORS: No specific risk factors are known.

MECHANISM: Not established.

CLINICAL EVALUATION: Chlorpromazine can enhance the hypoprothrombinemic effect of acenocoumarol in animals.[1] Studies in humans are lacking, but no case reports have appeared describing effects of chlorpromazine on anticoagulant therapy.

RELATED DRUGS: No information is available.

MANAGEMENT OPTIONS: No specific action is required, but be alert for evidence of the interaction.

REFERENCES:

1. Weiner M. Effect of centrally active drugs on the action of coumarin anticoagulants. *Nature.* 1966;212:1599.

5   Acetaminophen (eg, *Tylenol*)

Amantadine (eg, *Symmetrel*)

SUMMARY: Chronic amantadine administration has no effect on acetaminophen plasma concentrations.

RISK FACTORS: No specific risk factors are known.

MECHANISM: No interaction.

CLINICAL EVALUATION: The effect of chronic amantadine dosing (200 mg/day) on the pharmacokinetics of a single dose of acetaminophen was compared to the pharmacokinetics of a single dose of amantadine and acetaminophen in 5 healthy subjects.[1] No change in acetaminophen pharmacokinetics were noted during chronic amantadine administration.

RELATED DRUGS: No information is available.

MANAGEMENT OPTIONS: No interaction.

REFERENCES:

1. Aoki FY, et al. Effects of chronic amantadine hydrochloride ingestion on its and acetaminophen pharmacokinetics in young adults. *J Clin Pharmacol.* 1992;32:24.

4   Acetaminophen (eg, *Tylenol*)

Aspirin

SUMMARY: Although acetaminophen may alter the pharmacokinetics of aspirin slightly, the clinical importance of this effect is questionable.

RISK FACTORS: No specific risk factors are known.

MECHANISM: Not established.

CLINICAL EVALUATION: A study of 21 subjects who were given various combinations of aspirin and acetaminophen demonstrated that acetaminophen increased blood concentrations of unhydrolyzed aspirin but not total salicylate.[1] It was proposed that the increase in unhydrolyzed aspirin would increase the therapeutic effect; however, it also has been suggested that combinations of aspirin with either acetaminophen or phenacetin may increase the likelihood of analgesic nephropathy.[2] Neither of these possibilities has been proven clinically.

RELATED DRUGS: It has been suggested that combinations of aspirin with phenacetin also may increase the likelihood of analgesic nephropathy.[2]

MANAGEMENT OPTIONS: No specific action is required, but be alert for evidence of the interaction.

REFERENCES:

1. Cotty VF, et al. Augmentation of human blood acetylsalicylate concentrations by the simultaneous administration of acetaminophen with aspirin. *Toxicol Appl Pharmacol.* 1977;41:7.

2. Wilson DR, et al. Declining evidence of analgesic nephropathy in Canada. *Can Med Assoc J.* 1982;127:500.

Acetaminophen (eg, *Tylenol*)

Chloramphenicol (eg, *Chloromycetin*)

SUMMARY: Acetaminophen has been reported to increase, decrease, or have no effect on the clearance of chloramphenicol. More study is needed.

RISK FACTORS: No specific risk factors are known.

MECHANISM: Not established.

CLINICAL EVALUATION: Chloramphenicol has been reported to prolong the half-life of acetaminophen,[1] have no effect on acetaminophen,[2,4] and increase the clearance of acetaminophen.[3] The reasons for the disparate results in these studies probably result from differences in study design, number of subjects, assay techniques, or route of acetaminophen administration. Until clinical evidence of excessive or insufficient chloramphenicol effect associated with acetaminophen administration is reported, the clinical significance of this interaction will remain speculative.

RELATED DRUGS: No information is available.

MANAGEMENT OPTIONS: No specific action is required, but be alert for evidence of the interaction.

REFERENCES:

1. Buchanan N, et al. Interaction between chloramphenicol and paracetamol. *BMJ*. 1979;3:307.
2. Kearns GL, et al. Absence of a pharmacokinetic interaction between chloramphenicol and acetaminophen in children. *J Pediatr*. 1985;107:134.
3. Spika JS, et al. Interaction between chloramphenicol and acetaminophen. *Arch Dis Child*. 1986;61:1121.
4. Stein CM, et al. Lack of effect of paracetamol on the pharmacokinetics of chloramphenicol. *Br J Clin Pharmacol*. 1989;27:262.

Acetaminophen (eg, *Tylenol*)

Cholestyramine (eg, *Questran*)

SUMMARY: Cholestyramine markedly reduces plasma acetaminophen concentrations and probably reduces acetaminophen therapeutic response.

RISK FACTORS: No specific risk factors are known.

MECHANISM: Cholestyramine inhibits the GI absorption of acetaminophen.

CLINICAL EVALUATION: In 4 healthy subjects, coadministration of cholestyramine 12 g orally markedly reduced plasma levels of acetaminophen 2 g orally.[1] The magnitude of the effect appears sufficient to reduce the therapeutic response to acetaminophen.

RELATED DRUGS: Colestipol (*Colestid*) probably would reduce plasma acetaminophen concentrations also, but clinical studies are lacking.

MANAGEMENT OPTIONS:

➡ *Circumvent/Minimize.* Give acetaminophen 2 hours before or 6 hours after cholestyramine.

➥ *Monitor.* Monitor patients for reduced acetaminophen effects if this combination is given.

REFERENCES:
   1. Dordoni B, et al. Reduction of absorption of paracetamol by activated charcoal and cholestyramine: a possible therapeutic measure. *BMJ.* 1973;3:86.

 Acetaminophen (eg, *Tylenol*)

Cimetidine (eg, *Tagamet*)

SUMMARY: Although some evidence suggests that cimetidine protects against the hepatotoxicity of acetaminophen overdoses, this has not been a consistent finding.

RISK FACTORS: No specific risk factors are known.

MECHANISM: Cimetidine purportedly protects against the hepatotoxic effects of over-doses of acetaminophen by reducing the formation of a reactive acetaminophen metabolite; however, most studies have failed to confirm this mechanism.

CLINICAL EVALUATION: In isolated case reports and some animal studies, cimetidine seemed to protect against the hepatotoxicity of acetaminophen overdoses;[1-6] however, studies in humans have been conflicting. Some studies in normal subjects and patients suggest that cimetidine inhibits the formation of reactive (hepato-toxic) metabolites of acetaminophen.[7,8] In other studies involving healthy subjects, however, cimetidine did not affect the formation of these metabolites.[9-11] The reason for the disparate results is unclear, but it is probably because of differences in hepatic glutathione status, smoking or drinking habits among the subjects, and study design. Thus, the evidence for a protective effect of cimetidine in acetamino-phen overdose cases is not convincing. Because it would not be ethical to give cimetidine in place of acetylcysteine to patients with acetaminophen overdose, it will be difficult to assess the protective role of cimetidine in this situation.

Although cimetidine modestly reduced the plasma clearance of acetaminophen in one study; most studies of the effect of cimetidine on the disposition of therapeu-tic doses of acetaminophen have found no significant effect.[6,8,11,12] Cimetidine is, therefore, unlikely to affect the dosage requirements for acetaminophen.

RELATED DRUGS: Ranitidine (eg, *Zantac*) probably has minimal effects on acetaminophen response. Little is known regarding the effect of famotidine (eg, *Pepcid*) or nizati-dine (*Axid*) on acetaminophen, but there is no reason to suspect that they would interact.

MANAGEMENT OPTIONS: No specific action is required, but be alert for evidence of the interaction.

REFERENCES:
   1. Jackson JE. Cimetidine protects against acetaminophen toxicity. *Life Sci.* 1982;31:31.
   2. Rudd GD, et al. Prevention of acetaminophen-induced hepatic necrosis by cimetidine in mice. *Res Commun Chem Pathol Pharmacol.* 1981;32:369.
   3. Donn KH, et al. Prevention of acetaminophen-induced hepatic injury by cimetidine. *Clin Pharmacol Ther.* 1982;31:218.
   4. Rudd GD, et al. The hepatoprotective effect of cimetidine following acetaminophen overdose. *Clin Pharmacol Ther.* 1984;35:270.
   5. Mitchell MC, et al. Cimetidine protects against acetaminophen hepatotoxicity in rats. *Gastroenterology.* 1981;81:1052.

6. Abernethy DR, et al. Differential effect of cimetidine on drug oxidation (antipyrine and diazepam) vs conjugation (acetaminophen and lorazepam): prevention of acetaminophen toxicity by cimetidine. *J Pharmacol Exp Ther.* 1983;224:508.

7. Mitchell MC, et al. Selective inhibition of acetaminophen oxidation and toxicity by cimetidine and other histamine H_2-receptor antagonists in vivo and in vitro in the rat and man. *J Clin Invest.* 1984;73:383.

8. Vendemiale G, et al. Effect of acute and chronic cimetidine administration on acetaminophen metabolism in humans. *Am J Gastroenterol.* 1987;82:1031.

9. Critchley JAJH, et al. Is there a place for cimetidine or ethanol in the treatment of paracetamol poisoning? *Lancet.* 1983;1:1375.

10. Miners JO, et al. Determinants of acetaminophen metabolism: effect of inducers and inhibitors of drug metabolism on acetaminophen's metabolic pathways. *Clin Pharmacol Ther.* 1984;35:481.

11. Slattery JT, et al. Lack of effect of cimetidine on acetaminophen disposition in humans. *Clin Pharmacol Ther.* 1989;46:591.

12. Chen MM, et al. Cimetidine-acetaminophen interaction in humans. *J Clin Pharmacol.* 1985;25:227.

Acetaminophen (eg, *Tylenol*)

Contraceptives, Oral (eg, *Ortho-Novum*)

SUMMARY: Acetaminophen tends to increase plasma concentrations of ethinyl estradiol, while oral contraceptives reduce plasma acetaminophen concentrations; the clinical importance of these changes is not established.

RISK FACTORS: No specific risk factors are known.

MECHANISM: Acetaminophen probably reduces the sulfation of ethinyl estradiol in the GI mucosa, thus increasing the plasma concentration of the estrogen. Oral contraceptives appear to enhance the glucuronidation of acetaminophen.

CLINICAL EVALUATION: In 6 healthy women receiving oral contraceptives, the pharmacokinetics of ethinyl estradiol were studied with and without pretreatment of a single 1 g dose of acetaminophen.[1] Acetaminophen was associated with a modest increase in serum ethinyl estradiol concentrations. The clinical importance of these increases in estrogen levels is not established, but it is reasonable to assume that periodic use of acetaminophen may result in fluctuating levels of ethinyl estradiol. Several studies have shown that women taking oral contraceptives have considerably higher clearance of acetaminophen than those not taking these agents.[2-5] The magnitude of the reduction in plasma acetaminophen concentrations is probably sufficient to inhibit the effect of acetaminophen in at least some patients. It does not appear necessary for women on oral contraceptives to avoid taking acetaminophen, but patients on the combination may develop increased ethinyl estradiol concentrations or decreased acetaminophen concentrations.

RELATED DRUGS: Little is known regarding the effect of acetaminophen on estrogens other than ethinyl estradiol. Conjugated estrogens (eg, *Premarin*), however, did not appear to affect acetaminophen pharmacokinetics in a study that compared 12 women taking conjugated estrogen with 18 women who were not.[6]

MANAGEMENT OPTIONS: No specific action is required, but be alert for evidence of the interaction.

REFERENCES:
1. Rogers SM, et al. Paracetamol interaction with oral contraceptive steroids. *Br J Clin Pharmacol.* 1987;23:615P.

2. Abernethy DR, et al. Increased metabolic clearance of acetaminophen with oral contraceptive use. *Obstet Gynecol.* 1982;60:338.

3. Mitchell MC, et al. Effects of oral contraceptive steroids on acetaminophen metabolism and elimination. *Clin Pharmacol Ther.* 1983;34:48.

4. Miners JO, et al. Influence of sex and oral contraceptive steroids on paracetamol metabolism. *Br J Clin Pharmacol.* 1983;16:503.

5. Ochs HR, et al. Differential effects of isoniazid and oral contraceptive steroids on antipyrine oxidation and acetaminophen conjugation. *Pharmacology.* 1984;28:188.

6. Scavone JM, et al. Acetaminophen pharmacokinetics in women receiving conjugated estrogen. *Eur J Clin Pharmacol.* 1990;38:97.

4 Acetaminophen (eg, *Tylenol*)

Diazepam (eg, *Valium*)

SUMMARY: Acetaminophen may reduce diazepam bioavailability, but the clinical importance of this effect is probably minimal.

RISK FACTORS: No specific risk factors are known.

MECHANISM: Not established.

CLINICAL EVALUATION: Acetaminophen 3 g/day for 5 days somewhat reduced the 96-hour urinary excretion of diazepam and its metabolites in 4 subjects following a single 10 mg dose of diazepam.[1] The effect was greater in 2 women. Additional study is needed to confirm these results and to define the magnitude of the interaction.

RELATED DRUGS: The effect of acetaminophen on other benzodiazepines is not established.

MANAGEMENT OPTIONS: No specific action is required, but be alert for evidence of the interaction.

REFERENCES:
1. Mulley BA, et al. Interactions between diazepam and paracetamol. *J Clin Pharm.* 1978;3:25.

3 Acetaminophen (eg, *Tylenol*)

Ethanol (Ethyl Alcohol)

SUMMARY: Substantial evidence indicates that chronic, excessive alcohol ingestion increases the toxicity of high therapeutic doses or overdoses of acetaminophen, while preliminary evidence indicates that acute alcohol intoxication protects against acetaminophen overdose toxicity.

RISK FACTORS:

 Dosage Regimen. The increased risk of acetaminophen hepatotoxicity occurs primarily with excessive doses of acetaminophen in the presence of chronic, excessive alcohol ingestion.

MECHANISM: Enzyme induction from prolonged intake of large amounts of alcohol may enhance the formation of hepatotoxic metabolites of acetaminophen, while lowering the serum acetaminophen concentration.

CLINICAL EVALUATION: Data from acetaminophen overdoses in chronic alcoholics indicate that these individuals are more susceptible to acetaminophen-induced hepatotoxicity.[1-5,7] Also, there is growing evidence that alcohol abuse can predispose patients who chronically take large therapeutic doses of acetaminophen to hepatotoxicity. Indeed, some of the reported cases of acetaminophen hepatotoxicity have involved the use of therapeutic doses of acetaminophen rather than intentional overdoses.[2,3,7,13] Alcohol-acetaminophen hepatotoxicity may be misdiagnosed in many cases.[15] Also, overdoses of acetaminophen in alcoholics may result in lower than expected serum acetaminophen concentrations, resulting in a failure to use needed acetylcysteine. This may have contributed to the death of at least 1 patient.[16]

In contrast to chronic alcohol abuse, acute alcohol intoxication tends to inhibit hepatic microsomal drug metabolism. Thus, acute alcohol intoxication might be expected to reduce the formation of toxic acetaminophen metabolites. Animal studies indicate that acute ethanol administration tends to be protective against the hepatotoxicity of large acetaminophen doses.[8,9] Ethanol intoxication may have contributed to a favorable outcome in a patient who took 60 g of acetaminophen.[10] Finally, the bioavailability of acetaminophen may be lower in alcoholics as compared to nonalcoholics because first-pass metabolism is increased.[6,12] This may partly explain the tendency of alcoholics to take large quantities of acetaminophen for therapeutic purposes.[2,3,14]

RELATED DRUGS: No information is available.

MANAGEMENT OPTIONS:

➡ *Circumvent/Minimize.* Warn patients who chronically ingest large amounts of alcohol (eg, several drinks a day or more) to avoid taking large or prolonged doses of acetaminophen.

➡ *Monitor.* When monitoring serum acetaminophen following acute acetaminophen overdose in alcohol abusers, be aware that acetylcysteine may be indicated even if the serum acetaminophen concentration is below the "action line" on the standard nomogram. This is probably because of the ability of alcohol to enhance acetaminophen metabolism. (Some have recommended that the serum acetaminophen threshold for acetylcysteine therapy should be reduced by as much as 70% in patients who chronically ingest large amounts of alcohol.)[11]

REFERENCES:

1. Emby DJ, et al. Hepatotoxicity of paracetamol enhanced by ingestion of alcohol: report of two cases. *S Afr Med J.* 1977;51:208.

2. Barker JD Jr, et al. Chronic excessive acetaminophen use and liver damage. *Ann Intern Med.* 1977;87:299.

3. McClain CJ, et al. Potentiation of acetaminophen hepatotoxicity by alcohol. *JAMA.* 1980;244:251.

4. Johnson MW, et al. Alcoholism, nonprescription drugs and hepatotoxicity. The risk from unknown acetaminophen ingestion. *Am J Gastroenterol.* 1981;76:530.

5. McJunkin B, et al. Fatal massive hepatic necrosis following acetaminophen overdose. *JAMA.* 1976;236:1874.

6. Dietz AJ Jr, et al. Acetaminophen kinetics in the alcoholic. *Clin Pharmacol Ther.* 1982;31:218.

7. Licht J, et al. Apparent potentiation of acetaminophen hepatotoxicity by alcohol. *Ann Intern Med.* 1980;92:511.

8. Sato C, et al. Prevention of acetaminophen-induced hepatotoxicity by acute ethanol administration in the rat: comparison with carbon tetrachloride-induced hepatotoxicity. *J Pharmacol Exp Ther.* 1981;218:805.

9. Sato C, et al. Mechanism of the preventive effect of ethanol on acetaminophen-induced hepatotoxicity. *J Pharmacol Exp Ther.* 1981;218:811.

10. Lyons L, et al. Treatment of acetaminophen overdosage with N-acetylcysteine. *N Engl J Med.* 1977;296:174.

11. McClements BM, et al. Management of paracetamol poisoning complicated by enzyme induction due to alcohol or drugs. *Lancet.* 1990;1:1526.

12. Skinner MH, et al. Acetaminophen metabolism in recovering alcoholics. *Clin Pharmacol Ther.* 1990;47:160.
13. Wootton FT, et al. Acetaminophen hepatotoxicity in the alcoholic. *South Med J.* 1990;83:1047.
14. Seifert CF, et al. Patterns of acetaminophen use in alcoholic patients. *Pharmacotherapy.* 1993;13:391.
15. Kumar S, et al. Failure of physicians to recognize acetaminophen hepatotoxicity in chronic alcoholics. *Arch Intern Med.* 1991;151:1189.
16. Cheung L, et al. Acetaminophen treatment nomogram. *New Engl J Med.* 1994;330:1907.

4   Acetaminophen (eg, *Tylenol*)

Exenatide (*Byetta*)

SUMMARY: Exenatide slows gastric emptying for at least 4 hours after administration; reduced and delayed peak acetaminophen plasma concentrations may result in diminished analgesic effect.

RISK FACTORS: No specific risk factors are known.

MECHANISM: Exenatide slows gastric emptying, thus delaying acetaminophen delivery to the small intestine for absorption.

CLINICAL EVALUATION: Forty subjects received acetaminophen 1 g alone or from 1 hour before to 4 hours after a single subcutaneous injection of placebo or exenatide 10 mcg.[1] The mean peak concentration of acetaminophen was reduced between 37% and 56% by the administration of exenatide. The mean time to reach peak concentration was increased from 0.6 to 4.2 hours. The mean area under the plasma concentration-time curve of acetaminophen was modestly reduced by about 25%. The effect of exenatide on acetaminophen was still present when the acetaminophen was administered 4 hours after the exenatide. The delayed gastric emptying caused by exenatide could delay or reduce the efficacy of some drugs for which a rapid onset of action is desirable, such as analgesics or hypnotics.

RELATED DRUGS: None known.

MANAGEMENT OPTIONS:

➥ *Monitor.* Instruct patients taking exenatide to take other orally administered drugs 1 hour prior to exenatide dosing to avoid delayed absorption of the oral medication.

REFERENCES:
1. Blasé E, et al. Pharmacokinetics of an oral drug (acetaminophen) administered at various times in relation to subcutaneous injection of exenatide (exendin-4) in healthy subjects. *J Clin Pharmacol.* 2005;45:570-577.

5   Acetaminophen (eg, *Tylenol*)

Interferon Alfa-2a (*Roferon-A*)

SUMMARY: A study in healthy subjects suggests that acetaminophen does not interfere with the biologic response to interferon, but it also does not appear to alleviate the side effects of interferon.

RISK FACTORS: No specific risk factors are known.

MECHANISM: No interaction.

CLINICAL EVALUATION: Eight healthy subjects received intramuscular recombinant human interferon 18×10^6 units with acetaminophen 650 mg every 4 hours given 1 day before and for 6 additional days after the interferon.[1] Responses to interferon plus acetaminophen were compared with those of a group of subjects receiving interferon alone. Acetaminophen did not reduce interferon-induced fever, chills, headache, myalgia, or fatigue, nor did it affect the biologic response to interferon as measured by induction of 2'–5'-oligoadenylate synthetase or resistance to vesicular stomatitis virus infection.

RELATED DRUGS: No information is available.

MANAGEMENT OPTIONS: No interaction.

REFERENCES:

1. Witter FR, et al. Effects of prednisone, aspirin, and acetaminophen on an in vivo biologic response to interferon in humans. *Clin Pharmacol Ther*. 1988;44:239-243.

Acetaminophen (eg, *Tylenol*)

Isoniazid (eg, *Nydrazid*)

SUMMARY: Acetaminophen concentrations were increased by isoniazid; cases of hepatotoxicity have been reported following administration of isoniazid and acetaminophen.

RISK FACTORS: No specific risk factors are known.

MECHANISM: Isoniazid appears to reduce the oxidative metabolism of acetaminophen during coadministration. Acetaminophen metabolism transiently increases for a day or two after isoniazid is discontinued. No mechanism is known for the reported hepatotoxicity during the administration of isoniazid and acetaminophen.

CLINICAL EVALUATION: A 19-year-old woman ingested an approximate total single dose of acetaminophen 11.5 g.[1] She had been taking isoniazid 300 mg/day and oral contraceptives for several months before the ingestion. Despite the apparent low concentrations of acetaminophen (15 mcmol/mL 13 hours after ingestion), the patient developed severe acute liver toxicity and uremia. While acetaminophen doses greater than 7.5 g are known to cause hepatotoxicity, one study suggests that isoniazid induced the metabolism of acetaminophen to toxic metabolites. Additional anecdotal cases of hepatic toxicity following the concurrent ingestion of isoniazid and acetaminophen have been reported.[2] However, studies have demonstrated that isoniazid 300 mg/day for 7 days reduced the oxidative metabolism of acetaminophen to hepatotoxic metabolites during isoniazid administration.[3,4] A temporary increase in oxidative metabolism occurs over 1 to 2 days after isoniazid is discontinued. Case reports of increased hepatotoxicity caused by combined isoniazid and acetaminophen are unlikely to be the result of isoniazid-induced production of toxic metabolites of acetaminophen.

RELATED DRUGS: No information is available.

MANAGEMENT OPTIONS:

➥ *Circumvent/Minimize.* Until further data are available, patients taking isoniazid should limit their use of acetaminophen. Aspirin or a nonsteroidal anti-inflammatory drug may be used instead of acetaminophen.

➡️ *Monitor.* Until further data are available, monitor patients taking isoniazid and acetaminophen for hepatotoxicity.

REFERENCES:

1. Murphy R, et al. Severe acetaminophen toxicity in a patient receiving isoniazid. *Ann Intern Med.* 1990;113:799-800.
2. Moulding TS, et al. Acetaminophen, isoniazid, and hepatic toxicity. *Ann Intern Med.* 1991;114:431.
3. Epstein MM, et al. Inhibition of the metabolism of paracetamol by isoniazid. *Br J Clin Pharmacol.* 1991;31:139-142.
4. Zand R, et al. Inhibition and induction of cytochrome P450E1-catalyzed oxidation by isoniazid in humans. *Clin Pharmacol Ther.* 1993;54:142-149.

 Acetaminophen (eg, *Tylenol*)

Metoclopramide (eg, *Reglan*)

SUMMARY: Metoclopramide may hasten the onset of the effect of acetaminophen, but the clinical importance of this effect is minimal.

RISK FACTORS: No specific risk factors are known.

MECHANISM: Metoclopramide may increase the absorption rate of acetaminophen by stimulating gastric emptying.[1]

CLINICAL EVALUATION: Although the absorption rate of acetaminophen is increased by metoclopramide in healthy subjects,[1,2] the amount of acetaminophen absorbed did not appear to be affected. Theoretically, the therapeutic benefits of acetaminophen may occur more rapidly in patients taking metoclopramide, but the difference in onset time is not likely to be noticeable by most patients.

RELATED DRUGS: Cisapride[†] (*Propulsid*) may have a similar effect on acetaminophen.

MANAGEMENT OPTIONS: No specific action is required, but be alert for evidence of the interaction.

REFERENCES:

1. Nimmo J, et al. Pharmacological modification of gastric emptying: effects of propantheline and metoclopramide on paracetamol absorption. *Br Med J.* 1973;1:587-589.
2. Nimmo J. The influence of metoclopramide on drug absorption. *Postgrad Med J.* 1973;49(suppl 4):25-29.

† Available from the manufacturer on a limited-access protocol.

 Acetaminophen (eg, *Tylenol*)

Phenobarbital (eg, *Solfoton*)

SUMMARY: Barbiturates may enhance the hepatotoxic potential of overdoses (and possibly large therapeutic doses) of acetaminophen; it is also possible that barbiturates reduce the therapeutic response to acetaminophen.

RISK FACTORS:

➡️ *Dosage Regimen.* The danger of hepatotoxicity is primarily with overdoses or large or prolonged use of acetaminophen.

MECHANISM: Barbiturates appear to enhance the metabolism of acetaminophen. With excessive doses of acetaminophen, enzyme inducers such as barbiturates may increase the formation of toxic acetaminophen metabolites.[6]

CLINICAL EVALUATION: With acetaminophen overdoses, long-term barbiturate therapy would be expected to increase the conjugation of acetaminophen to its nontoxic glucuronide metabolite, and also to increase the oxidative biotransformation of acetaminophen to hepatotoxic metabolites. The overall effect of these 2 opposing mechanisms is not predictable, but phenobarbital pretreatment appears to increase the hepatotoxicity of toxic acetaminophen doses. Phenobarbital increases the hepatotoxicity and nephrotoxicity of acetaminophen overdose in rats,[2,3] and isolated case reports suggest that this also occurs in humans.[4,5,7] Following acetaminophen overdoses in patients on barbiturates, serum acetaminophen concentrations may be relatively low, leading to the erroneous conclusion that acetylcysteine (a specific antidote for acetaminophen toxicity) is not necessary.[8]

The fate of acetaminophen 1 g orally and IV was compared in 6 healthy subjects and 6 epileptic patients receiving chronic anticonvulsant therapy (eg, barbiturates, carbamazepine, primidone).[1] The acetaminophen bioavailability from an oral dose was less and the serum half-life of acetaminophen was shorter after the IV dose in the epileptic patients. Although clinical evidence is lacking, patients taking enzyme-inducing drugs may experience a reduced therapeutic response to acetaminophen. This might increase the likelihood that such patients would take excessive amounts of acetaminophen, which in turn could increase the risk of acetaminophen toxicity.

RELATED DRUGS: Enzyme inducers other than phenobarbital (eg, other barbiturates, carbamazepine [eg, *Tegretol*], phenytoin [eg, *Dilantin*], primidone [eg, *Mysoline*], rifabutin [eg, *Mycobutin*], and rifampin [eg, *Rifadin*]) may interact similarly.

MANAGEMENT OPTIONS:

➡ *Circumvent/Minimize.* Patients on barbiturate therapy should probably avoid taking large or prolonged doses of acetaminophen. With acute acetaminophen overdoses, acetylcysteine may be indicated even if the serum acetaminophen concentration is below the "action line" on the standard nomogram. (Some have recommended that the serum acetaminophen threshold for acetylcysteine therapy should be reduced by as much as 70% in patients who are taking enzyme inducers such as barbiturates.)[8]

➡ *Monitor.* Monitor patients for reduced acetaminophen effect. In patients taking large or prolonged doses of acetaminophen, watch for evidence of hepatotoxicity.

REFERENCES:
1. Perucca E, et al. Paracetamol disposition in normal subjects treated with antiepileptic drugs. *Br J Clin Pharmacol.* 1979;7:201.
2. Pessayre E, et al. Additive effects of inducers and fasting on acetaminophen hepatotoxicity. *Biochem Pharmacol.* 1980;29:2219.
3. McLean AEM, et al. Dietary factors in renal and hepatic toxicity of paracetamol. *J Int Med Res.* 1976;4(Suppl.4):79.
4. Wilson JT, et al. Death in an adolescent following an overdose of acetaminophen and phenobarbital. *Am J Dis Child.* 1978;132:466.
5. Boyer TD, et al. Acetaminophen-induced hepatic necrosis and renal failure. *JAMA.* 1971;218:440.
6. Neuvonen PJ, et al. Antipyretic analgesics in patients on antiepileptic drug therapy. *Eur J Clin Pharmacol.* 1979;15:263.
7. Minton NA, et al. Fatal paracetamol poisoning in an epileptic. *Hum Toxicol.* 1988;7:33.
8. McClements BM, et al. Management of paracetamol poisoning complicated by enzyme induction due to alcohol or drugs. *Lancet.* 1990;1:1526.

Acetaminophen (eg, *Tylenol*)

Phenytoin (eg, *Dilantin*)

SUMMARY: Phenytoin may enhance the hepatotoxic potential of overdoses (and possibly large therapeutic doses) of acetaminophen; it is also possible that phenytoin reduces the therapeutic response to acetaminophen.

RISK FACTORS: No specific risk factors are known.

MECHANISM: Enzyme inducers such as phenytoin appear to enhance the hepatic metabolism of acetaminophen to hepatotoxic metabolites.

CLINICAL EVALUATION: There is growing evidence that enzyme inducers such as phenytoin can increase the hepatotoxicity of acetaminophen overdoses by increasing the production of toxic acetaminophen metabolites. Following acetaminophen overdoses in patients receiving phenytoin, serum acetaminophen concentrations may be relatively low, leading to the erroneous conclusion that acetylcysteine is not necessary.[3] Isolated cases have been reported that suggest phenytoin can enhance the hepatotoxicity of acetaminophen in overdose situations.[3,4] Patients on combination anticonvulsant therapy that includes phenytoin tend to have reduced acetaminophen bioavailability and half-life.[1] Thus, it is possible that because of the phenytoin-induced reductions in acetaminophen serum concentration, acetaminophen may not be as effective in patients receiving phenytoin. This might increase the likelihood that such patients would take excessive amounts of acetaminophen, which in turn could increase the risk of acetaminophen toxicity. Acetaminophen 1.5 g/day did not significantly affect serum phenytoin concentrations in 9 epileptic patients on chronic phenytoin therapy.[2]

RELATED DRUGS: Other enzyme-inducing anticonvulsants such as carbamazepine (eg, *Tegretol*), phenobarbital (eg, *Solfoton*), and primidone (eg, *Mysoline*) probably also increase acetaminophen hepatotoxicity.

MANAGEMENT OPTIONS:

➡ ***Circumvent/Minimize.*** Patients on phenytoin therapy should probably avoid taking large or prolonged doses of acetaminophen. In cases of acute acetaminophen overdoses, acetylcysteine may be indicated even if the serum acetaminophen concentration is below the "action line" on the standard nomogram. (Some have recommended that the serum acetaminophen threshold for acetylcysteine therapy should be reduced by as much as 70% in patients who are taking enzyme inducers such as phenytoin.)[3]

➡ ***Monitor.*** Monitor patients taking this combination for evidence of hepatotoxicity.

REFERENCES:

1. Perucca E, et al. Paracetamol disposition in normal subjects and in patients treated with antiepileptic drugs. *Br J Clin Pharmacol.* 1971;7:201.
2. Neuvonen PJ, et al. Antipyretic analgesics in patients on antiepileptic drug therapy. *Eur J Clin Pharmacol.* 1979;15:263.
3. McClements BM, et al. Management of paracetamol poisoning complicated by enzyme induction due to alcohol or drugs. *Lancet.* 1990;1:1526.
4. Minton NA, et al. Fatal paracetamol poisoning in an epileptic. *Hum Toxicol.* 1988;7:33.

Acetaminophen (eg, *Tylenol*) 4

Propantheline (eg, *Pro-Banthine*)

SUMMARY: Anticholinergics may delay the onset of the response to acetaminophen, but the clinical importance of this effect is not established.

RISK FACTORS: No specific risk factors are known.

MECHANISM: Anticholinergics slow gastric emptying, thus reducing the rate of acetaminophen absorption from the intestine.

CLINICAL EVALUATION: Acetaminophen 1.5 g orally given to 6 patients with and without pretreatment with propantheline 30 mg IV.[1,2] The rate of acetaminophen absorption was considerably slower in the presence of propantheline than in its absence, but the extent of acetaminophen absorption did not appear to be affected. Oral administration of propantheline is likely to have a similar effect. Because acetaminophen is often used for acute relief of pain or fever, anticholinergics would be expected to delay the onset of the therapeutic response to acetaminophen; however, this has not been studied clinically. This interaction is unlikely to be clinically important in a patient receiving acetaminophen several times daily, because the extent of absorption is unaffected.

RELATED DRUGS: Other agents with anticholinergic activity such as tricyclic antidepressants, antihistamines, and neuroleptics also probably delay acetaminophen absorption.

MANAGEMENT OPTIONS: No specific action is required, but be alert for evidence of the interaction.

REFERENCES:
1. Nimmo J, et al. Pharmacological modification of gastric emptying: effects of propantheline and metoclopramide on paracetamol absorption. *BMJ*. 1973;1:587.
2. Nimmo J. The influence of metoclopramide on drug absorption. *Postgrad Med J*. 1973;49(July Suppl.):25.

Acetaminophen (eg, *Tylenol*) 4

Propranolol (eg, *Inderal*)

SUMMARY: Propranolol administration increased acetaminophen serum concentrations, but the clinical importance of this effect is not established.

RISK FACTORS:

➥ **Dosage Regimen.** Doses of propranolol more than 80 mg/day may increase the risk of interaction.

MECHANISM: Propranolol appears to inhibit the metabolism of acetaminophen.

CLINICAL EVALUATION: Ten healthy subjects received 1500 mg of acetaminophen following 4 days of treatment with a placebo or propranolol 160 mg/day.[1] Propranolol reduced the clearance of acetaminophen 14% and increased its half-life 25%. In another study of 6 healthy subjects receiving a lower propranolol dose (80 mg/day), a change in acetaminophen clearance was not observed.[2] The clinical significance of this interaction is unknown, but it appears to be limited.

RELATED DRUGS: Metoprolol (eg, *Lopressor*) and perhaps other beta blockers might similarly affect acetaminophen.

MANAGEMENT OPTIONS: No specific action is required, but be alert for evidence of the interaction.

REFERENCES:

1. Baraka OZ, et al. The effect of propranolol on paracetamol metabolism in man. *Br J Clin Pharmacol.* 1990;29:261.
2. Sanchez-Martinez V, et al. Lack of effect of propranolol on the kinetics of paracetamol in man. *Br J Clin Pharmacol.* 1985;20:548P.

---

5 Acetaminophen (eg, *Tylenol*)

Ranitidine (eg, *Zantac*)

SUMMARY: Some have suggested that ranitidine enhances acetaminophen hepatotoxicity, but a controlled study in humans indicates that no interaction occurs.

RISK FACTORS: No specific risk factors are known.

MECHANISM: No interaction.

CLINICAL EVALUATION: A patient receiving acetaminophen and ranitidine manifested hepatotoxicity, but the liver damage could have been caused by the drug acting alone or a nondrug cause.[1] Studies of this interaction in animals and in vitro have been conflicting; some suggest that ranitidine increases the hepatotoxicity of acetaminophen,[2,3] while others have failed to find an effect.[4,5] In a double-blind, placebo-controlled study of healthy subjects given 1000 mg acetaminophen with and without ranitidine 600 mg/day for 4 days, ranitidine did not affect the formation of hepatotoxic acetaminophen metabolites.[6] Thus, it appears that ranitidine is unlikely to enhance the hepatotoxicity of acetaminophen.

RELATED DRUGS: Cimetidine (eg, *Tagamet*) might protect against acetaminophen hepatotoxicity, but more study is needed (see Acetaminophen-Cimetidine monograph). Little is known regarding the effect of famotidine (eg, *Pepcid*) or nizatidine (*Axid*) on acetaminophen, but there is no reason to suspect that they would interact.

MANAGEMENT OPTIONS: No interaction.

REFERENCES:

1. Bredfeldt JE, et al. Ranitidine, acetaminophen, and hepatotoxicity. *Ann Intern Med.* 1984;101:719.
2. Leonard TB, et al. Ranitidine-acetaminophen interaction: effects on acetaminophen-induced hepatotoxicity in Fischer 344 rats. *Hepatology.* 1985;5:480.
3. Rogers SA, et al. Inhibition by ranitidine of acetaminophen conjugation and its possible role in ranitidine potentiation of acetaminophen induced hepatotoxicity. *J Pharmacol Exp Ther.* 1988;245:887.
4. Mitchell MC, et al. Selective inhibition of acetaminophen oxidation and toxicity by cimetidine and other histamine H_2-receptor antagonists in vivo and in vitro in the rat and man. *J Clin Invest.* 1984;73:383.
5. Speeg KV, et al. Ranitidine and acetaminophen hepatotoxicity. *Ann Intern Med.* 1984;100:315.
6. Jack D, et al. Ranitidine and paracetamol metabolism. *Lancet.* 1985;2:1067.

Acetaminophen (eg, *Tylenol*)

Sucralfate (eg, *Carafate*)

SUMMARY: A preliminary study in healthy subjects indicates that sucralfate does not affect the GI absorption of acetaminophen.

RISK FACTORS: No specific risk factors are known.

MECHANISM: No interaction.

CLINICAL EVALUATION: In a double-blind crossover study, 6 healthy subjects were given a single oral 1 g dose of acetaminophen with and without a single oral 1 g dose of sucralfate.[1] Sucralfate did not affect the bioavailability of acetaminophen as measured by salivary acetaminophen concentrations over 4 hours.

RELATED DRUGS: No information is available.

MANAGEMENT OPTIONS: No interaction.

REFERENCES:
1. Kamali F, et al. A double-blind placebo controlled study to examine effects of sucralfate on paracetamol absorption. *Br J Clin Pharmacol.* 1985;19:113.

Acetaminophen (eg, *Tylenol*)

Warfarin (eg, *Coumadin*)

SUMMARY: Repeated doses of acetaminophen may increase the hypoprothrombinemic response to oral anticoagulants like warfarin in some patients.

RISK FACTORS:

➡ ***Dosage Regimen.*** Although the dose relationship is not clearly established, an interaction appears more likely with daily acetaminophen doses of more than 2 g/day for at least 1 week. Maximal effects on the hypoprothrombinemic response have occurred 1 to 3 weeks after starting acetaminophen.[1-3,6,9] Occasional doses of acetaminophen do not appear likely to interact.

MECHANISM: Not established.

CLINICAL EVALUATION: In 12 patients stabilized on various anticoagulants (including warfarin), acetaminophen 2.6 g/day was associated with a gradual increase in the prothrombin time, reaching a 5.4 second increase by the end of the third week.[1] In 50 other patients (also on various oral anticoagulants), 2 weeks of acetaminophen 2.6 g/day and 2 weeks of placebo were given in a crossover study.[1] By the end of the second week, the prothrombin time had increased by 3.7 seconds compared with placebo. Fifteen healthy subjects were stabilized on warfarin to achieve a prothrombin time of 1.35 to 1.5 times control.[2] Two weeks each of acetaminophen 4 g/day and placebo were then given in a crossover study. Acetaminophen was associated with an increase in the prothrombin time more than 1.75 times control in 7 of 15 subjects compared to 1 with placebo, and it was associated with an increase to more than 2 times control in 5 of the 15 subjects compared to 0 with placebo. Initial effects on the prothrombin time were detected after approximately 7 days of acetaminophen, while the mean time to maximal effect on the prothrombin time was 12.5 days.

In another study, 10 of 20 patients on chronic oral anticoagulants (11 on phenprocoumon, 9 on acenocoumarol) were given acetaminophen 2 g/day for 3 weeks, and the other 10 were given placebo.[3] The hypoprothrombinemic response modestly increased in the patients given acetaminophen, and the anticoagulant dose had to be reduced in 5 of the 10 patients given acetaminophen (compared to 1 with placebo). A preliminary report of a case-control study also suggests that acetaminophen can increase warfarin effect, especially if large doses of acetaminophen are used.[10] A 66-year-old woman developed hematuria, gingival bleeding, and a prothrombin time of 96 seconds (control: 10 seconds) after taking a codeine-acetaminophen combination for about 10 days, but a causal relationship was not established.[4] In one study of 10 outpatients stabilized on warfarin, acetaminophen 3.2 g/day for 2 weeks had no effect on the prothrombin-time response.[5] Similarly, acetaminophen (4 g/day) had no effect on the pharmacokinetics of a single dose of warfarin in healthy subjects.[11]

It is not known why the results of the latter 2 studies differ from those cited above, but the bulk of the evidence suggests that acetaminophen is capable of increasing the hypoprothrombinemic response to warfarin and other oral anticoagulants. A combination product containing acetaminophen and propoxyphene (eg, *Darvocet-N*) has been associated with an enhanced hypoprothrombinemic response and bleeding in a few patients,[7,8] but acetaminophen's role in these cases was not established.

RELATED DRUGS: Although most data on this interaction involve warfarin, limited clinical information suggests that other oral anticoagulants such as acenocoumarol and phenprocoumon may interact with acetaminophen as well. Most alternative analgesics (eg, aspirin, NSAIDs) would not be suitable alternatives to acetaminophen in patients receiving oral anticoagulants.

MANAGEMENT OPTIONS:

➥ *Circumvent/Minimize.* Warn patients receiving warfarin or other oral anticoagulants to limit their intake of acetaminophen-containing products. Although a "safe" amount cannot be determined with certainty, it would be prudent to limit acetaminophen intake to 2 g/day or less for no more than a few days. Aspirin-containing products should not be used as alternatives; acetaminophen lacks the adverse effects of aspirin on the gastric mucosa and platelets, and it is considered safer than aspirin in anticoagulated patients.

➥ *Monitor.* Monitor patients taking amounts of acetaminophen larger than recommended above for enhanced hypoprothrombinemic response and the anticoagulant dose adjusted as needed.

REFERENCES:

1. Antlitz AM, et al. Potentiation of oral anticoagulant therapy by acetaminophen. *Curr Ther Res.* 1968;10:501.
2. Rubin RN, et al. Potentiation of anticoagulant effect of warfarin by acetaminophen (*Tylenol*). *Clin Res.* 1984;32:698a.
3. Boeijinga JJ, et al. Interaction between paracetamol and coumarin anticoagulants. *Lancet.* 1982;1:506.
4. Bartle WR, et al. Potentiation of warfarin anticoagulant by acetaminophen. *JAMA.* 1991;265:1260.
5. Udall JA. Drug interference with warfarin therapy. *Clin Med.* 1970;77:20.
6. Antlitz AM, et al. A double-blind study of acetaminophen used in conjunction with oral anticoagulant therapy. *Curr Ther Res.* 1969;11:360.
7. Orme M, et al. Warfarin and distalgesic interaction. *BMJ.* 1976;1:200.
8. Jones RV. Warfarin and distalgesic interaction. *BMJ.* 1976;1:460.
9. Kaye L. Warfarin and paracetamol. *Pharmaceutical J.* 1991;246:692.

10. Weibert RT. Warfarin-acetaminophen interaction. ASHP Midyear Clinical Meeting, Dec. 1994.
11. Kwan D, et al. The effects of acute and chronic acetaminophen dosing on the pharmacodynamics and pharmacokinetics of (R)- and (S) warfarin. *Clin Pharmacol Ther*. 1995;57:212.

Acetaminophen (eg, *Tylenol*)

Zidovudine (*Retrovir*)

SUMMARY: Preliminary reports suggested that acetaminophen may increase zidovudine-induced bone marrow suppression, but it appears that no interaction occurs.

RISK FACTORS: No specific risk factors are known.

MECHANISM: Not established. Acetaminophen does not appear to inhibit zidovudine metabolism and may even increase its clearance, but a pharmacodynamic interaction cannot be ruled out.

CLINICAL EVALUATION: Zidovudine has been reported to cause a higher frequency of neutropenia when administered with acetaminophen.[1] However, no details about the patients or drug doses were provided, and zidovudine is a known bone marrow toxin in the absence of acetaminophen.[2] Several groups have examined the potential for acetaminophen to interact with zidovudine.[3-5,8] None have found a significant difference in zidovudine clearance following acetaminophen 325 to 650 mg every 4 hours for 3 to 7 days; however, the issue of a pharmacodynamic interaction was not addressed. One study reported a 33% increase in zidovudine clearance after 7 days of acetaminophen 650 mg every 4 hours.[6] Naproxen (eg, *Naprosyn*) 500 mg twice daily for 5 days had no effect on zidovudine pharmacokinetics and could be used as an alternative to acetaminophen.[7] In addition, a case of acute hepatotoxicity has been reported in a patient taking zidovudine 200 mg twice daily who was administered less than 3.5 g of acetaminophen over 36 hours.[9] Causation was not established and other causes could not be ruled out.

RELATED DRUGS: No information is available.

MANAGEMENT OPTIONS: No specific action is required, but be alert for evidence of the interaction.

REFERENCES:

1. Richman DD, et al. The toxicity of azidothymidine (AZT) in the treatment of patients with AIDS and AIDS-related complex. *N Engl J Med*. 1987;317:192.
2. Gill PS, et al. Azidothymidine associated with bone marrow failure in the acquired immunodeficiency syndrome (AIDS). *Ann Intern Med*. 1987;107:502
3. Koda RT, et al. Effect of acetaminophen (ACET) on the pharmacokinetics of zidovudine (AZT). Fifth International Conference on AIDS. Quebec; 1989:203.
4. Pazin GJ, et al. Interactive pharmacokinetics of zidovudine and acetaminophen. Fifth International Conference on AIDS. Quebec; 1989:203.
5. Steffe EM, et al. The effect of acetaminophen on zidovudine metabolism in HIV-infected patients. *J Acquir Immune Defic Syndr*. 1990;3:691.
6. Sattler FR, et al. Acetaminophen does not impair clearance of zidovudine. *Ann Intern Med*. 1991;114:937.
7. Sahai J, et al. Lack of pharmacokinetic interaction between naproxen and zidovudine. *Clin Pharmacol Ther*. 1992;51:184.
8. Burger DM, et al. Pharmacokinetics of zidovudine and acetaminophen in a patient on chronic acetaminophen therapy. *Ann Pharmacother*. 1994;28:327.
9. Shriner K, et al. Severe hepatotoxicity in a patient receiving both acetaminophen and zidovudine. *Am J Med*. 1992;93:94.

2　Acetazolamide (*Diamox*)

Aspirin

SUMMARY: Aspirin increases the plasma concentrations of acetazolamide, leading to CNS toxicity.

RISK FACTORS: No specific risk factors are known.

MECHANISM: Salicylates displace acetazolamide from plasma protein-binding sites and inhibit its renal excretion, leading to the accumulation of acetazolamide. Acetazolamide also may increase renal elimination of salicylate through alkalinization of the urine.

CLINICAL EVALUATION: Two patients receiving chronic aspirin therapy for osteoarthritis developed CNS symptoms (including lethargy, confusion, incontinence, and somnolence) after acetazolamide was initiated for glaucoma.[3] Total acetazolamide concentration (and percentage unbound) was 20.8 mcg/mL (37.1%) in 1 patient and 12.4 mcg/mL (10.7%) in the other. The therapeutic acetazolamide concentration is 5 to 10 mcg/mL; normally, approximately 5% is unbound. In vivo binding studies confirmed a salicylate-induced reduction in acetazolamide binding.[5] In 4 healthy subjects, a reduction in unbound acetazolamide renal clearance was observed, varying from 14% at a salicylate concentration of 62 mcg/mL to approximately 60% when the salicylate concentration exceeded 200 mcg/mL. CNS toxicity secondary to salicylate administration may contribute to the symptoms accompanying this interaction, particularly if acidosis is present.[1,2,4]

RELATED DRUGS: Theoretically, salicylates other than aspirin would also interact with acetazolamide. The effect of salicylates on carbonic anhydrase inhibitors other than acetazolamide is not established.

MANAGEMENT OPTIONS:

➡ *Avoid Unless Benefit Outweighs Risk.* Avoid concurrent use of salicylates and acetazolamide if possible, particularly in patients with renal dysfunction.

➡ *Monitor.* If the combination is used, monitor the patient carefully for symptoms of CNS toxicity, such as lethargy, confusion, somnolence, tinnitus, and anorexia.

REFERENCES:

1. Hill JB. Experimental salicylate poisoning: observations on effects of altering blood pH on tissue and plasma salicylate concentrations. *Pediatrics.* 1971;47:658.

2. Anderson CJ, et al. Toxicity of combined therapy with carbonic anhydrase inhibitors and aspirin. *Am J Ophthalmol.* 1978;86:516.

　Acetazolamide (eg, *Diamox*)

Cyclosporine (eg, *Neoral*)

SUMMARY: Acetazolamide appeared to increase cyclosporine concentrations, leading to cyclosporine toxicity in 1 patient, but a causal relationship was not established.

RISK FACTORS: No specific risk factors are known.

MECHANISM: Not established.

CLINICAL EVALUATION: A cardiac transplant patient was maintained on cyclosporine 5.2 mg/kg/day for 4 months with serum trough radioimmunoassay cyclosporine concentrations of 290 ng/mL.[1] Acetazolamide 250 mg 4 times daily, timolol (eg, *Timoptic*) 0.5%, and prednisolone (eg, *AK–Pred*) 1% drops were added for the treatment of glaucoma. One month later, the patient was noted to be drowsy, anorectic, and in metabolic acidosis with a serum creatinine nearly twice preacetazolamide levels. Whole blood cyclosporine concentrations were elevated to 1736 ng/mL. Cyclosporine concentrations fell to 150 ng/mL 10 days after the discontinuation of acetazolamide and cyclosporine. Renal function returned to preacetazolamide levels. Nonetheless, a causal relationship could not be proven and a contribution of other drugs to the reaction could not be ruled out.

RELATED DRUGS: The effect of acetazolamide on tacrolimus (*Prograf*) is not established, nor is the effect of carbonic anhydrase inhibitors other than acetazolamide on cyclosporine.

MANAGEMENT OPTIONS: No specific action is required, but be alert for evidence of the interaction.

REFERENCES:

1. Keogh A, et al. Acetazolamide and cyclosporine. *Transplantation.* 1988;46:478.

Acetazolamide (eg, *Diamox*)

Methenamine (eg, *Urised*)

SUMMARY: Acetazolamide interferes with the urinary antibacterial activity of methenamine compounds.

RISK FACTORS: No specific risk factors are known.

MECHANISM: Acetazolamide tends to render the urine alkaline. During therapy with methenamine compounds, the urine must be kept at a pH level of approximately 5.5 or lower to effect proper conversion of methenamine to free formaldehyde. Acetazolamide administration could increase the urine pH and prevent the conversion of methenamine to formaldehyde.

CLINICAL EVALUATION: Acetazolamide is an effective urinary alkalinizer and would be expected to antagonize the effect of methenamine compounds. Although little clinical evidence exists, acetazolamide could alkalinize the urine effectively and would be expected to inhibit the effect of methenamine compounds that require a urine pH less than 5.5 for optimal effect.[1-3]

RELATED DRUGS: Other drugs that alkalinize the urine, such as sodium bicarbonate or large doses of antacids, would be expected to have a similar effect on methenamine compounds.

MANAGEMENT OPTIONS:

➡ *Monitor.* Monitor patients to keep the urine pH at approximately 5.5 or lower during methenamine use.

REFERENCES:

1. Product Information. Methenamine Mandelate (*Mandelamine*). Warner Chilcott. 1997.

2. Kevorkian CG, et al. Methenamine mandelate with acidification: an effective urinary antiseptic in patients with neurogenic bladder. *Mayo Clin Proc.* 1984;59:523.

3. Pearman JW, et al. The antimicrobial activity of urine of paraplegic patients receiving methenamine mandelate. *Invest Urol.* 1978;16:91.

Acetazolamide (*Diamox*)

Phenytoin (*Dilantin*)

SUMMARY: Acetazolamide may increase the risk of osteomalacia in patients receiving anticonvulsants.

RISK FACTORS: No specific risk factors are known.

MECHANISM: Several mechanisms for enhanced anticonvulsant osteomalacia caused by acetazolamide have been proposed.[1-3] Among these are acetazolamide-induced increases in urinary excretion of calcium and phosphates and the tendency of acetazolamide to cause systemic acidosis.

CLINICAL EVALUATION: Acetazolamide appeared to accelerate phenytoin (and other anticonvulsant)-induced osteomalacia in several patients.[1,3] In 2 patients with severe osteomalacia, stopping acetazolamide was associated with a considerable decrease in the rate of urinary calcium excretion.[3] Although more evidence is needed, the clinical and biochemical data suggest that acetazolamide can worsen phenytoin and other anticonvulsant-induced osteomalacia.

RELATED DRUGS: Other carbonic anhydrase inhibitors when prescribed with an anticonvulsant could increase the risk of osteomalacia.

MANAGEMENT OPTIONS:

➡ ***Monitor.*** Give special attention to early detection of osteomalacia to patients receiving acetazolamide (or other carbonic anhydrase inhibitors) in addition to an anticonvulsant such as phenytoin, phenobarbital, or primidone. If osteomalacia does occur under these conditions, stopping the acetazolamide and instituting replacement therapy with phosphate or vitamin D may be beneficial.[1,3]

REFERENCES:

1. Matsuda I, et al. Renal tubular acidosis and skeletal demineralization in patients on long-term anticonvulsant therapy. *J Pediatr.* 1975;87:202.
2. Mallette LE. Anticonvulsants, acetazolamide, and osteomalacia. *N Engl J Med.* 1975;293:668.
3. Mallette LE. Acetazolamide-accelerated anticonvulsant osteomalacia. *Arch Intern Med.* 1977;137:1013.

Acetazolamide (eg, *Diamox*)

Primidone (eg, *Mysoline*)

SUMMARY: A few case reports suggest that acetazolamide may reduce primidone serum concentrations and its anticonvulsant effect.

RISK FACTORS: No specific risk factors are known.

MECHANISM: Acetazolamide may reduce the GI absorption of primidone.[1]

CLINICAL EVALUATION: A patient receiving primidone and acetazolamide developed increased seizure activity and undetectable concentrations of primidone and phenobarbital.[1] Subsequent study of this patient showed that primidone was absorbed in the absence of acetazolamide. In 2 other patients given primidone with and without acetazolamide, acetazolamide delayed the absorption of primidone in 1 patient but had no effect on the other.

RELATED DRUGS: The effect of other carbonic anhydrase inhibitors on primidone is unknown.

MANAGEMENT OPTIONS:

➡ *Monitor.* It appears unnecessary to avoid the concomitant use of acetazolamide and primidone. However, until this interaction is better described, monitor patients receiving primidone and acetazolamide for a decreased primidone effect.

REFERENCES:

1. Syversen BG, et al. Acetazolamide-induced interference with primidone absorption. *Arch Neurol.* 1977;34:80.

Acetazolamide (eg, *Diamox*)

Procainamide (eg, *Pronestyl*)

SUMMARY: Acetazolamide does not appear to alter procainamide elimination.

RISK FACTORS: No specific risk factors are known.

MECHANISM: Urinary pH changes resulting from acetazolamide administration do not change procainamide renal excretion.

CLINICAL EVALUATION: Although it had been suspected that procainamide might undergo pH-dependent urinary excretion, several studies have failed to document this effect.[1-3] The active metabolite of procainamide (N-acetylprocainamide) probably also is unaffected by urinary pH changes.[3]

RELATED DRUGS: No information is available.

MANAGEMENT OPTIONS: No interaction.

REFERENCES:

1. Galeazzi RL, et al. The renal elimination of procainamide. *Clin Pharmacol Ther.* 1976;19:55.
2. Meyer N, et al. A study of the influence of pH on the buccal absorption and renal excretion of procainamide. *Eur J Clin Pharmacol.* 1974;7:287.
3. Reidenberg MM, et al. Polymorphic acetylation of procainamide in man. *Clin Pharmacol Ther.* 1975;17:722.

Acetazolamide (eg, *Diamox*)

Quinidine (eg, *Quinora*)

SUMMARY: Alkalinization of the urine by acetazolamide tends to increase plasma quinidine concentrations.

RISK FACTORS: No specific risk factors are known.

MECHANISM: Acetazolamide tends to render the urine alkaline, resulting in an increased proportion of nonionized quinidine. Thus, renal tubular reabsorption of quinidine is increased and serum concentrations may be increased.

CLINICAL EVALUATION: In a study of 4 subjects, the average quinidine excretion was 115 mg/L when urine pH was less than 6, but only 13 mg/L when urine pH was more than 7.5.[2] Because up to 50% of quinidine is cleared by the kidneys, quinidine toxicity may result when coadministered with agents that increase urine pH, particularly in patients with acidic urine.[1]

RELATED DRUGS: Other drugs that alkalinize the urine (eg, sodium bicarbonate) would produce similar effects on quinidine serum concentrations. Acetazolamide may increase quinine concentrations.

MANAGEMENT OPTIONS:

➡ **Monitor.** Initiation, discontinuation, or a change in dose of acetazolamide in a patient receiving quinidine may necessitate a change in the quinidine dose. Monitor for altered quinidine response of urine pH changes.

REFERENCES:

1. Knouss RF, et al. Variation in quinidine excretion with changing urine pH. *Ann Intern Med.* 1968;68:1157.
2. Gerhardt RE, et al. Quinidine excretion in aciduria and alkaluria. *Ann Intern Med.* 1969;71:927.

 4   Acetazolamide (eg, *Diamox*)

Quinine

SUMMARY: Acetazolamide administration may increase quinine serum concentrations.

RISK FACTORS: No specific risk factors are known.

MECHANISM: The urinary alkalinization produced by acetazolamide may increase the proportion of quinine present in the nonionized form, thus promoting renal tubular reabsorption of the quinine.

CLINICAL EVALUATION: Alkalinization of the urine reduces the urinary output of quinine from 17.4% of the administered dose (with acid urine) to 8.9% (with alkaline urine).[1] The increased quinine blood concentration that would be expected to accompany the decreased urinary excretion could increase the therapeutic efficacy of quinine as well as its dose-related adverse effects.

RELATED DRUGS: Other drugs that alkalinize the urine (eg, sodium bicarbonate) will produce similar effects on quinine elimination. Acetazolamide may increase quinidine concentrations.

MANAGEMENT OPTIONS: No specific action is required, but be alert for evidence of the interaction.

REFERENCES:

1. Haag HB, et al. The effect of urinary pH on the elimination of quinine in man. *J Pharmacol.* 1943;79:136.

 3   Acetohexamide

Potassium

SUMMARY: Treatment of hypokalemia with potassium may result in a tendency toward hypoglycemia.

RISK FACTORS: No specific risk factors are known.

MECHANISM: Not established. However, potassium loss is known to impair glucose tolerance,[1-3] while replacement of potassium in patients with a potassium deficit may improve their glucose tolerance.[3,4]

CLINICAL EVALUATION: Potentiation of the hypoglycemic effect of acetohexamide was observed in 8 of 11 patients given potassium chloride (30 mL/day of 25% solution for 1 week).[5] However, no mention was made of the potassium status of these patients before potassium chloride therapy. Diabetic patients with hypokalemia who receive potassium replacement may have improved glucose control.

RELATED DRUGS: A similar reaction may occur with all hypoglycemic agents.

MANAGEMENT OPTIONS:

➡ *Monitor.* The effect of potassium on the response to antidiabetic agents is unlikely to be large enough to warrant any precautionary measures. However, monitor hypokalemic diabetic patients treated with potassium supplementation for reduced blood glucose.

REFERENCES:

1. Levine R. Mechanisms of insulin secretion. *N Engl J Med.* 1970;283:522-526.
2. Grunfeld C, et al. Hypokalemia and diabetes mellitus. *Am J Med.* 1983;75:553-554.
3. Helderman JN, et al. Prevention of the glucose intolerance of thiazide diuretics by maintenance of body potassium. *Diabetes.* 1983;32:106-111.
4. Spergel G, et al. The effect of potassium on the impaired glucose tolerance in chronic uremia. *Metabolism.* 1967;16:581.
5. Gershberg H, et al. Antidiabetic effect of acetohexamide. Effect of potassium supplements. *N Y State J Med.* 1969;69:1287-1291.

Acetylcysteine (eg, *Mucomyst*)

Nitroglycerin

SUMMARY: Drugs containing sulfhydryl groups may potentiate the effects of nitrates.

RISK FACTORS: No specific risk factors are known.

MECHANISM: Nitrates cause vasodilation by interacting with sulfhydryl groups to increase cyclic guanylic acid, which induces vascular smooth muscle relaxation. Acetylcysteine is a sulfhydryl group donor and may enhance the activity of nitrates.

CLINICAL EVALUATION: Acetylcysteine 100 mg/kg intravenous (IV) increased the peripheral[1] and coronary[2] dilation caused by nitroglycerin. Acetylcysteine also can reverse nitrate tolerance in patients with coronary artery disease and congestive heart failure.[3-5] However, acetylcysteine 200 to 400 mg orally 3 times a day did not prevent the attenuation of transdermal nitroglycerin-induced hemodynamic changes over 4 days.[6,7] The IV infusion of acetylcysteine 225 mg/kg/day did not alter the development of tolerance to an IV infusion of nitroglycerin 1.5 mcg/kg/min over 24 hours in 13 patients with heart failure.[8] The differences in the effect of acetylcysteine on nitroglycerin tolerance between these reports may be caused by the large differences in acetylcysteine dosage regimens. The effects may be more prominent when large concentrations of both nitroglycerin and acetylcysteine are present. The clinical significance of these effects is unknown.

RELATED DRUGS: A study in rats found that captopril (eg, *Capoten*), which contains a sulfhydryl group, potentiated the effects of isosorbide dinitrate on coronary blood flow.[9]

MANAGEMENT OPTIONS: No specific action is required, but be alert for evidence of the interaction.

REFERENCES:

1. Horowitz JD, et al. Potentiation of the cardiovascular effect of nitroglycerin by N-acetylcysteine. *Circulation.* 1983;68:1247-1253.

2. Winniford MD, et al. Potentiation of nitroglycerin-induced coronary dilatation by N-acetylcysteine. *Circulation*. 1986;73:138-142.

3. Torresi J, et al. Prevention and reversal of tolerance to nitroglycerin with N-acetylcysteine. *J Cardiovasc Pharmacol*. 1985;7:777-783.

4. May DC, et al. In vivo induction and reversal of nitroglycerin tolerance in human coronary arteries. *N Engl J Med*. 1987;317:805-809.

5. Packer M, et al. Prevention and reversal of nitrate tolerance in patients with congestive heart failure. *N Engl J Med*. 1987;317:799-804.

6. Hogan JC, et al. N-acetylcysteine fails to attenuate haemodynamic tolerance to glyceryl trinitrate in healthy volunteers. *Br J Clin Pharmacol*. 1989;28:421-426.

7. Hogan JC, et al. Chronic administration of N-acetylcysteine to prevent nitrate tolerance in patients with stable angina pectoris. *Br J Clin Pharmacol*. 1990;30:573-577.

8. Dupuis J, et al. Tolerance to intravenous nitroglycerin in patients with congestive heart failure: role of increased intravascular volume, neurohumoral activation and lack of prevention with N-acetylcysteine. *J Am Coll Cardiol*. 1990;16:923-931.

9. Lawson DL, et al. Captopril-induced reversal of nitroglycerin tolerance: role of sulfhydryl group vs ACE-inhibitory activity. *J Cardiovasc Pharmacol*. 1981;17:411-418.

4   N-Acetylprocainamide (*NAPA*)

Procainamide (eg, *Pronestyl*)

SUMMARY: N-acetylprocainamide (NAPA) accumulation will result in increased procainamide serum concentrations and enhanced electrophysiologic effects.

RISK FACTORS:

 Concurrent Diseases. Patients with renal failure are at risk.

 Pharmacogenetics. Patients who are fast acetylators of procainamide are at risk.

MECHANISM: NAPA, a metabolite of procainamide, reduces procainamide renal and total body clearance. It appears to compete with procainamide for active renal tubular secretion.

CLINICAL EVALUATION: Ten patients with ventricular arrhythmias received 6-hour intravenous infusions of procainamide (8 to 14 mg/min) alone, procainamide and NAPA (dosed to produce a serum concentration of 8 mcg/mL), and NAPA alone.[1] The coadministration of NAPA significantly increased procainamide's half-life from 275 to 340 minutes without changing its volume of distribution. Both renal and total clearance of procainamide tended to be diminished by the infusion of NAPA (49% and 16% reductions, respectively).

RELATED DRUGS: No information is available.

MANAGEMENT OPTIONS: No specific action is required, but be alert for evidence of the interaction.

REFERENCES:

1. Funck-Brentano C, et al. Pharmacokinetic and pharmacodynamic interaction of N-acetyl procainamide and procainamide in humans. *J Cardiovasc Pharmacol*. 1989;14:364-373.

Acitretin (*Soriatane*)

Ethanol (Ethyl Alcohol) AVOID

SUMMARY: Ethanol can result in the conversion of acitretin to etretinate, and the latter substance may remain in the body for years, thus increasing the risk of teratogenic effects. Women on acitretin should totally abstain from alcohol.

RISK FACTORS:

➥ *Gender.* The teratogenic risk applies only to women.

MECHANISM: Alcohol appears to promote the transesterification of acitretin to etretinate in the body.

CLINICAL EVALUATION: While no published data are available for evaluation, the manufacturer of acitretin has made available some data on this interaction.[1] Acitretin, a known teratogen, has a mean half-life of approximately 50 hours. Thus, almost all of the drug would be eliminated from the body within 2 months after stopping the drug. If alcohol is ingested with acitretin; however, some of it is converted to etretinate (a teratogen that can remain in the body for years). Thus, alcohol can markedly enhance the duration of the teratogenic potential of acitretin.[1]

RELATED DRUGS: It is not known if other drugs or substances can also promote the conversion of acitretin to etretinate.

MANAGEMENT OPTIONS:

➥ *AVOID COMBINATION.* Warn women on acitretin to totally abstain from alcohol during and for at least 2 months after stopping the drug.

REFERENCES:
   1. Product information. Acitretin (*Soriatane*). Roche Pharmaceuticals. 1997.

Acitretin (*Soriatane*)

Methotrexate (*Mexate*)

SUMMARY: Combined use of acitretin and methotrexate reportedly increases the risk of hepatotoxicity.

RISK FACTORS: No specific risk factors are known.

MECHANISM: Possible additive hepatotoxicity.

CLINICAL EVALUATION: While no published data are available for evaluation, the manufacturer of acitretin has made available some data on this interaction.[1] The manufacturer of acitretin states that concurrent use of acitretin and methotrexate may increase the risk of hepatotoxicity, but no data were presented.[1] Nonetheless, both acitretin and methotrexate can result in hepatotoxicity when given alone, and it is reasonable to assume that a person on both drugs would have a higher risk.

RELATED DRUGS: No information is available.

MANAGEMENT OPTIONS:

➥ *Avoid Unless Benefit Outweighs Risk.* Although the risk of hepatotoxicity with concurrent use of acitretin and methotrexate is unknown, the manufacturer states that the combination should be avoided.

➥ **Monitor.** If the combination is used, monitor for clinical and laboratory evidence of hepatotoxicity.

REFERENCES:
1. Product information. Acitretin (*Soriatane*). Roche Pharmaceuticals. 1997.

 Acitretin (*Soriatane*)

AVOID **Norethindrone (*Micronor*)**

SUMMARY: Acitretin appears to inhibit the contraceptive efficacy of progestin "minipill" preparations and the latter should not be used in patients receiving acitretin.

RISK FACTORS: No specific risk factors are known.

MECHANISM: Not established.

CLINICAL EVALUATION: While no published data are available for evaluation, the manufacturer of acitretin has made available some data on this interaction.[1] The manufacturer states that acitretin has been "established" to interfere with the contraceptive effect of progestin "minipill" preparations.[1] Although no data were given, it is clear that this contraceptive is inappropriate given that acitretin is a known teratogen.

RELATED DRUGS: The effect of acitretin on other progestin contraceptives (eg, implants, injectables) or standard combined oral contraceptives is unknown.

MANAGEMENT OPTIONS:

➥ **AVOID COMBINATION.** Progestin "minipill" contraceptives should not be relied upon to prevent pregnancy in patients taking acitretin. Instead, suggest the use of at least 2 reliable forms of contraception at the same time to prevent pregnancy during acitretin therapy.

REFERENCES:
1. Product information. Acitretin (*Soriatane*). Roche Pharmaceuticals. 1997.

 Acitretin (*Soriatane*)

Vitamin A

SUMMARY: Since acitretin is a retinoid (a vitamin A derivative), it is recommended that large doses of vitamin A be avoided.

RISK FACTORS: No specific risk factors are known.

MECHANISM: Additive.

CLINICAL EVALUATION: While no published data are available for evaluation, the manufacturer of acitretin has made available some data on this interaction.[1] Although the manufacturer cautions against ingestion of large amounts of vitamin A, the recommendation appears to be based upon theoretical considerations rather than observed adverse consequences.[1] Nonetheless, the caution appears reasonable until more information is available.

RELATED DRUGS: Large doses of vitamin A should probably also be avoided with other retinoids such as etretinate (*Tegison*).

MANAGEMENT OPTIONS:

➡ *Circumvent/Minimize.* The manufacturer recommends against taking vitamin A in doses greater than the minimum recommended daily allowances while taking acitretin.

REFERENCES:

1. Product information. Acitretin (*Soriatane*). Roche Pharmaceuticals. 1997.

Acyclovir (eg, *Zovirax*)

Cimetidine (eg, *Tagamet*)

SUMMARY: Preliminary evidence suggests that cimetidine moderately increases acyclovir concentrations; the clinical significance of this interaction is probably limited.

RISK FACTORS: No specific risk factors are known.

MECHANISM: Cimetidine reduces the rate but not extent of the conversion of valacyclovir to acyclovir. Acyclovir renal clearance is reduced by cimetidine coadministration.

CLINICAL EVALUATION: Twelve healthy men subjects received valacyclovir (*Valtrex*), a prodrug of acyclovir, 1 g alone and again following 800 mg doses of cimetidine given 8 hours and 1 hour before the dose of valacyclovir.[1] The area under the concentration-time curve of valacyclovir during the 3 hours after its administration was increased more than 80% following cimetidine. The area under the concentration-time curve of acyclovir was also increased (23%) following cimetidine. Cimetidine reduced the renal clearance of acyclovir 22%. On the basis of this preliminary report, it is unlikely that these changes in valacyclovir pharmacokinetics would alter patient response. This is because of the wide therapeutic range of acyclovir. The effects of chronic cimetidine dosing await further studies.

RELATED DRUGS: Other H_2-receptor antagonists would theoretically be less likely to interact with acyclovir.

MANAGEMENT OPTIONS: No specific action is required, but be alert for evidence of the interaction.

REFERENCES:

1. Rolan PE, et al. The effects of cimetidine and probenecid on the conversion of a valine ester of acyclovir, 256U, to acyclovir and acyclovir renal clearance in healthy volunteers. *Br J Clin Pharmacol.* 1993;35:533P.

Acyclovir (eg, *Zovirax*)

Probenecid (*Benemid*)

SUMMARY: Probenecid appears to increase acyclovir concentrations moderately; the clinical significance of this interaction is probably limited.

RISK FACTORS: No specific risk factors are known.

MECHANISM: Acyclovir renal clearance is reduced by probenecid coadministration.

CLINICAL EVALUATION: Twelve healthy men received 1 g valacyclovir (*Valtrex*), a prodrug of acyclovir, alone and again 1 hour after a dose of probenecid (1 g).[1] The area under the concentration-time curve (AUC) of valacyclovir during the 3 hours after its administration was increased 22% following probenecid administration. The AUC of acyclovir increased by 46% following probenecid, while its renal clearance fell 33%. An earlier study found a 32% decrease in acyclovir renal clearance and a 40% increase in its AUC following a 1 g probenecid dose.[2] On the basis of these changes in valacyclovir and acyclovir pharmacokinetics, it is unlikely that a single dose of probenecid will significantly alter patient response. This is because of the wide therapeutic range of acyclovir. The effects of chronic probenecid dosing await further studies.

RELATED DRUGS: No information is available.

MANAGEMENT OPTIONS: No specific action is required, but be alert for evidence of the interaction.

REFERENCES:
1. Rolan PE, et al. The effects of cimetidine and probenecid on the conversion of a valine ester of acyclovir, 256U, to acyclovir and acyclovir renal clearance in healthy volunteers. *Br J Clin Pharmacol.* 1993;35:533P.
2. Laskin OL, et al. Effects of probenecid on the pharmacokinetics and elimination of acyclovir in humans. *Antimicrob Agents Chemother.* 1982;21:804.

 ## Acyclovir (eg, *Zovirax*)

Zidovudine (*Retrovir*)

SUMMARY: A single case of severe lethargy and fatigue has been reported following the coadministration of acyclovir and zidovudine; acyclovir does not appear to change zidovudine concentrations.

RISK FACTORS: No specific risk factors are known.

MECHANISM: Not established.

CLINICAL EVALUATION: A patient with herpes simplex was taking acyclovir 250 mg every 8 hours IV for 3 days before his first dose of zidovudine 200 mg.[1] Within 1 hour after ingestion of zidovudine, he complained of severe lethargy and fatigue. The symptoms persisted during the 3 remaining days of acyclovir therapy and resolved when acyclovir was discontinued. The patient remained on zidovudine and was rechallenged with a single IV acyclovir dose. Again he developed severe fatigue and lethargy. In a pharmacokinetic evaluation of low- and high-dose zidovudine in 41 patients with human immunodeficiency virus, concomitant high-dose acyclovir produced no alterations in zidovudine pharmacokinetics or side effects.[2]

RELATED DRUGS: No information is available.

MANAGEMENT OPTIONS: No specific action is required, but be alert for evidence of the interaction.

REFERENCES:
1. Bach MC. Possible drug interaction during therapy with azidothymidine and acyclovir for AIDS. *N Engl J Med.* 1987;317:547.
2. Tartaglione TA, et al. Pharmacokinetic evaluation of low- and high-dose zidovudine plus high-dose acyclovir in patients with symptomatic human immunodeficiency virus infection. *Antimicrob Agents Chemother.* 1991;35:2225.

Adenosine (*Adenocard*) 4

Caffeine

SUMMARY: Caffeine reduces the hemodynamic effects of adenosine; the clinical significance of these effects is not known.

RISK FACTORS: No specific risk factors are known.

MECHANISM: Caffeine is an adenosine antagonist that can affect several of the hemodynamic effects of adenosine.

CLINICAL EVALUATION: Adenosine infusion 0.12 mg/kg/min significantly increased systolic blood pressure and heart rate but reduced diastolic blood pressure.[1,2] Pretreatment with caffeine 3 mg/kg IV bolus followed by 0.6 mg/kg/hr significantly reduced the adenosine-induced increase in heart rate and systolic blood pressure. Adenosine-induced increases in forearm blood flow were attenuated by concomitant caffeine infusion.[3] The clinical significance of this interaction will require studies in patients treated with adenosine for arrhythmias. The effects of dietary caffeine on adenosine are unknown but are likely to be less.

RELATED DRUGS: Theophylline (eg, *Slo-Phyllin*) produces a similar effect on adenosine hemodynamics.

MANAGEMENT OPTIONS: No specific action is required, but be alert for evidence of the interaction.

REFERENCES:
1. Smits P, et al. Cardiovascular effects of two xanthines and the relation to adenosine antagonism. *Clin Pharmacol Ther.* 1989;45:593.
2. Smits P, et al. Evidence for an antagonism between caffeine and adenosine in the human cardiovascular system. *J Cardiovasc Pharmacol.* 1987;10:136.
3. Smits P, et al. Caffeine and theophylline attenuate adenosine-induced vasodilation in humans. *Clin Pharmacol Ther.* 1990;48:410.

Adenosine (eg, *Adenocard*)

Dipyridamole (eg, *Persantine*)

SUMMARY: Dipyridamole increases the serum concentrations of endogenous and exogenous adenosine, thereby potentiating its pharmacologic effects.

RISK FACTORS: No specific risk factors are known.

MECHANISM: Dipyridamole inhibits both cellular uptake and metabolism of adenosine, resulting in increased serum concentrations and pharmacologic effects of adenosine.

CLINICAL EVALUATION: Adenosine is a potent nucleoside with negative dromotropic effects (ie, it slows conduction) in the atrioventricular (AV) node. AV conduction was prolonged in subjects without heart disease who received dipyridamole 0.56 mg/kg IV bolus followed by 5 mcg/kg/min.[1] Dipyridamole 100 mg orally every 6 hours for 5 days increased endogenous adenosine concentrations 60%.[2] Serum adenosine concentrations were increased after 2 days and were higher with increasing dipyridamole concentrations. In 5 patients with supraventricular tachycardia, dipyridamole 0.56 mg/kg IV bolus followed by 5 mcg/kg/min reduced the amount of exogenous adenosine (from 68 mg/kg to 17 mg/kg) that was needed to terminate the tachycardia[2] and alter myocardial conduction.[3] Dipyridamole may potentiate the hemodynamic effects of adenosine 75% to 90%.[4,5] Asystole was reported in a patient taking dipyridamole who received diagnostic adenosine.[6] A 79-year-old woman on amlodipine, lisinopril, and *Aggrenox* (dipyridamole plus low dose aspirin) was given IV adenosine (140 mcg/kg/min). After 2 minutes she developed profound bradycardia (36 beats per minute) and dizziness.[7] The test was aborted, and 2 minutes after stopping the adenosine her heart rate increased to 60 beats per minute.

RELATED DRUGS: No information is available.

MANAGEMENT OPTIONS:

➡ *Circumvent/Minimize.* Patients taking dipyridamole should receive reduced doses of adenosine for the treatment of arrhythmias or diagnostic tests.

➡ *Monitor.* Be alert for bradycardia and prolonged AV conduction when dipyridamole and adenosine are coadministered. The enhancement of adenosine effects on AV conduction (eg, bradycardia) by dipyridamole may be reversed by aminophylline.

REFERENCES:

1. Lerman BB, et al. Electrophysiologic effects of dipyridamole on atrioventricular nodal conduction and supraventricular tachycardia. *Circulation.* 1989;80:1536-1543.
2. German DC, et al. Oral dipyridamole increases plasma adenosine levels in human beings. *Clin Pharmacol Ther.* 1989;45:80-84.
3. Watt AH, et al. Intravenous adenosine in the treatment of supraventricular tachycardia; a dose-ranging study and interaction with dipyridamole. *Br J Clin Pharmacol.* 1986;21:227-230.
4. Biaggioni I, et al. Cardiovascular effects of adenosine infusion in man and their modulation by dipyridamole. *Life Sci.* 1986;39:2229-2236.
5. Conradson TB, et al. Cardiovascular effects of infused adenosine in man: potentiation by dipyridamole. *Acta Physiol Scand.* 1987;129:387-391.
6. McCollam PL, et al. Adenosine-related ventricular asystole. *Ann Intern Med.* 1993;118:315-316.
7. Littmann L, et al. Adenosine and *Aggrenox*: a hazardous combination. *Ann Intern Med.* 2002;137:W1.

Adenosine (eg, *Adenocard*)

Nicotine (eg, *Nicorette*)

SUMMARY: Nicotine increases the hemodynamic and atrioventricular (AV) blocking effects of adenosine, resulting in low blood pressure and change in heart rate.

RISK FACTORS: No specific risk factors are known.

MECHANISM: Not established. The decrease in diastolic pressure may have resulted from reduced peripheral resistance, and probably cardiac output, during combination therapy. Thus, nicotine appears to enhance the hemodynamic effects of adenosine.

CLINICAL EVALUATION: Adenosine 0.07 mg/kg/min IV and nicotine chewing gum 2 mg were administered alone and together to 10 healthy subjects.[1] Adenosine alone increased the heart rate and decreased skin temperature; nicotine alone increased both heart rate and blood pressure, but it also reduced skin temperature. The combination of nicotine and adenosine increased the heart rate more (14.9 vs 5.5 bpm) and increased the diastolic blood pressure less (1.1 vs 4 mm Hg) than nicotine alone. In another study, nicotine gum 2 mg enhanced the severity of adenosine-induced chest pain and AV block in healthy subjects receiving repeated 2.65 mg doses of adenosine.[2] The clinical significance of this interaction requires more study in patients.

RELATED DRUGS: It is likely that other nicotine products would produce similar effects on adenosine.

MANAGEMENT OPTIONS:

➤ *Monitor.* Monitor cigarette smokers and those using nicotine gum or transdermal patches for a greater hemodynamic response to adenosine than nonsmokers. Enhanced hypotension or chest pain may result.

REFERENCES:

1. Smits P, et al. Nicotine enhances the circulatory effects of adenosine in human beings. *Clin Pharmacol Ther.* 1989;46:272-278.
2. Sylven C, et al. Nicotine enhances angina pectoris-like chest pain and atrioventricular blockade provoked by intravenous bolus of adenosine in healthy volunteers. *J Cardiovasc Pharmacol.* 1990;16:962–965.

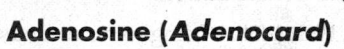

Adenosine (*Adenocard*)

Theophylline (eg, *Slo-Phyllin*)

SUMMARY: Theophylline inhibits the hemodynamic effects of adenosine and may increase adenosine dosage requirements.

RISK FACTORS: No specific risk factors are known.

MECHANISM: Theophylline acts as an adenosine antagonist capable of blunting the vasodilation caused by adenosine.[1]

CLINICAL EVALUATION: In a study on the effect of IV adenosine on forearm arteriolar blood flow, theophylline 1 mcg/mL/min IV blunted the vasodilation induced by adenosine.[2] Similar results have been reported with intra-arterial theophylline infusions.[3] Aminophylline can reverse dipyridamole-induced slowing of AV conduction.[4,5] These data suggest that theophylline, like caffeine, has the potential to alter the antiarrhythmic effects of adenosine.[6] Adenosine may reverse respiratory effects of theophylline by antagonizing the bronchodilating activity of theophylline.[7]

RELATED DRUGS: Caffeine produces similar effects on adenosine hemodynamics.

MANAGEMENT OPTIONS:

➤ *Circumvent/Minimize.* Patients maintained on theophylline may require greater than normal doses of adenosine to control arrhythmias.

➤ *Monitor.* Watch for decreased therapeutic response to adenosine when theophylline is initiated and for adenosine toxicity (eg, bradycardia) when theophylline is discontinued.

REFERENCES:

1. Fredholm BB. On the mechanism of action of theophylline and caffeine. *Acta Med Scand.* 1985;217:149-153.
2. Taddei S, et al. Theophylline antagonizes the vasorelaxant action of adenosine in human forearm arterioles of hypertensive patients. *Clin Pharmacol Ther.* 1990;47:144.
3. Smits P, et al. Caffeine and theophylline attenuate adenosine-induced vasodilation in humans. *Clin Pharmacol Ther.* 1990;48:410-418.
4. Lerman BB, et al. Electrophysiologic effects of dipyridamole on atrioventricular nodal conduction and supraventricular tachycardia. *Circulation.* 1989;80:1536-1543.

5. Heller GV, et al. Pretreatment with theophylline does not affect adenosine-induced thallium-201 myocardial imaging. *Am Heart J.* 1993;126:1077-1083.

6. Product information. Adenosine (*Adenocard*). Lyphomed, Inc. 1989.

7. Minton NA, et al. Pharmacodynamic interactions between infused adenosine and oral theophylline. *Hum Exp Toxicol.* 1991;10:411-418.

Albuterol (eg, *Proventil*)

Digoxin (eg, *Lanoxin*)

SUMMARY: Acute administration of albuterol modestly decreases serum digoxin concentrations; the clinical significance of this action is unknown.

RISK FACTORS: No specific risk factors are known.

MECHANISM: Not established. Albuterol may increase digoxin binding to muscle sodium-potassium adenosine triphosphatase, possibly resulting in a fall in digoxin serum concentration.

CLINICAL EVALUATION: A single intravenous (IV) dose of albuterol 4 mcg/kg or saline was administered to 10 healthy subjects following 10 days of digoxin 0.5 mg daily.[1] Albuterol administration caused a 16% reduction in serum digoxin concentrations 30 minutes after dosing. Digoxin concentrations slowly returned to baseline over the next 1.5 hours. Serum potassium concentrations declined a maximum of 14% ten minutes after the albuterol injection. In a similar study that used a single oral dose of albuterol 3 mg, maximum effects included a 16% decrease in serum digoxin and a 14% reduction in serum potassium concentrations.[2] The clinical significance of long-term administration of albuterol on serum digoxin concentrations is unknown.

RELATED DRUGS: Other beta-agonists may produce a similar effect when administered IV.

MANAGEMENT OPTIONS: No specific action is required, but be alert for evidence of the interaction.

REFERENCES:

1. Edner M, et al. Effect of salbutamol on digoxin concentration in serum and skeletal muscle. *Eur J Clin Pharmacol.* 1989;36(3):235-238.

2. Edner M, et al. Oral salbutamol decreases serum digoxin concentration. *Eur J Clin Pharmacol.* 1990;38(2):195-197.

Alendronate (eg, *Fosamax*)

Naproxen (eg, *Naprosyn*)

SUMMARY: Concurrent use of alendronate (or other bisphosphonates) and naproxen (or other nonsteroidal anti-inflammatory drugs [NSAIDs]) may increase the risk of peptic ulcers.

RISK FACTORS:

➡ *Habits.* Smokers are likely to be at greater risk.

MECHANISM: Not established. Bisphosphonates and NSAIDs may have additive toxic effects on the GI tract.

CLINICAL EVALUATION: Twenty-six healthy subjects took 10-day treatments of alendronate and naproxen 500 mg twice daily alone and together in a randomized, crossover trial.[1] Gastric ulcers occurred in 8% of subjects with alendronate alone, 12% of subjects with naproxen alone, and 38% of subjects when both drugs were given. Another study in patients taking long-term NSAID therapy for rheumatoid arthritis found GI ulcers in 31% of patients also taking bisphosphonates and in 17% taking NSAIDs alone.[2] Some other studies also suggest that combining NSAIDs and bisphosphonates increases the risk of GI toxicity over either drug taken alone.[3]

On the other hand, several other studies found little evidence of increased GI toxicity in patients taking bisphosphonates alone compared with patients taking bisphosphonates with NSAIDs.[4-6] The differing results are probably due to different end points (endoscopy vs adverse events), different types of subjects, different dosage regimens of bisphosphonates, and different durations of the studies. Also, some of the patients were at lower risk (eg, those taking proton pump inhibitors), while others were at higher risk (eg, smokers).

In summary, the evidence suggests that using bisphosphonates and NSAIDs together increases the risk of peptic ulcers compared with taking either drug alone, but may not increase other kinds of adverse GI outcomes (eg, upper GI bleeding). Nonetheless, additional research (especially prospective studies) is needed to resolve this issue.

RELATED DRUGS: Other biphosphonates, such as etidronate (eg, *Didronel*), ibandronate (*Boniva*), and risedronate (*Actonel*), may interact similarly with NSAIDs. Theoretically, an interaction would be less likely when giving bisphosphonates cyclically (eg, weekly, monthly) or if the biphosphonate is given parenterally. NSAIDs other than naproxen are expected to interact with bisphosphonates, including aspirin, diclofenac (eg, *Voltaren*), diflunisal, etodolac, fenoprofen (eg, *Nalfon*), flurbiprofen, ibuprofen (eg, *Motrin*), indomethacin (eg, *Indocin*), ketoprofen, ketorolac, meclofenamate, mefenamic acid (*Ponstel*), meloxicam (eg, *Mobic*), nabumetone, oxaprozin (eg, *Daypro*), piroxicam (eg, *Feldene*), sulindac (eg, *Clinoril*), and tolmetin.

MANAGEMENT OPTIONS:

➥ *Consider Alternative.* Consider using an alternative to the NSAID, if possible.

➥ *Circumvent/Minimize.* Cyclic use of bisphosphonates (eg, weekly, monthly) may reduce the risk of GI toxicity. Proton pump inhibitors, such as dexlansoprazole (*Dexilant*), esomeprazole (*Nexium*), lansoprazole (eg, *Prevacid*), omeprazole (eg, *Prilosec*), pantoprazole (eg, *Protonix*), or rabeprazole (*Aciphex*), probably reduce the risk of peptic ulcers caused by this combination.

➥ *Monitor.* Be alert for evidence of peptic ulcer or GI bleeding, but keep in mind that the absence of symptoms does not guarantee that there is no GI toxicity.

REFERENCES:

1. Graham DY, et al. Alendronate and naproxen are synergistic for development of gastric ulcers. *Arch Intern Med.* 2001;161(1):107-110.

2. Miyake K, et al. Biphosphonate increases risk of gastroduodenal ulcer in rheumatoid arthritis patients on long-term nonsteroidal antiinflammatory drug therapy. *J Gastroenterol.* 2009;44(2):113-120.

3. Anastasilakis AD, et al. Oral biphosphonate adverse effects in 849 patients with metabolic bone diseases. *Hormones.* 2007;6(3):233-241.

4. Bauer DC, et al. Upper gastrointestinal tract safety profile of alendronate: the Fracture Intervention Trial. *Arch Intern Med.* 2000;160(4):517-525.

5. Cryer B, et al. Upper gastrointestinal tolerability of once weekly alendronate 70 mg with concomitant non-steroidal anti-inflammatory drug use. *Aliment Pharmacol Ther.* 2005;21(5):599-607.

6. Etminan M, et al. Risk of upper gastrointestinal bleeding with oral bisphosphonates and non steroidal anti-inflammatory drugs: a case-control study. *Aliment Pharmacol Ther.* 2009;29(11):1188-1192.

Alendronate (eg, *Fosamax*)

Parathyroid Hormone

SUMMARY: Controlled studies suggest that alendronate may inhibit the therapeutic effect of parathyroid hormone in osteoporosis; the combination is not recommended.

RISK FACTORS: No specific risk factors are known.

MECHANISM: Not established.

CLINICAL EVALUATION: Evidence from controlled studies in patients with osteoporosis suggests that parathyroid hormone alone is more effective than parathyroid hormone with alendronate.[1] Alendronate appears to inhibit the therapeutic effect of parathyroid hormone. However, using bisphosphonates after finishing a course of parathyroid hormone may prove to be a reasonable approach.[1]

RELATED DRUGS: The efficacy of parathyroid hormone is also expected to be inhibited by other bisphosphonates such as etidronate (eg, *Didronel*), pamidronate (eg, *Aredia*), risedronate (*Actonel*), and tiludronate (*Skelid*).

MANAGEMENT OPTIONS:

➡ ***Avoid Unless Benefit Outweighs Risk.*** Based on current evidence, avoid alendronate and other bisphosphonates in combination with parathyroid hormone.

REFERENCES:
1. Khosla S. Parathyroid hormone plus alendronate—a combination that does not add up. *New Engl J Med.* 2003;349(13):1277-1279.

 Alfentanil (eg, *Alfenta*)

Cimetidine (eg, *Tagamet*)

SUMMARY: Cimetidine appears to substantially increase serum concentrations of alfentanil, but it is not known how often this interaction leads to adverse effects.

RISK FACTORS: No specific risk factors are known.

MECHANISM: Not established. Cimetidine probably inhibits the hepatic metabolism of alfentanil.

CLINICAL EVALUATION: Nineteen intensive care unit patients were given a single intravenous (IV) dose of alfentanil 125 mcg/kg after pretreatment with one of the following: an oral antacid, cimetidine 1,200 mg/day IV for 48 hours, or ranitidine 300 mg/day IV for 48 hours. Cimetidine increased the alfentanil half-life 75% and reduced its clearance 64%.[1] Pharmacodynamic effects of alfentanil were not measured. Ranitidine did not affect the pharmacokinetics of alfentanil.

RELATED DRUGS: Preliminary evidence suggests that ranitidine (eg, *Zantac*) does not affect the pharmacokinetics of alfentanil. The effect of famotidine (eg, *Pepcid*) and nizatidine (eg, *Axid*) on alfentanil is not established, but, theoretically, they are not expected to interact.

MANAGEMENT OPTIONS:

➡ ***Consider Alternative.*** Consider using H_2-receptor antagonists other than cimetidine.

➡ **Monitor.** If alfentanil is used in a patient receiving cimetidine, monitor for excessive or prolonged alfentanil effect. Adjust the alfentanil dose as needed.

REFERENCES:
1. Keinlen J, et al. Pharmacokinetics of alfentanil in patients treated with either cimetidine or ranitidine. *Drug Invest.* 1993;6(5):257-262.

Alfentanil (*Alfenta*)

Diltiazem (eg, *Cardizem*)

SUMMARY: Diltiazem increases alfentanil plasma concentrations and may prolong sedation and respiratory depression.

RISK FACTORS: No specific risk factors are known.

MECHANISM: Diltiazem appears to inhibit the metabolism (CYP3A4) of alfentanil.

CLINICAL EVALUATION: Thirty patients undergoing coronary artery bypass surgery were given midazolam (0.1 mg/kg induction followed by 1 mcg/kg/min) and alfentanil (50 mcg/kg induction and 1 mcg/kg/min maintenance) for anesthesia.[1] Fifteen of the patients were selected to receive placebo and 15 received diltiazem 60 mg orally 2 hours before induction and an infusion of 0.1 mg/kg/hr started at induction and continued for 23 hours. Mean total IV diltiazem dose was 169 mg. The 2 groups of patients were similar in other aspects of their surgeries. Coadministration of diltiazem prolonged the half-life of alfentanil from a mean of 169 to 254 minutes. The area under the concentration-time curve of alfentanil was increased by 24% in the diltiazem group. The awakening time was not statistically increased in the diltiazem group (125 vs 17 minutes) but time to extubation was prolonged by an average of 2.5 hours.

RELATED DRUGS: Diltiazem is likely to affect other analgesics that are metabolized by CYP3A4 including fentanyl (*Sublimaze*) and sufentanil (*Sufenta*). Verapamil (*Calan*) and mibefradil (*Posicor*) may inhibit the metabolism of alfentanil.

MANAGEMENT OPTIONS:

➡ **Consider Alternative.** The use of a dihydropyridine calcium channel blocker (eg, amlodipine [*Norvasc*] or felodipine [*Plendil*]) would probably avoid the interaction.

➡ **Monitor.** Monitor patients receiving diltiazem and alfentanil for prolonged sedation and respiratory depression.

REFERENCES:
1. Ahonen J, et al. Effect of diltiazem on midazolam and alfentanil disposition in patients undergoing coronary artery bypass grafting. *Anesthesiology.* 1996;85:1246.

Alfentanil (*Alfenta*)

Erythromycin (eg, *E-Mycin*)

SUMMARY: Patients taking erythromycin may experience prolonged anesthesia or increased respiratory depression when given alfentanil.

RISK FACTORS: No specific risk factors are known.

MECHANISM: Not established. Erythromycin or a metabolite may inhibit the clearance of alfentanil.

CLINICAL EVALUATION: The mean alfentanil clearance was reduced 25% and its half-life increased from 84 to 131 minutes after 7 days of erythromycin administration.[1] The delay in the appearance of this interaction is probably caused by the time required for 1 or more erythromycin metabolites to accumulate and inhibit the metabolism of alfentanil.[2] A 32-year-old patient taking erythromycin experienced prolonged respiratory depression following surgery that used alfentanil, nitrous oxide, and pancuronium.[3] Repeated doses of naloxone over several hours were required to reverse the effects of alfentanil.

RELATED DRUGS: Other macrolides such as troleandomycin (*TAO*) or clarithromycin (*Biaxin*) also may inhibit alfentanil. Azithromycin (*Zithromax*) and dirithromycin (*Dynabac*) would be unlikely to inhibit alfentanil metabolism.

MANAGEMENT OPTIONS:

➡ *Circumvent/Minimize.* Erythromycin has no effect on sufentanil serum concentrations.[4] Consider using azithromycin or dirithromycin with alfentanil.

➡ *Monitor.* Until further information is available, monitor patients taking erythromycin for enhanced effects following usual doses of alfentanil.

REFERENCES:

1. Bartkowski RR, et al. Inhibition of alfentanil metabolism by erythromycin. *Clin Pharmacol Ther.* 1989;46:99.
2. Mansuy D. Formation of reactive intermediates and metabolites: effects of macrolide antibiotics on cytochrome P-450. *Pharmacol Ther.* 1987;33:41.
3. Barkowski RR, et al. Prolonged alfentanil effect following erythromycin administration. *Anesthesiology.* 1990;73:566.
4. Barkowski RR, et al. Sufentanil disposition. Is it affected by erythromycin? *Anesthesiology.* 1993;78:260.

Alfentanil (eg, *Alfenta*)

Fluconazole (eg, *Diflucan*)

SUMMARY: Fluconazole increases alfentanil plasma concentrations; increased or prolonged respiratory depression may result.

RISK FACTORS: No specific risk factors are known.

MECHANISM: Fluconazole inhibits the hepatic metabolism (CYP3A4) of alfentanil.

CLINICAL EVALUATION: Nine healthy subjects were administered fluconazole 400 mg orally or as an intravenous (IV) infusion over 60 minutes. One hour later, alfentanil 20 mcg/kg was administered IV over 2 minutes.[1] The administration of IV fluconazole produced area under the concentration-time curve and peak fluconazole concentrations that were approximately 12% to 15% greater than those resulting from oral fluconazole administration. Mean alfentanil clearance decreased 55% and 60% following oral and IV fluconazole, respectively. Alfentanil's half-life was prolonged by fluconazole from 1.5 to 2.5 hours. Respiratory rate was reduced following fluconazole pretreatment compared with alfentanil alone. The effects of multiple doses of fluconazole on alfentanil are unknown, but a greater reduction in alfentanil clearance with increased pharmacologic effect might be expected.

RELATED DRUGS: Other antifungal agents (eg, ketoconazole [eg, *Nizoral*], itraconazole [eg, *Sporanox*]) that are known to inhibit CYP3A4 may decrease alfentanil metabolism.

Other analgesics such as fentanyl (eg, *Sublimaze*) and sufentanil (eg, *Sufenta*) may be affected by fluconazole or other antifungal agents that inhibit CYP3A4.

MANAGEMENT OPTIONS:

➡ *Monitor.* Be alert for altered opioid effects, including increased or prolonged respiratory depression, when alfentanil is administered to patients taking drugs known to inhibit CYP3A4 activity.

REFERENCES:

1. Palkama VJ, et al. The effect of intravenous and oral fluconazole on the pharmacokinetics and pharmacodynamics of intravenous alfentanil. *Anesth Analg.* 1998;87(1):190-194.

Alfentanil (eg, *Alfenta*)

Rifampin (eg, *Rifadin*)

SUMMARY: Rifampin administration markedly reduces alfentanil plasma concentrations; attenuation of alfentanil's therapeutic effect is expected.

RISK FACTORS: No specific risk factors are known.

MECHANISM: Rifampin increases the systemic clearance of alfentanil and reduces its bioavailability by inducing the metabolism (probably CYP3A4) of alfentanil.

CLINICAL EVALUATION: Ten subjects were administered alfentanil 15 mcg/kg intravenously (IV) or 60 mcg/kg orally alone and following rifampin 600 mg daily for 5 days.[1] After oral alfentanil administration, pretreatment with rifampin increased the clearance of alfentanil 145%, reduced the area under the plasma concentration-time curve (AUC) of alfentanil 63%, and shortened its half-life from 1.1 to 0.65 hours. The AUC of alfentanil after oral administration was reduced from 23 to 1 ng/hr/mL. In another study, rifampin in a similar dose increased the systemic clearance of alfentanil by a similar amount.[2] The magnitude of rifampin's effect on IV alfentanil pharmacokinetics suggests that some patients taking rifampin will have a diminished response to alfentanil.

RELATED DRUGS: Rifabutin (*Mycobutin*) is also known to induce CYP3A4 and may reduce alfentanil plasma concentrations in a similar manner. It is likely that the metabolism of fentanyl (eg, *Sublimaze*) would also be induced by rifampin.

MANAGEMENT OPTIONS:

➡ *Consider Alternative.* Consider using an analgesic that is not a CYP3A4 substrate (eg, morphine [eg, *MS Contin*]) for patients taking rifampin.

➡ *Monitor.* Be alert for reduced analgesic efficacy when alfentanil is administered to patients taking rifampin.

REFERENCES:

1. Kharasch ED, et al. Intravenous and oral alfentanil as in vivo probes for hepatic and first-pass cytochrome P450 3A activity: noninvasive assessment by use of pupillary miosis. *Clin Pharmacol Ther.* 2004;76(5):452-466.

2. Kharasch ED, et al. The role of cytochrome P450 3A4 in alfentanil clearance. Implications for interindividual variability in disposition and perioperative drug interactions. *Anesthesiology.* 1997;87(1):36-50.

Alfentanil (eg, _Alfenta_)

Troleandomycin†

SUMMARY: Troleandomycin administration increases alfentanil plasma concentrations; increased narcotic effects are likely to occur.

RISK FACTORS: No specific risk factors are known.

MECHANISM: Troleandomycin is known to inhibit CYP3A4, the enzyme responsible for alfentanil metabolism.

CLINICAL EVALUATION: Ten subjects were administered alfentanil 15 mcg/kg intravenously (IV) or 60 mcg/kg orally alone and following troleandomycin 500 mg twice daily for 2 days.[1] Troleandomycin pretreatment increased the mean area under the plasma concentration-time curve of alfentanil over 6-fold and about 20-fold following IV and oral administration of alfentanil, respectively. Alfentanil half-life was prolonged from 1.1 to 6.6 hours after troleandomycin administration. A similar dose of troleandomycin reduced the clearance of alfentanil nearly 80% after IV dosing.[2] These large increases in alfentanil concentrations are likely to increase the narcotic effect and prolong the drug response.

RELATED DRUGS: Erythromycin (eg, _Ery-Tab_) and clarithromycin (eg, _Biaxin_) also will inhibit the metabolism of alfentanil. It is also likely that troleandomycin will inhibit the metabolism of fentanyl (eg, _Sublimaze_).

MANAGEMENT OPTIONS:

➡ **_Consider Alternative._** Consider using an analgesic that is not a CYP3A4 substrate (eg, morphine [eg, _MS Contin_]) for patients taking troleandomycin. Azithromycin (eg, _Zithromax_) and dirithromycin† do not appear to significantly affect CYP3A4 activity and are not expected to inhibit alfentanil's metabolism.

➡ **_Monitor._** Be alert for increased narcotic effect (eg, sedation, respiratory depression) when alfentanil is administered to patients taking troleandomycin.

REFERENCES:
 1. Kharasch ED, et al. Intravenous and oral alfentanil as in vivo probes for hepatic and first-pass cytochrome P450 3A activity: noninvasive assessment by use of pupillary miosis. _Clin Pharmacol Ther._ 2004;76(5):452-466.
 2. Kharasch ED, et al. The role of cytochrome P450 3A4 in alfentanil clearance. Implications for interindividual variability in disposition and perioperative drug interactions. _Anesthesiology._ 1997;87(1):36-50.

† Not available in the United States.

 Alfuzosin (_Uroxatral_)

Atenolol (eg, _Tenormin_)

SUMMARY: Single-dose study in healthy subjects suggests that combining alfuzosin and atenolol may increase the risk of hypotensive episodes.

RISK FACTORS: No specific risk factors are known.

MECHANISM: Alfuzosin and atenolol probably have additive hypotensive effects; the mechanism(s) for the increased plasma concentrations of both drugs is not established.

CLINICAL EVALUATION: Eight healthy subjects received a single dose of atenolol (100 mg) with and without concurrent single-dose alfuzosin (2.5 mg of an immediate-release tablet).[1] Atenolol area under the plasma concentration-time curve (AUC) was increased 14%, and alfuzosin AUC was increased 21%. The mean blood pressure was also significantly reduced by the combination. The clinical significance of these findings must await studies with multiple doses of both drugs using the commercially available alfuzosin extended-release tablets. Until then, assume that some patients will manifest additive hypotensive effects.

RELATED DRUGS: The extent to which alfuzosin interacts with other beta-adrenergic blockers is not established, but expect additive hypotensive effects.

MANAGEMENT OPTIONS:

➡ *Monitor.* Monitor blood pressure in patients receiving alfuzosin with atenolol or other beta-adrenergic blockers.

REFERENCES:
1. *Uroxatral* [package insert]. Bridgewater, NJ: Sanofi-Aventis US; 2007.

Alfuzosin (*Uroxatral*)

Cimetidine (eg, *Tagamet*)

SUMMARY: Cimetidine slightly increases alfuzosin plasma concentrations, but the clinical importance is probably minimal.

RISK FACTORS: No specific risk factors are known.

MECHANISM: Not established. Cimetidine may inhibit alfuzosin metabolism.

CLINICAL EVALUATION: Multiple doses of cimetidine (1,000 mg/day) resulted in a 20% increase in alfuzosin area under the concentration-time curve.[1] An interaction of this magnitude is unlikely to cause adverse reactions, but an occasional patient might be affected.

RELATED DRUGS: If the mechanism of the interaction is reduced alfuzosin metabolism, famotidine (eg, *Pepcid*), nizatidine (eg, *Axid*), and ranitidine (eg, *Zantac*) are unlikely to interact because they have minimal effects on drug metabolism.

MANAGEMENT OPTIONS: No specific action is required, but be alert for evidence of the interaction.

REFERENCES:
1. *Uroxatral* [package insert]. Bridgewater, NJ: Sanofi-Aventis US; 2007.

Alfuzosin (*Uroxatral*)

Diltiazem (eg, *Cardizem*)

SUMMARY: Alfuzosin and diltiazem inhibit each other's metabolism; increased plasma concentrations may occur.

RISK FACTORS: No specific risk factors are known.

MECHANISM: Diltiazem inhibits CYP3A4, the enzyme that metabolizes alfuzosin. Alfuzosin appears to inhibit the metabolism (CYP3A4) of diltiazem.

CLINICAL EVALUATION: While information is limited, the manufacturer of alfuzosin reports that the coadministration of diltiazem 240 mg daily with alfuzosin resulted in a mean increase of 1.3-fold in area under the plasma concentration-time curve (AUC) of alfuzosin.[1] Alfuzosin increased the AUC of diltiazem 1.4-fold. It is possible that this magnitude of change in plasma concentrations could result in the development of hypotension and bradycardia in some patients.

RELATED DRUGS: Verapamil (eg, *Isoptin*) is also an inhibitor of CYP3A4 and may increase alfuzosin concentrations in a similar manner. It is also possible that alfuzosin will inhibit the metabolism of verapamil and other calcium channel antagonists that are metabolized by CYP3A4.

MANAGEMENT OPTIONS:

➡ *Monitor.* If alfuzosin and diltiazem are coadministered, be alert for hypotensive episodes and bradycardia.

REFERENCES:

1. *Uroxatral* [package insert]. New York, NY: Sanofi-Synthelabo, Inc; 2004.

 Alfuzosin (*Uroxatral*)

AVOID Doxazosin (eg, *Cardura*)

SUMMARY: Alfuzosin is contraindicated with doxazosin or other alpha-adrenergic blockers.

RISK FACTORS: No specific risk factors are known.

MECHANISM: Theoretically, alfuzosin combined with other alpha-adrenergic blockers may result in additive alpha-blockade.

CLINICAL EVALUATION: The product information for alfuzosin states that, although no data are available, concurrent use with other alpha-adrenergic blockers is contraindicated.[1]

RELATED DRUGS: Other alpha-adrenergic blockers, including prazosin (eg, *Minipress*), tamsulosin (*Flomax*), and terazosin (eg, *Hytrin*), are also contraindicated with alfuzosin.

MANAGEMENT OPTIONS:

➡ *AVOID COMBINATION.* The combination of alfuzosin and doxazosin is contraindicated.

REFERENCES:

1. *Uroxatral* [package insert]. Bridgewater, NJ: Sanofi-Aventis US; 2007.

 Alfuzosin (*Uroxatral*)

Ketoconazole (eg, *Nizoral*)

SUMMARY: Ketoconazole increases alfuzosin plasma concentrations; toxicity, including hypotension and dizziness, may occur.

RISK FACTORS: No specific risk factors are known.

MECHANISM: Ketoconazole inhibits CYP3A4, the enzyme responsible for the metabolism of alfuzosin.

CLINICAL EVALUATION: While information is limited, the manufacturer of alfuzosin reports that coadministration of ketoconazole 400 mg daily with alfuzosin resulted in a mean increase in area under the plasma concentration-time curve for alfuzosin of 3.2-fold.[1] This magnitude of effect could produce toxicity in some patients.

RELATED DRUGS: Other antifungal agents that inhibit CYP3A4 (eg, itraconazole [eg, *Sporanox*], fluconazole [eg, *Diflucan*], voriconazole [*Vfend*]) also may interact with alfuzosin.

MANAGEMENT OPTIONS:

➥ *Consider Alternative.* Terbinafine (eg, *Lamisil*) does not inhibit CYP3A4 activity and is not expected to interact with alfuzosin.

➥ *Monitor.* Watch for excessive alfuzosin response in patients taking CYP3A4 inhibitors such as ketoconazole.

REFERENCES:

1. *Uroxatral* [package insert]. New York, NY: Sanofi-Synthelabo, Inc; 2004.

Alfuzosin (eg, *Uroxatral*)

Ritonavir (*Norvir*) AVOID

SUMMARY: Potent CYP3A4 inhibitors substantially increase alfuzosin plasma concentrations; ritonavir is a potent CYP3A4 and contraindicated with alfuzosin.

RISK FACTORS: No specific risk factors are known.

MECHANISM: Alfuzosin is metabolized primarily by CYP3A4, and ritonavir is a potent CYP3A4 inhibitor.

CLINICAL EVALUATION: Because potent CYP3A4 inhibitors such as ketoconazole (eg, *Nizoral*) can produce several-fold increases in alfuzosin plasma concentrations, the manufacturer states the concurrent use of alfuzosin with other potent CYP3A4 inhibitors such as ritonavir is contraindicated.[1]

RELATED DRUGS: Other drugs used for HIV that inhibit CYP3A4 and may interact with alfuzosin include atazanavir (*Reyataz*), darunavir (*Prezista*), delavirdine (*Rescriptor*), indinavir (*Crixivan*), nelfinavir (*Viracept*), and saquinavir (*Invirase*).

MANAGEMENT OPTIONS:

➥ *AVOID COMBINATION.* Given that excessive hypotension may occur and that ritonavir is contraindicated in the product information, avoid concurrent use.

REFERENCES:

1. *Uroxatral* [package insert]. Bridgewater, NJ: Sanofi-Aventis US; 2007.

Alfuzosin (eg, *Uroxatral*) 5

Warfarin (eg, *Coumadin*)

SUMMARY: Alfuzosin does not appear to affect warfarin.

RISK FACTORS: None (no interaction).

MECHANISM: None (no interaction).

CLINICAL EVALUATION: The manufacturer states that an immediate-release formulation of alfuzosin (5 mg twice daily for 6 days) did not affect the pharmacodynamic response to a single dose of warfarin.[1]

RELATED DRUGS: No information is available.

MANAGEMENT OPTIONS: No interaction.

REFERENCES:

1. *Uroxatral* [package insert]. Bridgewater, NJ: Sanofi-Aventis US; 2007.

 Aliskiren (*Tekturna*)

Amlodipine (eg, *Norvasc*)

SUMMARY: The coadministration of amlodipine produces a small increase in aliskiren plasma concentrations.

RISK FACTORS: No specific risk factors are known.

MECHANISM: Unknown. Competitive inhibition of aliskiren metabolism by CYP3A4 is possible.

CLINICAL EVALUATION: Aliskiren 300 mg daily and amlodipine 10 mg daily were each administered for 2 weeks alone and in combination to 25 healthy subjects.[1] During the coadministration of aliskiren and amlodipine, the mean area under the plasma concentration-time curve of aliskiren was increased 29%. Peak aliskiren concentrations were unchanged and no half-life value was reported. Aliskiren had no effect on amlodipine pharmacokinetics. Subjects generally tolerated the combination well. Given the wide therapeutic range for aliskiren, this interaction is expected to have limited clinical significance.

RELATED DRUGS: None known. Diltiazem (eg, *Cardizem*) and verapamil (eg, *Calan*) may interact with aliskiren by inhibiting its metabolism via CYP3A4.

MANAGEMENT OPTIONS:

➡ **Monitor.** Patients receiving aliskiren and amlodipine may have some increase in hypotensive effect, which may be desirable. Monitor for evidence of hypotension or adverse reactions, including headache, dizziness, and fatigue.

REFERENCES:

1. Vaidyanathan S, et al. Lack of pharmacokinetic interactions of aliskiren, a novel direct renin inhibitor for the treatment of hypertension, with the antihypertensives amlodipine, valsartan, hydrochlorothiazide (HCTZ) and ramipril in healthy volunteers. *Int J Clin Pract*. 2006;60(11):1343-1356.

 Aliskiren (*Tekturna*)

Itraconazole (eg, *Sporanox*)

SUMMARY: Itraconazole can markedly increase the plasma concentration of aliskiren; some patients may experience excessive hypotension or hyperkalemia.

RISK FACTORS: No specific risk factors are known.

MECHANISM: Itraconazole inhibits the P-glycoprotein and perhaps the CYP3A4-mediated first-pass metabolism of aliskiren.

CLINICAL EVALUATION: Following a 200 mg first dose, 11 subjects received itraconazole 100 mg twice daily or placebo for 5 days.[1] On the third day, each subject was administered a single dose of aliskiren 150 mg. Compared with placebo, itraconazole treatment resulted in a mean 6.5-fold (range, 2.6- to 20.5-fold) increase in the area under the concentration-time curve of aliskiren, but did not alter the aliskiren elimination half-life. Aliskiren reduction in plasma renin activity was enhanced during itraconazole treatment.

RELATED DRUGS: Ketoconazole (eg, *Nizoral*) also has been noted to increase aliskiren concentrations. Other antifungal agents that inhibit P-glycoprotein (eg, posaconazole [*Noxafil*]) or CYP3A4 (eg, fluconazole [eg, *Diflucan*], posaconazole, voriconazole [*Vfend*]) may also increase aliskiren plasma concentrations.

MANAGEMENT OPTIONS:

➡ *Consider Alternative.* Terbinafine (eg, *Lamisil*) could be considered as an alternative antifungal agent because it does not affect CYP3A4 activity. Amphotericin, caspofungin (*Cancidas*), and anidulafungin (*Eraxis*) do not appear to inhibit CYP3A4.

➡ *Monitor.* Monitor patients stabilized on aliskiren for increased hypotensive effect during itraconazole coadministration.

REFERENCES:
1. Tapaninen T, et al. Itraconazole, a P-glycoprotein and CYP3A4 inhibitor, markedly raises the plasma concentrations and enhances the renin-inhibiting effect of aliskiren. *J Clin Pharmacol.* 2011;51(3):359-367.

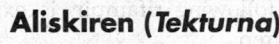

Aliskiren (*Tekturna*)

Ketoconazole (eg, *Nizoral*)

SUMMARY: Ketoconazole administration can increase aliskiren concentrations; some patients may develop adverse reactions.

RISK FACTORS: No specific risk factors are known.

MECHANISM: Ketoconazole is known to inhibit the activity of CYP3A4, the enzyme reported to be primarily responsible for aliskiren metabolism.

CLINICAL EVALUATION: While specific data are limited, the coadministration of ketoconazole 200 mg twice daily increased the plasma concentration of aliskiren (dose not reported) by approximately 80%.[1] Pending further data, observe patients receiving aliskiren and ketoconazole for increased aliskiren effect and potential adverse reactions, including headache, dizziness, and fatigue.

RELATED DRUGS: Fluconazole (eg, *Diflucan*), itraconazole (eg, *Sporanox*), posaconazole (*Noxafil*), and voriconazole (*Vfend*) also inhibit the activity of CYP3A4 and are expected to increase the plasma concentrations of aliskiren.

MANAGEMENT OPTIONS:

➡ *Consider Alternative.* Terbinafine (eg, *Lamisil*) may be an alternative antifungal agent because it does not affect CYP3A4 activity. Amphotericin, caspofungin (*Cancidas*), and anidulafungin (*Eraxis*) do not appear to inhibit CYP3A4.

➡ *Monitor.* Carefully monitor patients stabilized on aliskiren for increased hypotensive effect and adverse reactions when ketoconazole or other potent CYP3A4 inhibitors are coadministered.

REFERENCES:
1. *Tekturna* [package insert]. East Hanover, NJ: Novartis Pharmaceuticals; 2007.

Aliskiren (*Tekturna*)

Rifampin (eg, *Rifadin*)

SUMMARY: Rifampin administration reduces the plasma concentration of aliskiren and reduces its pharmacodynamic effects.

RISK FACTORS: No specific risk factors are known.

MECHANISM: Rifampin appears to induce intestinal P-glycoprotein, resulting in a lower bioavailability of aliskiren, and may also enhance the CYP3A4 metabolism of aliskiren.

CLINICAL EVALUATION: Twelve subjects were administered placebo or rifampin 600 mg daily for 5 days.[1] On day 6, each subject took a single dose of aliskiren 150 mg. The mean area under the concentration-time curve of aliskiren was reduced 56% following rifampin dosing. Aliskiren half-life was not significantly changed. The pharmacodynamic response to aliskiren, as measured by plasma renin concentration, was reduced 61% following rifampin. The reduction in aliskiren concentration following rifampin is expected to reduce the antihypertensive efficacy of aliskiren.

RELATED DRUGS: Rifabutin (*Mycobutin*) and rifapentine (*Priftin*) are known to induce CYP3A4 and P-glycoprotein and are likely to affect aliskiren in a similar manner as rifampin.

MANAGEMENT OPTIONS:

➡ ***Monitor.*** Monitor patients taking aliskiren for altered hypotensive response if rifampin is added to or discontinued from their drug regimen.

REFERENCES:
1. Tapaninen T, et al. Rifampicin reduces the plasma concentrations and the renin-inhibiting effect of aliskiren. *Eur J Clin Pharmacol.* 2010;66(5):497-502.

4 Aliskiren (*Tekturna*)

Valsartan (*Diovan*)

SUMMARY: The coadministration of valsartan produces a small decrease in aliskiren plasma concentrations.

RISK FACTORS: No specific risk factors are known.

MECHANISM: Unknown.

CLINICAL EVALUATION: Aliskiren 300 mg daily and valsartan 320 mg daily were each administered for 2 weeks alone and in combination to 19 healthy subjects.[1] During the coadministration of aliskiren and valsartan, the mean area under the plasma concentration-time curve of aliskiren was decreased 26%. Peak aliskiren concentrations were decreased 28% and no half-life value was reported. Aliskiren had no effect on valsartan pharmacokinetics. Subjects generally tolerated the combination well. Given the wide therapeutic range for aliskiren, this interaction is expected to have limited clinical significance.

RELATED DRUGS: None known.

MANAGEMENT OPTIONS:

➡ *Monitor.* Patients receiving aliskiren and valsartan may have some decrease in hypotensive effect, although this is likely to be minimal and offset by the hypotensive effects of valsartan.

REFERENCES:

1. Vaidyanathan S, et al. Lack of pharmacokinetic interactions of aliskiren, a novel direct renin inhibitor for the treatment of hypertension, with the antihypertensives amlodipine, valsartan, hydrochlorothiazide (HCTZ) and ramipril in healthy volunteers. *Int J Clin Pract.* 2006;60(11):1343-1356.

Aliskiren (*Tekturna*) 4

Verapamil (eg, *Isoptin*)

SUMMARY: Verapamil may increase the plasma concentration of aliskiren; increased hypotensive response is possible.

RISK FACTORS: No specific risk factors are known.

MECHANISM: Verapamil inhibits the P-glycoprotein and perhaps the CYP3A4-mediated first-pass metabolism of aliskiren.

CLINICAL EVALUATION: Eighteen subjects received a single dose of aliskiren 300 mg alone and after verapamil 240 mg sustained release for 8 days.[1] Coadministration of verapamil resulted in a mean 2-fold increase in the area under the concentration-time curve of aliskiren, but did not alter aliskiren half-life. The single dose of aliskiren did not significantly alter verapamil concentrations measured on day 7 (before aliskiren) and day 8 (with aliskiren) of verapamil dosing. Some patients stabilized on aliskiren may experience enhanced hypotensive effects during the administration of verapamil.

RELATED DRUGS: Diltiazem (eg, *Cardizem*) may also increase aliskiren plasma concentrations. Note that calcium channel blockers that do not inhibit CYP3A4 or P-glycoprotein (eg, felodipine) may produce a pharmacodynamic interaction with aliskiren, resulting in enhanced hypotensive effects.

MANAGEMENT OPTIONS:

➡ *Monitor.* Monitor patients stabilized on aliskiren for increased hypotensive effect during verapamil coadministration.

REFERENCES:

1. Rebello S, et al. Effect of verapamil on the pharmacokinetics of aliskiren in healthy participants. *J Clin Pharmacol.* 2011;51(2):218-228.

Allopurinol (eg, *Zyloprim*)

Ampicillin

SUMMARY: The prevalence of ampicillin rash increases in patients taking allopurinol.

RISK FACTORS: No specific risk factors are known.

MECHANISM: Not established.

CLINICAL EVALUATION: In an epidemiological study of adverse drug reactions, an association between ampicillin rash and allopurinol administration was detected.[1,2] Analysis of the data indicated that allopurinol or hyperuricemia appeared to predispose patients receiving ampicillin to the development of rash. More study is needed to determine if allopurinol itself produces this effect.

RELATED DRUGS: No information is available.

MANAGEMENT OPTIONS: No specific action is required, but be alert for evidence of the interaction.

REFERENCES:

1. Excess of ampicillin rashes associated with allopurinol or hyperuricemia. A report from the Boston Collaborative Drug Surveillance Program, Boston University Medical Center. *N Engl J Med.* 1972;286(10):505-507.

2. Ampicillin rashes. *N Engl J Med.* 1972;286(22):1217-1218.

Allopurinol (eg, *Zyloprim*)

Antacids

SUMMARY: Aluminum hydroxide appeared to inhibit the response to allopurinol considerably in several patients.

RISK FACTORS: No specific risk factors are known.

MECHANISM: Aluminum hydroxide probably inhibits the GI absorption of allopurinol.

CLINICAL EVALUATION: Hyperuricemia failed to respond to allopurinol 300 mg/day in 3 patients on long-term hemodialysis when allopurinol and aluminum hydroxide were administered simultaneously.[1] When allopurinol was given 3 hours before the aluminum hydroxide, the serum uric acid concentration declined in all 3 patients, suggesting improved allopurinol absorption. When 1 patient was rechallenged with simultaneous administration of the 2 drugs, the serum uric acid concentration increased substantially. Therefore, aluminum hydroxide probably reduced the absorption of allopurinol in these patients. Controlled studies are needed to determine the incidence and magnitude of this interaction and to determine the effect of other antacids on allopurinol absorption.

RELATED DRUGS: Pending additional information, consider all aluminum-containing antacids capable of inhibiting allopurinol absorption. Although little is known regarding magnesium- or calcium-containing antacids, assume that they also inhibit allopurinol absorption until proven otherwise.

MANAGEMENT OPTIONS:

➡ ***Circumvent/Minimize.*** Until more information is available, administer allopurinol at least 3 hours before or 6 hours after aluminum hydroxide.

➡ ***Monitor.*** Monitor patients for reduced allopurinol response. The same precautions would apply to other antacids until information on their effect on allopurinol is available.

REFERENCES:

1. Weissman I, Krivoy N. Interaction of aluminum hydroxide and allopurinol in patients on chronic hemodialysis. *Ann Intern Med.* 1987;107(5):787.

Allopurinol (eg, *Zyloprim*) | 5

Atenolol (eg, *Tenormin*)

SUMMARY: Allopurinol does not alter atenolol excretion.

RISK FACTORS: No specific risk factors are known.

MECHANISM: No interaction.

CLINICAL EVALUATION: In 6 healthy subjects, allopurinol 300 mg/day did not affect the disposition of atenolol 100 mg/day.[1]

RELATED DRUGS: No information is available.

MANAGEMENT OPTIONS: No interaction.

REFERENCES:

1. Schäfer-Korting M, et al. Atenolol interaction with aspirin, allopurinol, and ampicillin. *Clin Pharmacol Ther.* 1983;33(3):283-288.

Allopurinol (eg, *Zyloprim*)

Azathioprine (eg, *Imuran*)

SUMMARY: Allopurinol increases the concentration of the active metabolites of azathioprine, potentially increasing both the risk of toxicity and therapeutic efficacy.

RISK FACTORS: No specific risk factors are known.

MECHANISM: Azathioprine metabolism is complex. It is first metabolized to 6-mercaptopurine (6-MP), which is in turn metabolized by xanthine oxidase (XO) to a largely inactive product, and by other enzymes to active products that account for both the efficacy and toxicity of azathioprine and 6-MP. Thus, inhibition of XO results in formation of more active metabolites.

CLINICAL EVALUATION: This interaction has been known since 1970 and has resulted in a number of life-threatening and fatal reactions, usually due to bone marrow suppression.[1-9] In most cases, it has taken a few weeks or months for the adverse reactions to appear. Severe adverse reactions often occurred when allopurinol was added to azathioprine by a prescriber who was unaware of the interaction. Nonetheless, in patients with inflammatory bowel disease with inadequate azathioprine response, the addition of low-dose allopurinol (with substantial reductions in azathioprine dose and careful monitoring) may improve azathioprine efficacy without increasing toxicity.[10] Some evidence suggests that allopurinol may actually reduce the formation of hepatotoxic metabolites of azathioprine and reduce the risk of azathioprine-induced hepatoxicity.[11] Given the potentially serious nature of adverse outcomes, the combination of azathioprine and allopurinol should only be used by prescribers who are aware of the risks and benefits and able to take appropriate precautions; adequate monitoring must be performed to minimize the risk.

RELATED DRUGS: Allopurinol also increases the risk of 6-MP toxicity.

MANAGEMENT OPTIONS:

➡ ***Use Alternative.*** If allopurinol is used for gout, consider using an alternative treatment.

➥ *Circumvent/Minimize.* If allopurinol is started in a patient taking azathioprine, it is generally recommended that the azathioprine dose be reduced to 25% to 33% of the original dose. Lower than usual doses of allopurinol have also been recommended.

➥ *Monitor.* If the combination is used, close monitoring is essential. Weekly complete blood cell counts have been recommended by several researchers; some have recommended monitoring of plasma azathioprine metabolite concentrations before and after allopurinol is started. Instruct patients to be alert for evidence of infection, bleeding, or other signs of bone marrow suppression.

REFERENCES:

1. Hypertension and the lupus syndrome. *Am J Med.* 1970;49(4):519-528.
2. Nies AS, Oates JA. Clinicopathologic conference: hypertension and the lupus syndrome—revisited. *Am J Med.* 1971;51(6):812-814.
3. Zazgornik J, et al. Increased danger of bone marrow damage in simultaneous azathioprine-allopurinol therapy. *Int J Clin Pharmacol Ther Toxicol.* 1981;19(3):96-97.
4. Jeurissen ME, et al. Pancytopenia related to azathioprine in rheumatoid arthritis. *Ann Rheum Dis.* 1988;47(6):503-505.
5. Venkat Raman G, et al. Azathioprine and allopurinol: a potentially dangerous combination. *J Intern Med.* 1990;228(1):69-71.
6. Kennedy DT et al. Azathioprine and allopurinol: the price of an avoidable drug interaction. *Ann Pharmacother.* 1996;30(9):951-954.
7. Cummins D, et al. Myelosuppression associated with azathioprine-allopurinol interaction after heart and lung transplantation. *Transplantation.* 1996;61(11):1661-1662.
8. McConnell PJ. The $181,000 adverse drug reaction. *Hosp Pharm.* 2004;39:648-652.
9. Gearry RB, et al. Azathioprine and allopurinol: A two-edged interaction. *J Gastroenterol Hepatol.* 2010;25(4):653-655.
10. Sparrow MP, et al. Effect of allopurinol on clinical outcomes in inflammatory bowel disease nonresponders to azathioprine or 6-mercaptopurine. *Clin Gastroenterol Hepatol.* 2007;5(2):209-214.
11. Ansari A, et al. Long-term outcome of using allopurinol co-therapy as a strategy for overcoming thiopurine hepatotoxicity in treating inflammatory bowel disease. *Aliment Pharmacol Ther.* 2008;28(6):734-741.

 Allopurinol (eg, *Zyloprim*)

Captopril (eg, *Capoten*)

SUMMARY: Isolated case reports indicate that patients on allopurinol and angiotensin-converting enzyme (ACE) inhibitors such as captopril or enalapril may be predisposed to hypersensitivity reactions including Stevens-Johnson syndrome, anaphylaxis, skin eruptions, fever, and arthralgias, but a causal relationship has not been established.

RISK FACTORS:

➥ *Concurrent Diseases.* Impaired renal function has been proposed as a risk factor, but more study is needed.

MECHANISM: Not established.

CLINICAL EVALUATION: A 71-year-old man with hypertension, chronic renal failure, and CHF developed fatal Stevens-Johnson syndrome approximately 10 days after allopurinol 200 mg/day was added to his captopril therapy 50 mg/day.[1] A subsequent report described a 69-year-old man with diabetes, chronic renal failure, CHF, and hypertension who developed fever, arthralgia, and myalgia 1 month after 300 mg/day of allopurinol was added to captopril therapy 37.5 mg/day.[2] Two other patients reportedly developed Stevens-Johnson syndrome 3 to 5 weeks after allopurinol was added to long-term captopril therapy.[1] A 50-year-old man on enalapril (*Vasotec*) took one 100 mg allopurinol tablet and within 20 minutes developed anaphylaxis with pruritus, urticaria, severe chest pain, severe nausea, cyanosis, hypotension, and tachycardia. Cardiac enzymes and the electrocardiogram were consistent with a myocardial infarction.[6] Allopurinol can produce severe hypersensitivity reactions in the absence of captopril, especially in patients with renal failure and concurrent diuretic therapy.[3-5] Three of the patients described above were receiving diuretics and had impaired renal function; thus, the reactions could have been caused by allopurinol alone or to the combination of allopurinol and diuretics. However, in 1 case, the reaction improved when the captopril was stopped and allopurinol continued;[2] this is consistent with the view that the captopril contributed to the reaction.

RELATED DRUGS: It is not known whether ACE inhibitors other than captopril and enalapril would produce similar reactions if combined with allopurinol.

MANAGEMENT OPTIONS:

➥ *Avoid Unless Benefit Outweighs Risk.* Although it is not firmly established that these reactions resulted from the combined effects of ACE inhibitors and allopurinol, the severity of the potential reactions suggests that the combinations generally should be avoided until more information is available.

➥ *Monitor.* Monitor patients receiving the combination carefully for hypersensitivity reactions. Prompt discontinuation of the offending drugs is important.

REFERENCES:
1. Pennell DJ, et al. Fatal Stevens-Johnson syndrome in a patient on captopril and allopurinol. *Lancet*. 1984;1:463.
2. Sanamta A, et al. Fever, myalgia, and arthralgia in a patient on captopril and allopurinol. *Lancet*. 1984;1:679.
3. Lupton GP, et al. The allopurinol hypersensitivity syndrome. *J Am Acad Dermatol*. 1979;1:365.
4. Burkle WS. Allopurinol hypersensitivity. *Drug Intell Clin Pharm*. 1979;13:218.
5. Al-Kawas FH, et al. Allopurinol hepatotoxicity. Report of two cases and review of the literature. *Ann Intern Med*. 1981;95:588.
6. Ahmad S. Allopurinol and enalapril: drug induced anaphylactic coronary spasm and acute myocardial infarction. *Chest*. 1995;108:586.

Allopurinol (eg, *Zyloprim*)

Chlorpropamide (eg, *Diabinese*)

SUMMARY: Limited data suggest an interaction between allopurinol and chlorpropamide can result in an increased chlorpropamide effect.

RISK FACTORS: No specific risk factors are known.

MECHANISM: Allopurinol or its metabolites may compete with chlorpropamide for renal tubular secretion.

CLINICAL EVALUATION: A preliminary report briefly described 7 patients who received concomitant therapy with allopurinol and chlorpropamide.[1] Two of these patients had a markedly prolonged chlorpropamide half-life (more than 200 hours). In 2 other patients, the half-life appeared to be slightly prolonged. In the remaining 3 patients, who had only been on allopurinol for 1 or 2 days, the chlorpropamide half-life was within normal limits.

RELATED DRUGS: No information is available.

MANAGEMENT OPTIONS: No specific action is required, but be alert for evidence of an interaction.

REFERENCES:
1. Petitpierre B, et al. Behavior of chlorpropamide in renal insufficiency and under the effect of associated drug therapy. *Int J Clin Pharmacol Ther Toxicol.* 1972;6:120.

Allopurinol (eg, *Zyloprim*)

Cyclophosphamide (eg, *Cytoxan*)

SUMMARY: Some evidence indicates that allopurinol increases cyclophosphamide toxicity, but this has not been a consistent finding.

RISK FACTORS: No specific risk factors are known.

MECHANISM: Not established.

CLINICAL EVALUATION: Epidemiological information indicated that allopurinol might increase the frequency of bone marrow depression in patients receiving cyclophosphamide.[1] Of 58 patients receiving cyclophosphamide, bone marrow depression occurred in 57.7% of those also receiving allopurinol and in 18.8% of those not receiving allopurinol. In a subsequent study of 143 patients with malignant lymphoma, allopurinol did not appear to affect the bone marrow suppression of cytotoxic therapy.[2] In another study,[3] four patients who had been receiving allopurinol had a longer mean cyclophosphamide half-life than patients not receiving allopurinol, but the fraction of cyclophosphamide appearing as alkylating metabolites in the urine was the same in both groups. In yet another pharmacokinetic study, allopurinol did not affect the half-life of cyclophosphamide, but it did increase the concentration of cyclophosphamide metabolites in the serum.[4]

RELATED DRUGS: No information is available.

MANAGEMENT OPTIONS:

➡ **Monitor.** It has been proposed that the appropriateness of routine prophylactic use of allopurinol in patients receiving cytotoxic drugs be re-evaluated. When it is necessary to give allopurinol and cyclophosphamide concomitantly, be alert for evidence of excessive cyclophosphamide effect.

REFERENCES:
1. Boston Collaborative Drug Surveillance Program. Allopurinol and cytotoxic drugs. Interaction in relation to bone marrow depression. *JAMA.* 1974;227:1036.
2. Stolbach L, et al. Evaluation of bone marrow toxic reaction in patients treated with allopurinol. *JAMA.* 1982;247:334.
3. Bagley CM Jr, et al. Clinical pharmacology of cyclophosphamide. *Cancer Res.* 1973;33:226.
4. Witten J, et al. The pharmacokinetics of cyclophosphamide in man after treatment with allopurinol. *Acta Pharmacol et Toxicol.* 1980;46:392–94.

Allopurinol (eg, *Zyloprim*)

Cyclosporine (eg, *Sandimmune*)

SUMMARY: Case reports suggest that allopurinol may increase cyclosporine blood concentrations and increase the risk of cyclosporine toxicity.

RISK FACTORS: No specific risk factors are known.

MECHANISM: Not established.

CLINICAL EVALUATION: Isolated cases of increased cyclosporine blood concentrations and cyclosporine toxicity have been reported following the use of allopurinol.[1,2] Although more study is needed, the potential severity of the reactions dictates caution.

RELATED DRUGS: The effect of allopurinol on tacrolimus (eg, *Prograf*) is not established. Given the similarity in the metabolism of cyclosporine and tacrolimus, it is possible that allopurinol affects them similarly.

MANAGEMENT OPTIONS:

➡ *Circumvent/Minimize.* Adjustments of cyclosporine dosage may be needed.

➡ *Monitor.* Monitor for altered cyclosporine concentrations and renal function if allopurinol is initiated, discontinued, or changed in dosage.

REFERENCES:

1. Stevens SL, et al. Cyclosporine toxicity associated with allopurinol. *South Med J.* 1992;85(12):1265-1266.
2. Gorrie M, et al. Allopurinol interaction with cyclosporin. *BMJ.* 1994;308(6921):113.

Allopurinol (eg, *Zyloprim*)

Mercaptopurine (eg, *Purinethol*)

SUMMARY: Allopurinol increases the concentration of the active metabolites of 6-mercaptopurine, potentially increasing both the risk of toxicity and therapeutic efficacy.

RISK FACTORS: No specific risk factors are known.

MECHANISM: Mercaptopurine metabolism is complex. It is metabolized by xanthine oxidase (XO) to a largely inactive product, and by other enzymes to active products that account for both the efficacy and toxicity of mercaptopurine. Thus, inhibition of XO results in formation of more active metabolites. (Azathioprine is rapidly converted to mercaptopurine in the body, so the interactions of azathioprine and mercaptopurine are essentially identical.)

CLINICAL EVALUATION: The interaction of mercaptopurine or azathioprine with allopurinol has been known since the early 1970s and has resulted in a number of life-threatening and fatal reactions, usually due to bone marrow suppression.[1-10] In most cases, it has taken a few weeks or months for the adverse reactions to appear. Severe adverse reactions often occurred when allopurinol was added to mercaptopurine or azathioprine by a prescriber who was unaware of the interaction. Nonetheless, in patients with inflammatory bowel disease with inadequate mercaptopurine or azathioprine response, the addition of low-dose allopurinol (with substantial reductions in mercaptopurine or azathioprine dose and careful monitoring) may improve efficacy without increasing toxicity.[11] Some evidence suggests that allopurinol may actually reduce the formation of hepatotoxic metabolites of mercaptopurine and azathioprine and reduce the risk of hepatotoxicity.[12] Given the potentially serious nature of adverse outcomes, the combination of mercaptopurine or azathioprine with allopurinol should only be used by prescribers who are aware of the risks and benefits and able to take appropriate precautions; adequate monitoring must be performed to minimize the risk.

RELATED DRUGS: Allopurinol also increases the risk of azathioprine (eg, *Imuran*) toxicity.

MANAGEMENT OPTIONS:

➨ *Use Alternative.* If allopurinol is being used for gout, consider using an alternative treatment.

➨ *Circumvent/Minimize.* If allopurinol is started in a patient taking mercaptopurine, it is generally recommended that the mercaptopurine dose be reduced to 25% to 33% of the original dose. Lower than usual doses of allopurinol have also been recommended.

➨ *Monitor.* If the combination is used, close monitoring is essential. Weekly complete blood cell counts have been recommended by several researchers and some have recommended monitoring of plasma mercaptopurine metabolite concentrations before and after allopurinol is started. Instruct patients to be alert for evidence of infection, bleeding, or other signs of bone marrow suppression.

REFERENCES:

1. Hypertension and the lupus syndrome. *Am J Med.* 1970;49(4):519-528.
2. Nies AS, Oates JA. Clinicopathologic conference: hypertension and the lupus syndrome—revisited. *Am J Med.* 1971;51(6):812-814.
3. Case records of the Massachusetts General Hospital. Weekly clinicopathological exercises. Case 4–1972. *N Engl J Med.* 1972;286(4):205-212.
4. Zazgornik J, et al. Increased danger of bone marrow damage in simultaneous azathioprine-allopurinol therapy. *Int J Clin Pharmacol Ther Toxicol.* 1981;19(3):96-97.
5. Jeurissen ME, et al. Pancytopenia related to azathioprine in rheumatoid arthritis. *Ann Rheum Dis.* 1988;47(6):503-505.
6. Venkat Raman G, et al. Azathioprine and allopurinol: a potentially dangerous combination. *J Intern Med.* 1990;228(1):69-71.
7. Kennedy DT, et al. Azathioprine and allopurinol: the price of an avoidable drug interaction. *Ann Pharmacother.* 1996;30(9):951-954.
8. Cummins D, et al. Myelosuppression associated with azathioprine-allopurinol interaction after heart and lung transplantation. *Transplantation.* 1996;61(11):1661-1662.
9. McConnell PJ. The $181,000 adverse drug reaction. *Hosp Pharm.* 2004;39:648-652.
10. Gearry RB, et al. Azathioprine and allopurinol: a two-edged interaction. *J Gastroenterol Hepatol.* 2010;25(4):653-655.
11. Sparrow MP, et al. Effect of allopurinol on clinical outcomes in inflammatory bowel disease nonresponders to azathioprine or 6-mercaptopurine. *Clin Gastroenterol Hepatol.* 2007;5(2):209-214.
12. Ansari A, et al. Long-term outcome of using allopurinol co-therapy as a strategy for overcoming thiopurine hepatotoxicity in treating inflammatory bowel disease. *Aliment Pharmacol Ther.* 2008;28(6):734-741.

4   Allopurinol (eg, *Zyloprim*)

Phenytoin (eg, *Dilantin*)

SUMMARY: Allopurinol appeared to increase serum phenytoin concentrations in one child; more study is needed.

RISK FACTORS: No specific risk factors are known.

MECHANISM: Allopurinol may inhibit the hepatic metabolism of phenytoin.

CLINICAL EVALUATION: Allopurinol appeared to inhibit the metabolism of phenytoin in one patient,[1] but the incidence and magnitude of this purported interaction are not established. Allopurinol inhibits the hepatic metabolism of other drugs and theoretically also could affect phenytoin metabolism.

RELATED DRUGS: No information is available.

MANAGEMENT OPTIONS: No specific action is required, but be alert for evidence of the interaction.

REFERENCES:
1. Yokochi K, et al. Phenytoin-allopurinol interaction: Michaelis-Menten kinetic parameters of phenytoin with and without allopurinol in a child with Lesch-Nyhan syndrome. *Ther Drug Monit.* 1982;4(4):353-357.

Allopurinol (eg, *Zyloprim*)

Probenecid

SUMMARY: Although concurrent use of allopurinol and probenecid may alter the disposition of both drugs, the combination generally results in additive lowering of the serum uric acid level.

RISK FACTORS: No specific risk factors are known.

MECHANISM: Allopurinol (or one of its metabolites) appears to inhibit the metabolism of probenecid.[1,2] Probenecid appears to enhance the renal elimination of the active metabolite of allopurinol.[3]

CLINICAL EVALUATION: The clinical significance of these mechanisms has not been established, and combined therapy with probenecid and allopurinol has been used to advantage. An occasional patient may manifest toxic symptoms or lack of response caused by the increased plasma probenecid levels and decreased plasma alloxanthine levels. In one study, 2 of 5 subjects developed a 50% increase in probenecid half-life with allopurinol administration; in the other 3 subjects, there was little change.[2] Although the likelihood of adverse reactions from this combination appears small, reconsider the need for the use of 2 hypouricemic drugs.

RELATED DRUGS: No information is available.

MANAGEMENT OPTIONS: No specific action is required, but be alert for evidence of the interaction.

REFERENCES:
1. Tjandramaga TB, et al. Interaction of probenecid and allopurinol in gouty subjects. *Fed Proc.* 1971;30:392.
2. Horwitz D, et al. The influence of allopurinol and size of dose on the metabolism of phenylbutazone in patients with gout. *Eur J Clin Pharmacol.* 1977;12(2):133-136.
3. Elion GB, et al. Renal clearance of oxipurinol, the chief metabolite of allopurinol. *Am J Med.* 1968;45(1):69-77.

Allopurinol (eg, Zyloprim)

Theophylline (eg, Slo-Phyllin)

SUMMARY: Allopurinol, especially in large doses, may increase serum theophylline concentrations, but the incidence of theophylline toxicity in patients receiving the combination is not known.

RISK FACTORS:

➥ **Dosage Regimen.** Allopurinol doses at least 600 mg/day may inhibit the hepatic metabolism of theophylline.

MECHANISM: Pharmacokinetic studies suggest that allopurinol inhibits the hepatic metabolism of theophylline. This mechanism is consistent with a 44% increase in aminopyrine half-life in 5 subjects given allopurinol.[1] (Aminopyrine is used as a marker for alteration in hepatic oxidative drug metabolism.) Although allopurinol did not affect the spectrophotometric determination of theophylline in vitro,[7] the possibility that allopurinol therapy may falsely increase serum concentrations has not been strictly ruled out.

CLINICAL EVALUATION: A 62-year-old woman with chronic obstructive pulmonary disease on chronic therapy with 450 mg/day of theophylline developed a 38% increase in peak plasma theophylline concentrations about three days after allopurinol was added to her therapy (dose not stated).[1] Two other cases of possible allopurinol-induced inhibition of theophylline metabolism have been reported.[2,3] Studies in healthy subjects suggest that the interaction is dose related. In 5 healthy nonsmokers, allopurinol 300 mg/day for 7 days did not affect the clearance of theophylline 5 mg/kg IV.[4] In another study of 10 healthy subjects, theophylline clearance was slightly lower following allopurinol 300 mg/day for 7 days, but the effect was not statistically significant; a steady-state study in 4 subjects gave similar results.[5] However, in 12 healthy subjects receiving a large dose of allopurinol (600 mg/day for 14 days) the area under the theophylline serum concentration-time curve (AUC) increased by 27% and theophylline clearance declined by 21%.[6] The effect on theophylline AUC and clearance was slightly greater by day 28 of allopurinol (34% increase in AUC and 25% decrease in clearance).

RELATED DRUGS: No information is available.

MANAGEMENT OPTIONS:

➥ **Monitor.** Monitor for evidence of altered theophylline effect if allopurinol therapy is initiated or discontinued, especially if large doses of allopurinol are used. Alteration of theophylline dose may be needed.

REFERENCES:

1. Barry M, et al. Allopurinol influences aminophenazone elimination. *Clin Pharmacokinet.* 1990;19:167.

2. Jacobs MH, et al. Theophylline toxicity due to impaired theophylline degradation. *Am Rev Resp Dis.* 1974;110:342.

3. Marlin GE, et al. Assessment of combined oral theophylline and inhaled beta-adrenoceptor agonist bronchodilator therapy. *Br J Clin Pharmacol.* 1978;5:45.

4. Vozeh S, et al. Influence of allopurinol on theophylline disposition in adults. *Clin Pharmacol Ther.* 1980;27:194.

5. Grygiel JJ, et al. Effects of allopurinol on theophylline metabolism and clearance. *Clin Pharmacol Ther.* 1979;26:660.

6. Manfredi RL, et al. Inhibition of theophylline metabolism by longterm allopurinol administration. *Clin Pharmacol Ther.* 1981;29:224.

7. Matheson LE, et al. Drug interference with the Schack and Waxler plasma theophylline assay. *Am J Hosp Pharm.* 1977;34:496.

Allopurinol (eg, *Zyloprim*)

Vidarabine (*Vira-A*)

SUMMARY: Allopurinol may increase vidarabine toxicity.

RISK FACTORS: No specific risk factors are known.

MECHANISM: Vidarabine is rapidly metabolized to arabinosyl/hypoxanthine (ara-Hx), a metabolite that has some antiviral activity. A portion of the ara-Hx is further metabolized by xanthine oxidase to xanthine arabinoside. Allopurinol may inhibit this second metabolic step, resulting in accumulation of ara-Hx.

CLINICAL EVALUATION: Two patients with chronic lymphocytic leukemia were receiving allopurinol when vidarabine 300 mg daily for viral infection was added to their regimen.[1] After 4 days of concomitant therapy, both developed neurotoxicity, including tremors of the extremities and facial muscles and confusion. No dechallenge information was provided, and a causal relationship remains to be established. Note that vidarabine alone can cause CNS toxicity, particularly in patients with renal or hepatic failure.

RELATED DRUGS: No information is available.

MANAGEMENT OPTIONS:

➡ *Monitor.* Until additional information regarding this interaction is available, carefully monitor patients receiving allopurinol and vidarabine for signs of vidarabine toxicity.

REFERENCES:

1. Friedman HM, et al. Adenine arabinoside and allopurinol-possible adverse drug interaction. *N Engl J Med.* 1981;304:423.

Allopurinol (eg, *Zyloprim*)

Warfarin (eg, *Coumadin*)

SUMMARY: Although the evidence is conflicting, allopurinol appears to enhance the hypoprothrombinemic response to oral anticoagulants in some patients; bleeding episodes have been reported in some cases.

RISK FACTORS: No specific risk factors are known.

MECHANISM: Not established. Allopurinol may inhibit the hepatic metabolism of oral anticoagulants.

CLINICAL EVALUATION: Allopurinol 2.5 mg/kg twice daily for 14 days prolonged the half-life of a single dose of dicumarol in 6 healthy medical students.[1] However, in a subsequent study of healthy subjects, only 1 of 3 developed a prolonged dicumarol half-life during allopurinol administration, and warfarin disposition was not affected.[2] Another study demonstrated a decrease in warfarin elimination in only 1 of 6 subjects given allopurinol.[3] Two patients on chronic phenprocoumon therapy developed excessive hypoprothrombinemia and bleeding following initiation of allopurinol therapy.[4] These findings, along with several case reports of enhanced response to warfarin,[5-8] indicate that occasional patients on oral anticoagulants and allopurinol will develop enhanced anticoagulant effect. However, factors that predispose patients to this interaction have not been established.

RELATED DRUGS: Although data are limited, assume that all oral anticoagulants interact with allopurinol until proven otherwise.

MANAGEMENT OPTIONS:

➥ *Monitor.* Watch for an alteration in the hypoprothrombinemic response to oral anticoagulants when allopurinol is started, stopped, or changed in dosage; adjust oral anticoagulant dosage as needed.

REFERENCES:

1. Vesell ES, et al. Impairment of drug metabolism in man by allopurinol and nortriptyline. *N Engl J Med.* 1970;283:1484.
2. Pond SM, et al. The effects of allopurinol and clofibrate on the elimination of coumarin anticoagulants in man. *Aust NZ J Med.* 1975;5:324.
3. Rawlins MD, et al. Influence of allopurinol on drug metabolism in man. *Br J Pharmacol.* 1973;48:693.
4. Jahnchen E, et al. Interaction of allopurinol with phenprocoumon in man. *Klin Wochenschr.* 1977;55:759.
5. Self TH, et al. Drug-enhancement of warfarin activity. *Lancet.* 1975;2:557.
6. Weart CW. Coumarin and allopurinol: a drug interaction case report. Contributed paper, 32nd annual meeting ASHP, 1975.
7. McInnes GT, et al. Acute adverse reactions attributed to allopurinol in hospitalized patients. *Ann Rheum Dis.* 1981;40:245.
8. Barry M, et al. Allopurinol influences aminophenazone elimination. *Clin Pharmacokinet.* 1990;19:167.

Almotriptan (*Axert*)

Ketoconazole (eg, *Nizoral*)

SUMMARY: Ketoconazole administration increases the plasma concentration of almotriptan; increased side effects caused by vasoconstriction may occur in some patients.

RISK FACTORS:

➥ *Pharmacogenetics.* Since almotriptan is metabolized by CYP3A4, CYP2D6 and monoamine oxidase, the effect of a CYP3A4 inhibitor like ketoconazole may be greater in patients who are deficient in CYP2D6 and do not have this metabolic pathway for almotriptan elimination.

MECHANISM: Ketoconazole appears to inhibit the CYP3A4 metabolism of almotriptan resulting in reduced oral clearance. The noted reduction in renal clearance following ketoconazole might be a result of reduced renal tubular secretion of almotriptan.

CLINICAL EVALUATION: A single 12.5 mg oral dose of almotriptan was administered alone and on day 2 of a 3-day regimen of ketoconazole 400 mg once daily.[1] Compared with almotriptan alone, the coadministration of ketoconazole resulted in a mean increase in almotriptan area under the concentration-time curve and peak concentrations of 57% and 60%, respectively. The mean oral and renal clearance of almotriptan were significantly reduced by ketoconazole coadministration. Increased risk of almotriptan side effects (eg, ischemia, arrhythmia, hypertension) may occur in patients taking almotriptan and ketoconazole.

RELATED DRUGS: Itraconazole (*Sporanox*), voriconazole (*Vfend*), and fluconazole (*Diflucan*) are known to inhibit CYP3A4 and could increase almotriptan plasma concentrations.

MANAGEMENT OPTIONS:

➡ *Consider Alternative.* Terbinafine (*Lamisil*) does not inhibit CYP3A4 but it does inhibit CYP2D6. It is unknown how much CYP2D6 contributes to the metabolism of almotriptan. Although data are lacking, other selective serotonin 1B/1D receptor antagonists (naratriptan [*Amerge*], sumatriptan [*Imitrex*], rizatriptan [*Maxalt*], zolmitriptan [*Zomig*]) that do not rely on CYP3A4 for their metabolism may not be affected in a similar manner by ketoconazole.

➡ *Monitor.* Carefully monitor patients taking chronic antifungal therapy if almotriptan is administered. Almotriptan doses should probably start with 6.25 mg and repeated only with caution.

REFERENCES:

1. Fleishaker JC, et al. Effect of ketoconazole on the clearance of the antimigraine compound, almotriptan, in humans. *Clin Pharmacol Ther.* 2001;69:P25.

Almotriptan (*Axert*)

Verapamil (eg, *Calan*)

SUMMARY: Verapamil produced a modest increase in almotriptan concentrations; limited patient adverse effects.

RISK FACTORS:

➡ *Pharmacogenetics.* Because almotriptan is metabolized by CYP3A4, CYP2D6 and monoamine oxidase, the effect of a CYP3A4 inhibitor like verapamil may be greater in patients who are deficient in CYP2D6 and do not have this metabolic pathway for almotriptan elimination.

MECHANISM: Verapamil appears to increase the bioavailability of almotriptan, perhaps by inhibiting the CYP3A4 metabolism of almotriptan.

CLINICAL EVALUATION: Twelve healthy subjects received a single oral 12.5 mg dose of almotriptan alone and on the seventh day of sustained release verapamil 120 mg twice daily.[1] With verapamil pretreatment, the mean area under the concentration-time curve of almotriptan was increased 20% compared with almotriptan administered alone. No change in almotriptan half-life was observed. The modest degree of change in almotriptan concentrations will be unlikely to affect drug response in most patients.

RELATED DRUGS: Diltiazem (*Cardizem*) is likely to increase almotriptan concentrations to a similar degree.

MANAGEMENT OPTIONS:

➡ *Consider Alternative.* Dihydropyridine calcium channel blockers would be unlikely to cause a significant increase in almotriptan plasma concentrations. Although data are lacking, other selective serotonin 1B/1D receptor antagonists (naratriptan [*Amerge*], sumatriptan [*Imitrex*], rizatriptan [*Maxalt*], zolmitriptan [*Zomig*]) that do not rely on CYP3A4 for their metabolism may not be affected in a similar manner by verapamil.

➡ *Monitor.* Monitor patients taking verapamil who are administered almotriptan for increased almotriptan effects.

REFERENCES:
1. Fleishaker JC, et al. Pharmacokinetic interaction between verapamil and almotriptan in healthy volunteers. *Clin Pharmacol Ther.* 2000;67:498-503.

 Alprazolam (*Xanax*)

Contraceptives, Oral

SUMMARY: Oral contraceptives may increase serum concentrations of alprazolam, chlordiazepoxide, diazepam, triazolam, and possibly other benzodiazepines that undergo oxidative metabolism. The serum concentrations of benzodiazepines that undergo glucoronide conjugation (eg, lorazepam, oxazepam, temazepam) may be reduced by oral contraceptives.

RISK FACTORS: No specific risk factors are known.

MECHANISM: Oral contraceptives appear to inhibit the oxidative metabolism and enhance the glucoronide conjugation of benzodiazepines.[1-3]

CLINICAL EVALUATION: The disposition of diazepam (*Valium*) 10 mg IV in 8 women receiving oral contraceptives (50 mcg estrogen) was compared with that in 8 women who were not receiving oral contraceptives. The women receiving oral contraceptives had a longer mean diazepam half-life (69 vs 47 hours) and a lower total metabolic clearance (0.27 vs 0.45 mL/min/kg). The metabolism of triazolam (*Halcion*) may also be inhibited by low-dose oral contraceptives.[4] The mean half-life of chloridazepoxide (*Librium*) was 24.3 hours in 7 women receiving oral contraceptives (50 to 100 mcg estrogen) and 14.8 hours in 11 women who were not receiving oral contraceptives. Although the difference was not statistically significant, it seems likely that oral contraceptives inhibit chlordiazepoxide metabolism. Women taking low-dose oral contraceptives had small increases in alprazolam plasma concentrations in 1 study,[4] but another study found little effect.[5] Nevertheless, the adverse psychomotor effects of a single dose of alprazolam were found to be greater in women on oral contraceptives than in control subjects.[6]

The metabolism of other benzodiazepines may be increased in the presence of oral contraceptives. The half-life of lorazepam (*Ativan*) 2 mg IV was shorter (4.8 vs 13.4 hours) and lorazepam clearance was higher (302 vs 78 mL/min) in 8 women receiving oral contraceptives than in 9 similar women who were not on oral contraceptives. Likewise, comparison of the disposition of oral oxazepam (*Serax*) 45 mg in 8 women receiving oral contraceptives and in 9 comparable women who were not receiving oral contraceptives showed that the oxazepam half-life was shorter (6.8 vs 12.4 hours) and its clearance was higher (191 vs 81 mL/min) in those taking oral contraceptives. In another report, low-dose oral contraceptives also enhanced elimination of temazepam (*Restoril*), which like lorazepam and oxazepam, undergoes glucoronide conjugation.[4]

RELATED DRUGS: Although the interaction between oral contraceptives and other benzodiazepines is not established, oral contraceptives theoretically would be expected to increase the effect of benzodiazepines that undergo oxidative metabolism in the liver, including chlordiazepoxide, diazepam, triazolam, halazepam (*Paxipam*), prazepam (*Centrax*), clorazepate (*Tranxene*), and flurazepam (*Dalmane*). (Also see Clinical Evaluation.)

MANAGEMENT OPTIONS: No specific action is required, but be alert for evidence of the interaction.

REFERENCES:

1. Roberts RK, et al. Disposition of chlordiazepoxide: sex differences and effects of oral contraceptives. *Clin Pharmacol Ther.* 1979;25:826.

2. Abernethy DR, et al. Impairment of diazepam metabolism by low-dose estrogen-containing oral contraceptive steroids. *N Engl J Med.* 1982;306:791.

3. Patwardhan R, et al. Induction of glucoronidation by oral contraceptive steroids (OCs). *Clin Res.* 1981;29:861A.

4. Stoehr GP, et al. Effect of oral contraceptives on triazolam, temazepam, alprazolam, and lorazepam kinetics. *Clin Pharmacol Ther.* 1984;36:683.

5. Scavone JM, et al. Alprazolam pharmacokinetics in women on low-dose oral contraceptives. *J Clin Pharmacol.* 1988;28:454.

6. Kroboth PD, et al. Pharmacodynamic evaluation of the benzodazepine-oral contraceptive interaction. *Clin Pharmacol Ther.* 1985;38:525.

Alprazolam (eg, *Xanax*)

Digoxin (eg, *Lanoxin*)

SUMMARY: A case report indicates that alprazolam may increase digoxin serum concentrations, but this has not been a consistent finding.

RISK FACTORS:

➡ **Dosage Regimen.** Alprazolam doses greater than 0.5 mg/day may increase digoxin serum concentrations.

MECHANISM: Not established.

CLINICAL EVALUATION: The serum concentration of digoxin increased from 1.6 ng/mL to 4.3 ng/mL in a single patient after the addition of alprazolam 1 mg at bedtime[2] and was accompanied by symptoms of digoxin toxicity. Digoxin concentrations returned to normal after discontinuation of alprazolam. Alprazolam 1 mg produced significant increases in digoxin concentrations in 3 elderly patients while 0.5 mg had less effect.[3] In a study of 8 healthy subjects, a single dose of IV digoxin alone and 1 day after a 5-day course of alprazolam demonstrated no evidence of an interaction between the drugs.[1] Final evaluation of this interaction will require studies that evaluate chronic digoxin and alprazolam administration.

RELATED DRUGS: No information is available.

MANAGEMENT OPTIONS:

➡ **Monitor.** Pending further information, monitor patients stabilized on digoxin for increased digoxin concentrations and effect when alprazolam is added to their therapy.

REFERENCES:

1. Ochs HR, et al. Effect of alprazolam on digoxin kinetics and creatinine clearance. *Clin Pharmacol Ther.* 1985;38:595.

2. Tollefson G, et al. Alprazolam-related digoxin toxicity. *Am J Psych.* 1984;141:1612.

3. Guven H, et al. Age-related digoxin-alprazolam interaction. *Clin Pharmacol Ther.* 1993;54:42.

Alprazolam (*Xanax*)

Erythromycin (eg, *E-Mycin*)

SUMMARY: Erythromycin increases the plasma concentration and half-life of alprazolam. An increase in alprazolam effects may occur in some patients.

RISK FACTORS: No specific risk factors are known.

MECHANISM: Erythromycin probably inhibits the hepatic metabolism of alprazolam by inactivating CYP3A4, the enzyme likely to be responsible for alprazolam metabolism.

CLINICAL EVALUATION: Twelve healthy subjects were administered placebo or erythromycin 400 mg 3 times daily for 10 days.[1] On day 8, a single oral 0.8 mg dose of alprazolam was administered with the placebo or erythromycin. Compared with placebo, erythromycin increased the mean area under the concentration-time curve of alprazolam 147% and extended its half-life from 16 hours to 40 hours. Because alprazolam undergoes little first-pass metabolism (approximately 8%), the mean peak alprazolam concentrations were not significantly increased by erythromycin. Psychomotor function tests were not changed by the coadministration of alprazolam and erythromycin. This finding does not exclude the possibility that patients maintained on chronic alprazolam might experience increased effects during erythromycin treatment.

RELATED DRUGS: Erythromycin is known to increase the plasma concentrations of other benzodiazepines including triazolam (*Halcion*) and midazolam (*Versed*). Clarithromycin (*Biaxin*) or troleandomycin (*TAO*) may produce similar reductions in the clearance of alprazolam.

MANAGEMENT OPTIONS:

➡ *Consider Alternative.* Selection of a noninhibiting macrolide (eg, azithromycin [*Zithromax*] or dirithromycin [*Dynabac*]) is likely to limit changes in alprazolam pharmacokinetics. Anxiolytics not metabolized by CYP3A4 such as lorazepam (*Ativan*) or temazepam (*Restoril*) could be substituted for alprazolam.

➡ *Monitor.* Monitor patients taking alprazolam chronically for increased sedation during erythromycin administration.

REFERENCES:

1. Yasui N, et al. A kinetic and dynamic study of oral alprazolam with and without erythromycin in humans: in vivo evidence for the involvement of CYP3A4 in alprazolam metabolism. *Clin Pharmacol Ther*. 1996;59:514.

Alprazolam (eg, *Xanax*)

Fluoxetine (eg, *Prozac*)

SUMMARY: In healthy subjects, fluoxetine appears to increase alprazolam plasma concentrations, resulting in an increase in alprazolam-induced psychomotor impairment.

RISK FACTORS: No specific risk factors are known.

MECHANISM: Not established. Fluoxetine may inhibit the hepatic metabolism of alprazolam.

CLINICAL EVALUATION: Twelve healthy subjects received a single oral dose of alprazolam 1 mg with and without fluoxetine 40 mg/day for 3 to 7 days.[1] Fluoxetine was associated with a 21% reduction in alprazolam clearance and a 26% increase in the area under the alprazolam plasma concentration-time curve. In another double-blind, parallel study of 80 healthy subjects, alprazolam 1 mg 4 times/day and fluoxetine 60 mg/day were given alone and together for 4 days.[2] Fluoxetine was associated with a 33% increase in the average alprazolam plasma concentrations and a corresponding increase in alprazolam-induced psychomotor impairment. However, alprazolam did not affect the plasma concentrations of fluoxetine.

RELATED DRUGS: The effect of selective serotonin reuptake inhibitors other than fluoxetine on alprazolam is not established, but fluvoxamine is known to inhibit CYP3A4, an isozyme important in the metabolism of alprazolam.

MANAGEMENT OPTIONS:

➥ *Circumvent/Minimize.* Use conservative doses of alprazolam in the presence of fluoxetine until patient response is assessed. Advise patients receiving combined therapy to watch for excessive sedation.

➥ *Monitor.* Monitor for altered alprazolam effect if fluoxetine is initiated, discontinued, or changed in dosage. Adjust alprazolam dose as needed.

REFERENCES:

1. Greenblatt DJ, et al. Fluoxetine impairs clearance of alprazolam but not of clonazepam. *Clin Pharmacol Ther.* 1992;52:479-485.
2. Lasher TA, et al. Pharmacokinetic pharmacodynamic evaluation of the combined administration of alprazolam and fluoxetine. *Psychopharmacology.* 1991;104:323-327.

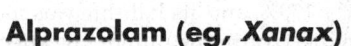

Alprazolam (eg, *Xanax*)

Fluvoxamine

SUMMARY: Fluvoxamine increases alprazolam plasma concentrations and may increase alprazolam sedation.

RISK FACTORS:

➥ *Pharmacogenetics.* The increases in alprazolam concentrations were greater in patients with higher CYP2C19 activity (0 or 1 mutated allele) than in patients with low CYP2C19 activity (2 mutated alleles).[1]

MECHANISM: Fluvoxamine appears to inhibit the cytochrome P450 metabolism of alprazolam, but the relative contribution of the individual isozymes is not yet established.

CLINICAL EVALUATION: Twenty-three patients received alprazolam with and without concurrent fluvoxamine therapy.[1] Plasma concentrations of alprazolam were 58% higher when the patients were receiving concurrent fluvoxamine compared with alprazolam alone. The magnitude of this effect is expected to increase the CNS depressant effect of alprazolam. In patients with no mutated or 1 mutated allele for CYP2C19, some developed more than a 100% increase in plasma alprazolam concentrations. However, none of the patients with 2 mutated alleles for CYP2C19 developed more than a 50% increase.

RELATED DRUGS: Fluoxetine (eg, *Prozac*) also can increase alprazolam plasma concentrations, but other selective serotonin reuptake inhibitors (SSRIs) would theoretically be less likely to interact.

MANAGEMENT OPTIONS:

➡ *Consider Alternative.* Theoretically, fluvoxamine is less likely to interact with benzodiazepines that are largely glucuronidated, such as temazepam (eg, *Restoril*), oxazepam (eg, *Serax*), estazolam (eg, *ProSom*), and lorazepam (eg, *Ativan*). SSRIs that are theoretically unlikely to interact with alprazolam include citalopram (eg, *Celexa*), escitalopram (*Lexapro*), paroxetine (eg, *Paxil*), and sertraline (*Zoloft*).

➡ *Monitor.* Be alert for evidence of excessive sedation in patients who receive alprazolam and fluvoxamine (or fluoxetine) concurrently.

REFERENCES:
1. Suzuki Y, et al. Effects of concomitant fluvoxamine on the metabolism of alprazolam in Japanese psychiatric patients: interaction with CYP2C19 mutated alleles. *Eur J Clin Pharmacol.* 2003;58:829-833.

Alprazolam (eg, *Xanax*)

Itraconazole (*Sporanox*)

SUMMARY: Itraconazole administration increases alprazolam plasma concentrations and pharmacologic effects.

RISK FACTORS: No specific risk factors are known.

MECHANISM: Itraconazole inhibits the metabolism (CYP3A4) of alprazolam, resulting in elevated plasma concentrations.

CLINICAL EVALUATION: Ten healthy men received a single oral dose of alprazolam 0.8 mg on day 4 of a total of 6 days of itraconazole 200 mg daily or placebo.[1] The mean area under the plasma concentration-time curve of alprazolam was increased nearly 170%, and its half-life was increased from 15.7 to 40.3 hours following itraconazole coadministration. The effect of alprazolam on psychomotor function was increased following pretreatment with itraconazole compared with placebo. Increased side effects (eg, sedation, ataxia) should be expected if alprazolam is administered with itraconazole.

RELATED DRUGS: Itraconazole is known to affect other anxiolytics (eg, midazolam [eg, *Versed*], triazolam [eg, *Halcion*]), in a similar manner. Ketoconazole (eg, *Nizoral*), fluconazole (eg, *Diflucan*), and voriconazole (*Vfend*) is expected to reduce the metabolism of alprazolam.

MANAGEMENT OPTIONS:

➡ *Consider Alternative.* Select a benzodiazepine that is not metabolized by CYP3A4, such as oxazepam (eg, *Serax*) or lorazepam (eg, *Ativan*). Terbinafine (*Lamisil*) does not inhibit CYP3A4 and is not expected to interact with alprazolam.

➡ *Monitor.* Monitor patients taking itraconazole and alprazolam for signs of increased benzodiazepine effect, including sedation and reduced psychomotor performance.

REFERENCES:
1. Yasui N, et al. Effect of itraconazole on the single oral dose pharmacokinetics and pharmacodynamics of alprazolam. *Psychopharmacology.* 1998;139:269-273.

Alprazolam (*Xanax*) [4]

Kava

SUMMARY: A patient became semi-comatose after taking alprazolam and kava, but a causal relationship was not established.

RISK FACTORS: No specific risk factors are known.

MECHANISM: Not established. The reaction may have been due to additive CNS depression, but an effect of kava on cytochrome P450 isozymes cannot be ruled out (in vitro studies suggest an inhibitory effect of kava on CYP3A4).

CLINICAL EVALUATION: A 54-year-old man became lethargic and disoriented after ingesting kava in the presence of alprazolam therapy.[1] A causal relationship was not established, but the reaction is consistent with the known pharmacodynamic properties of the drugs. Because herbal medications are generally not standardized, different herbal brands may interact differently because of varying amounts of active ingredient or additional ingredients not on the label (and in some cases no active ingredients at all). Moreover, different lots of the same brand may vary substantially.

RELATED DRUGS: Theoretically, additive sedative effects would be expected when any benzodiazepine is given with kava. Nevertheless, little interaction was detected in healthy subjects given bromazepam with and without concurrent kava.[2]

MANAGEMENT OPTIONS: No specific action is required, but be alert for evidence of the interaction.

REFERENCES:

1. Almeida J, Grimsley EW. Coma from the health food store: interaction between kava and alprazolam. *Ann Intern Med*. 1996;125:940-941.
2. Herberg KW. Safety-related performance after intake of kava-extract, bromazepam and their combination. *Z Allegemeinmedizin*. 1996;72:973-977.

Alprazolam (eg, *Xanax*) [4]

Lithium (eg, *Eskalith*)

SUMMARY: Alprazolam only slightly increased serum lithium concentrations in healthy subjects. Evidence suggests that the interaction is unlikely to be clinically important.

RISK FACTORS: No specific risk factors are known.

MECHANISM: Alprazolam appears to inhibit GI absorption and renal clearance of lithium. The reduced renal clearance may be caused by alprazolam-induced reductions in urine flow rates.

CLINICAL EVALUATION: Ten healthy subjects were given lithium 900 to 1,500 mg/day for 15 days; alprazolam 1 mg twice daily was added for the last 4 days.[1] Coadministration with alprazolam was associated with a 28% reduction in renal lithium clearance; however, lithium steady-state serum concentrations increased only slightly. The minor effect of alprazolam on serum lithium concentrations may be because of its additional ability to inhibit the GI absorption of lithium (as suggested by a reduction in the percentage of lithium dose recovered from 24-hour urine collections). Because this study had a longitudinal rather than a crossover design, the possibility that the minimal changes observed in steady-state serum concentrations were caused by changes in lithium disposition over time cannot be ruled out. Administration of alprazolam for more than 4 days might have a greater effect on lithium disposition. Nevertheless, the results of this study suggest that alprazolam is unlikely to have a clinically important effect on lithium pharmacokinetics.

RELATED DRUGS: The effect of other benzodiazepines on lithium is not established.

MANAGEMENT OPTIONS: No specific action is required, but be alert for evidence of the interaction.

REFERENCES:
1. Evans RL, et al. Evaluation of the interaction of lithium and alprazolam. *J Clin Psychopharmacol.* 1990;10:355-359.

 Alprazolam (eg, *Xanax*)

St. John's Wort

SUMMARY: St. John's wort may decrease alprazolam response, but the clinical importance of this effect is not established.

RISK FACTORS: No specific risk factors are known.

MECHANISM: St. John's wort appears to increase the metabolism of alprazolam by CYP3A4.

CLINICAL EVALUATION: Healthy subjects were given a single oral dose of alprazolam 2 mg with and without pretreatment with St. John's wort for 14 days.[1] St. John's wort was associated with a 2-fold decrease in alprazolam half-life and area under the concentration-time curve. The magnitude of this effect is expected to somewhat reduce the effect of alprazolam.

RELATED DRUGS: Midazolam (eg, *Versed*) and triazolam (eg, *Halcion*) also are metabolized by CYP3A4 and are expected to interact with St. John's wort.

MANAGEMENT OPTIONS: No specific action is required, but be alert for evidence of the interaction.

REFERENCES:
1. Markowitz JS, et al. Effect of St John's wort on drug metabolism by induction of cytochrome P450 3A4 enzyme. *JAMA.* 2003;290:1500-1504.

 Alprenolol

Pentobarbital (eg, *Nembutal*)

SUMMARY: Barbiturates may reduce the plasma concentrations of some beta-blockers.

RISK FACTORS: No specific risk factors are known.

MECHANISM: Barbiturates stimulate the metabolism of beta-blockers.

CLINICAL EVALUATION: In 6 healthy subjects, pretreatment with pentobarbital 0.1 g/day for 10 days significantly reduced plasma concentrations of alprenolol and its active metabolite (4-hydroxyalprenolol) approximately 40%.[1-3] Reduced alprenolol concentrations resulted in increased pulse rates and blood pressure in patients with hypertension.[2]

RELATED DRUGS: Pentobarbital also reduced the area under the concentration-time curve for metoprolol (eg, *Lopressor*) 32%.[4] In 68 patients receiving propranolol (eg, *Inderal*) or sotalol (eg, *Betapace*), the 3 patients on enzyme inducers (phenobarbital or phenytoin) had a higher plasma clearance of propanolol than did the other patients.[5] Sotalol, which undergoes minimal metabolism, was not influenced by the inducers. Atenolol (eg, *Tenormin*) and nadolol (eg, *Corgard*), which are excreted primarily unchanged by the kidneys, are unlikely to interact with barbiturates. Phenobarbital (eg, *Solfoton*) and other barbiturates probably will increase the metabolism of beta-blockers that are extensively metabolized.

MANAGEMENT OPTIONS:

➡ *Consider Alternative.* Beta-blockers excreted primarily unchanged by the kidneys (eg, atenolol, nadolol) are unlikely to interact with barbiturates and could be used to avoid the interaction.

➡ *Monitor.* Watch for evidence of altered response to beta-blockers metabolized by the liver (eg, propranolol, metoprolol, alprenolol) when barbiturate therapy is initiated or discontinued.

REFERENCES:

1. Alvan G, et al. Effect of pentobarbital on the disposition of alprenolol. *Clin Pharmacol Ther*. 1977;22:316-321.
2. Seideman P, et al. Decreased plasma concentrations and clinical effects of alprenolol during combined treatment with pentobarbitone in hypertension. *Br J Clin Pharmacol*. 1987;23:267-271.
3. Collste P, et al. Influence of pentobarbital on effect and plasma levels of alprenolol and 4-hydroxy-alprenolol. *Clin Pharmacol Ther*. 1979;25:423-427.
4. Haglund K, et al. Influence of pentobarbital on metoprolol plasma levels. *Clin Pharmacol Ther*. 1979;26:326-329.
5. Sotaniemi EA, et al. Plasma clearance of propranolol and sotalol and hepatic drug-metabolizing enyzme activity. *Clin Pharmacol Ther*. 1979;26:153-161.

Altretamine (*Hexalen*)

Imipramine (eg, *Tofranil*)

SUMMARY: Altretamine appears to increase the incidence of orthostatic hypotension caused by tricyclic antidepressants or MAO inhibitors.

RISK FACTORS: No specific risk factors are known.

MECHANISM: Not established.

CLINICAL EVALUATION: Four instances of symptomatic orthostatic hypotension were reported in patients older than 60 years of age receiving altretamine and antidepressants.[1] Two patients received antidepressants (phenelzine [*Nardil*] or imipramine) prior to and during treatment with altretamine. Two other patients began treatment with antidepressants (amitriptyline [eg, *Elavil*] or imipramine) while receiving altretamine. All developed dizziness and lightheadedness; 1 patient experienced a syncopal episode. The patients had significant postural hypotension that resolved upon discontinuation of antidepressants. One patient continued to manifest depressive symptoms and began treatment with nortriptyline while on altretamine; orthostatic hypotension symptoms did not return. Because this is the only published report of this interaction, it is not known whether it is only significant in elderly patients.

RELATED DRUGS: Theoretically, other tricyclic antidepressants or MAO inhibitors might interact with altretamine.

MANAGEMENT OPTIONS:

➡ *Consider Alternative.* Antidepressants which are normally associated with a low incidence of orthostatic hypotension, such as nortriptyline or selective serotonin reuptake inhibitors, could be considered.

➡ *Circumvent/Minimize.* Warn patients requiring an antidepressant and receiving altretamine about orthostatic hypotension.

➡ *Monitor.* Monitor for orthostatic hypotension in patients receiving altretamine with either tricyclic antidepressants or MAO inhibitors.

REFERENCES:

1. Bruckner HW, et al. Orthostatic hypotension as a complication of hexamethylmelamine antidepressant interaction. *Cancer Treat Rep.* 1983;67:516.

Aluminum

Cyclosporine (eg, *Sandimmune*)

SUMMARY: Clinical observations in pediatric patients suggest that aluminum hydroxide reduces cyclosporine blood concentrations, but additional study is needed.

RISK FACTORS: No specific risk factors are known.

MECHANISM: Not established. Aluminum hydroxide might bind with cyclosporine in the GI tract.

CLINICAL EVALUATION: Concurrent use of aluminum hydroxide gel appeared to reduce cyclosporine blood concentrations in an 8-month-old boy. When cyclosporine blood concentrations were assessed in 7 other children on cyclosporine with or without concurrent aluminum hydroxide, the antacid substantially increased cyclosporine dosage requirements.[1] Although controlled studies are needed to confirm these findings, the evidence suggests that aluminum hydroxide may reduce cyclosporine response.

RELATED DRUGS: The effect of other antacids on cyclosporine is not established, but assume that they may interact until it is proven otherwise.

MANAGEMENT OPTIONS:

➡ *Circumvent/Minimize.* Until more information is available, it would be prudent to give cyclosporine at least 2 hours before or 6 hours after aluminum hydroxide or other antacids.

➡ *Monitor.* Monitor for reduced cyclosporine blood concentrations if aluminum hydroxide or other antacids are given concurrently.

REFERENCES:

1. Ichisawa M, et al. The effect of dried aluminum hydroxide gel on the blood concentration of cyclosporine-A. *Jpn J Hosp Pharm.* 1997;23:407.

Amantadine (eg, *Symmetrel*)

Bupropion (eg, *Wellbutrin*)

SUMMARY: Bupropion may increase the risk of amantadine neurotoxicity, but more study is needed to establish a causal relationship.

RISK FACTORS: No specific risk factors are known.

MECHANISM: Not established. It is proposed that amantadine and bupropion have additive central dopaminergic effects.

CLINICAL EVALUATION: In a group of 8 elderly nursing home residents on bupropion, 6 were given amantadine for influenza prophylaxis.[1] Three of the 6 residents developed neurotoxicity, including restlessness, agitation, tremors, ataxia, dizziness, vertigo, and confusion. Two patients required hospitalization, but all reactions resolved within 72 hours of discontinuing both drugs. While it is plausible that the reactions resulted from a combined effect of the 2 drugs, it is not possible to exclude amantadine alone as a cause of the reactions.

RELATED DRUGS: No information is available.

MANAGEMENT OPTIONS:

➡ **Circumvent/Minimize.** If amantadine use is short-term for influenza, consider stopping the bupropion temporarily during the amantadine therapy.

➡ **Monitor.** If the combination is used, monitor for evidence of neurotoxicity. If neurotoxicity occurs, temporary discontinuation of both drugs may be required.

REFERENCES:

1. Trappler B, et al. Bupropion-amantadine-associated neurotoxicity. *J Clin Psychiatry*. 2000;61:61-62.

Amantadine (eg, *Symmetrel*) **5**

Cigarette Smoking

SUMMARY: Cigarette smoking has no effect on amantadine elimination.

RISK FACTORS: No specific risk factors are known.

MECHANISM: No interaction.

CLINICAL EVALUATION: Ten nonsmoking and 10 smoking (more than 20 cigarettes/day) subjects received amantadine 3 mg/kg as a single oral dose.[1] Amantadine clearance and half-life were similar in smokers and nonsmokers. The apparent volume of distribution of amantadine was larger in smokers; however, this difference is without apparent clinical significance.

RELATED DRUGS: The effect of cigarette smoking on other antivirals is unknown.

MANAGEMENT OPTIONS: No interaction.

REFERENCES:

1. Wong LT, et al. Chronic tobacco smoking and gender as variables affecting amantadine disposition in healthy subjects. *Br J Clin Pharmacol*. 1995;39:81-84.

Amantadine (eg, *Symmetrel*)

Quinidine (eg, *Quinora*)

SUMMARY: Quinidine causes a modest increase in amantadine serum concentrations; the clinical significance of this interaction appears to be limited.

RISK FACTORS: No specific risk factors are known.

MECHANISM: Amantadine is a drug that undergoes active renal tubular secretion and possibly could compete with quinidine for renal excretion. In such a situation, each drug would inhibit the clearance of the other. Quinidine does appear to inhibit the renal secretion of amantadine, causing an accumulation of amantadine in the serum.

CLINICAL EVALUATION: Eighteen healthy subjects, including 9 subjects between 27 and 39 years of age, and 9 subjects older than 60 years of age ingested amantadine syrup 3 mg/kg at 8 pm.[1] The following morning they received in random order either placebo, quinidine 200 mg, or quinine 200 mg. Amantadine renal clearance was measured for 4 hours beginning 2 hours after the quinidine dose. Quinidine reduced the renal clearance of amantadine only in men. The cause of this gender-specific response is unclear. Age was not associated with quinidine-induced reduction in amantadine renal clearance. The effect of amantadine on the renal clearance of quinidine was not measured, but the authors noted that the quinidine clearance in their subjects was approximately 50% less than that reported in other healthy subjects. The clinical significance of this interaction awaits further study, although the mean reduction in amantadine renal clearance appears to be approximately 25%. Studies with chronic doses of quinidine and in patients with reduced renal function would be useful to assess the potential of this interaction to cause adverse effects.

RELATED DRUGS: Quinine produces a similar reduction in amantadine renal clearance. Because rimantadine (*Flumadine*) is primarily metabolized in the liver, it would be less likely to be affected by quinidine.

MANAGEMENT OPTIONS: No specific action is required, but be alert for evidence of the interaction.

REFERENCES:
1. Gaudry SE, et al. Gender and age as factors in the inhibition of renal clearance of amantadine by quinine and quinidine. *Clin Pharmacol Ther.* 1993;54:23-27.

4 **Amantadine (eg, *Symmetrel*)**

Quinine

SUMMARY: Quinine causes a modest increase in amantadine serum concentrations; the clinical significance of this interaction appears to be limited.

RISK FACTORS: No specific risk factors are known.

MECHANISM: Quinine appears to inhibit the renal secretion of amantadine, causing an accumulation of amantadine in the serum; amantadine also may inhibit the clearance of quinine.

CLINICAL EVALUATION: Eighteen healthy subjects, including 9 subjects between 27 and 39 years of age and 9 subjects older than 60 years of age, ingested amantadine syrup 3 mg/kg at 8 pm.[1] The following morning, they received in random order either placebo or quinine 200 mg. Amantadine renal clearance was measured for 4 hours beginning 2 hours after the quinine dose. Quinine reduced the renal clearance of amantadine approximately 30%. Age was not associated with quinine-induced reduction in amantadine renal clearance. The effect of amantadine on the renal clearance of quinine was not measured, but the authors noted that the quinine clearance in their subjects was approximately 50% less than that reported in other normal subjects. The clinical significance of this interaction awaits further study.

RELATED DRUGS: Quinidine produces a similar reduction in amantadine renal clearance. Since rimantadine (*Flumadine*) is primarily metabolized in the liver, quinine would not be expected to influence its serum concentration.

MANAGEMENT OPTIONS: No specific action is required, but be alert for evidence of the interaction.

REFERENCES:
1. Gaudry SE, et al. Gender and age as factors in the inhibition of renal clearance of amantadine by quinine and quinidine. *Clin Pharmacol Ther.* 1993;54:23-27.

Amantadine (eg, *Symmetrel*)

Triamterene (*Dyrenium*)

SUMMARY: Triamterene/hydrochlorothiazide (eg, *Dyazide*) has been reported to increase serum concentrations and toxicity of amantadine.

RISK FACTORS: No specific risk factors are known.

MECHANISM: Not established. There is some evidence that the combination formulation of triamterene/hydrochlorothiazide can reduce the renal excretion of amantadine. Because this interaction has not been reported with thiazides, the triamterene appears to be responsible.

CLINICAL EVALUATION: A 61-year-old man developed evidence of amantadine toxicity (eg, ataxia, agitation, hallucinations) 1 week after starting triamterene/hydrochlorothiazide therapy.[1] The symptoms resolved after discontinuing both drugs. When amantadine was restarted, no symptoms occurred until the triamterene/hydrochlorothiazide also was restarted. The coadministration of this fixed-combination diuretic was associated with a reduction in the renal excretion of amantadine and an increase in serum amantadine concentration from 156 ng/mL to 243 ng/mL. Although the triamterene/hydrochlorothiazide combination product probably was responsible for the amantadine toxicity in this patient, it is unclear how often this interaction would occur in other patients receiving this combination. The available data do not indicate whether the triamterene or the hydrochlorothiazide component was responsible for the interaction.

RELATED DRUGS: It is possible that rimantadine (eg, *Flumadine*) is similarly affected by triamterene.

MANAGEMENT OPTIONS:

➡ *Circumvent/Minimize.* Amantadine dosage may need to be reduced when triamterene is coadministered.

➡ *Monitor.* In patients receiving amantadine, use triamterene or thiazides with caution and watch for signs of amantadine toxicity including nausea, dizziness, and dry mouth.

REFERENCES:

1. Wilson TW, et al. Amantadine-dyazide interaction. *Can Med Assoc J.* 1983;129(9):974-975.

Amantadine (eg, *Symmetrel*)

Trihexyphenidyl (eg, *Trihexy*)

SUMMARY: Trihexyphenidyl and other anticholinergic drugs may potentiate CNS adverse reactions of amantadine.

RISK FACTORS: No specific risk factors are known.

MECHANISM: Not established. An additive anticholinergic effect of amantadine and trihexyphenidyl or benztropine is possible.

CLINICAL EVALUATION: Amantadine can potentiate the anticholinergic effects of trihexyphenidyl.[1-3] Confusion and hallucinations, which are characteristic of excessive anticholinergic activity, have been reported in patients taking maximally tolerated doses of trihexyphenidyl and benztropine who also received amantadine.

RELATED DRUGS: It is possible that rimantadine (eg, *Flumadine*) would be similarly affected by trihexyphenidyl. Amantadine also can potentiate the anticholinergic effects of other anticholinergic drugs such as benztropine (eg, *Cogentin*).[1-3]

MANAGEMENT OPTIONS:

➡ *Circumvent/Minimize.* Although more information is needed, consider reducing high-dose anticholinergic therapy before administering amantadine.

➡ *Monitor.* Be alert for confusion and hallucinations when amantadine is combined with other anticholinergics.

REFERENCES:

1. Schwab RS, et al. Amantadine in the treatment of Parkinson's disease. *JAMA.* 1969;208(7):1168-1170.
2. Parkes JD, et al. Treatment of Parkinson's disease with amantadine and levodopa. A one-year study. *Lancet.* 1971;1(7709):1083-1086.
3. Postma JU, et al. Visual hallucinations and delirium during treatment with amantadine (*Symmetrel*). *J Am Geriatr Soc.* 1975;23(5):212-215.

Amantadine (eg, *Symmetrel*)

Trimethoprim/Sulfamethoxazole (eg, *Bactrim*)

SUMMARY: A patient taking amantadine developed mental confusion several days after the addition of trimethoprim/sulfamethoxazole therapy.

RISK FACTORS: No specific risk factors are known.

MECHANISM: Both amantadine and trimethoprim are secreted by the renal tubules; each can inhibit the renal clearance of the other, resulting in accumulation of toxic plasma concentrations.

CLINICAL EVALUATION: Parkinson disease was stabilized in an elderly man who was treated with amantadine 100 mg twice daily.[1] Treatment with 1 tablet of trimethoprim/sulfamethoxazole twice daily was begun for bronchitis. After 72 hours of coadministration, the patient was combative and complained of mental confusion. His mental status returned to normal within 24 hours after the amantadine and antibiotics were discontinued.

RELATED DRUGS: No information is available.

MANAGEMENT OPTIONS: No specific action is required, but be alert for evidence of the interaction.

REFERENCES:

1. Speeg KV, et al. Toxic delirium in a patient taking amantadine and trimethoprim-sulfamethoxazole. *Am J Med Sci.* 1989;298(6):410-412.

Ambrisentan (*Letairis*)
Ketoconazole (eg, *Nizoral*)

SUMMARY: Ketoconazole administration produces a modest increase in ambrisentan plasma concentrations; little change in clinical response is likely to be observed.

RISK FACTORS: No specific risk factors are known.

MECHANISM: Ambrisentan is partially metabolized by CYP3A4. This enzyme is known to be inhibited by ketoconazole.

CLINICAL EVALUATION: Sixteen healthy men received ambrisentan 10 mg alone and on day 4 of a 7-day regimen of ketoconazole 400 mg daily.[1] The geometric mean of the peak concentration and area under the concentration-time curve of ambrisentan increased by 20% and 35%, respectively, during the administration of ketoconazole. The half-life of ambrisentan was increased from 12.9 to 15.2 hours following ketoconazole coadministration. Although this was a single dose study, the reported magnitude of reduction in ambrisentan clearance is not expected to result in an increased risk of adverse reactions.

RELATED DRUGS: Fluconazole (eg, *Diflucan*), itraconazole (eg, *Sporanox*), posaconazole (*Noxafil*), and voriconazole (*Vfend*) also inhibit the activity of CYP3A4 and are expected to increase the plasma concentrations of ambrisentan in a similar manner. Bosentan (*Tracleer*) plasma concentrations are also increased by ketoconazole.

MANAGEMENT OPTIONS:

➡ *Monitor.* Monitor patients stabilized on ambrisentan for any change in response if ketoconazole is added to their therapy.

REFERENCES:

1. Richards DB, et al. Effect of ketoconazole on the pharmacokinetic profile of ambrisentan. *J Clin Pharmacol.* 2009;49(6):719-724.

Amiloride (*Midamor*)

Candesartan (*Atacand*)

SUMMARY: Combining amiloride with candesartan or other angiotensin II receptor blockers (ARBs) may increase the risk of hyperkalemia, especially in patients with 1 or more risk factors.

RISK FACTORS:

➡ **Other Drugs.** The addition of other hyperkalemic drugs may increase the risk of hyperkalemia in patients taking amiloride and ARBs. Hyperkalemic drugs include angiotension-converting enzyme (ACE) inhibitors, COX-2 inhibitors, cyclosporine, nonselective beta-adrenergic blockers, nonsteroidal anti-inflammatory drugs, pentamidine, potassium supplements, tacrolimus, and trimethoprim.

➡ **Concurrent Diseases.** Diseases that increase the risk of hyperkalemia for this interaction include diabetes and significant renal impairment.

➡ **Diet/Food.** A diet high in potassium may increase the risk of hyperkalemia from this interaction. Salt substitutes may contain potassium.

MECHANISM: Both amiloride and ARBs tend to increase serum potassium, and their effects are additive.

CLINICAL EVALUATION: Forty-four cases of life-threatening hyperkalemia have been described in patients receiving either ARBs or ACE inhibitors in combination with spironolactone.[1] It is likely that amiloride would also increase the risk of hyperkalemia when combined with ARBs or ACE inhibitors, especially in patients with 1 or more risk factors.

RELATED DRUGS: Amiloride is expected to increase the risk of hyperkalemia when combined with other ARBs, including eprosartan (*Teveten*), irbesartan (*Avapro*), losartan (*Cozaar*), telmisartan (*Micardis*), and valsartan (*Diovan*).

MANAGEMENT OPTIONS:

➡ **Monitor.** In patients receiving amiloride and an ARB, monitor serum potassium and renal function, particularly if the patient has 1 or more risk factors.

REFERENCES:
1. Wrenger E, et al. Interaction of spironolactone with ACE inhibitors or angiotensin receptor blockers: analysis of 44 cases. *BMJ.* 2003;327(7407):147-149.

Amiloride (*Midamor*)

Cimetidine (eg, *Tagamet*)

SUMMARY: Amiloride reduces the serum concentration of cimetidine, while cimetidine causes no change in the plasma concentration of amiloride. The clinical importance of this interaction is not established.

RISK FACTORS: No specific risk factors are known.

MECHANISM: Amiloride reduces the absorption of cimetidine. Although cimetidine reduces the renal clearance of amiloride, it also reduces the absorption of amiloride; therefore, the plasma concentration of amiloride is unaffected.

CLINICAL EVALUATION: Eight healthy subjects received 5 mg amiloride alone for 7 days, 400 mg cimetidine every 12 hours alone for 4 days, and 5 mg amiloride plus

400 mg cimetidine every 12 hours for 12 days.[1] Cimetidine administration appeared to reduce the absorption of amiloride 18% and reduce its renal clearance 17% compared with amiloride administered alone. These 2 effects tend to offset each other so that no change in the amiloride area under the concentration-time curve (AUC) was observed. However, amiloride significantly reduced cimetidine AUC (14%), maximum concentration (28%), and absorption (26%). No significant changes were observed in 24-hour urine volume or in sodium or potassium excretion during the administration of any single drug or combination of drugs. While no clinically significant effects were noted in healthy subjects, the effects of this interaction in patients await further study. Higher doses of amiloride or cimetidine may increase the magnitude of this interaction.

RELATED DRUGS: It is not known whether H_2-receptor antagonists other than cimetidine interact with amiloride.

MANAGEMENT OPTIONS: No specific action is required, but be alert for evidence of the interaction.

REFERENCES:

1. Somogyi AA, et al. Renal tubular secretion of amiloride and its inhibition by cimetidine in humans and in an animal model. *Drug Metab Dispos.* 1989;17:190-196.

Amiloride (*Midamor*)

Digoxin (eg, *Lanoxin*)

SUMMARY: Amiloride has little net effect on digoxin plasma concentrations, but it appears to reduce the inotropic effect of digoxin.

RISK FACTORS: No specific risk factors are known.

MECHANISM: Amiloride appears to increase the renal clearance and reduce the nonrenal clearance of digoxin. Amiloride also may inhibit the inotropic effect of digoxin.

CLINICAL EVALUATION: Six healthy subjects were given a single IV dose of digoxin 15 mcg/kg with and without pretreatment with amiloride 10 mg/day for 8 days.[1] Amiloride administration was associated with an almost 2-fold increase in renal digoxin clearance, while the nonrenal clearance of digoxin was markedly reduced. The net effect of amiloride therapy was to decrease the total body digoxin clearance and increase serum digoxin concentrations slightly. In this same study, an evaluation of myocardial contractility indicated that amiloride suppressed the positive inotropic effect of digoxin. Other investigators have not noted a reduced inotropic effect of digoxin following amiloride administration.[2]

RELATED DRUGS: Digitoxin[†] may be similarly affected by amiloride.

MANAGEMENT OPTIONS: No specific action is required, but be alert for evidence of the interaction.

REFERENCES:

1. Waldorff S, et al. Amiloride-induced changes in digoxin dynamics and kinetics: abolition of digoxin-induced inotropism with amiloride. *Clin Pharmacol Ther.* 1981;30:172-176.

2. Richter JP, et al. The acute effects of amiloride and potassium canrenoate on digoxin-induced positive inotropism in healthy volunteers. *Eur J Clin Pharmacol.* 1993;45:195-196.

† Not available in the United States.

Amiloride (*Midamor*)

Enalapril (eg, *Vasotec*)

SUMMARY: Combining amiloride with enalapril or other ACE inhibitors increases the risk of hyperkalemia, especially in patients with 1 or more risk factors.

RISK FACTORS:

➡ ***Other Drugs.*** In patients on amiloride and ACE inhibitors, the addition of other hyperkalemic drugs can increase the risk. Such drugs include potassium supplements, nonselective beta-adrenergic blockers, cyclosporine, tacrolimus, NSAIDs, COX-2 inhibitors, trimethoprim, and pentamidine.

➡ ***Concurrent Diseases.*** Diseases that increase the risk of hyperkalemia for this interaction include diabetes and significant renal impairment.

➡ ***Diet/Food.*** A diet high in potassium may increase the risk of hyperkalemia from this interaction. Some salt substitutes contain potassium.

MECHANISM: Both amiloride and ACE inhibitors tend to increase serum potassium, and their effects are additive.

CLINICAL EVALUATION: Five diabetic patients on ACE inhibitors developed severe hyperkalemia (2 died) after being started on amiloride-hydrochlorothiazide combination.[1] Most of the cases of hyperkalemia in patients receiving concurrent therapy with potassium-sparing diuretics and ACE inhibitors have involved spironolactone.[2-6] However, it seems likely that amiloride poses the same risk of hyperkalemia when combined with ACE inhibitors in predisposed patients.

RELATED DRUGS: Amiloride would also be expected to interact with other ACE inhibitors, including benazepril (*Lotensin*), captopril (eg, *Capoten*), fosinopril (*Monopril*), lisinopril (eg, *Prinivil*), moexipril (eg, *Univasc*), quinapril (*Accupril*), ramipril (*Altace*), and trandolapril (*Mavik*).

MANAGEMENT OPTIONS:

➡ ***Monitor.*** In patients receiving amiloride and an ACE inhibitor, monitor serum potassium and renal function, particularly if the patient has 1 or more of the risk factors listed above.

REFERENCES:

1. Chiu TF, et al. Rapid life-threatening hyperkalemia after addition of amiloride HCl/ hydrochlorothiazide to angiotensin-converting enzyme inhibitor therapy. *Ann Emerg Med.* 1997;30:612-615.
2. Schepkens H, et al. Life-threatening hyperkalemia during combined therapy with angiotensin-converting enzyme inhibitors and spironolactone. *Am J Med.* 2001;110:438-441.
3. Berry C, McMurray J. Life-threatening hyperkalemia during combined therapy with angiotensin-converting enzyme inhibitors and spironolactone. *Am J Med.* 2001;111:587.
4. Blaustein DA, et al. Estimation of glomerular filtration rate to prevent life-threatening hyperkalemia due to combined therapy with spironolactone and angiotensin-converting enzyme inhibition or angiotensin receptor blockade. *Am J Cardiol.* 2002;90:662-663.
5. Wrenger E, et al. Interaction of spironolactone with ACE inhibitors or angiotensin receptor blockers: analysis of 44 cases. *BMJ.* 2003;327:147-149.
6. Weber EW, et al. Incidence of hyperkalemia in chronic heart failure patients taking spironolactone in a VA medical center. *Pharmacotherapy.* 2003;23:391.

Amiloride (*Midamor*)
Quinidine

SUMMARY: Coadministration of amiloride with quinidine appears to increase the risk of arrhythmias in patients with ventricular tachycardia.

RISK FACTORS: No specific risk factors are known.

MECHANISM: Both quinidine and amiloride appear to block myocardial sodium channels, resulting in prolonged ventricular conduction.

CLINICAL EVALUATION: Ten patients with inducible ventricular tachycardia received quinidine (variable dosage to therapeutic concentration) alone and during 3 days of combination treatment with amiloride 5 or 10 mg/day.[1] No change in quinidine concentrations was noted in 6 patients in whom pre- and postamiloride-quinidine concentrations were available. Seven of the 10 patients had adverse outcomes to the combination therapy, including loss of quinidine efficacy and ventricular arrhythmias. Electrocardiograms showed more prolonged ventricular conduction without changes in ventricular refractoriness during concomitant therapy compared with the effects of quinidine monotherapy.

RELATED DRUGS: No information is available.

MANAGEMENT OPTIONS:

➡ *Consider Alternative.* Until more information is available, patients taking quinidine should avoid the use of amiloride. Thiazides have not been reported to produce proarrhythmic effects with quinidine.

➡ *Monitor.* If amiloride and quinidine are coadministered, carefully monitor patients for evidence of prolonged ventricular conduction (QRS prolongation) in excess of QRS changes produced by quinidine monotherapy.

REFERENCES:
    1. Wang L, et al. Amiloride-quinidine interaction: adverse outcomes. *Clin Pharmacol Ther*. 1994;56:659-667.

Aminoglutethimide (*Cytadren*)
Dexamethasone (eg, *Decadron*)

SUMMARY: Aminoglutethimide enhances the elimination of dexamethasone (and probably other corticosteroids), resulting in a marked reduction in corticosteroid response.

RISK FACTORS: No specific risk factors are known.

MECHANISM: Aminoglutethimide is known to induce hepatic microsomal enzymes[1] and appears to enhance the metabolism of dexamethasone.

CLINICAL EVALUATION: Patients receiving aminoglutethimide for breast cancer required large doses of dexamethasone (eg, 1.5 to 3 mg/day) to produce adrenal suppression.[2] Subsequent investigation revealed that aminoglutethimide reduced the half-life of dexamethasone to less than 50% of that seen before aminoglutethimide therapy.[2] A 51–year-old woman whose brain edema was controlled on dexamethasone 6 mg/day developed a recurrence of the edema 1 week after starting aminoglutethimide 250 mg/day.[3] She responded to discontinuation of the aminoglutethimide and a temporary increase in the dexamethasone dose.

RELATED DRUGS: Theoretically, the metabolism of corticosteroids other than dexamethasone (eg, hydrocortisone [eg, *Cortef*], cortisone, prednisone [eg, *Deltasone*], prednisolone [eg, *Prelone*], methylprednisolone [eg, *Medrol*]) also would be enhanced by aminoglutethimide, but it is not known whether they would be affected to the same degree as dexamethasone.

MANAGEMENT OPTIONS:

➥ *Monitor.* Dexamethasone dosage requirements are likely to increase considerably (eg, up to at least 2-fold) in the presence of aminoglutethimide. Give careful attention to dexamethasone response when aminoglutethimide is initiated, discontinued, or changed in dosage.

REFERENCES:

1. Kvinssland S, et al. Aminoglutethimide as an inducer of microsomal enzymes. Part 1: Pharmacological aspects. *Breast Cancer Res Treat.* 1986;7(suppl):573-576.
2. Santen RJ, et al. Successful medical adrenalectomy with amino-glutethimide. Role of altered drug metabolism. *JAMA.* 1974;230:1661-1665.
3. Halpern J, et al. A call for caution in the use of aminoglutethimide: negative interaction with dexamethasone and beta blocker treatment. *J Med.* 1984;15:59-63.

Aminoglutethimide (*Cytadren*)

Digitoxin†

SUMMARY: Aminoglutethimide administration reduced the serum concentration of digitoxin in several patients.

RISK FACTORS: No specific risk factors are known.

MECHANISM: Aminoglutethimide is known to stimulate the hepatic oxidation of several drugs, including itself.[1] Digitoxin is partially metabolized by oxidation. The metabolism of digitoxin via this oxidative pathway appears to be markedly increased by the administration of aminoglutethimide.

CLINICAL EVALUATION: Five patients receiving digitoxin were treated with aminoglutethimide: 4 with 250 mg 4 times daily and 1 with 125 mg twice daily for metastatic breast cancer.[2] Digitoxin clearance was significantly increased (an average of 109%) after 4 to 8 weeks of aminoglutethimide administration. The clearance of a single 1000 mg dose of antipyrine was increased 81% in 6 other patients being treated with aminoglutethimide, providing further evidence of aminoglutethimide's ability to increase oxidative metabolism. (Antipyrine has been used as a marker of oxidative metabolism.) Thus, based upon limited data from a few patients, the administration of aminoglutethimide would be expected to significantly reduce the serum concentrations of digitoxin.

RELATED DRUGS: Because the primary route of elimination is renal, digoxin (eg, *Lanoxin*), is not likely to interact with aminoglutethimide to the same degree as digitoxin.

MANAGEMENT OPTIONS:

➥ *Consider Alternative.* Theoretically, the substitution of digoxin for digitoxin would reduce the likelihood of an interaction.

➡ **Monitor.** Monitor digitoxin concentrations for several weeks when patients are maintained on digitoxin following the addition of aminoglutethimide. Increased digitoxin doses may be required to maintain the serum concentrations in the therapeutic range following aminoglutethimide administration.

REFERENCES:

1. Lonning PE, et al. Mechanisms of action of aminoglutethimide as endocrine therapy of breast cancer. *Drugs*. 1988;35:685-710.

2. Lonning E, et al. Effect of aminoglutethimide on antipyrine, theophylline, and digitoxin disposition in breast cancer. *Clin Pharmacol Ther*. 1984;36:796-802.

† Not available in the United States.

Aminoglutethimide (*Cytadren*)

Medroxyprogesterone (*Provera*)

SUMMARY: Aminoglutethimide substantially lowers plasma medroxyprogesterone concentrations, but more study is needed to determine the degree to which this reduces the therapeutic response.

RISK FACTORS: No specific risk factors are known.

MECHANISM: Aminoglutethimide is known to induce hepatic microsomal enzymes[1] and appears to enhance the metabolism of medroxyprogesterone.

CLINICAL EVALUATION: Seven postmenopausal patients with metastatic breast cancer were given oral medroxyprogesterone acetate 500 mg 3 times daily.[2] After 2 weeks, aminoglutethimide 250 mg twice daily was added; 2 weeks later the aminoglutethimide dose was increased to 250 mg 4 times daily. Plasma medroxyprogesterone concentrations were reduced approximately 50% by the 250 mg twice daily dose of aminoglutethimide; increasing the dose to 250 mg 4 times daily did not increase the magnitude of the interaction. In the presence of aminoglutethimide, plasma medroxyprogesterone concentrations were generally less than 100 ng/mL, a level that has little adrenal suppressive effect and may be insufficient for optimal therapeutic effect. In the absence of outcome studies, it is difficult to optimally manage this interaction. Some have proposed that medroxyprogesterone-induced adrenal suppression may be necessary for optimal therapeutic response.[2] Thus, lack of an effect of medroxyprogesterone on serum cortisol caused by aminoglutethimide may be an indication that the medroxyprogesterone effect is less than optimal. Clinical trials comparing the therapeutic outcome of medroxyprogesterone therapy alone with medroxyprogesterone plus aminoglutethimide are needed to determine whether this interaction adversely affects the therapeutic response.

RELATED DRUGS: It is not known to what extent aminoglutethimide enhances the metabolism of progestins other than medroxyprogesterone, but consider the possibility.

MANAGEMENT OPTIONS:

➡ **Monitor.** Monitor for altered medroxyprogesterone effect if aminoglutethimide is initiated, discontinued, or changed in dosage.

REFERENCES:

1. Kvinnsland S, et al. Aminoglutethimide as an inducer of microsomal enzymes. Part 1. Pharmacological aspects. *Breast Cancer Res Treat*. 1986;7(Suppl.).73.

2. Van Deijk WA, et al. Influence of aminoglutethimide on plasma levels of medroxyprogesterone acetate: its correlation with serum cortisol. *Cancer Treat Rep*. 1985;69:85.

Aminoglutethimide (*Cytadren*)

Tamoxifen (*Nolvadex*)

SUMMARY: Aminoglutethimide reduces tamoxifen concentrations and may reduce its clinical effect.

RISK FACTORS: No specific risk factors are known.

MECHANISM: Aminoglutethimide appears to increase the metabolism of tamoxifen and its metabolites.

CLINICAL EVALUATION: Six women with breast cancer were studied.[1] The pharmacokinetics of tamoxifen alone 20 to 90 mg/day, aminoglutethimide alone 250 mg 4 times daily, and the combination of tamoxifen with aminoglutethimide for 6 weeks were evaluated. During aminoglutethimide administration, the patients also received cortisone acetate. Tamoxifen clearance after oral administration was increased from 189 mL/min when administered alone to 608 mL/min during aminoglutethimide therapy. The concentrations of tamoxifen metabolites also were markedly reduced by aminoglutethimide. Aminoglutethimide plasma concentrations were not altered by tamoxifen.

RELATED DRUGS: No information is available.

MANAGEMENT OPTIONS:

➡ *Avoid Unless Benefit Outweighs Risk.* Generally, do not administer aminoglutethimide with tamoxifen since it lowers tamoxifen concentrations and does not enhance the response of breast cancer patients to tamoxifen therapy.

➡ *Monitor.* If the combination is used, monitor tamoxifen response carefully.

REFERENCES:
1. Lien EA, et al. Decreased serum concentrations of tamoxifen and its metabolites induced by aminoglutethimide. *Cancer Res.* 1990;50:5851.

 Aminoglutethimide (*Cytadren*)

Theophylline (eg, *Slo-Phyllin*)

SUMMARY: Preliminary evidence from a limited number of patients indicates that aminoglutethimide reduces the serum concentration of theophylline.

RISK FACTORS: No specific risk factors are known.

MECHANISM: Aminoglutethimide stimulates the hepatic oxidation of several drugs, including itself,[1] and appears to increase the oxidative metabolism of theophylline.

CLINICAL EVALUATION: Three patients receiving sustained-release theophylline 200 mg twice daily were treated with aminoglutethimide 250 mg 4 times daily for metastatic breast cancer.[2] Theophylline clearance was increased by an average of 32% (range: 18% to 43%) after 2 to 12 weeks of aminoglutethimide administration. The clearance of a single 1000 mg dose of antipyrine was increased by 81% in 6 other patients being treated with aminoglutethimide, providing further evidence of aminoglutethimide's ability to increase oxidative metabolism. (Antipyrine has been used as a marker of oxidative metabolism.) Thus, based upon data reported from only a few patients, aminoglutethimide would be expected to reduce the serum concentrations of theophylline.

RELATED DRUGS: No information is available.

MANAGEMENT OPTIONS:

➡ *Monitor.* Patients maintained on theophylline should have their theophylline concentrations monitored for several weeks following the initiation or discontinuation of aminoglutethimide. Adjustment of theophylline doses may be required for some patients to maintain their serum concentrations in the therapeutic range following the initiation or discontinuation of aminoglutethimide.

REFERENCES:

1. Lonning PE, et al. Mechanisms of action of aminoglutethimide as endocrine therapy of breast cancer. *Drugs.* 1988;35:685.

2. Lonning PE, et al. Effect of aminoglutethimide on antipyrine, theophylline, and digitoxin disposition in breast cancer. *Clin Pharmacol Ther.* 1984;6:796.

Aminoglutethimide (*Cytadren*)

Warfarin (eg, *Coumadin*)

SUMMARY: Aminoglutethimide enhances the elimination of warfarin and other oral anticoagulants and can considerably reduce the hypoprothrombinemic response.

RISK FACTORS:

➡ *Dosage Regimen.* The interaction appears to be dose related. In one study, plasma warfarin clearance was increased 41% by 250 mg/day of aminoglutethimide and 91% by 1000 mg/day of aminoglutethimide.[5]

MECHANISM: Aminoglutethimide is known to induce hepatic microsomal enzymes[1] and appears to enhance the metabolism of oral anticoagulants.

CLINICAL EVALUATION: Several patients manifested a marked increase in dosage requirements for warfarin or acenocoumarol (*Sintrom*) after beginning therapy with aminoglutethimide.[2-4] One report described the effect of 2, 4, and 8 weeks of aminoglutethimide (250 or 1000 mg/day) on warfarin pharmacokinetics in 9 women with metastatic breast cancer.[5] No additional increase in warfarin clearance was noted at 4 and 8 weeks.

RELATED DRUGS: Although the reports involved warfarin and acenocoumarol, it is likely that other oral anticoagulants interact similarly with aminoglutethimide.

MANAGEMENT OPTIONS:

➡ *Monitor.* In patients receiving warfarin or other oral anticoagulants, monitor the hypoprothrombinemic response carefully if aminoglutethimide is initiated, discontinued, or changed in dosage; oral anticoagulant dosage requirements are likely to change substantially. Warn patients accordingly.

REFERENCES:

1. Kvinssland S, et al. Aminoglutethimide as an inducer of microsomal enzymes. Part 1. Pharmacological aspects. *Breast Cancer Res Treat.* 1986;7(Suppl):73.

2. Murray RML, et al. Medical adrenalectomy with aminoglutethimide in the management of advanced breast cancer. *Med J Aust.* 1981;1:179.

3. Bruning PF. Aminoglutethimide and oral anticoagulant therapy. *Lancet.* 1983;2:582.

4. Lonning PE, et al. Aminoglutethimide and warfarin. A new important drug interaction. *Cancer Chemother Pharmacol.* 1984;12:10.

5. Lonning PE, et al. The influence of a graded dose schedule of aminoglutethimide on the disposition of the optical enantiomers of warfarin in patients with breast cancer. *Cancer Chemother Pharmacol.* 1986;17:177.

Aminosalicylic Acid (PAS)

Digoxin (eg, *Lanoxin*)

SUMMARY: A small reduction in digoxin serum concentrations may result from coadministration with aminosalicylic acid (PAS).

RISK FACTORS: No specific risk factors are known.

MECHANISM: PAS may reduce digoxin absorption, possibly by affecting the function of intestinal absorbing cells.

CLINICAL EVALUATION: The bioavailability of a single, oral dose of digoxin (as measured by cumulative urinary digoxin excretion) was reduced by 20% following PAS.[1] It is not known whether this interaction would be seen under more typical clinical conditions. Further, a 20% reduction in digoxin absorption may not be clinically important in many patients. Monitor patients receiving PAS and digoxin for reduced digoxin response.

RELATED DRUGS: None known.

MANAGEMENT OPTIONS: No specific action required, but be alert for evidence of the interaction.

REFERENCES:

1. Brown DD, et al. Decreased bioavailability of digoxin due to hypocholesterolemic interventions. *Circulation.* 1978;58:164.

Aminosalicylic Acid (PAS)

Diphenhydramine (eg, *Benadryl*)

SUMMARY: Diphenhydramine can reduce the serum concentration of aminosalicylic acid.

RISK FACTORS: No specific risk factors are known.

MECHANISM: Diphenhydramine appears to impair the GI absorption of PAS.

CLINICAL EVALUATION: Studies in rats and healthy subjects have shown that pretreatment with parenteral diphenhydramine lowers plasma concentrations of orally administered aminosalicylic acid.[1] Although the decreases in PAS blood concentrations were not large, the total amount of PAS absorbed appeared to be decreased. Thus, it is possible that the magnitude of this interaction could become larger with multiple dosing of diphenhydramine.

RELATED DRUGS: No information is available.

MANAGEMENT OPTIONS: No specific action is required, but be alert for evidence of the interaction.

REFERENCES:

1. Lavigne J-G, et al. Inhibition of the GI absorption of paminosalicylate (PAS) in rats and humans by diphenhydramine. *Clin Pharmacol Ther.* 1973;14:404.

Aminosalicylic Acid (PAS)

Phenytoin (eg, *Dilantin*)

SUMMARY: Aminosalicylic acid reportedly increases serum phenytoin concentrations, but supporting clinical evidence is minimal.

RISK FACTORS: No specific risk factors are known.

MECHANISM: PAS could inhibit phenytoin metabolism or increase the blood concentrations of coadministered isoniazid, which in turn would impair phenytoin metabolism.[1,2]

CLINICAL EVALUATION: More study of patients receiving PAS and phenytoin in the absence of isoniazid is needed to assess the clinical significance of the interaction between these two drugs. From current evidence, PAS alone appears unlikely to impair phenytoin metabolism.

RELATED DRUGS: No information is available.

MANAGEMENT OPTIONS: No specific action is required, but be alert for evidence of the interaction.

REFERENCES:

1. Kutt H, et al. Depression of parahydroxylation of diphenylhydantoin by antituberculosis chemotherapy. *Neurology.* 1966;16:594.
2. Kutt H, et al. Inhibition of diphenylhydantoin metabolism in rats and rat liver microsomes by antitubercular drugs. *Neurology.* 1968;18:706.

Aminosalicylic Acid (PAS) ▼3

Rifampin (eg, *Rifadin*)

SUMMARY: Aminosalicylic acid reduces serum concentrations of rifampin.

RISK FACTORS: No specific risk factors are known.

MECHANISM: PAS can impair GI absorption of rifampin, apparently because of bentonite present in the PAS granules.

CLINICAL EVALUATION: A preliminary study in 30 patients indicated that when PAS granules and rifampin are given together, serum rifampin concentrations are considerably lower than when rifampin is given alone.[1] A subsequent study in 6 volunteers indicated that the inhibition of rifampin absorption is because of the bentonite present in the PAS granules and not PAS itself.[2]

RELATED DRUGS: Other drugs containing bentonite probably inhibit rifampin absorption.

MANAGEMENT OPTIONS:

➡ ***Circumvent/Minimize.*** Separate doses of PAS and rifampin by 8 to 12 hours if possible.

➡ ***Monitor.*** Monitor rifampin concentrations if it is administered with bentonite.

REFERENCES:

1. Boman G, et al. Drug interaction: decreased serum concentrations of rifampicin when given with P.A.S. *Lancet.* 1971;1:800.
2. Boman G, et al. Mechanism of the inhibitory effect of PAS granules on the absorption of rifampicin: absorption of rifampicin by an excipient, bentonite. *Eur J Clin Pharmacol.* 1975;8:293.

Aminosalicylic Acid (PAS)

Vitamin B$_{12}$ (Cyanocobalamin)

SUMMARY: Long-term aminosalicylic acid administration potentially could result in vitamin B$_{12}$ deficiency.

RISK FACTORS: No specific risk factors are known.

MECHANISM: Not established. The decreased vitamin B$_{12}$ absorption induced by aminosalicylic acid may be because of the mild malabsorption syndrome that occurs in some aminosalicylic acid–treated patients.

CLINICAL EVALUATION: Prolonged administration of large doses of aminosalicylic acid is likely to be necessary to induce vitamin B$_{12}$ deficiency anemia.[1-3] Because vitamin B$_{12}$ for anemia treatment generally is given parenterally, PAS is unlikely to interfere with the therapeutic effect. Schilling tests of vitamin B$_{12}$ absorption may be affected.

RELATED DRUGS: No information is available.

MANAGEMENT OPTIONS: No specific action is required, but be alert for evidence of the interaction.

REFERENCES:
1. Palva IP, et al. Drug-induced malabsorption of vitamin B$_{12}$. V. Intestinal pH and absorption of vitamin B$_{12}$ during treatment with paraminosalicylic acid. *Scand J Haematol.* 1972;9(1):5-7.
2. Halsted CH, et al. Intestinal malabsorption caused by aminosalicylic acid therapy. *Arch Intern Med.* 1972;130(6):935-939.
3. Heinivaara O, et al. Malabsorption of vitamin B$_{12}$ during treatment with para-aminosalicylic acid. A preliminary report. *Acta Med Scand.* 1964;175:469-471.

4 **Aminosalicylic Acid (PAS)**

Warfarin (eg, *Coumadin*)

SUMMARY: Aminosalicylic acid was associated with an excessive hypoprothrombinemic response to warfarin in one patient, but a causal relationship was not established.

RISK FACTORS: No specific risk factors are known.

MECHANISM: Aminosalicylic acid reportedly decreases prothrombin formation by the liver.[1]

CLINICAL EVALUATION: In one patient, the administration of aminosalicylic acid appeared to enhance the hypoprothrombinemic effect of warfarin.[2] This patient also was receiving isoniazid (eg, *Nydrazid*). Therefore, the possibility that isoniazid (or some other factor) was involved cannot be ruled out. One case of possible isoniazid-induced enhancement of the hypoprothrombinemic response to warfarin has been reported.[3]

RELATED DRUGS: Little is known regarding the effect of aminosalicylic acid on oral anticoagulants other than warfarin.

MANAGEMENT OPTIONS: No specific action is required, but be alert for evidence of the interaction.

REFERENCES:

1. Weinstein L. Drugs used in chemotherapy of leprosy and tuberculosis. In: Goodman LS, Gilman A, eds. *The Pharmacological Basis of Therapeutics*. 4th ed. New York, NY: Macmillan; 1970:1320-1324.

2. Self TH. Interaction of warfarin and aminosalicylic acid. *JAMA*. 1973;223(11):1285.

3. Rosenthal AR, et al. Interaction of isoniazid and warfarin. *JAMA*. 1977;238(20):2177.

Amiodarone (eg, *Cordarone*)

Aprindine† (*Fibocil*)

SUMMARY: Amiodarone may increase the plasma concentrations of aprindine.

RISK FACTORS: No specific risk factors are known.

MECHANISM: Amiodarone is likely to inhibit the metabolism of aprindine.

CLINICAL EVALUATION: Two patients on long-term aprindine therapy experienced increased serum aprindine concentrations, nausea, ataxia, and light-headedness following initiation of amiodarone therapy (1,200 mg/day, then 400 to 600 mg/day).[1] More data are needed to establish the incidence and magnitude of this purported interaction.

RELATED DRUGS: No information is available.

MANAGEMENT OPTIONS:

➡ *Circumvent/Minimize.* Patients receiving both drugs may require less aprindine than those receiving aprindine alone.

➡ *Monitor.* Watch for evidence of altered aprindine response when amiodarone therapy is initiated or discontinued.

REFERENCES:

1. Southworth W, et al. Possible amiodarone-aprindine interaction. *Am Heart J*. 1982;104(2, pt 1):323.

† Not available in the United States.

Amiodarone (eg, *Cordarone*)

Aripiprazole (*Abilify*)

SUMMARY: Amiodarone is expected to markedly increase aripiprazole serum concentrations; the interaction is based largely on theoretical considerations.

RISK FACTORS:

➡ *Pharmacogenetics.* Patients who are normal (rapid) metabolizers for CYP2D6 are likely to be most affected by this interaction. However, because amiodarone inhibits both pathways for aripiprazole metabolism (CYP2D6 and CYP3A4), some increase in aripiprazole concentrations may still occur in patients with low CYP2D6 activity.

MECHANISM: Aripiprazole is metabolized by CYP2D6 and CYP3A4; amiodarone inhibits both of these isozymes. The CYP2D6 genotype has been shown to affect serum concentrations of aripiprazole; the lower the CYP2D6 activity, the higher the concentrations of aripiprazole.[1,2]

CLINICAL EVALUATION: Because amiodarone inhibits CYP2D6 and CYP3A4, theoretically, it should produce dramatic increases in aripiprazole serum concentrations.[3] Clinical studies are needed to confirm this potential interaction.

RELATED DRUGS: Quinidine is a potent CYP2D6 inhibitor, and has been shown to more than double aripiprazole serum concentrations. Another antiarrhythmic agent, propafenone (eg, *Rythmol*), also inhibits CYP2D6 and theoretically would increase aripirazole serum concentrations.

MANAGEMENT OPTIONS:

➥ *Use Alternative.* If possible, use an alternative to one of the drugs.

➥ *Monitor.* If the combination is used, monitor for altered aripiprazole effect if amiodarone is started, stopped, or changed in dosage. Keep in mind that aripiprazole and its active metabolite, dehydroaripiprazole, have long half-lives, and in some cases it may take weeks to achieve new aripiprazole steady-state serum concentrations.

REFERENCES:

1. Hendset M, et al. Impact of the CYP2D6 genotype on steady-state serum concentrations of aripiprazole and dehydroaripiprazole. *Eur J Clin Pharmacol.* 2007;63(12):1147-1151.
2. Kim JR, et al. Population pharmacokinetic modeling of aripiprazole and its active metabolite, dehydroaripiprazole, in psychiatric patients. *Br J Clin Pharmacol.* 2008;66(6):802-810.
3. *Abilify* [package insert]. Princeton, NJ: Bristol-Myers Squibb; 2010.

Amiodarone (eg, *Cordarone*)

Carvedilol (eg, *Coreg*)

SUMMARY: Amiodarone increases the plasma concentration of carvedilol; increased alpha- and beta-blocker effect may occur in some patients.

RISK FACTORS: No specific risk factors are known.

MECHANISM: Amiodarone and its metabolite inhibit CYP2D6, CYP3A4, and CYP2C9. Each of these enzymes is involved in the metabolism of carvedilol. S-carvedilol is thought to be more dependent on CYP2C9 than the R-enantiomer. Additionally, carvedilol is a substrate for P-glycoprotein that also is inhibited by amiodarone.

CLINICAL EVALUATION: Carvedilol plasma concentrations were determined in 52 patients taking carvedilol (mean dose, 0.179 mg/kg) and in a separate group of patients taking carvedilol (mean dose, 0.144 mg/kg) plus amiodarone (dose not stated) twice daily.[1] The mean plasma concentration of S-carvedilol in the patients receiving concurrent amiodarone increased nearly 100%. The concentration of R-carvedilol was not significantly different in the 2 groups. In a separate study, 6 of the 52 patients stabilized on carvedilol (mean dosage, 12 mg/day) had amiodarone (mean dosage, 117 mg/day) added to their therapy for 2 weeks. Following the addition of amiodarone, the mean S-carvedilol concentrations increased 115%. R-carvedilol concentrations did not change significantly.

RELATED DRUGS: Amiodarone can inhibit the metabolism of other beta-blockers that are metabolized by CYP2D6, such as metoprolol (eg, *Lopressor*) or timolol (eg, *Blocadren*).

MANAGEMENT OPTIONS:

➥ *Monitor.* Pending further study of this interaction, watch for altered alpha- and beta-blocking effects if amiodarone therapy is added or removed.

REFERENCES:

1. Fukumoto K, et al. Stereoselective effect of amiodarone on the pharmacokinetics of racemic carvedilol. *Drug Metab Pharmacokinet.* 2005;20(6):423-427.

Amiodarone (eg, *Cordarone*)

Cholestyramine (eg, *Questran*)

SUMMARY: Cholestyramine can decrease amiodarone plasma concentrations and antiarrhythmic efficacy.

RISK FACTORS: No specific risk factors are known.

MECHANISM: Cholestyramine appears to increase the elimination of amiodarone by reducing its enterohepatic circulation.

CLINICAL EVALUATION: Eleven patients received single doses of amiodarone with cholestyramine 4 g, followed by cholestyramine 4 g administered at 90-minute intervals after the amiodarone.[1] Plasma amiodarone concentrations measured 7 hours after amiodarone plus cholestyramine dosing were reduced 50%, compared with amiodarone plasma concentrations after the administration of amiodarone alone. The half-life of amiodarone (normally approximately 50 to 60 days) was reduced to approximately 30 days. When administered to cholestyramine-treated patients, loss of amiodarone antiarrhythmic efficacy is possible.

RELATED DRUGS: Colestipol (eg, *Colestid*) also is likely to decrease amiodarone plasma concentrations.

MANAGEMENT OPTIONS:

➥ *Monitor.* Observe patients receiving cholestyramine and amiodarone for increased amiodarone dosage requirements. Discontinuation of cholestyramine may result in excessive accumulation of amiodarone and toxicity (eg, arrhythmia, pneumonitis, thyroid abnormalities).

REFERENCES:

1. Nitsch J, et al. Acceleration of amiodarone elimination by cholestyramine [in German]. *Dtsch Med Wochenschr.* 1986;111(33):1241-1244.

Amiodarone (eg, *Cordarone*)

Cimetidine (eg, *Tagamet*)

SUMMARY: Cimetidine administration to patients stabilized on amiodarone can increase amiodarone serum concentrations and possibly enhance amiodarone toxicity.

RISK FACTORS: No specific risk factors are known.

MECHANISM: Not established. Cimetidine may inhibit the cytochrome P450 hepatic metabolism of amiodarone or the uptake of amiodarone by hepatocytes.

CLINICAL EVALUATION: Twelve patients receiving amiodarone 200 mg/day for 6 months or longer were administered cimetidine 300 mg 4 times daily for 1 week.[1] The average amiodarone serum concentrations following cimetidine administration were approximately 35% higher than before cimetidine administration. Eight of the 12 patients exhibited an increase in amiodarone serum concentrations. Because amiodarone has a very long half-life (50 days), 7 days of cimetidine coadministration may not accurately reflect the magnitude of this interaction. The serum concentrations of amiodarone would be expected to continue to rise for many weeks after the addition of cimetidine. The offset of the interaction also would be prolonged as amiodarone concentrations decline slowly following the discontinuation of cimetidine.

RELATED DRUGS: The effects of other H_2-receptor antagonists, such as ranitidine (eg, *Zantac*), famotidine (eg, *Pepcid*), and nizatidine (*Axid*), on amiodarone are unknown, but they probably would not affect amiodarone metabolism.

MANAGEMENT OPTIONS:

➡ *Monitor.* Monitor amiodarone serum concentrations in amiodarone-treated patients following the institution of cimetidine. Many weeks may be required for the maximum effects of this interaction to become evident. It also may take several weeks for amiodarone concentrations to return to normal after cimetidine is discontinued.

REFERENCES:

    1. Landau S, et al. Cimetidine-amiodarone interaction. *J Clin Pharmacol*. 1988;38:909.

4   Amiodarone (eg, *Cordarone*)

Clonazepam (eg, *Klonopin*)

SUMMARY: Benzodiazepine toxicity occurred in a patient taking amiodarone who was prescribed clonazepam. While causation cannot be established, it appears to be consistent with the known properties of the drugs involved.

RISK FACTORS: No specific risk factors are known.

MECHANISM: This patient's symptoms may have been caused by amiodarone-induced reduction in the metabolism of clonazepam resulting in the accumulation of toxic concentrations. Amiodarone-induced hypothyroidism is known to occur in some patients taking the antiarrhythmic and can reduce the metabolism of drugs that undergo oxidative metabolism. It is possible the worsening heart failure also contributed to reduced clonazepam clearance. The exact mechanism of this interaction requires further investigation. Because of amiodarone's long half-life, several weeks may be required to observe the full extent of an interaction with clonazepam.

CLINICAL EVALUATION: A 78-year-old man with heart failure had been treated for 4 months with amiodarone for ventricular tachycardia when he developed paresthesias on the bottom of his feet and myoclonus of the lower extremities.[1] Clonazepam 0.5 mg/day was initiated for restless leg syndrome. Two months later during an episode of worsening heart failure, the patient developed symptoms of clonazepam toxicity including slurred speech, ataxia, confusion, urinary incontinence, and dry mouth. Laboratory tests demonstrated hypothyroidism. Clonazepam was discontinued and his mental status improved over 5 days.

RELATED DRUGS: No information is available.

MANAGEMENT OPTIONS: No specific action is required, but be alert for evidence of the interaction.

REFERENCES:

1. Witt DM, et al. Amiodarone-clonazepam interaction. *Ann Pharmacother.* 1993;27:1463.

Amiodarone (eg, *Cordarone*)

Codeine

SUMMARY: Amiodarone inhibits CYP2D6, and theoretically would interfere with the bioactivation of codeine to morphine, but the extent to which it inhibits the analgesic effect of codeine is not established.

RISK FACTORS:

➥ *Pharmacogenetics.* Only patients with the extensive metabolizer CYP2D6 phenotype (EMs) would be expected to experience this interaction. Poor metabolizers (PMs) do not have the gene for production of CYP2D6, so there would be no CYP2D6 for the amiodarone to inhibit. About 8% of whites are deficient in CYP2D6, but the deficiency is rare in Asians, usually 2% or less.

MECHANISM: Codeine exerts its analgesic effects (and probably also its side effects) primarily through its metabolic conversion to morphine by the isozyme, CYP2D6.[1,2] Thus, patients genetically deficient in CYP2D6 or receiving CYP2D6 inhibitors such as amiodarone are likely to produce little or no morphine during codeine administration.

CLINICAL EVALUATION: Amiodarone is known to inhibit CYP2D6. Since several studies have shown that another CYP2D6 inhibitor, quinidine, inhibits the analgesic effect of codeine,[3-6] amiodarone might be expected to inhibit codeine analgesia as well. Nonetheless, clinical studies are needed to determine the clinical importance of this potential interaction.

RELATED DRUGS: The analgesic effect of dihydrocodeine (*Synalgos-DC*) and hydrocodone (*Vicodin*) also may be dependent on conversion to morphine-like active metabolites, and early evidence suggests that CYP2D6 inhibitors can reduce their analgesic efficacy. Whether amiodarone affects these drugs is unknown. Tramadol (*Ultram*) appears to be partially dependent upon CYP2D6 for analgesic activity, but theoretically would be less affected than codeine by amiodarone. Early pharmacodynamic evidence suggests that oxycodone (eg, *Percodan*) does not require conversion by CYP2D6 to an active metabolite. Theoretically, oxycodone would not be affected by amiodarone, but more study is needed.

MANAGEMENT OPTIONS: No specific action is required, but be alert for evidence of the interaction.

REFERENCES:

1. Sindrup SH, et al. Codeine increases pain thresholds to copper vapor laser stimuli in extensive but not poor metabolizers of sparteine. *Clin Pharmacol Ther.* 1990;48:686.

2. Poulsen L, et al. Codeine and morphine in extensive and poor metabolizers of sparteine: pharmacokinetics, analgesic effect and side effects. *Eur J Clin Pharmacol.* 1996;51:289.

3. Desmeules J, et al. Impact of environmental and genetic factors on codeine analgesia. *Eur J Clin Pharmacol.* 1991;41:23.

4. Sindrup SH, et al. The effect of quinidine on the analgesic effect of codeine. *Eur J Clin Pharmacol.* 1992;42:587.

5. Sindrup SH, et al. Impact of quinidine on plasma and cerebrospinal fluid concentrations of codeine and morphine after codeine intake. *Eur J Clin Pharmacol*. 1996;49:503.

6. Caraco Y, et al. Pharmacogenetic determination of the effects of codeine and prediction of drug interactions. *J Pharmacol Exp Ther*. 1996;278:1165.

 ## Amiodarone (eg, *Cordarone*)

Colchicine

SUMMARY: Based on the interactive properties of the 2 drugs, it is likely that amiodarone substantially increases colchicine plasma concentrations. Avoid the combination when possible.

RISK FACTORS: No specific risk factors are known.

MECHANISM: Colchicine is a P-glycoprotein substrate, and amiodarone is a P-glycoprotein inhibitor, so colchicine plasma concentrations are likely to increase.[1,2]

CLINICAL EVALUATION: Although the interaction is based primarily on theoretical considerations, it is likely that amiodarone would increase the risk of colchicine toxicity. Given that colchicine toxicity can be fatal, even a theoretical interaction warrants close attention.

RELATED DRUGS: Other antiarrhythmic agents and cardiovascular drugs that inhibit P-glycoprotein include propafenone (eg, *Rythmol*), quinidine, and the calcium channel blockers diltiazem (eg, *Cardizem*), nicardipine (eg, *Cardene*), and verapamil (eg, *Calan*).

MANAGEMENT OPTIONS:

➥ *Avoid Unless Benefit Outweighs Risk.* Given that colchicine toxicity can be life-threatening, use amiodarone only if it is likely to provide therapeutic benefits that cannot be achieved with noninteracting alternatives.

➥ *Use Alternative.* If possible, use an alternative to amiodarone that does not inhibit P-glycoprotein, or use an alternative to colchicine.

➥ *Monitor.* If the combination must be used, monitor carefully for colchicine toxicity such as diarrhea, vomiting, fever, abdominal pain, and muscle pain. Advise the patient to immediately contact their health care provider if any of these symptoms occur. Colchicine-induced pancytopenia can result in infections, bleeding, and anemia, and is often the cause of death in fatal cases.

REFERENCES:

1. Rautio J, et al. In vitro p-glycoprotein inhibition assays for assessment of clinical drug interaction potential of new drug candidates: a recommendation for probe substrates. *Drug Metab Dispos*. 2006;34(5):786-792.

2. Bates SE, et al. A pilot study of amiodarone with infusional doxorubicin or vinblastine in refractory breast cancer. *Cancer Chemother Pharmacol*. 1995;35(6):457-463.

Amiodarone (eg, *Cordarone*)

Cyclophosphamide

SUMMARY: A man taking amiodarone developed pulmonary toxicity after receiving a single high dose of cyclophosphamide; monitor patients for lung toxicity.

RISK FACTORS: Not established.

MECHANISM: Both amiodarone and cyclophosphamide can individually cause pulmonary toxicity, and it is possible that the effects can be additive when they are given together.

CLINICAL EVALUATION: A 59-year-old man on chronic amiodarone therapy developed pulmonary toxicity after a single high dose of cyclophosphamide (4,000 mg/m^2).[1] While taking amiodarone, he had previously received several cycles of chemotherapy with lower doses of cyclophosphamide (1,400 mg daily for 4 days) without developing overt pulmonary toxicity. Because both amiodarone and cyclophosphamide can cause lung damage, the toxicity may have resulted from the combined effects of both drugs.

RELATED DRUGS: Other antineoplastic drugs may also cause pulmonary toxicity (eg, bleomycin [eg, *Blenoxane*]), and it is possible that amiodarone may have additive effects with these as well.

MANAGEMENT OPTIONS:

➡ ***Monitor.*** In patients receiving amiodarone, monitor for pulmonary toxicity if cyclophosphamide is given concurrently.

REFERENCES:

1. Bhagat R, et al. Amiodarone and cyclophosphamide: potential for enhanced lung toxicity. *Bone Marrow Transplant.* 2001;27(10):1109-1111.

Amiodarone (eg, *Cordarone*)

Cyclosporine (eg, *Sandimmune*)

SUMMARY: An increase in cyclosporine concentrations following the addition of amiodarone therapy has been reported.

RISK FACTORS: No specific risk factors are known.

MECHANISM: Amiodarone appears to inhibit the clearance of cyclosporine.

CLINICAL EVALUATION: Cyclosporine clearance appears to be reduced by approximately 50% following the addition of amiodarone.[1-3] While little specific detail of this interaction is available, amiodarone is known to inhibit the metabolism of a number of drugs. The significance of this purported interaction requires more study.

RELATED DRUGS: It is possible that tacrolimus (*Prograf*) also may be affected by amiodarone.

MANAGEMENT OPTIONS:

➡ **Monitor.** Watch for increased cyclosporine concentrations and evidence of toxicity (renal dysfunction) in patients started on amiodarone therapy.

REFERENCES:

1. Nicolau DP, et al. Amiodarone-cyclosporine interaction in heart transplant patient. *J Heart Lung Transplant*. 1992;11:564.
2. Chitwood KK, et al. Cyclosporine-amiodarone interaction. *Ann Pharmacother*. 1993;27:569.
3. Mamprin F, et al. Amiodarone-cyclosporine interaction in cardiac transplantation. *Am Heart J*. 1992;123:1725.

Amiodarone (eg, *Cordarone*)

Dextromethorphan (eg, *Benylin-DM*)

SUMMARY: Dextromethorphan concentrations may increase during chronic amiodarone administration; the clinical significance of this interaction is unknown.

RISK FACTORS:

➡ **Pharmacogenetics.** Rapid dextromethorphan (CYP2D6) metabolizers will have an increased risk of the interaction.

MECHANISM: Amiodarone appears to inhibit hepatic cytochrome P4502D6 activity and reduce the metabolism of dextromethorphan.

CLINICAL EVALUATION: Eight patients with arrhythmias received amiodarone 1000 mg/day for 10 days followed by 200 or 400 mg/day.[1] Each patient took 40 mg of dextromethorphan before amiodarone was initiated and again after an average of 76 days of amiodarone therapy. The ratio of the concentration of dextromethorphan to the concentration of its metabolite, dextrorphan, was measured. The chronic administration of amiodarone increased the ratio of dextromethorphan to dextrorphan and increased the amount of dextromethorphan excreted in the urine. The clinical significance of this interaction is not known.

RELATED DRUGS: No information available.

MANAGEMENT OPTIONS: No specific action is required, but be alert for evidence of the interaction.

REFERENCES:

1. Funck-Brentano C, et al. Influence of amiodarone on genetically determined drug metabolism in humans. *Clin Pharmacol Ther*. 1991;50:259.

Amiodarone (eg, *Cordarone*)

Digoxin (eg, *Lanoxin*)

SUMMARY: Amiodarone can cause digoxin to accumulate in the serum to concentrations that often are associated with toxicity.

RISK FACTORS: No specific risk factors are known.

MECHANISM: Amiodarone reduces the renal and nonrenal clearance of digoxin and also increases its bioavailability.[4-10] Amiodarone and digoxin may both depress the sinus node, resulting in bradycardia.[3] Amiodarone-induced hypothyroidism also could reduce the clearance of digoxin.[9]

CLINICAL EVALUATION: Patients receiving digoxin and amiodarone can experience signs and symptoms of digoxin toxicity (eg, arrhythmias, CNS disturbances, GI upset). Because of the long half-life of amiodarone (50 days), the interaction with digoxin usually is noted after several days to weeks of concurrent therapy, especially if no loading dose of amiodarone is given.[1,2,7] This drug interaction appears to be related to the dose of amiodarone; digoxin serum concentrations several times higher than the preamiodarone levels can be encountered.[7,8]

RELATED DRUGS: The effect of amiodarone on digitoxin (*Crystodigin*) is not established but probably would be similar.

MANAGEMENT OPTIONS:

➥ *Circumvent/Minimize.* Digoxin doses probably will need to be reduced when amiodarone is added to therapy.

➥ *Monitor.* Monitor patients for changes in digoxin serum concentrations when amiodarone is initiated or discontinued during concurrent therapy. Several weeks may be required before new steady-state digoxin concentrations are achieved.

REFERENCES:

1. Moysey JO, et al. Amiodarone increases plasma digoxin concentrations. *BMJ.* 1981;282:272.
2. Klein HO, et al. Asystole produced by the combination of amiodarone and digoxin. *Am Heart J.* 1987;113(Part 1):399.
3. McGovern B, et al. Sinus arrest during treatment with amiodarone. *BMJ.* 1982;284:160.
4. Santostasi G, et al. Effects of amiodarone on oral and intravenous digoxin kinetics in healthy subjects. *J Cardiovasc Pharmacol.* 1987;9:385.
5. Fenster PE, et al. Pharmacokinetic evaluation of the digoxin-amiodarone interaction. *J Am Coll Cardiol.* 1985;5:108.
6. Nademanee K, et al. Amiodarone-digoxin interaction: clinical significance, time course of development, potential pharmacokinetic mechanisms and therapeutic implications. *J Am Coll Cardiol.* 1984;4:111.
7. Johnston A, et al. The digoxin-amiodarone interaction. *Br J Clin Pharmacol.* 1987;24:253P.
8. Koren G, et al. Digoxin toxicity associated with amiodarone therapy in children. *J Pediatr.* 1984;104:467.
9. Ben-chetrit E, et al. Case report: amiodarone-associated hypothyroidism—a possible cause of digoxin intoxication. *Am J Med Sci.* 1985;289:114.
10. Robinson K, et al. The digoxin-amiodarone interaction. *Cardiovasc Drugs Ther.* 1989;3:25.

Amiodarone (eg, *Cordarone*)

Diltiazem (eg, *Cardizem*)

SUMMARY: Amiodarone and diltiazem may result in cardiotoxicity with bradycardia and decreased cardiac output.

RISK FACTORS: No specific risk factors are known.

MECHANISM: Not established. Both amiodarone and diltiazem have the potential to decrease sinoatrial and atrioventricular nodal conduction and to decrease myocardial contractility. These effects may be additive when diltiazem and amiodarone are administered together.

CLINICAL EVALUATION: A 61-year-old patient with cardiomyopathy, congestive heart failure, atrial fibrillation, and ventricular tachycardia was treated with diltiazem 90 mg every 6 hours to control the ventricular response to the atrial fibrillation.[1] After 4 days of therapy, an amiodarone loading dose of 600 mg every 12 hours was added for persistent ventricular arrhythmias. Four days later, the patient developed sinus arrest, low cardiac output, and oliguria. Both drugs were discontinued, and pressor agents plus ventricular pacing were needed to stabilize the patient's hemodynamic status. After sinus rhythm and baseline hemodynamic function returned, amiodarone was reinstituted at 400 mg/day without further decompensation.

RELATED DRUGS: Verapamil (eg, *Calan*) may produce similar effects when used with amiodarone. Dihydropyridine calcium channel blockers (eg, nifedipine [eg, *Procardia*], amlodipine [eg, *Norvasc*], felodipine) are unlikely to interact with amiodarone.

MANAGEMENT OPTIONS:

➡ *Monitor.* Until more information is available, monitor patients receiving amiodarone for signs of cardiac toxicity when diltiazem is coadministered.

REFERENCES:

1. Lee TH, et al. Sinus arrest and hypotension with combined amiodarone-diltiazem therapy. *Am Heart J.* 1985;109(1):163-164.

Amiodarone (eg, *Cordarone*)

Disopyramide (eg, *Norpace*)

SUMMARY: Disopyramide and amiodarone have additive depressant effects on cardiac conduction.

RISK FACTORS: No specific risk factors are known.

MECHANISM: Both drugs prolong impulse conduction through the myocardium. A pharmacokinetic interaction has not been investigated.

CLINICAL EVALUATION: The combination of amiodarone and disopyramide can be beneficial in the treatment of ventricular arrhythmias;[1] however, excessive prolongation of the QT interval could result in arrhythmias, including torsades de pointes.[2] The potential for this combination to result in an arrhythmia is unknown but probably limited.

RELATED DRUGS: Use amiodarone with caution with any drug that may prolong the QT interval.

MANAGEMENT OPTIONS: No specific action is required, but be alert for evidence of the interaction.

REFERENCES:

1. James MA, et al. Combined therapy with disopyramide and amiodarone: a report of 11 cases. *Int J Cardiol.* 1986;13(2):248-252.
2. Tartini R, et al. Dangerous interaction between amiodarone and quinidine. *Lancet.* 1982;1(8285):1327-1329.

Amiodarone (eg, *Cordarone*)

Donepezil (eg, *Aricept*)

SUMMARY: The combination of amiodarone and donepezil may produce bradycardia in susceptible patients; amiodarone may interact similarly with other cholinesterase inhibitors.

RISK FACTORS: No specific risk factors are known.

MECHANISM: Donepezil and other cholinesterase inhibitors increase vagal tone, predisposing to bradycardia. Amiodarone may produce additive effects.

CLINICAL EVALUATION: The French Pharmacovigilance Database received 45 spontaneous reports of adverse effects in patients receiving amiodarone and cholinesterase inhibitors (donepezil, galantamine, rivastigmine).[1] After evaluation by clinical pharmacologists, 11 were thought to be adverse drug interactions. Of the 73 patients who received cholinesterase inhibitors along with amiodarone or other bradycardic drugs, 5 deaths were due to syncope, bradycardia, arrhythmias, or cardiac arrest. Although additional study is needed to establish the clinical importance of these interactions, the potential severity of the reactions dictates caution.

RELATED DRUGS: Amiodarone would be expected to interact with all cholinesterase inhibitors, including donepezil and galantamine (eg, *Razadyne*). Theoretically, dronedarone (*Multaq*) may also interact with cholinesterase inhibitors.

MANAGEMENT OPTIONS:

➡ *Consider Alternative.* If appropriate, use an alternative to either the cholinesterase inhibitor or amiodarone.

➡ *Monitor.* If the combination is used, monitor for bradycardia, hypotension, and syncope.

REFERENCES:

1. Tavassoli N, et al. Drug interactions with cholinesterase inhibitors: an analysis of the French Pharmacovigilance Database and a comparison of two national drug formularies (Vidal, British National Formulary). *Drug Saf.* 2007;30(11):1063-1071.

Amiodarone (eg, *Cordarone*) 4

Fentanyl (eg, *Sublimaze*)

SUMMARY: Patients taking amiodarone may be at increased risk for cardiovascular complications following general anesthesia.

RISK FACTORS: No specific risk factors are known.

MECHANISM: Not established.

CLINICAL EVALUATION: Sixteen surgical patients maintained on amiodarone received fentanyl and other drugs, such as diazepam (eg, *Valium*), enflurane (eg, *Ethrane*), isoflurane (*Forane*), morphine, and halothane (*Fluothane*). Perioperative complications (ie, cardiac conduction defects, low cardiac output states, and low systemic vascular resistance) were greater in this patient group than in a comparable group of 30 patients not taking amiodarone who underwent cardiac surgery.[1] Other complications following general anesthesia in patients taking amiodarone have been reported.[2,3] It cannot be ascertained whether these adverse effects are the result of amiodarone interactions with other perioperative medications or amiodarone alone.

RELATED DRUGS: No information is available.

MANAGEMENT OPTIONS: No specific action is required, but be alert for evidence of the interaction.

REFERENCES:

1. Liberman BA, et al. Anaesthesia and amiodarone. *Can Anaesth Soc J.* 1985;32(6).629-638.

2. MacKinnon G, et al. Should oral amiodarone be used for sustained ventricular tachycardia in patients requiring open heart surgery? *Can J Surg.* 1983;26(4):355-357.

3. Gallagher JD, et al. Amiodarone-induced complications during coronary artery surgery. *Anesthesiology.* 1981;55(2):186-188.

Amiodarone (eg, *Cordarone*)

Flecainide (eg, *Tambocor*)

SUMMARY: When amiodarone is administered in conjunction with flecainide, the dose of flecainide required to maintain therapeutic plasma concentrations may be one-third less than that required when flecainide is administered alone.

RISK FACTORS: No specific risk factors are known.

MECHANISM: Amiodarone appears to inhibit the metabolic clearance of flecainide.

CLINICAL EVALUATION: Amiodarone 600 mg twice daily for 10 to 14 days was followed by a 600 mg/day maintenance dosage in 8 patients whose arrhythmias were controlled by various stable doses of flecainide.[1] Flecainide doses had to be decreased to maintain concentrations in the therapeutic range subsequent to amiodarone therapy. The mean dose-adjusted flecainide concentrations increased nearly 50% after the addition of amiodarone. Detailed data from 2 patients indicate that the interaction has a rapid onset (days) and may require several weeks to achieve maximum effect. Amiodarone 400 mg/day for 5 days reduced the metabolic and renal clearance of flecainide in healthy subjects.[2]

RELATED DRUGS: Amiodarone may affect encainide in a similar manner.

MANAGEMENT OPTIONS:

➡ *Circumvent/Minimize.* Until more information is available, consider reducing the dose of flecainide by 33% to 50% when it is used in patients who already are being treated with amiodarone.

➡ *Monitor.* Observe patients for signs and symptoms consistent with altered flecainide serum concentrations when amiodarone is added to or discontinued from the regimens of patients taking flecainide. Because amiodarone has a long half-life, monitor patients for several weeks.

REFERENCES:

1. Shea P, et al. Flecainide and amiodarone interaction. *J Am Coll Cardiol.* 1986;7(5):1127-1130.
2. Funck-Brentano C, et al. Variable disposition kinetics and electrocardiographic effects of flecainide during repeated dosing in humans: contribution of genetic factors, dose-dependent clearance, and interaction with amiodarone. *Clin Pharmacol Ther.* 1994;55(3):256-269.

Amiodarone (eg, *Cordarone*)

Grapefruit Juice

SUMMARY: Grapefruit juice administration appears to increase amiodarone plasma concentrations; some patients may experience an increase in amiodarone side effects.

RISK FACTORS: No specific risk factors are known.

MECHANISM: Grapefruit juice inhibits CYP3A4, resulting in a reduction in the first-pass metabolism of amiodarone and an increase in plasma concentrations.

CLINICAL EVALUATION: Eleven healthy subjects received a single dose of oral amiodarone in 300 mL of water or grapefruit juice.[1] Additional 300 mL doses of grapefruit juice were administered at 3 and 9 hours after amiodarone. The 2 doses of amiodarone were separated by 6 to 8 months to allow for the long half-life of amiodarone. The mean area under the plasma concentration-time curve of amiodarone was increased 50% and peak concentration increased 84% when administered with grapefruit juice compared with water. The half-life of amiodarone did not change. A smaller dose of grapefruit juice is likely to produce a lesser effect on amiodarone concentrations.

RELATED DRUGS: None known.

MANAGEMENT OPTIONS:

➡ **Monitor.** Caution patients stabilized on amiodarone to avoid excessive amounts of grapefruit juice. Monitor for altered amiodarone response (eg, electrocardiogram) if grapefruit juice is coadministered.

REFERENCES:

1. Libersa CC, et al. Dramatic inhibition of amiodarone metabolism induced by grapefruit juice. *Brit J Clin Pharmacol.* 2000;49(4):373-378.

Amiodarone (eg, *Cordarone*)

Indinavir (*Crixivan*)

SUMMARY: Indinavir appears to increase amiodarone concentrations; increased effects on cardiac conduction may occur in some patients.

RISK FACTORS: No specific risk factors are known.

MECHANISM: Indinavir may inhibit the CYP3A4 metabolism of amiodarone, resulting in increased plasma concentrations.

CLINICAL EVALUATION: A patient stabilized on amiodarone 200 mg daily received zidovudine 200 mg 3 times daily, lamivudine 150 mg twice daily, and indinavir 800 mg 3 times daily for 4 weeks.[1] Amiodarone concentrations increased from 0.9 to 1.3 mg/L during antiretroviral treatment. Following discontinuation of the antiretrovirals, the amiodarone concentration declined to 0.8 mg/L over the next 2 months. While no change in amiodarone response was observed in this patient, the magnitude of this interaction could produce increased effects in some patients.

RELATED DRUGS: Nelfinavir (*Viracept*), saquinavir (*Invirase*), and ritonavir (*Norvir*) also inhibit CYP3A4 and may reduce amiodarone metabolism.

MANAGEMENT OPTIONS:

➡ **Monitor.** Carefully monitor patients receiving amiodarone for increased antiarrhythmic effects during indinavir administration.

REFERENCES:

1. Lohman JJ, et al. Antiretroviral therapy increases serum concentrations of amiodarone. *Ann Pharmacother.* 1999;33(5):645-646.

Amiodarone (eg, *Cordarone*)

Iohexol (*Omnipaque*)

SUMMARY: The administration of iohexol to patients taking amiodarone appears to result in a prolongation of the QTc; the potential for arrhythmias to occur is unknown.

RISK FACTORS: No specific risk factors are known.

MECHANISM: Unknown.

CLINICAL EVALUATION: A retrospective study compared 21 patients taking amiodarone who underwent cardiac catheterization with iohexol contrast media with 21 other catheterization patients not taking amiodarone.[1] An electrocardiogram was taken prior to catheterization and the day after the procedure. In patients not taking amiodarone, the QTc was the same before catheterization and the day after. The mean QTc in patients taking amiodarone significantly increased from 433 msec before catheterization to 480 msec on the day following. Six of the 21 patients taking amiodarone had QTc above 500 msec following cardiac catheterization, while none demonstrated QTc above 500 msec before the procedure. Prolonged QT interval may predispose patients to arrhythmias, including torsades de pointes.

RELATED DRUGS: Other drugs that prolong the QTc (eg, quinidine, procainamide [eg, *Procanbid*], disopyramide [eg, *Norpace*], dofetilide [*Tikosyn*], sotalol [eg, *Betapace*]) also may interact with iohexol.

MANAGEMENT OPTIONS:

➡ *Monitor.* Monitor the electrocardiogram for prolongation of the QT interval when iohexol is administered to patients receiving drugs known to cause QT prolongation.

REFERENCES:
1. Goernig M, et al. Iohexol contrast medium induces QT prolongation in amiodarone patients. *Br J Clin Pharmacol.* 2004;58(1):96-98.

Amiodarone (eg, *Cordarone*)

Lidocaine (eg, *Xylocaine*)

SUMMARY: It appears that a minimal pharmacokinetic interaction occurs between lidocaine and amiodarone. Additive suppression of sinus node conduction may be possible when lidocaine is administered to patients being treated with amiodarone.

RISK FACTORS: No specific risk factors are known.

MECHANISM: Amiodarone and lidocaine depress the sinus node.

CLINICAL EVALUATION: A 64-year-old man with sick sinus syndrome developed severe sinus bradycardia following local anesthesia with 15 mL of lidocaine 2% while on amiodarone therapy (600 mg/day).[1] Another patient receiving lidocaine for an arrhythmia had an apparent 50% decrease in lidocaine clearance after amiodarone was administered.[2] Causation was not established in this report. In a study of 15 patients, 1 month of amiodarone (mean concentration, 1.8 mg/L [normal, 1 to 2.5 mg/L]) had no effect on the pharmacokinetics of a single dose of lidocaine.[3]

More study is needed to determine the presence of a pharmacodynamic interaction and its potential clinical significance.

RELATED DRUGS: No information is available.

MANAGEMENT OPTIONS: No specific action is required, but be alert for evidence of the interaction.

REFERENCES:
1. Keidar S, et al. Sinoatrial arrest due to lidocaine injection in sick sinus syndrome during amiodarone administration. *Am Heart J.* 1982;104(6):1384-1385.
2. Siegmund JB, et al. Amiodarone interaction with lidocaine. *J Cardiovasc Pharmacol.* 1993;21(4):513-515.
3. Nattel S, et al. Absence of pharmacokinetic interaction between amiodarone and lidocaine. *Am J Cardiol.* 1994;73(1):92-94.

Amiodarone (eg, *Cordarone*)

Methotrexate (eg, *Rheumatrex*)

SUMMARY: A patient stabilized on methotrexate for psoriasis developed skin erosions following the addition of amiodarone.

RISK FACTORS: No specific risk factors are known.

MECHANISM: Not established.

CLINICAL EVALUATION: A patient being treated with methotrexate 17.5 mg weekly for psoriasis received amiodarone for atrial fibrillation.[1] This patient received amiodarone 600 mg/day for 2 weeks at which time the psoriatic plaques became red, tender, and ulcerated, and many eroded together. The erosions healed following discontinuation of methotrexate. Causation was not established.

RELATED DRUGS: No information is available.

MANAGEMENT OPTIONS: No specific action is required, but be alert for evidence of the interaction.

REFERENCES:
1. Reynolds NJ, et al. Methotrexate induced skin necrosis: a drug interaction with amiodarone? *BMJ.* 1989;299(6705):980-981.

Amiodarone (eg, *Cordarone*)

Metoprolol (eg, *Lopressor*)

SUMMARY: Amiodarone administration can increase the plasma concentration of metoprolol and enhance its effects on cardiac conduction.

RISK FACTORS:

➡ *Pharmacogenetics.* Patients who are rapid metabolizers for CYP2D6 will have a larger reduction in metoprolol clearance during amiodarone coadministration than poor metabolizers.

MECHANISM: Amiodarone inhibits the metabolism of metoprolol via CYP2D6 and enhances its effects on cardiac conduction.

CLINICAL EVALUATION: The coadministration of amiodarone and metoprolol has been noted to result in a 2-fold increase in metoprolol plasma concentration.[1] In another study, the metoprolol plasma concentration dose ratio was increased by approximately 50% in patients receiving both drugs.[2] Case reports of patients experiencing bradycardia, hypotension, and cardiac arrest following coadministration of amiodarone and metoprolol or propranolol have been published.[3,4]

RELATED DRUGS: Other beta-blockers metabolized by CYP2D6 (eg, carvedilol [eg, *Coreg*], propranolol [eg, *Inderal LA*], timolol) are expected to interact in a similar manner with amiodarone. Dronedarone (*Multaq*) is also known to be an inhibitor of CYP2D6 and can increase the plasma concentration of metoprolol.

MANAGEMENT OPTIONS:

➡ *Consider Alternative.* Beta-blockers that are not substrates for CYP2D6, such as atenolol (eg, *Tenormin*), may have less risk of adverse reactions when administered with dronedarone, but carefully monitor patients nevertheless.

➡ *Monitor.* Monitor patients taking amiodarone and metoprolol for decreased heart rate and cardiac output.

REFERENCES:

1. Werner D, et al. Effect of amiodarone on the plasma levels of metoprolol. *Am J Cardiol.* 2004;94(10):1319-1321.

2. Fukumoto K, et al. Effect of amiodarone on the serum concentration/dose ratio of metoprolol in patients with cardiac arrhythmia. *Drug Metab Pharmacokinet.* 2006;21(6):501-505.

3. Leor J, et al. Amiodarone and beta-adrenergic blockers: an interaction with metoprolol but not with atenolol. *Am Heart J.* 1988;116(1, pt 1):206-207.

4. Derrida JP, et al. Amiodarone and propranolol, a dangerous combination? *Nouv Presse Med.* 1979;8(17):1429.

Amiodarone (eg, *Cordarone*)

Phenytoin (eg, *Dilantin*)

SUMMARY: The serum concentration of phenytoin can be increased considerably during concomitant amiodarone therapy and the serum concentration of amiodarone can be reduced by phenytoin coadministration.

RISK FACTORS: No specific risk factors are known.

MECHANISM: Amiodarone inhibits the hepatic metabolism of phenytoin, while phenytoin appears to increase the metabolism of amiodarone.

CLINICAL EVALUATION: The serum concentration of phenytoin in a patient stabilized on phenytoin 300 mg/day increased from 14.1 mcg/mL to 41 mcg/mL 4 weeks after the addition of amiodarone. Ataxia and nystagmus were noted. Five days after phenytoin was discontinued, the serum phenytoin concentration was 24.1 mcg/mL. Other reports have noted increased phenytoin serum concentrations (60% to approximately 200%) or reduced phenytoin clearance 2 to 4 weeks after amiodarone was administered.[1-4] Phenytoin protein binding was not changed by amiodarone administration. Five healthy subjects were administered amiodarone 200 mg/day for 7 weeks, and the serum amiodarone concentrations steadily increased during the first 5 weeks. When phenytoin was added during the final 2 weeks of the study, amiodarone serum concentrations decreased to approximately 35% to 50% below predicted values.[5] Similar results were obtained in subjects taking phenytoin for 2 weeks before and after 6 weeks of amiodarone 200 mg/day.[6]

RELATED DRUGS: Mephenytoin (*Mesantoin*) has been reported not to interact with amiodarone.

MANAGEMENT OPTIONS:

➡ *Monitor.* Patients being treated with phenytoin should have their phenytoin serum concentrations monitored carefully when amiodarone is added to or removed from their drug regimen. This drug interaction may take several weeks to become fully apparent. In addition, monitor patients taking amiodarone for reduced anti-arrhythmic efficacy, and monitor amiodarone serum concentrations if phenytoin is added to their drug regimen.

REFERENCES:

1. Gore JM, et al. Interaction of amiodarone and diphenylhydantoin. *Am J Cardiol.* 1984;54:1145.
2. MacGovern B, et al. Possible interaction between amiodarone and phenytoin. *Ann Intern Med.* 1984;101:650.
3. Shackleford EJ, et al. Amiodarone-phenytoin interaction. *Drug Intell Clin Pharm.* 1987;21:921.
4. Nolan PE Jr., et al. Pharmacokinetic interaction between intravenous phenytoin and amiodarone in healthy volunteers. *Clin Pharmacol Ther.* 1989;46:43.
5. Nolan PE, et al. Evidence for an effect of phenytoin on the pharmacokinetics of amiodarone. *J Clin Pharmacol.* 1990;30:1112.
6. Nolan PE, et al. Steady-state interaction between amiodarone and phenytoin in normal subjects. *Am J Cardiol.* 1990;65:1252.

Amiodarone (eg, *Cordarone*)

Procainamide (eg, *Procan SR*)

SUMMARY: Amiodarone increases procainamide concentrations and may enhance toxicity.

RISK FACTORS: No specific risk factors known.

MECHANISM: Amiodarone appears to inhibit both the hepatic and renal clearance of procainamide.

CLINICAL EVALUATION: Amiodarone 1200 mg/day for 5 to 7 days followed by 600 mg/day increased procainamide concentrations in 11 of 12 patients studied. The mean increase in procainamide concentration was 57%, and N-acetylprocainamide concentrations increased by 32%. Several patients developed signs of toxicity, such as arrhythmias and hypotension, within 5 days of concomitant use of amiodarone and procainamide.[2] A 23% reduction in single-dose IV procainamide clearance and a 38% increase in half-life were noted in 8 patients treated with amiodarone 1600 mg/day for 1 to 2 weeks.[1] Electrophysiologic effects appeared to be additive.

RELATED DRUGS: No information is available.

MANAGEMENT OPTIONS:

➡ *Circumvent/Minimize.* Procainamide dosages may need to be reduced by 25% to avoid toxicity.

➡ *Monitor.* Monitor procainamide concentrations and the patient observed for hypotension or arrhythmias when amiodarone is added to therapy.

REFERENCES:

1. Windle J, et al. Pharmacokinetic and electrophysiologic interaction of amiodarone and procainamide. *Clin Pharmacol Ther.* 1987;41:603.
2. Saal AK, et al. Effect of amiodarone on serum quinidine and procainamide levels. *Am J Cardiol.* 1984;53:1264.

Amiodarone (eg, *Cordarone*)

Quinidine (eg, *Quinora*)

SUMMARY: Amiodarone increases quinidine plasma concentrations, and the combination can excessively prolong cardiac conduction.

RISK FACTORS: No specific risk factors are known.

MECHANISM: Amiodarone appears to reduce quinidine clearance. A pharmacodynamic interaction resulting in prolonged myocardial conduction also may be involved.

CLINICAL EVALUATION: A patient on long-term quinidine therapy (1200 mg/day) developed atypical ventricular tachycardia (torsades de pointes) and a prolonged QT interval shortly after an injection of amiodarone.[1] These effects did not recur when quinidine was subsequently administered alone. Another patient receiving quinidine 1200 mg/day and amiodarone 200 mg/day developed atypical ventricular tachycardia following routine bicycle ergometry. Eleven patients receiving quinidine therapy were given amiodarone 1200 mg/day for 5 to 7 days followed by 600 mg/day. The plasma quinidine concentrations increased by approximately 32%.[2] Short-course quinidine therapy has been used in patients treated with chronic amiodarone for atrial fibrillation without precipitating ventricular tachycardia.[3] The pharmacokinetics of quinidine were not studied in patients receiving concurrent amiodarone.

RELATED DRUGS: No information is available.

MANAGEMENT OPTIONS:

➥ **Monitor.** When amiodarone is added to quinidine therapy, monitor the cardiac status (eg, QT interval prolongation) and plasma quinidine concentrations.

REFERENCES:

1. Tartini R, et al. Dangerous interaction between amiodarone and quinidine. *Lancet.* 1982;1:1327.
2. Saal AK, et al. Effect of amiodarone on serum quinidine and procainamide levels. *Am J Cardiol.* 1984;53:1264.
3. Kerin NZ, et al. The effectiveness and safety of the simultaneous administration of quinidine and amiodarone in the conversion of chronic atrial fibrillation. *Am Heart J.* 1993;125:1017.

Amiodarone (eg, *Cordarone*)

Rifampin (eg, *Rifadin*)

SUMMARY: Rifampin reduces amiodarone plasma concentrations; a reduction or loss of therapeutic efficacy may result.

RISK FACTORS: No specific risk factors are known.

MECHANISM: Rifampin appears to induce the metabolism of amiodarone, perhaps via CYP3A4, resulting in an increased clearance and lower serum concentration.

CLINICAL EVALUATION: A 33-year-old woman was treated with amiodarone 400 mg/day for atrial and ventricular arrhythmias.[1] Serum concentrations of amiodarone and its active metabolite desethylamiodarone (DEA) were 0.5 and 0.7 mg/L, respectively. Secondary to a methicillin-resistant staphylococcal infection, the patient was treated with doxycycline (eg, *Vibramycin*) 200 mg/day and rifampin 600 mg/day. No other drugs known to affect amiodarone metabolism were administered.

Six weeks after the addition of rifampin, the amiodarone concentration had fallen to 0.3 mg/L, and DEA was not detectable. The patient complained of palpitations; atrial arrhythmias were present. An increase in the amiodarone dose to 400 mg twice daily resulted in an amiodarone and DEA concentration of 0.4 and 0.6 mg/L, respectively. Following the discontinuation of rifampin, amiodarone and DEA concentrations increased to 1.2 and 1 mg/L, respectively. The amiodarone dose was later reduced to 600 mg/day, with resulting amiodarone and DEA concentrations of 1.3 and 1.7 mg/L, respectively. The administration of rifampin with amiodarone may result in a reduction of amiodarone's antiarrhythmic efficacy.

RELATED DRUGS: Rifabutin (*Mycobutin*) may affect amiodarone in a similar manner.

MANAGEMENT OPTIONS:

➥ *Consider Alternative.* An alternative antiarrhythmic agent could be considered for patients receiving rifampin. However, rifampin is known to induce the metabolism of quinidine (eg, *Quinora*), disopyramide (eg, *Norpace*), propafenone (*Rythmol*), and verapamil (eg, *Isoptin*).

➥ *Monitor.* Monitor amiodarone and DEA concentrations in patients receiving concurrent rifampin or rifabutin.

REFERENCES:
1. Zarembski DG, et al. Impact of rifampin on serum amiodarone concentrations in a patient with congenital heart disease. *Pharmacotherapy.* 1999;19:249-51.

Amiodarone (eg, *Cordarone*)

Simvastatin (*Zocor*)

SUMMARY: Amiodarone appears likely to increase the risk of simvastatin toxicity.

RISK FACTORS: No specific risk factors are known.

MECHANISM: Amiodarone is known to inhibit both CYP3A4 and CYP2D6. The first-pass metabolism of simvastatin is primarily via CYP3A4 while both enzymes contribute to the systemic metabolism of simvastatin.

CLINICAL EVALUATION: A patient with hypertension, hyperlipidemia, and diabetes mellitus was taking amiodarone 200 mg for 6 weeks and simvastatin 80 mg for nearly 4 weeks before being admitted with weakness, muscle pain, and dark urine.[1] Serum creatine kinase and myoglobin were elevated. Following discontinuation of simvastatin and amiodarone, the patient slowly improved over the next few weeks. Several other cases of rhabdomyolysis have been reported in patients taking simvastatin and amiodarone.[2,3]

RELATED DRUGS: The metabolism of lovastatin (eg, *Mevacor*) and, to a lesser extent, atorvastatin (*Lipitor*) may be reduced by amiodarone. Fluvastatin (*Lescol*) is metabolized by CYP2C9, an enzyme that also is inhibited by amiodarone.

MANAGEMENT OPTIONS:

➥ *Use Alternative.* Avoid the concurrent use of amiodarone and simvastatin. If amiodarone must be administered, select a statin that is not a CYP3A4 substrate. Pravastatin (*Pravachol*) and rosuvastatin (*Crestor*) are less likely to be affected by amiodarone.

REFERENCES:

1. Ricaurte B, et al. Simvastatin-amiodarone interaction resulting in rhabdomyolysis, azotemia, and possible hepatotoxicity. *Ann Pharmacother.* 2006;40:753-757.

2. Roten L, et al. Rhabdomyolysis in association with simvastatin and amiodarone. *Ann Pharmacother.* 2004;38:978-981.

3. de Denus S, et al. Amiodarone's role in simvastatin-associated rhabdomyolysis. *Am J Health Syst Pharm.* 2003;60:1791-1792.

Amiodarone (eg, *Cordarone*)

Sotalol (eg, *Betapace*)

SUMMARY: A patient given amiodarone following chronic sotalol therapy developed hypotension and bradycardia, but a causal relationship for an interaction between the drugs was not established.

RISK FACTORS: No specific risk factors are known.

MECHANISM: Not established. Sotalol may inhibit the normal compensatory response to amiodarone-induced vasodilation, resulting in enhanced hypotensive effects. Both drugs may slow the heart rate.

CLINICAL EVALUATION: A 59-year-old patient with nonsustained ventricular tachycardia was treated with sotalol 160 mg twice daily.[1] Because of increasing episodes of arrhythmia, sotalol was discontinued and, 4 hours later, an infusion of amiodarone 50 mg/hr was started. After 5 hours of the infusion, the patient became profoundly hypotensive, and her heart rate decreased to 60 beats/min. The amiodarone infusion was discontinued and inotropic agents were required for the next 18 hours. Oral amiodarone therapy was initiated 24 hours later without further hemodynamic instability. Rechallenge with sotalol and amiodarone was not attempted. Because amiodarone may produce hypotension, causation was not clearly established.

RELATED DRUGS: Beta-blockers, including metoprolol (eg, *Lopressor*) and propranolol (eg, *Inderal*), have been noted to produce bradycardia when administered with amiodarone.

MANAGEMENT OPTIONS:

➡ *Circumvent/Minimize.* Avoid the administration of amiodarone for several days in patients previously receiving drugs that depress myocardial conduction and contractility.

➡ *Monitor.* Until further information is available, carefully monitor patients receiving sotalol (and perhaps other beta-blockers) and amiodarone for hemodynamic depression.

REFERENCES:

1. Warren R, et al. Serious interaction of sotalol with amiodarone and flecainide. *Med J Aust.* 1990;152:277.

Amiodarone (eg, *Cordarone*)

Theophylline (eg, *Theo-24*)

SUMMARY: Amiodarone may increase the concentration of theophylline, resulting in toxicity.

RISK FACTORS: No specific risk factors are known.

MECHANISM: Amiodarone is known to be an enzyme inhibitor and may inhibit the metabolism of theophylline.

CLINICAL EVALUATION: The theophylline serum concentration in an 86-year-old man taking sustained-release theophylline 300 mg twice daily increased from 93.2 mmol/L (normal range, 55 to 110 mmol/L) to 194.2 mmol/L after amiodarone 600 mg/day was started.[1] Symptoms included tachycardia, nervousness, and tremors that resolved 2 days after theophylline was discontinued. The patient expired from a cardiorespiratory arrest before this potential interaction could be further evaluated.

RELATED DRUGS: No information is available.

MANAGEMENT OPTIONS:

➡ ***Monitor.*** Carefully observe patients maintained on theophylline for the development of theophylline toxicity (eg, nausea, tachycardia, nervousness, tremor, seizures) following the addition of amiodarone. One or more weeks may be required for the onset and offset of this interaction because of the long half-life of amiodarone.

REFERENCES:

1. Soto J, et al. Possible theophylline-amiodarone interaction. *DICP.* 1990;24:1115.

Amiodarone (eg, *Cordarone*)

Thioridazine   `AVOID`

SUMMARY: Amiodarone may increase thioridazine serum concentrations and produce additive prolongation of the QT interval, thus increasing the risk of ventricular arrhythmias; avoid concurrent use.

RISK FACTORS:

➡ ***Pharmacogenetics.*** Only patients with the extensive metabolizer CYP2D6 phenotype would be expected to experience increased thioridazine serum concentrations. Poor metabolizers do not have the gene for production of CYP2D6 and would likely already have high serum concentrations of thioridazine. Approximately 8% of whites are deficient in CYP2D6, but the deficiency is rare in Asians (usually 1% or less).

➡ ***Hypokalemia.*** The corrected QT interval (QTc) may be prolonged in patients with hypokalemia, thus increasing the risk of this interaction. Any other factor that may prolong the QTc interval increases the risk of this interaction.

MECHANISM: Amiodarone is an inhibitor of CYP2D6 and probably inhibits the hepatic metabolism of thioridazine. Also, amiodarone and thioridazine prolong the QT interval, and additive effects may be seen.

CLINICAL EVALUATION: In a double-blind, randomized, crossover study of the pharmaco-dynamic effects of thioridazine alone, 9 healthy subjects received single oral doses of thioridazine 10 and 50 mg compared with placebo.[1] The dose of thioridazine 50 mg increased the QTc on the electrocardiogram by 23 msec, and the 10 mg dose increased QTc by 9 msec. These results suggest that thioridazine produces a dose-related slowing of cardiac repolarization. Thus, drugs such as amiodarone that inhibit CYP2D6 are expected to reduce the metabolism of thioridazine and increase the risk of excessive prolongation of the QTc and ventricular arrhythmias. Although this interaction is based primarily on theoretical considerations, the potential severity of the interaction dictates that the combination should be avoided. Moreover, the manufacturer's product information for *Mellaril*† stated that combined use of thioridazine with CYP2D6 inhibitors or with drugs that pro-long the QT interval is contraindicated.[2] Amiodarone does both, so it clearly would be contraindicated based on the product information.

RELATED DRUGS: Other antiarrhythmics such as disopyramide (eg, *Norpace*), procain-amide (eg, *Procanbid*), and quinidine can increase the QT interval and may increase the risk of arrhythmias. Also, propafenone (eg, *Rythmol*) and quinidine are known inhibitors of CYP2D6 and may increase thioridazine serum concentra-tions. Although a number of antipsychotic drugs such as thioridazine have been shown to prolong the QT interval, clinical evidence suggests that thioridazine may produce the greatest risk.

MANAGEMENT OPTIONS:

➡ *AVOID COMBINATION.* Although the risk of this combination is not well established, it would be prudent to avoid concurrent use.

REFERENCES:

1. Hartigan-Go K, et al. Concentration-related pharmacodynamic effects of thioridazine and its metabo-lites in humans. *Clin Pharmacol Ther.* 1996;60:543-553.

2. 'Dear Doctor or Pharmacist' [letter]. East Hanover, NJ: Novartis Pharmaceuticals; July 7, 2000.

† Not available in the United States.

Amiodarone (eg, *Cordarone*)

Warfarin (eg, *Coumadin*)

SUMMARY: Amiodarone enhances the hypoprothrombinemic response to warfarin.

RISK FACTORS: No specific risk factors are known.

MECHANISM: Amiodarone reduces the metabolism of oral anticoagulants, probably by inhibiting CYP2C9. Amiodarone-induced hyperthyroidism can further enhance the anticoagulant effect because hyperthyroidism itself is associated with increased susceptibility to oral anticoagulant–induced hypoprothrombinemia. Amiodarone-induced hypothyroidism would tend to reduce warfarin effect.

CLINICAL EVALUATION: Patients on chronic warfarin or acenocoumarol therapy have expe-rienced excessive hypoprothrombinemia and bleeding episodes following initia-tion of amiodarone therapy.[1-3] Amiodarone can increase the prothrombin time or international normalized ratio (INR) 30% to 100%. Warfarin clearance may be reduced up to 65%, probably in a concentration-dependent manner.[3-5] These changes can lead to warfarin dose reductions of 25% to 40% or more as the amiodarone dosage is increased from 100 to 400 mg/day. Following the initiation of amiodarone therapy, the increased warfarin effect may begin within a week. Because of amiodarone's long half-life, up to 8 weeks may be required for the effect of amiodarone on warfarin to be fully expressed.[4,5] Similarly, many weeks may be required for the effect of amiodarone on warfarin to disappear after amiodarone is discontinued.

RELATED DRUGS: Acenocoumarol[†] interacts in a similar manner with amiodarone.

MANAGEMENT OPTIONS:

➥ *Circumvent/Minimize.* A decrease in the warfarin dose by 33% to 50% may be necessary to maintain the INR within the therapeutic range.

➥ *Monitor.* When amiodarone is administered to patients requiring oral anticoagulant therapy, carefully monitor the hypoprothrombinemic response. Because the onset and offset of this interaction is delayed, continue to closely monitor for 1 or 2 months following the initiation or discontinuation of amiodarone.

REFERENCES:

1. Hamer A, et al. The potentiation of warfarin anticoagulation by amiodarone. *Circulation.* 1982;65:1025-1029.
2. Fondevila C, et al. Amiodarone potentiates acenocoumarin. *Thromb Res.* 1989;53:203-208.
3. Sanoski CA, Bauman JL. Clinical observations with the amiodarone/warfarin interaction: dosing relationships with long-term therapy. *Chest.* 2002;121:19-23.
4. O'Reilly RA, et al. Interaction of amiodarone with racemic warfarin and its separated enantiomorphs in humans. *Clin Pharmacol Ther.* 1987;42:290-294.
5. Kerin NZ, et al. The incidence, magnitude, and time course of the amiodarone-warfarin interaction. *Arch Intern Med.* 1988;148:1779-1781.

† Not available in the United States.

Amitriptyline (eg, *Elavil*)

Bethanidine

SUMMARY: Amitriptyline and other tricyclic antidepressants (TCAs) inhibit the antihypertensive effect of bethanidine.

RISK FACTORS: No specific risk factors are known.

MECHANISM: TCAs probably inhibit the uptake of bethanidine by adrenergic neurons.[3]

CLINICAL EVALUATION: Amitriptyline,[5] desipramine (*Norpramin*),[2,4] and imipramine (*Tofranil*)[5] have been shown to reduce bethanidine's antihypertensive effect in several patients. The antagonism occurs fairly rapidly (within a few hours) and lasts for several days following discontinuation of desipramine. In a preliminary report, doxepin (*Adapin*) antagonized the antihypertensive effect of bethanidine, but the effect was not marked and developed slowly.[1] Desipramine is apparently a stronger antagonist of bethanidine than doxepin, even at doxepin doses of 300 mg/day.[1]

RELATED DRUGS: Desipramine and imipramine have been shown to reduce bethanidine's antihypertensive effect. Assume that all TCAs inhibit bethanidine effect until proven otherwise. TCAs also may inhibit the antihypertensive effect of clonidine (*Catapres*), guanabenz (*Wytensin*), guanethidine (*Ismelin*), guanfacine (*Tenex*), guanadrel (*Hylorel*), and debrisoquin. The effect of selective serotonin reuptake inhibitors on bethanidine is not established.

MANAGEMENT OPTIONS:

➡ *Use Alternative.* Avoid combined therapy with TCAs and bethanidine. Doxepin might be less likely to interact than other TCAs. If tricyclics are to be used, consider selecting an alternative antihypertensive agent. But, keep in mind that TCAs also may inhibit the effect of clonidine, guanabenz, guanfacine, guanethidine, and debrisoquin.

REFERENCES:

1. Oates JA, et al. Effect of doxepin on the norepinephrine pump. A preliminary report. *Psychosomatics.* 1969;10:12.

2. Mitchell JR, et al. Antagonism of the antihypertensive action of guanethidine sulfate by desipramine hydrochloride. *JAMA.* 1967;202:973.

3. Feagin OT, et al. Uptake and release of guanethidine and bethanidine by the adrenergic neuron. *J Clin Invest.* 1969;48:23a.

4. Mitchell JR, et al. Guanethidine and related agents. III. Antagonism by drugs which inhibit the norepinephrine pump in man. *J Clin Invest.* 1970;49:1596.

5. Skinner C, et al. Antagonism of the hypotensive action of bethanidine and debrisoquine by tricyclic antidepressants. *Lancet.* 1969;2:564.

4   Amitriptyline (*Elavil*)

Chlordiazepoxide (eg, *Librium*)

SUMMARY: Isolated case reports indicate that chlordiazepoxide may increase tricyclic antidepressant (TCA) side effects, but a causal relationship is not established.

RISK FACTORS: No specific risk factors are known.

MECHANISM: The drugs probably exhibit additive CNS depressant effects.

CLINICAL EVALUATION: Additive sedation or enhanced atropine-like effects may occur with concomitant use of chlordiazepoxide and a TCA. Several case reports have appeared describing this interaction;[1-3] however, the drugs have been used concomitantly in clinical trials without mention of serious complications. Thus, it would appear that if the interaction does occur, it is clinically important in a very small proportion of patients and is not especially severe. Kline[4] states that it is safe to combine chlordiazepoxide with TCAs.

RELATED DRUGS: Most studies indicate that TCA plasma concentrations are not affected by the administration of benzodiazepines such as diazepam (eg, *Valium*), chlordiazepoxide, or nitrazepam (*Mogadon*).[5,6]

MANAGEMENT OPTIONS: No specific action is required, but be alert for evidence of the interaction.

REFERENCES:

1. Abdou FA. Elavil-Librium combination. *Am J Psychiatry.* 1964;120:1204.

2. Kane FJ Jr, et al. A toxic reaction to combined Elavil-Librium therapy. *Am J Psychiatry.* 1963;119:1179.

3. Beresford TP, et al. Adverse reactions to a benzodiazepine-tricyclic antidepressant compound. *J Clin Psychopharmacol.* 1981;1:392.

4. Kline NS. Psychochemotherapeutic drug combinations (Questions and Answers). *JAMA.* 1969;210:1928.

5. Gram LF, et al. Influence of neuroleptics and benzodiazepines on metabolism of tricyclic antidepressants in man. *Am J Psychiatry.* 1974;131:863.

6. Moody JP, et al. Pharmacokinetic aspects of protriptyline plasma levels. *Eur J Clin Pharmacol.* 1977;11:51.

Amitriptyline (*Elavil*)

Cigarette Smoking

SUMMARY: Smokers may have lower plasma concentrations of various tricyclic antidepressants (TCAs), but the clinical importance is not established.

RISK FACTORS: No specific risk factors are known.

MECHANISM: Not established. Cigarette smoking may enhance the hepatic metabolism of some TCAs.

CLINICAL EVALUATION: Although no difference in the steady-state plasma concentrations of nortriptyline was observed between smokers and nonsmokers in one study,[1] two subsequent studies involving large numbers of patients demonstrated lower plasma concentrations of amitriptyline, desipramine (*Norpramin*), imipramine (*Tofranil*), and nortriptyline (*Pamelor*) in smokers.[2,3] Smokers may have a higher percentage of unbound plasma nortriptyline than nonsmokers.[4] Thus, it is possible that the plasma concentration of unbound antidepressant is not significantly affected, even though the total plasma level may be reduced. Although a precise relationship between TCA plasma concentrations and therapeutic effect is not established, the magnitude of the decreases in plasma drug concentrations associated with smoking appears large enough to decrease antidepressant efficacy in some patients. Since it is likely that the enhanced metabolism of TCAs in smokers is caused by substances in smoke other than nicotine, patients who switch from cigarette smoking to nicotine gum or patches theoretically may manifest an increase in their plasma TCA concentrations.

RELATED DRUGS: Two studies demonstrated reduced desipramine, imipramine, and nortriptyline concentrations in smokers.[2,3]

MANAGEMENT OPTIONS: No specific action is required, but be alert for evidence of the interaction.

REFERENCES:

1. Norman TR, et al. Cigarette smoking and plasma nortriptyline levels. *Clin Pharmacol Ther.* 1977;21:453.
2. Linnoila M, et al. Effect of alcohol consumption and cigarette smoking on antidepressant levels of depressed patients. *Am J Psychiatry.* 1981;138:841.
3. Perel JM, et al. Pharmacodynamics of imipramine and clinical outcome in depressed patients. In: Gottschalk L, Merlis S, eds. *Pharmacokinetics of Psychoactive Drugs.* New York: Spectrum; 1975:186–98.
4. Perry PJ, et al. The effects of smoking on nortriptyline plasma levels in depressed patients. *Drug Intell Clin Pharm.* 1983;17:449.

Amitriptyline (*Elavil*)

Disulfiram (*Antabuse*)

SUMMARY: Combined use of amitriptyline and disulfiram has resulted in isolated cases of dementia, but a causal relationship is not established.

RISK FACTORS: No specific risk factors are known.

MECHANISM: Not established. Disulfiram is known to inhibit cytochrome P450 isozymes (eg, CYP1A2, CYP2C9), so it is possible that it inhibits the hepatic metabolism of some tricyclic antidepressants (TCAs).

CLINICAL EVALUATION: Two patients on disulfiram therapy developed acute organic brain syndrome following the addition of amitriptyline therapy.[1] Symptoms included confusion, disorientation, hallucinations, and memory loss, but a cause and effect relationship between the drug interaction and the symptoms was not established. Also, amitriptyline is said to enhance the alcohol reaction in patients taking disulfiram.[2-5] However, controlled studies are needed to confirm this finding.

RELATED DRUGS: The effect of disulfiram on other TCAs is not established.

MANAGEMENT OPTIONS: No specific action is required, but be alert for evidence of the interaction.

REFERENCES:
1. Maany I, et al. Possible toxic interaction between disulfiram and amitriptyline. *Arch Gen Psychiatry.* 1982;39:743.
2. Pullar-Strecker H. Drug interactions in alcoholism treatment. *Lancet.* 1969;1:735.
3. MacCallum WAG. Drug interactions in alcoholism treatment. *Lancet.* 1969;1:313.
4. Burnett GB, et al. Drug interactions in alcoholism treatment. *Lancet.* 1969;1:415.
5. Glatt MM. Drug interactions in alcoholism treatment. *Lancet.* 1969;1:627.

 Amitriptyline

Donepezil (eg, *Aricept*)

SUMMARY: Amitriptyline has anticholinergic properties and may inhibit the therapeutic effect of donepezil in Alzheimer disease.

RISK FACTORS: No specific risk factors are known.

MECHANISM: Donepezil is a cholinesterase inhibitor and its efficacy is likely to be inhibited by anticholinergic agents, such as amitriptyline.[1]

CLINICAL EVALUATION: In a preliminary study of 69 patients with Alzheimer disease receiving donepezil 10 mg/day and followed for 2 years, 16 patients received concurrent therapy with anticholinergic drugs and 53 patients did not.[2] Mental functioning, as measured by the Mini-Mental State Exam (MMSE), was significantly lower in the patients receiving concomitant anticholinergic drugs. Also, the French Pharmacovigilance Database received 118 spontaneous reports of adverse effects in patients receiving anticholinergic drugs with cholinesterase inhibitors (donepezil, galantamine, rivastigmine). After evaluation by clinical pharmacologists, 24 were thought to be adverse drug interactions.[3] Although additional study is needed to establish the clinical importance of these interactions, the evidence is consistent with the known pharmacological effects of the drugs.

RELATED DRUGS: All cholinesterase inhibitors used to treat Alzheimer disease (donepezil, galantamine [eg, *Razadyne*], rivastigmine [eg, *Exelon*]) are expected to interact similarly with amitriptyline, as well as other antidepressants with anticholinergic effects, such as clomipramine (eg, *Anafranil*), doxepin (eg, *Silenor*), imipramine (eg, *Tofranil*), nortriptyline (eg, *Aventyl*), protriptyline (eg, *Vivactil*), and trimipramine (eg, *Surmontil*).

MANAGEMENT OPTIONS:

➥ **Consider Alternative.** Use an alternative to the amitriptyline. Antidepressants with little or no anticholinergic activity include bupropion (*Wellbutrin*), mirtazapine

(*Remeron*), trazodone (*Desyrel*), selective serotonin reuptake inhibitors as a class, and serotonin-norepinephrine reuptake inhibitors as a class.

➡ **Monitor.** If amitriptyline (or other anticholinergic antidepressant) is used with done-pezil or other cholinesterase inhibitors, be alert for evidence of reduced mental functioning.

REFERENCES:

1. *Aricept* [package insert]. New York, NY: Pfizer; 2011.
2. Lu CJ, Tune LE. Chronic exposure to anticholinergic medications adversely affects the course of Alzheimer disease. *Am J Geriatr Psychiatry.* 2003;11(4):458-461.
3. Tavassoli N, et al. Drug interactions with cholinesterase inhibitors: an analysis of the French Pharma-covigilance Database and a comparison of two national drug formularies (Vidal, British National Formulary). *Drug Saf.* 2007;30(11):1063-1071.

Amitriptyline (eg, *Elavil*)

Ethanol (Ethyl Alcohol)

SUMMARY: Combined use of ethanol and tricyclic antidepressants (TCAs), such as amitriptyline, may result in additive impairment of motor skills; abstinent alcoholics may eliminate TCAs more rapidly than nonalcoholics.

RISK FACTORS: No specific risk factors are known.

MECHANISM: The mechanisms for this interaction are: 1) Depression of the CNS by combined cyclics and ethanol may account for the additive adverse effects on psychomotor performance.[1,2] 2) Acute ethanol ingestion may inhibit the first-pass hepatic metabolism of cyclic antidepressants.[3] 3) Prolonged intake of large amounts of alcohol appears to stimulate the hepatic metabolism of cyclic antidepressants.[4,5] 4) The anticholinergic effect of cyclic antidepressants may delay gastric emptying, thus delaying the absorption of ethanol.[6]

CLINICAL EVALUATION: Amitriptyline adds to the deleterious effect of ethanol on motor skill tests early in the course of therapy.[7-9] In 6 subjects, a modest amount of ethanol (0.5 mL/kg) produced additive impairment of manual dexterity when combined with single doses of amitriptyline 50 mg or trazodone (eg, *Desyrel*) 100 mg.[10] GI complications of cyclic antidepressants are reportedly more frequent when ethanol is consumed concomitantly.[11] In a study of the pharmacokinetics of imipramine and desipramine in 15 recently detoxified alcoholics and 14 healthy subjects, imipramine (eg, *Tofranil*) clearance was 3 times higher in the detoxified alcoholics than in the nonalcoholics.[4] Desipramine (eg, *Norpramin*) elimination also was increased in the detoxified alcoholics, but not to the same degree as imipramine. Amitriptyline elimination may be enhanced in alcoholic patients.[5] The magnitude of the increases in TCA elimination in abstinent alcoholics appears large enough to increase antidepressant dosage requirements in such patients (especially with imipramine). It is not known how long the effect of ethanol on TCA metabolism persists, but it seems unlikely that it would last more than a few months.

RELATED DRUGS: Doxepin (eg, *Sinequan*) adds to the deleterious effect of ethanol on motor skills.[7-9] However, the evidence for doxepin is conflicting; some evidence suggests that it is less likely to interact.[12] Trazodone also produced additive impairment of manual dexterity in the presence of alcohol.[10] Nortriptyline (eg, *Pamelor*) and clomipramine (eg, *Anafranil*) are less sedating than amitriptyline, which may account for reports that they are less likely to enhance the adverse effects of ethanol on psychomotor skills.[6] Imipramine and desipramine elimination is increased in detoxified alcoholics.[4,5]

MANAGEMENT OPTIONS:

➡ *Circumvent/Minimize.* Inform patients receiving tricyclic or related antidepressants that ethanol may produce a greater-than-expected impairment in psychomotor skills, especially during the first week of treatment. This warning probably is more important for the more sedative tricyclics, such as amitriptyline and, possibly, doxepin.

➡ *Monitor.* In abstinent alcoholics, monitor for an inadequate antidepressant effect and adjust the antidepressant dosage as needed. Measurement of antidepressant serum concentrations may be useful in selected cases.

REFERENCES:

1. Lockett MF, et al. Combining the antidepressant drugs. *BMJ.* 1965;1:921.
2. Laurie W. Alcohol as a cause of sudden unexpected death. *Med J Aust.* 1971;1:1224-1227.
3. Dorian P, et al. Amitriptyline and ethanol: pharmacokinetic and pharmacodynamic interaction. *Eur J Clin Pharmacol.* 1983;25:325-331.
4. Ciraulo DA, et al. Clinical pharmacokinetics of imipramine and desipramine in alcoholics and normal volunteers. *Clin Pharmacol Ther.* 1988;43:509-518.
5. Sandoz M, et al. Biotransformation of amitriptyline in alcoholic depressive patients. *Eur J Clin Pharmacol.* 1983;24:615-621.
6. Hall RC, et al. The effect of desmethylimipramine on the absorption of alcohol and paracetamol. *Postgrad Med J.* 1976;52:139-142.
7. Landauer AA, et al. Alcohol and amitriptyline effects on skills related to driving behavior. *Science.* 1969;163:1467-1468.
8. Seppala T, et al. Effect of tricyclic antidepressants and alcohol on psychomotor skills related to driving. *Clin Pharmacol Ther.* 1975;17:515-522.
9. Seppala T. Psychomotor skills during acute and two-week treatment with mianserin (ORG GB 94) and amitriptyline, and their combined effects with alcohol. *Ann Clin Res.* 1977;9:66-72.
10. Warrington SJ, et al. Evaluation of possible interactions between ethanol and trazodone or amitriptyline. *Neuropsychobiology.* 1986;15(Suppl 1):31-37.
11. Milner G. Gastrointestinal side effects and psychotropic drugs. *Med J Aust.* 1969;2:153-155. Review.
12. Milner G, et al. The effects of doxepin, alone and together with alcohol, in relation to driving safety. *Med J Aust.* 1973;1:837-841.

Amitriptyline (eg, *Elavil*)

Fluconazole (*Diflucan*)

SUMMARY: Fluconazole repeatedly resulted in syncope in a boy receiving amitriptyline, but it is not known how often this combination would result in adverse effects.

RISK FACTORS: No specific risk factors are known.

MECHANISM: Not established. Fluconazole inhibits CYP2C19 and CYP3A4 and may reduce the hepatic metabolism of amitriptyline.

CLINICAL EVALUATION: A 12-year-old boy on amitriptyline 100 mg/day developed several episodes of syncope, beginning 4 days after starting fluconazole 200 mg/day.[1] Later, after the amitriptyline dose was increased to 150 mg/day, fluconazole 200 mg/day was again started. Four days later he again lost consciousness, but the episode resolved spontaneously. Subsequent episodes of syncope occurred when fluconazole was given in the presence of amitriptyline. Because the patient had received fluconazole and amitriptyline alone without syncope, it appears that the episodes were caused by the combined effects of amitriptyline and fluconazole. Although this case was well documented, additional clinical information is needed to assess the incidence and magnitude of this interaction.

RELATED DRUGS: Other tricyclic antidepressants are metabolized by CYP2C19 or CYP3A4; theoretically, these may interact with fluconazole, but little clinical information is available.

MANAGEMENT OPTIONS:

➤ *Monitor.* Monitor for altered amitriptyline effect if fluconazole is initiated, discontinued, or changed in dosage.

REFERENCES:

1. Robinson RF, et al. Syncope associated with concurrent amitriptyline and fluconazole therapy. *Ann Pharmacother*. 2000;34:1406-1409.

Amitriptyline (eg, *Elavil*)

Fluoxetine (eg, *Prozac*)

SUMMARY: Fluoxetine increases amitriptyline serum concentrations and markedly increases the serum concentrations of its active metabolite, nortriptyline. The death of a man was attributed to fluoxetine-induced amitriptyline toxicity, but a causal relationship was not established.

RISK FACTORS: No specific risk factors are known.

MECHANISM: Fluoxetine appears to inhibit the metabolism of amitriptyline and its active metabolite, nortriptyline, by hepatic CYP2D6.

CLINICAL EVALUATION: A steady-state study of patients on amitriptyline and fluoxetine reported a 2-fold increase in amitriptyline levels and a 9-fold increase in nortriptyline levels compared with patients receiving the same dose of amitriptyline without fluoxetine.[1] A 36-year-old man died at home approximately 6 weeks after he started taking amitriptyline 150 mg/day and fluoxetine 40 mg/day.[2] The death did not appear to be a suicide, and it was proposed that the fatal event was a cardiac arrhythmia from fluoxetine-induced toxic amitriptyline serum concentrations. The explanation is certainly plausible, but it is difficult to establish a causal relationship with certainty since the body was not found until several weeks after his death.

RELATED DRUGS: Because fluoxetine-induced inhibition of CYP2D6 is the likely mechanism, one would expect paroxetine (*Paxil*), which is also a potent CYP2D6 inhibitor, to interact with amitriptyline in a similar manner. Sertraline (*Zoloft*) is only a weak CYP2D6 inhibitor and would theoretically be less likely to interact. Fluvoxamine (eg, *Luvox*) has little or no effect on CYP2D6, but its ability to inhibit other cytochrome P450 isozymes might affect the metabolism of tricyclic antidepressants.

MANAGEMENT OPTIONS:

➤ *Monitor.* Although combinations of tricyclic antidepressants and selective serotonin reuptake inhibitors are frequently used with positive results, the patient's response to the tricyclic antidepressant must be carefully monitored if a selective serotonin reuptake inhibitor is initiated, discontinued, or changed in dosage.

REFERENCES:

1. el-Yazigi A, et al. Steady-state kinetics of fluoxetine and amitriptyline in patients treated with a combination of these drugs as compared with those treated with amitriptyline alone. *J Clin Pharmacol.* 1995;35:17-21.

2. Preskorn SH, et al. Fatality associated with combined fluoxetine-amitriptyline therapy. *JAMA.* 1997;277:1682.

Amitriptyline (eg, *Elavil*)

Guanfacine (eg, *Tenex*)

SUMMARY: Limited clinical information and theoretical considerations suggest that tricyclic antidepressants (TCAs) can inhibit the antihypertensive response to guanfacine.

RISK FACTORS: No specific risk factors are known.

MECHANISM: Not established.

CLINICAL EVALUATION: Because guanfacine, like clonidine (*Catapres*), is a centrally acting alpha$_2$-agonist, one would expect that TCAs inhibit the antihypertensive response to guanfacine and exacerbate the hypertensive response following withdrawal of guanfacine. A 38-year-old woman well controlled on guanfacine 2 mg at night started taking amitriptyline 75 mg for neuralgia.[1] Her blood pressure increased over the next week and returned to former levels within 2 weeks after amitriptyline was discontinued. A later trial of imipramine (*Tofranil*) 50 mg/day also was associated with an increase in blood pressure that returned to baseline when imipramine was discontinued. The magnitude of the increases in diastolic and systolic blood pressure in this patient was not especially large (usually approximately 8 to 12 mm Hg). Although this would not adversely affect most patients in the short term, such an increase would not be desirable over months or years. Moreover, the doses of TCAs used in this patient were considerably less than many patients with depression receive; larger doses of TCAs may produce a greater inhibition of the antihypertensive response.

RELATED DRUGS: Theoretically, any combination of a TCA and a centrally acting alpha agonist (eg, clonidine [eg, *Catapres*], guanabenz [eg, *Wytensin*]) would interact.

MANAGEMENT OPTIONS:

➡ *Consider Alternative.* If tricyclics are to be used, consider selecting an alternative antihypertensive agent. But, keep in mind that TCAs also may inhibit the effect of clonidine, guanabenz, guanethidine, bethanidine, and debrisoquin.

➡ *Monitor.* Until more clinical evidence is available, monitor for reduced antihypertensive response when TCAs are added to guanfacine therapy. If guanfacine is withdrawn in the presence of TCAs, monitor for exaggerated rebound hypertension.

REFERENCES:

1. Buckley M, et al. Antagonism of antihypertensive effect of guanfacine by tricyclic antidepressants. *Lancet.* 1991;337:1173-1174.

Amitriptyline (*Elavil*)

Isoproterenol (*Isuprel*)

SUMMARY: Isolated case reports indicate that the combined use of isoproterenol and tricyclic antidepressants (TCAs) may predispose patients to cardiac arrhythmias, but the clinical importance of this interaction is not established.

RISK FACTORS:

➤ ***Dosage Regimen.*** It is possible that the risk is primarily in patients who take large doses of isoproterenol.

MECHANISM: Not established. Both drugs, especially in high doses, are known to increase the risk of arrhythmias in predisposed patients.

CLINICAL EVALUATION: A patient taking amitriptyline and isoproterenol concurrently died secondary to complications of a cardiac arrhythmia.[1] Although the cause of death was attributed to the combined effects of these 2 drugs, the patient apparently was using excessive quantities of isoproterenol before the onset of the arrhythmia. Thus, it is difficult to ascertain whether the death resulted from the isoproterenol alone or from the isoproterenol-amitriptyline combination. In a study of the effects of isoproterenol with and without TCA pretreatment, there was little evidence for an interaction, although 1 of the 4 patients developed tachycardia while on the combination.[2]

RELATED DRUGS: Little is known regarding the effect of beta agonists other than isoproterenol (eg, albuterol [eg, *Proventil*], metaproterenol [*Alupent*], terbutaline [eg, *Brethaire*]) in patients receiving TCAs. To the extent that these agents have less cardiac effects than isoproterenol, one would expect a reduced likelihood of cardiac interactions with TCAs.

MANAGEMENT OPTIONS:

➤ ***Circumvent/Minimize.*** Avoid excessive use of isoproterenol or other beta-agonists in any case, but it may be particularly important in patients receiving TCAs.

➤ ***Monitor.*** Although this interaction is not well documented, it would be prudent to monitor for cardiac arrhythmias if isoproterenol or other beta-agonists (especially in large doses) are used with TCAs.

REFERENCES:
1. Kadar D. Amitriptyline and isoproterenol: fatal drug combinations. *Can Med Assoc J.* 1975;112:556.
2. Boakes AJ, et al. Interactions between sympathomimetic amines and antidepressant agents in man. *BMJ.* 1973;1:311.

Amitriptyline (*Elavil*)

Lithium (eg, *Eskalith*)

SUMMARY: Although lithium and tricyclic antidepressants (TCAs) are frequently used together with good results, there is some evidence that their concurrent use may increase the risk for neurotoxicity (eg, tremors, ataxia, seizures), particularly in the elderly.

RISK FACTORS:

➤ ***Effects of Age.*** Elderly patients may be at higher risk.

MECHANISM: Not established. The neurotoxicity may be a result of combined effects of lithium and TCAs on certain neurotransmitters in the brain. Both lithium and TCAs lower the seizure threshold; an additive effect is possible.

CLINICAL EVALUATION: Lithium and TCAs are frequently used together with good results and without excessive adverse effects in patients with refractory depression and panic disorder.[1-3,7] However, there is some evidence that some elderly patients may not tolerate this combination as well as younger patients. In 1 uncontrolled study of 9 patients given combined lithium antidepressant therapy, the 5 patients under age 65 tolerated the combination well, while severe neurologic side effects (requiring discontinuation of lithium) developed in 4 elderly patients.[4] The toxicity included symptoms such as tremor, memory difficulties, disorganized thinking, and ataxia. However, given the lack of controls, one cannot rule out the possibility that the reactions were caused by lithium alone. Others also have reported neurological side effects in geriatric patients on lithium and antidepressants.[5] Also, a patient on 300 mg/day of amitriptyline developed grand mal seizures after the addition of 900 mg/day of lithium (plasma lithium concentration (0.8 to 0.9 mEq/L).[6] The seizures recurred following rechallenge.

RELATED DRUGS: TCAs other than amitriptyline probably have a similar effect when combined with lithium.

MANAGEMENT OPTIONS:

➥ *Circumvent/Minimize.* Limited information suggests that using low doses of lithium may reduce the risk of neurotoxicity in geriatric patients without compromising its therapeutic effect.

➥ *Monitor.* Until further information is available, cautiously use lithium and TCAs in elderly patients. Monitor for evidence of neurotoxicity such as tremors, disorders of mentation, ataxia, and seizures.

REFERENCES:

1. Price LH, et al. Variability of response to lithium augmentation in refractory depression. *Am J Psychiatry.* 1986;143:1387.
2. Feder R. Lithium augmentation of clomipramine. *J Clin Psychiatry.* 1988;49:11.
3. Camara EG. Lithium potentiation of antidepressant treatment in panic disorder. *J Clin Psychopharmacol.* 1990;10:225.
4. Austin LS, et al. Toxicity resulting from lithium augmentation of antidepressant treatment in elderly patients. *J Clin Psychiatry.* 1990;51:344.
5. Lafferman J, et al. Lithium augmentation for treatment-resistant depression in the elderly. *J Geriatric Psychiatry Neurol.* 1988;1:49.
6. Solomon JG. Seizures during lithium-amitriptyline therapy. *Postgrad Med.* 1979;66:145.
7. Kushnir SL. Lithium: antidepressant combinations in the treatment of depressed, physically ill geriatric patients. *Am J Psychiatry.* 1986;143:378.

 Amitriptyline (eg, *Elavil*)

Methyldopa (eg, *Aldomet*)

SUMMARY: The bulk of the evidence indicates that tricyclic antidepressants (TCAs) have minimal effects on the antihypertensive response to methyldopa.

RISK FACTORS: No specific risk factors are known.

MECHANISM: Not established.

CLINICAL EVALUATION: A hypertensive patient controlled on methyldopa therapy developed worsening of the hypertension when amitriptyline also was given.[1] In animal studies, TCAs have been shown to block hypotensive responses to methyldopa.[2-4] This is in contrast to reports in humans. Most patients on methyldopa do not seem to be adversely affected by TCAs; however, certain predisposed patients may manifest decreased control of hypertension.

RELATED DRUGS: Desipramine (*Norpramin*) 75 mg/day did not antagonize the hypotensive effect of methyldopa in 3 patients.[5] Moreover, it did not affect the response to a single 750 mg dose of methyldopa in 5 healthy subjects.[6] The effect of other TCAs on methyldopa is not established.

MANAGEMENT OPTIONS: No specific action is required, but be alert for evidence of the interaction.

REFERENCES:

1. White AG. Methyldopa and amitriptyline. *Lancet*. 1965;2:441.
2. Kale AK, et al. Modification of the central hypotensive effect of alpha-methyldopa by reserpine, imipramine and tranylcypromine. *Eur J Pharmacol*. 1970;9:120-123.
3. van Spanning HW, et al. The interaction between alpha-methyldopa and tricyclic antidepressants. *Int J Pharmacol Biopharm*. 1975;11:65-67.
4. van Zwieten PA. Interaction between centrally acting hypotensive drugs and tricyclic antidepressants. *Arch Int Pharmacodyn Ther*. 1975;214:12-30.
5. Mitchell JR, et al. Guanethidine and related agents. Antagonism by drugs which inhibit the norepinephrine pump in man. *J Clin Invest*. 1970;49:1596-1604.
6. Reid JL, et al. The effects of desmethylimipramine on the pharmacological actions of alpha-methyldopa in man. *Eur J Clin Pharmacol*. 1979;16:75-80.

Amitriptyline (eg, *Elavil*)
Orlistat (*Xenical*)

SUMMARY: Orlistat did not affect amitriptyline pharmacokinetics in healthy subjects.

RISK FACTORS: No specific risk factors are known.

MECHANISM: None (no interaction).

CLINICAL EVALUATION: In a randomized crossover study in 20 healthy subjects, orlistat (120 mg 3 times daily for 6 days), did not affect amitriptyline pharmacokinetics.

RELATED DRUGS: No information available.

MANAGEMENT OPTIONS: No interaction.

REFERENCES:

1. Zhi J, et al. Pharmacokinetic evaluation of the possible interaction between selected concomitant medications and orlistat at steadystate in healthy subjects. *J Clin Pharmacol*. 2002;42:1011-1019.

Amitriptyline (eg, *Elavil*)

Propantheline (eg, *Pro-Banthine*)

SUMMARY: Combined use of anticholinergic tricyclic antidepressants (TCAs) such as amitriptyline and anticholinergics such as propantheline may result in excessive anticholinergic effects.

RISK FACTORS:

➡ **Effects of Age.** The elderly possibly are at greater risk.

MECHANISM: TCAs may display additive anticholinergic effects with other drugs having anticholinergic activity.[1,2]

CLINICAL EVALUATION: Combined use of TCAs and other anticholinergics is not uncommon, at least in the elderly.[3] The adverse effects of excessive cholinergic blockade usually are minor (eg, dry mouth, constipation). However, consider the possibility of precipitating adynamic ileus, urinary retention, or acute glaucoma, especially in older patients.

RELATED DRUGS: Additive anticholinergic effects are more likely to be associated with TCAs possessing significant anticholinergic activity (eg, amitriptyline, nortriptyline [*Pamelor*], imipramine [*Tofranil*], trimipramine [*Surmontil*], doxepin [*Sinequan*], and maprotiline [*Ludiomil*]). Antidepressants with modest anticholinergic effects (eg, trazodone [*Desyrel*], protriptyline [*Vivactil*], desipramine [*Norpramin*], and amoxapine [*Asendin*]) are less likely to interact. Nevertheless, 1 patient receiving an anticholinergic (isopropamide iodide) developed acute urinary retention on 2 occasions when trazodone was taken.[4] A number of other drugs (eg, antihistamines, neuroleptics, disopyramide [*Norpace*], antiparkinsonian drugs, glutethimide, and meperidine [*Demerol*]) possess anticholinergic activity.

MANAGEMENT OPTIONS:

➡ **Consider Alternative.** If additive anticholinergic effects become troublesome, consider use of an antidepressant with low anticholinergic activity. Also, an alternative drug often can be found for the agent that is adding to the anticholinergic effect of the TCA.

➡ **Circumvent/Minimize.** A method has been described by which drug-induced dry mouth may be treated with a pilocarpine syrup.[5] Pyridoxine may prevent some of the anticholinergic side effects of TCAs.[6]

➡ **Monitor.** Serious complications are unlikely to occur if alert to the possibility of excessive anticholinergic activity.

REFERENCES:

1. Kessell A, et al. Side effects with a new hypnotic: drug potentiation. *Med J Aust.* 1967;2:1194.
2. Milner G. Gastro-intestinal side effects and psychotropic drugs. *Med J Aust.* 1969;2:153-155.
3. Blazer DG, et al. The risk of anticholinergic toxicity in the elderly: a study of prescribing practices in two populations. *J Gerontol.* 1983;38:31-35.
4. Chan CH, et al. Anticholinergic side effects of trazodone combined with another pharmacologic agent. *Am J Psychiatry.* 1990;147:533.
5. Ayd FJ. Rx tip: relieving drug-induced oral and pharyngeal dryness. *Int Drug Ther Newsl.* 1967;2:24.
6. Arnold SE, et al. Tricyclic antidepressant and peripheral anticholinergic activity. *Psychopharmacology.* 1981;74:325-328.

Amitriptyline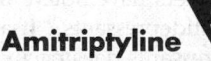

St. John's Wort

SUMMARY: Preliminary evidence suggests that St. John's wort may reduce amitriptyline serum concentrations, but the extent to which this would reduce the therapeutic effect of amitriptyline is unknown.

RISK FACTORS: No specific risk factors are known.

MECHANISM: Not established. St. John's wort appears to be an enzyme inducer and may enhance the metabolism of amitriptyline and nortriptyline (eg, *Pamelor*).

CLINICAL EVALUATION: Twelve patients with depression were given St. John's wort (900 mg of hypericum extract daily) with amitriptyline 75 mg twice daily for 14 days or more.[1] Amitriptyline area under the plasma concentration-time curve (AUC) decreased 22%, and the AUC of its active metabolite, nortriptyline, decreased 41%. Although this was a preliminary report and confirmation is needed, the results are consistent with other reports of reduced drug plasma concentrations caused by St. John's wort. Because St. John's wort appears to have some antidepressant activity, the clinical outcome of this interaction is not clear. More study is needed to assess the clinical importance of this interaction.

RELATED DRUGS: Most tricyclic antidepressants are probably susceptible to enzyme induction; therefore, assume that they would interact with St. John's wort until proven otherwise. In fact, nortriptyline plasma concentrations (derived from amitriptyline) were substantially reduced in this study.

MANAGEMENT OPTIONS: No specific action is required, but be alert for evidence of the interaction.

REFERENCES:
1. Roots I, et al. Interaction of a herbal extract from St. John's wort with amitriptyline and its metabolites. *Clin Pharmacol Ther.* 2000;67:159.

Amitriptyline

Tramadol (eg, *Ultram*)

SUMMARY: A patient on amitriptyline developed fatal serotonin toxicity after receiving tramadol, but it was not possible to rule out that it was the tramadol alone that caused the reaction.

RISK FACTORS: No specific risk factors are known.

MECHANISM: Probably additive serotonergic effects. Both drugs are serotonergic, although amitriptyline is generally considered to have only modest serotonergic effects.

CLINICAL EVALUATION: A 79-year-old woman on amitriptyline 75 mg/day was started on tramadol for sciatic pain.[1,2] Three days later, she was admitted with confusion and hallucinations, and subsequently developed sweating, fever, myoclonus, and muscle rigidity. This progressed to seizures, worsening fever and rigidity, coma, and death. The symptoms are consistent with a diagnosis of fatal serotonin toxicity.[3,4] Nonetheless, one cannot strictly rule out the possibility that the reaction was primarily due to the tramadol with the amitriptyline playing little or no role.

RELATED DRUGS: Clomipramine and imipramine generally have more serotonergic effects than amitriptyline, and they are expected to increase the risk of serotonin toxicity when combined with tramadol.

MANAGEMENT OPTIONS:

➡ **Monitor.** If the combination is used, monitor for symptoms of serotonin toxicity, including myoclonus, rigidity, tremor, hyperreflexia, seizures, confusion, agitation, hypomania, incoordination, fever, sweating, shivering, and coma.

REFERENCES:

1. Kitson R, et al. Tramadol and severe serotonin syndrome [letter]. *Anaesthesia.* 2005;60(9):934-935.

2. Gillman K. A response to Tramadol and severe serotonin syndrome [letter]. *Anaesthesia.* 2006;61(1):76.

3. Isbister GK, et al. Serotonin toxicity: a practical approach to diagnosis and treatment. *Med J Aust.* 2007;187(6):361-365.

4. Boyer EW, et al. The serotonin syndrome. *N Engl J Med.* 2005;352(11):1112-1120.

 Amitriptyline

Warfarin (eg, *Coumadin*)

SUMMARY: Although some evidence suggests that tricyclic antidepressants (TCAs) may increase the hypoprothrombinemic effect of dicumarol and warfarin, the clinical importance is not established.

RISK FACTORS: No specific risk factors are known.

MECHANISM: Impairment of dicumarol metabolism by cyclic antidepressants was proposed by Vesell et al,[1] but not confirmed by others.[2] The bioavailability of dicumarol may be increased by TCA-induced slowing of intestinal motility.[2] Animal studies indicate that amitriptyline and nortriptyline (eg, *Pamelor*) inhibit the hepatic metabolism of warfarin.[3]

CLINICAL EVALUATION: A clinically significant alteration in anticoagulant response to warfarin caused by amitriptyline has been reported, but few details were presented.[4] Others have noted anticoagulant control is less stable in patients receiving cyclic antidepressants.[5] If an interaction between oral anticoagulants and cyclic antidepressants does occur, it is probably significant only in an occasional patient.

RELATED DRUGS: In healthy volunteers, nortriptyline was found to inhibit dicumarol† metabolism[1]; however, this was not confirmed in subsequent work.[2] Warfarin metabolism also appeared to be unaffected by nortriptyline. In another study, mianserin† did not affect the anticoagulant response to phenprocoumon in 60 patients.[6]

MANAGEMENT OPTIONS: No specific action is required, but be alert for evidence of the interaction.

REFERENCES:

1. Vesell ES, et al. Impairment of drug metabolism in man by allopurinol and nortriptyline. *N Engl J Med.* 1970;283(27):1484-1488.

2. Pond SM, et al. Effects of tricyclic antidepressants on drug metabolism. *Clin Pharmacol Ther.* 1975;18(2):191-199.

3. Loomis CW, et al. Drug interactions of amitriptyline and nortriptyline with warfarin in the rat. *Res Commun Chem Pathol Pharmacol.* 1980;30(1):41-58.

4. Koch-Weser J. Hemorrhagic reactions and drug interactions in 500 warfarin-treated patients. *Clin Pharmacol Ther.* 1973;14:139-146.

5. Williams JR, et al. Effect of concomitantly administered drugs on the control of long term anticoagulant therapy. *Q J Med.* 1976;45(177):63-73.

6. Kopera H, et al. Phenprocoumon requirement, whole blood coagulation time, bleeding time and plasma gamma-GT in patients receiving mianserin. *Eur J Clin Pharmacol.* 1978;13(5):351-356.

† Not available in the United States.

Amlodipine (eg, *Norvasc*)

Benazepril (eg, *Lotensin*)

SUMMARY: The combined use of benazepril and amlodipine does not appear to affect the pharmacokinetics of either drug, but additive hypotensive effects may occur.

RISK FACTORS: No specific risk factors are known.

MECHANISM: No pharmacokinetic interaction was observed; theoretically, additive hypotensive effects may occur.

CLINICAL EVALUATION: In a 3-way, Latin square, randomized, crossover study, 12 healthy subjects received benazepril and amlodipine alone and in combination. Neither drug affected the pharmacokinetics of the other.[1] Four subjects developed a headache after combined therapy, but the combination was otherwise well tolerated. Although pharmacodynamic effects were not measured, other combinations of angiotensin-converting enzyme (ACE) inhibitors and calcium channel blockers have been used to advantage for their additive effects in patients with hypertension.

RELATED DRUGS: Combinations of ACE inhibitors and calcium channel blockers appear to have additive antihypertensive effects.

MANAGEMENT OPTIONS: No specific action is required, but be alert for evidence of the interaction.

REFERENCES:
1. Sun JX, et al. Pharmacokinetic interaction study between benazepril and amlodipine in healthy subjects. *Eur J Clin Pharmacol.* 1994;47(3):285-289.

Amlodipine (eg, *Norvasc*)

Diltiazem (eg, *Cardizem*)

SUMMARY: Diltiazem administration resulted in an increase in amlodipine plasma concentrations and hypotensive effect.

RISK FACTORS: No specific risk factors are known.

MECHANISM: Diltiazem is known to inhibit the activity of CYP3A4, the enzyme that metabolizes amlodipine. Additive pharmacodynamic effect (vasodilation) may also play a role in the increased hypotensive effects.

CLINICAL EVALUATION: Eight patients with hypertension were administered amlodipine 5 mg with and without pretreatment with diltiazem 180 mg daily for 3 days.[1] The coadministration of diltiazem increased the area under the concentration-time curve and peak amlodipine concentration 57%. The amlodipine half-life was not changed by diltiazem administration. The combination of amlodipine and diltiazem produced a greater reduction in blood pressure than amlodipine alone.

Although the combination may be uncommonly used, expect an increased hypotensive effect.

RELATED DRUGS: Diltiazem has been noted to increase the plasma concentration of immediate-release nifedipine (eg, *Procardia*) and enhance the hypotensive effects of other calcium channel blockers.

MANAGEMENT OPTIONS:

➡ *Monitor.* If diltiazem and amlodipine are coadministered, monitor for enhanced hypotensive effects.

REFERENCES:

1. Sasaki M, et al. Influence of diltiazem on the pharmacokinetics of amlodipine in elderly hypertensive patients. *Eur J Clin Pharmacol.* 2001;57(1):85-86.

Amlodipine (eg, *Norvasc*)

Erythromycin (eg, *Ery-Tab*)

SUMMARY: Erythromycin and clarithromycin (eg, *Biaxin*) may increase calcium channel blocker plasma concentrations, possibly leading to enhanced pharmacodynamic effects, such as hypotension.

RISK FACTORS: No specific risk factors are known.

MECHANISM: Erythromycin and clarithromycin inhibit the CYP3A4 metabolism of calcium channel blockers.

CLINICAL EVALUATION: A case-crossover study of patients older than 66 years of age taking calcium channel blockers found a nearly 6-fold increase in the risk of hospitalization for hypotension if erythromycin was coadministered.[1] The administration of clarithromycin resulted in nearly a 4-fold increase in the risk of hypotension. The increased risk was noted for patients taking dihydropyridine calcium channel blockers (amlodipine, nifedipine [eg, *Procardia*], and felodipine) as well as diltiazem (eg, *Cardizem*) and verapamil (eg, *Isoptin*). The study was not able to determine the incidence of bradycardia that may have occurred in patients taking diltiazem or verapamil. Azithromycin (eg, *Zithromax*) did not increase the risk of hypotension in patients taking calcium channel blockers.

RELATED DRUGS: Telithromycin (*Ketek*), a ketolide antibiotic, would be expected to interact in a similar manner with calcium channel blockers.

MANAGEMENT OPTIONS:

➡ *Consider Alternative.* Consider azithromycin as an alternative for erythromycin or clarithromycin. In the treatment of hypertension, consider other alternatives to calcium channel blockers, including angiotensin-converting enzyme inhibitors, beta-blockers, or alpha-blockers. Consider holding the administration of the calcium channel blocker during short courses of erythromycin or clarithromycin.

➡ *Monitor.* Monitor patients maintained on calcium channel blockers for excess hypotensive response during the administration of erythromycin or clarithromycin.

REFERENCES:

1. Wright AJ, et al. The risk of hypotension following co-prescription of macrolide antibiotics and calcium-channel blockers. *CMAJ.* 2011;183(3):303-307.

Amlodipine (eg, *Norvasc*)

Grapefruit Juice

SUMMARY: Amlodipine administration with grapefruit juice causes a small increase in amlodipine plasma concentrations that is unlikely to produce measurable changes in patient response.

RISK FACTORS: No specific risk factors are known.

MECHANISM: First-pass metabolism of amlodipine is primarily mediated by the intestinal enzyme CYP3A4. Grapefruit juice reduces the activity of CYP3A4, increasing amlodipine's bioavailability.

CLINICAL EVALUATION: Twelve healthy subjects were administered a single dose of amlodipine 5 mg with 250 mL of water or grapefruit juice.[1] Compared with administration with water, grapefruit juice increased the mean area under the concentration-time curve of amlodipine 14% and the mean peak amlodipine concentration 15%. Both changes were statistically significant but are likely to be of minimal clinical significance. No change in blood pressure or heart rate response was noted. The half-life of amlodipine was unchanged by grapefruit juice.

RELATED DRUGS: The bioavailability of several other dihydropyridine calcium channel blockers (eg, nifedipine [eg, *Procardia*], felodipine, nitrendipine†) is affected by grapefruit juice. Calcium channel blockers with rapid absorption or extensive first-pass clearance, such as felodipine, are more likely to be affected to a greater extent by concomitant grapefruit juice.

MANAGEMENT OPTIONS: No specific action is required, but be alert for evidence of the interaction.

REFERENCES:

1. Josefsson M, et al. Effect of grapefruit juice on the pharmacokinetics of amlodipine in healthy volunteers. *Eur J Clin Pharmacol.* 1996;51(2):189-193.

† Not available in the United States.

Amlodipine (eg, *Norvasc*) 4

Ibuprofen (eg, *Advil*)

SUMMARY: Ibuprofen administration produced a mild reduction in the hypotensive effect of amlodipine.

RISK FACTORS: No specific risk factors are known.

MECHANISM: Not established.

CLINICAL EVALUATION: Twelve patients with mild hypertension received amlodipine 10 mg/day for 1 month.[1] Amlodipine reduced the mean systolic and diastolic blood pressures approximately 22 and 14 mm Hg, respectively. Ibuprofen 400 mg 3 times daily was then added for 3 days. During ibuprofen administration, the mean systolic pressure increased by approximately 8 mm Hg and the diastolic increased by 4 mm Hg. The effect of long-term ibuprofen on amlodipine hypotensive effects was not studied. The intermittent administration of a nonsteroidal anti-inflammatory drug (NSAID) would be less likely to offset the antihypertensive effect of amlodipine.

RELATED DRUGS: Other NSAIDs may affect amlodipine in a similar manner. Ibuprofen 200 mg 3 times daily had no effect on the hypotensive effect of verapamil (eg, *Calan*) in patients with essential hypertension, but it may affect some patients taking other calcium channel blockers.[2]

MANAGEMENT OPTIONS: No specific action is required, but be alert for evidence of the interaction.

REFERENCES:
1. Minuz P, et al. Amlodipine and haemodynamic effects of cyclo-oxygenase inhibition. *Br J Clin Pharmacol.* 1995;39(1):45-50.

2. Houston MC, et al. The effects of nonsteroidal anti-inflammatory drugs on blood pressures of patients with hypertension controlled by verapamil. *Arch Intern Med.* 1995;155(10):1049-1054.

 ## Amlodipine (eg, *Norvasc*)

Indomethacin (eg, *Indocin*)

SUMMARY: Indomethacin does not appear to inhibit the antihypertensive effects of amlodipine.

RISK FACTORS: No specific risk factors are known.

MECHANISM: None (no interaction).

CLINICAL EVALUATION: In a double-blind crossover study of patients on amlodipine (n = 24) and enalapril (n = 25), indomethacin 50 mg twice daily or placebo was given for 3 weeks. The antihypertensive effect of amlodipine was not affected.[1]

RELATED DRUGS: Theoretically, the antihypertensive effect of amlodipine would not be affected by other NSAIDs, but little information is available.

MANAGEMENT OPTIONS: No interaction.

REFERENCES:
1. Morgan TO, et al. Effect of indomethacin on blood pressure in elderly people with essential hypertension well controlled on amlodipine or enalapril. *Am J Hypertens.* 2000;13(11):1161-1167.

 ## Amlodipine (eg, *Norvasc*)

Telaprevir (*Incivek*)

SUMMARY: The coadministration of telaprevir increases the plasma concentration of amlodipine; adverse reactions, including hypotension, may be more likely to occur.

RISK FACTORS: No specific risk factors are known.

MECHANISM: Telaprevir inhibits the CYP3A4-mediated metabolism of amlodipine.

CLINICAL EVALUATION: While specific data are limited, the manufacturer of telaprevir states that the coadministration of telaprevir 750 mg every 8 hours for 10 days increased the mean area under the plasma concentration-time curve (AUC) of amlodipine by nearly 3-fold.[1] Pending further data, observe patients receiving telaprevir and amlodipine for increased amlodipine response.

RELATED DRUGS: Boceprevir (*Victrelis*) also inhibits CYP3A4 and is expected to alter amlodipine metabolism. Atazanavir (*Reyataz*), darunavir (*Prezista*), fosamprenavir (*Lexiva*), indinavir (*Crixivan*), nelfinavir (*Viracept*), ritonavir (*Norvir*), and saquinavir (*Invirase*) also inhibit the activity of CYP3A4 and are expected to increase the plasma concentration of amlodipine. The metabolism of other calcium channel blockers such as diltiazem (*Cardizem*), verapamil (*Calan*), or nifedipine (*Procardia*) may be reduced in a similar manner by telaprevir.

MANAGEMENT OPTIONS:

➡ *Monitor.* Monitor patients stabilized on amlodipine for adverse effects (eg, hypotension, edema) if telaprevir is coadministered.

REFERENCES:

1. *Incivek* [package insert]. Cambridge, MA: Vertex Pharmaceuticals Inc; 2011.

Ammonium Chloride

Aspirin

SUMMARY: Ammonium chloride may decrease renal salicylate excretion in some patients, but the effect is usually small.

RISK FACTORS:

➡ *Dosage Regimen.* Increases in serum salicylate would occur primarily in patients receiving large doses of salicylate (eg, at least 3 g/day in an adult).

MECHANISM: Sufficient doses of ammonium chloride can acidify the urine, thus increasing the renal tubular reabsorption of salicylate and possibly increasing plasma salicylate concentrations. This would occur only with relatively large doses of salicylate, since renal elimination of unchanged salicylate is minimal at smaller doses.[1,2]

CLINICAL EVALUATION: In patients receiving large doses of salicylate, urinary acidification with ammonium chloride can increase serum salicylate.[3,4] However, if the urine is acidic before the ammonium chloride therapy (as it usually is), the changes are likely to be small.

RELATED DRUGS: This interaction also would occur with ingestion of salicylates other than aspirin (eg, diflunisal [eg, *Dolobid*], salsalate [eg, *Disalcid*]).

MANAGEMENT OPTIONS: No specific action is required, but be alert for evidence of the interaction.

REFERENCES:

1. Levy G, et al. Salicylate accumulation kinetics in man. *N Engl J Med.* 1972;287:430.
2. Levy G, et al. Urine pH and salicylate therapy. *JAMA.* 1971;217:81.
3. Klinenberg JR, et al. Effect of corticosteroids on blood salicylate concentration. *JAMA.* 1965;194:601.
4. Hansten PD, et al. Effect of antacids and ascorbic acid on serum salicylate concentration. *J Clin Pharmacol.* 1980;20:326.

Ammonium Chloride

Chlorpropamide (eg, *Diabinese*)

SUMMARY: Acidification of the urine may increase chlorpropamide serum concentrations; the clinical importance of these changes is unknown.

RISK FACTORS: No specific risk factors are known.

MECHANISM: Large doses of ammonium chloride acidify the urine, which decreases the ionization of chlorpropamide. Renal tubular reabsorption of the unionized form decreases urinary excretion of chlorpropamide.

CLINICAL EVALUATION: In 6 healthy subjects given chlorpropamide 250 mg orally, pretreatment with ammonium chloride (urine pH: 4.7 to 5.5) increased chlorpropamide half-life from 50 to 69 hours.[1] The extent to which ammonium chloride-induced acidification of the urine enhances the hypoglycemic effect of chlorpropamide is not established. The extent to which urine is acidified by ammonium chloride is likely to be greatest in patients with alkaline urine. A clinically important increase in serum chlorpropamide level is more likely to be observed in this group.

RELATED DRUGS: No information is available.

MANAGEMENT OPTIONS: No specific action is required, but be alert for evidence of the interaction.

REFERENCES:
1. Neuvonen PJ, et al. Effects of charcoal, sodium bicarbonate, and ammonium chloride on chlorpropamide kinetics. *Clin Pharmacol Ther.* 1983;33:386.

 ## Ammonium Chloride

Ephedrine

SUMMARY: Ammonium chloride tends to enhance ephedrine elimination, but the clinical importance of this effect is not established.

RISK FACTORS: No specific risk factors are known.

MECHANISM: Urine acidification by ammonium chloride enhances the ionization of ephedrine, resulting in decreased renal tubular reabsorption and increased urinary excretion of ephedrine.

CLINICAL EVALUATION: In normal subjects given single doses of ephedrine, acidification of the urine with ammonium chloride considerably increased urinary excretion rates of ephedrine.[1] The clinical importance of this effect is not established.

RELATED DRUGS: Several other sympathomimetics (eg, amphetamine [*Adderall*], pseudoephedrine [eg, *Sudafed*]) also undergo pH-dependent urinary excretion.

MANAGEMENT OPTIONS: No specific action is required, but be alert for evidence of the interaction.

REFERENCES:
1. Wilkinson GR, et al. Absorption metabolism and excretion of the ephedrines in man. I. The influence of urinary pH and urine volume output. *J Pharmacol Exp Ther.* 1968;162:139.

 ## Ammonium Chloride

Methadone (eg, *Dolophine*)

SUMMARY: Ammonium chloride tends to increase methadone elimination, but the clinical importance of this effect is not established.

RISK FACTORS: No specific risk factors are known.

MECHANISM: Methadone is a weak base that is more ionized (and thus more easily excreted) when the urine is acidic (eg, by ammonium chloride administration).

CLINICAL EVALUATION: Renal methadone clearance is considerably greater when the urine is acidic.[1,2] The magnitude of the increase appears sufficient to affect the response to methadone, but the clinical importance is not established.

RELATED DRUGS: The effect of urinary acidification on other narcotic analgesics is not established, but those that are metabolized extensively by the liver probably would be minimally affected.

MANAGEMENT OPTIONS: No specific action is required, but be alert for evidence of the interaction.

REFERENCES:
1. Baselt RC, et al. Urinary excretion of methadone in man. *Clin Pharmacol Ther*. 1972;13:64.
2. Bellward GD, et al. Methadone maintenance: effect of urinary pH on renal clearance in chronic high and low doses. *Clin Pharmacol Ther*. 1977;22:92.

Ammonium Chloride

Procainamide (eg, *Procan SR*)

SUMMARY: Ammonium chloride does not appear to alter procainamide elimination.

RISK FACTORS: No specific risk factors are known.

MECHANISM: Urinary pH changes resulting from ammonium chloride administration do not change procainamide renal excretion.

CLINICAL EVALUATION: Although it had been suspected that procainamide might undergo pH-dependent urinary excretion, urinary acidification with ammonium chloride administration does not affect renal procainamide excretion.[1,2] The active metabolite of procainamide (N-acetylprocainamide) also is unaffected by urinary pH changes.[3]

RELATED DRUGS: No information is available.

MANAGEMENT OPTIONS: No interaction.

REFERENCES:
1. Galeazzi RL, et al. The renal elimination of procainamide. *Clin Pharmacol Ther*. 1976;19:55.
2. Meyer N, et al. A study of the influence of pH on the buccal absorption and renal excretion of procainamide. *Eur J Clin Pharmacol*. 1974;7:287.
3. Reidenberg MM, et al. Polymorphic acetylation of procainamide in man. *Clin Pharmacol Ther*. 1975;17:722.

Ammonium Chloride

Pseudoephedrine (eg, *Sudafed*)

SUMMARY: Ammonium chloride tends to increase pseudoephedrine elimination, but the clinical importance of this effect is not established.

RISK FACTORS: No specific risk factors are known.

MECHANISM: Urine acidification by ammonium chloride enhances the ionization of pseudoephedrine resulting in decreased renal tubular reabsorption and increased urinary excretion of pseudoephedrine.

CLINICAL EVALUATION: In 3 volunteers given a single 180 mg dose of pseudoephedrine, urine acidification with ammonium chloride reduced the half-life of pseudoephedrine.[1] Although the reduction in plasma pseudoephedrine concentrations appeared sufficient to inhibit the clinical response, it is unknown how often this would occur under clinical conditions.

RELATED DRUGS: Several other sympathomimetics (eg, amphetamine, ephedrine) also undergo pH-dependent urinary excretion.

MANAGEMENT OPTIONS: No specific action is required, but be alert for evidence of the interaction.

REFERENCES:

1. Kuntzman RG, et al. The influence of urinary pH on the plasma halflife of pseudoephedrine in man and dog and a sensitive assay for its determination in human plasma. *Clin Pharmacol Ther.* 1971;12:62.

Ammonium Chloride

Spironolactone (*Aldactone*)

SUMMARY: Spironolactone may produce systemic acidosis when administered with ammonium chloride.

RISK FACTORS: No specific risk factors are known.

MECHANISM: The inhibition of aldosterone by spironolactone may impair the ability of the kidney to secrete hydrogen ions so that, in the presence of acidifying doses of ammonium chloride, systemic acidosis occurs.

CLINICAL EVALUATION: One case report described a patient who developed acidosis after treatment with spironolactone, ammonium chloride, and potassium chloride; the authors suggested that the combination of spironolactone and ammonium chloride was at least partially responsible.[1] The hyperkalemia caused by the spironolactone and potassium chloride may have contributed to the acidosis. A subsequent study in 4 normal volunteers showed that spironolactone pretreatment prevented urinary acidification by ammonium chloride[2] that is consistent with the ability of this combination to produce acidosis.

RELATED DRUGS: The effect of potassium-sparing diuretics other than spironolactone on ammonium chloride is not established.

MANAGEMENT OPTIONS:

➥ **Monitor.** Monitor for acidosis if spironolactone is used with acidifying doses of ammonium chloride.

REFERENCES:

1. Mashford ML, et al. Spironolactone and ammonium and potassium chloride. *BMJ.* 1972;4:299.
2. Manuel MA, et al. An effect of spironolactone on urinary acidification in normal man. *Arch Intern Med.* 1974;134:472.

Amobarbital (*Amytal*)

Phenmetrazine† (*Preludin*)

SUMMARY: Amobarbital may inhibit the anorexiant effect of phenmetrazine.

RISK FACTORS: No specific risk factors are known.

MECHANISM: Not established.

CLINICAL EVALUATION: Amobarbital 90 mg/day appeared to inhibit the weight-reducing ability of phenmetrazine in 50 patients, but the clinical importance of this effect is not established.[1]

RELATED DRUGS: It is not known whether other combinations of barbiturates and anorexiants would interact in a similar manner.

MANAGEMENT OPTIONS: No specific action is required, but be alert for evidence of the interaction.

REFERENCES:

1. Hadler AJ. Phenmetrazine vs. phenmetrazine with amobarbital for weight reduction; double-blind study. *Curr Ther Res.* 1969;11:750.

† Not available in the United States.

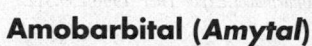

Amobarbital (*Amytal*)

Tranylcypromine (*Parnate*)

SUMMARY: Limited clinical evidence suggests that tranylcypromine may prolong the effect of amobarbital, but little is known about other combinations of nonselective monoamine oxidase inhibitors (MAOIs) and barbiturates.

RISK FACTORS: No specific risk factors are known.

MECHANISM: MAOIs may inhibit the metabolism of barbiturates; however, this mechanism has not been established.[2]

CLINICAL EVALUATION: A patient receiving tranylcypromine 30 mg/day for 3 weeks became semicomatose for 36 hours following the administration of amobarbital 250 mg IM.[1] Subsequent animal studies indicated that tranylcypromine may prolong amobarbital hypnosis. However, little is known concerning the effect of normal oral doses of barbiturates in patients receiving MAOI drugs.

RELATED DRUGS: Little is known about possible effects of other nonselective MAOIs such as isocarboxazid (*Marplan*) and phenelzine (*Nardil*) on barbiturates, but consider the possibility that the barbiturate effect may be increased.

MANAGEMENT OPTIONS:

➡ **Monitor.** Until more is known about this interaction, monitor for increased barbiturate effect if nonselective MAOIs are given concurrently.

REFERENCES:

1. Domino EF, et al. Barbiturate intoxication in patient treated with a MAO inhibitor. *Am J Psychiatry.* 1962;118:941.
2. Sjoqvist F. Psychotropic drugs (2). Interaction between monoamine oxidase (MAO) inhibitors and other substances. *Proc R Soc Med.* 1965;58:967.

Amoxicillin (*Amoxil*)   **4**

Nifedipine (eg, *Procardia*)

SUMMARY: Nifedipine increases the absorption of amoxicillin; this effect is unlikely to adversely affect patients.

RISK FACTORS: No specific risk factors are known.

MECHANISM: Nifedipine appears to enhance the active transport mechanism in the intestinal epithelial cells which are responsible for amoxicillin absorption.

CLINICAL EVALUATION: Eight normal subjects received amoxicillin 1 g orally alone as well as 30 minutes following nifedipine 20 mg.[1] The bioavailability of amoxicillin increased from 65.3% to 79.2%, the absorption rate increased by 70%, the area under the concentration-time curve increased 22%, and peak concentration increased 33% after nifedipine was given. Because of the relative safety of amoxicillin, this interaction is unlikely to be clinically significant.

RELATED DRUGS: No information is available.

MANAGEMENT OPTIONS: No specific action is required, but be alert for evidence of the interaction.

REFERENCES:

1. Westphal J-R, et al. Nifedipine enhances amoxicillin absorption kinetics and bioavailability in humans. *J Pharmacol Exper Ther*. 1990;255:312.

3

Amphotericin B (*Fungizone*)

Cyclosporine (eg, *Sandimmune*)

SUMMARY: The administration of amphotericin B and cyclosporine probably increases the nephrotoxicity of both drugs.

RISK FACTORS: No specific risk factors are known.

MECHANISM: Both cyclosporine and amphotericin B are known to produce nephrotoxicity, and their combined use may result in additive or synergistic nephrotoxicity.

CLINICAL EVALUATION: In a group of 47 patients undergoing bone marrow transplants, 21 received cyclosporine alone, 16 received methotrexate (eg, *Mexate*) plus amphotericin B, and 10 received cyclosporine plus amphotericin B.[1] The serum creatinine concentration doubled within 14 to 30 days in 38% of the patients on cyclosporine alone, doubled within 5 days in 19% of the patients on methotrexate plus amphotericin B, but doubled or tripled within 5 days in 80% of the patients who received cyclosporine plus amphotericin B. All patients also were receiving other nephrotoxic drugs. Until more information is available, concurrent amphotericin B and cyclosporine is assumed to exhibit additive or synergistic nephrotoxicity.

RELATED DRUGS: No information is available.

MANAGEMENT OPTIONS:

➡ ***Circumvent/Minimize.*** Alternative immunosuppression or antifungal therapy may be required to avoid or reverse renal toxicity.

➡ ***Monitor.*** Patients receiving both cyclosporine and amphotericin B should have their renal function monitored carefully.

REFERENCES:

1. Kennedy MS, et al. Acute renal toxicity with combined use of amphotericin B and cyclosporine after marrow transplantation. *Transplantation*. 1983;35:211.

Amphotericin B (*Fungizone*)

Digoxin (eg, *Lanoxin*)

SUMMARY: Digitalis toxicity may be enhanced by amphotericin B-induced hypokalemia.

RISK FACTORS:

➡ *Concurrent Diseases.* Diseases or drugs that cause hypokalemia may increase the risk of digitalis toxicity.

MECHANISM: The hypokalemia that may occur following systemic amphotericin B therapy may facilitate the development of digitalis toxicity.

CLINICAL EVALUATION: Hypokalemia during amphotericin B therapy is common and may be severe.[1,2] Digitalis toxicity may be exacerbated by amphotericin-induced hypokalemia.

RELATED DRUGS: Digitoxin (*Crystodigin*) also will be affected by amphotericin B-induced hypokalemia.

MANAGEMENT OPTIONS:

➡ *Monitor.* Closely follow the potassium status of patients on digitalis who receive amphotericin B therapy. Promptly treat any potassium deficit that develops.

REFERENCES:

1. Miller RP, et al. Amphotericin B toxicity. A follow-up report of 53 patients. *Ann Intern Med.* 1969;71:1089.
2. Cushard WG, et al. Blastomycosis of bone. Treatment with intramedullary amphotericin B. *J Bone Joint Surg.* 1969;51A:704.

Amphotericin B (*Fungizone*)

Gentamicin (*Garamycin*)

SUMMARY: The combination of aminoglycosides and amphotericin B may enhance the potential for nephrotoxicity.

RISK FACTORS:

➡ *Concurrent Diseases.* Renal dysfunction may increase the risk of nephrotoxicity.

MECHANISM: The nephrotoxicity of amphotericin B and aminoglycosides may be synergistic.

CLINICAL EVALUATION: In 4 patients receiving gentamicin, the addition of amphotericin B was associated with deterioration of renal function.[1] Since neither drug was being used in a dose likely to be nephrotoxic, the authors assumed that synergistic nephrotoxicity occurred in these patients. Additional study is required to establish a causal relationship.

RELATED DRUGS: Other aminoglycosides may produce nephrotoxicity with amphotericin.

MANAGEMENT OPTIONS:

➡ *Consider Alternative.* The use of an alternative antibiotic or antifungal agent without nephrotoxicity would be prudent.

➡ **Monitor.** Closely monitor patients on combined therapy with an aminoglycoside and amphotericin B for deterioration of renal function.

REFERENCES:
1. Churchill DN, et al. Nephrotoxicity associated with combined gentamicin-amphotericin B therapy. *Nephron.* 1977;19:176.

Amphotericin B (*Fungizone*)

Succinylcholine (eg, *Anectine*)

SUMMARY: Prolonged muscle relaxation may accompany the use of amphotericin B and neuromuscular blocking agents.

RISK FACTORS: No specific risk factors are known.

MECHANISM: The hypokalemia that may occur following amphotericin B therapy may enhance the effect of curariform drugs.

CLINICAL EVALUATION: Hypokalemia caused by amphotericin B is well documented and is likely to be of sufficient magnitude to enhance the response to muscle relaxants including succinylcholine, atracurium (*Tracrium*), and vecuronium (*Norcuron*).[1,2]

RELATED DRUGS: Other drugs causing hypokalemia may cause a similar reaction with muscle relaxants like atracurium and vecuronium.

MANAGEMENT OPTIONS:

➡ **Monitor.** Carefully check the potassium balance of patients on amphotericin B before use of neuromuscular blocking agents.

REFERENCES:
1. Miller RP, et al. Amphotericin B toxicity. A follow-up report of 53 patients. *Ann Intern Med.* 1969;71:1089.
2. Cushard WG, et al. Blastomycosis of bone. Treatment with intramedullary amphotericin B. *J Bone Joint Surg.* 1969;51A:704.

Ampicillin (eg, *Principen*)

Atenolol (eg, *Tenormin*)

SUMMARY: Ampicillin may reduce atenolol serum concentrations, and a reduction of beta-blocking effect is possible.

RISK FACTORS:

➡ **Dosage Regimen.** Ampicillin doses greater than 1 g appear to decrease the bioavailability of atenolol.

MECHANISM: Ampicillin appears to decrease the bioavailability of atenolol, particularly at higher ampicillin doses (1 g).

CLINICAL EVALUATION: In 6 healthy subjects, oral atenolol 100 mg was given with and without oral ampicillin 1 g in single-dose and 6-day studies.[1] The bioavailability of atenolol was 60% when given alone, 36% with a single dose of ampicillin, and 24% with combined therapy for 6 days. Atenolol inhibition of exercise tachycardia was reduced after ampicillin. A dose of ampicillin 1 g coadministered with atenolol 50 mg resulted in a 51% reduction in the area under the plasma concentration-time curve (AUC) of atenolol; ampicillin 250 mg 4 times daily resulted in an 18% reduction in the AUC.[2]

RELATED DRUGS: No information is available.

MANAGEMENT OPTIONS:

➥ *Monitor.* Until more data are available, monitor for evidence of altered atenolol response when large doses of ampicillin are coadministered.

REFERENCES:

1. Schafer-Körting M, et al. Atenolol interaction with aspirin, allopurinol, and ampicillin. *Clin Pharmacol Ther.* 1983;33(3):283-288.

2. McLean AJ, et al. Dose-dependence of atenolol-ampicillin interaction. *Br J Clin Pharmacol.* 1984;18(6):969-971.

Ampicillin (eg, *Principen*)

Contraceptives, Oral

SUMMARY: Ampicillin is likely to occasionally decrease oral contraceptive efficacy.

RISK FACTORS: No specific risk factors are known.

MECHANISM: Ampicillin may interrupt the enterohepatic circulation of estrogen by reducing the bacterial hydrolysis of conjugated estrogen in the GI tract.

CLINICAL EVALUATION: Ampicillin has been associated with a reduction in urinary excretion of endogenous estrogens in women not receiving oral contraceptives, and there also have been numerous reports of menstrual irregularities and unplanned pregnancies in patients receiving oral contraceptives.[1-4] However, in a study of 11 subjects observed for 2 months, oral ampicillin did not appear to interfere with the ability of an oral contraceptive (containing estrogen 50 mcg) to suppress ovulation.[5] In another study of 13 women taking oral contraceptives, ampicillin lowered plasma ethinyl estradiol concentrations in only 2 women.[6] Nevertheless, the data are consistent with the supposition that ampicillin occasionally decreases oral contraceptive efficacy.

RELATED DRUGS: The effect of other penicillins on oral contraceptives is not well established; however, reports of contraceptive failure have been noted with the concomitant use of a variety of antibiotics.

MANAGEMENT OPTIONS:

➥ *Circumvent/Minimize.* Because ampicillin often is given in relatively short courses, patients should continue to take oral contraceptives and use supplementary contraception during cycles in which ampicillin is used.

➥ *Monitor.* Inform patients that spotting or breakthrough bleeding may be an indication that an interaction between ampicillin and an oral contraceptive is occurring.

REFERENCES:

1. Boehm FH, et al. The effect of ampicillin administration on urinary estriol and serum estradiol in the normal pregnant patient. *Am J Obstet Gynecol.* 1974;119(1):98-103.

2. Sybulski S, et al. Effect of ampicillin administration on estradiol, estriol, and cortisol levels in maternal plasma and on estriol levels in urine. *Am J Obstet Gynecol.* 1976;124(4):379-381.

3. Adlercreutz H, et al. Effect of ampicillin administration on plasma conjugated and unconjugated estrogen and progesterone levels in pregnancy. *Am J Obstet Gynecol.* 1977;128(3):266-271.

4. DeSano EA Jr, et al. Possible interactions of antihistamines and antibiotics with oral contraceptive effectiveness. *Fertil Steril.* 1982;37(6):853-854.

5. Friedman CI, et al. The effect of ampicillin on oral contraceptive effectiveness. *Obstet Gynecol.* 1980;55(1):33-37.

6. Back DJ, et al. The effects of ampicillin oral contraceptive steroids in women. *Br J Clin Pharmacol.* 1982;14(1):43-48.

4 Ampicillin (eg, *Principen*)

Probenecid

SUMMARY: Probenecid increases penicillin concentrations.

RISK FACTORS: No specific risk factors are known.

MECHANISM: Probenecid appears to compete with the renal tubular secretion of penicillins.[1] It also may decrease the volume of distribution of penicillin.[2]

CLINICAL EVALUATION: Probenecid is known to increase the serum concentrations of most penicillins, including penicillin G (eg, *Pfizerpen*), ampicillin (eg, *Principen*), and nafcillin.[3,4] This effect usually is employed to potentiate the antibacterial effect of the penicillin but theoretically could lead to increased toxicity if large intravenous penicillin doses are given.

RELATED DRUGS: All penicillins that are secreted by the kidneys (eg, penicillin G, ampicillin, nafcillin) are likely to be affected by probenecid.

MANAGEMENT OPTIONS: No specific action is required, but be alert for evidence of the interaction.

REFERENCES:

1. Weiner IM, et al. On the mechanism of action of probenecid on renal tubular secretion. *Bull Johns Hopkins Hosp.* 1960;106:333-346.

2. Gibaldi M, et al. Apparent effect of probenecid on the distribution of penicillins in man. *Clin Pharmacol Ther.* 1968;9(3):345-349.

3. Blum RA, et al. Effect of probenecid on the pharmacokinetics of oral carbenicillin. *Pharm Res.* 1988;5:151.

4. Itoh T, et al. Stereoselective renal tubular secretion of carbenicillin. *Antimicrob Agents Chemother.* 1993;37(11):2327-2332.

Amprenavir†

Atorvastatin (*Lipitor*)

SUMMARY: The administration of amprenavir increases the plasma concentration of atorvastatin; some patients may require a reduction in atorvastatin dose.

RISK FACTORS: No specific risk factors are known.

MECHANISM: Amprenavir appears to inhibit the metabolism of atorvastatin via the CYP3A4 pathway.

CLINICAL EVALUATION: While specific data are limited, the manufacturer of amprenavir notes that the coadministration of amprenavir 1,400 mg twice daily, or the combination of amprenavir 700 mg twice daily plus ritonavir 100 mg twice daily, for 2 weeks prior to a 4-day course of atorvastatin 10 mg daily increased the mean area under the plasma concentration-time curve of atorvastatin 130% to 150%.[1]

Pending further data, observe patients receiving atorvastatin and amprenavir for increased atorvastatin effect.

RELATED DRUGS: Lovastatin (eg, *Mevacor*) and simvastatin (eg, *Zocor*) are also metabolized by CYP3A4, and are expected to interact with amprenavir in a similar manner.

MANAGEMENT OPTIONS:

➡ *Consider Alternative.* Theoretically, pravastatin (eg, *Pravachol*), rosuvastatin (*Crestor*), or fluvastatin (*Lescol*) are less likely to interact with amprenavir.

➡ *Monitor.* Monitor patients taking atorvastatin (particularly doses of more than 40 mg) for muscle pain or weakness if amprenavir is coadministered.

REFERENCES:

1. *Agenerase* [package insert]. Research Triangle Park, NC: GlaxoSmithKline; 2006.

† Not available in the United States.

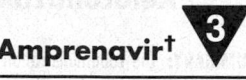

Amprenavir†

Delavirdine (*Rescriptor*)

SUMMARY: Chronic dosing of delavirdine increases amprenavir concentrations, while chronic amprenavir administration decreases delavirdine plasma concentrations. Careful monitoring of patients taking a combination of these drugs is necessary.

RISK FACTORS: No specific risk factors are known.

MECHANISM: Delavirdine inhibits the CYP3A4 metabolism of amprenavir, resulting in a large increase in amprenavir plasma concentrations. A single dose of amprenavir reduced CYP3A4 activity. However, chronic administration of amprenavir appeared to induce the metabolism (CYP3A4) of delavirdine, resulting in a reduction in delavirdine concentrations. The effect, if any, of P-glycoprotein on the mechanism of this interaction is unknown.

CLINICAL EVALUATION: Healthy volunteers (N = 12) received a single dose of amprenavir 1,200 mg alone and again following delavirdine 600 mg twice daily for 7 days.[1] In a second study, 11 healthy volunteers received amprenavir 1,200 mg/day alone for 7 days, delavirdine 600 mg twice daily alone for 7 days, and a combination of amprenavir 600 mg twice daily with delavirdine 600 mg twice daily for 7 days. The mean area under the concentration-time curve (AUC) of amprenavir was increased 4-fold following delavirdine pretreatment. Amprenavir half-life increased from 6 to 12 hours, and the mean oral clearance of amprenavir was decreased 75% during delavirdine coadministration.

The administration of a single dose of amprenavir resulted in a small decrease (17%) in delavirdine oral clearance during multiple dosing. However, the multiple dosing of amprenavir 600 mg twice daily produced significant reductions in delavirdine AUC and half-life (47% and 52%, respectively). The changes observed in this study are sufficient to produce altered patient response to these drugs.

RELATED DRUGS: Delavirdine may reduce the clearance, and thus increase the plasma concentration, of other antiretroviral drugs metabolized by CYP3A4. The chronic administration of amprenavir may reduce the concentration of other antiretrovirals metabolized by CYP3A4.

MANAGEMENT OPTIONS:

➥ **Monitor.** Monitor plasma concentrations, antiviral response, and drug toxicity when combinations of antiretroviral drugs are administered or when one drug is discontinued from a combination regimen. The apparent mixed effect on CYP3A4 activity demonstrated by amprenavir will produce different effects on object drugs, depending on the duration of amprenavir administration.

REFERENCES:

1. Tran JQ, et al. Pharmacokinetic interaction between amprenavir and delavirdine: evidence of induced clearance by amprenavir. *Clin Pharmacol Ther.* 2002;72(6):615-626.

† Not available in the United States.

Amprenavir†

Ketoconazole (eg, *Nizoral*)

SUMMARY: The coadministration of ketoconazole and amprenavir results in an increase in both drugs' plasma concentrations; the risk of adverse patient response may be limited.

RISK FACTORS: No specific risk factors are known.

MECHANISM: Ketoconazole and amprenavir are both substrates and inhibitors of CYP3A4. When administered together, they appear to inhibit each other's metabolism. Inhibition of P-glycoprotein by ketoconazole and amprenavir may also contribute to the increase in plasma concentrations observed.

CLINICAL EVALUATION: Twelve subjects received single doses of amprenavir 1,200 mg, ketoconazole 400 mg, and the combination.[1] The mean area under the plasma concentration-time curve (AUC) for amprenavir was increased 31% when coadministered with ketoconazole. The AUC for ketoconazole increased 44% during coadministration of amprenavir. The administration of multiple doses is expected to increase the magnitude of the interaction. However, because these drugs inhibit their own metabolism with chronic administration, the added effect of a second inhibitor may be somewhat limited during steady-state dosing.

RELATED DRUGS: Other antifungal agents, including itraconazole (eg, *Sporanox*), voriconazole (*Vfend*), and fluconazole (eg, *Diflucan*), also inhibit CYP3A4 and are expected to increase amprenavir plasma concentrations. Terbinafine (eg, *Lamisil*) does not inhibit CYP3A4 and is not expected to affect amprenavir metabolism. Several other protease inhibitors, including indinavir (*Crixivan*), ritonavir (*Norvir*), saquinavir (*Invirase*), and nelfinavir (*Viracept*), are metabolized by CYP3A4 and are likely to have their metabolism reduced by coadministration of ketoconazole.

MANAGEMENT OPTIONS:

➥ **Consider Alternative.** Consider terbinafine as an alternative antifungal in patients taking amprenavir.

➥ **Monitor.** Monitor patients taking both ketoconazole and amprenavir for increased amprenavir concentrations. The incidence of oral paresthesias or GI upset may be increased.

REFERENCES:

1. Polk RE, et al. Pharmacokinetic interaction between ketoconazole and amprenavir after single doses in healthy men. *Pharmacotherapy.* 1999;19(12):1378-1384.

† Not available in the United States.

Amprenavir† 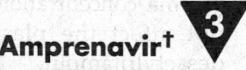 4

Methadone (eg, *Dolophine*)

SUMMARY: Amprenavir causes a small reduction in methadone plasma concentrations; most patients will not require a methadone dose adjustment.

RISK FACTORS: No specific risk factors are known.

MECHANISM: Unknown. Amprenavir may reduce the absorption or increase the elimination of methadone.

CLINICAL EVALUATION: Nineteen methadone-maintained subjects received their usual methadone dose alone and after concurrently taking amprenavir 1,200 mg daily for 10 days.[1] The coadministration of amprenavir resulted in a mean 13% decrease in the area under the concentration-time curve (AUC) of the active R-methadone enantiomer. The inactive S-methadone enantiomer's AUC was reduced 40%. No subject demonstrated evidence of opioid withdrawal nor required a methadone dose adjustment. A similar study design using fosamprenavir (*Lexiva*) 700 mg twice daily plus ritonavir 100 mg twice daily demonstrated a similar 18% reduction in the AUC of R-methadone.[2] These studies are in general agreement (mean 35% reduction of methadone concentration) with an earlier study that did not differentiate between the enantiomers of methadone.[3]

RELATED DRUGS: Ritonavir (*Norvir*) has been noted to reduce methadone plasma concentrations.

MANAGEMENT OPTIONS:

➡ *Monitor.* Observe patients taking methadone who require amprenavir for reduced methadone efficacy.

REFERENCES:

1. Hendrix CW, et al. Pharmacokinetics and pharmacodynamics of methadone enantiomers after coadministration with amprenavir in opioid-dependent subjects. *Pharmacotherapy.* 2004;24(9):1110-1121.
2. Cao YJ, et al. Pharmacokinetics and pharmacodynamics of methadone enantiomers after coadministration with fosamprenavir-ritonavir in opioid-dependent subjects. *Pharmacotherapy.* 2008;28(7):863-874.
3. Bart PA, et al. Methadone blood concentrations are decreased by the administration of abacavir plus amprenavir. *Ther Drug Monit.* 2001;23(5):553-555.

† Not available in the United States.

Amprenavir† ▼ 3

Rifabutin (*Mycobutin*)

SUMMARY: Amprenavir administration significantly increased the plasma concentration of rifabutin; monitor patients for increased rifabutin adverse reactions.

RISK FACTORS: No specific risk factors are known.

MECHANISM: Amprenavir appears to inhibit the CYP3A4 metabolism of rifabutin and its metabolite.

CLINICAL EVALUATION: Six healthy subjects received amprenavir 1,200 mg twice daily for 4 days followed by rifabutin 300 mg daily for 18 days with concurrent amprenavir on days 14 to 18.[1] The coadministration of amprenavir increased the mean area under the concentration-time curve (AUC) of rifabutin nearly 3-fold and increased the AUC of 25-O-desactylrifabutin over 13-fold. These marked increases in the plasma concentrations of rifabutin and its metabolite were accompanied by adverse reactions, including flu-like symptoms and leukopenia. Rifabutin did not affect the plasma concentration of amprenavir.

RELATED DRUGS: Atazanavir (*Reyataz*), darunavir (*Prezista*), indinavir (*Crixivan*), nelfinavir (*Viracept*), saquinavir (*Invirase*), and ritonavir (*Norvir*) also inhibit the activity of CYP3A4 and are expected to increase the plasma concentrations of rifabutin. Rifampin (eg, *Rimactane*) has been noted to reduce the plasma concentration of amprenavir.

MANAGEMENT OPTIONS:

➡ *Monitor.* If rifabutin is coadministered with amprenavir, monitor the plasma concentration of rifabutin and adjust doses as needed to prevent adverse reactions.

REFERENCES:
1. Polk RE, et al. Pharmacokinetic interaction between amprenavir and rifabutin or rifampin in healthy males. *Antimicrob Agents Chemother.* 2001;45(2):502-508.

† Not available in the United States.

Amprenavir†

Rifampin (eg, *Rimactane*)

SUMMARY: Rifampin markedly reduced the plasma concentration of amprenavir; reduction in antiviral activity is likely to occur in some patients.

RISK FACTORS: No specific risk factors are known.

MECHANISM: Rifampin appears to induce the CYP3A4 metabolism of amprenavir, increase P-glycoprotein activity, or both.

CLINICAL EVALUATION: Eleven healthy subjects received amprenavir 1,200 mg twice daily for 4 days followed by rifampin 600 mg daily for 18 days with concurrent amprenavir on days 14 through 18.[1] The coadministration of rifampin reduced the mean area under the concentration-time curve of amprenavir over 80% and the minimum concentration of amprenavir over 90%. Rifampin increased the mean oral clearance of amprenavir over 5-fold. These marked reductions in amprenavir plasma concentrations would likely reduce its antiviral efficacy. Amprenavir did not affect the plasma concentration of rifampin or its metabolite 25-O-desactylrifampin.

RELATED DRUGS: Other protease inhibitors (eg, nelfinavir [*Viracept*], saquinavir [*Invirase*], and ritonavir [*Norvir*]) are similarly affected by rifampin. Rifabutin does not appear to significantly alter the pharmacokinetics of amprenavir.

MANAGEMENT OPTIONS:

➡ *Consider Alternative.* If possible, avoid the use of rifampin in patients taking amprenavir.

➥ *Monitor.* If rifampin is coadministered with amprenavir, monitor the plasma concentration of amprenavir and adjust doses as needed.

REFERENCES:

1. Polk RE, et al. Pharmacokinetic interaction between amprenavir and rifabutin or rifampin in healthy males. *Antimicrob Agents Chemother.* 2001;45(2):502-508.

† Not available in the United States.

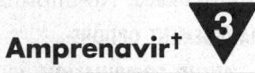

Amprenavir†

Tipranavir (*Aptivus*)

SUMMARY: The coadministration of amprenavir with tipranavir/ritonavir may result in lower plasma concentrations of amprenavir and reduced antiviral effect.

RISK FACTORS: No specific risk factors are known.

MECHANISM: Unknown. Amprenavir is considered to be a substrate of CYP3A4 and P-glycoprotein. The combination of tipranavir/ritonavir has inhibited CYP3A4 and induced P-glycoprotein. These offsetting effects may account for the reduction in amprenavir plasma concentrations, possibly by reducing its bioavailability via P-glycoprotein induction.

CLINICAL EVALUATION: While specific data are limited, the manufacturer of tipranavir notes that coadministration of tipranavir 500 mg with ritonavir 100 mg twice daily and amprenavir 600 mg with ritonavir 100 mg twice daily decreased the mean area under the plasma concentration-time curve of amprenavir 44%, compared with administration of amprenavir/ritonavir alone.[1]

RELATED DRUGS: Tipranavir/ritonavir also has been reported to reduce the plasma concentrations of lopinavir (*Kaletra*) and saquinavir (*Invirase*).

MANAGEMENT OPTIONS:

➥ *Monitor.* Carefully monitor patients being treated with tipranavir/ritonavir and amprenavir for any change in antiviral efficacy.

REFERENCES:

1. *Aptivus* [package insert]. Ridgefield, CT: Boehringer Ingelheim Pharmaceuticals Inc; 2007.

† Not available in the United States.

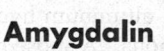

Amygdalin

Vitamin C AVOID

SUMMARY: A patient taking high-dose vitamin C developed life-threatening cyanide toxicity after a single dose of amygdalin. Avoid the combination.

RISK FACTORS: No specific risk factors are known.

MECHANISM: The mechanism is not established. High-dose vitamin C may promote the hydrolysis of amygdalin to cyanide and/or reduce body stores of cysteine, which facilitates the detoxification of cyanide.

CLINICAL EVALUATION: A 68-year-old woman with carcinoma of the bladder taking vitamin C 4,800 mg daily developed cyanide toxicity soon after her first dose of amygdalin.[1] She developed severe lactic acidosis and seizures that responded to the cyanide antidote, hydroxocobalamin. A causal relationship cannot be established based on one case report, and it is not possible to rule out the possibility that the amygdalin alone was responsible for the reaction. High-dose vitamin C may increase the risk of amygdalin-induced cyanide toxicity, but more data are needed. Theoretically, low-dose vitamin C (such as that found in multivitamin preparations) is not expected to increase amygdalin toxicity, but no data are available.

RELATED DRUGS: No information is available.

MANAGEMENT OPTIONS:

➡ *AVOID COMBINATION.* Given its lack of efficacy and potential toxicity, avoid amygdalin use with or without vitamin C. Warn patients who insist on taking amygdalin to avoid high-dose vitamin C.

REFERENCES:

   1. Bromley J, et al. Life-threatening interaction between complementary medicines: cyanide toxicity following ingestion of amygdalin and vitamin C. *Ann Pharmacother.* 2005;39(9):1566-1569.

Antacids

Aspirin

SUMMARY: Some antacids can decrease serum salicylate concentrations in patients receiving large doses of salicylates; in some patients, this effect may be sufficient to require salicylate dosage adjustments.

RISK FACTORS:

➡ *Dosage Regimen.* The lowering of serum salicylate concentrations by antacids is likely to occur only in patients receiving large doses of salicylate (eg, several grams per day), since it is only with such doses that the renal excretion of unchanged salicylic acid is an important elimination pathway.

MECHANISM: Antacid-induced alkalinization of the urine reduces renal tubular reabsorption of salicylate, which in turn may result in reduced serum salicylate concentrations.[5] It also has been proposed that antacids might cause premature disruption of the coating of enteric-coated aspirin or perhaps increase gastric emptying resulting in earlier release of the aspirin in the intestine.[1,4]

CLINICAL EVALUATION: A study of 3 children with rheumatic fever who were receiving large doses of salicylate indicated that coadministration of an antacid (magnesium and aluminum hydroxide) was associated with reduced serum salicylate concentrations.[2] A subsequent study of 9 healthy subjects given choline salicylate (daily dose equivalent to 3.75 gm of aspirin) showed that magnesium and aluminum hydroxide were associated with reduced steady-state salicylate levels.[3] Moreover, not all antacids appear to affect urine pH to the same extent as magnesium-aluminum hydroxides,[8,9] so the magnitude of the changes in serum salicylate would depend on the specific antacid used. A study of 9 healthy subjects showed that magnesium and aluminum hydroxide (*Maalox*) resulted in an earlier peak urinary excretion rate of aspirin administered in enteric-coated form (*Ecotrin*).[1] This may indicate earlier or more rapid release of aspirin, the clinical significance of which is not yet established. Antacids do not appear to affect the bioavailability of aspirin. In 6 healthy subjects, the bioavailability of aspirin tablets was not affected by coadministration of 300 mg of aluminum hydroxide.[6] Similarly, the bioavailability of aspirin formulations containing antacids such as magnesium-aluminum hydroxides or magnesium carbonate appears to be equivalent to unbuffered aspirin.[7]

RELATED DRUGS: Salicylates other than aspirin also would be affected by increases in urine pH.

MANAGEMENT OPTIONS:

➡ *Monitor.* In patients receiving large doses of salicylates (eg, for arthritis), be alert for alteration in serum salicylate concentrations if antacids are initiated, discontinued, or changed in dosage. Adjustments in salicylate dosage may be required in some cases.

REFERENCES:

1. Feldman S, et al. Effect of antacid on absorption of enteric-coated aspirin. *JAMA.* 1974;227:660.
2. Levy G, et al. Decreased serum salicylate concentrations in children with rheumatic fever treated with antacid. *N Engl J Med.* 1975;293:323.
3. Hansten PD, et al. Effect of antacids and ascorbic acid on serum salicylate concentration. *J Clin Pharmacol.* 1980;24:326.
4. Strickland-Hodge B, et al. The effects of antacids on enteric coated salicylate preparations. *Rheumatol Rehab.* 1976;15:148.
5. Shastri RA. Effect of antacids on salicylate kinetics. *Int J Clin Pharmacol Ther Toxicol.* 1985;23:480.
6. Kaniwa N, et al. The bioavailabilities of aspirin from an aspirin aluminum and aspirin tablets and the effects of food and aluminum hydroxide gel. *J Pharm Dyn.* 1981;4:860.
7. Nayak RK, et al. Effect of antacids on aspirin dissolution and bioavailability. *J Pharmacokinet Biopharm.* 1977;5:597.
8. Gibaldi M, et al. Effect of antacids on pH of urine. *Clin Pharmacol Ther.* 1974;16:520.
9. Gibaldi M, et al. Time course and dose dependency of antacid effect on urine pH. *J Pharmaceut Sci.* 1975;64:2003.

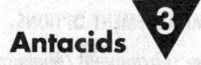

Antacids 3

Atenolol (*Tenormin*)

SUMMARY: The GI absorption of atenolol may be reduced by coadministration of aluminum or magnesium antacids, but the clinical importance is not established.

RISK FACTORS: No specific risk factors are known.

MECHANISM: Not established. Presumably, antacids bind atenolol in the gut.

CLINICAL EVALUATION: Two studies in healthy human subjects indicate that magnesium-aluminum, calcium, or aluminum antacids may reduce the bioavailability of atenolol.[1,2] The impact of these findings on the therapeutic response to atenolol has not been assessed.

RELATED DRUGS: Other beta-adrenergic blockers also may be affected by antacids.

MANAGEMENT OPTIONS:

➡ *Circumvent/Minimize.* Take atenolol at least 2 hours before or 6 hours after the antacid, and try to maintain a relatively constant interval and sequence of administration of the two drugs.

➡ **Monitor.** Monitor for altered atenolol effect if antacid therapy is initiated, discontinued, or changed in dosage; adjust atenolol dose as needed.

REFERENCES:
1. Regardh CG, et al. The effect of antacid, metoclopramide, and propantheline on the bioavailability of metoprolol and atenolol. *Biopharm Drug Dispos.* 1981;2:79.
2. Kirch W, et al. Interaction of atenolol with furosemide and calcium and aluminum salts. *Clin Pharmacol Ther.* 1981;30:429.

Antacids

Atevirdine

SUMMARY: Atevirdine administration contiguous with antacid dosing reduces atevirdine concentrations; reduced antiviral efficacy could result.

RISK FACTORS: No specific risk factors are known.

MECHANISM: Not established.

CLINICAL EVALUATION: A single 600 mg dose of atevirdine was administered alone and 10 minutes following 30 mL of *Maalox TC* suspension in 11 patients with human immunodeficiency virus.[1] The area under the concentration-time curve of atevirdine was reduced by about 40%, and the peak concentration was 60% lower. This degree of interaction would be expected to reduce the efficacy of atevirdine in some patients.

RELATED DRUGS: The effect of other antacids on atevirdine is unknown, but consider all antacids to interact until more information is available.

MANAGEMENT OPTIONS:

➡ **Circumvent/Minimize.** Avoid the administration of atevirdine and antacids. Until more information is available, separate doses of atevirdine and antacids by 2 to 3 hours.

➡ **Monitor.** If patients receiving atevirdine are administered antacids, monitor for reduced antiviral effects.

REFERENCES:
1. Borin MT, et al. Effects of food and antacid on bioavailability of atevirdine mesylate (ATV) in HIV+ patients. *Clin Pharmacol Ther.* 1994;55:194.

Antacids

Cefpodoxime Proxetil (*Vantin*)

SUMMARY: Antacids reduce the bioavailability and serum concentrations of cefpodoxime proxetil and could reduce the efficacy of the antibiotic.

RISK FACTORS: No specific risk factors are known.

MECHANISM: The dissolution of cefpodoxime proxetil is reduced as the pH is increased.

CLINICAL EVALUATION: Ten healthy subjects ingested 200 mg cefpodoxime proxetil after an overnight fast and in conjunction with 10 mL of magnesium and aluminum hydroxides (*Maalox 70*) administered twice, at 2 hours and at 15 minutes before the cefpodoxime.[1] The peak concentration and area under the concentration-time curve of cefpodoxime were reduced about 40% by *Maalox 70*. The administration of 12.6 g sodium bicarbonate or 7.68 gm aluminum hydroxide 10 minutes before cefpodoxime produced similar results.[2]

RELATED DRUGS: Theoretically, any drug that substantially increases gastric pH also would reduce cefpodoxime absorption. This would include H_2-receptor antagonists (eg, cimetidine [eg, *Tagamet*], famotidine [eg, *Pepcid*], nizatidine [*Axid*], ranitidine [*Zantac*]), proton pump inhibitors (eg, omeprazole [*Prilosec*], lansoprazole [*Prevacid*]) and other antacids.

MANAGEMENT OPTIONS:

➡ *Circumvent/Minimize.* Advise patients taking cefpodoxime to take the antibiotic between meals, preferably on an empty stomach. Do not administer antacids for at least 2 hours before or after administration of cefpodoxime.

➡ *Monitor.* Be alert for evidence of reduced cefpodoxime response if antacids are used concurrently.

REFERENCES:

1. Saathoff N, et al. Pharmacokinetics of cefpodoxime proxetil and interactions with an antacid and an H_2-receptor antagonist. *Antimicrob Agents Chemother.* 1992;36:796.
2. Hughes GS, et al. The effects of gastric pH and food on the pharmacokinetics of a new oral cephalosporin, cefpodoxime proxetil. *Clin Pharmacol Ther.* 1989;46:647.

Antacids

Chlordiazepoxide (eg, *Librium*)

SUMMARY: A magnesium-aluminum hydroxide antacid did not affect the bioavailability of chlordiazepoxide in healthy subjects.

RISK FACTORS: No specific risk factors are known.

MECHANISM: Not established. The delayed absorption of chlordiazepoxide may result from binding with the antacid in the gut.

CLINICAL EVALUATION: In 10 healthy subjects the absorption of oral chlordiazepoxide 25 mg was delayed by concomitant magnesium hydroxide-aluminum hydroxide (*Maalox*), but the bioavailability was not affected.[1]

RELATED DRUGS: The effect of antacids other than magnesium-aluminum hydroxide on chlordiazepoxide is not established, but it may be similar.

MANAGEMENT OPTIONS: No specific action is required, but be alert for evidence of the interaction.

REFERENCES:

1. Greenblatt DJ, et al. Influence of magnesium and aluminum hydroxide mixture on chlordiazepoxide absorption. *Clin Pharmacol Ther.* 1976;19:234.

Antacids

Chloroquine (*Aralen*)

SUMMARY: Magnesium antacids may cause a small reduction in the serum concentration of chloroquine, but the clinical importance of this effect is not established.

RISK FACTORS: No specific risk factors are known.

MECHANISM: Not established. Magnesium trisilicate may bind with chloroquine in the gut.

CLINICAL EVALUATION: In 6 healthy subjects, magnesium trisilicate 1 g reduced the area under the plasma chloroquine concentration-time curve by 18%.[1] Whether the magnitude of this reduction would be sufficient to reduce the therapeutic effect of chloroquine is not established.

RELATED DRUGS: The effect of antacids other than magnesium trisilicate on chloroquine absorption has not been established.

MANAGEMENT OPTIONS: No specific action is required, but be alert for evidence of the interaction.

REFERENCES:

1. McElnay JC, et al. In vitro experiments on chloroquine and pyrimethamine absorption in the presence of antacid constituents or kaolin. *J Trop Med Hyg*. 1982;85:153.

 4   Antacids

Chlorpromazine (eg, *Thorazine*)

SUMMARY: Limited clinical information indicates that antacids may reduce the absorption of chlorpromazine, but the degree to which this reduces the therapeutic response to chlorpromazine is not established.

RISK FACTORS: No specific risk factors are known.

MECHANISM: Antacids have a large surface area and probably adsorb chlorpromazine in the GI tract.

CLINICAL EVALUATION: In one study of 10 patients receiving large doses of chlorpromazine, the coadministration of aluminum hydroxide (*Aludrox*) resulted in 10% to 45% decreases in urinary chlorpromazine excretion.[1] Information from another study indicates that an antacid containing magnesium trisilicate and aluminum hydroxide may decrease blood concentrations of chlorpromazine given as an oral suspension.[2] Thus, it is possible that a decreased therapeutic response to chlorpromazine may occur; one possible case has been reported.[2] In one other preliminary report, antacids did not affect the absorption of chlorpromazine.[3] Until further studies are performed, assume that antacids are capable of reducing the GI absorption of chlorpromazine (and possibly other neuroleptics).

RELATED DRUGS: The effect of antacids on other neuroleptics is not established.

MANAGEMENT OPTIONS: No specific action is required, but be alert for evidence of the interaction.

REFERENCES:

1. Forrest FM, et al. Modification of chlorpromazine metabolism by some other drugs frequently administered to psychiatric patients. *Biol Psychiatry*. 1970;2:53.

2. Fann WE. Chlorpromazine: effects of antacids on its gastrointestinal absorption. *J Clin Pharmacol*. 1973;13:388.

3. Pinell OC, et al. Drug-drug interaction of chlorpromazine and antacid. *Clin Pharmacol Ther*. 1978;23:125.

Antacids 4

Cimetidine (eg, *Tagamet*)

SUMMARY: Although simultaneous administration of antacids with cimetidine reduces cimetidine serum concentrations, the clinical importance of this effect is questionable.

RISK FACTORS: No specific risk factors are known.

MECHANISM: Antacids inhibit the extent of absorption of cimetidine, possibly by adsorbing cimetidine in the GI tract.

CLINICAL EVALUATION: In several studies involving both patients and normal subjects, coadministration of aluminum and/or magnesium antacids decreased the extent of cimetidine absorption and decreased serum cimetidine concentrations.[1-3] The reductions in cimetidine serum concentrations are usually modest and the acid-neutralizing effect of the antacids would be expected to offset the reduction in cimetidine levels. Also, the interaction between these drugs is minimal when cimetidine is given with a meal and the antacid is given 1 hour after the meal. Thus, it seems unlikely that the therapeutic response to cimetidine would be adversely affected.

RELATED DRUGS: Ranitidine (*Zantac*), famotidine (*Pepcid*), and nizatidine (*Axid*) absorption may also be reduced by antacids; however, as with cimetidine, the clinical importance of this effect is probably minimal.

MANAGEMENT OPTIONS: No specific action is required, but be alert for evidence of the interaction.

REFERENCES:
1. Steinberg WM, et al. Antacids inhibit absorption of cimetidine. *N Engl J Med.* 1982;307:400.
2. Russell WL, et al. Effect of antacids on predicted steady-state cimetidine concentrations. *Dig Dis Sci.* 1984;29:385.
3. Bodemar G, et al. Diminished absorption of cimetidine caused by antacids. *Lancet.* 1979;1:444.

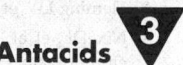

Antacids

Ciprofloxacin (*Cipro*)

SUMMARY: Antacids reduce the serum concentration of ciprofloxacin and may inhibit its efficacy.

RISK FACTORS:

➡ *Dosage Regimen.* The effects of antacids on quinolone absorption appear to be greater when large antacid doses are administered.

➡ *Diet/Food.* Binding interactions in the GI tract tend to be greater in the fasting state than if there is food in the stomach.

MECHANISM: The probable mechanism involves chelation between the antacid cations and the 4-oxo and 3-carboxyl groups of the quinolone, resulting in decreased bioavailability of the antibiotic.[6]

CLINICAL EVALUATION: When an aluminum-magnesium hydroxide antacid (*Maalox*) was administered every 2 hours for 24 hours before ciprofloxacin, the peak serum concentration and urinary excretion of unmetabolized drug were reduced by more than 90%.[1] In other reports, ciprofloxacin serum concentrations were reduced 40% to 70% when antacids were coadministered.[2,3,5] Ciprofloxacin administered with 100 mL magnesium citrate reduced the absorption by 80%.[10] Antacids administered 6 hours before or 2 hours after ciprofloxacin had little effect on serum concentrations.[4] Calcium may inhibit ciprofloxacin absorption less than magnesium-aluminumhydroxides. In healthy subjects the bioavailability of 250 mg ciprofloxacin was 35% when given alone and 29% when given with 500 mg calcium carbonate.[11] Other sources of calcium, including a high-calcium breakfast (729 mg calcium)[7] and nasogastric tube feedings with Osmolite[8] had no effect on ciprofloxacin pharmacokinetics.

RELATED DRUGS: The absorption of other quinolones is also reduced by antacids, but the absorption of lomefloxacin (*Maxaquin*) and ofloxacin (*Floxacin*) appears somewhat less affected by cations (eg, antacids) than ciprofloxacin. Since ranitidine (*Zantac*) does not appear to affect ciprofloxacin absorption,[4,9] one would assume that other H_2-receptor antagonists (eg, cimetidine [*Tagamet*], famotidine [*Pepcid*], nizatidine [*Axid*]) and proton pump inhibitors (eg, omeprazole [*Prilosec*], lansoprazole [*Prevacid*]) also would have no effect. Sucralfate (*Carafate*) dramatically reduces ciprofloxacin absorption.

MANAGEMENT OPTIONS:

➡ ***Consider Alternative.*** Since it may be difficult to separate the doses of magnesium-aluminum-hydroxide antacids and ciprofloxacin sufficiently to prevent their interaction, consider using H_2-receptor antagonists or proton pump inhibitors.

➡ ***Circumvent/Minimize.*** If antacids are used with oral ciprofloxacin, give the ciprofloxacin at least 2 hours before or 6 hours after the antacid.

➡ ***Monitor.*** Monitor for reduced ciprofloxacin response if antacids are also taken.

REFERENCES:

1. Hoffken G, et al. Reduced enteral absorption of ciprofloxacin in the presence of antacids. *Eur J Clin Microbiol.* 1985;4:345.

2. Preheim LC, et al. Ciprofloxacin and antacids. *Lancet.* 1986;2:48.

3. Fleming LW, et al. Ciprofloxacin and antacids. *Lancet.* 1986:2:294.

4. Nix DE, et al. Effects of aluminum and magnesium antacids and ranitidine on the absorption of ciprofloxacin. *Clin Pharmacol Ther.* 1989;46:700.

5. Frost RW, et al. Effect of aluminum hydroxide and calcium carbonate antacids on ciprofloxacin bioavailability. *Clin Pharmacol Ther.* 1989;45:165.

6. Hoffken G, et al. Pharmacokinetics and bioavailability of ciprofloxacin and ofloxacin: effect of food and antacid intake. *Rev Infect Dis.* 1988;10:S138.

7. Frost RW, et al. Ciprofloxacin pharmacokinetics after a standard or high-fat/high-calcium breakfast. *J Clin Pharmacol.* 1989;29:953.

8. Yek JHJ, et al. Relative bioavailability in healthy volunteers of ciprofloxacin administration through a nasogastric tube with and without enteral feeding. *Antimicrob Agents Chemother.* 1989;22:1118.

9. Watson WA, et al. Effects of timing of Maalox administration and ranitidine on ciprofloxacin (*Cipro*) absorption. *Pharm Res.* 1988:5(Suppl):S164.

10. Brouwers JRBJ, et al. Important reduction of ciprofloxacin absorption by sucralfate and magnesium citrate solution. *Drug Invest.* 1990;2:197.

11. Navarro AS, et al. Comparative study of the influence of CA^{2+} on absorption parameters of ciprofloxacin and ofloxacin. *J Antimicrob Chemother.* 1994;34:119.

Antacids **3**

Dextroamphetamine (eg, *Dextrostat*)

SUMMARY: Large sodium bicarbonate doses can inhibit the elimination and increase the effect of dextroamphetamine.

RISK FACTORS: No specific risk factors are known.

MECHANISM: Alkalinization of the urine by sufficient doses of sodium bicarbonate increases the proportion of nonionized dextroamphetamine resulting in increased renal tubular reabsorption of the amphetamine.

CLINICAL EVALUATION: This interaction is well documented. Excretion of dextroamphetamine is extremely small in those with highly alkaline urine, which prolongs the effect of the amphetamine.[1-3] Individuals abusing dextroamphetamine have made use of this property by ingesting sodium bicarbonate along with amphetamine.

RELATED DRUGS: Any drug that substantially alkalinizes the urine (eg, carbonic anhydrase inhibitors) would be expected to inhibit amphetamine elimination. Some antacids other than sodium bicarbonate (eg, aluminum-, magnesium-, and calcium-containing antacids) may slightly alkalinize the urine, but their effect on dextroamphetamine excretion is probably not large. Sympathomimetic amines other than dextroamphetamine have been shown to demonstrate pH dependent urinary excretion.

MANAGEMENT OPTIONS:

➡ *Monitor.* Monitor for altered dextroamphetamine effect if sodium bicarbonate is initiated, discontinued or changed in dosage. Alteration in dextroamphetamine dose may be necessary.

REFERENCES:
1. Anggard E, et al. Amphetamine metabolism in amphetamine psychosis. *Clin Pharmacol Ther.* 1973;14:870.
2. Rowland M. Amphetamine blood and urine levels in man. *J Pharm Sci.* 1969;58:508.
3. Milne MD. Influence of acid-base balance on efficacy and toxicity of drugs. *Proc R Soc Med.* 1965;58:961.

Antacids **4**

Dicumarol

SUMMARY: Dicumarol absorption may be enhanced by coadministration of magnesium hydroxide, but the clinical importance of this effect is not clear; warfarin absorption does not appear to be affected by magnesium or aluminum hydroxides.

RISK FACTORS: No specific risk factors are known.

MECHANISM: The coadministration of magnesium hydroxide and dicumarol may result in the formation of a magnesium chelate of dicumarol that is more readily absorbed than dicumarol itself.

CLINICAL EVALUATION: In 1 study, peak plasma concentrations of dicumarol occurred earlier and were higher when the dicumarol was given with magnesium hydroxide than when it was given with water.[1] In the same study, aluminum hydroxide did not appear to affect dicumarol blood concentrations.

RELATED DRUGS: Warfarin (eg, *Coumadin*) plasma concentrations do not appear to be affected by aluminum hydroxide,[1] magnesium hydroxide,[1] or a mixture of the 2 antacids.[2] Little is known regarding the effect of other types of antacids (eg, calcium carbonate) on oral anticoagulants or the effect of antacids on oral anticoagulants other than dicumarol and warfarin.

MANAGEMENT OPTIONS: No specific action is required, but be alert for evidence of the interaction.

REFERENCES:

1. Ambre JJ, et al. Effect of coadministration of aluminum and magnesium hydroxides on absorption of anticoagulants in man. *Clin Pharmacol Ther*. 1973;14:231.

2. Robinson DS, et al. Interaction of warfarin and nonsystemic gastrointestinal drugs. *Clin Pharmacol Ther*. 1971;12:491.

 Antacids

Diflunisal (*Dolobid*)

SUMMARY: Aluminum-containing antacids tend to reduce diflunisal bioavailability under fasting conditions.

RISK FACTORS:

➡ *Diet/Food.* The binding of diflunisal to antacids appears to occur in patients with no food in their stomachs, but not after a meal. Neither aluminum hydroxide nor magnesium-aluminum hydroxide affected diflunisal bioavailability in the fed state.

MECHANISM: Some antacids reduce the extent of absorption of diflunisal, possibly by adsorption of diflunisal in the GI tract.

CLINICAL EVALUATION: In single-dose studies in fasting healthy subjects, aluminum hydroxide reduced diflunisal bioavailability by approximately 25% to 40%[1,2] and magnesium-aluminum hydroxide reduced diflunisal bioavailability by approximately 15% to 20%.[3] Repeated doses of magnesium-aluminum hydroxide lowered diflunisal bioavailability by approximately 30%;[3] magnesium hydroxide slightly increased diflunisal bioavailability.[1]

RELATED DRUGS: Antacids may delay or reduce the absorption of other nonsteroidal anti-inflammatory drugs, but the clinical importance is probably not large.

MANAGEMENT OPTIONS: No specific action is required, but be alert for evidence of the interaction.

REFERENCES:

1. Tobert JA, et al. Effect of antacids on the bioavailability of diflunisal in the fasting and postprandial states. *Clin Pharmacol Ther*. 1981;30:385.

2. Verbeeck R, et al. Effect of aluminum hydroxide on diflunisal absorption. *Br J Clin Pharmacol*. 1979;7:519.

3. Holmes GI, et al. Effects of Maalox on the bioavailability of diflunisal. *Clin Pharmacol Ther*. 1979;25:229.

Antacids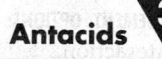

Enoxacin (*Penetrex*)

SUMMARY: Antacids reduce the serum concentration of enoxacin and may inhibit its efficacy.

RISK FACTORS:

➡ **Dosage Regimen.** The effects of antacids on quinolone absorption appear to be greater when large antacid doses are administered.

➡ **Diet/Food.** Binding interactions in the GI tract tend to be greater in the fasting state than if there is food in the stomach.

MECHANISM: The probable mechanism involves chelation between the antacid cations and the 4-oxo and 3-carboxyl groups of the quinolone, resulting in a decreased bioavailability of the antibiotic. Alkalinization of the stomach also may reduce enoxacin bioavailability.

CLINICAL EVALUATION: Enoxacin absorption was reduced by 73% and 49% when antacids were administered one-half hour and 2 hours before enoxacin, respectively.[1] Ranitidine (*Zantac*) was reported to cause a 25% to 40% reduction in enoxacin bioavailability.[1,2] Re-acidification of the stomach avoided the interaction.[2]

RELATED DRUGS: The absorption of other quinolones also is reduced by antacids. Given the effect of ranitidine on enoxacin absorption, other H₂-receptor antagonists (eg, cimetidine [*Tagamet*], famotidine [*Pepcid*], nizatidine [*Axid*]) and proton pump inhibitors (eg, omeprazole [*Prilosec*], lansoprazole [*Prevacid*]) should be expected to reduce enoxacin absorption as well.

MANAGEMENT OPTIONS:

➡ **Circumvent/Minimize.** If antacids are used with oral enoxacin, give the enoxacin at least 2 hours before or 6 hours after the antacid.

➡ **Monitor.** Monitor for reduced enoxacin response if antacids are also taken.

REFERENCES:

1. Grasela TH, et al. Inhibition of enoxacin absorption by antacids or ranitidine. *Antimicrob Agents Chemother.* 1989;33:615.

2. Lebsack M, et al. Impact of gastric pH on ranitidine-enoxacin drugdrug interaction. *J Clin Pharmacol.* 1988;28:939.

Antacids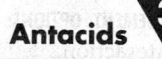

Ephedrine

SUMMARY: Large doses of sodium bicarbonate may increase serum concentrations of ephedrine.

RISK FACTORS: No specific risk factors are known.

MECHANISM: Sodium bicarbonate-induced alkalinization of the urine decreases the ionization of ephedrine, thus enhancing renal tubular reabsorption.

CLINICAL EVALUATION: A study in normal subjects given single doses of ephedrine showed that urinary excretion of ephedrine is reduced when the urine is alkaline.[1] Short-term urinary alkalinization with sodium bicarbonate is unlikely to be important clinically, but ephedrine toxicity is possible if the urine remains alkaline for several days or longer.

RELATED DRUGS: Any drug that substantially alkalinizes the urine (eg, carbonic anhydrase inhibitors) would be expected to inhibit ephedrine elimination. Some antacids other than sodium bicarbonate (eg, aluminum-, magnesium-, and calcium-containing antacids) may slightly alkalinize the urine, but their effect on ephedrine excretion is probably not large. Sympathomimetic amines other than ephedrine have been shown to demonstrate pH dependent urinary excretion.

MANAGEMENT OPTIONS:

➡ **Monitor.** Monitor for evidence of ephedrine toxicity (eg, nervousness, insomnia, excitability) if the urine remains alkaline for more than a day or two. Monitor for altered ephedrine effect if sodium bicarbonate therapy is initiated, discontinued, or changed in dosage; adjust ephedrine dose as needed.

REFERENCES:

1. Wilkinson GR, et al. Absorption, metabolism and excretion of the ephedrines in man I. The influence of urinary pH and urine volume output. *J Pharmacol Exp Ther*. 1968;162:139.

4   Antacids

Erythromycin (eg, *E-Mycin*)

SUMMARY: Antacids can increase the apparent half-life of erythromycin; but the clinical importance of the effect is probably minimal.

RISK FACTORS: No specific risk factors are known.

MECHANISM: Not established.

CLINICAL EVALUATION: Eight healthy subjects received erythromycin stearate 500 mg alone or immediately before 30 mL of aluminum and magnesium hydroxides (*Mylanta*).[1] No significant differences were noted in the erythromycin area under the concentration-time curve, time to peak concentration, or peak concentration. The apparent half-life of erythromycin was increased by 54%. This increase in half-life following antacid administration may represent a prolongation of erythromycin absorption, but the effect is not likely to be clinically important.

RELATED DRUGS: Sucralfate (*Carafate*) 1 g taken with erythromycin ethylsuccinate 400 mg did not alter the plasma concentration of erythromycin.[2]

MANAGEMENT OPTIONS: No specific action is required, but be alert for evidence of the interaction.

REFERENCES:

1. Yamreudeewong W, et al. Effect of antacid coadministration on the bioavailability of erythromycin stearate. *Clin Pharm*. 1989;8:352.

2. Miller LC, et al. Effect of concurrent sucralfate administration on the absorption of erythromycin. *J Clin Pharmacol*. 1990;30:39.

Antacids **4**

Famotidine (*Pepcid*)

SUMMARY: Famotidine bioavailability may be reduced by large doses of antacids containing magnesium and aluminum hydroxides, but the clinical importance of this effect is probably small.

RISK FACTORS: No specific risk factors are known.

MECHANISM: Not established. Antacids may adsorb famotidine in the gut.

CLINICAL EVALUATION: Eight healthy fasting subjects received a 40 mg famotidine tablet under the following 3 conditions in a randomized crossover study: famotidine alone, famotidine with concurrent antacid, and antacid 2 hours after the famotidine.[1] The antacid consisted of 30 mL of *Mylanta* II, a high potency antacid containing magnesium and aluminum hydroxides plus simethicone. Concurrent antacid reduced the peak famotidine plasma concentrations by 33% and reduced the area under the famotidine plasma concentration-time curve by 37%. Administration of the antacid 2 hours after the famotidine slightly reduced famotidine bioavailability, but the effect did not reach statistical significance. One cannot rule out the possibility that simethicone may have contributed to the observed reduction in famotidine absorption. Although the magnitude of the reduction in famotidine absorption in this study would be expected to reduce famotidine effects, the acid neutralizing effect of the antacids would be expected to offset somewhat the effect of reduction in famotidine levels. Moreover, the relative benefits of famotidine alone vs famotidine plus concurrent antacid in patients with acid-peptic disease is not established. Indeed, the manufacturer of famotidine states that antacids may be given with famotidine.[2]

RELATED DRUGS: Although different types or doses of antacids may not produce the same degree of interaction, assume that all antacids interfere with famotidine bioavailability until proven otherwise. Cimetidine (eg, *Tagamet*), ranitidine (*Zantac*), and nizatidine (*Axid*) absorption also may be reduced by antacids; however, as with famotidine, the clinical importance of this effect is probably minimal.

MANAGEMENT OPTIONS: No specific action is required, but be alert for evidence of the interaction.

REFERENCES:
1. Barzaghi N, et al. Impaired bioavailability of famotidine given concurrently with a potent antacid. *J Clin Pharmacol.* 1989;29:670.
2. Product information. Antacids (*Pepcid*). 1990

Antacids (eg, *Maalox*)

Fleroxacin†

SUMMARY: Limited data demonstrate a small effect of aluminum hydroxide on fleroxacin concentrations.

RISK FACTORS:

➥ *Dosage Regimen.* The effects of antacids on quinolone absorption appear to be greater when large doses of antacids are administered.

➥ *Diet/Food.* Binding interactions in the GI tract tend to be greater in the fasting state than if there is food in the stomach.

MECHANISM: The probable mechanism involves chelation between the antacid cations and the 4-oxo and 3-carboxyl groups of the quinolone, resulting in a decreased bioavailability of the antibiotic.

CLINICAL EVALUATION: Six healthy subjects received a single dose of fleroxacin 200 mg alone and followed by 1 g of dried aluminum hydroxide gel 0.5, 12, 24, and 36 hours later.[1] The peak fleroxacin concentration was reduced 24%; the area under the fleroxacin concentration-time curve was not reduced significantly (16%). The clinical significance of antacid interactions with fleroxacin requires further study.

RELATED DRUGS: The absorption of other quinolones also is reduced by antacids. H_2-receptor antagonists (eg, cimetidine [eg, *Tagamet*], famotidine [eg, *Pepcid*], nizatidine [eg, *Axid*], ranitidine [eg, *Zantac*]) and proton pump inhibitors (eg, lansoprazole [eg, *Prevacid*], omeprazole [eg, *Prilosec*]) are not known to affect fleroxacin absorption.

MANAGEMENT OPTIONS:

➥ *Consider Alternative.* Because it may be difficult to separate the doses of antacid and fleroxacin sufficiently to prevent an interaction, the use of H_2-receptor antagonists or proton pump inhibitors may be necessary for severe infections when patients require gastric acid reduction.

➥ *Circumvent/Minimize.* If antacids are used with oral fleroxacin, give the fleroxacin at least 2 hours before or 6 hours after the antacid.

➥ *Monitor.* Monitor for reduced fleroxacin response if antacids are coadministered.

REFERENCES:

1. Shiba K, et al. Interactions of fleroxacin with dried aluminum hydroxide gel and probenecid. *Rev Infect Dis.* 1989;11(suppl 5):S1097-S1098.

† Not available in the United States.

Antacids (eg, *Maalox*)

Fluconazole (eg, *Diflucan*)

SUMMARY: Antacid administration does not alter fluconazole pharmacokinetics.

RISK FACTORS: No specific risk factors are known.

MECHANISM: No interaction.

CLINICAL EVALUATION: Fourteen healthy subjects received a single dose of fluconazole 100 mg fasting or following 20 mL of aluminum and magnesium hydroxides.[1] The antacid had no effect on fluconazole pharmacokinetics.

RELATED DRUGS: Antacids reduce the absorption of ketoconazole (eg, *Nizoral*) and itraconazole (eg, *Sporanox*).

MANAGEMENT OPTIONS: No interaction.

REFERENCES:

1. Thorpe JE, et al. Effect of oral antacid administration on the pharmacokinetics of oral fluconazole. *Antimicrob Agents Chemother.* 1990;34(10):2032-2033.

Antacids (eg, *Maalox*)
Gatifloxacin[†]

SUMMARY: Antacids can lower the absorption of gatifloxacin, resulting in reduced serum concentrations and possibe loss of antibiotic efficacy.

RISK FACTORS: No specific risk factors are known.

MECHANISM: Gatifloxacin forms a complex with the cations found in many antacids, reducing its bioavailability.

CLINICAL EVALUATION: Gatifloxacin 400 mg orally was administered alone, 2 hours after, concurrently, and 2 and 4 hours before 20 mL of *Maalox* was given to 24 healthy subjects.[1] Compared with gatifloxacin administered alone, the coadministration of the antacid resulted in a 64% reduction in the area under the concentration-time curve (AUC) of gatifloxacin. Giving the antacid 2 hours before the gatifloxacin lowered its AUC 42%. Administration of the antacid 2 hours after the gatifloxacin reduced the gatifloxacin AUC 17.5%, while waiting 4 hours after the gatifloxacin dose to give the antacid produced no significant change in the gatifloxacin serum concentrations. Avoid the administration of antacids within 2 hours of a dose of gatifloxacin.

RELATED DRUGS: Aluminum- and magnesium-containing antacids inhibit the absorption of other quinolone antibiotics, including ciprofloxacin (eg, *Cipro*), ofloxacin, and trovafloxacin.[†]

MANAGEMENT OPTIONS:

➥ **Consider Alternative.** Advise patients taking quinolone antibiotics to use other acid-suppressant drugs, such as H_2-antagonists or proton pump inhibitors.

➥ **Circumvent/Minimize.** Administration of the gatifloxacin more than 2 hours before the antacid will minimize the magnitude of the interaction.

➥ **Monitor.** Monitor patients taking gatifloxacin and antacid products containing di- or trivalent cations for adequate antibiotic response.

REFERENCES:

1. Lober S, et al. Pharmacokinetics of gatifloxacin and interaction with an antacid containing aluminum and magnesium. *Antimicrob Agents Chemother.* 1999;43(5):1067-1071.

† Not available in the United States.

Antacids (eg, *Maalox*)

Gemifloxacin (*Factive*)

SUMMARY: Antacids can reduce the plasma concentrations of gemifloxacin; loss of antibiotic efficacy may occur.

RISK FACTORS: No specific risk factors are known.

MECHANISM: Aluminum- and magnesium-containing antacids bind with gemifloxacin in the gut, inhibiting its absorption.

CLINICAL EVALUATION: Sixteen healthy subjects received a single oral dose of gemifloxacin 320 mg with water and 3 hours after 20 mL of *Maalox*, or 10 minutes or 2 hours before *Maalox* administration.[1,2] When gemifloxacin was taken 10 minutes before the antacid, its mean area under the concentration-time curve (AUC) was reduced 85%. Taking gemifloxacin 3 hours after or 2 hours before the antacid resulted in no significant change in gemifloxacin AUC. As with other quinolones, administer gemifloxacin at least 2 hours before any antacid to maintain maximal absorption. In another study, the simultaneous administration of calcium carbonate 1,000 mg resulted in a modest (21%) reduction in gemifloxacin AUC.[3] Separation of the calcium carbonate dose by 2 hours, either before or after the gemifloxacin, avoided the interaction. In a study of 27 healthy subjects, administration of gemifloxacin 3 hours after a single dose of sucralfate (eg, *Carafate*) 2 g resulted in a 53% decrease in the AUC of gemifloxacin.[4] Giving the gemifloxacin 2 hours before the sucralfate avoided the interaction.

RELATED DRUGS: Nearly all quinolones have been reported to have lower bioavailability when administered with antacids containing aluminum and magnesium ions.

MANAGEMENT OPTIONS:

➡ *Circumvent/Minimize.* Administer gemifloxacin 2 hours before any antacid containing magnesium or aluminum ions.

➡ *Monitor.* Monitor patients receiving gemifloxacin and antacids for adequate anti-infective response.

REFERENCES:

1. *Factive* [package insert]. Waltham, MA: Oscient Pharmaceuticals; 2008.
2. Allen A, et al. Effect of *Maalox* on the bioavailability of oral gemifloxacin in healthy volunteers. *Chemotherapy.* 1999;45(6):504-511.
3. Pletz MW, et al. Effect of calcium carbonate on bioavailability of orally administered gemifloxacin. *Antimicrob Agents Chemother.* 2003;47(7):2158-2160.
4. Allen A, et al. The effect of ferrous sulphate and sucralfate on the bioavailability of oral gemifloxacin in healthy volunteers. *Int J Antimicrob Agents.* 2000;15(4):283-289.

Antacids (eg, *Maalox*)

Glipizide (eg, *Glucotrol*)

SUMMARY: Magnesium hydroxide or sodium bicarbonate may enhance the rate of absorption of glipizide, but the clinical importance has not been established.

RISK FACTORS: No specific risk factors are known.

MECHANISM: Not established.

CLINICAL EVALUATION: In healthy subjects, magnesium hydroxide enhanced the rate of absorption of glipizide and increased the maximal reduction in glucose levels 35%.[1] In another study, sodium bicarbonate enhanced glipizide absorption rate and maximal reduction in glucose 50%.[2] Nonetheless, the bioavailability of glipizide was not affected by either antacid. The extent to which the increase in maximal reduction in glucose levels would result in symptoms is not clear, but it is possible that some patients would be affected adversely. Aluminum hydroxide did not appear to affect the rate or extent of glipizide absorption.[2]

RELATED DRUGS: H_2-receptor antagonists (eg, cimetidine [eg, *Tagamet*], famotidine [eg, *Pepcid*], nizatidine [eg, *Axid*], ranitidine [eg, *Zantac*]) also have been reported to increase the hypoglycemic effect of glipizide. Glyburide (eg, *DiaBeta*) absorption also appears to be increased by elevating gastric pH.

MANAGEMENT OPTIONS:

➥ *Circumvent/Minimize.* Until more information is available, it is recommended to give glipizide 2 hours before or after antacids.

➥ *Monitor.* Monitor for altered hypoglycemic effect of glipizide if antacids are initiated, discontinued, or changed in dosage, or if the dosage interval between the antacid and glipizide is changed.

REFERENCES:

1. Kivisto KT, et al. Enhancement of absorption and effect of glipizide by magnesium hydroxide. *Clin Pharmacol Ther*. 1991;49(1):39-43.

2. Kivisto KT, et al. Differential effects of sodium bicarbonate and aluminum hydroxide on the absorption and activity of glipizide. *Eur J Clin Pharmacol*. 1991;40(4):383-386.

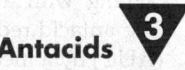

Antacids

Glyburide (eg, *DiaBeta*)

SUMMARY: Antacid (aluminum-magnesium hydroxides) increased glyburide serum concentrations, but the clinical importance of this effect is not established.

RISK FACTORS: No specific risk factors are known.

MECHANISM: Antacids appear to increase the absorption of glyburide, perhaps because of increasing gastric pH.

CLINICAL EVALUATION: Eight healthy subjects were given glyburide 2.5 mg and a standardized breakfast with and without 10 mL of aluminum and magnesium hydroxides (*Maalox*).[1] The antacid resulted in a significant increase in the glyburide area under the concentration-time curve (25%) and peak serum concentration (32%). No differences were observed in glucose, C-peptide, or insulin concentrations. More study is needed using larger doses of both drugs and patients with diabetes as subjects.

RELATED DRUGS: If the increased glyburide levels are caused by increased gastric pH, all antacids would be expected to interact, as would H_2-receptor antagonists (eg, cimetidine [eg, *Tagamet*], famotidine [eg, *Pepcid*], nizatidine [eg, *Axid*]) and proton pump inhibitors (eg, lansoprazole [*Prevacid*], omeprazole [eg, *Prilosec*]). Ranitidine does not alter glyburide pharmacokinetics.

MANAGEMENT OPTIONS:

➥ *Circumvent/Minimize.* Because the interaction is most likely caused by the increased gastric pH, one would expect that giving the glyburide at least 2 hours before or after the antacid should minimize the effect. If antacids are taken regularly, maintain a relatively constant interval between the antacid and glyburide so that any interaction will remain relatively constant.

➥ *Monitor.* Monitor for altered hypoglycemic effect of glyburide if antacids are initiated, discontinued, changed in dosage, or if the dosing interval between the antacid and glyburide is changed.

REFERENCES:

1. Zuccaro P, et al. Influence of antacids on the bioavailability of glibenclamide. *Drugs Exp Clin Res.* 1989;15:165-169.

Antacids (eg, magnesium carbonate [eg, *Marblen*])

Halofantrine (*Halfan*)

SUMMARY: Magnesium carbonate, and possibly other antacids, may reduce the bioavailability of halofantrine.

RISK FACTORS: No specific risk factors are known.

MECHANISM: Magnesium carbonate probably binds halofantrine in the GI tract, reducing its absorption.

CLINICAL EVALUATION: Seven healthy subjects took a single oral dose of halofantrine 500 mg with and without coadministration of magnesium carbonate 1000 mg.[1] The antacid reduced halofantrine area under the plasma concentration-time curve (AUC) by a mean of 28% and reduced halofantrine peak plasma concentrations by 49%. The magnitude of the reductions in halofantrine plasma concentrations was highly variable among subjects, and it seems likely that the interaction would reduce halofantrine efficacy in at least some patients. In vitro studies found aluminum hydroxide and magnesium trisilicate to bind halofantrine more strongly than magnesium carbonate.

RELATED DRUGS: Although the effect of other antacids on halofantrine bioavailability is not established, assume that they interact until proven otherwise.

MANAGEMENT OPTIONS:

➥ *Consider Alternative.* Theoretically, H_2-receptor antagonists other than cimetidine (eg, *Tagamet*) would be unlikely to interact with halofantrine.

➥ *Circumvent/Minimize.* Although the effect of spacing doses of halofantrine and antacids is not known, it would be prudent to give the halofantrine at least 2 hours before or 6 hours after the antacid.

REFERENCES:

1. Aideloje SO, et al. Altered halofantrine by an antacid, magnesium carbonate. *Eur J Pharm Biopharm.* 1998;46:299-303.

Antacids

Indomethacin (*Indocin*)

SUMMARY: Antacids may reduce the absorption of indomethacin slightly, but reduced indomethacin therapeutic response has not been established.

RISK FACTORS: No specific risk factors are known.

MECHANISM: Some antacids appear to inhibit the absorption of indomethacin, possibly by adsorbing indomethacin in the GI tract.

CLINICAL EVALUATION: In studies in normal volunteers, aluminum- and magnesium-containing antacids slightly decrease the GI absorption of indomethacin.[1-3] Antacids are sometimes used in an attempt to minimize the adverse effects of indomethacin on the gastric mucosa. Although the benefit of such use of antacids is not clearly established, the magnitude of the reduction in serum indomethacin concentration is unlikely to reduce its therapeutic effect significantly.

RELATED DRUGS: Antacids may delay or reduce the absorption of other NSAIDs, but the clinical importance is probably not large.

MANAGEMENT OPTIONS: No specific action is required, but be alert for evidence of the interaction.

REFERENCES:
1. Emori HW, et al. Indomethacin serum concentrations in man: effects of dosage, food, and antacid. *Ann Rheum Dis*. 1976;35:333.
2. Garnham JC, et al. Different effects of sodium bicarbonate and aluminum hydroxide on absorption of indomethacin in man. *Postgrad Med J*. 1977;53:126.
3. Galeazzi RL. The effect of an antacid on the bioavailability of indomethacin. *Eur J Clin Pharmacol*. 1977;12:65.

Antacids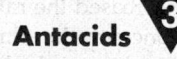

Iron

SUMMARY: Some antacids reduce the GI absorption of iron; inhibition of the hematological response to iron has been reported.

RISK FACTORS: No specific risk factors are known.

MECHANISM: Not established. Magnesium trisilicate presumably forms poorly soluble substances with oral iron, thus decreasing iron absorption.[2] Antacids containing carbonate reportedly may have a similar effect.[1]

CLINICAL EVALUATION: Patients with iron deficiency anemia may not respond to oral iron therapy as expected when antacids such as magnesium trisilicate are given concomitantly.[2] In a study of 9 patients, magnesium trisilicate markedly impaired the absorption of simultaneously administered ferrous sulfate.[2] In patients with iron deficiency anemia, absorption of ferrous sulfate was reduced by approximately 50% to 60% when 1 gm sodium bicarbonate or 500 mg calcium carbonate was given concurrently. Although 5 mL of *Mylanta II* did not reduce iron absorption significantly,[4] many patients take considerably more than 5 mL; thus, it cannot be concluded that magnesium-aluminum hydroxide antacids such as *Mylanta* do not affect the absorption of iron. In in vitro studies, iron availability is reduced in the presence of certain antacids.[3]

RELATED DRUGS: Until more information is available, assume that all antacids can reduce iron absorption.

MANAGEMENT OPTIONS:

➡ *Circumvent/Minimize.* Space antacids containing magnesium trisilicate, calcium carbonate, or sodium bicarbonate as far apart as possible from oral iron preparations. Until further information is available, observe the same precaution with other antacids.

➡ *Monitor.* Monitor for reduced iron response if antacids are also taken.

REFERENCES:

1. Azarnoff DL, et al. Drug interactions. *Pharmacol Physicians*. 1970;4 (Feb):1.
2. Hall GJL, et al. Inhibition of iron absorption by magnesium trisilicate. *Med J Aust*. 1969;2:95.
3. Coste JF, et al. In vitro interactions of oral hematinics and antacid suspensions. *Curr Ther Res*. 1977;22:205.
4. O'Neil-Cutting MA, et al. The effect of antacids on the absorption of simultaneously ingested iron. *JAMA*. 1986;255:1468.

 Antacids

Isoniazid (INH; eg, *Nydrazid*)

SUMMARY: Some antacids may reduce the plasma concentration of INH.

RISK FACTORS: No specific risk factors are known.

MECHANISM: Not established. Antacids may bind with isoniazid in the GI tract.

CLINICAL EVALUATION: In a study of 11 patients with tuberculosis, aluminum hydroxide gel decreased the rate and amount of INH absorbed as measured by the plasma drug concentration-time curve.[1] The effect of magaldrate on INH plasma concentrations was less marked. Curiously, one alcoholic patient demonstrated a marked increase in INH plasma concentrations when aluminum hydroxide or magaldrate was given. In healthy subjects, the antacids in didanosine tablets (containing magnesium and aluminum) did not affect the bioavailability of INH.[2]

RELATED DRUGS: Until more information is available, assume that all antacids can reduce INH absorption.

MANAGEMENT OPTIONS:

➡ *Circumvent/Minimize.* Give isoniazid 2 hours before or 6 hours after antacids.

➡ *Monitor.* Monitor for reduced isoniazid response if antacids are also used.

REFERENCES:

1. Hurwitz A, et al. Effects of antacids on gastrointestinal absorption of isoniazid in rat and man. *Am Rev Respir Dis*. 1974;109:41.
2. Gallicano K, et al. Effect of antacids in didanosine tablet on bioavailability of isoniazid. *Antimicrob Agents Chemother*. 1994;38:894.

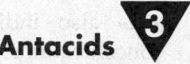

Antacids

Itraconazole (eg, *Sporanox*)

SUMMARY: Antacids markedly reduce the plasma concentration of itraconazole; loss of efficacy may occur.

RISK FACTORS: No specific risk factors are known.

MECHANISM: Itraconazole requires an acidic media for dissolution. Increasing the pH of the stomach will inhibit the dissolution and absorption of itraconazole.

CLINICAL EVALUATION: Twelve subjects received a single dose of itraconazole 200 mg with 240 mL of water alone and 5 minutes after ingesting 30 mL of an antacid suspension containing aluminum hydroxide and magnesium hydroxide.[1] The pretreatment with antacid reduced the mean area under the plasma concentration-time curve of itraconazole 66% and the peak itraconazole concentration 71%. This large reduction in the itraconazole plasma concentration associated with antacid ingestion will likely lead to a reduction in its antifungal efficacy.

RELATED DRUGS: Any drug that suppresses gastric acidity, including H_2-receptor blockers, antacids, and proton pump inhibitors, would be expected to reduce the bioavailability of itraconazole. The bioavailability of ketoconazole (eg, *Nizoral*) is also reduced by alkalinization of the stomach.

MANAGEMENT OPTIONS:

➡ **Consider Alternative.** Fluconazole (eg, *Diflucan*), voriconazole (*Vfend*), and terbinafine (*Lamisil*) are not affected by changes in gastric pH.

➡ **Circumvent/Minimize.** Administer itraconazole at least 2 hours prior to any antacid product. This will allow for dissolution of the itraconazole to be completed before the gastric pH is increased. Separation of doses will not be effective for systemic inhibitors of gastric acid secretion. The administration of acidic beverages (eg, *Coke*, *Pepsi*) can enhance the absorption of itraconazole, but some reduction in absorption is still likely to occur.

➡ **Monitor.** Be alert for reduced antifungal efficacy when antacids are administered with itraconazole.

REFERENCES:

1. Lohitnavy M, et al. Reduced oral itraconazole bioavailability by antacid suspension. *J Clin Pharm Ther.* 2005;30:201-206.

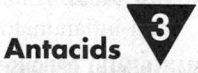

Antacids

Ketoconazole (*Nizoral*)

SUMMARY: Antacids may reduce ketoconazole concentrations.

RISK FACTORS: No specific risk factors are known.

MECHANISM: Ketoconazole requires an acidic environment to be absorbed; antacids reduce GI absorption of ketoconazole by increasing the pH within the GI tract.[3]

CLINICAL EVALUATION: In 12 healthy subjects, a simulated achlorhydric state induced by 300 mg of cimetidine and 2 g of sodium bicarbonate reduced ketoconazole absorption to 8% of that seen with ketoconazole alone.[2] Evidence from a few other subjects also indicates that antacids considerably reduce ketoconazole plasma concentrations.[1]

RELATED DRUGS: Any agents that substantially increase gastric pH (eg, H$_2$-receptor antagonists, proton pump inhibitors, and antacids containing aluminum, magnesium, or calcium) are likely to reduce the absorption of ketoconazole. Itraconazole absorption is similarly reduced by increased gastric pH, but fluconazole (*Diflucan*) is not.

MANAGEMENT OPTIONS:

➡ *Circumvent/Minimize.* Avoid antacids 2 hours before or after administration of ketoconazole.

➡ *Monitor.* Monitor for reduced ketoconazole effect if antacids are also given.

REFERENCES:

1. Van Der Meer JWM, et al. The influence of gastric acidity on the bioavailability of ketoconazole. *J Antimicrob Chemother.* 1980;6:552.

2. Lelawongs P, et al. Effect of food and gastric acidity on absorption of orally administered ketoconazole. *Clin Pharm.* 1988;7:228.

3. Carlson JA, et al. Effect of pH on disintegration and dissolution of ketoconazole tablets. *Am J Hosp Pharm.* 1983;40:1334.

5 Antacids

Ketorolac (*Toradol*)

SUMMARY: A single-dose study in healthy subjects suggests that magnesium-aluminum hydroxides do not affect the absorption of ketorolac.

RISK FACTORS: No specific risk factors are known.

MECHANISM: No interaction.

CLINICAL EVALUATION: Twelve healthy subjects received 10 mg ketorolac orally with and without coadministration of an unspecified dose of aluminum-magnesium hydroxide (*Maalox*).[1] The area under the plasma concentration-time curve was 11% lower in the presence of the antacid, but the change was not statistically significant. Thus, it appears unlikely that the therapeutic response to ketorolac would be affected by the use of magnesium-aluminum hydroxides (and probably other antacids).

RELATED DRUGS: Antacids may delay or reduce the absorption of other nonsteroidal anti-inflammatory drugs, but the clinical importance is probably not large.

MANAGEMENT OPTIONS: No interaction.

REFERENCES:

1. Mroszczak EJ, et al. Ketorolac tromethamine pharmacokinetics and metabolism after intravenous, intramuscular, and oral administration in humans and animals. *Pharmacotherapy.* 1990;10(Suppl. 6):33S.

Levodopa (eg, *Larodopa*)

SUMMARY: Antacids may increase levodopa bioavailability in some patients, but in most patients this effect is probably not clinically important.

RISK FACTORS: No specific risk factors are known.

MECHANISM: Not established. The acceleration of gastric emptying by antacids may decrease the amount of levodopa degraded in the stomach, leaving more to be absorbed in the small intestine.[1-4] Antacids may differ in their ability to speed gastric emptying; aluminum hydroxide gel may actually slow gastric emptying.

CLINICAL EVALUATION: Some parkinsonian patients have an improved response to levodopa following administration of antacids.[5-7] These patients may have slow gastric emptying resulting in excessive breakdown of levodopa in the stomach. Certain antacids may enhance gastric emptying in some of these patients, thus increasing the amount of levodopa absorbed. Patients on levodopa with normal gastric emptying probably would not be affected significantly by antacid administration.

RELATED DRUGS: Theoretically, other agents that enhance GI motility (eg, metoclopramide [*Reglan*], cisapride [*Propulsid*]) also may increase the bioavailability of levodopa in certain patients. However, metoclopramide is best avoided in patients with parkinsonism.

MANAGEMENT OPTIONS: No specific action is required, but be alert for evidence of the interaction.

REFERENCES:

1. Fermaglich J, et al. Effect of gastric motility on levodopa. *Dis Nerv Syst.* 1972;33:624.
2. Rivera-Calimlim L, et al. L-DOPA absorption and metabolism by the human stomach. *Pharmacologist.* 1970;12:269.
3. Dujovne CA, et al. The stomach as an important factor in the metabolism and effectiveness of L-DOPA in parkinsonian patients. *Gastroenterology.* 1970;58:1039.
4. Rivera-Calimlim L, et al. L-DOPA absorption and metabolism by the human stomach. *J Clin Invest.* 1970;49:79a
5. Rivera-Calimlim L, et al. L-DOPA treatment failure: explanation and correction. *BMJ.* 1970;4:93.
6. Leon A, et al. The effect of antacid administration on the absorption and metabolism of levodopa. *J Clin Pharmacol.* 1972;12:263.
7. Jenkins R, et al. Gastric acidity and levodopa in parkinsonism. *JAMA.* 1973;223:81.

 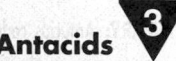

Levofloxacin (*Levaquin*)

SUMMARY: Antacids containing aluminum, calcium, or magnesium may reduce the plasma concentrations of levofloxacin. A reduction in antibiotic effect may occur.

RISK FACTORS: No specific risk factors are known.

MECHANISM: Divalent cations found in antacids can chelate with levofloxacin, reducing its bioavailability.

CLINICAL EVALUATION: While no specific data have been reported, the manufacturer of levofloxacin has cautioned against the coadministration of levofloxacin and antacids. Binding of levofloxacin by antacid cations in the GI tract may limit the absorption of levofloxacin. A loss of therapeutic effect may occur.

RELATED DRUGS: Antacids are known to reduce the absorption of other quinolone antibiotics including ciprofloxacin (*Cipro*) and lomefloxacin (*Maxaquin*). Other drugs that contain divalent cations (eg, sucralfate [*Carafate*], iron) would be expected to interact with levofloxacin in a similar manner.

MANAGEMENT OPTIONS:

➡ *Circumvent/Minimize.* Administration of levofloxacin 2 hours prior to the cation-containing drug will ensure optimal absorption of the quinolone.

➡ *Monitor.* Monitor patients taking levofloxacin for a reduced therapeutic response if antacids are coadministered.

REFERENCES:

1. Product information. Levofloxacin (*Levaquin*). McNeil Pharmaceutical. 1997.

 Antacids

Lithium (eg, *Eskalith*)

SUMMARY: Aluminum-magnesium hydroxide does not appear to interact with lithium carbonate.

RISK FACTORS: No specific risk factors are known.

MECHANISM: No interaction.

CLINICAL EVALUATION: In a study of 6 healthy subjects, an aluminum-magnesium hydroxide antacid did not affect lithium absorption.[1]

RELATED DRUGS: The effect of antacids other than aluminum-magnesium hydroxide is not established.

MANAGEMENT OPTIONS: No interaction.

REFERENCES:

1. Goode DL, et al. Effect of antacid on the bioavailability of lithium carbonate. *Clin Pharm.* 1984;3:284.

 Antacids

Lomefloxacin (*Maxaquin*)

SUMMARY: Antacids reduce the serum concentration of lomefloxacin and may inhibit its efficacy.

RISK FACTORS:

➡ *Dosage Regimen.* The effects of antacids on quinolone absorption appear to be greater when large antacid doses are administered.

➡ *Diet/Food.* Binding interactions in the GI tract tend to be greater in the fasting state than if there is food in the stomach.

MECHANISM: The probable mechanism involves chelation between the antacid cations and the 4-oxo and 3-carboxyl groups of the quinolone, resulting in a decreased bioavailability of the antibiotic.

CLINICAL EVALUATION: Twenty-four healthy subjects received lomefloxacin 400 mg alone and with 30 mL aluminum and magnesium hydroxides (eg, *Maalox*), 12 hours before antacid and 4 hours after antacid.[1] The area under the lomefloxacin concentration time curve was reduced 48% with antacid coadministration. Separation of the doses prevented any changes in quinolone concentrations.

RELATED DRUGS: The absorption of other quinolones also is reduced by antacids. Lomefloxacin absorption appears somewhat less affected by cations (eg, antacids) than ciprofloxacin (*Cipro*) or norfloxacin (*Noroxin*). H_2-receptor antagonists (eg, cimetidine [eg, *Tagamet*], famotidine [*Pepcid*], nizatidine [*Axid*], ranitidine [*Zantac*]) and proton pump inhibitors (eg, omeprazole [*Prilosec*], lansoprazole [*Prevacid*]) are not known to affect lomefloxacin absorption.

MANAGEMENT OPTIONS:

➡ *Consider Alternative.* Because it may be difficult to separate the doses of antacid and lomefloxacin sufficiently to prevent their interaction, the use of H_2-receptor antagonists or proton pump inhibitors may be necessary for severe infections when patients require gastric acid reduction.

➡ *Circumvent/Minimize.* If antacids are used with oral lomefloxacin, give the lomefloxacin at least 2 hours before or 6 hours after the antacid.

➡ *Monitor.* Monitor for reduced lomefloxacin response if antacids are also taken.

REFERENCES:

1. Kunka RL, et al. Effect of antacid on the pharmacokinetics of lomefloxacin. *Pharm Res.* 1988;10(suppl): S165.

Antacids 4

Metoprolol (eg, *Lopressor*)

SUMMARY: A magnesium-aluminum containing antacid had little effect on metoprolol absorption.

RISK FACTORS: No specific risk factors are known.

MECHANISM: Not established.

CLINICAL EVALUATION: The bioavailability of metoprolol may actually increase slightly with magnesium-aluminum antacid coadministration.[1]

RELATED DRUGS: Antacids delay the absorption of propranolol (*Inderal*).

MANAGEMENT OPTIONS: No specific action is required, but be alert for evidence of the interaction.

REFERENCES:

1. Regardh CG, et al. The effect of antacid, metoclopramide, and propantheline on the bioavailability of metoprolol and atenolol. *Biopharm Drug Dispos.* 1981;2:79.

Antacids 4

Metronidazole (eg, *Flagyl*)

SUMMARY: The coadministration of a single dose of aluminum hydroxide antacid reduced the bioavailability of metronidazole in healthy subjects, but the clinical importance of this effect is not established.

RISK FACTORS: No specific risk factors are known.

MECHANISM: Not established.

CLINICAL EVALUATION: Five healthy subjects took a single oral dose of metronidazole 500 mg alone and following a single 30 mL dose of an aluminum hydroxide suspension that also contained simethicone.[1] Metronidazole bioavailability was reduced by approximately 15% by the administration of this particular antacid/simethicone product. While this change is not likely to be clinically significant, it would be important to study the effects of repeated doses of antacids, with or without simethicone, on the bioavailability of metronidazole.

RELATED DRUGS: No information is available.

MANAGEMENT OPTIONS: No specific action is required, but be alert for evidence of the interaction.

REFERENCES:
    1. Molokhia AM, et al. Effect of concomitant oral administration of some adsorbing drugs on the bio-availability of metronidazole. *Drug Dev Ind Pharm.* 1987;13:1229.

Antacids (eg, *Maalox*)

Moxifloxacin (*Avelox*)

SUMMARY: The administration of antacid (eg, *Maalox*) reduced the plasma concentrations of moxifloxacin; some loss of efficacy may result.

RISK FACTORS: No specific risk factors are known.

MECHANISM: Moxifloxacin appears to chelate with the di- and trivalent cations such as magnesium or aluminum found in the antacid. Antacids may interfere with the GI circulation of moxifloxacin.

CLINICAL EVALUATION: Twelve healthy subjects took a single dose of moxifloxacin 400 mg orally alone or simultaneously with 10 mL of *Maalox* suspension containing 600 mg magnesium hydroxide and 900 mg aluminum hydroxide.[1] The same doses were also administered with the antacid given 4 hours before or 2 hours after the moxifloxacin. When moxifloxacin was administered simultaneously with *Maalox*, the area under the concentration-time curve (AUC) of moxifloxacin was reduced 59% compared with the AUC measured during moxifloxacin administration alone. Peak moxifloxacin concentration was reduced 61%. Giving the antacid 4 hours prior to or 2 hours after the moxifloxacin reduced the AUC of moxifloxacin 23% and 26% of the control value, respectively. Peak moxifloxacin concentrations were minimally affected when the doses of antacid and moxifloxacin were separated. The half-life of moxifloxacin was reduced 2 to 3 hours with antacid administration. The reduction in moxifloxacin concentrations following simultaneous antacid administration could reduce its antimicrobial efficacy.

RELATED DRUGS: Other quinolone antibiotics such as ciprofloxacin (*Cipro*) and lomefloxacin (*Maxaquin*) are affected in a similar manner by antacids. Other antacids containing di- or trivalent cations would be expected to affect moxifloxacin in a similar manner.

MANAGEMENT OPTIONS:

➡ *Consider Alternative.* Because it may be difficult to separate the doses of antacid and moxifloxacin sufficiently to prevent the interaction, consider using H_2-receptor antagonists or proton pump inhibitors to reduce gastric acidity.

➡ *Circumvent/Minimize.* If antacids are used with moxifloxacin, administer the moxifloxacin at least 2 hours before or 6 hours after the antacid.

➡ *Monitor.* Watch for reduced antibiotic efficacy if moxifloxacin and antacids are coadministered.

REFERENCES:

1. Stass H, et al. Evaluation of the influence of antacids and H_2 antagonists on the absorption of moxifloxacin after oral administration of a 400 mg dose to health volunteers. *Clin Pharmacokinet.* 2001;40(suppl 1):39.

Antacids (eg, *Maalox*)

Naproxen (eg, *Naprosyn*)

SUMMARY: Some antacids may delay the absorption of naproxen, but their effect on the extent of naproxen absorption is unknown.

RISK FACTORS: No specific risk factors are known.

MECHANISM: Not established.

CLINICAL EVALUATION: A study in 14 healthy subjects indicated that magnesium oxide and aluminum hydroxide may delay naproxen absorption;[1] however, plasma naproxen levels were not measured long enough to determine whether the completeness of naproxen absorption was affected. Sodium bicarbonate appeared to increase the absorption rate of naproxen; magnesium-aluminum hydroxide (eg, *Maalox*) seemed to have minimal effects. The clinical significance of these findings cannot be determined until studies assess whether the bioavailability of naproxen is affected by antacids.

RELATED DRUGS: Antacids may delay or reduce the absorption of other nonsteroidal anti-inflammatory drugs, but the clinical importance is probably not large.

MANAGEMENT OPTIONS: No specific action is required, but be alert for evidence of the interaction.

REFERENCES:

1. Segre EJ, et al. Effects of antacids on naproxen absorption. *N Engl J Med.* 1974;291:582.

Antacids

Norfloxacin (*Noroxin*)

SUMMARY: Antacids reduce the serum concentration of norfloxacin and probably inhibit its efficacy.

RISK FACTORS:

➡ *Dosage Regimen.* The effects of antacids on quinolone absorption appear to be greater when large antacid doses are coadministered.

➡ *Diet/Food.* Binding interactions in the GI tract tend to be greater in the fasting state than if there is food in the stomach.

MECHANISM: The probable mechanism involves chelation between the antacid cations and the 4-oxo and 3-carboxyl groups of the quinolone, resulting in a decreased bioavailability of the antibiotic.

CLINICAL EVALUATION: Norfloxacin absorption is markedly inhibited by aluminum and magnesium antacids.[1-3] *Maalox* administered within 5 minutes of norfloxacin resulted in a 98% reduction in the area under the concentration-time curve (AUC) of the antibiotic.[1] Giving the antacid 2 hours after the norfloxacin reduced the AUC by only 23%.

RELATED DRUGS: The absorption of other quinolones also is reduced by antacids, but the absorption of lomefloxacin (*Maxaquin*) and ofloxacin (*Floxin*) appears somewhat less affected by cations (eg, antacids) than norfloxacin. H_2-receptor antagonists (eg, cimetidine [eg, *Tagamet*], famotidine [*Pepcid*], nizatidine [*Axid*], ranitidine [*Zantac*]) and proton pump inhibitors (eg, omeprazole [*Prilosec*], lansoprazole [*Prevacid*]) are not known to affect norfloxacin absorption.

MANAGEMENT OPTIONS:

➡ *Consider Alternative.* Since it may be difficult to separate the doses of antacid and norfloxacin sufficiently to prevent their interaction, the use of H_2-receptor antagonists or proton pump inhibitors may be necessary for severe infections when patients require gastric acid reduction.

➡ *Circumvent/Minimize.* If antacids are used with oral norfloxacin, give the norfloxacin at least 3 hours before or 6 hours after the antacid.

➡ *Monitor.* Monitor for reduced norfloxacin response if antacids are also given.

REFERENCES:

1. Nix DE, et al. Inhibition of norfloxacin absorption by antacids. *Antimicrob Agents Chemother.* 1990;34:432.
2. Noyes M, et al. Norfloxacin and absorption of magnesium-aluminum. *Ann Intern Med.* 1988;109:168.
3. Campbell NRC, et al. Norfloxacin interaction with antacids and minerals. *Br J Clin Pharmacol.* 1992;33:115.

Antacids

Ofloxacin (*Floxin*)

SUMMARY: Antacids reduce the serum concentration of ofloxacin and may inhibit its efficacy.

RISK FACTORS:

➡ *Dosage Regimen.* Larger doses of antacids produce a greater reduction in ofloxacin absorption.

➡ *Diet/Food.* Binding interactions in the GI tract tend to be greater in the fasting state than if there is food in the stomach.

MECHANISM: The probable mechanism involves chelation between the antacid cations and the 4-oxo and 3-carboxyl groups of the quinolone, resulting in a decreased bioavailability of the antibiotic.

CLINICAL EVALUATION: Ofloxacin absorption was minimally affected by 1 tablet of magnesium-aluminum hydroxide (*Maalox*), while large doses significantly (50% to 70%) reduced its absorption.[1,2] Administration of ofloxacin 2 hours after a dose of antacid reduced the absorption by about 20%.[3] Nine healthy subjects received

200 mg ofloxacin alone and with 11 gm colloidal aluminum phosphate.[4] The antacid did not affect the amount of ofloxacin excreted in the urine. The administration of 500 mg doses of magnesium trisilicate, aluminum hydroxide, calcium carbonate, sodium bicarbonate, and potassium citrate with 200 mg ofloxacin had little effect on ofloxacin salivary concentrations.[5] In healthy subjects 500 mg calcium carbonate did not appear to affect the bioavailability of 200 mg ofloxacin.[6]

RELATED DRUGS: The absorption of other quinolones also is reduced by antacids. Ofloxacin absorption appears somewhat less affected by cations (eg, antacids) than ciprofloxacin (*Cipro*) or norfloxacin (*Noroxin*). H$_2$-receptor antagonists (eg, cimetidine [eg, *Tagamet*], famotidine [*Pepcid*], nizatidine [*Axid*], ranitidine [*Zantac*]) and proton pump inhibitors (eg, omeprazole [*Prilosec*], lansoprazole [*Prevacid*]) are not known to affect ofloxacin absorption.

MANAGEMENT OPTIONS:

➡ *Consider Alternative.* Calcium antacids, at least in small doses, appear to have little effect on the absorption of ofloxacin. Also consider the use of H$_2$-receptor antagonists or proton pump inhibitors in place of antacids.

➡ *Circumvent/Minimize.* If antacids are used with oral ofloxacin, give the ofloxacin at least 2 hours before or 6 hours after the antacid.

➡ *Monitor.* Monitor for reduced ofloxacin response if antacids are also given.

REFERENCES:

1. Maesen FPV, et al. Ofloxacin and antacids. *J Antimicrob Chemother*. 1987;19:848.
2. Hoffken G, et al. Pharmacokinetics and bioavailability of ciprofloxacin and ofloxacin: effect of food and antacid intake. *Rev Infect Dis*. 1988;10:S138.
3. Flor D, et al. Effects of magnesium-aluminum hydroxide and calcium carbonate antacids on bioavailability of ofloxacin. *Antimicrob Agents Chemother*. 1990;34:2436.
4. Cabarga MM, et al. Effects of two cations on gastrointestinal absorption of ofloxacin. *Antimicrob Agents Chemother*. 1991;35:2102.
5. Akerele JO, et al. Influence of oral coadministered metallic drugs on ofloxacin pharmacokinetics. *J Antimicrob Chemother*. 1991;28:87.
6. Navarro AS, et al. Comparative study of the influence of Ca^{2+} on absorption parameters of ciprofloxacin and ofloxacin. *J Antimicrob Chemother*. 1994;34:119.

Antacids **5**

Paroxetine (*Paxil*)

SUMMARY: A preliminary study in healthy subjects suggests that aluminum hydroxide has minimal effects on the absorption of paroxetine.

RISK FACTORS: No specific risk factors are known.

MECHANISM: No interaction.

CLINICAL EVALUATION: Seven healthy subjects were given a single oral dose of paroxetine with and without aluminum hydroxide (15 mL 3 times daily the day before paroxetine and twice daily on the day of paroxetine).[1] The exact timing of the administration of the paroxetine in relation to the aluminum hydroxide in the study day was not stated. Although there was a trend toward an increased area under the plasma paroxetine concentration-time curve in the presence of aluminum hydroxide, there were not significant changes in any of paroxetine's pharmacokinetic parameters. Nonetheless, since two of the subjects dropped out of the study, the statistical analysis had relatively low power.

RELATED DRUGS: The effect of other more commonly used antacids (ie, aluminum-magnesium hydroxides) on paroxetine is not established, but the lack of effect of aluminum hydroxide lowers the likelihood that other antacids will interact. The effect of antacids on selective serotonin reuptake inhibitors other than paroxetine is not established.

MANAGEMENT OPTIONS: No interaction.

REFERENCES:

1. Greb WH, et al. Absorption of paroxetine under various dietary conditions and following antacid intake. *Acta Psychiatr Scand.* 1989;80(Suppl. 350):99.

Antacids

Pefloxacin

SUMMARY: Antacids reduce the serum concentration of pefloxacin and may inhibit its efficacy.

RISK FACTORS:

➡ **Dosage Regimen.** The effects of antacids on quinolone absorption appear to be greater when large antacid doses are coadministered.

➡ **Diet/Food.** Binding interactions in the GI tract tend to be greater in the fasting state than if there is food in the stomach.

MECHANISM: The probable mechanism involves chelation between the antacid cations and the 4-oxo and 3-carboxyl groups of the quinolone, resulting in a decreased bioavailability of the antibiotic.

CLINICAL EVALUATION: In a randomized crossover study in healthy subjects, a magnesium-aluminum hydroxide suspension reduced the bioavailability of a single 400 mg dose of pefloxacin to 44% of control.[1]

RELATED DRUGS: The absorption of other quinolones also is reduced by antacids. H_2-receptor antagonists (eg, cimetidine [eg, *Tagamet*], famotidine [*Pepcid*], nizatidine [*Axid*], ranitidine [*Zantac*]) and proton pump inhibitors (eg, omeprazole [*Prilosec*], lansoprazole [*Prevacid*]) are not known to affect pefloxacin absorption.

MANAGEMENT OPTIONS:

➡ **Consider Alternative.** Since it may be difficult to separate the doses of antacid and pefloxacin sufficiently to prevent their interaction, the use of H_2-receptor antagonists or proton pump inhibitors may be considered in place of the antacid.

➡ **Circumvent/Minimize.** If antacids are used with oral pefloxacin, give the pefloxacin at least 2 hours before or 6 hours after the antacid.

➡ **Monitor.** Monitor for reduced pefloxacin effect if antacids are also given.

REFERENCES:

1. Jaehde U, et al. Effect of an antacid containing magnesium and aluminum on absorption, metabolism and mechanism of renal elimination of pefloxacin in humans. *Antimicrob Agents Chemother.* 1994;38:1129.

Antacids **3**

Penicillamine (*Cuprimine*)

SUMMARY: Magnesium-aluminum hydroxides may reduce the bioavailability of penicillamine.

RISK FACTORS: No specific risk factors are known.

MECHANISM: Antacids may reduce the absorption of penicillamine, possibly by adsorbing penicillamine in the GI tract.

CLINICAL EVALUATION: Six healthy subjects were given penicillamine 500 mg orally with and without 30 mL of an antacid containing magnesium-aluminum hydroxides and simethicone (*Maalox Plus*).[1] The antacid reduced urinary recovery of penicillamine, indicating that penicillamine bioavailability was reduced.

RELATED DRUGS: The effect of antacids other than magnesium aluminum hydroxides on penicillamine absorption is not established.

MANAGEMENT OPTIONS:

➡ *Circumvent/Minimize.* Until more is known about this interaction, it would be prudent to give penicillamine 2 hours before or 6 hours after antacids.

➡ *Monitor.* Monitor for reduced penicillamine response if antacids are also given.

REFERENCES:

1. Osman MA, et al. Reduction in oral penicillamine absorption by food, antacid, and ferrous sulfate. *Clin Pharmacol Ther.* 1983;33:465.

Antacids **4**

Phenytoin (eg, *Dilantin*)

SUMMARY: Antacids can reduce phenytoin absorption, but the clinical importance remains to be established.

RISK FACTORS: No specific risk factors are known.

MECHANISM: Antacids may impair the GI absorption of phenytoin.

CLINICAL EVALUATION: Antacids containing aluminum and/or magnesium impaired the GI absorption of phenytoin in some studies[1,2] but not in others.[3,4] If the interaction does occur, it probably occurs under specific circumstances that relate to dose, type of antacid, or time of administration of antacid and phenytoin doses.

RELATED DRUGS: No information available.

MANAGEMENT OPTIONS: No specific action is required, but be alert for evidence of the interaction.

REFERENCES:

1. Kulshrestha VK, et al. Interaction between phenytoin and antacids. *Br J Clin Pharmacol.* 1978;6:177.
2. Garnett WR, et al. Bioavailability of phenytoin administered with antacids. *Ther Drug Monit.* 1979;1:435.
3. O'Brien WM, et al. Failure of antacids to alter the pharmacokinetics of phenytoin. *Br J Clin Pharmacol.* 1978;6:276.
4. Chapron DJ, et al. Effect of calcium and antacids on phenytoin bioavailability. *Arch Neurol.* 1979;36:436.

Antacids

Prednisone

SUMMARY: Antacids may impair the absorption of prednisone and other corticosteroids, but the evidence is conflicting and the clinical importance of this effect is questionable.

RISK FACTORS: No specific risk factors are known.

MECHANISM: Not established. Antacids may bind with corticosteroids in the GI tract.

CLINICAL EVALUATION: Although some clinical studies have shown that aluminum or magnesium antacids may reduce the absorption of corticosteroids such as prednisone and dexamethasone,[1,2] other studies have found no effect of antacids on prednisolone absorption.[3,4] Even if the interaction does occur, a patient on consistent doses of both a corticosteroid and an antacid may not be adversely affected since the corticosteroid dose would probably be titrated to the appropriate level in the presence of the antacid.

RELATED DRUGS: Little is known regarding other combinations of antacids and corticosteroids.

MANAGEMENT OPTIONS: No specific action is required, but be alert for evidence of the interaction.

REFERENCES:
1. Naggar VF, et al. Effect of concomitant administration of magnesium trisilicate on GI absorption of dexamethasone in humans. *J Pharm Sci.* 1978;67:1029.
2. Urbine M, et al. Decreased bioavailability of prednisone due to antacids in patients with chronic active liver disease and in healthy volunteers. *Gastroenterology.* 1981;30:661.
3. Lee DAH, et al. The effect of concurrent administration of antacids on prednisolone absorption. *Br J Clin Pharmacol.* 1979;8:92.
4. Tanner AR, et al. Concurrent administration of antacids and prednisolone: effect on serum levels of prednisolone. *Br J Clin Pharmacol.* 1979;7:397.

4 Antacids

Propranolol (*Inderal*)

SUMMARY: Aluminum hydroxide may delay the GI absorption of propranolol, but the clinical importance of the effect is probably minimal.

RISK FACTORS: No specific risk factors are known.

MECHANISM: Not established. It may be because of delayed gastric emptying caused by the aluminum hydroxide.[2]

CLINICAL EVALUATION: Aluminum hydroxide gel appears to delay the absorption of propranolol in healthy human subjects.[1]

RELATED DRUGS: Antacids have been reported to increase metoprolol (*Lopressor*) absorption.

MANAGEMENT OPTIONS: No specific action is required, but be alert for evidence of the interaction.

REFERENCES:

1. Dobbs JH, et al. Effects of aluminum hydroxide on the absorption of propranolol. *Curr Ther Res.* 1977;21:887.
2. Hurwitz A, et al. Effects of antacids on gastric emptying. *Gastroenterology.* 1976;71:268.

Antacids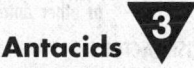

Pseudoephedrine (eg, *Sudafed*)

SUMMARY: Sodium bicarbonate in doses sufficient to alkalinize the urine may inhibit the elimination of pseudoephedrine markedly.

RISK FACTORS: No specific risk factors are known.

MECHANISM: Alkalinization of the urine with sodium bicarbonate results in less ionization of pseudoephedrine, thus increasing its renal tubular reabsorption and reducing its urinary excretion.

CLINICAL EVALUATION: Alkalinization of the urine with sodium bicarbonate approximately doubled the half-life of pseudoephedrine in 3 normal subjects given a single pseudoephedrine 180 mg dose.[2] Similar results were found in a subsequent study of 8 healthy subjects given a single 5 mg/kg dose of oral pseudoephedrine; urine alkalinization with sodium bicarbonate increased the half-life from 1.9 to 21 hours.[1]

RELATED DRUGS: Any drug that significantly alkalinizes the urine (eg, carbonic anhydrase inhibitors) would be expected to reduce the urinary excretion of pseudoephedrine. Nonsystemic antacids such as magnesium-aluminum hydroxides also may alkalinize the urine somewhat, but the extent to which this reduced pseudoephedrine elimination is not established. Sympathomimetic amines other than pseudoephedrine (eg, amphetamines, ephedrine) also have been shown to undergo pH dependent urinary excretion.

MANAGEMENT OPTIONS:

➡ *Consider Alternative.* If more than an occasional dose of sodium bicarbonate is used, consider using alternative antacid. (See Related Drugs.)

➡ *Monitor.* Monitor for enhanced pseudoephedrine effect (eg, anxiety, tremor, palpitations, psychiatric changes) if large doses of sodium bicarbonate are taken concurrently.

REFERENCES:

1. Brater DC, et al. Renal excretion of pseudoephedrine. *Clin Pharmacol Ther.* 1980;28:690.
2. Kuntzman RG, et al. The influence of urinary pH on the plasma halflife of pseudoephedrine in man and dog and a sensitive assay for its determination in human plasma. *Clin Pharmacol Ther.* 1971;12:62.

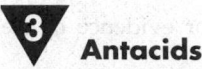

Antacids

Quinidine

SUMMARY: Antacids capable of increasing urine pH (eg, magnesium-aluminum hydroxides) may increase serum quinidine concentrations. Aluminum hydroxide probably does not impair GI quinidine absorption, but the effect of other antacids is not established.

RISK FACTORS:

➥ **Diet/Food.** Diets that increase urine pH (eg, large amounts of citrus juices) may add to the effect of antacids.

MECHANISM: Some antacids can increase urinary pH. This increases the proportion of nonionized quinidine, resulting in increased renal tubular reabsorption.[1]

CLINICAL EVALUATION: The effects of 7 days of administration of 5 antacids on urinary pH were studied in 11 subjects.[1] Aluminum hydroxide suspension (*Amphojel*) 10 mL 4 times daily and dihydroxyaluminum glycinate (*Robalate*) 5 mL 4 times daily had no effect on urine pH. Magnesium hydroxide (*Milk of Magnesia*) 5 mL 4 times daily and calcium carbonate-glycine (*Titralac*) 5 mL 4 times daily increased urine pH approximately ½ unit, while aluminum and magnesium hydroxide suspension (*Maalox*) 5 mL 4 times daily increased urine pH by almost 1 unit. Subjects receiving an aluminum and magnesium hydroxide-containing tablet (*Mylanta*) developed an increased urine pH; 1 patient developed quinidine intoxication following the use of *Mylanta* tablets (approximately 8/day for 1 week) in addition to large quantities of citrus fruit juice. Studies in humans and dogs indicate that aluminum hydroxide does not reduce the extent of quinidine absorption,[2-4] but magnesium oxide did reduce the amount of quinidine absorbed in dogs.[2]

RELATED DRUGS: H$_2$-receptor antagonists (eg, famotidine [*Pepcid*], nizatidine [*Axid*], ranitidine [*Zantac*]) and proton pump inhibitors (eg, omeprazole [*Prilosec*], lansoprazole [*Prevacid*]) are not known to affect urine pH significantly, but cimetidine (eg, *Tagamet*) inhibits the hepatic metabolism of quinidine and may increase its serum concentrations significantly.

MANAGEMENT OPTIONS:

➥ **Monitor.** Monitor for altered quinidine effect if antacids are initiated, discontinued or changed in dosage. Current evidence does not suggest that it is necessary to space doses of quinidine from antacids.

REFERENCES:

1. Gibaldi M, et al. Effect of antacids on pH of urine. *Clin Pharmacol Ther.* 1974;16:520.
2. Remon JP, et al. Interaction of antacids with antiarrhythmics. V. Effect of aluminum hydroxide and magnesium oxide on the bioavailability of quinidine, procainamide and propranolol in dogs. *Arzneimittelforsch.* 1983;33:117.
3. Romankiewicz JA, et al. The noninterference of aluminum hydroxide gel with quinidine sulfate absorption: an approach to control quinidine-induced diarrhea. *Am Heart J.* 1978;96:518.
4. Mauro VF, et al. Effect of aluminum hydroxide gel on quinidine gluconate absorption. *DICP.* 1990;24:252.

Ranitidine (*Zantac*)

SUMMARY: Large doses of aluminum-magnesium antacids can reduce the bioavailability of ranitidine, but the clinical importance of this effect is not established; smaller amounts of antacid do not appear to affect ranitidine bioavailability significantly.

RISK FACTORS: No specific risk factors are known.

MECHANISM: Not established. Antacids may adsorb ranitidine in the gut.

CLINICAL EVALUATION: Six healthy, fasting subjects received ranitidine 150 mg orally with and without concurrent ingestion of 30 mL of *Mylanta II*, a high potency antacid containing magnesium and aluminum hydroxides plus simethicone.[1] The antacid reduced the area under the ranitidine plasma concentration-time curve by 34%. A similar reduction in ranitidine bioavailability was observed in 10 fasting subjects given 150 mg of ranitidine with and without 11 g of aluminum phosphate.[2] Conversely, ranitidine bioavailability was not reduced in 12 fasting subjects given 30 mL of *Maalox* (which contains about half as much aluminum and magnesium hydroxide as *Mylanta II*).[3] Ranitidine bioavailability was also unaffected in 11 nonfasting subjects given ranitidine 150 mg with and without an aluminum hydroxide/magnesium carbonate antacid (2 tablets 1 and 3 hours after the ranitidine).[4]

Thus, high doses of some antacids may reduce the absorption of ranitidine. Although the magnitude of the reduction in ranitidine absorption using high doses of antacids would be expected to reduce ranitidine effects, the acid neutralizing effect of the antacids would be expected to offset the effect of reduction in ranitidine levels. Moreover, the relative benefits of ranitidine alone vs ranitidine plus concurrent antacid in patients with acid-peptic disease is not established.

Ranitidine may also promote bezoar formation in patients taking antacids. A patient receiving oral ranitidine 150 mg twice daily and 300 mL/day of *Maalox TC*, a magnesium-aluminum hydroxide antacid, developed small bowel obstruction from an antacid bezoar.[5] Ranitidine-induced reduction in gastric secretion could have predisposed these patients to concretion of the large doses of antacid; therefore, any H_2-receptor antagonist should be capable of producing a similar effect.

RELATED DRUGS: Other H_2-receptor antagonists (eg, cimetidine [eg, *Tagamet*], famotidine [*Pepcid*], nizatidine [*Axid*]) appear to be similarly affected by antacids.

MANAGEMENT OPTIONS: No specific action is required, but be alert for evidence of the interaction.

REFERENCES:

1. Mihaly GW, et al. High dose of antacid (*Mylanta II*) reduces bioavailability of ranitidine. *BMJ*. 1982;285:998.
2. Albin H, et al. Effect of aluminum phosphate on the bioavailability of ranitidine. *Eur J Clin Pharmacol*. 1987;32:97.
3. Donn KH, et al. The effects of antacid and propantheline on the absorption of oral ranitidine. *Pharmacotherapy*. 1984;4:89.
4. Frislid K, et al. High dose of antacid reduces bioavailability of ranitidine. *BMJ*. 1983;286:1358.
5. Burruss GL, et al. Small bowel obstruction from an antacid bezoar: a ranitidine-antacid interaction? *South Med J*. 1986;79:917.

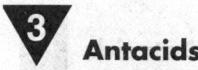

Antacids

Sodium Polystyrene Sulfonate Resin (*Kayexalate*)

SUMMARY: Combined use of magnesium- or calcium-containing antacids with sodium polystyrene sulfonate resin may result in systemic alkalosis.

RISK FACTORS: No specific risk factors are known.

MECHANISM: Sodium polystyrene sulfonate resin probably binds the magnesium or calcium present in antacids and prevents magnesium or calcium from combining with bicarbonate ions in the small intestine. Thus, the neutralization of bicarbonate ions by the magnesium or calcium from the antacid is impaired, resulting in systemic alkalosis.

CLINICAL EVALUATION: A study of 11 patients demonstrated considerable elevation of plasma bicarbonate following the concomitant use of sodium polystyrene sulfonate resin with a magnesium-containing (*Maalox*) or calcium-containing (calcium carbonate) antacid.[1] In a subsequent study, this interaction was used to advantage in the treatment of a patient with metabolic acidosis.[2] Also, a patient receiving magnesium hydroxide (*Milk of Magnesia*) and sodium polystyrene sulfonate resin developed severe alkalosis, presumably as a result of this interaction.[3] The extent to which aluminum-containing antacids interact with sodium polystyrene sulfonate resin is unknown.

RELATED DRUGS: Theoretically, H_2–receptor antagonists (eg, cimetidine [eg, *Tagamet*], famotidine [*Pepcid*], nizatidine [*Axid*], ranitidine [*Zantac*]) and proton pump inhibitors (eg, lansoprazole [*Prevacid*], omeprazole [*Prilosec*]) would not be expected to interact with sodium polystyrene sulfonate resin.

MANAGEMENT OPTIONS:

➡ **Consider Alternative.** Consider use of alternative to antacids (see Related Drugs).

➡ **Circumvent/Minimize.** Separating the time of administration of doses of antacid from the oral sodium polystyrene sulfonate resin would theoretically avoid the interaction; since it is not known how much of a separation would be necessary to avoid the interaction, separate doses by as much time as possible. Administering sodium polystyrene sulfonate resin rectally also would be expected to avoid this interaction.

➡ **Monitor.** If antacids and sodium polystyrene sulfonate resin are used concurrently, be alert for clinical or laboratory evidence of alkalosis.

REFERENCES:

1. Schroeder ET. Alkalosis resulting from combined administration of a nonsystemic antacid and a cation-exchange resin. *Gastroenterology*. 1969;56:868.

2. Fernandez PC, et al. Metabolic acidosis reversed by the combination of magnesium hydroxide and a cation-exchange resin. *N Engl J Med*. 1972;286:23.

3. Ziessman HA. Alkalosis and seizure due to a cation-exchange resin and magnesium hydroxide. *South Med J*. 1976;69:497.

Antacids ▼ 3

Tetracycline

SUMMARY: Cotherapy with a tetracycline and an antacid containing divalent or trivalent cations (aluminum, calcium, magnesium) can reduce the serum concentration and efficacy of the tetracycline.

RISK FACTORS: No specific risk factors are known.

MECHANISM: Antacids containing divalent or trivalent cations impair the absorption of orally-administered tetracyclines. This effect has been attributed to chelation of the cation by the tetracycline. Antacids may also affect the dissolution of the tetracycline.

CLINICAL EVALUATION: Even though the interaction between aluminum-, magnesium-, or calcium-containing antacids and tetracyclines is well documented and well known,[1,3-7] one study indicated that more than 5% of patients receiving tetracycline also receive such antacids.[2] The area under the concentration-time curve of doxycycline (*Vibramycin*) 200 mg IV was reduced by 30% during aluminum hydroxide 30 mL 4 times daily.[8] The simultaneous administration of a tetracycline and these antacids may decrease serum tetracycline concentrations considerably.

RELATED DRUGS: H_2-receptor antagonists (eg, cimetidine [eg, *Tagamet*], famotidine [*Pepcid*], nizatidine [*Axid*], ranitidine [*Zantac*]) and proton pump inhibitors (eg, lansoprazole [*Prevacid*], omeprazole [*Prilosec*]) are not known to affect tetracycline.

MANAGEMENT OPTIONS:

➥ *Circumvent/Minimize.* Take oral tetracyclines 2 hours before or 6 hours after antacids. This may not completely avoid the interaction, but it should minimize it.

➥ *Monitor.* Monitor for reduced tetracycline response if antacids are also used.

REFERENCES:

1. Scheiner J, et al. Experimental study of factors inhibiting absorption and effective therapeutic levels of declomycin. *Surg Gynecol Obstet.* 1962;114:9.
2. Anon. Risk of drug interaction may exist in 1 of 13 prescriptions (Medical News). *JAMA.* 1972;220:1287.
3. Jaffe JM, et al. Effect of altered urinary pH on tetracycline and doxycycline excretion in humans. *J Pharmacokinet Biopharm.* 1973;1:267.
4. Jaffe JM, et al. Influence of repetitive dosing and altered urinary pH on doxycycline excretion human. *J Pharm Sci.* 1974;63:1256.
5. Chin TF, et al. Drug diffusion and bioavailability: tetracycline metallic chelation. *Am J Hosp Pharm.* 1975;32:625.
6. Neuvonen PJ. Interactions with the absorption of tetracyclines. *Drugs.* 1976;11:45.
7. Rosenblatt JE, et al. Comparison of *in vitro* activity and clinical pharmacology of doxycycline with other tetracyclines. *Antimicrob Agents Chemother.* 1966:134.
8. Nix DE, et al. Effect of oral aluminum containing antacids on the disposition of intravenous doxycycline. *Pharm Res.* 1988;5(Suppl.):S174.

Antacids

Ticlopidine (*Ticlid*)

SUMMARY: A magnesium-aluminum hydroxide antacid produced a small decrease in ticlopidine bioavailability, but the clinical importance of this effect is probably minimal.

RISK FACTORS: No specific risk factors are known.

MECHANISM: Antacids probably adsorb ticlopidine in the GI tract, thus impairing its absorption.

CLINICAL EVALUATION: In a study of healthy subjects, 30 mL of a magnesium-aluminum hydroxide antacid (*Maalox*) reduced the bioavailability of a single 250 mg dose of ticlopidine by about 20%.[1]

RELATED DRUGS: The effect of antacids other than magnesium aluminum hydroxides on ticlopidine absorption is not established, but assume that the interaction is similar until data are available.

MANAGEMENT OPTIONS: No specific action is required, but be alert for evidence of the interaction.

REFERENCES:
   1. Shah J, et al. Effect of food and antacid on absorption of orally administered ticlopidine hydrochloride. *J Clin Pharmacol*. 1990;30:733.

4 **Antacids (eg, *Mylanta*)**

Tipranavir (*Aptivus*)

SUMMARY: Antacids containing aluminum and magnesium modestly reduce the plasma concentration of tipranavir; chronic coadministration may reduce the efficacy of tipranavir.

RISK FACTORS: No specific risk factors are known.

MECHANISM: Unknown.

CLINICAL EVALUATION: While specific data are limited, the manufacturer of tipranavir notes that the coadministration of tipranavir 500 mg with ritonavir 200 mg twice daily and 20 mL of aluminum hydroxide and magnesium hydroxide–based liquid antacid decreased the mean area under the plasma concentration-time curve of tipranavir 27%, compared with tipranavir/ritonavir administered alone.[1]

RELATED DRUGS: Other antacids may have a similar effect on tipranavir plasma concentrations.

MANAGEMENT OPTIONS:

➡ *Monitor.* Watch for reduced tipranavir plasma concentrations and antiviral effect if antacids are coadministered.

REFERENCES:
   1. *Aptivus* [package insert]. Ridgefield, CT: Boehringer Ingelheim Pharmaceuticals, Inc; 2007.

Antacids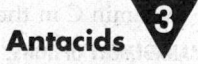

Tocainide (*Tonocard*)

SUMMARY: In a report involving healthy subjects, antacids that increase urine pH were found to increase tocainide serum concentrations. The degree to which this effect increases the potential for adverse reactions is unknown.

RISK FACTORS: No specific risk factors are known.

MECHANISM: Tocainide is a weak base that exhibits pH-dependent renal excretion. Alkalinization of the urine will increase the proportion of nonionized tocainide, enhance the reabsorption of tocainide, and increase serum concentrations.

CLINICAL EVALUATION: The effects of urinary alkalinization (secondary to short-term antacid therapy) on tocainide pharmacokinetics was studied in 6 healthy subjects.[1] Each subject took 30 mL of antacid (*Mylanta*) 4 times daily for 48 hours before and 48 hours after a 600 mg oral dose of tocainide. The antacid significantly increased the urine pH (from 5.9 to 6.9). Tocainide clearance was significantly reduced (21%) while the area under the tocainide serum concentration-time curve and the peak tocainide concentration increased by nearly 30%. The change in tocainide pharmacokinetics could have an effect on patient response, but no pharmacodynamic effects were measured. Additional studies will be required to determine the potential for adverse reactions.

RELATED DRUGS: No information is available.

MANAGEMENT OPTIONS:

➥ *Monitor.* Monitor patients taking tocainide more closely for excessive tocainide effect when antacids are coadministered.

REFERENCES:
1. Meneilly GP et al. The effect of antacid induced urinary alkalinization on the pharmacokinetics of tocainide. *Pharmacotherapy*. 1988;8:120.

Antacids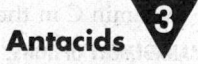

Trovafloxacin (*Trovan*)

SUMMARY: Antacids reduce the bioavailability of trovafloxacin; a loss of therapeutic efficacy may occur in some patients.

RISK FACTORS: No specific risk factors are known.

MECHANISM: Antacids adsorb quinolone antibiotics and prevent their absorption.

CLINICAL EVALUATION: While no published data are available for evaluation, the manufacturer of trovafloxacin has made available some data on this interaction.[1] Like other quinolone antibiotics, the absorption of trovafloxacin is reduced when administered with antacids containing di-and trivalent cations. The AUC of trovafloxacin administered 30 minutes after an antacid containing magnesium hydroxide and aluminum hydroxide was reduced 66%. Calcium carbonate (1000 mg) administered with trovafloxacin reduced trovafloxacin AUC by 17%.

RELATED DRUGS: Antacids containing di- and trivalent cations similarly affect other quinolones such as ciprofloxacin (*Cipro*) and ofloxacin (*Floxin*).

MANAGEMENT OPTIONS:

➥ *Consider Alternative.* Consider the use of an OTC H_2-receptor antagonist.

➥ *Circumvent/Minimize.* Administer the antibiotic at least 2 hours before the antacid. If possible, avoid antacids during trovafloxacin administration.

➥ *Monitor.* Observe patients receiving trovafloxacin who also take antacids for a potential reduction in antibiotic effect.

REFERENCES:

1. Product information. Trovafloxacin (*Trovan*). Pfizer Inc. 1998.

 Antacids

Vitamin C

SUMMARY: Preliminary evidence from healthy subjects and animal studies suggests that vitamin C increases the amount of aluminum absorbed from aluminum hydroxide, but the clinical importance is not established.

RISK FACTORS: No specific risk factors are known.

MECHANISM: Not established.

CLINICAL EVALUATION: Thirteen healthy subjects received aluminum hydroxide 900 mg 3 times daily with and without concurrent vitamin C 2 g 3 times daily.[1] Vitamin C was associated with about a 3-fold increase in urinary aluminum elimination, suggesting increased aluminum absorption. This is consistent with studies showing that vitamin C increased the aluminum concentration in the liver, brain, and bone of rats given aluminum hydroxide.[2] The extent to which vitamin C would increase the toxicity of aluminum-containing antacids in patients with severe renal impairment is not established.

RELATED DRUGS: Theoretically, any aluminum-containing antacid would interact with vitamin C in the same way.

MANAGEMENT OPTIONS:

➥ *Circumvent/Minimize.* The degree to which separating the doses of aluminum from vitamin C would circumvent the interaction is unknown, but taking the ascorbic acid at least 2 hours before or 4 hours after the aluminum antacid would be prudent.

➥ *Monitor.* There are no specific monitoring recommendations.

REFERENCES:

1. Domingo JL, et al. Effect of ascorbic acid on gastrointestinal aluminum absorption. *Lancet*. 1991;338:1467.

2. Domingo JL, et al. Influence of some dietary constituents on aluminum absorption and retention in rats. *Kidney Int*. 1991;39:598.

Antipyrine

Ciprofloxacin (*Cipro*)

SUMMARY: Ciprofloxacin reduces the clearance of antipyrine and probably other drugs that are metabolized in metabolic pathways similar to antipyrine.

RISK FACTORS:

➡ ***Dosage Regimen.*** Ciprofloxacin doses more than 250 mg/day are likely to reduce antipyrine clearance.

MECHANISM: Antipyrine hepatic metabolism is reduced by ciprofloxacin administration. This reduction of antipyrine metabolism indicates that ciprofloxacin can inhibit the oxidative metabolism of other drugs in the liver.

CLINICAL EVALUATION: Antipyrine clearance was reduced by 10% and 38% following ciprofloxacin 250 mg/day and 1000 mg/day, respectively.[1,2] Several other studies reported reductions in the clearance of antipyrine of 22% to 70% following ciprofloxacin doses of 500 to 750 mg twice daily.[1,3,4] These studies demonstrate the dose dependency of this interaction and the potential for ciprofloxacin to interact with other drugs undergoing hepatic oxidation.

RELATED DRUGS: Ofloxacin 200 mg every 12 hours for 7 days did not alter the antipyrine clearance in 12 healthy subjects.[5] Other quinolones reported to inhibit drug metabolism include enoxacin (*Penetrex*), norfloxacin (*Noroxin*), pipemidic acid, and pefloxacin.

MANAGEMENT OPTIONS:

➡ ***Monitor.*** While antipyrine is not used clinically, monitor patients receiving drugs that undergo similar hepatic oxidative metabolism (eg, theophylline) for reduced clearance if ciprofloxacin is prescribed.

REFERENCES:

1. Ludwig E, et al. The effect of ciprofloxacin on antipyrine metabolism. *J Antimicrob Chemother*. 1988;22:61.
2. Ludwig E, et al. Metabolic interactions of ciprofloxacin. *Diagn Microbiol Infect Dis*. 1990;13:135.
3. Waite NM, et al. The effect of ciprofloxacin on antipyrine pharmacokinetics in young and elderly healthy subjects. *Pharmacotherapy*. 1989;9:183.
4. Tan KKC, et al. Effect of ciprofloxacin on the pharmacokinetics of antipyrine. *Br J Clin Pharmacol*. 1989;27:235.
5. Graber H, et al. Ofloxacin does not influence antipyrine metabolism. *Rev Infect Dis*. 1989;11(Suppl. 5):S1093.

Antipyrine 4

Ethanol (Ethyl Alcohol)

SUMMARY: Chronic ingestion of large amounts of ethanol enhances the elimination of antipyrine.

RISK FACTORS: No specific risk factors are known.

MECHANISM: Chronic ethanol abuse can induce hepatic microsomal enzymes resulting in enhanced antipyrine metabolism.

CLINICAL EVALUATION: Enhanced metabolism of antipyrine occurs following the ingestion of large amounts of ethanol over a prolonged period (1 mL/kg/day for 21 days),[2] but not with more moderate ethanol intake.[1] Conversely, acute intoxication with ethanol would be expected to inhibit drug metabolism, including that of antipyrine. Also, in chronic alcoholics with significant liver damage, the ethanol-induced enzyme induction may be offset by a diminished drug metabolizing capacity of the liver.[3] Since antipyrine seldom is used clinically, the primary significance of these findings relates to the concomitant use of ethanol and other drugs metabolized by hepatic microsomal enzymes.

RELATED DRUGS: No information is available.

MANAGEMENT OPTIONS: No specific action is required, but be alert for evidence of the interaction.

REFERENCES:

1. Vestal RE, et al. Antipyrine metabolism in man: influence of age, alcohol, caffeine, and smoking. *Clin Pharmacol Ther.* 1975;18:425.
2. Vesell ES, et al. Genetic and environmental factors affecting ethanol metabolism in man. *Clin Pharmacol Ther.* 1971;12:192.
3. Sotaniemi EA, et al. Histological changes in the liver and indices of drug metabolism in alcoholics. *Eur J Clin Pharmacol.* 1977;11:295.

4 Antipyrine

Fusidic Acid

SUMMARY: The clearance of antipyrine was increased during chronic fusidic acid administration; the clinical significance of this interaction remains to be determined.

RISK FACTORS: No specific risk factors are known.

MECHANISM: It appears that fusidic acid increases the metabolism of antipyrine.

CLINICAL EVALUATION: In a preliminary study, 28 days of fusidic acid administration (500 mg/day) increased antipyrine clearance by almost 20%, and its half-life decreased from 12.3 to 9.4 hours.[1] After 14 days of fusidic acid administration, no effect was observed on antipyrine metabolism. The cause of the slow onset of this interaction (more than 14 days of fusidic acid administration) is unknown. The effect of fusidic acid on the metabolism of other drugs is unknown, but consider its potential to increase the metabolism of drugs during long-term therapy.

RELATED DRUGS: Other drugs metabolized similarly to antipyrine (eg, theophylline [eg, *Slo-Phyllin*]) might also be affected by fusidic acid administration.

MANAGEMENT OPTIONS: No specific action is required, but be alert for evidence of the interaction.

REFERENCES:

1. Spatz D, et al. Effect of fusidic acid on antipyrine pharmacokinetic parameters. *Br J Clin Pharmacol.* 1993;35:545P.

4 Antipyrine

Moricizine (*Ethmozine*)

SUMMARY: Moricizine reduced the serum concentrations of antipyrine.

RISK FACTORS: No specific risk factors are known.

MECHANISM: Moricizine appears to increase the metabolism of antipyrine by stimulating the hepatic cytochrome P450 enzyme system.

CLINICAL EVALUATION: Twelve healthy subjects received antipyrine 500 mg before and after 7 days of moricizine 250 mg every 8 hours.[1] Six subjects received another dose of antipyrine following an additional 6 days of moricizine. Antipyrine half-life was reduced to 21% and 28% of baseline following 7 and 13 days of moricizine treatment, respectively. Since antipyrine is a marker for cytochrome P450 metabolism, other drugs sharing this pathway of hepatic metabolism are likely to be influenced similarly by moricizine administration.

RELATED DRUGS: Moricizine may enhance the metabolism of other drugs metabolized by P450 such as theophylline (eg, *Slo-Phyllin*).

MANAGEMENT OPTIONS: No specific action is required, but be alert for evidence of the interaction.

REFERENCES:

1. Pieniaszek HJ Jr, et al. Enzyme induction by moricizine: time course and extent in healthy volunteers. *J Clin Pharmacol*. 1989;29:832.

Antipyrine

Omeprazole (*Prilosec*)

SUMMARY: Large doses of omeprazole can slightly inhibit the elimination of antipyrine.

RISK FACTORS:

➠ *Dosage Regimen.* Large doses of omeprazole are required (30 mg/day had no effect) to inhibit antipyrine elimination.

MECHANISM: Omeprazole appears to inhibit the hepatic microsomal metabolism of antipyrine.

CLINICAL EVALUATION: Ten healthy subjects were given antipyrine 1 g orally with and without omeprazole pretreatment (30 and 60 mg/day for 14 days).[1] The 60 mg/day dose of omeprazole increased antipyrine half-life by 10% and reduced its clearance by 14%, but the 30 mg/day dose did not affect antipyrine metabolism. Although antipyrine is rarely used as a drug, these data suggest that omeprazole is an inhibitor of hepatic drug metabolism. The effect on antipyrine was slight, but the magnitude of the effect of omeprazole on the metabolism of other drugs cannot be predicted until specifically studied.

RELATED DRUGS: Available evidence suggests that lansoprazole (*Prevacid*) is less likely than omeprazole to inhibit drug metabolism.

MANAGEMENT OPTIONS: No specific action is required, but be alert for evidence of the interaction.

REFERENCES:

1. Henry DA, et al. Omeprazole: effects on oxidative drug metabolism. *Br J Clin Pharmacol*. 1984 18:195.

4   Antipyrine

Phenobarbital (eg, *Donnatal*)

SUMMARY: Barbiturates enhance the elimination of antipyrine.

RISK FACTORS: No specific risk factors are known.

MECHANISM: Barbiturates appear to enhance the metabolism of antipyrine because of induction of hepatic microsomal enzymes.[1]

CLINICAL EVALUATION: In a study of 19 healthy subjects, amobarbital decreased antipyrine half-life 35%.[2] Another study of this interaction in fraternal and identical twins indicated that genetic influences may be important in the degree to which phenobarbital enhances the metabolism of antipyrine.[3] Although the therapeutic effect of antipyrine might be decreased by barbiturate coadministration, antipyrine is seldom prescribed for systemic use.

RELATED DRUGS: All barbiturates would be expected to enhance the hepatic metabolism of antipyrine.

MANAGEMENT OPTIONS: No specific action is required, but be alert for evidence of the interaction.

REFERENCES:

1. Kampffmeyer HG. Elimination of phenacetin and phenazone by man before and after treatment with phenobarbital. *Eur J Clin Pharmacol.* 1971;3:113.
2. Stevenson JH, et al. Changes in human drug metabolism after longterm exposure to hypnotics. *Br Med J.* 1972;4:322.
3. Vesell ES, et al. Genetic control of the phenobarbital-induced shortening of plasma antipyrine half-lives in man. *J Clin Invest.* 1969;48:2202.

Antipyrine

Propranolol (eg, *Inderal*)

SUMMARY: Propranolol and, to a lesser extent, metoprolol and atenolol are capable of increasing antipyrine serum concentrations.

RISK FACTORS: No specific risk factors are known.

MECHANISM: Several beta blockers appear to reduce the hepatic clearance of antipyrine.

CLINICAL EVALUATION: In healthy volunteers, propranolol reduced antipyrine clearance 30% to 40%.[1-3] Antipyrine clearance was reduced 18% by metoprolol (eg, *Lopressor*).[1] Similar reductions in antipyrine clearance were noted following propranolol 80 mg twice daily or atenolol (eg, *Tenormin*) 50 mg twice daily.[4] In a study of 125 hypertensive patients taking chronic beta blockers, propranolol, pindolol (eg, *Viskin*), nadolol (eg, *Corgard*), metoprolol (eg, *Lopressor*), acebutolol (eg, *Sectral*), and atenolol significantly increased antipyrine half-life, while labetalol (eg, *Normodyne*) reduced antipyrine half-life.[5] Propranolol consistently has the greatest effect in studies comparing the effects of multiple beta blockers. Because antipyrine is seldom used therapeutically, the primary significance of these findings relates to possible inhibition of metabolism of other drugs by beta blockers.

RELATED DRUGS: Other drugs metabolized by the cytochrome P450 system may be affected similarly by beta blocker administration.

MANAGEMENT OPTIONS:

➥ **Monitor.** Watch for increased effect of hepatically metabolized drugs when beta blockers, particularly propranolol, are coadministered.

REFERENCES:

1. Bax ND, et al. Inhibition of antipyrine metabolism by beta-adrenoreceptor antagonists. *Br J Clin Pharmacol.* 1981;12:779.
2. Bax ND, et al. Penbutolol and propranolol: a comparison of their effects on antipyrine clearance in man. *Br J Clin Pharmacol.* 1985;19:593.
3. Greenblatt DJ. Impairment of antipyrine clearance in humans by propranolol. *Circulation.* 1978;57:1161.
4. Perrild H, et al. Differential effect of continuous administration of beta-adrenoreceptor antagonists on antipyrine and phenytoin clearance. *Br J Clin Pharmacol.* 1989;28:551.
5. Adamska-Dyniewska H, et al. The effect of six beta-adrenolytics and labetalol on hepatic biotransformation studied by antipyrine test, in man. *Int J Clin Pharmacol Ther Toxicol.* 1986;24:303.

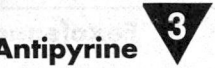

Antipyrine 3

Verapamil (eg, *Calan*)

SUMMARY: Verapamil and diltiazem can increase antipyrine serum concentrations and inhibit the metabolism of other hepatically-eliminated drugs.

RISK FACTORS: No specific risk factors are known.

MECHANISM: Verapamil and diltiazem appear to inhibit hepatic oxidative metabolism, particularly by the CYP1A2 and CYP3A4 enzymes.

CLINICAL EVALUATION: Diltiazem (eg, *Cardizem*) 120 to 180 mg/day and verapamil 80 mg every 8 hours significantly reduced the clearance of oral antipyrine;[1,2] nifedipine (eg, *Procardia*) does not change antipyrine clearance.[1,3,4] In other reports, verapamil or diltiazem decreased antipyrine clearance 11% to 33%.[5-10] Although changes in antipyrine metabolism are of little clinical importance, antipyrine is used as an indicator drug for the study of oxidative metabolism.

RELATED DRUGS: Other drugs that undergo oxidative metabolism by the hepatic cytochrome P450 enzyme system also may have reduced clearance in the presence of verapamil or diltiazem.

MANAGEMENT OPTIONS:

➥ **Consider Alternative.** Nifedipine or other dihydropyridine calcium channel blockers have little effect on the hepatic metabolism of other drugs.

➥ **Circumvent/Minimize.** Dose reduction may be appropriate for other drugs whose metabolism is reduced by the calcium channel blockers verapamil and diltiazem.

➥ **Monitor.** If verapamil or diltiazem are administered with other drugs that undergo hepatic metabolism, monitor for increased object drug effects and toxicity.

REFERENCES:

1. Bauer LA, et al. Changes in antipyrine and indocyanine green kinetics during nifedipine, verapamil and diltiazem therapy. *Clin Pharmacol Ther.* 1986;40:239.
2. Ohashi K, et al. The effect of diltiazem on hepatic drug oxidation assessed by antipyrine and trimethadione. *J Clin Pharmacol.* 1991;31:1132.

3. Dickinson TH, et al. Effects of nifedipine on hepatic drug oxidation. *Pharmacology*. 1988;36:405.

4. Edeki T, et al. An examination of a possible pharmacokinetic interaction between nifedipine and antipyrine. *Eur J Clin Pharmacol*. 1990;39:405.

5. Bach D, et al. The effect of verapamil on antipyrine pharmacokinetics and metabolism in man. *Br J Clin Pharmacol*. 1986;21:655.

6. Egan JM, et al. Effect of chronic oral verapamil on antipyrine metabolism. *Clin Pharmacol Ther*. 1986;39:191.

7. Carrum BA, et al. Diltiazem treatment impairs hepatic drug oxidation: studies of antipyrine. *Clin Pharmacol Ther*. 1986;40:140.

8. Rumiantsev DO, et al. The effect of oral verapamil therapy on antipyrine clearance. *Br J Clin Pharmacol*. 1986;22:606.

9. Rocci ML, et al. Comparative evaluation of the effects of labetalol, verapamil and diltiazem on antipyrine and indocyanine green clearances. *J Clin Pharmacol*. 1989;29:891.

10. Bottorff MB, et al. The effects of encainide versus diltiazem on the oxidative metabolic pathways of antipyrine. *Pharmacotherapy*. 1989;9:315.

Apple Juice

Fexofenadine (*Allegra*)

SUMMARY: Ingestion of large amounts of apple juice reduces the absorption of fexofenadine and may reduce fexofenadine efficacy.

RISK FACTORS: No specific risk factors are known.

MECHANISM: In vitro studies suggest that apple juice inhibits organic anion transporting polypeptide, a transporter involved in the intestinal absorption of fexofenadine.

CLINICAL EVALUATION: In a randomized crossover study in 10 healthy subjects, a single oral 120 mg fexofenadine dose was given with water and apple juice (1.2 L over 3 hours).[1] Apple juice was associated with a 73% reduction in fexofenadine plasma concentrations. The magnitude of this effect appears sufficient to reduce the efficacy of fexofenadine in at least some patients. The amount of apple juice used in this study was larger than most people consume; smaller amounts of apple juice would probably have less effect.

RELATED DRUGS: Orange and grapefruit juice also appear to reduce fexofenadine bioavailability.

MANAGEMENT OPTIONS:

➡ *Circumvent/Minimize.* Until more data are available, take fexofenadine with water rather than apple juice or other fruit juices.

REFERENCES:

1. Dresser GK, et al. Fruit juices inhibit organic anion transporting polypeptide-mediated drug uptake to decrease the oral availability of fexofenadine. *Clin Pharmacol Ther*. 2002;71:11-20.

Aprepitant (*Emend*) 2

Cisapride†

SUMMARY: Theoretically, aprepitant may increase the risk of cisapride-induced ventricular arrhythmias; the combination should generally be avoided.

RISK FACTORS: No specific risk factors are known.

MECHANISM: Aprepitant theoretically would inhibit the metabolism of cisapride by CYP3A4.

CLINICAL EVALUATION: Because aprepitant appears to be a moderate CYP3A4 inhibitor, the manufacturer states that its use with cisapride is contraindicated.[1] Elevated cisapride serum concentrations have been associated with life-threatening ventricular arrhythmias (torsades de pointes). Although there are no clinical data to support an interaction between aprepitant and cisapride, theoretical considerations suggest that it is possible.

RELATED DRUGS: No information is available.

MANAGEMENT OPTIONS:

➥ **Avoid Unless Benefit Outweighs Risk.** Although the interaction is theoretical, the fact that the combination is listed as contraindicated in the product information must be considered.

➥ **Monitor.** If the combination is used, monitor the electrocardiogram for evidence of cisapride toxicity (QT prolongation).

REFERENCES:

1. *Emend* [package insert]. White House Station, NJ: Merck & Company; 2003.

† Available only through an investigational limited access program.

Aprepitant (*Emend*) 3

Contraceptives, Oral

SUMMARY: Aprepitant may reduce ethinyl estradiol serum concentrations, but it is not known if oral contraceptive efficacy is reduced.

RISK FACTORS: No specific risk factors are known.

MECHANISM: Not established. Aprepitant may act as an enzyme inducer, increasing metabolism of ethinyl estratiol.

CLINICAL EVALUATION: Aprepitant (100 mg/day for 14 days) given with an oral contraceptive (ethinyl estradiol 35 mcg plus norethindrone 1 mg) decreased ethinyl estradiol area under the concentration-time curve 43%.[1] The effect of 3 days of aprepitant (the usual dosage) on oral contraceptives is not established, but one should assume that reduced contraceptive efficacy is a possibility.

RELATED DRUGS: No information is available.

MANAGEMENT OPTIONS:

➡ *Circumvent/Minimize.* Consider using additional or alternative contraception during therapy with aprepitant.

REFERENCES:

1. *Emend* [package insert]. White House Station, NJ: Merck & Company; 2003.

Aprepitant (*Emend*)

Dexamethasone (eg, *Decadron*)

SUMMARY: Aprepitant increases dexamethasone serum concentrations; a reduction in dexamethasone dose is recommended.

RISK FACTORS: No specific risk factors are known.

MECHANISM: Aprepitant is a moderate inhibitor of CYP3A4 and probably reduces the intestinal and hepatic metabolism of dexamethasone.

CLINICAL EVALUATION: In a randomized crossover study, 20 subjects received dexamethasone in a standard regimen for chemotherapy-induced nausea and vomiting, with and without concurrent aprepitant.[1] Aprepitant more than doubled the dexamethasone area under the concentration-time curve.

RELATED DRUGS: Aprepitant also increases serum concentrations of methylprednisolone (eg, *Medrol*). Theoretically, other corticosteroids that undergo extensive CYP3A4 metabolism, such as budesonide (eg, *Entocort EC*), would also interact with aprepitant. Prednisone and prednisolone appear to be less affected by CYP3A4 inhibitors than dexamethasone and methylprednisolone.

MANAGEMENT OPTIONS:

➡ *Circumvent/Minimize.* The manufacturer of aprepitant recommends a 50% reduction in the dose of dexamethasone when aprepitant is used concurrently.[2]

REFERENCES:

1. McCrea JB, et al. Effects of the neurokinin 1 receptor antagonist aprepitant on the pharmacokinetics of dexamethasone and methylprednisolone. *Clin Pharmacol Ther.* 2003;74:17-24.

2. *Emend* [package insert]. White House Station, NJ: Merck & Company; 2003.

Aprepitant (*Emend*)

Diltiazem (eg, *Cardizem*)

SUMMARY: Aprepitant increases diltiazem concentrations; diltiazem increases aprepitant concentrations. The clinical effect of this dual interaction is unknown but is likely to be limited.

RISK FACTORS: No specific risk factors are known.

MECHANISM: Both aprepitant and diltiazem are metabolized by CYP3A4 and are known to inhibit CYP3A4. It would appear from the limited data available that diltiazem and aprepitant inhibited the metabolism of the other. The clinical outcome of this interaction with typical administration of aprepitant is unknown but is likely to be modest.

CLINICAL EVALUATION: A group of hypertensive patients were administered diltiazem 120 mg 3 times daily, aprepitant 230 mg/day, and the combination for 5 days.[1] The area under the concentration-time curve (AUC) of aprepitant was increased 2-fold by diltiazem. Additionally, the AUC of diltiazem was increased 1.7-fold by aprepitant. No pharmacodynamic changes were noted with the increase in diltiazem serum concentrations in these patients.

RELATED DRUGS: Verapamil (eg, *Calan*) is also a CYP3A4 substrate and inhibitor. It would be expected to interact in a similar manner to diltiazem. Dihydropyridine calcium channel blockers (eg, amlodipine [*Norvasc*], felodipine [*Plendil*], nifedipine [eg, *Procardia*]) are substrates of CYP3A4 and would be affected by aprepitant. However, they are not CYP3A4 inhibitors and would not be expected to alter the metabolism of aprepitant.

MANAGEMENT OPTIONS:

➥ *Monitor.* Monitor patients taking both diltiazem and aprepitant for increased effects of both drugs.

REFERENCES:

1. *Emend* [package insert]. White House Station, NJ: Merck & Company; 2003.

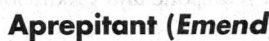

Aprepitant (*Emend*)

Ketoconazole (eg, *Nizoral*)

SUMMARY: Ketoconazole coadministration may produce large increases in aprepitant serum concentrations; aprepitant side effects may occur.

RISK FACTORS: No specific risk factors are known.

MECHANISM: Ketoconazole inhibits the metabolism of aprepitant by CYP3A4.

CLINICAL EVALUATION: Ketoconazole 400 mg/day was administered for 10 days.[1] On the fifth day of administration, a single 125 mg dose of aprepitant was given. Compared with aprepitant administered alone, pretreatment with ketoconazole produced a 5-fold increase in the mean area under the concentration-time curve of aprepitant and prolonged the half-life about 3-fold. Increased side effects from aprepitant is expected if coadministered with ketoconazole.

RELATED DRUGS: Itraconazole (*Sporanox*), and to a lesser extent voriconazole (*Vfend*) and fluconazole (*Diflucan*), inhibit CYP3A4 and would be expected to reduce aprepitant's metabolism.

MANAGEMENT OPTIONS:

➥ *Consider Alternative.* Terbinafine (*Lamisil*) does not inhibit CYP3A4 and should be considered as an alternative antifungal agent in patients receiving aprepitant. Other antiemetics, including ondansetron (*Zofran*) and dexamethasone, are also metabolized by CYP3A4.

➥ *Monitor.* Monitor patients receiving ketoconazole and aprepitant for increased side effects including fatigue, dizziness, and diarrhea.

REFERENCES:

1. *Emend* [package insert]. White House Station: Merck & Company; 2003.

Aprepitant (*Emend*)

Methylprednisolone (eg, *Medrol*)

SUMMARY: Aprepitant increases methylprednisolone serum concentrations; a reduction in methylprednisolone dose is recommended.

RISK FACTORS: No specific risk factors are known.

MECHANISM: Aprepitant is a moderate inhibitor of CYP3A4, and probably reduces the intestinal and hepatic metabolism of methylprednisolone.

CLINICAL EVALUATION: In a randomized crossover study, 10 subjects received methylprednisolone (IV on day 1, orally on days 2 and 3) with and without concurrent aprepitant.[1] Aprepitant increased the IV methylprednisolone area under the concentration-time curve (AUC) 1.3-fold and the oral methylprednisolone AUC 2.5-fold.

RELATED DRUGS: Aprepitant also increases serum concentrations of dexamethasone (eg, *Decadron*). Theoretically, other corticosteroids that undergo extensive CYP3A4 metabolism, such as budesonide (eg, *Entocort EC*), would also interact with aprepitant. Prednisone and prednisolone appear to be less affected by CYP3A4 inhibitors than dexamethasone and methylprednisolone.

MANAGEMENT OPTIONS:

➡ *Circumvent/Minimize.* The manufacturer of aprepitant recommends a 25% reduction in the dose of IV methylprednisolone and a 50% reduction in the dose of oral methylprednisolone when aprepitant is used concurrently.[2]

REFERENCES:
1. McCrea JB, et al. Effects of the neurokinin 1 receptor antagonist aprepitant on the pharmacokinetics of dexamethasone and methylprednisolone. *Clin Pharmacol Ther*. 2003;74:17-24.
2. *Emend* [package insert]. White House Station, NJ: Merck & Company; 2003.

Aprepitant (*Emend*)

Midazolam (eg, *Versed*)

SUMMARY: Aprepitant increases midazolam serum concentrations, but the clinical importance of this effect is not established.

RISK FACTORS: No specific risk factors are known.

MECHANISM: Aprepitant appears to inhibit the metabolism of midazolam by CYP3A4.

CLINICAL EVALUATION: Healthy subjects received a single oral 2 mg dose of midazolam with and without concurrent aprepitant for 5 days.[1] Midazolam area under the concentration-time curve was increased 2- to 3-fold, and midazolam half-life was about doubled. The magnitude of this effect appears to be sufficient to increase the central nervous system depressant effects of oral midazolam, but theoretically, parenteral midazolam would not be affected to the same extent.

RELATED DRUGS: Alprazolam (eg, *Xanax*) and triazolam (eg, *Halcion*) are also metabolized by CYP3A4 and would be expected to interact with aprepitant.

MANAGEMENT OPTIONS:

➡ *Monitor.* Monitor for increased central nervous system depression with midazolam (especially orally) if aprepitant is given concurrently.

REFERENCES:

1. Majumdar AK, et al. Effects of aprepitant on cytochrome P450 3A4 activity using midazolam as a probe. *Clin Pharmacol Ther.* 2003;74:150-156.

Aprepitant (*Emend*)

Paroxetine (eg, *Paxil*)

SUMMARY: Paroxetine serum concentrations may be lower in the presence of aprepitant, but the clinical importance is not known.

RISK FACTORS: No specific risk factors are known.

MECHANISM: Not established.

CLINICAL EVALUATION: Aprepitant may modestly decrease paroxetine serum concentrations.[1] Given the lack of details about the study, it is not possible to determine the clinical importance of the interaction.

RELATED DRUGS: No information is available.

MANAGEMENT OPTIONS: No specific action is required, but be alert for evidence of the interaction.

REFERENCES:

1. *Emend* [package insert]. White House Station, NJ: Merck & Company; 2003.

Aprepitant (*Emend*)

Pimozide (*Orap*)

SUMMARY: Theoretically, aprepitant may increase the risk of pimozide-induced ventricular arrhythmias; the combination should generally be avoided.

RISK FACTORS: No specific risk factors are known.

MECHANISM: Theoretically, aprepitant would inhibit the metabolism of pimozide by CYP3A4.

CLINICAL EVALUATION: Because aprepitant appears to be a moderate CYP3A4 inhibitor, the manufacturer states that its use with pimozide is contraindicated.[1] Elevated pimozide serum concentrations have been associated with life-threatening ventricular arrhythmias (torsades de pointes). Although there are no clinical data to support an interaction between aprepitant and pimozide, theoretical considerations suggest that it is possible.

RELATED DRUGS: No information is available.

MANAGEMENT OPTIONS:

➡ *Avoid Unless Benefit Outweighs Risk.* Although the interaction is theoretical, the fact that the combination is listed as contraindicated in the product information must be considered.

➡ *Monitor.* If the combination is used, monitor the electrocardiogram for evidence of pimozide toxicity (QT prolongation).

REFERENCES:
1. *Emend* [package insert]. White House Station, NJ: Merck & Company; 2003.

Aprepitant (*Emend*)

Rifampin (eg, *Rifadin*)

SUMMARY: Rifampin coadministration markedly lowers the serum concentration of aprepitant; loss of antiemetics effect may occur.

RISK FACTORS: No specific risk factors are known.

MECHANISM: Rifampin induces CYP3A4, CYP1A2, and CYP2C19, the enzymes responsible for aprepitant metabolism.

CLINICAL EVALUATION: Rifampin 600 mg/day was administered for 14 days.[1] On day 9 of rifampin administration, a single 375 mg dose of aprepitant was given. The coadministration of rifampin resulted in a greater than 11-fold reduction in the mean area under the concentration-time curve of aprepitant. The mean half-life of aprepitant was reduced nearly 3-fold by rifampin. This large reduction in aprepitant serum concentrations will likely prevent aprepitant from demonstrating any efficacy.

RELATED DRUGS: Rifabutin (*Mycobutin*) is also an inducer of CYP3A4 and would be expected to reduce aprepitant serum concentrations, although perhaps to a lesser degree than rifampin.

MANAGEMENT OPTIONS:

➡ *Monitor.* Patients taking rifampin may require very large doses of aprepitant, as well as higher doses of dexamethasone and ondansetron (*Zofran*), to control nausea and vomiting.

REFERENCES:
1. *Emend* [package insert]. White House Station, NJ: Merck & Company; 2003.

Aprepitant (*Emend*)

Tolbutamide (eg, *Orinase*)

SUMMARY: Aprepitant administration resulted in a modest reduction in the serum concentration of tolbutamide; limited changes in blood sugar would be expected as a result.

RISK FACTORS: No specific risk factors are known.

MECHANISM: Aprepitant appears to be an inducer of CYP2C9, the enzyme that metabolized tolbutamide. Induction of tolbutamide's systemic clearance by aprepitant would be expected.

CLINICAL EVALUATION: Aprepitant 125 mg administered on day 1 and 80 mg administered on day 2 reduced the mean area under the concentration-time curve of single doses of tolbutamide 500 mg 23%, 28%, and 15% on days 4, 8, and 15, respectively.[1] The effect of aprepitant on tolbutamide metabolism appears to be modest and, because of the short duration of aprepitant dosing, limited to the week to

10 days after the last dose of aprepitant. Patients using aprepitant for nausea and vomiting may not have usual caloric intake and may be somewhat less susceptible to the reduced tolbutamide concentrations.

RELATED DRUGS: Other hypoglycemic drugs metabolized by CYP2C9 (eg, chlorpropamide [eg, *Diabinese*], glimepiride [*Amaryl*], glipizide [eg, *Glucotrol*], glyburide [eg, *Diabeta*]) are likely to be affected by aprepitant in a similar manner.

MANAGEMENT OPTIONS:

➡ *Monitor.* Monitor patients taking tolbutamide for any reduction in glycemic control following aprepitant administration.

REFERENCES:
    1. *Emend* [package insert]. White House Station, NJ: Merck & Company; 2003.

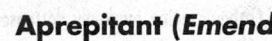

Aprepitant (*Emend*)

Warfarin (eg, *Coumadin*)

SUMMARY: Aprepitant may modestly reduce the hypoprothrombinemic effect of warfarin; monitor anticoagulant response.

RISK FACTORS: No specific risk factors are known.

MECHANISM: Not established. Evidence suggests that aprepitant is a modest inducer of CYP2C9, and S-warfarin is a CYP2C9 substrate.

CLINICAL EVALUATION: Based on a study of healthy subjects stabilized on warfarin, 3 days of treatment with aprepitant modestly reduced the hypoprothrombinemic response to warfarin (as measured 5 days after completing the aprepitant).[1]

RELATED DRUGS: The effect of aprepitant on other oral anticoagulants is not established. Theoretically, acenocoumarol[†] would interact similarly.

MANAGEMENT OPTIONS:

➡ *Monitor.* In patients on long-term warfarin, monitor the international normalized ratio closely for 2 weeks after the 3-day course of aprepitant is initiated.

REFERENCES:
    1. *Emend* [package insert]. White House Station, NJ: Merck & Company; 2003.

    † Not available in the United States.

Aprotinin (*Trasylol*)

Succinylcholine (eg, *Anectine*)

SUMMARY: Aprotinin may enhance the effect of neuromuscular blockers, but the clinical importance of this effect is unknown.

RISK FACTORS: No specific risk factors are known.

MECHANISM: Not established.

CLINICAL EVALUATION: Apnea followed the use of aprotinin in 3 patients who had recently received muscle relaxants (eg, succinylcholine, tubocurarine).[1] These findings, however, were not supported in subsequent animal studies.[2]

RELATED DRUGS: No information is available.

MANAGEMENT OPTIONS: No specific action is required, but be alert for evidence of the interaction.

REFERENCES:

1. Chasapakis G, et al. Possible interaction between muscle relaxants and the kallikrein-trypsin inactivator "Trasylol." *Br J Anaesth.* 1966;38(10):838-839.

2. Ambrus JL, et al. Effect of the protease inhibitor *Trasylol* on cholinesterase levels and on susceptibility to succinylcholine. *Res Commun Chem Pathol Pharmacol.* 1970;1(1):141-148.

Aripiprazole (*Abilify*)

Carbamazepine (eg, *Tegretol*)

SUMMARY: Carbamazepine markedly decreases aripiprazole serum concentrations, and is likely to inhibit aripiprazole efficacy.

RISK FACTORS:

➡ *Pharmacogenetics.* The magnitude of this interaction is likely to be larger in patients who have reduced or absent CYP2D6 activity, because in such patients CYP3A4 is likely to be more important in the elimination of aripiprazole.

MECHANISM: Aripiprazole is metabolized by CYP3A4 and CYP2D6; carbamazepine is a potent inducer of CYP3A4 and is likely to substantially enhance aripiprazole metabolism.

CLINICAL EVALUATION: In 9 patients receiving aripiprazole, the addition of carbamazepine for 4 to 6 weeks was associated with a 71% reduction in aripiprazole area under the plasma concentration-time curve.[1] In another study of 18 patients with schizophrenia on aripiprazole who were given carbamazepine for 1 week, carbamazepine was associated with approximately a 65% reduction in aripiprazole plasma concentrations.[2] It is likely that a greater reduction in aripiprazole would have been found if the carbamazepine had been given for more than 1 week. Information from a therapeutic drug monitoring program also found carbamazepine to be associated with marked reductions in aripiprazole serum concentrations.[3,4] It is likely that this interaction would result in subtherapeutic aripiprazole plasma concentrations in a majority of patients.

RELATED DRUGS: Other CYP3A4 inducers are also expected to substantially reduce aripiprazole plasma concentrations; they include efavirenz (*Sustiva*), nevirapine (*Viramune*), oxcarbazepine (eg, *Trileptal*), phenytoin (eg, *Dilantin*), primidone (eg, *Mysoline*), rifabutin (*Mycobutin*), rifampin (eg, *Rifadin*), rifapentine (*Priftin*), and St. John's wort.

MANAGEMENT OPTIONS:

➡ *Consider Alternative.* If possible, use an alternative to one of the drugs.

➡ *Circumvent/Minimize.* The *Abilify* product information states that the dose of aripiprazole should be doubled if it is used with CYP3A4 inducers, such as carbamazepine.[5]

➡ *Monitor.* If the combination is used, monitor for altered aripiprazole effect if carbamazepine or another enzyme inducer is started, stopped, or changed in dosage. Keep in mind that aripiprazole and its active metabolite, dehydroaripiprazole, have long half-lives, and in some cases it may take weeks to achieve new aripiprazole steady-state serum concentrations.

REFERENCES:

1. Citrome L, et al. Pharmacokinetics of aripiprazole and concomitant carbamazepine. *J Clin Psychopharmacol.* 2007;27(3):279-283.

2. Nakamura A, et al. Pharmacokinetic and pharmacodynamic interactions between carbamazepine and aripiprazole in patients with schizophrenia. *Ther Drug Monit.* 2009;31(5):575-578.

3. Waade RB, et al. Influence of comedication on serum concentrations of aripiprazole and dehydroaripiprazole. *Ther Drug Monit.* 2009;31(2):233-238.

4. Castberg I, et al. Effects of comedication on the serum levels of aripiprazole: evidence from a routine therapeutic drug monitoring service. *Pharmacopsychiatry.* 2007;40(3):107-110.

5. *Abiliby* [package insert]. Princeton, NJ: Bristol-Myers Squibb; 2010.

Aripiprazole (*Abilify*)

Clozapine (eg, *Clozaril*)

SUMMARY: A patient taking clozapine developed evidence of neuroleptic malignant syndrome (NMS) after aripiprazole was added to his therapy, but a causal relationship was not established.

RISK FACTORS: No specific risk factors are known.

MECHANISM: Not established.

CLINICAL EVALUATION: A 27-year-old man with schizophrenia taking clozapine 300 mg/day was started on aripiprazole, increasing to 30 mg/day over 15 days.[1] After 12 days of taking aripiprazole 30 mg/day, he developed evidence of NMS (eg, confusion, hyperthermia, extrapyramidal rigidity, markedly elevated creatine phosphokinase). Both drugs were stopped, and he responded to intensive care over the next few days. This case is rated "possible" using the Drug Interaction Probability Scale.[2] More information is needed to determine if the combination of aripiprazole and clozapine increases the risk of NMS.

RELATED DRUGS: No information is available.

MANAGEMENT OPTIONS: No specific action is required, but be alert for evidence of the interaction.

REFERENCES:

1. Dassa D, et al. Neuroleptic malignant syndrome with the addition of aripiprazole to clozapine. *Prog Neuropsychopharmacol Biol Psychiatry.* 2010;34(2):427-428.

2. Horn JR, et al. Proposal for a new tool to evaluate drug interaction cases. *Ann Pharmacother.* 2007;41(4):674-680.

Aripiprazole (*Abilify*)

Escitalopram (*Lexapro*)

SUMMARY: Escitalopram may slightly increase aripiprazole serum concentrations.

RISK FACTORS:

➡ **Pharmacogenetics.** The magnitude of this interaction is likely to be larger in patients who are normal (rapid) metabolizers of CYP2D6, compared with those with reduced or absent CYP2D6 activity.

MECHANISM: Aripiprazole undergoes a significant amount of metabolism via CYP2D6, and escitalopram is a weak inhibitor of CYP2D6. The CYP2D6 genotype has been shown to affect serum concentrations of aripiprazole; the lower the CYP2D6 activity, the higher the concentrations of aripiprazole.[1,2]

CLINICAL EVALUATION: Information from a therapeutic drug monitoring program found escitalopram to be associated with an increase of approximately 20% in aripiprazole serum concentrations.[3] In most patients, this would not result in adverse consequences.

RELATED DRUGS: Fluoxetine (eg, *Prozac*) and paroxetine (eg, *Paxil*) are potent inhibitors of CYP2D6, and both have been associated with substantial elevations in aripiprazole serum concentrations; theoretically, other CYP2D6-inhibitor antidepressants, such as bupropion (eg, *Wellbutrin*) and duloxetine (*Cymbalta*), would have a similar effect. Fluvoxamine is a moderate inhibitor of CYP3A4 and may inhibit the CYP3A4 metabolism of aripiprazole. Antidepressants with generally weak inhibitory effects on CYP2D6 include citalopram (eg, *Celexa*), desvenlafaxine (*Pristiq*), and sertraline (eg, *Zoloft*). Venlafaxine (eg, *Effexor*) and mirtazapine (eg, *Remeron*) have little or no effect on CYP2D6 and are unlikely to interact with aripiprazole.

MANAGEMENT OPTIONS: No specific action is required, but be alert for evidence of the interaction.

REFERENCES:
1. Hendset M, et al. Impact of the CYP2D6 genotype on steady-state serum concentrations of aripiprazole and dehydroaripiprazole. *Eur J Clin Pharmacol.* 2007;63(12):1147-1151.
2. Kim JR, et al. Population pharmacokinetic modeling of aripiprazole and its active metabolite, dehydroaripiprazole, in psychiatric patients. *Br J Clin Pharmacol.* 2008;66(6):802-810.
3. Waade RB, et al. Influence of comedication on serum concentrations of aripiprazole and dehydroaripiprazole. *Ther Drug Monit.* 2009;31(2):233-238.

Aripiprazole (*Abilify*)

Fluoxetine (eg, *Prozac*)

SUMMARY: Fluoxetine may increase aripiprazole serum concentrations and increase the risk of aripiprazole toxicity.

RISK FACTORS:

➡ ***Pharmacogenetics.*** The magnitude of this interaction is likely to be larger in patients who are normal (rapid) metabolizers of CYP2D6, compared with those with reduced or absent CYP2D6 activity.

MECHANISM: Aripiprazole undergoes a significant metabolism via CYP2D6, and fluoxetine is a potent inhibitor of CYP2D6. The CYP2D6 genotype has been shown to affect serum concentrations of aripiprazole; the lower the CYP2D6 activity, the higher the concentrations of aripiprazole.[1,2]

CLINICAL EVALUATION: Information from a therapeutic drug monitoring program found fluoxetine to be associated with elevated aripiprazole serum concentrations.[3,4] The extent to which this increases the risk of aripiprazole toxicity is not established.

RELATED DRUGS: Paroxetine (eg, *Paxil*) also inhibits CYP2D6 and has been associated with elevated aripiprazole serum concentrations; theoretically, other CYP2D6-inhibitor antidepressants, such as bupropion (eg, *Wellbutrin*) and duloxetine (*Cym-*

balta), would have a similar effect. Fluvoxamine is a moderate inhibitor of CYP3A4 and may inhibit the CYP3A4 metabolism of aripiprazole.

MANAGEMENT OPTIONS:

➡️ *Use Alternative.* If possible, use an alternative to one of the drugs. Antidepressants with generally weak inhibitory effects on CYP2D6 include citalopram (eg, *Celexa*), desvenlafaxine (*Pristiq*), escitalopram (*Lexapro*), and sertraline (eg, *Zoloft*). Venlafaxine (eg, *Effexor*) and mirtazapine (eg, *Remeron*) have little or no effect on CYP2D6 and are unlikely to interact with aripiprazole.

➡️ *Circumvent/Minimize.* The *Abilify* package insert states that the dose of aripiprazole should be reduced to one-half the normal dose if it is used with CYP2D6 inhibitors, such as fluoxetine.[5]

➡️ *Monitor.* If the combination is used, monitor for altered aripiprazole effect if fluoxetine is started, stopped, or changed in dosage. Keep in mind that aripiprazole and its active metabolite, dehydroaripiprazole, have long half-lives, and in some cases it may take weeks to achieve new aripiprazole steady-state serum concentrations.

REFERENCES:

1. Hendset M, et al. Impact of the CYP2D6 genotype on steady-state serum concentrations of aripiprazole and dehydroaripiprazole. *Eur J Clin Pharmacol.* 2007;63(12):1147-1151.

2. Kim JR, et al. Population pharmacokinetic modeling of aripiprazole and its active metabolite, dehydroaripiprazole, in psychiatric patients. *Br J Clin Pharmacol.* 2008;66(6):802-810.

3. Waade RB, et al. Influence of comedication on serum concentrations of aripiprazole and dehydroaripiprazole. *Ther Drug Monit.* 2009;31(2):233-238.

4. Castberg I, et al. Effects of comedication on the serum levels of aripiprazole: evidence from a routine therapeutic drug monitoring service. *Pharmacopsychiatry.* 2007;40(3):107-110.

5. *Abilify* "package insert]. Princeton, NJ: Bristol-Myers Squibb; 2010.

Aripiprazole (*Abilify*)
Itraconazole (eg, *Sporanox*)

SUMMARY: Itraconazole increases the plasma concentration of aripiprazole and its active metabolite; some patients may experience increased adverse reactions.

RISK FACTORS:

➡️ *Pharmacogenetics.* Patients who are poor metabolizers for CYP2D6 may be at increased risk.

MECHANISM: Itraconazole is known to inhibit the activity of one of the enzymes (CYP3A4) that metabolizes aripiprazole and its active metabolite.

CLINICAL EVALUATION: Twenty-four healthy subjects received a single dose of aripiprazole 3 mg alone and on day 7 of 21 days of itraconazole 100 mg daily.[1] The mean area under the concentration-time curve (AUC) of aripiprazole increased by nearly 50% during itraconazole administration. Larger doses of itraconazole may produce a greater effect on aripiprazole pharmacokinetics. The effect of itraconazole on the AUC of aripiprazole tended to be greater in patients who had reduced CYP2D6 activity compared with those with normal activity. This is due to the partial metabolism of aripiprazole by CYP2D6. Although no CYP2D6 poor metabolizers were included in the study, these patients are most dependent on CYP3A4 for the metabolism of aripiprazole and would be expected to demonstrate the largest reduction in aripiprazole metabolism when a CYP3A4 inhibitor is coadministered. Itraconazole administration produced a similar effect on the active metabolite of aripiprazole. Some patients may require a dose adjustment of aripiprazole if itraconazole is initiated or discontinued.

RELATED DRUGS: Ketoconazole (eg, *Nizoral*), fluconazole (eg, *Diflucan*), posaconazole (*Noxafil*), and voriconazole (*Vfend*) also inhibit the activity of CYP3A4 and would be expected to increase the plasma concentrations of aripiprazole.

MANAGEMENT OPTIONS:

➡ **Monitor.** Observe patients on aripiprazole for altered response if itraconazole or another CYP3A4 inhibitor is initiated or discontinued.

REFERENCES:

1. Kubo M, et al. Influence of itraconazole coadministration and CYP2D6 genotype on the pharmacokinetics of the new antipsychotic aripiprazole. *Drug Metab Pharmacokinet*. 2005;20(1):55-64.

Aripiprazole (*Abilify*)

Ketoconazole (eg, *Nizoral*)

SUMMARY: Ketoconazole increases the plasma concentrations of aripiprazole and its active metabolite; aripiprazole dose reductions may be required.

RISK FACTORS:

➡ **Pharmacogenetics.** Patients who are poor metabolizers for CYP2D6 are likely to be most affected by this interaction.

MECHANISM: Aripiprazole is metabolized by CYP3A4 and CYP2D6. Ketoconazole inhibits the CYP3A4 metabolism of aripiprazole.

CLINICAL EVALUATION: While published data are limited, the manufacturer reports that ketoconazole 200 mg/day for 14 days increased the area under the concentration-time curve of a single dose of aripiprazole 63%.[1] The concentration of the major metabolite of aripiprazole, dehydroaripiprazole (that has an affinity for the D_2 receptor similar to that of the parent compound), also was increased 77%. The effects of higher doses of ketoconazole on aripiprazole have not been reported. The manufacturer recommends reducing the dose of aripiprazole 50% in patients taking drugs that are potent CYP3A4 inhibitors. Because of the long half-life (75 to 95 hours) for aripiprazole and its metabolite, the maximum effect of the interaction is likely to be delayed for up to 10 to 14 days.

RELATED DRUGS: Itraconazole (eg, *Sporanox*) is a potent CYP3A4 inhibitor that is likely to produce similar increases in aripiprazole concentrations. Other antifungal agents that are known to inhibit CYP3A4 include fluconazole (eg, *Diflucan*) and voriconazole (*Vfend*). Terbinafine (eg, *Lamisil*) would not represent a suitable alternative antifungal agent because it inhibits CYP2D6, the other pathway for aripiprazole metabolism.

MANAGEMENT OPTIONS:

➡ *Monitor.* Observe patients maintained on aripiprazole for altered response if a potent inhibitor of CYP3A4 is added to or discontinued from therapy. Aripiprazole dosage adjustments may be required.

REFERENCES:

1. *Abilify* [package insert]. Princeton, NJ: Bristol-Myers Squibb; 2002.

Aripiprazole (*Abilify*)

Lorazepam (eg, *Ativan*)

SUMMARY: The combination of parenteral aripiprazole and lorazepam may increase the risk of sedation and orthostatic hypotension.

RISK FACTORS: No specific risk factors are known.

MECHANISM: Aripiprazole and lorazepam may have additive pharmacodynamic effects.

CLINICAL EVALUATION: In a study of 40 healthy subjects given single parenteral doses of aripiprazole 15 mg and lorazepam 2 mg, there was no effect on the pharmacokinetics of either drug. However, the combination was associated with increased sedation and orthostatic hypotension.[1] It is not clear whether the usual oral route of administration of both drugs would result in similar effects.

RELATED DRUGS: Theoretically, other benzodiazepines may produce a similar effect when combined with aripiprazole.

MANAGEMENT OPTIONS: No specific action is required, but be alert for evidence of the interaction.

REFERENCES:

1. *Abiliby* [package insert]. Princeton, NJ: Bristol-Myers Squibb; 2010.

Aripiprazole (*Abilify*)

Paroxetine (eg, *Paxil*)

SUMMARY: Paroxetine may increase aripiprazole serum concentrations.

RISK FACTORS:

➡ *Pharmacogenetics.* The magnitude of this interaction is likely to be larger in patients who are normal ("rapid") metabolizers of CYP2D6, compared with those with reduced or absent CYP2D6 activity.

MECHANISM: Aripiprazole undergoes a significant amount of metabolism via CYP2D6, and paroxetine is a potent inhibitor of CYP2D6. The CYP2D6 genotype has been shown to affect serum concentrations of aripiprazole; the lower the CYP2D6 activity, the higher the concentrations of aripiprazole.[1,2]

CLINICAL EVALUATION: Information from a therapeutic drug monitoring program found paroxetine to be associated with elevated aripiprazole serum concentrations.[3] The increased ariprazole concentrations were moderate, but may cause excessive aripiprazole levels in some patients.

RELATED DRUGS: Fluoxetine (eg, *Prozac*) also inhibits CYP2D6, and it has also been associated with elevated aripiprazole serum concentrations; theoretically, other CYP2D6-inhibitor antidepressants, such as bupropion (eg, *Wellbutrin*) and duloxetine (*Cymbalta*), would have a similar effect. Fluvoxamine is a moderate inhibitor of CYP3A4, and may inhibit the CYP3A4 metabolism of aripiprazole.

MANAGEMENT OPTIONS:

➡ *Use Alternative.* If possible, use an alternative to one of the drugs. Antidepressants with generally weak inhibitory effects on CYP2D6 include citalopram (eg, *Celexa*), desvenlafaxine (*Pristiq*), escitalopram (*Lexapro*), and sertraline (eg, *Zoloft*). Venlafaxine (*Effexor*) and mirtazapine (eg, *Remeron*) have little or no effect on CYP2D6 and are unlikely to interact with aripiprazole.

➡ *Circumvent/Minimize.* The *Abilify* product information states that the dose of aripiprazole should be reduced to one-half the normal dose if it is used with CYP2D6 inhibitors, such as paroxetine.[4]

➡ *Monitor.* If the combination is used, monitor for altered aripiprazole effect if paroxetine is started, stopped, or changed in dosage. Keep in mind that aripiprazole and its active metabolite, dehydroaripiprazole, have long half-lives, and in some cases it may take weeks to achieve new aripiprazole steady-state serum concentrations.

REFERENCES:
1. Waade RB, et al. Influence of comedication on serum concentrations of aripiprazole and dehydroaripiprazole. *Ther Drug Monit.* 2009;31(2):233-238.
2. Hendset M, et al. Impact of the CYP2D6 genotype on steady-state serum concentrations of aripiprazole and dehydroaripiprazole. *Eur J Clin Pharmacol.* 2007;63(12):1147-1151.
3. Kim JR, et al. Population pharmacokinetic modeling of aripiprazole and its active metabolite, dehydroaripiprazole, in psychiatric patients. *Br J Clin Pharmacol.* 2008;66(6):802-810.
4. *Abiliby* [package insert]. Princeton, NJ: Bristol-Myers Squibb; 2010.

Aripiprazole (*Abilify*)

Quinidine

SUMMARY: Quinidine increases the plasma concentrations of aripiprazole and its active metabolite; aripiprazole dose reductions may be required.

RISK FACTORS:

➡ *Pharmacogenetics.* Patients who are rapid metabolizers for CYP2D6 are likely to be most affected by this interaction. Quinidine will have a minimal effect on aripiprazole in poor metabolizers of CYP2D6.

MECHANISM: Aripiprazole is metabolized by CYP3A4 and CYP2D6. Quinidine inhibits the CYP2D6 metabolism of aripiprazole.

CLINICAL EVALUATION: While published data are limited, the manufacturer reports that quinidine 166 mg/day for 13 days increased the area under the concentration-time curve of a single dose of aripiprazole 112%.[1] The concentration of the major metabolite of aripiprazole, dehydroaripiprazole (that has an affinity for the D2 receptor similar to that of the parent compound), was decreased 35%. The effects of higher doses of quinidine on aripiprazole have not been reported. The manufacturer recommends reducing the dose of aripiprazole 50% in patients taking drugs that are potent CYP2D6 inhibitors. Because of the long half-life (75 to

95 hours) for aripiprazole and its metabolite, the maximum effect of the interaction is likely to be delayed for up to 10 to 14 days.

RELATED DRUGS: Other antiarrhythmic agents that inhibit CYP2D6 (eg, amiodarone [eg, *Cordarone*], propafenone [eg, *Rythmol*]) also would be expected to inhibit the metabolism of aripiprazole.

MANAGEMENT OPTIONS:

➡ *Monitor.* Observe patients maintained on aripiprazole for altered response if a potent inhibitor of CYP2D6 is added to or discontinued from therapy. Aripiprazole dosage adjustments may be required.

REFERENCES:

> 1. *Abilify* [package insert]. Princeton, NJ: Bristol-Myers Squibb; 2002.

Aripiprazole (*Abilify*)

Sertraline (eg, *Zoloft*)

SUMMARY: Sertraline appears to have little effect on aripiprazole serum concentrations, but a case of myxedema coma occurred in a patient taking the combination.

RISK FACTORS: No specific risk factors are known.

MECHANISM: Not established.

CLINICAL EVALUATION: A 41-year-old man developed myxedema coma while taking aripiprazole and sertraline, but it was not possible to determine whether the myxedema was due to a drug interaction, one of the drugs alone, or some other factor.[1] More study is needed to determine whether the combination of aripiprazole and sertraline increases the risk of myxedema coma. Information from a therapeutic drug monitoring program found no effect of sertraline on aripiprazole serum concentrations in 11 patients.[2] Although the number of patients was small, these results are consistent with other data suggesting that sertraline is only a weak inhibitor of CYP2D6.

RELATED DRUGS: No information available.

MANAGEMENT OPTIONS: No specific action is required, but be alert for evidence of the interaction.

REFERENCES:

> 1. Church CO, et al. Myxedema coma associated with combination aripiprazole and sertraline therapy. *Ann. Pharmacother*. 2009;43(12):2113-2116.
>
> 2. Waade RB, et al. Influence of comedication on serum concentrations of aripiprazole and dehydroaripiprazole. *Ther Drug Monit*. 2009;31(2):233-238.

Aripiprazole (*Abilify*)

Venlafaxine (eg, *Effexor*)

SUMMARY: Available evidence indicates that venlafaxine does not affect aripiprazole serum concentrations.

RISK FACTORS: No interaction.

MECHANISM: No interaction.

CLINICAL EVALUATION: Information from a therapeutic drug monitoring program found no effect of venlafaxine on aripiprazole serum concentrations in 18 patients.[1] Although the number of patients was small, these results are consistent with other data suggesting that venlafaxine has little or no effect on CYP2D6. Mirtazapine (12 patients) also appeared to have no effect on aripiprazole.

RELATED DRUGS: Antidepressants with generally weak inhibitory effects on CYP2D6 include citalopram (eg, *Celexa*), desvenlafaxine (*Pristiq*), and escitalopram (*Lexapro*). Mirtazapine (eg, *Remeron*) has little or no effect on CYP2D6 and does not interact with aripiprazole. Fluoxetine (eg, *Prozac*) and paroxetine (eg, *Paxil*) are potent inhibitors of CYP2D6, and have been associated with substantial elevations in aripiprazole serum concentrations; theoretically, other CYP2D6-inhibitor antidepressants, such as bupropion (eg, *Wellbutrin*) and duloxetine (*Cymbalta*), would have a similar effect. Fluvoxamine is a moderate inhibitor of CYP3A4, and may inhibit the CYP3A4 metabolism of aripiprazole.

MANAGEMENT OPTIONS: No interaction.

REFERENCES:

1. Waade RB, et al. Influence of comedication on serum concentrations of aripiprazole and dehydroaripiprazole. *Ther Drug Monit.* 2009;31(2):233-238.

Aspirin

Caffeine

SUMMARY: Caffeine may increase the absorption of aspirin slightly, but the clinical importance of this effect is probably small.

RISK FACTORS: No specific risk factors are known.

MECHANISM: Caffeine appears to increase the GI absorption of aspirin but does not appear to affect salicylate elimination.

CLINICAL EVALUATION: Twelve healthy subjects were given 650 mg aspirin with and without coadministration of 120 mg of caffeine citrate (equivalent to 60 mg caffeine base).[1] Caffeine administration was associated with a more rapid absorption of aspirin and a small (12.4%) increase in aspirin bioavailability; the elimination phase of aspirin was not affected. These small changes in salicylate pharmacokinetics are not likely to be clinically important.

RELATED DRUGS: The effect of caffeine on salicylates other than aspirin is not established.

MANAGEMENT OPTIONS: No specific action is required, but be alert for evidence of the interaction.

REFERENCES:

1. Yoovathaworn KC, et al. Influence of caffeine on aspirin pharmacokinetics. *Eur J Drug Metab Pharmacokinet.* 1986;11:71.

Aspirin ▼ ③

Captopril (*Capoten*)

SUMMARY: Aspirin appears to inhibit both the antihypertensive effects of captopril and other angiotensin-converting enzyme (ACE) inhibitors and the favorable hemodynamic effects of ACE inhibitors in patients with CHF.

RISK FACTORS:

➥ **Dosage Regimen.** The inhibitory effect of aspirin on ACE inhibitors is probably dose related.

MECHANISM: The observed inhibition of ACE inhibitor response is probably caused by aspirin-induced inhibition of prostaglandin synthesis. Prostaglandins appear to be involved in the favorable effects of ACE inhibitors in hypertension and congestive heart failure.

CLINICAL EVALUATION: The effect of aspirin on ACE inhibitors has been studied in patients with hypertension and in patients with CHF.

Patients with Hypertension. In a study of 8 hypertensive patients, aspirin 600 mg every 6 hours reduced the hypotensive response to a single dose of captopril (25 to 100 mg) in 50% of the patients.[1] In another study of 15 hypertensive patients, a small dose of aspirin (75 mg/day) for 2 weeks did not affect the antihypertensive effect of captopril (25 mg twice daily).[3] Additional study is needed to assess the clinical significance of analgesic or anti-inflammatory doses of aspirin in hypertensive patients on chronic captopril therapy. Occasional aspirin doses probably have little negative effect on the antihypertensive effect of ACE inhibitors.

Patients with CHF. In 18 patients with severe but stable CHF, a single 350 mg dose of aspirin inhibited the favorable hemodynamic effects of 10 mg of enalapril (*Vasotec*) in a double-blind, randomized, crossover study.[4] However, a smaller single dose of aspirin (236 mg) did not affect the hemodynamic effects of 25 mg captopril in 13 patients with CHF who were on chronic ACE inhibitor therapy.[5] Additional study is needed to assess the clinical significance of multiple analgesic or anti-inflammatory doses of aspirin in CHF patients on chronic therapy with ACE inhibitors.

Other studies. A 66-year-old woman on captopril developed acute renal failure after starting aspirin for osteoarthritis.[2] Renal function promptly improved when the captopril and aspirin were discontinued. Although the renal failure may have resulted from the combined use of captopril and aspirin, one cannot rule out the possibility that it was caused by the aspirin alone. A study in healthy subjects found no effect of aspirin (single 325 mg dose) on the pharmacokinetics of benazepril.[6]

RELATED DRUGS: The effect of aspirin is probably similar for all ACE inhibitors. Other nonsteroidal anti-inflammatory drugs probably also inhibit ACE inhibitor effect, although it is possible that sulindac (*Clinoril*) interacts to a lesser degree. The effect of salicylates other than aspirin on ACE inhibitors is not established; theoretically, nonacetylated salicylates may be less likely to interact since they tend to have less inhibitory effect on prostaglandin synthesis.

MANAGEMENT OPTIONS:

➡ *Consider Alternative.* Acetaminophen is not known to affect ACE inhibitor response and may be a suitable alternative to aspirin as an analgesic or antipyretic.

➡ *Monitor.* If more than occasional doses of aspirin are used in a patient on an ACE inhibitor, monitor for worsening of disease (hypertension or CHF). Be alert for evidence of reduced renal function.

REFERENCES:

1. Moore TJ, et al. Contribution of prostaglandins to the antihypertensive action of captopril in essential hypertension. *Hypertension.* 1981;3:168.

2. Seelig CB, et al. Nephrotoxicity associated with concomitant ACE inhibitor and NSAID therapy. *South Med J.* 1990;83:1144.

3. Smith SR, et al. Effect of low-dose aspirin on thromboxane production and the antihypertensive effect of captopril. *J Am Soc Nephrol.* 1993;4:1133.

4. Hall D, et al. Counteraction of the vasodilator effects of enalapril by aspirin in severe heart failure. *J Am Coll Cardiol.* 1992;20:1549.

5. van Wijngaarden J, et al. Effects of acetylsalicylic acid on peripheral hemodynamics in patients with chronic heart failure treated with angiotensin-converting enzyme inhibitors. *J Cardiovasc Pharmacol.* 1994;23:240.

6. Sioufi A, et al. The absence of a pharmacokinetic interaction between aspirin and the angiotensin-converting enzyme inhibitor benazepril in healthy volunteers. *Biopharm Drug Disposit.* 1994;15:451.

Aspirin

Chlorpropamide (*Diabinese*)

SUMMARY: Salicylate administration may enhance the hypoglycemic response to sulfonylureas, particularly chlorpropamide.

RISK FACTORS: No specific risk factors are known.

MECHANISM: Large doses of salicylates may have an intrinsic effect on carbohydrate metabolism resulting from an increase in the effects of insulin in noninsulin-dependent diabetics.[2,5] Sodium salicylate displaces tolbutamide and chlorpropamide from plasma protein-binding sites and temporarily increases unbound (active) sulfonylurea concentrations;[3] however, the most probable mechanism involves salicylate inhibition of prostaglandin E synthesis in noninsulin-dependent diabetic patients.[2,5] Prostaglandin E inhibits glucose-induced insulin secretion; inhibition of prostaglandin E by salicylates would increase the insulin response to hyperglycemia in noninsulindependent diabetics. Salicylates do not appear to alter the serum concentrations of chlorpropamide.[2]

CLINICAL EVALUATION: Aspirin administration enhances the hypoglycemic response to chlorpropamide; in some cases this effect has been seen at serum salicylate concentrations of 10 mg/dl or lower.[2] Cases have been reported in which aspirin appeared to have contributed to hypoglycemic coma in patients receiving sulfonylureas.[1,4] Large doses of salicylates may enhance the hypoglycemic effect of sulfonylureas or insulin through an intrinsic hypoglycemic effect; small doses of salicylates probably have minimal effects on antidiabetic drugs, with the possible exception of chlorpropamide.

RELATED DRUGS: Similar cases of hypoglycemia have been reported with tolbutamide (*Orinase*).[4] Aspirin also has been noted to reduce glyburide (*DiaBeta*) serum concentrations while enhancing its hypoglycemic effects.[6] More study in diabetic patients is needed to evaluate this interaction.

MANAGEMENT OPTIONS:

➡ **Monitor.** Be alert for evidence of altered response to oral hypoglycemics and insulin when salicylate therapy is started or stopped. Monitor blood glucose concentrations and watch for symptoms of hyper- or hypoglycemia.

REFERENCES:

1. Peaston MJT, et al. A case of combined poisoning with chlorpropamide, acetylsalicylic acid and paracetamol. *Br J Clin Pract.* 1968;22:30.
2. Richardson T, et al. Enhancement by sodium salicylate of the blood glucose lowering effect of chlorpropamide—drug interaction or summation of similar effects? *Br J Clin Pharmacol.* 1986;22:43.
3. Wishinsky H, et al. Protein interactions of sulfonylurea compounds. *Diabetes.* 1962;2(Suppl.):18.
4. Cherner R, et al. Prolonged tolbutamide-induced hypoglycemia. *JAMA.* 1963;185:883.
5. Guigliano D, et al. Effects of salicylate, tolbutamide, and prostaglandin E2 on insulin responses to glucose in non insulin-dependent diabetes mellitus. *J Clin Endocrinol Metab.* 1985;61:160.
6. Kubacka RT, et al. Effects of aspirin and ibuprofen on the pharmacokinetics and pharmacodynamics of in healthy subjects. *Ann Pharmacother.* 1996;30:20.

Aspirin 4

Cimetidine (eg, *Tagamet*)

SUMMARY: Cimetidine may produce a small increase in serum salicylate concentrations, but the magnitude of the effect is unlikely to be clinically important in most patients.

RISK FACTORS: No specific risk factors are known.

MECHANISM: Not established. Cimetidine may increase aspirin bioavailability and may inhibit salicylate elimination.

CLINICAL EVALUATION: Cimetidine has been shown to increase serum salicylate concentrations and bioavailability slightly following the administration of enteric-coated aspirin.[1,2] In another study of 6 subjects, cimetidine appeared to increase the absorption rate of aspirin in 3 subjects, but there was no significant change in the group as a whole.[3] The type of aspirin used was not stated. In 11 healthy subjects, cimetidine 1 g/day for 4 days was associated with reduced clearance of salicylic acid after single 1 g doses of aspirin.[4] The area under the salicylic acid plasma concentration-time curve was increased approximately 23% in the presence of cimetidine. Thus, the evidence suggests that cimetidine produces a small increase in plasma salicylic acid concentrations.

RELATED DRUGS: The effect of other H₂-receptor antagonists such as ranitidine (*Zantac*), famotidine (*Pepcid*), and nizatidine (*Axid*) on salicylates is unknown.

MANAGEMENT OPTIONS: No specific action is required, but be alert for evidence of the interaction.

REFERENCES:

1. Paton TW, et al. Effect of cimetidine on bioavailability of entericcoated aspirin tablets. *Clin Pharm.* 1983;2:165.
2. Willoughby JS, et al. The effect of cimetidine on enteric-coated ASA disposition. *Clin Pharmacol Ther.* 1982;33:268.
3. Khoury W, et al. The effect of cimetidine on aspirin absorption. *Gastroenterology.* 1979;76:1169.
4. Tranvska Z, et al. The effect of cimetidine on the pharmacokinetics of salicylic acid. *Drugs Exp Clin Res.* 1985;11:703.

Aspirin

Diclofenac (*Voltaren*)

SUMMARY: Aspirin may reduce plasma diclofenac concentrations but does not appear to interfere with its therapeutic effect.

RISK FACTORS: No specific risk factors are known.

MECHANISM: Aspirin increases the plasma clearance of diclofenac, possibly by decreasing diclofenac plasma protein binding.[1]

CLINICAL EVALUATION: In 5 healthy subjects, aspirin and diclofenac mutually depressed serum concentrations of the other drug.[1] In a subsequent study, 6 healthy subjects received 50 mg diclofenac orally and IV with and without oral coadministration of 900 mg aspirin.[2] Aspirin reduced the area under the plasma concentration-time curve of oral diclofenac by 31% and of IV diclofenac by 27%. In a study of the clinical importance of this interaction, 36 patients with rheumatoid arthritis received diclofenac, aspirin, or a combination of the 2 in a crossover study.[3] The therapeutic response to diclofenac alone was similar to that of diclofenac plus aspirin. A larger study would be necessary to determine whether the combination results in an increase in adverse effects over either agent alone.

RELATED DRUGS: The effect of salicylates other than aspirin on diclofenac is not established. Aspirin interacts with many nonsteroidal anti-inflammatory drugs, but most of these interactions appear to have limited clinical importance.

MANAGEMENT OPTIONS: No specific action is required, but be alert for evidence of the interaction.

REFERENCES:

1. Muller FO, et al. Pharmacokinetic and pharmacodynamic implications of long-term administration of nonsteroidal anti-inflammatory agents. *Int J Clin Pharmacol*. 1977;15:397.

2. Willis JV, et al. A study of the effect of aspirin on the pharmacokinetics of oral and intravenous diclofenac sodium. *Eur J Clin Pharmacol*. 1980;18:415.

3. Bird HA, et al. A study to determine the clinical relevance of the pharmacokinetic interaction between aspirin and diclofenac. *Agents Actions*. 1986;18:447.

4 **Aspirin**

Diflunisal (*Dolobid*)

SUMMARY: Aspirin may reduce plasma diflunisal concentrations slightly, but it is unlikely that this effect is clinically significant.

RISK FACTORS: No specific risk factors are known.

MECHANISM: Not established. It is likely that diflunisal and salicylates compete for plasma protein binding sites.

CLINICAL EVALUATION: Preliminary evidence suggests that aspirin 600 mg 4 times daily lowers the plasma concentration of diflunisal 250 mg twice daily by only 13%.[1] It is not likely that this change would affect the therapeutic response to diflunisal adversely.

RELATED DRUGS: The effect of salicylates other than aspirin or diflunisal is not established. Aspirin interacts with many nonsteroidal anti-inflammatory drugs, but most of these interactions appear to have limited clinical importance.

MANAGEMENT OPTIONS: No specific action is required, but be alert for evidence of the interaction.

REFERENCES:

1. Tempero KF, et al. Diflunisal: a review of pharmacokinetic and pharmacodynamic properties, drug interactions, and special tolerability studies in humans. *Br J Clin Pharmacol.* 1977;4:31S.

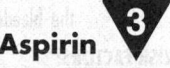

Aspirin

Diltiazem (*Cardizem*)

SUMMARY: Diltiazem appears to enhance the antiplatelet activity of aspirin, but the clinical importance of this effect is not established.

RISK FACTORS: No specific risk factors are known.

MECHANISM: Not established.

CLINICAL EVALUATION: Five healthy subjects received aspirin 40 mg/day for 3 days, diltiazem 60 mg every 8 hours for 7 doses, and both drugs for 3 days.[1] Both diltiazem and aspirin inhibited in vitro platelet aggregation. Bleeding time increased from 304 seconds to 573 seconds following aspirin, but diltiazem did not increase bleeding time significantly. Bleeding times increased to more than 15 minutes during aspirin plus diltiazem administration in 2 of the 5 subjects. Other investigators have noted that diltiazem administered alone appears to have a minimal effect on platelet aggregation;[5,6,7] however, it enhanced aspirin inhibition of platelet aggregation.[3] Diltiazem 60 mg appears to have an additive effect in inhibiting platelet aggregation when given with other drugs (eg, propranolol 40 mg).[4] Patients have developed bruising or petechiae following the combination of aspirin with either verapamil (*Calan*)[8] or diltiazem.[2]

RELATED DRUGS: Verapamil (*Calan*) may interact similarly; patients have developed bruising or petechiae following coadministration with aspirin.

MANAGEMENT OPTIONS:

➡ **Monitor.** Until further information is available, monitor patients for prolonged bleeding times when diltiazem or verapamil is coadministered with aspirin.

REFERENCES:

1. Ring ME, et al. Effects of oral diltiazem on platelet function: alone and in combination with "low dose" aspirin. *Thromb Res.* 1986;44:391.

2. Ring ME, et al. Clinically significant antiplatelet effects of calciumchannel blockers. *J Clin Pharmacol.* 1986;26:719.

3. Altman R, et al. Diltiazem potentiates the inhibitory effect of aspirin on platelet aggregation. *Clin Pharmacol Ther.* 1988;44:320.

4. Ring ME, et al. Antiplatelet effects of oral diltiazem, propranolol, and their combination. *Br J Clin Pharmacol.* 1987;24:615.

5. Yamauchi K, et al. Effects of diltiazem hydrochloride on cardiovascular response, platelet aggregation and coagulating activity during exercise testing in systemic hypertension. *Am J Card.* 1986;57:609.

6. Cremer KF, et al. Effects of diltiazem, dipyridamole, and their combination on hemostasis. *Clin Pharmacol Ther.* 1984;34:641.

7. Kiyomoto A, et al. Inhibition of platelet aggregation by diltiazem: comparison with verapamil and nifedipine and inhibitory potencies of diltiazem metabolites. *Circ Res.* 1983;52(Suppl.):115.

8. Verzino E, et al. Verapamil-aspirin interaction. *Annals Pharmacother.* 1994;28:536.

Aspirin

Ethanol (Ethyl Alcohol)

SUMMARY: Ethanol appears to enhance aspirin-induced gastric mucosal damage and aspirin-induced prolongation of the bleeding time.

RISK FACTORS:

➡ ***Diet/Food.*** Theoretically, more concentrated alcohol (eg, hard liquor) on an empty stomach would be more likely to enhance gastric mucosal damage from aspirin.

MECHANISM: Ethanol appears to increase the GI bleeding produced by aspirin. Aspirin and ethanol individually damage the gastric mucosal barrier, and their combined use appears to result in additive or synergistic effects. Also, the ability of aspirin to prolong the bleeding time is enhanced by ethanol administration.[7]

CLINICAL EVALUATION: Available evidence indicates that ethanol ingestion produces about a 2-fold increase in the minor gastric bleeding that regularly occurs with aspirin administration.[1-6] It has not been established whether ethanol increases the likelihood of upper GI hemorrhage because of aspirin, but indirect evidence indicates that it may.[8] The clinical significance of the ethanol-induced increase in the bleeding time response to aspirin is not known, but the effect may be large enough in some patients to result in spontaneous bleeding. In 5 healthy subjects given 0.3 g/kg alcohol 1 hour after a standard breakfast, blood alcohol concentrations were significantly higher when the subjects were given 1000 mg aspirin 1 hour before the alcohol.[9] It is unknown whether this increase in blood alcohol would be seen under other circumstances (eg, alcohol ingested in the evening, on an empty stomach, in different doses).

RELATED DRUGS: Theoretically, salicylate preparations which are less likely to produce gastric mucosal injury (eg, effervescent buffered salicylates [*Alka-Seltzer*], enteric-coated aspirin [eg, *Ecotrin*], and nonacetylated salicylates) would be less likely to produce additive gastric mucosal damage when administered in the presence of alcohol. Also, salicylate-induced prolongation of the bleeding time can be avoided by using nonacetylated salicylates such as choline salicylate (*Arthropan*), salsalate (*Disalcid*), choline magnesium salicylate, and sodium salicylate; ethanol induced potentiation of the salicylate-induced prolongation of the bleeding time by ethanol would not be a factor with these nonacetylated salicylates.

MANAGEMENT OPTIONS:

➡ ***Consider Alternative.*** Some forms of salicylate appear to be less likely to produce gastric mucosal injury than standard aspirin tablets. Such products include effervescent buffered products, enteric-coated products, and the nonacetylated salicylates. Theoretically, these preparations would be less likely to produce additive gastric mucosal damage with alcohol than standard aspirin tablets. (Also see Related Drugs for additional alternatives.)

➡ *Circumvent/Minimize.* Although concomitant use of ethanol and aspirin is not necessarily contraindicated, consider the possibility of enhanced GI bleeding. When possible, avoid aspirin use within 8 to 10 hours of heavy alcohol use.

➡ *Monitor.* Be alert for evidence of GI bleeding (eg, melena, black stools).

REFERENCES:

1. Goulston K, et al. Alcohol, aspirin and gastrointestinal bleeding. *BMJ.* 1968;4:664.

2. Bouchier IND, et al. Determination of faecal blood-loss after combined alcohol and sodium-acetylsalicylate intake. *Lancet.* 1969;1:178.

3. Mould G. Faecal blood-loss after sodium acetylsalicylate taken with alcohol. *Lancet.* 1969;1:1268.

4. Wood PHN. Faecal blood-loss after sodium acetylsalicylate taken with alcohol. *Lancet.* 1969;1:677.

5. Dobbing J. Faecal blood-loss after sodium acetylsalicylate taken with alcohol. *Lancet.* 1969;1:527.

6. DeSchepper PJ, et al. Gastrointestinal blood loss after diflunisal and after aspirin: effect of ethanol. *Clin Pharmacol Ther.* 1978;23:669.

7. Deykin D, et al. Ethanol potentiation of aspirin-induced prolongation of the bleeding time. *N Engl J Med.* 1982;306:852.

8. Needham CD, et al. Aspirin and alcohol in gastrointestinal haemorrhage. *Gut.* 1971;12:819.

9. Roine R, et al. Aspirin increases blood alcohol concentrations in humans after ingestion of ethanol. *JAMA.* 1990;264:2406.

Aspirin 4

Fenoprofen (eg, *Nalfon*)

SUMMARY: Aspirin may lower plasma fenoprofen concentrations somewhat, but the effect has not been shown to be clinically significant.

RISK FACTORS: No specific risk factors are known.

MECHANISM: Not established.

CLINICAL EVALUATION: In healthy subjects ingesting fenoprofen and aspirin, the area under the fenoprofen concentration-time curve was reduced by single doses of aspirin and more so by multiple aspirin doses.[1,2] There was also evidence the half-life of fenoprofen was decreased by multiple doses (but not single doses) of aspirin. However, the clinical significance of these findings remains to be determined.

RELATED DRUGS: The effect of salicylates other than aspirin on fenoprofen is not established.

MANAGEMENT OPTIONS: No specific action is required, but be alert for evidence of the interaction.

REFERENCES:

1. Rubin A, et al. Interactions of aspirin with nonsteroidal antiinflammatory drugs in man. *Arthritis Rheum.* 1973;16:635-645.

2. Gruber CM Jr. Clinical pharmacology of fenoprofen: a review. *J Rheumatol.* 1976;2:8-17.

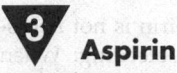 **Aspirin**

Fluoxetine (eg, *Prozac*)

SUMMARY: The combined use of selective serotonin reuptake inhibitors (SSRIs) or clomipramine with aspirin appears to increase the risk of upper GI bleeding.

RISK FACTORS: No specific risk factors are known.

MECHANISM: Serotonin appears to play a role in platelet function, but platelets do not synthesize serotonin. SSRIs inhibit the uptake of serotonin by platelets, and this may add to the antiplatelet effects of aspirin. Also, aspirin impairs the defenses of the gastric mucosa, which can lead to gastric erosions and bleeding.

CLINICAL EVALUATION: In a population-based cohort study of 26,005 antidepressant users, SSRIs without aspirin or NSAIDs increased the risk of serious GI bleeding by 3.6-fold, but patients on both an SSRI and low-dose aspirin had over a 5-fold increase in risk.[1] The increase in GI bleeding risk appeared to correlate with the potency of the antidepressant as a serotonin reuptake inhibitor. Antidepressants with less serotonergic effect than SSRIs, such as imipramine (*Tofranil*), amitriptyline (*Elavil*), and doxepin (*Adapin*), appeared somewhat less likely to be associated with GI bleeding than SSRIs or clomipramine (*Anafranil*), although the risk was increased. Antidepressants with minimal serotonergic effects, such as desipramine (*Norpramin*), trimipramine (*Surmontil*), nortriptyline (*Aventyl*), maprotiline (*Ludiomil*), and mianserin, did not appear to increase the risk of GI bleeding.[1]

Given the plausible biological mechanism (see Mechanism), and the consistent findings from 2 studies, one should assume the combination of SSRIs or clomipramine with aspirin increases the relative risk of upper GI bleeding. Nonetheless, note that the absolute risk of GI bleeding was not high; GI bleeding occurred in only 20 of 2640 patients receiving SSRIs or clomipramine with low-dose aspirin.[1] Given the low absolute risk, there may be situations in which the benefit of the combination would outweigh the risk.

RELATED DRUGS: Assume all other drugs that inhibit serotonin reuptake (citalopram [*Effexor*], clomipramine [*Anafranil*], fluvoxamine [*Luvox*], nefazodone [*Serzone*], paroxetine [*Paxil*], sertraline [*Zoloft*], and venlafaxine [*Effexor*]) would interact with aspirin. The risk of using SSRIs with other platelet inhibitors such as clopidogrel (*Plavix*) or ticlopidine (*Ticlid*) is not known, but it is possible that the risk of GI bleeding would be increased.

MANAGEMENT OPTIONS:

➡ *Consider Alternative.* For analgesia, consider using a nonaspirin analgesic such as acetaminophen. If a salicylate is needed, consider a nonacetylated salicylate such as choline magnesium trisalicylate (*Trilisate*), salsalate (*Disalcid*), or magnesium salicylate (*Doan's*) since these products have minimal effects on platelets and the gastric mucosa. It is not known whether COX-2 inhibitors such as celecoxib (*Celebrex*), rofecoxib (*Vioxx*), or valdecoxib (*Bextra*) would be less likely to cause GI bleeding with SSRIs. Antidepressants with less effect on serotonin (see Clinical Evaluation) may reduce the risk of GI bleeding when combined with aspirin.

➥ **Monitor.** Patients receiving both a SSRI and aspirin should be alert for evidence of GI bleeding.

REFERENCES:
1. Dalton SO, et al. Use of selective serotonin reuptake inhibitors and risk of upper gastrointestinal tract bleeding: a population-based cohort study. *Arch Intern Med.* 2003;163:59-64.

Aspirin 4

Flurbiprofen (eg, *Ansaid*)

SUMMARY: Aspirin may lower serum flurbiprofen concentrations considerably, but it does not appear to interfere with its therapeutic effect.

RISK FACTORS: No specific risk factors are known.

MECHANISM: Not established. Aspirin and flurbiprofen may compete for plasma protein binding sites.

CLINICAL EVALUATION: In healthy subjects, multiple doses of aspirin 900 mg 4 times daily and flurbiprofen 50 mg 4 times daily resulted in a 65% reduction in the area under the flurbiprofen plasma concentration-time curve.[1] In another study, 15 patients with rheumatoid arthritis were given 2 courses of 150 mg/day flurbiprofen for 2 weeks, one with and one without concurrent therapy with aspirin 3 g/day.[2] Although aspirin markedly reduced the area under the flurbiprofen serum concentration-time curve, there was no reduction in the antirheumatic response to flurbiprofen. The latter may be explained by an aspirin-induced displacement of flurbiprofen from plasma protein binding which would increase the free fraction of flurbiprofen and maintain adequate unbound flurbiprofen concentrations in the plasma. Also, the anti-inflammatory effect of the aspirin could have compensated for the reduction in flurbiprofen serum concentrations. In another study, 6 healthy subjects were given the following treatments on 3 separate occasions: flurbiprofen 100 mg alone, aspirin 325 mg alone, both drugs together.[3] Platelet aggregation at 2, 8, and 24 hours was inhibited to the same degree by all 3 treatments. However, a study of chronic dosing of these agents is needed to ensure that there are no additive or antagonistic effects on platelet functions.

RELATED DRUGS: The effect of salicylates other than aspirin on flurbiprofen is not established. Aspirin interacts with many nonsteroidal anti-inflammatory drugs, but most of these interactions appear to have limited clinical importance.

MANAGEMENT OPTIONS: No specific action is required but be alert for evidence of the interaction.

REFERENCES:
1. Kaiser DG, et al. Pharmacokinetics of flurbiprofen. *Am J Med.* 1986;80(3A):10-15.
2. Brooks PM, et al. Flurbiprofen-aspirin interaction: a double-blind crossover study. *Curr Med Res Opin.* 1977;5:53-57.
3. Pincus KT, et al. Effect of flurbiprofen and aspirin on platelet aggregation. *Clin Pharm.* 1991;10:935-938.

Aspirin

Ginkgo

SUMMARY: A patient on low-dose aspirin developed ocular hemorrhage after starting *Ginkgo biloba*, but the contribution of ginkgo to the bleeding was not established.

RISK FACTORS: No specific risk factors are known.

MECHANISM: In vitro evidence suggests that ginkgo inhibits platelet aggregation, but the clinical relevance of this effect is not established.

CLINICAL EVALUATION: A 70-year-old man taking aspirin 325 mg/day developed spontaneous bleeding from the iris into the anterior chamber.[1] He stopped taking ginkgo but continued the aspirin; there was no recurrence of the bleeding during the 3 months of follow-up. Nonetheless, it is not possible to determine if ginkgo contributed to the bleeding. Other cases of bleeding (eg, subdural hematoma) have been reported in patients receiving ginkgo in the absence of aspirin, but again a cause-and-effect relationship was not established.[2]

RELATED DRUGS: No information is available.

MANAGEMENT OPTIONS:

➡ *Use Alternative.* Although the risk of serious bleeding associated with the addition of ginkgo to aspirin therapy is not established, the combination should generally be avoided, because a) the benefit of ginkgo as a "memory aid" is questionable and b) the potential adverse outcome of the interaction is life-threatening.

REFERENCES:
1. Rosenblatt M, et al. Spontaneous hyphema associated with ingestion of Ginkgo biloba extract. *N Engl J Med.* 1997;336:1108.
2. Matthews MK Jr. Association of Ginkgo biloba with intracerebral hemorrhage. *Neurology.* 1998;50:1933-1934.

4 Aspirin

Gold (*Myochrysine*)

SUMMARY: Gold purportedly may increase the likelihood of aspirin-induced hepatotoxicity, but convincing evidence is lacking.

RISK FACTORS: No specific risk factors are known.

MECHANISM: Not established.

CLINICAL EVALUATION: In 1 study, aspirin 3.9 g/day was given with and without gold to patients with rheumatoid arthritis.[1] Serum aspartate aminotransferase levels were higher in the patients also receiving gold, leading the authors to conclude that gold therapy may predispose to aspirin hepatotoxicity.

RELATED DRUGS: No information is available.

MANAGEMENT OPTIONS: No specific action is required, but be alert for evidence of the interaction.

REFERENCES:
1. Davis JD, et al. Fenoprofen, aspirin, and gold induction in rheumatoid arthritis. *Clin Pharmacol Ther.* 1977;21:52-61.

Aspirin (eg, *Bayer*)

Griseofulvin (eg, *Grifulvin V*)

SUMMARY: Griseofulvin administration markedly reduced the plasma concentration of salicylate in a patient taking chronic aspirin therapy.

RISK FACTORS: No specific risk factors are known.

MECHANISM: Not established. Griseofulvin may reduce the absorption of aspirin, increase salicylate elimination, or both. The rapid onset of this interaction, however, suggests griseofulvin-inhibition of aspirin absorption rather than an induction of salicylate metabolism.

CLINICAL EVALUATION: An 8-year-old child with rheumatic fever was being treated with aspirin 147 mg/kg/day in 4 divided doses.[1] Four days after treatment began, his plasma salicylate concentration was 30.6 mg/dL 5.5 hours after the last aspirin dose. On day 6, griseofulvin suspension 10 mg/kg was started, and the aspirin dose was reduced to 100 mg/kg/day. Other medications remained constant. On day 8, salicylate concentrations obtained 1.5 and 10.5 hours after a dose were undetectable (less than 0.2 mg/dL). The griseofulvin suspension was discontinued on day 9. By day 11, the salicylate plasma concentration increased to 16.9 mg/dL 9.5 hours after the aspirin dose. Griseofulvin interference with the immunoassay for salicylate was ruled out. The magnitude of this interaction can be expected to inhibit the therapeutic effect of aspirin.

RELATED DRUGS: No information is available.

MANAGEMENT OPTIONS:

➡ *Circumvent/Minimize.* Until the mechanism of this interaction is established, consider the administration of an alternative antifungal agent in patients receiving aspirin.

➡ *Monitor.* Based on an initial case report, monitor patients stabilized on aspirin therapy for loss of efficacy following the coadministration of griseofulvin.

REFERENCES:

1. Phillips KR, et al. Griseofulvin significantly decreases serum salicylate concentrations. *Pediatr Infect Dis J.* 1993;12:350-352.

Aspirin (eg, *Bayer*)

Ibuprofen (eg, *Advil*)

SUMMARY: Ibuprofen appears to inhibit the antiplatelet effect of aspirin and may reduce its cardioprotective effects.

RISK FACTORS: No specific risk factors are known.

MECHANISM: Ibuprofen may block access of aspirin to the active site on platelet cyclooxygenase.

CLINICAL EVALUATION: In a crossover study in healthy subjects, aspirin 81 mg/day for 6 days was given 2 hours before or 2 hours after ibuprofen 400 mg.[1] Aspirin-induced inhibition of platelet aggregation was blocked when ibuprofen was given 2 hours before aspirin, but not when it was given 2 hours after aspirin. Ibuprofen also blocked aspirin-induced inhibition of platelet aggregation when it was given in multiple daily doses (400 mg given 2, 7, and 12 hours after aspirin). Ibuprofen-induced inhibition of the antiplatelet effects of aspirin had been previously reported with larger doses of aspirin (650 mg).[2] Occasional use of ibuprofen appears unlikely to have much effect on the antiplatelet effect of aspirin.[3] Aspirin may reduce serum ibuprofen concentrations in patients with rheumatoid arthritis, but the therapeutic response does not appear to be affected.[4]

RELATED DRUGS: Agents that do not appear to affect the antiplatelet effects of aspirin include diclofenac (eg, *Voltaren*) and acetaminophen (eg, *Tylenol*).[1] The effect of other nonsteroidal antiinflammatory drugs and cyclooxygenase-2 inhibitors on the ability of aspirin to inhibit platelet aggregation is not established.

MANAGEMENT OPTIONS:

➡ *Use Alternative.* Based on current evidence, diclofenac, rofecoxib, and acetaminophen do not interfere with the antiplatelet effects of aspirin.

➡ *Circumvent/Minimize.* Giving ibuprofen 2 hours after aspirin does not appear to affect the antiplatelet effect of aspirin. Nonetheless, if ibuprofen is given in multiple daily doses (eg, 3 times daily), giving it after aspirin does not appear to circumvent the interaction.

REFERENCES:

1. Catella-Lawson F, et al. Cyclooxygenase inhibitors and the antiplatelet effects of aspirin. *N Engl J Med.* 2001;345:1809-1817.
2. Rao GH, et al. Ibuprofen protects platelet cyclooxygenase from irreversible inhibition by aspirin. *Arteriosclerosis.* 1983;3:383-388.
3. Hudson M, et al. Ibuprofen may abrogate the benefits of aspirin when used for secondary prevention of myocardial infarction. *J Rheumatol.* 2005;32:1589-1593.
4. Grennan DM, et al. The aspirin-ibuprofen interaction in rheumatoid arthritis. *Br J Clin Pharmacol.* 1979;8:497-503.

4　Aspirin (eg, *Bayer*)

Imipramine (eg, *Tofranil*)

SUMMARY: Aspirin appeared to increase the toxicity of imipramine, but additional data is needed to establish a causal relationship.

RISK FACTORS: No specific risk factors are known.

MECHANISM: Aspirin appeared to increase free imipramine plasma concentrations, suggesting that aspirin displaced imipramine from plasma protein binding.

CLINICAL EVALUATION: Evidence from a study in 20 depressed patients suggested that addition of aspirin 1,000 mg daily for 2 days increased the incidence of imipramine-induced adverse effects. A placebo-controlled study is needed to confirm these preliminary results and to determine whether this purported interaction is clinically important.

RELATED DRUGS: No information is available.

MANAGEMENT OPTIONS: No specific action is required, but be alert for evidence of the interaction.

REFERENCES:

1. Juarez-Olguin H, et al. Clinical evidence of an interaction between imipramine and acetylsalicylic acid on protein binding in depressed patients. *Clin Neuropharmacol.* 2002;25:32-36.

Aspirin (eg, *Bayer*) 4

Indomethacin (eg, *Indocin*)

SUMMARY: Aspirin may reduce serum concentrations of indomethacin, but it probably does not inhibit the therapeutic response to indomethacin in patients with rheumatoid arthritis.

RISK FACTORS: No specific risk factors are known.

MECHANISM: Not established. Some evidence suggests that aspirin inhibits the GI absorption of indomethacin, but aspirin-induced displacement of indomethacin from plasma protein binding sites would also account for the reduction in plasma indomethacin concentrations.[1-5]

CLINICAL EVALUATION: Using C-indomethacin,[6] aspirin was found to decrease serum and urine concentrations of indomethacin and to increase fecal excretion.[7] In another study of 10 healthy subjects, 1200 mg of aspirin 3 times daily resulted in a 20% reduction in plasma indomethacin concentrations after a single dose, but the reduction was not as large when the indomethacin was given in multiple doses.[8] Subsequent study seemed to discount the existence of this interaction,[9] but the timing of the doses and the blood sampling were such that an interaction could have escaped detection. When the indomethacin was given rectally and the aspirin was given orally, no interaction could be detected.[10] Rubin et al,[11] observed that oral aspirin decreased peak indomethacin plasma concentrations, although the area under the plasma concentration-time curve was not significantly affected. Thus, oral aspirin appears to have some inhibitory effect on the GI absorption of indomethacin. Although 1 clinical study indicated that 1500 mg/day of aspirin inhibited the anti-inflammatory response to indomethacin,[12] subsequent double-blind clinical studies indicated that aspirin had no effect[13] or actually increased[14] the anti-inflammatory response to indomethacin in patients with rheumatic diseases. Thus, the bulk of the evidence indicates that aspirin is unlikely to affect the anti-inflammatory effects of indomethacin adversely in patients with rheumatic disease. Also, preliminary evidence indicates that sodium salicylate may reduce indomethacin-induced GI blood loss.[15]

RELATED DRUGS: The effect of salicylates other than aspirin on indomethacin is not established.

MANAGEMENT OPTIONS: No specific action is required, but be alert for evidence of the interaction.

REFERENCES:

1. Yesair DW, et al. Comparative effects of salicylic acid, phenylbutazone, probenecid and other anions on the metabolism, distribution and excretion of indomethacin by rats. *Biochem Pharmacol.* 1970;19:1591-1600.

2. Brooks PM, et al. Indomethacin-aspirin interaction: a clinical appraisal. *Br Med J.* 1975;3:69.

3. Kaldestad E, et al. Interaction of indomethacin and acetylsalicylic acid as shown by the serum concentrations of indomethacin and salicylate. *Eur J Clin Pharmacol.* 1975;9:199-207.

4. Lei BW, et al. The influence of aspirin on the absorption and disposition of indomethacin. *Clin Pharmacol Ther.* 1976;19:110.

5. Barraclough DR, et al. Salicylate therapy and drug interaction in rheumatoid arthritis. *Aust N Z J Med.* 1975;5:518-523.

6. Kendall MJ, et al. Xylose test: effect of aspirin and indomethacin. *Br Med J.* 1971;1:553.

7. Jeremy R, et al. Interaction between aspirin and indomethacin in the treatment of rheumatoid arthritis. *Med J Aust.* 1970;2:127-129.

8. Kwan KC, et al. Effects of concomitant aspirin administration on the pharmacokinetics of indomethacin in man. *J Pharmacokinet Biopharm*. 1978;6:451-476.

9. Champion GD, et al. The effect of aspirin on serum indomethacin. *Clin Pharmacol Ther*. 1972;13:239-244.

10. Lindquist B, et al. Effect of concurrent administration of aspirin and indomethacin on serum concentrations. *Clin Pharmacol Ther*. 1974;15:247-252.

11. Rubin A, et al. Interactions of aspirin with nonsteroidal antiinflammatory drugs in man. *Arthritis Rheum*. 1973;16:635-645.

12. Pawlotsky Y, et al. Comparative interaction of aspirin with indomethacin and sulindac in chronic rheumatic diseases. *Eur J Rheumatol Inflamm*. 1978;1:18.

13. Torgyan S, et al. A comparative study with indomethacin and combined indomethacin-sodium salicylate in rheumatoid arthritis. *Int J Clin Pharmacol Biopharm*. 1979;17:439-441.

14. Alvan G, et al. Clinical effects of indomethacin and additive clinical effect of indomethacin during salicylate maintenance therapy. *Scand J Rheumatol Suppl*. 1981;39:29-32.

15. Torgyan S, et al. Reduction of indomethacin-induced gastrointestinal blood loss by sodium salicylate in man. *Int J Clin Pharmacol Biopharm*. 1978;16:610-611.

 Aspirin

Intrauterine Contraceptive Devices (IUDs)

SUMMARY: Aspirin has been reported to decrease the efficacy of IUDs, but a causal relationship has not been established.

RISK FACTORS: No specific risk factors are known.

MECHANISM: Not established. The contraceptive efficacy of IUDs may be related to an inflammatory reaction which would be inhibited by aspirin.

CLINICAL EVALUATION: Isolated cases of unwanted pregnancy during IUD use have occurred in women taking aspirin[1] or other antiinflammatory drugs such as corticosteroids.[2,3] However, it has not been established that the anti-inflammatory drugs were responsible for the contraceptive failure.

RELATED DRUGS: If this interaction is real, it would be expected to occur with other anti-inflammatory drugs as well such as nonsteroidal anti-inflammatory drugs and salicylates.

MANAGEMENT OPTIONS:

➡ *Circumvent/Minimize.* Although this interaction is not well documented, women using intrauterine contraceptive devices should consider using another form of contraception during short-term therapy with salicylates or other anti-inflammatory drugs. If the anti-inflammatory drug is used chronically, consider the possibility that the IUD failure rate may be increased somewhat when selecting a contraceptive method.

➡ *Monitor.* Since pregnancy is the potential outcome, monitoring guidelines are not applicable.

REFERENCES:

1. Buhler M, et al. Successive pregnancies in women fitted with intrauterine devices who take antiinflammatory drugs. *Lancet*. 1983;1:483.

2. Inkeles DM, et al. Unexpected pregnancy in a woman using an intrauterine device and receiving steroid therapy. *Ann Ophthalmol*. 1982;14:975.

3. Zerner J, et al. Failure of an intrauterine device concurrent with administration of corticosteroids. *Fertil Steril*. 1976;27:1467.

Aspirin

Kaolin-Pectin

SUMMARY: Kaolin-pectin slightly reduces the bioavailability of aspirin, but the effect is not likely to be clinically important.

RISK FACTORS: No specific risk factors are known.

MECHANISM: Not established. Kaolin-pectin probably binds with aspirin in the GI tract.

CLINICAL EVALUATION: In 10 healthy subjects, 30 and 60 mL of kaolin-pectin slightly reduced the bioavailability of 975 mg of aspirin, as measured by urinary salicylate excretion.[1] However, the 5% to 10% reduction in aspirin bioavailability is unlikely to reduce the therapeutic response to aspirin.

RELATED DRUGS: The effect of kaolin-pectin on salicylates other than aspirin is not established, but it is probably similar to aspirin.

MANAGEMENT OPTIONS: No specific action is required, but be alert for evidence of the interaction.

REFERENCES:
1. Juhl RP. Comparison of kaolin-pectin and activated charcoal for inhibition of aspirin absorption. *Am J Hosp Pharm.* 1979;36:1097.

Aspirin 4

Ketoprofen (*Orudis*)

SUMMARY: Aspirin lowers plasma ketoprofen concentrations but has not been shown to interfere with its therapeutic effect.

RISK FACTORS: No specific risk factors are known.

MECHANISM: Not established.

CLINICAL EVALUATION: Six healthy subjects were given 50 mg of ketoprofen every 6 hours for 13 doses with and without 975 mg of aspirin with each ketoprofen dose.[1] The aspirin substantially reduced plasma ketoprofen concentrations and increased plasma ketoprofen clearance. Aspirin similarly reduces the plasma concentrations of several nonsteroidal anti-inflammatory drugs (NSAIDs) but does not appear to interfere with their therapeutic effect. Thus, it seems unlikely that aspirin adversely affects the therapeutic response to ketoprofen.

RELATED DRUGS: The effect of salicylates other than aspirin on ketoprofen is not established. Aspirin interacts with many NSAIDs, but most of these interactions appear to have limited clinical importance.

MANAGEMENT OPTIONS: No specific action is required, but be alert for evidence of the interaction.

REFERENCES:
1. Williams RL, et al. Ketoprofen-aspirin interactions. *Clin Pharmacol Ther.* 1981;30:226.

4　Aspirin

Levamisole (*Ergamisol*)

SUMMARY: Although a case of possible levamisole-induced increase in plasma salicylate concentration has been reported, no interaction was found in a study of healthy subjects.

RISK FACTORS: No specific risk factors are known.

MECHANISM: Not established.

CLINICAL EVALUATION: Although 1 patient appeared to develop an increase in plasma salicylate concentrations because of levamisole therapy,[1] a subsequent study of 9 healthy subjects given aspirin 3.9 g/day for 3 weeks found no effect of levamisole (50 mg/day for 7 days) on plasma salicylate concentrations.[2] Although a controlled study of patients receiving salicylates is needed to determine whether an interaction occurs, current evidence suggests that an interaction is unlikely.

RELATED DRUGS: Little is known regarding the effect of levamisole on salicylates other than aspirin.

MANAGEMENT OPTIONS: No specific action is required, but be alert for evidence of the interaction.

REFERENCES:
1. Laidlaw DA. Rheumatoid arthritis improved by treatment with levamisole and L-histidine. *Med J Aust.* 1976;2:382.
2. Rumble RH, et al. Interaction between levamisole and aspirin in man. *Br J Clin Pharmacol.* 1979;7:631.

5　Aspirin

Lithium (eg, *Eskalith*)

SUMMARY: Salicylates appear to have minimal effects on plasma lithium concentrations in healthy subjects.

RISK FACTORS: No specific risk factors are known.

MECHANISM: No interaction.

CLINICAL EVALUATION: Ten healthy women were given lithium in doses sufficient to produce steady-state plasma lithium concentrations between 0.5 and 0.8 mEq/L.[1] The subjects then received placebo followed by indomethacin 50 mg 3 times daily or aspirin 1 g 4 times daily and then placebo again. The indomethacin resulted in a 40% increase in plasma lithium concentrations, but aspirin had no effect. In another study of 6 healthy women with steady-state plasma lithium concentrations between 0.6 and 0.8 mmol/L, renal lithium clearance was unaffected by IV aspirin and only slightly reduced by IV salicylic acid.[2] Thus, the majority of the evidence from healthy subjects suggests that aspirin and other salicylates have minimal effects on lithium elimination. It seems likely that patients receiving lithium would be similarly unaffected, but studies on patients on chronic lithium therapy are needed to confirm this.[3,4]

RELATED DRUGS: No information is available.

MANAGEMENT OPTIONS: No interaction.

REFERENCES:

1. Reimann IW, et al. Indomethacin but not aspirin increases plasma lithium ion levels. *Arch Gen Psychiatry.* 1983;40:283.
2. Reimann IW, et al. Influence of intravenous acetylsalicylic acid and sodium salicylate on human renal function and lithium clearance. *Eur J Clin Pharmacol.* 1985;29:435.
3. Bendz H, et al. Aspirin increases serum lithium ion levels. *Arch Gen Psychiatry.* 1984;41:310.
4. Rerman I. Aspirin increases serum lithium ion levels. Reply. *Arch Gen Psychiatry.* 1984;41:310.

Aspirin 4

Meclofenamate (*Meclomen*)

SUMMARY: Aspirin may decrease total plasma meclofenamate concentrations somewhat, but it is unlikely that the therapeutic response to meclofenamate will be reduced; the combination may cause more damage to the gastric mucosa than either drug alone.

RISK FACTORS: No specific risk factors are known.

MECHANISM: Not established. Aspirin probably displaces meclofenamate from plasma protein binding sites.

CLINICAL EVALUATION: Each of 4 groups of 10 healthy subjects received one of the following treatments in a 28-day study: meclofenamate 100 mg 3 times daily; aspirin 600 mg 3 times daily; meclofenamate for 14 days and meclofenamate plus aspirin for 14 days; aspirin for 14 days and aspirin plus meclofenamate for 14 days.[1] GI blood loss was more than doubled with the combination of meclofenamate and aspirin compared to either agent alone. Total plasma meclofenamate concentrations were somewhat lower in the presence of aspirin compared to meclofenamate alone, but plasma salicylate concentrations were not affected by meclofenamate. However, unbound meclofenamate concentrations were not measured. If the mechanism of the reduction in total meclofenamate concentrations is displacement from plasma protein binding sites by salicylate, unbound meclofenamate would be expected to be about the same as when meclofenamate was given alone. Thus, the therapeutic response to meclofenamate would not be expected to change. Moreover, even if the unbound concentration of meclofenamate did decrease, the anti-inflammatory effect of aspirin would be expected to offset this effect. Resolution of this issue will require studies in patients receiving meclofenamate therapeutically.

RELATED DRUGS: The effect of salicylates other than aspirin on meclofenamate is not established. Aspirin interacts with many nonsteroidal anti-inflammatory drugs, but most of these interactions appear to have limited clinical importance.

MANAGEMENT OPTIONS: No specific action is required, but be alert for evidence of the interaction.

REFERENCES:

1. Baragar FD, et al. Drug interaction studies with sodium meclofenamate (Meclomen). *Curr Ther Res.* 1978;23:S51.

② Aspirin

Methotrexate (eg, *Rheumatrex*)

SUMMARY: Case reports, limited pharmacokinetic and epidemiological reports, and animal studies all indicate that salicylates may enhance methotrexate toxicity.

RISK FACTORS:

➦ **Dosage Regimen.** The risk of adverse effects from this interaction is primarily in patients receiving antineoplastic doses of methotrexate rather than the lower doses used to treat rheumatoid arthritis, psoriasis, and related diseases.

MECHANISM: Methotrexate undergoes renal tubular secretion that appears to be blocked by salicylates. Salicylates have also been shown to displace methotrexate from plasma proteinbinding sites, but the significance of this is not clear.[4]

CLINICAL EVALUATION: Study in humans has shown a decreased clearance (approximately 35%) of methotrexate following salicylate administration as well as a decrease in plasma protein binding of approximately 30%.[1] Both of these factors would tend to increase the amount of active methotrexate and, therefore, toxicity. In another study[7] 2 patients receiving methotrexate and salicylate rapidly developed pancytopenia and died. A subsequent retrospective review of 176 patients who had received methotrexate infusions revealed that 66 patients also received salicylate in a dose greater than 600 mg/day. Of the 7 patients who rapidly developed a severe pancytopenia, 6 were in the group who had received salicylates. Studies in mice also indicated that salicylates can enhance methotrexate toxicity.[7] One patient with psoriatic arthritis has been described who developed methotrexate hepatotoxicity while also taking moderate doses of aspirin for arthritis.[5] Also, 2 elderly patients with psoriasis developed signs of excessive methotrexate effect with concomitant aspirin therapy.[6] Another patient has been briefly described in whom aspirin ingestion was associated with a prolonged methotrexate half-life.[3] Taking all of the evidence together, it appears that some patients on methotrexate are adversely affected by concomitant salicylate therapy. Statements to the contrary[2] appear to arise from an inadequate review or analysis of the literature.

RELATED DRUGS: All salicylates are likely to interact with methotrexate.

MANAGEMENT OPTIONS:

➦ **Avoid Unless Benefit Outweighs Risk.** Aspirin should generally be avoided in patients taking antineoplastic doses of methotrexate. The manufacturer of methotrexate also recommends that salicylates be avoided in patients receiving methotrexate. Remind patients receiving methotrexate of the many nonprescription mixtures that contain salicylates.

➦ **Monitor.** If the combination is used, anticipate that a reduction in methotrexate dosage may be required. Serum methotrexate determinations would be helpful, and also monitor for excessive methotrexate effect (eg, GI toxicity, stomatitis, bone marrow suppression, hepatotoxicity, infection).

REFERENCES:

1. Liegler DG, et al. The effect of organic acids on renal clearance of methotrexate in man. *Clin Pharmacol Ther.* 1969;10:849.
2. Taylor JR, et al. Effect of sodium salicylate and indomethacin on methotrexate-serum albumin binding. *Arch Dermatol.* 1977;113:588.

3. Aherne GW, et al. Prolongation and enhancement of serum methotrexate concentrations by probenecid. *BMJ*. 1978;1:1097.

4. Dixon RL, et al. Plasma protein binding of methotrexate and its displacement by various drugs. *Fed Proc*. 1965;24:454.

5. Dubin HV, et al. Liver disease associated with methotrexate treatment of psoriatic patients. *Arch Dermatol*. 1970;102:498.

6. Baker H. Intermittent high dose oral methotrexate therapy in psoriasis. *Br J Dermatol*. 1970;82:65.

7. Mandel MA. The synergistic effect of salicylates on methotrexate toxicity. *Plast Reconstr Surg*. 1976;57:733.

Aspirin

Metoprolol (eg, *Lopressor*)

SUMMARY: Metoprolol may increase peak salicylate serum concentrations, but it is unknown whether this increases the risk of salicylate toxicity.

RISK FACTORS: No specific risk factors are known.

MECHANISM: A modest increase in the rate of salicylate absorption without a change in the amount of salicylate absorbed could account for the changes reported.

CLINICAL EVALUATION: Six healthy volunteers were given metoprolol 100 mg twice daily for 6 days, acetylsalicylic acid (ASA) 500 mg 3 times daily for 6 days, and the combination of both agents for 6 days.[1] Metoprolol pharmacokinetics were not altered by ASA administration; however, the maximum serum concentrations of ASA were increased by approximately 30% during metoprolol coadministration. The area under the ASA concentration-time curve and half-life were not altered by metoprolol.

RELATED DRUGS: No information is available.

MANAGEMENT OPTIONS: No specific action is required, but be alert for evidence of the interaction.

REFERENCES:

1. Spahn H, et al. Pharmacokinetics of salicylates administered with metoprolol. *Arzneimittelforschung*. 1986;36:1697.

Aspirin

Midazolam (*Versed*)

SUMMARY: The onset of action of midazolam may be more rapid in patients who have been pretreated with aspirin; the clinical importance of this finding is unknown.

RISK FACTORS: No specific risk factors are known.

MECHANISM: Not established.

CLINICAL EVALUATION: Of 205 surgical patients undergoing induction with midazolam, 78 were pretreated with 1 g of aspirin (given IV as 1.8 g of lysine acetyl salicylate) in a nonblinded manner.[1] Of the 127 patients receiving midazolam alone, 60% were "asleep" within 3 minutes; with aspirin pretreatment 81% were "asleep" within 3 minutes. Although this study suggests that aspirin (and presumably other salicylates) may speed the action of midazolam, it is not known whether this would increase the risk of adverse reactions to midazolam.

RELATED DRUGS: The effect of salicylates other than aspirin on midazolam is unknown, but it is probably similar. The effect of aspirin or other salicylates on benzodiazepines other than midazolam is unknown.

MANAGEMENT OPTIONS: No specific action is required, but be alert for evidence of the interaction.

REFERENCES:
1. Dundee JW, et al. Aspirin and probenecid pretreatment influences the potency of thiopentone and the onset of action of midazolam. *Eur J Anaesthesiol.* 1986;3:247.

Aspirin (eg, *Bayer*)

Milnacipran (*Savella*)

SUMMARY: The combined use of aspirin with serotonin-norepinephrine reuptake inhibitors (SNRIs), such as milnacipran, has been associated with an increased risk of GI bleeding.

RISK FACTORS: No specific risk factors are known.

MECHANISM: SNRI and selective serotonin reuptake inhibitors (SSRIs) appear to inhibit platelet function by inhibiting the uptake of serotonin by platelets. When this effect is combined with the platelet inhibition and GI toxicity of aspirin, an increased risk of GI bleeding may occur.

CLINICAL EVALUATION: This interaction is based largely on epidemiological studies with SNRIs and SSRIs other than milnacipran, and it is not known how often adverse outcomes would be observed. Nonetheless, given the potential severity of the GI bleeding, consider this risk when deciding whether to use this combination.[1]

RELATED DRUGS: Theoretically, salicylates with minimal effects on platelets, such as salsalate, choline magnesium trisalicylate, and magnesium salicylate (eg, *Doans Pills*), would be less likely to interact with milnacipran.

MANAGEMENT OPTIONS:

➥ *Consider Alternative.* If possible, use an alternative to one of the drugs.

➥ *Monitor.* If the combination is used, monitor for evidence of GI bleeding.

REFERENCES:
1. *Savella* [package insert]. St. Louis, MO: Forest Pharmaceuticals; 2010.

Aspirin

Naproxen (eg, *Naprosyn*)

SUMMARY: Aspirin may reduce plasma naproxen concentrations slightly, but the therapeutic response to naproxen is probably not reduced.

RISK FACTORS: No specific risk factors are known.

MECHANISM: Aspirin may compete with naproxen for plasma protein-binding sites thereby increasing the renal clearance of naproxen.[1]

CLINICAL EVALUATION: In healthy subjects, aspirin has been shown to produce a small decrease in plasma naproxen concentrations,[1] but the magnitude of the change is probably insufficient to affect the therapeutic response to naproxen. A double-blind study of 36 patients with rheumatoid arthritis indicated that naproxen plus aspirin was more effective than aspirin alone.[2] However, since the combination of naproxen and aspirin was not compared with naproxen alone, it is not possible to determine whether the response to naproxen is affected by aspirin.

RELATED DRUGS: The effect of salicylates other than aspirin on naproxen is not established. Aspirin interacts with many nonsteroidal anti-inflammatory drugs, but most of these interactions appear to have limited clinical importance.

MANAGEMENT OPTIONS: No specific action is required, but be alert for evidence of the interaction.

REFERENCES:

1. Segre EJ, et al. Naproxen-aspirin interactions in man. *Clin Pharmacol Ther.* 1974;15:374.
2. Willkens RF, et al. Combination therapy with naproxen and aspirin in rheumatoid arthritis. *Arthritis Rheum.* 1976;19:677.

Aspirin 4

Nicotinic Acid (Niacin)

SUMMARY: Aspirin reduces the cutaneous flushing associated with nicotinic acid administration and increases plasma nicotinic acid concentrations; the clinical importance of the latter effect is not established.

RISK FACTORS: No specific risk factors are known.

MECHANISM: Glycine conjugation is an important elimination pathway for both nicotinic acid and salicylic acid, and it is proposed that competitive inhibition of metabolism may occur.

CLINICAL EVALUATION: Six subjects received a constant infusion of nicotinic acid (0.075 to 0.1 mg/kg/min) for 6 hours, with 1 g of aspirin given orally 2 hours after starting the infusion.[1] Aspirin reduced the clearance of nicotinic acid by about 45% and substantially increased plasma nicotinic acid concentrations. Nevertheless, the degree to which salicylates increase the risk of nicotinic acid toxicity is not established. Moreover, it is not known whether the use of aspirin to mitigate nicotinic acid-induced flushing or inhibit platelet function would increase and prolong plasma nicotinic acid concentrations.[2]

RELATED DRUGS: The effect of salicylates other than aspirin on niacin pharmacokinetics is not established, but it may be similar to aspirin.

MANAGEMENT OPTIONS: No specific action is required, but be alert for evidence of the interaction.

REFERENCES:

1. Ding RW, et al. Pharmacokinetics of nicotinic acid-salicylic acid interaction. *Clin Pharmacol Ther.* 1989;46:642.
2. Wilkin JK, et al. Aspirin blocks nicotinic acid-induced flushing. *Clin Pharmacol Ther.* 1982;31:478.

Aspirin

Nitroglycerin

SUMMARY: Some evidence indicates that analgesic doses of aspirin increase the plasma concentration of nitroglycerin and enhance its pharmacologic effects.

RISK FACTORS: No specific risk factors are known.

MECHANISM: Prostaglandin inhibitors, including aspirin, may reduce liver blood flow[2] and could reduce the metabolism of nitroglycerin.

CLINICAL EVALUATION: Seven healthy subjects received 0.8 mg of nitroglycerin by sublingual spray alone, 1 hour after 1 g of aspirin, and 30 hours after the fourth dose of aspirin 500 mg administered every 48 hours.[1] Compared to nitroglycerin alone, pretreatment with 1 g of aspirin significantly increased plasma nitroglycerin concentrations and heart rate while significantly reducing diastolic blood pressure, end-diastolic diameter, and end-systolic diameter. The smaller doses of aspirin had no significant effect on nitroglycerin pharmacokinetics or pharmacodynamics. Forty healthy subjects received 0.4 mg of nitroglycerin sublingually alone and 1 to 2 hours after 650 mg aspirin.[3] Aspirin administration had little effect on the hemodynamic response (blood pressure, heart rate) to nitroglycerin. The clinical significance of this interaction appears limited.

RELATED DRUGS: Other prostaglandin inhibitors (eg, NSAIDs) may have a similar effect.

MANAGEMENT OPTIONS: No specific action is required, but be alert for evidence of the interaction.

REFERENCES:
1. Weber S, et al. Influence of aspirin on the hemodynamic effects of sublingual nitroglycerin. *J Cardiovasc Pharmacol.* 1983;5:874.
2. Feely J, et al. Effects of inhibitors of prostaglandin synthesis on hepatic drug clearance. *Br J Clin Pharmacol.* 1983;15:109.
3. Levin RI, et al. The effect of aspirin on the hemodynamic response to nitroglycerin. *Am Heart J.* 1988;116:77.

4 **Aspirin**

Omeprazole (*Prilosec*)

SUMMARY: An omeprazole-induced increase in gastric pH appears to cause enteric-coated salicylates to dissolve more quickly than usual. An increase in gastric side effects may result.

RISK FACTORS: No specific risk factors are known.

MECHANISM: An increase in gastric pH results in the premature dissolution of enteric coatings designed to dissolve in the higher pH of the small intestine.

CLINICAL EVALUATION: Eight healthy subjects received a single 500 mg dose of uncoated aspirin or enteric-coated sodium salicylate alone and after 4 days of pretreatment with omeprazole 20 mg/day.[1] Omeprazole administration did not affect the pharmacokinetics of the uncoated aspirin. Three of the 8 subjects demonstrated equal times to peak (t_{max}) salicylate concentrations following the administration of both formulations of salicylate administered alone. Omeprazole did not affect the t_{max} of either formulation in these 3 subjects. In the remaining 5 subjects, omeprazole coadministration reduced the t_{max} of the enteric-coated formulation from 4 to 2.7 hours but did not affect the t_{max} of the uncoated formulation. No other changes were noted in the pharmacokinetics of either formulation following omeprazole pretreatment. The apparent premature loss of enteric coating in patients with gastric acid suppression may increase the risk of gastric irritation from salicylate-containing products. The clinical significance of this change awaits further study.

RELATED DRUGS: Other proton pump inhibitors (eg, lansoprazole [*Prevacid*], pantoprazole [*Protonix*], and rabeprazole [*Aciphex*]) would be expected to produce the same changes in the absorption of enteric-coated salicylate products.

MANAGEMENT OPTIONS:

➡ *Monitor.* Monitor patients taking enteric-coated salicylate products to avoid gastric irritation for potential early dissolution of the formulation, resulting in gastric exposure to salicylate and possibly increased gastric side effects.

REFERENCES:

1. Nefesoglu FZ, et al. Interaction of omeprazole with enteric-coated salicylate tablets. *Int J Clin Pharmacol Ther.* 1998;10:549-53.

Aspirin

Para-Aminobenzoic Acid (PABA)

SUMMARY: PABA may increase serum salicylate concentrations, but there is little evidence to suggest that the combination increases the risk of salicylate toxicity.

RISK FACTORS: No specific risk factors are known.

MECHANISM: PABA appears to block the formation of salicyluric acid from salicylic acid, resulting in increased salicylate serum concentrations.[1]

CLINICAL EVALUATION: PABA has been combined with salicylates in a number of proprietary analgesic mixtures. Excessive salicylate concentrations probably do not occur often as a result of this interaction.

RELATED DRUGS: One would expect salicylates other than aspirin to interact similarly with PABA.

MANAGEMENT OPTIONS: No specific action is required, but be alert for evidence of the interaction.

REFERENCES:

1. Smith MJH, et al. *The Salicylates. A Critical Bibliographic Review.* New York: Interscience Publishers; 1966:34–43.

Aspirin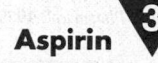

Pentazocine (*Talwin*)

SUMMARY: A patient on chronic therapy with aspirin and large doses of pentazocine developed papillary necrosis, but a causal relationship between this drug combination and the papillary necrosis was not established.

RISK FACTORS: No specific risk factors are known.

MECHANISM: It has been proposed that pentazocine reduced renal blood flow, thus potentiating the adverse effects of aspirin on the kidney.[1]

CLINICAL EVALUATION: A 49-year-old man with chronic alcoholism with cirrhosis, chronic pancreatitis, chemical diabetes mellitus, and cholelithiasis was admitted for renal papillary necrosis.[1] He had been taking aspirin 1.8 to 2.4 g/day for over 4 years and large doses of pentazocine (800 to 850 mg/day) for 6 months. The authors propose that this drug combination may have produced the papillary necrosis. When the pentazocine was discontinued and aspirin was continued, clinical episodes of renal papillary necrosis did not recur. Thus, on two occasions, before and after pentazocine coadministration, aspirin alone did not result in papillary necrosis. This suggests that if the papillary necrosis was drug induced, it may have been caused by pentazocine alone or in combination with aspirin. In the absence of additional cases; however, it is not possible to establish a causal relationship.

RELATED DRUGS: The effect of salicylates other than aspirin combined with pentazocine is not established.

MANAGEMENT OPTIONS:

➥ *Monitor.* Until more information is available, be alert for evidence of renal papillary necrosis (eg, passing tissue via the urethra) in patients receiving large doses of pentazocine combined with aspirin.

REFERENCES:

1. Muhalwas KK, et al. Renal papillary necrosis caused by long-term ingestion of pentazocine and aspirin. *JAMA.* 1981;246:867.

5   Aspirin

Piroxicam (*Feldene*)

SUMMARY: Aspirin does not appear to affect piroxicam pharmacokinetics in healthy subjects.

RISK FACTORS: No specific risk factors are known.

MECHANISM: No interaction.

CLINICAL EVALUATION: In a study of 16 healthy subjects given piroxicam (40 mg on day 1, 20 mg on days 2 to 5), aspirin (972 mg 4 times daily on days 4 and 5) had minimal effects on piroxicam pharmacokinetics.[1] However, the risk vs benefit of adding salicylates to piroxicam therapy is not well established.

RELATED DRUGS: Aspirin interacts with many nonsteroidal anti-inflammatory drugs, but most of these interactions appear to have limited clinical importance.

MANAGEMENT OPTIONS: No interaction.

REFERENCES:

1. Hobbs DC, et al. Piroxicam pharmacokinetics in man: aspirin and antacid interaction studies. *J Clin Pharmacol.* 1979;19:720.

Aspirin ▼ 3

Prednisone (eg, *Meticorten*)

SUMMARY: Prednisone and other corticosteroids may enhance the elimination of salicylates markedly, resulting in subtherapeutic salicylate concentrations in some patients. Discontinuing corticosteroids during high-dose salicylate therapy may result in salicylate toxicity.

RISK FACTORS:

➧ *Dosage Regimen.* Patients taking large (antiarthritic) salicylate doses are at greater risk.

MECHANISM: Not established. Although corticosteroids have been associated with an increased glomerular filtration rate,[4,5] this is unlikely to have a large effect on salicylate elimination. Corticosteroids may enhance the metabolism of salicylates.[7] Aspirin decreases corticosteroid conjugation, but the clinical significance of this effect is unknown.[2]

CLINICAL EVALUATION: Decreasing the corticosteroid dose in patients who are also on large doses of salicylates may cause the serum salicylate concentration to increase with possible salicylate intoxication. One report described 4 cases that may represent examples of this effect.[1] In another study, systemic corticosteroid therapy appeared to lower serum salicylate concentrations to below the desired therapeutic range in several patients.[7] An 11-year-old boy receiving chronic aspirin therapy developed a 67% drop in serum salicylate concentrations after the addition of prednisone 15 mg/day.[3] Intra-articular corticosteroids significantly reduced steady-state plasma salicylate concentrations in 10 patients.[6] Also remember that GI ulceration may be more likely in patients receiving both salicylates and corticosteroids than in patients receiving either drug alone.

RELATED DRUGS: Salicylates other than aspirin also can be expected to interact similarly with corticosteroids.

MANAGEMENT OPTIONS:

➧ *Monitor.* Corticosteroids and salicylates are frequently administered together, and their concomitant use is not contraindicated. However, salicylate dose requirements may be higher in the presence of corticosteroids, and watch patients for salicylate intoxication if the corticosteroid dose is reduced. Keep in mind the possibility that concomitant therapy may increase the incidence or severity of GI ulceration.

REFERENCES:

1. Klinenberg JR, et al. Effect of corticosteroids on blood salicylate concentration. *JAMA.* 1965;194:601.
2. Elliott HC. Reduced adrenocortical steroid excretion rates in man following aspirin administration. *Metabolism.* 1962;11:1015.
3. Koren G, et al. Corticosteroids-salicylate interaction—a case of juvenile rheumatoid arthritis. *Ther Drug Monit.* 1987;9:177.
4. George CRP. Nonspecific enhancement of glomerular filtration by corticosteroids. *Lancet.* 1974;2:728.
5. Polak A, et al. Nonspecific enhancement of glomerular filtration by corticosteroids. *Lancet.* 1974;2:841.
6. Edelman J, et al. The effect of intra-articular steroids on plasma salicylate concentrations. *Br J Clin Pharmacol.* 1986;21:301.
7. Graham GG, et al. Patterns of plasma concentrations and urinary excretion of salicylate in rheumatoid arthritis. *Clin Pharmacol Ther.* 1977;22:410.

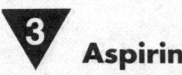

Aspirin

Probenecid (*Benemid*)

SUMMARY: Salicylates inhibit the uricosuric activity of probenecid, but they do not appear to affect the ability of probenecid to inhibit the renal elimination of penicillins.

RISK FACTORS:

➥ ***Dosage Regimen.*** Doses of salicylate that do not produce serum salicylate concentrations more than 5 mg/dL do not appear to affect probenecid uricosuria significantly. Thus, occasional analgesic doses of salicylate may be insufficient to interact with probenecid.

MECHANISM: Not established.

CLINICAL EVALUATION: Probenecid uricosuria may be inhibited considerably by large doses of salicylates.[1,3] Also, probenecid appears to inhibit the uricosuria that usually follows large doses of salicylates. Six patients were given an IV dose of 500,000 units of penicillin G alone, after 24 hours pretreatment with probenecid 0.5 g every 6 hours, and after 1 g aspirin given with each dose of probenecid.[2] Aspirin did not interfere with the ability of probenecid to inhibit renal elimination of penicillin G (and presumably other penicillins).

RELATED DRUGS: All salicylates probably interact with probenecid in a similar manner.

MANAGEMENT OPTIONS:

➥ ***Circumvent/Minimize.*** Avoid more than occasional small doses of salicylates in patients receiving probenecid as a uricosuric agent. Available evidence suggests that patients receiving probenecid to prolong serum penicillin levels do not have to avoid salicylates.

➥ ***Monitor.*** Monitor for reduced probenecid uricosuric effect if salicylates are given concurrently.

REFERENCES:

1. Pascale LR, et al. Inhibition of the uricosuric action of Benemid by salicylate. *J Lab Clin Med*. 1955;45:771.

2. Boger WP, et al. Probenecid and salicylates: the question of interaction in terms of penicillin excretion. *J Lab Clin Med*. 1955;45:478.

3. Regal, RE. Aspirin and uricosurics: interaction revisited. *Drug Intell Clin Pharm*. 1987;21:219.

4   Aspirin

Spironolactone (*Aldactone*)

SUMMARY: Aspirin may reduce the natriuresis following spironolactone administration, but potassium retention is not reduced.

RISK FACTORS: No specific risk factors are known.

MECHANISM: There is evidence that aspirin reduces the active renal tubular secretion of canrenone, the active metabolite of spironolactone.[3] This reduction in tubular secretion of canrenone is thought to reduce the pharmacologic activity of administered spironolactone.

CLINICAL EVALUATION: Aspirin somewhat inhibits the natriuresis produced by spironolactone.[1-3] However, neither the effect of spironolactone on urinary potassium excretion,[3] nor the antihypertensive response to spironolactone 4 appears to be affected by aspirin. The clinical importance of the interaction between spironolactone and aspirin is still not clear, but in most cases it is probably minimal.

RELATED DRUGS: No information is available.

MANAGEMENT OPTIONS: No specific action is required, but be alert for evidence of the interaction.

REFERENCES:

1. Tweeddale MG, et al. Antagonism of spironolactone-induced natriuresis by aspirin in man. *N Engl J Med*. 1973;289:198.

2. Elliott HC. Reduced adrenocortical steroid excretion rates in man following aspirin administration. *Metabolism*. 1962;11:1015.

3. Ramsay LE, et al. Influence of acetylsalicylic acid on the renal handling of a spironolactone metabolite in healthy subjects. *Eur J Clin Pharmacol*. 1976;10:43.

4. Hollifield JW. Failure of aspirin to antagonize the antihypertensive effect of spironolactone in low-renin hypertension. *South Med J*. 1976;69:1034.

Aspirin 5

Sucralfate (*Carafate*)

SUMMARY: A study of healthy subjects indicates that sucralfate does not affect the GI absorption of aspirin; it seems likely that other salicylates would be similarly unaffected.

RISK FACTORS: No specific risk factors are known.

MECHANISM: No interaction.

CLINICAL EVALUATION: In a randomized crossover study, 12 healthy subjects were given a single oral 650 mg dose of aspirin with and without sucralfate 1 g 4 times daily for 2 days.[1] Sucralfate did not affect the bioavailability of aspirin. In another crossover study of 12 healthy subjects, sucralfate had no effect on the steady-state bioavailability of choline magnesium trisalicylate (*Trilisate*).[2]

RELATED DRUGS: The effect of sucralfate on other salicylates is not established, but it seems unlikely that their bioavailability would be reduced by sucralfate.

MANAGEMENT OPTIONS: No interaction.

REFERENCES:

1. Lau AH, et al. Evaluation of potential drug interaction between sucralfate and aspirin. *Clin Pharmacol Ther*. 1986;39:151.

2. Schneider D, et al. Influence of sucralfate on choline magnesium trisalicylate bioavailability. *J Clin Pharmacol*. 1989;29:845.

Aspirin 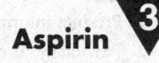 3

Sulfinpyrazone (*Anturane*)

SUMMARY: Salicylates inhibit the uricosuric effect of sulfinpyrazone.

RISK FACTORS: No specific risk factors are known.

MECHANISM: Not established.

CLINICAL EVALUATION: Sulfinpyrazone uricosuria may be inhibited considerably by large doses of salicylates.[1-3] The amount of salicylate required to inhibit sulfinpyrazone uricosuria is not well established, but it seems unlikely that occasional salicylate use would interact. Sulfinpyrazone also appears to inhibit the uricosuria that usually follows large doses of salicylates.

RELATED DRUGS: All salicylates probably interact with sulfinpyrazone in a similar manner.

MANAGEMENT OPTIONS:

➡ *Circumvent/Minimize.* Avoid more than occasional small doses of salicylates in patients receiving sulfinpyrazone.

➡ *Monitor.* Monitor for reduced uricosuric effect of sulfinpyrazone if salicylates are given concurrently.

REFERENCES:

1. Smith MJH, et al. The Salicylates. *A Critical Bibliographic Review.* New York: Interscience Publishers; 1966:86–90.

2. Oyer JH, et al. Suppression of salicylate-induced uricosuria by phenylbutazone. *Am J Med Sci.* 1966;251:1.

3. Yu TF, et al. Mutual suppression of the uricosuric effects of sulfinpyrazone and salicylate: a study in interactions between drugs. *J Clin Invest.* 1963;42:1330.

---

4   Aspirin

Sulindac (*Clinoril*)

SUMMARY: Limited clinical evidence indicates that aspirin may reduce plasma concentrations of sulindac and may produce additive GI toxicity; the clinical importance of these effects is not established.

RISK FACTORS: No specific risk factors are known.

MECHANISM: Not established.

CLINICAL EVALUATION: Although aspirin reportedly reduces the plasma concentrations of the active sulfide metabolite of sulindac,[1] available evidence indicates that aspirin does not affect the anti-inflammatory response to sulindac appreciably.[1,2] However, a possible increase in the incidence of adverse GI effects with the combination compared to sulindac alone has prompted the manufacturers of sulindac to recommend against combining it with aspirin.[1]

RELATED DRUGS: The effect of salicylates other than aspirin on sulindac is not established. Aspirin interacts with many nonsteroidal anti-inflammatory drugs, but most of these interactions appear to have limited clinical importance.

MANAGEMENT OPTIONS: No specific action is required, but be alert for evidence of the interaction.

REFERENCES:

1. Product information. Sulindac (*Clinoril*). Merck & Co., Inc. 1992.

2. Pawlotsky Y, et al. Comparative interaction of aspirin with indomethacin and sulindac in chronic rheumatic diseases. *Eur J Rheumatol Inflamm.* 1978;1:18.

Aspirin

Tenoxicam

SUMMARY: Aspirin may decrease total plasma tenoxicam concentrations substantially, but it is unlikely that the therapeutic response to tenoxicam will be reduced.

RISK FACTORS: No specific risk factors are known.

MECHANISM: Aspirin appears to displace tenoxicam from plasma protein binding sites.

CLINICAL EVALUATION: Five healthy subjects received multiple doses of tenoxicam (20 mg/day) with and without multiple doses of aspirin (2.6 to 3.9 g/day).[1] Aspirin was associated with a 57% reduction in total plasma steady-state tenoxicam concentrations. Aspirin was also associated with more than a doubling of the unbound tenoxicam concentrations in the plasma. Since the reduction in total tenoxicam concentrations appears to be caused by displacement of tenoxicam from plasma protein binding sites by salicylate, the unbound tenoxicam concentration would be expected to be about the same as when tenoxicam is given alone. Thus, the therapeutic response to tenoxicam would not be expected to change. Moreover, even if the unbound concentration of tenoxicam did decrease, the anti-inflammatory effect of aspirin would be expected to offset this effect. Resolution of this issue will require studies in patients receiving tenoxicam therapeutically.

RELATED DRUGS: The effect of salicylates other than aspirin on tenoxicam is not established. Aspirin interacts with many nonsteroidal anti-inflammatory drugs, but most of these interactions appear to have limited clinical importance.

MANAGEMENT OPTIONS: No specific action is required, but be alert for evidence of the interaction.

REFERENCES:
1. Day RO, et al. The effect of concurrent aspirin upon plasma concentrations of tenoxicam. *Br J Clin Pharmacol.* 1988;26:455.

Aspirin

Tolmetin (*Tolectin*)

SUMMARY: Aspirin caused a small decrease in tolmetin concentrations, but it is unlikely that the therapeutic response to tolmetin will be reduced.

RISK FACTORS: No specific risk factors are known.

MECHANISM: Aspirin appears to displace tolmetin from plasma protein binding sites.

CLINICAL EVALUATION: Eleven healthy subjects received tolmetin 400 mg orally with and without aspirin 975 mg 4 times daily for 16 days.[1] Aspirin was associated with a 17% increase in tolmetin clearance and a reduction in plasma tolmetin concentrations. Since the reduction in total tolmetin concentrations appears to be caused by displacement of tolmetin from plasma protein binding sites by the salicylate, one would expect the unbound tolmetin concentration to be about the same as when tolmetin is given alone. Thus, the therapeutic response to tolmetin would not be expected to change. Moreover, even if the unbound concentration of tolmetin did decrease, the anti-inflammatory effect of aspirin would be expected to offset this effect. Resolution of this issue will require studies in patients receiving tolmetin therapeutically.

RELATED DRUGS: The effect of salicylates other than aspirin on tolmetin is not established. Aspirin interacts with many nonsteroidal anti-inflammatory drugs, but most of these interactions appear to have limited clinical importance.

MANAGEMENT OPTIONS: No specific action is required, but be alert for evidence of the interaction.

REFERENCES:
    1. Cressman WA, et al. Absorption and excretion of tolmetin in man. *Clin Pharmacol Ther*. 1976;19:224.

 Aspirin

Warfarin (eg, *Coumadin*)

SUMMARY: Aspirin (even in small doses) increases the risk of bleeding in anticoagulated patients by inhibiting platelet function and possibly by producing gastric erosions. Larger aspirin doses (eg, more than 3 g/day) may also enhance the hypoprothrombinemic response to warfarin. Nonetheless, the benefit of low-dose aspirin plus warfarin appears to outweigh the increased risk of bleeding in selected patients.

RISK FACTORS:

➡ **Dosage Regimen.** In most patients, more than 3 g/day of aspirin is likely to have an intrinsic hypoprothrombinemic effect that would be additive with that of oral anticoagulants; the aspirin dosage required for this effect varies from patient to patient.

MECHANISM: Large doses of salicylates tend to have an intrinsic hypoprothrombinemic effect. It is also possible that salicylates displace oral anticoagulants from plasma protein-binding sites, but the significance of this mechanism is questionable. Probably more important is the ability of aspirin to impair platelet function and produce GI bleeding (occurring less than 2 g/day of aspirin).

CLINICAL EVALUATION: Many reports have addressed the interaction of aspirin and oral anticoagulants.[5-15] A study in 534 patients with prosthetic heart valves showed that excessive bleeding was approximately 3 times more common with warfarin plus aspirin (500 mg/day) than with warfarin plus dipyridamole (400 mg/day) or warfarin alone.[1] In another study, 2 of 11 patients on warfarin and dipyridamole developed enhanced hypoprothrombinemia during the first few days of aspirin therapy (1 g/day).[2] Others also have noted bleeding episodes that may have been caused by concurrent therapy with aspirin and oral anticoagulants.[3,4] Low dose aspirin (100 to 150 mg/day) appears to increase the risk of minor bleeding in patients on warfarin, but the risk may be more than offset by the benefit.[17,18]

RELATED DRUGS: Nonacetylated salicylates (eg, choline salicylate, magnesium salicylate, salsalate, sodium salicylate) are probably safer with oral anticoagulants than aspirin, since such salicylates have minimal effects on platelet function and the gastric mucosa. Enteric-coated aspirin tends to produce less gastric mucosal damage,[16] but it would still be capable of increasing the hypoprothrombinemic response (if given in large doses) and inhibiting platelet function (in any dose).

MANAGEMENT OPTIONS:

➥ *Avoid Unless Benefit Outweighs Risk.* Combine aspirin with an oral anticoagulant only when used intentionally for additive anticoagulant effects. If the aspirin is being used as an analgesic or antipyretic, acetaminophen is probably safer to use with oral anticoagulants. If a salicylate is needed, nonacetylated salicylates are probably safer (see Related Drugs). Warn patients that many nonprescription products contain aspirin and advise them to read the ingredients carefully.

➥ *Monitor.* If aspirin is used with oral anticoagulants, note that the increased bleeding risk is usually not accompanied by an increase in the hypoprothrombinemic response, especially when small doses of aspirin are used. Thus, direct particular attention to early detection of bleeding, especially from the GI tract.

REFERENCES:

1. Chesbro JH, et al. Trial of combined warfarin plus dipyridamole or ASA therapy in prosthetic heart valve replacement: danger of ASA compared with dipyridamole. *Am J Cardiol.* 1983;51:1537.

2. Donaldson DR, et al. Assessment of the interaction of warfarin with aspirin and dipyridamole. *Thromb Haemost.* 1982;47:77.

3. Starr KJ, et al. Drug interactions in patients on long-term oral anticoagulant and antihypertensive adrenergic neuron-blocking drugs. *BMJ.* 1972;4:133.

4. Deckert FW. Ascorbic acid and warfarin. *JAMA.* 1973;223:440.

5. Udall JA. Drug interference with warfarin therapy. *Clin Med.* 1970;77:20.

6. Chignell CF, et al. Optical studies of drug-protein complexes. V. The interaction of phenylbutazone, flufenamic acid, and dicumarol with acetylsalicylic acid-treated human serum albumin. *Mol Pharmacol.* 1971;7:229.

7. Coldwell BB, et al. Effect of aspirin on the fate of bishydroxycoumarin in the rat. *J Pharm Pharmacol.* 1971;23:226.

8. Anon. Aspirin and gastrointestinal bleeding. *JAMA.* 1969;207:2430. Editorial.

9. Barrow MV, et al. Salicylate hypoprothrombinemia in rheumatoid arthritis with liver disease. *Arch Intern Med.* 1967;120:620.

10. Holmes EL. Pharmacology of the fenamates. IV. Toleration of normal human subjects. *Ann Phys Med.* (Suppl). 1967;9:36.

11. O'Reilly RA, et al. Impact of aspirin and chlorthalidone on the pharmacodynamics of oral anticoagulant drugs in man. *Ann NY Acad Sci.* 1971;179:173.

12. Fausa O. Salicylate-induced hypoprothrombinemia: a report of four cases. *Acta Med Scand.* 1970;188:403.

13. Anon. Aspirin and bleeding. *JAMA.* 1971;218:89. Editorial.

14. O'Brien JR, et al. A comparison of an effect of different anti-inflammatory drugs on human platelets. *J Clin Pathol.* 1970;23:522.

15. Trunet P, et al. The role of iatrogenic disease in admissions to intensive care. *JAMA.* 1980;244:2617.

16. Hawthorne AB, et al. Aspirin-induced gastric mucosal damage: prevention by enteric-coating and relation to prostaglandin synthesis. *Br J Clin Pharmacol.* 1991;32:77.

17. Turpie AGG, et al. A comparison of aspirin with placebo in patients treated with warfarin after heart-valve replacement. *New Engl J Med.* 1993;329:524.

18. Hurlen M, et al. Comparison of bleeding complications of warfarin and warfarin plus acetylsalicylic acid: a study in 3166 outpatients. *J Int Med.* 1994;236:299.

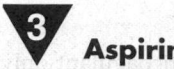 **Aspirin**

Zafirlukast (*Accolate*)

SUMMARY: The manufacturer reports that aspirin can increase plasma concentrations of zafirlukast; adjustments in zafirlukast dose may be needed.

RISK FACTORS: No specific risk factors are known.

MECHANISM: Not established.

CLINICAL EVALUATION: Coadministration of multiple doses of zafirlukast (40 mg/day) and aspirin (650 mg 4 times daily) resulted in about a 45% increase in zafirlukast mean plasma concentrations. The clinical importance of an increase in zafirlukast plasma concentrations of this magnitude is not clear.[1]

RELATED DRUGS: No information is available.

MANAGEMENT OPTIONS:

➡ *Monitor.* Monitor for altered zafirlukast effect if aspirin is initiated, discontinued, or changed in dosage. Adjust zafirlukast dose as needed.

REFERENCES:

1. Product information. Zafirlukast (*Accolate*). Zeneca Pharmaceuticals. 1997.

 Astemizole† (*Hismanal*)

AVOID **Erythromycin (eg, *E-Mycin*)**

SUMMARY: Preliminary reports indicate that erythromycin and astemizole administration can cause QT interval prolongation and arrhythmia.

RISK FACTORS: No specific risk factors are known.

MECHANISM: It appears that erythromycin inhibits the metabolism (CYP3A4) of astemizole.

CLINICAL EVALUATION: Several patients taking astemizole and erythromycin developed syncope with torsades de pointes arrhythmias.[1,2] One of the patients was also taking ketoconazole. Her serum potassium and magnesium concentrations were below normal. In vitro studies note the inhibition of astemizole metabolism by erythromycin, ketoconazole, and itraconazole.[3] Astemizole can cause arrhythmias in overdose cases.[4,5]

RELATED DRUGS: Ketoconazole (*Nizoral*) and itraconazole (*Sporanox*) interact similarly in vitro. Troleandomycin (*TAO*) and clarithromycin (*Biaxin*) also may inhibit astemizole metabolism. Terfenadine (*Seldane*) is also known to interact with erythromycin.

MANAGEMENT OPTIONS:

➡ *AVOID COMBINATION.* It would be prudent to avoid giving the 2 drugs together. The use of sedating antihistamines or perhaps loratadine (*Claritin*) or cetirizine (*Zyrtec*) instead of astemizole would be preferred in patients taking erythromycin, ketoconazole, or itraconazole.

REFERENCES:

1. Gelb LN, ed. *FDA Medical Bull.* 1993;23:2.
2. Goss JE, et al. Torsades de pointes associated with astemizole (*Hismanal*) therapy. *Arch Intern Med.* 1993;153:2705.

3. Lavriisen K, et al. The interaction of ketoconazole, itraconazole and erythromycin with the in vitro metabolism of antihistamines in human liver microsomes. *Allergy*. 1993;48(Suppl.):34.

4. Snook J, et al. Torsades de pointes ventricular tachycardia associated with astemizole overdose. *Br J Clin Pract*. 1988;42:257.

5. Bishop R, et al. Prolonged Q-T interval following astemizole overdose. *Arch Emerg Med*. 1989;6:63.

† Not available in the United States.

Astemizole† (Hismanal)

Fluvoxamine (Luvox) AVOID

SUMMARY: Fluvoxamine appears to inhibit the enzyme that metabolizes astemizole, which theoretically could result in increased serum astemizole concentrations and cardiac arrhythmias; avoid the combination.

RISK FACTORS: No specific risk factors are known.

MECHANISM: Theoretically, fluvoxamine may inhibit the firstpass hepatic metabolism of astemizole by cytochrome P450 3A4.

CLINICAL EVALUATION: Fluvoxamine has been shown to substantially inhibit the metabolism of alprazolam, a drug that is metabolized by CYP3A4.[1] Thus, fluvoxamine may also inhibit the metabolism of other drugs metabolized by CYP3A4, such as astemizole. Astemizole undergoes extensive first-pass hepatic metabolism by CYP3A4, and inhibitors of CYP3A4, such as ketoconazole, have been shown to increase astemizole serum concentrations, leading to electrocardiographic changes (QT prolongation) and, in some cases, life-threatening ventricular arrhythmias (torsades de pointes). Although it is not known whether fluvoxamine would inhibit the metabolism of astemizole enough to increase the risk of arrhythmias, it is theoretically possible.

RELATED DRUGS: Terfenadine (*Seldane*) is also metabolized by CYP3A4 and can cause the same types of cardiac arrhythmias when combined with CYP3A4 inhibitors; thus, it may also interact adversely with fluvoxamine. Loratadine (*Claritin*) and cetirizine (*Zyrtec*) do not appear to produce cardiotoxicity when combined with CYP3A4 inhibitors.

MANAGEMENT OPTIONS:

➡ *AVOID COMBINATION.* Although this interaction is based largely upon theoretical considerations, avoid the combination of astemizole and fluvoxamine.[2] The potential adverse effects of the interaction can be life-threatening, and astemizole is generally used for symptomatic relief of allergic disorders. Theoretically, loratadine would be a safer nonsedating antihistamine in the presence of fluvoxamine.

REFERENCES:

1. Fleishaker JC, et al. A pharmacokinetic and pharmacodynamic evaluation of the combined administration of alprazolam and fluvoxamine. *Eur J Clin Pharmacol*. 1994;46:35.

2. Product information. Fluvoxamine (*Luvox*). Solvay Pharmaceuticals. 1996.

† Not available in the United States.

Astemizole† (*Hismanal*)

AVOID **Ketoconazole (*Nizoral*)**

SUMMARY: Ketoconazole administration can cause astemizole concentrations to increase and result in QT interval prolongation and arrhythmia.

RISK FACTORS: No specific risk factors are known.

MECHANISM: Ketoconazole inhibits the metabolism (CYP3A4) of astemizole resulting in the accumulation of cardiotoxic drug concentrations.

CLINICAL EVALUATION: A patient taking ketoconazole, erythromycin, and astemizole developed syncope with torsades de pointes arrhythmias.[1] No further data are available regarding this case. Erythromycin could have contributed to the interaction reported in this patient (see erythromycin-astemizole interaction). Unpublished studies in humans indicate that ketoconazole inhibits astemizole metabolism. In vitro studies note the inhibition of astemizole metabolism by erythromycin, ketoconazole, and itraconazole.[2] It appears likely that ketoconazole-induced increases in astemizole concentrations could result in arrhythmias, since astemizole has been noted to cause arrhythmias in overdose cases.[3,4]

RELATED DRUGS: Other antifungal agents (eg, miconazole [*Monistat*], itraconazole [*Sporanox*], fluconazole [*Diflucan*]) are likely to increase astemizole concentrations. Terfenadine (*Seldane*) concentrations have been noted to increase when it is administered with antifungal agents. Cetirizine (*Zyrtec*) and loratadine (*Claritin*) appear to be less likely to produce side effects when administered with ketoconazole.

MANAGEMENT OPTIONS:

➡ ***AVOID COMBINATION.*** It would be prudent to avoid giving the 2 drugs together. The use of sedating antihistamines or perhaps loratadine or cetirizine instead of astemizole would seem to be preferred in patients taking ketoconazole or other oral antifungal agents. If ketoconazole and astemizole are coadministered, monitor for cardiac arrhythmias.

REFERENCES:

1. Gelb LN, ed. *FDA Medical Bull.* 1993;23:2.
2. Lavriisen K, et al. The interaction of ketoconazole, itraconazole and erythromycin with the in vitro metabolism of antihistamines in human liver microsomes. *Allergy.* 1993;48(Suppl.):34.
3. Snook J, et al. Torsades de pointes ventricular tachycardia associated with astemizole overdose. *Br J Clin Pract.* 1988;42:257.
4. Bishop R, et al. Prolonged Q-T interval following astemizole overdose. *Arch Emerg Med.* 1989;6:63.

† Not available in the United States.

 Astemizole† (*Hismanal*)

Mibefradil (*Posicor*)

SUMMARY: Mibefradil is likely to increase astemizole serum concentrations; cardiac arrhythmias may result. Pending further information on this interaction, avoid the concomitant use of mibefradil and astemizole.

RISK FACTORS: No specific risk factors are known.

MECHANISM: Mibefradil is known to inhibit the activity of CYP3A4, the enzyme responsible for the metabolism of astemizole. Astemizole accumulation can result in cardiac effects (prolonged QTc intervals) and arrhythmias.

CLINICAL EVALUATION: While no published data are available for evaluation, the manufacturer of mibefradil has made available some information on this interaction.[1] Mibefradil is known to increase terfenadine (*Seldane*) plasma concentrations and it is likely that astemizole would be similarly affected. Until specific studies defining the magnitude of this potential interaction are available, avoid the coadministration of astemizole and mibefradil.

RELATED DRUGS: Mibefradil administration causes an accumulation of terfenadine resulting in prolonged QTc intervals. Other calcium channel blockers (eg, amlodipine [*Norvasc*], nifedipine [*Procardia*], nicardipine [*Cardene*]) would not be expected to change astemizole plasma concentrations. The metabolism of fexofenadine (*Allegra*), cetirizine (*Zyrtec*), and loratadine (*Claritin*) would be unlikely to be affected by mibefradil coadministration.

MANAGEMENT OPTIONS:

➡ **Use Alternative.** Because of the risk of a possibly serious arrhythmia, avoid the combination of mibefradil and astemizole (or terfenadine). Use available noninteracting antihistamines in patients receiving mibefradil.

REFERENCES:

1. Product information. Mibefradil (*Posicor*). Roche Laboratories, Inc. 1997.

† Not available in the United States.

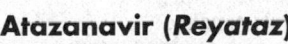

Atazanavir (*Reyataz*)

Clarithromycin (eg, *Biaxin*)

SUMMARY: The coadministration of atazanavir and clarithromycin results in elevated plasma concentrations of both drugs; increased side effects may occur.

RISK FACTORS: No specific risk factors are known.

MECHANISM: Clarithromycin and atazanavir inhibit CYP3A4, the enzyme responsible for the metabolism of both drugs.

CLINICAL EVALUATION: Clarithromycin 500 mg twice daily and atazanavir 400 mg once daily were administered alone and concurrently.[1] Clarithromycin administration produced a mean increase in the area under the plasma concentration-time curve (AUC) of atazanavir of 28% (range, 16% to 43%). The AUC of clarithromycin was increased an average of 94% during atazanavir coadministration. Monitor patients receiving clarithromycin and atazanavir for signs of toxicity, including dizziness, elevated liver function tests, nausea, or prolonged atrioventricular conduction.

RELATED DRUGS: Erythromycin can be expected to affect atazanavir in a similar manner. Many other protease inhibitors are substrates for CYP3A4 and will have increased plasma concentrations during coadministration with clarithromycin.

MANAGEMENT OPTIONS:

➡ **Consider Alternative.** Azithromycin (*Zithromax*) is not expected to affect atazanavir plasma concentrations.

➥ *Monitor.* Monitor patients receiving clarithromycin and atazanavir for evidence of increased plasma concentrations.

REFERENCES:

    1. *Reyataz* [package insert]. Princeton, NJ: Bristol-Myers Squibb Company; 2004.

Atazanavir (*Reyataz*)

Diltiazem (eg, *Cardizem*)

SUMMARY: Atazanavir increases diltiazem plasma concentrations; watch for increased calcium channel blocker effect.

RISK FACTORS: No specific risk factors are known.

MECHANISM: Atazanavir inhibits CYP3A4, the enzyme known to metabolize diltiazem.

CLINICAL EVALUATION: Diltiazem 180 mg daily and atazanavir 400 mg once daily were administered alone and concurrently.[1] Diltiazem administration did not alter the area under the plasma concentration-time curve (AUC) of atazanavir. The AUC of diltiazem was increased an average of 125% during atazanavir coadministration. Monitor patients receiving diltiazem and atazanavir for signs of toxicity, including prolonged atrioventricular conduction, dizziness, and hypotension.

RELATED DRUGS: Atazanavir is likely to increase the concentration of other calcium channel blockers, including, felodipine (*Plendil*), nifedipine (eg, *Procardia*), and verapamil (eg, *Calan*). Many other protease inhibitors, such as ritonavir (*Norvir*) and indinavir (*Crixivan*), are inhibitors of CYP3A4 and will increase the plasma concentration of diltiazem.

MANAGEMENT OPTIONS:

➥ *Consider Alternative.* If possible, consider selection of a noncalcium channel blocker in patients requiring atazanavir.

➥ *Monitor.* Monitor patients receiving diltiazem and atazanavir for increased calcium channel blocker effect.

REFERENCES:

    1. *Reyataz* [package insert]. Princeton, NJ: Bristol-Myers Squibb Company; 2004.

Atazanavir (*Reyataz*)

Efavirenz (*Sustiva*)

SUMMARY: Efavirenz administration markedly reduces the plasma concentration of atazanavir; loss of antiviral effect may occur.

RISK FACTORS: No specific risk factors are known.

MECHANISM: Efavirenz is an inducer of the CYP3A4 enzymes responsible for the metabolism of atazanavir.

CLINICAL EVALUATION: Twenty-seven subjects received atazanavir 400 mg daily for 20 days.[1] On days 7 through 20, efavirenz 600 mg daily also was administered. The mean area under the plasma concentration-time curve (AUC) of atazanavir was reduced 74%, and the peak atazanavir concentration was reduced nearly 60%. When the same study was repeated with the addition of ritonavir (*Norvir*) 100 mg daily on days 7 through 20, the AUC of atazanavir was increased 39%. The addition of ritonavir reversed the efavirenz-induced metabolism of atazanavir.

RELATED DRUGS: Efavirenz is known to reduce the plasma concentrations of ritonavir and indinavir (*Crixivan*). Other protease inhibitors metabolized by CYP3A4 will likely be affected in a similar manner by efavirenz.

MANAGEMENT OPTIONS:

➡ *Monitor.* Monitor patients taking atazanavir for reduced plasma concentrations and possible reduced antiviral efficacy during efavirenz coadministration.

REFERENCES:

1. *Sustiva* [package insert]. Princeton, NJ: Bristol-Myers Squibb Company; 2005.

Atazanavir (*Reyataz*)

Ergotamine (*Ergomar*)

SUMMARY: Elevated ergotamine concentrations and toxicity may occur if atazanavir and ergotamine are coadministered.

RISK FACTORS: No specific risk factors are known.

MECHANISM: Atazanavir is known to be an inhibitor of CYP3A4, the enzyme responsible for the metabolism of ergotamine.

CLINICAL EVALUATION: While specific data are lacking, the manufacturer of atazanavir contraindicates the coadministration of ergotamine and atazanavir.[1] The coadministration of ergotamine and atazanavir could lead to hypertension or cyanosis.

RELATED DRUGS: Other ergot drugs, including dihydroergotamine (eg, *D.H.E. 45*) and methylergonovine (*Methergine*), are likely to be affected in a similar manner by atazanavir. Other protease inhibitors, such as ritonavir (*Norvir*), indinavir (*Crixivan*), amprenavir (*Agenerase*), nelfinavir (*Viracept*), and saquinavir (eg, *Fortovase*), can be expected to interact with ergotamine in a similar manner.

MANAGEMENT OPTIONS:

➡ *Use Alternative.* Do not administer atazanavir or any protease inhibitor known to inhibit the activity of CYP3A4 to patients receiving ergotamine.

➡ *Monitor.* If atazanavir is coadministered with ergotamine, monitor for evidence of excess vasoconstriction.

REFERENCES:

1. *Reyataz* [package insert]. Princeton, NJ: Bristol-Myers Squibb Company; 2004.

Atazanavir (*Reyataz*)

Esomeprazole (*Nexium*)

SUMMARY: Esomeprazole coadministration may reduce atazanavir plasma concentrations; some loss of antiviral efficacy is expected.

RISK FACTORS: No specific risk factors are known.

MECHANISM: Unknown. It appears that gastric acid is necessary for the absorption of atazanavir.

CLINICAL EVALUATION: A 65-year-old man with HIV was taking atazanavir 300 mg and ritonavir 100 mg daily with stavudine 30 mg twice daily.[1] In the evening, he took esomeprazole 40 mg daily. His atazanavir plasma concentrations were low, even following a doubling of the atazanavir and ritonavir dosage. The atazanavir was switched to fosamprenavir (eg, *Lexiva*) with attainment of adequate amprenavir plasma concentrations. No dechallenge of the esomeprazole was attempted. Several retrospective studies and case reports have noted mixed effects of proton pump inhibitors on atazanavir concentrations.[2-4] These reports are limited by their designs and inadequate control of variables. Pending further controlled pharmacokinetic studies, consider the potential for reduced atazanavir concentrations when acid suppressants are administered. The serious risk to patients of this interaction demands avoidance of coadministration if possible and careful monitoring if the drugs are coadministered.

RELATED DRUGS: Indinavir (*Crixivan*) absorption also is reduced by inhibition of gastric acid secretion. Omeprazole (eg, *Prilosec*) and lansoprazole (*Prevacid*) are known to affect atazanavir absorption. Pantoprazole (eg, *Protonix*) and rabeprazole (*Aciphex*) are expected to interact with atazanavir. H_2-receptor antagonists (eg, ranitidine [eg, *Zantac*], famotidine [eg, *Pepcid*]) and antacids (eg, *Maalox*) also may reduce atazanavir concentrations.

MANAGEMENT OPTIONS:

➠ *Monitor.* Monitor atazanavir plasma concentrations and adjust the atazanavir dose to reach therapeutic atazanavir concentrations in patients who require therapy with both esomeprazole and atazanavir.

REFERENCES:

1. Kiser JJ, et al. Effects of esomeprazole on the pharmacokinetics of atazanavir and fosamprenavir in a patient with human immunodeficiency virus infection. *Pharmacotherapy.* 2006;26(4):511-514.
2. Khanlou H, et al. Co-administration of atazanavir with proton-pump inhibitors and H_2 blockers. *J Acquir Immune Defic Syndr.* 2005;39(4):503.
3. Guiard-Schmid JB, et al. Lack of interaction between atazanavir and proton pump inhibitors in HIV-infected patients treated with ritonavir-boosted atazanavir. *J Acquir Immune Defic Syndr.* 2006;41(3):393-394.
4. Furtek KJ, et al. Proton pump inhibitor therapy in atazanavir-treated patients: contraindicated? *J Acquir Immune Defic Syndr.* 2006;41(3):394-396.

Atazanavir (*Reyataz*)

Etravirine (*Intelence*)

SUMMARY: The coadministration of atazanavir and etravirine increases the plasma concentration of etravirine, but reduces the concentration of atazanavir.

RISK FACTORS: No specific risk factors are known.

MECHANISM: Etravirine appears to increase the metabolism of atazanavir (via CYP3A4), while atazanavir inhibits the CYP3A4 metabolism of etravirine.

CLINICAL EVALUATION: While specific data are limited, the manufacturer of etravirine states that the coadministration of etravirine 800 mg twice daily and atazanavir 400 mg daily resulted in an approximate 50% increase in the mean area under the plasma concentration-time curve (AUC) of etravirine.[1] Trough etravirine concentrations increased 58%. Atazanavir's mean AUC was reduced 17%, and its trough concentration declined 47% during coadministration. The effects of coadministration were similar when atazanavir 300 mg plus ritonavir 100 mg daily were coadministered with etravirine. Pending further data, observe patients receiving etravirine and atazanavir for increased etravirine effect and reduced atazanavir response.

RELATED DRUGS: Etravirine may reduce the concentration of other protease inhibitors that are substrates for CYP3A4, such as darunavir (*Prezista*), indinavir (*Crixivan*), nelfinavir (*Viracept*), saquinavir (*Invirase*), and ritonavir (*Norvir*). The plasma concentration of etravirine may be increased by other CYP3A4 inhibitors, including indinavir, nelfinavir, saquinavir, and fosamprenavir (*Lexiva*).

MANAGEMENT OPTIONS:

➡ *Monitor.* Monitor patients taking etravirine and atazanavir for increased and decreased plasma concentration, respectively.

REFERENCES:

1. *Intelence* [package insert]. Raritan, NJ: Tibotec Therapeutics; 2008.

Atazanavir (*Reyataz*) 4

Famotidine (eg, *Pepcid*)

SUMMARY: Famotidine can reduce the bioavailability of atazanavir; separation of doses will mitigate most of the interaction.

RISK FACTORS: No specific risk factors are known.

MECHANISM: Atazanavir solubility requires an acidic media in the stomach; famotidine-induced acid suppression will reduce the solubility of atazanavir and lower its bioavailability.

CLINICAL EVALUATION: A number of studies on the effect of famotidine on the absorption of atazanavir have been conducted.[1,2] When atazanavir and famotidine (40 mg twice daily) are administered simultaneously, the area under the concentration-time curve (AUC) of atazanavir is reduced by up to 40%. Administering the atazanavir 2 hours before the famotidine avoided the reduction in the absorption of atazanavir. Lower doses of famotidine (20 mg twice daily) produced only small reductions in the absorption of atazanavir.

RELATED DRUGS: Fosamprenavir (*Lexiva*), indinavir (*Crixivan*), nelfinavir (*Viracept*), and tipranavir (*Aptivus*) have also been reported to have reduced absorption in the presence of gastric acid inhibitors. Other H_2-receptor antagonists (cimetidine [eg, *Tagamet*], ranitidine [eg, *Zantac*], and nizatidine [eg, *Axid*]) as well as proton pump inhibitors and antacids may also reduce the absorption of atazanavir.

MANAGEMENT OPTIONS:

➡ *Monitor.* Separating the doses of H_2-receptor antagonists and atazanavir by giving atazanavir at least 2 hours before the H_2-receptor antagonist will reduce the magnitude of the interaction. If acid suppressants are given with atazanavir, monitor patients for reduced antiviral activity.

REFERENCES:

1. *Reyataz* [package insert]. Princeton, NJ: Bristol-Myers Squibb; 2011.
2. Wang X, et al. Effects of the H_2-receptor antagonist famotidine on the pharmacokinetics of atazanavir-ritonavir with or without tenofovir in HIV-infected patients. *AIDS Patient Care STDs*. 2011;25(9):509-515.

② Atazanavir (*Reyataz*)

Lansoprazole (eg, *Prevacid*)

SUMMARY: Lansoprazole coadministration markedly reduced atazanavir plasma concentrations; loss of antiviral efficacy is expected.

RISK FACTORS: No specific risk factors are known.

MECHANISM: Unknown. It appears that gastric acid is necessary for the absorption of atazanavir.

CLINICAL EVALUATION: Healthy subjects received a single dose of atazanavir 400 mg alone or following 2 doses of lansoprazole 60 mg administered 24 hours apart.[1] Following the 2 lansoprazole doses, the mean area under the concentration-time curve and peak plasma concentration of atazanavir were reduced approximately 95%. This reduction in atazanavir concentrations would likely result in a loss of antiviral effect. Several retrospective and case reports have noted mixed effects of proton pump inhibitors on atazanavir concentrations.[2-4] These reports are limited by their designs and inadequate control of variables. Pending further controlled pharmacokinetic studies, consider the potential for reduced atazanavir concentrations when acid suppressants are administered. The serious risk to patients from this interaction demands avoidance of coadministration if possible and careful monitoring if the drugs are coadministered.

RELATED DRUGS: Indinavir (*Crixivan*) absorption also is reduced by the inhibition of gastric acid secretion. Omeprazole (eg, *Prilosec*) and esomeprazole (*Nexium*) are known to affect atazanavir absorption. Pantoprazole (eg, *Protonix*) and rabeprazole (*Aciphex*) also are expected to interact with atazanavir. H_2-receptor antagonists (eg, ranitidine [eg, *Zantac*], famotidine [eg, *Pepcid*]) and antacids (eg, *Maalox*) also may reduce atazanavir concentrations.

MANAGEMENT OPTIONS:

➡ *Monitor.* Monitor atazanavir plasma concentrations and adjust the atazanavir dose to reach therapeutic atazanavir concentrations in patients who require both lansoprazole and atazanavir.

REFERENCES:

1. Tomilo DL, et al. Inhibition of atazanavir oral absorption by lansoprazole gastric acid suppression in healthy volunteers. *Pharmacotherapy.* 2006;26(3):341-346.

2. Khanlou H, et al. Co-administration of atazanavir with proton-pump inhibitors and H_2 blockers. *J Acquir Immune Defic Syndr.* 2005;39(4):503.

3. Guiard-Schmid JB, et al. Lack of interaction between atazanavir and proton pump inhibitors in HIV-infected patients treated with ritonavir-boosted atazanavir. *J Acquir Immune Defic Syndr.* 2006;41(3):393-394.

4. Furtek KJ, et al. Proton pump inhibitor therapy in atazanavir-treated patients: contraindicated? *J Acquir Immune Defic Syndr.* 2006;41(3):394-396.

Atazanavir (*Reyataz*)

Lovastatin (eg, *Mevacor*)

SUMMARY: Atazanavir administration can produce elevated concentrations of lovastatin; myopathy or rhabdomyolysis may occur.

RISK FACTORS: No specific risk factors are known.

MECHANISM: Atazanavir inhibits the metabolism of lovastatin via the enzyme CYP3A4.

CLINICAL EVALUATION: While specific data are limited, the manufacturer of atazanavir states that the coadministration of atazanavir and lovastatin is contraindicated.[1] Pending further data, observe patients receiving atazanavir and lovastatin for evidence of lovastatin toxicity.

RELATED DRUGS: Simvastatin (eg, *Zocor*) and atorvastatin (*Lipitor*) are also metabolized by CYP3A4, and they also interact with atazanavir. Other protease inhibitors that are known to inhibit CYP3A4 (eg, darunavir [*Prezista*], indinavir [*Crixivan*], nelfinavir [*Viracept*], ritonavir [*Norvir*], saquinavir [*Invirase*]) are expected to increase systemic exposure to lovastatin.

MANAGEMENT OPTIONS:

➡ *Use Alternative.* Compared with lovastatin, atorvastatin plasma concentrations may be increased to a lesser extent by atazanavir. Theoretically, pravastatin (eg, *Pravachol*) and possibly rosuvastatin (*Crestor*) or fluvastatin (*Lescol*) are less likely to interact with atazanavir.

➡ *Monitor.* Counsel patients taking lovastatin to report any muscle pain or weakness, particularly when they are also taking a CYP3A4 inhibitor.

REFERENCES:
1. *Reyataz* [package insert]. Princeton, NJ: Bristol-Myers Squibb Company; 2008.

Atazanavir (*Reyataz*) ▼

Maraviroc (*Selzentry*)

SUMMARY: The coadministration of atazanavir can increase the concentration of maraviroc; some patients may experience increased adverse reactions.

RISK FACTORS: No specific risk factors are known.

MECHANISM: Atazanavir appears to inhibit the CYP3A4 metabolism of maraviroc.

CLINICAL EVALUATION: Twelve healthy men received maraviroc 300 mg twice daily on days 1 through 14, with atazanavir 400 mg daily on days 1 through 7 and then atazanavir 300 mg/ritonavir 100 mg on days 8 through 14 or placebo.[1] The coadministration of atazanavir resulted in a mean increase in the area under the concentration-time curve (AUC) and peak concentration of maraviroc of 357% and 209%, respectively. The combination of atazanavir/ritonavir produced a greater increase in maraviroc concentrations than atazanavir alone, with the mean maraviroc AUC increasing by more than 480%. These increases in maraviroc concentrations are likely to produce an increase in adverse reactions (eg, dizziness, pyrexia, rash) in some patients. Maraviroc doses may require reduction.

RELATED DRUGS: Darunavir (*Prezista*), fosamprenavir (*Lexiva*), indinavir (*Crixivan*), nelfinavir (*Viracept*), ritonavir (*Norvir*), and saquinavir (*Invirase*) also inhibit the activity of CYP3A4 and are expected to increase the plasma concentrations of maraviroc.

MANAGEMENT OPTIONS:

➥ *Monitor.* Monitor patients taking maraviroc for changing maraviroc response if atazanavir is initiated or discontinued from their drug regimen.

REFERENCES:

1. Abel S, et al. Effects of CYP3A4 inhibitors on the pharmacokinetics of maraviroc in healthy volunteers. *Br J Clin Pharmacol.* 2008;65(suppl 1):27-37.

Atazanavir (*Reyataz*)

Nevirapine (*Viramune*)

SUMMARY: Nevirapine administration produces a reduction in atazanavir concentrations; some reduction in antiviral effect may occur.

RISK FACTORS: No specific risk factors are known.

MECHANISM: Nevirapine appears to induce the metabolism of atazanavir via CYP3A4.

CLINICAL EVALUATION: Patients being treated for HIV infection with atazanavir/ritonavir combination therapy were administered nevirapine at varying periods of time.[1,2] The mean clearance of atazanavir was increased 54% during coadministration of nevirapine.[1] In another study, the mean trough atazanavir concentration was reduced 52% during the coadministration of nevirapine. Some reduction in the efficacy of atazanavir may occur. In this study, it is likely that ritonavir mitigated the potential magnitude of the interaction by partially inhibiting the metabolism of atazanavir.

RELATED DRUGS: None known.

MANAGEMENT OPTIONS:

➥ *Monitor.* Monitor patients being treated with atazanavir/ritonavir combinations for reduced atazanavir plasma concentrations and response during concurrent nevirapine therapy.

REFERENCES:

1. Dailly E, et al. Influence of tenofovir, nevirapine and efavirenz on ritonavir-boosted atazanavir pharmacokinetics in HIV-infected patients. *Eur J Clin Pharmacol.* 2006;62(7):523-526.
2. Winston A, et al. Atazanavir trough plasma concentration monitoring in a cohort of HIV-1-positive individuals receiving highly active antiretroviral therapy. *J Antimicrob Chemother.* 2005;56(2):380-387.

Atazanavir (*Reyataz*)

Omeprazole (eg, *Prilosec*)

SUMMARY: Omeprazole markedly reduces atazanavir plasma concentrations; loss of efficacy is likely to occur.

RISK FACTORS: No specific risk factors are known.

MECHANISM: Unknown. It appears that gastric acid is necessary for the absorption of atazanavir.

CLINICAL EVALUATION: The administration of omeprazole 40 mg daily reduced atazanavir's mean area under the plasma concentration-time curve 76%, peak concentration 72%, and trough concentration 78%.[1] In this study, atazanavir was coadministered with ritonavir 100 mg daily. Neither increasing the atazanavir dosage to 400 mg daily nor the coadministration of 8 oz of cola returned atazanavir concentrations to noninteraction levels. Consider loss of antiviral efficacy in patients taking both agents.

RELATED DRUGS: Esomeprazole (*Nexium*), lansoprazole (*Prevacid*), pantoprazole (eg, *Protonix*), and rabeprazole (*AcipHex*) are expected to interact with atazanavir in a similar manner. H_2-receptor antagonists (eg, famotidine [eg, *Pepcid*], ranitidine [eg, *Zantac*]) and antacids (eg, *Maalox*) also may reduce atazanavir concentrations. Indinavir (*Crixivan*) and fosamprenavir (*Lexiva*) absorption is reduced by gastric acid inhibition.

MANAGEMENT OPTIONS:

➡ *Monitor.* Monitor atazanavir plasma concentrations and adjust the atazanavir dose to reach therapeutic atazanavir concentrations in patients who require both omeprazole and atazanavir.

REFERENCES:

1. *Reyataz* [package insert]. Princeton, NJ: Bristol-Myers Squibb Company; 2004.

Atazanavir (*Reyataz*)

Raltegravir (*Isentress*)

SUMMARY: Atazanavir administration increases the plasma concentration of raltegravir; some patients may develop increased adverse reactions, including headache, GI upset, and pyrexia.

RISK FACTORS: No specific risk factors are known.

MECHANISM: Raltegravir is metabolized by UDP-glucuronosyltransferase; atazanavir inhibits this glucuronidation of raltegravir.

CLINICAL EVALUATION: While specific data are limited, the manufacturer of raltegravir states that the coadministration of atazanavir 400 mg daily prior to a single dose of raltegravir 100 mg increased the mean area under the plasma concentration-time curve (AUC) of raltegravir approximately 70%.[1] When ritonavir 100 mg was combined with atazanavir 300 mg, the increase in the AUC of raltegravir was 40%. Pending further data, observe patients receiving raltegravir and atazanavir for increased raltegravir effect.

RELATED DRUGS: None known.

MANAGEMENT OPTIONS:

➡ *Monitor.* Monitor patients taking raltegravir and atazanavir for signs of increased raltegravir plasma concentration.

REFERENCES:

1. *Isentress* [package insert]. Whitehouse Station, NJ: Merck & Co; 2010.

Atazanavir (*Reyataz*)

Ramelteon (*Rozerem*)

SUMMARY: Ramelteon is very sensitive to inhibition of CYP1A2; theoretically, atazanavir increases ramelteon plasma concentrations.

RISK FACTORS: No specific risk factors are known.

MECHANISM: Ramelteon is metabolized primarily by CYP1A2, and atazanavir is a CYP1A2 inhibitor.

CLINICAL EVALUATION: In healthy subjects, administration of the potent CYP1A2 inhibitor fluvoxamine 100 mg twice daily for 3 days produced a 190-fold increase in ramelteon area under the plasma concentration-time curve from time zero to infinity and a 70-fold increase in the ramelteon maximal plasma concentrations.[1] The ramelteon product information states that ramelteon should be administered with caution to patients taking CYP1A2 inhibitors.[1]

RELATED DRUGS: No information is available.

MANAGEMENT OPTIONS:

➡ **Monitor.** If atazanavir and ramelteon are used concurrently, monitor patients for excessive ramelteon effects.

REFERENCES:

1. *Rozerem* [package insert]. Lincolnshire, IL: Takeda Pharmaceuticals; 2006.

Atazanavir (*Reyataz*)

Rifabutin (*Mycobutin*)

SUMMARY: Atazanavir administration increases the plasma concentration of rifabutin; observe patients for evidence of rifabutin toxicity.

RISK FACTORS: No specific risk factors are known.

MECHANISM: Atazanavir appears to inhibit the CYP3A4 mediated metabolism of rifabutin.

CLINICAL EVALUATION: While specific data are limited, the manufacturer of atazanavir notes that the coadministration of rifabutin 300 mg on days 1 to 10 and then 150 mg on days 11 to 20 prior to atazanavir 600 mg daily increased the mean area under the plasma concentration-time curve (AUC) of rifabutin by approximately 110%.[1] The administration of atazanavir 300 mg plus ritonavir 100 mg daily for 17 days with rifabutin 150 mg twice daily resulted in an increase in the AUC of rifabutin of approximately 50%.[2] Reducing the dosage of rifabutin to 150 mg 3 times weekly normalized the levels of rifabutin during atazanavir coadministration. Rifabutin does not appear to alter the plasma concentration of atazanavir.

RELATED DRUGS: Darunavir (*Prezista*), fosamprenavir (*Lexiva*), indinavir (*Crixivan*), nelfinavir (*Viracept*), ritonavir (*Norvir*), and saquinavir (*Invirase*) also inhibit the activity of CYP3A4 and are expected to increase the plasma concentrations of rifabutin. Rifampin (eg, *Rifadin*) is known to markedly reduce atazanavir concentrations; the effects of rifapentine (*Priftin*) on atazanavir are unknown, but it may also reduce atazanavir concentration.

MANAGEMENT OPTIONS:

➥ *Monitor.* Monitor for evidence of rifabutin toxicity (eg, neutropenia) in patients who are coadministered rifabutin and atazanavir or atazanavir/ritonavir.

REFERENCES:

1. *Reyataz* [package insert]. Princeton, NJ: Bristol-Myers Squibb; 2011.

2. Zhang J, et al. Determination of rifabutin dosing regimen when administered in combination with ritonavir-boosted atazanavir. *J Antimicrob Chemother.* 2011;66(9):2075-2082.

Atazanavir (*Reyataz*)

Rifampin (eg, *Rifadin*)

SUMMARY: Rifampin markedly reduces atazanavir plasma concentrations; failure of its antiviral effect is likely.

RISK FACTORS: No specific risk factors are known.

MECHANISM: Rifampin appears to induce the metabolism of atazanavir via CYP3A4.

CLINICAL EVALUATION: Several clinical studies have reported marked reductions in the plasma concentration of atazanavir when coadministered with rifampin.[1-3] Atazanavir concentrations were reduced by more than 50% during rifampin coadministration, even when atazanavir was administered with ritonavir. Inadequate atazanavir concentrations are likely to result. Avoid the coadministration of rifampin and atazanavir.

RELATED DRUGS: The plasma concentrations of other protease inhibitors metabolized by CYP3A4 (eg, indinavir [*Crixivan*], ritonavir [*Norvir*], saquinavir [*Invirase*]) are also reduced by rifampin administration. Rifabutin (*Mycobutin*) and rifapentine (*Priftin*) may exhibit a similar effect on atazanavir plasma concentrations.

MANAGEMENT OPTIONS:

➥ *Monitor.* Monitor atazanavir concentrations to ensure adequate antiviral levels if atazanavir and rifampin are coadministered.

REFERENCES:

1. Burger DM, et al. Effect of rifampin on steady-state pharmacokinetics of atazanavir with ritonavir in healthy volunteers. *Antimicrob Agents Chemother.* 2006;50(10):3336-3342.

2. Acosta EP, et al. Effect of concomitantly administered rifampin on the pharmacokinetics and safety of atazanavir administered twice daily. *Antimicrob Agents Chemother.* 2007;51(9):3104-3110.

3. Mallolas J, et al. Pharmacokinetic interaction between rifampin and ritonavir-boosted atazanavir in HIV-infected patients. *HIV Med.* 2007;8(2):131-134.

Atazanavir (*Reyataz*)

Simvastatin (eg, *Zocor*)

SUMMARY: Atazanavir administration can produce elevated concentrations of simvastatin; myopathy or rhabdomyolysis may occur.

RISK FACTORS: No specific risk factors are known.

MECHANISM: Atazanavir inhibits the metabolism of simvastatin via the enzyme CYP3A4.

CLINICAL EVALUATION: While specific data are limited, the manufacturer of atazanavir states that the coadministration of atazanavir and simvastatin is contraindicated.[1] A case report noted a patient who developed rhabdomyolysis while receiving atazanavir 400 mg daily, amiodarone 200 mg daily, and simvastatin 80 mg daily.[2] Because amiodarone is also known to inhibit the elimination of simvastatin, the role of atazanavir in this case is unclear. Pending further data, observe patients receiving atazanavir and simvastatin for evidence of simvastatin toxicity.

RELATED DRUGS: Lovastatin (eg, *Mevacor*) and atorvastatin (*Lipitor*) are also metabolized by CYP3A4 and may interact with atazanavir. Other protease inhibitors that are known to inhibit CYP3A4 (eg, darunavir [*Prezista*], indinavir [*Crixivan*], nelfinavir [*Viracept*], ritonavir [*Norvir*], saquinavir [*Invirase*]) are expected to increase systemic exposure to simvastatin.

MANAGEMENT OPTIONS:

➡ **Use Alternative.** Atorvastatin plasma concentrations are likely to be increased to a lesser extent by atazanavir than simvastatin. Theoretically, pravastatin (eg, *Pravachol*) and possibly rosuvastatin (*Crestor*) or fluvastatin (*Lescol*) are less likely to interact with atazanavir.

➡ **Monitor.** Advise patients taking simvastatin to report any muscle pain or weakness, particularly when they are also taking a CYP3A4 inhibitor.

REFERENCES:

1. *Reyataz* [package insert]. Princeton, NJ: Bristol-Myers Squibb Company; 2008.
2. Schmidt GA, et al. Severe rhabdomyolysis and acute renal failure secondary to concomitant use of simvastatin, amiodarone, and atazanavir. *J Am Board Fam Med.* 2007;20(4):411-416.

4 | Atazanavir (*Reyataz*)

Tenofovir (*Viread*)

SUMMARY: Tenofovir administration produces a modest reduction in atazanavir concentrations; some reduction in antiviral effect may occur.

RISK FACTORS: No specific risk factors are known.

MECHANISM: Unknown.

CLINICAL EVALUATION: Patients being treated for HIV infection with atazanavir/ritonavir combination therapy were also administered tenofovir 300 mg daily for at least 2 weeks.[1,2] The mean clearance of atazanavir was increased 20% to 33% during coadministration of tenofovir; the half-life of atazanavir was not changed. Some reduction in the efficacy of atazanavir may occur. In this study, it is likely that ritonavir mitigated the potential magnitude of the interaction by partially inhibiting the metabolism of atazanavir.

RELATED DRUGS: None known.

MANAGEMENT OPTIONS:

➡ **Monitor.** Monitor patients being treated with atazanavir/ritonavir combinations for reduced atazanavir plasma concentrations and response if tenofovir is administered.

REFERENCES:

1. Taburet AM, et al. Interactions between atazanavir-ritonavir and tenofovir in heavily pretreated human immunodeficiency virus-infected patients. *Antimicrob Agents Chemother.* 2004;48(6):2091-2096.
2. Dailly E, et al. Influence of tenofovir, nevirapine and efavirenz on ritonavir-boosted atazanavir pharmacokinetics in HIV-infected patients. *Eur J Clin Pharmacol.* 2006;62(7):523-526.

Atenolol (eg, *Tenormin*)

Dipyridamole (eg, *Persantine*)

SUMMARY: Several patients developed bradycardia following the administration of dipyridamole and atenolol.

RISK FACTORS: No specific risk factors are known.

MECHANISM: Dipyridamole inhibits the metabolism of adenosine, an inhibitor of sino-atrial and atrioventricular conduction. Because beta-adrenergic blocking drugs share the same negative chronotropic and dromotropic effects, an additive pharmacodynamic mechanism is probably responsible.

CLINICAL EVALUATION: Two patients receiving dipyridamole 0.56 mg/kg intravenously during diagnostic testing for coronary artery disease developed bradycardia.[1] One of the patients was taking atenolol 50 mg/day, and the other patient was taking metoprolol (eg, *Lopressor*) 100 mg twice daily. Bradycardia began within 3 minutes and in 1 case progressed to asystole. Both patients were treated with aminophylline; atropine also was administered to the patient with asystole. Bradycardia and asystole have been noted rarely in trials of dipyridamole and appear to occur most often in patients taking concomitant beta-blockers.[2,3]

RELATED DRUGS: This interaction is expected to occur with all beta-blockers. A similar interaction is expected with adenosine (eg, *Adenocard*) and beta-blockers.

MANAGEMENT OPTIONS:

➡ *Circumvent/Minimize.* Discontinuation of atenolol or other beta-blockers before the administration of dipyridamole may be the most appropriate approach.

➡ *Monitor.* Because of the potentially serious outcome of this interaction, carefully observe patients taking beta-blockers or other drugs known to have negative chronotropic or dromotropic effects for signs of bradycardia following dipyridamole injections.

REFERENCES:

1. Roach PJ, et al. Asystole and bradycardia during dipyridamole stress testing in patients receiving beta blockers. *Int J Cardiol*. 1993;42(1):92-94.
2. Blumenthal MS, et al. Cardiac arrest during dipyridamole imaging. *Chest*. 1988;93(5):1103-1104.
3. Picano E, et al. Safety of intravenous high-dose dipyridamole echocardiography. The Echo-Persantine International Cooperative Study Group. *Am J Cardiol*. 1992;70(2):252-258.

Atenolol (eg, *Tenormin*)

Fingolimod (*Gilenya*)

SUMMARY: The combined administration of fingolimod and atenolol may lead to bradycardia.

RISK FACTORS: No specific risk factors are known.

MECHANISM: Both fingolimod and atenolol can reduce heart rate; an additive effect may be seen.

CLINICAL EVALUATION: Twenty-five healthy subjects were administered a single oral dose of fingolimod 5 mg alone, atenolol 50 mg daily for 5 days, or fingolimod on day 5 of the atenolol administration.[1] The combination of fingolimod plus atenolol resulted in a 15% lower heart rate than that observed with fingolimod alone.

Because the effect of fingolimod on heart rate is greatest during the first month of therapy with fingolimod, be alert for this interaction following the initiation of fingolimod therapy.

RELATED DRUGS: Other beta-blockers are likely to have an effect similar to that reported with atenolol. Bradycardia or heart block may occur if other drugs that have a negative chronotropic or dromotropic effect (amiodarone [eg, *Cordarone*], diltiazem [eg, *Cardizem*], verapamil [eg, *Calan*]) are coadministered.[2]

MANAGEMENT OPTIONS:

➡ *Monitor.* In patients taking fingolimod and drugs known to slow the heart rate or atrioventricular conduction, monitor for bradycardia, particularly during the first month of fingolimod administration.

REFERENCES:

1. Kovarik JM, et al. The effect on heart rate of combining single-dose fingolimod with steady-state atenolol or diltiazem in healthy subjects. *Eur J Clin Pharmacol*. 2008;64(5):457-463.

2. *Gilenya* [package insert]. East Hanover, NJ: Novartis Pharmaceuticals Corporation; 2010.

Atenolol (eg, *Tenormin*)

Orlistat (eg, *Xenical*)

SUMMARY: The administration of atenolol with orlistat had no effect on the pharmacokinetics of atenolol.

RISK FACTORS: No specific risk factors are known.

MECHANISM: No interaction.

CLINICAL EVALUATION: A single dose of atenolol 100 mg was administered alone and after 7 days of orlistat 50 mg 3 times daily to 6 healthy subjects.[1] The orlistat was taken during meals. Atenolol peak concentrations, half-life, and area under the concentration-time curve were unchanged by orlistat administration. No changes in blood pressure, pulse rate, or electrocardiogram were noted.

RELATED DRUGS: The effect of orlistat with other beta-blockers is unknown.

MANAGEMENT OPTIONS: No interaction.

REFERENCES:

1. Weber C, et al. Effect of the lipase inhibitor orlistat on the pharmacokinetics of four different antihypertensive drugs in healthy volunteers. *Eur J Clin Pharmacol*. 1996;51(1):87-90.

Atenolol (eg, *Tenormin*)

Propantheline

SUMMARY: Anticholinergic drugs can block beta-blocker–induced bradycardia and may increase atenolol concentrations.

RISK FACTORS: No specific risk factors are known.

MECHANISM: Anticholinergic agents can increase the heart rate and may increase atenolol bioavailability, possibly by slowing GI motility.

CLINICAL EVALUATION: In 6 healthy subjects, atenolol 100 mg orally was given with and without propantheline 30 mg orally 1.5 hours before atenolol.[1] Propantheline slowed the absorption rate of atenolol, but atenolol bioavailability increased 36%.

If this effect is sustained under conditions of multiple dosing, expect the atenolol response to be enhanced. However, this has not been studied.

RELATED DRUGS: The bradycardiac effects of other beta-blockers also may be reduced by propantheline.

MANAGEMENT OPTIONS: No specific action is required, but be alert for evidence of the interaction.

REFERENCES:

1. Regardh CG, et al. The effect of antacid, metoclopramide, and propantheline on the bioavailability of metoprolol and atenolol. *Biopharm Drug Dispos*. 1981;2(1):79-87.

Atenolol (eg, *Tenormin*)

Rifampin (eg, *Rifadin*)

SUMMARY: Rifampin reduces the plasma concentrations of atenolol; some patients may experience an increase in blood pressure or angina.

RISK FACTORS: No significant risk factors are known.

MECHANISM: Rifampin increases the renal excretion of atenolol.

CLINICAL EVALUATION: Nine healthy volunteers received a single dose of atenolol 100 mg following 5 days of placebo or rifampin 600 mg daily.[1] The mean area under the plasma concentration-time curve of atenolol was reduced approximately 20% following rifampin. Atenolol renal clearance was increased approximately 10% during rifampin administration. The reduction in heart rate and diastolic blood pressure observed following atenolol and placebo was significantly blunted after rifampin pretreatment. In another report, a patient with angina reported decreased exercise tolerance when rifampin was added to his regimen.[2]

RELATED DRUGS: None known.

MANAGEMENT OPTIONS:

➡ *Monitor.* Monitor patients taking atenolol for reduced therapeutic effect if rifampin is coadministered.

REFERENCES:

1. Lilja JJ, et al. Effect of rifampicin on the pharmacokinetics of atenolol. *Basic Clin Pharmacol Toxicol*. 2006;98(6):555-558.
2. Goldberg SV, et al. Rifamycin treatment of tuberculosis in a patient receiving atenolol: less interaction with rifabutin than with rifampin. *Clin Infect Dis*. 2003;37(4):607-608.

Atenolol (eg, *Tenormin*)

Rivastigmine (eg, *Exelon*)

SUMMARY: The combination of atenolol and rivastigmine may produce bradycardia and atrioventricular block in susceptible patients. Any other combination of a beta-adrenergic blocker and a cholinesterase inhibitor may produce a similar effect.

RISK FACTORS: No specific risk factors are known.

MECHANISM: Rivastigmine and other cholinesterase inhibitors increase vagal tone, predisposing to bradycardia. Atenolol and other beta-adrenergic blockers also slow the heart rate, and the effects may be additive.

CLINICAL EVALUATION: A 65-year-old woman taking atenolol and rivastigmine was admitted with a history of syncope.[1] She developed episodes of bradycardia (heart rates in the low 40s), but after discontinuation of both drugs her bradycardia resolved. It is possible that the bradycardia was due to either drug alone, because bradycardia and atrioventricular block have been reported with rivastigmine alone.[2] Nonetheless, given the ability of beta-blockers to slow the heart rate, it is likely that atenolol contributed to the reaction. Also, the French Pharmacovigilance Database received 83 spontaneous reports of adverse effects in patients receiving beta-blockers and cholinesterase inhibitors (donepezil, galantamine, rivastigmine).[3] After evaluation by clinical pharmacologists, 33 were thought to be adverse drug interactions. Of the 73 patients who received cholinesterase inhibitors along with beta-blockers or other bradycardic drugs, 5 deaths were due to syncope, bradycardia, arrhythmias, or cardiac arrest. Although additional study is needed to establish the clinical importance of these interactions, the potential severity of the reactions dictates caution.

RELATED DRUGS: All beta-blockers are expected to interact similarly with rivastigmine, including acebutolol (eg, *Sectral*), betaxolol (eg, *Kerlone*), bisoprolol (eg, *Zebeta*), esmolol (eg, *Brevibloc*), carteolol, carvedilol (eg, *Coreg*), labetalol (eg, *Trandate*), levobunolol (eg, *Betagan*), metoprolol (eg, *Lopressor*), nadolol (eg, *Corgard*), nebivolol (*Bystolic*), penbutolol (*Levatol*), pindolol, propranolol (eg, *Inderal*), sotalol (eg, *Betapace*), and timolol (eg, *Betimol*). All of these beta-blockers are also expected to interact with the other cholinesterase inhibitors, such as donepezil (eg, *Aricept*) and galantamine (eg, *Razadyne*).

MANAGEMENT OPTIONS:

➡ *Consider Alternative.* If appropriate, use an alternative to either the cholinesterase inhibitor or the beta-blocker.

➡ *Circumvent/Minimize.* In patients who require both drugs, the interaction has been circumvented in some cases by inserting a cardiac pacemaker.

➡ *Monitor.* If the combination is used, monitor for bradycardia, hypotension, and syncope.

REFERENCES:

1. Paulison B, Léos CL. Potential cardiotoxic reaction involving rivastigmine and beta-blockers: a case report and a review of the literature. *Cardiovasc Toxicol.* 2010;10(4):306-310.

2. Kayrak M, et al. Complete atrioventricular block associated with rivastigmine therapy. *Am J Health Syst Pharm.* 2008;65(11):1051-1053.

3. Tavassoli N, et al. Drug interactions with cholinesterase inhibitors: an analysis of the French Pharmacovigilance Database and a comparison of two national drug formularies (Vidal, British National Formulary). *Drug Saf.* 2007;30(11):1063-1071.

4   Atenolol (eg, *Tenormin*)

Tamsulosin (*Flomax*)

SUMMARY: Tamsulosin does not appear to affect the antihypertensive response to atenolol.

RISK FACTORS: No specific risk factors are known.

MECHANISM: Theoretically, additive hypotension could occur, but does not appear to be a problem clinically.

CLINICAL EVALUATION: Eight hypertensive subjects stabilized on atenolol for at least 3 months were given tamsulosin 0.4 mg/day for 7 days followed by 0.8 mg/day for 7 days.[1] According to the manufacturer, tamsulosin did not produce any clinically significant effects on blood pressure or pulse rate compared with placebo.

RELATED DRUGS: Tamsulosin did not affect hypotensive response to nifedipine (eg, *Adalat*) or enalapril.

MANAGEMENT OPTIONS: No specific action is required, but be alert for evidence of the interaction.

REFERENCES:
1. *Flomax* [package insert]. Ridgefield, CT: Boehringer Ingelheim; 2009.

Atenolol (eg, *Tenormin*)

Valsartan (*Diovan*)

SUMMARY: A 40-year-old pregnant woman taking valsartan and atenolol miscarried at 33 weeks' gestation; it is possible that the drugs played a role in the fetal death.

RISK FACTORS: No specific risk factors are known.

MECHANISM: Valsartan, like angiotensin-converting enzyme inhibitors, may compromise fetal renal perfusion, resulting in pulmonary hypoplasia. Beta-blockers have been associated with placental hypoplasia.

CLINICAL EVALUATION: A 40-year-old woman on valsartan and atenolol became pregnant. The valsartan was discontinued at 24 weeks' gestation, when the pregnancy was diagnosed, but fetal death was documented at 33 weeks' gestation.[1] The fetus had small, hypoplastic lungs and an extremely small placenta. The combined effects of valsartan and atenolol may have contributed to the fetal death.

RELATED DRUGS: Theoretically, other combinations of angiotensin II receptor antagonists and beta-blockers could also result in fetal compromise.

MANAGEMENT OPTIONS:

➥ *Avoid Unless Benefit Outweighs Risk.* If possible, avoid use of angiotensin II receptor antagonists and beta-blockers in pregnant women.

REFERENCES:
1. Briggs GG, et al. Fatal fetal outcome with the combined use of valsartan and atenolol. *Ann Pharmacother*. 2001;35(7-8):859-861.

Atenolol (eg, *Tenormin*)

Warfarin (eg, *Coumadin*)

SUMMARY: Atenolol, bisoprolol, and metoprolol appear to have no effect on the response to warfarin or acenocoumarol.

RISK FACTORS: No specific risk factors are known.

MECHANISM: No interaction.

CLINICAL EVALUATION: In 6 healthy subjects, single doses of warfarin 15 mg were given alone or after 3 days of propranolol 80 mg twice daily, metoprolol (eg, *Lopressor*) 100 mg twice daily, or atenolol 100 mg/day.[1] Metoprolol and atenolol had no significant effect on the warfarin area under the concentration-time curve. Metoprolol 100 mg twice daily or atenolol 100 mg/day were administered to 5 patients on chronic acenocoumarol[†] for 3 weeks.[2] No changes in prothrombin times were observed. Bisoprolol (eg, *Zebeta*) 10 mg/day for 10 days did not affect the hypo-prothrombinemic response to warfarin in 12 healthy men.[3] Atenolol did not inter-act with phenprocoumon in 1 report.[4]

RELATED DRUGS: The effect of other beta-adrenergic blockers on oral anticoagulants has not been established.

MANAGEMENT OPTIONS: No interaction.

REFERENCES:

1. Bax ND, et al. The effect of beta-adrenoceptor antagonists on the pharmacokinetics and pharmacody-namics of warfarin. *Br J Clin Pharmacol.* 1984;17(suppl 1):85S.

2. Mantero F, et al. Effect of atenolol and metoprolol on the anticoagulant activity of acenocoumarin. *Br J Clin Pharmacol.* 1984;17(suppl 1):94S-96S.

3. Warrington SJ, et al. Bisoprolol: studies of potential interactions with theophylline and warfarin in healthy volunteers. *J Cardiovasc Pharmacol.* 1990;16(suppl 5):S164-S168.

4. Spahn H, et al. Pharmacokinetic and pharmacodynamic interactions between phenprocoumon and atenolol or metoprolol. *Br J Clin Pharmacol.* 1984;17(suppl 1):97S-102S.

† Not available in the United States.

 Atevirdine[†]

Fluconazole (eg, *Diflucan*)

SUMMARY: Fluconazole administration causes an increase in the serum concentration of atevirdine; the clinical signifi-cance of this is unknown.

RISK FACTORS: No specific risk factors are known.

MECHANISM: Fluconazole may inhibit the metabolism of atevirdine or increase its bio-availability.

CLINICAL EVALUATION: The effects of fluconazole 400 mg/day administered for several weeks on the kinetics of atevirdine were studied in patients with HIV.[1] Compared with administration alone, fluconazole reduced the clearance of orally adminis-tered atevirdine 39%. The clinical significance of this change is unknown.

RELATED DRUGS: Other imidazole antifungal agents (eg, itraconazole [eg, *Sporanox*], keto-conazole [eg, *Nizoral*]) may interact in a similar manner with atevirdine.

MANAGEMENT OPTIONS:

➡ *Monitor.* Until further information is available, monitor patients receiving atevird-ine who are prescribed fluconazole for increased atevirdine levels.

REFERENCES:

1. Borin MT, et al. The effect of fluconazole (FLU) on the pharmacokinetics of atevirdine mesylate (ATV) in HIV+ patients. *Clin Pharmacol Ther.* 1994;55(2):193.

† Not available in the United States.

Atomoxetine (*Strattera*)

Tranylcypromine (eg, *Parnate*) AVOID

SUMMARY: Combined use of atomoxetine and tranylcypromine is contraindicated.

RISK FACTORS: No specific risk factors are known.

MECHANISM: Not established. The interaction is based on the theoretical risk of giving a drug that inhibits the presynaptic norepinephrine transporter (atomoxetine) along with a nonselective monoamine oxidase inhibitor (MAOI) that increases norepinephrine stores in neurons (tranylcypromine).

CLINICAL EVALUATION: Although the interaction is based on theoretical considerations, the potential severity of the reaction indicates that the combination be avoided. The manufacturer of atomoxetine lists MAOIs as absolutely contraindicated with atomoxetine.[1]

RELATED DRUGS: Atomoxetine is also contraindicated with other nonselective MAOIs, such as isocarboxazid (*Marplan*) and phenelzine (*Nardil*).

MANAGEMENT OPTIONS:

➠ *AVOID COMBINATION.* Do not coadminister atomoxetine with tranylcypromine or other nonselective MAOIs. Discontinue either the atomoxetine or the MAOI for 2 weeks before the other drug is given.

REFERENCES:

1. *Strattera* [package insert]. Indianapolis, IN: Eli Lilly and Company; 2004.

Atorvastatin (*Lipitor*)

Azithromycin (eg, *Zithromax*)

SUMMARY: No interaction.

RISK FACTORS: No specific risk factors are known.

MECHANISM: No interaction.

CLINICAL EVALUATION: Twelve healthy subjects received atorvastatin 10 mg/day for 8 days.[1] On days 6 to 8, azithromycin 500 mg/day was added. The mean area under the atorvastatin concentration-time curve, peak plasma concentration, and time to peak concentration were unchanged following 3 days of azithromycin dosing.

RELATED DRUGS: Clarithromycin (eg, *Biaxin*) and erythromycin (eg, *Ery-Tab*) are known to reduce the metabolism of atorvastatin. Azithromycin is unlikely to alter the pharmacokinetics of any of the statin drugs including fluvastatin (*Lescol*), lovastatin (eg, *Mevacor*), pravastatin (eg, *Pravachol*), rosuvastatin (*Crestor*), or simvastatin (eg, *Zocor*).

MANAGEMENT OPTIONS: No interaction.

REFERENCES:

1. Amsden GW, et al. A study of the interaction potential of azithromycin and clarithromycin with atorvastatin in healthy volunteers. *J Clin Pharmacol.* 2002;42(4):444-449.

5   Atorvastatin (*Lipitor*)

Cimetidine (eg, *Tagamet*)

SUMMARY: Cimetidine does not affect atorvastatin pharmacokinetics or pharmacodynamics.

RISK FACTORS: No specific risk factors are known.

MECHANISM: No interaction.

CLINICAL EVALUATION: In a randomized crossover study, 12 healthy subjects received atorvastatin (10 mg/day for 2 weeks) with and without concurrent cimetidine 300 mg 4 times/day.[1] Cimetidine had no effect on atorvastatin pharmacokinetics or on atorvastatin-induced reduction of LDL-cholesterol. These findings are consistent with the fact that cimetidine has little effect on CYP3A4, the isozyme primarily responsible for the metabolism of atorvastatin.

RELATED DRUGS: Famotidine (eg, *Pepcid*), nizatidine (eg, *Axid*), and ranitidine (eg, *Zantac*) theoretically are unlikely to interact with atorvastatin; however, clinical studies are needed.

MANAGEMENT OPTIONS: No interaction.

REFERENCES:
1. Stern RH, et al. Cimetidine does not alter atorvastatin pharmacokinetics or LDL-cholesterol reduction. *Eur J Clin Pharmacol.* 1998;53(6):475-478.

Atorvastatin (*Lipitor*)

Clarithromycin (eg, *Biaxin*)

SUMMARY: Clarithromycin increases atorvastatin plasma concentrations; an increase in effects and possibly adverse reactions may occur.

RISK FACTORS: No specific risk factors are known.

MECHANISM: Clarithromycin inhibits the activity of the enzyme (CYP3A4) known to metabolize atorvastatin, resulting in increased plasma concentrations.

CLINICAL EVALUATION: Twelve healthy subjects received atorvastatin 10 mg/day for 8 days.[1] On days 6 to 8, clarithromycin 500 mg/day was added. The mean area under the atorvastatin concentration-time curve and peak atorvastatin plasma concentration increased 81% and 56%, respectively, following the addition of clarithromycin. It is possible that a longer duration of clarithromycin administration would increase the magnitude of its effects on atorvastatin plasma concentrations. While an increased antihyperlipidemic effect of atorvastatin might be seen during coadministration with clarithromycin, an occasional patient may experience added adverse reactions.

RELATED DRUGS: Erythromycin (eg, *Ery-Tab*) is known to reduce the metabolism of atorvastatin. Azithromycin does not affect the metabolism of atorvastatin. Clarithromycin is likely to reduce the metabolism of lovastatin (eg, *Mevacor*) and simvastatin (eg, *Zocor*), resulting in elevated plasma concentrations.

MANAGEMENT OPTIONS:

➡ *Circumvent/Minimize.* During treatment with clarithromycin, withholding atorvastatin dosing may avoid any potential adverse reactions.

➡ *Monitor.* Monitor for any evidence of atorvastatin adverse reactions, such as myopathy, during the coadministration of clarithromycin.

REFERENCES:

1. Amsden GW, et al. A study of the interaction potential of azithromycin and clarithromycin with atorvastatin in healthy volunteers. *J Clin Pharmacol.* 2002;42(4):444-449.

Atorvastatin (*Lipitor*)

Clopidogrel (*Plavix*)

SUMMARY: Atorvastatin may inhibit the antiplatelet effects of clopidogrel, but it is not known if the therapeutic effect is reduced.

RISK FACTORS: No specific risk factors are known.

MECHANISM: Clopidogrel is a prodrug, and CYP3A4 appears to be the primary isozyme involved in formation of the active metabolite.[1] In vitro studies showed atorvastatin substantially inhibited the metabolism of clopidogrel, presumably through inhibition of CYP3A4. Pravastatin (*Pravachol*) is not a substrate or inhibitor of cytochrome P450 isozymes and does not appear to interact.

CLINICAL EVALUATION: The effect of clopidogrel on platelet aggregation was studied in 44 patients undergoing coronary artery stent implantation.[2] Nineteen patients were also taking atorvastatin (10, 20, or 40 mg/day), 9 were taking pravastatin (40 mg/day), and 16 were not taking a statin. Atorvastatin therapy was associated with a dose-dependent reduction in the ability of clopidogrel to inhibit platelet aggregation. With clopidogrel alone, platelet aggregation was 34%, but with 10, 20, and 40 mg/day of atorvastatin, platelet aggregation increased to 58%, 74%, and 89% of control, respectively. Thus, 40 mg/day of atorvastatin almost completely reversed the antiplatelet effects of clopidogrel. Conversely, another study of 25 patients receiving clopidogrel found no effect of statins on the ability of clopidogrel to inhibit platelet aggregation.[3] Of the 25 patients, 9 were receiving atorvastatin, 6 were receiving fluvastatin (*Lescol*), 4 were receiving pravastatin, 3 were receiving cerivastatin, 2 were receiving lovastatin (eg, *Mevacor*), and 1 was receiving simvastatin (*Zocor*). The authors stated that "analysis according to individual statin use" also did not reveal any effect of statins on clopidogrel, although no data were presented. Another study in 77 patients taking low-dose aspirin also failed to find any effect of any statin (atorvastatin, fluvastatin, lovastatin, pravastatin, simvastatin) on the antiplatelet effect of a high loading dose (600 mg) of clopidogrel.[4] Finally, atorvastatin had no effect on the antiplatelet effect or therapeutic efficacy of clopidogrel in a study of 45 patients with acute coronary syndromes.[5] Additional study is needed to determine if this interaction is clinically important, ideally with assessment of clinical outcome rather than just platelet aggregation. Pravastatin did not affect the antiplatelet activity of clopidogrel.[2]

RELATED DRUGS: No information is available.

MANAGEMENT OPTIONS: No specific action is required, but be alert for evidence of the interaction.

REFERENCES:

1. Clarke TA, et al. The metabolism of clopidogrel is catalyzed by human cytochrome P450 3A and is inhibited by atorvastatin. *Drug Metab Dispos.* 2003;31:53-59.

2. Lau WC, et al. Atorvastatin reduces the ability of clopidogrel to inhibit platelet aggregation: a new drug-drug interaction. *Circulation.* 2003;107:32-37.

3. Serebruany VL, et al. Statins do not affect platelet inhibition with clopidogrel during coronary stenting. *Atherosclerosis.* 2001;159:239-241.

4. Muller I, et al. Effects of statins on platelet inhibition by a high loading dose of clopidogrel. *Circulation.* 2003;108:2195-2197.

5. Mitsios JV, et al. Atorvastatin does not affect the antiplatelet potency of clopidogrel when it is administered concomitantly for 5 weeks in patients with acute coronary syndromes. *Circulation.* 2004;109:1335-1338.

4 — Atorvastatin (*Lipitor*)

Cyclosporine (eg, *Neoral*)

SUMMARY: Cyclosporine increases atorvastatin concentrations, and 1 patient on cyclosporine developed rhabdomyolysis after starting atorvastatin; monitor for evidence of skeletal muscle damage.

RISK FACTORS: Not established. Cyclosporine may inhibit the hepatic uptake of atorvastatin by transporters, such as OATP-C, and also may inhibit the metabolism of atorvastatin by CYP3A4.

MECHANISM: Not established. It is possible that cyclosporine increases atorvastatin plasma concentrations through inhibition of CYP3A4, P-glycoprotein, or other transport protein.

CLINICAL EVALUATION: A 40-year-old woman received a renal transplant 4 years earlier and was on chronic therapy with cyclosporine 125 mg/day in addition to azathioprine (eg, *Imuran*), diltiazem (eg, *Cardizem*), furosemide (eg, *Lasix*), prednisone (eg, *Deltasone*), and multivitamins.[1] Two months after starting atorvastatin 10 mg/day, she developed nausea, diarrhea, muscle pain, and such extreme muscular weakness that she was unable to walk. Her creatine kinase was elevated at 1,846 units/L. She responded to hydration and discontinuation of atorvastatin. Although it is not possible to rule out the possibility that the myositis was caused by atorvastatin alone, it seems likely that the cyclosporine contributed. In addition, because diltiazem is a CYP3A4 inhibitor, it could have contributed to elevated atorvastatin serum concentrations.

A study in renal transplant patients found a 6-fold higher HMG-inhibitory activity of atorvastatin with concurrent cyclosporine therapy compared with historic controls without cyclosporine.[2] Another study in heart transplant patients found atorvastatin to be relatively safe when used in moderate doses (mean atorvastatin dose was about 20 mg/day).[3] Thus, some patients may be at higher risk of atorvastatin-induced myopathy if cyclosporine is given concurrently, but the risk can be mitigated somewhat by avoiding large doses of atorvastatin.

RELATED DRUGS: Cyclosporine can increase the serum concentrations of fluvastatin (*Lescol*), lovastatin (eg, *Mevacor*), pravastatin (eg, *Pravachol*), rosuvastatin (*Crestor*), and simvastatin (eg, *Zocor*), although the risk of adverse reactions appears to differ depending on the statin. Pravastatin, for example, is frequently used in transplant patients without evidence of adverse drug interactions.

MANAGEMENT OPTIONS: No specific action is required, but be alert for evidence of the interaction.

REFERENCES:

1. Maltz HC, et al. Rhabdomyolysis associated with concomitant use of atorvastatin and cyclosporine. *Ann Pharmacother.* 1999;33:1176-1179.

2. Asberg A, et al. Bilateral pharmacokinetic interaction between cyclosporine A and atorvastatin in renal transplant recipients. *Am J Transplant.* 2001;1:382-386.

3. Patel DN, et al. Safety and efficacy of atorvastatin in heart transplant recipients. *J Heart Lung Transplant.* 2002;21:204-210.

Atorvastatin (*Lipitor*)

Digoxin (eg, *Lanoxin*)

SUMMARY: Atorvastatin administration produces a small increase in digoxin concentrations; toxicity is unlikely.

RISK FACTORS: No specific risk factors are known.

MECHANISM: Not established.

CLINICAL EVALUATION: While no published data are available for evaluation, the manufacturer of atorvastatin has made some information on the interaction available.[1] Multiple-dose regimens of atorvastatin (dose not stated) increased steady-state digoxin concentrations about 20%. In most patients, this magnitude of change in digoxin concentration is unlikely to produce any clinically noticeable effects.

RELATED DRUGS: Fluvastatin (*Lescol*) and pravastatin (eg, *Pravachol*) appear to have minimal effects on digoxin plasma concentrations.[2,3]

MANAGEMENT OPTIONS: No specific action is required, but be alert for evidence of the interaction.

REFERENCES:

1. *Lipitor* [package insert]. New York, NY: Pfizer; 1997.

2. Triscari J, et al. Steady state concentrations of pravastatin and digoxin when given in combination. *Br J Clin Pharmacol.* 1993;36:263-265.

3. Garnett WR, et al. Pharmacokinetic effects of fluvastatin in patients chronically receiving digoxin. *Am J Med.* 1994;96:84S-86S.

Atorvastatin (*Lipitor*)

Efavirenz (*Sustiva*)

SUMMARY: Atorvastatin plasma concentrations are reduced during efavirenz coadministration; some reduction in the lipid-lowering effect of atorvastatin may occur.

RISK FACTORS: No specific risk factors are known.

MECHANISM: Efavirenz is an inducer of CYP3A4, the primary pathway of atorvastatin metabolism.

CLINICAL EVALUATION: Fourteen healthy subjects received atorvastatin 10 mg daily for 4 days both before and following 14 days of efavirenz 600 mg daily.[1] The mean area under the plasma concentration-time curve of atorvastatin following efavirenz was 42% lower than when the atorvastatin was administered alone. The low-density lipoprotein (LDL)-lowering effect of atorvastatin tended to be less following efavirenz pretreatment. Monitor patients requiring efavirenz therapy who are taking atorvastatin for reduced hypolipemic efficacy.

RELATED DRUGS: Nevirapine (*Viramune*) is also known to induce CYP3A4 and would be likely to reduce atorvastatin plasma concentrations. Lovastatin (eg, *Mevacor*) and simvastatin (eg, *Zocor*) would probably be affected in a similar manner.

MANAGEMENT OPTIONS:

➡ *Consider Alternative.* Ezetimibe (*Zetia*) is not known to be affected by CYP3A4 inducers.

➡ *Monitor.* Monitor LDL concentrations in patients stabilized on atorvastatin following the addition or discontinuation of efavirenz.

REFERENCES:

1. Gerber JG, et al. Effect of efavirenz on the pharmacokinetics of simvastatin, atorvastatin, and pravastatin: results of AIDS Clinical Trials Group 5108 Study. *J Acquir Immune Defic Syndr.* 2005;39:307-312.

Atorvastatin (*Lipitor*)

Erythromycin (eg, *Ery-Tab*)

SUMMARY: Erythromycin increases atorvastatin plasma concentrations; an increase in effect and adverse reactions may occur.

RISK FACTORS: No specific risk factors are known.

MECHANISM: Erythromycin inhibits the activity of the enzyme (CYP3A4) known to metabolize atorvastatin, resulting in increased plasma concentrations.

CLINICAL EVALUATION: Eleven healthy subjects received a single dose of atorvastatin 10 mg before and on day 8 of an 11-day regimen of erythromycin 500 mg 4 times/day.[1] The mean area under the atorvastatin concentration-time curve and peak atorvastatin plasma concentration increased 33% and 38%, respectively, following the addition of erythromycin. While an increased antihyperlipidemic effect of atorvastatin might be seen during coadministration with erythromycin, added adverse reactions also may be experienced.

RELATED DRUGS: Clarithromycin (eg, *Biaxin*) is known to reduce the metabolism of atorvastatin. Azithromycin does not affect the metabolism of atorvastatin. Erythromycin is likely to reduce the metabolism of lovastatin (eg, *Mevacor*) and simvastatin (eg, *Zocor*), resulting in elevated plasma concentrations.

MANAGEMENT OPTIONS:

➡ *Circumvent/Minimize.* During treatment with erythromycin, withholding atorvastatin may avoid any potential adverse reactions.

➡ *Monitor.* Monitor patients for any evidence of atorvastatin adverse reactions, such as myopathy, during coadministration of erythromycin.

REFERENCES:

1. Siedlik PH, et al. Erythromycin coadministration increases plasma atorvastatin concentrations. *J Clin Pharmacol.* 1999;39(5):501-504.

Atorvastatin (*Lipitor*)

Etravirine (*Intelence*)

SUMMARY: The coadministration of atorvastatin and etravirine reduced the plasma concentration of atorvastatin. Some reduction in atorvastatin lipid-lowering effect may occur.

RISK FACTORS: No specific risk factors are known.

MECHANISM: Etravirine appears to increase the metabolism of atorvastatin via CYP3A4.

CLINICAL EVALUATION: While specific data are limited, the manufacturer of etravirine notes that the coadministration of etravirine 800 mg twice daily and atorvastatin 40 mg daily resulted in an approximate 40% decrease in the mean area under the plasma concentration-time curve (AUC) of atorvastatin.[1] Atorvastatin administration did not alter the AUC of etravirine. Pending further data, monitor patients receiving etravirine and atorvastatin for reduced atorvastatin response.

RELATED DRUGS: Lovastatin (eg, *Mevacor*) and simvastatin (eg, *Zocor*) are also metabolized by CYP3A4 and are likely to interact with etravirine in a similar manner.

MANAGEMENT OPTIONS:

➡ **Monitor.** Monitor patients taking etravirine and atorvastatin for reduced atorvastatin response.

REFERENCES:
1. *Intelence* [package insert]. Raritan, NJ: Tibotec Therapeutics; 2008.

Atorvastatin (*Lipitor*)

Gemfibrozil (eg, *Lopid*)

SUMMARY: Gemfibrozil increases the plasma concentrations of atorvastatin; increased risk of myopathy may result.

RISK FACTORS: No specific risk factors are known.

MECHANISM: Gemfibrozil inhibits the organic anion-transporting polypeptide (OATP1B1) that is partially responsible for the uptake of atorvastatin into hepatic cells. Reduced cellular uptake limits the ability of hepatic enzymes to metabolize atorvastatin.

CLINICAL EVALUATION: Ten healthy subjects received a single dose of atorvastatin 20 mg on day 3 of a 5-day regimen of gemfibrozil 600 mg or placebo twice daily.[1] The mean area under the concentration-time curve of atorvastatin was increased 24% during gemfibrozil coadministration. Although this increase was rather modest, a case of muscle toxicity (myopathy and rhabdomyolysis) has been reported during combined atorvastatin and gemfibrozil administration.[2] Myopathy has been reported during monotherapy with atorvastatin and gemfibrozil.

RELATED DRUGS: Myopathy has also been reported following combined therapy with gemfibrozil and lovastatin (eg, *Mevacor*) or simvastatin (eg, *Zocor*).[3-5] Other statins have also been reported to produce muscle toxicity when used with gemfibrozil, although pravastatin and fluvastatin may be least likely to interact.

MANAGEMENT OPTIONS:

➡ *Monitor.* Monitor patients receiving gemfibrozil with atorvastatin or another HMG-CoA reductase inhibitor for evidence of myopathy such as muscle pain or weakness.

REFERENCES:

1. Backman JT, et al. Rifampin markedly decreases and gemfibrozil increases the plasma concentrations of atorvastatin and its metabolites. *Clin Pharm Ther*. 2005;78(2):154-167.

2. Duell PB, et al. Rhabdomyolysis after taking atorvastatin with gemfibrozil. *Am J Cardiol*. 1998;81(3):368-369.

3. Pierce LR, et al. Myopathy and rhabdomyolysis associated with lovastatin-gemfibrozil combination therapy. *JAMA*. 1990;264(1):71-75.

4. Tal A, et al. Rhabdomyolysis associated with simvastatin-gemfibrozil therapy. *South Med J*. 1997;90(5):546-547.

5. Federman DG, et al. Fatal rhabdomyolysis caused by lipid-lowering therapy. *South Med J*. 2001;94(10):1023-1026.

Atorvastatin (*Lipitor*)

Itraconazole (*Sporanox*)

SUMMARY: Itraconazole administration increases the serum concentration of atorvastatin; increased toxicity (myopathy) could result.

RISK FACTORS: No specific risk factors are known.

MECHANISM: Itraconazole is known to inhibit the activity of CYP3A4, the enzyme known to metabolize atorvastatin. This would result in a decrease in the systemic clearance of atorvastatin and an increase in its bioavailability because of reduced intestinal metabolism.

CLINICAL EVALUATION: Ten healthy subjects received itraconazole 200 mg or placebo every day for 5 days.[1] On the fourth day of itraconazole administration, a single atorvastatin dose (40 mg) was administered. The area under the concentration-time curve (AUC) of atorvastatin increased approximately 3-fold following itraconazole. The serum concentrations of 2 active hydroxy metabolites of atorvastatin were reduced. The AUC of atorvastatin plus its active metabolites was increased 1.6 times compared with placebo. The clinical significance of these increases is unknown; however, an increased risk of side effects such as myopathy cannot be ruled out.

RELATED DRUGS: Other antifungal drugs that inhibit CYP3A4 enzyme activities such as ketoconazole (eg, *Nizoral*) or fluconazole (*Diflucan*) would be expected to have a similar effect on atorvastatin. Itraconazole inhibits the metabolism of lovastatin (eg, *Mevacor*). Cerivastatin[†] and simvastatin (*Zocor*) are metabolized by CYP3A4 and would probably be affected by itraconazole. Pravastatin (*Pravachol*) and fluvastatin (*Lescol*) may be less likely to interact with itraconazole. Terbinafine (*Lamisil*) may have limited effect on the metabolism of HMG-CoA reductase inhibitors.

MANAGEMENT OPTIONS:

➡ *Circumvent/Minimize.* Pravastatin or fluvastatin can be administered to patients receiving itraconazole. Terbinafine may have a limited effect on HMG-CoA reductase inhibitors such as atorvastatin.

➡ **Monitor.** Monitor patients receiving atorvastatin and itraconazole for signs of myalgia and myopathy.

REFERENCES:
1. Kantola T, et al. Effect of itraconazole on the pharmacokinetics of atorvastatin. *Clin Pharmacol Ther.* 1998;64:58-65.

† Not available in the United States.

Atorvastatin (*Lipitor*)

Midazolam (eg, *Versed*)

SUMMARY: A parallel study suggested that atorvastatin may prolong the effect of midazolam, but the clinical importance of this effect is not established.

RISK FACTORS: Not established.

MECHANISM: Not established. Atorvastatin may impair the metabolism of midazolam.

CLINICAL EVALUATION: Seven patients on atorvastatin and 7 matched controls were given IV midazolam prior to elective surgery.[1] On average, the patients on atorvastatin developed 41% higher midazolam area under the plasma concentration-time curve. The magnitude of this increase would probably prolong the sedation and respiratory depression of midazolam. However, this was a parallel design study, and more research is needed to determine whether the interaction would result in adverse consequences.

RELATED DRUGS: No information is available.

MANAGEMENT OPTIONS: No specific action is required, but be alert for evidence of the interaction.

REFERENCES:
1. McDonnell CG, et al. The effects of concurrent atorvastatin therapy on the pharmacokinetics of intravenous midazolam. *Anaesthesia.* 2003;58:899-904.

Atorvastatin (*Lipitor*)

Nelfinavir (*Viracept*)

SUMMARY: Nelfinavir administration increases atorvastatin concentrations moderately; some patients may experience increased side effects.

RISK FACTORS: No specific risk factors are known.

MECHANISM: Nelfinavir may inhibit the activity of CYP3A4 or P-glycoprotein resulting in a decrease in the elimination of atorvastatin.

CLINICAL EVALUATION: Fifteen healthy subjects received atorvastatin 10 mg daily for 14 days. Nelfinavir 1,250 mg twice daily was then added, and both drugs were taken for an additional 14 days.[1] The coadministration of nelfinavir resulted in a mean increase in the atorvastatin area under the concentration-time curve of 74% (range, -3% to 361%) and a mean increase in atorvastatin's peak concentration of 122%. No significant changes in the cholesterol-lowering effects of atorvastatin were noted during the 2-week coadministration of nelfinavir. While no subjects experienced side effects thought to be related to increased atorvastatin concentrations, some patients might be at increased risk for myopathy.

RELATED DRUGS: Other protease inhibitors such as ritonavir (*Norvir*), amprenavir (*Agenerase*), indinavir (*Crixivan*), and saquinavir (eg, *Invirase*) would be expected to affect atorvastatin in a similar manner. The clearance of other statins that are metabolized by CYP3A4 would likely be reduced by nelfinavir. Lovastatin (eg, *Mevacor*) and simvastatin (*Zocor*) may be affected to a greater degree than atorvastatin because of their greater susceptibility to CYP3A4 inhibitors.

MANAGEMENT OPTIONS:

➡ *Consider Alternative.* Because pravastatin (*Pravachol*) and fluvastatin (*Lescol*) are not metabolized by CYP3A4, consider using 1 of these agents in patients taking protease inhibitors.

➡ *Monitor.* Monitor patients taking atorvastatin and protease inhibitors for side effects including myopathy and myoglobinuria. It would be advisable to begin with a low dose of atorvastatin and slowly titrate the dose to the desired response.

REFERENCES:

1. Hsyu PH, et al. Pharmacokinetic interactions between nelfinavir and 3-hydroxy-3-methylglutaryl coenzyme A reductase inhibitors atorvastatin and simvastatin. *Antimicrob Agents Chemother.* 2001;45:3445-3450.

Atorvastatin (*Lipitor*)

Orlistat (*Xenical*)

SUMMARY: Orlistat did not affect atorvastatin pharmacokinetics in healthy subjects.

RISK FACTORS: No specific risk factors are known.

MECHANISM: None (no interaction).

CLINICAL EVALUATION: In a randomized crossover study in 32 healthy subjects, orlistat (120 mg 3 times daily for 6 days) did not affect atorvastatin pharmacokinetics.[1]

RELATED DRUGS: *Xenical* product information states that orlistat does not affect the pharmacokinetics of pravastatin.

MANAGEMENT OPTIONS: No interaction.

REFERENCES:

1. Zhi J, et al. Pharmacokinetic evaluation of the possible interaction between selected concomitant medications and orlistat at steady state in healthy subjects. *J Clin Pharmacol.* 2002;42:1011-1019.

Atorvastatin (*Lipitor*)

Rifampin (eg, *Rifadin*)

SUMMARY: Rifampin reduces the plasma concentrations of atorvastatin; a reduction of atorvastatin's lipid-lowering effect may occur.

RISK FACTORS: No specific risk factors are known.

MECHANISM: Rifampin induces the CYP3A4 metabolism of atorvastatin.

CLINICAL EVALUATION: Ten healthy subjects received a single dose of atorvastatin 40 mg following rifampin 600 mg or placebo once daily for 5 days.[1] The mean area under the plasma concentration-time curve of atorvastatin was reduced 80% following rifampin. The mean half-life of atorvastatin was reduced from 10.3 to 2.7 hours by rifampin pretreatment. While this study did not evaluate the hypolipidemic effect of atorvastatin, rifampin coadministration is likely to markedly reduce the efficacy of atorvastatin.

RELATED DRUGS: Rifampin is known to reduce the plasma concentrations of simvastatin (eg, *Zocor*), fluvastatin (*Lescol*), and pravastatin (eg, *Pravachol*). The plasma concentrations of lovastatin (eg, *Mevacor*) and rosuvastatin (*Crestor*) also are likely to be reduced by rifampin. Rifabutin (*Mycobutin*) may lower atorvastatin plasma concentrations.

MANAGEMENT OPTIONS:

➥ *Consider Alternative.* Based on available data, rifampin appears to affect pravastatin less than other statin drugs. However, monitor for possible reduced pravastatin efficacy and adjust dose as necessary. Rifabutin may affect atorvastatin in a similar manner.

➥ *Monitor.* Monitor patients taking atorvastatin for a reduction in lipid-lowering effect if rifampin is coadministered. Atorvastatin doses may need to be increased.

REFERENCES:
1. Backman JT, et al. Rifampin markedly decreases and gemfibrozil increases the plasma concentrations of atorvastatin and its metabolites. *Clin Pharmacol Ther.* 2005;78(2):154-167.

Atorvastatin (*Lipitor*)

Telaprevir (*Incivek*)

SUMMARY: The coadministration of telaprevir increases the plasma concentration of atorvastatin; adverse reactions, including weakness or muscle pain, may be more likely to occur.

RISK FACTORS: No specific risk factors are known.

MECHANISM: Telaprevir inhibits the CYP3A4-mediated metabolism and P-glycoprotein elimination of atorvastatin

CLINICAL EVALUATION: While specific data are limited, the manufacturer of telaprevir notes that the administration of telaprevir 750 mg every 8 hours for 7 days increased the mean area under the plasma concentration-time curve of atorvastatin by approximately 8-fold.[1] Pending further data, observe patients receiving telaprevir and atorvastatin for atorvastatin adverse reactions.

RELATED DRUGS: Atazanavir (*Reyataz*), darunavir (*Prezista*), fosamprenavir (*Lexiva*), indinavir (*Crixivan*), nelfinavir (*Viracept*), and saquinavir (*Invirase*) also inhibit the activity of CYP3A4 and are expected to increase the plasma concentrations of atorvastatin. Telaprevir is likely to produce marked increases the plasma concentration of simvastatin (eg, *Zocor*) and lovastatin (eg, *Mevacor*).

MANAGEMENT OPTIONS:

➥ *Avoid Unless Benefit Outweighs Risk.* Generally avoid the coadministration of telaprevir with atorvastatin, simvastatin, or lovastatin.

➡ **Monitor.** Monitor patients stabilized on atorvastatin for adverse reactions if telaprevir is coadministered.

REFERENCES:

1. *Incivek* [package insert]. Cambridge, MA: Vertex Pharmaceuticals; 2011.

Atorvastatin (*Lipitor*)

Tipranavir (*Aptivus*)

SUMMARY: The long-term administration of tipranavir plus ritonavir resulted in a large increase in atorvastatin plasma concentrations; some increase in the risk of atorvastatin toxicity may be experienced.

RISK FACTORS: No specific risk factors are known.

MECHANISM: The ritonavir component of tipranavir and ritonavir therapy is known to inhibit the enzyme (CYP3A4) primarily responsible for the metabolism of atorvastatin.

CLINICAL EVALUATION: A single dose of atorvastatin 40 mg was administered alone, and a 10 mg dose was administered after 20 days of tipranavir 500 mg and ritonavir 200 mg twice daily.[1] The mean dose-adjusted area under the plasma concentration-time curve of atorvastatin was increased more than 9-fold by the tipranavir and ritonavir combination. Anticipate an increase in atorvastatin adverse reactions.

RELATED DRUGS: Lovastatin (eg, *Mevacor*) and simvastatin (eg, *Zocor*) are also metabolized by CYP3A4 and are likely to have a very large increase in their plasma concentrations if administered with tipranavir. The labeling for tipranavir recommends not using lovastatin or simvastatin in patients receiving tipranavir.[1] Atorvastatin plasma concentrations may be elevated by other protease inhibitors, such as indinavir (*Crixivan*), saquinavir (*Invirase*), and nelfinavir (*Viracept*).

MANAGEMENT OPTIONS:

➡ **Consider Alternative.** Theoretically, pravastatin (eg, *Pravachol*) and possibly rosuvastatin (*Crestor*) or fluvastatin (*Lescol*) are less likely to interact with tipranavir.

➡ **Monitor.** Monitor patients treated with atorvastatin and tipranavir with ritonavir for signs of muscle pain or weakness.

REFERENCES:

1. *Aptivus* [package insert]. Ridgefield, CT: Boehringer Ingelheim Pharmaceuticals, Inc; 2007.

Atorvastatin (*Lipitor*)

Verapamil (eg, *Calan*)

SUMMARY: Atorvastatin coadministered with verapamil produces a modest increase in verapamil plasma concentrations; some patients may experience increased verapamil effects.

RISK FACTORS: No specific risk factors are known.

MECHANISM: Atorvastatin appears to increase the relative bioavailability of verapamil via inhibition of CYP3A4, P-glycoprotein (P-gp), or both.

CLINICAL EVALUATION: Twelve healthy subjects received a single dose of verapamil 60 mg alone or with a single dose of atorvastatin 40 mg.[1] The mean area under the concentration-time curve (AUC) of verapamil was increased 43% and its peak concentration 22% when atorvastatin was coadministered. Although no half-life values were provided for verapamil, it appears that most of the change in its AUC was due to an increase in bioavailability instead of a reduction in its systemic clearance. No change in heart rate or blood pressure was noted during concomitant dosing. Because of the single-dose study design, clinical significance will need to be assessed during long-term administration of both drugs. Because the mechanism of this interaction may be caused by competition for CYP3A4 or P-gp, separation of the doses may reduce the magnitude of the interaction. No data were provided on the potential effect of verapamil on atorvastatin.

RELATED DRUGS: The effect of other statins on verapamil is unknown. A similar interaction may be expected for statins that are substrates for CYP3A4 and P-gp. Verapamil has been reported to reduce the metabolism of simvastatin.

MANAGEMENT OPTIONS:

➡ *Monitor.* Monitor patients stabilized on verapamil for changes in heart rate or blood pressure if atorvastatin is initiated or discontinued .

REFERENCES:

1. Choi DH, et al. Drug interaction between oral atorvastatin and verapamil in healthy subjects: effects of atorvastatin on the pharmacokinetics of verapamil and norverapamil. *Eur J Clin Pharmacol.* 2008;64(5):445-449.

Atovaquone (*Mepron*)

Zidovudine (eg, *Retrovir*)

SUMMARY: Atovaquone administration results in a modest increase in zidovudine serum concentrations; the clinical significance is unknown.

RISK FACTORS: No specific risk factors are known.

MECHANISM: Atovaquone appears to inhibit the glucuronidation of zidovudine.

CLINICAL EVALUATION: Fourteen men with HIV received oral zidovudine 200 mg every 8 hours for 2 days, oral atovaquone 750 mg every 12 hours for 12 days, and zidovudine plus atovaquone for 12 days, in random order.[1] During the dosing of both drugs, the area under the concentration-time curve of zidovudine increased 31%, and its clearance after oral administration was reduced 25%, compared with the values obtained following zidovudine administration alone. The formation of the glucuronide metabolite of zidovudine also was reduced significantly during atovaquone administration. Zidovudine administration had no effect on atovaquone serum concentrations. The clinical significance of this interaction is unknown. The inhibition of zidovudine metabolism by the glucuronidation pathway could result in an increase in the formation of other metabolites with increased hematologic toxicity.

RELATED DRUGS: No information is available.

MANAGEMENT OPTIONS: No specific action is required, but be alert for evidence of the interaction.

REFERENCES:

1. Lee BL, et al. Atovaquone inhibits the glucuronidation and increases the plasma concentrations of zidovudine. *Clin Pharmacol Ther.* 1996;59(1):14-21.

 Atracurium

Clindamycin (eg, *Cleocin*)

SUMMARY: Clindamycin can enhance the activity of neuromuscular blockers such as atracurium, but the evidence for this effect is limited.

RISK FACTORS:

➥ *Dosage Regimen.* Large doses of clindamycin are more likely to enhance neuromuscular blocker activity.

MECHANISM: Clindamycin may have some neuromuscular blocking activity.

CLINICAL EVALUATION: In vitro studies have indicated that clindamycin may have neuromuscular blocking activity and may enhance the effect of neuromuscular blockers,[1,2] including succinylcholine (eg, *Anectine*), atracurium, and vecuronium. Only isolated clinical examples of such an effect of clindamycin have been reported.[3,4] A very large dose of clindamycin (2,400 mg) appeared to produce prolonged neuromuscular block in a patient who had recovered from the effects of succinylcholine.[5]

RELATED DRUGS: Clindamycin also may enhance the effect of other neuromuscular blockers, including succinylcholine and vecuronium.

MANAGEMENT OPTIONS: No specific action is required, but be alert for evidence of the interaction.

REFERENCES:

1. Becker LD, Miller RD. Clindamycin enhances a nondepolarizing neuromuscular blockade. *Anesthesiology.* 1976;45(1):84-87.
2. Rubbo JT, et al. Comparative neuromuscular effects of lincomycin and clindamycin. *Anesth Analg.* 1977;56(3):329-332.
3. Avery D, Finn R. Succinylcholine-prolonged apnea associated with clindamycin and abnormal liver function tests. *Dis Nerv Syst.* 1977;38(6):473-475.
4. Jedeikin R, et al. Prolongation of neuromuscular blocking effect of vecuronium by antibiotics. *Anaesthesia.* 1987;42(8):858-860.
5. al Ahdal O, Bevan DR. Clindamycin-induced neuromuscular blockade. *Can J Anaesth.* 1995;42(7):614-617.

Atracurium (eg, *Tracrium*)

Gentamicin

SUMMARY: Aminoglycoside antibiotics such as gentamicin potentiate the respiratory suppression produced by neuromuscular blockers such as atracurium.

RISK FACTORS:

➡ *Concurrent Diseases.* Patients with renal function impairment are probably at greater risk.

➡ *Dosage Regimen.* Elevated aminoglycoside concentrations may lead to respiratory suppression.

MECHANISM: Aminoglycosides can produce a neuromuscular blockade that may enhance the blockade of succinylcholine, atracurium, and vecuronium.

CLINICAL EVALUATION: A number of cases have been reported in which aminoglycoside (eg, gentamicin, tobramycin [eg, *TOBI*]) antibiotics produced respiratory paralysis, alone and in combination with neuromuscular blockers (eg, succinylcholine [eg, *Anectine*], atracurium, vecuronium [eg, *Norcuron*]).[1-5] This may occur following administration of the antibiotic by a variety of routes (eg, intramuscular, intravenous, intraperitoneal, intrapleural, beneath skin flaps). Extended ventilation may be required until the respiratory muscle block dissipates.

RELATED DRUGS: Other aminoglycosides (eg, tobramycin) also may produce enhanced neuromuscular blockade when administered in combination with neuromuscular blockers (eg, succinylcholine, vecuronium).

MANAGEMENT OPTIONS:

➡ *Avoid Unless Benefit Outweighs Risk.* Administer aminoglycoside antibiotics with extreme caution during surgery or in the immediate postoperative period.

➡ *Monitor.* Watch for respiratory depression; mechanical ventilation or treatment with anticholinesterase agents or calcium may be necessary.

REFERENCES:

1. Kronenfeld MA, et al. Recurrence of neuromuscular blockade after reversal of vecuronium in a patient receiving polymyxin/amikacin sternal irrigation. *Anesthesiology.* 1986;65(1):93-94.
2. Warner WA, et al. Neuromuscular blockade associated with gentamicin therapy. *JAMA.* 1971;215(7):1153-1154.
3. Wright EA, et al. Antibiotic-induced neuromuscular blockade. *Ann N Y Acad Sci.* 1971;183:358-368.
4. Levanen J, et al. Complete respiratory paralysis caused by a large dose of streptomycin and its treatment with calcium chloride. *Ann Clin Res.* 1975;7(1):47-49.
5. Lippmann M, et al. Neuromuscular blocking effects of tobramycin, gentamicin, and cefazolin. *Anesth Analg.* 1982;61(9):767-770.

Attapulgite (eg, *Diasorb*)

Promazine†

SUMMARY: Limited data indicate that attapulgite may reduce serum promazine concentrations.

RISK FACTORS: No specific risk factors are known.

MECHANISM: Attapulgite appears to inhibit the GI absorption of promazine.

CLINICAL EVALUATION: Repeated studies in a single subject demonstrated that an antidiarrheal mixture of attapulgite and pectin could impair the absorption of promazine as measured by urinary promazine excretion.[1]

RELATED DRUGS: The effect of attapulgite on other phenothiazines is not established, but consider the possibility that their absorption is also inhibited.

MANAGEMENT OPTIONS:

➡ *Circumvent/Minimize.* Although clinical evidence is very limited, it would be prudent to give phenothiazines 2 hours before or 6 hours after attapulgite.

➡ *Monitor.* Monitor for reduced phenothiazine effect if the combination is given.

REFERENCES:

1. Sorby DL, et al. Effects of adsorbents on drug absorption. II. Effect of an antidiarrhea mixture on promazine absorption. *J Pharm Sci.* 1966;55:504.

† Not available in the United States.

 Azapropazone†

Methotrexate (eg, *Rheumatrex*)

SUMMARY: A patient on chronic methotrexate developed evidence of methotrexate toxicity several days after starting azapropazone.

RISK FACTORS:

➡ *Concurrent Diseases.* Particular caution is suggested in patients with preexisting renal function impairment who may be more susceptible to nonsteroidal anti-inflammatory drug (NSAID)–induced renal failure.

➡ *Dosage Regimen.* The risk of adverse reactions from this interaction is primarily in patients receiving antineoplastic doses of methotrexate, rather than the lower doses used to treat rheumatoid arthritis, psoriasis, and related diseases.

MECHANISM: It is widely held that NSAIDs interfere with renal secretion of methotrexate, either by inhibiting tubular secretion of methotrexate or by reducing renal blood flow by inhibiting prostaglandin synthesis. Alterations in plasma protein binding have also been proposed, but this is unlikely to be clinically significant because methotrexate is normally only 50% to 70% bound to plasma proteins. Pharmacokinetic studies involving several different NSAIDs have failed to consistently identify an alteration in methotrexate pharmacokinetics by NSAIDs[1-8]; however, even in studies in which methotrexate pharmacokinetics remained unchanged overall, occasional patients appeared to exhibit reduced clearance of methotrexate after NSAID administration.[1,3]

CLINICAL EVALUATION: A 30-year-old woman with psoriasis was stabilized on methotrexate 25 mg per week with no undue toxicity.[9] A 9-day course of azapropazone therapy was started for joint pain, and a dose of methotrexate was given on day 8 of azapropazone therapy. Six days after the methotrexate dose, the patient was admitted with a 4-day history of bloody diarrhea, oral and genital ulcerations, and sore throat. The patient had a fever, oral and vaginal candidiasis, and a grossly hypocellular bone marrow, but she survived with supportive therapy. The case is complicated by the fact that the patient also was receiving small doses of aspirin (300 mg/day), which may have contributed somewhat to the enhanced methotrexate response. Although one cannot be certain that azapropazone was primarily responsible for the excessive methotrexate effects, a cause and effect relationship is supported by the fact that the patient had been on the same dose of methotrexate for 4 years with no toxicity and also by the temporal relationship between the addition of the azapropazone and the toxic response.

RELATED DRUGS: Several other NSAIDs also have been shown to increase methotrexate serum concentrations, although the magnitude varies depending on which NSAID is used and at what dose.

MANAGEMENT OPTIONS:

➥ *Avoid Unless Benefit Outweighs Risk.* Until more information is available on this interaction, avoid azapropazone (as well as other NSAIDs) in patients receiving antineoplastic doses of methotrexate. Although decreasing the methotrexate dosage is expected to reduce the likelihood of toxicity, the magnitude of the required reduction in methotrexate dosage has not been established. Rarely, low-dose methotrexate may interact adversely with an NSAID, as described in the Clinical Evaluation.

➥ *Monitor.* Many patients receiving methotrexate for rheumatoid arthritis will require an NSAID for symptomatic treatment. Closely monitor patients for evidence of increased methotrexate toxicity.

REFERENCES:

1. Ahern M, et al. Methotrexate kinetics in rheumatoid arthritis: is there an interaction with nonsteroidal antiinflammatory drugs? *J Rheumatol.* 1988;15(9):1356-1360.
2. Furst DE, et al. Effect of aspirin and sulindac on methotrexate clearance. *J Pharm Sci.* 1990;79(9):782-786.
3. Dupuis LL, et al. Methotrexate-nonsteroidal antiinflammatory drug interaction in children with arthritis. *J Rheumatol.* 1990;17(11):1469-1473.
4. Liegler DG, et al. The effect of organic acids on renal clearance of methotrexate in man. *Clin Pharmacol Ther.* 1969;10(6):849-857.
5. Skeith KJ, et al. Lack of significant interaction between low dose methotrexate and ibuprofen or flurbiprofen in patients with arthritis. *J Rheumatol.* 1990;17(8):1008-1010.
6. Stewart CF, et al. Effect of aspirin (ASA) on the disposition of methotrexate (MTX) in patients with rheumatoid arthritis (RA). *Clin Pharmacol Ther.* 1990;47:139.
7. Taylor JR, et al. Effect of sodium salicylate and indomethacin on methotrexate-serum albumin binding. *Arch Dermatol.* 1977;113(5):588-591.
8. Tracy FS, et al. The effect of NSAIDS on methotrexate disposition in patients with rheumatoid arthritis. *Clin Pharmacol Ther.* 1990;47:138.
9. Daly HM, et al. Methotrexate toxicity precipitated by azapropazone. *Br J Dermatol.* 1986;114(6):733-735.

† Not available in the United States.

Azapropazone

Warfarin (eg, *Coumadin*)

SUMMARY: Azapropazone appeared to enhance the hypoprothrombinemic effect of warfarin markedly in one patient, but more study is needed to confirm this effect.

RISK FACTORS:

➥ *Concurrent Diseases.* Patients with peptic ulcer disease or a history of GI bleeding are probably at greater risk.

MECHANISM: Not established. In vitro protein-binding studies indicate that azapropazone can displace warfarin from human serum albumin,[1] but protein displacement alone is unlikely to produce large changes in warfarin response. Thus, additional mechanisms may be involved.

CLINICAL EVALUATION: A patient stabilized on warfarin developed hematemesis and a markedly prolonged prothrombin time after receiving azapropazone 1.2 g/day for 4 days;[2] azapropazone appeared to be responsible for the bleeding episode in this patient. Additional studies are needed to determine the incidence and magnitude of this interaction. The fact that the chemical structure of azapropazone resembles phenylbutazone, a drug that markedly increases warfarin response, lends credence to this interaction. In a retrospective cohort study, hospitalizations for hemorrhagic peptic ulcer disease were about 13 times higher in patients receiving warfarin plus a nonsteroidal anti-inflammatory drug (NSAID) than in patients receiving neither drug.[3]

RELATED DRUGS: All NSAIDs inhibit platelet function, cause gastric erosions, and probably increase the risk of GI bleeding. Phenylbutazone (*Butazolidin*) markedly increases warfarin response. Some NSAIDs, however, such as ibuprofen (eg, *Advil*), naproxen (eg, *Naprosyn*), and diclofenac (*Voltaren*) may be less likely to increase oral anticoagulant-induced hypoprothrombinemia than other NSAIDs.

MANAGEMENT OPTIONS:

➡ ***Avoid Unless Benefit Outweighs Risk.*** Since all NSAIDs probably increase the risk of GI bleeding in patients on oral anticoagulants, use the combination only after careful consideration of the benefit vs risk. If a NSAID must be used with an oral anticoagulant it would be prudent to use NSAIDs that are unlikely to affect the hypoprothrombinemic response to oral anticoagulants (see Related Drugs). If the NSAID is being used as an analgesic or antipyretic, acetaminophen is probably safer to use with oral anticoagulants. Nonacetylated salicylates (eg, choline salicylate, magnesium salicylate, salsalate, sodium salicylate) are probably also safer with oral anticoagulants than NSAIDs, since such salicylates have minimal effects on platelet function and the gastric mucosa.

➡ ***Monitor.*** If any NSAID is used with an oral anticoagulant, monitor the prothrombin time carefully and watch for evidence of bleeding, especially from the GI tract.

REFERENCES:

1. McElnay JC, et al. Interaction between azapropazone and warfarin. *BMJ*. 1977;2:773.
2. Powell-Jackson PR. Interaction between azapropazone and warfarin. *BMJ*. 1977;1:1193.
3. Shorr RI, et al. Concurrent use of nonsteroidal anti-inflammatory drugs and oral anticoagulants places elderly persons at high risk for hemorrhagic peptic ulcer disease. *Arch Intern Med*. 1993;153:1665.

Azathioprine (*Imuran*)

Captopril (*Capoten*)

SUMMARY: Preliminary evidence indicates the likelihood of neutropenia may be greater with the combined use of captopril and azathioprine than with the use of either drug alone.

RISK FACTORS: No specific risk factors are known.

MECHANISM: Not established. Additive bone marrow suppression may be involved.

CLINICAL EVALUATION: Several patients have developed leukopenia following combined therapy with captopril and azathioprine.[1-4] Since both drugs can cause leukopenia under certain conditions, it is possible that the bone marrow suppression was additive in these patients. In support of this hypothesis, the white cell count of 1 patient who had developed leukopenia while on captopril plus azathioprine recovered when he was placed on either drug alone and declined again when the drugs were given together.[4] Another patient who developed neutropenia with combined captopril and azathioprine was not affected by captopril alone.[2] Although these cases are suggestive of a combined effect of captopril and azathioprine, a causal relationship has not been established.

RELATED DRUGS: Given that azathioprine is converted to mercaptopurine in the body, one would expect mercaptopurine (6-MP) to interact with angiotensin-converting enzyme (ACE) inhibitors in a similar manner. Little is known regarding the combined use of azathioprine or mercaptopurine with ACE inhibitors other than captopril.

MANAGEMENT OPTIONS:

➡ *Monitor.* Although evidence for an interaction between azathioprine and captopril is only preliminary, it would be prudent to monitor for laboratory and clinical evidence of bone marrow suppression in patients on both drugs.

REFERENCES:

1. Elijovisch F, et al. Captopril associated granulocytopenia in hypertension after renal transplantation. *Lancet.* 1980;1:927.
2. Edwards CRW, et al. Successful reintroduction of captopril following neutropenia. *Lancet.* 1981;1:723.
3. Case DB, et al. Successful low dose captopril rechallenge following drug-induced leukopenia. *Lancet.* 1981;1:1362.
4. Kirchertz EF, et al. Successful low dose captopril rechallenge following drug-induced leukopenia. *Lancet.* 1981;1:1363.

Azathioprine (*Imuran*)   **4**

Cyclophosphamide (eg, *Cytoxan*)

SUMMARY: Cyclophosphamide has been reported to cause hepatotoxicity when given immediately after azathioprine therapy.

RISK FACTORS: No specific risk factors are known.

MECHANISM: Not established.

CLINICAL EVALUATION: Reports of this possible interaction are limited to a series of 4 patients with collagen vascular diseases who received cyclophosphamide preceded by treatment with azathioprine and developed varying degrees of hepatic dysfunction.[1] Two patients became jaundiced, and all developed elevated liver function tests within 2 to 5 weeks of stopping azathioprine and starting cyclophosphamide. Liver biopsies in 2 patients showed hepatic necrosis. Liver function tests returned to normal upon discontinuation of cyclophosphamide. Whether this interaction occurs frequently, if at all, is unclear, especially since azathioprine alone is known to cause hepatic dysfunction in some patients. Furthermore, in a retrospective review of 320 cardiac transplant patients, 29 of whom developed hepatotoxicity suspected to be because of azathioprine, substitution of cyclophosphamide for azathioprine resulted in improvement of hepatic dysfunction.[2]

RELATED DRUGS: No information is available.

MANAGEMENT OPTIONS: No specific action is required, but be alert for evidence of the interaction.

REFERENCES:

1. Shaunak S, et al. Cyclophosphamide-induced liver necrosis: a possible interaction with azathioprine. *Quart J Med.* 1988;67:309.
2. Wagoner LE, et al. Cyclophosphamide as an alternative to azathioprine in cardiac transplant recipients with suspected azathioprine-induced hepatotoxicity. *Transplantation.* 1993;56:1415.

 Azathioprine (eg, *Imuran*)

AVOID **Febuxostat (*Uloric*)**

SUMMARY: Febuxostat theoretically increases the risk of serious azathioprine toxicity; avoid the combination.

RISK FACTORS: No specific risk factors are known.

MECHANISM: Azathioprine is metabolized by xanthine oxidase and febuxostat is a xanthine oxidase inhibitor; plasma concentrations of azathioprine are likely to increase.

CLINICAL EVALUATION: A 66-year-old woman taking azathioprine developed marked pancytopenia several weeks after febuxostat was initiated. She responded quickly to discontinuation of the 2 drugs and supportive therapy.[1] Although this interaction is based largely on theoretical considerations, an interaction is likely to occur and azathioprine toxicity is potentially fatal. Another xanthine oxidase inhibitor (allopurinol) has been used intentionally with azathioprine to improve efficacy and reduce hepatotoxicity in patients with inflammatory bowel disease, but this is only done with azathioprine dose reductions and careful monitoring for bone marrow suppression.[2,3]

RELATED DRUGS: Any other xanthine oxidase inhibitor (eg, allopurinol) is likely to increase the effect of both azathioprine and mercaptopurine.

MANAGEMENT OPTIONS:

➡ *AVOID COMBINATION.* Avoid concurrent use of azathioprine and febuxostat.

REFERENCES:

1. Kaczmorski S, et al. Gout and transplantation: new treatment option same old drug interaction. *Transplantation.* 2011;92(3):e13-e14.
2. Sparrow MP, et al. Effect of allopurinol on clinical outcomes in inflammatory bowel disease nonresponders to azathioprine or 6-mercaptopurine. *Clin Gastroenterol Hepatol.* 2007;5(2):209-214.
3. Ansari A, et al. Long-term outcome of using allopurinol co-therapy as a strategy for overcoming thiopurine hepatotoxicity in treating inflammatory bowel disease. *Aliment Pharmacol Ther.* 2008;28(6):734-741.

Azathioprine (eg, *Imuran*)

Infliximab (*Remicade*)

SUMMARY: The combination of azathioprine and infliximab may increase the risk of opportunistic infection over either drug alone, especially if corticosteroids are given concurrently. Some evidence suggests that combining infliximab with azathioprine or mercaptopurine (6-MP) may increase the risk of lymphoma.

RISK FACTORS:

➡ *Effects of Age.* In patients receiving azathioprine or 6-MP concurrently with infliximab, people older than 50 years may be at greater risk of opportunistic infections,[1] while lymphoma has occurred mostly in adolescent or young adult males taking infliximab with azathioprine or 6-MP.[2]

MECHANISM: Both azathioprine and infliximab can increase the risk of opportunistic infections, and their effects may be additive.

CLINICAL EVALUATION: In a case-control study of patients with inflammatory bowel disease, 100 consecutive patients with opportunistic infections were compared with 200 matched controls. Therapy with azathioprine/6-MP, infliximab, or corticosteroids were individually associated with increased odds for infection (odds ratios of approximately 3), whereas use of 2 or 3 of these agents concurrently was associated with an odds ratio of almost 15.[1] A 41-year-old man with ulcerative colitis developed life-threatening infective endocarditis after infliximab was added to his therapy with azathioprine and prednisolone.[3] Finally, the product information states that a rare, fatal lymphoma (hepatosplenic T-cell lymphoma) has been reported in younger males with inflammatory bowel disease who received azathioprine or 6-MP with infliximab.[2] Make a careful assessment of benefit versus risk before using infliximab with azathioprine or 6-MP, particularly if the patient is also taking corticosteroids.

RELATED DRUGS: Azathioprine acts by being metabolized to 6-MP, so 6-MP is likely to interact with infliximab in the same way as azathioprine.

MANAGEMENT OPTIONS:

➡ *Circumvent/Minimize.* If possible, avoid the concurrent use of azathioprine or 6-MP with infliximab, particularly if the patient is also receiving corticosteroids.

➡ *Monitor.* If the combination is used, monitor the patient carefully for opportunistic infections and evidence of other potential adverse reactions such as lymphoma.

REFERENCES:

1. Toruner M, et al. Risk factors for opportunistic infections in patients with inflammatory bowel disease. *Gastroenterology.* 2008;134(4):929-936.

2. *Remicade* [package insert]. Horsham, PA: Janssen Biotech Inc; 2011.

3. Baumgart DC. How many lives does an ulcerative colitis patient have? *Lancet.* 2010;376(9744):928.

Azathioprine (eg, *Imuran*)

Mesalamine (eg, *Asacol*)

SUMMARY: Mesalamine appears to increase the concentrations of azathioprine's active metabolites and may increase the risk of bone marrow suppression.

RISK FACTORS: No specific risk factors are known.

MECHANISM: Mesalamine appears to alter azathioprine metabolism, but the exact details are not established.

CLINICAL EVALUATION: In a small nonrandomized study of 34 patients with Crohn disease receiving azathioprine or mercaptopurine (6-MP), the addition of mesalamine 4 g/day or sulfasalazine 4 g/day was associated with an increase in leukopenia and an increase in the concentrations of 6-thioguanine nucleotides (6-TGN), active metabolites that may increase the risk of bone marrow suppression.[1] Similar results were found in a study of 16 patients taking long-term azathioprine in whom 6-TGN concentrations decreased modestly after the concurrent mesalamine or sulfasalazine was discontinued.[2] In a retrospective study of 199 patients with Crohn disease, 104 patients who received azathioprine plus mesalamine had more adverse reactions than the 95 patients who received azathioprine alone.[3] Finally, in a prospective study in 22 patients with inflammatory bowel disease, administration of 5-aminosalicylate increased the concentration of active 6-TGN metabolites.[4] Although these studies were not entirely consistent, mesalamine was assumed to affect azathioprine therapeutic response and adverse reactions; therefore, monitor patients accordingly.

RELATED DRUGS: Sulfasalazine (eg, *Azulfidine*) is likely to interact with azathioprine in a manner similar to mesalamine. Mercaptopurine (*Purinethol*) interacts in the same way as azathioprine with mesalamine and sulfasalazine.

MANAGEMENT OPTIONS:

➡ *Monitor.* Because the clinical outcome of combining azathioprine and mesalamine may differ from patient to patient, carefully monitor patients for efficacy and adverse effects when mesalamine or sulfasalazine is started or stopped in a patient taking azathioprine or 6-MP.

REFERENCES:

1. Lowry PW, et al. Leucopenia resulting from a drug interaction between azathioprine or 6-mercaptopurine and mesalamine, sulphasalazine, or balsalazide. *Gut*. 2001;49(5):656-664.

2. Dewit O, et al. Interaction between azathioprine and aminosalicylates: an in vivo study in patients with Crohn's disease. *Aliment Pharmacol Ther*. 2002;16(1):79-85.

3. Shah JA, et al. Should azathioprine and 5-aminosalicylates be coprescribed in inflammatory bowel disease? An audit of adverse events and outcome. *Eur J Gastroenterol Hepatol*. 2008;20(3):169-173.

4. de Graaf P, et al. Influence of 5-aminosalicylic acid on 6-thioguanosine phosphate metabolite levels: a prospective study in patients under steady thiopurine therapy. *Br J Pharmacol*. 2010;160(5):1083-1091.

Azathioprine (eg, *Imuran*)

Phenprocoumon†

SUMMARY: Two patients developed reduced phenprocoumon effect after azathioprine was started; monitor hypoprothrombinemic response.

RISK FACTORS: No specific risk factors are known.

MECHANISM: Not established.

CLINICAL EVALUATION: Two patients with systemic lupus erythematosus who were anticoagulated on phenprocoumon developed a gradual reduction in hypoprothrombinemic response after azathioprine was added.[1]

RELATED DRUGS: Theoretically, azathioprine's active metabolite, mercaptopurine (6-MP), is expected to reduce phenprocoumon response. Both azathioprine and mercaptopurine have been reported to reduce the anticoagulant response to warfarin (eg, *Coumadin*).

MANAGEMENT OPTIONS:

➥ *Monitor.* Monitor for altered phenprocoumon response if azathioprine is initiated, discontinued, or changed in dosage. Adjust phenprocoumon dosage as needed.

REFERENCES:

1. Jeppesen U, et al. Clinically important interaction between azathioprine (*Imurel*) and phenprocoumon (*Marcoumar*). *Eur J Clin Pharmacol.* 1997;52(6):503-504.

† Not available in the United States.

Azathioprine (eg, *Imuran*)

Prednisolone (eg, *Millipred*)

SUMMARY: The combination of azathioprine with prednisolone or other corticosteroids appears to substantially increase the risk of opportunistic infection over either drug alone; consider the benefit versus risk of using the combination, particularly in patients with inflammatory bowel disease.

RISK FACTORS:

➥ *Effects of Age.* In patients receiving azathioprine concurrently with corticosteroids, people older than 50 years may be at greater risk of opportunistic infections.[1]

MECHANISM: Both azathioprine and corticosteroids can increase the risk of opportunistic infections, and their effects may be additive.

CLINICAL EVALUATION: In a case-control study of patients with inflammatory bowel disease, 100 consecutive patients with opportunistic infections were compared with 200 matched controls. Therapy with azathioprine, mercaptopurine (6-MP), or corticosteroids was individually associated with an approximate 3-fold increase in infection, whereas use of azathioprine or 6-MP with corticosteroids was associated with an approximate 15-fold increase in infection.[1] A 41-year-old man with ulcerative colitis developed life-threatening infective endocarditis after infliximab was added to his therapy with azathioprine and prednisolone.[2] Thus, the clinical evidence suggests that the combination of azathioprine and corticosteroids increases the risk of opportunistic infections.

RELATED DRUGS: Azathioprine is metabolized to 6-MP, so 6-MP is likely to interact with corticosteroids in the same way as azathioprine.

MANAGEMENT OPTIONS:

➥ *Circumvent/Minimize.* Carefully assess benefit versus risk before using any combination of azathioprine/6-MP, corticosteroids, and infliximab.

➥ *Monitor.* If the combination is used, monitor the patient carefully for evidence of opportunistic infections.

REFERENCES:

1. Toruner M, et al. Risk factors for opportunistic infections in patients with inflammatory bowel disease. *Gastroenterology.* 2008;134(4):929-936.

2. Baumgart DC. How many lives does an ulcerative colitis patient have? *Lancet.* 2010;376(9744):928.

 ## Azathioprine (eg, *Imuran*)

Ribavirin (eg, *Rebetol*)

SUMMARY: Ribavirin appears to increase the risk of azathioprine-induced bone marrow suppression; the combination should generally be avoided.

RISK FACTORS: No specific risk factors are known.

MECHANISM: Ribavirin is known to inhibit inosine monophosphate dehydrogenase (IMPDH), one of the enzymes responsible for the metabolism of azathioprine. Theoretically, this would increase azathioprine toxicity by shunting azathioprine metabolism to myelotoxic methylated metabolites.[1]

CLINICAL EVALUATION: Eight patients with inflammatory bowel disease developed severe pancytopenia following concurrent use of azathioprine and ribavirin. The maximal bone marrow suppression occurred on average approximately 1 month after the ribavirin was added to azathioprine (in 7 patients), and approximately 3 weeks after azathioprine was added to ribavirin (in 1 patient). No bone marrow suppression was observed after the reintroduction of ribavirin or azathioprine alone.[1] Another report describes a 39-year-old man taking ribavirin who developed pancytopenia 12 weeks after starting azathioprine.[2] Given the plausible mechanism and the clinical data, ribavirin likely increases the risk of azathioprine toxicity.

RELATED DRUGS: Azathioprine is simply a prodrug for mercaptopurine; mercaptopurine is expected to interact similarly with ribavirin.

MANAGEMENT OPTIONS:

➥ *Circumvent/Minimize.* Withdrawal of azathioprine or mercaptopurine during ribavirin therapy has been recommended to reduce the risk of toxicity. If the combination is used, a reduced dose of azathioprine or mercaptopurine is likely to be necessary.

➥ *Monitor.* If the combination is used, monitor carefully for bone marrow suppression and other evidence of toxicity.

REFERENCES:

1. Peyrin-Biroulet L, et al. Interaction of ribavirin with azathioprine metabolism potentially induces myelosuppression. *Aliment Pharmacol Ther.* 2008;28(8):984-993.

2. Chaparro M, et al. Azathioprine plus ribavirin treatment and pancytopenia. *Aliment Pharmacol Ther.* 2009;30(9):962-963.

Azathioprine (eg, *Imuran*)

Warfarin (eg, *Coumadin*)

SUMMARY: Azathioprine appeared to inhibit the hypoprothrombinemic response to warfarin in 1 patient; more information is needed to establish the clinical importance.

RISK FACTORS: No specific risk factors are known.

MECHANISM: Not established.

CLINICAL EVALUATION: A 52-year-old woman taking prednisone, aspirin, and azathioprine required large doses of warfarin (14 to 17 mg/day).[1] When the azathioprine was discontinued, she developed epistaxis over several weeks and presented to the emergency department with hematemesis. Her prothrombin time had doubled to approximately 32 seconds. She was subsequently maintained on a warfarin dosage of 5 mg/day in the absence of azathioprine.

RELATED DRUGS: Mercaptopurine (6-MP) also has been reported to inhibit the hypoprothrombinemic response to warfarin.

MANAGEMENT OPTIONS:

➡ **Monitor.** Monitor for altered oral anticoagulant effect if azathioprine is initiated, discontinued, or changed in dosage. Adjust the anticoagulant dosage as needed.

REFERENCES:

1. Singleton JD, Conyers L. Warfarin and azathioprine: an important drug interaction. *Am J Med*. 1992;92(2):217.

Azithromycin (eg, *Zithromax*)

Carbamazepine (eg, *Tegretol*)

SUMMARY: Azithromycin does not alter the plasma concentration of carbamazepine.

RISK FACTORS: No specific risk factors are known.

MECHANISM: No interaction.

CLINICAL EVALUATION: Azithromycin 500 mg/day for 3 days had no significant effect on the plasma concentrations of carbamazepine and carbamazepine 10,11-epoxide.[1]

RELATED DRUGS: Other macrolide antibiotics (eg, clarithromycin [eg, *Biaxin*], erythromycin [eg, *Ery-Tab*]) may inhibit carbamazepine metabolism.

MANAGEMENT OPTIONS: No interaction.

REFERENCES:

1. Rapeport WG, et al. Lack of an interaction between azithromycin and carbamazepine. *Br J Clin Pharmacol*. 1992;33:551P.

Azithromycin (eg, *Zithromax*)

Cimetidine (eg, *Tagamet*)

SUMMARY: A single dose of cimetidine does not influence azithromycin concentrations.

RISK FACTORS: No specific risk factors are known.

MECHANISM: No interaction.

CLINICAL EVALUATION: Cimetidine 800 mg 2 hours before azithromycin caused no changes in azithromycin pharmacokinetics.[1] A multiple-dose, crossover study is needed to confirm these findings.

RELATED DRUGS: Other H_2-receptor antagonists (eg, famotidine [eg, *Pepcid*], nizatidine [eg, *Axid*], ranitidine [eg, *Zantac*]) are not expected to interact with azithromycin.

MANAGEMENT OPTIONS: No interaction.

REFERENCES:

1. Foulds G, et al. The effects of an antacid or cimetidine on the serum concentrations of azithromycin. *J Clin Pharmacol.* 1991;31(2):164-167.

 Azithromycin (eg, *Zithromax*)

Digoxin (eg, *Lanoxin*)

SUMMARY: A case report noted elevated digoxin concentrations following azithromycin administration; causation was not established.

RISK FACTORS: No specific risk factors are known.

MECHANISM: Unknown. Macrolide antibiotics, including erythromycin and clarithromycin, appear to alter digoxin pharmacokinetics by inhibiting P-glycoprotein. It is unknown if azithromycin also inhibits P-glycoprotein.

CLINICAL EVALUATION: A 31-month-old child was treated with digoxin following surgical repair of tetralogy of Fallot.[1] He was treated with azithromycin empirically for fever. Three days later, he developed cardiac arrhythmias, diarrhea, and anorexia. Digoxin plasma concentration at 9 hours postdose was noted to be 2.4 mcg/L. Several days prior to initiation of azithromycin, the patient's digoxin concentration at 11 hours postdose was 1.8 mcg/L. Digoxin was held for a day and then restarted at a lower dose. Cardiac rhythm returned to normal, and all signs of digoxin toxicity abated. Pending additional study, monitor patients receiving digoxin during azithromycin coadministration.

RELATED DRUGS: Erythromycin (eg, *Ery-Tab*) and clarithromycin (eg, *Biaxin*) are known to increase digoxin concentrations. Digitoxin[†] concentration may also be affected by azithromycin.

MANAGEMENT OPTIONS:

➡ *Monitor.* Monitor patients stabilized on digoxin for signs of digoxin toxicity (eg, arrhythmias, malaise, nausea, visual changes). Monitor digoxin plasma concentrations following the addition or discontinuation of azithromycin.

REFERENCES:

1. Ten Eick AP, et al. Possible drug interaction between digoxin and azithromycin in a young child. *Clin Drug Invest.* 2000;20:61-64.

† Not available in the United States.

Azithromycin (eg, *Zithromax*) 5

Sildenafil (eg, *Viagra*)

SUMMARY: Azithromycin does not affect sildenafil concentrations.

RISK FACTORS: No specific risk factors are known.

MECHANISM: No interaction.

CLINICAL EVALUATION: Twenty-four healthy subjects received a single dose of sildenafil 100 mg.[1] They were randomly assigned to 3 days of placebo or azithromycin 100 mg/day. On day 4, all subjects again received a single dose of sildenafil 100 mg. The administration of placebo or azithromycin had no effect on any of sildenafil's pharmacokinetic parameters compared with those measured following sildenafil administered alone. No change in the concentration of sildenafil's primary metabolite was noted in either group. Azithromycin does not appear to alter the metabolism of sildenafil.

RELATED DRUGS: Erythromycin (eg, *Ery-Tab*) has been reported to increase sildenafil plasma concentrations. Clarithromycin (eg, *Biaxin*) is expected to affect sildenafil in a similar manner. Although no data are available, dirithromycin[†] would not be expected to inhibit sildenafil metabolism.

MANAGEMENT OPTIONS: No interaction.

REFERENCES:
1. Muirhead GJ, et al. The effects of steady-state erythromycin and azithromycin on the pharmacokinetics of sildenafil in healthy volunteers. *Br J Clin Pharmacol.* 2002;53(suppl 1):37S-43S.

† Not available in the United States.

Azithromycin (*Zithromax*) 5

Terfenadine[†] (*Seldane*)

SUMMARY: Azithromycin does not appear to interact with terfenadine.

RISK FACTORS: No specific risk factors are known.

MECHANISM: No interaction.

CLINICAL EVALUATION: Azithromycin 250 mg/day for 5 days had no effect on the area under the concentration-time curve of terfenadine carboxylate, terfenadine's active metabolite.[1] Terfenadine was not detectable in the plasma of any subject during either phase of the study. Unlike other macrolide antibiotics, azithromycin does not appear to alter the metabolism of terfenadine and may offer an acceptable alternative to other macrolide antibiotics for patients taking terfenadine or astemizole (*Hismanal*).

RELATED DRUGS: Azithromycin, and perhaps dirithromycin (*Dynabac*), would not be expected to interact with other antihistamines. Troleandomycin (*TAO*), erythromycin (eg, *Ery-Tab*), and clarithromycin (*Biaxin*) inhibit terfenadine metabolism.

MANAGEMENT OPTIONS: No interaction.

REFERENCES:
1. Honig PK, et al. Comparison of the effect of the macrolide antibiotics erythromycin, clarithromycin and azithromycin on terfenadine steady-state pharmacokinetics and electrocardiographic parameters. *Drug Invest.* 1994;7:148.

† Not available in the United States.

---

5   Azithromycin (*Zithromax*)

Theophylline (eg, *Slo-Phyllin*)

SUMMARY: Azithromycin does not appear to alter theophylline concentrations.

RISK FACTORS: No specific risk factors are known.

MECHANISM: No interaction.

CLINICAL EVALUATION: No significant changes in sustained-release theophylline plasma concentrations were observed during 5 days of azithromycin administration.[1]

RELATED DRUGS: Other macrolides (eg, erythromycin [eg, *Ery-Tab*], clarithromycin [*Biaxin*]) can inhibit theophylline metabolism.

MANAGEMENT OPTIONS: No interaction.

REFERENCES:
1. Coates PE, et al. A double blind, placebo controlled, parallel group study to investigate the effect of orally administered azithromycin on the plasma concentration profile of theophylline. Data on file, 1991;Pfizer Labs, Inc.

---

5   Azithromycin (*Zithromax*)

Triazolam (*Halcion*)

SUMMARY: Azithromycin did not affect triazolam plasma concentrations or pharmacologic effects.

RISK FACTORS: No specific risk factors are known.

MECHANISM: No interaction.

CLINICAL EVALUATION: Twelve subjects received azithromycin 500 mg on day 1 and 250 mg on day 2.[1] Following the second dose of azithromycin, a single 0.125 mg oral dose of triazolam was administered. No change in triazolam pharmacokinetics was observed following azithromycin administration. The pharmacologic response (eg, sedation, fatigue, mental ability) to triazolam was not affected by azithromycin.

RELATED DRUGS: Erythromycin (eg, *E-Mycin*), clarithromycin (*Biaxin*), and troleandomycin (*Tao*) are known to inhibit triazolam metabolism.

MANAGEMENT OPTIONS: No interaction.

REFERENCES:
1. Greenblatt DJ, et al. Inhibition of triazolam clearance by macrolide antimicrobial agents: in vitro correlates and dynamic consequences. *Clin Pharmacol Ther.* 1998;64:278.

Azithromycin (*Zithromax*) 5

Warfarin (eg, *Coumadin*)

SUMMARY: Although isolated cases of increased warfarin effect have been reported with azithromycin, the bulk of the evidence suggests that the drugs do not interact.

RISK FACTORS: No specific risk factors are known.

MECHANISM: No interaction.

CLINICAL EVALUATION: Although isolated cases of purported azithromycin-induced increases in warfarin effect have been reported, such an interaction is not consistent with the known interactive properties of the 2 drugs. Indeed, a retrospective review of 26 patients receiving the 2 drugs did not reveal any effect of azithromycin on the hypoprothrombinemic response to warfarin.[1] The evaluation of interactions between warfarin and antibiotics is complicated by the fact that the infection itself (caused by release of endogenous substances and fever) may affect warfarin metabolism or clotting factor catabolism.

RELATED DRUGS: Erythromycin and clarithromycin (*Biaxin*) have been reported to increase the hypoprothrombinemic response to warfarin in some patients.

MANAGEMENT OPTIONS: No specific action is required, but be alert for evidence of altered warfarin response when any drug is started or stopped.

REFERENCES:
1. Beckey NP, et al. Retrospective evaluation of a potential interaction between azithromycin and warfarin in patients stabilized on warfarin. *Pharmacotherapy.* 2000;20:1055.

Azithromycin (*Zithromax*) 5

Zidovudine (*Retrovir*)

SUMMARY: Single doses of azithromycin had no effect on zidovudine concentrations.

RISK FACTORS: No specific risk factors are known.

MECHANISM: No interaction.

CLINICAL EVALUATION: Azithromycin 1 g was administered to HIV-infected patients once weekly for 5 weeks, 2 hours before their morning zidovudine dose.[1] Azithromycin administration had no effect on the plasma concentration of zidovudine or its glucuronide metabolite.

RELATED DRUGS: Clarithromycin (*Biaxin*) has been noted to reduce zidovudine serum concentrations.

MANAGEMENT OPTIONS: No interaction.

REFERENCES:
1. Chave JP, et al. Once-a-week azithromycin in AIDS patients: tolerability, kinetics, and effects on zidovudine disposition. *Antimicrob Agents Chemother.* 1992;36:1013.

4 Azlocillin (*Azlin*)

Ciprofloxacin (*Cipro*)

SUMMARY: Azlocillin administration increases ciprofloxacin serum concentrations; the clinical significance of this interaction is unclear.

RISK FACTORS: No specific risk factors are known.

MECHANISM: Azlocillin appears to interfere with the renal tubular secretion of ciprofloxacin and may alter the hepatic uptake or biliary secretion of ciprofloxacin.

CLINICAL EVALUATION: Six healthy subjects were given IV doses of ciprofloxacin 4 mg/kg and azlocillin 60 mg/kg alone and concurrently.[1] The pharmacokinetics of azlocillin were unchanged by coadministration of ciprofloxacin. However, the mean total body clearance of ciprofloxacin was reduced 35%; half-life did not change because of a reduction in volume of distribution.

RELATED DRUGS: Other antibiotics secreted by the kidney (eg, penicillins, imipenem [*Primaxin*]) potentially could interact with ciprofloxacin.

MANAGEMENT OPTIONS: No specific action is required, but be alert for evidence of the interaction.

REFERENCES:
1. Barriere SL, et al. Alteration in the pharmacokinetic disposition of ciprofloxacin by simultaneous administration of azlocillin. *Antimicrob Agents Chemother*. 1990;34:823.

Baicalin 4

Bupropion (eg, *Wellbutrin*)

SUMMARY: Baicalin appears to increase the plasma concentrations of hydroxybupropion, the active metabolite of bupropion; the clinical importance of this effect is not established.

RISK FACTORS: No specific risk factors are known.

MECHANISM: Unknown.

CLINICAL EVALUATION: Seventeen healthy subjects were given a single dose of bupropion 150 mg with and without pretreatment with baicalin (500 mg 3 times/day for 14 days).[1] Baicalin did not affect the pharmacokinetics of bupropion itself, but produced a substantial 87% increase in the plasma concentrations of the active metabolite, hydroxybupropion. The clinical importance of this interaction is not known. Baicalin might increase the efficacy of bupropion without increasing its toxicity, but this study was not designed to test this possibility.[1]

RELATED DRUGS: No information is available.

MANAGEMENT OPTIONS: No specific action is required, but be alert for evidence of the interaction.

REFERENCES:
1. Fan L, et al. Induction of cytochrome P450 2B6 activity by the herbal medicine baicalin as measured by bupropion hydroxylation. *Eur J Clin Pharmacol.* 2009;65(4):403-409.

Benztropine (eg, *Cogentin*)

Donepezil (eg, *Aricept*)

SUMMARY: Benztropine is an anticholinergic drug, and may inhibit the therapeutic effect of donepezil in Alzheimer disease.

RISK FACTORS: No specific risk factors are known.

MECHANISM: Donepezil is a cholinesterase inhibitor and thus increases cholinergic activity; its efficacy is likely to be inhibited by anticholinergic drugs, such as benztropine.[1]

CLINICAL EVALUATION: In a preliminary study of 69 patients with Alzheimer disease receiving donepezil 10 mg/day and followed for 2 years, 16 patients received concurrent therapy with anticholinergic drugs and 53 patients did not.[2] Mental functioning, as measured by the Mini-Mental State Exam (MMSE), was significantly lower in the patients receiving concomitant anticholinergic drugs. Also, the French Pharmacovigilance Database received 118 spontaneous reports of adverse effects in patients receiving anticholinergic drugs with cholinesterase inhibitors (eg, donepezil, galantamine, rivastigmine). After evaluation by clinical pharmacologists, 24 were thought to be adverse drug interactions.[3] Although additional study is needed to establish the clinical importance of these interactions, the evidence is consistent with the known pharmacological effects of the drugs.

RELATED DRUGS: All cholinesterase inhibitors used to treat Alzheimer disease (donepezil, galantamine [eg, *Razadyne*], rivastigmine [eg, *Exelon*]) are expected to interact similarly with benztropine and other anticholinergic antiparkinson drugs, such as biperiden,† procyclidine,† and trihexyphenidyl. Amantadine may also have anticholinergic effects, although that does not appear to be its primary mechanism of action in Parkinson disease.

MANAGEMENT OPTIONS:

➡ *Consider Alternative.* If possible, use an alternative to the benztropine or other anticholinergic antiparkinson drugs (see Related Drugs).

➡ *Monitor.* If benztropine or other anticholinergic antiparkinson drugs are used with donepezil or another cholinesterase inhibitor, be alert for evidence of reduced mental functioning.

REFERENCES:

1. *Aricept* [package insert]. New York, NY: Pfizer; 2011.
2. Lu CJ, Tune LE. Chronic exposure to anticholinergic medications adversely affects the course of Alzheimer disease. *Am J Geriatr Psychiatry.* 2003;11(4):458-461.
3. Tavassoli N, et al. Drug interactions with cholinesterase inhibitors: an analysis of the French Pharmacovigilance Database and a comparison of two national drug formularies (Vidal, British National Formulary). *Drug Saf.* 2007;30(11):1063-1071.

† Not available in the United States.

Benztropine (eg, *Cogentin*)

Haloperidol (eg, *Haldol*)

SUMMARY: Benztropine and other anticholinergics may inhibit the therapeutic response to neuroleptics; excess anticholinergic effects may occur.

RISK FACTORS: No specific risk factors are known.

MECHANISM: The following potential mechanisms exist for interactions between neuroleptics and anticholinergic agents: 1) inhibition of the antipsychotic effect of the neuroleptics; 2) additive anticholinergic effects; and 3) possible inhibition of GI absorption of neuroleptics by anticholinergics.[1-4]

CLINICAL EVALUATION: There is some evidence benztropine and other anticholinergic agents may inhibit the therapeutic response to neuroleptics, possibly through a direct inhibitory effect. In a study of 10 schizophrenic patients, the addition of benztropine to haloperidol increased "social avoidance behavior."[5] Some of the other therapeutic effects of haloperidol (eg, cognitive, perceptual) did not appear to be adversely affected.

The additive anticholinergic effects of neuroleptics and anticholinergics also may result in paralytic ileus[6,7] or heat stroke,[8-10] either one of which may be fatal. However, it is unknown whether the risk of ileus or heat stroke is higher in patients taking neuroleptics plus anticholinergics than in patients taking either drug alone. In 1 patient, abrupt withdrawal of an anticholinergic (benztropine) in the presence of continuing haloperidol therapy resulted in nausea and vomiting.[11] When benztropine was restarted, nausea and vomiting recurred only when a placebo was substituted for benztropine on day 13.

RELATED DRUGS: Many combinations of antipsychotics and anticholinergics probably interact by 1 or more of the mechanisms described above. Trihexyphenidyl (*Artane*) apparently had a similar inhibitory effect on the therapeutic response to haloperidol in schizophrenic patients. However, there is also evidence that anticholinergics may reduce the GI absorption of chlorpromazine (eg, *Thorazine*). For example, tri-hexyphenidyl has been shown to reduce plasma chlorpromazine concentrations in schizophrenic patients,[12] and orphenadrine (eg, *Norflex*) has been shown to reduce plasma concentrations and the pharmacologic response of chlorpromazine.[13]

MANAGEMENT OPTIONS:

➡ *Circumvent/Minimize.* Do not use anticholinergics routinely in patients receiving neuroleptics. When the combination is needed, patients should take precautions to avoid heat stroke.

➡ *Monitor.* If the combination is used, be alert for evidence of reduced neuroleptic effects and for symptoms that may signal the onset of a dynamic ileus (eg, constipation, abdominal pain, distension).

REFERENCES:

1. Rivera-Calimlim L, et al. Clinical response and plasma levels: effect of dose, dosage schedules and drug interactions on plasma chlorpromazine levels. *Am J Psychiatry.* 1976;133(6):646-652.

2. Gershon S, et al. Interaction between some anticholinergic agents and phenothiazines. *Clin Pharmacol Ther.* 1965;6(6):749-756.

3. Alpert M, et al. Anticholinergic exacerbation of phenothiazine-induced extrapyramidal syndrome. *Am J Psychiatry.* 1976;133(9):1073-1075.

4. Rivera-Calimlim L. Chlorpromazine-trihexyphenidyl interaction. *Drug Ther.* 1976;6:196.

5. Singh MM, et al. Reversal of some therapeutic effects of an antipsychotic agent by an antiparkinsonisn drug. *J Nerv Ment Dis.* 1973;157(1):50-58.

6. Giordano J, et al. Fatal paralytic ileus complicating phenothiazine therapy. *South Med J.* 1975;68(3):351-353.

7. Warnes J, et al. A dynamic ileus during psychoactive medication: a report of three fatal and five severe cases. *Can Med Assoc J.* 1967;96:1112-1113.

8. Mann SC, et al. Psychotropic drugs, summer heat and humidity, and hyperpyrexia: a danger restated. *Am J Psychiatry.* 1978;135(9):1097-1100.

9. Hyperpyrexia from drug combinations. *JAMA.* 1973;225(10):1250.

10. Zelman S, et al. Heat stroke in phenothiazine-treated patients: a report of three fatalities. *Am J Psychiatry.* 1970;126(12):1787-1790.

11. Schaffer CB, et al. A case report of vomiting related to the interactions of antipsychotic and benztropine. *Am J Psychiatry.* 1981;138(6):833-835.

12. Rivera-Calimlim L, et al. Effects of mode of management on plasma chlorpromazine in psychiatric patients. *Clin Pharmacol Ther.* 1973;14(6):978-986.

13. Loga S, et al. Interactions of orphenadrine and phenobarbitone with chlorpromazine: plasma concentrations and effects in man. *Br J Clin Pharmacol.* 1975;2(3):197-208.

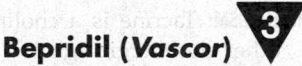

Bepridil (*Vascor*)

Digoxin (eg, *Lanoxin*)

SUMMARY: Bepridil increases digoxin serum concentrations; digoxin toxicity may result.

RISK FACTORS: No specific risk factors are known.

MECHANISM: Bepridil appears to inhibit the elimination of digoxin.

CLINICAL EVALUATION: Bepridil 300 mg/day increased digoxin concentrations 34% and enhanced the reduction in heart rate caused by digoxin.[1]

RELATED DRUGS: Verapamil (eg, *Calan*), diltiazem (eg, *Cardizem*), and nitrendipine (*Baypress*) appear to reduce digoxin elimination. Digitoxin (*Crystodigin*) is likely to be similarly affected.

MANAGEMENT OPTIONS:

➡ **Consider Alternative.** Nifedipine (eg, *Procardia*),[2-5] isradipine (*DynaCirc*),[6] nicardipine (eg, *Cardene*),[7] felodipine (*Plendil*),[8] and amlodipine (*Norvasc*)[9] do not appear to increase digoxin concentrations.

➡ **Circumvent/Minimize.** Digoxin dosages may need to be reduced when bepridil is added to a patient stabilized on digoxin.

➡ **Monitor.** Monitor patients for evidence of increased serum digitalis effects (eg, bradycardia, heart block, GI upset, mental changes) in the presence of bepridil therapy.

REFERENCES:

1. Belz GG, et al. Digoxin and bepridil: pharmacokinetic and pharmacodynamic interactions. *Clin Pharmacol Ther.* 1986;39(1):65-71.
2. Kuhlmann J. Effects of nifedipine and diltiazem on plasma levels and renal excretion of beta-acetyldigoxin. *Clin Pharmacol Ther.* 1985;37(2):150-156.
3. Schwartz JB, et al. Effect of nifedipine on serum digoxin concentration and renal digoxin clearance. *Clin Pharmacol Ther.* 1984;36(1):19-24.
4. Belz GG, et al. Digoxin plasma concentrations and nifedipine. *Lancet.* 1981;1(8224):844-845.
5. Hutt HJ, et al. Dose-dependence of the nifedipine/digoxin interaction? *Arch Toxicol Suppl.* 1986;9:209-212.
6. Rodin SM, et al. Comparative effects of verapamil and isradipine on steady-state digoxin kinetics. *Clin Pharmacol Ther.* 1988;43(6):668-672.
7. Debruyne D, et al. Nicardipine does not significantly affect serum digoxin concentrations at the steady state of patients with congestive heart failure. *Int J Clin Pharmacol Res.* 1989;9(1):15-19.
8. Kirch W, et al. The felodipine/digoxin interaction. A placebo-controlled study in patients with heart failure. *Br J Clin Pharmacol.* 1988;26:644P.
9. Schwartz JB. Effects of amlodipine on steady-state digoxin concentrations and renal digoxin clearance. *J Cardiovasc Pharmacol.* 1988;12(1):1-5.

Bethanechol (eg, *Urecholine*)

Tacrine (*Cognex*)

SUMMARY: Increased cholinergic effects may be seen when tacrine is combined with other cholinergic agents, like bethanechol.

RISK FACTORS: No specific risk factors are known.

MECHANISM: Tacrine is a cholinergic agent and is likely to have additive effects with other cholinergic agents.[1]

CLINICAL EVALUATION: Although this interaction is based primarily on theoretical considerations, it is likely tacrine would have additive effects with other drugs in the same pharmacologic class. This would include direct-acting cholinergics such as bethanechol as well as anticholinesterase agents.

RELATED DRUGS: Tacrine probably has additive effects with all cholinergic agents, including direct-acting cholinergics, as well as anticholinesterase agents, such as ambenonium (*Mytelase*), edrophonium (eg, *Tensilon*), neostigmine (eg, *Prostigmin*), and pyridostigmine (eg, *Mestinon*).

MANAGEMENT OPTIONS:

➡ **Monitor.** Monitor patients for excessive cholinergic response if tacrine is used with other cholinergic medications. Theoretically, it would be possible to reduce the dose of the cholinomimetic agent if tacrine is used concurrently without compromising the therapeutic response.

REFERENCES:

1. Taylor P. Agents acting at the neuromuscular junction and autonomic ganglia. In: Hardman JG, et al, eds. *Goodman and Gilman's The Pharmacological Basis of Therapeutics.* 9th ed. New York: Pergamon Press;1996;177–197.

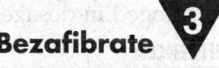

Bezafibrate

Dicumarol

SUMMARY: A patient on dicumarol developed increased anticoagulant response and GI bleeding after bezafibrate was added to her therapy.

RISK FACTORS: No specific risk factors are known.

MECHANISM: Not established.

CLINICAL EVALUATION: A 55-year-old woman on chronic anticoagulation therapy with dicumarol was started on bezafibrate 800 mg/day.[1] Two weeks later she was admitted to the hospital with an INR of 26 and severe upper GI bleeding. She was treated successfully with fresh-frozen plasma, vitamin K, and packed red cells. The magnitude of the interaction in this patient may have been increased by her chronic renal failure and the large dose of bezafibrate.

RELATED DRUGS: Both clofibrate (*Atromid-S*) and gemfibrozil (eg, *Lopid*) have been reported to increase dicumarol response. Bezafibrate has also been reported to increase the effect of warfarin (eg, *Coumadin*)[2] and phenprocoumon.

MANAGEMENT OPTIONS:

➡ *Monitor.* Monitor patients receiving dicumarol or other anticoagulants for altered hypoprothrombinemic response if bezafibrate therapy is started, stopped, or changed in dosage.

REFERENCES:

1. Blum A, et al. Severe gastrointestinal bleeding induced by a probable hydroxycoumarin-bezafibrate interaction. *Isr J Med Sci.* 1992;28:47-49.
2. Beringer TR. Warfarin potentiation with bezafibrate. *Postgrad Med J.* 1997;73:657-658.

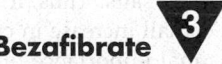

Bezafibrate

Warfarin (eg, *Coumadin*)

SUMMARY: Isolated cases of enhanced warfarin response have been reported in patients given bezafibrate concurrently.

RISK FACTORS: No specific risk factors are known.

MECHANISM: Not established.

CLINICAL EVALUATION: Two patients developed an increased hypoprothrombinemic response to warfarin during concurrent bezafibrate therapy.[1] In both cases, the changes in warfarin response appeared after changes in the bezafibrate dose. There was a positive dechallenge in 1 case.

RELATED DRUGS: Both clofibrate (*Atromid-S*) and gemfibrozil (eg, *Lopid*) have been reported to increase warfarin response. Bezafibrate has also been reported to increase the effect of dicumarol[2] and phenprocoumon.

MANAGEMENT OPTIONS:

➡ *Monitor.* Monitor patients receiving warfarin or other anticoagulants for altered hypoprothrombinemic response if bezafibrate therapy is started, stopped, or changed in dosage.

REFERENCES:

1. Beringer TR. Warfarin potentiation with bezafibrate. *Postgrad Med J.* 1997;73:657-658.

2. Blum A, et al. Severe gastrointestinal bleeding induced by a probable hydroxycoumarin-bezafibrate interaction. *Isr J Med Sci.* 1992;28:47-49.

4   Bile Salts

Cyclosporine (eg, *Neoral*)

SUMMARY: Bile salts appear to produce small increases in cyclosporine bioavailability, but the clinical importance of this effect is probably not large.

RISK FACTORS: No specific risk factors are known.

MECHANISM: Bile salts seem to increase the GI absorption of cyclosporine; however, the precise mechanism for this interaction requires more study.

CLINICAL EVALUATION: In a single-dose study, bile salt tablets (400 mg cholic acid, 100 mg dehydrocholic acid) increased the bioavailability of cyclosporine 22% in 11 healthy subjects. However, no interaction was detected when multiple doses of cyclosporine were given with bile salt tablets (200 mg cholic acid, 50 mg dehydrocholic acid) to 19 clinically stable transplant patients.[1] The results of these studies are not necessarily contradictory because the impact of food on cyclosporine was carefully controlled in the study of healthy subjects but not in the study of renal transplant patients. The dose of bile salts given to the 2 groups also differed. In another study of 15 renal transplant recipients, cyclosporine bioavailability was slightly greater when the drug was taken with bile salts (900 mg ursodeoxycholic acid) and a low-fat breakfast than when taken with a low-fat breakfast alone.[2] A high-fat breakfast produced about the same increase in cyclosporine bioavailability as the bile salts. Thus, if the effect of meals is controlled, bile salts appear to produce a small increase in cyclosporine bioavailability, but the effect appears to be of minimal importance under multiple dosing conditions.

RELATED DRUGS: No information is available.

MANAGEMENT OPTIONS: No specific action is required, but be alert for evidence of the interaction.

REFERENCES:

1. Lindhold A, et al. The effect of food and bile acid administration on the relative bioavailability of cyclosporin. *Br J Clin Pharmacol.* 1990;29:541.

2. Shriner DA, et al. Influence of dietary fat and bile salts on oral cyclosporine absorption in renal transplant patients. *Pharmacotherapy.* 1991;11:277.

Bismuth (eg, *Pepto-Bismol*)

Doxycycline (eg, *Vibramycin*)

SUMMARY: Bismuth can reduce the bioavailability of doxycycline significantly and could result in reduced antibacterial efficacy.

RISK FACTORS: No specific risk factors are known.

MECHANISM: Bismuth appears to inhibit the absorption of doxycycline from the GI tract.

CLINICAL EVALUATION: Six healthy subjects took a single dose of doxycycline 200 mg alone, with 60 mL of bismuth, with 60 mL of bismuth administered 2 hours before or after the doxycycline, or 60 mL of bismuth subsalicylate administered every 6 hours for 5 doses with the doxycycline given immediately following the final dose.[1] Compared with doxycycline administered alone, no effect was observed on doxycycline pharmacokinetic parameters when the bismuth was administered 2 hours after doxycycline. Administration of bismuth 2 hours before doxycycline resulted in a 32% reduction in peak doxycycline concentrations and a 22% decrease in relative bioavailability.[2] When both drugs were administered together, the relative bioavailability was reduced 37%, while 5 doses of bismuth before the doxycycline administration resulted in a 51% reduction in doxycycline bioavailability.

RELATED DRUGS: Tetracycline (*Actisite*) absorption is also affected by bismuth.

MANAGEMENT OPTIONS:

➥ ***Use Alternative.*** Patients taking tetracyclines for the treatment of infections should avoid bismuth. The use of doxycycline to prevent traveler's diarrhea should not include coadministration of bismuth.

REFERENCES:

1. Albert KS, et al. Decreased tetracycline bioavailability caused by a bismuth subsalicylate antidiarrheal mixture. *J Pharmaceut Sci.* 1979;68:586-588.
2. Ericsson CD, et al. Influence of subsalicylate bismuth on absorption of doxycycline. *JAMA.* 1982;247:2266-2267.

Bismuth (eg, *Pepto-Bismol*)

Omeprazole (eg, *Prilosec*)

SUMMARY: Omeprazole appears to increase the systemic absorption of bismuth from tripotassium dicitrato bismuthate, but the clinical importance of this effect is not established.

RISK FACTORS: No specific risk factors are known.

MECHANISM: The GI absorption of bismuth appears to be increased substantially if gastric pH is increased.[1,2]

CLINICAL EVALUATION: Six healthy subjects received a single oral dose of tripotassium dicitrato bismuthate 240 mg with and without pretreatment with omeprazole 40 mg/day for 7 days.[1] Omeprazole increased the bismuth area under the concentration-time curve almost 3-fold. It is not known whether this effect increases the risk of bismuth toxicity or interferes with the ability of bismuth to eradicate *Helicobacter pylori*.

Although some have recommended a 50% or more reduction of bismuth dosage in the presence of agents that increase gastric pH, it is not known whether such reductions would also reduce the ability of bismuth to eradicate *H. pylori*.

RELATED DRUGS: The effect of omeprazole on other bismuth preparations is not established, but consider the possibility that they would interact with omeprazole in the same way. Given the proposed mechanism, lansoprazole (eg, *Prevacid*) is likely to interact similarly with bismuth.

MANAGEMENT OPTIONS: No specific action is required, but be alert for evidence of the interaction.

REFERENCES:

1. Treiber G, et al. Omeprazole-induced increase in the absorption of bismuth from tripotassium dicitrato bismuthate. *Clin Pharmacol Ther.* 1994;55(5):486-491.
2. Nwokolo CU, et al. The effect of histamine H$_2$-receptor blockade on bismuth absorption from three ulcer-healing compounds. *Gastroenterology.* 1991;101(4):889-894.

Bismuth (eg, *Pepto-Bismol*)

Tetracycline

SUMMARY: Bismuth can significantly reduce the bioavailability of tetracycline and may cause reduced antibacterial efficacy.

RISK FACTORS: No specific risk factors are known.

MECHANISM: Bismuth appears to inhibit the absorption of tetracyclines from the GI tract.

CLINICAL EVALUATION: Fifteen healthy subjects received a single dose of tetracycline 250 mg alone and with bismuth 60 mL suspension.[1] The tetracycline area under the concentration-time curve and peak serum concentration were reduced 33% and 27%, respectively. Based on urinary recovery and renal clearance, tetracycline bioavailability was reduced 34% when it was administered with bismuth subsalicylate.

RELATED DRUGS: Doxycycline (eg, *Vibramycin*) absorption is also affected by bismuth.

MANAGEMENT OPTIONS:

➥ *Use Alternative.* Patients taking tetracyclines for the treatment of infections should avoid bismuth. The use of doxycycline to prevent traveler's diarrhea should not include coadministration of bismuth.

REFERENCES:

1. Albert KS, et al. Decreased tetracycline bioavailability caused by a bismuth subsalicylate antidiarrheal mixture. *J Pharm Sci.* 1979;68(5):586-588.

Bortezomib (*Velcade*)

Itraconazole (eg, *Sporanox*)

SUMMARY: Itraconazole administration may increase bortezomib concentrations, leading to an increase risk of adverse reactions, including thrombocytopenia and neuropathy.

RISK FACTORS: No specific risk factors are known.

MECHANISM: Itraconazole is known to inhibit CYP3A4, the primary enzyme responsible for the metabolism of bortezomib.

CLINICAL EVALUATION: Three patients with multiple myeloma who were receiving bortezomib and dexamethasone were treated with concomitant itraconazole.[1] All 3 patients developed peripheral neuropathy and thrombocytopenia during concurrent therapy with itraconazole and bortezomib. No bortezomib plasma concentrations were reported. The neuropathy improved after bortezomib was discontinued. Based on the pharmacologic properties of bortezomib and itraconazole, it appears that itraconazole administration may have produced elevated plasma concentrations of bortezomib that led to toxicity. Controlled studies are needed to define the magnitude of this interaction.

RELATED DRUGS: Ketoconazole (eg, *Nizoral*), fluconazole (eg, *Diflucan*), posaconazole (*Noxafil*), and voriconazole (*Vfend*) also inhibit the activity of CYP3A4 and are expected to increase the plasma concentrations of bortezomib.

MANAGEMENT OPTIONS:

➥ **Monitor.** Carefully monitor patients receiving bortezomib for adverse reactions if itraconazole is added to their regimen.

REFERENCES:
    1. Iwamoto T, et al. Drug interaction between itraconazole and bortezomib: exacerbation of peripheral neuropathy and thrombocytopenia induced by bortezomib. *Pharmacotherapy.* 2010;30(7):661-665.

Bortezomib (*Velcade*)

Ketoconazole (eg, *Nizoral*)

SUMMARY: Ketoconazole increases the plasma concentration of bortezomib; the effect of this increase on the adverse reaction profile of bortezomib appears to be modest.

RISK FACTORS:

➥ **Pharmacogenetics.** Patients who are poor metabolizers for CYP2C19 may be at increased risk.

MECHANISM: Ketoconazole inhibits CYP3A4, the enzyme thought to be primarily responsible for bortezomib metabolism.

CLINICAL EVALUATION: Patients with solid tumors who were receiving bortezomib 1 mg/m^2 intravenously twice weekly were randomly assigned to receive ketoconazole 400 mg for 4 days during 1 of 2 cycles of bortezomib therapy.[1] The administration of ketoconazole resulted in an increase of 35% in the mean area under the concentration-time curve of bortezomib. No increase in toxicity of bortezomib was noted in this short-term trial. Bortezomib is also metabolized by CYP2C19 and CYP1A2; these pathways may mitigate the effects of CYP3A4 inhibition caused by ketoconazole.

RELATED DRUGS: Fluconazole (eg, *Diflucan*), itraconazole (eg, *Sporanox*), posaconazole (*Noxafil*), and voriconazole (*Vfend*) also inhibit the activity of CYP3A4 and are expected to increase the plasma concentrations of bortezomib.

MANAGEMENT OPTIONS:

➥ *Monitor.* Be alert for signs of excessive bortezomib effect (eg, peripheral neuropathy, hearing loss) in patients receiving ketoconazole.

REFERENCES:

1. Venkatakrishnan K, et al. Effect of the CYP3A inhibitor ketoconazole on the pharmacokinetics and pharmacodynamics of bortezomib in patients with advanced solid tumors: a prospective, multicenter, open-label, randomized, two-way crossover drug-drug interaction study. *Clin Ther.* 2009;(31, pt 2):2444-2458.

Bosentan (*Tracleer*)

Ketoconazole (eg, *Nizoral*)

SUMMARY: Ketoconazole administration increases the plasma concentrations of bosentan; some increase in bosentan vasodilator effect may occur.

RISK FACTORS: No specific risk factors are known.

MECHANISM: Bosentan is metabolized by CYP3A4 and CYP2C9. Ketoconazole inhibits the CYP3A4 metabolism of bosentan.

CLINICAL EVALUATION: Bosentan 62.5 mg was administered twice daily for 5 days followed by a single dose the morning of blood sampling.[1] The same dosing schedule was repeated with the addition of ketoconazole 200 mg once daily. The mean peak plasma concentration and area under the concentration-time curve of bosentan were increased 2.1- and 2.3-fold, respectively, during ketoconazole coadministration. The moderate magnitude of the increase in bosentan plasma concentration associated with concurrent ketoconazole may increase the risk of adverse reactions (eg, headache, nausea) in some patients.

RELATED DRUGS: Other azole antifungal agents that inhibit CYP3A4, including itraconazole (eg, *Sporanox*), fluconazole (eg, *Diflucan*), and voriconazole (*Vfend*) (which also inhibits CYP2C9), may increase the plasma concentrations of bosentan.

MANAGEMENT OPTIONS:

➥ *Monitor.* Monitor patients requiring concurrent ketoconazole and bosentan for excessive vasodilator effects, including headache and hypotension.

REFERENCES:

1. van Giersbergen PL, et al. Single- and multiple-dose pharmacokinetics of bosentan and its interaction with ketoconazole. *Br J Clin Pharmacol.* 2002;53(6):589-595.

Bosentan (*Tracleer*)

Tadalafil (eg, *Cialis*)

SUMMARY: Bosentan administration resulted in a modest reduction in tadalafil plasma concentrations; some loss of tadalafil efficacy may occur.

RISK FACTORS: No specific risk factors are known.

MECHANISM: Bosentan is known to induce CYP3A4, the enzyme that metabolizes tadalafil; reduced bioavailability, increased clearance, or both may result.

CLINICAL EVALUATION: Fifteen healthy men were administered tadalafil 40 mg daily, bosentan 125 mg twice daily, or the combination for 10 consecutive days.[1] The mean area under the concentration-time curve of tadalafil was reduced approximately 40%, while its peak plasma concentration declined approximately 25% during bosentan coadministration. Some patients may have a reduced response to tadalafil administration if bosentan is coadministered.

RELATED DRUGS: Sildenafil (eg, *Viagra*) and vardenafil (*Levitra*) are likely to be affected in a similar manner by bosentan.

MANAGEMENT OPTIONS:

➡ *Monitor.* Monitor for reduced efficacy of tadalafil when bosentan is coadministered.

REFERENCES:

1. Wrishko RE, et al. Pharmacokinetic interaction between tadalafil and bosentan in healthy male subjects. *J Clin Pharmacol*. 2008;48(5):610-618.

Bosentan (*Tracleer*)

Warfarin (eg, *Coumadin*)

SUMMARY: A patient taking warfarin developed reduced anticoagulant effect after starting bosentan; monitor international normalized ratio (INR) carefully in patients receiving the combination.

RISK FACTORS: No specific risk factors are known.

MECHANISM: Not established. Bosentan has been shown to be an enzyme inducer and probably increases the metabolism of warfarin via CYP2C9 and CYP3A4.

CLINICAL EVALUATION: A 35-year-old woman stabilized on long-term warfarin therapy was started on bosentan 62.5 mg twice daily.[1] Ten days later, her INR was found to be subtherapeutic and continued to be subtherapeutic for 5 weeks, despite weekly increases in the warfarin dose. Although only 1 case has been reported, theoretical considerations suggest that bosentan is likely to reduce warfarin response.

RELATED DRUGS: No information is available.

MANAGEMENT OPTIONS:

➡ *Monitor.* In patients receiving warfarin, be alert for alterations in INR if bosentan is started, stopped, or changed in dosage.

REFERENCES:

1. Murphey LM, et al. Bosentan and warfarin interaction. *Ann Pharmacother*. 2003;37(7-8):1028-1031.

Bromazepam†

Itraconazole (eg, *Sporanox*)

SUMMARY: Itraconazole administration did not produce a significant change in the plasma concentrations of bromazepam.

RISK FACTORS: No specific risk factors are known.

MECHANISM: No interaction.

CLINICAL EVALUATION: Eight healthy subjects received itraconazole 200 mg once daily or placebo for 6 days.[1] On day 4 of itraconazole administration, a single oral dose of bromazepam 3 mg was given. The mean area under the plasma concentration-time curve of bromazepam was not significantly increased (9%) by itraconazole compared with placebo.

RELATED DRUGS: The plasma concentrations of other anxiolytic agents, including midazolam, triazolam (eg, *Halcion*), and alprazolam (eg, *Xanax*), are increased by itraconazole.

MANAGEMENT OPTIONS: No interaction.

REFERENCES:
1. Oda M, et al. The effect of itraconazole on the pharmacokinetics and pharmacodynamics of bromazepam in healthy volunteers. *Eur J Clin Pharmacol*. 2003;59(8-9):615-619.

† Not available in the United States.

Bromfenac (*Xibrom*)

Cimetidine (eg, *Tagamet*)

SUMMARY: The manufacturer reports cimetidine can increase bromfenac serum concentrations, but the clinical importance of this effect is not established.

RISK FACTORS: No specific risk factors are known.

MECHANISM: Not established.

CLINICAL EVALUATION: The manufacturer reports cimetidine can produce a moderate increase in bromfenac serum concentrations, but details were not given.[1]

RELATED DRUGS: Theoretically, famotidine (eg, *Pepcid*), nizatidine (eg, *Axid*), and ranitidine (eg, *Zantac*) are unlikely to interact with bromfenac, but clinical studies are needed for confirmation.

MANAGEMENT OPTIONS: No specific action is required, but be alert for evidence of the interaction.

REFERENCES:
1. *Duract* [package insert]. Madison, NJ: Wyeth Laboratories; 1997.

Bromfenac

Lithium (eg, *Eskalith*)

SUMMARY: Because nonsteroidal anti-inflammatory drugs (NSAIDs) can increase lithium serum concentrations, bromfenac, theoretically, could also do so.

RISK FACTORS: No specific risk are factors known.

MECHANISM: Several NSAIDs have been shown to reduce renal lithium excretion. Theoretically, bromfenac would produce a similar effect but studies are lacking.

CLINICAL EVALUATION: NSAIDs tend to increase lithium serum concentrations and can cause lithium toxicity. Bromfenac probably produces a similar effect, but clinical studies are needed for confirmation.[1]

RELATED DRUGS: Other NSAIDs, except perhaps sulindac (eg, *Clinoril*), tend to increase lithium serum concentrations.

MANAGEMENT OPTIONS:

➡ *Monitor.* Be alert for evidence of lithium toxicity (eg, nausea, vomiting, diarrhea, anorexia, coarse tremor, slurred speech, vertigo, confusion, lethargy; in severe cases, seizures, stupor, coma, cardiovascular collapse). Adjust lithium dose as needed.

REFERENCES:
1. Product information. Bromfenac (*Duract*). Wyeth Laboratories, 1997.

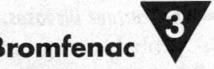

Bromfenac

Phenytoin (eg, *Dilantin*)

SUMMARY: Study in healthy subjects found a substantial reduction in bromfenac plasma concentrations in the presence of phenytoin, but the clinical importance of this effect is not established.

RISK FACTORS: No specific risk factors are known.

MECHANISM: Not established. Phenytoin probably increases the hepatic metabolism of bromfenac.

CLINICAL EVALUATION: Twelve healthy subjects received multiple doses of bromfenac and phenytoin alone and together. Phenytoin reduced the bromfenac area under the plasma concentration-time curve 43%.[1,2] An interaction of this magnitude would be expected to reduce the therapeutic effect of bromfenac in at least some patients. Nonetheless, studies in patients are required for confirmation. Bromfenac only slightly increased bound and unbound phenytoin serum concentrations.

RELATED DRUGS: Other enzyme inducers (eg, aminoglutethimide [*Cytadren*], barbiturates, carbamazepine [eg, *Tegretol*], griseofulvin, primidone [eg, *Mysoline*], rifabutin [*Mycobutin*], rifampin [eg, *Rifadin*], troglitazone [*Rezulin*]) may also reduce bromfenac plasma concentrations.

MANAGEMENT OPTIONS:

➡ *Monitor.* Monitor for reduced therapeutic effect of bromfenac if phenytoin is given concurrently. Adjust bromfenac dose as needed.

REFERENCES:
1. Gumbhir K, et al. Evaluation of pharmacokinetic interaction between bromfenac and phenytoin in healthy men. *J Clin Pharmacol.* 1997;37:160.
2. Product information. Bromfenac (*Duract*). Wyeth Laboratories, 1997.

Bromfenac

Warfarin (eg, *Coumadin*)

SUMMARY: Bromfenac does not appear to affect the hypoprothrombinemic response to warfarin, but cotherapy requires caution because of possible detrimental effects of bromfenac on gastric mucosa and platelet function.

RISK FACTORS:

➡ **Concurrent Diseases.** Patients with peptic ulcer disease or a history of GI bleeding are probably at greater risk for this interaction.

➡ **Dosage Regimen.** The risk of severe GI toxicity from bromfenac and other nonsteroidal anti-inflammatory drugs (NSAIDs) is directly related to the duration of NSAID therapy.

MECHANISM: Although bromfenac may not affect the hypoprothrombinemic response to warfarin, bromfenac-induced gastric erosions and inhibition of platelet function theoretically could increase the risk of bleeding in anticoagulated patients.

CLINICAL EVALUATION: The manufacturer states that bromfenac does not affect warfarin pharmacokinetics or anticoagulant response, but no data were presented.[1]

RELATED DRUGS: All NSAIDs inhibit platelet function, cause gastric erosions, and increase the risk of GI bleeding. Thus, any combination of an oral anticoagulant with an NSAID would theoretically increase the risk of bleeding.

MANAGEMENT OPTIONS:

➡ **Avoid Unless Benefit Outweighs Risk.** Because all NSAIDs increase the risk of GI bleeding in patients on oral anticoagulants, use the combination only after careful consideration of the benefit versus risk. If the NSAID is being used as an analgesic or antipyretic, acetaminophen (eg, *Tylenol*) is probably safer to use with oral anticoagulants. Nonacetylated salicylates (eg, choline salicylate [*Arthropan*], magnesium salicylate [eg, *Magan*], salsalate, sodium salicylate [eg, *Disalcid*]) also are probably safer with oral anticoagulants than standard NSAIDs since they have minimal effects on platelet function and the gastric mucosa.

➡ **Monitor.** Monitor the prothrombin time carefully and watch for evidence of bleeding, especially from the GI tract, if any NSAID is used with an oral anticoagulant.

REFERENCES:

1. Product information. Bromfenac (*Duract*). Wyeth Laboratories, 1997.

 Bromocriptine (*Parlodel*)

Erythromycin (eg, *E-Mycin*)

SUMMARY: Bromocriptine concentrations are markedly increased following erythromycin administration; the clinical significance is unknown.

RISK FACTORS: No specific risk factors are known.

MECHANISM: Not established. However, it appears that erythromycin increases the bioavailability of bromocriptine, reduces its clearance, or has both effects on bromocriptine pharmacokinetics.

CLINICAL EVALUATION: Bromocriptine clearance after oral administration was reduced 71% and peak serum concentrations increased 460% following erythromycin administration compared with bromocriptine administration alone.[1] The clinical significance of this interaction is unknown, but large increases in bromocriptine concentrations could lead to toxicity.

RELATED DRUGS: Troleandomycin (*TAO*) and clarithromycin (*Biaxin*) may also inhibit the metabolism of bromocriptine.

MANAGEMENT OPTIONS:

➡ *Monitor.* Observe patients maintained on bromocriptine for bromocriptine toxicity (eg, hypotension, headache, nausea) during coadministration of erythromycin.

REFERENCES:

1. Nelson MV, et al. Pharmacokinetic evaluation of erythromycin and caffeine administered with bromocriptine in normal subjects. *Clin Pharmacol Ther.* 1990;47:694.

Bromocriptine (*Parlodel*)

Ethanol (*Ethyl Alcohol*)

SUMMARY: Ethanol intolerance has been reported in some patients receiving bromocriptine; more study is needed.

RISK FACTORS: No specific risk factors are known.

MECHANISM: Not established.

CLINICAL EVALUATION: Preliminary clinical evidence indicates that the combined use of ethanol and bromocriptine may increase the likelihood of GI side effects or alcohol intolerance.[1,2]

RELATED DRUGS: No information is available.

MANAGEMENT OPTIONS: No specific action is required, but be alert for evidence of the interaction.

REFERENCES:

1. Wass JA, et al. Long-term treatment of acromegaly with bromocriptine. *BMJ.* 1977;1:875.
2. Ayres J, et al. Alcohol increases bromocriptine's side effects. *N Engl J Med.* 1980;302:806.

Bromocriptine (eg, *Parlodel*)

Isometheptene (eg, *Midrin*) AVOID

SUMMARY: A patient on bromocriptine developed hypertension and ventricular tachycardia after taking isometheptene; avoid the combination until additional data are available.

RISK FACTORS: No specific risk factors are known.

MECHANISM: Not established. The combination may result in vasospasm, probably as a result of combined pharmacodynamic effects.

CLINICAL EVALUATION: A 39-year-old woman was given bromocriptine 2.5 mg twice daily for treatment of postpartum breast engorgement.[1] She was admitted 4 days postpartum with headache and a blood pressure of 188/80 mm Hg. She then was started on *Midrin* (isometheptene 65 mg, acetaminophen 325 mg, dichloralphenazone 100 mg). She took 2 *Midrin* capsules and was discharged with instructions to take 1 additional *Midrin* capsule every hour for 6 doses or until the headache resolved. After she had taken 3 doses of *Midrin*, her headache worsened dramatically and she returned to the emergency room. Her blood pressure was 164/100 mm Hg, and she developed frequent premature ventricular complexes and runs of ventricular tachycardia. She was given supportive treatment and recovered completely. Although bromocriptine in the absence of sympatho-mimetics has been associated with hypertension, seizures, and MI,[2,3] it is possible that isometheptene contributed to the reaction in this patient.

RELATED DRUGS: Assume that all sympathomimetics are capable of interacting adversely with bromocriptine.

MANAGEMENT OPTIONS:

➡ *AVOID COMBINATION.* Even though a causal relationship for this interaction has not been established conclusively, it would be prudent to avoid isometheptene (and other sympathomimetics) in patients receiving bromocriptine.

REFERENCES:

1. Kulig K, et al. Bromocriptine-associated headache: possible life-threatening sympathomimetic interaction. *Obstet Gynecol*. 1991;78:941.

2. Gittelman DK. Bromocriptine associated with postpartum hypertension, seizures, and pituitary hemorrhage. *Gen Hosp Psychiatry*. 1991;13:278.

3. Ruch A, et al. Postpartum myocardial infarction in a patient receiving bromocriptine. *Obstet Gynecol*. 1989;74:448.

4. Chan JC, et al. Postpartum hypertension, bromocriptine and phenylpropanolamine. *Drug Invest*. 1994;8:254.

---

4 Bromocriptine (eg, *Parlodel*)

Lansoprazole (*Prevacid*)

SUMMARY: Lansoprazole appeared to inhibit the effect of bromocriptine in a patient with Parkinson disease, but a causal relationship was not established.

RISK FACTORS: No specific risk factors are known.

MECHANISM: Not established.

CLINICAL EVALUATION: A 73-year-old man with Parkinson disease was on chronic therapy with bromocriptine 20 mg 4 times/day and levodopa/benserazide 400 mg/100 mg 4 times/day.[1] Two days after he started lansoprazole 15 mg/day, he developed acute worsening of his Parkinson disease (akinesia and frequent falls). The symptoms resolved one day after stopping the lansoprazole, and subsequent use of omeprazole did not produce the same reaction. Additional data are needed to establish whether lansoprazole can inhibit the effect of bromocriptine.

RELATED DRUGS: The effect of other proton pump inhibitors on bromocriptine is not known. This case would suggest that omeprazole does not interact with bromocriptine, but more data are needed.

MANAGEMENT OPTIONS: No specific action is required, but be alert for evidence of the interaction.

REFERENCES:

1. Angles A, et al. Interaction between lansoprazole and bromocriptine in a patient with Parkinson's disease. *Therapie*. 2002;57:408-410.

Bromocriptine (*Parlodel*)

Tacrolimus (*Prograf*)

SUMMARY: Drug interaction studies using human liver microsomes in vitro suggest that bromocriptine inhibits the metabolism of tacrolimus; watch for excessive tacrolimus if the drugs are used concurrently.

RISK FACTORS: No specific risk factors are known.

MECHANISM: Tacrolimus is metabolized by cytochrome P450 3A4 (CYP3A4), and bromocriptine appears to inhibit this process.

CLINICAL EVALUATION: Thirty-four drugs were tested for interactions with tacrolimus using in vitro human liver microsomal preparations.[1] Bromocriptine was found to inhibit tacrolimus metabolism. Although the clinical importance of this finding is not established, in vitro human microsomal studies have been remarkably accurate in predicting which drugs will interact in the clinical setting.

RELATED DRUGS: The effect of bromocriptine on cyclosporine (eg, *Neoral*) is not established, but cyclosporine and tacrolimus tend to have similar drug interactions.

MANAGEMENT OPTIONS: No specific action is required, but be alert for evidence of the interaction.

REFERENCES:

1. Christians U, et al. Identification of drugs inhibiting the in vitro metabolism of tacrolimus by human liver microsomes. *Br J Clin Pharmacol.* 1996;41:187.

Bromocriptine (*Parlodel*)

Thioridazine (eg, *Mellaril*)

SUMMARY: Phenothiazines probably inhibit the ability of bromocriptine to lower serum prolactin concentrations in patients with pituitary adenomas. Theoretically, bromocriptine should inhibit the antipsychotic effects of phenothiazines, but clinical evidence suggests that this may be uncommon.

RISK FACTORS: No specific risk factors are known.

MECHANISM: Neuroleptics block dopamine receptors, while bromocriptine is a dopamine agonist.[2] Thus, their effects may be mutually inhibitory.

CLINICAL EVALUATION: In a 40-year-old man with schizophrenia and a large prolactin-secreting pituitary adenoma, serum prolactin concentrations fell dramatically following initiation of bromocriptine therapy and discontinuation of neuroleptic therapy.[1] During the third month of bromocriptine therapy, his psychiatric symptoms returned and he was started on thioridazine 25 mg twice daily. His prolactin levels increased more than 2-fold, and his peripheral vision deteriorated. After thioridazine was discontinued, the prolactin concentration returned to the prethioridazine level. Two months later, while still on bromocriptine, another course of thioridazine in doses up to 200 mg/day resulted in a 4- to 5-fold increase in serum prolactin concentrations; again these levels fell to prethioridazine levels after thioridazine was discontinued. Thus, there is little doubt that in this patient thioridazine inhibited the prolactin-lowering ability of bromocriptine.

Theoretically, bromocriptine should be capable of inhibiting the antipsychotic effects of neuroleptics, but the clinical evidence is conflicting. Psychosis recurred in 1 schizophrenic woman receiving molindone (*Moban*) 100 mg/day and imipramine (eg, *Tofranil*) 200 mg/day after she was given bromocriptine 2.5 mg 3 times daily for 5 days.[3] Another schizophrenic patient on fluphenazine (eg, *Prolixin*) did not develop an exacerbation of psychiatric symptoms when bromocriptine in doses up to 20 mg/day were given for 6 weeks to treat a pituitary adenoma.[4] There was no evidence of reduced tumor size after the bromocriptine therapy, but it is not known whether the antipsychotic drugs interfered with any tumor-shrinking effect of bromocriptine. In a double-blind study, 16 psychiatric patients stabilized on neuroleptics were given 30 to 60 mg/day of bromocriptine. Bromocriptine did not appear to worsen their psychiatric disorders.[6] A review of several studies of concurrent use of neuroleptics and bromocriptine suggests that clinically stable patients maintained on neuroleptics are unlikely to manifest an exacerbation of their psychiatric illness with the addition of bromocriptine.[6]

RELATED DRUGS: It is likely that a similar interference with bromocriptine response would be seen with other phenothiazines and related neuroleptics such as haloperidol (eg, *Haldol*), chlorprothixene (*Taractan*), pimozide (*Orap*), thiothixene (eg, *Navane*), loxapine (eg, *Loxitane*), and molindone (*Moban*). Whether neuroleptics (eg, clozapine [eg, *Clozaril*]) that have less effect on serum prolactin concentrations would be less likely to interfere with the prolactin-lowering effect of bromocriptine is unknown.[5]

MANAGEMENT OPTIONS:

➡ *Consider Alternative.* When possible, avoid the combined use of bromocriptine and neuroleptics.

➡ *Monitor.* When they are used concurrently, monitor the patient carefully for reduced effect of both drugs.

REFERENCES:

1. Robbins RJ, et al. Interactions between thioridazine and bromocriptine in a patient with a prolactin-secreting pituitary adenoma. *Am J Med*. 1984;76:921.

2. Langer G, et al. The prolactin response to neuroleptic drugs. A test of dopaminergic blockade: neuro-endocrine studies in normal men. *J Clin Endocrinol Metab*. 1977;45:996.

3. Frye PE, et al. Bromocriptine associated with symptom exacerbation during neuroleptic treatment of schizoaffective schizophrenia. *J Clin Psychiatry*. 1982;43:252.

4. Kellner C, et al. Concurrent use of bromocriptine and fluphenazine. *J Clin Psychiatry*. 1985;46:455. Letter.

5. Ereshefsky L, et al. Clozapine: an atypical antipsychotic agent. *Clin Pharm*. 1989;8:691.

6. Perovich RM, et al. The behavioral toxicity of bromocriptine in patients with psychiatric illness. *J Clin Psychopharmacol*. 1989;9:417.

Budesonide (eg, *Entocort EC*)

Grapefruit Juice

SUMMARY: Grapefruit juice doubled the bioavailability of orally administered budesonide; increased budesonide toxicity may occur.

RISK FACTORS: No specific risk factors are known.

MECHANISM: Grapefruit juice is likely to inhibit the presystemic metabolism of budesonide by intestinal CYP3A4.

CLINICAL EVALUATION: In an open crossover study, 8 healthy subjects received budesonide (enteric-coated or immediate-release) with and without pretreatment with grapefruit juice 200 mL 3 times daily for 4 days.[1] The grapefruit juice was associated with an approximate doubling of the bioavailability of both forms of budesonide, although the budesonide systemic clearance was not affected. The magnitude of this interaction is likely to increase the risk of budesonide toxicity and adrenal suppression. Inhalation of budesonide theoretically would not interact with grapefruit juice because the site of this interaction appears to be CYP3A4 in the intestine.

RELATED DRUGS: Other corticosteroids that are metabolized by CYP3A4 include dexamethasone (eg, *Baycadron*), fluticasone (eg, *Flonase*), and methylprednisolone (eg, *Medrol*). Theoretically, grapefruit juice would increase the oral bioavailability of these agents, but not when the corticosteroid is given by other routes.

MANAGEMENT OPTIONS:

➥ *Consider Alternative.* Orange juice does not appear to inhibit CYP3A4 and can be used in place of grapefruit juice.

➥ *Monitor.* If grapefruit juice is ingested with oral budesonide, monitor for excessive budesonide effects.

REFERENCES:

1. Seidegard J, et al. Grapefruit juice interaction with oral budesonide: equal effect on immediate-release and delayed-release formulations. *Pharmazie.* 2009;64(7):461-465.

Budesonide (eg, *Pulmicort*)

Itraconazole (eg, *Sporanox*)

SUMMARY: Itraconazole decreases the metabolism of inhaled budesonide; increased adverse reactions may occur in patients taking both drugs on a long-term basis.

RISK FACTORS: No specific risk factors are known.

MECHANISM: Itraconazole inhibits the CYP3A4 metabolism of budesonide.

CLINICAL EVALUATION: Budesonide 1,000 mcg was administered by inhalation as 5 doses of 200 mcg over 2 minutes to 10 healthy subjects on the final day of 5 days of either placebo or itraconazole 200 mg/day.[1] The administration of itraconazole resulted in a mean increase of budesonide area under the concentration-time curve of 4.2-fold (range, 1.75 to 9.8), and peak concentration of 1.6-fold. Budesonide half-life increased from 1.6 to 6.2 hours following itraconazole coadministration. Budesonide-induced suppression of cortisol was increased by itraconazole. Short-term itraconazole administered to patients stabilized on budesonide is not expected to produce an increase in adverse effects.

In another study, 11 of 25 patients with cystic fibrosis on long-term treatment with budesonide and itraconazole had evidence of adrenal insufficiency.[2] Cases of Cushing syndrome following combined use of itraconazole with inhaled budesonide have also been reported.[3-5]

RELATED DRUGS: Ketoconazole has been reported to enhance the cortisol suppression associated with budesonide administration.[6] Fluconazole (eg, *Diflucan*), ketoconazole (eg, *Nizoral*), posaconazole (*Noxafil*), and voriconazole (*Vfend*) also inhibit the activity of CYP3A4 and are expected to increase the plasma concentrations of budesonide. Other corticosteroids that are metabolized by CYP3A4 and also may interact with CYP3A4 inhibitors include dexamethasone (eg, *Baycadron*), fluticasone (eg, *Flonase*), and methylprednisolone (eg, *Medrol*).

MANAGEMENT OPTIONS:

➡ *Monitor.* If budesonide and itraconazole are used concurrently, monitor for Cushing syndrome (eg, moon face, acne, easy bruising, increased facial hair, buffalo hump). Other evidence of corticosteroid toxicity includes increased blood glucose, hypertension, bone fractures, muscle weakness, cataracts, glaucoma, mood swings, and poor wound healing.

REFERENCES:

1. Raaska K, et al. Plasma concentrations of inhaled budesonide and its effects on plasma cortisol are increased by the cytochrome P4503A4 inhibitor itraconazole. *Clin Pharmacol Ther.* 2002;72(4):362-369.
2. Skov M, et al. Iatrogenic adrenal insufficiency as a side-effect of combined treatment of itraconazole and budesonide. *Eur Respir J.* 2002;20(1):127-133.
3. Bolland MJ, et al. Cushing's syndrome due to interaction between inhaled corticosteroids and itraconazole. *Ann Pharmacother.* 2004;38(1):46-49.
4. Main KM, et al. Cushing's syndrome due to pharmacological interaction in a cystic fibrosis patient. *Acta Paediatr.* 2002;91(9):1008-1011.
5. De Wachter E, et al. Rapidly developing Cushing syndrome in a 4-year-old patient during combined treatment with itraconazole and inhaled budesonide. *Eur J Pediatr.* 2003;162(7-8):488-489.
6. Falcoz C, et al. Effects of CYP4503A inhibition by ketoconazole on systemic activity of inhaled fluticasone propionate and budesonide. *Eur Respir J.* 1997;10(suppl 25):175-176.

Budesonide (eg, *Entocort EC*)

Ketoconazole (eg, *Nizoral*)

SUMMARY: Ketoconazole increases orally administered budesonide plasma concentrations; increased systemic steroid effects are likely to occur.

RISK FACTORS: No specific risk factors are known.

MECHANISM: Ketoconazole inhibits the CYP3A4 metabolism of budesonide, markedly increasing its bioavailability and plasma concentrations.

CLINICAL EVALUATION: A single oral dose of budesonide 3 mg was taken alone, on the morning of the fourth day of ketoconazole 200 mg daily in the morning, and on the fourth day of ketoconazole 200 mg daily but 12 hours before the last ketoconazole dose.[1] During coadministration of ketoconazole and budesonide, the mean area under the concentration-time curve (AUC) increased 6.8 times (range, 3.9 to 14). With the 12-hour separation between the doses, the mean AUC increased approximately 4 times. This large increase in the bioavailability of oral budesonide may produce unwanted systemic effects in patients taking oral budesonide for inflammatory bowel disease. Ketoconazole has been reported to enhance the cortisol suppression associated with budesonide administration.[2]

RELATED DRUGS: Itraconazole (eg, *Sporanox*) is known to increase budesonide plasma concentrations; voriconazole (*Vfend*) and fluconazole (eg, *Diflucan*) also inhibit CYP3A4 and are expected to affect budesonide.

MANAGEMENT OPTIONS:

➡ *Monitor.* Monitor patients stabilized on oral budesonide for altered systemic steroid effect and disease response if ketoconazole is initiated or discontinued.

REFERENCES:

1. Seidegard J. Reduction of the inhibitory effect of ketoconazole on budesonide pharmacokinetics by separation of their time of administration. *Clin Pharmacol Ther.* 2000;68(1):13-17.

2. Falcoz C, et al. Effects of CYP4503A inhibition by ketoconazole on systemic activity of inhaled fluticasone propionate and budesonide. *Eur Respir J.* 1997;10(suppl 25):175-176.

Budesonide (eg, *Pulmicort*)

Ritonavir (*Norvir*)

SUMMARY: Ritonavir may increase the effect of budesonide, leading to Cushing syndrome and other evidence of corticosteroid toxicity.

RISK FACTORS: No specific risk factors are known.

MECHANISM: Ritonavir appears to inhibit the CYP3A4 metabolism of budesonide.

CLINICAL EVALUATION: One report describes 3 children with perinatally acquired HIV infection who developed Cushing syndrome during combined therapy with ritonavir and inhaled budesonide.[1] Another report describes a 37-year-old woman with asthma who, after having ritonavir added to her inhaled fluticasone, developed evidence of Cushing syndrome.[2] The fluticasone was discontinued and the symptoms resolved within 2 months. These cases are consistent with the known interactive properties of budesonide and ritonavir.

RELATED DRUGS: Other protease inhibitors, including atazanavir (*Reyataz*), darunavir (*Prezista*), fosamprenavir (*Lexiva*), indinavir (*Crixivan*), nelfinavir (*Viracept*), and saquinavir (*Invirase*), also inhibit the activity of CYP3A and are expected to increase the plasma concentration of budesonide. Other corticosteroids that are metabolized by CYP3A4 and also may interact with CYP3A4 inhibitors include dexamethasone (eg, *Baycadron*), fluticasone (eg, *Flonase*), and methylprednisolone (eg, *Medrol*). A case of Cushing syndrome has also been reported following epidural triamcinolone in a patient receiving ritonavir.[3]

MANAGEMENT OPTIONS:

➡ *Consider Alternative.* Consider using an alternative to one of the drugs (see Related Drugs).

➡ *Monitor.* If budesonide and ritonavir are used concurrently, monitor for Cushing syndrome (eg, moon face, acne, easy bruising, increased facial hair, buffalo hump). Other evidence of corticosteroid toxicity includes increased blood glucose, hypertension, bone fractures, muscle weakness, cataracts, glaucoma, mood swings, and poor wound healing.

REFERENCES:

1. Gray D, et al. Adrenal suppression and Cushing's syndrome secondary to ritonavir and budesonide. *S Afr Med J.* 2010;100(5):296-297.

2. Kedem E, et al. Iatrogenic Cushing's syndrome due to coadministration of ritonavir and inhaled budesonide in an asthmatic human immunodeficiency virus infected patient. *J Asthma.* 2010;47(7):830-831.

3. Ramanathan R, et al. Iatrogenic Cushing syndrome after epidural triamcinolone injections in an HIV type 1-infected patient receiving therapy with ritonavir-lopinavir. *Clin Infect Dis.* 2008;47(12):e97-e99.

Bumetanide (eg, *Bumex*)

Indomethacin (eg, *Indocin*)

SUMMARY: Indomethacin administration reduces the diuretic and antihypertensive efficacy of bumetanide.

RISK FACTORS: No specific risk factors are known.

MECHANISM: Indomethacin inhibits prostaglandin synthesis, resulting in a tendency for the patient to retain sodium.

CLINICAL EVALUATION: Indomethacin reduces the natriuretic and diuretic response to bumetanide in healthy subjects and patients with hypertension.[1-4]

RELATED DRUGS: Prostaglandin inhibitors other than indomethacin (eg, other nonsteroidal anti-inflammatory drugs [NSAIDs]) may have a similar effect on bumetanide, but few data are available. However, aspirin may be less likely to interact with bumetanide. Furosemide (eg, *Lasix*) is also affected by indomethacin.

MANAGEMENT OPTIONS:

➡ **Consider Alternative.** Aspirin may be less likely than NSAIDs to interfere with the response to bumetanide and, thus, may be a possible substitute for indomethacin. Because furosemide also is affected by indomethacin, it is not a viable alternative.

➡ **Monitor.** Monitor for reduced diuretic and natriuretic response to bumetanide in the presence of indomethacin or other NSAIDs.

REFERENCES:

1. Brater DC, et al. Interaction studies with bumetanide and furosemide. Effects of probenecid and of indomethacin on response to bumetanide in man. *J Clin Pharmacol.* 1981;21(11-12 pt 2):647-653.
2. Brater DC, et al. Indomethacin and the response to butanimide. *Clin Pharmacol Ther.* 1980;27:421.
3. Kaufman J, et al. Bumetanide-induced diuresis and natriuresis: effect of prostaglandin synthetase inhibition. *J Clin Pharmacol.* 1981;21(11-12 pt 2):663-667.
4. Pedrinelli R, et al. Influence of indomethacin on the natriuretic and renin-stimulating effect of bumetanide in essential hypertension. *Clin Pharmacol Ther.* 1980;28:722-731.

Bumetanide (eg, *Bumex*)

Probenecid

SUMMARY: Probenecid can slightly reduce bumetanide-induced diuresis; however, the clinical significance is likely to be minimal.

RISK FACTORS: No specific risk factors are known.

MECHANISM: Not established.

CLINICAL EVALUATION: Bumetanide diuresis may be reduced slightly in the presence of probenecid,[1] although this has not been a consistent finding.[2]

RELATED DRUGS: Probenecid also appears to have minimal effects on the response to furosemide (eg, *Lasix*).

MANAGEMENT OPTIONS: No specific action is required, but be alert for evidence of the interaction.

REFERENCES:

1. Velasquez MT, et al. Effect of probenecid on the natriuresis and renin release induced by bumetanide in man. *J Clin Pharmacol.* 1981;21(11-12 pt 2):657-662.
2. Brater DC, et al. Interaction studies with bumetanide and furosemide. Effects of probenecid and of indomethacin on response to bumetanide in man. *J Clin Pharmacol.* 1981;21(11-12 pt 2):647-653.

Bumetanide (eg, *Bumex*) 5

Warfarin (eg, *Coumadin*)

SUMMARY: Bumetanide does not appear to interact with warfarin.

RISK FACTORS: No specific risk factors are known.

MECHANISM: No interaction.

CLINICAL EVALUATION: In 2 studies involving a total of 21 healthy subjects, bumetanide 1 to 2 mg/day did not affect the disposition of or the hypoprothrombinemic response to warfarin.[1,2] Studies in patients who need the diuretic effect of bumetanide are required to confirm that no interaction occurs.

RELATED DRUGS: Other loop diuretics and thiazides also appear to have minimal effects on warfarin response.

MANAGEMENT OPTIONS: No interaction.

REFERENCES:

1. Nilsson CM, et al. The effect of furosemide and bumetanide on warfarin metabolism and anticoagulant response. *J Clin Pharmacol.* 1978;18:91-94.

2. Nipper H, et al. The effect of bumetanide on the serum disappearance of warfarin sodium. *J Clin Pharmacol.* 1981;21:654-656.

Bunazosin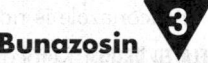

Enalapril (eg, *Vasotec*)

SUMMARY: Limited evidence suggests that patients receiving angiotensin-converting enzyme (ACE) inhibitors such as enalapril can have an exaggerated, first-dose hypotensive response to alpha-blockers such as bunazosin.

RISK FACTORS: No specific risk factors are known.

MECHANISM: Additive hypotensive effects are produced by the addition of ACE inhibitors.

CLINICAL EVALUATION: After a severe first-dose, hypotensive episode caused by an alpha-blocker (bunazosin) was observed in a patient taking enalapril, 6 healthy subjects were given bunazosin and enalapril, alone and together.[1] Bunazosin plus 2.5 mg of enalapril reduced systolic and diastolic blood pressure 19 and 22 mm Hg, while bunazosin plus 10 mg enalapril resulted in 27 and 28 mm Hg reductions. Thus, it appears that the first-dose hypotensive effect of bunazosin may be enhanced by enalapril.

RELATED DRUGS: Theoretically, one would expect this interaction to occur with any combination of an ACE inhibitor (eg, benazepril [*Lotensin*], captopril [eg, *Capoten*], lisinopril [eg, *Prinivil*]) with alpha-blockers such as prazosin (eg, *Minipress*), terazosin (eg, *Hytrin*), doxazosin (eg, *Cardura*), and trimazosin.

MANAGEMENT OPTIONS:

➡ *Circumvent/Minimize.* In patients receiving ACE inhibitors, undertake initiation of therapy with bunazosin or other alpha-blockers with caution and with conservative doses. Taking the initial doses of the alpha-blocker at bedtime would be prudent.

➡ **Monitor.** Be alert for evidence of excessive hypotension.

REFERENCES:
1. Baba T, et al. Enhancement by an ACE inhibitor of first-dose hypotension caused by an alpha 1-blocker. *N Engl J Med.* 1990;322:1237.

Bupivacaine (eg, *Sensorcaine*)

Itraconazole (*Sporanox*)

SUMMARY: A small increase in bupivacaine serum concentrations may occur in patients taking itraconazole; the clinical significance is likely to be limited.

RISK FACTORS: No specific risk factors are known.

MECHANISM: Itraconazole reduces the clearance of bupivacaine. It is not clear if this is the result of itraconazole-induced inhibition of CYP3A4 or an active transporter of bupivacaine.

CLINICAL EVALUATION: Seven volunteers received bupivacaine 0.3 mg IV over 60 minutes 4 days following pretreatment with either placebo or itraconazole 200 mg once daily.[1] The clearance of both R- and S-bupivacaine was reduced about 20% to 25% by itraconazole. Bupivacaine half-life was not altered following itraconazole dosing. No evidence of toxicity or electrocardiogram changes were noted. Based on the limited magnitude of change in bupivacaine clearance, coadministration with itraconazole is not likely to produce adverse effects in most patients.

RELATED DRUGS: Ketoconazole (eg, *Nizoral*), voriconazole (*Vfend*), and fluconazole (*Diflucan*) are CYP3A4 inhibitors and may reduce the clearance of bupivacaine.

MANAGEMENT OPTIONS:

➡ **Monitor.** When administering bupivacaine to patients taking itraconazole, be alert for possible increased cardiotoxicity.

REFERENCES:
1. Palkama VJ, et al. Effect of itraconazole on the pharmacokinetics of bupivacaine enantiomers in healthy volunteers. *Br J Anaesth.* 1999;83:659-661.

Bupropion (eg, *Wellbutrin*)

Clopidogrel (*Plavix*)

SUMMARY: Clopidogrel increases plasma concentrations of bupropion and reduces concentrations of its active metabolite; it is possible that these changes would decrease the efficacy and increase the toxicity of bupropion.

RISK FACTORS: No specific risk factors are known.

MECHANISM: Clopidogrel appears to be a potent mechanism-based inhibitor of CYP2B6, the enzyme responsible for the metabolism of bupropion.[1]

CLINICAL EVALUATION: In healthy subjects given a single dose of bupropion 150 mg with and without pretreatment with clopidogrel 75 mg/day for 4 days, clopidogrel was associated with a 60% increase in bupropion plasma concentrations and a 52% reduction in plasma concentrations of hydroxybupropion, the active metabolite of bupropion. Theoretically, the efficacy of bupropion may be reduced because of reduction in the concentration of the active metabolite, and the risk of toxicity may increase because of increased concentration of the parent drug. The study was not designed to address these possibilities, but both are plausible.

RELATED DRUGS: Ticlopidine appears to interact with bupropion similarly, but likely to a greater extent than clopidine.

MANAGEMENT OPTIONS:

➡ *Consider Alternative.* Prasugrel (*Effient*) appears to interact minimally with bupropion.

➡ *Monitor.* If the combination is used, monitor for reduced bupropion efficacy and increased bupropion toxicity.

REFERENCES:

1. Richter T, et al. Potent mechanism-based inhibition of human CYP2B6 by clopidogrel and ticlopidine. *J Pharmacol Exp Ther*. 2004;308(1):189-197.

2. Turpeinen M, et al. Effect of clopidogrel and ticlopidine on cytochrome P450 2B6 activity as measured by bupropion hydroxylation. *Clin Pharmacol Ther*. 2005;77(6):553-559.

Bupropion (eg, *Wellbutrin*)
Cyclosporine (eg, *Neoral*)

SUMMARY: A boy receiving cyclosporine following a heart transplant developed a marked decrease in cyclosporine concentrations during bupropion administration, but a causal relationship was not established.

RISK FACTORS: No specific risk factors are known.

MECHANISM: Not established.

CLINICAL EVALUATION: A 10-year-old boy taking cyclosporine following a heart transplant developed a marked reduction in cyclosporine blood concentrations after starting bupropion 75 mg twice daily.[1] It was not certain that the patient adhered to the cyclosporine dosing schedule, so a causal relationship was not established.

RELATED DRUGS: No information is available.

MANAGEMENT OPTIONS: No specific action is required, but be alert for evidence of the interaction.

REFERENCES:

1. Lewis BR, et al. Pharmacokinetic interactions between cyclosporine and bupropion or methylphenidate. *J Child Adolesc Psychopharmacol*. 2001;11(2):193-198.

Bupropion (eg, *Wellbutrin*)
Desipramine (eg, *Norpramin*)

SUMMARY: Bupropion produces marked increases in desipramine plasma concentrations; increased desipramine toxicity may occur.

RISK FACTORS:

➡ *Pharmacogenetics.* Only patients who have CYP2D6 activity (ie, extensive metabolizers and, to a lesser extent, intermediate metabolizers) are expected to experience this interaction. Poor metabolizers do not have the gene for production of CYP2D6 and, therefore, have no CYP2D6 for bupropion to inhibit.

MECHANISM: Bupropion inhibits the CYP2D6 metabolism of desipramine.[1-3]

CLINICAL EVALUATION: In a study of 15 subjects, bupropion 150 mg twice daily produced a marked (5-fold) increase in desipramine plasma concentrations.[4] Bupropion is a potent inhibitor of CYP2D6; the increase in desipramine plasma concentration is likely to increase the risk of desipramine toxicity. Bupropion has a long half-life, and the interaction was still detectible 1 week after the last dose of bupropion.

RELATED DRUGS: Several other tricyclic antidepressants are also metabolized by CYP2D6, and are expected to interact with bupropion, including: amitriptyline, amoxapine, clomipramine (eg, *Anafranil*), doxepin (eg, *Silenor*), imipramine (eg, *Tofranil*), nortriptyline (eg, *Pamelor*), protriptyline (eg, *Vivactil*), and trimipramine (eg, *Surmontil*). Most of these antidepressants have other metabolic pathways in addition to CYP2D6, and the magnitude of the interactions with bupropion may be less than with desipramine, for which CYP2D6 is essentially the only important pathway for metabolism.

MANAGEMENT OPTIONS:

➡ *Consider Alternative.* Most of the tricyclic antidepressants listed under Related Drugs have less of an interaction with bupropion than desipramine.

➡ *Monitor.* If bupropion is used with desipramine or other tricyclic antidepressants, monitor for adverse tricyclic effects such as dry mouth, constipation, blurred vision, tachycardia, and urinary retention. Adjust the tricyclic antidepressant dose as needed.

REFERENCES:

1. Kotlyar M, et al. Inhibition of CYP2D6 activity by bupropion. *J Clin Psychopharmacol.* 2005;25(3):226-229.
2. Güzey C, et al. Change from the CYP2D6 extensive metabolizer to the poor metabolizer phenotype during treatment with bupropion. *Ther Drug Monit.* 2002;24(3):436-437.
3. Reese MJ, et al. An in vitro mechanistic study to elucidate the desipramine/bupropion clinical drug-drug interaction. *Drug Metab Dispos.* 2008;36(7):1198-1201.
4. *Wellbutrin* [package insert]. Research Triangle Park, NC: GlaxoSmithKline; 2010.

Bupropion (eg, *Wellbutrin*)

Dextromethorphan

SUMMARY: Bupropion substantially increases dextromethorphan plasma concentrations; in 1 case this may have lead to serotonin syndrome.

RISK FACTORS:

➡ *Pharmacogenetics.* Only patients who have CYP2D6 activity (ie, extensive metabolizers and, to a lesser extent, intermediate metabolizers) are expected to experience this interaction. Poor metabolizers do not have the gene for production of CYP2D6 and, therefore, have no CYP2D6 for bupropion to inhibit.

MECHANISM: Dextromethorphan is a CYP2D6 substrate and has serotonergic effects. Bupropion is a potent CYP2D6 inhibitor and is known to inhibit dextromethorphan metabolism and substantially increase dextromethorphan plasma concentrations.[1,2] Bupropion may increase dextromethorphan plasma concentrations sufficiently to produce serotonin syndrome.

CLINICAL EVALUATION: A 43-year-old man on long-term bupropion therapy and who had recently used dextromethorphan underwent a molar extraction under local anesthesia with 144 mg of lidocaine 2% with epinephrine 1:100,000.[3] Soon after the procedure, he developed clear evidence of serotonin syndrome (ie, confusion, restlessness, agitation, tachycardia, fever, rigidity, myoclonus). He was hospitalized in the intensive care unit, but gradually responded to supportive therapy. The fact that the patient had recently increased his bupropion dose and had taken dextromethorphan before the procedure suggests that this combination was the most likely cause of his serotonin syndrome. Whether the lidocaine and epinephrine contributed to the reaction is not clear.

RELATED DRUGS: No information is available.

MANAGEMENT OPTIONS:

➥ **Consider Alternative.** Dextromethorphan is of dubious efficacy in the treatment of coughs, so benefit-risk considerations suggest the use of alternative agents in patients receiving bupropion.

➥ **Monitor.** If dextromethorphan is used in patients on bupropion therapy, monitor for evidence of serotonin syndrome (ie, myoclonus, rigidity, tremor, hyperreflexia, fever, sweating, seizures, confusion, agitation, incoordination, coma).

REFERENCES:

1. Kotlyar M, et al. Inhibition of CYP2D6 activity by bupropion. *J Clin Psychopharmacol.* 2005;25(3):226-229.
2. Güzey C, et al. Change from the CYP2D6 extensive metabolizer to the poor metabolizer phenotype during treatment with bupropion. *Ther Drug Monit.* 2002;24(3):436-437.
3. Szakaly B, et al. Serotonin syndrome in the oral and maxillofacial surgery office: a review of the literature and report of a case. *J Oral Maxillofac Surg.* 2008;66(9):1949-1952.

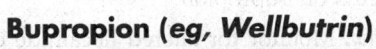

Bupropion (eg, Wellbutrin)

Efavirenz (Sustiva)

SUMMARY: Efavirenz administration reduces the plasma concentration of bupropion; partial loss of therapeutic effect may occur in some patients.

RISK FACTORS: No specific risk factors are known.

MECHANISM: It appears that efavirenz is an inducer of the enzyme CYP2B6, the primary enzyme responsible for bupropion metabolism.

CLINICAL EVALUATION: Thirteen healthy subjects received a single dose of sustained-release bupropion 150 mg before and after 2 weeks of efavirenz 600 mg daily.[1] The mean area under the concentration-time curve of bupropion was reduced 55% by pretreatment with efavirenz. The peak bupropion concentration was reduced 34% and its half-life decreased from 8.6 to 4.7 hours following efavirenz. The reduction in the plasma concentration of bupropion could reduce its efficacy.

RELATED DRUGS: None known.

MANAGEMENT OPTIONS:

➥ **Monitor.** Monitor patients stabilized on bupropion for altered response if efavirenz therapy is initiated or discontinued.

REFERENCES:

1. Robertson SM, et al. Efavirenz induces CYP2B6-mediated hydroxylation of bupropion in healthy subjects. *J Acquir Immune Defic Syndr.* 2008;49(5):513-519.

Bupropion (eg, *Wellbutrin*)

Flecainide (eg, *Tambocor*)

SUMMARY: Theoretically, bupropion increases flecainide plasma concentrations, but the clinical importance is not established.

RISK FACTORS:

➦ **Pharmacogenetics.** Only patients who have CYP2D6 activity (ie, extensive metabolizers and, to a lesser extent, intermediate metabolizers) are expected to experience this interaction. Poor metabolizers do not have the gene for production of CYP2D6 and, therefore, have no CYP2D6 for bupropion to inhibit.

MECHANISM: Bupropion is likely to inhibit the CYP2D6 metabolism of flecainide.

CLINICAL EVALUATION: This interaction is based primarily on theoretical considerations. Nonetheless, bupropion is a potent inhibitor of CYP2D6 and is likely to increase flecainide plasma concentrations.[1-3]

RELATED DRUGS: Other antiarrhythmics that are also metabolized by CYP2D6 include mexiletine and propafenone (eg, *Rythmol*); they are also expected to interact with bupropion.

MANAGEMENT OPTIONS:

➦ **Circumvent/Minimize.** Consider using conservative initial doses of flecainide in patients on bupropion.

➦ **Monitor.** Monitor for altered flecainide effects if bupropion is started, stopped, or changed in dosage.

REFERENCES:

1. Kotlyar M, et al. Inhibition of CYP2D6 activity by bupropion. *J Clin Psychopharmacol.* 2005;25(3):226-229.
2. Güzey C, et al. Change from the CYP2D6 extensive metabolizer to the poor metabolizer phenotype during treatment with bupropion. *Ther Drug Monit.* 2002;24(3):436-437.
3. *Wellbutrin* [package insert]. Research Triangle Park, NC: GlaxoSmithKline; 2010.

4   Bupropion (eg, *Wellbutrin*)

Guanfacine (eg, *Tenex*)

SUMMARY: A 10-year-old girl taking bupropion and guanfacine experienced a generalized tonic-clonic seizure, but a causal relationship between the drug combination and the seizure was not established.

RISK FACTORS: No specific risk factors are known.

MECHANISM: Not established.

CLINICAL EVALUATION: A 10-year-old girl was receiving bupropion 100 mg 3 times daily for treatment of attention deficit hyperactivity disorder.[1] Guanfacine 0.5 mg twice daily was added and then increased to 0.5 mg 3 times daily. Ten days after increasing the guanfacine to 3 times daily, she had a generalized tonic-clonic seizure. The cause of the seizure in this patient is not clear. Bupropion is associated with an increased rate of seizures, but it is not possible to determine the role that guanfacine played in the reaction.

RELATED DRUGS: No information is available.

MANAGEMENT OPTIONS: No specific action is required, but be alert for evidence of the interaction.

REFERENCES:
1. Tilton P. Bupropion and guanfacine. *J Am Acad Child Adolesc Psychiatry*. 1998;37(7):682-683.

Bupropion (eg, *Wellbutrin*)

Levodopa

SUMMARY: Bupropion given with levodopa may increase the risk of adverse reactions, but the clinical importance is not established.

RISK FACTORS: No specific risk factors are known.

MECHANISM: Not established.

CLINICAL EVALUATION: Some evidence suggests that combining bupropion with levodopa may increase adverse outcomes, but no details were provided.[1] More clinical study is needed to assess if this results from a drug interaction between bupropion and levodopa.

RELATED DRUGS: Combining bupropion with amantadine purportedly also increases the risk of adverse reactions.

MANAGEMENT OPTIONS: No specific action is required, but be alert for evidence of the interaction.

REFERENCES:
1. *Wellbutrin* [package insert]. Research Triangle Park, NC: GlaxoSmithKline; 2010.

Bupropion (eg, *Wellbutrin*)

Metoprolol (eg, *Lopressor*)

SUMMARY: A patient taking metoprolol and diltiazem developed bradycardia after starting bupropion, but the clinical importance of this interaction is not established.

RISK FACTORS:

➡ **Pharmacogenetics.** Only patients with the extensive metabolizer CYP2D6 phenotype are expected to experience this interaction. Poor metabolizers do not have the gene for production of CYP2D6 and, therefore, have no CYP2D6 for bupropion to inhibit. Approximately 8% of white patients are deficient in CYP2D, but the deficiency is rare in Asian patients, usually less than 2%.

MECHANISM: Bupropion likely inhibits the CYP2D6 metabolism of metoprolol.

CLINICAL EVALUATION: A 56-year-old man stabilized on metoprolol 150 mg/day and diltiazem 480 mg/day developed severe bradycardia after bupropion 150 mg twice daily was added for smoking cessation.[1] Bupropion-induced increase in metoprolol concentrations was a likely factor, but the relatively high dose of diltiazem almost certainly contributed as well. The risk of concurrent use of bupropion and metoprolol in patients not receiving calcium channel blockers is not known.

RELATED DRUGS: Bupropion also may inhibit the metabolism of other beta-adrenergic blockers that are metabolized by CYP2D6, such as propranolol (eg, *Inderal LA*) and timolol (eg, *Betimol*).

MANAGEMENT OPTIONS: No specific action is required, but be alert for evidence of the interaction.

REFERENCES:

1. McCollum DL, et al. Severe sinus bradycardia after initiation of bupropion therapy: a probable drug-drug interaction with metoprolol. *Cardiovasc Drugs Ther.* 2004;18(4):329-330.

Bupropion (eg, *Wellbutrin*)

Mexiletine

SUMMARY: Theoretically, bupropion would increase mexiletine plasma concentrations, but the clinical importance is not established.

RISK FACTORS:

➤ *Pharmacogenetics.* Only patients who have CYP2D6 activity (ie, extensive metabolizers and, to a lesser extent, intermediate metabolizers) are expected to experience this interaction. Poor metabolizers do not have the gene for production of CYP2D6 and, therefore, have no CYP2D6 for bupropion to inhibit.

MECHANISM: Bupropion is likely to inhibit the CYP2D6 metabolism of mexiletine.

CLINICAL EVALUATION: This interaction is based primarily on theoretical considerations. Nonetheless, bupropion is a potent inhibitor of CYP2D6 and is likely to increase mexiletine plasma concentrations.[1-3]

RELATED DRUGS: Other antiarrhythmics that are also metabolized by CYP2D6 include flecainide (eg, *Tambocor*) and propafenone (eg, *Rythmol*); they are also expected to interact with bupropion.

MANAGEMENT OPTIONS:

➤ *Circumvent/Minimize.* Consider using conservative initial doses of mexiletine in patients taking bupropion.

➤ *Monitor.* Monitor for altered mexiletine effects if bupropion is started, stopped, or changed in dosage.

REFERENCES:

1. Kotlyar M, et al. Inhibition of CYP2D6 activity by bupropion. *J Clin Psychopharmacol.* 2005;25(3):226-229.
2. Güzey C, et al. Change from the CYP2D6 extensive metabolizer to the poor metabolizer phenotype during treatment with bupropion. *Ther Drug Monit.* 2002;24(3):436-437.
3. *Wellbutrin* [package insert]. Research Triangle Park, NC: GlaxoSmithKline; 2010.

4 Bupropion (eg, *Wellbutrin*)

Nelfinavir (*Viracept*)

SUMMARY: In vitro studies suggest an interaction between bupropion and nelfinavir, but no evidence of adverse outcomes was found in a small retrospective clinical study.

RISK FACTORS: No risk factors are known.

MECHANISM: Unknown.

CLINICAL EVALUATION: The records of 6 patients who had taken bupropion with nelfinavir were reviewed after in vitro studies found inhibition of bupropion hydroxylation with nelfinavir.[1,2] No evidence of adverse interaction (eg, seizures) was detected, which might have been expected given the low rate of bupropion-induced seizures, the small number of patients observed, and the retrospective nature of the study. Additional study is needed to determine if this purported interaction results in adverse outcomes.

RELATED DRUGS: No information is available.

MANAGEMENT OPTIONS: No specific action is required, but be alert for evidence of the interaction.

REFERENCES:

1. Hesse LM, et al. Ritonavir, efavirenz, and nelfinavir inhibit CYP2B6 activity in vitro: potential drug interactions with bupropion. *Drug Metab Dispos.* 2001;29(2):100-102.

2. Park-Wyllie LY, et al. Concurrent use of bupropion with CYP2B6 inhibitors, nelfinavir, ritonavir and efavirenz: a case series. *AIDS.* 2003;17(4):638-640.

Bupropion (eg, *Wellbutrin*) 4

Nortriptyline (eg, *Pamelor*)

SUMMARY: A patient taking nortriptyline developed toxicity when bupropion was added to her therapy; the case was well documented, but more information is needed to determine the clinical importance of this interaction.

RISK FACTORS:

➡ *Pharmacogenetics.* Only patients with the extensive metabolizer CYP2D6 phenotype can be expected to experience this interaction. Poor metabolizers do not have the gene for production of CYP2D6 and, therefore, have no CYP2D6 for bupropion to inhibit. Approximately 8% of white patients are deficient in CYP2D6, but the deficiency is rare in Asian patients, usually no more than 2%.

MECHANISM: Bupropion is known to inhibit CYP2D6, and it likely increases nortriptyline plasma concentrations by interfering with the hepatic CYP2D6 metabolism of nortriptyline.

CLINICAL EVALUATION: An 83-year-old woman on nortriptyline 75 mg/day developed a 185% increase in nortriptyline plasma concentrations after starting bupropion 150 mg twice daily.[1] There was a positive dechallenge and rechallenge, and the elevated nortriptyline concentrations were associated with signs of nortriptyline toxicity, such as lethargy, confusion, and falling. It is likely that an adverse drug interaction between bupropion and nortriptyline occurred in this case, but more study is needed to determine the magnitude of this interaction.

RELATED DRUGS: The manufacturer of bupropion states that bupropion doubled the serum concentrations of desipramine (eg, *Norpramin*) in 15 subjects, but details of the study were not presented. Most tricyclic antidepressants are metabolized by CYP2D6 to at least some extent and are expected to interact with bupropion.

MANAGEMENT OPTIONS: No specific action is required, but be alert for evidence of the interaction.

REFERENCES:

1. Weintraub D. Nortriptyline toxicity secondary to interaction with bupropion sustained-release. *Depress Anxiety.* 2001;13(1):50-52.

Bupropion (eg, *Wellbutrin*)

AVOID **Phenelzine (eg, *Nardil*)**

SUMMARY: The manufacturer of bupropion lists concurrent use of monoamine oxidase inhibitors (MAOIs), such as phenelzine, as contraindicated.

RISK FACTORS: No specific risk factors are known.

MECHANISM: Not established. Bupropion has little effect on serotonin reuptake, so theoretically it would not have additive serotonergic effects with MAOIs.

CLINICAL EVALUATION: Phenelzine reportedly increased the acute toxicity of bupropion in animals, but no details were provided.[1]

RELATED DRUGS: Other MAOIs would theoretically also interact with bupropion, including isocarboxazid (*Marplan*), methylene blue, and tranylcypromine (eg, *Parnate*).

MANAGEMENT OPTIONS:

➡ *AVOID COMBINATION.* Avoid concurrent use of bupropion with phenelzine or other MAOIs.

REFERENCES:
1. *Wellbutrin* [package insert]. Research Triangle Park, NC: GlaxoSmithKline; 2010.

 Bupropion (eg, *Wellbutrin*)

Prasugrel (*Effient*)

SUMMARY: Prasugrel may produce small increases in bupropion plasma concentrations, but adverse reactions are unlikely.

RISK FACTORS: No specific risk factors are known.

MECHANISM: Prasugrel appears to inhibit the CYP2B6 metabolism of bupropion.

CLINICAL EVALUATION: In healthy subjects, prasugrel produced an 18% increase in bupropion area under the plasma concentration-time curve.[1] This effect is small and not likely to be clinically important.

RELATED DRUGS: Both clopidogrel (*Plavix*) and ticlopidine have been shown to produce substantial increases in bupropion plasma concentrations and to reduce plasma concentrations of its active metabolite, hydroxybupropion.

MANAGEMENT OPTIONS: No specific action is required, but be alert for evidence of the interaction.

REFERENCES:
1. Farid NA, et al. Prasugrel, a new thienopyridine antiplatelet drug, weakly inhibits cytochrome P450 2B6 in humans. *J Clin Pharmacol.* 2008;48(1):53-59.

Bupropion (eg, *Wellbutrin*)

Propafenone (eg, *Rythmol*)

SUMMARY: Theoretically, bupropion will increase propafenone plasma concentrations, but the clinical importance is not established.

RISK FACTORS:

➡ ***Pharmacogenetics.*** Only patients who have CYP2D6 activity (ie, extensive metabolizers and, to a lesser extent, intermediate metabolizers) are expected to experience this interaction. Poor metabolizers do not have the gene for production of CYP2D6 and, therefore, have no CYP2D6 for bupropion to inhibit.

MECHANISM: Bupropion is likely to inhibit the CYP2D6 metabolism of propafenone.

CLINICAL EVALUATION: This interaction is based primarily on theoretical considerations. Nonetheless, bupropion is a potent inhibitor of CYP2D6 and is likely to increase propafenone plasma concentrations.[1-3]

RELATED DRUGS: Other antiarrhythmics that are also metabolized by CYP2D6 include flecainide (eg, *Tambocor*) and mexiletine; they are also expected to interact with bupropion.

MANAGEMENT OPTIONS:

➡ ***Circumvent/Minimize.*** Consider using conservative initial doses of propafenone in patients on bupropion.

➡ ***Monitor.*** Monitor for altered propafenone effects if bupropion is started, stopped, or changed in dosage.

REFERENCES:

1. Kotlyar M, et al. Inhibition of CYP2D6 activity by bupropion. *J Clin Psychopharmacol.* 2005;25(3):226-229.
2. Güzey C, et al. Change from the CYP2D6 extensive metabolizer to the poor metabolizer phenotype during treatment with bupropion. *Ther Drug Monit.* 2002;24(3):436-437.
3. *Wellbutrin* [package insert]. Research Triangle Park, NC: GlaxoSmithKline; 2010.

Bupropion (eg, *Wellbutrin*)

Rifampin (eg, *Rifadin*)

SUMMARY: Rifampin reduces bupropion plasma concentrations; expect some loss of therapeutic effect.

RISK FACTORS: No specific risk factors are known.

MECHANISM: Rifampin appears to increase bupropion metabolism by induction of CYP2B6, the enzyme responsible for bupropion's metabolism.

CLINICAL EVALUATION: Sixteen healthy subjects received a single dose of sustained-release bupropion 150 mg with water and following rifampin 600 mg daily for 7 days.[1] Rifampin was continued for 3 days after bupropion administration. The mean area under the concentration-time curve of bupropion decreased 3-fold (range, 2.7- to 3.5-fold), and its half-life decreased from 15.9 to 8.2 hours after rifampin pretreatment. The efficacy of bupropion may be reduced by coadministration of rifampin.

RELATED DRUGS: While no data are available, rifabutin may also induce the metabolism of bupropion.

MANAGEMENT OPTIONS:

➡ *Monitor.* Monitor patients using bupropion for loss of therapeutic effect if rifampin is administered.

REFERENCES:

1. Loboz KK, et al. Cytochrome P450 2B6 activity as measured by bupropion hydroxylation: effect of induction by rifampin and ethnicity. *Clin Pharmacol Ther.* 2006;80(1):75-84.

 Bupropion (eg, *Wellbutrin*)

Ritonavir (*Norvir*)

SUMMARY: In vitro studies suggest an interaction between bupropion and ritonavir, but no evidence of adverse outcomes was found in a small retrospective clinical study.

RISK FACTORS: No risk factors are known.

MECHANISM: Unknown.

CLINICAL EVALUATION: After in vitro studies found inhibition of bupropion hydroxylation with ritonavir, the records of 2 patients who had taken bupropion with ritonavir were reviewed.[1,2] No evidence of adverse interaction (eg, seizures) was detected, which might have been expected given the low rate of bupropion-induced seizures, the small number of patients observed, and the retrospective nature of the study. Additional study is needed to determine if this purported interaction results in adverse outcomes.

RELATED DRUGS: No information is available.

MANAGEMENT OPTIONS: No specific action is required, but be alert for evidence of the interaction.

REFERENCES:

1. Hesse LM, et al. Ritonavir, efavirenz, and nelfinavir inhibit CYP2B6 activity in vitro: potential drug interactions with bupropion. *Drug Metab Dispos.* 2001;29(2):100-102.

2. Park-Wyllie LY, et al. Concurrent use of bupropion with CYP2B6 inhibitors, nelfinavir, ritonavir and efavirenz: a case series. *AIDS.* 2003;17(4):638-640.

 Bupropion (eg, *Wellbutrin*)

Sertraline (eg, *Zoloft*)

SUMMARY: Bupropion may increase sertraline plasma concentrations, possibly increasing the risk of serotonin syndrome.

RISK FACTORS:

➡ *Pharmacogenetics.* Only patients who have CYP2D6 activity (ie, extensive metabolizers and, to a lesser extent, intermediate metabolizers) are expected to experience this interaction. Poor metabolizers do not have the gene for production of CYP2D6 and, therefore, have no CYP2D6 for bupropion to inhibit.

MECHANISM: Bupropion is a potent inhibitor of CYP2D6 and is likely to inhibit the CYP2D6 metabolism of sertraline.[1,2]

CLINICAL EVALUATION: A 62-year-old woman developed evidence of serotonin syndrome (ie, myoclonus, agitation, confusion, lethargy, gait difficulties) after 3 weeks of therapy with bupropion and sertraline.[3] The reaction may have been due to the combination of bupropion and sertraline; no other cause for serotonin syndrome was found. Nonetheless, bupropion has been used in combination with selective serotonin reuptake inhibitors (SSRIs) and serotonin-norepinephrine reuptake inhibitors (SNRIs) with good results (with careful monitoring) in patients with refractory depression.[4]

RELATED DRUGS: Several other SSRIs and SNRIs are also metabolized at least partially by CYP2D6 and are expected to interact with bupropion. These include duloxetine (*Cymbalta*), fluoxetine (eg, *Prozac*), fluvoxamine (eg, *Luvox*), paroxetine (eg, *Paxil*), trazodone (eg, *Oleptro*), and venlafaxine (eg, *Effexor*).

MANAGEMENT OPTIONS:

➥ *Monitor.* If bupropion is used with sertraline or other SSRIs or SNRIs, monitor for symptoms of serotonin syndrome, including myoclonus, rigidity, tremor, hyperreflexia, fever, sweating, seizures, confusion, agitation, incoordination, and coma.

REFERENCES:

1. Kotlyar M, et al. Inhibition of CYP2D6 activity by bupropion. *J Clin Psychopharmacol.* 2005;25(3):226-229.
2. Güzey C, et al. Change from the CYP2D6 extensive metabolizer to the poor metabolizer phenotype during treatment with bupropion. *Ther Drug Monit.* 2002;24(3):436-437.
3. Munhoz RP. Serotonin syndrome induced by a combination of bupropion and SSRIs. *Clin Neuropharmacol.* 2004;27(5):219-222.
4. Zisook S, et al. Use of bupropion in combination with serotonin uptake inhibitors. *Biol Psychiatry.* 2006;59(3):203-210.

Bupropion (eg, *Wellbutrin*)
Ticlopidine

SUMMARY: Ticlopidine markedly increases plasma concentrations of bupropion and markedly reduces concentrations of its active metabolite; these changes may decrease the efficacy and increase the toxicity of bupropion.

RISK FACTORS: No specific risk factors are known.

MECHANISM: Ticlopidine appears to be a potent mechanism-based inhibitor of CYP2B6, the enzyme responsible for the metabolism of bupropion.[1]

CLINICAL EVALUATION: In healthy subjects given a single dose of bupropion 150 mg with and without pretreatment with ticlopidine 250 mg twice daily for 4 days, ticlopidine was associated with an 85% increase in bupropion plasma concentrations and an 84% reduction in plasma concentrations of hydroxybupropion, the active metabolite of bupropion.[2] These findings suggest that ticlopidine may reduce the efficacy of bupropion because of reduction in concentration of the active metabolite, and may increase the risk of toxicity because of increased concentration of the parent drug. The study was not designed to address these possibilities, but both are plausible given the large magnitude of the interaction.

RELATED DRUGS: Clopidogrel (*Plavix*) appears to interact with bupropion similarly, but probably to a lesser extent than ticlopidine.

MANAGEMENT OPTIONS:

➥ *Consider Alternative.* Prasugrel (*Effient*) appears to interact minimally with bupropion.

➥ *Monitor.* If the combination is used, monitor for reduced bupropion efficacy and increased bupropion toxicity.

REFERENCES:

1. Richter T, et al. Potent mechanism-based inhibition of human CYP2B6 by clopidogrel and ticlopidine. *J Pharmacol Exp Ther.* 2004;308(1):189-197.

2. Turpeinen M, et al. Effect of clopidogrel and ticlopidine on cytochrome P450 2B6 activity as measured by bupropion hydroxylation. *Clin Pharmacol Ther.* 2005;77(6):553-559.

4   Bupropion (eg, *Wellbutrin*)

Venlafaxine (eg, *Effexor*)

SUMMARY: Bupropion may increase venlafaxine plasma concentrations; increased venlafaxine toxicity may occur.

RISK FACTORS:

➥ *Pharmacogenetics.* Only patients who have CYP2D6 activity (ie, extensive metabolizers and, to a lesser extent, intermediate metabolizers) are expected to experience this interaction. Poor metabolizers do not have the gene for production of CYP2D6 and, therefore, have no CYP2D6 for bupropion to inhibit.

MECHANISM: Bupropion is a potent inhibitor of CYP2D6 and is likely to inhibit the CYP2D6 metabolism of venlafaxine.[1,2]

CLINICAL EVALUATION: Case reports suggest that bupropion increases venlafaxine plasma concentrations, increasing both efficacy and the risk of adverse reactions.[3] Bupropion has a long half-life, and the interaction is likely to persist for up to a week after bupropion is stopped. Nonetheless, bupropion has been used in combination with selective serotonin reuptake inhibitors (SSRIs) and serotonin-norepinephrine reuptake inhibitors (SNRIs) with good results (with careful monitoring) in patients with refractory depression.[4]

RELATED DRUGS: Several other SSRIs and SNRIs are also metabolized at least partially by CYP2D6 and are expected to interact with bupropion. These include duloxetine (*Cymbalta*), fluoxetine (eg, *Prozac*), fluvoxamine (eg, *Luvox*), paroxetine (eg, *Paxil*), sertraline (eg, *Zoloft*), and trazodone (eg, *Oleptro*).

MANAGEMENT OPTIONS:

➥ *Monitor.* If bupropion is used with venlafaxine or other SSRI or SNRI, monitor for symptoms of serotonin syndrome including myoclonus, rigidity, tremor, hyperreflexia, fever, sweating, seizures, confusion, agitation, incoordination, and coma.

REFERENCES:

1. Kotlyar M, et al. Inhibition of CYP2D6 activity by bupropion. *J Clin Psychopharmacol.* 2005;25(3):226-229.

2. Güzey C, et al. Change from the CYP2D6 extensive metabolizer to the poor metabolizer phenotype during treatment with bupropion. *Ther Drug Monit.* 2002;24(3):436-437.

3. Paslakis G, et al. Clinically relevant pharmacokinetic interaction between venlafaxine and bupropion: a case series. *J Clin Psychopharmacol.* 2010;30(4):473-474.

4. Zisook S, et al. Use of bupropion in combination with serotonin uptake inhibitors. *Biol Psychiatry.* 2006;59(3):203-210.

Buspirone (*BuSpar*)

Cimetidine (eg, *Tagamet*)

SUMMARY: Cimetidine has only minor effects on the pharmacokinetics of buspirone and its active metabolite, but the combination may produce a higher incidence of minor side effects (eg, lightheadedness) than buspirone alone.

RISK FACTORS:

➡ ***Dosage Regimen.*** In most patients, clinically important inhibition of hepatic drug metabolism by cimetidine requires doses of 400 mg/day or more.

MECHANISM: Not established. Cimetidine may inhibit the hepatic metabolism of the active metabolite of buspirone.

CLINICAL EVALUATION: The effect of 1 g/day of cimetidine on the pharmacokinetic and pharmacodynamic effects of buspirone 45 mg/day was studied in 10 healthy subjects.[1] Cimetidine had little effect on the pharmacokinetics of buspirone itself but did significantly increase the maximum serum concentration of its active metabolite. Although side effects (especially lightheadedness) were more common with the combination of buspirone and cimetidine than with buspirone alone, none of the subjects' psychomotor or cognitive performances were affected significantly. Thus, cimetidine induced some changes in the pharmacokinetics of buspirone, but the alterations were not of sufficient magnitude to produce important clinical difficulties.

RELATED DRUGS: Little is known regarding the effect of other H_2-receptor antagonists such as famotidine (eg, *Pepcid*), nizatidine (*Axid*), and *ranitidine* (*eg*, Zantac) on buspirone; theoretically, they would not interact.

MANAGEMENT OPTIONS: No specific action is required, but be alert for evidence of the interaction.

REFERENCES:
1. Gammans RE, et al. Lack of interaction between cimetidine and buspirone. *Pharmacotherapy*. 1987;7:72.

Buspirone (*BuSpar*) ▼3

Citalopram (*Celexa*)

SUMMARY: A patient on excessive doses of buspirone and citalopram developed evidence of serotonin syndrome; the risk of this reaction in patients on therapeutic doses is not established.

RISK FACTORS:

➡ ***Dosage Regimen.*** Based on limited clinical data, it appears that large doses of one or both drugs increases the risk of interaction.

MECHANISM: Buspirone is a serotonin agonist (5-HT_{1A}) and citalopram is a selective serotonin reuptake inhibitor. Thus, the combination may result in excessive serotonergic effect.

CLINICAL EVALUATION: A 69-year-old woman on chronic therapy with buspirone 10 mg/day and citalopram 40 mg/day began to take higher doses than prescribed. After a few days she was admitted with evidence of serotonin syndrome (eg, agitation, hyperactivity, tremor, confusion, disorientation, uncontrolled movements of arms and legs, hallucinations).[1] She also had hyponatremia with a serum sodium of 121 mmol/L. The drugs were discontinued, and the reaction resolved in approximately 5 days. Note that the patient only had difficulty after taking excessive doses. Hence, it is not clear how often this would occur in patients taking therapeutic doses. Moreover, one cannot rule out the possibility that the reaction was caused by the citalopram alone rather than a drug interaction with buspirone.

RELATED DRUGS: The effect of buspirone with other serotonin reuptake inhibitors is not established.

MANAGEMENT OPTIONS:

➡ *Monitor.* Be alert for evidence of serotonin syndrome. Serotonin syndrome can result in neurotoxicity (eg, myoclonus, tremors, rigidity, incoordination, restlessness, hyperreflexia, seizures, coma), psychiatric symptoms (eg, agitation, confusion, hypomania), and temperature regulation abnormalities (eg, fever, sweating). Fatalities have occurred.

REFERENCES:

1. Spigset O, et al. Combined serotonin syndrome and hyponatreamia caused by a citalopram-buspirone interaction. *Int Clin Psychopharmacol.* 1997;12:61.

Buspirone (*BuSpar*)

Diltiazem (*eg, Cardizem*)

SUMMARY: Diltiazem administration increases the concentration of buspirone; increased side effects could result in some patients.

RISK FACTORS: No specific risk factors are known.

MECHANISM: Buspirone is metabolized by CYP3A4 and undergoes significant first-pass metabolism, presumably in the wall of the small intestine and liver, and has a bioavailability of 5%. Diltiazem inhibits the CYP3A4 enzymes, resulting in an increase in the bioavailability, and thus, plasma concentration, of buspirone.

CLINICAL EVALUATION: Nine healthy subjects received diltiazem 60 mg 3 times daily or matching placebo for 5 doses. A single 10 mg oral dose of buspirone was then administered. Compared with placebo, diltiazem administration increased the mean area under the concentration-time curve (AUC) of buspirone 5.3-fold. The range of increase in buspirone AUC varied from 3.3- to 7.4-fold. The mean peak concentration of buspirone was increased from 2.6 ng/ml after placebo to 10.3 ng/ml following diltiazem. No change in buspirone half-life was noted. Pharmacodynamic changes following diltiazem pretreatment were limited to a subjective increase in overall buspirone effect. Some patients may exhibit increased buspirone effects such as sedation.

RELATED DRUGS: Verapamil (eg, *Calan*) also produces an increase in buspirone concentrations. Although no data are available, dihydropyridine calcium channel blockers (eg, amlodipine [*Norvasc*], felodipine [*Plendil*], nifedipine [eg, *Procardia*]) would not be expected to interact with buspirone.

MANAGEMENT OPTIONS:

➡ **Consider Alternative.** Use of a dihydropyridine calcium channel blocker would probably avert this interaction. An alternative anxiolytic agent that does not undergo CYP3A4 metabolism, such as diazepam (eg, *Valium*) or lorazepam (eg, *Ativan*), could be selected.

➡ **Monitor.** Monitor patients receiving the combination of buspirone and diltiazem for increased buspirone effects, such as sedation.

REFERENCES:

1. Lamberg TS, et al. Effects of verapamil and diltiazem on the pharmacokinetics and pharmacodynamics of buspirone. *Clin Pharmacol Ther.* 1998;63:640.

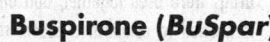

Buspirone (*BuSpar*)

Erythromycin (eg, *E-Mycin*)

SUMMARY: Erythromycin administration results in a large increase in buspirone concentrations; increased buspirone side effects are likely to result.

RISK FACTORS: No specific risk factors are known.

MECHANISM: Erythromycin inhibits the first-pass elimination of buspirone by reducing the activity of the isozyme (CYP3A4) responsible for its metabolism. The absence of a change in buspirone half-life indicates little change in its systemic clearance.

CLINICAL EVALUATION: Eight healthy subjects received buspirone following 4 days of placebo or erythromycin 500 mg 3 times daily.[1] Following erythromycin administration, buspirone peak plasma concentrations increased 5-fold and the area under the concentration-time curve increased nearly 6-fold compared with placebo treatment. Buspirone half-life was not significantly increased during erythromycin treatment. The increases in buspirone plasma concentrations were reflected in an increase in pharmacodynamic effects as measured by impaired psychomotor testing. Because erythromycin is metabolized to a nitrosoalkane that inactivates CYP3A4, the administration of erythromycin for more than 4 days may increase the magnitude of this interaction. Patients receiving buspirone are likely to suffer increased side effects (eg, sedation or dizziness) during erythromycin coadministration.

RELATED DRUGS: Other macrolide antibiotics that inhibit CYP3A4 such as clarithromycin (*Biaxin*) and troleandomycin (*TAO*) are likely to produce similar effects on buspirone pharmacokinetics. Noninhibiting macrolides include azithromycin (*Zithromax*) and dirithromycin (*Dynabac*). Other anxiolytics such as midazolam (*Versed*), alprazolam (eg, *Xanax*), and triazolam (eg, *Halcion*) are known to be inhibited by erythromycin. Anxiolytics not metabolized by CYP3A4 include lorazepam (eg, *Ativan*) and temazepam (eg, *Restoril*).

MANAGEMENT OPTIONS:

➡ **Consider Alternative.** Consider the use of a noninhibiting macrolide (see Related Drugs) for patients taking buspirone. Anxiolytics not metabolized by CYP3A4 (see Related Drugs) could be substituted for buspirone.

➡ **Monitor.** Monitor patients receiving buspirone for increased sedation if erythromycin is administered.

REFERENCES:
1. Kivisto KT, et al. Plasma buspirone concentrations are greatly increased by erythromycin and itraconazole. *Clin Pharmacol Ther.* 1997;62:348.

Buspirone (*BuSpar*)

Fluoxetine (*Prozac*)

SUMMARY: Isolated cases of reduced therapeutic response to buspirone or fluoxetine have been reported when the drugs were used together, and one patient on the combination developed a grand mal seizure. More study is needed to establish a causal relationship.

RISK FACTORS: No specific risk factors are known.

MECHANISM: Not established.

CLINICAL EVALUATION: A 35-year-old man with severe anxiety and depression was receiving buspirone 60 mg/day.[1] Because of worsening depression, he was given a 3-week trial of trazodone 200 mg/day, with little benefit. A trial of fluoxetine 20 mg/day was then begun, but within 2 days his anxiety had increased considerably. Increasing the buspirone dose to 80 mg/day for 1 week was not helpful, and stopping the buspirone did not affect his anxiety. A 24-year-old man with obsessive-compulsive disorder receiving fluoxetine 80 mg/day developed a grand mal seizure during the third week after starting buspirone 30 mg/day.[2] A 31-year-old woman on fluoxetine 20 mg/day for 4 weeks developed a marked worsening of her obsessive-compulsive symptoms within a few days of starting buspirone 10 mg/day.[3] Additional study is needed to establish whether the adverse effects noted in these patients resulted from an interaction between buspirone and fluoxetine or from some other cause.

RELATED DRUGS: The effect of combining buspirone with other selective serotonin reuptake inhibitors is not established.

MANAGEMENT OPTIONS:

➡ **Monitor.** Until more information is available, monitor patients for altered response to either buspirone or fluoxetine when they are used together.

REFERENCES:
1. Bodkin JA, et al. Fluoxetine may antagonize the anxiolytic action of buspirone. *J Clin Psychopharmacol.* 1989;9:150. Letter.
2. Grady TA, et al. Seizure associated with fluoxetine and adjuvant buspirone therapy. *J Clin Psychopharmacol.* 1992;12:70. Letter.
3. Tanquary J, et al. Paradoxical reaction to buspirone augmentation of fluoxetine. *J Clin Psychopharmacol.* 1990;10:377. Letter.

Buspirone (*BuSpar*) 4

Fluvoxamine (*Luvox*)

SUMMARY: Fluvoxamine increases buspirone serum concentrations, but the risk of buspirone toxicity appears small.

RISK FACTORS: No specific risk factors are known.

MECHANISM: Buspirone undergoes extensive first-pass metabolism by CYP3A4 in the small intestine, resulting in low bioavailability. Fluvoxamine appears to be a moderate inhibitor of CYP3A4, thus increasing the bioavailability of buspirone.

CLINICAL EVALUATION: In a randomized, crossover study of 10 healthy subjects, a single oral dose of buspirone 10 mg was given with and without pretreatment with fluvoxamine 100 mg/day for 5 days.[1] Fluvoxamine increased the buspirone area under the plasma concentration-time curve 2.4-fold, but buspirone half-life was not affected. Nonetheless, fluvoxamine did not increase the pharmacodynamic effects of buspirone, which probably attests to buspirone's relative lack of dose-dependent toxicity. Some patients may be at greater risk of buspirone toxicity than the young, healthy volunteers in this study.

RELATED DRUGS: Fluoxetine (*Prozac*) appears to be a weak inhibitor of CYP3A4, and theoretically would only have a small effect on buspirone. Other selective serotonin reuptake inhibitors, such as paroxetine (*Paxil*), sertraline (*Zoloft*), and citalopram (*Celexa*) appear to have minimal effects on CYP3A4 and would not be expected to interact.

MANAGEMENT OPTIONS: No specific action is required, but be alert for evidence of the interaction.

REFERENCES:
1. Lamberg TS, et al. The effect of fluvoxamine on the pharmacokinetics and pharmacodynamics of buspirone. *Eur J Clin Pharmacol.* 1998;54:761–76.

Buspirone (eg, *BuSpar*)

Grapefruit Juice

SUMMARY: Repeated doses of grapefruit juice markedly increase buspirone serum concentrations and also may enhance the subjective effect of buspirone.

RISK FACTORS: No specific risk factors are known.

MECHANISM: Buspirone undergoes extensive first-pass metabolism by CYP3A4 in the small intestine and liver, resulting in low bioavailability. Grapefruit juice inhibits intestinal CYP3A4, thus increasing the bioavailability of buspirone.

CLINICAL EVALUATION: Ten healthy subjects received a single oral dose of buspirone 10 mg with and without repeated doses of grapefruit juice 200 mL, double strength.[1] Grapefruit juice increased the mean area under the plasma buspirone concentration-time curve more than 9-fold, but the effect was highly variable (range, 3- to more than 20-fold). The subjects ingested a large amount of grapefruit juice; the effect of a more "normal amount" of grapefruit juice on buspirone would probably be less than that observed in this study. Most psychomotor tests of buspirone effect were not significantly affected by the addition of grapefruit juice, with the exception of subjective drug effect. Although buspirone has a relatively wide therapeutic index, it is likely that at least some patients would be adversely affected by this interaction. This is particularly true given the large variability in the magnitude of the interaction from person to person. One should also consider the possibility that some patients may be more at risk than the young, healthy volunteers in this study.

RELATED DRUGS: Grapefruit juice also may increase the serum concentrations of benzodiazepines that are metabolized by CYP3A4 (eg, alprazolam [eg, *Xanax*], midazolam [eg, *Versed*], triazolam [eg, *Halcion*]), but only when the benzodiazepine is given orally.

MANAGEMENT OPTIONS:

➡ **Consider Alternative.** Orange juice does not inhibit CYP3A4 and would not be expected to interact with buspirone.

➡ **Circumvent/Minimize.** Advise patients to take buspirone at least 2 hours before or 6 to 8 hours after grapefruit juice.

➡ **Monitor.** If buspirone is taken with grapefruit juice, monitor for increased buspirone effect (eg, sedation, psychomotor impairment).

REFERENCES:
1. Lilja JJ, et al. Grapefruit juice substantially increases plasma concentrations of buspirone. *Clin Pharmacol Ther*. 1998;64:655–660.

Buspirone (eg, *BuSpar*)

Itraconazole (*Sporanox*)

SUMMARY: Itraconazole administration results in a large increase in buspirone concentrations; increased buspirone side effects are likely to result.

RISK FACTORS: No specific risk factors are known.

MECHANISM: Itraconazole inhibits the first-pass elimination of buspirone by reducing the activity of the isozyme (CYP3A4) responsible for its metabolism. The absence of a change in buspirone half-life indicates little change in its systemic clearance.

CLINICAL EVALUATION: Eight healthy subjects received buspirone following 4 days of placebo or 100 mg itraconazole twice daily.[1] Following itraconazole administration, buspirone peak plasma concentrations increased 13-fold and the area under the concentration-time curve increased approximately 19-fold compared with placebo treatment. Buspirone half-life was not significantly increased during itraconazole treatment. The increases in buspirone plasma concentrations were reflected in an increase in pharmacodynamic effects as measured by impaired psychomotor testing. Patients receiving buspirone are likely to suffer increased side effects (eg, sedation, dizziness) during itraconazole coadministration.

RELATED DRUGS: Other azole antifungals that inhibit CYP3A4 such as ketoconazole (eg, *Nizoral*) are likely to produce similar effects on buspirone pharmacokinetics. Noninhibiting antifungals include terbinafine (*Lamisil*). Other anxiolytics such as midazolam (eg, *Versed*) and triazolam (eg, *Halcion*) are known to be inhibited by itraconazole. Anxiolytics not metabolized by CYP3A4 include lorazepam (eg, *Ativan*) and temazepam (eg, *Restoril*).

MANAGEMENT OPTIONS:

➡ *Consider Alternative.* Consider the use of a noninhibiting antifungal (see Related Drugs) for patients taking buspirone. Anxiolytics not metabolized by CYP3A4 (see Related Drugs) could be substituted for buspirone.

➡ *Monitor.* Monitor patients receiving buspirone for increased sedation if itraconazole is administered.

REFERENCES:
  1. Kivisto KT, et al. Plasma buspirone concentrations are greatly increased by erythromycin and itraconazole. *Clin Pharmacol Ther.* 1997;62:348-354.

Buspirone (eg, *BuSpar*)

Rifampin (eg, *Rifadin*)

SUMMARY: Rifampin markedly reduces the serum concentration of buspirone; loss of efficacy is likely to result.

RISK FACTORS: No specific risk factors are known.

MECHANISM: Rifampin induces the metabolism of buspirone by CYP3A4 enzymes.

CLINICAL EVALUATION: Ten healthy subjects received either placebo or rifampin 600 mg/day for 5 days.[1] On day 6, a single 30 mg buspirone dose was orally administered. Rifampin reduced the area under the concentration-time curve of buspirone 93%. Buspirone half-life was reduced from 2.8 to 1.3 hours following rifampin administration. The pharmacodynamic effects of buspirone were reduced by pretreatment with rifampin.

RELATED DRUGS: No information is available.

MANAGEMENT OPTIONS:

➡ *Consider Alternative.* Because of the significant reduction in buspirone when administered with rifampin, consider an alternative antianxiety drug that is not metabolized by CYP3A4 (eg, lorazepam [eg, *Ativan*] or temazepam [eg, *Restoril*]).

➡ *Monitor.* Monitor patients taking buspirone for loss of efficacy following the coadministration of rifampin.

REFERENCES:
  1. Lamberg TS, et al. Concentrations and effects of buspirone are considerably reduced by rifampin. *Br J Clin Pharmacol.* 1998;45:381-385.

Buspirone (eg, *Buspar*)

Ritonavir (*Norvir*)

SUMMARY: Reduction of buspirone metabolism by ritonavir appears to have resulted in the development of Parkinson-like side effects.

RISK FACTORS: No specific risk factors are known.

MECHANISM: Ritonavir and indinavir are inhibitors of CYP3A4, the enzyme responsible for buspirone metabolism.

CLINICAL EVALUATION: A 54-year-old HIV-positive patient had been receiving buspirone 70 mg/day in divided doses for several years.[1] Combination therapy with ritonavir 400 mg twice daily, indinavir (*Crixivan*) 400 mg twice daily, didanosine (*Videx*) 400 mg/day, and stavudine (*Zerit*) 40 mg twice daily was initiated. Other chronic medications being taken at the time included alprazolam, amitriptyline, citalopram co-trimoxazole, valacyclovir, warfarin, modafinil, and levothyroxine. About 4 weeks after the addition of the antiretroviral drugs, the patient developed symptoms of Parkinson disease, including dizziness, ataxia, shuffling gait, rigidity, and tremor. Ritonavir and indinavir were discontinued and amprenavir (*Agenerase*) initiated. Buspirone dose was reduced to 45 mg/day in divided doses. Two weeks later, the patient's Parkinson symptoms had resolved while on the reduced dose of buspirone and amprenavir.

RELATED DRUGS: Several other protease inhibitors, including indinavir (*Crixivan*), amprenavir (*Agenerase*), and saquinavir (eg, *Fortovase*) have been reported to inhibit the activity of CYP3A4. Other anxiolytics metabolized by CYP3A4 (eg, alprazolam [eg, *Xanax*], midazolam [eg, *Versed*]) may be affected in a similar manner by ritonavir.

MANAGEMENT OPTIONS:

➥ *Monitor.* Monitor patients receiving buspirone for evidence of elevated serum concentrations if ritonavir or other CYP3A4 inhibitors are coadministered.

REFERENCES:

1. Clay PG, et al. Pseudo-Parkinson disease secondary to ritonavir-buspirone interaction. *Ann Pharmacother.* 2003;37:202-205.

Buspirone (eg, *BuSpar*)

Trazodone (eg, *Desyrel*)

SUMMARY: A patient on buspirone and trazodone developed myoclonic movements, possibly as a result of additive serotonergic effects; a causal relationship was not established.

RISK FACTORS: No specific risk factors are known.

MECHANISM: Not established. Buspirone and trazodone are serotonergics; additive effects are theoretically possible.

CLINICAL EVALUATION: A 74-year-old man who had numerous medical conditions and was taking many medications was admitted for major depression and anxiety.[1] He was given trazodone 600 mg/day, buspirone 5 mg 3 times/day, and haloperidol (eg, *Haldol*) 1 mg 3 times/day. After approximately 1 week he developed myoclonic movements of the face and arms, but there was no muscular rigidity and no mention of other evidence of serotonin syndrome. All 3 of the drugs were stopped. Treatment with the anticholinergic agent, benztropine, did not improve the myoclonus, but the abnormal movement did stop after 3 doses of the serotonin antagonist, cyproheptadine. This patient had only 1 of the typical findings of serotonin syndrome (myoclonus), and as such would not satisfy Sternbach's criteria for the diagnosis of serotonin syndrome.[2] Nonetheless, it is possible that the myoclonus resulted from excessive serotonin activity caused by the combined therapy of buspirone and trazodone. This contention is supported by the apparent response of the myoclonus to a serotonin antagonist. Whether the myoclonus would have stopped on its own without the cyproheptadine is impossible to determine.

RELATED DRUGS: No information is available.

MANAGEMENT OPTIONS:

➡ *Monitor.* Be alert for evidence of serotonin syndrome in patients receiving buspirone and trazodone. Serotonin syndrome can result in neurotoxicity (eg, myoclonus, tremors, rigidity, incoordination, hyperreflexia, seizures, coma), psychiatric symptoms (eg, agitation, confusion, hypomania, restlessness), and autonomic dysfunction (fever, sweating, tachycardia, hypertension).

REFERENCES:

1. Goldberg RJ, et al. Serotonin syndrome from trazodone and buspirone. *Psychosomatics.* 1992;33:235-236.
2. Sternbach H. The serotonin syndrome. *Am J Psychiatry.* 1991;148:705-713.

Buspirone (*BuSpar*)

Verapamil (eg, *Calan*)

SUMMARY: Verapamil administration increases the concentration of buspirone; increased side effects could result in some patients.

RISK FACTORS: No specific risk factors are known.

MECHANISM: Buspirone is metabolized by CYP3A4 and undergoes significant first-pass metabolism, presumably in the wall of the small intestine and liver, and has a bioavailability of 5%. Verapamil inhibits the CYP3A4 enzymes, resulting in an increase in the bioavailability, and thus plasma concentration, of buspirone.

CLINICAL EVALUATION: Nine healthy subjects received verapamil 80 mg 3 times daily or matching placebo for 5 doses. A single 10 mg oral dose of buspirone was then administered. Compared with placebo, verapamil administration increased the mean area under the concentration-time curve (AUC) of buspirone 3.5-fold. The range of increase in buspirone AUC varied from 1.9- to 6.4-fold. The mean peak concentration of buspirone increased from 2.6 ng/mL after placebo to 8.8 ng/mL following verapamil. No change in buspirone half-life was noted. Pharmacodynamic changes following verapamil pretreatment were limited to a subjective increase in overall buspirone effect. Some patients may exhibit increased buspirone effects such as sedation.

RELATED DRUGS: Diltiazem (eg, *Cardizem*) also produces an increase in buspirone concentrations. Although no data are available, dihydropyridine calcium channel blockers (eg, amlodipine [*Norvasc*], felodipine [*Plendil*], nifedipine [eg, *Procardia*]) would not be expected to interact with buspirone.

MANAGEMENT OPTIONS:

➡ *Consider Alternative.* Use of a dihydropyridine calcium channel blocker would probably avoid this interaction. An alternative anxiolytic agent that does not undergo CYP3A4 metabolism, such as diazepam (eg, *Valium*) or lorazepam (eg, *Ativan*), could be selected.

➡ *Monitor.* Monitor patients receiving the combination of buspirone and verapamil for increased buspirone effects such as sedation.

REFERENCES:

1. Lamberg TS, et al. Effects of verapamil and diltiazem on the pharmacokinetics and pharmacodynamics of buspirone. *Clin Pharmacol Ther.* 1998;63:640.

5 Busulfan (eg, *Myleran*)

Fluconazole (*Diflucan*)

SUMMARY: No interaction.

RISK FACTORS: No specific risk factors are known.

MECHANISM: No interaction.

CLINICAL EVALUATION: Thirteen bone marrow transplant patients who received busulfan and fluconazole were compared with 26 bone marrow transplant patients receiving busulfan but not fluconazole.[1] The patients received a variety of transplant conditioning regimens but in each the dose of busulfan was 1 mg/kg every 6 hours. Fluconazole dose was 6 mg/kg once daily. The patients taking both fluconazole and busulfan had similar busulfan pharmacokinetics as those taking only busulfan.

RELATED DRUGS: Itraconazole (*Sporanox*) appears to reduce busulfan's elimination. The effect of ketoconazole (*Nizoral*) on busulfan pharmacokinetics is unknown but may be similar to the effect observed following itraconazole.

MANAGEMENT OPTIONS:

 Monitor. No interaction.

REFERENCES:

1. Buggia I, et al. Itraconazole can increase systemic exposure to busulfan in patients given bone marrow transplantation. *Anticancer Res.* 1996;16:2083.

4 Busulfan (eg, *Myleran*)

Itraconazole (*Sporanox*)

SUMMARY: Itraconazole produces a small increase in busulfan plasma concentrations; the clinical effect is likely to be limited.

RISK FACTORS: No specific risk factors are known.

MECHANISM: Unknown. Busulfan does not appear to be dependent upon the cytochrome P450 system for its metabolism.

CLINICAL EVALUATION: Thirteen bone marrow transplant patients who received busulfan and itraconazole were compared with 26 bone marrow transplant patients receiving busulfan but not itraconazole.[1] The patients received a variety of transplant conditioning regimens but in each, the dose of busulfan was 1 mg/kg every 6 hours. Itraconazole dose was 6 mg/kg once daily. The oral clearance of busulfan was approximately 18% lower in the patients receiving itraconazole, and steady-state busulfan concentrations were 24% higher compared with the patients only receiving busulfan. Busulfan's half-life was 17% greater in patients concurrently receiving itraconazole.

RELATED DRUGS: Fluconazole (*Diflucan*) does not appear to alter busulfan's pharmacokinetics. The effect of ketoconazole (*Nizoral*) on busulfan pharmacokinetics is unknown but may be similar to the effect observed following itraconazole.

MANAGEMENT OPTIONS:

➡ *Monitor.* Monitor patients receiving itraconazole and busulfan for evidence of busulfan toxicity (eg, hepatic veno-occlusive disease, hepatic toxicity, bone marrow hypoplasia).

REFERENCES:

1. Buggia I, et al. Itraconazole can increase systemic exposure to busulfan in patients given bone marrow transplantation. *Anticancer Res.* 1996;16:2083.

Cabergoline (eg, *Dostinex*)

Clarithromycin (eg, *Biaxin*)

SUMMARY: Clarithromycin administration increases cabergoline plasma concentrations; increased response or adverse reactions may occur.

RISK FACTORS: No significant risk factors are known.

MECHANISM: Unknown. Clarithromycin may inhibit the metabolism (CYP3A) or efflux (P-glycoprotein) of cabergoline.

CLINICAL EVALUATION: In a study of 10 healthy subjects, the administration of clarithromycin 200 mg twice daily for 6 days increased the mean area under the concentration-time curve (AUC) by 2.6-fold following a single dose of cabergoline.[1] In a second study, 7 patients with Parkinson disease taking cabergoline were coadministered clarithromycin for 6 days.[1] Compared with cabergoline taken alone, the addition of clarithromycin increased the mean plasma concentration of cabergoline, drawn 3 hours after dosing, by 1.7-fold. Several of the patients reported better symptom control following the coadministration of clarithromycin.

RELATED DRUGS: Erythromycin (*Ery-Tab*) and troleandomycin[†] would be likely to inhibit the metabolism of cabergoline in a similar manner.

MANAGEMENT OPTIONS:

➡ ***Consider Alternative.*** Azithromycin (*Zithromax*) and dirithromycin[†] do not inhibit CYP3A4 and may be considered as alternatives to clarithromycin in patients receiving cabergoline.

➡ ***Monitor.*** Monitor patients taking cabergoline who receive clarithromycin for adverse reactions (eg, nausea, vomiting, headache, dizziness).

REFERENCES:
1. Nakatsuka A, et al. Effect of clarithromycin on the pharmacokinetics of cabergoline in healthy controls and in patients with Parkinson's disease. *J Pharmacol Sci*. 2006;100:59-64.

† Not available in the United States.

Cabergoline (eg, *Dostinex*)

Itraconazole (eg, *Sporanox*)

SUMMARY: Cabergoline plasma concentrations will increase with the coadministration of itraconazole; increased response or toxicity may result.

RISK FACTORS: No significant risk factors are known.

MECHANISM: Unknown. Itraconazole may inhibit the metabolism (CYP3A) or efflux (P-glycoprotein) of cabergoline.

CLINICAL EVALUATION: A patient with Parkinson disease was taking cabergoline 4 mg daily and selegiline 5 mg twice daily.[1] Itraconazole 200 mg twice daily for 7 days was prescribed for toenail fungal infection. Following itraconazole administration, the patient reported some improvement in his Parkinson symptoms that gradually returned to pre-itraconazole levels over the following weeks. The plasma concentration of cabergoline increased over 3-fold following a week of itraconazole therapy. The concentration of cabergoline gradually declined over several weeks following the discontinuation of itraconazole. A second patient taking cabergoline, carbidopa, and selegiline experienced reduced parkinsonian symptoms and some adverse reactions (hyperkinesia) during coadministration of itraconazole. In both cases, repeated periods of itraconazole administration produced similar clinical improvement in the patient's condition.

RELATED DRUGS: Other antifungal agents that inhibit CYP3A4 (eg, ketoconazole [eg, *Nizoral*], voriconazole [*Vfend*], posaconazole [*Noxafil*], fluconazole [eg, *Diflucan*]) are expected to affect cabergoline in a similar manner.

MANAGEMENT OPTIONS:

➡ *Consider Alternative.* Terbinafine (eg, *Lamisil*) may be considered as an alternative antifungal agent because it does not affect CYP3A4 activity.

➡ *Monitor.* Monitor patients taking cabergoline who receive itraconazole for adverse reactions (eg, nausea, vomiting, headache, dizziness).

REFERENCES:

1. Christensen J, et al. Cabergoline plasma concentration is increased during concomitant treatment with itraconazole. *Mov Disord.* 2002;17:1360-1362.

Caffeine

Cimetidine (eg, *Tagamet*)

SUMMARY: Cimetidine substantially increases serum caffeine concentrations, but the clinical importance of this effect is not established.

RISK FACTORS:

➡ *Dosage Regimen.* In most patients, clinically important inhibition of hepatic drug metabolism by cimetidine requires doses of 400 mg/day or more.

MECHANISM: Cimetidine appears to inhibit the hepatic metabolism of caffeine.

CLINICAL EVALUATION: Five healthy nonsmoking subjects received a single oral dose of caffeine 300 mg with and without pretreatment with 6 days of oral cimetidine 200 mg 3 times daily and 400 mg at bedtime or placebo in random order.[1] Cimetidine pretreatment was associated with a 31% reduction in caffeine clearance and a 60% increase in caffeine half-life. In another study of 6 smokers and 6 nonsmokers, caffeine 2 mg/kg was given orally with and without pretreatment with cimetidine 300 mg every 6 hours for 4 days. Cimetidine reduced caffeine clearance 31% in smokers and 42% in nonsmokers; cimetidine increased caffeine half-life 45% in smokers and 96% in nonsmokers. Although cimetidine substantially increased plasma caffeine concentrations in these studies, the clinical importance of this effect is not established. Serious toxicity in patients with elevated plasma caffeine concentrations appears minimal; however, some patients could possibly develop adverse CNS or cardiovascular effects (eg, nervousness, anxiety, insomnia, tachycardia).

RELATED DRUGS: The interaction of other H_2-receptor agonists such as ranitidine (eg, *Zantac*), famotidine (eg, *Pepcid*), and nizatidine (eg, *Axid*) with caffeine is not established. Theoretically, they would be unlikely to affect caffeine metabolism.

MANAGEMENT OPTIONS: No specific action is required, but be alert for evidence of the interaction.

REFERENCES:

1. Broughton LJ, et al. Decreased systemic clearance of caffeine due to cimetidine. *Br J Clin Pharmacol.* 1981;12:155-159.

 Caffeine

Ciprofloxacin (eg, *Cipro*)

SUMMARY: Ciprofloxacin increases caffeine concentrations and may enhance its adverse reactions.

RISK FACTORS:

➡ *Dosage Regimen.* Ciprofloxacin dosages of 250 mg or more twice daily can increase the risk of interaction.

MECHANISM: Ciprofloxacin inhibits the N-demethylation of caffeine by hepatic enzymes (CYP1A2).

CLINICAL EVALUATION: Twelve healthy volunteers received 3 different daily doses of ciprofloxacin for 4 days as follows: 100, 250, and 500 mg twice daily.[1] The area under the concentration-time curve of caffeine was increased 16.8%, 57. 1%, and 57. 8% by the above doses, respectively. The increase following the 100 mg twice-daily dosage was not statistically significant. Other studies have demonstrated ciprofloxacin-induced reduction in caffeine clearance of up to 75%.[2-4] Increased caffeine effects would be expected in patients taking ciprofloxacin.

RELATED DRUGS: Quinolones reported to inhibit caffeine metabolism include ciprofloxacin, enoxacin,† norfloxacin (*Noroxin*), and pipemidic acid. Quinolones reported to have no effect on caffeine include rufloxacin†, ofloxacin (eg, *Floxin*), and lomefloxacin (*Maxaquin*).[5]

MANAGEMENT OPTIONS:

➡ *Consider Alternative.* Ofloxacin or lomefloxacin may be used.

➡ *Circumvent/Minimize.* Patients who are taking ciprofloxacin should minimize their intake of caffeine.

➡ *Monitor.* Treatment with ciprofloxacin may cause significant increases in caffeine concentrations; advise patients of the potential for enhanced caffeine effects (eg, tachycardia, tremors, increased blood pressure).

REFERENCES:

1. Harder S, et al. 4-quinolones inhibit biotransformation of caffeine. *Eur J Clin Pharmacol.* 1988;35:651-656.

2. Healy DP, et al. Interaction between oral ciprofloxacin and caffeine in normal volunteers. *Antimicrob Agents Chemother.* 1989;33:474-478.

3. Staib AH, et al. Gyrase inhibitors impair caffeine metabolism in man. *Methods Find Exp Clin Pharmacol.* 1987;9:193-198.

4. Stille W, et al. Decrease of caffeine elimination in man during coadministration of 4-quinolones. *J Antimicrob Chemother.* 1987;20:729-734.

5. Cesana M, et al. Effect of single doses of rufloxacin on the disposition of theophylline and caffeine after single administration. *Int J Clin Pharmacol Ther Toxicol.* 1991;29:133-138.

† Not available in the United States.

Caffeine 4

Clozapine (eg, *Clozaril*)

SUMMARY: A schizophrenic man developed a transient exacerbation of his psychosis when clozapine was taken with caffeinated beverages, but a causal relationship was not established.

RISK FACTORS: No specific risk factors are known.

MECHANISM: Not established. Both clozapine and caffeine are metabolized by cytochrome P4501A2, and it is possible that they compete for metabolism in the liver.[1] It has been proposed that classic dopamine D_2 receptor antagonists such as haloperidol (eg, *Haldol*) are able to block the dopamine agonist effects of caffeine, but clozapine is unable to do so.[2] Thus, caffeine may inhibit the antipsychotic effect of clozapine.

CLINICAL EVALUATION: A 39-year-old schizophrenic man who was receiving haloperidol 30 mg/day and procyclidine (*Kemadrin*) 30 mg/day also consumed 5 to 10 cups of caffeinated coffee daily. He had used coffee for many years in an attempt to counteract the sedative effects of various neuroleptics that he had taken. He then was switched to clozapine in a gradually increasing dose from 75 up to 200 mg/day. When he reached a clozapine dose of 150 mg/day, he noticed that when he took his clozapine with 2 cups of coffee, he experienced a temporary return of psychotic and other symptoms (ie, anxiety, agitation, insomnia, weakness, headaches, abdominal pain, generalized stiffness, strong paranoid ideation). These reactions did not occur when he was advised to take his clozapine with water instead of coffee. Later at a clozapine dose of 200 mg/day, he had a similar reaction when he took his clozapine with caffeinated *Diet Coke*. The subsequent use of decaffeinated *Diet Coke* did not produce the reaction. The temporal relationship observed in this case is consistent with caffeine-induced inhibition of clozapine effect. Also, the fact that caffeine did not affect previous neuroleptics would suggest that neither the patient nor the physicians would have been looking for such an effect. Nonetheless, a causal relationship is difficult to assess because a blinded dechallenge and rechallenge were not attempted. If, as the authors suggest, caffeine directly inhibits the antipsychotic effect of clozapine in the brain, this inhibitory effect may have been potentiated by clozapine-induced inhibition of caffeine metabolism (resulting in higher than expected plasma caffeine concentrations). However, some of the observed symptoms are consistent with high serum levels of caffeine (eg, anxiety, agitation, insomnia).

RELATED DRUGS: No information is available.

MANAGEMENT OPTIONS: No specific action is required, but be alert for evidence of the interaction.

REFERENCES:
1. Bertilsson L, et al. Clozapine disposition covaries with CYP1A2 activity determined by a caffeine test. *Br J Clin Pharmacol.* 1994;38:471.
2. Vainer JL, et al. Interaction between caffeine and clozapine. *J Clin Psychopharmacol.* 1994;14:228.

4   Caffeine

Contraceptives, Oral (eg, *Ortho-Novum*)

SUMMARY: Patients on oral contraceptives may have higher plasma caffeine concentrations than those who are not on oral contraceptives.

RISK FACTORS: No specific risk factors are known.

MECHANISM: Oral contraceptives probably reduce the hepatic metabolism of caffeine.

CLINICAL EVALUATION: The pharmacokinetics of caffeine 250 mg orally in 9 women taking oral contraceptives (estrogen content varied from 35 to 80 mcg) were compared with 9 women who were not. The half-life of caffeine was longer (10.7 vs 6.2 hours) and the total plasma clearance was lower in women taking oral contraceptives.[1] In another study of 9 women, 229 mg caffeine was given before, 2 weeks after, and 6 weeks after starting an oral contraceptive.[2] Six women took a contraceptive with 50 mcg estrogen and 3 took 30 mcg of estrogen. Caffeine plasma concentrations were considerably higher than the control levels after 2 weeks of the oral contraceptive therapy, and by 6 weeks, the area under the caffeine plasma concentration-time curve had more than doubled. Thus, caffeine may be expected to have a somewhat greater pharmacodynamic effect in women taking oral contraceptives. Some women may need to moderate their caffeine intake.

RELATED DRUGS: No information is available.

MANAGEMENT OPTIONS: No specific action is required, but be alert for evidence of the interaction.

REFERENCES:

1. Patwardhan RV, et al. Impaired elimination of caffeine by oral contraceptive steroids. *J Lab Clin Med*. 1980;95:603.
2. Rietveld EC, et al. Rapid onset of an increase in caffeine residence time in young women due to oral contraceptive steroids. *Eur J Clin Pharmacol*. 1984;26:371.

Caffeine

Enoxacin (*Penetrex*)

SUMMARY: Enoxacin significantly increases caffeine serum concentrations and may increase caffeine side effects.

RISK FACTORS:

➤ **Dosage Regimen.** Increasing enoxacin doses from 100 to 400 mg twice daily can increase the risk of interaction.

MECHANISM: Enoxacin inhibits the N-demethylation of caffeine by hepatic enzymes.

CLINICAL EVALUATION: The area under the concentration-time curve of caffeine was doubled by the administration of enoxacin 100 mg twice daily for 4 days. It was increased 3-fold by 200 mg twice daily, and nearly 5-fold following 400 mg twice daily for 4 days.[1-3] Increased caffeine effects were reported during enoxacin and caffeine administration.[3]

RELATED DRUGS: Quinolones reported to inhibit caffeine metabolism include ciprofloxacin (*Cipro*), enoxacin (*Penetrex*), norfloxacin (*Noroxin*), and pipemidic acid. Quinolones reported to have no effect on caffeine include ofloxacin (*Floxin*), lomefloxacin (*Maxaquin*), and rufloxacin.[4]

MANAGEMENT OPTIONS:

➡ *Consider Alternative.* Ofloxacin or lomefloxacin could be used.

➡ *Circumvent/Minimize.* Patients taking enoxacin should limit their intake of caffeine.

➡ *Monitor.* Treatment with enoxacin may cause significant increases in caffeine concentrations; advise patients of the potential for enhanced caffeine effects (eg, tachycardia, tremors, increased blood pressure).

REFERENCES:

1. Harder S, et al. 4-Quinolones inhibit biotransformation of caffeine. *Eur J Clin Pharmacol.* 1988;35:651.
2. Staib AH, et al. Gyrase inhibitors impair caffeine metabolism in man. *Methods Find Exp Clin Pharmacol.* 1987;9:193.
3. Peloquin CA, et al. Pharmacokinetics and clinical effects of caffeine alone and in combination with oral enoxacin. *Rev Infect Dis.* 1989;11 (Suppl. 5):S1095.
4. Cesana M, et al. Effect of single doses of rufloxacin on the disposition of theophylline and caffeine after single administration. *Int J Clin Pharmacol Ther Toxicol.* 1991;29:133.

Caffeine

Ephedrine

SUMMARY: In healthy subjects, the combination of ephedrine and caffeine increased systolic blood pressure more than either drug alone, but the clinical importance of this effect may be minimal in most patients.

RISK FACTORS: No specific risk factors are known.

MECHANISM: The effect appears to be pharmacodynamic rather than pharmacokinetic, but the exact nature of the interaction is not known.

CLINICAL EVALUATION: In a randomized, double-blind, placebo-controlled, crossover study of 16 healthy subjects, caffeine and ephedrine were given alone and in combination.[1] The combination produced higher increases in systolic blood pressure than either drug alone, but in most people the effect would have minimal clinical consequences.

RELATED DRUGS: No information is available.

MANAGEMENT OPTIONS: No specific action is required, but be alert for evidence of the interaction.

REFERENCES:

1. Haller CA, et al. Enhanced stimulant and metabolic effects of combined ephedrine and caffeine. *Clin Pharmacol Ther.* 2004;75:259-273.

Caffeine

Ethanol (Ethyl Alcohol)

SUMMARY: Caffeine does not appear to reverse the adverse psychomotor effects of ethanol intoxication.

RISK FACTORS: No specific risk factors are known.

MECHANISM: Not established.

CLINICAL EVALUATION: In a study of 68 healthy subjects, ethanol 0.75 g/kg body weight and caffeine 300 mg per 70 kg body weight were given alone and in combination, followed by measurement of psychomotor skills.[1] Caffeine failed to reverse the detrimental effects of ethanol on performance with the exception of the reaction-time tests. Thus, caffeine is ineffective as an agent to help patients "sober up" following excessive ethanol ingestion.

RELATED DRUGS: No information is available.

MANAGEMENT OPTIONS: No specific action is required, but be alert for evidence of the interaction.

REFERENCES:
1. Franks HM, et al. The effect of caffeine on human performance, alone and in combination with ethanol. *Psychopharmacologia.* 1975;45:177-181.

 Caffeine

Fluconazole (eg, *Diflucan*)

SUMMARY: Fluconazole increases the plasma concentration of caffeine.

RISK FACTORS:

➡ **Dosage Regimen.** High doses of fluconazole (more than 200 mg/day) can increase the risk of interaction.

MECHANISM: Fluconazole appears to inhibit the metabolism of caffeine in a concentration-dependent manner.

CLINICAL EVALUATION: Five elderly and 6 young, healthy subjects received fluconazole 200 and 400 mg/day, respectively, for 10 days.[1] Caffeine clearance was reduced 32% in the young subjects and 17% in the elderly. Fluconazole concentrations correlated with the degree of caffeine inhibition. While this interaction has limited clinical significance, be alert for increased caffeine effects.

RELATED DRUGS: Theoretically, other azole antifungal agents may interact in a similar manner with caffeine.

MANAGEMENT OPTIONS:

➡ **Monitor.** Be alert for increased caffeine effects such as tachycardia and nervousness.

REFERENCES:
1. Nix DE, et al. The effect of fluconazole on the pharmacokinetics of caffeine in young and elderly subjects. *Clin Pharmacol Ther.* 1992;51:183.

4 **Caffeine**

Melatonin

SUMMARY: Caffeine may increase melatonin serum concentrations, but the clinical importance of this effect is not established.

RISK FACTORS: No specific risk factors are known.

MECHANISM: Caffeine may inhibit the metabolism of melatonin by CYP1A2.

CLINICAL EVALUATION: Twelve healthy subjects were given melatonin 6 mg alone and with caffeine (200 mg 1 hour before and 1 and 3 hours after the melatonin).[1] Caffeine more than doubled the melatonin area under the concentration-time curve, but the clinical consequences of this effect are probably minimal.

RELATED DRUGS: No information is available.

MANAGEMENT OPTIONS: No specific action is required, but be alert for evidence of the interaction.

REFERENCES:

1. Härtter S, et al. Effects of caffeine intake on the pharmacokinetics of melatonin, a probe drug for CYP1A2 activity. *Br J Clin Pharmacol.* 2003;56:679-682.

Caffeine

Menthol

SUMMARY: Menthol does not appear to affect caffeine metabolism, but may delay caffeine absorption.

RISK FACTORS: No specific risk factors are known.

MECHANISM: Not established. The mechanism by which menthol delays the absorption of caffeine is not known.

CLINICAL EVALUATION: A randomized crossover study consisted of 11 healthy subjects given a single oral dose of caffeine 200 mg with and without coadministration of menthol 100 mg.[1] Menthol had no effect on the caffeine area under the plasma concentration-time curve, half-life, or oral clearance, but did increase the time to maximal caffeine concentrations from 44 to 76 minutes.

RELATED DRUGS: No information is available.

MANAGEMENT OPTIONS: No specific action is required, but be alert for evidence of the interaction.

REFERENCES:

1. Gelal A, et al. Influence of menthol on caffeine disposition and pharmacodynamics in healthy female volunteers. *Eur J Clin Pharmacol.* 2003;59(5-6):417-422.

Caffeine

Methotrexate (eg, *Trexall*)

SUMMARY: Preliminary clinical evidence suggests that caffeine may inhibit the therapeutic effect of methotrexate in rheumatoid arthritis.

RISK FACTORS: No specific risk factors are known.

MECHANISM: Not established. The mechanism of action of methotrexate in rheumatoid arthritis may be through increasing adenosine concentrations. Adenosine is thought to have anti-inflammatory effects in rheumatoid arthritis. Xanthines, such as theophylline and caffeine, are known to be adenosine receptor antagonists, and thus might be expected to inhibit methotrexate effect.

CLINICAL EVALUATION: In a study of methotrexate therapy in 39 patients with rheumatoid arthritis, patients were divided into low-, medium-, and high-caffeine intake groups.[1] Patients with high-caffeine intake (estimated to be more than 180 mg/

day) experienced significantly less improvement in joint pain and morning stiffness with methotrexate therapy than patients with low-caffeine intake (estimated to be less than 120 mg/day). Although this was a small preliminary study, a previous abstract had been published with similar results. Until more information is available, the possibility that caffeine may inhibit the effect of methotrexate in rheumatoid arthritis should be considered.

RELATED DRUGS: Theophylline also antagonizes adenosine and would be expected to interact with methotrexate in the same way as caffeine.

MANAGEMENT OPTIONS:

➡ *Circumvent/Minimize.* In patients with rheumatoid arthritis who do not respond adequately to methotrexate, ask about caffeine intake. If caffeine intake is high, a trial of reduced intake is recommended.

REFERENCES:
1. Nesher G, et al. Effect of caffeine consumption on efficacy of methotrexate in rheumatoid arthritis. *Arthritis Rheum.* 2003;48(2):571-572.

 Caffeine

Nifedipine (eg, *Procardia*)

SUMMARY: Caffeine does not appear to alter the response to nifedipine. Nifedipine reverses the pressor effect of caffeine while verapamil may not.

RISK FACTORS: No specific risk factors are known.

MECHANISM: Not established. It is possible that verapamil inhibits caffeine metabolism. This could account for greater apparent effect of caffeine on verapamil than that seen with nifedipine, although further study is needed to clarify the mechanisms involved.

CLINICAL EVALUATION: Ten healthy subjects received 300 mg caffeine or placebo followed by nifedipine 10 mg 60 minutes later.[1] Caffeine significantly increased standing blood pressure, while nifedipine reduced it. Nifedipine reversed the hypertensive effects of caffeine, but caffeine did not reverse the hypotensive effect of nifedipine.

RELATED DRUGS: In another study,[2] healthy subjects were pretreated with placebo or verapamil (eg, *Calan*) 80 mg 3 times/day and given enough coffee to produce a plasma caffeine concentration of approximately 6 mcg/mL. Pretreatment with verapamil had no effect on the hypertensive effect of coffee. The clinical significance of this effect is unknown, but patients with hypertension should probably avoid large amounts of caffeine while taking verapamil and, perhaps, other calcium channel blockers.

MANAGEMENT OPTIONS: No specific action is required, but be alert for evidence of the interaction.

REFERENCES:
1. van Nguyen P, et al. Cardiovascular effects of caffeine and nifedipine. *Clin Pharmacol Ther.* 1988;44:315-319.
2. Smits P, et al. Influence of slow calcium-channel blockade on the cardiovascular effects of coffee. *Eur J Clin Pharmacol.* 1986;30:171-175.

Caffeine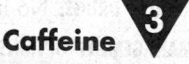

Norfloxacin (*Noroxin*)

SUMMARY: Norfloxacin increases caffeine serum concentrations; the clinical significance of these changes is probably limited.

RISK FACTORS:

➥ **Dosage Regimen.** Norfloxacin doses of greater than or equal to 800 mg twice daily can increase the risk of interaction.

MECHANISM: Norfloxacin inhibits the N-demethylation of caffeine by hepatic enzymes when administered in high doses.

CLINICAL EVALUATION: Norfloxacin 400 mg twice daily for 4 days resulted in no statistically significant (16.4%) increase in the area under the caffeine concentration-time curve in 12 healthy subjects receiving 230 mg orally.[1] The mean oral clearance of caffeine 350 mg oral was significantly reduced (from 9.70 to 6.27 L/hr) after pretreatment with norfloxacin 800 mg.[2]

RELATED DRUGS: Quinolones reported to inhibit caffeine metabolism included ciprofloxacin (*Cipro*), enoxacin (*Penetrex*), norfloxacin (*Noroxin*), and pipemidic acid. Quinolones having no effect on caffeine included ofloxacin (*Floxin*), lomefloxacin (*Maxaquin*), and rufloxacin.[3]

MANAGEMENT OPTIONS:

➥ **Consider Alternative.** Ofloxacin or lomefloxacin could be used.

➥ **Circumvent/Minimize.** Patients taking norfloxacin should limit their intake of caffeinated beverages.

➥ **Monitor.** When high doses of norfloxacin (eg, greater than or equal to 800 mg twice daily) are administered, monitor patients for enhanced caffeine effects (eg, tachycardia, tremors, increased blood pressure).

REFERENCES:

1. Harder S, et al. 4-quinolones inhibit biotransformation of caffeine. *Eur J Clin Pharmacol*. 1988;35:651-656.
2. Carbo M, et al. Effect of quinolones on caffeine disposition. *Clin Pharmacol Ther*. 1989;45:234-240.
3. Cesana M, et al. Effect of single doses of rufloxacin on the disposition of theophylline and caffeine after single administration. *Int J Clin Pharmacol Ther Toxicol*. 1991;29:133-138.

Caffeine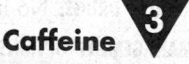

Pipemidic Acid

SUMMARY: Pipemidic acid produces a large increase in caffeine serum concentrations and may increase caffeine side effects.

RISK FACTORS: No specific risk factors are known.

MECHANISM: Pipemidic acid inhibits the N-demethylation of caffeine by hepatic enzymes.

CLINICAL EVALUATION: The administration of pipemidic acid 400 mg twice daily for 4 days significantly (180%) increased the area under the concentration-time curve of caffeine.[1] The clearance of caffeine was reduced in other studies by doses of pipemidic acid from 100 mg 3 times daily to 800 mg twice daily.[2] Increased caffeine effects would be expected in patients taking pipemidic acid.

RELATED DRUGS: Quinolones reported to inhibit caffeine metabolism include ciprofloxacin (*Cipro*), enoxacin (*Penetrex*), norfloxacin (*Noroxin*), and pipemidic acid. Quinolones reported to have no effect on caffeine include ofloxacin (*Floxin*), lomefloxacin (*Maxaquin*), and rufloxacin.[3]

MANAGEMENT OPTIONS:

➥ *Consider Alternative.* Ofloxacin or lomefloxacin could be used.

➥ *Circumvent/Minimize.* Patients taking pipemidic acid should limit their intake of caffeinated beverages.

➥ *Monitor.* When caffeine and pipemidic acid are administered, monitor patients for enhanced caffeine effects (eg, tachycardia, tremors, increased blood pressure).

REFERENCES:

1. Harder S, et al. 4-Quinolones inhibit biotransformation of caffeine. *Eur J Clin Pharmacol.* 1988;35:651.
2. Carbo M, et al. Effect of quinolones on caffeine disposition. *Clin Pharmacol Ther.* 1989;45:234.
3. Cesana M, et al. Effect of single doses of rufloxacin on the disposition of theophylline and caffeine after single administration. *Int J Clin Pharmacol Ther Toxicol.* 1991;29:133.

 Calcitonin (eg, *Calcimar*)

Lithium (eg, *Eskalith*)

SUMMARY: Preliminary evidence suggests that calcitonin may modestly decrease lithium serum concentrations, but the clinical importance of this effect is not established.

RISK FACTORS: No specific risk factors are known.

MECHANISM: Not established. Preliminary evidence suggests that calcitonin decreases lithium renal elimination, but an additional effect on lithium GI absorption has not been ruled out.

CLINICAL EVALUATION: Four women with manic depressive illness who had been stabilized on lithium for 10 years or longer received subcutaneous salmon calcitonin 100 units/day for 3 days.[1] Lithium serum concentrations decreased in all 4 patients, with an average decrease of approximately 17%. Lithium renal clearance was assessed in 2 of the 4 patients, and was decreased in both cases.

RELATED DRUGS: No information is available.

MANAGEMENT OPTIONS: No specific action is required, but be alert for evidence of the interaction.

REFERENCES:

1. Passiu G, et al. Calcitonin decreases lithium plasma levels in man. Preliminary report. *Int J Clin Pharmacol Res.* 1998;18(4):179-81.

Calcium 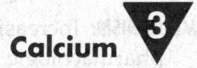 3

Digoxin (eg, *Lanoxin*)

SUMMARY: Elevated calcium concentrations following parenteral administration have been associated with acute digoxin toxicity.

RISK FACTORS:

➡ ***Route of Administration.*** Administration of IV calcium can increase the risk of interaction.

MECHANISM: Calcium ion and digitalis have some similar effects on the myocardium. The positive inotropic effect of digitalis is probably mediated via an effect on calcium.

CLINICAL EVALUATION: Parenteral calcium may precipitate cardiac arrhythmias in patients receiving digitalis glycosides.[1,2] The deaths of 2 digitalized patients apparently caused by IV administration of calcium preparations were reported in 1936, but subsequent clinical descriptions of this interaction are lacking. Nevertheless, use calcium cautiously in patients taking digoxin or digitoxin (*Crystodigin*).

RELATED DRUGS: A similar interaction would be expected with digitoxin.

MANAGEMENT OPTIONS:

➡ ***Circumvent/Minimize.*** Do not administer calcium IV to patients taking digoxin.

➡ ***Monitor.*** If calcium is administered IV, give slowly or in small amounts to avoid high serum calcium concentrations. Monitor patients for arrhythmias.

REFERENCES:

1. Schick D, et al. Current concepts of therapy with digitalis glycosides. Part II. *Am Heart J.* 1974;87:391.
2. Nola GT, et al. Assessment of the synergistic relationship between serum calcium and digitalis. *Am Heart J.* 1970;79:499.

Calcium 3

Thiazides

SUMMARY: The use of large doses of calcium with thiazides can result in the development of the milk-alkali syndrome.

RISK FACTORS:

➡ ***Dosage Regimen.*** Excessive doses of calcium appear to increase the risk of interaction.

MECHANISM: The ingestion of large amounts of calcium and the inhibition of renal calcium excretion by thiazides can result in the development of hypercalcemia. The continued use of calcium and thiazides results in metabolic alkalosis caused by enhanced tubular bicarbonate reabsorption.

CLINICAL EVALUATION: A patient with a history of hypertension, hypothyroidism, heartburn, back pain, and kidney stones was admitted with complaints of dizziness and weakness of 2 months duration.[1] His medications included chlorothiazide (eg, *Diuril*) 500 mg, calcium 7.5 to 10 g, and thyroid 120 mg/day for several years. His abnormal laboratory values included an elevated serum calcium of 6.8 mEq/L (normal: less than 5.2 mEq/L), an elevated serum creatinine of 7.2 mg/dL, and hypokalemia. He also had metabolic alkalosis with respiratory compensation, an abnormal electrocardiogram (ECG), and a calcified granuloma on chest X-ray. A previous case of hypercalcemia involving a patient who ingested calcium 5 to 7.5 g/day for several weeks together with 50 mg/day of hydrochlorothiazide (eg, *Esidrix*) has been reported.[2] The patient's signs and symptoms were similar and included obtundation, metabolic alkalosis, ECG changes, fatigue, hypercalcemia (19.7 mg/dL), and renal failure. Both patients responded to the discontinuation of the thiazide and calcium and treatment with sodium chloride, potassium, and furosemide (eg, *Lasix*). Over several weeks, the laboratory values and physical findings returned to normal.

RELATED DRUGS: No information is available.

MANAGEMENT OPTIONS:

➡ *Circumvent/Minimize.* Caution patients against excessive or prolonged self-administration of calcium, particularly if they are taking thiazides.

➡ *Monitor.* Monitor patients taking thiazides and calcium concurrently for evidence of hypercalcemia.

REFERENCES:

1. Gora ML, et al. Milk-alkali syndrome associated with use of chlorothiazide and calcium carbonate. *Clin Pharm.* 1989;8:227.
2. Hakim R, et al. Severe hypercalcemia associated with hydrochlorothiazide and calcium carbonate therapy. *Can Med Assoc J.* 1979;8:591.

Calcium

Verapamil (eg, *Calan*)

SUMMARY: Calcium administration may inhibit the activity of verapamil and other calcium channel blockers.

RISK FACTORS: No specific risk factors are known.

MECHANISM: Increasing the extracellular calcium concentration may antagonize the pharmacologic response to calcium channel blockers.

CLINICAL EVALUATION: In a patient with atrial fibrillation controlled by verapamil, the arrhythmia recurred following administrations of calcium adipinate 1.2 g/day and calciferol 3,000 units/day.[1] Calcium infusions have been used successfully to treat verapamil overdoses.[2,3] Thus, calcium may reduce the response to verapamil and probably other calcium channel blockers. However, the amount of calcium required and the magnitude of this effect cannot be determined from available data. In 1 study of 16 patients with multifocal atrial tachycardia, calcium gluconate 1 g intravenously given to 5 patients reduced verapamil-induced hypotension without inhibiting the antiarrhythmic effect of verapamil.[4] One gram of calcium chloride had no effect on verapamil-induced prolongation of atrioventricular conduction in healthy subjects;[5] however, it blunted the hypotensive effect of nifedipine (eg, *Procardia*) without altering its anti-ischemic activity in patients with angina.[6,7]

RELATED DRUGS: Calcium can be expected to reduce the effects of all calcium channel blockers.

MANAGEMENT OPTIONS:

➥ **Monitor.** Watch for evidence of reduced response, particularly hypotensive effects, when large doses of calcium products are given concurrently to patients receiving calcium channel blockers.

REFERENCES:

1. Bar-Or D, et al. Calcium and calciferol antagonise effect of verapamil in atrial fibrillation. *Br Med J.* 1981;282:1585-1586.

2. Perkins CM. Serious verapamil poisoning: treatment with intravenous calcium gluconate. *Br Med J.* 1978;2:1127.

3. Woie L, et al. Successful treatment of suicidal verapamil poisoning with calcium gluconate. *Eur Heart J.* 1981;2:239-242.

4. Salerno DM, et al. Intravenous verapamil for treatment of multifocal atrial tachycardia with and without calcium pretreatment. *Ann Intern Med.* 1987;107:623-628.

5. Schoen MD, et al. Clarification of the interaction between IV calcium chloride and IV verapamil. *Pharmacotherapy.* 1990;10:244.

6. O'Quinn SV, et al. Influence of calcium on the hemodynamic and antiischemic effects of nifedipine observed during treadmill exercise testing. *Pharmacotherapy.* 1990;10:247.

7. Wohns DH, et al. Influence of calcium administration on the short-term hemodynamic and anti-ischemic effects of nifedipine. *J Am Coll Cardiol.* 1991;18:1070-1076.

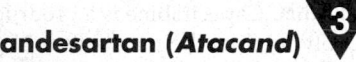

Candesartan (*Atacand*)
Lithium (eg, *Eskalith*)

SUMMARY: A patient developed lithium toxicity after starting candesartan, but it is not known how often this combination would produce adverse consequences.

RISK FACTORS: No specific risk factors are known.

MECHANISM: Not established. Candesartan may reduce the renal elimination of lithium.

CLINICAL EVALUATION: A 58-year-old woman stabilized on chronic lithium therapy (900 mg/day) was started on candesartan 16 mg/day.[1] About 7 weeks later, she developed evidence of lithium toxicity (eg, confusion, disorientation, agitation, ataxia) and lithium levels had increased markedly from approximately 0.7 to 3.25 mmol/L. After the toxicity was treated in the intensive care unit, she was again stabilized on lithium 900 mg/day in the absence of candesartan. The fact that other angiotensin II receptor antagonists have also been associated with lithium toxicity, the magnitude of the increases in lithium serum concentrations suggests that this interaction may be clinically important.

RELATED DRUGS: Both losartan (*Cozaar*)[2] and valsartan (*Diovan*)[3] have also been reported to produce lithium toxicity, so it is possible that all angiotensin II receptor antagonists interact with lithium. Angiotensin-converting enzyme (ACE) inhibitors have also been reported to cause lithium toxicity.

MANAGEMENT OPTIONS:

➥ **Consider Alternative.** In patients taking lithium, consider using alternatives to angiotensin II receptor antagonists such as candesartan. Note that ACE inhibitors appear to interact with lithium in a similar manner and may not be suitable as noninteracting alternatives.

➥ **Monitor.** If candesartan or other angiotensin II receptor antagonists are used concurrently with lithium, be alert for evidence of lithium toxicity (eg, nausea, vomiting, diarrhea, anorexia, coarse tremor, slurred speech, vertigo, confusion, lethargy; in severe cases, seizures, stupor, coma, cardiovascular collapse). Adjust lithium dose as needed.

REFERENCES:

1. Zwanzger P, et al. Lithium intoxication after administration of AT1 blockers. *J Clin Psychiatry.* 2001;62:208-209.

2. Blanche P, et al. Lithium intoxication in an elderly patient after combined treatment with losartan. *Eur J Clin Pharmacol.* 1997;52:501.

3. Leung M, et al. Potential drug interaction between lithium and valsartan. *J Clin Psychopharmacol.* 2000;20:392-393.

Capecitabine (*Xeloda*)

Phenytoin (eg, *Dilantin*)

SUMMARY: Isolated cases and theoretical considerations indicate that capecitabine can increase phenytoin serum concentrations.

RISK FACTORS: No specific risk factors are known.

MECHANISM: Capecitabine is a prodrug for fluorouracil (eg, *Adrucil*), and the latter probably inhibits the metabolism of phenytoin by CYP2C9.

CLINICAL EVALUATION: A patient on phenytoin developed phenytoin toxicity after capecitabine was started.[1] Capecitabine is an oral prodrug for fluorouracil, a drug that is known to increase the plasma concentrations of phenytoin and other drugs metabolized by CYP2C9. Although clinical evidence is meager, theoretical consideration suggests that capecitabine is likely to increase phenytoin plasma concentrations.

RELATED DRUGS: Fluorouracil (5-FU), the active metabolite of capecitabine, is known to increase phenytoin concentrations.

MANAGEMENT OPTIONS:

➡ *Monitor.* In patients given phenytoin and capecitabine, monitor phenytoin plasma concentrations and be alert for evidence of phenytoin toxicity. Adjustments in phenytoin dose may be needed if capecitabine is initiated, discontinued, or changed in dosage.

REFERENCES:

1. Brickell K, et al. Phenytoin toxicity due to fluoropyrimidines (5FU/capecitabine): three case reports. *Br J Cancer.* 2003;89:615-616.

Capecitabine (*Xeloda*)

Warfarin (eg, *Coumadin*)

SUMMARY: Capecitabine appears to increase warfarin effect; monitor anticoagulant response.

RISK FACTORS: No specific risk factors are known.

MECHANISM: Capecitabine is a prodrug for fluorouracil (eg, *Adrucil*), and the latter appears to inhibit the metabolism of warfarin by CYP2C9.

CLINICAL EVALUATION: Two patients on warfarin developed international normalized ratios (INRs) above 10, as well as GI bleeding after capecitabine was added to their therapy.[1] This is consistent with a study reported by the manufacturer in which capecitabine was associated with substantial increases in warfarin effect in 4 cancer patients.[2] In another case, a woman stabilized on long-term warfarin developed severe bleeding and an INR of 8.6 about a month after starting capecitabine.[3] This information, in addition to the data on increased warfarin response from fluorouracil, suggests that capecitabine is capable of increasing warfarin response.

RELATED DRUGS: Fluorouracil (5-FU), the active metabolite of capecitabine, is known to increase the anticoagulant response to warfarin.

MANAGEMENT OPTIONS:

➡ *Monitor.* Monitor for altered warfarin response if capecitabine is initiated, discontinued, or changed in dosage; adjustments in warfarin dosage may be needed. If warfarin is started during capecitabine therapy, begin with conservative doses of warfarin.

REFERENCES:

1. Copur MS, et al. An adverse interaction between warfarin and capecitabine: a case report and review of the literature. *Clin Colorectal Cancer*. 2001;1:182-184.

2. *Xeloda* [package insert]. Nutley, NJ: Roche Laboratories; April 2003.

3. Isaacs K, Haim N. Adverse interaction between capecitabine and warfarin resulting in altered coagulation parameters and bleeding: case report and review of the literature. *J Chemother*. 2005;17:339-342.

Captopril (eg, *Capoten*) Digitoxin[†]

SUMMARY: Captopril does not appear to affect the pharmacokinetics or pharmacodynamics of digitoxin.

RISK FACTORS: No specific risk factors are known.

MECHANISM: No interaction.

CLINICAL EVALUATION: In 12 healthy subjects taking chronic digitoxin 0.07 mg/day, captopril 25 mg twice daily for 19 days had no effect on the pharmacokinetics or pharmacodynamics of digitoxin.[1]

RELATED DRUGS: No information is available, but it is unlikely that digoxin (eg, *Lanoxin*) would be affected by captopril.

MANAGEMENT OPTIONS: No interaction.

REFERENCES:

1. de Mey C, et al. Captopril does not interact with pharmacodynamics and pharmacokinetics of digitoxin in healthy man. *Eur J Clin Pharmacol*. 1992;43:445-447.

† Not available in the United States.

Captopril (eg, *Capoten*)

Insulin

SUMMARY: Captopril and other angiotensin-converting enzyme (ACE) inhibitors appear to enhance insulin sensitivity. Nonetheless, ACE inhibitors are used intentionally in patients with diabetes and hypertension or heart failure.

RISK FACTORS: No specific risk factors are known.

MECHANISM: ACE inhibitors may increase insulin-mediated glucose uptake by altering skeletal muscle blood flow or serum electrolytes.

CLINICAL EVALUATION: Several studies have demonstrated an increase in insulin sensitivity in nondiabetic patients during ACE inhibitors administration.[1,2] Other studies have found similar results in diabetic patients.[3,4] Combination therapy with ACE inhibitors and insulin or oral hypoglycemics in diabetic patients has resulted in symptomatic hypoglycemia.[3,5] Two epidemiologic studies of diabetic patients treated with insulin or oral hypoglycemic agents who were admitted to a hospital with hypoglycemia have been reported.[6,7] In both studies, the coadministration of ACE inhibitors was associated with about a 3 times greater risk of developing hypoglycemia.

RELATED DRUGS: While not all ACE inhibitors have been studied, assume that enalapril (eg, *Vasotec*), benazepril (eg, *Lotensin*), fosinopril (eg, *Monopril*), ramipril (*Altace*), quinapril (eg, *Accupril*), trandolapril (*Mavik*), and moexipril (*Univasc*) also may affect glycemic control in patients with diabetes mellitus. Oral hypoglycemic agents, including chlorpropamide (eg, *Diabinese*), tolbutamide (eg, *Orinase*), tolazamide (eg, *Tolinase*), repaglinide (*Prandin*), metformin (eg, *Glucophage*), glimepiride (*Amaryl*), glyburide (eg, *DiaBeta*), and glipizide (eg, *Glucotrol*), are expected to interact in a similar manner with ACE inhibitors.

MANAGEMENT OPTIONS:

➡ *Consider Alternative.* While data are limited, it appears that all angiotensin II receptor inhibitors may not have the same effect on insulin sensitivity.[1] Pending further clinical trials, accompany the use of these agents (eg, losartan [*Cozaar*], candesartan [*Atacand*]) with blood glucose monitoring in patients with diabetes mellitus. Also consider antihypertensive drugs from different classes.

➡ *Monitor.* Monitor patients for altered hypoglycemic effect if ACE inhibitor therapy is initiated, discontinued, or changed in dose; adjust insulin and oral hypoglycemic dosages as necessary.

REFERENCES:

1. Fogari R, et al. Comparative effects of lisinopril and losartan on insulin sensitivity in the treatment of non diabetic hypertensive patients. *Br J Clin Pharmacol.* 1998;46:467-471.
2. Paolisso G, et al. Lisinopril administration improves insulin action in aged patients with hypertension. *J Hum Hypertens.* 1995;9:541-546.
3. Rett K, et al. Role of angiotensin-converting enzyme inhibitors in early antihypertensive treatment in non-insulin dependent diabetes mellitus. *Postgrad Med J.* 1988;64(suppl 3):69-74; 90-92.
4. Vuorinen-Markkola H, et al. Antihypertensive therapy with enalapril improves glucose storage and insulin sensitivity in hypertensive patients with non-insulin-dependent diabetes mellitus. *Metabolism.* 1995;44:85-89.

5. Arauz-Pacheco C, et al. Hypoglycemia induced by angiotensin-converting enzyme inhibitors in patients with non-insulin-dependent diabetes receiving sulfonylurea therapy. *Am J Med*. 1990;89:811-813.

6. Herings RM, et al. Hypoglycemia associated with use of inhibitors of angiotensin converting enzyme. *Lancet*. 1995;345:1195-1198.

7. Morris AD, et al. ACE inhibitor use is associated with hospitalization for severe hypoglycemia in patients with diabetes. *Diabetes Care*. 1997;20:1363-1367.

Carbamazepine (eg, *Tegretol*)

Cimetidine (eg, *Tagamet*)

SUMMARY: Cimetidine may transiently increase plasma carbamazepine concentrations, but the effect appears to dissipate after 1 week of cimetidine therapy.

RISK FACTORS:

➡ ***Dosage Regimen.*** In most patients, clinically important inhibition of hepatic drug metabolism by cimetidine requires dosages of at least 400 mg/day.

MECHANISM: Cimetidine probably inhibits the hepatic metabolism of carbamazepine, although an effect on carbamazepine bioavailability has not been ruled out. Carbamazepine could stimulate the metabolism of cimetidine, but clinical evidence is lacking.

CLINICAL EVALUATION: An 89-year-old woman on long-term carbamazepine therapy 600 mg/day developed evidence of carbamazepine toxicity (severe dizziness) 2 days after starting cimetidine 400 mg/day.[1] Subsequent concurrent use of carbamazepine 800 mg/day and cimetidine 1 g/day resulted in severe neurologic symptoms (somnolence, dizziness, nystagmus, and twitching) and carbamazepine blood concentrations in the toxic range. The use of cimetidine 1 g/day in this elderly woman, who had reduced renal function, probably resulted in relatively high serum cimetidine concentrations that would increase the magnitude of a cimetidine-carbamazepine interaction and raise the possibility that cimetidine-induced neurologic toxicity contributed to the symptoms. Subsequent studies using single doses[2,3] and 15 days[4] of carbamazepine confirmed a cimetidine-induced inhibition of carbamazepine elimination; however, cimetidine did not appear to affect carbamazepine disposition in 2 studies involving patients with steady-state carbamazepine concentrations.[5,6] The discrepancy seems to have been resolved by a study that observed a transient increase in plasma carbamazepine 2 days after starting cimetidine 1,200 mg/day in 8 healthy subjects on long-term carbamazepine 600 mg/day. This was followed by a return of carbamazepine concentrations to pre-cimetidine values by day 7 of cimetidine therapy.[7] Six of the 8 subjects developed adverse reactions (eg, nausea, drowsiness, fatigue, ataxia) during the first few days after cimetidine was initiated. Cimetidine apparently increases serum carbamazepine concentrations for the first few days of cimetidine therapy, but the interaction dissipates by day 7 of treatment.

RELATED DRUGS: Ranitidine (eg, *Zantac*) does not appear to affect the elimination of single doses of carbamazepine.[2,8] The effect of famotidine (eg, *Pepcid*) and nizatidine (eg, *Axid*) on carbamazepine is unknown, but they are not expected to interact.

MANAGEMENT OPTIONS:

➡ **Consider Alternative.** The use of ranitidine, famotidine, or nizatidine in place of cimetidine is likely to minimize the risk of carbamazepine toxicity.

➡ **Monitor.** Warn patients receiving carbamazepine of the possibility of adverse reactions (eg, drowsiness, dizziness, nausea, vomiting, ataxia, headache, nystagmus, blurred vision) during the first few days of cimetidine therapy. Based upon current evidence, patients on long-term therapy with both cimetidine and carbamazepine do not appear to be at increased risk for adverse reactions. Nevertheless, monitor patients for altered responses to carbamazepine if cimetidine is discontinued or changed in dosage.

REFERENCES:

1. Telerman-Toppet N, et al. Cimetidine interaction with carbamazepine. *Ann Intern Med.* 1981;94(4, pt 1):544.
2. Webster LK, et al. Effect of cimetidine and ranitidine on carbamazepine and sodium valproate pharmacokinetics. *Eur J Clin Pharmacol.* 1984;27(3):341-343.
3. Dalton MJ, et al. The influence of cimetidine on single-dose carbamazepine pharmacokinetics. *Epilepsia.* 1985;26(2):127-130.
4. MacPhee GJ, et al. Effects of cimetidine on carbamazepine auto- and hetero-induction in man. *Br J Clin Pharmacol.* 1984;18(3):411-419.
5. Sonne J, et al. Lack of interaction between cimetidine and carbamazepine. *Acta Neurol Scand.* 1983;68(4):253-256.
6. Levine M, et al. Differential effect of cimetidine on serum concentrations of carbamazepine and phenytoin. *Neurology.* 1985;35(4):562-565.
7. Dalton MJ, et al. Cimetidine and carbamazepine: a complex drug interaction. *Epilepsia.* 1986;27(5):553-558.
8. Dalton MJ, et al. Ranitidine does not alter single-dose carbamazepine pharmacokinetics in healthy adults. *Drug Intell Clin Pharm.* 1985;19(12):941-944.

Carbamazepine (eg, *Tegretol*)

Ciprofloxacin (eg, *Cipro*)

SUMMARY: Ciprofloxacin administration increases carbamazepine plasma concentrations; some patients may experience carbamazepine adverse reactions.

RISK FACTORS: No specific risk factors are known.

MECHANISM: Unknown. Ciprofloxacin may be inhibiting the metabolism of carbamazepine via CYP3A4.

CLINICAL EVALUATION: Eight healthy subjects received a single dose of carbamazepine 200 mg alone and concurrently with a single dose of ciprofloxacin 500 mg.[1] Compared with carbamazepine alone, the concurrent ciprofloxacin dose increased the mean maximum carbamazepine plasma concentration and its area under the concentration-time curve approximately 50%. The half-life of carbamazepine increased from 38 to 50 hours. Because this study was a single-dose design, it is difficult to estimate what the effect of long-term ciprofloxacin would have on steady-state carbamazepine concentrations.

RELATED DRUGS: None known.

MANAGEMENT OPTIONS:

➡ *Monitor.* Pending further study, monitor patients stabilized on carbamazepine for signs of carbamazepine toxicity (eg, dizziness, drowsiness, nausea) if ciprofloxacin is coadministered.

REFERENCES:

1. Shahzadi A, et al. Therapeutic effects of ciprofloxacin on the pharmacokinetics of carbamazepine in healthy adult male volunteers. *Pak J Pharm Sci.* 2011;24(1):63-68.

Carbamazepine (eg, *Tegretol*)

Citalopram (eg, *Celexa*)

SUMMARY: Isolated case reports suggest that carbamazepine reduces citalopram serum concentrations, but the clinical importance of this effect is not established.

RISK FACTORS: No specific risk factors are known.

MECHANISM: Carbamazepine probably enhances the metabolism of citalopram.

CLINICAL EVALUATION: Two patients developed marked increases in citalopram serum concentrations when they were switched from carbamazepine (an enzyme inducer) to oxcarbazepine (eg, *Trileptal*) (not an enzyme inducer).[1] In the first case, a 31-year-old man who clearly had subtherapeutic citalopram serum concentrations achieved therapeutic concentrations when carbamazepine was discontinued. The second case involved a 42-year-old woman whose citalopram serum concentrations increased from 164 nmol/L to an excessive level of 560 nmol/L when carbamazepine was discontinued. Although more study of this interaction is needed to establish its clinical importance, the magnitude of effect suggests that carbamazepine may inhibit the therapeutic response to citalopram.

RELATED DRUGS: The effect of carbamazepine on selective serotonin reuptake inhibitors other than citalopram is not established, but it is possible that their metabolism is affected by carbamazepine. The metabolism of carbamazepine may be inhibited by fluoxetine (eg, *Prozac*) and fluvoxamine (eg, *Luvox*), but paroxetine (eg, *Paxil*) and sertraline (eg, *Zoloft*) may be less likely to affect carbamazepine metabolism.

MANAGEMENT OPTIONS:

➡ *Monitor.* Monitor for reduced citalopram effect (eg, decreased effectiveness for indicated uses such as depression) if carbamazepine is given concurrently.

REFERENCES:

1. Lewis CF, et al. Dystonia associated with trazodone and sertraline. *J Clin Psychopharmacol.* 1997;17(1):64-65.

Carbamazepine (eg, *Tegretol*)

Clarithromycin (eg, *Biaxin*)

SUMMARY: Clarithromycin administration appears to increase carbamazepine concentrations; carbamazepine toxicity could result.

RISK FACTORS: No specific risk factors are known.

MECHANISM: It appears that clarithromycin inhibits the metabolism (CYP3A4) of carbamazepine.

CLINICAL EVALUATION: Clarithromycin 250 mg twice daily increased carbamazepine concentrations and reduced the concentration of carbamazepine epoxide.[1] The apparent reduction in carbamazepine metabolism could lead to increased concentrations and toxicity. However, to the extent that the concentration of the epoxide metabolite was reduced, adverse reactions might be reduced. Other cases of increased carbamazepine occurring after the addition of clarithromycin and omeprazole have been noted.[2]

RELATED DRUGS: Erythromycin and troleandomycin[†] are known to inhibit the metabolism of carbamazepine. Azithromycin (eg, *Zithromax*) and dirithromycin[†] are unlikely to decrease carbamazepine metabolism.

MANAGEMENT OPTIONS:

➥ *Consider Alternative.* Azithromycin does not appear to affect carbamazepine metabolism.

➥ *Monitor.* Until further information is available, carefully monitor patients maintained on carbamazepine for changing serum concentrations following the addition of clarithromycin.

REFERENCES:

1. Albani F, et al. Clarithromycin-carbamazepine interaction: a case report. *Epilepsia.* 1993;34(1):161-162.
2. Metz DC, et al. *Helicobacter pylori* gastritis therapy with omeprazole and clarithromycin increases serum carbamazepine levels. *Dig Dis Sci.* 1995;40(4):912-915.

† Not available in the United States.

5   Carbamazepine (eg, *Tegretol*)

Clonazepam (eg, *Klonopin*)

SUMMARY: Clonazepam does not appear to interact with carbamazepine.

RISK FACTORS: No specific risk factors are known.

MECHANISM: Not established.

CLINICAL EVALUATION: Clonazepam did not affect carbamazepine serum concentrations in patients with seizure disorders.[1]

RELATED DRUGS: None known.

MANAGEMENT OPTIONS: No interaction.

REFERENCES:

1. Johannessen SI, et al. Lack of effect of clonazepam on serum levels of diphenylhydantoin, phenobarbital and carbamazepine. *Acta Neurol Scand.* 1977;55:506.

Carbamazepine (eg, *Tegretol*)

Clozapine (eg, *Clozaril*)

SUMMARY: Carbamazepine appears to considerably reduce clozapine plasma concentrations, but the clinical importance of this effect is not established.

RISK FACTORS: No specific risk factors are known.

MECHANISM: Not established. Carbamazepine probably enhances the hepatic microsomal metabolism of clozapine.

CLINICAL EVALUATION: Data from a therapeutic drug monitoring service were used to determine the effect of coadministered drugs on clozapine serum concentrations.[1] Patients receiving carbamazepine and clozapine had, on average, a 50% lower ratio of concentration/dose (C/D) for clozapine than those not receiving carbamazepine. In 8 patients, clozapine plasma concentrations were measured in the presence and absence of carbamazepine therapy. In every case, the clozapine C/D ratio was lower in the presence of carbamazepine therapy. Patients receiving larger doses of carbamazepine manifested a larger decrease in the C/D ratio. Some patients manifested marked reductions in clozapine concentrations during concurrent carbamazepine therapy. In 6 patients, clozapine concentrations decreased 40% to 50% after receiving 6 months of carbamazepine treatment.[2]

RELATED DRUGS: Other enzyme-inducing anticonvulsants such as phenytoin (eg, *Dilantin*), primidone (eg, *Mysoline*), and barbiturates may have a similar effect.

MANAGEMENT OPTIONS:

➡ *Monitor.* Although more information is needed, monitor for altered clozapine response if carbamazepine therapy is initiated, discontinued, or changed in dosage.

REFERENCES:

1. Jerling M, et al. Fluvoxamine inhibition and carbamazepine induction of the metabolism of clozapine: evidence from a therapeutic drug monitoring service. *Ther Drug Monit.* 1994;16:368.
2. Tiihonen J, et al. Carbamazepine induced changes in plasma levels of neuroleptics. *Pharmacopsychiatry.* 1995;28:26.

Carbamazepine (eg, *Tegretol*)

Colestipol (*Colestid*)

SUMMARY: Single-dose studies in healthy subjects suggest that colestipol only slightly reduces the bioavailability of carbamazepine.

RISK FACTORS: No specific risk factors are known.

MECHANISM: Colestipol probably binds somewhat with carbamazepine in the GI tract.

CLINICAL EVALUATION: Six healthy subjects received a single oral 400 mg dose of carbamazepine with and without coadministration of 10 g colestipol.[1] The bioavailability of carbamazepine as measured by area under the plasma concentration-time curve was reduced 10% by colestipol. Although chronic dosing studies in patients are needed to rule out a clinically significant effect on carbamazepine bioavailability, this study suggests that colestipol does not have an important effect on carbamazepine absorption. In the same study, carbamazepine bioavailability was unaffected by coadministration of 10 g of cholestyramine.[1]

RELATED DRUGS: Cholestyramine (eg, *Questran*) 8 g did not affect the bioavailability of carbamazepine in 6 healthy subjects.[1]

MANAGEMENT OPTIONS: No specific action is required, but be alert for evidence of the interaction.

REFERENCES:

1. Neuvonen PJ, et al. Effects of resins and activated charcoal on the absorption of digoxin, carbamazepine and furosemide. *Br J Clin Pharmacol*. 1988;25:229.

Carbamazepine (eg, *Tegretol*)

Contraceptives, Oral (eg, *Ortho-Novum*)

SUMMARY: Carbamazepine and other enzyme-inducing anticonvulsants, such as barbiturates, phenytoin, and primidone, can inhibit the effect of oral contraceptives, resulting in menstrual irregularities and unplanned pregnancies.

RISK FACTORS:

➡ **Dosage Regimen.** Oral contraceptives with lower doses of hormones can increase the risk of interaction.

MECHANISM: Anticonvulsant-induced enzyme induction probably enhances the metabolism of oral contraceptives.[2]

CLINICAL EVALUATION: A woman receiving a low-dose oral contraceptive became pregnant after carbamazepine therapy was instituted.[1] A number of unplanned pregnancies have occurred in women taking anticonvulsants and oral contraceptives concurrently.[2-4] In a retrospective study, 3 of 41 women developed unplanned pregnancies while on oral contraceptives and anticonvulsants; none of the women with seizure disorders on oral contraceptives alone became pregnant.[5] Anticonvulsants also have been associated with unplanned pregnancies and low norgestrel plasma concentrations in women receiving norgestrel (progestrin-only contraception) subdermal capsules.[6] Although oral contraceptives purportedly can induce seizures,[7] a study of 20 patients with seizure disorders failed to show an effect of oral contraceptives on seizure frequency compared with placebo.[8] Single-dose pharmacokinetics of oral doses of ethinyl estradiol and levonorgestrel were studied in women before and 8 to 12 weeks after initiating carbamazepine (n = 4) or phenytoin (eg, *Dilantin*) (n = 6). Carbamazepine decreased the area under the plasma concentration-time curve (AUC) of ethinyl estradiol 42% and levonorgestrel 40%. Phenytoin decreased the AUC of ethinyl estradiol 49% and levonorgestrel 40%.[9] Valproic acid does not appear to affect the pharmacokinetics of oral contraceptives;[10] clinical evidence and theoretical considerations suggest that benzodiazepine anticonvulsants would be unlikely to affect oral contraceptive efficacy.

RELATED DRUGS: See Clinical Evaluation.

MANAGEMENT OPTIONS:

➡ **Consider Alternative.** Consider an other means of contraception instead of, or in addition to, oral contraceptives when pregnancy is to be avoided in women receiving carbamazepine or other enzyme-inducing anticonvulsants such as phenobarbital (eg, *Solfoton*), phenytoin, and primidone (eg, *Mysoline*). Although an oral contraceptive with a higher estrogen content would be preferable for some women who are being treated with enzyme-inducing anticonvulsants, individualize based upon patient response (eg, lack of breakthrough bleeding).

➡ **Monitor.** Spotting or breakthrough bleeding in patients taking oral contraceptives and enzyme-inducing anticonvulsants could indicate that the drugs are interacting, although lack of breakthrough bleeding does not ensure contraceptive protection.

REFERENCES:

1. Rapport DJ, et al. Interactions between carbamazepine and birth control pills. *Psychosomatics*. 1989;30:462.
2. Kenyon IE. Unplanned pregnancy in an epileptic. *BMJ*. 1972;1:686.
3. Janz D, et al. Anti-epileptic drugs and failure of oral contraceptives. *Lancet*. 1974;1:1113.
4. Laengner H, et al. Antiepileptic drugs and failure of oral contraceptives. *Lancet*. 1974;2:600.
5. Coulam CG, et al. Do anticonvulsants reduce the efficacy of oral contraceptives? *Epilepsia*. 1979;20:519.
6. Haukkamaa M. Contraception by Norplant subdermal capsules is not reliable in epileptic patients on anticonvulsant treatment. *Contraception*. 1986;33:559.
7. McArthrur J. Oral contraceptives and epilepsy (Notes and Comments). *BMJ*. 1967;3:162.
8. Espir M, et al. Epilepsy and oral contraception. *BMJ*. 1969;1:294.
9. Crawford P, et al. The interaction of phenytoin and carbamazepine with combined oral contraceptive steroids. *Br J Clin Pharmacol*. 1990;30:892.
10. Crawford P, et al. The lack of effect on sodium valproate on the pharmacokinetics of oral contraceptive steroids. *Contraception*. 1986;33:23.
11. Mattson RH, et al. Use of oral contraceptives by women with epilepsy. *JAMA*. 1986;256:238.
12. Robertson YR, et al. Interactions between oral contraceptives and other drugs; a review. *Curr Med Res Opin*. 1976;3:647.

Carbamazepine (eg, *Tegretol*)
Cyclosporine (eg, *Neoral*)

SUMMARY: Carbamazepine can substantially reduce blood cyclosporine concentrations; adjustments in cyclosporine dosage may be required.

RISK FACTORS: No specific risk factors are known.

MECHANISM: Carbamazepine probably increases the hepatic metabolism or presystemic clearance of cyclosporine.

CLINICAL EVALUATION: Several cases have been reported of reduced blood cyclosporine concentrations in patients receiving carbamazepine concurrently.[1-4] The blood cyclosporine concentrations were decreased markedly, resulting in subtherapeutic (and in some cases undetectable) concentrations. The blood cyclosporine concentrations decreased over several days after the initiation of carbamazepine; however, up to 2 to 3 weeks were needed for the interaction to dissipate after the carbamazepine was discontinued.

RELATED DRUGS: Other enzyme-inducing anticonvulsants such as phenobarbital, phenytoin (eg, *Dilantin*), and primidone (eg, *Mysoline*) appear to reduce blood cyclosporine concentrations,[5] but in some cases valproic acid (eg, *Depakene*) was successfully substituted for carbamazepine without evidence of interaction.[2,4] Tacrolimus (*Prograf*) probably is affected similarly by enzyme inducers.

MANAGEMENT OPTIONS:

➡ *Consider Alternative.* The interaction can be avoided (based upon limited clinical evidence) when valproic acid can be substituted for carbamazepine.

➡ *Monitor.* Be alert for evidence of altered cyclosporine effect if carbamazepine therapy is initiated or discontinued; monitor blood cyclosporine concentrations carefully.

REFERENCES:
1. Alvarez JS, et al. Effect of carbamazepine on cyclosporin blood level. *Nephron.* 1991;58:235.
2. Schofield OMV, et al. Cyclosporine A in psoriasis: interaction with carbamazepine. *Br J Dermatol.* 1990;122:425.
3. Lele P, et al. Cyclosporine and tegretol—another drug interaction. *Kidney Int.* 1985;27:344.
4. Hillebrand G, et al. Valproate for epilepsy in renal transplant recipients receiving cyclosporine. *Transplantation.* 1987;43:915.
5. Yee GC, et al. Pharmacokinetic drug interactions with cyclosporine (Part I). *Clin Pharmacokinet.* 1990;19:319.

 Carbamazepine (eg, *Tegretol*)

Danazol (*Danocrine*)

SUMMARY: Danazol predictably increases serum carbamazepine concentrations substantially and induces carbamazepine toxicity (eg, dizziness, nausea, drowsiness, ataxia) in some patients receiving both drugs.

RISK FACTORS: No specific risk factors are known.

MECHANISM: Danazol inhibits the hepatic oxidative metabolism of carbamazepine.

CLINICAL EVALUATION: Observation of a marked increase in plasma carbamazepine concentrations and mild carbamazepine toxicity in a patient who had been started on danazol prompted a detailed study of this interaction.[1] During danazol coadministration (600 mg/day) in this patient, carbamazepine half-life more than doubled and carbamazepine plasma clearance was reduced by more than half when compared with the predanazol values. In 5 other epileptic patients, danazol increased steady-state plasma carbamazepine concentrations 50% to 100%, but clinical evidence of carbamazepine toxicity was lacking. In another study of 6 patients on chronic carbamazepine therapy, danazol 400 to 600 mg/day was associated with an almost 2-fold increase in serum carbamazepine concentrations.[2] Five of the 6 patients exhibited symptoms of carbamazepine toxicity (eg, lethargy, ataxia, dizziness, blurred vision, drowsiness) within 7 to 30 days of starting danazol, necessitating dosage reductions of 100 to 200 mg/day. Thus, danazol generally increases plasma carbamazepine concentrations approximately 2-fold, but clinical evidence of carbamazepine toxicity is not always evident, especially because the toxicity appears to be delayed.

RELATED DRUGS: No information is available.

MANAGEMENT OPTIONS:

➡ *Avoid Unless Benefit Outweighs Risk.* If possible, avoid danazol in patients receiving carbamazepine.

➡ *Monitor.* Monitor patients on carbamazepine for evidence of carbamazepine toxicity for several weeks after danazol is initiated. Carbamazepine dosage may need to be reduced. Stopping danazol therapy may result in decreasing carbamazepine serum concentrations and response, necessitating an increase in carbamazepine dosage.

REFERENCES:

1. Kramer G, et al. Carbamazepine-danazol drug interaction: its mechanism examined by a stable isotope technique. *Ther Drug Monit.* 1986;8:387.

2. Zielinski JJ, et al. Clinically significant danazol-carbamazepine interaction. *Ther Drug Monit.* 1987;9:24.

Carbamazepine (eg, *Tegretol*)

Darunavir (*Prezista*)/Ritonavir (*Norvir*)

SUMMARY: The coadministration of darunavir/ritonavir and carbamazepine results in an increase in the plasma concentrations of carbamazepine; some patients may experience carbamazepine adverse reactions.

RISK FACTORS: No specific risk factors are known.

MECHANISM: Darunavir/ritonavir appears to inhibit the elimination of carbamazepine, probably via the CYP3A4 enzyme.

CLINICAL EVALUATION: While specific data are limited, the manufacturer of darunavir notes that the coadministration of darunavir/ritonavir 600/100 mg twice daily with carbamazepine 200 mg twice daily to 16 subjects increased the mean area under the plasma concentration-time curve of carbamazepine by about 45%.[1] Pending further data, observe patients receiving darunavir/ritonavir and carbamazepine for evidence of carbamazepine toxicity, including dizziness, ataxia, and nausea.

RELATED DRUGS: Atazanavir (*Reyataz*), indinavir (*Crixivan*), nelfinavir (*Viracept*), and saquinavir (*Invirase*) also inhibit the activity of CYP3A4 and are expected to increase the plasma concentrations of carbamazepine.

MANAGEMENT OPTIONS:

➡ *Monitor.* Carefully monitor patients taking carbamazepine for alterations in their carbamazepine plasma concentrations and therapeutic response if darunavir/ritonavir is added to, or withdrawn from, their drug regimen.

REFERENCES:

1. *Prezista* [package insert]. Raritan, NJ: Tibotec Therapeutics; 2008.

Carbamazepine (eg, *Tegretol*)

Diltiazem (eg, *Cardizem*)

SUMMARY: Diltiazem increases carbamazepine serum concentrations, and frequently results in carbamazepine toxicity.

RISK FACTORS: No specific risk factors are known.

MECHANISM: Diltiazem inhibits carbamazepine metabolism, probably by inhibiting intestinal and hepatic CYP3A4. The first-pass metabolism of oral diltiazem can be increased dramatically by enzyme induction, and carbamazepine, a known enzyme inducer, is expected to produce a similar effect.

CLINICAL EVALUATION: A number of case reports have appeared in which diltiazem was associated with carbamazepine toxicity.[1-5] In one case, increased serum concentrations of carbamazepine were noted 3 days after diltiazem 60 mg 3 times daily was started.[1] In another case, diltiazem-induced carbamazepine toxicity resolved when the carbamazepine dose was reduced 60%.[2] In a retrospective study, carbamazepine toxicity was observed in 10 of 15 patients given concurrent diltiazem or verapamil (eg, *Calan*), but not with concurrent nifedipine (eg, *Procardia*). Thus, it appears that carbamazepine toxicity is likely if diltiazem is used concurrently, unless the carbamazepine dosage is reduced.

RELATED DRUGS: Verapamil can produce carbamazepine toxicity, but limited evidence suggests that nifedipine is less likely to do so. Felodipine undergoes extensive first-pass metabolism and is highly susceptible to enzyme induction; thus, it may be difficult to achieve therapeutic felodipine concentrations in the presence of carbamazepine. (See also Carbamazepine/Verapamil, Carbamazepine/Nifedipine, and Carbamazepine/Felodipine.)

MANAGEMENT OPTIONS:

➡ **Avoid Unless Benefit Outweighs Risk.** Given the high likelihood of carbamazepine toxicity with concurrent use and the possibility of reduced diltiazem effect, avoid the combination if possible. (See Related Drugs.)

➡ **Monitor.** If the combination is used, monitor for carbamazepine toxicity (eg, nausea, vomiting, dizziness, drowsiness, headache, diplopia, confusion). Toxic symptoms are likely to occur within 2 to 3 days of starting diltiazem.

REFERENCES:

1. Brodie MJ, et al. Carbamazepine neurotoxicity precipitated by diltiazem. *Br Med J (Clin Res Ed)*. 1986;292(6529):1170-1171.

2. Eimer M, et al. Elevated serum carbamazepine concentrations following diltiazem initiation. *Drug Intell Clin Pharm*. 1987;21(4):340-342.

3. Bahls FH, et al. Interactions between calcium channel blockers and the anticonvulsants carbamazepine and phenytoin. *Neurology*. 1991;41(5):740-742.

4. Gadde K, et al. Diltiazem effect on carbamazepine levels in manic depression. *J Clin Psych Opharmacol*. 1990;10(5):378-379.

5. Ahmad S. Diltiazem-carbamazepine interaction. *Am Heart J*. 1990;120(6 pt 1):1485-1486.

Carbamazepine (eg, *Tegretol*)

Doxycycline (eg, *Vibramycin*)

SUMMARY: Doxycycline serum concentrations may be reduced by carbamazepine.

RISK FACTORS: No specific risk factors are known.

MECHANISM: Carbamazepine appears to stimulate the hepatic metabolism of doxycycline.

CLINICAL EVALUATION: The half-life of doxycycline was shorter in 5 patients on chronic carbamazepine therapy (8.4 hours) than in 9 control patients (15.1 hours).[1] The effect of this shortened half-life of the clinical antibacterial effect of doxycycline has not been assessed, but the magnitude of the difference in half-life suggests that carbamazepine is likely to reduce the efficacy of doxycycline.

RELATED DRUGS: The effect of carbamazepine on other tetracyclines has not been established, but an interaction does not seem likely because these agents are largely excreted renally.

MANAGEMENT OPTIONS:

➡ **Monitor.** Be alert for a decreased clinical response to doxycycline when carbamazepine and doxycycline are used concomitantly.

REFERENCES:

1. Penttila O, et al. Interaction between doxycycline and some antiepileptic drugs. *Br Med J.* 1974;2(5917):470-472.

Carbamazepine (eg, *Tegretol*)

Erythromycin (eg, *Ery-Tab*)

SUMMARY: Erythromycin markedly increases serum carbamazepine concentrations; numerous cases of carbamazepine toxicity have been reported in patients receiving both drugs.

RISK FACTORS: No specific risk factors are known.

MECHANISM: Erythromycin inhibits the hepatic metabolism of carbamazepine.

CLINICAL EVALUATION: Numerous case reports have appeared describing carbamazepine toxicity following the addition of erythromycin therapy.[1-8] Serum carbamazepine concentrations usually increase 2- to 4-fold, although 1 patient developed an almost 6-fold increase in serum carbamazepine following intravenous erythromycin.[7] Carbamazepine toxicity usually occurs within the first day or two of erythromycin therapy. The interaction may be dose related, with larger doses of erythromycin producing larger increases in serum carbamazepine.[4,7]

RELATED DRUGS: Troleandomycin[+] and clarithromycin (eg, *Biaxin*) also may produce carbamazepine toxicity. Azithromycin (eg, *Zithromax*) and dirithromycin[+] are not likely to cause carbamazepine toxicity.

MANAGEMENT OPTIONS:

➡ **Consider Alternative.** If possible, avoid erythromycin and troleandomycin in patients receiving carbamazepine. Azithromycin does not appear to affect carbamazepine.

➡ **Monitor.** If erythromycin is used in patients receiving carbamazepine, monitor for evidence of carbamazepine toxicity (eg, dizziness, drowsiness, nausea, vomiting, ataxia, headache, nystagmus, blurred vision), and reduce the dose of carbamazepine if necessary. Carbamazepine dosage may need to be increased when erythromycin is stopped.

REFERENCES:

1. Mesdjian E, et al. Carbamazepine intoxication due to triacetyloleandomycin administration in epileptic patients. *Epilepsia.* 1980;21(5):489-496.

2. Hedrick R, et al. Carbamazepine-erythromycin interaction leading to carbamazepine toxicity in four epileptic children. *Ther Drug Monit.* 1983;5(4):405-407.

3. Jaster PJ, et al. Erythromycin-carbamazepine interaction. *Neurology* 1986;36(4):594-595.

4. Goulden KJ, et al. Severe carbamazepine intoxication after coadministration of erythromycin. *J Pediatr.* 1986;109(1):135-138.

5. Berrettini WH. A case of erythromycin-induced carbamazepine toxicity. *J Clin Psychiatry.* 1986;47(3):147.

6. Macnab AJ, et al. Heart block secondary to erythromycin-induced carbamazepine toxicity. *Pediatrics.* 1987;80(6):951-953.

7. Mitsch RA. Carbamazepine toxicity precipitated by intravenous erythromycin. *Drug Intell Clin Pharm.* 1989;23(11):878-879.

8. Wong YY, et al. Effect of erythromycin on carbamazepine kinetics. *Clin Pharmacol Ther.* 1983;33(4):460-464.

† Not available in the United States.

 Carbamazepine (eg, *Tegretol*)

Felbamate (*Felbatol*)

SUMMARY: Felbamate modestly reduces plasma carbamazepine concentrations and increases plasma concentrations of carbamazepine-10,11-epoxide, the active metabolite of carbamazepine, resulting in signs of carbamazepine toxicity. Carbamazepine appears to decrease serum felbamate concentrations. The clinical importance of these changes is not established.

RISK FACTORS: No specific risk factors are known.

MECHANISM: The mechanism of the effect of felbamate on carbamazepine is not established, but it may stimulate the metabolism of carbamazepine. Carbamazepine probably stimulates the hepatic metabolism of felbamate.

CLINICAL EVALUATION: The clinical importance of felbamate-induced reductions in serum carbamazepine concentrations is not yet established. Because the decrease in carbamazepine concentrations is offset by an increase in the concentrations of the active metabolite, carbamazepine-10,11-epoxide, an alteration of carbamazepine dose may not be necessary. Carbamazepine-10,11-epoxide contributes significantly to the therapeutic and, possibly, the toxic effects of carbamazepine. Doses of carbamazepine may need to be reduced to prevent toxicity. In a double-blind, placebo-controlled, crossover study in 32 patients, addition of felbamate was associated with a 20% reduction in serum carbamazepine concentrations and a 28% increase in oral carbamazepine clearance.[1] In a report of 19 patients, felbamate was associated with a 17% reduction in serum carbamazepine concentrations and a 33% increase in carbamazepine-epoxide concentrations.[2] Felbamate therapy was initiated in 22 patients receiving carbamazepine monotherapy in a double-blind study. Carbamazepine concentrations fell 25% with the addition of felbamate. In a subset of 4 patients, the ratio of carbamazepine-epoxide to carbamazepine increased from 0.2 to 0.43.[3] In 8 patients receiving carbamazepine or phenytoin (eg, *Dilantin*), the half-life of felbamate was 14 hours, which is shorter than that seen in healthy subjects (20 hours).[4] When phenytoin and then carbamazepine were tapered in 4 patients receiving all 3 drugs (felbamate, carbamazepine, and phenytoin), felbamate clearance decreased and a dose reduction was required.[5]

RELATED DRUGS: No information is available.

MANAGEMENT OPTIONS:

➡ *Monitor.* Serum concentrations of carbamazepine epoxide are not usually clinically available; therefore, monitor patients for signs of carbamazepine toxicity that may occur concurrently with reductions in serum carbamazepine. Symptoms of carbamazepine toxicity include ataxia, blurred vision, dizziness, drowsiness, headache, nausea, nystagmus, and vomiting. It is not clear whether an alteration in felbamate dosage is needed when carbamazepine therapy is initiated or discontinued.

REFERENCES:

1. Graves NM, et al. Effect of felbamate on phenytoin and carbamazepine serum concentrations. *Epilepsia*. 1989;30(2):225-229.

2. Graves NM, et al. The effect of felbamate on the major metabolites of carbamazepine. *Pharmacotherapy*. 1989;9:196.

3. Albani F, et al. Effect of felbamate on plasma levels of carbamazepine and its metabolites. *Epilepsia* 1991;32(1):130-132.

4. Wilensky AJ, et al. Pharmacokinetics of W-554 (ADD 03055) in epileptic patients. *Epilepsia*. 1985;26(6):602-606.

5. Wagner ML, et al. Discontinuation of phenytoin and carbamazepine in patients receiving felbamate. *Epilepsia*. 1991;32(3):398-406.

Carbamazepine (eg, *Tegretol*)

Felodipine

SUMMARY: Felodipine bioavailability may be reduced dramatically in the presence of carbamazepine therapy.

RISK FACTORS: No specific risk factors are known.

MECHANISM: Felodipine undergoes extensive first-pass metabolism by CYP3A4, an isozyme whose activity can be increased substantially by carbamazepine and other enzyme inducers.

CLINICAL EVALUATION: In a parallel study, the area under the serum concentration-time curve (AUC) of felodipine in 10 patients with epilepsy on anticonvulsants (carbamazepine, phenytoin, or phenobarbital) was only 6% of that found in healthy subjects.[1] Although it is not possible to completely separate the effect of carbamazepine from the other anticonvulsants, it is likely that carbamazepine is capable of substantially reducing felodipine serum concentrations. Carbamazepine is known to induce CYP3A4, so it would be expected to reduce the bioavailability and increase the metabolism of substrates for this isozyme such as felodipine. If further study confirms that carbamazepine can reduce felodipine AUC more than 90%, a dramatic reduction in felodipine therapeutic response would be expected.

RELATED DRUGS: Most calcium channel blockers have reduced bioavailability in the presence of enzyme inducers, but felodipine is probably one of the most markedly affected. Some calcium channel blockers (eg, diltiazem [eg, *Cardizem*], verapamil [eg, *Calan*]) can produce carbamazepine toxicity. (Also see Carbamazepine/Diltiazem, Carbamazepine/Verapamil, and Carbamazepine/Nifedipine monographs.)

MANAGEMENT OPTIONS:

➡ *Avoid Unless Benefit Outweighs Risk.* Because it may prove difficult to achieve therapeutic felodipine concentrations in the presence of carbamazepine, even if the felodipine dose is increased, it may be prudent to avoid concurrent use when possible. Keep in mind that the metabolism of most, if not all, calcium channel blockers is enhanced by enzyme inducers, and some calcium channel blockers (eg, diltiazem, verapamil) regularly produce carbamazepine toxicity.

➡️ **Monitor.** If felodipine or another calcium channel blocker is used with carbamazepine, monitor for reduced calcium channel blocker response.

REFERENCES:

1. Capewell S, et al. Gross reduction in felodipine bioavailability in patients taking anticonvulsants. *Br J Clin Pharmacol.* 1987;24:243P.

Carbamazepine (eg, *Tegretol*)

Fexofenadine (eg, *Allegra*)

SUMMARY: Carbamazepine reduces plasma concentrations of fexofenadine; reduced fexofenadine efficacy may occur.

RISK FACTORS: No specific risk factors are known.

MECHANISM: Carbamazepine probably reduces the intestinal absorption of fexofenadine by increasing the activity of intestinal P-glycoprotein.

CLINICAL EVALUATION: In a randomized, crossover study, 12 healthy subjects received a single dose of fexofenadine 60 mg with and without pretreatment with carbamazepine 300 mg/day for 7 days.[1] Carbamazepine was associated with a 43% reduction in fexofenadine area under the plasma concentration-time curve. An interaction of this magnitude is likely to reduce the efficacy of fexofenadine in some patients.

RELATED DRUGS: Other anticonvulsants that also may increase P-glycoprotein activity include barbiturates, oxcarbazepine (eg, *Trileptal*), phenytoin (eg, *Dilantin*), and primidone (eg, *Mysoline*).

MANAGEMENT OPTIONS:

➡️ **Consider Alternative.** Consider using an antihistamine other than fexofenadine, although some other antihistamines may also be substrates for P-glycoprotein, such as cetirizine (eg, *Zyrtec*), desloratadine (*Clarinex*), loratadine (eg, *Claritin*), and possibly others.

➡️ **Monitor.** If carbamazepine or other enzyme inducers are used with fexofenadine, monitor for altered fexofenadine effect if the inducer is started, stopped, or changed in dosage.

REFERENCES:

1. Yamada S, et al. Effects of the P-glycoprotein inducer carbamazepine on fexofenadine pharmacokinetics. *Ther Drug Monit.* 2009;31(6):764-768.

Carbamazepine (eg, *Tegretol*)

Fluconazole (eg, *Diflucan*)

SUMMARY: Fluconazole administration may result in elevated carbamazepine concentrations with signs of toxicity.

RISK FACTORS:

➡️ **Dosage Regimen.** Fluconazole dosages of 200 mg/day and higher have been noted to produce more profound inhibition of CYP3A4.

MECHANISM: Fluconazole inhibits the activity of the enzyme (CYP3A4) that metabolizes carbamazepine.

CLINICAL EVALUATION: A patient with a history of seizures had been taking carbamazepine 400 mg 3 times daily for more than 5 years.[1] His most recent carbamazepine concentration was 11.1 mcg/mL. Following the development of a skin rash thought to be candidiasis, he was started on fluconazole 150 mg/day, ciprofloxacin (eg, *Cipro*) 250 mg twice daily, and methylprednisolone (eg, *Medrol*) 60 mg intravenously followed by oral steroid in tapering doses. The ciprofloxacin was stopped after 2 days of therapy. Three days after starting therapy, he was lethargic and had a carbamazepine concentration of 24.5 mcg/mL. Fluconazole was discontinued and carbamazepine was withheld for 1 day. This therapy resulted in a gradual resolution of symptoms and a reduction in carbamazepine concentration to 12.4 mcg/mL. The patient's carbamazepine concentration was 11.7 mcg/mL 4 days after restarting carbamazepine 400 mg 3 times daily. While fluconazole would be likely to affect carbamazepine clearance, an additional effect of methylprednisolone (perhaps competitive CYP3A4 inhibition) cannot be ruled out. Carbamazepine's autoinduction of its metabolism by CYP3A4 may make it particularly sensitive to CYP3A4 inhibitors.

RELATED DRUGS: Ketoconazole (eg, *Nizoral*) and itraconazole (eg, *Sporanox*) would be expected to inhibit carbamazepine metabolism. Fluconazole is known to inhibit the metabolism of phenytoin (eg, *Dilantin*), particularly when fluconazole dosages exceed 200 mg/day.

MANAGEMENT OPTIONS:

➡ ***Consider Alternative.*** Terbinafine (eg, *Lamisil*) is an antifungal agent that does not affect the activity of CYP3A4. Depending on the indication for carbamazepine, an alternative, such as gabapentin (eg, *Neurontin*), could be considered.

➡ ***Monitor.*** Carefully monitor patients stabilized on carbamazepine for increased carbamazepine concentrations and adverse reactions (eg, sedation, lethargy) if fluconazole is added to their therapy.

REFERENCES:
    1. Nair DR, et al. Potential fluconazole-induced toxicity. *Ann Phamacother*. 1999;33(7-8):790-792.

Carbamazepine (eg, *Tegretol*)

Fluoxetine (*Prozac*)

SUMMARY: Case reports describe carbamazepine toxicity, parkinsonism, and serotonin syndrome with concurrent use of fluoxetine, but data from pharmacokinetic studies are conflicting; one study found increased carbamazepine plasma concentrations, and another did not.

RISK FACTORS: No specific risk factors are known.

MECHANISM: Fluoxetine may inhibit the hepatic metabolism of carbamazepine, but the formation of carbamazepine epoxide is not inhibited.[6] Increases in carbamazepine epoxide concentrations may contribute to signs of carbamazepine toxicity, but more study is needed to confirm this effect.

CLINICAL EVALUATION: A 55-year-old woman receiving 1000 mg/day of carbamazepine developed symptoms of carbamazepine toxicity (diplopia, blurred vision, tremor, vertigo) and a 33% increase in carbamazepine plasma concentration one week after starting fluoxetine 20 mg/day.[1] The symptoms resolved with a reduction in the carbamazepine dose. In a similar case, a 45-year-old woman developed a worsening of multiple sclerosis symptoms (including ataxia) and new symptoms of carbamazepine toxicity (nausea, vomiting, vertigo, and tinnitus) 10 days after starting 20 mg/day of fluoxetine.[1] The carbamazepine plasma concentration increased 63%. Two other patients stabilized on carbamazepine developed parkinsonism 3 and 9 days after starting fluoxetine 20 mg/day.[2] However, neither of these patients developed increased serum carbamazepine concentrations. Another patient developed a "toxic serotonin syndrome" (eg, shivering, agitation, incoordination, hyperreflexia, myoclonus) after fluoxetine 20 mg/day was added to her carbamazepine therapy (200 mg/day).[3]

Six healthy subjects received carbamazepine 400 mg/day for 28 days, with fluoxetine 20 mg/day added for the last 7 days.[4] Fluoxetine increased the area under the plasma carbamazepine concentration-time curve 27% and reduced carbamazepine intrinsic clearance 46%. However, in another study of 8 patients stabilized on carbamazepine 800 to 1600 mg/day, the addition of fluoxetine 20 mg/day for 3 weeks did not affect the steady-state plasma concentrations of carbamazepine or its epoxide metabolite.[5] The reasons for the disparate results are not clear. It is possible that the larger doses of carbamazepine in the latter study enhanced the metabolism of fluoxetine, thus mitigating this drug interaction. More study is needed to resolve this issue.

RELATED DRUGS: Fluvoxamine (*Luvox*) inhibits CYP3A4 and would be expected to inhibit carbamazepine metabolism. The effect of paroxetine (*Paxil*) and sertraline (*Zoloft*) on CYP3A4 is not established (but is being studied).

MANAGEMENT OPTIONS:

➡ *Monitor.* Until additional information is available to resolve this interaction, monitor for altered carbamazepine response if fluoxetine is initiated, discontinued, or changed in dosage. Also be alert for evidence of parkinsonism or a serotonin syndrome in patients receiving the combination.

REFERENCES:

1. Pearson HJ. Interaction of fluoxetine with carbamazepine. *J Clin Psychiatry*. 1990;51:126.
2. Gernaat HBPE, et al. Fluoxetine and parkinsonism in patients taking carbamazepine. *Am J Psychiatry*. 1991;148:1604.
3. Dursun SM, et al. Toxic serotonin syndrome after fluoxetine plus carbamazepine. *Lancet*. 1993;342:442.
4. Grimsley SR, et al. Increased carbamazepine plasma concentrations after fluoxetine coadministration. *Clin Pharmacol Ther*. 1991;50:10.
5. Spina E, et al. Carbamazepine coadministration with fluoxetine or fluvoxamine. *Ther Drug Monit*. 1993;15:247.
6. Gidal BE, et al. Evaluation of the effect of fluoxetine on the formation of carbamazepine epoxide. *Ther Drug Monit*. 1993;15:405.

Carbamazepine (eg, *Tegretol*)

Fluvoxamine (*Luvox*)

SUMMARY: Case reports suggest that fluvoxamine can increase plasma carbamazepine concentrations to toxic levels, while one study in epileptic patients found no effect of fluvoxamine on carbamazepine. More study is needed to resolve these conflicting results.

RISK FACTORS: No specific risk factors are known.

MECHANISM: Unknown. It has been proposed that fluvoxamine inhibits the hepatic metabolism of carbamazepine, but confirmation is needed.

CLINICAL EVALUATION: Three patients stabilized on carbamazepine manifested increased carbamazepine plasma concentrations and symptoms of carbamazepine toxicity when fluvoxamine was added to their therapy.[1] In one case there was a positive rechallenge and dechallenge, supporting the authors' contention that the fluvoxamine was responsible for the carbamazepine toxicity. However, in a subsequent study of 7 patients stabilized on carbamazepine 800 to 1600 mg/day, the addition of fluvoxamine 100 mg/day for 3 weeks did not affect carbamazepine steady-state plasma concentrations.[2] The reasons for the disparate results are not immediately clear. In both reports fluvoxamine was started in patients stabilized on long-term carbamazepine therapy, and the doses of the drugs were similar. It is possible that the carbamazepine toxicity observed in the first report was because of factors other than fluvoxamine, but it is also possible that the interaction occurs only in certain predisposed individuals. Clearly, additional study is needed to resolve this issue.

RELATED DRUGS: Isolated reports suggest that fluoxetine (*Prozac*) and sertraline (*Zoloft*) may increase carbamazepine serum concentrations, but a causal relationship was not established. Preliminary evidence suggests that paroxetine (*Paxil*) does not affect carbamazepine plasma concentrations, but more study is needed.

MANAGEMENT OPTIONS:

➡ *Monitor.* Until additional information is available to resolve this interaction, monitor for altered carbamazepine response if fluvoxamine is initiated, discontinued, or changed in dosage.

REFERENCES:

1. Fritze J, et al. Interaction between carbamazepine and fluvoxamine. *Acta Psychiatr Scand.* 1991;84:583.
2. Spina E, et al. Carbamazepine coadministration with fluoxetine of fluvoxamine. *Ther Drug Monit.* 1993;15:247.

Carbamazepine (eg, *Tegretol*)

Grapefruit Juice

SUMMARY: Grapefruit juice may increase carbamazepine plasma concentrations; avoid grapefruit juice or monitor for evidence of carbamazepine toxicity.

RISK FACTORS: No specific risk factors are known.

MECHANISM: Grapefruit juice probably inhibits the CYP3A4 metabolism of carbamazepine in the small intestine.

CLINICAL EVALUATION: A 58-year-old man on carbamazepine 1000 mg/day developed carbamazepine toxicity (eg, visual disturbances) and toxic carbamazepine levels after starting to eat 1 whole yellow grapefruit a day.[1] Because the patient would not stop the grapefruit, the carbamazepine dose was lowered to 800 mg/day with good results. Previous pharmacokinetic study in 10 epileptic patients showed increased carbamazepine steady-state plasma concentrations with concurrent use of grapefruit juice.[2]

RELATED DRUGS: No information is available.

MANAGEMENT OPTIONS:

➡ *Consider Alternative.* Orange juice is unlikely to affect the pharmacokinetics of carbamazepine.

➡ *Monitor.* If grapefruit juice is taken concurrently with carbamazepine, monitor for evidence of carbamazepine toxicity (eg, nausea, vomiting, dizziness, drowsiness, headache, diplopia, confusion). Adjust carbamazepine dosage as needed.

REFERENCES:

1. Bonin B, et al. Effect of grapefruit intake on carbamazepine bioavailability: a case report. *Thérapie.* 2001;56:69-71.

2. Garg SK, et al. Effect of grapefruit juice on carbamazepine bioavailability in patients with epilepsy. *Clin Pharmacol Ther.* 1998;64:286-288.

Carbamazepine (eg, *Tegretol*)

Haloperidol (eg, *Haldol*)

SUMMARY: Carbamazepine appears to decrease serum haloperidol concentrations and inhibit the response to haloperidol in some patients.

RISK FACTORS: No specific risk factors are known.

MECHANISM: Carbamazepine probably stimulates the hepatic metabolism of haloperidol.

CLINICAL EVALUATION: Seven psychotic men maintained on stable doses of haloperidol (mean dose, 19.2 mg/day) were given carbamazepine (mean dose, 614 mg/day).[1] Plasma haloperidol concentrations measured 9 days or more after carbamazepine concentrations reached steady state were reduced by a mean of 60%. The psychotic symptoms in 3 patients were exacerbated in association with the lowered haloperidol concentrations, and in 2 patients the deterioration was marked. In another study, carbamazepine reduced haloperidol serum concentrations approximately 50% in 6 patients with schizophrenia, but a worsening of symptoms was seen in only 1 patient.[6] Two other patients improved when carbamazepine was added, a finding which might be related to a therapeutic response to carbamazepine or a reduction of excessive haloperidol serum concentrations. In two other studies, haloperidol serum concentrations were reduced in association with carbamazepine therapy;[2,3] no effect was noted in 2 other studies.[4,5] Although the bulk of the evidence indicates that haloperidol plasma concentrations are reduced by carbamazepine therapy, only some patients manifest a clinically significant deterioration.

RELATED DRUGS: The effect of carbamazepine on other butyrophenones is not established.

MANAGEMENT OPTIONS:

➡ *Monitor.* Be alert for evidence of reduced haloperidol effect if carbamazepine is given concurrently.

REFERENCES:

1. Arana GW, et al. Does carbamazepine-induced reduction of plasma haloperidol levels worsen psychotic symptoms? *Am J Psychiatry.* 1986;143:650.

2. Jann MW, et al. Effects of carbamazepine on plasma haloperidol levels. *J Clin Psychopharmacol.* 1985;5:106.

3. Kidron R, et al. Carbamazepine-induced reduction of blood levels of haloperidol in chronic schizophrenia. *Biol Psychiatry*. 1985;20:219.

4. Forsman A, et al. Applied pharmacokinetics of haloperidol in man. *Curr Ther Res Clin Exp*. 1977;21:396.

5. Klein E, et al. Carbamazepine and haloperidol vs. placebo and haloperidol in excited psychoses; a controlled study. *Arch Gen Psychiatry*. 1984;41:165.

6. Kahn EM, et al. Change in haloperidol level due to carbamazepine: a complicating factor in combined medication for schizophrenia. *J Clin Psychopharmacol*. 1990;10:54.

Carbamazepine (eg, *Tegretol*)

Imipramine (eg, *Tofranil*)

SUMMARY: Preliminary evidence suggests that carbamazepine reduces serum concentrations of imipramine; other cyclic antidepressants probably are affected similarly.

RISK FACTORS: No specific risk factors are known.

MECHANISM: Carbamazepine probably enhances the hepatic microsomal metabolism of cyclic antidepressants. Carbamazepine is a known enzyme inducer, and the metabolism of cyclic antidepressants is enhanced by enzyme inducers such as barbiturates.[1]

CLINICAL EVALUATION: In a retrospective study of 36 children with attention deficit hyperactivity disorder, half of the children received imipramine alone and the other half received imipramine plus chronic carbamazepine.[2] The plasma concentrations of imipramine were similar in the 2 groups, but the mean imipramine dosage in the group receiving imipramine plus carbamazepine was about twice that of the group receiving imipramine alone. Moreover, in 12 children matched for imipramine dosage, the total plasma concentration of imipramine plus its metabolite desipramine (eg, *Norpramin*) in children receiving carbamazepine was approximately 50% of that observed in children receiving imipramine alone. Although this study was retrospective, the results are consistent with the known properties of both drugs. The clinical significance of a decreased imipramine concentration in this interaction is unknown because many of the cyclic antidepressants have one or more active metabolite(s). In the case of imipramine, not only is desipramine active, so are the 2 major hydroxylated metabolites.[3]

RELATED DRUGS: Because cyclic antidepressants are metabolized primarily by the liver, one would expect most of them to be affected by carbamazepine. In one retrospective analysis, patients on concurrent carbamazepine therapy had significantly lower concentration/dose ratios of amitriptyline (eg, *Elavil*) (n = 10) and nortriptyline (eg, *Pamelor*) (n = 8) when compared with patients on monotherapy.[5] In addition, carbamazepine increased the oral clearance of single doses of desipramine 30% in 6 normal volunteers.[4] The effect of carbamazepine on other cyclic antidepressants is not known, but because most of them are extensively metabolized by the liver, they probably would also be affected by carbamazepine therapy.

MANAGEMENT OPTIONS:

➡️ *Monitor.* Patients on chronic carbamazepine therapy may require larger than expected doses of cyclic and related antidepressants. Monitor patients for altered response to these antidepressants if carbamazepine therapy is started or stopped.

REFERENCES:

1. Moody JP, et al. Pharmacokinetic aspects of protriptyline plasma levels. *Eur J Clin Pharmacol.* 1977;11:51.

2. Brown CS, et al. Possible influence of carbamazepine on plasma imipramine concentration in children with attention-deficit hyperactivity disorder. *J Clin Psychopharmacol.* 1990;10:359.

3. De La Fuente JM. Carbamazepine-induced low plasma levels of tricyclic antidepressants. *J Clin Psychopharmacol.* 1991;12:67.

4. Spina E, et al. The effect of carbamazepine on the 2-hydroxylation of desipramine. *Psychopharmacology.* 1995;117:413.

5. Jerling M, et al. The use of therapeutic drug monitoring data to document kinetic drug interactions: an example with amitriptyline and nortriptyline. *Ther Drug Monit.* 1994;16:1.

 Carbamazepine (eg, *Tegretol*)

Irinotecan

SUMMARY: Irinotecan may exhibit reduced efficacy in patients receiving carbamazepine or other enzyme-inducing anticonvulsants; increased irinotecan dosage may be required.

RISK FACTORS: No specific risk factors are known.

MECHANISM: Carbamazepine probably enhances the metabolism of irinotecan to inactive metabolites, but its effects on ABC transporters also may be involved.

CLINICAL EVALUATION: In a study of 102 patients given irinotecan, some were taking concurrent enzyme-inducing anticonvulsants, such as carbamazepine, and others were not.[1] Those taking anticonvulsants had substantially lower plasma concentrations of irinotecan and SN-38. Given the magnitude of the reduction in irinotecan and SN-38 concentrations, expect a reduction in the efficacy of irinotecan in such patients.

RELATED DRUGS: Enzyme-inducing anticonvulsants other than carbamazepine, such as barbiturates, oxcarbazepine (*Trileptal*), phenytoin, and primidone, also may reduce irinotecan effect.

MANAGEMENT OPTIONS:

➡️ *Circumvent/Minimize.* Patients receiving carbamazepine or other enzyme-inducing anticonvulsants may require larger doses of irinotecan. Check the latest prescribing information before starting irinotecan therapy in patients on enzyme-inducing anticonvulsants.

➡️ *Monitor.* Monitor for altered irinotecan response if enzyme-inducing anticonvulsants are given concurrently; where available, pharmacokinetic monitoring may be useful.

REFERENCES:

1. Kuhn JG. Influence of anticonvulsants on the metabolism and elimination of irinotecan. *Oncology.* 2002;16:(8 suppl 7):33-40.

Carbamazepine (eg, *Tegretol*)

Isoniazid (INH; eg, *Nydrazid*)

SUMMARY: Isoniazid appears to increase serum carbamazepine concentrations in most patients; symptoms of carbamazepine toxicity may occur. The interaction seems most likely to occur with INH doses of at least 200 mg/day, with toxicity occurring within day 1 or 2 of INH therapy.

RISK FACTORS:

➥ **Dosage Regimen.** INH doses higher than 200 mg/day can increase the risk of interaction.

MECHANISM: INH probably inhibits carbamazepine metabolism. Carbamazepine purportedly stimulates the production of hepatotoxic isoniazid metabolites.

CLINICAL EVALUATION: In several studies, patients taking carbamazepine developed symptoms of carbamazepine toxicity (eg, ataxia, disorientation, drowsiness, lethargy) following administration of INH.[1-3] These symptoms subsided when the carbamazepine dose was reduced. Study in 1 patient indicated that INH 300 mg/day reduced carbamazepine clearance 45%, while a daily dose of INH 150 mg had little effect.

RELATED DRUGS: No information is available.

MANAGEMENT OPTIONS:

➥ **Monitor.** Isoniazid is likely to reduce the dosage requirements for carbamazepine in a majority of patients. Watch for symptoms of carbamazepine toxicity (ataxia, blurred vision, dizziness, drowsiness, headache, nausea, nystagmus, vomiting), and monitor serum carbamazepine concentrations if possible. Monitor for evidence of reduced serum carbamazepine concentrations when INH is discontinued or dosage is reduced.

REFERENCES:

1. Block SH. Carbamazepine-isoniazid interaction. *Pediatrics.* 1982;69:494-495.
2. Valsalan VC, et al. Carbamazepine intoxication caused by interaction with isoniazid. *Br Med J.* 1982;285:261-262.
3. Wright JM, et al. Isoniazid-induced carbamazepine toxicity and vice versa: a double drug interaction. *N Engl J Med.* 1982;307:1325.

Carbamazepine (eg, *Tegretol*)

Isotretinoin (eg, *Accutane*)

SUMMARY: In 1 patient, isotretinoin decreased the area under the concentration-time curve (AUC) of carbamazepine and carbamazepine epoxide, the active metabolite of carbamazepine. The clinical importance of this effect is unknown.

RISK FACTORS: No specific risk factors are known.

MECHANISM: Isotretinoin may decrease the bioavailability or increase the clearance of carbamazepine.

CLINICAL EVALUATION: In 1 patient, a 10% decrease in the AUC of carbamazepine was observed after a 2-week course of isotretinoin 0.5 mg/kg/day. After an additional 4 weeks of therapy (1 mg/kg/day), a 24% decrease in the AUC was observed. The

AUC of the active metabolite of carbamazepine, carbamazepine epoxide, also decreased 21% and 44% after the 0.5 and 1 mg/kg/day isotretinoin doses, respectively.[1]

RELATED DRUGS: No information is available.

MANAGEMENT OPTIONS:

➡ *Monitor.* Be alert for evidence of a reduced response to carbamazepine if isotretinoin is given concurrently. Until the clinical significance of this interaction is determined, monitor plasma concentrations of carbamazepine more frequently when the 2 drugs are given concurrently.

REFERENCES:

1. Marsden JR. Effect of isotretinoin on carbamazepine pharmacokinetics. *Br J Dermatol*. 1988;119:403-404.

Carbamazepine (eg, *Tegretol*)

Ketoconazole (eg, *Nizoral*)

SUMMARY: The administration of ketoconazole to patients stabilized on carbamazepine may increase carbamazepine concentrations; toxicity could result.

RISK FACTORS: No specific risk factors are known.

MECHANISM: Ketoconazole is known to decrease the activity of 1 of the enzymes (CYP3A4) thought to be primarily responsible for the metabolism of carbamazepine.

CLINICAL EVALUATION: Eight patients with epilepsy were stabilized on carbamazepine at doses ranging from 400 to 800 mg/day. Each patient received a 10-day course of ketoconazole 200 mg/day. Mean plasma carbamazepine concentrations increased from 5.6 mcg/mL prior to the addition of ketoconazole to 7.2 mcg/mL after 10 days of ketoconazole treatment. Carbamazepine concentrations returned to pre-ketoconazole levels after the discontinuation of ketoconazole. No significant changes in carbamazepine epoxide were noted at any time during or after ketoconazole coadministration. This modest increase in carbamazepine concentrations may be partially explained by the low concentrations of ketoconazole (mean, 1 mcg/mL; range, 0.6 to 1.3 mcg/mL) observed in patient samples obtained 1 hour after ketoconazole administration. Because carbamazepine is known to induce the enzyme that metabolizes ketoconazole (CYP3A4), the effect of adding ketoconazole to patients stabilized on carbamazepine may be tempered by a carbamazepine-induced reduction in ketoconazole plasma concentrations.

RELATED DRUGS: Other antifungal agents that are known to inhibit CYP3A4 (eg, fluconazole [eg, *Diflucan*], itraconazole [eg, *Sporanox*]) also would be expected to increase carbamazepine concentrations.

MANAGEMENT OPTIONS:

➡ *Consider Alternative.* Consider the use of an alternative antifungal agent such as terbinafine (*Lamisil*) that does not inhibit CYP3A4 activity.

➡ *Circumvent/Minimize.* Adjust the carbamazepine dosage to maintain therapeutic concentrations when ketoconazole is coadministered.

➡ *Monitor.* Monitor patients receiving carbamazepine and ketoconazole for increased carbamazepine concentrations and possible toxicity. Consider the potential for reduced ketoconazole efficacy.

REFERENCES:

1. Spina E, et al. Elevation of plasma carbamazepine concentrations by ketoconazole in patients with epilepsy. *Ther Drug Monit.* 1997;19:535-538.

Carbamazepine (eg, *Tegretol*)

Lamotrigine (eg, *Lamictal*)

SUMMARY: Lamotrigine may increase the carbamazepine epoxide to carbamazepine ratio, resulting in signs of carbamazepine toxicity. Carbamazepine reduces the concentrations of lamotrigine. The clinical importance of these changes in not established.

RISK FACTORS: No specific risk factors are known.

MECHANISM: The mechanism of the effect of lamotrigine on the carbamazepine epoxide to carbamazepine ratio is not established. Carbamazepine stimulates the hepatic metabolism of lamotrigine.

CLINICAL EVALUATION: Case reports have suggested that lamotrigine increases the carbamazepine epoxide to carbamazepine ratio, resulting in signs of carbamazepine toxicity (eg, dizziness, nausea, diplopia).[1,2] This suggests that lamotrigine may decrease the metabolic disposition of carbamazepine epoxide. However, in a limited single-dose pharmacokinetic study of carbamazepine epoxide in 10 controls and 10 patients taking lamotrigine, similar oral clearance and elimination half-lives of the epoxide were found in the 2 groups.[3] Carbamazepine stimulates the metabolism of lamotrigine, resulting in reductions in the elimination half-life of lamotrigine in a dose-dependent manner.[4]

The clinical importance of the effect of lamotrigine on serum concentrations of carbamazepine and carbamazepine epoxide is not yet established. The carbamazepine epoxide contributes significantly to the therapeutic and, possibly, the toxic effects of carbamazepine.

RELATED DRUGS: No information is available.

MANAGEMENT OPTIONS:

➡ *Monitor.* Serum concentrations of carbamazepine epoxide usually are not clinically available; therefore, patients need to be monitored for signs of carbamazepine toxicity that may occur concurrently with reductions in serum carbamazepine. Symptoms of carbamazepine toxicity include drowsiness, dizziness, nausea, vomiting, ataxia, headache, nystagmus, and blurred vision. Doses of carbamazepine may need to be reduced. It is not clear whether an alteration in lamotrigine dosage is needed when carbamazepine therapy is initiated or discontinued.

REFERENCES:

1. Warner T, et al. Lamotrigine-induced carbamazepine toxicity: an interaction with carbamazepine-10,11-epoxide. *Epilepsy Res.* 1992;11(2):147-150.

2. Graves N, et al. Effect of lamotrigine on the carbamazepine epoxide concentrations. *Epilepsia.* 1991,32(suppl 3):13.

3. Pisani F, et al. Single-dose pharmacokinetics of carbamazepine-10,11-epoxide in patients on lamotrigine monotherapy. *Epilepsy Res.* 1994;19(3):245-248.
4. Jawad S, et al. Lamotrigine: single-dose pharmacokinetics and initial 1 week experience in refractory epilepsy. *Epilepsy Res.* 1987;1(3):194-201.

Carbamazepine (eg, *Tegretol*)

Lapatinib (*Tykerb*)

SUMMARY: Coadministration of carbamazepine markedly decreases the plasma concentration of lapatinib; some loss of efficacy is expected.

RISK FACTORS: No specific risk factors are known.

MECHANISM: Carbamazepine induces the enzyme (CYP3A4) known to primarily metabolize lapatinib. Carbamazepine also induces P-glycoprotein, a transporter of lapatinib. Both of these mechanisms may lead to reduced lapatinib plasma concentrations.

CLINICAL EVALUATION: Twenty-four healthy subjects received a single dose of lapatinib 250 mg alone or following a 21-day escalating dose of carbamazepine (200 mg twice a day for the last 17 days).[1] Following carbamazepine administration, the mean area under the concentration-time curve of lapatinib was decreased more than 70%, while its half-life remained unchanged. Because lapatinib has been reported to inhibit its own metabolism, long-term lapatinib dosing may alter the magnitude of this interaction.

RELATED DRUGS: Dasatinib (*Sprycel*), erlotinib (*Tarceva*), gefitinib (*Iressa*), imatinib (*Gleevec*), nilotinib (*Tasigna*), pazopanib (*Votrient*), sorafenib (*Nexavar*), and sunitinib (*Sutent*) may be affected in a similar manner. Other enzyme-inducing anticonvulsants, such as phenobarbital, phenytoin (eg, *Dilantin*), primidone (eg, *Mysoline*), and oxcarbazepine (eg, *Trileptal*), are also expected to reduce lapatinib plasma concentrations.

MANAGEMENT OPTIONS:
➡ **Consider Alternative.** Consider valproic acid (eg, *Depakote*) or other noninducing anticonvulsants as an alternative.
➡ **Monitor.** Observe patients taking lapatinib who require carbamazepine for reduced lapatinib efficacy.

REFERENCES:
1. Smith DA, et al. Effects of ketoconazole and carbamazepine on lapatinib pharmacokinetics in healthy subjects. *Br J Clin Pharmacol.* 2009;67(4):421-426.

Carbamazepine (eg, *Tegretol*)

Lithium (eg, *Lithobid*)

SUMMARY: Several cases of neurotoxicity (in the absence of toxic serum lithium concentrations) have been reported in patients receiving lithium and carbamazepine, but the combination has been used to advantage in some manic patients. Lithium reverses carbamazepine-induced leukopenia, but additive antithyroidal effects can occur.

RISK FACTORS: No specific risk factors are known.

MECHANISM: Not established.

CLINICAL EVALUATION: Five of 10 patients on long-term lithium therapy developed ataxia, dizziness, confusion, and restlessness within a few days after starting carbamazepine 300 to 600 mg/day.[1] Similar symptoms occurred in another patient taking the combination of lithium and carbamazepine but not with either drug alone.[2] The combination of lithium and carbamazepine improved acute manic symptoms in 3 patients more than either drug alone.[3] Lithium plus carbamazepine was used to apparent advantage in another patient with rapid-cycling bipolar affective disorder.[4] Carbamazepine possibly increases the effect of lithium, producing toxicity in some patients and improved response in others. In 23 patients with affective disorders, the addition of lithium to carbamazepine resulted in a reversal, past baseline, of carbamazepine-induced neutropenia. The increase in white blood cells was predominantly comprised of neutrophils. The combination also resulted in greater decreases in thyroxine (T_4) and free T_4 than were observed with carbamazepine alone.[5]

RELATED DRUGS: No information is available.

MANAGEMENT OPTIONS:

➡ *Monitor.* Be alert for evidence of lithium toxicity when carbamazepine is given concurrently. Because the carbamazepine might increase the effect of lithium without increasing plasma lithium concentrations, it is not yet established whether plasma lithium concentrations are useful in monitoring this interaction.

REFERENCES:

1. Ghose K. Effect of carbamazepine in polyuria associated with lithium therapy. *Pharmakopsychiatr Neuropsychopharmakol.* 1978;11(5):241-245.
2. Chaudhry RP, et al. Lithium and carbamazepine interaction: possible neurotoxicity. *J Clin Psychiatry.* 1983;44(1):30-31.
3. Lipinski JF, et al. Possible synergistic action between carbamazepine and lithium carbonate in the treatment of three acutely manic patients. *Am J Psychiatry.* 1982;139(7):948-949.
4. Laird KL, et al. The use of carbamazepine and lithium in controlling a case of chronic rapid cycling. *Pharmacotherapy.* 1987;7(4):130-132.
5. Kramlinger KG, et al. Addition of lithium carbonate to carbamazepine: hematological and thyroid effects. *Am J Psychiatry.* 1990;147(5):615-620.

Carbamazepine (eg, *Tegretol*)

Mebendazole (eg, *Vermox*)

SUMMARY: Carbamazepine decreases plasma mebendazole concentrations. This may be most important when large oral doses of mebendazole are used for the treatment of *Echinococcus multilocularis* or *Echinococcus granulosus* (hydatid disease).

RISK FACTORS: No specific risk factors are known.

MECHANISM: Mebendazole appears to undergo metabolism by hepatic microsomal enzymes.[2,3] Carbamazepine, a known hepatic microsomal enzyme inducer, probably enhances the metabolism of mebendazole. Other enzyme-inducing agents would be expected to produce a similar effect.

CLINICAL EVALUATION: When mebendazole is used to treat intestinal helminths, such as whipworms or hookworms, the rate of hepatic mebendazole metabolism probably has little bearing on the therapeutic outcome. However, when mebendazole is used to treat tissue-dwelling organisms, such as those causing hydatid disease, lowered plasma mebendazole levels caused by enzyme induction could impair the therapeutic response. In a group of patients receiving mebendazole in addition to several other drugs, those patients on carbamazepine or phenytoin (eg, *Dilantin*) had considerably lower plasma concentrations of mebendazole than those patients not receiving enzyme inducers.[1] Several of these patients who could not be adequately treated with mebendazole while on carbamazepine or phenytoin were switched to valproic acid (eg, *Depakene*), resulting in a therapeutically significant increase in plasma mebendazole concentrations in each case.

RELATED DRUGS: Theoretically, carbamazepine could affect thiabendazole (*Mintezol*) in a similar manner.

MANAGEMENT OPTIONS:

➡ *Consider Alternative.* No special precautions appear necessary during cotherapy with carbamazepine in patients receiving mebendazole to treat intestinal helminths. However, in patients receiving mebendazole for tissue-dwelling organisms, avoid enzyme-inducing drugs if possible. If carbamazepine is being used for seizures in such patients, valproic acid could be considered as an alternative to carbamazepine, because it does not appear to reduce plasma mebendazole concentrations.

➡ *Monitor.* If carbamazepine is used with mebendazole (for tissue-dwelling organisms), monitor for reduced mebendazole effect.

REFERENCES:
1. Luder PJ, et al. Treatment of hydatid disease with high oral doses of mebendazole. Long-term follow-up of plasma mebendazole levels and drug interactions. *Eur J Clin Pharmacol.* 1986;31:443.
2. Witassek F, et al. Chemotherapy of larval echinococcus with mebendazole: microsomal liver function and cholestasis as determinants of plasma drug level. *Eur J Clin Pharmacol.* 1983;25:85.
3. Bekhti A, et al. A correlation between serum mebendazole concentrations and the aminopyrine breath test. Implications in the treatment of hydatid disease. *Br J Clin Pharmacol* 1986;21:223.

Carbamazepine (eg, *Tegretol*)

Methadone (eg, *Dolophine*)

SUMMARY: Carbamazepine may decrease serum methadone concentrations, thereby increasing symptoms associated with narcotic withdrawal.

RISK FACTORS: No specific risk factors are known.

MECHANISM: Not established. Carbamazepine is a known enzyme inducer and probably enhances the hepatic metabolism of methadone.

CLINICAL EVALUATION: In 37 patients receiving methadone maintenance, trough serum methadone concentrations were considerably lower in the 10 patients who were receiving enzyme-inducing drugs such as barbiturates (5 patients), phenytoin (4 patients), or carbamazepine (1 patient).[1] Low serum methadone concentrations tend to be associated with an increased likelihood of withdrawal symptoms.

RELATED DRUGS: Other enzyme-inducing drugs (eg, barbiturates, phenytoin [eg, *Dilantin*]) may interact similarly.

MANAGEMENT OPTIONS:

➡ *Monitor.* Patients receiving enzyme inducers such as carbamazepine may require larger doses of methadone than patients who are not on enzyme inducers.

Observe for symptoms of methadone withdrawal such as lacrimation, rhinorrhea, sweating, restlessness, insomnia, and piloerection.

REFERENCES:

1. Bell J, et al. The use of serum methadone levels in patients receiving methadone maintenance. *Clin Pharmacol Ther.* 1988;43:623.

Carbamazepine (eg, *Tegretol*)
Methylphenidate (eg, *Ritalin*)

SUMMARY: Isolated cases suggest that carbamazepine may reduce methylphenidate's effect in attention deficit disorders.

RISK FACTORS: No specific risk factors are known.

MECHANISM: Not established. Carbamazepine may increase the hepatic metabolism of methylphenidate.

CLINICAL EVALUATION: A 7-year-old boy with attention deficit disorder (ADD) was receiving carbamazepine 1000 mg/day for grand mal epilepsy.[1] His ADD failed to respond to methylphenidate 20 mg every 4 hours and thiothixene (eg, *Navane*) 10 mg/day; serum concentrations of both drugs were found to be undetectable. His methylphenidate was increased to 30 mg every 4 hours and thiothixene was increased to 20 mg/day without any benefit or toxicity. A 13-year-old girl with attention deficit hyperactivity disorder (ADHD) on methylphenidate 20 mg 3 times a day was started on carbamazepine 200 mg/day.[2] Her methylphenidate serum concentrations progressively decreased as the carbamazepine dose was titrated upward, accompanied by an increase in her ADHD symptoms. She eventually required an increase in her methylphenidate dose to 60 mg 3 times a day to achieve the same benefit as before administration of carbamazepine.

RELATED DRUGS: No information is available.

MANAGEMENT OPTIONS:

➡ *Monitor.* Watch for evidence of reduced methylphenidate response if carbamazepine is given concurrently. Substantially increasing the methylphenidate dose to overcome the interaction may be necessary.

REFERENCES:

1. Behar D, et al. Extreme reduction of methylphenidate levels by carbamazepine. *J Am Acad Child Adolesc Psychiatry.* 1998;37:1128.

2. Schaller JL, et al. Carbamazepine and methylphenidate in ADHD. *J Am Acad Child Adolesc Psychiatry.* 1999;38:112.

Carbamazepine (eg, *Tegretol*)
Metronidazole (eg, *Flagyl*)

SUMMARY: Metronidazole may increase carbamazepine plasma concentrations resulting in symptoms of toxicity (eg, dizziness, nausea, diplopia).

RISK FACTORS: No specific risk factors are known.

MECHANISM: Not established. Metronidazole is known to inhibit the metabolism of some drugs; thus, it may inhibit the metabolism of carbamazepine.

CLINICAL EVALUATION: A patient taking 1000 mg/day of carbamazepine had a plasma concentration of 9 mcg/ml.[1] Her plasma carbamazepine concentration increased to 14.3 mcg/ml during the administration of metronidazole. Four days after initiation of the metronidazole, the patient reported dizziness, diplopia, and nausea. A month later (although not stated, apparently after stopping the metronidazole), her carbamazepine concentration on 1000 mg/day was 7.1 mcg/ml.

RELATED DRUGS: No information is available.

MANAGEMENT OPTIONS:

➡ **Monitor.** Until more definitive studies of this interaction are available, monitor patients receiving carbamazepine for altered response and plasma concentrations if metronidazole therapy is initiated or discontinued.

REFERENCES:
1. Patterson BD. Possible interaction between metronidazole and carbamazepine. *Ann Pharmacother.* 1994;28:1303.

Carbamazepine (eg, *Tegretol*)

Midazolam (*Versed*)

SUMMARY: Carbamazepine markedly reduces the effect of oral midazolam, but parenteral midazolam is likely to be less affected.

RISK FACTORS:

➡ **Route of Administration.** Because the majority of the interaction is likely caused by increased presystemic metabolism of oral midazolam by the gut wall and liver, parenteral midazolam is likely to be much less affected.

MECHANISM: Carbamazepine appears to enhance the presystemic metabolism of oral midazolam in the gut wall and liver by CYP3A4, thus reducing midazolam bioavailability. The subsequent hepatic metabolism of midazolam by CYP3A4 also may be reduced.

CLINICAL EVALUATION: The pharmacokinetics and pharmacodynamics of a single 15 mg oral dose of midazolam were compared in patients receiving carbamazepine 700 to 900 mg/day or phenytoin (eg, *Dilantin*) vs healthy subjects not receiving enzyme inducers.[1] The midazolam area under the plasma concentration-time curve was dramatically lower in those receiving carbamazepine or phenytoin (7% of value in control subjects); midazolam half-life also was substantially lower. The pharmacodynamic response to midazolam was markedly reduced as measured by various objective and subjective methods. Nonetheless, if parenteral midazolam is given in multiple doses or continuously to patients on enzyme inducers, larger midazolam doses may be required because of enhanced hepatic metabolism.

RELATED DRUGS: Triazolam (eg, *Halcion*) and alprazolam (eg, *Xanax*) and to some extent diazepam (eg, *Valium*) also are metabolized by CYP3A4 and would be expected to interact with enzyme inducers in a manner similar to midazolam.

MANAGEMENT OPTIONS:

➡ *Consider Alternative.* When midazolam is used orally as a sedative-hypnotic (as it is in several countries) patients receiving enzyme inducers such as carbamazepine are unlikely to respond unless very large doses of midazolam are used. Thus, it may be preferable to use alternative sedative-hypnotics in such patients.

➡ *Monitor.* Although parenteral midazolam is likely to be much less affected, monitor for inadequate midazolam effect and increase its dose if needed.

REFERENCES:
1. Backman JT, et al. Concentrations and effects of oral midazolam are greatly reduced in patients treated with carbamazepine or phenytoin. *Epilepsia.* 1996;37:253.

Carbamazepine (eg, *Tegretol*) 4

Nifedipine (eg, *Procardia*)

SUMMARY: Limited clinical evidence suggests that nifedipine has little effect on carbamazepine serum concentrations, but carbamazepine theoretically would reduce nifedipine serum concentrations by increasing its metabolism.

RISK FACTORS: No specific risk factors are known.

MECHANISM: The first-pass metabolism of nifedipine can be increased by enzyme induction, and one would expect carbamazepine, a known enzyme inducer, to produce a similar effect.

CLINICAL EVALUATION: The bioavailability of nifedipine, as with most calcium channel blockers, is reduced by enzyme inducers. In 15 healthy subjects, phenobarbital 100 mg/day for 2 weeks resulted in an almost 3-fold increase in nifedipine apparent clearance and a 61% reduction in nifedipine area under the concentration-time curve.[1] One would expect carbamazepine also to reduce nifedipine serum concentrations, but little information is available. Conversely, nifedipine does not appear to affect carbamazepine serum concentrations. In a retrospective study, carbamazepine toxicity was observed in 10 of 15 patients given concurrent verapamil (eg, *Calan*) or diltiazem (eg, *Cardizem*), but not with concurrent nifedipine.[2] Similarly, a patient who developed carbamazepine toxicity with verapamil and diltiazem, was able to take nifedipine without toxicity.[3] Thus, available evidence suggests that nifedipine does not inhibit carbamazepine metabolism, but prospective pharmacokinetic studies are needed for confirmation.

RELATED DRUGS: Most calcium channel blockers, like nifedipine, have reduced bioavailability in the presence of enzyme inducers. Felodipine (*Plendil*) undergoes extensive first-pass metabolism and is highly susceptible to enzyme induction; thus, it may be difficult to achieve therapeutic felodipine concentrations in the presence of carbamazepine. Some calcium channel blockers (eg, diltiazem and verapamil) can produce carbamazepine toxicity. (Also see Carbamazepine/Diltiazem, Carbamazepine/Verapamil, and Carbamazepine/Felodipine monographs.)

MANAGEMENT OPTIONS: No specific action is required, but be alert for evidence of the interaction (eg, failure to respond to nifedipine as expected).

REFERENCES:
1. Schellens JHM, et al. Influence of enzyme induction and inhibition on the oxidation of nifedipine, sparteine, mephenytoin and antipyrine in humans as assessed by a cocktail study design. *J Pharmacol Exp Ther.* 1989;249:638.

2. Beattie B, et al. Verapamil-induced carbamazepine neurotoxicity. *Eur Neurol*. 1988;28:104.

3. Bahls F, et al. Interactions between calcium channel blockers and the anticonvulsants carbamazepine and phenytoin. *Neurol*. 1991;41:740.

 Carbamazepine (eg, *Tegretol*)

Omeprazole (eg, *Prilosec*)

SUMMARY: Omeprazole may increase carbamazepine plasma concentrations; however, studies are conflicting.

RISK FACTORS: No specific risk factors are known.

MECHANISM: Omeprazole may inhibit the metabolism of carbamazepine.

CLINICAL EVALUATION: Nine patients received a single dose of carbamazepine before and after 2 weeks of omeprazole. Omeprazole decreased the plasma clearance of carbamazepine 40% and increased the elimination half-life 100%.[1] In another retrospective analysis, trough carbamazepine plasma concentrations were compared in 20 patients on chronic carbamazepine therapy before and during concomitant omeprazole therapy. Omeprazole did not appear to cause a significant change in carbamazepine concentrations.[2] The effect of long-term treatment with carbamazepine may be different because carbamazepine induces its own metabolism. More study is needed to resolve this issue.

RELATED DRUGS: The effect of lansoprazole (*Prevacid*) on carbamazepine is not established; in general, lansoprazole has little effect on drug-metabolizing enzymes.

MANAGEMENT OPTIONS:

➡ **Monitor.** Until additional information is available, monitor for altered carbamazepine response if omeprazole is initiated, discontinued, or dosage is changed. Carbamazepine toxicity can result in ataxia, blurred vision, dizziness, drowsiness, headache, nausea, nystagmus, and vomiting.

REFERENCES:

1. Naidu MU, et al. Effect of multiple dose omeprazole on the pharmacokinetics of carbamazepine. *Drug Invest*. 1994;7:8.

2. Bottiger Y, et al. No effect on plasma carbamazepine concentration with concomitant omeprazole treatment. *Clin Drug Invest*. 1995;9:180.

 Carbamazepine (eg, *Tegretol*)

Oxybutynin (eg, *Ditropan*)

SUMMARY: A patient developed carbamazepine toxicity after oxybutynin was started; the interaction is consistent with the known interactive properties of the 2 drugs.

RISK FACTORS: No specific risk factors are known.

MECHANISM: Not established. Carbamazepine is metabolized partially by CYP2C8, and there is some evidence that oxybutynin is a CYP2C8 inhibitor.[1] It is possible that oxybutynin inhibits the CYP2C8 metabolism of carbamazepine.

CLINICAL EVALUATION: A 37-year-old woman with a spinal cord lesion was stabilized on carbamazepine 1,000 mg daily, and then was given oxybutynin and dantroline.[2] She developed carbamazepine toxicity with dizziness and vomiting. The oxybutynin and dantroline were stopped, but she developed carbamazepine toxicity again when oxybutynin was restarted. The role of dantroline in causing the carbamazepine toxicity cannot completely be ruled out, but oxybutynin seems to be the cause.

RELATED DRUGS: No information is available.

MANAGEMENT OPTIONS:

➡ *Monitor.* Monitor patients on carbamazepine for carbamazepine toxicity if oxybutynin is given concurrently. Evidence of carbamazepine toxicity includes ataxia, blurred vision, dizziness, drowsiness, headache, nausea, nystagmus, and vomiting.

REFERENCES:

1. Walsky RL, et al. Examination of 209 drugs for inhibition of cytochrome P450 2C8. *J Clin Pharmacol.* 2005;45:68-78.
2. Vander T, et al. Carbamazepine toxicity following oxybutynin and dantroline administration: a case report. *Spinal Cord.* 2005;43:252-255.

Carbamazepine (eg, *Tegretol*)

Paroxetine (eg, *Paxil*)

SUMMARY: Preliminary study in epileptic patients suggests that paroxetine does not affect carbamazepine plasma concentrations.

RISK FACTORS: No specific risk factors are known.

MECHANISM: No interaction.

CLINICAL EVALUATION: In 6 epileptic patients stabilized on chronic carbamazepine therapy 600 to 900 mg/day, placebo was added for 7 days, followed by paroxetine 10 mg/day for 3 days, 20 mg/day for 3 days, and 30 mg/day for 10 days.[1] Paroxetine did not affect steady-state carbamazepine plasma concentrations, and no seizures occurred during the trial.

RELATED DRUGS: No information is available.

MANAGEMENT OPTIONS: No interaction.

REFERENCES:

1. Andersen BB, et al. No influence of the antidepressant paroxetine on carbamazepine, valproate and phenytoin. *Epilepsy Res.* 1991;10:201-204.

Carbamazepine (eg, *Tegretol*) 5

Phenelzine (*Nardil*)

SUMMARY: In a single case report, addition of phenelzine to a combination of carbamazepine and doxepin (eg, *Sinequan*) did not alter the patient's mean steady-state carbamazepine plasma concentration.

RISK FACTORS: No specific risk factors are known.

MECHANISM: No interaction.

CLINICAL EVALUATION: In a case report, a 70-year-old woman receiving a combination of carbamazepine and doxepin was started on the nonselective monoamine oxidase inhibitor (MAOI) phenelzine 45 mg/day. Before phenelzine was initiated, the patient had a carbamazepine plasma concentration of 47 mcmol/L. There were no signs of toxicity and her carbamazepine plasma concentration remained unchanged with the combination of drugs.[1] Nonetheless, more study is needed to ensure that phenelzine does not affect carbamazepine disposition. It is not known whether MAOIs other than phenelzine have any effect on carbamazepine.

RELATED DRUGS: No information is available.

MANAGEMENT OPTIONS: No interaction.

REFERENCES:

1. Yatham LN, et al. Is the carbamazepine-phenelzine combination safe? *Am J Psychiatry.* 1990;147:367.

 4   Carbamazepine (eg, *Tegretol*)

Phenobarbital

SUMMARY: Although phenobarbital (and presumably other barbiturates) may lower serum carbamazepine concentrations, a reduction in the anticonvulsant effect of carbamazepine is not likely. Whether other effects of carbamazepine might be reduced by barbiturates is unknown.

RISK FACTORS: No specific risk factors are known.

MECHANISM: Phenobarbital stimulates the metabolism of carbamazepine by hepatic microsomal enzymes.[1] Phenobarbital also induces the formation[2] and elimination of the active metabolite of carbamazepine, carbamazepine-10,11-epoxide.[3]

CLINICAL EVALUATION: In a study of 123 patients receiving carbamazepine, those patients who also were receiving phenobarbital tended to have lower plasma concentrations of carbamazepine (mean, 5.5 mg/L) than those who received carbamazepine alone (mean, 6.7 mg/L).[1] Similar differences in plasma concentrations of carbamazepine were found in a group of 43 children.[4] Those on carbamazepine alone had higher carbamazepine plasma concentrations than those receiving carbamazepine plus other anticonvulsants (usually phenobarbital or phenytoin [eg, *Dilantin*]). In a study of 113 patients with epilepsy receiving carbamazepine, those patients receiving concurrent phenobarbital had significantly higher ratios of carbamazepine-epoxide to carbamazepine. Phenobarbital also induces the metabolism of carbamazepine-epoxide. The elimination half-life (mean) of carbamazepine-epoxide was 4.3 hours in 6 patients with epilepsy receiving phenobarbital and 6.7 hours in 6 drug-free volunteers.[3] Although the clinical significance of this effect is unclear, recent data suggest that carbamazepine-epoxide contributes significantly to the therapeutic effect of carbamazepine (but it is not measured clinically).[5]

RELATED DRUGS: Little is known regarding the effect of barbiturates other than phenobarbital on carbamazepine, but they probably also reduce carbamazepine serum concentrations. Theoretically, administration of a barbiturate in doses capable of inducing enzymes but not sufficient to exert significant anticonvulsant effect (eg, a nightly hypnotic barbiturate) might be more likely to interfere with the anticonvulsant effect of carbamazepine. However, this has not been studied clinically.

MANAGEMENT OPTIONS: No specific action is required, but be alert for evidence of the interaction.

REFERENCES:

1. Christiansen J, et al. Influence of phenobarbital and diphenylhydantoin on plasma carbamazepine levels in patients with epilepsy. *Acta Neurol Scand.* 1973;49:543.
2. Ramsay E, et al. Carbamazepine metabolism in humans. Effect of concurrent anticonvulsant therapy. *Ther Drug Monit.* 1990;12:235.
3. Spina E, et al. Effect of phenobarbital on the pharmacokinetics of carbamazepine-10,11-epoxide, an active metabolite of carbamazepine. *Ther Drug Monit.* 1991;13:109.
4. Rane A, et al. Kinetics of carbamazepine and its 10,11-epoxide metabolite in children. *Clin Pharmacol Ther.* 1976;19:276.
5. Tomson T, et al. Carbamazepine-10,11-epoxide in epilepsy. A pilot study. *Arch Neurol.* 1990;46:888.

Carbamazepine (eg, *Tegretol*)

Phenytoin (eg, *Dilantin*)

SUMMARY: Combined use of phenytoin and carbamazepine may decrease the serum concentrations of both drugs. In some patients, however, phenytoin concentrations may increase or stay the same when carbamazepine is added.

RISK FACTORS: No specific risk factors are known.

MECHANISM: Carbamazepine appears to enhance phenytoin metabolism by induction of hepatic microsomal enzymes; carbamazepine also may be a competitive inhibitor of phenytoin metabolism. Phenytoin appears to increase the metabolism of carbamazepine.[5]

CLINICAL EVALUATION: In a preliminary study, carbamazepine appeared to decrease serum phenytoin concentrations in 3 of 7 patients.[2] In another part of this study, phenytoin half-life was decreased in all 5 patients; lowered phenytoin serum concentrations were noted during carbamazepine administration in yet another study.[6] In other studies, carbamazepine serum concentrations have been lower when phenytoin or other anticonvulsants have been given concomitantly than when carbamazepine was given alone.[1,3,4] Thus, in a patient receiving both drugs, the potential exists for decreased plasma concentrations of phenytoin[2] and carbamazepine.[1] Nevertheless, the combination frequently is used to advantage in patients with seizures.

In a study of 32 patients receiving a constant phenytoin dose, the mean phenytoin concentration increased from 14.1 ± 3.5 mcg/ml to 19.3 ± 3.6 mcg/ml when the carbamazepine dose was gradually increased. When the phenytoin dose was gradually lowered in 22 patients, carbamazepine concentrations increased approximately 28%.[7] The enzyme inhibitory effect of carbamazepine also has been shown in 6 healthy volunteers who received phenytoin with and without carbamazepine. Another study found a 35% increase in phenytoin steady-state concentrations when carbamazepine was used concurrently.[8]

RELATED DRUGS: No information is available.

MANAGEMENT OPTIONS:

➥ *Monitor.* During coadministration of phenytoin and carbamazepine, serum concentrations of carbamazepine and phenytoin could decrease or phenytoin serum concentrations could increase. Monitor plasma concentrations of both phenytoin and carbamazepine during dosage changes. Also clinically monitor patients to determine if a change of dosage of either drug is required.

REFERENCES:

1. Christiansen J, et al. Influence of phenobarbital and diphenylhydantoin on plasma carbamazepine levels in patients with epilepsy. *Acta Neurol Scand.* 1973;49:543.
2. Hansen JM, et al. Carbamazepine-induced acceleration of diphenylhydantoin and warfarin metabolism in man. *Clin Pharmacol Ther.* 1971;12:539.
3. Cereghino JJ, et al. The efficacy of carbamazepine combinations in epilepsy. *Clin Pharmacol Ther.* 1975;18:733.
4. Rane A, et al. Kinetics of carbamazepine and its 10,11-epoxide metabolite in children. *Clin Pharmacol Ther.* 1976;19:276.
5. Windorfer A. Drug interaction during anticonvulsive therapy. *Int J Clin Pharmacol.* 1976;14:236.
6. Levy RH, et al. Pharmacokinetics of carbamazepine in normal man. *Clin Pharmacol Ther.* 1977;17:657.
7. Zielinski JJ, et al. Dual effects of carbamazepine-phenytoin interaction. *Ther Drug Monit.* 1987;9:21.
8. Brown TR, et al. Carbamazepine increases phenytoin serum concentrations and reduces phenytoin clearance. *Neurology.* 1988;38:1146.

 Carbamazepine (eg, *Tegretol*)

Propoxyphene (eg, *Darvon-N*)

SUMMARY: Propoxyphene markedly increases plasma carbamazepine concentrations; carbamazepine toxicity is likely to occur in most patients receiving both drugs.

RISK FACTORS: No specific risk factors are known.

MECHANISM: Propoxyphene inhibits the oxidative metabolism of carbamazepine.

CLINICAL EVALUATION: Several reports show that propoxyphene increases plasma carbamazepine. The effect is rapid, usually taking place over 2 to 3 days. After clinical observations suggested an interaction between carbamazepine and propoxyphene, 7 patients taking carbamazepine were given propoxyphene 65 mg 3 times daily.[1] Plasma carbamazepine concentrations rose considerably after propoxyphene administration, and some patients developed signs of carbamazepine toxicity (eg, ataxia, dizziness, drowsiness, headache, nausea). In another study, all 6 patients taking long-term carbamazepine 600 to 800 mg/day therapy experienced increased serum carbamazepine concentrations (mean increase, 66%) following the addition of propoxyphene 65 mg 3 times daily.[2] Three elderly patients developed carbamazepine toxicity after starting propoxyphene therapy. Two of these patients became comatose, and serum carbamazepine concentrations were about 3 times higher than those usually associated with acceptable therapeutic serum concentrations.[3] Another patient developed 200% to 300% increases in serum carbamazepine concentrations following propoxyphene administration.[4] Although an occasional dose of propoxyphene is unlikely to cause carbamazepine toxicity, regular dosing of propoxyphene for more than 1 to 2 days appears to produce carbamazepine toxicity in most patients.

RELATED DRUGS: Other analgesics have not been shown to interact with carbamazepine.

MANAGEMENT OPTIONS:

➡ ***Use Alternative.*** Use analgesics other than propoxyphene in patients receiving carbamazepine.

REFERENCES:

1. Dam M, et al. Interaction of propoxyphene with carbamazepine. *Lancet.* 1977;2(8036):509.

2. Hansen BS, et al. Influence of dextropropoxyphene on steady state serum levels and protein binding of three antiepileptic drugs in man. *Acta Neurol Scand.* 1980;61(6):357-367.

3. Yu YL, et al. Interaction between carbamazepine and dextropropoxyphene. *Postgrad Med J.* 1986;62(725):231-233.

4. Kubacka RT, et al. Carbamazepine-propoxyphene interaction. *Clin Pharm.* 1983;2(2):104.

Carbamazepine (eg, *Tegretol*)

Quinidine

SUMMARY: Carbamazepine reduces the plasma concentrations of quinidine; some patients may experience a loss of antiarrhythmic efficacy.

RISK FACTORS: No specific risk factors are known.

MECHANISM: Carbamazepine induces the activity of CYP3A4, an enzyme that is known to metabolize quinidine.

CLINICAL EVALUATION: Nine healthy subjects received carbamazepine 800 mg for 17 days.[1] A single dose of quinidine 200 mg was administered before and following the carbamazepine. The administration of carbamazepine resulted in a marked increase in the formation of 3-hydroxyquinidine, a major metabolite of quinidine. The half-life of quinidine was reduced 32% following carbamazepine. These changes in quinidine pharmacokinetics may result in a reduction of its antiarrhythmic activity.

RELATED DRUGS: Oxcarbazepine (*Trileptal*) also increases the metabolism of quinidine, although to a lesser extent.

MANAGEMENT OPTIONS:

➡ **Monitor.** Monitor quinidine plasma concentrations whenever carbamazepine or oxcarbazepine is added or removed from a patient's drug regimen.

REFERENCES:
1. Andreasen AH, et al. A comparative pharmacokinetic study in healthy volunteers of the effect of carbamazepine and oxcarbazepine on CYP3A4. *Epilepsia.* 2007;48(3):490-496.

Carbamazepine (eg, *Tegretol*)

Risperidone (*Risperdal*)

SUMMARY: Carbamazepine appears to reduce risperidone plasma concentrations; adjust the risperidone dose as needed.

RISK FACTORS: No specific risk factors are known.

MECHANISM: Carbamazepine probably enhances the metabolism of risperidone.

CLINICAL EVALUATION: Two patients stabilized on carbamazepine and risperidone developed parkinsonian symptoms (eg, fixed facial expression, muscle rigidity, small shuffling steps) after carbamazepine was stopped.[1] The symptoms of both patients resolved after the risperidone dose was reduced. These finding are consistent with previous studies, suggesting that carbamazepine reduces risperidone plasma concentrations.[2]

RELATED DRUGS: No information is available.

MANAGEMENT OPTIONS: Be alert for evidence of altered risperidone effect if carbamazepine is initiated, discontinued, or changed in dosage.

REFERENCES:

1. Takahashi H, et al. Development of parkinsonian symptoms after discontinuation of carbamazepine in patients concurrently treated with risperidone: two case reports. *Clin Neuropharmacol.* 2001;24(6):358-360.

2. Spina E, et al. Plasma concentrations of risperidone and 9-hydroxyrisperidone: effect of comedication with carbamazepine or valproate. *Ther Drug Monit.* 2000;22(4):481-485.

Carbamazepine (eg, *Tegretol*)

Ritonavir (*Norvir*)

SUMMARY: Ritonavir administration appears to increase carbamazepine concentrations; carbamazepine toxicity may result.

RISK FACTORS: No specific risk factors are known.

MECHANISM: Acute administration of ritonavir is known to inhibit the enzyme (CYP3A4) that metabolizes carbamazepine.

CLINICAL EVALUATION: A patient with HIV and a history of seizures was stabilized on phenobarbital (eg, *Solfoton*) 250 mg/day in divided doses, phenytoin (eg, *Dilantin*) 500 mg/day in divided doses, and carbamazepine 400 mg 3 times daily.[1] His antiretroviral therapy was changed from stavudine (*Zerit*), lamivudine (*Epivir*), and indinavir (*Crixivan*) to ritonavir 300 mg twice daily, saquinavir (*Invirase*) 400 mg twice daily, and nevirapine (*Viramune*) 200 mg/day. Two days later, he developed symptoms consistent with carbamazepine toxicity, including vertigo, drowsiness, diplopia, and ataxia. Plasma carbamazepine concentrations had doubled to 16.6 mg/L. The carbamazepine dosage was reduced to 200 mg 3 times daily, and ritonavir was discontinued and replaced with nelfinavir 1,000 mg twice daily. Carbamazepine concentrations returned to normal and toxic symptoms cleared over the next 2 days. The patient was stabilized on the new regimen without further problems. Although not studied, carbamazepine is an inducer of CYP3A4 and could decrease the concentration of protease inhibitors, including ritonavir.

RELATED DRUGS: Nelfinavir (*Viracept*), saquinavir, and indinavir also inhibit CYP3A4 and may reduce carbamazepine metabolism.

MANAGEMENT OPTIONS:

➧ *Monitor.* Monitor patients stabilized on carbamazepine for altered serum concentrations and signs of carbamazepine toxicity if ritonavir is started or discontinued. Also, be alert for reduced antiviral response in patients taking ritonavir and carbamazepine.

REFERENCES:

1. Mateu-de Antonio J, et al. Ritonavir-induced carbamazepine toxicity. *Ann Pharmacother.* 2001;35(1):125-126.

Carbamazepine (eg, *Tegretol*)

Simvastatin (*Zocor*)

SUMMARY: Carbamazepine markedly reduced simvastatin serum concentrations in healthy subjects; simvastatin efficacy is likely to be reduced.

RISK FACTORS: No specific risk factors are known.

MECHANISM: Carbamazepine increases CYP3A4 activity and probably decreases simvastatin bioavailability.

CLINICAL EVALUATION: Twelve healthy subjects took a single oral dose of simvastatin 80 mg with and without pretreatment with carbamazepine 600 mg daily except 200 mg daily for the first 2 days.[1] Carbamazepine reduced the area under the serum concentration-time curve of both simvastatin and simvastatin acid about 80%. The magnitude of this effect can be expected to reduce the efficacy of simvastatin.

RELATED DRUGS: Lovastatin (eg, *Mevacor*) and atorvastatin (*Lipitor*) also are metabolized by CYP3A4 and may also interact with carbamazepine. Theoretically, pravastatin (*Pravachol*), and possibly rosuvastatin (*Crestor*) and fluvastatin (*Lescol*), are less likely to interact with carbamazepine.

MANAGEMENT OPTIONS:

➥ *Consider Alternative.* Using a statin other than atorvastatin, lovastatin, or simvastatin may reduce the risk of interaction.

➥ *Circumvent/Minimize.* Increasing the simvastatin dose would theoretically circumvent the interaction.

➥ *Monitor.* When carbamazepine is used with any statin, monitor for impairment of cholesterol-lowering effect.

REFERENCES:

1. Ucar M, et al. Carbamazepine markedly reduces serum concentrations of simvastatin and simvastatin acid. *Eur J Clin Pharmacol.* 2004;59:879-882.

Carbamazepine (eg, *Tegretol*)

Theophylline (eg, *Theolair*)

SUMMARY: Carbamazepine may reduce serum theophylline concentrations, thus increasing theophylline dosage requirements.

RISK FACTORS: No specific risk factors are known.

MECHANISM: Carbamazepine probably stimulates the hepatic metabolism of theophylline.

CLINICAL EVALUATION: In an 11-year-old girl maintained on theophylline, the administration of carbamazepine was associated with subtherapeutic theophylline levels and worsening asthma symptoms.[1] The theophylline half-life was about 3 hours while she was receiving carbamazepine and approximately 6 hours when she was not receiving carbamazepine. Theophylline clearance in another patient receiving theophylline and carbamazepine 600 mg/day was reduced from 0.139 to 0.069 L/

kg/hr when carbamazepine was discontinued.[2] A boy receiving theophylline and carbamazepine developed intractable seizures and severe permanent brain damage 2 to 3 weeks after the carbamazepine was discontinued. These findings are consistent with the known ability of carbamazepine to produce enzyme induction and the known susceptibility of theophylline to enzyme induction. Additional studies are needed to determine the incidence and magnitude of this interaction.

RELATED DRUGS: No information is available.

MANAGEMENT OPTIONS:

➡ **Monitor.** Be alert for evidence of altered theophylline serum levels when carbamazepine is initiated, discontinued, or changed in dosage.

REFERENCES:

1. Rosenberry KR, et al. Reduced theophylline half-life induced by carbamazepine therapy. *J Pediatr.* 1983;102:472.

2. Phenytoin-theophylline-quinidine interactions. *N Engl J Med.* 1983;308:724.

 Carbamazepine (eg, *Tegretol*)

Thioridazine (eg, *Mellaril*)

SUMMARY: Preliminary results suggest that there is no effect of thioridazine on plasma concentrations of carbamazepine and its active metabolite, carbamazepine-epoxide.

RISK FACTORS: No specific risk factors are known.

MECHANISM: No interaction.

CLINICAL EVALUATION: Steady-state concentrations of carbamazepine and carbamazepine-epoxide were unchanged after thioridazine 100 to 200 mg/day was added to the therapy of patients receiving chronic carbamazepine treatment.[1] Theoretically, carbamazepine could enhance thioridazine elimination because it is an enzyme inducer; however, clinical evidence is lacking.

RELATED DRUGS: No information is available.

MANAGEMENT OPTIONS: No interaction.

REFERENCES:

1. Spina E, et al. No effect of thioridazine on plasma concentrations of carbamazepine and its active metabolite carbamazepine-10,11-epoxide. *Ther Drug Monit.* 1990;12:511.

 Carbamazepine (eg, *Tegretol*)

Thyroid

SUMMARY: Carbamazepine appears to increase the elimination of thyroid and may increase the requirements for thyroid in hypothyroid patients.

RISK FACTORS: No specific risk factors are known.

MECHANISM: Carbamazepine, like other enzyme inducers, appears to enhance the metabolism of thyroxine (T_4) and triiodothyronine (T_3). Carbamazepine also can interfere with the increase in circulating thyrotropin (TSH) that normally occurs in response to reduced serum concentrations of thyroids. This observation is consistent with the effects of other enzyme inducers; phenytoin (eg, *Dilantin*) and rifampin (eg, *Rifadin*) increase thyroxine replacement requirements in hypothyroid patients.[1,2] Moreover, carbamazepine has been associated with reductions in serum concentrations of total thyroxine, free thyroxine, and triiodothyronine in people without pre-existing hypothyroidism (eg, healthy subjects, patients with epilepsy or affective illness).[3-6] Curiously, the reductions in circulating thyroid hormones in these latter groups generally have not been associated with increases in serum thyrotropin or clinical evidence of hypothyroidism. This raises the question of whether determinations of serum thyroxine (free or total) or serum triiodothyronine are accurate reflections of thyrometabolic status in patients receiving carbamazepine.

CLINICAL EVALUATION: Initiation of carbamazepine therapy to hypothyroid patients maintained on levothyroxine reduces circulating thyroid concentrations.[7]

RELATED DRUGS: Other enzyme inducers (eg, phenytoin, rifampin) also appear to interact similarly.

MANAGEMENT OPTIONS:

➡ *Monitor.* If carbamazepine therapy is initiated or discontinued in hypothyroid patients receiving thyroid replacement therapy, be alert for clinical and laboratory evidence of altered circulating thyroid concentrations. Adjust thyroid dosage as needed.

REFERENCES:

1. Blackshear JL, et al. Thyroxine replacement requirements in hypothyroid patients receiving phenytoin. *Ann Intern Med*. 1983;99:341.
2. Isley WL. Effect of rifampin therapy on thyroid function tests in a hypothyroid patient on replacement L-thyroxine. *Ann Intern Med*. 1987;107:517.
3. Connell JM, et al. Changes in circulating thyroid hormones during short-term hepatic enzyme induction with carbamazepine. *Eur J Clin Pharmacol*. 1984;26:453.
4. Cathro DM, et al. Sub-normal serum thyroxine levels associated with carbamazepine and valproic acid treatment. *Nebr Med J*. 1985;70:235.
5. Roy-Byrne PP, et al. Carbamazepine and thyroid function in affectively ill patients. Clinical and theoretical implications. *Arch Gen Psychiatry*. 1984;41:1150.
6. Joffe RT, et al. The effects of carbamazepine on the thyrotropin response to thyrotropin-releasing hormone. *Psychiatry Res*. 1984;12:161.
7. Aanderud S, et al. The influence of carbamazepine on thyroid hormones and thyroxine binding globulin in hypothyroid patients substituted with thyroxine. *Clin Endocrinol*. 1981;15:247.

Carbamazepine (eg, *Tegretol*)

Troleandomycin (*TAO*)

SUMMARY: Troleandomycin may increase plasma carbamazepine concentrations; carbamazepine toxicity has occurred in some patients receiving both drugs.

RISK FACTORS: No specific risk factors are known.

MECHANISM: Troleandomycin inhibits the metabolism of carbamazepine.

CLINICAL EVALUATION: Eight patients maintained on carbamazepine developed signs of carbamazepine intoxication within 24 hours after starting troleandomycin therapy.[1] Plasma carbamazepine concentrations in 2 of the patients were increased. In another study of epileptic patients receiving carbamazepine, troleandomycin 8 to 33 mg/kg body weight/day was associated with increased plasma carbamazepine concentrations and evidence of carbamazepine toxicity.[2]

RELATED DRUGS: Erythromycin (eg, *E-Mycin*) and clarithromycin (*Biaxin*) appear to inhibit carbamazepine metabolism. Azithromycin (*Zithromax*) and dirithromycin (*Dynabac*) would be unlikely to interact with carbamazepine.

MANAGEMENT OPTIONS:

➡ *Consider Alternative.* Avoid concomitant use of troleandomycin and carbamazepine if possible. Azithromycin does not appear to alter carbamazepine metabolism.

➡ *Monitor.* When both drugs are used, monitor for evidence of carbamazepine toxicity (dizziness, drowsiness, nausea, vomiting, ataxia, headache, nystagmus, blurred vision), and measure plasma carbamazepine concentrations as needed. Monitor for evidence of reduced serum carbamazepine concentrations when troleandomycin is discontinued or reduced in dosage.

REFERENCES:

1. Dravet C, et al. Interaction between carbamazepine and triacetyloleandomycin. *Lancet*. 1977;2:810.
2. Mesdjian E, et al. Carbamazepine intoxication due to triacetyloleandomycin administration in epileptic patients. *Epilepsia*. 1980;21:489.

Carbamazepine (eg, *Tegretol*)

Valproic Acid (eg, *Depakene*)

SUMMARY: Valproic acid can increase, decrease, or have no effect on carbamazepine serum concentrations.[1] Plasma concentrations of carbamazepine-epoxide, the active metabolite, also can increase. Carbamazepine decreases plasma concentrations of valproic acid and larger doses of valproic acid are required to maintain therapeutic steady-state concentrations.[2,3]

RISK FACTORS: No specific risk factors are known.

MECHANISM: Valproic acid can affect carbamazepine in 3 ways. First, by inhibiting the metabolism of carbamazepine, increased carbamazepine plasma concentrations can result. Secondly, valproic acid can displace carbamazepine from plasma proteins resulting in decreased total carbamazepine concentrations. Thirdly, valproic acid inhibits the epoxide hydrolase enzyme responsible for metabolism of carbamazepine-epoxide. Carbamazepine induces the metabolism of valproic acid.

CLINICAL EVALUATION: In one study of 5 patients maintained on carbamazepine, carbamazepine concentrations decreased or showed no change when valproic acid was added.[4] In a study of 14 children, the addition of carbamazepine to valproic acid therapy resulted in high concentrations of carbamazepine-epoxide. This was associated with marked side effects in 9 of the children.[5] When a group of patients receiving carbamazepine monotherapy (n = 31) was compared with patients receiving carbamazepine plus valproic acid (n = 12), there was no difference in carbamazepine concentrations, but the ration of carbamazepine-epoxide to carbamazepine was doubled.[6] Carbamazepine decreased valproic acid plasma concentrations and its discontinuation had resulted in increased valproic acid concentrations and toxicity.[3]

RELATED DRUGS: No information is available.

MANAGEMENT OPTIONS:

→ *Monitor.* The unpredictability of the effect of valproic acid on total carbamazepine plasma concentrations and carbamazepine-epoxide (which is not routinely monitored) makes interpretation of carbamazepine plasma concentrations difficult when the 2 drugs are used concurrently. Carbamazepine-epoxide contributes significantly to the therapeutic and, possibly, the toxic effects of carbamazepine. Monitor patients for symptoms of carbamazepine toxicity and measure serum carbamazepine concentrations. Symptoms of carbamazepine toxicity include drowsiness, dizziness, nausea, vomiting, ataxia, headache, nystagmus, and blurred vision. Monitor for a decreased therapeutic response to carbamazepine when valproic acid is discontinued or reduced in dosage. An increase in valproic acid dose may be needed if carbamazepine is added. Monitor for evidence of valproic acid toxicity if carbamazepine is discontinued or reduced in dosage.

REFERENCES:

1. Acid DJ, et al. Sodium valproate in the treatment of intractable seizure disorders; a clinical and electroencephalographic study. *Neurology.* 1978;28:152.
2. Kondo T, et al. The effects of phenytoin and carbamazepine on serum concentrations of monounsaturated metabolites of valproic acid. *Br J Clin Pharmacol.* 1990;29:116-19.
3. Jann MW, et al. Increased valproate serum concentrations upon carbamazepine cessation. *Epilepsia.* 1988;29:578.
4. Wilder BJ, et al. Valproic acid: interaction with other anticonvulsant drugs. *Neurology.* 1978;28:892.
5. Rambeck B, et al. Valproic acid-induced carbamazepine-10,11-epoxide toxicity in children and adolescents. *Eur Neurol.* 1990;30:79.
6. Ramsey RE, et al. Carbamazepine metabolism in humans: effect of concurrent anticonvulsant therapy. *Ther Drug Monit.* 1990;12:235.

Carbamazepine (eg, *Tegretol*)

Verapamil (eg, *Calan*)

SUMMARY: Verapamil increases carbamazepine serum concentrations, and frequently results in carbamazepine toxicity.

RISK FACTORS: No specific risk factors are known.

MECHANISM: Verapamil inhibits carbamazepine metabolism, probably by inhibiting intestinal and hepatic cytochrome P4503A4. Also, the first-pass metabolism of oral verapamil can be dramatically increased by enzyme induction, and one would expect carbamazepine, a known enzyme inducer, to produce a similar effect.

CLINICAL EVALUATION: In 6 patients on carbamazepine, the addition of verapamil 120 mg 3 times daily resulted in carbamazepine neurotoxicity in all patients within 3 days, accompanied by a mean 40% reduction in carbamazepine apparent clearance.[1] Case reports of verapamil-induced carbamazepine neurotoxicity also have appeared.[2,3] In a retrospective study, carbamazepine toxicity was observed in 10 of 15 patients given concurrent verapamil or diltiazem, but not with concurrent nifedipine (eg, *Procardia*).[4] Thus, it appears that carbamazepine toxicity is likely if verapamil is used concurrently unless carbamazepine dosage is reduced.

RELATED DRUGS: Diltiazem also can produce carbamazepine toxicity, but limited evidence suggests that nifedipine is less likely to do so. Felodipine (*Plendil*) undergoes extensive first-pass metabolism and is highly susceptible to enzyme induction; thus, it may be difficult to achieve therapeutic felodipine concentrations in the presence of carbamazepine. (Also see Carbamazepine/Diltiazem, Carbamazepine/Nifedipine, and Carbamazepine/Felodipine monographs.)

MANAGEMENT OPTIONS:

➥ *Avoid Unless Benefit Outweighs Risk.* Given the high likelihood of carbamazepine toxicity with concurrent use and the possibility of reduced verapamil effect, it would be best to avoid the combination if possible. (See Related Drugs section for possible alternative calcium channel blockers.)

➥ *Monitor.* If the combination is used, monitor for carbamazepine toxicity (eg, nausea, vomiting, dizziness, drowsiness, headache, diplopia, and confusion). Toxic symptoms are likely to occur within 2 to 3 days of starting the verapamil.

REFERENCES:

1. Macphee GJ, et al. Verapamil potentiates carbamazepine neurotoxicity: a clinically important inhibitory interaction. *Lancet.* 1986;1:700.

2. Price WA. Verapamil-carbamazepine neurotoxicity. *J Clin Psych.* 1988;49:80.

3. Beattie B, et al. Verapamil-induced carbamazepine neurotoxicity. *Eur Neurol.* 1988;28:104.

4. Bahls F, et al. Interactions between calcium channel blockers and the anticonvulsants carbamazepine and phenytoin. *Neurol.* 1991;41:740.

Carbamazepine (eg, *Tegretol*)

Warfarin (eg, *Coumadin*)

SUMMARY: Carbamazepine inhibits the hypoprothrombinemic response to oral anticoagulants; adjustments in anticoagulant dosage may be required during cotherapy.

RISK FACTORS: No specific risk factors are known.

MECHANISM: Carbamazepine appears to enhance warfarin metabolism by inducing hepatic microsomal enzymes.

CLINICAL EVALUATION: In 3 patients taking warfarin, both the serum warfarin levels and the prothrombin time decreased when carbamazepine therapy was given; in 2 of these patients, the warfarin half-life also decreased.[1] Another report describes a patient on chronic warfarin therapy whose hypoprothrombinemic response reversed completely after carbamazepine 400 mg/day was added.[2] Three other patients reportedly also developed reduced anticoagulant response when carbamazepine was added to stabilized warfarin therapy.[3]

RELATED DRUGS: Oral anticoagulants other than warfarin are likely to be similarly affected by carbamazepine.

MANAGEMENT OPTIONS:

➥ *Monitor.* Monitor patients taking oral anticoagulants for altered hypoprothrombinemic response to warfarin if carbamazepine therapy is initiated, discontinued, or changed in dosage; adjust the anticoagulant dose as needed.

REFERENCES:

1. Hansen JM, et al. Carbamazepine-induced acceleration of diphenylhydantoin and warfarin metabolism in man. *Clin Pharmacol Ther.* 1971;12:539.

2. Kendall AG, et al. Warfarin-carbamazepine interaction. *Ann Intern Med.* 1981;94:280.

3. Massey EW. Effect of carbamazepine on coumadin metabolism. *Ann Neurol.* 1983;13:691.

Carbamazepine (*Tegretol*)

Ziprasidone (*Geodon*)

SUMMARY: Carbamazepine moderately reduces ziprasidone serum concentrations, but the clinical importance of this effect is not established.

RISK FACTORS: No specific risk factors are known.

MECHANISM: Carbamazepine probably enhances the CYP3A4 metabolism of ziprasidone in the liver and possibly the small intestine.

CLINICAL EVALUATION: In a randomized, parallel study, 25 healthy subjects received multiple doses of ziprasidone before and after 24 days of carbamazepine or placebo.[1] Carbamazepine reduced ziprasidone area under the serum concentration-time curve 36%. The extent to which this would reduce the efficacy of ziprasidone is not known, but note that the 36% is a mean value. Thus, it is possible that some patients will have a sufficient reduction in ziprasidone serum concentrations to impair the therapeutic response.

RELATED DRUGS: Other anticonvulsants such as phenytoin (eg, *Dilantin*), primidone (*Mysoline*), and phenobarbital (eg, *Solfoton*) increase CYP3A4 activity, and would be expected to reduce ziprasidone effect.

MANAGEMENT OPTIONS:

➡ **Monitor.** Monitor for reduced ziprasidone efficacy if carbamazepine is used concurrently. Adjustment of ziprasidone dose may be needed if carbamazepine therapy is initiated, discontinued, or changed in dosage.

REFERENCES:
1. Miceli JJ, et al. The effect of carbamazepine on the steady-state pharmacokinetics of ziprasidone in healthy volunteers. *Br J Clin Pharmacol.* 2000;49 (suppl 1):65S-70S.

Carbenicillin (*Geocillin*)

Gentamicin (eg, *Garamycin*)

SUMMARY: Carbenicillin and some penicillins inactivate gentamicin and other aminoglycosides in vitro and, in certain patients with severe renal dysfunction, in vivo. The effect of the aminoglycoside can be reduced.

RISK FACTORS:

➡ **Route of Administration.** In vitro mixing of the antibiotics before administration can increase the risk of interaction.

➡ **Concurrent Diseases.** Patients with severe renal dysfunction are at increased risk.

➡ **Assay Delay.** Delay in aminoglycoside assay when penicillin is present in serum can increase the risk of interaction.

MECHANISM: Both carbenicillin and ticarcillin (and probably the related extended spectrum penicillins: azlocillin, mezlocillin [*Mezlin*], and piperacillin [*Pipracil*]) chemically inactivate aminoglycosides, such as gentamicin and tobramycin.

CLINICAL EVALUATION: Good evidence exists for the in vitro inactivation of gentamicin and tobramycin (eg, *Nebcin*) by carbenicillin or ticarcillin (*Ticar*), but such inactivation is unlikely in vivo in patients with normal renal function.[1,2,6] In patients with severe renal impairment, clinical evidence indicates that carbenicillin, piperacillin, or ticarcillin may inactivate gentamicin and tobramycin, in vivo, causing a reduction of their antimicrobial efficacy.[3-10] In addition, aminoglycoside serum assays may be affected by penicillin therapy, especially if the assay of the serum sample is delayed.

RELATED DRUGS: Other extended spectrum penicillins are likely to inactivate some aminoglycosides. (See Clinical Evaluation.)

MANAGEMENT OPTIONS:

➡ *Consider Alternative.* Choose an alternative antibiotic for the aminoglycoside or penicillin. Amikacin and netilmicin may be less likely than other aminoglycosides to interact with extended-spectrum penicillins; however, observe the same precautions with all combinations of aminoglycosides and extended-spectrum penicillins.

➡ *Circumvent/Minimize.* Avoid mixing antibiotics in vitro (eg, in the same IV bag or line).

➡ *Monitor.* If the antibiotics must be coadministered, monitor serum gentamicin (or other aminoglycoside) concentrations for evidence of the interaction (note potential for in vitro serum inactivation) and doses adjusted accordingly.

REFERENCES:

1. Riff LJ, et al. Laboratory and clinical conditions for gentamicin inactivation by carbenicillin. *Arch Intern Med.* 1972;130:887.

2. McLaughlin JE, et al. Clinical and laboratory evidence for inactivation of gentamicin by carbenicillin. *Lancet.* 1971;1:261.

3. Ervin FR, et al. Inactivation of gentamicin by penicillins in patients with renal failure. *Antimicrob Agents Chemother.* 1976;9:1004.

4. Weibert RT, et al. Carbenicillin-gentamicin interaction in acute renal failure. *Am J Hosp Pharm.* 1977;34:1137.

5. Davies M, et al. Interactions of carbenicillin and ticarcillin with gentamicin. *Antimicrob Agents Chemother.* 1975;7:431.

6. Henderson JL, et al. *In vitro* inactivation of gentamicin, tobramycin, and netilmicin by carbenicillin, azlocillin, or mezlocillin. *Am J Hosp Pharm.* 1981;38:1167.

7. Matzke GR, et al. Effect of ticarcillin on gentamicin and tobramycin pharmacokinetics in a patient with end-stage renal disease. *Pharmacotherapy.* 1984;4:158.

8. Halstenson CE, et al. Effect of concomitant administration of piperacillin on the disposition of netilmicin and tobramycin in patients with end-stage renal disease. *Antimicrob Agents Chemother.* 1990;34:128.

9. Uber WE, et al. *In vivo* inactivation of tobramycin by piperacillin. *DICP, Ann Pharmacother.* 1991;25:357.

10. Halstenson CE, et al. Effect of concomitant administration of piperacillin on the dispositions of isepanicin and gentamicin in patients with end-stage renal disease. *Antimicrob Agents Chemother.* 1992;36:1832.

Carbenicillin (*Geocillin*)

Methotrexate

SUMMARY: Administration of carbenicillin and other penicillins may increase methotrexate serum concentrations and may potentiate methotrexate toxicity.

RISK FACTORS: No specific risk factors are known.

MECHANISM: Large doses of penicillin may interfere with the active renal tubular secretion of methotrexate.

CLINICAL EVALUATION: A patient receiving high-dose methotrexate with folinic acid rescue developed considerably elevated serum methotrexate levels following carbenicillin administration 30 g/day.[1] This effect also has been observed during mezlocillin (*Mezlin*) administration with methotrexate.[2] Low doses of methotrexate may produce toxicity when administered with various penicillins.[3] While causation is not clear in these cases, use the combination of penicillins and methotrexate only with careful monitoring.

RELATED DRUGS: Other penicillins administered in large doses could have similar effects on methotrexate.

MANAGEMENT OPTIONS:

➡ *Monitor.* Monitor patients for evidence of enhanced methotrexate effect and possible toxicity (eg, mucositis, leukopenia) when large doses of carbenicillin or other penicillins are given concurrently.

REFERENCES:

1. Gibson DL, et al. Midyear Clinical Meeting Abstracts. American Society of Hospital Pharmacists. New Orleans; 1981:305 Dec 6–10.
2. Dean R, et al. Possible methotrexate-mezlocillin interaction. *Am J Pediatr Hematol Oncol.* 1992;141:88.
3. Mayall B, et al. Neutropenia due to low-dose methotrexate therapy for psoriasis and rheumatoid arthritis may be fatal. *Med J Aust.* 1991;155:480.

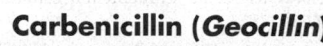

Carbenicillin (*Geocillin*)

Tobramycin (eg, *Nebcin*)

SUMMARY: Carbenicillin and some other penicillins inactivate tobramycin and other aminoglycosides in vitro and, in certain patients with severe renal dysfunction, in vivo. the effect of the aminoglycoside can be reduced.

RISK FACTORS:

➡ *Route of Administration.* In vitro mixing of the antibiotics before administration can increase the risk of interaction.

➡ *Concurrent Diseases.* Patients with severe renal dysfunction are at increased risk.

➡ *Assay Delay.* Delay in aminoglycoside assay when penicillin is present in serum can increase the risk of interaction.

MECHANISM: Carbenicillin and ticarcillin (*Ticar*) (and probably the related extended spectrum penicillins: azlocillin, mezlocillin [*Mezlin*], and piperacillin [*Pipracil*]) chemically inactivate aminoglycosides, such as tobramycin and gentamicin (eg, *Garamycin*).

CLINICAL EVALUATION: Good evidence exists for the in vitro inactivation of tobramycin and gentamicin by carbenicillin or ticarcillin, but such inactivation is unlikely in vivo in patients with normal renal function.[1,2,6] In patients with severe renal impairment, clinical evidence indicates that carbenicillin, piperacillin, or ticarcillin may inactivate tobramycin and gentamicin in vivo, causing a reduction of their antimicrobial efficacy.[3-5,7,8-10] In addition, aminoglycoside serum assays may be affected by penicillin therapy, especially if the assay of the serum sample is delayed.

RELATED DRUGS: Other extended spectrum penicillins (eg, ticarcillin, piperacillin) are likely to inactivate some aminoglycosides (eg, gentamicin). Amikacin (eg, *Amikin*) and netilmicin (*Netromycin*) may be less likely to interact with extended spectrum penicillins.

MANAGEMENT OPTIONS:

➡ **Consider Alternative.** Choose an alternative antibiotic for the aminoglycoside or the penicillin. Amikacin and netilmicin may be less likely than other aminoglycosides to interact with extended spectrum penicillins; however, observe the same precautions with all combinations of aminoglycosides and extended spectrum penicillins.

➡ **Circumvent/Minimize.** Avoid mixing antibiotics in vitro (eg, in the same IV bag or line).

➡ **Monitor.** If the antibiotics must be coadministered, evaluations of serum tobramycin (or other aminoglycoside) concentrations should consider the possibility of the interaction (note potential) for in vitro serum inactivational and adjust doses accordingly.

REFERENCES:

1. Riff LJ, et al. Laboratory and clinical conditions for gentamicin inactivation by carbenicillin. *Arch Intern Med.* 1972;130:887.
2. McLaughlin JE, et al. Clinical and laboratory evidence for inactivation of gentamicin by carbenicillin. *Lancet.* 1971;1:261.
3. Ervin FR, et al. Inactivation of gentamicin by penicillins in patients with renal failure. *Antimicrob Agents Chemother.* 1976;9:1004.
4. Weibert RT, et al. Carbenicillin-gentamicin interaction in acute renal failure. *Am J Hosp Pharm.* 1977;34:1137.
5. Davies M, et al. Interactions of carbenicillin and ticarcillin with gentamicin. *Antimicrob Agents Chemother.* 1975;7:431.
6. Henderson JL, et al. In vitro inactivation of gentamicin, tobramycin, and netilmicin by carbenicillin, azlocillin, or mezlocillin. *Am J Hosp Pharm.* 1981;38:1167.
7. Matzke GR, et al. Effect of ticarcillin on gentamicin and tobramycin pharmacokinetics in a patient with end-stage renal disease. *Pharmacotherapy.* 1984;4:158.
8. Halstenson CE, et al. Effect of concomitant administration of piperacillin on the disposition of netilmicin and tobramycin in patients with end-stage renal disease. *Antimicrob Agents Chemother.* 1990;34:128.
9. Uber WE, et al. In vivo inactivation of tobramycin by piperacillin. *DICP. Ann Pharmacother.* 1991;25:357.
10. Halstenson CE, et al. Effect of concomitant administration of piperacillin on the disposition of isepanicin and gentamicin in patients with end-stage renal disease. *Antimicrob Agents Chemother.* 1992;36:1832.

Carbenoxolone

Chlorthalidone (eg, *Hygroton*)

SUMMARY: Severe hypokalemia may result from the coadministration of carbenoxolone and chlorthalidone.

RISK FACTORS: No specific risk factors are known.

MECHANISM: Chlorthalidone and carbenoxolone may have additive potassium-wasting effects.

CLINICAL EVALUATION: A patient receiving carbenoxolone and chlorthalidone with no potassium supplementation developed a severe potassium deficiency with associated rhabdomyolysis and acute tubular necrosis.[1]

RELATED DRUGS: The combination of carbenoxolone with other potassium-wasting diuretics such as furosemide (eg, *Lasix*), bumetanide (eg, *Bumex*), metolazone (eg, *Zaroxolyn*), or thiazides would most likely produce a similar effect, especially in the absence of potassium supplementation.

MANAGEMENT OPTIONS:

➡ *Monitor.* Closely monitor the potassium status of patients receiving carbenoxolone and a potassium-wasting. Potassium supplementation may be necessary.

REFERENCES:

1. Descamps C. Rhabdomyolysis and acute tubular necrosis associated with carbenoxolone and diuretic treatment. *BMJ.* 1977;1:272.

Carboplatin (*Paraplatin*)

Gentamicin (eg, *Garamycin*)

SUMMARY: The combination of carboplatin and aminoglycoside antibiotics causes more hearing loss than would be expected with either agent alone.

RISK FACTORS: No specific risk factors are known.

MECHANISM: Not established. Because carboplatin and aminoglycosides may cause ototoxicity, the effect may be additive when the 2 are used together.

CLINICAL EVALUATION: In a dose-escalation trial of carboplatin, significant hearing loss, documented by audiometry, occurred in 5 patients, all of whom had prior or recent exposure to aminoglycosides, and 4 of whom were receiving concurrent aminoglycosides.[1] Because this trial involved high doses of carboplatin, it is not known whether this is a clinically relevant interaction at more conventional doses.

RELATED DRUGS: It is likely that other aminoglycosides such as amikacin (eg, *Amikin*), kanamycin (eg, *Kantrex*), netilmicin (*Netromycin*), streptomycin, and tobramycin (eg, *Nebcin*) also may result in additive ototoxicity with carboplatin.

MANAGEMENT OPTIONS:

➡ *Consider Alternative.* Consider alternatives to aminoglycosides in patients receiving high doses of carboplatin.

➡ *Monitor.* If aminoglycosides are used, be alert for evidence of ototoxicity.

REFERENCES:

1. Lee EJ, et al. Phase I and pharmacokinetic trial of carboplatin in refractory adult leukemia. *J Natl Cancer Inst.* 1988;80:131-35.

Carisoprodol (eg, *Soma*)

Oxycodone (eg, *Oxycontin*)

SUMMARY: A patient on oxycodone became unconscious after adding an excessive dose of carisoprodol.

RISK FACTORS: No specific risk factors are known.

MECHANISM: Both carisoprodol and oxycodone are CNS depressants, and their effects may be additive.

CLINICAL EVALUATION: A 49-year-old woman on long-term therapy with oxycodone 40 mg twice daily started taking carisoprodol 1,400 mg/day.[1] A week later, she began taking carisoprodol at a dosage of 2,800 to 3,500 mg/day. She was found unconscious on the floor, but rapidly returned to alertness when given naloxone 2 mg. The excessive CNS depression most likely resulted from oxycodone plus an excessive dose of carisoprodol.

RELATED DRUGS: Carisoprodol is expected to increase the CNS depression of other opiates in addition to oxycodone.

MANAGEMENT OPTIONS:

➥ *Monitor.* Use carisoprodol and oxycodone (or other opiates) concomitantly only with careful monitoring for excessive CNS depression.

REFERENCES:

1. Reeves RR, et al. Possible dangerous interaction of *Oxycontin* and carisoprodol. *Am Fam Physician.* 2003;67(11):2273.

Carmustine (eg, *BiCNU*)

Cimetidine (eg, *Tagamet*)

SUMMARY: Epidemiological evidence indicates that cimetidine increases the myelotoxicity of carmustine.

RISK FACTORS: No specific risk factors are known.

MECHANISM: Not established. Cimetidine might inhibit the metabolism of carmustine, or the 2 drugs may have additive effects on the bone marrow.

CLINICAL EVALUATION: Patients receiving carmustine plus cimetidine appear to manifest a greater degree of bone marrow suppression than those receiving carmustine alone.[1,2]

RELATED DRUGS: Little is known regarding the effect of cimetidine on the myelosuppressive effect of other cytotoxic drugs, but be alert for such effects. Isolated reports indicate that chloramphenicol (eg, *Chloromycetin*)[3] and phenytoin (eg, *Dilantin*)[4,5] may be more myelosuppressive in the presence of cimetidine. A similar interaction has been reported with lomustine (*CeeNU*), another nitrosourea.[6] Severe myelosuppression developed in a 55-year-old man receiving lomustine and cimetidine and resolved rapidly upon discontinuation of cimetidine. Myelosuppression from subsequent doses of lomustine, after the cimetidine had been discontinued, was less severe. The effect of other H_2-receptor antagonists, such as famotidine (eg, *Pepcid*), nizatidine (eg, *Axid*), and ranitidine (eg, *Zantac*), on carmustine is not established; theoretically, they may be less likely to interact.

MANAGEMENT OPTIONS:

➥ *Consider Alternative.* Theoretically, other H_2-receptor antagonists are less likely to interact.

➥ *Monitor.* Until more is known regarding the incidence and magnitude of this potential interaction, monitor carefully for evidence of excessive bone marrow suppression when cimetidine is used concurrently with carmustine or other myelosuppressive drugs.

REFERENCES:

1. Selker RG, et al. Bone-marrow depression with cimetidine plus carmustine. *N Engl J Med.* 1978;299(15):834.

2. Volkin RL, et al. Potentiation of carmustine-cranial irradiation-induced myelosuppression by cimetidine. *Arch Intern Med.* 1982;142(2):243-245.

3. Farber BF, et al. Rapid development of aplastic anemia after intravenous chloramphenicol and cimetidine therapy. *South Med J.* 1981;74(10):1257-1258.

4. Sazie E, et al. Severe granulocytopenia with cimetidine and phenytoin. *Ann Intern Med.* 1980;93(1):151-152.

5. Al-Kawas FH, et al. Cimetidine and agranulocytosis. *Ann Intern Med.* 1979;90(6):992-993.

6. Hess WA, et al. Combination of lomustine and cimetidine in the treatment of a patient with malignant glioblastoma: a case report. *Cancer Treat Rep.* 1985;69(6):733.

Carvedilol (eg, *Coreg*)

Cimetidine (eg, *Tagamet*)

SUMMARY: Cimetidine administration produces a modest increase in carvedilol plasma concentrations; some patients may experience increased beta-blockade.

RISK FACTORS: No specific risk factors are known.

MECHANISM: Cimetidine may inhibit 1 or more of carvedilol's metabolic pathways (eg, CYP1A2, CYP2D6), but the exact mechanism is unknown.

CLINICAL EVALUATION: While specific data are limited, the manufacturer of carvedilol states that the coadministration of cimetidine 1,000 mg daily increased the mean area under the plasma concentration-time curve of carvedilol by approximately 30%.[1] Pending further data, observe patients receiving carvedilol and cimetidine for increased beta-blocker effects, such as hypotension or bradycardia.

RELATED DRUGS: Other beta-blockers metabolized by CYP2D6 (eg, metoprolol [eg, *Lopressor*], propranolol, timolol) are expected to interact in a similar manner with cimetidine. The H_2-receptor antagonists ranitidine (eg, *Zantac*), famotidine (eg, *Pepcid*), and nizatidine (eg, *Axid*) are not expected to interact with carvedilol.

MANAGEMENT OPTIONS:

➡ **Monitor.** Monitor patients stabilized on carvedilol for altered beta-blocker response if cimetidine is added to or removed from their drug regimen.

REFERENCES:

1. *Coreg* [package insert]. Research Triangle Park, NC: GlaxoSmithKline; 2008.

Carvedilol (eg, *Coreg*)

Cyclosporine (eg, *Neoral*)

SUMMARY: Carvedilol appears to increase the plasma concentration of cyclosporine; some reduction in the dose of cyclosporine may be required.

RISK FACTORS: No specific risk factors are known.

MECHANISM: Carvedilol has been demonstrated to inhibit P-glycoprotein in animal and in vitro models.[1,2] This mechanism would be consistent with increased bioavailability of cyclosporine or reduced elimination during carvedilol coadministration.

CLINICAL EVALUATION: When 21 renal transplant patients taking oral cyclosporine and atenolol were converted from atenolol to carvedilol (maximum dose, 50 mg daily), it was noted that their cyclosporine plasma concentrations increased over the several months of the study.[3] The dose of cyclosporine was reduced by an average of 20% to maintain therapeutic cyclosporine concentrations. Another report noted a 10% reduction in cyclosporine dosage following the addition of carvedilol to patients with cardiac transplants.[4] This report also stated that the coadministration of metoprolol did not alter cyclosporine dose requirements. Although the average magnitude of the effect of carvedilol on cyclosporine appears somewhat limited, interpatient variability warrants close monitoring of cyclosporine concentrations.

RELATED DRUGS: While sirolimus (*Rapamune*) and tacrolimus (*Prograf*) are both substrates of P-glycoprotein, it is unknown if carvedilol affects their pharmacokinetics.

MANAGEMENT OPTIONS:

➡ *Consider Alternative.* Other beta-blockers that do not inhibit P-glycoprotein (eg, metoprolol [eg, *Lopressor*]) could be considered for patients taking cyclosporine.

➡ *Monitor.* Monitor cyclosporine concentrations if carvedilol is added to or removed from a patient's drug regimen.

REFERENCES:
1. Amioka K, et al. Carvedilol increases ciclosporin bioavailability by inhibiting P-glycoprotein–mediated transport. *J Pharm Pharmacol.* 2007;59(10):1383-1387.

2. Bachmakov I, et al. Characterization of beta-adrenoceptor antagonists as substrates and inhibitors of the drug transporter P-glycoprotein. *Fundam Clin Pharmacol.* 2006;20(3):273-282.

3. Kaijser M, et al. Elevation of cyclosporin A blood levels during carvedilol treatment in renal transplant patients. *Clin Transplant.* 1997;11(6):577-581.

4. Bader FM, et al. The effect of beta-blocker use on cyclosporine level in cardiac transplant recipients. *J Heart Lung Transplant.* 2005;24(12):2144-2147.

Carvedilol (eg, *Coreg*)

Digoxin (eg, *Lanoxin*)

SUMMARY: Carvedilol appears to modestly increase digoxin concentrations. Some patients may require a reduction in digoxin dose to avoid toxicity.

RISK FACTORS: No specific risk factors are known.

MECHANISM: Carvedilol may increase the absorption of digoxin (reduced intestinal wall edema or inhibition of intestinal P-glycoprotein) and/or reduce its renal elimination (renal tubular P-glycoprotein inhibition). In vitro studies have demonstrated carvedilol inhibition of digoxin transport via P-glycoprotein.[1,2]

CLINICAL EVALUATION: Several studies have examined the effects of both short- and long-term carvedilol dosing on digoxin pharmacokinetics.[3-6] The mean area under the concentration-time curve of digoxin was increased 14% to 20%.[3,5] A study of 8 children noted an average 50% decrease in the oral clearance of digoxin when administered with carvedilol.[6] It is not clear why children may be more sensitive than adults to carvedilol and digoxin coadministration; however, children have been reported to have a higher baseline digoxin clearance than adults.

RELATED DRUGS: It is possible that carvedilol would have a similar effect on digitoxin concentrations. No other beta-blockers have been identified as inhibitors of P-glycoprotein transporters.

MANAGEMENT OPTIONS:

➡ **Monitor.** Check digoxin concentrations in patients whenever carvedilol is added to or deleted from drug regimens. Watch for signs of digoxin toxicity, including arrhythmias, anorexia, nausea, or visual changes.

REFERENCES:

1. Takara K, et al. Interaction of digoxin with antihypertensive drugs via MDR1. *Life Sci.* 2002;70(13):1491-1500.
2. Kakumoto M, et al. Effects of carvedilol on MDR1-mediated multidrug resistance: comparison with verapamil. *Cancer Sci.* 2003;94(1):81-86.
3. De Mey C, et al. Carvedilol increases the systemic bioavailability of oral digoxin. *Br J Clin Pharmacol.* 1990;29(4):486-490.
4. Grunden JW, et al. Augmented digoxin concentrations with carvedilol dosing in mild-moderate heart failure. *Am J Ther.* 1994;1(2):157-161.
5. Wermeling DP, et al. Effects of long-term oral carvedilol on the steady-state pharmacokinetics of oral digoxin in patients with mild to moderate hypertension. *Pharmacotherapy.* 1994;14(5):600-606.
6. Ratnapalan S, et al. Digoxin-carvedilol interactions in children. *J Pediatr.* 2003;142(5):572-574.

Carvedilol (eg, *Coreg*)

Fluoxetine (eg, *Prozac*)

SUMMARY: Fluoxetine increases the plasma concentrations of carvedilol; the clinical significance is unknown, but increased cardiovascular effects, such as hypotension or bradycardia, may result.

RISK FACTORS: Extensive metabolizers of CYP2D6 will be affected to a greater degree than poor CYP2D6 metabolizers.

MECHANISM: Fluoxetine is a CYP2D6 inhibitor and reduces the metabolism of R-carvedilol to a greater extent than S-carvedilol because the R-enantiomer is more dependent on CYP2D6 for its metabolism.

CLINICAL EVALUATION: Ten patients with heart failure taking carvedilol 25 to 50 mg/day were administered fluoxetine 20 mg or placebo for 30 days.[1] The area under the concentration-time curve (AUC) of the R-enantiomer of carvedilol was increased approximately 78%, while the AUC of the S-enantiomer was not significantly affected by fluoxetine coadministration. The oral clearance of R-carvedilol and S-carvedilol were reduced 56% and 44%, respectively. The clinical significance of these changes is unclear; however, an increase in carvedilol's alpha- and beta-blocking effects may be seen.

RELATED DRUGS: Paroxetine (eg, *Paxil*) is also a potent inhibitor of CYP2D6 and is likely to affect carvedilol in a similar manner. Fluoxetine may also inhibit the metabolism of other beta-blockers that are metabolized by CYP2D6, including metoprolol (eg, *Lopressor*), propranolol (eg, *Inderal*), and timolol.

MANAGEMENT OPTIONS:

➡ *Consider Alternative.* Other selective serotonin reuptake inhibitor antidepressants, such as citalopram (eg, *Celexa*) or nefazodone, do not inhibit CYP2D6 and would be less likely to alter carvedilol plasma concentrations. If not treating heart failure, a beta-blocker that does not undergo CYP2D6 metabolism, such as atenolol (eg, *Tenormin*), could be considered.

➡ *Monitor.* Watch for increased alpha- or beta-blocking effects if carvedilol is coadministered with fluoxetine.

REFERENCES:

1. Graff DW, et al. Effect of fluoxetine on carvedilol stereo-specific pharmacokinetics in patients with heart failure. *Clin Pharmacol Ther.* 1999;65(2):148.

 ## 4   Carvedilol (eg, *Coreg*)

Rifampin (eg, *Rifadin*)

SUMMARY: Rifampin reduces the plasma concentrations of carvedilol; a reduction in efficacy may result.

RISK FACTORS: No specific risk factors are known.

MECHANISM: Rifampin induces the metabolism of carvedilol, most likely by increasing CYP2C9 activity. Rifampin may also increase CYP2D6 activity to a limited degree.

CLINICAL EVALUATION: Although published data are lacking, the manufacturer of carvedilol reports that rifampin 600 mg/day for 12 days reduced the carvedilol area under the concentration-time curve by approximately 70%.[1] Carvedilol is primarily metabolized by CYP2D6 and CYP2C9. The S-enantiomer of carvedilol has beta-blocking activity, while both the R- and S-enantiomers have alpha-blocking properties. S-carvedilol undergoes more extensive first-pass metabolism than the R-enantiomer, while R-carvedilol is more dependent on CYP2D6 for its metabolism. Based on these differences between the enantiomers, rifampin may have a greater effect on S-carvedilol than on R-carvedilol. This could result in a shift in carvedilol's activity away from beta blockade to a more predominant alpha-blocker. However, no data are provided by the manufacturer on the effect of rifampin on the individual isomers of carvedilol. The clinical effect, if any, of this change in pharmacologic activity is unknown.

RELATED DRUGS: Rifabutin (*Mycobutin*) is also expected to increase the metabolism of carvedilol.

MANAGEMENT OPTIONS:

➡ *Monitor.* Pending further data, monitor for reduced carvedilol efficacy if it is administered with rifampin or other enzyme inducers.

REFERENCES:

1. *Coreg* [package insert]. Research Triangle Park, NC: GlaxoSmithKline; 1998.

Caspofungin (*Cancidas*)

Cyclosporine (eg, *Neoral*)

SUMMARY: Acute cyclosporine dosing increases caspofungin plasma concentrations; monitor for increased caspofungin side effects.

RISK FACTORS: No specific risk factors are known.

MECHANISM: Unknown.

CLINICAL EVALUATION: While only limited details are currently available, the manufacturer of caspofungin notes that the mean area under the plasma concentration-time curve of caspofungin was increased 35% following one 4 mg/kg or two 3 mg/kg doses of cyclosporine compared with caspofungin administered alone.[1] The effect of chronic cyclosporine dosing on caspofungin plasma concentrations is not known. Caspofungin does not alter cyclosporine plasma concentrations.[1] Pending further data, monitor patients receiving this combination for increased caspofungin concentrations.

RELATED DRUGS: No information is available.

MANAGEMENT OPTIONS:

➡ *Monitor.* Monitor patients receiving cyclosporine and caspofungin for increased caspofungin effect including elevated liver enzymes, flushing, or nausea.

REFERENCES:
1. *Cancidas* [package insert]. White House Station, NJ: Merck & Co, Inc.; 2005.

Caspofungin (*Cancidas*)

Rifampin (eg, *Rifadin*)

SUMMARY: Rifampin decreases caspofungin plasma concentrations; monitor for reduced caspofungin efficacy.

RISK FACTORS: No specific risk factors are known.

MECHANISM: Unknown. It appears that rifampin is a modest inducer of caspofungin elimination.

CLINICAL EVALUATION: A 14-day course of caspofungin 50 mg intravenously once daily was administered alone and with rifampin 600 mg orally once daily.[1] When caspofungin and rifampin were initiated on the same day, caspofungin area under the concentration-time curve (AUC) was increased about 60% on the first day of concomitant administration. After 14 days of concurrent therapy or when rifampin was initiated before caspofungin, no significant change in caspofungin AUC was noted. With concurrent rifampin therapy, caspofungin trough plasma concentrations were about 30% lower compared with caspofungin administered alone. The reduction in caspofungin trough concentrations may reduce its antifungal efficacy. Caspofungin administration did not alter rifampin plasma concentrations.

RELATED DRUGS: No data is available.

MANAGEMENT OPTIONS:

➡ *Circumvent/Minimize.* The manufacturer suggests increasing the dose of caspofungin to 70 mg daily during coadministration with rifampin.

➡ **Monitor.** Observe patients for loss of caspofungin efficacy during concomitant administration of rifampin.

REFERENCES:
1. Stone JA, et at. Potential for interactions between caspofungin and nelfinavir or rifampin. *Antimicrob Agents Chemother*. 2004;48:4306-4314.

Caspofungin (*Cancidas*)

Tacrolimus (*Prograf*)

SUMMARY: Caspofungin administration caused a modest reduction in the plasma concentration of tacrolimus.

RISK FACTORS: No specific risk factors are known.

MECHANISM: Unknown.

CLINICAL EVALUATION: While only limited details are available, the manufacturer of caspofungin notes that tacrolimus plasma concentrations were decreased 20% to 25% following 10 days of caspofungin 70 mg/daily compared with tacrolimus administered alone.[1] Some patients may experience reduced tacrolimus efficacy during the administration of caspofungin.

RELATED DRUGS: Micafungin does not appear to alter the plasma concentrations of tacrolimus.

MANAGEMENT OPTIONS:

➡ **Monitor.** Monitor tacrolimus plasma concentrations during concurrent caspofungin administration.

REFERENCES:
1. *Cancidas* [package insert]. White House Station, NJ: Merck & Co, Inc.; 2005.

Cefamandole (*Mandol*)

Ethanol (Ethyl Alcohol)

SUMMARY: Cefamandole and some other cephalosporins may cause a disulfiram-like reaction when administered with ethanol.

RISK FACTORS: No specific risk factors are known.

MECHANISM: The disulfiram-like reactions caused by some cephalosporins may be the result of acetaldehyde accumulation.

CLINICAL EVALUATION: Several cephalosporins (eg, cefamandole, cefoperazone [*Cefobid*], cefotetan [*Cefotan*], moxalactam) have produced disulfiram-like reactions (eg, flushing, nausea, headache, tachycardia) following the ingestion of alcohol.[1-6] The reactions have been mild in most cases, but in a few patients, the reactions have been severe, necessitating the use of fluids and dopamine to correct hypotension. The reaction closely resembles the disulfiram-alcohol reaction with respect to onset, symptoms, and severity.

RELATED DRUGS: Cefoperazone, cefotetan, and moxalactam also produce disulfiram reactions following alcohol ingestion.

MANAGEMENT OPTIONS:

➡ *Circumvent/Minimize.* Counsel patients to avoid alcohol while taking the cephalosporins noted and for 2 to 3 days after discontinuing the cephalosporin.

➡ *Monitor.* If ethanol is administered to a patient taking cefamandole or other cephalosporins, be alert for flushing, nausea, headache, or tachycardia.

REFERENCES:

1. Neu HC, et al. Interaction between moxalactam and alcohol. *Lancet.* 1980;1:1422.
2. Portier H, et al. Interaction between cephalosporins and alcohol. *Lancet.* 1980;2:263.
3. Drummer S, et al. Antabuse-like effect of beta-lactam antibiotics. *N Engl J Med.* 1980;303:1417-1418.
4. Elenbaas RM, et al. On the disulfiram-like activity of moxalactam. *Clin Pharmacol Ther.* 1982;32:347-355.
5. Buening MK, et al. Disulfiram-like reaction to beta-lactams. *JAMA.* 1981;245:2027.
6. Kline SS, et al. Cefotetan-induced disulfiram-type reactions and hypoprothrombinemia. *Antimicrob Agents Chemother.* 1987;31:1328-1331.

Cefixime (*Suprax*)

Nifedipine (eg, *Procardia*)

SUMMARY: Nifedipine increases the serum concentration of cefixime; this effect is unlikely to produce adverse effects.

RISK FACTORS: No specific risk factors are known.

MECHANISM: Nifedipine appears to enhance the active transport mechanism in the intestinal epithelial cells that is responsible for cefixime absorption.

CLINICAL EVALUATION: The peak serum concentration of cefixime was increased 46% by nifedipine 20 mg and its area under the concentration-time curve increased 69%.[1] The bioavailability of cefixime was 31% when administered with placebo and 53% when administered with nifedipine. The absorption rate of cefixime was increased by nifedipine administration. While the wide therapeutic ratio for cefixime limits the clinical significance of this interaction, nifedipine might affect other drugs that have absorption characteristics similar to cefixime.

RELATED DRUGS: No information is available.

MANAGEMENT OPTIONS: No specific action is required, but be alert for evidence of the interaction.

REFERENCES:

1. Duverne C, et al. Modification of cefixime bioavailability by nifedipine in humans: involvement of the dipeptide carrier system. *Antimicrob Agents Chemother.* 1992;36:2462.

Cefpodoxime Proxetil (*Vantin*)

Ranitidine (eg, *Zantac*)

SUMMARY: Serum concentrations of cefpodoxime proxetil are reduced by coadministration of agents that increase gastric pH; antibiotic efficacy may be reduced.

RISK FACTORS: No specific risk factors are known.

MECHANISM: Increasing the gastric pH appears to reduce the dissolution or absorption of cefpodoxime proxetil.

CLINICAL EVALUATION: The area under the cefpodoxime serum concentration-time curve (AUC) was reduced 29% and its peak concentration fell 33% following ranitidine administration.[1] Similar reductions in AUC and peak concentrations were observed following the administration of 12.6 g sodium bicarbonate or 7.68 g aluminum hydroxide 10 minutes before the cefpodoxime. Similarly, cefuroxime axetil (eg, *Ceftin*) AUC was reduced more than 40% by the coadministration of ranitidine 300 mg.[2] The AUC of cefpodoxime was reduced 40% during famotidine (eg, *Pepcid*) administration.[5] The clinical importance of these changes is unknown, but reduction in efficacy is possible in some patients.

RELATED DRUGS: Cefuroxime axetil concentrations are reduced by ranitidine. Cefetamet pivoxil and cefixime (*Suprax*) appear to be unaffected by concurrent ranitidine administration. Other H_2-receptor antagonists (eg, cimetidine [eg, *Tagamet*], nizatidine [*Axid*]), antacids, and proton pump inhibitors (eg, omeprazole [*Prilosec*], lansoprazole [*Prevacid*]) would be expected to have similar effects.

MANAGEMENT OPTIONS:

➡ *Consider Alternative.* Cefetamet pivoxil pharmacokinetics were not affected by *Maalox* or ranitidine administration;[3] similarly, cefixime pharmacokinetics were unaffected by antacids.[4] Pending determination of the clinical importance of the changes in serum concentrations, patients receiving cefpodoxime proxetil or cefuroxime axetil should avoid agents that increase gastric pH.

➡ *Monitor.* If the drugs are used together, watch for diminished antibiotic effect.

REFERENCES:
1. Hughes GS, et al. The effects of gastric pH and food on the pharmacokinetics of a new oral cephalosporin, cefpodoxime proxetil. *Clin Pharmacol Ther.* 1989;46:674.
2. Sommers DEK, et al. Influence of food and reduced gastric acidity on the bioavailability of bacampicillin and cefuroxime axetil. *Br J Clin Pharmacol.* 1984;18:535.
3. Blouin RA, et al. Influence of antacid and ranitidine on the pharmacokinetics of oral cefetamet pivoxil. *Antimicrob Agents Chemother.* 1990;34:1744.
4. Petitjean O, et al. Study of a possible pharmacokinetic interaction between cefixime and two antacids. *Presse Med.* 1989;18:1596.
5. Saathoff N, et al. Pharmacokinetics of cefpodoxime proxetil and interactions with an antacid and an H_2-receptor antagonist. *Antimicrob Agents Chemother.* 1992;36:796.

Cefprozil (*Cefzil*)

Metoclopramide (eg, *Reglan*)

SUMMARY: Metoclopramide causes a small reduction in the plasma concentrations of cefprozil compared with those produced when cefprozil is administered in the fasting state. The clinical significance of this interaction appears limited.

RISK FACTORS: No specific risk factors are known.

MECHANISM: Metoclopramide increases the rate of cefprozil's gastric emptying but it does not appear to alter the amount of cefprozil absorbed.

CLINICAL EVALUATION: A single 30 mg dose of metoclopramide taken 0.5 hours before 250 mg cefprozil reduced the peak cefprozil concentration 12% (not significant) and reduced the time-to-peak concentration from 1.5 to 1 hours.[1] The area under the plasma concentration-time curve of cefprozil was not altered by metoclopramide.

RELATED DRUGS: Cisapride (available only through an investigational limited access program) might affect cefprozil in a similar manner.

MANAGEMENT OPTIONS: No specific action is required, but be alert for evidence of the interaction.

REFERENCES:

1. Shukla UA, et al. Pharmacokinetic interactions of cefprozil with food, propantheline, metoclopramide, and probenecid in healthy volunteers. *J Clin Pharmacol.* 1992;32:725.

Cefprozil (*Cefzil*)

Propantheline (eg, *Pro-Banthine*)

SUMMARY: The peak plasma concentrations of cefprozil are reduced and delayed when cefprozil is administered with propantheline compared with the fasting state. The clinical significance of this interaction appears limited.

RISK FACTORS: No specific risk factors are known.

MECHANISM: Propantheline slows gastric emptying and retards the absorption of cefprozil. It does not appear to reduce the amount of cefprozil absorbed.

CLINICAL EVALUATION: A single 30 mg dose of propantheline produced a 20% reduction in the peak cefprozil concentration and doubled the time to peak concentration from 1.5 to 3 hours.[1] The area under the plasma concentration-time curve of cefprozil was not altered. Propantheline's effects were similar on both isomers (cis and trans) of cefprozil. The clinical significance of this interaction is limited because the rate of cefprozil absorption, but not its extent, is reduced by propantheline.

RELATED DRUGS: Other drugs with anticholinergic activity might affect cefprozil in a similar manner.

MANAGEMENT OPTIONS: No specific action is required, but be alert for evidence of the interaction.

REFERENCES:

1. Shukla UA, et al. Pharmacokinetic interactions of cefprozil with food, propantheline, metoclopramide, and probenecid in healthy volunteers. *J Clin Pharmacol.* 1992;32:725.

Ceftazidime (*Fortaz*)

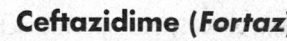

Chloramphenicol (eg, *Chloromycetin*)

SUMMARY: Chloramphenicol may inhibit the antibacterial activity of ceftazidime.

RISK FACTORS: No specific risk factors are known.

MECHANISM: A bacteriostatic drug such as chloramphenicol presumably may interfere with the action of a bactericidal agent such as a cephalosporin. Because cephalosporins act by inhibiting cell wall synthesis, agents that inhibit protein synthesis (eg, chloramphenicol) theoretically could reduce the bactericidal effect of cephalosporins.

CLINICAL EVALUATION: A 2.5-month-old infant was treated with IV chloramphenicol 100 mg/kg/day and ceftazidime 100 mg/kg/day for meningitis.[1] The minimum bactericidal concentration of ceftazidime was 0.5 mg/L. Four days later, the infant was clinically unimproved, and *S. enteritidis* was again cultured from the cerebrospinal fluid. Repeated titrations of varying concentrations of ceftazidime and chloramphenicol against the infecting organism demonstrated antagonism of ceftazidime by chloramphenicol. When concentrations of chloramphenicol were 4 mg/L or more, the bactericidal concentration for ceftazidime increased from 0.5 to 16 mg/L. Chloramphenicol was discontinued and the patient recovered after 7 additional days of ceftazidime monotherapy.

RELATED DRUGS: Other cephalosporins or antibiotics that inhibit bacterial cell wall synthesis also may be inhibited.

MANAGEMENT OPTIONS:

➡ *Consider Alternative.* Although definitive data are unavailable regarding the interaction of bactericidal and bacteriostatic antibiotics, it would be appropriate to avoid such combinations until they are proven to be without harm.

➡ *Monitor.* If chloramphenicol is used with a cephalosporin, carefully monitor the patient for continuing signs and symptoms of an interaction.

REFERENCES:
1. French, et al. Antagonism of ceftazidime by chloramphenicol *in vitro* and *in vivo* during treatment of gram negative meningitis. *BMJ.* 1985;291:636.

4   Ceftizoxime (*Cefizox*)

Probenecid (*Benemid*)

SUMMARY: Probenecid increases the serum concentration of ceftizoxime and other renally eliminated cephalosporins; the clinical significance is unknown, but increased efficacy or toxicity could result.

RISK FACTORS: No specific risk factors are known.

MECHANISM: Probenecid inhibits the renal excretion of cephalosporins.

CLINICAL EVALUATION: Probenecid reduces the renal clearance of most cephalosporins, resulting in increased serum concentrations.[1-4] It may be possible to reduce the dose of the cephalosporin when probenecid is administered. Because of the wide therapeutic window of cephalosporins, toxicity is unlikely.

RELATED DRUGS: Probenecid reduces renal clearance of most cephalosporins.

MANAGEMENT OPTIONS: No specific action is required, but be alert for evidence of the interaction.

REFERENCES:
1. Meister FL, et al. Reduction of ceftizoxime dosing interval by coadministration of probenecid. *Clin Pharmacol Ther.* 1986;39:210.
2. Mischler TW, et al. Influence of probenecid and food on the bioavailability of cephradine in normal male subjects. *J Clin Pharmacol.* 1974;14:604.

4   Ceftriaxone (*Rocephin*)

Diclofenac (eg, *Voltaren*)

SUMMARY: Diclofenac reduces the renal clearance of ceftriaxone and increases its biliary excretion. The clinical effects of this interaction are unknown.

RISK FACTORS: No specific risk factors are known.

MECHANISM: Not established.

CLINICAL EVALUATION: Patients taking diclofenac 50 mg every 12 hours had a 320% increase in the biliary excretion of ceftriaxone and a 56% reduction in ceftriaxone renal excretion.[1] The clinical significance of this interaction is probably limited.

RELATED DRUGS: Other nonsteroidal anti-inflammatory drugs may alter the renal excretion of other cephalosporins.

MANAGEMENT OPTIONS: No specific action is required, but be alert for evidence of the interaction.

REFERENCES:

1. Merle-Melet M, et al. Effects of diclofenac on ceftriaxone pharmacokinetics in humans. *Antimicrob Agents Chemother*. 1992;36:2331.

Ceftriaxone (*Rocephin*)
Verapamil (eg, *Calan*)

SUMMARY: The administration of a combination of ceftriaxone and clindamycin (eg, *Cleocin*) with verapamil has been reported to cause verapamil toxicity in a patient. The evidence for this interaction is poor.

RISK FACTORS: No specific risk factors are known.

MECHANISM: The authors of this report suggest that ceftriaxone or clindamycin displace verapamil from its protein-binding sites, causing an acute increase in verapamil concentration and cardiac toxicity.[1] This mechanism appears to be unlikely since the antibiotics are acidic drugs bound to albumin and verapamil is a basic drug bound to alpha$_1$-acid glycoprotein. Thus, the potential for protein-binding displacement would be very small. In addition, the relatively low protein binding of the active enantiomer of verapamil (88%) would tend to minimize any opportunity for a protein binding displacement reaction to produce a clinically relevant change in effect.

CLINICAL EVALUATION: A 59-year-old man was taking sustained-release verapamil 240 mg every 12 hours, methyldopa (eg, *Aldomet*) 250 mg every 12 hours, and phenytoin (eg, *Dilantin*) 300 mg/day for several years. He was treated with IV ceftriaxone 1 g and clindamycin 900 mg for pneumonia. Shortly after the antibiotics were administered, the patient developed bradycardia and heart block. Sixteen hours later, he converted to normal sinus rhythm. Verapamil concentrations were measured 20 hours after his last dose and found to be 212 ng/mL. Estimate the patient's verapamil concentration to be approximately 800 ng/ml at the time of admission. This concentration of verapamil is compatible with concentrations observed to cause junctional rhythms in subjects administered verapamil.[2] Thus, it seems probable that the adverse effect observed in this patient was not related to the coadministration of verapamil with ceftriaxone or clindamycin, but rather was caused by simple verapamil toxicity. No rechallenge with verapamil was reported.

RELATED DRUGS: No information is available.

MANAGEMENT OPTIONS: No specific action is required, but be alert for evidence of the interaction.

REFERENCES:

1. Kishore K, et al. Acute verapamil toxicity in a patient with chronic toxicity: possible interaction with ceftriaxone and clindamycin. *Ann Pharmacother*. 1993;26:877.
2. Horn JR, et al. Comment: pitfalls in reporting drug interactions. *Ann Pharmacother*. 1993;27:1545.

Cefuroxime (eg, Ceftin)

Ranitidine (eg, Zantac)

SUMMARY: Serum concentrations of cefpodoxime proxetil and cefuroxime axetil are reduced by coadministration of agents that increase gastric pH; antibiotic efficacy may be reduced.

RISK FACTORS: No specific risk factors are known.

MECHANISM: It appears that increasing the gastric pH reduces the dissolution or absorption of cefpodoxime proxetil and cefuroxime axetil.

CLINICAL EVALUATION: The area under the cefpodoxime (*Vantin*) serum concentration-time curve (AUC) was reduced 29%, and its peak concentration fell 33% following ranitidine administration.[1] Similar reductions in AUC and peak concentrations were observed following the administration of 12.6 mg sodium bicarbonate or 7.68 g aluminum hydroxide (eg, *Amphojel*) 10 minutes before cefpodoxime. Cefuroxime axetil AUC was reduced more than 40% by the coadministration of ranitidine 300 mg.[2] The AUC of cefpodoxime was reduced 40% during famotidine (eg, *Pepcid*) administration.[3] The clinical importance of these changes is unknown, but a reduction in efficacy is possible in some patients.

RELATED DRUGS: Cefpodoxime concentrations are reduced following ranitidine administration. Cefetamet pivoxil and cefixime (*Suprax*) appear to be unaffected by ranitidine coadministration.[4] Other H_2-receptor antagonists (eg, cimetidine [eg, *Tagamet*], famotidine [eg, *Pepcid*], nizatidine [eg, *Axid*]), antacids,[5] and proton pump inhibitors (eg, omeprazole [eg, *Prilosec*], lansoprazole [*Prevacid*]) are expected to have similar effects.

MANAGEMENT OPTIONS:

➡ *Consider Alternative.* Cefetamet pivoxil pharmacokinetics were not affected by *Maalox* or ranitidine administration; similarly, cefixime (*Suprax*) pharmacokinetics were unaffected by antacids. Pending determination of the clinical importance of the changes in serum concentrations, patients receiving cefpodoxime proxetil or cefuroxime axetil should avoid agents that increase gastric pH.

➡ *Monitor.* If the drugs are used together, watch for diminished antibiotic effect.

REFERENCES:

1. Hughes GS, et al. The effects of gastric pH and food on the pharmacokinetics of a new oral cephalosporin, cefpodoxime proxetil. *Clin Pharmacol Ther.* 1989;46:674-685.

2. Sommers DK, et al. Influence of food and reduced gastric acidity on the bioavailability of bacampicillin and cefuroxime axetil. *Br J Clin Pharmacol.* 1984;18:535-539.

3. Saathoff N, et al. Pharmacokinetics of cefpodoxime proxetil and interactions with an antacid and an H_2 receptor antagonist. *Antimicrob Agents Chemother.* 1992;36:796-800.

4. Blouin RA, et al. Influence of antacid and ranitidine on the pharmacokinetics of oral cefetamet pivoxil. *Antimicrob Agents Chemother.* 1990;34:1744-1748.

5. Petitjean O, et al. Pharmacokinetic interaction of cefixime and 2 antacids. Preliminary results [in French]. *Presse Med.* 1989;18:1596-1598.

Celecoxib (*Celebrex*)
Clopidogrel (*Plavix*)

SUMMARY: An elderly woman developed intracerebral hemorrhage after starting clopidogrel and celecoxib therapy, but a causal relationship was not established.

RISK FACTORS: No specific risk factors are known.

MECHANISM: Not established.

CLINICAL EVALUATION: An 86-year-old woman developed intracerebral hemorrhage 3 weeks after starting therapy with both clopidogrel 75 mg/day and celecoxib 200 mg/day.[1] It was not possible to rule out clopidogrel alone as the cause of the bleeding episode, and more clinical data are needed to establish a causal relationship.

RELATED DRUGS: No information is available.

MANAGEMENT OPTIONS: No specific action is required, but be alert for evidence of the interaction.

REFERENCES:
1. Fisher AA, et al. Intracerebral hemorrhage following possible interaction between celecoxib and clopidogrel. *Ann Pharmacother*. 2001;35:1567-1569.

Celecoxib (*Celebrex*)
Lithium (eg, *Eskalith*)

SUMMARY: Celecoxib has been associated with elevated lithium serum concentrations; monitor for lithium toxicity.

RISK FACTORS: No specific risk factors are known.

MECHANISM: Celecoxib probably reduces renal lithium clearance, presumably through inhibition of COX-2.

CLINICAL EVALUATION: Several cases of lithium toxicity have been reported following the use of celecoxib.[1,2] Given the nature of the case reports, a causal relationship cannot be conclusively established. Nonetheless, the fact that nonsteroidal anti-inflammatory drugs (inhibitors of COX-1 and COX-2) are known to cause lithium toxicity suggests that COX-2 inhibitors may produce a similar effect.

RELATED DRUGS: All COX-2 inhibitors, including rofecoxib (*Vioxx*) and valdecoxib (*Bextra*), appear to increase lithium serum concentrations. Some evidence suggests that rofecoxib produces the largest increases, but confirmation is needed.

MANAGEMENT OPTIONS:

➠ *Monitor.* If celecoxib is initiated in patients receiving lithium, monitor lithium concentrations and for evidence of lithium toxicity (eg, nausea, vomiting, diarrhea, anorexia, coarse tremor, slurred speech, vertigo, confusion, lethargy; in severe cases, seizures, stupor, coma, cardiovascular collapse).

REFERENCES:
1. Gunja N, et al. Lithium toxicity: a potential interaction with celecoxib. *Intern Med J*. 2002;32:494.
2. Phelan KM, et al. Lithium interaction with the cyclooxygenase 2 inhibitors rofecoxib and celecoxib and other nonsteroidal anti-inflammatory drugs. *J Clin Psychiatry*. 2003;64:1328-1334.

4   Celecoxib (*Celebrex*)

Rifampin (eg, *Rifadin*)

SUMMARY: Rifampin administration reduces celecoxib plasma concentrations; the effect on analgesic activity is unknown, but some reduction in celecoxib efficacy is expected.

RISK FACTORS: No specific risk factors are known.

MECHANISM: Rifampin appears to induce the hepatic metabolism of celecoxib, probably by increasing CYP2C9 activity.

CLINICAL EVALUATION: Celecoxib 200 mg twice daily and rifampin 600 mg daily or placebo were administered to 8 subjects for 11 days.[1] The area under the concentration-time curve of celecoxib was reduced nearly 50% by rifampin coadministration compared with placebo. While no estimate was made in this study of the analgesic effect of celecoxib, it is expected that some patients would have a reduced response to celecoxib following treatment with rifampin.

RELATED DRUGS: Rifabutin (*Mycobutin*) does not appear to be as potent an inducer as rifampin and is less likely to produce large reductions in the plasma concentrations of celecoxib. The effect of rifampin on rofecoxib (*Vioxx*) is unknown, but a similar response may be expected.

MANAGEMENT OPTIONS:

➡ *Monitor.* While no specific action is required, be alert for reduced celecoxib effect if rifampin is coadministered.

REFERENCES:

1. Porras AG, et al. The effects of metabolic induction by rifampin on the elimination of celecoxib and the effect of celecoxib on CYP2D6 metabolism. *Clin Pharmacol Ther*. 2001;69:P58.

4   Celecoxib (*Celebrex*)

Warfarin (eg, *Coumadin*)

SUMMARY: Isolated cases of increased warfarin response following celecoxib have been reported, but study in healthy subjects suggests that celecoxib does not affect the pharmacokinetics or hypoprothrombinemic response to warfarin.

RISK FACTORS: No specific risk factors are known.

MECHANISM: Not established.

CLINICAL EVALUATION: A 73-year-old woman on chronic warfarin 5 mg/day developed bleeding with an international normalized ratio (INR) of 5.7, five weeks after starting celecoxib.[1] No other cause for the excessive hypoprothrombinemia was found, but a causal relationship was not clear. Similar cases of increased warfarin response, usually in the elderly, have been reported to the FDA. However, a randomized parallel study in 24 healthy subjects found no effect of celecoxib 200 mg twice daily for 7 days on the pharmacokinetics or prothrombin time response to multiple-dose warfarin.[2] In the absence of any well-documented cases in the literature, one cannot conclude that celecoxib increases the hypoprothrombinemic response to warfarin. Nonetheless, one cannot rule out the possibility that an interaction may occur in an occasional predisposed patient.

RELATED DRUGS: Rofecoxib (*Vioxx*) is like celecoxib in that it does not affect platelets and is probably less likely than standard NSAIDs to adversely affect the GI tract. Preliminary evidence suggests that rofecoxib slightly increases the hypoprothrombinemic response to warfarin.

MANAGEMENT OPTIONS: No specific action is required, but be alert for evidence of the interaction.

REFERENCES:

1. Mersfelder TL, et al. Warfarin and celecoxib interaction. *Ann Pharmacother*. 2000;34:325.
2. Karim A, et al. Celecoxib does not significantly alter the pharmacokinetics or hypoprothrombinemic effect of warfarin in healthy subjects. *J Clin Pharmacol*. 2000;40:655.

Charcoal 2

Digoxin (eg, *Lanoxin*)

SUMMARY: Activated charcoal significantly reduces digoxin serum concentrations, and, apparently to a lesser extent, digitoxin[†] serum concentrations.

RISK FACTORS: No specific risk factors are known.

MECHANISM: Activated charcoal appears to adsorb digoxin in the GI tract, thus preventing absorption and enterohepatic circulation.

CLINICAL EVALUATION: Six healthy subjects were administered digoxin 0.25 mg alone and within 5 minutes of ingesting 8 g of activated charcoal.[1] The charcoal reduced the absorption of digoxin 96%. Similar results have been reported following 10 and 50 g doses of charcoal.[2,3] Charcoal 2 g 3 times daily for 12 days reduced digoxin and digitoxin serum concentrations 30% and 18%, respectively.[3] If charcoal interferes with the enterohepatic circulation of digitalis glycosides, separation of the doses of charcoal and digitalis will not avoid the interaction completely.

RELATED DRUGS: Digitalis concentrations are also reduced by charcoal coadministration, but to an apparently lesser extent than digoxin.

MANAGEMENT OPTIONS:

➡ *Avoid Unless Benefit Outweighs Risk.* Do not administer activated charcoal to patients taking digoxin because loss of the therapeutic effect of digoxin is likely. This combination might be beneficial in patients with digitalis glycoside intoxication.

➡ *Monitor.* Monitor patients taking digoxin or digitoxin for reduced glycoside concentrations if charcoal is coadministered.

REFERENCES:

1. Neuvonen PJ, et al. Effects of resins and activated charcoal on the absorption of digoxin, carbamazepine and frusemide. *Br J Clin Pharmacol*. 1988;25(2):229.
2. Reissell P, et al. Effect of administration of activated charcoal and fibre on absorption, excretion and steady-state blood levels of digoxin and digitoxin. Evidence for intestinal secretion of the glycosides. *Acta Med Scand Suppl*. 1982; 668:88-90.
3. Neuvonen PJ, et al. Reduction of absorption of digoxin, phenytoin and aspirin by activated charcoal in man. *Eur J Clin Pharmacol*. 1978;13(3):213-218.

† Not available in the United States.

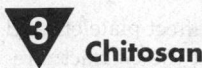 **Chitosan**

Valproic Acid (eg, *Depakene*)

SUMMARY: Isolated cases suggest that chitosan may reduce valproic acid serum concentrations, leading to seizures.

RISK FACTORS: No specific risk factors are known.

MECHANISM: Not established. It is proposed that the tertiary amino group on the chitosan may bind with the anionic group on the valproic acid.

CLINICAL EVALUATION: A 35-year-old woman on valproate and phenobarbital who had not had seizures for 3 years developed a sudden reappearance of seizures a few days after starting chitosan as a dietary supplement.[1] The seizures abated after the chitosan was stopped, but 3 months later she resumed taking chitosan and the seizures recurred within 5 days. The valproate serum concentration was undetectable, while the phenobarbital concentration was therapeutic. Chitosan was stopped, and within 4 days, the valproate concentrations returned to baseline. In another case, a 29-year-old woman on valproate with no seizures for 2 years developed seizure recurrence after taking chitosan for 1 week.[1] Valproate serum concentrations were undetectable, and the seizures abated after the chitosan was discontinued. Both of these cases are rated "probable" using the Drug Interaction Probability Scale (DIPS),[2] although the first case was clearly stronger.

RELATED DRUGS: No information is available.

MANAGEMENT OPTIONS:

➡ ***Monitor.*** If a patient on valproic acid starts taking chitosan, monitor for reduced valproic acid response; serum valproic acid determinations may be useful.

REFERENCES:

1. Striano P, et al. Chitosan may decrease serum valproate and increase the risk of seizure reappearance. *BMJ.* 2009;339:b3751.
2. Horn JR, et al. Proposal for a new tool to evaluate drug interaction cases. *Ann Pharmacother.* 2007;41(4):674-680.

 Chitosan

Warfarin (eg, *Coumadin*)

SUMMARY: A patient on warfarin therapy developed an increased international normalized ratio (INR) on 2 occasions when he took chitosan concomitantly.

RISK FACTORS: No specific risk factors are known.

MECHANISM: Not established. It is possible that the chitosan reduced the GI absorption of vitamin K, thus enhancing the anti–vitamin K activity of warfarin.

CLINICAL EVALUATION: An 83-year-old man on long-term warfarin therapy developed a marked increase in his INR on 2 occasions after self-medicating with chitosan.[1] There was a positive dechallenge after the second course of chitosan. This case is rated "probable" using the Drug Interaction Probability Scale (DIPS).[2] Although more study is needed to determine if chitosan affects warfarin response, the potential severity of the interaction warrants attention.

RELATED DRUGS: No information is available.

MANAGEMENT OPTIONS:

➡ *Monitor.* If chitosan is used concurrently with warfarin, monitor the warfarin response if chitosan is started, stopped, or changed in dosage.

REFERENCES:

1. Huang SS, et al. Chitosan potentiation of warfarin effect. *Ann Pharmacother.* 2007;41(11):1912-1914.

2. Horn JR, et al. Proposal for a new tool to evaluate drug interaction cases. *Ann Pharmacother.* 2007;41(4):674-680.

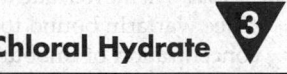

Chloral Hydrate

Ethanol (Ethyl Alcohol)

SUMMARY: Ethanol and chloral hydrate have at least additive CNS-depressant effects; combined use may be dangerous in patients performing tasks requiring alertness.

RISK FACTORS: No specific risk factors are known.

MECHANISM: In vitro studies indicate that a metabolite of chloral hydrate, trichloroethanol, inhibits the metabolism of ethanol. Ethanol, in turn, appears to stimulate the formation of trichloroethanol and inhibit its conjugation with glucuronide.[1-4]

CLINICAL EVALUATION: The coadministration of ethanol and chloral hydrate can elevate plasma trichloroethanol and blood ethanol.[4] Because all of these agents are CNS depressants, the combination of chloral hydrate and ethanol has at least additive (and probably synergistic) CNS depressant activity. Performance of a complex motor task is considerably more affected by chloral hydrate plus ethanol than by either agent alone.[5] Another type of reaction (eg, flushing, tachycardia, headache) occasionally occurs when ethanol is ingested by a patient who has been receiving chloral hydrate.[5,6] This vasodilation reaction probably occurs to a lesser extent in many other patients who do not manifest the full symptomatic reaction.

RELATED DRUGS: Alcohol would be expected to increase the CNS depression of all sedative-hypnotic drugs.

MANAGEMENT OPTIONS:

➡ *Circumvent/Minimize.* Warn patients taking chloral hydrate of the combined CNS depressant activity with ethanol. Patients with cardiovascular disease who are taking chloral hydrate should be careful about ingesting ethanol because of tachycardia and hypotension associated with the vasodilation reaction.

➡ *Monitor.* If the combination is used, monitor for excessive CNS depression, flushing, headache, and tachycardia.

REFERENCES:

1. Kaplan HL, et al. Chloral hydrate and alcohol metabolism in human subjects. *J Forensic Sci.* 1967;12(3):295-304.

2. Freeman J, et al. Reactions of chloral hydrate and ethanol with alcohol dehydrogenase from human liver. *Fed Proc.* 1970;29:275.

3. Gessner PK, et al. A study of the interaction of the hypnotic effects and of the toxic effects of chloral hydrate and ethanol. *J Pharmacol Exp Ther.* 1970;174(2):247-259.

4. Sellers EM, et al. Interaction of chloral hydrate and ethanol in man. I. Metabolism. *Clin Pharmacol Ther.* 1972;13(1):37-19.

5. Sellers EM, et al. Interaction of chloral hydrate and ethanol in man. II. Hemodynamics and performance. *Clin Pharmacol Ther.* 1972;13(1):50-58.

6. Chapman AH. Reaction to alcohol and chloral hydrate (Questions and Answers). *JAMA.* 1958;167:273.

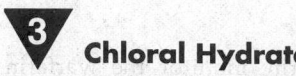

Chloral Hydrate

Warfarin (eg, *Coumadin*)

SUMMARY: Chloral hydrate may produce a transient increase in the hypoprothrombinemic response to warfarin.

RISK FACTORS: No specific risk factors are known.

MECHANISM: Trichloroacetic acid, a major metabolite of chloral hydrate, appears to displace warfarin bound to plasma proteins. This results in a transient increase in the concentration of unbound (active) plasma warfarin and also in its rate of metabolism. Dicumarol probably is affected similarly, although most studies involve subjects taking warfarin.[3-16]

CLINICAL EVALUATION: Several clinical studies show that chloral hydrate temporarily increases the hypoprothrombinemic effect of warfarin in some patients.[1-5] Reports to the contrary[6,7] have focused on the long-term effects, demonstrating that the 2 effects of trichloroacetic acid tend to counter-balance one another, leading to no net effect on the hypoprothrombinemic effect of warfarin. Although most patients appear to be minimally affected by this interaction, an occasional predisposed patient may develop a clinically important increase in hypoprothrombinemic response when chloral hydrate is added to the drug therapy.

RELATED DRUGS: Alternative sedative/hypnotic drugs unlikely to interact with oral anticoagulants include flurazepam (eg, *Dalmane*), chlordiazepoxide (eg, *Librium*), diazepam (eg, *Valium*), or diphenhydramine (eg, *Benadryl*). Barbiturates would not be suitable alternatives, because they can enhance oral anticoagulant metabolism.

MANAGEMENT OPTIONS:

➡ **Consider Alternative.** Even though the interaction between chloral hydrate and warfarin usually does not cause adverse effects, it is preferable to use hypnotic drugs that do not appear to interact with anticoagulants, such as flurazepam or diazepam.

➡ **Monitor.** When chloral hydrate is given to a patient receiving an oral anticoagulant, monitor the patient for excessive hypoprothrombinemia during the first several days of chloral hydrate therapy. However, long-term coadministration of the 2 drugs probably does not increase the hazard of bleeding significantly.

REFERENCES:

1. Sellers EM, et al. Potentiation of warfarin-induced hypoprothrombinemia by chloral hydrate. *N Engl J Med.* 1970;283:827.
2. Weiner M. Species differences in the effect of chloral hydrate on coumarin anticoagulants. *Ann NY Acad Sci.* 1971;179:226.
3. Sellers EM, et al. Kinetics and clinical importance of displacement of warfarin from albumin by acidic drugs. *Ann NY Acad Sci.* 1971;179:213.
4. Boston Collaborative Drug Surveillance Program. Interaction between chloral hydrate and warfarin. *N Engl J Med.* 1972;286:53.
5. Udall JA. Warfarin-chloral hydrate interaction: pharmacological activity and clinical significance. *Ann Intern Med.* 1974;81:341.
6. Griner PF, et al. Chloral hydrate and warfarin interaction: clinical significance? *Ann Intern Med.* 1971;74:540.
7. Udall JA. Chloral hydrate and warfarin therapy. *Ann Intern Med.* 1971;75:141.
8. Beliles RP, et al. Interaction of bishydroxycoumarin with chloral hydrate and trichloroethyl phosphate. *Toxicol Appl Pharmacol.* 974;27:225.

9. Udall JA. Drug interference with warfarin therapy. *Clin Med*. 1970;77:20.

10. Cucinell SA, et al. The effect of chloral hydrate on bishydroxycoumarin metabolism. *JAMA*. 1966;197:366.

11. Robinson DS, et al. Interaction of commonly prescribed drugs and warfarin. *Ann Intern Med*. 1970;72:853.

12. MacDonald MG, et al. The effects of phenobarbital, chloral betaine, and glutethimide administration of warfarin plasma levels and hypoprothrombinemic responses in man. *Clin Pharmacol Ther*. 1969;10:80.

13. Rickles FR, et al. Chloral hydrate and warfarin. *N Engl J Med*. 1972;286:611.

14. Anon. Chloral hydrate and oral anticoagulants. *Lancet*. 1972;1:524.

15. Udall JA. Clinical implications of warfarin interactions with five sedatives. *Am J Cardiol*. 1975;35:67.

16. Galinsky RE, et al. "Post hoc" and hypoprothrombinemia. *Ann Intern Med*. 1975;83:286.

Chloramphenicol (eg, *Chloromycetin*)

Chlorpropamide (eg, *Diabinese*)

SUMMARY: Chloramphenicol may increase the hypoglycemic effects of chlorpropamide.

RISK FACTORS: No specific risk factors are known.

MECHANISM: Chloramphenicol inhibits tolbutamide hepatic metabolism and seems to prolong the half-life of chlorpropamide.

CLINICAL EVALUATION: Chloramphenicol administration has been reported to increase the half-life of tolbutamide (eg, *Orinase*) and chlorpropamide.[1-4] Hypoglycemic episodes have been reported in patients taking chloramphenicol and oral hypoglycemic agents.

RELATED DRUGS: Chloramphenicol has been reported to increase the half-life of tolbutamide. The effect of chloramphenicol on other oral antidiabetics is unknown.

MANAGEMENT OPTIONS:

➡ *Monitor.* Monitor patients receiving tolbutamide or chlorpropamide who receive chloramphenicol concurrently for hypoglycemia.

REFERENCES:

1. Petitpierre B, et al. Behavior of chlorpropamide in renal insufficiency and under the effect of associated drug therapy. *Int J Clin Pharmacol Ther Toxicol*. 1972;6:120.

2. Christensen LK, et al. Inhibition of drug metabolism by chloramphenicol. *Lancet*. 1969;2:1397.

3. Petitpierre B, et al. Chlorpropamide and chloramphenicol. *Lancet*. 1970;1:789.

4. Brunova E, et al. Interaction of tolbutamide and chloramphenicol in diabetic patients. *Int J Clin Pharmacol*. 1977;15:7.

Chloramphenicol (eg, *Chloromycetin*)

Cyclophosphamide (eg, *Cytoxan*)

SUMMARY: Chloramphenicol could reduce the conversion of cyclophosphamide to its active metabolites, but the clinical importance is not established.

RISK FACTORS: No specific risk factors are known.

MECHANISM: Chloramphenicol presumably slows the metabolism of cyclophosphamide.

CLINICAL EVALUATION: Cyclophosphamide half-life was considerably prolonged following treatment with chloramphenicol, and the rate of production of cyclophosphamide metabolite appeared to be reduced.[1] Because cyclophosphamide metabolites are thought to be active therapeutically, chloramphenicol could theoretically reduce the activity of cyclophosphamide. Clinical studies are needed for confirmation.

RELATED DRUGS: No information is available.

MANAGEMENT OPTIONS: No specific action is required, but be alert for evidence of the interaction.

REFERENCES:

1. Faber OK, et al. The effect of chloramphenicol and sulphaphenazole on the biotransformation of cyclophosphamide in man. *Br J Clin Pharmacol*. 1975;2:281.

 ## Chloramphenicol (eg, *Chloromycetin*)

Dicumarol

SUMMARY: Chloramphenicol may enhance the hypoprothrombinemic response to dicumarol and possibly other oral anticoagulants.

RISK FACTORS:

➠ **Diet/Food.** Dietary deficiency of vitamin K[8] can increase the risk of interaction.

MECHANISM: The mechanisms for this interaction are: 1) Chloramphenicol has been shown to inhibit the metabolism of dicumarol, probably by inhibiting hepatic microsomal enzymes.[1] 2) Some people have proposed that chloramphenicol decreases vitamin K production by GI bacteria; however, bacterial production of vitamin K appears less important than dietary intake.[2-4] Moreover, chloramphenicol does not usually have much effect on bowel flora.[5] 3) Chloramphenicol may affect the production of prothrombin by an effect within the hepatic cell.[6] 4) Because fever enhances the catabolism of clotting factors,[7] the infection for which chloramphenicol is used theoretically could enhance oral anticoagulant hypoprothrombinemia, an effect that would dissipate as chloramphenicol lowered the fever.

CLINICAL EVALUATION: Chloramphenicol produced a 2- to 4-fold increase in the half-life of dicumarol in 4 patients.[1]

RELATED DRUGS: Although the effect of chloramphenicol on the metabolism of warfarin (eg, *Coumadin*) and other oral anticoagulants has not been established, theoretical considerations suggest that it would be similar to the effect on dicumarol. Warfarin would be expected to interact similarly with chloramphenicol because chloramphenicol is known to inhibit CYP2C9, the enzyme primarily responsible for warfarin metabolism.

MANAGEMENT OPTIONS:

➠ **Use Alternative.** Avoid concomitant use of chloramphenicol and dicumarol. Warfarin may not be an acceptable alternative anticoagulant.

REFERENCES:

1. Christensen LK, et al. Inhibition of drug metabolism by chloramphenicol. *Lancet*. 1969;2:1397.
2. O'Reilly RA, et al. Determinants of the response to oral anticoagulant drugs in man. *Pharmacol Rev* 1970;22:35.

3. Koch-Weser J, et al. Drug interactions with coumarin anticoagulants (First of two parts). *N Engl J Med.* 1971;285:487.

4. Koch-Weser J, et al. Drug interactions with coumarin anticoagulants (Second of two parts). *N Engl J Med.* 1971;285:547.

5. Finegold SM. Interaction of antimicrobial therapy and intestinal flora. *Am J Clin Nutr.* 1970;23:1466.

6. Kippel AP, et al. Hypoprothrombinemia secondary to antibiotic therapy and manifested by massive gastrointestinal hemorrhage. Report of three cases. *Arch Surg.* 1968;96:266.

7. Loeliger EA, et al. The biological disappearance rate of prothrombin and factors VII, IX and X from plasma in hypothyroidism, hyperthyroidism and during fever. *Thromb Diath Haemorrh.* 1964;10:267.

8. Ansell JE, et al. The spectrum of vitamin K deficiency. *JAMA.* 1977;238:40.

Chloramphenicol (eg, *Chloromycetin*)

Iron

SUMMARY: The response of anemic patients receiving iron therapy may be inhibited by chloramphenicol administration.

RISK FACTORS: No specific risk factors are known.

MECHANISM: Chloramphenicol is known to interfere with erythrocyte maturation in a considerable number of patients treated with the drug (not related to aplastic anemia, which is quite rare).[1]

CLINICAL EVALUATION: Chloramphenicol administration may inhibit the response to iron therapy in patients with iron deficiency anemia.

RELATED DRUGS: No information is available.

MANAGEMENT OPTIONS: No specific action is required, but be alert for evidence of the interaction.

REFERENCES:

1. Saidi P, et al. Effect of chloramphenicol on erythropoiesis. *J Lab Clin Med.* 1961;57:247.

Chloramphenicol (eg, *Chloromycetin*)

Penicillin G

SUMMARY: Chloramphenicol may inhibit the antibacterial activity of penicillins.

RISK FACTORS: No specific risk factors are known.

MECHANISM: A bacteriostatic drug, such as chloramphenicol, presumably may interfere with the action of a bactericidal agent, such as penicillin. Because penicillin acts by inhibiting cell wall synthesis, agents that inhibit protein synthesis (eg, chloramphenicol) theoretically could reduce the bactericidal effect of penicillin.

CLINICAL EVALUATION: Some have suggested that antibiotic antagonism occurs only under specific conditions of dose, order of therapy, or the infection that is being treated, and thus, probably plays a minor role clinically.[1 5] However, the potential for chloramphenicol-induced antagonism action in disease such as meningitis has not been adequately studied in humans and remains a possibility.

RELATED DRUGS: Other bactericidal antibiotics could interact with chloramphenicol in a similar manner.

MANAGEMENT OPTIONS:

➡ *Consider Alternative.* Avoid the use of chloramphenicol and penicillins except where the combination has been demonstrated to be beneficial.

➡ *Circumvent/Minimize.* Be sure that adequate amounts of each agent are being given and, if possible, begin administration of the penicillin a few hours or more before the chloramphenicol.

➡ *Monitor.* Observe patients for failure of antibiotic efficacy when the 2 agents are coadministered.

REFERENCES:

1. Garrod LP. Causes of failure in antibiotic treatment. *BMJ*. 1972;4:441.
2. De Ritis F, et al. Chloramphenicol combined with ampicillin in treatment of typhoid. *BMJ*. 1972;4:17.
3. Wallace JF, et al. Studies on the pathogenesis of meningitis. VI. Antagonism between penicillin and chloramphenicol in experimental pneumococcal meningitis. *J Lab Clin Med*. 1967;70:408.
4. Jawetz E. The use of combinations of antimicrobial drugs. *Ann Rev Pharmacol*. 1968;8:151.
5. Mills J, et al. Clinical use of antimicrobials. In: Katzung BG. Basic and Clinical Pharmacology. 4th ed. Los Altos: Lange Medical Publications; 1989;624–29.

Chloramphenicol (eg, *Chloromycetin*)

Phenobarbital

SUMMARY: Chloramphenicol can increase serum barbiturate concentrations, and barbiturates can reduce chloramphenicol concentrations.

RISK FACTORS: No specific risk factors are known.

MECHANISM: Barbiturates can enhance chloramphenicol metabolism, and chloramphenicol can inhibit barbiturate metabolism.

CLINICAL EVALUATION: Chloramphenicol appeared to enhance serum phenobarbital concentrations in 1 patient,[1] whereas serum chloramphenicol concentrations were lower than expected in patients receiving phenobarbital.[2] Determination of the incidence and magnitude of these interactions awaits additional studies.

RELATED DRUGS: Other barbiturates may be similarly affected by chloramphenicol and could reduce chloramphenicol concentrations as well.

MANAGEMENT OPTIONS:

➡ *Circumvent/Minimize.* Increased chloramphenicol dosage may be needed in some patients.

➡ *Monitor.* In patients receiving phenobarbital (and possibly other barbiturates), watch for evidence of reduced chloramphenicol effect. Also be alert for evidence of increased effect of phenobarbital (and possibly other barbiturates) when chloramphenicol is given concurrently.

REFERENCES:

1. Koup JR, et al. Interaction of chloramphenicol with phenytoin and phenobarbital. Case report. *Clin Pharmacol Ther*. 1978;24:571.
2. Bloxham RA, et al. Chloramphenicol and phenobarbitone. A drug interaction. *Arch Dis Child*. 1979;54:76.

Chloramphenicol (eg, *Chloromycetin*)

Phenytoin (eg, *Dilantin*)

SUMMARY: Chloramphenicol predictably increases serum phenytoin concentrations; symptoms of phenytoin toxicity have occurred. Phenytoin also may affect serum chloramphenicol concentrations, but results have been conflicting.

RISK FACTORS: No specific risk factors are known.

MECHANISM: Chloramphenicol appears to inhibit the metabolism of phenytoin by reducing microsomal enzyme activity in the liver.

CLINICAL EVALUATION: Chloramphenicol can increase plasma phenytoin concentrations considerably; phenytoin toxicity may occur.[1-6] Because of phenytoin's nonlinear pharmacokinetics, the degree of increase in plasma phenytoin concentration and onset of toxicity will vary widely. Phenytoin also can decrease[7] or increase[8] serum chloramphenicol concentrations.

RELATED DRUGS: No information is available.

MANAGEMENT OPTIONS:

➡ *Consider Alternative.* If possible, avoid chloramphenicol use in patients receiving phenytoin.

➡ *Monitor.* Watch patients who receive both phenytoin and chloramphenicol closely for signs of phenytoin toxicity (eg, nystagmus, lethargy, ataxia, rash).

REFERENCES:

1. Ballek RE, et al. Inhibition of diphenylhydantoin metabolism by chloramphenicol. *Lancet.* 1973;1:150.
2. Rose JQ, et al. Intoxication caused by interaction of chloramphenicol and phenytoin. *JAMA.* 1977;237:2630.
3. Koup JR, et al. Interaction of chloramphenicol with phenytoin and phenobarbital. Case report. *Clin Pharmacol Ther.* 1978;24:571.
4. Saltiel MS, et al. Phenytoin-chloramphenicol interaction. *Drug Intel Clin Pharm* 1980;14:221.
5. Greenlaw CW. Chloramphenicol-phenytoin drug interaction. *Drug Intell Clin Pharm* 1979;13:609.
6. Harper JM, et al. Phenytoin-chloramphenicol interaction: a retrospective study. *Drug Intel Clin Pharm.* 1970;13:425.
7. Powell DA, et al. Interactions among chloramphenicol, phenytoin, and phenobarbital in a pediatric patient. *J Pediatr.* 1981;98:1001.
8. Krasinski K, et al. Pharmacologic interactions among chloramphenicol, phenytoin and phenobarbital. *Pediatr Infect Dis.* 1982;1:232.

Chloramphenicol (eg, *Chloromycetin*)

Rifampin (eg, *Rifadin*)

SUMMARY: Rifampin can reduce chloramphenicol concentrations, potentially reducing its antibacterial efficacy.

RISK FACTORS: No specific risk factors are known.

MECHANISM: Rifampin probably stimulates the metabolism of chloramphenicol, resulting in lower serum chloramphenicol concentrations.

CLINICAL EVALUATION: Four days of rifampin therapy reduced the serum concentration of chloramphenicol 86% and 64% in 2 children being treated for meningitis.[1] Two additional cases reported a similar reduction in chloramphenicol concentrations during rifampin coadministration.[2] A reduction in the serum chloramphenicol concentration of this magnitude could reduce its efficacy in some situations.

RELATED DRUGS: No information is available.

MANAGEMENT OPTIONS:

➡ *Consider Alternative.* If possible, avoid rifampin use in patients receiving chloramphenicol.

➡ *Monitor.* Monitor chloramphenicol concentrations when rifampin is coadministered.

REFERENCES:

1. Prober CG. Effect of rifampin on chloramphenicol levels. *N Engl J Med.* 1985;312:788.
2. Kelly HW, et al. Interaction of chloramphenicol and rifampin. *J Pediatr.* 1988;12:817.

Chlordiazepoxide (eg, *Librium*)

Ketoconazole (eg, *Nizoral*)

SUMMARY: Ketoconazole increases chlordiazepoxide concentrations, but the degree to which chlordiazepoxide adverse effects are increased is not established.

RISK FACTORS: No specific risk factors are known.

MECHANISM: Ketoconazole may inhibit one of the oxidative metabolic pathways responsible for the metabolism of chlordiazepoxide.

CLINICAL EVALUATION: In a study of 6 healthy subjects, a single dose of ketoconazole 200 or 400 mg reduced the clearance of IV administered chlordiazepoxide 20% and its volume of distribution (Vd) 26%.[1] When 400 mg of ketoconazole was administered for 5 days, the clearance of chlordiazepoxide was reduced 38% without changes in its Vd. The reasons for the differences in Vd noted after single-dose versus multiple-dose ketoconazole are unknown. The reduction in clearance could produce significant increases in chlordiazepoxide concentrations in patients on chronic chlordiazepoxide therapy.

RELATED DRUGS: Other antifungal agents (eg, itraconazole [*Sporanox*], fluconazole [*Diflucan*]) are likely to increase chlordiazepoxide concentrations. Ketoconazole also inhibits the metabolism of alprazolam (eg, *Xanax*), midazolam (*Versed*), and triazolam (*Halcion*).

MANAGEMENT OPTIONS:

➡ *Monitor.* Observe patients on chronic chlordiazepoxide who receive ketoconazole for increased sedation.

REFERENCES:

1. Brown MW, et al. Effect of ketoconazole on hepatic oxidative drug metabolism. *Clin Pharmacol Ther.* 1985;37:290.

Chlordiazepoxide (eg, *Librium*) **4**

Phenelzine (*Nardil*)

SUMMARY: Limited case reports suggest that combined chlordiazepoxide-phenelzine therapy can result in edema.

RISK FACTORS: No specific risk factors are known.

MECHANISM: Not established.

CLINICAL EVALUATION: One case report describes a patient receiving phenelzine and chlordiazepoxide who developed massive edema. The authors proposed that the drug combination may have been responsible.[1] Subsequently, another patient who developed edema while receiving isocarboxazid (*Marplan*) and chlordiazepoxide was reported.[2] Although the drug combinations may have contributed to the edema in these 2 patients, the evidence for such an association is tentative.

RELATED DRUGS: Little is known regarding the effect of nonselective monoamine oxidase inhibitors on benzodiazepines other than chlordiazepoxide.

MANAGEMENT OPTIONS: No specific action is required, but be alert for evidence of the interaction.

REFERENCES:

1. Goonewardene A, et al. Gross edema occurring during treatment for depression. *BMJ.* 1977;2:879.
2. Pathak SK. Gross oedema during treatment for depression. *BMJ.* 1977;2:1220.

Chlordiazepoxide (eg, *Librium*) **5**

Warfarin (eg, *Coumadin*)

SUMMARY: Chlordiazepoxide does not appear to affect the response to warfarin.

RISK FACTORS: No specific risk factors are known.

MECHANISM: No interaction.

CLINICAL EVALUATION: Several studies have demonstrated a lack of interaction between chlordiazepoxide and oral anticoagulants.[1-4]

RELATED DRUGS: Other oral anticoagulants are not likely to interact with chlordiazepoxide.

MANAGEMENT OPTIONS: No interaction.

REFERENCES:

1. Whitfield JB, et al. Changes in plasma gamma-glutamyl transpeptidase activity associated with alterations in drug metabolism in man. *BMJ.* 1973;1:316.
2. Robinson DS, et al. Interaction of commonly prescribed drugs and warfarin. *Ann Intern Med.* 1970;72:853.
3. Lackner H, et al. The effect of Librium on hemostasis. *Am J Med Sci.* 1968;256:368.
4. DeCarolis PP, et al. Effect of tranquilizers on prothrombin time response to coumarin. *J Clin Pharmacol.* 1975;15:557.

Chlormethiazole

Cimetidine (eg, *Tagamet*)

SUMMARY: Cimetidine increases chlormethiazole (a sedative-hypnotic with anticonvulsant effects available in Europe) serum concentrations and may increase its pharmacologic effect. Study in patients is needed to establish the clinical significance of this interaction.

RISK FACTORS: No specific risk factors are known.

MECHANISM: Not established. Cimetidine may reduce the first-pass hepatic metabolism of chlormethiazole, thus enhancing its systemic availability after oral administration.

CLINICAL EVALUATION: Eight healthy subjects were given a single 1000 mg oral dose of chlormethiazole ethanedisulphonate (equivalent to 768 mg chlormethiazole base) before and after cimetidine 1000 mg/day for 1 week.[1] In the presence of cimetidine, the apparent clearance of chlormethiazole decreased 69% and its half-life increased 60%. Also, chlormethiazole-induced sedation appeared to be greater with chlormethiazole plus cimetidine than with chlormethiazole alone.

RELATED DRUGS: Ranitidine (eg, *Zantac*) does not appear to affect the pharmacokinetics of chlormethiazole; the effect of famotidine (eg, *Pepcid*) and nizatidine (*Axid*) on chlormethiazole is not established, but an interaction would not be expected.

MANAGEMENT OPTIONS:

➡ *Consider Alternative.* Ranitidine may be preferable to cimetidine in this situation because it does not appear to interact with chlormethiazole.

➡ *Monitor.* If the combination is used, be alert for altered chlormethiazole response (eg, sedation, respiratory depression) if cimetidine is initiated, discontinued, or changed in dosage.

REFERENCES:

1. Shaw G, et al. Cimetidine impairs the elimination of chlormethiazole. *Eur J Clin Pharmacol.* 1981;21:83.

Chlormethiazole

Ranitidine (eg, *Zantac*)

SUMMARY: Ranitidine does not appear to interact with chlormethiazole (a sedative-hypnotic with anticonvulsant effects available in Europe).

RISK FACTORS: No specific risk factors are known.

MECHANISM: No interaction,

CLINICAL EVALUATION: Six healthy subjects were given single 1000 mg doses of chlormethiazole ethanedsiulphonate (equivalent to 768 mg chlormethiazole base), orally and IV, with and without pretreatment with ranitidine 150 mg twice daily for 7 days.[1] Ranitidine did not affect oral or IV chlormethiazole clearance of half-life.

RELATED DRUGS: Cimetidine (eg, *Tagamet*) appears to inhibit chlormethiazole metabolism. The effect of famotidine (eg, *Pepcid*) and nizatidine (*Axid*) on chlormethiazole is not established, but an interaction would not be expected.

MANAGEMENT OPTIONS: No interaction.

REFERENCES:

1. Mashford ML, et al. Ranitidine does not affect chlormethiazole or indocyanine green disposition. *Clin Pharmacol Ther.* 1983;34;231.

Chloroquine (eg, *Aralen*)

Chlorpromazine (eg, *Thorazine*)

SUMMARY: Chlorpromazine concentrations are increased by chloroquine and other antimalarial agents; the clinical significance of these changes is unknown.

RISK FACTORS: No specific risk factors are known.

MECHANISM: It appears that the metabolism of chlorpromazine is reduced by the antimalarial agents chloroquine, amodiaquine, and sulfadoxine-pyrimethamine (*Fansidar*).

CLINICAL EVALUATION: The serum chlorpromazine concentrations of 15 patients maintained on chlorpromazine 400 to 500 mg/day were measured 3 hours after the morning dose.[1] The patients were then divided into 3 equal groups and administered single doses of chloroquine 400 mg, amodiaquine 600 mg, or 3 tablets of sulfadoxine-pyrimethamine 1 hour before their chlorpromazine dose. Chlorpromazine serum concentrations were increased 1.7 to 4.3 times control values following pretreatment with the antimalarial drugs. The clinical significance of these changes is unknown; however, increased side effects from chlorpromazine might be expected if increased serum concentrations persist.

RELATED DRUGS: Other phenothiazines may be similarly affected by chloroquine and other antimalarials.

MANAGEMENT OPTIONS:

➥ *Monitor.* Monitor patients maintained on chlorpromazine for increased neuroleptic effects if antimalarial agents are prescribed.

REFERENCES:

1. Makanjuola ROA, et al. Effects of antimalarial agents on plasma levels of chlorpromazine and its metabolites in schizophrenic patients. *Trop Geogr Med.* 1988;40:31.

Chloroquine (eg, *Aralen*)

Cimetidine (eg, *Tagamet*)

SUMMARY: Cimetidine appears to increase serum concentrations of chloroquine; the clinical significance is not established.

RISK FACTORS: No specific risk factors are known.

MECHANISM: Cimetidine appears to inhibit the metabolism of chloroquine.

CLINICAL EVALUATION: Five healthy subjects received 300 mg chloroquine alone and 5 other subjects received 300 mg chloroquine following 4 days of pretreatment with cimetidine 400 mg at bedtime.[1] The apparent clearance after an oral dose of chloroquine was 0.49 L/day/kg in the subjects taking chloroquine alone and 0.23 L/day/kg in those taking it after cimetidine. Chloroquine half-life was significantly prolonged (48%) in the subjects taking cimetidine. The clinical significance of this interaction is unknown.

RELATED DRUGS: H₂-receptor antagonists less likely to interfere with the metabolism of chloroquine (eg, ranitidine [eg, *Zantac*], famotidine [eg, *Pepcid*], or nizatidine [*Axid*]) could be used.

MANAGEMENT OPTIONS: No specific action is required, but be alert for evidence of the interaction.

REFERENCES:

1. Ette EI, et al. Chloroquine elimination in humans: effect of low-dose cimetidine. *J Clin Pharmacol.* 1987;27:813.

 4 Chloroquine (eg, *Aralen*)

Codeine

SUMMARY: Chloroquine inhibits CYP2D6, and theoretically would interfere with the bioactivation of codeine to morphine, but the extent to which it inhibits the analgesic effect of codeine is not established.

RISK FACTORS:

➡ **Pharmacogenetics.** Only patients with the extensive metabolizer CYP2D6 phenotype (EMs) would be expected to experience this interaction. Poor metabolizers (PMs) do not have the gene for production of CYP2D6, so there would be no CYP2D6 for the chloroquine to inhibit. Approximately 8% of whites are deficient in CYP2D6, but the deficiency is rare in Asians, usually less than 2%.

MECHANISM: Codeine exerts it analgesic effects (and probably also its side effects) primarily through its metabolic conversion to morphine by the isozyme, CYP2D6.[1,2] Thus, patients genetically deficient in CYP2D6 or receiving CYP2D6 inhibitors such as chloroquine are likely to produce little or no morphine during codeine administration.

CLINICAL EVALUATION: Chloroquine is known to inhibit CYP2D6. Since several studies have shown that another CYP2D6 inhibitor, quinidine (eg, *Quinora*), inhibits the analgesic effect of codeine,[3-6] chloroquine might be expected to inhibit codeine analgesia as well. Nonetheless, clinical studies are needed to determine the clinical importance of this potential interaction.

RELATED DRUGS: The analgesic effect of dihydrocodeine (eg, *Synalgos-DC*) and hydrocodone (eg, *Vicodin*) also may be dependent on conversion to morphine-like active metabolites, and early evidence suggests that CYP2D6 inhibitors can reduce their analgesic efficacy. Whether chloroquine affects these drugs is not known. Tramadol (*Ultram*) appears to be partially dependent upon CYP2D6 for analgesic activity, but theoretically would be less affected than codeine by chloroquine. Early pharmacodynamic evidence suggests that oxycodone (eg, *Percodan*) does not require conversion by CYP2D6 to an active metabolite. Theoretically, oxycodone would not be affected by chloroquine, but more study is needed.

MANAGEMENT OPTIONS: No specific action is required, but be alert for evidence of the interaction.

REFERENCES:

1. Sindrup SH, et al. Codeine increases pain thresholds to copper vapor laser stimuli in extensive but not poor metabolizers of sparteine. *Clin Pharmacol Ther.* 1990;48:686.

2. Poulsen L, et al. Codeine and morphine in extensive and poor metabolizers of sparteine: pharmacokinetics, analgesic effect and side effects. *Eur J Clin Pharmacol.* 1996;51:289.

3. Desmeules J, et al. Impact of environmental and genetic factors on codeine analgesia. *Eur J Clin Pharmacol.* 1991;41:23.

4. Sindrup SH, et al. The effect of quinidine on the analgesic effect of codeine. *Eur J Clin Pharmacol.* 1992;42:587.

5. Sindrup SH, et al. Impact of quinidine on plasma and cerebrospinal fluid concentrations of codeine and morphine after codeine intake. *Eur J Clin Pharmacol.* 1996;49:503.

6. Caraco Y, et al. Pharmacogenetic determination of the effects of codeine and prediction of drug interactions. *J Pharmacol Exp Ther.* 1996;278:1165.

Chloroquine (eg, *Aralen*)

Cyclosporine (eg, *Neoral*)

SUMMARY: Patients stabilized on cyclosporine may develop elevated cyclosporine concentrations following the addition of chloroquine. Signs and symptoms of cyclosporine toxicity may accompany the interaction.

RISK FACTORS: No specific risk factors are known.

MECHANISM: Chloroquine appears to inhibit the metabolism of cyclosporine.

CLINICAL EVALUATION: A 28-year-old kidney transplant patient was maintained on prednisone (eg, *Prelone*), azathioprine (eg, *Imuran*), and cyclosporine 70 mg/day with a cyclosporine concentration of 105 ng/ml.[1] Chloroquine 100 mg/day was initiated for malaria prophylaxis. Six days later, his cyclosporine concentration was 470 ng/ml and was accompanied by elevations in his blood pressure and serum creatinine. Chloroquine was discontinued with normalization of the laboratory values and blood pressure. A rechallenge with chloroquine was undertaken a month later with similar results. A second case report involved a 51-year-old kidney transplant patient stabilized on cyclosporine 3.4 mg/kg/day with a cyclosporine concentration of 148 ng/ml.[2] Chloroquine 900 mg/day was administered for 3 days. The cyclosporine concentration increased to 420 ng/ml and was accompanied by an increase in serum creatinine. Seven days after stopping the chloroquine, cyclosporine and creatinine concentrations returned to baseline values.

RELATED DRUGS: Tacrolimus (*Prograf*) may be affected similarly by coadministered chloroquine.

MANAGEMENT OPTIONS:

➡ *Circumvent/Minimize.* Cyclosporine dosages may require reduction during concomitant chloroquine treatment.

➡ *Monitor.* Carefully observe patients taking cyclosporine for increased cyclosporine concentrations if chloroquine is coadministered.

REFERENCES:

1. Finielz P, et al. Interaction between cyclosporin and chloroquine. *Nephron.* 1993;65:333.

2. Nampoory MRN, et al. Drug interaction of chloroquine with ciclosporin. *Nephron.* 1992;62:108.

Chloroquine (eg, *Aralen*)

Imipramine (eg, *Tofranil*)

SUMMARY: A single dose of imipramine did not alter chloroquine concentrations.

RISK FACTORS: No specific risk factors are known.

MECHANISM: No interaction.

CLINICAL EVALUATION: Six healthy subjects received 300 mg of chloroquine alone and with a single dose of imipramine 50 mg.[1] No changes in chloroquine pharmacokinetics were observed following imipramine coadministration. The effects of multiple imipramine doses are unknown.

RELATED DRUGS: No information is available.

MANAGEMENT OPTIONS: No interaction.

REFERENCES:

1. Onyeji CO, et al. Lack of pharmacokinetic interaction between chloroquine and imipramine. *Ther Drug Monit*. 1993;15:43.

Chloroquine (eg, *Aralen*)

Kaolin-Pectin

SUMMARY: Kaolin-pectin administration may reduce the serum concentrations of chloroquine; the clinical significance of these changes is unknown.

RISK FACTORS: No specific risk factors are known.

MECHANISM: Kaolin appears to reduce the GI absorption of chloroquine.

CLINICAL EVALUATION: Chloroquine 1 g was given orally with and without coadministration of oral kaolin 1 g in 6 healthy subjects.[1] Kaolin reduced the area under the plasma chloroquine concentration-time curve approximately 30%.

RELATED DRUGS: The effect of kaolin on hydroxychloroquine (eg, *Plaquenil*) absorption was not studied, but expect it to be similarly affected by kaolin.

MANAGEMENT OPTIONS: No specific action is required, but be alert for evidence of the interaction.

REFERENCES:

1. McElnay JC, et al. *In vitro* experiments on chloroquine and pyrimethamine absorption in the presence of antacid constituents or kaolin. *J Trop Med Hyg*. 1982;85:153.

Chloroquine (eg, *Aralen*)

Methotrexate

SUMMARY: Methotrexate concentrations are reduced by chloroquine coadministration; the clinical significance is unknown but some patients could experience reduced methotrexate efficacy.

RISK FACTORS: No specific risk factors are known.

MECHANISM: Not established. Chloroquine appears to reduce the absorption of methotrexate or increase its metabolism.

CLINICAL EVALUATION: Eleven patients taking methotrexate 15 mg/week for arthritis had their methotrexate concentrations measured while taking only methotrexate and after the addition of a single dose of chloroquine 250 mg.[1] Methotrexate peak concentrations were reduced 20% and its area under the concentration-time curve was reduced 28% following the chloroquine dose. The clinical significance of these changes is likely to be limited; however, the effects of multiple chloroquine dosing on methotrexate concentrations is not established.

RELATED DRUGS: Hydroxychloroquine (eg, *Plaquenil*) may affect methotrexate in a similar manner.

MANAGEMENT OPTIONS:

➡ **Monitor.** Until more information is available, monitor patients receiving methotrexate for loss of efficacy during chloroquine coadministration.

REFERENCES:
1. Seidman P, et al. Chloroquine reduces the bioavailability of methotrexate in patients with rheumatoid arthritis. *Arthritis Rheum*. 1994;37:830.

Chloroquine (eg, *Aralen*)

Metronidazole (eg, *Flagyl*)

SUMMARY: An acute dystonic reaction following intramuscular chloroquine administration to a patient maintained on metronidazole has been reported.

RISK FACTORS: No specific risk factors are known.

MECHANISM: Not established.

CLINICAL EVALUATION: A 30-year-old woman was treated with oral metronidazole 400 mg 3 times daily and ampicillin (eg, *Principen*) 500 mg every 6 hours.[1] Chloroquine 200 mg intramuscularly and promethazine 25 mg were administered on the sixth day of metronidazole therapy. Within 10 minutes, the patient developed acute dystonia with facial grimacing, coarse tremors, anxiety, and restlessness. The symptoms resolved over 2 hours following diazepam (eg, *Valium*) 5 mg intravenously. The patient had previously received chloroquine without dystonic symptoms; however, causation was not established. Note that promethazine itself also may cause extrapyramidal symptoms and may have contributed to this report.

RELATED DRUGS: No information is available.

MANAGEMENT OPTIONS: No specific action is required, but be alert for evidence of the interaction.

REFERENCES:
1. Achumba JI, et al. Chloroquine-induced acute dystonic reactions in the presence of metronidazole. *Drug Intell Clin Pharm*. 1988;22(4):308-310.

Chloroquine (eg, *Aralen*)

Praziquantel (*Biltricide*)

SUMMARY: Chloroquine administration reduces the plasma concentration of praziquantel; loss of efficacy may occur.

RISK FACTORS: No specific risk factors are known.

MECHANISM: Not established. It appears that the absorption of praziquantel is decreased by chloroquine administration.

CLINICAL EVALUATION: Eight healthy subjects received an oral dose of praziquantel 40 mg/kg alone and 2 hours after a single dose of chloroquine 600 mg.[1] While the half-life of praziquantel was unchanged, its area under the concentration-time curve was reduced 65% and peak concentrations were reduced 59%. Loss of praziquantel efficacy could result from this degree of reduction in plasma praziquantel concentrations.

RELATED DRUGS: Hydroxychloroquine (eg, *Plaquenil*) may affect praziquantel in a similar manner.

MANAGEMENT OPTIONS:

➡ *Monitor.* Until more information is available, monitor patients taking praziquantel and chloroquine concurrently for reduced plasma concentrations and possible loss of efficacy.

REFERENCES:

1. Masimirembwa CM, et al. The effect of chloroquine on the pharmacokinetics and metabolism of praziquantel in rats and in humans. *Biopharm Drug Dispos.* 1994;15(1):33-43.

Chloroquine (eg, *Aralen*)

Tamoxifen (eg, *Soltamox*)

SUMMARY: Theoretically, chloroquine may reduce the efficacy of tamoxifen in the treatment of breast cancer.

RISK FACTORS: No specific risk factors are known.

MECHANISM: Tamoxifen is metabolized to 2 active metabolites by CYP2D6, the most important of which is endoxifen. By reducing endoxifen formation, CYP2D6 inhibitors such as chloroquine may reduce tamoxifen efficacy.[1,2,3]

CLINICAL EVALUATION: A study in patients with breast cancer found substantial reductions in endoxifen plasma concentrations in patients taking potent CYP2D6 inhibitors such as fluoxetine and paroxetine.[4] Another tamoxifen study found a nearly 2-fold increase in the risk of breast cancer relapse in women with low CYP2D6 activity, either due to CYP2D6-inhibiting drugs or genetic deficiency.[5] Taken together, these and other results strongly suggest that CYP2D6 inhibitors reduce the efficacy of tamoxifen in the treatment of breast cancer. Chloroquine is a CYP2D6 inhibitor, and may inhibit the anticancer effects of tamoxifen.

RELATED DRUGS: Hydroxychloroquine (eg, *Plaquenil*) and quinine may also inhibit CYP2D6, and thus reduce the efficacy of tamoxifen.

MANAGEMENT OPTIONS:

➥ *Consider Alternative.* If possible, use an antimalarial other than chloroquine or hydroxychloroquine.

➥ *Monitor.* If a CYP2D6 inhibitor such as chloroquine is used with tamoxifen, cancer recurrence may be an indication that tamoxifen efficacy has been reduced. If this happens, consider discontinuing the CYP2D6 inhibitor.

REFERENCES:

1. Dezentjé VO, et al. Clinical implications of CYP2D6 genotyping in tamoxifen treatment for breast cancer. *Clin Cancer Res.* 2009;15(1):15-21.
2. Tan SH, et al. Pharmacogenetics in breast cancer therapy. *Clin Cancer Res.* 2008;14(24):8027-8041.
3. Newman WG, et al. Impaired tamoxifen metabolism reduces survival in familial breast cancer patients. *Clin Cancer Res.* 2008;14(18):5913-5918.
4. Borges S, et al. Quantitative effect of CYP2D6 genotype and inhibitors on tamoxifen metabolism: implication for optimization of breast cancer treatment. *Clin Pharmacol Ther.* 2006;80(1):61-74.
5. Goetz MP, et al. The impact of cytochrome P450 2D6 metabolism in women receiving adjuvant tamoxifen. *Breast Cancer Res Treat.* 2007;101(1):113-121.

Chlorpheniramine (eg, *Chlor-Trimeton*)

Phenytoin (eg, *Dilantin*)

SUMMARY: Chlorpheniramine therapy was associated with symptoms of phenytoin toxicity in 1 patient; more study is needed.

RISK FACTORS: No specific risk factors are known.

MECHANISM: Not established. Chlorpheniramine may inhibit the metabolism of phenytoin.

CLINICAL EVALUATION: A patient developed phenytoin intoxication (plasma concentration greater than 60 mcg/mL) following coadministration of chlorpheniramine 12 mg/day and phenytoin 300 mg/day.[1] A causal relationship between the chlorpheniramine administration and the toxic concentrations of phenytoin is possible, but additional study is needed.

RELATED DRUGS: No information is available.

MANAGEMENT OPTIONS: No specific action is required, but be alert for evidence of the interaction.

REFERENCES:

1. Pugh RN, et al. Interaction of phenytoin with chlorpheniramine. *Br J Clin Pharmacol.* 1975;2(2):173-175.

Chlorphentermine

Chlorpromazine

SUMMARY: Preliminary evidence indicates that chlorpromazine may inhibit the anorectic effect of chlorphentermine.

RISK FACTORS: No specific risk factors are known.

MECHANISM: Not established.

CLINICAL EVALUATION: In a crossover study with 30 obese psychiatric patients, neither chlorphentermine nor phenmetrazine resulted in weight loss in the presence of chlorpromazine therapy.[1] This suggests, but does not prove, that neuroleptics inhibit the anorectic effect of chlorphentermine.

RELATED DRUGS: Other anorexiants may be similarly affected, but little information is available.

MANAGEMENT OPTIONS: No specific action is required, but be alert for evidence of the interaction.

REFERENCES:
1. Sletten IW, et al. Weight reduction with chlorphentermine and phenmetrazine in obese psychiatric patients during chlorpromazine therapy. *Curr Ther Res Clin Exp.* 1967;9(11):570-575.

Chlorpromazine (eg, *Thorazine*)

Cigarette Smoking

SUMMARY: Preliminary evidence indicates that cigarette smokers have less drowsiness and hypotension from chlorpromazine than nonsmokers, but the clinical importance of these findings is unclear.

RISK FACTORS: No specific risk factors are known.

MECHANISM: Cigarette smoking may enhance the hepatic metabolism of neuroleptics.

CLINICAL EVALUATION: In an epidemiologic study of the frequency of drowsiness attributed to oral chlorpromazine, only 3% of heavy smokers (more than 20 cigarettes/day) developed drowsiness, while the frequency in light smokers (20 cigarettes/day or fewer) and nonsmokers was 11% and 16%, respectively.[1] In another study, the frequency of hypotension in patients on chlorpromazine was 0% in heavy smokers, 8% in light smokers, and 10% in nonsmokers.[2] Another study comparing the effect of chlorpromazine 75 mg in 8 cigarette smokers and 9 nonsmokers found a greater hypotensive and sedative effect in the nonsmokers.[3] In 1 patient, chlorpromazine serum levels and adverse effects increased when she stopped smoking; rechallenge and dechallenge produced the same results.[4] It seems unlikely that cigarette smoking would decrease the chlorpromazine side effects selectively, without affecting the therapeutic response to chlorpromazine. However, the effect of cigarette smoking on the efficacy of chlorpromazine has not been systematically studied.

RELATED DRUGS: Little is known regarding the effect of cigarette smoking on the response of other phenothiazines or neuroleptics. It is possible that some of them are similarly affected by cigarette smoking.

MANAGEMENT OPTIONS:

➥ *Monitor.* Be alert for evidence of increased neuroleptic dosage requirements in cigarette smokers and for reduced neuroleptic dosage requirements in patients who stop cigarette smoking.

REFERENCES:
1. Swett C Jr. Drowsiness due to chlorpromazine in relation to cigarette smoking. *Arch Gen Psychiatry.* 1974;31:211.
2. Swett C Jr, et al. Hypotension due to chlorpromazine: relation to cigarette smoking, blood pressure and dosage. *Arch Gen Psychiatry.* 1977;34:661.
3. Panguck EJ, et al. Cigarette smoking and chlorpromazine disposition and actions. *Clin Pharmacol Ther.* 1982;31:533.

4. Stimmel GL, et al. Chlorpromazine plasma levels, adverse effects, and tobacco smoking: case report. *J Clin Psychiatry*. 1983;44:420.

Chlorpromazine (eg, *Thorazine*) 4

Cimetidine (eg, *Tagamet*)

SUMMARY: Cimetidine has been reported to increase and decrease chlorpromazine effect; more study is needed.

RISK FACTORS: No specific risk factors are known.

MECHANISM: Not established. It is possible that cimetidine impairs the hepatic metabolism and GI absorption of chlorpromazine.

CLINICAL EVALUATION: In 8 patients on chlorpromazine 75 to 450 mg/day, administration of cimetidine 1 g/day for 7 days decreased steady-state chlorpromazine concentrations by a mean of 35%.[1] Conversely, the addition of cimetidine 400 mg twice daily to 2 schizophrenic patients resulted in excessive sedation over 5 to 7 days, necessitating a reduction in chlorpromazine dose.[2] When cimetidine was discontinued, the chlorpromazine dosage had to be increased to control the schizophrenic symptoms. Based upon theoretical considerations, increased chlorpromazine serum concentrations would be more likely than *decreased* concentrations. Pharmacokinetic studies involving both oral and parenteral chlorpromazine may be needed to resolve this issue.

RELATED DRUGS: Theoretically, other H_2-receptor antagonists such as famotidine (eg, *Pepcid*), nizatidine (*Axid*), and ranitidine (eg, *Zantac*) would be unlikely to affect the hepatic metabolism of chlorpromazine. Nonetheless, if cimetidine affects the GI absorption of chlorpromazine, other H_2-receptor antagonists may produce a similar effect. The effect of cimetidine on other phenothiazines or nonphenothiazine neuroleptics is unknown.

MANAGEMENT OPTIONS: No specific action is required, but be alert for evidence of the interaction.

REFERENCES:

1. Howes CA, et al. Reduced steady-state plasma concentrations of chlorpromazine and indomethacin in patients receiving cimetidine. *Eur J Clin Pharmacol*. 1983;24:99.
2. Byrne A, et al. Adverse interaction between cimetidine and chlorpromazine in two cases of chronic schizophrenia. *Br J Psychiatry*. 1989;155:413.

Chlorpromazine (eg, *Thorazine*)

Clonidine (eg, *Catapres*)

SUMMARY: Isolated cases of severe hypotensive episodes or delirium have been reported following the concurrent use of clonidine and chlorpromazine, but a causal relationship has not been established.

RISK FACTORS: No specific risk factors are known.

MECHANISM: Not established. Neuroleptics appear to have additive hypotensive effects with clonidine.

CLINICAL EVALUATION: A 51-year-old man with hypertension developed severe, symptomatic hypotension 70 minutes after receiving clonidine 0.1 mg, furosemide (eg, *Lasix*) 40 mg, and oral chlorpromazine 100 mg.[1] A similar case of hypotension occurred in an 88-year-old hypertensive woman 2.5 hours after she received 0.1 mg of oral clonidine followed in 30 minutes by 1 mg IM haloperidol (eg, *Haldol*). Both patients had evidence of mitral regurgitation. Although the possibility that the hypotensive episodes were caused by clonidine alone or clonidine plus furosemide cannot be ruled out, it seems likely that the neuroleptic agents contributed to the hypotensive effect. Neuroleptics alone can produce hypotension, especially following initial doses and in patients with mitral insufficiency.[2]

RELATED DRUGS: Other antipsychotics also may interact with clonidine. The combined use of clonidine and fluphenazine (eg, *Prolixin*) was associated with delirium (eg, confusion, disorientation, agitation) in a 33-year-old man,[3] but a causal relationship was not established. Additionally, the combined use of haloperidol and clonidine was associated with a case of hypotension.[1] Although little is known regarding the effect of centrally acting alpha-agonists other than clonidine such as guanabenz (*Wytensin*) and guanfacine (eg, *Tenex*), consider the possibility that they interact with neuroleptic drugs until clinical information is available.

MANAGEMENT OPTIONS:

➡ **Monitor.** Watch for additive hypotensive effects when clonidine and neuroleptics are used concurrently, especially when the neuroleptic is initiated in a patient with impaired cardiac function.

REFERENCES:

1. Gruncillo RJ, et al. Severe hypotension associated with concurrent clonidine and antipsychotic medication. *Am J Psychiatry*. 1985;142:274.
2. McEvoy GK, ed. AHFS Drug Information 89. Bethesda, MD: American Society of Hospital Pharmacists; 1995:1189.
3. Allen RM, et al. Delirium associated with combined fluphenazine-clonidine therapy. *J Clin Psychiatry*. 1979;40:236.

4   Chlorpromazine (eg, *Thorazine*)

Contraceptives, Oral (eg, *Ortho-Novum*)

SUMMARY: A woman on chlorpromazine developed high plasma concentrations and toxicity after starting a combination oral contraceptive, but a causal relationship was not established.

RISK FACTORS: No specific risk factors are known.

MECHANISM: Not established.

CLINICAL EVALUATION: A 21-year-old woman developed a dramatic (6-fold) increase in her chlorpromazine plasma concentrations after starting a combined oral contraceptive (ethinyl estradiol 50 mcg plus norgestrel 500 mcg).[1] The high chlorpromazine concentrations were associated with severe dyskinesias and tremor. Although the temporal relationship suggests that the oral contraceptive may have caused the increased chlorpromazine concentrations, the large magnitude of the effect raises questions as to the cause. Oral contraceptives typically produce only modest changes in the pharmacokinetics of other drugs, and an interaction of this magnitude seems unusual. Nonetheless, since chlorpromazine has a relatively low bioavailability, it is possible that the oral contraceptive produced a marked increase in bioavailability by interfering with the presystemic metabolism of chlorpromazine.

RELATED DRUGS: No information is available.

MANAGEMENT OPTIONS: No specific action is required, but be alert for evidence of the interaction.

REFERENCES:

1. Chetty M, et al. Oral contraceptives increase the plasma concentrations of chlorpromazine. *Ther Drug Monit.* 2001;23:556-558.

Chlorpromazine (eg, *Thorazine*)

Dextroamphetamine (eg, *Dexedrine*)

SUMMARY: Amphetamines may inhibit the antipsychotic effect of neuroleptics, and neuroleptics may inhibit the anorectic effect of amphetamines.

RISK FACTORS: No specific risk factors are known.

MECHANISM: Not established.

CLINICAL EVALUATION: Amphetamines have been shown to aggravate schizophrenic symptoms in patients receiving chlorpromazine.[1] The reverse interaction also may occur. Obese schizophrenic patients taking neuroleptics and other psychotherapeutic agents did not respond to dextroamphetamine therapy for weight reduction in 1 study and the expected amphetamine-induced alterations in sleep patterns were not seen.[2] On the positive side, chlorpromazine has been used successfully to treat amphetamine overdose.[3]

RELATED DRUGS: In an uncontrolled study in 8 patients, haloperidol (eg, *Haldol*) inhibited amphetamine-induced symptoms; thus, it may be of value in the treatment of amphetamine abuse.[4] The effect of haloperidol on the therapeutic response to amphetamines (eg, obesity) is unclear.

MANAGEMENT OPTIONS: No specific action is required, but be alert for evidence of the interaction.

REFERENCES:

1. Casey JF, et al. Combined drug therapy of chronic schizophrenics. *Am J Psychiatry.* 1961;117:997.
2. Modell W, et al. Failure of dextroamphetamine sulfate to influence eating and sleeping patterns in obese schizophrenic patients. Clinical and pharmacological significance. *JAMA.* 1965;193:275.
3. Espelin DE, et al. Amphetamine poisoning. Effectiveness of chlorpromazine. *N Engl J Med.* 1968;278:1361-1365.
4. Angrist B, et al. The antagonism of amphetamine-induced symptomatology by a neuroleptic. *Am J Psychiatry.* 1974;131:817-819.

Chlorpromazine (eg, *Thorazine*)

Diazoxide (eg, *Hyperstat*)

SUMMARY: Combined use of diazoxide and chlorpromazine was associated with hyperglycemia in a young child; more study is needed.

RISK FACTORS: No specific risk factors are known.

MECHANISM: Not established.

CLINICAL EVALUATION: A 2-year-old boy on chronic diazoxide and thiazide therapy for hypoglycemia developed severe hyperglycemia following a single 30 mg dose of chlorpromazine.[1] It was proposed that the chlorpromazine, acting in concert with the diazoxide and thiazide, was responsible for the hyperglycemia.

RELATED DRUGS: The effect of other phenothiazines combined with diazoxide is not established.

MANAGEMENT OPTIONS: No specific action is required, but be alert for evidence of the interaction.

REFERENCES:

1. Aynsley-Green A, et al. Enhancement by chlorpromazine of hyperglycemic action of diazoxide. *Lancet*. 1975;2:658-659.

Chlorpromazine

Donepezil (eg, *Aricept*)

SUMMARY: Chlorpromazine has anticholinergic properties and may inhibit the therapeutic effect of donepezil in Alzheimer disease.

RISK FACTORS: No specific risk factors are known.

MECHANISM: Donepezil is a cholinesterase inhibitor and its efficacy is likely to be inhibited by anticholinergic agents such as chlorpromazine.[1]

CLINICAL EVALUATION: In a preliminary study of 69 patients with Alzheimer disease receiving donepezil 10 mg/day and followed for 2 years, 16 patients received concurrent therapy with anticholinergic drugs and 53 patients did not.[2] Mental functioning, as measured by the Mini-Mental State Exam (MMSE), was significantly lower in the patients receiving concomitant anticholinergic drugs. Also, the French Pharmacovigilance Database received 118 spontaneous reports of adverse reactions in patients receiving anticholinergic drugs with cholinesterase inhibitors (eg, donepezil, galantamine, rivastigmine). After evaluation by clinical pharmacologists, 24 were thought to be adverse drug interactions.[3] Although additional study is needed to establish the clinical importance of these interactions, the evidence is consistent with the known pharmacological effects of the drugs.

RELATED DRUGS: All cholinesterase inhibitors used to treat Alzheimer disease (donepezil, galantamine [eg, *Razadyne*], rivastigmine [eg, *Exelon*]) are expected to interact similarly with chlorpromazine, as well as other antipsychotics with anticholinergic effects, such as clozapine (eg, *Clozaril*), olanzapine (eg, *Zyprexa*), quetiapine (*Seroquel*), thioridazine, and trifluoperazine.

MANAGEMENT OPTIONS:

➡ *Consider Alternative.* If possible, use an alternative to chlorpromazine or other antipsychotics with significant anticholinergic effects (see Related Drugs).

➡ *Monitor.* If chlorpromazine or other anticholinergic antipsychotic drug are used with donepezil or another cholinesterase inhibitor, be alert for evidence of reduced mental functioning.

REFERENCES:

1. *Aricept* [package insert]. New York, NY: Pfizer; 2011.
2. Lu CJ, Tune LE. Chronic exposure to anticholinergic medications adversely affects the course of Alzheimer disease. *Am J Geriatr Psychiatry*. 2003;11(4):458-461.

3. Tavassoli N, et al. Drug interactions with cholinesterase inhibitors: an analysis of the French Pharmacovigilance Database and a comparison of two national drug formularies (Vidal, British National Formulary). *Drug Saf.* 2007;30(11):1063-1071.

Chlorpromazine (eg, *Thorazine*)

Epinephrine (eg, *Adrenalin*)

SUMMARY: Chlorpromazine, and possibly some other phenothiazines, may reverse the pressor response of epinephrine.

RISK FACTORS: No specific risk factors are known.

MECHANISM: Neuroleptics block peripheral alpha-adrenergic receptors, thus inhibiting the alpha vasoconstricting effects of epinephrine and leaving the beta-vasodilator effect relatively unopposed.

CLINICAL EVALUATION: Most pharmacology textbooks state that in the presence of phenothiazine therapy, systemic doses of epinephrine paradoxically decrease the blood pressure; this is the so-called "epinephrine reversal" phenomenon. Epinephrine reversal caused by chlorpromazine pretreatment has been demonstrated in the blood vessels of the hand[1] and in dogs,[2] but has not been a consistent finding in patients receiving chlorpromazine as premedication for surgical anesthesia.[3] The degree to which patients receiving chronic therapy with chlorpromazine or other phenothiazines would manifest epinephrine reversal is not established, but consider it a possibility.

RELATED DRUGS: Neuroleptics such as thioridazine (eg, *Mellaril*) and clozapine (eg, *Clozaril*) could theoretically interact with epinephrine similarly, but other neuroleptics with a low incidence of postural hypotension may have less effect on alpha-adrenergic receptors and may be less likely to affect epinephrine response (eg, fluphenazine [eg, *Prolixin*], trifluoperazine [eg, *Stelazine*], haloperidol [eg, *Haldol*], loxapine [eg, *Loxitane*], molindone [*Moban*], and pimozide [*Orap*]).

MANAGEMENT OPTIONS:

➡ ***Consider Alternative.*** It has been suggested that in neuroleptic-treated patients with hypotension, alpha-adrenergic agonists with little beta-adrenergic activity (eg, phenylephrine [eg, *Neo-Synephrine*], levarterenol [*Levophed*]) would be more effective in increasing the blood pressure than epinephrine.[4,5]

➡ ***Monitor.*** Monitor the blood pressure when epinephrine is given to hypotensive patients receiving neuroleptics, particularly chlorpromazine, thioridazine, or clozapine.

REFERENCES:

1. Foster CA. Chlorpromazine: a study of its action on the circulation in man. *Lancet.* 1954;2:614.
2. Yagiela JA, et al. Drug interaction and vasoconstrictors used in local anesthetic solutions. *Oral Surg Oral Med Oral Pathol.* 1985;59:565.
3. Lear E, et al. A clinical study of mechanisms of action of chlorpromazine. *JAMA.* 1957;163:30.
4. Gonzales, ER. Catecholamine selection for vasopressor-dependent patients. *Clin Pharm.* 1988;7:493.
5. Alexander CS. Epinephrine not contraindicated in cardiac arrest attributed to phenothiazine. *JAMA.* 1976;236:405.

Chlorpromazine (eg, *Thorazine*)

Ethanol (Ethyl Alcohol)

SUMMARY: Patients receiving antipsychotic doses of chlorpromazine are probably more sensitive to the adverse effects of ethanol on psychomotor skills and behavior. Thioridazine may be less likely to induce this effect with ethanol, but the effects of other neuroleptics have not been well studied. More study also is needed to assess the ability of ethanol to induce extrapyramidal reactions in patients on neuroleptics.

RISK FACTORS: No specific risk factors are known.

MECHANISM: Ethanol and neuroleptics probably exhibit additive CNS depressant activity.

CLINICAL EVALUATION: Studies in normal subjects and patients indicate that chlorpromazine adds to the detrimental effects of ethanol on simulated driving[1] and other various measures of coordination and judgment.[1,2] Subjective assessments of impairment and observation of behavior also indicate that chlorpromazine plus ethanol has a greater effect than ethanol alone. It also has been proposed that ethanol may precipitate extrapyramidal reactions in patients receiving neuroleptics. Seven cases have been briefly described in which akathisia or dystonia followed ingestion of moderate to large amounts of ethanol in the presence of neuroleptic therapy.[4]

RELATED DRUGS: Thioridazine (eg, *Mellaril*) may be less likely to add to the detrimental effects of ethanol on psychomotor skills.[1,3] One would expect neuroleptics other than chlorpromazine to add to the psychomotor impairment of alcohol, but there may be differences in degree with different phenothiazines.

MANAGEMENT OPTIONS:

➡ *Circumvent/Minimize.* Patients receiving neuroleptics (especially large doses) should be aware that ethanol ingestion can impair motor performance and driving ability. The possibility that ethanol might precipitate extrapyramidal reactions in certain susceptible patients receiving neuroleptics is another reason to limit ethanol intake.

➡ *Monitor.* Be alert for evidence of excessive CNS depression if ethanol and phenothiazines are used together.

REFERENCES:

1. Milner G, et al. Alcohol, thioridazine and chlorpromazine effects on skills related to driving behaviour. *Br J Psychiatry.* 1971;118:351.
2. Zirkle GA, et al. Effects of chlorpromazine and alcohol on coordination and judgment. *JAMA.* 1959;168:1496.
3. Saario I. Psychomotor skills during subacute treatment with thioridazine and bromazepam, and their combined effects with alcohol. *Ann Clin Res.* 1976;8:117.
4. Lutz EG. Neuroleptic-induced akathisia and dystonia triggered by alcohol. *JAMA.* 1976;236:2422.

Chlorpromazine (eg, *Thorazine*)

Guanethidine (*Ismelin*)

SUMMARY: Phenothiazines may inhibit the antihypertensive response to guanethidine.

RISK FACTORS: No specific risk factors are known.

MECHANISM: Chlorpromazine appears to inhibit the uptake of guanethidine into the adrenergic neuron in a manner similar to that of the tricyclic antidepressants.[1-3,5]

CLINICAL EVALUATION: In several patients receiving guanethidine, considerable increases in mean blood pressure occurred a few days after starting therapy with chlorpromazine.[4,6,7] In all patients, the dose of chlorpromazine was 100 mg/day or more; it is not known whether smaller doses of chlorpromazine would have a similar effect.

RELATED DRUGS: Guanadrel (*Hylorel*) is pharmacologically similar to guanethidine and also may be inhibited by phenothiazines.

MANAGEMENT OPTIONS:

➥ *Consider Alternative.* Consider using an antihypertensive agent other than guanethidine (or drugs related to guanethidine such as guanadrel). Keep in mind that the intrinsic hypotensive effect of phenothiazines might enhance the effect of antihypertensives other than guanethidine or guanadrel.

➥ *Monitor.* If the combination is used, monitor blood pressure for evidence of the interaction. If guanethidine antagonism is noted, consider increasing the guanethidine dose, or using an alternative antihypertensive agent.

REFERENCES:

1. Day MD, et al. Antagonism of guanethidine and betrylium by various agents. *Lancet.* 1962;2:1282.
2. Ober KF, et al. Drug interactions with guanethidine. *Clin Pharmacol Ther.* 1973;14:190.
3. Tuck D, et al. Drug interactions: effect of chlorpromazine on the uptake of monoamines into adrenergic neurons in man. *Lancet.* 1972;2:492..
4. Reports of Suspected Adverse Reactions to Drugs. 1970, No. 700201-056-00101.
5. Lahti RA, et al. The tricyclic antidepressants: inhibition of norepinephrine uptake as related to potentiation of norepinephrine and clinical efficacy. *Biochem Pharmacol.* 1971;20:482.
6. Fann WE, et al. Chlorpromazine reversal of the antihypertensive action of guanethidine. *Lancet.* 1971;2:436.
7. Janowsky DS, et al. Antagonism of guanethidine by chlorpromazine. *Am J Psychiatry.* 1973;130:808.

Chlorpromazine (eg, *Thorazine*)

Hydroxyzine (eg, *Atarax*)

SUMMARY: Preliminary evidence indicates that hydroxyzine may inhibit the antipsychotic response to neuroleptics.

RISK FACTORS: No specific risk factors are known.

MECHANISM: Not established.

CLINICAL EVALUATION: Preliminary evidence from a double-blind trial in 19 psychotic patients indicates that hydroxyzine impairs the therapeutic response to neuroleptics,[1] but a causal relationship was not established.

RELATED DRUGS: No information is available.

MANAGEMENT OPTIONS: No specific action is required, but be alert for evidence of the interaction.

REFERENCES:

1. Ross, EK et al. The effect of hydroxyzine on phenothiazine therapy. *Dis Nerv Syst.* 1970;31:412.

 Chlorpromazine (eg, *Thorazine*)

Insulin

SUMMARY: Chlorpromazine administration may result in a loss of blood glucose control in diabetic patients.

RISK FACTORS:

→ ***Dosage Regimen.*** Chlorpromazine doses more than 100 mg are likely to increase the risk of interaction.

MECHANISM: Some have proposed that neuroleptics activate adrenergic mechanisms; however, the mechanism is unknown.[1]

CLINICAL EVALUATION: One study described 5 diabetic patients controlled on insulin in whom the disease became unstable during chlorpromazine therapy.[3] The effect appears to be dose related; chlorpromazine doses lower than 100 mg/day are less likely to affect glucose tolerance than higher doses.[2,4]

RELATED DRUGS: Little information is available on the effect of other neuroleptics on glucose tolerance.

MANAGEMENT OPTIONS: No specific action is required, but be alert for evidence of the interaction.

REFERENCES:

1. Jori A, et al. On the mechanism of the hyperglycemic effect of chlorpromazine. *J Pharm Pharmacol.* 1966;18:623.
2. Thonnard-Neumann E. Phenothiazines and diabetes in hospitalized women. *Am J Psychiatry.* 1968;124:978.
3. Arneson G. Phenothiazine derivatives and glucose metabolism. *J Neuropsychiatry.* 1964;5:181.
4. Erle G, et al. Effect of chlorpromazine on blood glucose and plasma insulin in man. *Eur J Clin Pharmacol.* 1977;11:15.

 Chlorpromazine (eg, *Thorazine*)

Levodopa (eg, *Larodopa*)

SUMMARY: Phenothiazines and related neuroleptic agents may inhibit the antiparkinsonian effect of levodopa.

RISK FACTORS: No specific risk factors are known.

MECHANISM: Neuroleptics block dopamine receptors in the brain and can produce extrapyramidal symptoms.

CLINICAL EVALUATION: The therapeutic response of patients with parkinsonism to levodopa may be inhibited by phenothiazines.[2-4] Chlorpromazine 200 mg/day for 3 days has been shown to inhibit stimulation of growth hormone secretion by levodopa.[1]

RELATED DRUGS: Levodopa also probably is inhibited by butyrophenones (eg, haloperidol [eg, *Haldol*]) and other neuroleptics.

MANAGEMENT OPTIONS:

➡ *Avoid Unless Benefit Outweighs Risk.* If possible, avoid administration of phenothiazines and other neuroleptics to patients receiving levodopa.

➡ *Monitor.* Monitor patients for reduced levodopa effect if phenothiazines are used.

REFERENCES:

1. Mims RB, et al. Inhibition of L-dopa-induced growth hormone stimulation by pyridoxine and chlorpromazine. *J Clin Endocrinol Metab.* 1975;40:256.
2. Yaryura-Tobias JA, et al. Action of L-dopa in a drug-induced extrapyramidalism. *Dis Nerv Syst.* 1970;31:60.
3. Yahr MD, et al. Drug therapy of parkinsonism. *N Engl J Med.* 1972;287:20.
4. Campbell JB. Long-term treatment of Parkinson's disease with levodopa. *Neurology.* 1970;20:18.

Chlorpromazine (eg, *Thorazine*)

Lithium (eg, *Eskalith*)

SUMMARY: Combined use of lithium and chlorpromazine may lower serum concentrations of both drugs. Rare cases of severe neurotoxicity have been reported in acute manic patients receiving lithium and phenothiazines, especially thioridazine.

RISK FACTORS:

➡ *Concurrent Diseases.* Patients with acute manic symptoms appear to be more likely to manifest neurotoxicity with the concurrent use of lithium and phenothiazines.

MECHANISM: Several pharmacokinetic interactions between neuroleptics and lithium have been described: lithium-induced reductions in plasma chlorpromazine concentrations; neuroleptic-induced increases in the uptake of lithium by the red cell and, perhaps, the brain; and chlorpromazine-induced increases in renal lithium excretion.

CLINICAL EVALUATION: The clinical outcome of the pharmacokinetic mechanisms is difficult to predict, but an altered response to either drug is possible when they are used concurrently. In addition to the pharmacokinetic interactions, clinical reports indicate that, in acute manic patients, concurrent therapy with lithium and phenothiazines (especially thioridazine [eg, *Mellaril*]) may increase the likelihood of neurotoxicity (eg, delirium, seizures, encephalopathy) or extrapyramidal symptoms.[1-3,5-12], In a retrospective study of 5 "severely agitated," elderly, bipolar patients on lithium, 3 rapidly developed neurotoxicity (disorientation, incoherence, fluctuating levels of consciousness) following the addition of chlorpromazine or haloperidol (eg, *Haldol*).[13] Two young men receiving neuroleptics (chlorpromazine or haloperidol) developed extrapyramidal symptoms within hours after lithium was added to their therapy.[14] In 1 patient, however, lithium-chlorpromazine neurotoxicity purportedly developed after 2 years of combined therapy.[16] It also has been suggested that chlorpromazine may reduce plasma lithium concentrations, and that the discontinuation of chlorpromazine in a patient taking lithium therapy may result in lithium toxicity.[4,15]

RELATED DRUGS: Consider the possibility that lithium interacts with other phenothiazines (especially thioridazine). The combined use of haloperidol and lithium has been implicated in the production of severe neurotoxic symptoms.

MANAGEMENT OPTIONS:

➥ *Monitor.* Monitor patients for neurotoxicity (eg, delirium, seizures, encephalopathy) with the concurrent use of lithium and phenothiazines (especially thioridazine) in patients with acute manic symptoms. Chronic therapy with these combinations appears less likely to result in an adverse interaction. Although the clinical importance of the pharmacokinetic interactions of phenothiazine and lithium is not well established, be alert for evidence of reduced phenothiazine response in the presence of lithium therapy.

REFERENCES:

1. Zall H, et al. Lithium carbonate: a clinical study. *Am J Psychiatry*. 1968;125:549.
2. Crammer JL, et al. Blood levels and management of lithium treatment. *BMJ*. 1974;3:650.
3. Kerzner B, et al. Lithium and chlorpromazine (CPZ) interaction. *Clin Pharmacol Ther*. 1976;19:109.
4. Sletten I, et al. The effect of chlorpromazine on lithium excretion in psychiatric subjects. *Curr Ther Res*. 1966;8:441.
5. Strayhorn JM, et al. Severe neurotoxicity despite "therapeutic" serum lithium levels. *Dis Nerv Syst*. 1977;38:107.
6. Rivera-Calimlim L, et al. Effect of lithium on plasma chlorpromazine levels. *Clin Pharmacol Ther*. 1978;23:451.
7. Ghadirian AM, et al. Neurological side effects of lithium: organic brain syndrome, seizures, extrapyramidal side effects, and EEG changes. *Compr Psychiatry*. 1981;21:327.
8. Spring S, et al. New data on lithium and haloperidol incompatibility. *Am J Psychiatry*. 1981;138:818.
9. Kamlana SH, et al. Lithium: some drug interactions. *Practitioner*. 1980;224:1291.
10. Addonizio G. Rapid induction of extrapyramidal side effects with combined use of lithium and neuroleptics. *J Clin Psychopharmacol*. 1985;5:296.
11. Yassa R. A case of lithium-chlorpromazine interaction. *J Clin Psychiatry*. 1986;47:90.
12. Bailine SH, et al. Neurotoxicity induced by combined lithium-thioridazine treatment. *Biol Psychiatry*. 1986;21:834.
13. Miller F, et al. Lithium-neuroleptic neurotoxicity in the elderly bipolar patient. *J Clin Psychopharmacol*. 1986;6:176.
14. Addonizio G, et al. Rapid induction of extrapyramidal side effects with combined use of lithium and neuroleptics. *J Clin Psychopharmacol*. 1985;5:296.
15. Pakes GE. Lithium toxicity with neuroleptics withdrawal. *Lancet*. 1979;2:701.
16. Yassa R. A case of lithium-chlorpromazine interaction. *J Clin Psychiatry*. 1986;47:90.

Chlorpromazine (eg, *Thorazine*)

Meperidine (eg, *Demerol*)

SUMMARY: The combination of chlorpromazine and meperidine may result in hypotension and excessive CNS depression.

RISK FACTORS: No specific risk factors are known.

MECHANISM: Unknown; probably additive pharmacodynamic effects.

CLINICAL EVALUATION: Ten healthy subjects were given a single dose of IM meperidine 26 mg/m² with and without concurrent IM chlorpromazine 30 mg/m².[1] Chlorpromazine did not alter meperidine pharmacokinetics, but did increase the urinary excretion of normeperidine. The meperidine-chlorpromazine combination also was associated with considerably more lethargy and a greater hypotensive response than the meperidine-placebo combination. Two of the subjects on meperidine and chlorpromazine developed severe orthostatic hypotension.

Although these toxic effects were associated with evidence of increased norme-peridine formation, the role of normeperidine in the production of these effects is unclear. For example, one cannot rule out the possibility that the adverse effects resulted from the combined pharmacologic effect of chlorpromazine and meperidine itself.

RELATED DRUGS: Whether other combinations of neuroleptics and narcotic analgesics would produce similar effects is unknown, but, in general, expect enhanced respiratory depression and hypotension with such combinations.

MANAGEMENT OPTIONS:

➡ *Monitor.* Be alert for evidence of excessive CNS depression, hypotension, and respiratory depression when meperidine and chlorpromazine are used concurrently. Until more information is available, caution is advised for other combinations of neuroleptics and narcotic analgesics.

REFERENCES:

1. Stambaugh JE, et al. Drug interaction: meperidine and chlorpromazine, a toxic combination. *J Clin Pharmacol.* 1981;21:140.
2. Swett C, et al. Hypotension due to chlorpromazine. *Arch Gen Psychiatry.* 1977;34:661.

Chlorpromazine (eg, *Thorazine*)

Orphenadrine (eg, *Norflex*)

SUMMARY: The combination of orphenadrine and chlorpromazine may result in lower serum chlorpromazine concentrations and excessive anticholinergic effects. Also, a patient on chlorpromazine and orphenadrine developed hypoglycemia; the clinical importance of this effect is unclear.

RISK FACTORS: No specific risk factors are known.

MECHANISM: Not established.

CLINICAL EVALUATION: The anticholinergic effect of orphenadrine may reduce the chlorpromazine plasma concentrations by inhibiting the GI absorption of the chlorpromazine.[1] A single case has been reported in which a patient receiving both orphenadrine and chlorpromazine developed severe symptomatic hypoglycemia.[3] Subsequent studies in this patient indicated that combined therapy with these agents may result in an enhanced hypoglycemic response to a tolbutamide test (1 g IV).

RELATED DRUGS: The effect of orphenadrine combined with other phenothiazines is not established. There was no mention of adverse effects caused by drug interaction in 6 patients who were receiving orphenadrine and fluphenazine (eg, *Prolixin*).[2]

MANAGEMENT OPTIONS:

➡ *Monitor.* In patients on concomitant neuroleptics and orphenadrine, be alert for evidence of excessive anticholinergic effects (especially ileus), reduced neuroleptic plasma concentrations, or hypoglycemia.

REFERENCES:

1. Loga S, et al. Interactions of orphenadrine and phenobarbitone with chlorpromazine: plasma concentrations and effects in man. *Br J Clin Pharmacol.* 1975;2:197.
2. Fleming P, et al. Levodopa in drug-induced extrapyramidal disorders. *Lancet.* 1970;2:1186.
3. Buckle RM, et al. Hypoglycaemic coma occurring during treatment with chlorpromazine and orphenadrine. *BMJ.* 1967;4:599.

4   Chlorpromazine (eg, *Thorazine*)

Phenmetrazine

SUMMARY: Chlorpromazine may inhibit the anorectic effect of phenmetrazine.

RISK FACTORS: No specific risk factors are known.

MECHANISM: Not established.

CLINICAL EVALUATION: A double-blind, controlled study in psychiatric patients indicated that chlorpromazine reduced the ability of phenmetrazine to produce weight loss.[1] Another study in 30 obese psychiatric patients yielded similar results.[2] Thus, it appears that chlorpromazine (and possibly other neuroleptics) can reduce the anorectic effect of phenmetrazine.

RELATED DRUGS: The effect of other phenothiazines on phenmetrazine is not established, but consider the possibility that they also interact.

MANAGEMENT OPTIONS: No specific action is required, but be alert for evidence of the interaction.

REFERENCES:

1. Reid AA. Pharmacological antagonism between chlorpromazine and phenmetrazine in mental hospital patients. *Med J Aust*. 1964;1:187.
2. Sletten IW, et al. Weight reduction with chlorphentermine and phenmetrazine in obese psychiatric patients during chlorpromazine therapy. *Curr Ther Res*. 1967;9:570.

Chlorpromazine (eg, *Thorazine*)

Phenobarbital

SUMMARY: Barbiturates may reduce some chlorpromazine concentrations, but the degree to which the therapeutic response to chlorpromazine is reduced is not established.

RISK FACTORS: No specific risk factors are known.

MECHANISM: Barbiturates probably increase the metabolism of chlorpromazine by inducing hepatic microsomal enzymes. The increased urinary excretion of the conjugated fraction of chlorpromazine following phenobarbital supports this view.

CLINICAL EVALUATION: Phenobarbital increases the urinary excretion of chlorpromazine[1] and also reduces plasma chlorpromazine concentrations.[2,3] In a crossover study involving 12 patients on chlorpromazine 300 mg/day, phenobarbital 150 mg/day was associated with considerable reductions in plasma chlorpromazine concentrations.[3] The therapeutic significance of these findings has not been determined, but it appears reasonable to assume that the antipsychotic effect of chlorpromazine may be somewhat reduced.

RELATED DRUGS: The effect of barbiturates on other neuroleptics is not established, but be aware of a possible reduction in the antipsychotic effect. There is also some evidence that thioridazine (eg, *Mellaril*) may reduce serum phenobarbital concentrations.[4] One patient undergoing withdrawal from barbiturates and methaqualone developed fatal hyperthermia after he was given haloperidol (eg, *Haldol*).[5] It was proposed that the tendency of sedative-hypnotic withdrawal to produce hyperpyrexia was markedly enhanced by the ability of the haloperidol to interfere with thermoregulation.

MANAGEMENT OPTIONS:

➡ **Monitor.** It does not seem necessary to avoid concomitant use of neuroleptics and barbiturates, but monitor patients for evidence of a reduced effect of either drug if the combination is used.

REFERENCES:

1. Forrest FM, et al. Modification of chlorpromazine metabolism by some other drugs frequently administered to psychiatric patients. *Biol Psychiatry*. 1970;2:53.
2. Curry SH, et al. Factors affecting chlorpromazine plasma levels in psychiatric patients. *Arch Gen Psychiatry*. 1970;22:209.
3. Loga S et, al. Interactions of orphenadrine and phenobarbitone with chlorpromazine: plasma concentrations and effects in a man. *Br J Clin Pharmacol*. 1975;2:197.
4. Gay PE, et al. Interaction between phenobarbital and thioridazine. *Neurology*. 1983;33:1631.
5. Greenblatt DJ, et al. Fatal hyperthermia following haloperidol therapy of sedative-hypnotic withdrawal. *J Clin Psychiatry*. 1978;39:673.

Chlorpromazine (eg, *Thorazine*)

Propranolol (eg, *Inderal*)

SUMMARY: Propranolol and some beta blockers and neuroleptics such as chlorpromazine can increase the plasma concentrations of each other, resulting in accentuated pharmacologic responses of both drugs.

RISK FACTORS: No specific risk factors are known.

MECHANISM: Chlorpromazine and propranolol each inhibit the metabolism of the other.[2,3,6,7] Propranolol also may inhibit the metabolism of other neuroleptics.[4,5,8] Furthermore, both the beta blockers and neuroleptics can cause hypotension, and propranolol can reverse some of the electrocardiographic abnormalities induced by neuroleptics.[1,3]

CLINICAL EVALUATION: Chlorpromazine 150 mg/day increased propranolol plasma concentrations and the degree of beta blockade.[6] Propranolol 8 to 10 mg/kg/day inhibited the metabolism of chlorpromazine and resulted in accumulation of chlorpromazine and its metabolites.[2,7] A schizophrenic patient on thiothixene (eg, *Navane*) developed delirium and seizures after the addition of propranolol (up to 1200 mg/day).[8] Plasma concentrations of thioridazine (eg, *Mellaril*) and its active metabolite were increased by up to 3 to 4 times the baseline levels in patients treated with propranolol 320 to 800 mg/day.[4,5] Propranolol had little effect on haloperidol (eg, *Haldol*) concentrations.[4] Chlorpromazine is known to have hypotensive activity and may enhance the effects of beta blockers.

RELATED DRUGS: Thiothixene and thioridazine concentrations increase in patients treated with propranolol, while propranolol appears to have little effect on haloperidol concentrations. While other pairs of beta blockers and neuroleptics may interact in a similar manner, the interaction may not occur with beta blockers excreted primarily by the kidneys, such as atenolol (eg, *Tenormin*) and nadolol (eg, *Corgard*).

MANAGEMENT OPTIONS:

➡ **Consider Alternative.** The use of beta blockers (eg, nadolol) that are renally eliminated may lessen the magnitude of this interaction.

➤ **Monitor.** Monitor patients receiving neuroleptics and beta blockers for enhanced effects of both drugs. The dosage of one or both drugs may require reduction.

REFERENCES:

1. Alvarez-Mena SC, et al. Phenothiazine-induced abnormalities. *JAMA.* 1973;224:1730.

2. Peet M, et al. Propranolol in schizophrenia. II. Clinical and biochemical aspects of combining propranolol with chlorpromazine. *Br J Psychiatry.* 1981;139:112.

3. Arita M, et al. Effects of phenothiazine and propranolol on ECG. The effects of propranolol on the electrocardiographic abnormalities induced by phenothiazine derivatives. *Jpn Circ J.* 1970;34:391.

4. Greendyke RM, et al. Plasma propranolol levels and their effect on plasma thioridazine and haloperidol concentrations. *J Clin Psychopharmacol.* 1987;7:178.

5. Silver JM, et al. Elevation of thioridazine plasma levels by propranolol. *Am J Psychiatry.* 1986;143:1290.

6. Vestal RE, et al. Inhibition of propranolol metabolism by chlorpromazine. *Clin Pharmacol Ther.* 1979;25:19.

7. Peet M, et al. Pharmacokinetic interaction between propranolol and chlorpromazine in schizophrenic patients. *Lancet.* 1980;2:978.

8. Miller FA. Adverse effects of combined propranolol and chlorpromazine therapy. *Am J Psychiatry.* 1982;139:1198.

4   Chlorpromazine (eg, *Thorazine*)

Tranylcypromine (*Parnate*)

SUMMARY: The combined use of monoamine oxidase inhibitors (MAOIs) and phenothiazines has been reported to cause increased extrapyramidal symptoms.

RISK FACTORS: No specific risk factors are known.

MECHANISM: Not established. MAOIs may inhibit the metabolism of neuroleptics.

CLINICAL EVALUATION: Nonselective MAOIs reportedly increase phenothiazine side effects (eg, extrapyramidal reactions).[1] However, in several reported studies, various combinations of these drugs were used to treat psychiatric disorders without any significant problems. In at least one of these studies using tranylcypromine plus trifluoperazine (eg, *Stelazine*), side effects of both agents were *decreased* by using them in combination.[2] Some have proposed that trifluoperazine protects against tyramine-induced hypertensive crises in patients receiving tranylcypromine. This effect, if it indeed occurs, may result from the alpha-adrenergic blocking effect of trifluoperazine. Thus, some combinations of MAOIs and neuroleptics may be beneficial, while other combinations may increase side effects.

RELATED DRUGS: See Clinical Evaluation.

MANAGEMENT OPTIONS: No specific action is required, but be alert for evidence of the interaction.

REFERENCES:

1. Sjoqvist F. Psychotropic drugs (2). Interaction between monoamine oxidase (MAO) inhibitors and other substances. *Proc R Soc Med.* 1965;58:967.

2. Hedberg DL, et al. Tranylcypromine-trifluoperazine combination in the treatment of schizophrenia. *Am J Psychiatry.* 1971;127:1141.

Chlorpromazine (eg, *Thorazine*)

Trazodone (eg, *Desyrel*)

SUMMARY: Isolated case reports suggest that concurrent therapy with trazodone and neuroleptics such as chlorpromazine may produce an additive hypotension.

RISK FACTORS: No specific risk factors are known.

MECHANISM: Both trazodone and neuroleptics individually can result in hypotension; additive effects may be seen with combined use.

CLINICAL EVALUATION: A 28-year-old man taking chlorpromazine developed hypotension and fell after trazodone (100 mg/day increasing to 300 mg/day) was added to his therapy. The blood pressure returned to baseline when trazodone was stopped. A similar hypotensive reaction was observed in a 20-year-old woman when 100 mg/day of trazodone was added to trifluoperazine (*Stelazine*) therapy; again, the hypotension resolved when the trazodone was discontinued.[1] Although it appears that the hypotension resulted from combined use of trazodone and neuroleptics, hypotension caused by trazodone alone cannot be ruled out.

RELATED DRUGS: Trifluoperazine (eg, *Stelazine*) appears to interact similarly.

MANAGEMENT OPTIONS:

➡ *Monitor.* Monitor patients for hypotension if trazodone and neuroleptics are used concurrently.

REFERENCES:
1. Asayesh K, et al. Combination of trazodone and phenothiazines; a possible additive hypotensive effect. *Can J Psychiatry.* 1986;31:857.

Chlorpropamide (eg, *Diabinese*)

Clofibrate (*Atromid-S*)

SUMMARY: Clofibrate may enhance the effects of oral hypoglycemic drugs in some patients.

RISK FACTORS: No specific risk factors are known.

MECHANISM: Clofibrate may enhance the activity of chlorpropamide and other sulfonylureas by displacing them from plasma protein binding sites, decreasing insulin resistance,[3] and competing with chlorpropamide for renal tubular secretion.[1]

CLINICAL EVALUATION: Some investigators have failed to detect an effect of clofibrate on the hypoglycemic response to sulfonylureas in diabetes,[4,6] whereas others have noted enhanced hypoglycemia.[2,3,5] Also, a study in 5 subjects given clofibrate plus chlorpropamide indicated that clofibrate may prolong chlorpropamide half-life.[1] In summary, certain diabetic patients appear to develop enhanced hypoglycemia when clofibrate is given with sulfonylureas, while other patients are not so affected.

RELATED DRUGS: Other sulfonylureas may be similarly affected by clofibrate.

MANAGEMENT OPTIONS:

➡ **Monitor.** Closely monitor patients treated with clofibrate and chlorpropamide or other sulfonylureas for hypoglycemia. This caution would apply especially when clofibrate is started or stopped in patients stabilized on a sulfonylurea.

REFERENCES:

1. Petitpierre B, et al. Behavior of chlorpropamide in renal insufficiency and under the effect of associated drug therapy. *Int J Clin Pharmacol Ther Toxicol.* 1972;6:120.

2. Daubresse JC, et al. Potentiation of hypoglycemic effect of sulfonylureas by clofibrate. *N Engl J Med.* 1976;294:613..

3. Ferrari C, et al. Potentiation of hypoglycemic response to intravenous tolbutamide by clofibrate. *N Engl J Med.* 1976;294:613.

4. Albert M, et al. Vascular symptomatic relief during administration of ethylchlorophenoxyisobutyrate (clofibrate). *Metabolism.* 1969;18:635.

5. Daubresse JC, et al. Clofibrate and diabetes control in patients treated with oral hypoglycaemic agents. *Br J Clin Pharmacol.* 1979;7:599.

6. Jain AK, et al. Potentiation of hypoglycemic effect of sulfonylureas by halofenate. *N Engl J Med.* 1975;239:1283.

 Chlorpropamide (eg, *Diabinese*)

Dicumarol

SUMMARY: Limited clinical evidence suggests that dicumarol and acenocoumarol may increase chlorpropamide serum concentrations, but the clinical importance is not established. Little is known about a possible interaction between chlorpropamide and warfarin (eg, *Coumadin*).

RISK FACTORS: No specific risk factors are known.

MECHANISM: Not established. Dicumarol may impair the hepatic metabolism or the renal excretion of chlorpropamide.[1]

CLINICAL EVALUATION: Increases in serum chlorpropamide concentrations following dicumarol therapy were noted in 3 diabetic patients,[1] and an increase in chlorpropamide half-life was noted in 1 patient following the administration of acenocoumarol.[2]

RELATED DRUGS: The effect of chlorpropamide on the response to oral anticoagulants, if any, is not known. It does not seem likely that oral anticoagulants would interact with insulin.

MANAGEMENT OPTIONS: No specific action is required, but be alert for evidence of the interaction.

REFERENCES:

1. Kristensen M, et al. Accumulation of chlorpropamide caused by dicumarol. *Acta Med Scand.* 1968;183:83.

2. Petitpierre B, et al. Behaviour of chlorpropamide in renal insufficiency and under the effect of associated drug therapy. *Int J Clin Pharmacol Ther Toxicol.* 1972;6:120.

Chlorpropamide (eg, *Diabinese*)

Erythromycin (eg, *E-Mycin*)

SUMMARY: A patient developed severe hepatic toxicity during the coadministration of erythromycin ethylsuccinate and chlorpropamide.

RISK FACTORS: No specific risk factors are known.

MECHANISM: Not established.

CLINICAL EVALUATION: A case of severe cholestatic hepatitis was reported in a patient receiving chlorpropamide and erythromycin ethylsuccinate 1 g/day.[1] During the second week of combined therapy, the patient developed a rash, jaundice, and hepatomegaly. Chlorpropamide and erythromycin were discontinued, but hepatic failure continued and the patient eventually died of liver and heart failure. While liver toxicity has been reported with both erythromycin and chlorpropamide, this case is unusual in that the hepatic damage did not reverse upon withdrawal of the drugs and the liver displayed significant hepatocellular damage. A causal relationship was not established. No information was provided on the hypoglycemic response to chlorpropamide during erythromycin administration.

RELATED DRUGS: No information is available.

MANAGEMENT OPTIONS:

➡ *Monitor.* Until more information is available on this potential interaction, monitor patients taking chlorpropamide and erythromycin for changes in hypoglycemic control and hepatotoxicity.

REFERENCES:

1. Geubel AP, et al. Prolonged cholestasis and disappearance of interlobular bile ducts following chlorpropamide and erythromycin ethylsuccinate: case of drug interaction? *Liver.* 1988;8:350.

Chlorpropamide (eg, *Diabinese*)

Ethanol (Ethyl Alcohol) AVOID

SUMMARY: Excessive ethanol intake may lead to altered glycemic control, most commonly hypoglycemia. An "*Antabuse*"-like reaction may occur in patients taking sulfonylureas.

RISK FACTORS: No specific risk factors are known.

MECHANISM: The mechanisms for this interaction are the following: 1) Ethanol may exhibit intrinsic hypoglycemic activity, although hyperglycemia also has been noted, 2) Chlorpropamide and, to a lesser extent, other sulfonylureas may provoke an "*Antabuse* reaction" (eg, flushing and headache) to ethanol.[10,11] A similar effect may occur with chlorpropamide, and 3) Ethanol may inhibit the antidiuretic effect of chlorpropamide when used to treat diabetes insipidus.[8]

CLINICAL EVALUATION: Acute ingestion of ethanol by patients on any antidiabetic agent carries the risk of severe hypoglycemia, especially in fasting patients.[1,2,7] The increased tolbutamide (eg, *Orinase*) metabolism in alcoholics probably decreases its hypoglycemic effect, although the intrinsic hypoglycemic activity of ethanol may counteract the effects somewhat. The ingestion of even small amounts of ethanol by patients taking chlorpropamide and other sulfonylureas has been reported to result in an *"Antabuse"*-like reaction that includes flushing and headache. The incidence of this reaction is probably uncommon. Finally, 2 patients receiving chlorpropamide for diabetes insipidus developed polyuria and polydipsia following ethanol intake, presumably because of ethanol inhibition of chlorpropamide-induced antidiuresis.[8]

RELATED DRUGS: Excessive ethanol may produce hypoglycemia in patients taking insulin or other oral hypoglycemic agents. Prolonged heavy intake of ethanol markedly decreases the half-life of tolbutamide, probably by inducing hepatic enzymes.[3,6,9] Ethanol ingestion may contribute to lactic acidosis in patients receiving phenformin.[4,5]

MANAGEMENT OPTIONS:

➡ *AVOID COMBINATION.* Because an *"Antabuse reaction"* may occur following ethanol ingestion in patients receiving sulfonylureas, inform patients of this possibility when therapy is initiated. Avoid ingestion of moderate to large amounts of ethanol by patients on antidiabetic drugs because of the possible adverse effects of alcohol on diabetic control.

REFERENCES:

1. Arky RA, et al. Irreversible hypoglycemia, a complication of alcohol and insulin. *JAMA.* 1968;206:575.
2. Hartling SG, et al. Interaction of ethanol and glipizide in humans. *Diabetes Care.* 1987;10:263.
3. Kater RMH, et al. Increased rate tolbutamide metabolism in alcoholic patients. *JAMA.* 1969;207:363.
4. Johnson HK, et al. Relationship of alcohol and hyperlactatemia in diabetic subjects treated with phenformin. *Am J Med.* 1968;45:98.
5. Kreisberg RA, et al. Hyperlacticacidemia in man: ethanol-phenformin synergism. *J Clin Endocrinol.* 1972;34:29.
6. Carulli N, et al. Alcohol-drugs interaction in man: alcohol and tolbutamide. *Eur J Clin Invest.* 1971;1:421.
7. Baruh S, et al. Fasting hypoglycemia. *Med Clin North Am.* 1973;57:1441.
8. Yamamoto LT. Diabetes insipidus and drinking alcohol. *N Engl J Med.* 1976;294:55.
9. Sotaniemi EA, et al. Half-life of intravenous tolbutamide in the serum of patients in medical wards. *Ann Clin Res.* 1974;6:146.
10. Assad MM, et al. Studies on the biochemical aspects of the "disulfiram like" reaction induced by oral hypoglycemics. *Eur Pharmacol.* 1976;35:301.
11. Wardle EN, et al. Alcohol and glibenclamide. *BMJ.* 1971;3:309.

5 Chlorpropamide (eg, *Diabinese*)

Lovastatin (*Mevacor*)

SUMMARY: No interaction.

RISK FACTORS: No specific risk factors are known.

MECHANISM: No interaction.

CLINICAL EVALUATION: Seven patients with type 2 diabetes mellitus and hypercholesterolemia were stabilized on chlorpropamide doses ranging from 125 to 750 mg/day. Lovastatin 20 mg twice daily was administered for 6 weeks. No change in chlorpropamide plasma concentrations or glycemic response was noted during lovastatin coadministration.

RELATED DRUGS: It appears unlikely that chlorpropamide would interact with any HMG-CoA reductase inhibitor. The effect of lovastatin on other hypoglycemic agents is unknown but would likely be similar to that of chlorpropamide.

MANAGEMENT OPTIONS: No interaction.

REFERENCES:

1. Johnson BF, et al. Effects of lovastatin in diabetic patients treated with chlorpropamide. *Clin Pharmacol Ther.* 1990;48:467.

Chlorpropamide (eg, *Diabinese*)

Probenecid (*Benemid*)

SUMMARY: Probenecid may increase chlorpropamide concentrations in some patients; however, the clinical significance of this is uncertain.

RISK FACTORS: No specific risk factors are known.

MECHANISM: Probenecid may inhibit the renal tubular secretion of chlorpropamide.[1]

CLINICAL EVALUATION: In 6 patients receiving probenecid 1 to 2 g/day, the average half-life of chlorpropamide was found to be 50 hours (usual half-life, 36 hours).[1] An earlier report[2] indicated that probenecid increased half-life of tolbutamide (eg, *Orinase*), but a later study failed to confirm this finding.[3] Thus, probenecid possibly increases the effect of chlorpropamide and probably has little effect on tolbutamide.

RELATED DRUGS: Probenecid probably has little effect on tolbutamide.

MANAGEMENT OPTIONS: No specific action is required, but be alert for evidence of the interaction.

REFERENCES:

1. Petitpierre B, et al. Behavior of chlorpropamide in renal insufficiency and under the effect of associated drug therapy. *Int J Clin Pharmacol Ther Toxicol.* 1972;6:120.

2. Stowers JM, et al. Clinical and pharmacological comparison of chlorpropamide and other sulfonyl-ureas. *Ann NY Acad Sci.* 1959;74:689.

3. Brook R, et al. Failure of probenecid to inhibit the rate of metabolism of tolbutamide in man. *Clin Pharmacol Ther.* 1968;9:314.

Chlorpropamide (eg, *Diabinese*)

Sucralfate (eg, *Carafate*)

SUMMARY: A single study in normal subjects indicates that sucralfate has minimal effects on the GI absorption of chlorpropamide.

RISK FACTORS: No specific risk factors are known.

MECHANISM: The mechanism for the slight reduction in chlorpropamide bioavailability is not established.

CLINICAL EVALUATION: In a randomized crossover study, 12 healthy subjects were given a single 250 mg oral dose of chlorpropamide with and without sucralfate 1 g 4 times daily for 3 days.[1] Sucralfate only slightly reduced the bioavailability of chlorpropamide. Although a multiple-dose study in patients on chlorpropamide is needed to rule out a clinically important reduction in chlorpropamide absorption, the results of the current study indicate that the combined use of chlorpropamide and sucralfate is unlikely to affect chlorpropamide response.

RELATED DRUGS: No information is available.

MANAGEMENT OPTIONS: No specific action is required, but be alert for evidence of the interaction.

REFERENCES:
1. Letendre PW, et al. Effect of sucralfate on the absorption and pharmacokinetics of chlorpropamide. *J Clin Pharmacol.* 1986;26:622.

Cholestyramine (eg, *Questran*)

Diclofenac (eg, *Voltaren*)

SUMMARY: Single dose studies in healthy subjects suggest that cholestyramine substantially reduces the bioavailability of diclofenac; reduced diclofenac effect may occur.

RISK FACTORS: No specific risk factors are known.

MECHANISM: Cholestyramine probably binds with diclofenac in the GI tract, thus inhibiting diclofenac absorption. Cholestyramine also may interfere with the enterohepatic circulation of diclofenac.

CLINICAL EVALUATION: Six healthy subjects took a single oral dose of diclofenac 100 mg alone and with cholestyramine 8 mg or colestipol in a randomized 3-way crossover study.[1] Cholestyramine reduced the diclofenac area under the plasma concentration-time curve 62%. Although the effect of chronic concurrent dosing of the 2 drugs was not studied, it is likely that a substantial reduction in diclofenac plasma concentrations would occur.

RELATED DRUGS: Cholestyramine also reduces the serum concentrations of other nonsteroidal anti-inflammatory drugs such as ketoprofen (eg, *Orudis*), piroxicam (eg, *Feldene*), and tenoxicam. Colestipol (*Colestid*) also appears to inhibit the absorption of diclofenac, but to a somewhat lesser extent.

MANAGEMENT OPTIONS:

➡ *Consider Alternative.* Colestipol appears to reduce diclofenac absorption to a lesser extent than cholestyramine, but it still would be prudent to give the diclofenac 2 hours before or 6 hours after the colestipol.

➡ *Circumvent/Minimize.* Giving diclofenac 2 hours before or 6 hours after the cholestyramine would be expected to optimize the absorption of the diclofenac. Nonetheless, because diclofenac undergoes enterohepatic circulation, reduced diclofenac plasma concentrations may occur even if dosing of the drugs is separated.

➡ *Monitor.* Monitor patients for reduced diclofenac effect, regardless of how far apart the doses are separated.

REFERENCES:
1. Al-balla SR, et al. The effects of cholestyramine and colestipol on the absorption of diclofenac in man. *Int J Clin Pharmacol Ther.* 1994;32;441.

Cholestyramine (eg, *Questran*)

Digoxin (*Lanoxin*)

SUMMARY: Cholestyramine appears to reduce the serum concentrations of digoxin and digitoxin (*Crystodigin*), but the clinical impact in chronically treated patients has not been adequately assessed.

RISK FACTORS: No specific risk factors are known.

MECHANISM: Cholestyramine appears to bind digoxin and digitoxin in the GI tract, thus interrupting the enterohepatic circulation of their cardiac glycosides and shortens their half-lives.

CLINICAL EVALUATION: A multiple-dose study in healthy subjects found a 32% reduction in the area under the digoxin concentration-time curve after cholestyramine 8 g/day.[1] Additional studies in healthy volunteers also have indicated that cholestyramine inhibits the absorption of digoxin[4,6] or reduces its half-life,[5] but some long-term studies have failed to demonstrate a consistent effect of cholestyramine on serum concentrations of digoxin.[3] In a study of 15 subjects, 7 received maintenance doses of cholestyramine following digitalization with digitoxin.[2] Serum concentrations were lower and the pharmacologic activity of digitoxin was diminished in those receiving cholestyramine. Cholestyramine also may accelerate digitoxin elimination in cases of digitoxin overdose.[5]

RELATED DRUGS: Digitoxin concentrations and pharmacologic activity were reduced after cholestyramine coadministration. Colestipol (*Colestid*) also has been noted to reduce digitalis glycoside concentrations.

MANAGEMENT OPTIONS:

➡ *Monitor.* Until more is known about this interaction, monitor patients on digitalis glycosides for underdigitalization when cholestyramine is coadministered. Giving the digitalis product 2 hours or more before the cholestyramine may lessen the magnitude of the interaction.

REFERENCES:

1. Brown DD, et al. A steady-state evaluation of the effects of propantheline bromide and cholestyramine on the bioavailability of digoxin when administered as tablets or capsules. *J Clin Pharmacol.* 1985;25:360.
2. Caldwell JH, et al. Interruption of the enterohepatic circulation of digitoxin by cholestyramine. *J Clin Invest.* 1971;50:2638.
3. Hall WH, et al. Effect of cholestyramine on digoxin absorption and excretion in man. *Am J Cardiol.* 1977;39:213.
4. Brown DD, et al. Decreased bioavailability of digoxin due to hypocholesterolemic interventions. *Circulation.* 1978;58:164.
5. Pieroni RE, et al. Use of cholestyramine resin in digitoxin toxicity. *JAMA.* 1981;245:1939.
6. Neuvonen PJ, et al. Effects of resins and activated charcoal on the absorption of digoxin, carbamazepine and furosemide. *Br J Clin Pharmacol.* 1988;25:229.

Cholestyramine (eg, *Questran*)

Furosemide (eg, *Lasix*)

SUMMARY: Study in healthy subjects suggests that cholestyramine markedly reduces the bioavailability and diuretic response of furosemide.

RISK FACTORS: No specific risk factors are known.

MECHANISM: Cholestyramine probably binds with furosemide in the GI tract, thus reducing its bioavailability.

CLINICAL EVALUATION: Six healthy subjects received a single oral 40 mg dose of furosemide with and without coadministration of cholestyramine 8 g.[1] The bioavailability of furosemide, as measured by area under the plasma concentration-time curve and total urinary elimination, was reduced 95% by cholestyramine. The reduction in furosemide bioavailability was accompanied by a 77% reduction in furosemide diuretic response. Thus, it appears that cholestyramine can dramatically reduce furosemide effects.

RELATED DRUGS: Colestipol (*Colestid*) also substantially reduces the bioavailability of furosemide. The effect of cholestyramine and colestipol on other loop diuretics is not established.

MANAGEMENT OPTIONS:

➡ *Circumvent/Minimize.* Although the ability to circumvent the interaction by separating doses of furosemide from cholestyramine has not been systematically studied, giving furosemide 2 hours before or 6 hours after the cholestyramine would be expected to minimize the interaction.

➡ *Monitor.* Monitor patients for altered furosemide response if cholestyramine therapy is initiated, discontinued, changed in dosage, or if the interval between doses of the 2 drugs is changed.

REFERENCES:

1. Neuvonen PJ, et al. Effects of resins and activated charcoal on the absorption of digoxin, carbamazepine and furosemide. *Br J Clin Pharmacol.* 1988;25:229.

Cholestyramine (eg, *Questran*)

Glipizide (eg, *Glucotrol*)

SUMMARY: Glipizide absorption is reduced by cholestyramine coadministration, but the clinical importance of this interaction is unknown.

RISK FACTORS: No specific risk factors are known.

MECHANISM: Cholestyramine probably binds glipizide in the GI tract, thereby inhibiting its absorption and possibly its enterohepatic circulation.

CLINICAL EVALUATION: Six healthy subjects received a single 5 mg dose of glipizide alone and with 8 g of cholestyramine in 150 ml of water.[1] The relative bioavailability of glipizide following cholestyramine administration was reduced on average 29% (range, 17% to 41%) compared with taking glipizide alone. The peak glipizide serum concentration was reduced 33%. Clinical studies are needed to assess whether cholestyramine reduces the hypoglycemic response to glipizide.

RELATED DRUGS: Cholestyramine does not appear to alter the absorption of tolbutamide (eg, *Orinase*).[2] While the use of tolbutamide could be considered, the effect of cholestyramine on other oral hypoglycemic agents is unknown. Colestipol (*Colestid*) might affect glipizide in a similar manner.

MANAGEMENT OPTIONS: No specific action is required, but be alert for evidence of the interaction.

REFERENCES:

1. Kivisto KT, et al. The effect of cholestyramine and activated charcoal on glipizide absorption. *Br J Clin Pharmacol*. 1990;30:733.

2. Hunninghake DB, et al. Effect of bile acid sequestering agents on the absorption of aspirin, tolbutamide and warfarin. *Fed Proc*. 1977;35:996.

Cholestyramine (eg, *Questran*)

Hydrocortisone (eg, *Hycort*)

SUMMARY: Cholestyramine may lower plasma concentrations of oral hydrocortisone, possibly reducing its therapeutic effect.

RISK FACTORS: No specific risk factors are known.

MECHANISM: Cholestyramine may inhibit the GI absorption of hydrocortisone.

CLINICAL EVALUATION: Ten healthy subjects were given hydrocortisone 50 mg orally with and without concurrent oral cholestyramine 4 to 8 g.[1] The 4 g dose of cholestyramine reduced the area under the hydrocortisone plasma concentration-time curve 35%; the effect was greater with the 8 g dose. Thus, it appears that cholestyramine reduces the extent of hydrocortisone absorption, but multiple-dose studies will be required to determine the clinical importance of these findings.

RELATED DRUGS: The effect of cholestyramine on other corticosteroids is not established, but because corticosteroids are closely related structurally, it is possible that cholestyramine affects their absorption as well. Colestipol (*Colestid*) probably interacts with corticosteroids in a manner similar to cholestyramine, but evidence is lacking.

MANAGEMENT OPTIONS:

➡ *Circumvent/Minimize.* Separate doses of oral hydrocortisone (and other corticosteroids) from cholestyramine as much as possible to minimize their mixing in the GI tract. Theoretically, giving the corticosteroid 2 hours before or 6 hours after the cholestyramine would optimize corticosteroid absorption. It also would be prudent to maintain a constant interval between the doses of corticosteroids and cholestyramine to minimize fluctuation of any interaction that does occur.

➡ *Monitor.* Monitor patients for evidence of reduced corticosteroid response and increase the dose as needed when these drugs are used concurrently.

REFERENCES:

1. Johansson C, et al. Interaction by cholestyramine on the uptake of hydrocortisone in the GI tract. *Acta Med Scand*. 1978;204:509.

Cholestyramine (eg, *Questran*)

Imipramine (eg, *Tofranil*)

SUMMARY: Cholestyramine may produce a modest reduction in imipramine plasma concentrations, but the clinical importance of this effect is not established.

RISK FACTORS: No specific risk factors are known.

MECHANISM: Cholestyramine probably binds with imipramine in the GI tract, thus reducing its absorption.

CLINICAL EVALUATION: Six depressed patients receiving imipramine 75 to 150 mg/day (usually twice daily) were given cholestyramine 4 g 3 times daily for 4 days).[1] Each dose of imipramine was taken simultaneously with the cholestyramine. Concurrent cholestyramine reduced steady-state imipramine plasma concentrations 25%; levels returned to baseline after the cholestyramine was discontinued. Cholestyramine also somewhat reduced plasma concentrations of desipramine (an imipramine metabolite), but the effect was not statistically significant. Although the reductions in imipramine plasma concentrations were not large in most patients, it is possible that some patients would manifest a reduction in antidepressant response.

RELATED DRUGS: Little is known about the effect of cholestyramine on antidepressants other than imipramine, but consider the possibility of reduced antidepressant plasma concentrations if cholestyramine is taken concurrently. Theoretically, the binding resin colestipol (*Colestid*) also may interact with tricyclic antidepressants (TCAs).

MANAGEMENT OPTIONS:

➡ *Circumvent/Minimize.* Although the ability to circumvent the interaction by separating doses of imipramine before cholestyramine has not been systematically studied, giving imipramine 2 hours before or 6 hours after the cholestyramine would be expected to minimize the interaction.

➡ *Monitor.* Monitor patients for altered TCA effect if cholestyramine is initiated, discontinued, or changed in dosage; adjust antidepressant dose as needed.

REFERENCES:

1. Spina E, et al. Decreased plasma concentrations of imipramine and desipramine following cholestyramine intake in depressed patients. *Ther Drug Monit*. 1994;16:432.

Cholestyramine (eg, *Questran*)

Iron

SUMMARY: Cholestyramine can inhibit iron absorption, but the clinical importance of this effect is unknown.

RISK FACTORS: No specific risk factors are known.

MECHANISM: Cholestyramine can bind iron in the GI tract, thus preventing its absorption.

CLINICAL EVALUATION: A single case report and animal studies indicate that cholestyramine can moderately impair the absorption of dietary iron.[1] The significance of these findings remains to be established.

RELATED DRUGS: The effect of colestipol (*Colestid*) on iron is not established.

MANAGEMENT OPTIONS: No specific action is required, but be alert for evidence of the interaction.

REFERENCES:
1. Thomas FB, et al. Inhibition of the intestinal absorption of inorganic and hemoglobin iron by cholestyramine. *J Lab Clin Med.* 1971;78:70.

Cholestyramine (eg, *Questran*)

Loperamide (eg, *Imodium*)

SUMMARY: Cholestyramine appeared to inhibit the effect of loperamide in 1 patient, but a causal relationship was not established.

RISK FACTORS: No specific risk factors are known.

MECHANISM: Cholestyramine may reduce the GI absorption of loperamide by binding it in the GI tract.

CLINICAL EVALUATION: In a patient with an ileostomy, cholestyramine appeared to inhibit the ability of loperamide to reduce fluid loss from the ileostomy.[1] More study is needed to assess the clinical importance of this interaction.

RELATED DRUGS: The effect of colestipol (*Colestid*) on loperamide is not established.

MANAGEMENT OPTIONS: No specific action is required, but be alert for evidence of the interaction.

REFERENCES:
1. Ti TY, et al. Probable interaction of loperamide and cholestyramine. *Can Med Assoc J.* 1978;119:607.

Cholestyramine (eg, *Questran*)

Lorazepam (eg, *Ativan*)

SUMMARY: The combination of cholestyramine and oral neomycin may reduce plasma concentrations of lorazepam, but the clinical importance of this effect is unknown.

RISK FACTORS:

➡ **Other Drugs.** Cholestyramine alone does not appear to affect lorazepam, but cholestyramine plus oral neomycin does.

MECHANISM: Not established. Cholestyramine may bind with lorazepam in the GI; oral neomycin may inhibit the bacterial hydrolysis of conjugated lorazepam in the intestine, thus interfering with the enterohepatic circulation of lorazepam.

CLINICAL EVALUATION: Seven healthy men were given lorazepam (oral and IV) with and without oral coadministration of cholestyramine 4 g every 4 hours plus neomycin (eg, *Mycifradin*) 1 g every 6 hours.[1] With oral administration of lorazepam, the cholestyramine plus neomycin resulted in a 26% reduction in lorazepam half-life and a 34% increase in the clearance of free lorazepam. Cholestyramine plus neomycin also increased the clearance of free lorazepam when the lorazepam was given IV, suggesting that lorazepam may undergo enterohepatic circulation. Neither cholestyramine nor oral neomycin alone affected lorazepam elimination.

Separation of the doses of lorazepam from the other 2 drugs may not circumvent the interaction, because of the apparent enterohepatic circulation of lorazepam.

RELATED DRUGS: The effect of cholestyramine plus neomycin on benzodiazepines other than lorazepam is not established. Because benzodiazepines are metabolized by a variety of pathways, one cannot assume that others will be affected by cholestyramine and neomycin until specific studies are available.

MANAGEMENT OPTIONS: No specific action is required, but be alert for evidence of the interaction.

REFERENCES:

1. Herman RJ, et al. Disposition of lorazepam in human beings: enterohepatic recirculation and first pass effect. *Clin Pharmacol Ther.* 1989;46:18.

Cholestyramine (eg, *Questran*)

Methotrexate

SUMMARY: Preliminary evidence indicates that cholestyramine binds methotrexate in the gut and thus may reduce serum methotrexate concentrations. The degree to which this effect reduces the therapeutic response to methotrexate is not established.

RISK FACTORS: No specific risk factors are known.

MECHANISM: Cholestyramine binds with methotrexate in vitro and appears to enhance the nonrenal elimination of methotrexate in vivo, possibly because of interruption of the enterohepatic circulation of methotrexate. Theoretically, one also would expect cholestyramine to reduce the bioavailability of orally administered methotrexate.

CLINICAL EVALUATION: Cholestyramine was first used to treat methotrexate toxicity in an 11-year-old with osteosarcoma. The first course of high-dose IV methotrexate resulted in severe colitis, so the subsequent 8 methotrexate cycles were given with cholestyramine 2 g every 6 hours from 6 to 48 hours after methotrexate. Serum methotrexate concentrations 24 hours after the methotrexate infusion were approximately 50% of the concentration measured after the first course of methotrexate given without cholestyramine. In another patient with osteosarcoma, severe methotrexate toxicity occurred after the twelfth methotrexate cycle. When cholestyramine 2 g every 6 hours was given, there was a sharp drop in the serum methotrexate concentration. In another case, cholestyramine 4 g/day was used to treat methotrexate intoxication in a 61-year-old woman with rheumatoid arthritis who developed renal insufficiency while receiving low-dose methotrexate, resulting in a decrease in the serum concentration of methotrexate.[2] In vitro investigation suggests that cholestyramine binds avidly with methotrexate, with almost 100% of methotrexate bound at a methotrexate/cholestyramine concentration ratio of 0.5 or lower.[1] Similarly, experiments in animals confirm that cholestyramine causes a decrease in the serum levels of methotrexate.[3]

RELATED DRUGS: The effect of colestipol (*Colestid*) on methotrexate is unknown, but it may be similar to that of cholestyramine.

MANAGEMENT OPTIONS:

➡ *Circumvent/Minimize.* Until clinical studies are performed, it would be prudent to separate oral doses of methotrexate from cholestyramine as much as possible.

➡ *Monitor.* Be alert for altered response to oral or parenteral methotrexate when cholestyramine is given concurrently.

REFERENCES:

1. Erttmann R, et al. Effect of oral cholestyramine on elimination of highdose methotrexate. *J Cancer Res Clin Oncol.* 1985;110:48.

2. Ellman MH, et al. Benefit of G-CSF for methotrexate-induced neutropenia in rheumatoid arthritis. *Am J Med.* 1992;92:337.

3. McAnena OJ, et al. Alteration of methotrexate metabolism in rats by administration of an elemental liquid diet. *Cancer.* 1987;59:1091.

Cholestyramine (eg, *Questran*)

Metronidazole (eg, *Flagyl*)

SUMMARY: Cholestyramine administration reduced the bioavailability of metronidazole in a single-dose study of healthy subjects.

RISK FACTORS: No specific risk factors are known.

MECHANISM: Not established. It is assumed that cholestyramine reduces the absorption of metronidazole.

CLINICAL EVALUATION: Five healthy subjects took a single oral dose of metronidazole 500 mg alone and with a single 4 g dose of cholestyramine.[1] Metronidazole bioavailability was reduced by an average of 21% subsequent to the administration of cholestyramine. Study the effects of repeated doses of cholestyramine on metronidazole bioavailability since a further reduction in bioavailability could be clinically significant.

RELATED DRUGS: Colestipol (*Colestid*) might affect metronidazole in a similar manner.

MANAGEMENT OPTIONS:

➡ *Circumvent/Minimize.* Advise patients to separate taking metronidazole from doses of cholestyramine as much as possible and take at least 2 hours before the cholestyramine.

➡ *Monitor.* If metronidazole and bile acid binding resins are coadministered, watch for reduced metronidazole efficacy.

REFERENCES:

1. Molokhia AM, et al. Effect of oral coadministration of some adsorbing drugs on the bioavailability of metronidazole. *Drug Dev Ind Pharm.* 1987;13:1229.

Cholestyramine (eg, *Questran*)

Piroxicam (eg, *Feldene*)

SUMMARY: Cholestyramine enhanced the elimination of piroxicam in one study, but the clinical importance of this effect is unknown.

RISK FACTORS: No specific risk factors are known.

MECHANISM: Cholestyramine probably binds piroxicam in the GI tract and interrupts its enterohepatic circulation. Cholestyramine is known to interfere with the enterohepatic circulation of other drugs such as oral anticoagulants.[1,2]

CLINICAL EVALUATION: Eight healthy subjects were given piroxicam 20 mg orally with and without subsequent administration of cholestyramine 4 g 3 times daily.[3] Even though the cholestyramine was not started until after the piroxicam was absorbed from the GI tract, piroxicam's half-life was reduced 40% and clearance was increased 52%. An even greater interaction would be expected if the cholestyramine was given before the piroxicam was completely absorbed. Although the magnitude of these changes in piroxicam disposition appears sufficient to inhibit its therapeutic effects, studies in patients will be needed to assess this possibility.

RELATED DRUGS: The elimination of IV tenoxicam, a nonsteroidal anti-inflammatory drug (NSAID) related to piroxicam, also was enhanced by cholestyramine in this study.[1] Although little is known regarding the effect of cholestyramine on other NSAIDs, it would not be surprising to find that some of them also interact. The effect of another binding resin, colestipol (*Colestid*), on the pharmacokinetics of piroxicam or other NSAIDs is not established, but some evidence suggests that colestipol binds drugs less avidly than cholestyramine.

MANAGEMENT OPTIONS:

➥ *Circumvent/Minimize.* Separate the doses of piroxicam and cholestyramine as much as possible.

➥ *Monitor.* Monitor the patient for inadequate piroxicam response. If an inadequate piroxicam response appears to be related to the use of cholestyramine, consider the use of an alternative hypolipidemic agent or NSAID therapy.

REFERENCES:

1. Meinertz T, et al. Interruption of the enterohepatic circulation of phenprocoumon by cholestyramine. *Clin Pharmacol Ther.* 1977;21:731.

2. Jahnchen E, et al. Enhanced elimination of warfarin during treatment with cholestyramine. *Br J Clin Pharmacol.* 1978;5:437.

3. Guentert TW, et al. Accelerated elimination of tenoxicam and piroxicam by cholestyramine. *Clin Pharmacol Ther.* 1988;43:179.

Cholestyramine (eg, *Questran*)

Pravastatin (*Pravachol*)

SUMMARY: Cholestyramine can inhibit the bioavailability of pravastatin, but this effect appears to be more than offset by the additive lipid-lowering effect of concurrent therapy.

RISK FACTORS: No specific risk factors are known.

MECHANISM: Cholestyramine and colestipol probably bind with pravastatin in the GI tract, thus reducing its absorption.

CLINICAL EVALUATION: Thirty-three patients with primary hypercholesterolemia were randomized to receive pravastatin 5, 10, or 20 mg twice daily for 8 weeks with cholestyramine 24 g/day added for the last 4 weeks.[1] Pravastatin was taken before the morning and evening meals (at least 1 hour before the cholestyramine), and the cholestyramine was taken with each meal. Although cholestyramine was associated with a 20% to 40% reduction in pravastatin serum concentrations (0 to 12 hour area under the concentration-time curve), it substantially enhanced the lipid-lowering effect of pravastatin. Thus, the additive hypolipidemic effect of the 2 drugs more than offset the reduction in pravastatin bioavailability. Moreover, because the recommended dosing of pravastatin is once at bedtime and binding resins are normally taken with meals, it does not seem likely that cholestyramine or colestipol would often interfere significantly with pravastatin absorption. In another study, *simultaneous* administration of pravastatin with cholestyramine or colestipol (*Colestid*) reduced the serum concentrations of pravastatin 40% to 50%.[2] Again, the lipid-lowering effect of the bile acid binding resins would be expected to offset the reduction in pravastatin serum concentrations.

RELATED DRUGS: Colestipol affects pravastatin similarly. Although little is known regarding the effect of bile acid binding resins on the absorption of other HMG-CoA reductase inhibitors such as lovastatin (*Mevacor*), simvastatin (*Zocor*), or fluvastatin (*Lescol*), they may be similarly affected.

MANAGEMENT OPTIONS:

➡ *Circumvent/Minimize.* Cholestyramine or colestipol-induced reduction in pravastatin bioavailability probably is minimized by giving the cholestyramine or colestipol with meals and the pravastatin at bedtime. Other dosing schedules also may be suitable, but it would be best to avoid giving bile acid binding resins at the same time as pravastatin or other HMG-CoA reductase inhibitors.

➡ *Monitor.* Monitor patients for reduced pravastatin effect if cholestyramine is also given.

REFERENCES:

1. Pan HY, et al. Pharmacokinetics and pharmacodynamics of pravastatin alone and with cholestyramine in hypercholesterolemia. *Clin Pharmacol Ther.* 1990;48:201.

2. Pan HY. Clinical pharmacology of pravastatin, a selective inhibitor of HMG-CoA reductase. *Eur J Clin Pharmacol.* 1991;40:S15.

Cholestyramine (eg, *Questran*) 5

Propranolol (eg, *Inderal*)

SUMMARY: Propranolol concentrations are not affected by coadministration with cholestyramine.

RISK FACTORS: No specific risk factors are known.

MECHANISM: No interaction.

CLINICAL EVALUATION: In 5 patients with hyperlipidemia, cholestyramine did not affect the blood concentrations of propranolol administered simultaneously.[1]

RELATED DRUGS: Colestipol (*Colestid*) might affect propranolol in a similar manner.

MANAGEMENT OPTIONS: No interaction.

REFERENCES:

1. Schwartz DE, et al. Bioavailability of propranolol following administration of cholestyramine. *Clin Pharmacol Ther.* 1982;31:268.

Cholestyramine (eg, *Questran*)

Thyroid

SUMMARY: Cholestyramine may reduce serum thyroid concentrations in patients receiving thyroid replacement therapy.

RISK FACTORS: No specific risk factors are known.

MECHANISM: Cholestyramine binds thyroxine and triiodothyronine in the intestine, thus impairing absorption of these thyroids. In vitro studies indicate that the binding is not easily reversed.

CLINICAL EVALUATION: Decreased thyroid absorption caused by cholestyramine was suspected in 1 patient and later documented in patients and volunteers using radioactive thyroxine.[1] Separating the doses of thyroid from the cholestyramine by 4 to 5 hours minimized, but did not completely eliminate, the interaction. In vitro studies showed triiodothyronine to be similarly bound by cholestyramine.

RELATED DRUGS: Until more information is available, assume that the absorption of all thyroid preparations can be reduced by cholestyramine administration. Although the effect of colestipol (*Colestid*) on thyroid absorption is not established, assume that it also interacts until proved otherwise.

MANAGEMENT OPTIONS:

➥ *Circumvent/Minimize.* The available evidence suggests that at least 4 to 5 hours should elapse between administration of cholestyramine and thyroid. Also, try to maintain a relatively constant interval between doses of the 2 drugs.

➥ *Monitor.* Even with the above precautions, monitor for altered thyroid response (eg, serum thyroid-stimulating hormone concentrations) when cholestyramine is initiated, discontinued, changed in dosage, or when the interval between doses of the 2 drugs is changed for more than a few days.

REFERENCES:
1. Northcutt RC, et al. The influence of cholestyramine on thyroxine absorption. *JAMA.* 1969;208:1857.

Cholestyramine (eg, *Questran*)

Valproic Acid (eg, *Depakene*)

SUMMARY: Cholestyramine inhibits the GI absorption of valproic acid, but it is not known how often this would result in a clinically important reduction in valproic acid effect.

RISK FACTORS: No specific risk factors are known.

MECHANISM: Cholestyramine probably binds with valproic acid in the GI tract.

CLINICAL EVALUATION: Six healthy subjects received a single oral dose of valproic acid 250 mg alone, with concurrent cholestyramine, and with cholestyramine administered 3 hours after the valproic acid.[1] Concurrent cholestyramine reduced the valproic acid area under the plasma concentration-time curve 15%, and reduced its peak plasma concentration 21%. However, the intersubject variability was large, and 1 subject had a 27% reduction in valproic acid bioavailability. Thus, an occasional patient may be adversely affected by this interaction. Cholestyramine given 3 hours after valproic acid had no effect on cholestyramine bioavailability.

RELATED DRUGS: Theoretically, one would expect colestipol (*Colestid*) also to inhibit the absorption of valproic acid.

MANAGEMENT OPTIONS:

➥ *Circumvent/Minimize.* Although the magnitude of the interaction appears small in most people, it would be prudent to take valproic acid at least 2 hours before or 6 hours after cholestyramine, and maintain a relatively constant interval between administration of the 2 drugs.

➡ *Monitor.* Even if the doses of the drugs are separated appropriately, it would be prudent to monitor for reduced effect, especially in the first few weeks of combined therapy.

REFERENCES:

1. Malloy MJ, et al. Effect of cholestyramine resin on single dose valproate pharmacokinetics. *Int J Clin Pharmacol Ther.* 1996;34:208.

Cholestyramine (eg, *Questran*)

Warfarin (eg, *Coumadin*)

SUMMARY: Cholestyramine may inhibit the hypoprothrombinemic response to warfarin, phenprocoumon, and possibly other oral anticoagulants; colestipol (*Colestid*) might be less likely to interact.

RISK FACTORS: No specific risk factors are known.

MECHANISM: Cholestyramine may bind oral anticoagulants in the GI tract, resulting in impaired absorption. The binding also may interfere with the enterohepatic circulation of oral anticoagulants.[1,2] Hypoprothrombinemia with bleeding has occurred rarely in patients treated with cholestyramine who are not on oral anticoagulant therapy; this is presumably caused by the inhibition of vitamin K absorption.

CLINICAL EVALUATION: Preliminary results indicated that when warfarin and cholestyramine were given concomitantly or 3 hours apart, warfarin absorption was decreased.[3] The clearance of IV phenprocoumon in healthy subjects was enhanced by the coadministration of cholestyramine 12 g/day,[1] indicating that phenprocoumon undergoes enterohepatic circulation that is impaired by cholestyramine. Similar results were found with IV warfarin and oral cholestyramine.[2] The possible hypoprothrombinemia that may follow cholestyramine therapy alone is unlikely to be an important clinical problem in most patients.[4]

RELATED DRUGS: Phenprocoumon interacts similarly. Some evidence suggests that colestipol (*Colestid*) is less likely than cholestyramine to interact with warfarin or phenprocoumon.[5,6]

MANAGEMENT OPTIONS:

➡ *Consider Alternative.* Consider hypolipidemic therapy, but keep in mind that other agents also may interact with oral anticoagulants (eg, clofibrate [*Atromid-S*], gemfibrozil [eg, *Lopid*], and lovastatin [*Mevacor*]).

➡ *Circumvent/Minimize.* Giving the anticoagulant at least 2 hours before or 6 hours after the binding resin probably minimizes the impairment of oral anticoagulant absorption. However, any anticoagulant that undergoes enterohepatic circulation (eg, warfarin, phenprocoumon) may be affected by cholestyramine therapy even if the doses are separated. The binding resin and the oral anticoagulant should consistently be given the same number of hours apart so that any interaction that does occur will be relatively consistent from day to day.

➡ *Monitor.* Monitor patients for altered response to oral anticoagulants if a binding resin is initiated, discontinued, changed in dosage, or if the interval between the resin and the anticoagulant is changed.

REFERENCES:

1. Meinertz T, et al. Interruption of the enterohepatic circulation of phenprocoumon by cholestyramine. *Clin Pharmacol Ther.* 1977;21:731.

2. Jahnchen E, et al. Enhanced elimination of warfarin during treatment with cholestyramine. *Br J Clin Pharmacol*. 1978;5:437.

3. Robinson DS, et al. Interaction of warfarin and nonsystemic gastrointestinal drugs. *Clin Pharmacol Ther*. 1971;12:491.

4. Gross L, et al. Hypoprothrombinemia and hemorrhage associated with cholestyramine therapy. *Ann Intern Med*. 1970;72:95.

5. Harvengt C, et al. Effect of colestipol, a new bile acid sequestrant, on the absorption of phenprocoumon in man. *Eur J Clin Pharmacol*. 1973;6:19.

6. Product information. Colestipol (*Colestid*). Upjohn Company. 1993.

5   Choline Salicylate (*Arthropan*)

Vitamin C (Ascorbic Acid)

SUMMARY: Ascorbic acid does not appear to affect serum salicylate concentrations in most patients.

RISK FACTORS: No specific risk factors are known.

MECHANISM: The renal elimination of large doses of salicylates is pH-dependent.[3,4] It previously was thought that vitamin C could render the urine acidic, thus increasing the renal tubular reabsorption of salicylate and increasing plasma salicylate concentrations. However, clinical studies have failed to confirm that vitamin C predictably acidifies the urine.[1,2]

CLINICAL EVALUATION: One study of 9 healthy subjects receiving choline salicylate (daily dose equivalent to 3.75 g aspirin) showed that vitamin C 3 g/day did not affect serum salicylate concentrations.[1] This is consistent with the findings that vitamin C 4 to 6 g/day did not consistently reduce urine pH.[2] Also, salicylate serum levels are not likely to be increased by urinary acidification if the patient has an acidic urine before administration of the acidifier.

RELATED DRUGS: Other salicylates also are unlikely to interact with vitamin C.

MANAGEMENT OPTIONS: No interaction.

REFERENCES:
1. Hansten PD, et al. Effect of antacids and ascorbic acid on serum salicylate concentration. *J Clin Pharmacol*. 1980;24:326.

2. McLeod DC, et al. Inefficacy of ascorbic acid as a urinary acidifier. *N Engl J Med*. 1977;296:1413.

3. Levy G, et al. Salicylate accumulation kinetics in man. *N Engl J Med*. 1972;287:430.

4. Levy G, et al. Urine pH and salicylate therapy. *JAMA*. 1971;217:81.

4   Cifenline (*Cipralan*)

Cimetidine (eg, *Tagamet*)

SUMMARY: Cimetidine may increase cifenline plasma concentrations, but the clinical significance of the interaction is not established.

RISK FACTORS: No specific risk factors are known.

MECHANISM: Not established. Cimetidine may inhibit the hepatic metabolism of cifenline, but other mechanisms have not been ruled out.

CLINICAL EVALUATION: Twelve healthy subjects received a single oral 160 mg dose of cifenline alone with cimetidine 300 mg 4 times daily for 48 hours and ranitidine (eg, *Zantac*) 150 mg twice daily for 48 hours in a 3-way crossover study.[1] Cimetidine reduced cifenline clearance 30%, and increased cifenline half-life and area under the plasma concentration-time curve 30% and 44%, respectively. Changes of this magnitude would be expected to increase the pharmacodynamic response to cifenline, but studies in patients are needed to assess the clinical importance of this interaction.

RELATED DRUGS: Ranitidine does not appear to affect cifenline pharmacokinetics. The effect of famotidine (eg, *Pepcid*) and nizatidine (*Axid*) on cifenline pharmacokinetics is unknown, but they would be unlikely to interact on a theoretical basis.

MANAGEMENT OPTIONS: No specific action is required, but be alert for evidence of the interaction.

REFERENCES:

1. Massarella JW, et al. The effects of cimetidine and ranitidine on the pharmacokinetics of cifenline. *Br J Clin Pharmacol.* 1991;31:481.

Cifenline (*Cipralan*) 5
Ranitidine (eg, *Zantac*)

SUMMARY: Ranitidine does not appear to affect the pharmacokinetics of cifenline.

RISK FACTORS: No specific risk factors are known.

MECHANISM: No interaction.

CLINICAL EVALUATION: Twelve healthy subjects received a single oral 160 mg dose of cifenline alone and ranitidine 150 mg twice daily for 48 hours in a crossover study.[1] Ranitidine did not affect cifenline's peak plasma concentration, time to peak plasma concentration, area under the plasma concentration-time curve, apparent clearance, half-life, or apparent volume of distribution.

RELATED DRUGS: The effect of famotidine (eg, *Pepcid*) and nizatidine (*Axid*) on cifenline pharmacokinetics is unknown, but they would be unlikely to interact on a theoretical basis. Cimetidine (eg, *Tagamet*) is known to increase cifenline plasma concentrations.

MANAGEMENT OPTIONS: No interaction.

REFERENCES:

1. Massarella JW, et al. The effects of cimetidine and ranitidine on the pharmacokinetics of cifenline. *Br J Clin Pharmacol.* 1991;31:481.

Cigarette Smoking
Contraceptives, Oral (eg, *Ortho-Novum*) AVOID

SUMMARY: Smoking increases the risk of oral contraceptive-induced adverse cardiovascular events.

RISK FACTORS:

➥ **Dosage Regimen.** Smoking more than 15 cigarettes/day places women at greater risk.

➥ **Effects of Age.** Women older than 35 years of age are at greater risk.

MECHANISM: Not established.

CLINICAL EVALUATION: Considerable epidemiologic evidence indicates that cigarette smoking increases the risk of cardiovascular adverse effects associated with oral contraceptive use (eg, stroke, MI, thromboembolism).[1-3] Smoking did not appear to alter the metabolism of ethinyl estradiol or levonorgestrel in 1 study,[4] but the clearance of ethinyl estradiol was increased in smokers in another study.[5] The smoking-induced increase in ethinyl estradiol metabolism might increase formation of toxic ethinyl estradiol metabolites or increase the risk of unintended pregnancy with low-dose oral contraceptives. However, both of these hypotheses need further study to assess their validity.

RELATED DRUGS: See Clinical Evaluation.

MANAGEMENT OPTIONS:

➥ *AVOID COMBINATION.* Encourage women taking oral contraceptives not to smoke; if they continue to smoke, consider suggesting an alternative form of contraception.

REFERENCES:

1. Goldbaum GM, et al. The relative impact of smoking and oral contraceptive use on women in the United States. *JAMA.* 1987;258:1339.

2. Fredricksen H, et al. Thromboembolism, oral contraceptives and cigarettes. *Public Health Rep.* 1970;85:197.

3. Product information. (*Ovulen*). Searle Laboratories. 1984.

4. Crawford FE, et al. Oral contraceptive steroid plasma concentrations in smokers and nonsmokers. *BMJ.* 1981;282:1829.

 Cigarette Smoking

Diazepam (eg, *Valium*)

SUMMARY: Smokers may be somewhat resistant to the effects of benzodiazepines.

RISK FACTORS:

➥ *Dosage Regimen.* Increased cigarette consumption enhances the effect on diazepam elimination.

➥ *Effects of Age.* Younger smokers are more affected.

MECHANISM: Not established. Smoking may enhance diazepam elimination.

CLINICAL EVALUATION: In an epidemiologic study of the incidence of drowsiness due to diazepam and chlordiazepoxide (eg, *Librium*), drowsiness was less likely to occur in smokers than in nonsmokers.[1] The results of studies of the effects of cigarette smoking on benzodiazepine pharmacokinetics have not been consistent. In some reports, the pharmacokinetics of diazepam and chlordiazepoxide were unaffected by cigarette smoking,[2,3] whereas in others, the clearances of diazepam and lorazepam (eg, *Ativan*) were increased in smokers.[4,5] Diazepam clearance appears more affected in younger smokers than in elderly smokers.[4]

RELATED DRUGS: The effect of cigarette smoking on other benzodiazepines is not established.

MANAGEMENT OPTIONS: No specific action is required, but be alert for evidence of the interaction.

REFERENCES:

1. Boston Collaborative Drug Surveillance Program: Clinical depression of the central nervous system caused by diazepam and chlordiazepoxide in relation to cigarette smoking and age. *N Engl J Med.* 1973;288:277.

2. Klotz U et al. The effects of age and liver disease on the disposition and elimination of diazepam in adult man. *J Clin Invest*. 1975;55:347.

3. Desmond PV, et al. No effect of smoking on metabolism of chlordiazepoxide. *N Engl J Med*. 1979;300:199.

4. Greenblatt DJ, et al. Diazepam disposition determinants. *Clin Pharmacol Ther*. 1980;27:301.

5. Greenblatt DJ, et al. Lorazepam kinetics in the elderly. *Clin Pharmacol Ther*. 1979;26:103.

Cigarette Smoking

Flecainide (*Tambocor*)

SUMMARY: Based on meta-analysis, cigarette smoking appears to reduce flecainide serum concentrations.

RISK FACTORS: No specific risk factors are known.

MECHANISM: Not established. Cigarette smoking may increase the hepatic metabolism of flecainide.

CLINICAL EVALUATION: Seven pharmacokinetic and 5 efficacy trials of flecainide were subjected to meta-analysis to determine the effect of cigarette smoking on flecainide clearance and dosage requirements.[1] While flecainide clearance values varied widely between pharmacokinetic studies, the overall clearance in smokers was 13.1 vs 8.5 ml/kg/min in nonsmokers. The half-life of flecainide was not different between groups, but the calculated volume of distribution was greater in smokers. Patients with premature ventricular contractions in the efficacy studies required significantly higher flecainide doses than nonsmokers, yet their flecainide serum concentrations were lower.

RELATED DRUGS: No information is available.

MANAGEMENT OPTIONS: No specific action is required, but be alert for evidence of the interaction.

REFERENCES:
1. Holtzman JL et al. Identification of drug interactions by meta-analysis of premarketing trials: the effect of smoking on the pharmacokinetics and dosage requirements for flecainide acetate. *Clin Pharmacol Ther*. 1989;46:1.

Cigarette Smoking **4**

Glutethimide

SUMMARY: Smoking may increase the effect of glutethimide, but confirmation is needed.

RISK FACTORS: No specific risk factors are known.

MECHANISM: Not established.

CLINICAL EVALUATION: In a study of 7 normal subjects, glutethimide had a greater detrimental effect on a tracking psychomotor test in smokers than in nonsmokers.[1] The results of pharmacokinetic studies in these subjects were consistent with an increase in glutethimide absorption in the smokers, but the number of subjects is too small to arrive at definite conclusions.

RELATED DRUGS: No information is available.

MANAGEMENT OPTIONS: No specific action is required, but be alert for evidence of the interaction.

REFERENCES:
1. Crow JW et al. Glutethimide and 4-OH glutethimide: pharmacokinetics and effect on performance in man. *Clin Pharmacol Ther*. 1978;22:458.

Cigarette Smoking

Insulin

SUMMARY: Cigarette smoking may increase glucose concentrations and decrease response to insulin administration.

RISK FACTORS: No specific risk factors are known.

MECHANISM: Cigarette smoking may result in release of endogenous substances that antagonize the hypoglycemic effect of insulin. Cigarette smoking also reduces the rate of insulin absorption following subcutaneous injection, probably as a result of smoking-induced peripheral vasoconstriction.[2]

CLINICAL EVALUATION: Diabetic patients who smoke heavily may have insulin requirements approximately 33% higher than nonsmokers.[1] Thus, consider smoking as a factor that can affect insulin requirements and the time course of insulin action.

RELATED DRUGS: No information is available.

MANAGEMENT OPTIONS:

➡ *Monitor.* Inform patients that a change in smoking habits may change the response to insulin.

REFERENCES:
1. Madsbad S, et al. Influence of smoking on insulin requirement and metabolic status in diabetes mellitus. *Diabetes Care*. 1980;3:41.
2. Klemp P, et al. Smoking reduces insulin absorption from subcutaneous tissue. *BMJ*. 1982;284:237.

 ## Cigarette Smoking

Lidocaine (eg, *Xylocaine*)

SUMMARY: Although IV lidocaine probably has a similar disposition in smokers and nonsmokers, cigarette smoking may alter lidocaine metabolism in an occasional patient.

RISK FACTORS: No specific risk factors are known.

MECHANISM: Cigarette smoking appears to increase the metabolism of lidocaine.

CLINICAL EVALUATION: The bioavailability of oral lidocaine is markedly reduced in smokers; however, the enzyme induction caused by smoking has relatively little effect on the disposition of IV lidocaine because it is highly extracted by the liver.[1] In addition, the ability of smoking to reduce hepatic blood flow may offset any effect of enzyme induction on lidocaine given IV.

RELATED DRUGS: No information is available.

MANAGEMENT OPTIONS: No specific action is required, but be alert for evidence of the interaction.

REFERENCES:

1. Huet P-M, et al. Effects of smoking and chronic hepatitis B on lidocaine and indocyanine green kinetics. *Clin Pharmacol Ther.* 1980;28:208.

Cigarette Smoking

Pentazocine (*Talwin*)

SUMMARY: Cigarette smokers may have higher dosage requirements for pentazocine than nonsmokers.

RISK FACTORS: No specific risk factors are known.

MECHANISM: Cigarette smoking may enhance the hepatic metabolism of pentazocine.

CLINICAL EVALUATION: In 1 study, smokers required larger doses of pentazocine than nonsmokers when pentazocine was used as a supplement for nitrous oxide anesthesia in 41 patients.[1] In another study of 70 healthy subjects, smokers metabolized 40% more pentazocine than nonsmokers as measured by cumulative urinary pentazocine excretion.[2] These results are consistent with a smoking-induced increase in the hepatic metabolism of pentazocine.

RELATED DRUGS: Little is known regarding the effect of smoking on other analgesics.

MANAGEMENT OPTIONS: No specific action is required, but be alert for evidence of the interaction.

REFERENCES:

1. Keeri-Szanto M, et al. Atmosphere pollution and pentazocine metabolism. *Lancet.* 1971;1:947.
2. Vaughan DP, et al. The influence of smoking on the intersubject variation in pentazocine elimination. *Br J Clin Pharmacol.* 1976;3:279.

Cigarette Smoking

Propoxyphene (eg, *Darvocet-N*)

SUMMARY: Cigarette smokers may have higher dosage requirements for propoxyphene than nonsmokers.

RISK FACTORS:

➥ *Dosage Regimen.* The effect appears to be proportional to the number of cigarettes smoked per day.

MECHANISM: Cigarette smoking may enhance the hepatic metabolism of propoxyphene.[1]

CLINICAL EVALUATION: In an epidemiologic study of propoxyphene efficacy, the drug was rated ineffective in 20% of heavy smokers (more than 20 cigarettes/day), 15% of light smokers (20 cigarettes/day or fewer), and 10% of nonsmokers.[2] These results are consistent with a smoking-induced reduction in propoxyphene effect, but confirmation is needed.

RELATED DRUGS: No information is available.

MANAGEMENT OPTIONS: No specific action is required, but be alert for evidence of the interaction.

REFERENCES:

1. Miller RR. Effects of smoking on drug action. *Clin Pharmacol Ther.* 1977;22:749.
2. Boston Collaborative Drug Surveillance Program. Decreased clinical efficacy of propoxyphene in cigarette smokers. *Clin Pharmacol Ther.* 1973;14:259.

Cigarette Smoking

Quinine

SUMMARY: Cigarette smokers have lower quinine serum concentrations than nonsmokers; clinical efficacy could be reduced.

RISK FACTORS: No specific risk factors are known.

MECHANISM: Cigarette smoking appears to increase the metabolism of quinine.

CLINICAL EVALUATION: Ten healthy nonsmokers and 10 healthy smokers each received a single 600 mg dose of quinine.[1] The area under the concentration-time curve of quinine was reduced 44% and the clearance after oral quinine administration was increased 77% in smokers compared to nonsmokers. The half-life of quinine was 7.5 hours in smokers and 12 hours in the nonsmokers. The renal clearance of quinine was similar in both groups. The increase in quinine metabolism associated with cigarette smoking could lead to subtherapeutic concentrations and loss of antimalarial efficacy. Smokers may appear to have quinine-resistant malaria or be more likely to develop true resistant strains of plasmodia because of subtherapeutic concentrations.

RELATED DRUGS: No information is available.

MANAGEMENT OPTIONS:

➡ *Circumvent/Minimize.* Smokers requiring quinine therapy for malaria may need increased quinine doses to achieve a cure.

➡ *Monitor.* Consider measurement of plasma quinine concentrations in smokers to ensure therapeutic plasma concentrations are attained.

REFERENCES:

1. Wanwimolruk S, et al. Cigarette smoking enhances the elimination of quinine. *Br J Clin Pharmacol.* 1993;36:610.

Cigarette Smoking

Tacrine (*Cognex*)

SUMMARY: Cigarette smoking appears to reduce tacrine plasma concentrations markedly and may increase tacrine dosage requirements.

RISK FACTORS: No specific risk factors are known.

MECHANISM: Cigarette smoking induces cytochrome P450 1A2 (CYP1A2), an isozyme that is involved in the metabolism of tacrine. Thus, it appears likely that smoking markedly increases the first pass metabolism of tacrine and also may increase tacrine systemic clearance somewhat.

CLINICAL EVALUATION: Seven smokers and 4 nonsmokers took a single oral 40 mg dose of tacrine.[1] The tacrine area under the plasma concentration-time curve was almost 10 times higher and the tacrine half-life was approximately 50% longer in non-smokers than in smokers. The manufacturer states that mean plasma tacrine concentrations in smokers are approximately 33% of the concentration in nonsmokers (presumably after multiple doses of tacrine).[2] Some evidence suggests that CYP1A2 converts tacrine into reactive metabolites that may cause cellular toxicity, but a study of tacrine hepatotoxicity in patients with Alzheimer's disease failed to show an increased risk of hepatotoxicity in smokers.[3] However, the study did not exonerate cigarette smoking as a risk factor completely, because the number of patients was not large, and they did not test for a dose effect of smoking.[4]

RELATED DRUGS: No information is available.

MANAGEMENT OPTIONS:

➡ **Monitor.** Monitor tacrine response, and keep in mind that smokers are likely to have higher tacrine dosage requirements than nonsmokers.

REFERENCES:

1. Welty D, et al. The effect of smoking on the pharmacokinetics and metabolism of Cognex in healthy volunteers. *Pharm Res.* 1993;10:S334.
2. Product information. Tacrine (*Cognex*). Parke-Davis. 1993.
3. Watkins PB, et al. Hepatotoxic effects of tacrine administration in patients with Alzheimer's disease. *JAMA.* 1994;271:992.
4. Winker MA. Tacrine for Alzheimer's disease: which patient, what dose? *JAMA.* 1994;271:1023. Editorial.

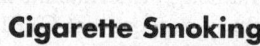

Cigarette Smoking

Theophylline (eg, *Theolair*)

SUMMARY: Cigarette smoking increases the elimination of theophylline, thus increasing theophylline dosage requirements.

RISK FACTORS: No specific risk factors are known.

MECHANISM: Cigarette smoking stimulates the hepatic metabolism (CYP1A2) of theophylline.

CLINICAL EVALUATION: The elimination of theophylline is considerably more rapid in smokers than in nonsmokers.[1,2] Cigarette smoking shortens theophylline half-life, increases total body theophylline clearance, and reduces theophylline serum levels. Adverse reactions to theophylline tend to occur less frequently in smokers than in nonsmokers,[3] which is consistent with smoking-induced reductions in serum theophylline. The smoking-induced increase in theophylline elimination tends to dissipate somewhat when patients stop smoking, but this occurs slowly over a period of months.[4,5]

RELATED DRUGS: No information is available.

MANAGEMENT OPTIONS:

➡ **Monitor.** Monitor theophylline response and serum concentrations. Keep in mind that patients who smoke cigarettes require considerably larger maintenance dosages of theophylline than nonsmokers in order to achieve adequate serum theophylline levels.

REFERENCES:

1. Jenne H, et al. Decreased theophylline half-life in cigarette smokers. *Life Sci.* 1975;17:195-198.
2. Jusko WJ, et al. Enhanced biotransformation of theophylline in marihuana and tobacco smokers. *Clin Pharmacol Ther.* 1978;24:405-410.
3. Pfeifer HJ, et al. Clinical toxicity of theophylline in relation to cigarette smoking. A report from the Boston Collaborative Drug Surveillance Program. *Chest.* 1978;73:455-459.
4. Hunt SN, et al. Effect of smoking on theophylline disposition. *Clin Pharmacol Ther.* 1976;19:546-551.
5. Powell JR, et al. The influence of cigarette smoking and sex on theophylline disposition. *Am Rev Respir Dis.* 1977;116:17-23.

 Cigarette Smoking

Thioridazine

SUMMARY: Cigarette smokers tend to have lower plasma concentrations of thioridazine and may require larger doses to achieve adequate therapeutic response.

RISK FACTORS: No specific risk factors are known.

MECHANISM: Cigarette smoking appears to increase the metabolism of thioridazine, probably by CYP1A2.

CLINICAL EVALUATION: In a study of 76 patients on thioridazine, the dose-corrected, steady-state plasma concentrations were 46% lower in smokers compared with nonsmokers.[1] Although thioridazine is known to be metabolized by CYP2D6, the results of this study suggest that CYP1A2 also may be involved.

RELATED DRUGS: Some evidence suggests that cigarette smoking also may reduce chlorpromazine (eg, *Thorazine*) effect, but little is known regarding the effect of smoking on other phenothiazines. Some other antipsychotics, such as clozapine (eg, *Clozaril*) and olanzapine (eg, *Zyprexa*), are metabolized by CYP1A2 and also can be expected to be affected by cigarette smoking.

MANAGEMENT OPTIONS:

➡ *Monitor.* Be alert for evidence of increased thioridazine dosage requirements in patients who smoke cigarettes. Other phenothiazines and neuroleptics may be similarly affected.

REFERENCES:

1. Berecz R, et al. Thioridazine steady-state plasma concentrations are influenced by tobacco smoking and CYP2D6, but not by the CYP2C9 genotype. *Eur J Clin Pharmacol.* 2003;59:45-50.

 Cigarette Smoking

Warfarin (eg, *Coumadin*)

SUMMARY: Cigarette smoking does not appear to have much effect on warfarin response in most patients, but the anticoagulant response should be monitored if smoking activity changes.

RISK FACTORS: No specific risk factors are known.

MECHANISM: Not established. Cigarette smoking is known to increase activity of CYP1A2, which is partially responsible for metabolism of R-warfarin.

CLINICAL EVALUATION: Studies of warfarin response in smokers versus nonsmokers have generally found little effect,[1,2] but isolated case reports suggest that smoking cessation may be followed by increased INR and necessitate reductions in warfarin dosage.[3,4] It is possible that the interaction is clinically important only in certain individuals.

RELATED DRUGS: No information is available.

MANAGEMENT OPTIONS: No specific action is required, but be alert for evidence of the interaction.

REFERENCES:

1. Mitchell AA. Smoking and warfarin dosage. *New Engl J Med.* 1972;287:1153-1154.
2. Weiner B, et al. Warfarin dosage following prosthetic valve replacement: effect of smoking history. *Drug Intell Clin Pharm.* 1984;18:904-906.
3. Colucci VJ. Increase in international normalized ratio associated with smoking cessation. *Ann Pharmacother.* 2001;35:385-386.
4. Evans M, Lewis GM. Increase in international normalized ratio after smoking cessation in a patient receiving warfarin. *Ann Pharmacother.* 2005;25:1656-1659.

Cilostazol (eg, *Pletal*)

Diltiazem (eg, *Cardizem*)

SUMMARY: Diltiazem may increase the effect of cilostazol; some increase in side effects may occur.

RISK FACTORS: No specific risk factors are known.

MECHANISM: Diltiazem appears to inhibit the CYP3A4-mediated metabolism of cilostazol.

CLINICAL EVALUATION: While data are limited, the manufacturer of cilostazol notes that diltiazem 180 mg increased the area under the plasma concentration-time curve of cilostazol 40%.[1] These increases could result in higher antiplatelet and vasodilatory effects as well as increased side effects (eg, diarrhea, headache) in some patients.

RELATED DRUGS: Verapamil (eg, *Calan*) can be expected to effect cilostazol in a similar manner.

MANAGEMENT OPTIONS:

➡ *Monitor.* Be alert for increased cilostazol effects if diltiazem is coadministered.

REFERENCES:

1. *Pletal* [package insert]. Rockville, MD: Otsuka America Pharmaceutical, Inc; 2004.

Cilostazol (eg, *Pletal*)

Erythromycin (eg, *Ery-Tab*)

SUMMARY: Erythromycin may increase the effect of cilostazol; some increase in side effects may occur.

RISK FACTORS: No specific risk factors are known.

MECHANISM: Erythromycin appears to inhibit the CYP3A4-mediated metabolism of cilostazol.

CLINICAL EVALUATION: While data are limited, the manufacturer of cilostazol notes that erythromycin 500 mg every 8 hours increased the area under the plasma concentration-time curve of cilostazol 73%.[1] These increases could result in higher antiplatelet and vasodilatory effects as well as increased side effects (eg, diarrhea, headache) in some patients.

RELATED DRUGS: Clarithromycin (eg, *Biaxin*) and troleandomycin[†] can be expected to effect cilostazol in a similar manner.

MANAGEMENT OPTIONS:

➠ *Consider Alternative.* Azithromycin (eg, *Zithromax*) and dirithromcyin (*Dynabac*) do not inhibit CYP3A4 and may be considered as alternatives to erythromycin in patients receiving cilostazol.

➠ *Monitor.* Be alert for increased cilostazol effects if erythromycin is coadministered.

REFERENCES:

1. *Pletal* [package insert]. Rockville, MD: Otsuka America Pharmaceutical, Inc; 2004.

† Not available in the United States.

Cilostazol (eg, *Pletal*)

Ketoconazole (eg, *Nizoral*)

SUMMARY: Ketoconazole may increase the effect of cilostazol; some increase in side effects may occur.

RISK FACTORS: No specific risk factors are known.

MECHANISM: Ketoconazole appears to inhibit the CYP3A4-mediated metabolism of cilostazol.

CLINICAL EVALUATION: While data are limited, the manufacturer of cilostazol notes that ketoconazole 400 mg daily for 2 days increased the area under the plasma concentration-time curve of cilostazol 117%.[1] These increases could result in higher antiplatelet and vasodilatory effects as well as increased side effects (eg, headache, diarrhea) in some patients.

RELATED DRUGS: Other antifungal agents that inhibit CYP3A4 (eg, itraconazole [eg, *Sporanox*], voriconazole [*Vfend*], fluconazole [eg, *Diflucan*]) can be expected to effect cilostazol in a similar manner.

MANAGEMENT OPTIONS:

➠ *Monitor.* Be alert for increased cilostazol effects if ketoconazole is coadministered.

REFERENCES:

1. *Pletal* [package insert]. Rockville, MD: Otsuka America Pharmaceutical, Inc; 2004.

 4   Cilostazol (eg, *Pletal*)

Omeprazole (eg, *Prilosec*)

SUMMARY: Omeprazole may increase the effect of cilostazol; some increase in side effects may occur.

RISK FACTORS: No specific risk factors are known.

MECHANISM: Omeprazole appears to inhibit the CYP2C19-mediated metabolism of cilostazol.

CLINICAL EVALUATION: Twenty subjects were administered omeprazole 40 mg daily for 11 days.[1] A single dose of cilostazol 100 mg was administered before omeprazole and on day 7 of omeprazole dosing. The mean area under the plasma concentration-time curve (AUC) for cilostazol was increased approximately 22% by omeprazole. The mean AUCs of 2 of cilostazol's active metabolites were increased 29% and 69% during the coadministration of omeprazole. These increases could result in higher antiplatelet and vasodilatory effects as well as increased side effects (eg, headache, diarrhea) in some patients.

RELATED DRUGS: Esomeprazole (*Nexium*) may affect cilostazol in a similar manner.

MANAGEMENT OPTIONS:

➡ *Monitor.* Be alert for increased cilostazol effects if omeprazole is coadministered.

REFERENCES:

1. Suri A, et al. Effect of omeprazole on the metabolism of cilostazol. *Clin Pharmacokinet.* 1999;37:53-59.

Cimetidine (eg, *Tagamet*)

Ciprofloxacin (eg, *Cipro*)

SUMMARY: Cimetidine increases ciprofloxacin and pefloxacin[†] serum concentrations; the significance of these changes appears to be limited.

RISK FACTORS: No specific risk factors are known.

MECHANISM: Cimetidine appears to reduce the metabolism of some quinolone antibiotics.

CLINICAL EVALUATION: The coadministration of cimetidine 800 mg reduced the clearance after oral administration of ciprofloxacin 18%.[1] Pending studies in patients, the increase in ciprofloxacin concentrations resulting from cimetidine administration appears to have limited clinical significance.

RELATED DRUGS: The nonrenal clearance of pefloxacin[†] was reduced nearly 25% by cimetidine administration.[2] Other H_2-receptor antagonists, such as ranitidine (eg, *Zantac*), famotidine (eg, *Pepcid*), and nizatidine (eg, *Axid*), are less likely to affect ciprofloxacin or pefloxacin.[†]

MANAGEMENT OPTIONS: No specific action is required, but be alert for evidence of the interaction.

REFERENCES:

1. Prince RA, et al. Effect of cimetidine on ciprofloxacin pharmacokinetics. *Pharmacotherapy.* 1990;10:234.
2. Sorgel F, et al. Effects of cimetidine on the pharmacokinetics of pefloxacin in healthy volunteers. *Rev Infect Dis.* 1988;10:137.

† Not available in the United States.

Cimetidine (eg, *Tagamet*)

Cisapride[†]

SUMMARY: Cimetidine substantially increased the bioavailability of cisapride in healthy subjects, but the clinical importance of the interaction is not established.

RISK FACTORS: No specific risk factors are known.

MECHANISM: Although the mechanism for the increased bioavailability of cisapride is not established, cimetidine-induced inhibition of cisapride metabolism seems the most likely.

CLINICAL EVALUATION: Eight healthy subjects each received three 1-week oral treatments as follows: cisapride 10 mg 3 times/day alone, cimetidine 400 mg 3 times/day alone, and cisapride plus cimetidine.[1] Cisapride bioavailability, as measured by the area under the plasma concentration-time curve, was increased 45% during cimetidine coadministration; cimetidine bioavailability was slightly reduced during cisapride administration. Possible interference of cimetidine with the cisapride assay was not addressed. The clinical importance of these changes is not established, but high levels of cisapride have been associated with ventricular arrhythmias. Cisapride and cimetidine were used together to treat severe gastroesophageal reflux disease in 1 trial with apparent good results, but the study was not large enough to rule out a rare, serious adverse interaction.[2]

RELATED DRUGS: The effect of other H_2-receptor antagonists, such as ranitidine (eg, *Zantac*), famotidine (eg, *Pepcid*), and nizatidine (eg, *Axid*), on cisapride pharmacokinetics is not established; theoretically, they would be less likely to affect cisapride metabolism than cimetidine.

MANAGEMENT OPTIONS:

➥ *Consider Alternative.* Although there is little evidence to suggest that the combination is dangerous, it would be prudent to use an alternative to cimetidine, such as ranitidine, famotidine, or nizatidine given the potential severity of the adverse interaction.

➥ *Monitor.* If the combination is used, monitor for evidence of ventricular arrhythmias (eg, fainting, palpitations).

REFERENCES:

1. Kirch W, et al. Cisapride-cimetidine interaction: enhanced cisapride bioavailability and accelerated cimetidine absorption. *Ther Drug Monit.* 1989;11:411-414.

2. Galmiche JP, et al. Combined therapy with cisapride and cimetidine in severe reflux oesophagitis: a double blind controlled trial. *Gut.* 1988;29:675-681.

† Available only through an investigational limited access program.

Cimetidine (eg, *Tagamet*)

Citalopram (eg, *Celexa*)

SUMMARY: Cimetidine appears to moderately increase citalopram serum concentrations, but it is not known how often this would result in adverse outcomes.

RISK FACTORS: No specific risk factors are known.

MECHANISM: Not established. Cimetidine may inhibit citalopram metabolism by CYP2C19.

CLINICAL EVALUATION: In a multiple-dose study of young, healthy subjects given citalopram 40 mg/day, cimetidine 400 mg twice daily for 7 days increased the citalopram area under the serum concentration-time curve 43%.[1] Given that citalopram is relatively well tolerated, the interaction may not frequently result in adverse outcomes. Nonetheless, some predisposed patients may be adversely affected by the interaction.

RELATED DRUGS: Famotidine (eg, *Pepcid*), nizatidine (eg, *Axid*), and ranitidine (eg, *Zantac*) theoretically are unlikely to interact with citalopram, but clinical studies are needed for confirmation. Omeprazole (eg, *Prilosec*) could interact with citalopram because of its ability to inhibit CYP2C19.

MANAGEMENT OPTIONS:

➡ *Consider Alternative.* Consider using an alternative H$_2$-receptor antagonist such as famotidine, nizatidine, or ranitidine.

➡ *Monitor.* If the combination is used, monitor for altered citalopram effect if cimetidine is initiated, discontinued, or changed in dosage; adjust citalopram dose as needed.

REFERENCES:

1. Priskorn M, et al. Pharmacokinetic interaction study of citalopram and cimetidine in healthy subjects. *Eur J Clin Pharmacol.* 1997;52:241-242.

Cimetidine (eg, *Tagamet*)

Clozapine (eg, *Clozaril*)

SUMMARY: A patient receiving clozapine developed increased serum clozapine concentrations and evidence of clozapine toxicity after starting cimetidine. Although this reaction was probably caused by an interaction between cimetidine and clozapine, the frequency and magnitude of this interaction is not established.

RISK FACTORS:

➡ *Dosage Regimen.* In most patients, clinically important inhibition of hepatic drug metabolism by cimetidine requires doses of 400 mg/day or more.

MECHANISM: Not established. Cimetidine probably inhibits the hepatic metabolism of clozapine.

CLINICAL EVALUATION: A 24-year-old man with schizophrenia was stabilized on clozapine 900 mg/day and a serum clozapine concentration of approximately 100 ng/mL.[1] After cimetidine therapy 800 mg/day was started for gastritis and gastroesophageal reflux, the serum clozapine increased to approximately 1600 ng/mL. After 3 months the cimetidine dose was increased to 1200 mg/day; 3 days later he complained of diaphoresis, dizziness, vomiting, weakness, and lightheadedness. The symptoms resolved gradually over 5 days after the cimetidine was discontinued and the clozapine dosage was reduced to 200 mg/day. Over the next week the clozapine dose was increased again to 900 mg/day. The patient was then maintained on ranitidine (eg, *Zantac*) 300 mg/day with good results and no recurrence of clozapine toxicity. While he was taking ranitidine, the serum clozapine concentration returned to approximately 1000 ng/mL. The temporal relationship between the initiation and discontinuation of cimetidine administration and the changes in clozapine serum concentrations and symptoms of clozapine toxicity make it probable that the cimetidine was responsible for the effects in this patient. Nonetheless, more study is needed to determine how often this interaction would result in adverse clinical effects.

RELATED DRUGS: Based on this case, it appears that ranitidine would be preferable to cimetidine in patients receiving clozapine. Theoretically, famotidine (eg, *Pepcid*) and nizatidine (eg, *Axid*) also would be unlikely to interact with clozapine.

MANAGEMENT OPTIONS:

➡ *Consider Alternative.* Until more information is available, avoid the use of cimetidine in patients receiving clozapine. Theoretically, famotidine and nizatidine would be unlikely to interact and can be considered as alternatives.

➡ *Monitor.* If the combination is used, monitor for altered clozapine effect if cimetidine is initiated, discontinued, or changed in dosage. Adjust clozapine dosage as needed.

REFERENCES:

   1. Szymanski S, et al. A case report of cimetidine-induced clozapine toxicity. *J Clin Psychiatry*. 1991;52:21-22.

 Cimetidine (eg, *Tagamet*)

Cyclosporine (eg, *Neoral*)

SUMMARY: Cimetidine may increase the serum creatinine in patients receiving cyclosporine, but the effect does not seem to be caused by reduced renal function. Cimetidine does not appear to affect blood cyclosporine concentrations.

RISK FACTORS: No specific risk factors are known.

MECHANISM: Cimetidine appears to compete with creatinine for renal tubular secretion. Available evidence suggests that cimetidine does not inhibit cyclosporine metabolism in humans, but more study is needed. Cimetidine inhibits cyclosporine elimination in rabbits.[1]

CLINICAL EVALUATION: Cimetidine has been reported to increase serum creatinine concentrations in kidney and heart transplant patients receiving cyclosporine, raising concern that cimetidine may increase the risk of cyclosporine-induced nephrotoxicity.[2] However, cimetidine also increases the serum creatinine in patients who are not receiving cyclosporine.[3] Moreover, when 11 cyclosporine-treated kidney transplant patients were given cimetidine 1200 mg/day for 7 days, creatinine clearance decreased, but inulin clearance and blood urea nitrogen were unaffected.[4] This suggests that cimetidine reduced the tubular secretion of creatinine but did not affect renal function adversely. Cyclosporine trough levels increased slightly during cimetidine therapy, but the changes were not statistically (or clinically) significant. In another report, a cyclosporine-treated renal transplant patient developed more than a doubling of her blood cyclosporine concentrations during treatment with cimetidine and metronidazole,[5] but careful analysis of the temporal relationship reveals that the effect could have been caused by the metronidazole alone.

RELATED DRUGS: Ranitidine (eg, *Zantac*) appears to have less effect on serum creatinine than does cimetidine, and its lack of effect on blood cyclosporine concentrations is better documented. Thus, ranitidine may be preferable to cimetidine in patients on cyclosporine. Other H$_2$-receptor antagonists, such as famotidine (eg, *Pepcid*) and nizatidine (eg, *Axid*), are probably similar to ranitidine when combined with cyclosporine, but little information is available.

MANAGEMENT OPTIONS: No specific action is required, but be alert for evidence of the interaction.

REFERENCES:

   1. D'Souza MJ, et al. Cyclosporine-cimetidine interaction. *Drug Metab Dispos*. 1988;16:57-59.

2. Jarowenko MV, et al. Ranitidine, cimetidine, and the cyclosporine–treated recipient. *Transplantation.* 1986;42:311-312.

3. Rocci ML Jr, et al. Creatinine serum concentrations and H₂-receptor antagonists. *Clin Nephrol.* 1984;22:214-215.

4. Pachon J, et al. Effects of H₂-receptor antagonists on renal function in cyclosporine-treated renal transplant patients. *Transplantation.* 1989;47:254-259.

5. Zylber-Katz E, et al. Cyclosporine interactions with metronidazole and cimetidine. *Drug Intell Clin Pharm.* 1988;22:504-505.

Cimetidine (eg, *Tagamet*) 4

Dapsone

SUMMARY: Cimetidine administration increases dapsone plasma concentrations and reduces the concentration of a toxic dapsone metabolite.

RISK FACTORS: No specific risk factors are known.

MECHANISM: Cimetidine inhibits the metabolism of dapsone to a toxic metabolite (N-hydroxylamine) that is known to cause methemoglobinemia during chronic dapsone therapy.

CLINICAL EVALUATION: The coadministration of cimetidine may offer some protection against dapsone-induced methemoglobinemia by inhibiting dapsone metabolism.[1,2] The potential toxicity of elevated dapsone concentrations is unknown.

RELATED DRUGS: Other H₂-receptor antagonists, such as ranitidine (eg, *Zantac*), famotidine (eg, *Pepcid*), and nizatidine (*Axid*), would not be expected to affect dapsone metabolism.

MANAGEMENT OPTIONS: No specific action is required, but be alert for evidence of the interaction.

REFERENCES:

1. Coleman MD, et al. The use of cimetidine as a selective inhibitor of dapsone N-hydroxylation in man. *Br J Clin Pharmacol.* 1990;30:761.

2. Coleman MD, et al. The use of cimetidine to reduce dapsone-dependent methaemoglobinaemia in dermatitis herpetiformis patients. *Br J Clin Pharmacol.* 1992;34:244.

Cimetidine (eg, *Tagamet*)

Desipramine (eg, *Norpramin*)

SUMMARY: Limited clinical evidence suggests that cimetidine increases serum desipramine concentrations. Given the proven effect of cimetidine on tricyclic antidepressants closely related to desipramine, it seems likely that desipramine is affected similarly.

RISK FACTORS:

➡ *Dosage Regimen.* In most patients, clinically important inhibition of hepatic drug metabolism by cimetidine requires doses of at least 400 mg/day.

MECHANISM: Cimetidine probably inhibits the hepatic metabolism of desipramine.

CLINICAL EVALUATION: A woman receiving 1200 mg/day of cimetidine unexpectedly developed severe anticholinergic symptoms (eg, severe dry mouth, urinary retention, blurred vision) when imipramine therapy 100 to 125 mg/day was started.[1]

Similar symptoms were seen when the imipramine was replaced by 125 mg/day of desipramine.

RELATED DRUGS: Theoretically, ranitidine (eg, *Zantac*), famotidine (eg, *Pepcid*), and probably nizatidine (*Axid*) would be less likely to interact with desipramine. Other clinical studies suggest that cimetidine also inhibits the elimination of other tricyclic antidepressants such as imipramine (eg, *Tofranil*) and nortriptyline (eg, *Pamelor*). Little clinical information is available on the effect of cimetidine on tricyclics such as amitriptyline (eg, *Elavil*), amoxapine (eg, *Asendin*), protriptyline, trimipramine (*Surmontil*), maprotiline (eg, *Ludiomil*), or trazodone (eg, *Desyrel*). However, theoretical considerations would indicate that their elimination also might be reduced by cimetidine therapy.

MANAGEMENT OPTIONS:

➡ **Consider Alternative.** Consider using an alternative to cimetidine. Ranitidine, famotidine, and probably nizatidine are less likely to interact.

➡ **Monitor.** Until more information is available, be alert or altered desipramine effect if cimetidine therapy is initiated, discontinued, or changed in dosage.

REFERENCES:
1. Miller DD, et al. Cimetidine-imipramine interaction: a case report. *Am J Psychiatry*. 1983;140:351.

Cimetidine (eg, *Tagamet*)

Diazepam (eg, *Valium*)

SUMMARY: Plasma levels of diazepam and several other benzodiazepines or their active metabolites can be increased by cimetidine, but the frequency of adverse effects associated with increased benzodiazepine concentration is unknown.

RISK FACTORS:

➡ **Dosage Regimen.** In most patients, clinically important inhibition of hepatic drug metabolism by cimetidine requires doses at least 400 mg/day.

➡ **Effects of Age.** The elderly can be more susceptible to the sedative effects of benzodiazepines.

MECHANISM: Cimetidine appears to inhibit the hepatic metabolism of some benzodiazepines.

CLINICAL EVALUATION: Although some studies have found an increased sedative effect of diazepam in the presence of cimetidine,[2] others have found that cimetidine has minimal effects on diazepam response.[1,7,8] Cimetidine reduces the plasma clearance of diazepam.[2,4,6]

RELATED DRUGS: Because clorazepate (eg, *Tranxene*), halazepam (*Paxipam*), and prazepam are metabolized to active desmethyldiazepam, they probably also interact with cimetidine. Clonazepam (eg, *Klonopin*) and flurazepam (eg, *Dalmane*) undergo oxidative metabolism in the liver, and their elimination would be expected to be reduced by cimetidine. Cimetidine also reduces plasma clearance of chlordiazepoxide (eg, *Librium*), desmethyldiazepam, and probably also alprazolam (eg, *Xanax*) and triazolam (*Halcion*).[3,5,6,9,10] The pharmacokinetics of benzodiazepines that undergo glucuronide conjugation, such as lorazepam (eg, *Ativan*), oxazepam (eg, *Serax*), and temazepam (eg, *Restoril*), do not appear to be affected by cimetidine therapy.[10,11] Ranitidine (eg, *Zantac*) appears to be less likely to interact with benzodiazepines than cimetidine; famotidine (eg, *Pepcid*) and probably nizatidine (*Axid*) also appear unlikely to interact.

MANAGEMENT OPTIONS:

➡ **Consider Alternative.** Consider using an alternative to cimetidine. Ranitidine, famotidine, and probably nizatidine appear less likely to interact.

➡ **Monitor.** Watch patients receiving benzodiazepines that undergo oxidative metabolism for evidence of altered benzodiazepine response when cimetidine is initiated, discontinued, or changed in dosage.

REFERENCES:

1. Greenblatt DJ, et al. Clinical importance of the interaction of diazepam and cimetidine. *N Engl J Med.* 1984;310:1639.
2. Klotz U, et al. Delayed clearance of diazepam due to cimetidine. *N Engl J Med.* 1980;302:1012.
3. Desmond PV, et al. Cimetidine impairs elimination of chlordiazepoxide (*Librium*) in man. *Ann Intern Med.* 1980;93:266.
4. Klotz U, et al. Elevation of steady-state diazepam levels by cimetidine. *Clin Pharmacol Ther.* 1981;30:513.
5. Patwardhan RV, et al. Lack of tolerance and rapid recovery of cimetidine-inhibited chlordiazepoxide (*Librium*) elimination. *Gastroenterology.* 1981;81:547.
6. Ruffalo RL, et al. Cimetidine-benzodiazepine drug interaction. *Am J Hosp Pharm.* 1981;38:1365.
7. Gough PA, et al. Influence of cimetidine on oral diazepam elimination with measurement of subsequent cognitive change. *Br J Clin Pharmacol.* 1982;14:739.
8. Greenblatt DJ, et al. The diazepam-cimetidine interaction: is it clinically important? *Clin Pharmacol Ther.* 1984;35:245.
9. Greenblatt DJ, et al. Old age, cimetidine, and disposition of alprazolam and triazolam. *Clin Pharmacol Ther.* 1983;33:253.
10. Klotz U, et al. Influence of cimetidine on the pharmacokinetics of desmethyldiazepam and oxazepam. *Eur J Clin Pharmacol.* 1980;18:517.
11. Patwardhan RV, et al. Cimetidine spares the glucuronidation of lorazepam and oxazepam. *Gastroenterology.* 1970;79:912.

Cimetidine (eg, *Tagamet*)

Digoxin (eg, *Lanoxin*)

SUMMARY: Cimetidine appears to have no consistent effect on digoxin serum concentrations.

RISK FACTORS: No specific risk factors are known.

MECHANISM: Not established. Although gastric acid appears to be involved in the degradation of digoxin in the GI tract,[6,7] it does not appear that cimetidine-induced increase in gastric pH has much effect on digoxin absorption.

CLINICAL EVALUATION: In 11 hospitalized patients receiving digoxin for congestive heart failure (CHF), the addition of cimetidine 600 to 1200 mg/day resulted in a 25% reduction in mean steady-state serum digoxin concentration.[4] However, no increase in the severity of CHF was noted. In other studies, cimetidine did not affect the pharmacokinetics of digoxin[1,5,8] or had minimal effect.[2]

RELATED DRUGS: A patient receiving digitoxin (*Crystodigin*) and quinidine developed digitoxin intoxication following initiation of cimetidine therapy.[3] The cimetidine probably increased the quinidine concentration which in turn increased the serum digitoxin concentration; however, the cimetidine also may have increased serum digitoxin concentrations directly by reducing its hepatic metabolism. Although no data are available, other H_2-receptor antagonists, such as ranitidine (eg, *Zantac*), famotidine (eg, *Pepcid*), and nizatidine (*Axid*), would not be expected to alter digoxin concentrations significantly.

MANAGEMENT OPTIONS: No specific action is required, but be alert for evidence of the interaction.

REFERENCES:

1. Garty M, et al. Effect of cimetidine on digoxin disposition in peptic ulcer patients. *Eur J Clin Pharmacol.* 1986;30:489.

2. Crome P, et al. Digoxin and cimetidine: investigation of the potential for a drug interaction. *Human Toxicol.* 1985;4:391.

3. Polish LB, et al. Digitoxin-quinidine interaction: potentiation during administration of cimetidine. *South Med J.* 1981;74:633.

4. Fraley DS, et al. Effect of cimetidine on steady-state serum digoxin concentrations. *Clin Pharm.* 1983;2:163.

5. Ochs HR, et al. Cimetidine impairs clearance of creatinine but not of digoxin. *Clin Pharmacol Ther.* 1983;33:218.

6. Gault H, et al. Influence of gastric pH on digoxin biotransformation. I. Intragastric hydrolysis. *Clin Pharmacol Ther.* 1980;27:16.

7. McGilveray IJ, et al. Digoxin dosage in patients with gastric hyperacidity. *Can Med Assoc J.* 1979;121:704.

8. Mouser B, et al. Effect of cimetidine on oral digoxin absorption. *DICP, Ann Pharmacother.* 1990;24:286.

Cimetidine (eg, *Tagamet*)

Diltiazem (eg, *Cardizem*)

SUMMARY: Cimetidine can increase the serum concentration of diltiazem; excessive diltiazem effects may be seen.

RISK FACTORS: No specific risk factors are known.

MECHANISM: The metabolism of diltiazem is reduced by cimetidine.

CLINICAL EVALUATION: Cimetidine 300 mg 4 times daily for 7 days significantly increased the area under the concentration-time curve (AUC) and peak concentration of diltiazem and its active metabolite. Although this study used a single dose of diltiazem, this interaction would be expected to lead to excessive diltiazem effects including bradycardia or hypotension during chronic dosing.[1]

RELATED DRUGS: Cimetidine also increases the concentrations of nifedipine (eg, *Procardia*), nisoldipine (*Sular*), nitrendipine, and verapamil (eg, *Calan*). Other H_2-receptor antagonists, such as ranitidine (eg, *Zantac*), famotidine (eg, *Pepcid*), and nizatidine (*Axid*), would be less likely to affect diltiazem concentrations.

MANAGEMENT OPTIONS:

➡ *Consider Alternative.* Ranitidine 150 mg twice daily does not appear to affect diltiazem concentrations.[1] Nizatidine and famotidine also would be unlikely to affect diltiazem pharmacokinetics.

➡ *Monitor.* Monitor patients receiving diltiazem carefully (eg, bradycardia, hypotension) when cimetidine is added or deleted from their drug regimen.

REFERENCES:

1. Winship LC, et al. The effect of ranitidine and cimetidine on singledose diltiazem pharmacokinetics. *Pharmacotherapy.* 1985;5:16.

Cimetidine (eg, *Tagamet*) 5

Disopyramide (eg, *Norpace*)

SUMMARY: Cimetidine does not alter the serum concentrations of disopyramide.

RISK FACTORS: No specific risk factors are known.

MECHANISM: No interaction.

CLINICAL EVALUATION: Seven healthy subjects received an IV bolus of disopyramide 150 mg before and after cimetidine 400 mg twice daily for 14 days.[1] The administration of cimetidine did not alter the pharmacokinetics of enantiomer or disopyramide. The effect of larger doses of cimetidine is unknown.

RELATED DRUGS: Other H$_2$-receptor antagonists, such as ranitidine (eg, *Zantac*), famotidine (eg, *Pepcid*), and nizatidine (*Axid*), would be unlikely to interact with disopyramide.

MANAGEMENT OPTIONS: No interaction.

REFERENCES:

1. Bonde J, et al. Stereoselective pharmacokinetics of disopyramide and interaction with cimetidine. *Br J Clin Pharmacol.* 1991;31:708.

Cimetidine (eg, *Tagamet*)

Dofetilide (*Tikosyn*)

SUMMARY: Cimetidine increases the concentration and effect of dofetilide; toxicity may result.

RISK FACTORS: No specific risk factors are known.

MECHANISM: Dofetilide is eliminated by renal elimination and hepatic (probably CYP3A4 and CYP2D6) metabolism.[1] Cimetidine reduces the renal and nonrenal clearance of dofetilide. Because of cimetidine's relatively modest inhibition of CYP3A4, the major effect of cimetidine is observed on the renal clearance of dofetilide. The reduced clearance of dofetilide results in increased plasma concentrations and myocardial conduction effect.

CLINICAL EVALUATION: Twenty healthy subjects received a single 500 mcg dose of dofetilide following 4 days of placebo or 100 or 400 mg of cimetidine twice daily. Following pretreatment with cimetidine 100 and 400 mg twice daily doses, the area under the concentration-time curve of dofetilide increased 11% and 48%, respectively. The renal clearance of dofetilide was reduced 13% and 33% by the 100 and 400 mg doses of cimetidine, respectively. The maximum effect on nonrenal dofetilide clearance was a 21% reduction following the 400 mg twice daily dose of cimetidine. The electrocardiographic effects of dofetilide (increase in QTc interval) were increased by cimetidine coadministration. Because the 100 mg twice daily cimetidine dose increase the QTc effect 22% above the effect of dofetilide alone, even OTC doses of cimetidine could alter dofetilide's effect on cardiac conduction. In a second study, dofetilide 500 mcg twice daily for 5 days was administered alone and following cimetidine 400 mg twice daily or placebo for 7 days.[3] Cimetidine increased the AUC of dofetilide 58% and reduced its renal clearance 44%. In this study, no significant change in QTc was noted between the 2 treatment arms.

Increased QTc intervals (prolongation of ventricular repolarization) may increase the risk for the development of arrhythmias during dofetilide therapy. Ranitidine (eg, *Zantac*) 150 mg twice daily did not affect dofetilide pharmacokinetics or pharmacodynamics.[2]

RELATED DRUGS: As noted above, ranitidine 150 mg twice daily had no effect on dofetilide. Effects of other H_2-receptor antagonists (eg, famotidine [eg, *Pepcid*], nizatidine [*Axid*]) on dofetilide elimination are unknown, but would likely be limited. Omeprazole (*Prilosec*) and an antacid (eg, *Maalox*) had no effect on dofetilide concentrations or pharmacodynamic effects.[4]

MANAGEMENT OPTIONS:

➡ *Circumvent/Minimize.* Patients receiving dofetilide should avoid using cimetidine, even in *otc* doses. Ranitidine would appear to be a safe alternative at doses of 150 mg or less twice daily.

➡ *Monitor.* Monitor patients carefully for increased QTc intervals if they take dofetilide with cimetidine.

REFERENCES:

1. Walker DK, et al. Significance of metabolism in the disposition and action of the antidysrhythmic drug, dofetilide. In vitro studies and correlation with in vivo date. *Drug Metab Dispos.* 1996;24(4):447-55.

2. Abel S, et al. Effect of cimetidine and ranitidine on pharmacokinetics and pharmacodynamics of a single dose of dofetilide. *Br J Clin Pharmacol.* 2000;49(1):64-71.

3. Vincent J, et al. Cimetidine inhibits renal elimination of dofetilide without altering QTc activity on multiple dosing. *Clin Pharmacol Ther.* 1998;63:210.

4. Vincent J, et al. Concurrent administration of omeprazole and antacid does not alter the pharmacokinetics and pharmacodynamics of dofetilide in healthy subjects. *Clin Pharmacol Ther.* 1996;59:182.

Cimetidine (eg, *Tagamet*)

Doxepin (eg, *Sinequan*)

SUMMARY: Cimetidine substantially increased serum concentrations of doxepin in healthy subjects, but it is not known how often this results in doxepin toxicity.

RISK FACTORS:

➡ *Dosage Regimen.* In most patients, clinically important inhibition of hepatic drug metabolism by cimetidine requires doses at least 400 mg/day.

MECHANISM: Cimetidine probably impairs the hepatic metabolism of doxepin.

CLINICAL EVALUATION: In 6 healthy men, cimetidine 600 mg twice daily was associated with about a doubling of steady-state plasma doxepin concentrations.[1] An interaction of this magnitude would be expected to increase the risk of doxepin toxicity, but studies in patients receiving the drugs therapeutically are needed to determine how often such toxicity would occur.

RELATED DRUGS: Ranitidine does not appear to interact with doxepin. In 6 healthy men, ranitidine (eg, *Zantac*) 150 mg twice daily had no effect on steady-state plasma doxepin concentrations.[1] Theoretically, famotidine (eg, *Pepcid*) and nizatidine (*Axid*) also would be unlikely to affect doxepin metabolism. Other clinical studies suggest that cimetidine also inhibits the elimination of other tricyclic antidepressants (TCAs) such as imipramine (eg, *Tofranil*), desipramine (eg, *Norpramin*), and nortriptyline (eg, *Pamelor*). Little clinical information is available on the effect of cimetidine on TCAs such as amitriptyline (eg, *Elavil*), amoxapine (eg, *Asendin*), protriptyline (eg, *Vivactil*), trimipramine (*Surmontil*), maprotiline (eg, *Ludiomil*), or trazodone (eg, *Desyrel*). However, theoretical considerations would indicate that their elimination also might be reduced by cimetidine therapy.

MANAGEMENT OPTIONS:

➡ **Consider Alternative.** Consider using an alternative to cimetidine, such as ranitidine, famotidine, or nizatidine.

➡ **Circumvent/Minimize.** In patients who are already receiving cimetidine and are about to begin a course of therapy with doxepin, consider using conservative doxepin doses until the patient's response to therapy can be evaluated.

➡ **Monitor.** In patients stabilized on doxepin who are then given cimetidine, be alert for evidence of doxepin toxicity (eg, severe dry mouth, blurred vision, urinary retention, tachycardia, constipation, postural hypotension). If cimetidine is discontinued or its dose substantially reduced in a patient stabilized on both doxepin and cimetidine, monitor the patient for an inadequate response to the doxepin.

REFERENCES:

1. Sutherland DL, et al. The influence of cimetidine versus ranitidine on doxepin pharmacokinetics. *Eur J Clin Pharmacol.* 1987;32:159.

2. Smedley HM. Malignant breast change in man given two drugs associated with breast hyperplasia. *Lancet.* 1981;2:638.

Cimetidine (eg, *Tagamet*)

Enoxacin (*Penetrex*)

SUMMARY: Cimetidine increases the plasma concentration following IV administration of enoxacin; the clinical significance of this interaction is likely to be limited.

RISK FACTORS: No specific risk factors are known.

MECHANISM: Cimetidine inhibits the renal secretion of enoxacin and may reduce enoxacin absorption.

CLINICAL EVALUATION: Ten healthy subjects received 400 mg enoxacin IV alone and following 1200 mg cimetidine or 300 mg ranitidine (eg, *Zantac*) for 4 days.[1] Enoxacin area under the concentration-time curve increased 28% and its renal clearance declined 25% during cimetidine coadministration. Ranitidine had no effect on IV enoxacin.

RELATED DRUGS: Ranitidine had no effect on serum concentrations following IV enoxacin but is known to reduce the absorption of oral enoxacin.[2] Cimetidine increases ciprofloxacin (*Cipro*) and pefloxacin concentrations. Theoretically, famotidine (eg, *Pepcid*) and nizatidine (*Axid*) might also reduce enoxacin absorption.

MANAGEMENT OPTIONS: No specific action is required, but be alert for evidence of the interaction.

REFERENCES:

1. Misiak PM, et al. Effects of oral cimetidine or ranitidine on the pharmacokinetics of intravenous enoxacin. *J Clin Pharmacol.* 1993;33:53.

2. Lebsack ME, et al. Effect of gastric acidity on enoxacin absorption. *Clin Pharmacol Ther.* 1992;52:252.

4   Cimetidine (eg, *Tagamet*)

Ethanol (Ethyl Alcohol)

SUMMARY: Cimetidine may produce small increases in blood alcohol concentrations under certain circumstances, but the effect is unlikely to be clinically important in most patients. Patients receiving cimetidine for peptic ulcers or gastroesophageal reflux should minimize their alcohol intake to avoid worsening their disease.

RISK FACTORS:

➡ ***Dosage Regimen.*** Cimetidine has a greater effect on blood alcohol if a small amount of alcohol is taken. An interaction with cimetidine is unlikely with 2 to 3 drinks or more.

➡ ***Diet/Food.*** Increased alcohol levels are more likely to occur after a meal.

➡ ***Gender.*** Men are more likely to experience increased alcohol levels.

➡ ***Time of Day.*** Evidence suggests the interaction is more likely to occur in the morning.

MECHANISM: Cimetidine may a) inhibit gastric alcohol dehydrogenase, thus increasing the bioavailability of alcohol, and b) inhibit the hepatic metabolism of alcohol.[16,17]

CLINICAL EVALUATION: Although some studies have shown an increase in blood alcohol concentrations with cimetidine pretreatment, other studies have failed to show an effect.[1-12] The disparate results are probably from differences in study design and type of subjects (see Risk Factors). A 55-year-old man on 1200 mg/day of cimetidine developed acute brain syndrome (disoriented, irritable, irrational) after drinking alcohol. He had consumed alcohol regularly before cimetidine therapy without developing such difficulties.[13] The possibility of a pharmacodynamic interaction between cimetidine and alcohol should also be considered. The CNS toxicity that can follow cimetidine use in susceptible people (eg, the elderly, patients with renal or hepatic disease) may interact adversely with the CNS effects of alcohol. Acute alcohol intoxication is known to inhibit drug metabolism; thus, alcohol-induced inhibition of cimetidine metabolism could increase the serum cimetidine concentration, which in turn would increase the likelihood of cimetidine-induced CNS toxicity. Cimetidine has been shown to attenuate cutaneous flushing and headaches that follow the use of certain alcoholic beverages in susceptible people.[14,15]

RELATED DRUGS: Other H$_2$-receptor antagonists (eg, ranitidine [eg, *Zantac*], famotidine [eg, *Pepcid*], nizatidine [*Axid*]) appear to have minimal effects on response to ethanol.

MANAGEMENT OPTIONS: No specific action is required, but be alert for evidence of the interaction.

REFERENCES:

1. Caballeria J, et al. Effects of cimetidine on gastric alcohol dehydrogenase activity and blood ethanol levels. *Gastroenterology.* 1989;96:388.

2. Hernandez-Munoz R, et al. Human gastric alcohol dehydrogenase; its inhibition by H$_2$-receptor antagonists, and its effect on the bioavailability of ethanol. *Alcohol Clin Exp Res.* 1990;14:946.

3. Roine R, et al. Effects of omeprazole, cimetidine and ranitidine on blood ethanol concentrations. *Gastroenterology.* 1990;98:A114.

4. Guram M, et al. Further evidence for an interaction between alcohol and certain H$_2$-receptor antagonists. *Alcohol Clin Exp Res.* 1991;15:1084.

5. Palmer RH, et al. Effects of various concomitant medications on gastric alcohol dehydrogenase and the first pass metabolism of ethanol. *Am J Gastroenterol.* 1991;86:1749.

6. Fraser AG, et al. The effect of ranitidine, cimetidine or famotidine on low-dose post-prandial alcohol absorption. *Aliment Pharmacol Ther.* 1991;5:263.

7. Terpin MM, et al. Antisecretive drugs and interactions of ethanol metabolism. *Ital J Gastroenterol.* 1990;22:266.

8. Etienne M, et al. Influence of anti-secretory drugs on gastric alcoholic dehydrogenase activity in man. *Gastroenterology.* 1991;100:A521.

9. DiPadova C, et al. Effects of ranitidine on blood alcohol levels after ethanol ingestion: comparison with other H_2-receptor antagonists. *JAMA.* 1992;267:3.

10. Hansten PD. Effects of H_2-receptor antagonists on blood alcohol levels. *JAMA.* 1992;267:2469.

11. Jonsson K, et al. Lack of an effect of omeprazole, cimetidine, and ranitidine on the pharmacokinetics of ethanol in fasting male volunteers. *Eur J Clin Pharmacol.* 1992;42:209.

12. Raufman JP, et al. Histamine-H_2-receptor antagonists do not alter serum ethanol levels in fed, non-alcoholic men. *Am J Gastroenterol.* 1992;87:1344.

13. Harkness LL, et al. Cimetidine psychotoxicity without significant medical illness: case report. *J Clin Psychiatry.* 1983;44:75.

14. Tan OT, et al. Blocking of alcohol-induced flush with a combination of H_1 and H_2 histamine antagonists. *Lancet.* 1979;2:365.

15. Glaser D, et al. Cimetidine and red-wine headaches. *Ann Intern Med.* 1983;98:413.

16. Gugler R. H_2-antagonists and alcohol: do they interact? *Drug Safety.* 1994;10:271.

17. Levitt MD. Review article: lack of clinical significance of the interaction between H_2-receptor antagonists and ethanol. *Aliment Pharmacol Ther.* 1993;7:131.

Cimetidine (eg, *Tagamet*) ▼ 3

Femoxetine

SUMMARY: Preliminary study in healthy subjects suggests that cimetidine markedly increases femoxetine serum concentrations, but an increase in adverse effects was not observed.

RISK FACTORS: No specific risk factors are known.

MECHANISM: Femoxetine undergoes extensive first-pass metabolism; it is converted into an active N-desmethyl metabolite as well as inactive hydroxy metabolites.[1] Because cimetidine has been reported to inhibit hepatic metabolism by both demethylation and hydroxylation, it is possible that cimetidine interferes with the metabolism of femoxetine.

CLINICAL EVALUATION: Six healthy subjects received oral femoxetine (a selective serotonin reuptake inhibitor) for 14 days with oral cimetidine added for the last 7 days.[1] The steady-state trough plasma concentrations of femoxetine were 140% higher in the presence of cimetidine therapy, but the serum concentrations of the active metabolite of femoxetine (norfemoxetine) were not affected significantly. The increased serum concentrations of femoxetine were not associated with a significant increase in adverse effects.

RELATED DRUGS: The effect of H_2-receptor antagonists other than cimetidine on femoxetine pharmacokinetics is unknown; theoretically, famotidine (eg, *Pepcid*), nizatidine (*Axid*), and ranitidine (eg, *Zantac*) would not be expected to interact.

MANAGEMENT OPTIONS:

➡ *Consider Alternative.* Theoretically, other H_2-receptor antagonists such as ranitidine, famotidine, or nizatidine would be less likely to interact with femoxetine; thus, their use may be preferred over cimetidine until more information is available on this interaction.

➡ *Monitor.* Patients receiving cimetidine may have lower dosage requirements for femoxetine. However, the results of this study suggest that femoxetine has little dosedependent toxicity. Nonetheless, it would be prudent to monitor for alterations in therapeutic and toxic effects of femoxetine if cimetidine is initiated, discontinued, or changed in dosage.

REFERENCES:
1. Schmidt J et al. Femoxetine and cimetidine: interaction in healthy volunteers. *Eur J Clin Pharmacol.* 1986;31:299.

Cimetidine (eg, *Tagamet*)

Flecainide (eg, *Tambocor*)

SUMMARY: Cimetidine increases the plasma concentration of flecainide, but the clinical importance of this effect is not established.

RISK FACTORS:

➡ *Concurrent Diseases.* Patients with renal failure are more likely to experience this interaction.

MECHANISM: Cimetidine inhibits the hepatic metabolism of flecainide.

CLINICAL EVALUATION: Eight healthy subjects took flecainide 200 mg before and after cimetidine doses of 200 mg 3 times daily with 400 mg at bedtime for 6 days. The mean area under the concentration-time curve increased 28% after the cimetidine, and the time required to reach the maximum flecainide concentration was prolonged from 1.8 hours to 3.6 hours.[1] The clinical significance of this increase in plasma flecainide concentration is unknown; however, plasma flecainide concentrations are likely to increase within a week.

RELATED DRUGS: Ranitidine (eg, *Zantac*), famotidine (eg, *Pepcid*), and nizatidine (*Axid*) are less likely to interact with flecainide because they have little or no effect on hepatic metabolism.

MANAGEMENT OPTIONS:

➡ *Monitor.* Monitor patients stabilized on flecainide (particularly those with renal disease) for increased flecainide effect if cimetidine is added to their therapy.

REFERENCES:
1. Tjamdra-Maga TB, et al. Altered pharmacokinetics of oral flecainide by cimetidine. *Br J Clin Pharmacol.* 1986;22:108.

Cimetidine (eg, *Tagamet*)

Fluconazole (*Diflucan*)

SUMMARY: Fluconazole concentrations were reduced slightly by the administration of cimetidine; the importance of this interaction is unknown.

RISK FACTORS: No specific risk factors are known.

MECHANISM: Not established. Fluconazole absorption seems to be reduced by increasing stomach pH.

CLINICAL EVALUATION: A single 400 mg dose of cimetidine reduced the area under the concentration-time curve (AUC) of fluconazole 13% and the peak concentration 20% in a study of 24 healthy subjects.[1] In these 24 healthy subjects, elevation of gastric pH to 6 with cimetidine had no effect on fluconazole pharmacokinetics.[2] The significance of this interaction during chronic cimetidine therapy is unknown, but it is likely to be limited because of the small change in AUC.

RELATED DRUGS: Other drugs (eg, omeprazole [*Prilosec*], ranitidine [eg, *Zantac*], nizatidine [*Axid*], famotidine [eg, *Pepcid*]) that increase the pH of the stomach also would be likely to reduce the absorption of fluconazole. Ketoconazole (eg, *Nizoral*) absorption also is affected by cimetidine.

MANAGEMENT OPTIONS: No specific action is required, but be alert for evidence of the interaction.

REFERENCES:
1. Lazar J, et al. Drug interactions with fluconazole. *Rev Infect Dis*. 1990;12(Suppl. 3):S327.
2. Blum RA, et al. Increased gastric pH and the bioavailability of fluconazole and ketoconazole. *Ann Intern Med*. 1991;114:755.

Cimetidine (eg, *Tagamet*)

Fluorouracil (FU; eg, *Adrucil*)

SUMMARY: Chronic cimetidine administration increases the serum concentration of fluorouracil, but it is unclear whether these changes will result in an alteration of the patient's response to FU.

RISK FACTORS: No specific risk factors are known.

MECHANISM: Not established. Cimetidine appears to interfere with the metabolism of FU.

CLINICAL EVALUATION: Patients with carcinoma who were receiving FU also received cimetidine.[1] In all trials, the FU dosage regimen was 15 mg/kg orally on day 1 and the same dose IV on days 2 through 5. This regimen was repeated at 4-week intervals. In 5 patients, a single 400 mg dose of cimetidine taken 90 minutes before the oral administration of FU had no effect on FU pharmacokinetics. Six patients, given cimetidine 1 g/day for 7 days before FU, had no change in the FU area under the concentration-time curve (AUC) following oral or IV FU. When 6 other patients received cimetidine 1 g/day for 4 weeks before FU therapy, the fluorouracil AUC was increased 72% and 27% following oral and IV FU administration, respectively. Although the FU clearance was reduced 28%, it was not statistically significant. An increase in FU toxicity or efficacy was not noted. A well-designed trial is needed to evaluate the potential clinical significance of this interaction.

RELATED DRUGS: The effect of other H_2-receptor antagonists on FU is not established.

MANAGEMENT OPTIONS: No specific action is required, but be alert for evidence of the interaction.

REFERENCES:
1. Harvey VJ, et al. The influence of cimetidine on the pharmacokinetics of 5-fluorouracil. *Br J Clin Pharmacol*. 1984;18:421.

Cimetidine (eg, *Tagamet*)

Imipramine (eg, *Tofranil*)

SUMMARY: Cimetidine can increase serum concentrations of imipramine substantially leading to imipramine toxicity in some patients.

RISK FACTORS:

➡ **Dosage Regimen.** In most patients, clinically important inhibition of hepatic drug metabolism by cimetidine requires doses of at least 400 mg/day.

MECHANISM: Cimetidine appears to inhibit the hepatic metabolism of imipramine. Preliminary evidence suggests that cimetidine also may increase the bioavailability of imipramine.[1,2]

CLINICAL EVALUATION: A woman receiving 1200 mg/day of cimetidine unexpectedly developed severe anticholinergic symptoms (eg, severe dry mouth, urinary retention, blurred vision) when imipramine therapy 100 to 125 mg/day was started.[3] Similar symptoms were seen when the imipramine was replaced by 125 mg/day of desipramine. The disposition of imipramine was then studied with and without cimetidine in this patient; the half-life and steady-state serum concentrations of imipramine were approximately doubled in the presence of cimetidine. In another case, a patient receiving 1200 mg/day of cimetidine and 300 mg/day of imipramine developed a 58% decrease in the steady-state serum concentration of imipramine 7 to 10 days after cimetidine was stopped; the serum concentration of imipramine then increased approximately 3-fold 5 to 7 days after cimetidine was resumed.[4] A preliminary report described 6 healthy subjects who were given imipramine with and without cimetidine.[1] Cimetidine increased the half-life of imipramine 43% and reduced imipramine clearance 41%. Furthermore, the bioavailability of imipramine was 40% when given alone and 75% when given in combination with cimetidine.

RELATED DRUGS: Ranitidine (eg, *Zantac*) does not appear to affect imipramine metabolism or pharmacokinetics.[5,6] Theoretically, it is unlikely that famotidine (eg, *Pepcid*) and nizatidine (*Axid*) will interact with imipramine because these H_2-receptor antagonists have little effect on drug metabolism. Cimetidine also may increase serum concentrations of desipramine (eg, *Norpramin*), doxepin (eg, *Sinequan*), and nortriptyline (eg, *Pamelor*).

MANAGEMENT OPTIONS:

➡ **Consider Alternative.** Consider using an alternative to cimetidine (eg, ranitidine, famotidine, nizatidine).

➡ **Circumvent/Minimize.** In patients who are already receiving cimetidine and are about to begin a course of therapy with imipramine, consider using conservative imipramine doses until the patient's response to therapy can be evaluated.

➡ **Monitor.** In patients stabilized on imipramine who are then given cimetidine, be alert for evidence of imipramine toxicity (eg, severe dry mouth, blurred vision, urinary retention, tachycardia, constipation, and postural hypotension). If cimetidine is discontinued or its dose substantially reduced in a patient stabilized on both imipramine and cimetidine, monitor the patient for an inadequate response to the cyclic antidepressant.

REFERENCES:

1. Abernethy DR, et al. Imipramine-cimetidine interaction: impairment of clearance and enhanced bioavailability. *Clin Pharmacol Ther.* 1983;33:237.

2. Henauer SA, et al. Cimetidine interaction with imipramine and nortriptyline. *Clin Pharmacol Ther.* 1984;35:183.

3. Miller DD, et al. Cimetidine-imipramine interaction: a case report. *Am J Psychiatry.* 1983;140:351.

4. Shapiro PA. Cimetidine-imipramine interaction: case report and comments. *Am J Psychiatry.* 1984;141:152.

5. Wells BG, et al. The effect of ranitidine and cimetidine on imipramine disposition. *Eur J Clin Pharmacol.* 1986;31:285.

6. Spine E, et al. Differential effects of cimetidine and ranitidine on imipramine demethylation and desmethylimipramine hydroxylation by human liver microsomes. *Eur J Clin Pharmacol.* 1986;30:239.

Cimetidine (eg, *Tagamet*)

Indinavir (*Crixivan*)

SUMMARY: No interaction.

RISK FACTORS: No specific risk factors are known.

MECHANISM: No interaction.

CLINICAL EVALUATION: While no published data are available for evaluation, the manufacturer of indinavir has made available some data on this interaction. Seven days of cimetidine 600 mg twice daily did not alter the serum concentrations resulting from a single dose of indinavir 400 mg.[1] The effect of larger cimetidine doses on indinavir serum concentrations is not known.

RELATED DRUGS: It is unlikely that ranitidine (eg, *Zantac*), nizatidine (eg, *Axid*), or famotidine (eg, *Pepcid*) would alter indinavir serum concentrations. The effect of cimetidine on other protease inhibitors is unknown but is likely to be similar to that seen with indinavir.

MANAGEMENT OPTIONS: No interaction.

REFERENCES:

1. *Crixivan* [package insert]. White House Station, NJ: Merck and Co.; 1996.

Cimetidine (eg, *Tagamet*)

Itraconazole (*Sporanox*)

SUMMARY: Itraconazole produces a small increase in cimetidine plasma concentrations; no adverse events are likely to occur. Cimetidine is likely to cause a marked reduction in itraconazole plasma concentrations that may lead to loss of antifungal efficacy.

RISK FACTORS: No specific risk factors are known.

MECHANISM: Itraconazole appears to inhibit the active tubular secretion of cimetidine, perhaps by inhibiting p-glycoprotein or other active transporters. Cimetidine reduction in gastric acidity will reduce itraconazole absorption.

CLINICAL EVALUATION: Eight healthy subjects received a 4-hour infusion of cimetidine alone and after 4 days of itraconazole 200 mg twice daily.[1] The mean area under the plasma concentration-time curve of cimetidine was increased just over 20%. Clearance of cimetidine was reduced about 25% following itraconazole pretreatment. The magnitude of change in cimetidine is unlikely to be of clinical significance. While not investigated in this study, cimetidine administration would probably reduce the bioavailability of itraconazole as has been observed with ketoconazole.[2] Both of these azole antifungal agents need gastric acidity for absorption, and any increase in gastric pH is likely to reduce absorption.

RELATED DRUGS: Ketoconazole (eg, *Nizoral*) would also be likely to produce a small increase in cimetidine plasma concentrations. The effect of itraconazole on other H_2-receptor antagonists is unknown. Other H_2-receptor antagonists (eg, ranitidine [eg, *Zantac*]), as well as proton pump inhibitors have been reported to reduce the absorption of itraconazole.[3]

MANAGEMENT OPTIONS:

➥ *Consider Alternative.* Evaluate patients requiring antifungal therapy during gastric acid suppression therapy for fluconazole (eg, *Diflucan*), voriconazole (*Vfend*), or terbinafine (eg, *Lamisil*) treatment.

➥ *Monitor.* No additional monitoring of cimetidine response appears to be necessary. However, marked reduction in itraconazole plasma concentrations are likely with cimetidine coadministration.

REFERENCES:

1. Karyekar CS, et al. Renal interaction between itraconazole and cimetidine. *J Clin Pharmacol.* 2004;44:919-927.

2. Blum RA, et al. Increased gastric pH and the bioavailability of fluconazole and ketoconazole. *Ann Intern Med.* 1991;114:755-757.

3. *Sporanox* [package insert]. Titusville, NJ: Janssen Pharmaceutica; 2004.

Cimetidine (eg, *Tagamet*)

Ketoconazole (eg, *Nizoral*)

SUMMARY: Cimetidine administration reduces ketoconazole concentrations.

RISK FACTORS: No specific risk factors are known.

MECHANISM: Cimetidine reduces the GI absorption of ketoconazole by increasing the pH of the GI tract.

CLINICAL EVALUATION: In 12 healthy subjects, a simulated achlorhydric state induced by cimetidine 300 mg and sodium bicarbonate 2 g reduced ketoconazole absorption to 8% of that seen with ketoconazole alone.[1] A similar reduction in ketoconazole bioavailability was seen with cimetidine-induced elevation of gastric pH to 6.[2] Evidence from a few other subjects also indicates that cimetidine significantly reduces ketoconazole plasma concentrations.[3]

RELATED DRUGS: Other oral imidazole antifungal agents (eg, fluconazole [eg, *Diflucan*]) may be affected similarly by cimetidine administration. Other H_2-receptor antagonists (eg, ranitidine [eg, *Zantac*], famotidine [eg, *Pepcid*], nizatidine [eg, *Axid*]) and proton pump inhibitors can be expected to reduce ketoconazole absorption.

MANAGEMENT OPTIONS:

➡ *Circumvent/Minimize.* Several recommendations have been made to avoid this inter-action in patients with elevated gastric pH. The product information for ketocona-zole suggests that each tablet be dissolved in 4 mL of an aqueous solution of 0.2 N hydrochloric acid, with the resulting mixture ingested with a straw (to avoid contact with teeth) and followed by a glass of water.[4] Another easy and equally effective method is to give 2 capsules of glutamic acid hydrochloride 15 minutes before ketoconazole.[1]

➡ *Monitor.* Until more is known about this interaction, be alert for evidence of reduced ketoconazole effect when cimetidine or other agents that increase gastric pH are coadministered.

REFERENCES:

1. Lelawongs P, et al. Effect of food and gastric acidity on absorption of orally administered ketocona-zole. *Clin Pharm.* 1988;7:228-235.
2. Blum RA, et al. Effect of increased gastric pH on the relative bioavailability of fluconazole and keto-conazole. *Pharm Res.* 1990;7:S52.
3. Van Der Meer JW, et al. The influence of gastric acidity on the bioavailability of ketoconazole. *J Anti-microb Chemother.* 1980;6:552-554.
4. *Nizoral* [package insert]. Titusville, NJ: Janssen Pharmaceutica; 1993.

Cimetidine (eg, *Tagamet*)

Lidocaine (eg, *Xylocaine*)

SUMMARY: Cimetidine modestly increases lidocaine serum concentrations, but it is not known how often this would cause lidocaine toxicity.

RISK FACTORS: No specific risk factors are known.

MECHANISM: Cimetidine inhibits lidocaine's hepatic drug metabolism. It also may alter the protein (tissue) binding and decrease the volume of distribution of lidocaine.[1-4]

CLINICAL EVALUATION: Single doses of cimetidine have decreased lidocaine clearance 12% to 30%.[1,2,5-8] Similar results were found in subsequent studies of patients receiv-ing lidocaine infusions[3,8] or topical lidocaine. In contrast, IV cimetidine had no effect on the disposition of lidocaine given as a continuous IV infusion in 7 pa-tients.[9] However, note that lidocaine clearance decreases with continuous dosing, even without cimetidine, and this can confound studies utilizing chronic lidocaine administration.[10] Lidocaine protein binding may be increased in patients with acute myocardial infarctions, which may blunt the effects of a decrease in lido-caine clearance by decreasing unbound lidocaine concentrations.

RELATED DRUGS: Ranitidine (eg, *Zantac*) may be a good alternative to cimetidine because it has minimal effect on lidocaine disposition.[4] For similar reasons, it is unlikely that famotidine (eg, *Pepcid*) and nizatidine (eg, *Axid*) would interact with lido-caine.

MANAGEMENT OPTIONS:

➡ *Consider Alternative.* Ranitidine, famotidine, or nizatidine are less likely to interact with lidocaine.

➥ **Monitor.** Monitor patients for lidocaine toxicity when cimetidine and lidocaine are given concurrently.

REFERENCES:

1. Jackson JE, et al. Effects of histamine-2 receptor blockade on lidocaine kinetics. *Clin Pharmacol Ther.* 1985;37:544-548.

2. Feely J, et al. Increased toxicity and reduced clearance of lidocaine by cimetidine. *Ann Intern Med.* 1982;96:592-594.

3. Feely J, et al. Reduction of liver blood flow and propranolol metabolism by cimetidine. *N Engl J Med.* 1981;304:692-695.

4. Jackson JE, et al. The effects of H₂-blockers on lidocaine disposition. *Clin Pharmacol Ther.* 1983;33:255.

5. Wing LM, et al. Lidocaine disposition— sex differences and effects of cimetidine. *Clin Pharmacol Ther.* 1984;35:695-701.

6. Bauer LA, et al. Cimetidine-induced decrease in lidocaine metabolism. *Am Heart J.* 1984;108:413-415.

7. Knapp AB, et al. The cimetidine-lidocaine interaction. *Ann Intern Med.* 1983;98:174.

8. Powell JR, et al. Effect of duration of lidocaine infusion and route of cimetidine administration on lidocaine pharmacokinetics. *Clin Pharm.* 1986;5:993-998.

9. Powell JR, et al. Lack of cimetidine-lidocaine interaction in patients with suspected myocardial infarction. *Drug Intell Clin Pharm.* 1983;17:445.

10. Bauer LA, et al. Influence of long-term infusion on lidocaine kinetics. *Clin Pharmacol Ther.* 1982;31:433-437.

4   Cimetidine (eg, *Tagamet*)

Loratadine (eg, *Claritin*)

SUMMARY: Preliminary results suggest that cimetidine can increase plasma concentrations of loratadine, but the clinical importance of this effect is probably minimal.

RISK FACTORS: No specific risk factors are known.

MECHANISM: Cimetidine probably inhibits the hepatic metabolism of loratadine, possibly through inhibition of CYP2D6.

CLINICAL EVALUATION: Preliminary results from study in humans found that cimetidine inhibits the clearance and increases the plasma concentrations of loratadine and its active metabolite, but there were no clinically relevant consequences associated with these pharmacokinetic changes.[1] Given that loratadine does not appear to produce cardiac arrhythmias (as terfenadine and astemizole can, albeit rarely), significant adverse effects from this combination are not expected.

RELATED DRUGS: Theoretically, H₂-receptor antagonists other than cimetidine, such as famotidine (eg, *Pepcid*), nizatidine (eg, *Axid*), and ranitidine (eg, *Zantac*), would not be expected to interact with loratadine. Cetirizine (*Zyrtec*), like loratadine, does not appear to result in ventricular arrhythmias and is eliminated primarily by the kidneys.

MANAGEMENT OPTIONS:

➥ **Consider Alternative.** To avoid the interaction, consider using an H₂-receptor antagonist other than cimetidine (eg, famotidine, nizatidine, ranitidine).

➥ **Monitor.** Although the risk of this combination does not appear large, be alert for adverse loratadine effects.

REFERENCES:

1. Brannan MD, et al. Effects of various cytochrome P450 inhibitors on the metabolism of loratadine. *Clin Pharmacol Ther.* 1995;57:193.

Cimetidine (eg, *Tagamet*)

Mebendazole (eg, *Vermox*)

SUMMARY: Cimetidine appears to increase mebendazole serum concentrations; the significance of this interaction is not established.

RISK FACTORS: No specific risk factors are known.

MECHANISM: Not established.

CLINICAL EVALUATION: Seven patients taking mebendazole for *Echinococcus* were given cimetidine 1 g/day for 8 weeks.[1] Five of 7 patients had increased mebendazole concentrations following cimetidine, although sparse specific kinetic data were presented. Eight patients taking mebendazole were administered cimetidine 400 mg 3 times daily for 30 days.[2] Mean peak mebendazole concentrations increased from 55 to 82 ng/mL. Several patients had an improved response to mebendazole with the increased concentrations. Limited data prevent a more complete assessment of this interaction.

RELATED DRUGS: No information is available.

MANAGEMENT OPTIONS: No specific action is required, but be alert for evidence of the interaction.

REFERENCES:
1. Luder PJ, et al. Treatment of hydatid disease with high oral doses of mebendazole. Long-term follow-up of plasma mebendazole levels and drug interactions. *Eur J Clin Pharmacol*. 1986;31:443-448.
2. Bekhti A, et al. Cimetidine increases serum mebendazole concentrations. Implications for treatment of hepatic hydatid cysts. *Br J Clin Pharmacol*. 1987;24:390-392.

Cimetidine (eg, *Tagamet*) 4

Mefloquine (eg, *Lariam*)

SUMMARY: Cimetidine administration increases mefloquine plasma concentrations; mefloquine toxicity could result in some patients.

RISK FACTORS: No specific risk factors are known.

MECHANISM: Unknown. Cimetidine appears to increase the absorption of mefloquine, perhaps by increasing gastric pH or affecting the first-pass metabolism of mefloquine.

CLINICAL EVALUATION: Six healthy subjects and 6 peptic ulcer patients received a single dose of mefloquine 500 mg alone and following cimetidine 400 mg bid for 3 days.[1] The mean area under the concentration-time curve of mefloquine increased 37% and 32% in the healthy subjects and ulcer patients, respectively. Mefloquine half-life was not changed by cimetidine pretreatment. No toxicity was observed in these single-dose studies; patients on chronic dosing may be at increased risk.

RELATED DRUGS: Other H_2-receptor antagonists (famotidine [eg, *Pepcid*], nizatidine [eg, *Axid*], and ranitidine [eg, *Zantac*]) and antacids also may increase mefloquine concentrations. Esomeprazole (*Nexium*), omeprazole (eg, *Prilosec*), pantoprazole (*Protonix*), and rabeprazole (*Aciphex*) also would be expected to interact with mefloquine.

MANAGEMENT OPTIONS:

➡ *Monitor.* Monitor patients stabilized on mefloquine for evidence of toxicity (abdominal pain, arrhythmias, sedation) following the coadministration of cimetidine.

REFERENCES:

1. Kolawole JA, et al. Mefloquine pharmacokinetics in healthy subjects and in peptic ulcer patients after cimetidine administration. *Eur J Drug Metab Pharmacokinet.* 2000;25:165-170.

Cimetidine (eg, *Tagamet*)

Melphalan (*Alkeran*)

SUMMARY: Cimetidine administration appears to reduce the serum concentrations of melphalan, but the clinical importance of this effect is not established.

RISK FACTORS: No specific risk factors are known.

MECHANISM: Not established. Cimetidine may inhibit the absorption of melphalan.

CLINICAL EVALUATION: Melphalan pharmacokinetics were compared in 7 patients following 5 days of placebo or cimetidine 200 mg 3 times daily and 400 mg at bedtime.[1] Cimetidine treatment resulted in a significant reduction in melphalan area under the concentration-time curve (35%) and a reduction in its half-life from 1.94 to 1.57 hours. No differences were observed in melphalan response (platelet count, white cell count, serum creatinine) during cimetidine administration.

RELATED DRUGS: Other inhibitors of gastric acid secretion also may reduce the serum concentrations of melphalan, but little clinical information is available.

MANAGEMENT OPTIONS:

➡ *Monitor.* Until further information is available, monitor patients treated with melphalan and cimetidine for reduced melphalan activity.

REFERENCES:

1. Sviland L, et al. Interaction of cimetidine with oral melphalan. *Cancer Chemother Pharmacol.* 1987;20:173-175.

Cimetidine (eg, *Tagamet*)

Meperidine (eg, *Demerol*)

SUMMARY: Cimetidine may increase the effect of meperidine and possibly other narcotic analgesics; morphine may be less likely to interact than other narcotics.

RISK FACTORS: No specific risk factors are known.

MECHANISM: Not established. The hepatic metabolism of certain narcotic analgesics may be inhibited by cimetidine, and the effects of histamine released in response to narcotic analgesics may be inhibited partially by cimetidine. The CNS effects of narcotic analgesics and cimetidine may be additive.

CLINICAL EVALUATION: In several cases, the respiratory depression and sedation accompanying the administration of narcotic analgesics might have been exacerbated by cimetidine.[1,2] In a study of 8 subjects, cimetidine 1,200 mg/day reduced the clearance of meperidine,[3] while ranitidine 300 mg/day did not.[4]

RELATED DRUGS: In vitro studies also indicate that cimetidine may inhibit the hepatic microsomal metabolism of meperidine and fentanyl.[5,6] Morphine disposition was not affected by cimetidine pretreatment in 7 healthy men,[7] probably because morphine undergoes glucuronidation, a metabolic process little affected by cimetidine. Cimetidine may inhibit some of the cardiovascular effects of histamine, which is released in response to administration of narcotic analgesics. Pharmacodynamic interactions between cimetidine and narcotic analgesics are also possible but not well studied. Ranitidine (eg, *Zantac*) is probably less likely to interact than cimetidine and thus may be preferable in patients receiving meperidine. Theoretically, famotidine (eg, *Pepcid*) and nizatidine (eg, *Axid*) also are less likely to interact than cimetidine.

MANAGEMENT OPTIONS:

➡ *Consider Alternative.* Ranitidine may be preferable in patients receiving meperidine, because it is less likely to interact.

➡ *Monitor.* Be alert for evidence of enhanced respiratory and CNS depression during combined therapy with cimetidine and narcotic analgesics until these interactions are more clearly established.

REFERENCES:

1. Fine A, et al. Potentially lethal interaction of cimetidine and morphine. *Can Med Assoc J.* 1981;124:1434-1436.
2. Lam AM, et al. Cimetidine and prolonged post-operative somnolence. *Can Anaesth Soc J.* 1981;28:450-452.
3. Guay DR, et al. Cimetidine alters pethidine disposition in man. *Br J Clin Pharmacol.* 1984;18:907-914.
4. Guay DR, et al. Ranitidine does not alter pethidine disposition in man. *Br J Clin Pharmacol.* 1985;20:55-59.
5. Knodell RG, et al. Drug metabolism by rat and human hepatic microsomes in response to interaction with H$_2$-receptor antagonists. *Gastroenterology.* 1982;82:84-88.
6. Lee HR, et al. Effect of histamine H$_2$-receptors on fentanyl metabolism. *Pharmacologist.* 1982;24:145.
7. Mojaverian P, et al. Cimetidine does not alter morphine disposition in man. *Br J Clin Pharmacol.* 1982;14:309.

Cimetidine (eg, *Tagamet*)

Metformin (*Glucophage*)

SUMMARY: Cimetidine administration increases metformin plasma concentrations; an increase in therapeutic effect or toxicity may occur.

RISK FACTORS:

➡ *Concurrent Diseases.* Patients with reduced renal function may be at an increased risk of elevated metformin concentrations during cimetidine administration.

MECHANISM: Cimetidine reduces the renal clearance of metformin by inhibiting its tubular secretion.

CLINICAL EVALUATION: Seven healthy subjects received single daily doses of metformin 250 mg for 10 days.[1] On days 6 through 10, subjects also received cimetidine 400 mg twice daily. Cimetidine 400 mg twice daily was administered alone for 2 days to each subject on a different occasion. Metformin plasma and urine concentrations were measured on days 5 and 10 of metformin dosing. The mean area under the concentration-time curve of metformin was increased 50% during cimetidine coadministration. The mean renal clearance of metformin was reduced 27% during cimetidine administration with the greatest effect occurring during the first 6 hours after the cimetidine dose. While no data are available, higher doses of cimetidine would be expected to increase the magnitude of this interaction. Increased metformin concentrations may increase its hypoglycemic effects or toxicity (lactic acidosis). Metformin administration did not affect cimetidine plasma concentrations.

RELATED DRUGS: Other drugs that may compete with metformin for secretion at the renal tubular organic cation system (eg, procainamide [eg, *Ponestyl*], trimethoprim [eg, *Proloprim*]) could result in a similar effect on metformin elimination. While no data are available, other acid suppressive agents [eg, famotidine (eg, *Pepcid*)] may be less likely to affect metformin renal elimination.

MANAGEMENT OPTIONS:

➥ *Consider Alternative.* Consider the use of an alternative H_2-antagonist such as famotidine in patients taking metformin. The effect of proton pump inhibitors such as omeprazole (*Prilosec*) on the renal tubular secretion of metformin is unknown.

➥ *Monitor.* Monitor patients taking metformin for lactic acidosis (eg, hyperventilation, tachycardia, nausea) if cimetidine is administered.

REFERENCES:
1. Somogyi A, et al. Reduction of metformin renal tubular secretion by cimetidine in man. *Br J Clin Pharmacol.* 1987;23:545.

 Cimetidine (eg, *Tagamet*)

Metronidazole (eg, *Flagyl*)

SUMMARY: Metronidazole serum concentrations may be increased by the coadministration of cimetidine, but the clinical importance is not established.

RISK FACTORS: No specific risk factors are known.

MECHANISM: Cimetidine appears to reduce the metabolic clearance of metronidazole.

CLINICAL EVALUATION: In a study with 6 healthy subjects, pretreatment with cimetidine 800 mg/day for 6 days increased the half-life of an IV dose of metronidazole from 6.2 to 7.9 hours and reduced its clearance 29%.[1] Some patients may develop adverse effects from increased metronidazole serum concentrations when cimetidine is coadministered.

RELATED DRUGS: Other H_2-receptor antagonists, such as ranitidine (eg, *Zantac*), famotidine (eg, *Pepcid*), and nizatidine (*Axid*), would be less likely to reduce metronidazole clearance.

MANAGEMENT OPTIONS: No specific action is required, but be alert for evidence of the interaction.

REFERENCES:
1. Gugler R, et al. Interaction between cimetidine and metronidazole. *N Engl J Med.* 1983;309:1158.

Cimetidine (eg, *Tagamet*) 5

Mexiletine (*Mexitil*)

SUMMARY: Cimetidine appears to have no clinically significant effect on mexiletine metabolism.

RISK FACTORS: No specific risk factors are known.

MECHANISM: Cimetidine has no effect on mexiletine clearance but may cause some alteration in absorption kinetics.

CLINICAL EVALUATION: Cimetidine 300 mg 4 times daily for 7 days caused no change in single-dose mexiletine clearance in healthy subjects;[1] however, cimetidine decreased the rate of absorption and reduced the peak mexiletine concentration 20%. No effect on mexiletine pharmacokinetics was observed after cimetidine 800 mg/day or ranitidine (eg, *Zantac*) 600 mg/day was administered to healthy subjects.[2] A similar dosage of cimetidine had no significant effect on the steady-state peak or trough mexiletine plasma concentrations in 11 patients on chronic mexiletine therapy.[3]

RELATED DRUGS: Other H_2-receptor antagonists (eg, ranitidine, famotidine [eg, *Pepcid*], nizatidine [*Axid*]) would be unlikely to interact with mexiletine.

MANAGEMENT OPTIONS: No interaction.

REFERENCES:
1. Klein AL, et al. Mexiletine kinetics in healthy subjects taking cimetidine. *Clin Pharmacol Ther.* 1985;37:669.
2. Brockmeyer NH, et al. Kinetics of oral and intravenous mexiletine: lack of effect of cimetidine and ranitidine. *Eur J Clin Pharmacol.* 1989;36:375.
3. Klein Al, et al. Usefulness and safety of cimetidine in patients receiving mexiletine for ventricular arrhythmia. *Am Heart J.* 1985;109:1281.

Cimetidine (eg, *Tagamet*) 4

Moclobemide

SUMMARY: Chronic cimetidine administration increases serum concentrations of the monoamine oxidase inhibitor (MAOI), moclobemide; the clinical importance of this effect is not established.

RISK FACTORS: No specific risk factors are known.

MECHANISM: Cimetidine inhibits the metabolism of moclobemide, thereby decreasing its clearance and increasing its bioavailability.

CLINICAL EVALUATION: Eight normal subjects received moclobemide 100 mg IV and orally alone and after 2 weeks of cimetidine 200 mg 5 times a day.[1] The clearance of IV moclobemide was reduced from a mean of 46.6 to 28.3 L/hr (39%) after cimetidine was given. The mean clearance of oral moclobemide decreased 52%, serum half-life and peak concentration increased, and absolute bioavailability increased from 54% to 68%. The subjects with the highest moclobemide clearance before cimetidine administration tended to experience the greatest absolute reduction in clearance after ingesting cimetidine. The clinical significance of this interaction is unknown; however, clearance changes of this magnitude may enhance moclobemide's clinical effects.

RELATED DRUGS: Theoretically, H_2-receptor antagonists other than cimetidine, such as ranitidine (eg, *Zantac*), famotidine (eg, *Pepcid*), and nizatidine (*Axid*), would not be expected to affect moclobemide metabolism. The effect of cimetidine on MAOIs other than moclobemide is not established.

MANAGEMENT OPTIONS: No specific action is required, but be alert for evidence of the interaction.

REFERENCES:

1. Schoerlin M-P, et al. Cimetidine alters the disposition kinetics of the monoamine oxidase-A inhibitor moclobemide. *Clin Pharmacol Ther*. 1991;49:32.

Cimetidine (eg, *Tagamet*)

Moricizine (*Ethmozine*)

SUMMARY: In a single-dose study in healthy subjects, cimetidine significantly increased moricizine serum concentrations.

RISK FACTORS: No specific risk factors are known.

MECHANISM: Cimetidine appears to reduce the hepatic clearance of moricizine.

CLINICAL EVALUATION: Eight healthy subjects received a single dose of moricizine 500 mg before and after 7 days of cimetidine 300 mg 4 times daily.[1] Cimetidine treatment reduced the clearance 48% after oral administration of moricizine. The increased serum concentrations of moricizine did not significantly alter the pharmacodynamic effects of moricizine on the cardiovascular system. However, the magnitude of change in moricizine clearance is likely to produce clinically significant changes in serum concentrations at steady state.

RELATED DRUGS: Theoretically, other histamine H_2-receptor antagonists such as ranitidine (eg, *Zantac*), famotidine (eg, *Pepcid*), and nizatidine (eg, *Axid*) are less likely to interact with moricizine.

MANAGEMENT OPTIONS:

➡ *Monitor.* Monitor patients taking moricizine for increased moricizine concentrations and increased cardiovascular effects if cimetidine is added.

REFERENCES:

1. Biollaz J, et al. Cimetidine inhibition of ethmozine metabolism. *Clin Pharmacol Ther*. 1985;37(6):665-668.

Cimetidine (eg, *Tagamet*)

Nebivolol (*Bystolic*)

SUMMARY: Cimetidine modestly increases the plasma concentration of nebivolol; excess beta-blockade may occur in some patients.

RISK FACTORS:

➡ *Pharmacogenetics.* Rapid metabolizers of nebivolol via CYP2D6 will be at increased risk of developing the interaction.

MECHANISM: Cimetidine is an inhibitor of CYP2D6, one of the pathways of metabolism for nebivolol.

CLINICAL EVALUATION: While specific data are limited, the manufacturer of nebivolol notes that the coadministration of cimetidine 400 mg twice daily resulted in a 23% increase in nebivolol plasma concentrations.[1] In a study of 20 healthy subjects, cimetidine 400 mg twice daily was administered for 24 hours before and 48 hours after a single dose of nebivolol 5 mg.[2] The mean area under the plasma concentration-time curve of nebivolol was increased nearly 50%, while the peak nebivolol plasma concentration was increased 23%. The coadministration of cimetidine did not change the heart rate or blood pressure response to nebivolol in these subjects. In a similar study with ranitidine 150 mg twice daily, no effect on nebivolol pharmacokinetics was observed.

RELATED DRUGS: Other beta-blockers metabolized by CYP2D6, including propranolol, metoprolol, and labetalol (eg, *Normodyne*), are affected in a similar manner by cimetidine.

MANAGEMENT OPTIONS:

➡ *Consider Alternative.* Consider beta-blockers that are not metabolized by CYP2D6 such as atenolol (eg, *Tenormin*) or acebutolol (eg, *Sectral*) in patients requiring cimetidine administration. Ranitidine (eg, *Zantac*) does not alter nebivolol plasma concentrations, and it is also unlikely that other H_2-receptor antagonists would.

➡ *Monitor.* Monitor patients receiving both nebivolol and cimetidine for evidence of excess beta-blockade.

REFERENCES:

1. *Bystolic* [package insert]. St. Louis, MO: Forest Pharmaceuticals; 2007.
2. Kamali F, et al. A pharmacokinetic and pharmacodynamic interaction study between nebivolol and the H_2-receptor antagonists cimetidine and ranitidine. *Br J Clin Pharmacol*. 1997;43(2):201-204.

Cimetidine (eg, *Tagamet*)

Nicotine (eg, *Nicorette*)

SUMMARY: Cimetidine increases blood nicotine concentrations, which may reduce the amount of nicotine gum or patches needed.

RISK FACTORS: No specific risk factors are known.

MECHANISM: The majority of nicotine is hydroxylated by CYP-450 enzymes in the liver, a process that appears to be inhibited by cimetidine. A small amount of nicotine (a weak base) is excreted unchanged in the urine; cimetidine and ranitidine (eg, *Zantac*) (and possibly other H_2-receptor antagonists) appear to interfere with this process.

CLINICAL EVALUATION: In a randomized, crossover study in 6 healthy subjects, nicotine 1 mcg/kg/min intravenously for 30 minutes was given with cimetidine 600 mg twice daily for 2 days, ranitidine 300 mg twice daily for 2 days, or placebo.[1] Cimetidine reduced nicotine clearance 30%, which would likely be sufficient to increase nicotine effect in smokers or in patients taking nicotine gum or nicotine patches. Only 2 of the 6 subjects developed a reduction in nicotine clearance with ranitidine, resulting in a mean 10% reduction in nicotine clearance for all 6 subjects.

RELATED DRUGS: Ranitidine may reduce nicotine clearance as mentioned previously. The effect of famotidine (eg, *Pepcid*) and nizatidine (eg, *Axid*) on nicotine elimination is unknown, but one would expect these drugs, like ranitidine, to interact minimally.

MANAGEMENT OPTIONS:

➡ *Circumvent/Minimize.* Patients on cimetidine therapy may not need to use as much nicotine gum or as many patches as those not on cimetidine. For smokers, it is possible that cimetidine therapy would allow a reduction in the number of cigarettes smoked while maintaining the same blood nicotine concentrations.

➡ *Monitor.* Be alert for evidence of excessive nicotine response.

REFERENCES:

1. Bendayan R, et al. Effect of cimetidine and ranitidine on the hepatic and renal elimination of nicotine in humans. *Eur J Clin Pharmacol.* 1990;38(2):165-169.

Cimetidine (eg, *Tagamet*)

Nifedipine (eg, *Procardia*)

SUMMARY: Cimetidine can increase the serum concentration of nifedipine; excessive nifedipine effects can occur.

RISK FACTORS: No specific risk factors are known.

MECHANISM: The metabolism of nifedipine is reduced by cimetidine. In addition, increases in gastric pH may be responsible for the increases in nifedipine bioavailability observed after administration of cimetidine or other H_2-receptor antagonists that do not affect the metabolism of nifedipine but increase its concentration (eg, ranitidine [eg, *Zantac*]).

CLINICAL EVALUATION: Several reports have noted a 60% to 90% increase in the nifedipine area under the concentration-time curve (AUC) following cimetidine administration.[1,2,3,4,5]

RELATED DRUGS: Ranitidine appears to have a smaller effect on nifedipine serum concentrations but may increase nifedipine AUC 13% to 48%.[1-7] If confirmed, other H_2-receptor antagonists (eg, famotidine [eg, *Pepcid*], nizatidine [eg, *Axid*]), omeprazole (eg, *Prilosec*), and lansoprazole (*Prevacid*) would be expected to have a similar effect. Increased nifedipine effects (eg, headache, hypotension) could occur. Cimetidine also increases the concentrations of diltiazem (eg, *Cardizem*), nisoldipine (*Sular*), nitrendipine, and verapamil (eg, *Calan*).

MANAGEMENT OPTIONS:

➡ *Monitor.* Carefully monitor patients receiving nifedipine when cimetidine or other drugs that alter gastric pH are added or removed from their drug regimen.

REFERENCES:

1. Kirch W, et al. Effect of cimetidine and ranitidine on the pharmacokinetics and anti-hypertensive effect of nifedipine [In German]. *Dtsch Med Wochenschr.* 1983;108(46):1757-1761.

2. Renwick AG, et al. Factors affecting the pharmacokinetics of nifedipine. *Eur J Clin Pharmacol.* 1987;32(4):351-355.

3. Smith SR, et al. Ranitidine and cimetidine; drug interactions with single and steady-state nifedipine administration. *Br J Clin Pharmacol.* 1987;23(3):311-315.

4. Adams LJ, et al. Effect of ranitidine on bioavailability of nifedipine. *Gastroenterology.* 1986;90:1320.

5. Kirch W, et al. Ranitidine increases bioavailability of nifedipine. *Clin Pharmacol Ther.* 1985;37:204.

6. Schwartz JB, et al. Effect of cimetidine or ranitidine administration of nifedipine pharmacokinetics and pharmacodynamics. *Clin Pharmacol Ther.* 1988;43(6):673-680.

7. Khan A, et al. The pharmacokinetics and pharmacodynamics of nifedipine at steady state during concomitant administration of cimetidine or high dose ranitidine. *Br J Clin Pharmacol.* 1991;32(4):519-522.

Cimetidine (eg, *Tagamet*)

Nimodipine (eg, *Nimotop*)

SUMMARY: Cimetidine can increase the serum concentration of nimodipine; the clinical significance of this interaction is unknown.

RISK FACTORS: No specific risk factors are known.

MECHANISM: Cimetidine appears to inhibit the metabolism or increase the bioavailability of nimodipine. Increased gastric pH may contribute to the increase in nimodipine concentration.

CLINICAL EVALUATION: Cimetidine 1,000 mg/day for 7 days increased the area under the concentration-time curve of nimodipine 30 mg 3 times daily approximately 75% in healthy subjects.[1] No changes in hemodynamic parameters (blood pressure and heart rate) were noted. Although more study is needed, the hypotensive effects of nimodipine could be increased in some patients.

RELATED DRUGS: Cimetidine also increases the concentrations of diltiazem (eg, *Cardizem*), nisoldipine (*Sular*), nifedipine (eg, *Procardia*), and verapamil (eg, *Calan*). Ranitidine (eg, *Zantac*) 300 mg/day for 5 days produced no change in the pharmacokinetics of nimodipine.[1] Other drugs that increase gastric pH (eg, omeprazole [eg, *Prilosec*]) may affect nimodipine similarly.

MANAGEMENT OPTIONS:

➥ **Monitor.** Monitor patients receiving nimodipine for excessive effects (eg, headache, hypotension) when cimetidine is added or removed from their drug regimen.

REFERENCES:

1. Mück W, et al. Influence of the H_2-receptor antagonists cimetidine and ranitidine on the pharmacokinetics of nimodipine in healthy volunteers. *Eur J Clin Pharmacol.* 1992;42(3):325-328.

Cimetidine (eg, *Tagamet*)

Nisoldipine (*Sular*)

SUMMARY: Cimetidine can increase the serum concentration of nisoldipine; excessive nisoldipine effects may be seen.

RISK FACTORS:

➥ **Route of Administration.** Oral administration of nisoldipine increases the likelihood of this interaction.

MECHANISM: Cimetidine increased the bioavailability of nisoldipine but did not alter the systemic clearance of nisoldipine or its hemodynamic effects. These changes may be the result of increased gastric pH.

CLINICAL EVALUATION: When cimetidine 1000 mg was administered to 8 healthy subjects for 1 day before nisoldipine 10 mg orally or 0.374 mg IV, the bioavailability of nisoldipine was increased from 3.9% to 5.7%; the peak serum concentration was increased 52%; and the volume of distribution was increased 38%.[1] No changes in pharmacodynamics were reported; the outcome of steady-state studies is unknown.

RELATED DRUGS: Cimetidine also increases the concentrations of diltiazem (eg, *Cardizem*), nifedipine (eg, *Procardia*), nitrendipine, and verapamil (eg, *Calan*). Other drugs that increase gastric pH (eg, famotidine [eg, *Pepcid*], nizatidine [*Axid*], ranitidine [eg, *Zantac*], omeprazole [*Prilosec*]) may affect nisoldipine in a similar manner.

MANAGEMENT OPTIONS:

➥ *Monitor.* Carefully monitor patients receiving nisoldipine for altered hypotensive effects when cimetidine or other drugs that alter gastric pH are added or deleted from their drug regimen.

REFERENCES:

1. van Harten J, et al. Pharmacokinetics and hemodynamic effects of nisoldipine and its interaction with cimetidine. *Clin Pharmacol Ther.* 1988;43:332.

Cimetidine (eg, *Tagamet*)

Nitrendipine (*Baypress*)

SUMMARY: Cimetidine can increase the serum concentration of nitrendipine; excessive nitrendipine effects may be seen.

RISK FACTORS: No specific risk factors are known.

MECHANISM: Cimetidine appears to inhibit the metabolism or increase the bioavailability of nitrendipine. It is possible that an increase in gastric pH also may increase nitrendipine concentrations.

CLINICAL EVALUATION: Cimetidine coadministration resulted in an average increase in nitrendipine area under the concentration-time curve (AUC) of 154%.[2] The increase in AUC was greater for the more active S-nitrendipine enantiomer resulting in a mean increase of 20% in the S/R-enantiomer ratio. Some patients could experience enhanced nitrendipine effects including hypotension or headache.

RELATED DRUGS: Cimetidine also increases the concentrations of diltiazem (eg, *Cardizem*), nisoldipine (*Sular*), nifedipine (eg, *Procardia*), and verapamil (eg, *Calan*). Ranitidine (eg, *Zantac*) 300 mg/day for 1 week increased the AUC of nitrendipine 50% without changing its hemodynamic effects.[1] Other drugs that increase gastric pH (eg, famotidine [eg, *Pepcid*], nizatidine [*Axid*], omeprazole [*Prilosec*]) may affect nitrendipine in a similar manner.

MANAGEMENT OPTIONS:

➥ *Monitor.* Carefully monitor patients receiving nitrendipine for altered hypotensive effects when cimetidine or other drugs that increase gastric pH are added or deleted from their drug regimen.

REFERENCES:

1. Halabi A, et al. Influence of ranitidine on kinetics of nitrendipine and on noninvasive hemodynamic parameters. *Ther Drug Monit.* 1990;12:303.

2. Soons PA, et al. Grapefruit juice and cimetidine inhibit stereoselective metabolism of nitrendipine in humans. *Clin Pharmacol Ther.* 1991;50:394.

Cimetidine (eg, *Tagamet*)

Nortriptyline (eg, *Pamelor*)

SUMMARY: Limited clinical evidence suggests that cimetidine increases serum nortriptyline concentrations; given the proven effect of cimetidine on tricyclic antidepressants closely related to nortriptyline, it seems likely that nortriptyline is affected similarly.

RISK FACTORS:

➡ ***Dosage Regimen.*** In most patients, clinically important inhibition of hepatic drug metabolism by cimetidine requires doses at least 400 mg/day.

MECHANISM: Cimetidine probably inhibits the hepatic metabolism of nortriptyline.

CLINICAL EVALUATION: In a man who was receiving cimetidine and nortriptyline, the steady-state serum concentration of nortriptyline decreased from 104 to 75 mg/L when the cimetidine was discontinued.[1] For this patient, the steady-state serum concentration of nortriptyline was, on average, 42% higher while he was taking cimetidine. In another study, 6 healthy men were given single oral 100 mg doses of imipramine or nortriptyline, with and without pretreatment with cimetidine 300 mg 4 times daily for 2 days.[2] Nortriptyline pharmacokinetics were affected only minimally by cimetidine pretreatment in this single-dose study, but plasma concentrations of the major metabolite of nortriptyline (10-hydroxynortriptyline) were substantially affected. Multiple-dose pharmacokinetic studies are needed to assess this interaction, preferably in patients receiving the drugs therapeutically. Moreover, the fact that cimetidine appears to increase serum concentrations of other cyclic antidepressants supports the possibility that nortriptyline is affected.

RELATED DRUGS: The evidence suggests that ranitidine (eg, *Zantac*) is unlikely to interact with cyclic antidepressants. Theoretically, it is unlikely that famotidine (eg, *Pepcid*) and nizatidine (*Axid*) will interact with cyclic antidepressants because these H_2-receptor antagonists have little effect on drug metabolism. Cimetidine also may increase serum concentrations of desipramine (eg, *Norpramin*), doxepin (eg, *Sinequan*), imipramine (eg, *Tofranil*), and protriptyline (eg, *Vivactil*).

MANAGEMENT OPTIONS:

➡ ***Consider Alternative.*** Consider using an alternative to cimetidine (eg, ranitidine, nizatidine, famotidine).

➡ ***Circumvent/Minimize.*** In patients who are already receiving cimetidine and are about to begin a course of therapy with nortriptyline, consider using conservative nortriptyline doses until the patient's response to therapy can be evaluated.

➡ ***Monitor.*** In patients stabilized on nortriptyline who are then given cimetidine, be alert for evidence of nortriptyline toxicity (eg, severe dry mouth, blurred vision, urinary retention, tachycardia, constipation, postural hypotension). If cimetidine is discontinued or its dose substantially reduced in a patient stabilized on both nortriptyline and cimetidine, monitor the patient for an inadequate nortriptyline response.

REFERENCES:

1. Miller DD, et al. Cimetidine's effect on steady-state serum nortriptyline concentrations. *Drug Intell Clin Pharm.* 1983;17:904.
2. Henauer SA, et al. Cimetidine interaction with imipramine and nortriptyline. *Clin Pharmacol Ther.* 1984;35:183.

Cimetidine (eg, *Tagamet*)

Paroxetine (*Paxil*)

SUMMARY: Preliminary evidence suggests that cimetidine substantially increases paroxetine serum concentrations, but the clinical importance of the interaction is not established.

RISK FACTORS: No specific risk factors are known.

MECHANISM: Not established. The pharmacokinetic changes in paroxetine are consistent with cimetidine-induced reduction in first-pass metabolism of paroxetine.

CLINICAL EVALUATION: In a study of 10 healthy subjects, a single oral 30 mg dose of paroxetine was given with and without pretreatment with cimetidine 200 mg 4 times daily for 8 days.[1] Cimetidine was associated with a 57% increase in the area under the paroxetine plasma concentration-time curve, but the change was not statistically significant because of high intersubject variability. In another study that was more typical of the clinical situation, 11 healthy subjects were given paroxetine for 28 days, with cimetidine added for the last 7 days.[2] Cimetidine increased the area under the paroxetine plasma concentration-time curve 51% and the maximal paroxetine plasma concentration 45%, but it produced no change in the paroxetine half-life or elimination rate constant. The elevated plasma paroxetine concentrations apparently were not associated with significant adverse effects, but additional study is needed to assess the clinical consequences of this interaction.

RELATED DRUGS: The effect of ranitidine (eg, *Zantac*), famotidine (eg, *Pepcid*), and nizatidine (*Axid*) on paroxetine pharmacokinetics is unknown; theoretically they would not be expected to interact.

MANAGEMENT OPTIONS:

➡ ***Consider Alternative.*** Theoretically, other H_2-receptor antagonists, such as ranitidine, famotidine, and nizatidine, would be less likely to interact with paroxetine; thus their use may be preferred over cimetidine until more information is available on this interaction.

➡ ***Monitor.*** Monitor patients for alterations in therapeutic and toxic effects of paroxetine if cimetidine is initiated, discontinued, or changed in dosage. Patients receiving cimetidine may require lower doses of paroxetine. However, determining whether to adjust the dose of paroxetine and by how much may not be easy, because the degree to which paroxetine produces dose-dependent adverse effects is not well established.

REFERENCES:

1. Greb WH, et al. The effect of liver enzyme inhibition by cimetidine and enzyme induction by phenobarbitone on the pharmacokinetics of paroxetine. *Acta Psychiatr Scand*. 1989;80(Suppl. 350):95.
2. Bannister SJ, et al. Evaluation of the potential for interactions of paroxetine with diazepam, cimetidine, warfarin, and digoxin. *Acta Psychiatr Scand*. 1989;80(Suppl. 350):102.

Cimetidine (eg, *Tagamet*)

Phenobarbital

SUMMARY: Phenobarbital slightly reduces plasma cimetidine concentrations, but the effect is of doubtful clinical importance.

RISK FACTORS: No specific risk factors are known.

MECHANISM: Not established. Phenobarbital (and presumably other barbiturates) may enhance the hepatic metabolism of cimetidine.

CLINICAL EVALUATION: In a study of healthy subjects, phenobarbital 100 mg/day for 3 weeks reduced plasma cimetidine concentration and enhanced total cimetidine clearance.[1] The magnitude of the changes was small and probably not sufficient to reduce the clinical response to cimetidine.

RELATED DRUGS: One would expect that other H_2-receptor antagonists also would be affected minimally by barbiturate coadministration. It is likely that this interaction would occur when other H_2-receptor antagonists, such as famotidine (eg, *Pepcid*), nizatidine (*Axid*), and ranitidine (eg, *Zantac*), are used with any barbiturate.

MANAGEMENT OPTIONS: No specific action is required, but be alert for evidence of the interaction.

REFERENCES:
1. Somogyi A, et al. Influence of phenobarbital treatment on cimetidine kinetics. *Eur J Clin Pharmacol.* 1981;19:343.

Cimetidine (eg, *Tagamet*) ▼

Phenytoin (eg, *Dilantin*)

SUMMARY: Cimetidine increases serum phenytoin concentrations; phenytoin intoxication occurs in some patients. Ranitidine may increase serum phenytoin concentrations in some patients, but the data are limited.

RISK FACTORS:

➡ *Dosage Regimen.* Cimetidine doses of 400 mg/day may increase serum phenytoin slightly, but larger cimetidine doses can produce greater increases.

MECHANISM: Cimetidine inhibits the hepatic metabolism of phenytoin.

CLINICAL EVALUATION: Numerous clinical studies in both patients and healthy subjects have shown that cimetidine increases serum phenytoin concentrations. Cimetidine doses of about 1 to 1.2 g/day increase serum phenytoin concentrations approximately 70%,[1-8] although there is considerable variation from patient to patient. When cimetidine is started in a patient maintained on phenytoin, serum phenytoin concentrations usually begin to increase after the first day or two of cimetidine therapy. A new steady-state serum phenytoin concentration may be achieved as soon as 4 to 5 days or as long as several weeks or more after starting cimetidine. Stopping cimetidine usually results in a return of serum phenytoin concentrations to precimetidine levels within approximately 2 weeks.

RELATED DRUGS: Ranitidine (eg, *Zantac*), famotidine (eg, *Pepcid*), and nizatidine (*Axid*) do not appear to affect phenytoin metabolism.[9,10] Case reports have suggested that ranitidine may increase serum phenytoin concentrations, but the cases were complicated by other confounding variables.[11-13]

MANAGEMENT OPTIONS:

➡ *Consider Alternative.* Ranitidine, famotidine, and nizatidine would be preferable to cimetidine in most patients receiving phenytoin.

➡ *Monitor.* Be alert for evidence of phenytoin toxicity (eg, nystagmus, ataxia, confusion) when cimetidine is given concurrently. In a patient well stabilized on both drugs, discontinuation of cimetidine may result in inadequate serum phenytoin concentrations.

REFERENCES:

1. Levine M, et al. Differential effect of cimetidine on serum concentrations of carbamazepine and phenytoin. *Neurology.* 1985;35:562.
2. Hetzel DJ, et al. Cimetidine interaction with phenytoin. *BMJ.* 1981;282:1512.
3. Neuvonen PJ, et al. Cimetidine-phenytoin interaction: effect on serum phenytoin concentration and antipyrine test. *Eur J Clin Pharmacol.* 1981;21:215.
4. Algozzine GJ, et al. Decreased clearance of phenytoin with cimetidine. *Ann Intern Med.* 1981;95:244.
5. Bartle WR, et al. Dose-dependent effect of cimetidine on phenytoin kinetics. *Clin Pharmacol Ther.* 1983;33:649.
6. Salem RB, et al. Effect of cimetidine on phenytoin serum levels. *Epilepsia.* 1983;24:284.
7. Iteogu MO, et al. Effect of cimetidine on single-dose phenytoin kinetics. *Clin Pharm.* 1983;2:302.
8. Phillips P, Hansky J. Phenytoin toxicity secondary to cimetidine administration. *Med J Aust.* 1984;141:602.
9. Watts RW, et al. Lack of interaction between ranitidine and phenytoin. *Br J Clin Pharmacol.* 1983;15:499.
10. Sambol NC, et al. Influence of famotidine (Fam) and cimetidine (Cim) on the disposition of phenytoin (Phe) and indocyanine green (ICG). *Clin Pharmacol Ther.* 1986;39:225.
11. Bramhall D, et al. Possible interaction of ranitidine with phenytoin. *Drug Intell Clin Pharm.* 1988;22:979.
12. Tse CST, et al. Phenytoin concentration elevation subsequent to ranitidine administration. *Ann Pharmacother.* 1993;27:1448.
13. Tse CST, et al. Phenytoin and ranitidine interaction. *Ann Intern Med.* 1994;120:892.

Cimetidine (eg, *Tagamet*)

Posaconazole (*Noxafil*)

SUMMARY: Cimetidine may reduce the plasma concentration of posaconazole after the administration of posaconazole suspension; some loss of antifungal efficacy is expected.

RISK FACTORS: No specific risk factors are known.

MECHANISM: Unknown. Product label refers to the mechanism as altered gastric pH.

CLINICAL EVALUATION: While specific data are limited, the manufacturer of posaconazole notes that the coadministration of cimetidine 400 mg twice daily with posaconazole tablets 200 mg daily for 10 days reduces the mean area under the plasma concentration time-curve (AUC) of posaconazole by about 40%.[1] While this study was done with posaconazole tablets, the approved formulation is a suspension for which no cimetidine interaction data are available. The label notes the mechanism of this interaction is considered "alteration of gastric pH," but then states that other H_2 receptor antagonists or proton pump inhibitors have no clinically relevant effect on posaconazole plasma concentrations. Because these statements appear to be in conflict, pending further data it would be prudent to assume other drugs that reduce gastric acidity will interact with posaconazole. The coadministration of antacid (*Mylanta*) 20 mL resulted in a small increase in the mean posaconazole (tablet) AUC when given fasting and produced a small decrease in posaconazole AUC in the nonfasting setting.[2] Studies with the oral suspension formulation of posaconazole are needed to assess the potential interaction with the available dosage formulation.

RELATED DRUGS: Pending additional data, it would be prudent to assume other drugs that lower gastric acidity may also reduce posaconazole plasma concentrations. The bioavailability of ketoconazole (eg, *Nizoral*) and itraconazole (eg, *Sporanox*) are known to be reduced by drugs that increase gastric pH.

MANAGEMENT OPTIONS:

➡ *Consider Alternative.* The manufacturer of posaconazole recommends avoiding the combination. Oral antifungal agents that are not affected by changes in gastric pH include voriconazole (*Vfend*), terbinafine (eg, *Lamisil*), and fluconazole (eg, *Diflucan*).

➡ *Monitor.* Be alert for reduced antifungal efficacy if posaconazole is coadministered with cimetidine.

REFERENCES:

1. *Noxafil* [package insert]. Kenilworth, NJ: Schering Corporation; 2006.
2. Courtney R, et al. Pharmacokinetics of posaconazole coadministered with antacid in fasting or non-fasting healthy men. *Antimicrob Agents Chemother*. 2004;48:804-808.

Cimetidine (eg, *Tagamet*)
Praziquantel (*Biltricide*)

SUMMARY: Cimetidine increases praziquantel concentrations; the clinical significance of these changes are unknown, but toxicity is possible.

RISK FACTORS: No specific risk factors are known.

MECHANISM: Cimetidine appears to inhibit the first-pass metabolism and systemic clearance of praziquantel.

CLINICAL EVALUATION: A patient with neurocysticercosis was being treated with phenytoin and phenobarbital for a seizure disorder.[1] Praziquantel 3600 mg/day was prescribed and produced a peak concentration of 350 ng/ml. Cimetidine 400 mg 4 times daily was added, and 1 week later his praziquantel peak concentration was increased to 826 ng/ml and its half-life increased from 1.7 to 3.3 hours. The area under the concentration-time curve of praziquantel was increased 4-fold during cimetidine administration. A single 800 mg dose of cimetidine produced a 55% to 65% increase in praziquantel concentration in 20 healthy subjects.[2] Praziquantel half-life was prolonged following cimetidine administration. No toxicity has been reported during praziquantel and cimetidine therapy.

RELATED DRUGS: Other H_2-receptor antagonists, such as ranitidine (eg, *Zantac*), famotidine (eg, *Pepcid*), and nizatidine (*Axid*), would be unlikely to affect the metabolism of praziquantel.

MANAGEMENT OPTIONS:

➡ **Consider Alternative.** In patients not receiving anticonvulsants, an alternative H_2-receptor antagonist (eg, ranitidine, famotidine, nizatidine) probably would avoid the interaction.

➡ **Monitor.** Monitor patients who receive cimetidine and praziquantel for increased praziquantel plasma concentrations and potential toxicity (eg, headache, nausea, dizziness).

REFERENCES:

1. Dachman WD, et al. Cimetidine-induced rise in praziquantel levels in a patient with neurocysticercosis being treated with anticonvulsants. *J Infect Dis.* 1994;169:689.

2. Metwally A, et al. Effect of cimetidine, bicarbonate and glucose on the bioavailability of different formulations of praziquantel. *Arzneimittelforschung.* 1995;45:460.

Cimetidine (eg, *Tagamet*)

Procainamide (eg, *Pronestyl*)

SUMMARY: Cimetidine may increase procainamide serum concentrations significantly; procainamide toxicity from this interaction has been reported.

RISK FACTORS:

➡ **Concurrent Diseases.** Patients with renal dysfunction are at particular risk.

MECHANISM: Cimetidine reduces the renal tubular secretion of procainamide and its major metabolite N-acetylprocainamide.[1,5]

CLINICAL EVALUATION: Procainamide and N-acetylprocainamide renal clearance (from 0 to 12 hours) were decreased more than 40%[1,7] and 24%,[1] respectively, following treatment with cimetidine in both healthy subjects and patients with arrhythmias. The area under the procainamide concentration-time curve increased 44% after cimetidine administration. The effect of cimetidine appears to be dose dependent.[6] The magnitude of these changes indicates that some patients may develop excessive concentrations of procainamide and NAPA in the presence of cimetidine. Patients with marked renal impairment and the elderly are probably most at risk, since they may have reduced renal clearance of all 3 drugs.[1-4]

RELATED DRUGS: Ranitidine (eg, *Zantac*) produces a small increase in procainamide concentrations; famotidine (eg, *Pepcid*) appears to have no effect. Theoretically, nizatidine (*Axid*) is unlikely to interact. Although no data exist, proton pump inhibitors (eg, omeprazole [*Prilosec*]) would be unlikely to alter procainamide clearance.

MANAGEMENT OPTIONS:

➡ **Consider Alternative.** Famotidine or nizatidine use would likely avoid the interaction.

➡ **Monitor.** Be alert for evidence of enhanced procainamide and NAPA response (eg, wide QRS, QT interval) in the presence of cimetidine therapy. A reduction in procainamide dose may be necessary.

REFERENCES:

1. Somogyi A, et al. Cimetidine-procainamide pharmacokinetic interaction in man: evidence of competition for tubular secretion of basic drugs. *Eur J Clin Pharmacol.* 1983;25:339.

2. Drayer DE, et al. Cumulation of N-acetylprocainamide, an active metabolite of procainamide, in patients with impaired renal function. *Clin Pharmacol Ther.* 1977;22:63.

3. Reidenberg MM, et al. Aging and renal clearance of procainamide and acetylprocainamide. *Clin Pharmacol Ther.* 1980;28:732.

4. Higbee MD, et al. Procainamide-cimetidine interaction: a potential toxic interaction in the elderly. *J Am Geriatr Soc.* 1984;32:162.

5. Christain CW Jr, et al. Cimetidine inhibits renal procainamide clearance. *Clin Pharmacol Ther.* 1984;36:221.

6. Lai MY, et al. Dose dependent effect of cimetidine on procainamide disposition in man. *Int J Clin Pharmacol Ther Toxicol.* 1988;26:118.

7. Bauer LA, et al. Procainamide-cimetidine drug interaction in elderly male patients. *J Am Geriatr Soc.* 1990;38:467.

Cimetidine (eg, *Tagamet*)

Propafenone (*Rythmol*)

SUMMARY: Cimetidine significantly increased propafenone concentration in 8 of 12 subjects stabilized on propafenone.

RISK FACTORS: No specific risk factors are known.

MECHANISM: Not established. Cimetidine appears to increase the concentration of propafenone in most subjects. The increase could be caused by reduced metabolism or increased bioavailability. Propafenone appears to increase the rate of cimetidine absorption without changing its clearance.

CLINICAL EVALUATION: Twelve healthy subjects were given propafenone 225 mg every 8 hours for 5 days, cimetidine 400 mg every 8 hours for 5 days, and both drugs for 5 days.[1] During coadministration of both drugs, the average propafenone concentration for all 12 subjects increased 21.5%. The propafenone serum concentration was reduced in 4 of the subjects (mean 8.9%) following cimetidine administration. The remaining 8 subjects averaged a 54% increase in propafenone concentration. Propafenone alone significantly increased the PR interval and QRS duration compared to baseline. Only the QRS duration was significantly prolonged during cimetidine coadministration. Propafenone also increased cimetidine peak serum concentration 14% (P < 0.05) and decreased the time to peak serum concentration, but it did not affect cimetidine steady-state concentrations.

RELATED DRUGS: The effects of other H_2-receptor antagonists on propafenone are unknown; ranitidine (eg, *Zantac*), nizatidine (*Axid*), and famotidine (eg, *Pepcid*) would be expected to have little effect on propafenone.

MANAGEMENT OPTIONS:

➡ *Monitor.* Until further information is available, carefully observe patients maintained on propafenone for increased propafenone response if cimetidine is added or for a reduced response if cimetidine is removed from their drug regimen.

REFERENCES:

1. Pritchett ELC, et al. Pharmacokinetic and pharmacodynamic interactions of propafenone and cimetidine. *J Clin Pharmacol.* 1988;28:619.

Cimetidine (eg, *Tagamet*)

Propranolol (eg, *Inderal*)

SUMMARY: Propranolol and other plasma concentrations of beta blockers that undergo significant hepatic metabolism (eg, metoprolol, labetalol) may be increased by cimetidine therapy.

RISK FACTORS: No specific risk factors are known.

MECHANISM: Cimetidine reduces the activity of the hepatic microsomal enzymes that metabolize propranolol and some other beta-adrenergic blockers. It has been proposed that cimetidine reduces propranolol metabolism by decreasing blood flow, but the contribution of this mechanism to the interaction is probably minimal. Cimetidine reduces the renal tubular secretion of pindolol (eg, *Visken*).

CLINICAL EVALUATION: In studies utilizing both single- and multiple-dose designs, cimetidine consistently and substantially increased plasma propranolol concentrations.[3-6,10] Peak and steady-state plasma propranolol concentrations generally increase approximately 50% to 100% in the presence of cimetidine, but the degree to which this increases the pharmacologic and toxic effects of propranolol is not well established.

RELATED DRUGS: Metoprolol (eg, *Lopressor*) pharmacokinetics (100 mg single dose) were not affected by cimetidine in one study,[7] but cimetidine substantially increased plasma concentrations of metoprolol 100 mg twice daily for 7 days in other studies.[3,4,11] The bioavailability of labetalol (eg, *Normodyne*) was increased 55% to 80% without significant change in systemic clearance after the administration of cimetidine 1.6 g/day for 3 days,[8,9] while the bioavailability of dilevalol increased 11% and the area under the concentration-time curve (AUC) increased 20% following cimetidine 1.2 g/day.[3] The renal clearance of pindolol (eg, *Visken*) was reduced approximately 30% and its AUC increased approximately 45% with cimetidine 400 mg twice daily coadministration.[12] Atenolol (eg, *Tenormin*),[3,4,7] penbutolol (*Levatol*),[2,3] and nadolol (eg, *Corgard*)[1] appear to be affected minimally by cimetidine therapy. Ranitidine (eg, *Zantac*) does not affect propranolol concentrations. Famotidine (eg, *Pepcid*) and nizatidine (*Axid*) would be unlikely to affect propranolol concentrations.

MANAGEMENT OPTIONS:

➡ *Consider Alternative.* Atenolol or nadolol could be administered instead of hepatically metabolized beta blockers. Ranitidine, famotidine, nizatidine, antacids, or sucralfate (eg, *Carafate*) also may be suitable alternatives to cimetidine, although beta blocker doses probably should be separated from antacids or sucralfate to minimize the possibility of impaired absorption of the beta blocker.

➡ *Monitor.* Be alert for evidence of altered response to propranolol, labetalol, and possibly other beta blockers when cimetidine therapy is initiated or discontinued.

REFERENCES:

1. Duchin KL, et al. Comparison of kinetic interaction of nadolol and propranolol with cimetidine. *Am Heart J.* 1984;108(Part 2):1084.

2. Spahn H, et al. Penbutolol pharmacokinetics: the influence of concomitant administration of cimetidine. *Eur J Clin Pharmacol.* 1986;29:555.

3. Mutschler E, et al. The interaction between H$_2$-receptor antagonists and beta-adrenoceptor blockers. *Br J Clin Pharmacol.* 1984;17:51S.

4. Kirch W, et al. Interaction of metoprolol, propranolol and atenolol with concurrent administration of cimetidine. *Klin Wochenschr.* 1982;60:1401.

5. Tomonori T, et al. The influence of diltiazem versus cimetidine on propranolol metabolism. *J Clin Pharmacol.* 1992;32:1099.

6. Reimann IW, et al. Cimetidine increases steady plasma levels of propranolol. *Br J Clin Pharmacol.* 1981;12:785.

7. Houtzagers JJR, et al. The effect of pretreatment with cimetidine on the bioavailability and disposition of atenolol and metoprolol. *Br J Clin Pharmacol.* 1982;14:67.

8. Daneshmend TK, et al. Cimetidine and bioavailability of labetalol. *Lancet.* 1981;1:565.

9. Daneshmend TK, et al. The effects of enzyme induction and enzyme inhibition of labetalol pharmacokinetics. *Br J Clin Pharmacol.* 1984;18:393.

10. Donn KH, et al. Stereoselectivity of cimetidine inhibition of propranolol oral clearance. *Clin Pharmacol Ther.* 1988;43:283.

11. Toon S, et al. The racemic metoprolol H2-antagonist interaction. *Clin Pharmacol Ther.* 1988;43:283.

12. Somogyi AA, et al. Stereoselective inhibition of pindolol renal clearance by cimetidine in humans. *Clin Pharmacol Ther.* 1992;51:379.

Cimetidine (eg, *Tagamet*)

Quinidine (eg, *Quinora*)

SUMMARY: Cimetidine coadministration elevates quinidine serum concentrations; watch for evidence of quinidine toxicity.

RISK FACTORS: No specific risk factors are known.

MECHANISM: Cimetidine inhibits the hepatic metabolism of quinidine and may reduce its renal clearance.

CLINICAL EVALUATION: In several case reports quinidine concentrations increased 50% after the addition of cimetidine.[1,2] In a study of 9 subjects, quinidine 400 mg was given before and after cimetidine 300 mg 4 times daily.[3] Cimetidine was associated with a 23% increase in the plasma half-life of quinidine. In other studies of normal subjects, cimetidine 1.2 g/day for 5 to 7 days increased the quinidine half-life approximately 55% and reduced quinidine clearance 35% to 40%.[4,5] The effect of cimetidine on quinidine renal clearance is unclear. Some have observed a reduction in renal clearance while others have seen no significant effect.[6]

RELATED DRUGS: While ranitidine (eg, *Zantac*) would not be expected to alter quinidine metabolism, a case of ventricular bigeminy during quinidine and ranitidine coadministration has been reported.[7]

MANAGEMENT OPTIONS:

➡ **Consider Alternative.** Other H_2-receptor antagonists, such as ranitidine, famotidine (eg, *Pepcid*), and nizatidine (*Axid*), are probably less likely to interact with quinidine than cimetidine.

➡ **Monitor.** Be alert for evidence of altered quinidine response when cimetidine is started or stopped. Serum quinidine determinations would be useful if the interaction is suspected.

REFERENCES:

1. Polish LB, et al. Digitoxin-quinidine interaction: potentiation during administration of cimetidine. *South Med J.* 1981;74:633-634.

2. Farringer JA, et al. Cimetidine-quinidine interaction. *Clin Pharm.* 1984;3:81-83.

3. Kolb KW, et al. The effect of cimetidine on urinary pH and quinidine clearance. American Society of Hospital Pharmacists Midyear Clinical Meeting; December, 1982.

4. Hardy BG, et al. Effect of cimetidine on the pharmacokinetics and pharmacodynamics of quinidine. *Am J Cardiol*. 1983;52:172-175.

5. MacKichan JJ, et al. Effect of cimetidine on quinidine bioavailability. *Biopharm Drug Dispos*. 1989;10:121-125.

6. Hardy BG, et al. Lack of effect of cimetidine on the metabolism of quinidine: effect on renal clearance. *Int J Clin Pharmacol Ther Toxicol*. 1988;26:388-391.

7. Iliopoulou A, et al. Quinidine-ranitidine adverse reaction. *Eur Heart J*. 1986;7:360.

5 Cimetidine (eg, *Tagamet*)

Repaglinide (*Prandin*)

SUMMARY: Cimetidine administration does not alter repaglinide plasma concentrations.

RISK FACTORS: No specific risk factors are known.

MECHANISM: No interaction.

CLINICAL EVALUATION: Repaglinide 2 mg/day was administered for 4 days alone and with cimetidine 400 mg twice daily to 14 healthy subjects.[1] The pharmacokinetic parameters of repaglinide were not altered during cimetidine coadministration. While not measured in this study, cimetidine would not be expected to alter the hypoglycemic of repaglinide.

RELATED DRUGS: Cimetidine has been reported to increase the concentrations of tolbutamide (*Orinase*), glipizide (*Glucotrol*), and glyburide (*Diabeta*). Other H_2-receptor antagonists would not be expected to affect repaglinide plasma concentrations.

MANAGEMENT OPTIONS: No interaction.

REFERENCES:
1. Hatorp V, et al. Drug interaction studies with repaglinide: repaglinide on digoxin or theophylline pharmacokinetics and cimetidine on repaglinide pharmacokinetics. *J Clin Pharmacol*. 2000;40:184-192.

4 Cimetidine (eg, *Tagamet*)

Rimantadine (*Flumadine*)

SUMMARY: Cimetidine causes a small increase in the plasma concentration of the antiviral agent, rimantadine; the clinical significance appears to be limited.

RISK FACTORS: No specific risk factors are known.

MECHANISM: Cimetidine appears to reduce the metabolic clearance of rimantadine.

CLINICAL EVALUATION: Rimantadine 100 mg was administered alone and with the first dose of a 5-day regimen of cimetidine 300 mg 4 times daily.[1] Rimantadine half-life increased significantly from 25 to 29 hours, and its apparent total body clearance was reduced 18% following cimetidine administration. The area under the rimantadine concentration-time curve increased 20% during cimetidine administration. The renal clearance of rimantadine was not altered by cimetidine. Confirmation of the apparent limited clinical significance of this interaction will require studies under steady-state conditions in patients being treated with rimantadine for influenza.

RELATED DRUGS: Because amantadine (eg, *Symmetrel*) is primarily eliminated by the kidneys, cimetidine would not be expected to cause significant increases in its serum concentrations. Other H_2-receptor antagonists, such as ranitidine (eg, *Zantac*), famotidine (eg, *Pepcid*), and nizatidine (*Axid*), would not be expected to affect rimantadine concentrations.

MANAGEMENT OPTIONS: No specific action is required, but be alert for evidence of the interaction.

REFERENCES:

1. Holazo AA, et al. Effect of cimetidine on the disposition of rimantadine in healthy subjects. *Antimicrob Agents Chemother*. 1989;33:820-823.

Cimetidine (eg, *Tagamet*)

Sildenafil (*Viagra*)

SUMMARY: Cimetidine may increase sildenafil plasma concentrations, but it is not known how often the combination would result in adverse consequences.

RISK FACTORS: No specific risk factors are known.

MECHANISM: Cimetidine probably inhibits the metabolism of sildenafil.

CLINICAL EVALUATION: In a study of 22 healthy men, cimetidine increased sildenafil area under the plasma concentration-time curve and maximum plasma concentration 56% and 54% respectively.[1] The combination was well tolerated in these subjects, but it seems likely that the combination would produce adverse effects in at least an occasional patient.

RELATED DRUGS: Theoretically, other H_2-receptor antagonists are unlikely to interact with sildenafil (eg, famotidine [eg, *Pepcid*], nizatidine [eg, *Axid*], and ranitidine [eg, *Zantac*]).

MANAGEMENT OPTIONS:

➡ *Consider Alternative.* Although the combination of cimetidine and sildenafil is probably safe in most patients, it would be prudent to use an alternative to cimetidine (see Related Drugs).

➡ *Monitor.* If sildenafil and cimetidine are used concurrently, monitor for excessive sildenafil effects such as hypotension.

REFERENCES:

1. Wilner K, et al. The effects of cimetidine and antacid on the pharmacokinetic profile of sildenafil citrate in healthy male volunteers. *Br J Clin Pharmacol*. 2002;53:31S-36S.

Cimetidine (eg, *Tagamet*)

Sucralfate (eg, *Carafate*)

SUMMARY: For most patients with peptic ulcers, the combined use of cimetidine and sucralfate appears to be no more effective than either drug alone; thus, for most patients, concurrent use increases risk without improving results.

RISK FACTORS: No specific risk factors are known.

MECHANISM: Drugs capable of reducing gastric acidity (eg, cimetidine) formerly were thought to interfere with the binding of sucralfate to ulcerated tissue; however, experimental evidence does not support such a mechanism. Also, sucralfate does not appear to alter cimetidine absorption.

CLINICAL EVALUATION: In vitro and animal studies indicate that cimetidine is not likely to inhibit binding of sucralfate to ulcerated tissue.[1,2] Sucralfate appears to have no effect on cimetidine bioavailability. In 3 human studies, cimetidine's bioavailability was similar in healthy subjects when they were given cimetidine both with or without sucralfate.[3-5] A study in dogs also found the extent of cimetidine absorption to be unaffected by sucralfate, although the systemic absorption of aluminum was approximately 30% higher with sucralfate plus cimetidine than with sucralfate alone.[6] The clinical significance of the increased aluminum absorption is unknown. Finally, in a double-blind study of 61 patients with duodenal ulcer, sucralfate, cimetidine, and a combination of the 2 were equally effective in ulcer healing, indicating that the drugs do not antagonize one another.[7] Although cimetidine and sucralfate do not appear to interact with each other, they both can interact with other drugs. Thus, combined use may increase the overall risk of drug interactions in the patient.

RELATED DRUGS: It seems unlikely that the action of any H_2-receptor antagonists (eg, ranitidine [eg, *Zantac*], famotidine [eg, *Pepcid*], nizatidine [eg, *Axid*]) would be affected by the concurrent use of sucralfate.

MANAGEMENT OPTIONS: No interaction.

REFERENCES:

1. DeChristoforo R. Cimetidine-sucralfate: drug interaction? *Hosp Pharm.* 1985;20:270.
2. Lacz JP, et al. Sucralfate binding in cimetidine treated rats. *Gastroenterology.* 1983;848:1220.
3. Albin H, et al. Effect of sucralfate on the bioavailability of cimetidine. *Eur J Clin Pharmacol.* 1986;30:493-494
4. D'Angio R, et al. Cimetidine absorption in humans during sucralfate coadministration. *Br J Clin Pharmacol.* 1986;21:515-520.
5. Beck CL, et al. Evaluation of potential cimetidine sucralfate interaction. *Clin Pharmacol Ther.* 1987;41:168.
6. Ritschel WA, et al. Cimetidine-sucralfate drug interaction. *Methods Find Exp Clin Pharmacol.* 1984;6:261-263.
7. Van Deventer G, et al. Comparison of sucralfate and cimetidine taken alone and in combination for treatment of active duodenal ulcer (DU). *Gastroenterology.* 1984;86:1287.

Cimetidine (eg, *Tagamet*)

Tacrine (*Cognex*)

SUMMARY: Cimetidine substantially increases tacrine plasma concentrations, but the degree to which it increases tacrine adverse reactions is not established.

RISK FACTORS:

➡ **Dosage Regimen.** In most patients, clinically important inhibition of hepatic drug metabolism by cimetidine requires dosages of 400 mg/day or higher.

MECHANISM: Cimetidine appears to reduce the extensive first-pass metabolism of tacrine, probably by inhibiting CYP1A2.[1] Anticholinesterase agents, such as tacrine, tend to increase gastric acid secretion and increase lower esophageal sphincter pressure.

CLINICAL EVALUATION: Eleven healthy subjects received a single oral dose of tacrine 40 mg with and without concurrent treatment with cimetidine 300 mg 4 times daily.[2] Cimetidine decreased tacrine apparent clearance 30%, but it did not affect tacrine half-life. Cimetidine increased the tacrine area under the plasma concentration-time curve 64%.[3] The magnitude of these changes appears large enough to increase the risk of tacrine adverse reactions (eg, cholinergic effects such as nausea, vomiting, and diarrhea). On the other hand, some evidence suggests that tacrine hepatotoxicity results from reactive tacrine metabolites.[4] Thus, theoretically, cimetidine actually might be expected to reduce the risk of tacrine hepatotoxicity. The ability of tacrine to increase gastric acid secretion is undesirable in patients receiving H_2-receptor antagonists, but the clinical importance of this effect is not established. It might be of greater importance in patients receiving H_2-receptor antagonists once daily at bedtime (eg, peptic ulcer treatment) because the gastric stimulatory effect of tacrine is unopposed during much of the day. In patients with gastroesophageal reflux disease (GERD), the twice-daily dosing of the H_2-receptor antagonists may be more effective in offsetting the acid stimulatory effect of tacrine. Moreover, it is likely that tacrine increases lower esophageal sphincter pressure, which is beneficial in GERD.

RELATED DRUGS: The effect of ranitidine (eg, *Zantac*), famotidine (eg, *Pepcid*), and nizatidine (eg, *Axid*) on tacrine metabolism is not established, but an interaction is not expected.

MANAGEMENT OPTIONS:

➡ *Consider Alternative.* Until the clinical importance of the cimetidine-tacrine interaction is established, consider using alternative H_2-receptor antagonists, such as ranitidine, famotidine, or nizatidine.

➡ *Monitor.* If cimetidine and tacrine are used concurrently, monitor for excessive cholinergic response (eg, nausea, vomiting, anorexia, diarrhea, abdominal pain) and adjust tacrine dosage as needed.

REFERENCES:

1. Spaldin V, et al. The effect of enzyme inhibition on the metabolism and activation of tacrine by human liver microsomes. *Br J Clin Pharmacol.* 1994;38(1):15-22.

2. de Vries TM, et al. Effect of cimetidine and low-dose quinidine on tacrine pharmacokinetics in humans. *Pharm Res.* 1993;10:S337.

3. *Cognex* [package insert]. New York, NY: Parke-Davis; 1993.

4. Madden S, et al. An investigation into the formation of stable, protein-reactive and cytotoxic metabolites from tacrine in vitro. Studies with human and rat liver microsomes. *Biochem Pharmacol.* 1993;46(1):13-20.

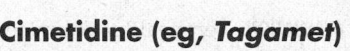

Cimetidine (eg, *Tagamet*)

Tamoxifen (eg, *Soltamox*)

SUMMARY: Theoretically, cimetidine may reduce the efficacy of tamoxifen in the treatment of breast cancer.

RISK FACTORS: No specific risk factors are known.

MECHANISM: Tamoxifen is metabolized to 2 active metabolites by CYP2D6, the most important of which is endoxifen. By reducing endoxifen formation, CYP2D6 inhibitors, such as cimetidine, may reduce tamoxifen efficacy.[1-3]

CLINICAL EVALUATION: A study in patients with breast cancer found substantial reductions in endoxifen plasma concentrations in patients taking potent CYP2D6 inhibitors, such as fluoxetine and paroxetine.[4] Another tamoxifen study found a nearly 2-fold increase in the risk of breast cancer relapse in women with low CYP2D6 activity, either due to CYP2D6-inhibiting drugs or genetic deficiency.[5] Taken together, these and other results strongly suggest that CYP2D6 inhibitors reduce the efficacy of tamoxifen in the treatment of breast cancer. Cimetidine is only a modest CYP2D6 inhibitor, so the extent to which it may inhibit the anticancer effects of tamoxifen is not known. Nonetheless, it is easy to avoid the use of cimetidine because there are a number of alternatives.

RELATED DRUGS: No information is available.

MANAGEMENT OPTIONS:

➡ *Consider Alternative.* Famotidine (eg, *Pepcid*), nizatidine (eg, *Axid*), and ranitidine (eg, *Zantac*) have minimal effects on drug metabolism and, theoretically, are unlikely to interact.

➡ *Monitor.* If a CYP2D6 inhibitor, such as cimetidine, is used with tamoxifen, cancer recurrence may be an indication that tamoxifen efficacy has been reduced. If this happens, consider discontinuing the CYP2D6 inhibitor.

REFERENCES:
1. Dezentjé VO, et al. Clinical implications of CYP2D6 genotyping in tamoxifen treatment for breast cancer. *Clin Cancer Res.* 2009;15(1):15-21.
2. Tan SH, et al. Pharmacogenetics in breast cancer therapy. *Clin Cancer Res.* 2008;14(24):8027-8041.
3. Newman WG, et al. Impaired tamoxifen metabolism reduces survival in familial breast cancer patients. *Clin Cancer Res.* 2008;14(18):5913-5918.
4. Borges S, et al. Quantitative effect of CYP2D6 genotype and inhibitors on tamoxifen metabolism: implication for optimization of breast cancer treatment. *Clin Pharmacol Ther.* 2006;80(1):61-74.
5. Goetz MP, et al. The impact of cytochrome P450 2D6 metabolism in women receiving adjuvant tamoxifen. *Breast Cancer Res Treat.* 2007;101(1):113-121.

Cimetidine (eg, *Tagamet*)

Tamsulosin (*Flomax*)

SUMMARY: Cimetidine can increase tamsulosin plasma concentrations.

RISK FACTORS: No specific risk factors are known.

MECHANISM: Not established. Cimetidine probably inhibits tamsulosin metabolism.

CLINICAL EVALUATION: Ten healthy volunteers received a single 0.4 mg dose of tamsulosin with and without pretreatment with cimetidine 400 mg every 6 hours for 6 days.[1] Tamsulosin area under the plasma concentration-time curve increased by 44% in the presence of cimetidine. The extent to which this would increase tamsulosin adverse effects is not known.

RELATED DRUGS: Assuming that the increased tamsulosin concentrations were caused by inhibition of tamsulosin metabolism by cimetidine, an interaction with famotidine (eg, *Pepcid*), nizatidine (eg, *Axid*), or ranitidine (eg, *Zantac*) is not expected.

MANAGEMENT OPTIONS:

➡ **Consider Alternative.** Using famotidine, nizatidine, or ranitidine is preferable because they are unlikely to interact.

➡ **Monitor.** If the combination is used, monitor for altered tamsulosin effect if cimetidine is initiated, discontinued, or changed in dosage.

REFERENCES:

1. *Flomax* [package insert]. Ridgefield, CT: Boehringer Ingelheim; 2009.

Cimetidine (eg, *Tagamet*) 4

Temafloxacin†

SUMMARY: Cimetidine increases temafloxacin serum concentrations, although the changes are not likely to be of clinical significance.

RISK FACTORS: No specific risk factors are known.

MECHANISM: Cimetidine appears to inhibit both the renal and metabolic clearances of temafloxacin, resulting in increased serum concentrations.

CLINICAL EVALUATION: Cimetidine 400 mg 3 times daily for 8 days caused an approximately 20% increase in the area under the serum concentration-time curve of temafloxacin.[1] Temafloxacin renal clearance was reduced 18%; apparent total clearance declined from 224 to 183 mL/min. In most patients, these changes in temafloxacin pharmacokinetics will be of minimal clinical significance.

RELATED DRUGS: Cimetidine also increases the concentrations of ciprofloxacin (eg, *Cipro*), enoxacin,† and pefloxacin.† Other H_2-receptor antagonists (eg, ranitidine [eg, *Zantac*], famotidine [eg, *Pepcid*], nizatidine [eg, *Axid*]) are likely to affect temafloxacin's metabolism.

MANAGEMENT OPTIONS: No specific action is required, but be alert for evidence of the interaction.

REFERENCES:

1. Sörgel F, et al. Effect of cimetidine on the pharmacokinetics of temafloxacin. *Clin Pharmacokinet.* 1992;22(suppl 1):75-82.

† Not available in the United States.

Cimetidine (eg, *Tagamet*) 5

Terfenadine†

SUMMARY: Neither cimetidine nor ranitidine affected terfenadine plasma concentrations in healthy subjects.

RISK FACTORS: No specific risk factors are known.

MECHANISM: No interaction.

CLINICAL EVALUATION: Two cohorts of 6 healthy subjects received terfenadine 60 mg twice daily for 8 days followed by 6 days of coadministration of cimetidine 600 mg twice daily for 1 week[1] or ranitidine (eg, *Zantac*) 150 mg twice daily for 7 days. Neither H_2-receptor antagonist produced any change in terfenadine pharmacokinetics or the subjects' electrocardiograms. Based on this study, cimetidine and ranitidine do not alter the pharmacokinetics of terfenadine and they are not likely to produce adverse reactions if administered to patients taking terfenadine.

RELATED DRUGS: Ranitidine did not alter the pharmacokinetics of terfenadine and they are not likely to produce adverse reactions when administered with terfenadine. Theoretically, other H$_2$-receptor antagonists (eg, famotidine [eg, *Pepcid*], nizatidine [eg, *Axid*]) are not expected to interact with terfenadine.

MANAGEMENT OPTIONS: No interaction.

REFERENCES:
1. Honig PK, et al. Effect of concomitant administration of cimetidine and ranitidine on the pharmacokinetics and electrocardiographic effects of terfenadine. *Eur J Clin Pharmacol.* 1993;45(1):41-46.

† Not available in the United States.

Cimetidine (eg, *Tagamet*)

Theophylline (eg, *Theo-24*)

SUMMARY: Cimetidine increases serum theophylline concentrations, resulting in symptoms of theophylline toxicity in some patients.

RISK FACTORS:

➡ **Dosage Regimen.** The magnitude of this interaction increases as the dose of cimetidine increases.

➡ **Habits.** Cimetidine may have a greater effect in patients who smoke and in those with high basal theophylline clearance.

MECHANISM: Cimetidine inhibits the hepatic metabolism of theophylline.[1]

CLINICAL EVALUATION: Cimetidine consistently reduces theophylline plasma clearance, increases theophylline half-life, and increases plasma theophylline levels.[2-8] Moreover, several case reports have described elevated plasma theophylline levels or theophylline toxicity during cimetidine therapy[9-17]; one of these reports described the death of an elderly man that may have been associated with cimetidine-induced theophylline toxicity.[17] Because cimetidine begins to reduce theophylline elimination as soon as therapeutic serum levels of cimetidine are achieved, a new steady-state serum theophylline level will usually be observed by the second day of cimetidine therapy. However, it may take longer in some patients (eg, those whose theophylline half-life is relatively long to begin with or those who develop a marked increase in theophylline half-life caused by cimetidine).

RELATED DRUGS: H$_2$-receptor antagonists other than cimetidine, such as famotidine (eg, *Pepcid*), nizatidine (eg, *Axid*), and ranitidine (eg, *Zantac*), are unlikely to affect theophylline pharmacokinetics.

MANAGEMENT OPTIONS:

➡ **Consider Alternative.** Ranitidine does not appear to affect theophylline disposition and so would be preferable to cimetidine in patients receiving theophylline. Famotidine and nizatidine are also unlikely to interact with theophylline.[18]

➡ **Monitor.** If cimetidine is used with theophylline, monitor for altered theophylline response if cimetidine therapy is initiated, discontinued, or dosage is changed; the dose of theophylline may need to be adjusted. In a patient already receiving cimetidine, initial doses of theophylline should be conservative until the dosage requirement is determined. Serum theophylline determinations would be useful in following this interaction.

REFERENCES:

1. Grygiel JJ, et al. Differential effects of cimetidine on theophylline metabolic pathways. *Eur J Clin Pharmacol.* 1984;265:335-340.

2. Jackson JE, et al. Cimetidine decreases theophylline clearance. *Am Rev Respir Dis.* 1981;23:615-617.

3. Reitberg DP, et al. Alteration of theophylline clearance and half-life by cimetidine in normal volunteers. *Ann Intern Med.* 1981;95:582-585.

4. Roberts RK, et al. Cimetidine impairs the elimination of theophylline and antipyrine. *Gastroenterology.* 1981;81:19-21.

5. Schwartz JI, et al. Impact of cimetidine on the pharmacokinetics of theophylline. *Clin Pharm.* 1982;1:534-538.

6. Lalonde RL, et al. The effects of cimetidine on theophylline pharmacokinetics at steady state. *Chest.* 1983;2:221-224.

7. Kelly JF, et al. The effect of cimetidine on theophylline metabolism in the elderly. *Clin Pharmacol Ther.* 1982;31:238.

8. Boehning W, et al. Effect of cimetidine and ranitidine on plasma theophylline in patients with chronic obstructive airways disease treated with theophylline and corticosteroids. *Eur J Clin Pharmacol.* 1990;38:43-45.

9. Fenje PC, et al. Interaction of cimetidine and theophylline in two infants. *Can Med Assoc J.* 1982;126:1178.

10. Cluxton RJ, et al. Cimetidine-theophylline interaction. *Ann Intern Med.* 1982;96:684.

11. Jackson JE, et al. More on cimetidine-theophylline interaction. *Drug Intell Clin Pharm.* 1981;15:809.

12. Hendeles L, et al. The interaction of cimetidine and theophylline. *Drug Intell Clin Pharm.* 1981;15:808.

13. Weinberger MM, et al. Decreased theophylline clearance due to cimetidine. *N Engl J Med.* 1981;304:672.

14. Campbell MA, et al. Cimetidine decreases theophylline clearance. *Ann Intern Med.* 1981;95:68-69.

15. Lofgren RP, et al. Cimetidine and theophylline. *Ann Intern Med.* 1982;96:378.

16. Bauman JH, et al. Cimetidine-theophylline interaction: report of four patients. *Ann Allergy.* 1982;48:100-102.

17. Anderson JR, et al. A fatal case of theophylline intoxication. *Arch Intern Med.* 1983;143:559-560.

18. Lin JH, et al. Comparative effect of famotidine and cimetidine on the pharmacokinetics of theophylline in normal volunteers. *Br J Clin Pharmacol.* 1987;24:669-672.

Cimetidine (eg, *Tagamet*)

Tizanidine (eg, *Zanaflex*)

SUMMARY: Tizanidine appears to be very susceptible to interactions with inhibitors of CYP1A2, and it is likely that cimetidine would substantially increase tizanidine concentrations.

RISK FACTORS: No specific risk factors are known.

MECHANISM: Cimetidine is known to inhibit CYP1A2, the enzyme responsible for the metabolism of tizanidine.

CLINICAL EVALUATION: In a study of healthy subjects, other potent inhibitors of CYP1A2 (fluvoxamine and ciprofloxacin) produced increases in tizanidine plasma concentrations accompanied by severe hypotension and CNS depression.[1,2] Given the severity of the interaction, consider the likelihood that all potent CYP1A2 inhibitors (eg, cimetidine) also would interact adversely with tizanidine.

RELATED DRUGS: None known.

MANAGEMENT OPTIONS:

➡ **Consider Alternative.** Other H_2-receptor antagonists (eg, famotidine [eg, *Pepcid*], nizatidine [eg, *Axid*], ranitidine [eg, *Zantac*]) do not inhibit CYP1A2 and would be unlikely to interact with tizanidine.

➡ **Monitor.** If the combination is used, monitor for hypotension and excessive CNS depression.

REFERENCES:

1. Granfors MT, et al. Fluvoxamine drastically increases concentrations and effects of tizanidine: a potentially hazardous interaction. *Clin Pharmacol Ther*. 2004;75:331-341.

2. Granfors MT, et al. Ciprofloxacin greatly increases concentrations and hypotensive effect of tizanidine by inhibiting its cytochrome P450 1A2-mediated presystemic metabolism. *Clin Pharmacol Ther*. 2004;76:598-606.

4 Cimetidine (eg, *Tagamet*)

Tocainide† (*Tonocard*)

SUMMARY: Tocainide plasma concentrations are reduced by cimetidine. The clinical effects of these changes are unknown.

RISK FACTORS: No specific risk factors are known.

MECHANISM: Not established. It appears that cimetidine reduces the absorption of tocainide.

CLINICAL EVALUATION: Seven healthy subjects were randomly administered cimetidine 300 mg 4 times daily, ranitidine (eg, *Zantac*) 150 mg twice daily, or a placebo for 2 days.[1] Subjects then were administered a single dose of tocainide 400 mg. The area under the tocainide concentration-time curve decreased 27% and the peak tocainide concentration fell 39.5% during cimetidine administration. The half-life of tocainide was not altered by cimetidine. Ranitidine had no significant effect on tocainide pharmacokinetics.

RELATED DRUGS: Ranitidine has no significant effect on tocainide. The effects of famotidine (eg, *Pepcid*) and nizatidine (eg, *Axid*) on tocainide disposition are unknown, but little effect would be expected.

MANAGEMENT OPTIONS: No specific action is required, but be alert for evidence of the interaction.

REFERENCES:

1. North DS, et al. The effect of histamine-2 receptor antagonists on tocainide pharmacokinetics. *J Clin Pharmacol*. 1988;28:640-643.

† Not available in the United States.

3 Cimetidine (eg, *Tagamet*)

Tolbutamide (eg, *Orinase*)

SUMMARY: Tolbutamide, glipizide, and glyburide serum concentrations may be increased by cimetidine. Cimetidine may have independent effects on serum glucose.

RISK FACTORS: No specific risk factors are known.

MECHANISM: The metabolism of tolbutamide, glipizide, and glyburide may be inhibited or their absorption enhanced by H_2-blockade. Cimetidine may decrease the metabolic clearance of glucose.[8]

CLINICAL EVALUATION: Cimetidine 800 to 1200 mg day has been reported to increase the area under the plasma concentration-time curve (AUC) of tolbutamide, glipizide (eg, *Glucotrol*), and glyburide (eg, *Micronase*).[1,4,5,9] However, in other studies, cimetidine 400 mg twice daily had no effect on tolbutamide pharmacokinetics,[2,3] and 400 mg 3 times daily for 3 days also had no effect on tolbutamide.[7] The significance of these changes on glucose tolerance in diabetic patients is unknown. Cimetidine, when administered alone to normal subjects, increased plasma glucose following an oral glucose load. The hyperglycemia persisted even when 5 mg glyburide was administered with the H_2-receptor antagonist. The significance of these changes in diabetic patients is unknown.

RELATED DRUGS: Ranitidine (eg, *Zantac*) does not alter tolbutamide pharmacokinetics. The effect of famotidine (eg, *Pepcid*) and nizatidine (*Axid*) on sulfonylureas is unknown, but they may interact if increased gastric pH is involved in the observed changes with cimetidine and ranitidine. Glipizide and glyburide interact similarly with cimetidine. Sucralfate (*Carafate*) produced a significant but small (8%) reduction in the chlorpropamide AUC in healthy subjects.[6]

MANAGEMENT OPTIONS:

➡ *Consider Alternative.* Sucralfate may be a good alternative therapy for the treatment of ulcer disease in diabetics because it appears unlikely to alter glycemic control to a clinically significant degree.

➡ *Monitor.* Observe diabetics stabilized on any hypoglycemic therapy in whom H_2-receptor antagonist therapy is initiated or discontinued for altered glycemic responses.

REFERENCES:
1. Catt EW, et al. Inhibition of tolbutamide elimination by cimetidine but not ranitidine. *J Clin Pharmacol.* 1986;26:372.
2. Stockley C, et al. Lack of inhibition of tolbutamide hydroxylation by cimetidine in man. *Eur J Clin Pharmacol.* 1986;31:235.
3. Dey NG, et al. The effect of cimetidine on tolbutamide kinetics. *Br J Clin Pharmacol.* 1983;16:438.
4. Feely J, et al. Potentiation of the hypoglycemic response to glipizide in diabetic patients by histamine H_2-receptor antagonists. *Br J Clin Pharmacol.* 1993;35:321.
5. Kubacka RT, et al. The paradoxical effect of cimetidine and ranitidine on glibenclamide pharmacokinetics and pharmacodynamics. *Br J Clin Pharmacol.* 1987;23:743.
6. Letendre PW, et al. Effect of sucralfate on the absorption and pharmacokinetics of chlorpropamide. *J Clin Pharmacol.* 1986;26:622.
7. Adebayo GI, et al. Lack of efficacy of cimetidine and ranitidine as inhibitors of tolbutamide metabolism. *Eur J Clin Pharmacol.* 1988;34:653.
8. Lahtela JT, et al. The effect of liver microsomal enzyme inducing and inhibiting drugs on insulin mediated glucose metabolism in man. *Br J Clin Pharmacol.* 1986;21:19.
9. Toon S, et al. Effects of cimetidine, ranitidine and omeprazole on tolbutamide pharmacokinetics. *J Pharm Pharmacol.* 1995;47:85.

4 Cimetidine (eg, *Tagamet*)

Triamterene (*Dyrenium*)

SUMMARY: Cimetidine alters triamterene pharmacokinetics but is not likely to alter its efficacy.

RISK FACTORS: No specific risk factors are known.

MECHANISM: Cimetidine appears to reduce the metabolism, renal excretion, and absorption of triamterene.

CLINICAL EVALUATION: Six healthy subjects received triamterene 100 mg/day for 4 days with and without cimetidine 400 mg every 12 hours; the cimetidine was continued for an additional 4 days.[1] Cimetidine significantly reduced the hydroxylation of triamterene (37%) and increased the area under the triamterene concentration-time curve (22%). Cimetidine tended to reduce triamterene's renal clearance (28%), but it did not change triamterene protein binding. In addition, the amount of triamterene and metabolites recovered in the urine was reduced 16%, implying a reduction of triamterene absorption. These pharmacokinetic changes did not result in significant changes in the natriuretic or potassium-sparing effects of triamterene. Triamterene did not alter cimetidine kinetics.

RELATED DRUGS: If an increased gastric pH reduces the absorption of triamterene, other H$_2$-receptor antagonists, such as ranitidine (eg, *Zantac*), famotidine (eg, *Pepcid*), and nizatidine (*Axid*), may reduce the concentration of triamterene.

MANAGEMENT OPTIONS: No specific action is required, but be alert for evidence of the interaction.

REFERENCES:
1. Muirhead MR, et al. Effect of cimetidine on renal and hepatic drug elimination: studies with triamterene. *Clin Pharmacol Ther.* 1986;40:400.

3 Cimetidine (eg, *Tagamet*)

Verapamil (eg, *Calan*)

SUMMARY: Cimetidine can increase the serum concentration of verapamil; excessive verapamil effects may be seen.

RISK FACTORS: No specific risk factors are known.

MECHANISM: The metabolism of verapamil appears to be reduced by cimetidine.

CLINICAL EVALUATION: In several studies, verapamil pharmacokinetics were affected by cimetidine dosing.[1-4] Cimetidine reduced the clearance of verapamil 35% in some patients, but in others cimetidine produced no change or an increase in verapamil clearance. All these studies utilized a single-dose verapamil protocol. Subjects who had higher baseline verapamil clearance seemed to have the greatest reduction in clearance following cimetidine administration.[4] Cimetidine has been reported to inhibit the metabolism of the more potent enantiomer of verapamil (S-verapamil) to a greater extent (150% vs 117%) than the less potent enantiomer.[5] This effect tends to cause a more pronounced pharmacologic response when cimetidine is coadministered.

RELATED DRUGS: Cimetidine also increases the concentrations of diltiazem (eg, *Cardizem*), nisoldipine (*Sular*), nifedipine (eg, *Procardia*), and nitrendipine. Ranitidine (eg,

Zantac), famotidine (eg, *Pepcid*), and nizatidine (*Axid*) would not be expected to alter verapamil metabolism.

MANAGEMENT OPTIONS:

➡ *Consider Alternative.* Although data is limited, other H_2-receptor antagonists (eg, ranitidine, famotidine, nizatidine) would be unlikely to inhibit the metabolism of verapamil.

➡ *Monitor.* Carefully monitor patients receiving verapamil for signs of toxicity (eg, hypotension, bradycardia, heart block) when cimetidine is added to their drug regimen.

REFERENCES:

1. Smith MS, et al. Influence of cimetidine on verapamil kinetics and dynamics. *Clin Pharmacol Ther.* 1984;36:551.

2. Wing LMH, et al. Verapamil disposition—effects of sulphinpyrazone and cimetidine. *Br J Clin Pharmacol.* 1985;19:385.

3. Abernethy DR, et al. Lack of interaction between verapamil and cimetidine. *Clin Pharmacol Ther.* 1985;38:342.

4. Loi C-M, et al. Effect of cimetidine on verapamil disposition. *Clin Pharmacol Ther.* 1985;37:654.

5. Mikus G, et al. Interaction of verapamil and cimetidine: stereochemical aspects of drug metabolism, drug disposition and drug action. *J Pharmacol Exper Ther.* 1990;253:1042.

Cimetidine (eg, *Tagamet*)

Voriconazole (*Vfend*)

SUMMARY: Cimetidine administration causes a modest increase in voriconazole plasma concentrations. No change in patient response is likely to occur.

RISK FACTORS: No specific risk factors are known.

MECHANISM: Unknown; however, cimetidine is known to inhibit several cytochrome enzymes, including CYP2C19, that are partially responsible for voriconazole's metabolism.

CLINICAL EVALUATION: Twelve healthy subjects received voriconazole 200 mg twice daily alone and concurrently with cimetidine 400 mg twice daily for 8 days.[1] The mean plasma voriconazole area under the plasma concentration-time curve was increased about 22% during cimetidine coadministration. Voriconazole half-life was unchanged by cimetidine administration. This change in voriconazole plasma concentration is unlikely to produce changes in patient response. It is possible that higher doses of cimetidine would produce a greater effect on voriconazole plasma concentrations.

RELATED DRUGS: Other H_2-receptor antagonists are unlikely to interact with voriconazole. Cimetidine administration does not affect fluconazole (eg, *Diflucan*) but does reduce the absorption of ketoconazole (eg, *Nizoral*) and itraconazole (*Sporanox*) by increasing gastric pH.

MANAGEMENT OPTIONS:

➡ *Monitor.* Because of the small magnitude of this interaction, no special precautions appear to be necessary to avoid patient harm.

REFERENCES:

1. Purkins L, et al. Histamine H_2-receptor antagonists have no clinically significant effect on the steady-state pharmacokinetics of voriconazole. *Br J Clin Pharmacol.* 2003;56:51-55.

Cimetidine (eg, *Tagamet*)

Warfarin (eg, *Coumadin*)

SUMMARY: Cimetidine may increase the hypoprothrombinemic response to oral anticoagulants; the effect is usually modest, but bleeding has occurred in some patients receiving both drugs.

RISK FACTORS:

➡ ***Dosage Regimen.*** The interaction between cimetidine and warfarin is dose related. For example, cimetidine doses of 800 mg nightly tend to affect warfarin less than larger doses given at least 2 times daily, and cimetidine 400 mg/day may be insufficient to produce clinically significant effects on warfarin in some patients.

MECHANISM: Cimetidine inhibits the hepatic metabolism of warfarin, affecting the metabolism of R-warfarin to a greater extent than the more active S-warfarin.[1-5]

CLINICAL EVALUATION: Cimetidine may produce a clinically important increase in the hypoprothrombinemic response to oral anticoagulants[6-11] As with many warfarin interactions, there is considerable variation in the magnitude of the interaction from one patient to another; most patients develop only modest changes in anticoagulant effect, while a few have large increases. In patients receiving warfarin, the addition of cimetidine usually results in a gradual increase in hypoprothrombinemia over 1 to 2 weeks; it takes approximately 1 week for the prothrombin time to return to pre-cimetidine levels when cimetidine is discontinued.

RELATED DRUGS: Ranitidine (eg, *Zantac*), famotidine (eg, *Pepcid*), and probably nizatidine (eg, *Axid*) are unlikely to affect the hypoprothrombinemic response to warfarin.[12,13] Phenprocoumon does not appear to be affected by cimetidine.[14] Omeprazole (eg, *Prilosec*), at least in doses of 20 mg/day, appears to produce a small increase in the hypoprothrombinemic response of warfarin. Cimetidine also inhibits the metabolism of acenocoumarol[15] and possibly other oral anticoagulants with the exception of phenprocoumon, which undergoes glucuronide conjugation. Cimetidine does not appear to affect glucuronidation of drugs in the liver.

MANAGEMENT OPTIONS:

➡ ***Use Alternative.*** Use ranitidine, famotidine, or nizatidine instead of cimetidine in patients receiving oral anticoagulants. If cimetidine is used, monitor for altered oral anticoagulant effect if cimetidine is initiated, discontinued, or changed in dosage. Adjust the anticoagulant dosage as needed.

REFERENCES:

1. Burnham D, et al. Effects of low cimetidine doses on steady-state warfarin pharmacokinetics and prothrombin time. *J Clin Pharmacol*. 1989;29:862.
2. Hunt BA, et al. Stereoselective alterations in the pharmacokinetics of warfarin enantiomers with two cimetidine dose regimens. *Pharmacotherapy*. 1989;9:184.
3. Toon S, et al. The warfarin-cimetidine interaction: stereochemical considerations. *Br J Clin Pharmacol*. 1986;21:245-246.
4. Choonara IA, et al. Stereoselective interaction between the R enantiomer of warfarin and cimetidine. *Br J Clin Pharmacol*. 1986;21:271-277.
5. Niopas I, et al. Further insight into the stereoselective interaction between warfarin and cimetidine in man. *Br J Clin Pharmacol*. 1991;32:508-511.
6. Flind AC. Cimetidine and oral anticoagulants. *Br Med J*. 1978;2:1367.
7. Serlin MJ, et al. Cimetidine: interaction with oral anticoagulants in man. *Lancet*. 1979;2:317-319.

8. Puurunen J, et al. Effect of cimetidine on microsomal drug metabolism in man. *Eur J Clin Pharmacol.* 1980;18:185-187.

9. Kerley B, et al. Cimetidine potentiation of warfarin action. *Can Med Assoc J.* 1982;126:116.

10. Silver BA, et al. Cimetidine potentiation of the hypoprothrombinemic effect of warfarin. *Ann Intern Med.* 1979;90:348-349.

11. Hetzel D, et al. Cimetidine interaction with warfarin. *Lancet.* 1979;2:639.

12. Serlin MJ, et al. Lack of effect of ranitidine on warfarin action. *Br J Clin Pharmacol.* 1981;12:791-794.

13. O'Reilly RA. Comparative interaction of cimetidine and ranitidine with racemic warfarin in man. *Arch Intern Med.* 1984;144:989-991.

14. Harenberg J, et al. Lack of effect of cimetidine on action of phenprocoumon. *Eur J Clin Pharmacol.* 1982;23:365-367.

15. Kroon C, et al. Interaction between single dose acenocoumarol and cimetidine or pentobarbitone: validation of a single dose model to predict interactions in steady state. *Br J Clin Pharmacol.* 1990;29:643P.

Cimetidine (eg, *Tagamet*)

Zidovudine (eg, *Retrovir*)

SUMMARY: While cimetidine reduces the renal secretion of zidovudine, no change in serum concentrations or response appears to result.

RISK FACTORS: No specific risk factors are known.

MECHANISM: Cimetidine appears to reduce the renal tubular secretion of zidovudine.

CLINICAL EVALUATION: Six subjects with HIV received 2 regimens: zidovudine 4 times daily (200 mg alternating with 100 mg) and zidovudine in combination with cimetidine 300 mg 4 times daily.[1] Each dosage regimen was administered for 7 days. During cimetidine administration, the renal clearance of zidovudine was reduced 56%. However, the serum concentration of zidovudine did not increase, partially because of an increase in the conversion of zidovudine to its glucuronide metabolite.

RELATED DRUGS: Ranitidine (eg, *Zantac*) does not affect zidovudine elimination. Other H_2-receptor antagonists (eg, nizatidine [eg, *Axid*], famotidine [eg, *Pepcid*]) are not expected to alter zidovudine renal elimination. Cimetidine also reduces the renal clearance of zalcitabine.[†]

MANAGEMENT OPTIONS: No specific action is required, but be alert for evidence of the interaction.

REFERENCES:
1. Fletcher CV, et al. The effect of cimetidine and ranitidine administration with zidovudine. *Pharmacotherapy.* 1995;15:701-708.

† Not available in the United States.

Cinacalcet (*Sensipar*)

Desipramine (eg, *Norpramin*)

SUMMARY: Cinacalcet increases desipramine plasma concentrations and may increase desipramine toxicity.

RISK FACTORS: No specific risk factors are known.

MECHANISM: Cinacalcet probably inhibits the CYP2D6 metabolism of desipramine.

CLINICAL EVALUATION: In a randomized crossover study, 17 healthy subjects (all CYP2D6 extensive metabolizers) received a single dose of desipramine 50 mg with and without pretreatment with cinacalcet (90 mg/day for 7 days).[1] Cinacalcet produced a 3.6-fold increase in desipramine area under the plasma concentration-time curve and increased adverse reactions from 33% to 86%. Thus, it appears that cinacalcet may increase the risk of desipramine toxicity.

RELATED DRUGS: Most tricyclic antidepressants are metabolized to some extent by CYP2D6, so cinacalcet may also increase plasma concentrations of other tricyclics to varying degrees.

MANAGEMENT OPTIONS:

➥ **Monitor.** Monitor for evidence of desipramine toxicity if it is used concurrently with cinacalcet; the dose of desipramine may need to be reduced.

REFERENCES:

1. Harris RZ, et al. Pharmacokinetics of desipramine HCl when administered with cinacalcet HCl. *Eur J Clin Pharmacol.* 2007;63:159-163.

 Cinacalcet (Sensipar)

Ketoconazole (eg, Nizoral)

SUMMARY: Ketoconazole increases the plasma concentration of cinacalcet; increased therapeutic response may occur.

RISK FACTORS: No specific risk factors are known.

MECHANISM: Cinacalcet is partially metabolized by CYP3A4. This enzyme is inhibited by ketoconazole.

CLINICAL EVALUATION: Although data are limited, the manufacturer of cinacalcet notes that coadministration of ketoconazole 200 mg twice daily for 7 days can increase the area under the plasma concentration-time curve of a single dose of cinacalcet 90 mg more than 2-fold.[1] This increase in plasma concentration may increase cinacalcet's effect on plasma parathyroid hormone, calcium, and phosphorus concentrations.

RELATED DRUGS: Itraconazole (eg, *Sporanox*), voriconazole (*Vfend*), and fluconazole (eg, *Diflucan*) may also inhibit the metabolism of cinacalcet.

MANAGEMENT OPTIONS:

➥ **Consider Alternative.** Evaluate patients requiring antifungal therapy during cinacalcet administration for terbinafine (eg, *Lamisil*) treatment.

➥ **Monitor.** Monitor the patient's response (eg, parathyroid hormone, calcium, and phosphorus concentrations) if ketoconazole therapy is initiated or discontinued.

REFERENCES:

1. *Sensipar* [package insert]. Thousand Oaks, CA: Amgen Inc; 2004.

Cinacalcet (*Sensipar*)

Tamoxifen (eg, *Soltamox*)

SUMMARY: Theoretically, cinacalcet may reduce the efficacy of tamoxifen in the treatment of breast cancer.

RISK FACTORS: No specific risk factors are known.

MECHANISM: Tamoxifen is metabolized to 2 active metabolites by CYP2D6, the most important of which is endoxifen. By reducing endoxifen formation, CYP2D6 inhibitors such as cinacalcet may reduce tamoxifen efficacy.[1-3]

CLINICAL EVALUATION: A study in patients with breast cancer found substantial reductions in endoxifen plasma concentrations in patients taking potent CYP2D6 inhibitors such as fluoxetine and paroxetine.[4] Another tamoxifen study found a nearly 2-fold increase in the risk of breast cancer relapse in women with low CYP2D6 activity, either due to CYP2D6-inhibiting drugs or genetic deficiency.[5] Taken together, these and other results strongly suggest that CYP2D6 inhibitors reduce the efficacy of tamoxifen in the treatment of breast cancer. Cinacalcet is a CYP2D6 inhibitor, and may inhibit the anticancer effects of tamoxifen.

RELATED DRUGS: No information is available.

MANAGEMENT OPTIONS:

➥ **Consider Alternative.** If possible, use an alternative to cinacalcet.

➥ **Monitor.** If a CYP2D6 inhibitor such as cinacalcet is used with tamoxifen, cancer recurrence may be an indication that tamoxifen efficacy has been reduced. If this happens, consider discontinuing the CYP2D6 inhibitor.

REFERENCES:

1. Dezentjé VO, et al. Clinical implications of CYP2D6 genotyping in tamoxifen treatment for breast cancer. *Clin Cancer Res.* 2009;15(1):15-21.
2. Tan SH, et al. Pharmacogenetics in breast cancer therapy. *Clin Cancer Res.* 2008;14(24):8027-8041.
3. Newman WG, et al. Impaired tamoxifen metabolism reduces survival in familial breast cancer patients. *Clin Cancer Res.* 2008;14(18):5913-5918.
4. Borges S, et al. Quantitative effect of CYP2D6 genotype and inhibitors on tamoxifen metabolism: implication for optimization of breast cancer treatment. *Clin Pharmacol Ther.* 2006;80(1):61-74.
5. Goetz MP, et al. The impact of cytochrome P450 2D6 metabolism in women receiving adjuvant tamoxifen. *Breast Cancer Res Treat.* 2007;101(1):113-121.

Cinacalcet (*Sensipar*)

Thioridazine

SUMMARY: Theoretically, cinacalcet may increase the risk of arrhythmias when combined with thioridazine, but the clinical importance is not established.

RISK FACTORS:

➥ **Pharmacogenetics.** Patients who are deficient in CYP2D6 are not expected to manifest this interaction.

MECHANISM: In vitro evidence suggests that cinacalcet is a potent CYP2D6 inhibitor. Because thioridazine is metabolized by CYP2D6, cinacalcet is expected to increase thioridazine serum concentrations.

CLINICAL EVALUATION: This interaction is based on in vitro and theoretical considerations, and it is not known if the combination actually poses a risk. Nonetheless, the potential severity of the interaction (serious ventricular arrhythmias and possible sudden death) dictates that the combination of cinacalcet and thioridazine be used only with appropriate monitoring.[1]

RELATED DRUGS: No information is available.

MANAGEMENT OPTIONS:

➡ **Monitor.** If the combination is used, monitor for evidence of arrhythmias (eg, syncope) and for prolonged QT intervals.

REFERENCES:

1. *Sensipar* [package insert]. Thousand Oaks, CA: Amgen Inc; 2004.

Ciprofloxacin (eg, *Cipro*)

Clozapine (eg, *Clozaril*)

SUMMARY: Ciprofloxacin administration increases clozapine concentrations; some patients may develop clozapine-induced adverse effects.

RISK FACTORS: No specific risk factors are known.

MECHANISM: Ciprofloxacin inhibits the activity of CYP1A2, the primary route of metabolism of clozapine.

CLINICAL EVALUATION: Seven schizophrenic patients taking clozapine dosages ranging from 150 to 450 mg daily were administered ciprofloxacin 250 mg twice daily or placebo for 7 days.[1] The mean plasma concentration of clozapine and its metabolite N-desmethylclozapine increased approximately 30% following ciprofloxacin. Individual increases in clozapine concentrations ranged from 6% to 57% with ciprofloxacin coadministration. While this study used low doses of ciprofloxacin, another report noted a patient taking ciprofloxacin 500 mg twice daily had an 80% increase in the patient's clozapine concentration during ciprofloxacin administration.[2] Thus, therapeutic doses of ciprofloxacin may elevate clozapine concentrations to levels that produce adverse reactions such as sedation.

RELATED DRUGS: Other quinolones known to inhibit CYP1A2 (eg, enoxacin†) may increase clozapine concentrations in a similar manner. Ciprofloxacin also may increase the concentrations of olanzapine (*Zyprexa*), a psychotropic agent that also is metabolized by CYP1A2.

MANAGEMENT OPTIONS:

➡ **Consider Alternative.** For patients taking clozapine, consider a quinolone that does not inhibit CYP1A2 (eg, ofloxacin [eg, *Floxin*], lomefloxacin [*Maxaquin*]).

➡ **Monitor.** Monitor patients stabilized on clozapine for increased adverse reactions if ciprofloxacin is coadministered.

REFERENCES:

1. Raaska K, et al. Ciprofloxacin increases serum clozapine and N-desmethylclozapine: a study in patients with schizophrenia. *Eur J Clin Pharmacol.* 2000;56(8):585-589.

2. Markowitz JS, et al. Fluoroquinolone inhibition of clozapine metabolism. *Am J Psychiatry.* 1997;154(6):881.

† Not available in the United States.

Ciprofloxacin (eg, *Cipro*)

Cyclophosphamide

SUMMARY: Ciprofloxacin plasma concentrations appear to be reduced by coadministration of chemotherapy agents.

RISK FACTORS: No specific risk factors are known.

MECHANISM: Not established. Chemotherapeutic agents may reduce ciprofloxacin absorption.

CLINICAL EVALUATION: Six patients with leukemia or lymphoma were administered ciprofloxacin 500 mg orally twice daily during chemotherapy and for 21 days after the completion of chemotherapy with cytosine arabinoside, cyclophosphamide, adriamycin, prednisolone, daunorubicin, vincristine, and mitoxantrone.[1] Two patients also were taking antacids, which are known to reduce ciprofloxacin absorption. Ciprofloxacin serum concentrations during the first 4 hours after administration decreased an average of 46.7% following chemotherapy. The small number of patients in this study precludes any meaningful conclusion regarding the clinical significance of this interaction.

RELATED DRUGS: The effects of chemotherapy on other quinolones is unknown, but other orally administered agents might be similarly affected.

MANAGEMENT OPTIONS: No specific action is required, but be alert for evidence of the interaction.

REFERENCES:
1. Johnson EJ, et al. Reduced absorption of oral ciprofloxacin after chemotherapy for haematological malignancy. *J Antimicrob Chemother.* 1990;25(5):837-842.

Ciprofloxacin (*Cipro*)

Cyclosporine (eg, *Neoral*)

SUMMARY: While most patients appear to be minimally affected by the combination of cyclosporine and ciprofloxacin, their combined use has been reported to cause nephrotoxicity in a few patients.

RISK FACTORS: No specific risk factors are known.

MECHANISM: Not established.

CLINICAL EVALUATION: Four days after starting ciprofloxacin 750 mg every 8 hours, a patient stabilized on cyclosporine developed acute renal failure.[1] The peak blood cyclosporine concentrations appeared to increase and creatinine concentrations peaked at 14.1 mg/dL 8 days after ciprofloxacin was started and returned to baseline over 2 weeks. While ciprofloxacin does not appear to have increased markedly in the cyclosporine concentrations, additive nephrotoxicity is suggested (but not proven) by the temporal relationship between ciprofloxacin administration and the development of renal failure. Other reports of nephrotoxicity with and without changes in cyclosporine concentrations during cyclosporine and ciprofloxacin coadministration have been reported.[6,7] The pharmacokinetics of cyclosporine were not altered in several studies involving ciprofloxacin doses of 500 to 750 mg twice daily.[2-5,8]

RELATED DRUGS: Norfloxacin (*Noroxin*) has been reported to increase cyclosporine concentrations; further study is needed. Ciprofloxacin might affect tacrolimus (*Prograf*) in a similar manner.

MANAGEMENT OPTIONS: No specific action is required, but be alert for evidence of the interaction.

REFERENCES:

1. Advent CK, et al. Synergistic nephrotoxicity due to ciprofloxacin and cyclosporine. *Am J Med.* 1988;85:452.
2. Tan KKC, et al. Co-administration of ciprofloxacin and cyclosporin: lack of evidence for a pharmacokinetic interaction. *Br J Clin Pharmacol.* 1989;28:185.
3. Kruger HU, et al. Investigation of potential interaction of ciprofloxacin with cyclosporine in bone marrow transplant recipients. *Antimicrob agents Chemother.* 1990;34:1048.
4. Van Buren DH, et al. Effect of ciprofloxacin on cyclosporine pharmacokinetics. *Transplantation.* 1990;50:888.
5. Lang J, et al. Cyclosporine pharmacokinetics in renal transplant patients receiving ciprofloxacin. *Am J Med.* 1989;87(Suppl. 5A):82S.
6. Elston RA, et al. Possible interaction of ciprofloxacin with cyclosporin A. *J Antimicrob Chemother.* 1988;21:679.
7. Nasir M, et al. Interaction between cyclosporin and ciprofloxacin. *Nephron.* 1991;57:245.
8. Robinson JA, et al. Patients receiving quinolones and cyclosporine after heart transplantation. *J Heart Transplant.* 1990;9:30.

Ciprofloxacin (*Cipro*)

Diazepam (eg, *Valium*)

SUMMARY: The plasma concentrations of diazepam are increased by ciprofloxacin; the clinical significance of this interaction is unknown.

RISK FACTORS: No specific risk factors are known.

MECHANISM: Ciprofloxacin inhibits the metabolism of diazepam. It is not known if it also competes at γ-aminobutyric acid (GABA) receptors with diazepam; however, quinolones are known to inhibit GABA receptors while diazepam is a GABA agonist.

CLINICAL EVALUATION: Ciprofloxacin 500 mg twice daily reduced diazepam clearance 37% and increased its half-life from 36.7 to 71.1 hours.[1] Ciprofloxacin did not appear to alter the pharmacodynamics of diazepam as measured by various psychometric testing. The clinical significance of this interaction remains to be determined with chronic dosing studies.

RELATED DRUGS: Other quinolones also may inhibit the metabolism of diazepam or compete with it at the GABA receptor. Other benzodiazepines may be inhibited by ciprofloxacin.

MANAGEMENT OPTIONS:

➡ *Monitor.* Patients stabilized on diazepam may experience increased plasma concentrations if ciprofloxacin is administered. Observe patients for any increased or prolonged diazepam effects (eg, sedation, ataxia).

REFERENCES:

1. Kamali F, et al. The influence of steady-state ciprofloxacin on the pharmacokinetics and pharmacodynamics of a single dose of diazepam in healthy volunteers. *Eur J Clin Pharmacol.* 1993;44:365.

Ciprofloxacin (*Cipro*)

Didanosine (*Videx*)

SUMMARY: The buffers contained in didanosine markedly reduce the plasma concentrations of ciprofloxacin and will likely reduce the efficacy of ciprofloxacin.

RISK FACTORS: No specific risk factors are known.

MECHANISM: Ciprofloxacin binding to the aluminum and magnesium ions in the didanosine buffering compound prevents absorption of ciprofloxacin.

CLINICAL EVALUATION: Twelve healthy subjects received ciprofloxacin 750 mg alone or immediately following 2 tablets of didanosine placebo.[1] The didanosine placebo contained the aluminum and magnesium buffer but no didanosine. Following coadministration of the didanosine placebo, the ciprofloxacin area under the concentration-time curve was decreased 98% and the peak ciprofloxacin concentration fell 93%. This reduction in ciprofloxacin concentrations will likely lead to therapeutic failure.

RELATED DRUGS: Other orally administered quinolones also would be expected to interact with didanosine. Drugs containing magnesium or aluminum will likely interact with ciprofloxacin in a similar manner.

MANAGEMENT OPTIONS:

➡ *Circumvent/Minimize.* To avoid this interaction, take ciprofloxacin at least 2 hours before didanosine. Ciprofloxacin administration up to 6 hours after the didanosine will probably not avoid the interaction because of the persistence of aluminum and magnesium in the gut.[2]

➡ *Monitor.* Monitor patient response to ciprofloxacin if this combination is administered.

REFERENCES:

1. Sahai J, et al. Cations in the didanosine tablet reduce ciprofloxacin bioavailability. *Clin Pharmacol Ther.* 1993;53:292.
2. Nix DE, et al. Effects of aluminum and magnesium antacids and ranitidine on the absorption of ciprofloxacin. *Clin Pharmacol Ther.* 1989;46:700.

Ciprofloxacin (eg, *Cipro*)

Erlotinib (*Tarceva*)

SUMMARY: Ciprofloxacin administration increased the plasma concentration of erlotinib; patients may experience an increase in adverse reactions, including rash or GI upset.

RISK FACTORS: No specific risk factors are known.

MECHANISM: Ciprofloxacin appears to reduce the metabolism of erlotinib, probably by inhibition of CYP1A2.

CLINICAL EVALUATION: While specific data are limited, the coadministration of ciprofloxacin (dose not stated) increased the mean area under the plasma concentration-time curve of erlotinib by about 40%.[1] Pending further data, patients receiving erlotinib and ciprofloxacin should be observed for increased erlotinib adverse reactions.

RELATED DRUGS: Enoxacin[†] would likely inhibit the metabolism of erlotinib in a similar manner.

MANAGEMENT OPTIONS:

➠ *Consider Alternative.* Quinolones that do not appear to inhibit CYP1A2 or CYP3A4 include ofloxacin (eg, *Floxin*), lomefloxacin,[†] and moxifloxacin (*Avelox*).

➠ *Monitor.* Be alert for GI adverse reactions or rash in patients taking erlotinib and ciprofloxacin.

REFERENCES:

1. *Tarceva* [package insert]. South San Francisco, CA: Genentech USA Inc; 2008.

† Not available in the United States.

 Ciprofloxacin (eg, *Cipro*)

Ethanol (Ethyl Alcohol)

SUMMARY: Ciprofloxacin does not appear to affect ethanol concentrations or pharmacodynamic effects.

RISK FACTORS: No specific risk factors are known.

MECHANISM: No interaction.

CLINICAL EVALUATION: Twelve healthy subjects received ciprofloxacin 500 mg twice daily or placebo for 3 days.[1] On day 4, a single oral dose of ethanol 30 g was administered to fasting subjects. Ciprofloxacin pretreatment had no effect on ethanol concentrations or psychomotor tests compared to pretreatment with placebo.

RELATED DRUGS: While no data are available, the other quinolones would not be expected to alter ethanol concentrations.

MANAGEMENT OPTIONS: No interaction.

REFERENCES:

1. Kamali F. No influence of ciprofloxacin on ethanol disposition. *Eur J Clin Pharmacol*. 1994;47:71.

 Ciprofloxacin (eg, *Cipro*)

Food

SUMMARY: The administration of ciprofloxacin with milk or yogurt reduces ciprofloxacin concentrations; the clinical significance is unknown but could result in therapeutic failure in some patients.

RISK FACTORS: No specific risk factors are known.

MECHANISM: The calcium ions in dairy products and antacids chelate to the quinolone molecule and reduce its absorption.

CLINICAL EVALUATION: Seven healthy subjects received ciprofloxacin 500 mg with 300 mL water, milk (360 mg calcium), or yogurt (450 mg calcium).[1] Compared with water, milk reduced ciprofloxacin's peak serum concentration and area under the plasma concentration-time curve (AUC) 36% and 33%, respectively. Results with yogurt were similar; peak concentration reduced 47% and AUC reduced 36%. The effect of a high-fat, high-calcium (729 mg) meal on ciprofloxacin 750 mg did not decrease ciprofloxacin absorption,[2] but nutritional supplements produce variable effects on ciprofloxacin absorption.[3-5] Milk and yogurt may be more effective in binding to ciprofloxacin when taken without other foods. Pancreatic enzymes (7 capsules) did not affect ciprofloxacin pharmacokinetics following a single 250 mg dose in patients with cystic fibrosis.[6]

RELATED DRUGS: Lomefloxacin (*Maxaquin*) and temafloxacin pharmacokinetics were not affected significantly by administration with meals.[7-9] Additionally, ofloxacin (eg, *Floxin*) appears to be similarly unaffected. Some of the other quinolones may be similarly affected.

MANAGEMENT OPTIONS:

➥ *Consider Alternative.* Lomefloxacin, ofloxacin, or temafloxacin could be considered for use instead of ciprofloxacin.

➥ *Circumvent/Minimize.* Counsel patients to avoid taking ciprofloxacin with milk or yogurt.

➥ *Monitor.* Watch for decreased quinolone efficacy if administered with milk or high calcium foods. Quinolone administration with foods not high in calcium appears to be acceptable.

REFERENCES:

1. Neuvonen PJ, et al. Interference of diary products with the absorption of ciprofloxacin. *Clin Pharmacol Ther*. 1991;50:498.
2. Frost RW, et al. Ciprofloxacin pharmacokinetics after a standard or high-fat/high-calcium breakfast. *J Clin Pharmacol*. 1989;29:953.
3. Noer BL, et al. The effect of enteral feedings on ciprofloxacin pharmacokinetics. *Pharmacotherapy*. 1990;10:58.
4. Piccolo ML, et al. Effect of coadministration of a nutritional supplement on ciprofloxacin absorption. *Am J Hosp Pharm*. 1994;51:2697.
5. Yuk JH, et al. Relative bioavailability in healthy volunteers of ciprofloxacin administered through a nasogastric tube with and without enteral feedings. *Antimicrob Agents Chemother*. 1989;33:1118.
6. Mack G, et al. Effects of enzyme supplementation on oral absorption of ciprofloxacin in patients with cystic fibrosis. *Antimicrob Agents Chemother*. 1991;35:1484.
7. Hooper WD, et al. Effect of food on absorption of lomefloxacin. *Antimicrob Agents Chemother*. 1990;34:1797.
8. Granneman GR, et al. The effect of food on the bioavailability of temafloxacin. *Clin Pharmacokinet*. 1992;22(Suppl. 1):48.
9. Lehto P, et al. Different effects of products containing metal ions on the absorption of lomefloxacin. *Clin Pharmacol Ther*. 1994;56:477.

Ciprofloxacin (eg, *Cipro*)

Foscarnet (*Foscavir*)

SUMMARY: The combination of ciprofloxacin and foscarnet has resulted in tonic-clonic seizure activity in 2 patients; the potential significance of this purported interaction requires additional study.

RISK FACTORS: No specific risk factors are known.

MECHANISM: Not established. Both ciprofloxacin and foscarnet have been reported to cause seizures. It is possible that this interaction represents a pharmacodynamic interaction between the 2 agents leading to increased seizure activity.

CLINICAL EVALUATION: Two patients with human immunodeficiency virus were receiving several drugs, including ciprofloxacin 750 mg twice daily.[1] Both developed seizures after foscarnet was added on several occasions. Foscarnet was discontinued and the patients had no further seizures. While neither of these cases provide causation of an interaction between foscarnet and ciprofloxacin, the temporal relationship and rechallenge suggests that administration of both agents may potentiate their individual epileptogenic activities.

RELATED DRUGS: Other quinolones potentially could produce a similar interaction with foscarnet.

MANAGEMENT OPTIONS:

➡ **Monitor.** Until further evidence of this purported interaction is available, monitor patients receiving foscarnet and ciprofloxacin for seizure activity.

REFERENCES:

1. Fan-Havard P, et al. Concurrent use of foscarnet and ciprofloxacin may increase the propensity for seizures. *Ann Pharmacother.* 1994;28:869.

Ciprofloxacin (eg, *Cipro*)

Glyburide (eg, *Diabeta*)

SUMMARY: Ciprofloxacin may increase the risk of hypoglycemic episodes in patients with diabetes who are taking oral hypoglycemic agents.

RISK FACTORS: No specific risk factors are known.

MECHANISM: Unknown. Limited evidence suggests that some quinolones may increase insulin release from the pancreas.[1] Other factors may also contribute such as reduced metabolism of the oral hypoglycemic agent by infection-induced cytokine activation.

CLINICAL EVALUATION: Several case reports have noted hypoglycemic episodes in patients with diabetes being treated with glyburide and ciprofloxacin.[2-4] Hypoglycemia often occurs within the first day or two of concurrent ciprofloxacin administration. While these cases appear to be rare, be alert for signs of hypoglycemia.

RELATED DRUGS: Several other quinolone antibiotics (eg, levofloxacin [*Levaquin*], gatifloxacin [*Tequin*], and moxifloxacin [*Maxaquin*]) have been associated with hypoglycemic episodes in diabetic patients taking oral hypoglycemic agents.

MANAGEMENT OPTIONS:

➡ **Monitor.** Diabetic patients with infections are likely to have unstable glucose control and should check their blood sugar more frequently until treatment of the infection is completed.

REFERENCES:

1. Gajjar DA, et al. Effect of multiple-dose gatifloxacin or ciprofloxacin on glucose homeostasis and insulin production in patients with noninsulin-dependent diabetes mellitus maintained with diet and exercise. *Pharmacotherapy.* 2000;20(6 pt 2):76S-86S.

2. Roberge RJ, et al. Glyburide-ciprofloxacin interaction with resistant hypoglycemia. *Ann Emerg Med.* 2000;36:160-163.

3. Whiteley MS, et al. Hypoglycemia in a diabetic patient, associated with ciprofloxacin therapy. *Pract Diabetes.* 1999;10:35.

4. Lin G, et al. Refractory hypoglycemia from ciprofloxacin and glyburide interaction. *J Toxicol Clin Toxicol.* 2004;42:295-297.

Ciprofloxacin (eg, *Cipro*)

Iron

SUMMARY: The administration of iron salts with ciprofloxacin lowers the antibiotic serum concentration and may lead to therapeutic failure.

RISK FACTORS: No specific risk factors are known.

MECHANISM: Iron salts inhibit ciprofloxacin absorption by binding to it in the GI tract.

CLINICAL EVALUATION: The administration of ferrous sulfate, ferrous fumarate, and ferrous gluconate has reduced the absorption of ciprofloxacin 40% to 65%.[1-5]

RELATED DRUGS: Other quinolones, including norfloxacin (*Noroxin*), have been reported to be affected similarly by iron.[5,6] Ofloxacin (eg, *Floxin*) absorption may be less affected by iron.[5,7]

MANAGEMENT OPTIONS:

➡ *Consider Alternative.* Patients taking ciprofloxacin (and probably other quinolones) should not take oral iron salts concurrently because serum ciprofloxacin concentrations may be subtherapeutic. Ofloxacin absorption may be less affected by iron.[5,7]

➡ *Circumvent/Minimize.* Giving IV iron or IV ciprofloxacin doses may avoid the interaction. If ciprofloxacin is administered orally, give it at least 2 hours before any oral iron product.

➡ *Monitor.* If the drugs are used together, watch for lessened antibiotic effect.

REFERENCES:

1. Polk RE, et al. Effect of ferrous sulfate and multivitamins with zinc on absorption of ciprofloxacin in normal volunteers. *Antimicrob Agents Chemother*. 1989;33:1841-1844.
2. LePennec MP, et al. Possible interaction of ciprofloxacin with ferrous sulfate. *J Antimicrob Chemother*. 1990;25:184-185.
3. Brouwers JR, et al. Decreased ciprofloxacin absorption with concomitant administration of ferrous fumarate. *Pharm Weekbl Sci*. 1990;12:182-183.
4. Kara M, et al. Clinical and chemical interactions between iron preparations and ciprofloxacin. *Br J Clin Pharmacol*. 1991;31:257-261.
5. Lehto P, et al. The effect of ferrous sulphate on the absorption of norfloxacin, ciprofloxacin and ofloxacin. *Br J Clin Pharmacol*. 1994;37:82-85.
6. Campbell NR, et al. Norfloxacin interaction with antacids and minerals. *Br J Clin Pharmacol*. 1992;33:115-116.
7. Akerele JO, et al. Influence of oral co-administered metallic drugs on ofloxacin pharmacokinetics. *J Antimicrob Chemother*. 1991;28:87-94.

Ciprofloxacin (*Cipro*)

Metoprolol (eg, *Lopressor*)

SUMMARY: Ciprofloxacin increases the concentration of metoprolol enantiomers; the greatest effect is on the enantiomer with the least beta-blocking activity.

RISK FACTORS: No specific risk factors are known.

MECHANISM: Ciprofloxacin appears to reduce the clearance of orally administered metoprolol.

CLINICAL EVALUATION: Ciprofloxacin 500 mg every 12 hours reduced the clearances of (+) and (−)metoprolol 38.5% and 12.5%, respectively.[1] The area under the concentration-time curve was increased 54% and 29% for (+) and (−)metoprolol, respectively. The majority of beta-blocking activity is produced by (−)metoprolol. Because ciprofloxacin has its greatest effect on (+)metoprolol, the potential clinical significance of this interaction is somewhat reduced. Studies defining the pharmacodynamic effects of this interaction are needed.

RELATED DRUGS: Quinolones reported to inhibit drug metabolism include ciprofloxacin, enoxacin (*Penetrex*), norfloxacin (*Noroxin*), pipemidic acid, and pefloxacin. These quinolones also may inhibit metoprolol metabolism. Other beta blockers (eg, propranolol [eg, *Inderal*]) may be affected similarly by ciprofloxacin administration.

MANAGEMENT OPTIONS:

➡ *Monitor.* Because patients stabilized on oral metoprolol might experience increased beta blockade during ciprofloxacin coadministration, monitor for bradycardia, heart failure, or prolonged atrioventricular conduction.

REFERENCES:
1. Waite NM, et al. Disposition of the (+) and (−) isomers of metoprolol following ciprofloxacin treatment. *Pharmacotherapy.* 1990;10:236.

4   Ciprofloxacin (*Cipro*)

Mexiletine (*Mexitil*)

SUMMARY: Ciprofloxacin increases the plasma concentration of mexiletine; the magnitude of this change is not likely to produce clinically important changes in most patients.

RISK FACTORS: No specific risk factors are known.

MECHANISM: CYP1A2 has been identified as the enzyme responsible for the metabolism of mexiletine. Ciprofloxacin is a known inhibitor of this enzyme and appears to reduce the clearance of mexiletine.

CLINICAL EVALUATION: Nine healthy nonsmoking subjects and 8 smoking subjects received mexiletine alone and after 3 days of a 5-day course of ciprofloxacin 750 mg twice daily.[1] While smokers had higher clearance after oral mexiletine administration than nonsmokers, the clearance after oral administration of mexiletine enantiomers was reduced by an average of 7% to 15% following ciprofloxacin in both smokers and nonsmokers. While no pharmacodynamic data were presented, the limited magnitude of the change in mexiletine clearance is not likely to produce adverse effects in most patients.

RELATED DRUGS: Some quinolones (eg, enoxacin [*Penetrex*]) may produce a similar interaction with mexiletine while other quinolones (eg, ofloxacin [*Floxin*]) would be less likely to interact.

MANAGEMENT OPTIONS: No specific action is required, but be alert for evidence of the interaction.

REFERENCES:
1. Labbe L, et al. Ciprofloxacin (Cipro) decreases mexiletine (Mex) clearance in smokers and nonsmokers. *Clin Pharmacol Ther.* 1995;57:210.

Ciprofloxacin (*Cipro*) 4

Olanzapine (*Zyprexa*)

SUMMARY: Ciprofloxacin increases olanzapine plasma concentrations; increased somnolence, dizziness, or orthostatic hypotension may occur.

RISK FACTORS: No specific risk factors are known.

MECHANISM: Ciprofloxacin appears to inhibit the metabolism of olanzapine, probably via the CYP1A2 pathway.

CLINICAL EVALUATION: A patient taking olanzapine 10 mg/day, nefazodone (*Serzone*) 100 mg twice daily, atenolol (eg, *Tenormin*) 25 mg/day, levothyroxine (eg, *Synthroid*) 0.025 mg/day, and phenytoin (eg, *Dilantin*) 100 mg twice daily was administered ciprofloxacin 250 mg twice daily for 7 days for a suspected UTI.[1] Trough olanzapine plasma concentration just prior to the last ciprofloxacin dose was 32.6 ng/ml. A repeat trough olanzapine concentration obtained 3 days after the last dose of ciprofloxacin was 14.6 mg/ml. The effect of larger doses of ciprofloxacin on olanzapine is unknown but a greater effect may occur.

RELATED DRUGS: Enoxacin (*Penetrex*) would probably affect olanzapine in a similar manner. Other quinolone antibiotics such as ofloxacin (*Floxin*) or levofloxacin (*Levaquin*) would be unlikely to alter olanzapine concentrations.

MANAGEMENT OPTIONS: No specific action is required, but monitor patients taking olanzapine for side effects when ciprofloxacin is coadministered.

REFERENCES:
1. Markowitz JS, et al. Suspected ciprofloxacin inhibition of olanzapine resulting in increased plasma concentration. *J Clin Psychopharmacol.* 1999;19(3):289-91.

Ciprofloxacin (*Cipro*)

Pentoxifylline (eg, *Trental*)

SUMMARY: Ciprofloxacin increases pentoxifylline plasma concentrations and may increase adverse effects.

RISK FACTORS: No specific risk factors are known.

MECHANISM: Ciprofloxacin reduces the metabolism of pentoxifylline.

CLINICAL EVALUATION: Six healthy subjects received a single dose of pentoxifylline 400 mg alone and after 3 days of ciprofloxacin 500 mg/day.[1] Following the administration of ciprofloxacin, peak pentoxifylline concentrations increased 36% while the area under the pentoxifylline concentration-time curve increased 13%. All of the subjects reported headaches following ciprofloxacin and pentoxifylline administration.

RELATED DRUGS: Other quinolones that inhibit metabolism (eg, enoxacin [*Penetrex*], norfloxacin [*Noroxin*], pipemidic acid, pefloxacin) would be expected to produce a similar reaction.

MANAGEMENT OPTIONS:

➡ *Monitor.* Monitor patients taking pentoxifylline for increased pentoxifylline effects and side effects (eg, flushing, nausea, headache) if ciprofloxacin is administered.

REFERENCES:

1. Cleary JD, et al. Ciprofloxacin (CIPRO) and pentoxifylline (PTF): a clinically significant drug interaction. *Pharmacotherapy.* 1992;12:259.

Ciprofloxacin (eg, *Cipro*)

Phenytoin (eg, *Dilantin*)

SUMMARY: Preliminary evidence suggests that ciprofloxacin administration may elevate plasma phenytoin concentrations modestly.

RISK FACTORS: No specific risk factors are known.

MECHANISM: Not established.

CLINICAL EVALUATION: Seven patients with epilepsy maintained on phenytoin monotherapy received ciprofloxacin 500 mg twice daily for 10 days. Phenytoin plasma concentrations increased on average 24% when evaluated on days 5 and 10 of ciprofloxacin treatment.[1] In another report, serum phenytoin concentration was increased following the addition of ciprofloxacin; causation was not established.[2] A study in 4 healthy subjects detected no change in phenytoin concentrations following 4 days of ciprofloxacin 500 mg twice daily.[3] The clinical significance of these changes is undetermined.

RELATED DRUGS: Other quinolones that inhibit metabolism (eg, enoxacin,[†] norfloxacin [*Noroxin*]) are expected to produce a similar reaction.

MANAGEMENT OPTIONS:

➡ *Monitor.* Until further data are available, monitor patients for phenytoin toxicity (eg, ataxia, confusion, dizziness, involuntary muscular movements, nystagmus, slurred speech) when ciprofloxacin is started. Serum phenytoin determinations also may be useful. When ciprofloxacin therapy is stopped in the presence of phenytoin therapy, monitor for reduced phenytoin effect.

REFERENCES:

1. Schroeder D, et al. Effect of ciprofloxacin on serum phenytoin concentrations in epileptic patients. *Pharmacotherapy.* 1991;11:276.
2. Hull RL. Possible phenytoin-ciprofloxacin interaction. *Ann Pharmacother.* 1993;27(10):1283.
3. Job ML, et al. Effect of ciprofloxacin on the pharmacokinetics of multiple-dose phenytoin serum concentrations. *Ther Drug Monit.* 1994;16(4):427-431.

† Not available in the United States.

Ciprofloxacin (eg, *Cipro*)

Probenecid

SUMMARY: Probenecid administration increases the plasma concentration of ciprofloxacin; some patients may experience increased adverse reactions.

RISK FACTORS: No specific risk factors are known.

MECHANISM: Probenecid inhibits the renal tubular secretion of ciprofloxacin.

CLINICAL EVALUATION: Twelve healthy subjects received a single intravenous dose of ciprofloxacin 200 mg alone and after probenecid 3 g administered in divided doses starting 10 hours before ciprofloxacin and ending 16 hours after the ciprofloxacin dose.[1] The mean area under the concentration-time curve of ciprofloxacin was increased approximately 75% during probenecid coadministration. The increase in ciprofloxacin concentration resulted from a reduction in its renal clearance by 65%.

RELATED DRUGS: Other quinolones, including norfloxacin (*Noroxin*) and enoxacin,[†] are affected by probenecid in a similar manner.

MANAGEMENT OPTIONS:

➥ *Monitor.* Monitor patients taking ciprofloxacin for potentially reduced efficacy in treating urinary tract infections as well as increased adverse reactions, including anxiety, dizziness, and headaches, if probenecid is coadministered.

REFERENCES:

1. Landersdorfer CB, et al. Competitive inhibition of renal tubular secretion of ciprofloxacin and metabolite by probenecid. *Br J Clin Pharmacol.* 2010;69(2):167-178.

† Not available in the United States.

Ciprofloxacin (eg, *Cipro*)

Quinidine

SUMMARY: Ciprofloxacin does not alter quinidine serum concentrations or electrophysiologic effects.

RISK FACTORS: No specific risk factors are known.

MECHANISM: No interaction.

CLINICAL EVALUATION: Seven healthy subjects received quinidine 400 mg alone and following ciprofloxacin 750 mg every 12 hours for 5 days.[1] Neither quinidine clearance nor QRS or QTc intervals were altered significantly (10% reduction) by ciprofloxacin administration.

RELATED DRUGS: No information is available.

MANAGEMENT OPTIONS: No interaction.

REFERENCES:

1. Bleske BE, et al. The effect of ciprofloxacin on the pharmacokinetic and ECG parameters of quinidine. *J Clin Pharmacol.* 1990;30(10):911-915.

Ciprofloxacin (eg, *Cipro*)

Ramelteon (*Rozerem*)

SUMMARY: Ramelteon is very sensitive to inhibition of CYP1A2; theoretically, ciprofloxacin produces substantial increases in ramelteon plasma concentrations.

RISK FACTORS: No specific risk factors are known.

MECHANISM: Ramelteon is metabolized primarily by CYP1A2, and ciprofloxacin is a moderate CYP1A2 inhibitor.

CLINICAL EVALUATION: In healthy subjects, administration of fluvoxamine 100 mg twice daily for 3 days produced a 190-fold increase in ramelteon plasma concentrations and a 70-fold increase in the ramelteon maximal plasma concentrations.[1] Although ciprofloxacin is less potent than fluvoxamine as a CYP1A2 inhibitor, substantial increases in ramelteon plasma concentrations are expected. The ramelteon package insert states that ramelteon should be administered with caution with CYP1A2 inhibitors.[1]

RELATED DRUGS: Enoxacin[†] is a more potent inhibitor of CYP1A2 than ciprofloxacin and should generally be avoided with ramelteon. Other fluoroquinolones, such as gatifloxacin (*Zymar*), levofloxacin (*Levaquin*), lomefloxacin,[†] moxifloxacin (*Avelox*), and ofloxacin (eg, *Floxin*), have little effect on CYP1A2 and theoretically are not expected to interact significantly with ramelteon.

MANAGEMENT OPTIONS:

➥ *Use Alternative.* If a fluoroquinolone is needed, avoid ciprofloxacin or enoxacin. Use an alternative that has little effect on CYP1A2 (see Related Drugs).

REFERENCES:

1. *Rozerem* [package insert]. Lincolnshire, IL: Takeda Pharmaceuticals; 2006.

† Not available in the United States.

Ciprofloxacin (eg, *Cipro*)

Rasagiline (*Azilect*)

SUMMARY: Ciprofloxacin increases the plasma concentration of rasagiline; some patients may experience increased adverse reactions.

RISK FACTORS: No specific risk factors are known.

MECHANISM: Ciprofloxacin inhibits the CYP1A2-mediated metabolism of rasagiline.

CLINICAL EVALUATION: Although data are limited, the manufacturer of rasagiline has noted that ciprofloxacin 500 mg twice daily increased the mean area under the plasma concentration-time curve of rasagiline 83%.[1] No change was observed in the half-life of rasagiline.

RELATED DRUGS: Quinolones known to inhibit CYP1A2 (eg, enoxacin[†]) are likely to interact with rasagiline.

MANAGEMENT OPTIONS:

➥ *Consider Alternative.* Consider quinolones that do not inhibit CYP1A2, such as levofloxacin (*Levaquin*), lomefloxacin,[†] or ofloxacin (eg, *Floxin*), as substitutes for ciprofloxacin in patients taking rasagiline.

➥ *Monitor.* Carefully monitor patients who receive ciprofloxacin and rasagiline, and are concurrently taking levodopa, for evidence of dyskinesia, hallucinations, and postural hypotension.

REFERENCES:

1. *Azilect* [package insert]. North Wales, PA: Teva Neuroscience Inc; 2006.

† Not available in the United States.

Ciprofloxacin (eg, *Cipro*) 5

Rifampin (eg, *Rifadin*)

SUMMARY: Ciprofloxacin concentrations do not appear to be altered by rifampin.

RISK FACTORS: No specific risk factors are known.

MECHANISM: No interaction.

CLINICAL EVALUATION: Twelve elderly patients received ciprofloxacin 750 mg every 12 hours for 14 days, and 6 of the patients also received rifampin 300 mg every 12 hours. No difference in total ciprofloxacin clearance (approximately 15% metabolic) was noted between the groups. Rifampin 600 mg/day had no effect on ciprofloxacin pharmacokinetics.[1,2] Rifampin did not affect ciprofloxacin pharmacokinetics, and ciprofloxacin did not alter rifampin pharmacokinetics.[2]

RELATED DRUGS: No information is available.

MANAGEMENT OPTIONS: No interaction.

REFERENCES:

1. Chandler MH, et al. Multiple-dose pharmacokinetics of concurrent oral ciprofloxacin and rifampin therapy in elderly patients. *Antimicrob Agents Chemother*. 1990;34:442-447.

2. Weinstein MP, et al. Crossover assessment of serum bactericidal activity and pharmacokinetics of ciprofloxacin alone and in combination in healthy elderly volunteers. *Antimicrob Agents Chemother*. 1991;35:2352-2358.

Ciprofloxacin (eg, *Cipro*)

Ropinirole (*Requip*)

SUMMARY: Ropinirole concentrations are increased during coadministration of ciprofloxacin; increased adverse reactions may result.

RISK FACTORS: No specific risk factors are known.

MECHANISM: Ciprofloxacin appears to inhibit the metabolism (CYP1A2) of ropinirole.

CLINICAL EVALUATION: While no published data are available for evaluation, the manufacturer of ropinirole has made some information on the interaction available.[1] The administration of ciprofloxacin 500 mg twice daily with ropinirole 2 mg 3 times daily increased the ropinirole area under the concentration-time curve 84%. The peak concentration of ropinirole was increased 60%. It is possible that these changes could increase the incidence of ropinirole-induced adverse reactions such as dizziness, nausea, somnolence, or syncope.

RELATED DRUGS: Some quinolone antibiotics (eg, enoxacin†) may also increase ropinirole concentrations. Ofloxacin (eg, *Floxin*) and lomefloxacin (*Maxaquin*) may be less likely to interact.

MANAGEMENT OPTIONS:

➥ **Consider Alternative.** Using ofloxacin or lomefloxacin instead of ciprofloxacin may avoid any significant increase in ropinirole concentrations.

➡ **Monitor.** Monitor patients taking ropinirole and ciprofloxacin for increased ropinirole effects and adverse reactions, including dizziness, nausea, and syncope.

REFERENCES:

1. *Requip* [package insert]. Research Triangle Park, NC: GlaxoSmithKline; 1997.

† Not available in the US.

Ciprofloxacin (eg, *Cipro*)

Ropivacaine (*Naropin*)

SUMMARY: Ciprofloxacin increases the plasma concentration of ropivacaine; an increase in adverse reactions may occur in patients receiving both drugs.

RISK FACTORS: No specific risk factors are known.

MECHANISM: Ciprofloxacin appears to inhibit the metabolism (CYP1A2) of ropivacaine.

CLINICAL EVALUATION: Nine healthy subjects received a single intravenous dose of ropivacaine 0.6 mg/kg following 2.5 days of placebo or ciprofloxacin 500 mg twice daily.[1] Ciprofloxacin increased the mean area under the plasma concentration-time curve of ropivacaine 22% and decreased the mean clearance of ropivacaine 30%.

RELATED DRUGS: Enoxacin† is also a potent CYP1A2 inhibitor and is likely to affect ropivacaine in a similar manner.

MANAGEMENT OPTIONS:

➡ **Consider Alternative.** Consider quinolones that do not inhibit CYP1A2, such as ofloxacin (eg, *Floxin*), levofloxacin (*Levaquin*), or lomefloxacin (*Maxaquin*), in patients who receive ropivacaine.

➡ **Monitor.** Closely monitor patients taking ciprofloxacin and ropivacaine for bradycardia, hypotension, nausea, and vomiting.

REFERENCES:

1. Jokinen MJ, et al. Effect of ciprofloxacin on the pharmacokinetics of ropivacaine. *Eur J Clin Pharmacol.* 2003;58:653-657.

† Not available in the US.

Ciprofloxacin (eg, *Cipro*)

Sildenafil (eg, *Viagra*)

SUMMARY: Ciprofloxacin administration increases sildenafil plasma concentrations; increased sildenafil adverse reactions are likely to occur.

RISK FACTORS: No specific risk factors are known.

MECHANISM: Ciprofloxacin appears to inhibit the metabolism of sildenafil, probably via the CYP3A4 pathway.

CLINICAL EVALUATION: Twelve healthy men received sildenafil 50 mg alone or 2 hours after taking a single dose of ciprofloxacin 500 mg.[1] The mean area under the plasma concentration-time curve of sildenafil was increased 112% by the coadministration of ciprofloxacin. Peak sildenafil concentrations increased 117%. Sildenafil's half-life increased from 2.5 to 3.4 hours with coadministration of ciprofloxacin. The effect of multiple doses of ciprofloxacin on sildenafil plasma concentrations is likely to be even greater.

RELATED DRUGS: Enoxacin[+] is likely to affect sildenafil in a similar manner. Ciprofloxacin may increase the plasma concentrations of vardenafil (*Levitra*) and tadalafil (*Cialis*).

MANAGEMENT OPTIONS:

➡ *Consider Alternative.* Consider quinolones that do not inhibit CYP3A4, such as levofloxacin (*Levaquin*), lomefloxacin (*Maxaquin*), or ofloxacin (eg, *Floxin*), as substitutes for ciprofloxacin in patients taking sildenafil.

➡ *Monitor.* Patients using sildenafil should be alert for adverse reactions (eg, dizziness, headache, hypotension) if ciprofloxacin is coadministered.

REFERENCES:

1. Hedaya MA, et al. The effect of ciprofloxacin and clarithromycin on sildenafil oral bioavailability in human volunteers. *Biopharm Drug Dispos.* 2006;27:103-110.

† Not available in the US.

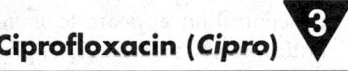

Ciprofloxacin (*Cipro*)

Sucralfate (eg, *Carafate*)

SUMMARY: The administration of sucralfate markedly reduced ciprofloxacin serum concentrations; loss of antibiotic effect may occur.

RISK FACTORS: No specific risk factors are known.

MECHANISM: Aluminum contained in sucralfate inhibits the absorption of ciprofloxacin.

CLINICAL EVALUATION: Ciprofloxacin 750 mg was administered alone and after 1 g doses of sucralfate 6 and 2 hours before ciprofloxacin dosing.[1] The combination produced an average 30% reduction in ciprofloxacin bioavailability. Other studies noted markedly reduced ciprofloxacin concentrations (up to 85%) when administered with sucralfate 1 g 4 times daily,[2,4] a single 2 g dose,[3] or 2 g every 12 hours.[5]

RELATED DRUGS: Sucralfate inhibits the absorption of fleroxacin, norfloxacin (*Noroxin*), and ofloxacin (*Floxin*). Antacids containing aluminum also inhibit ciprofloxacin absorption.

MANAGEMENT OPTIONS:

➡ *Consider Alternative.* If dosage separation is not possible, consider an alternative to sucralfate (eg, H_2-receptor antagonist, omeprazole, but not an antacid).

➡ *Circumvent/Minimize.* Avoid the coadministration of ciprofloxacin and sucralfate if possible. Administer ciprofloxacin several hours before sucralfate or 6 hours after.[5]

➡ *Monitor.* If sucralfate and a quinolone are coadministered, monitor the patient for reduced antibiotic efficacy.

REFERENCES:

1. Nix DE, et al. The effect of sucralfate pretreatment on the pharmacokinetics of ciprofloxacin. *Pharmacotherapy.* 1989;9:377.

2. Yuk JH, et al. Ciprofloxacin levels when receiving sucralfate. *JAMA.* 1989;262:901.

3. Brouwers JRBJ, et al. Important reduction of ciprofloxacin absorption by sucralfate and magnesium citrate solution. *Drug Invest.* 1990;2:197.

4. Garrelts JC, et al. Sucralfate significantly reduces ciprofloxacin concentrations in serum. *Antimicrob Agents Chemother*. 1990;34:931.

5. Van Slooten AD, et al. Combined use of ciprofloxacin and sucralfate. *DICP, Ann Pharmacother*. 1991;25:578.

Ciprofloxacin (*Cipro*)

Theophylline (eg, *Theolair*)

SUMMARY: Ciprofloxacin increases the serum concentration of theophylline and can induce theophylline toxicity.

RISK FACTORS:

➡ **Dosage Regimen.** High doses of ciprofloxacin place one at greater risk.

MECHANISM: Ciprofloxacin probably inhibits the N-demethylation (CYP1A2) of theophylline.

CLINICAL EVALUATION: In a number of case reports and clinical studies ciprofloxacin reduced theophylline clearance 15% to over 50%.[1-8,10] The serum theophylline concentration appears to increase over an approximately 3-day period after the antibiotic is started. Theophylline toxicity can occur and seizures have been reported with the combination, even when theophylline concentrations are within the therapeutic range.[9] Theophylline does not alter ciprofloxacin serum concentrations.[7]

RELATED DRUGS: Quinolones reported to inhibit the metabolism of drugs include enoxacin (*Penetrex*), norfloxacin (*Noroxin*), pipemidic acid, and pefloxacin.

MANAGEMENT OPTIONS:

➡ **Consider Alternative.** Quinolones reported to produce no or minor changes in theophylline kinetics include fleroxacin, flosequinan, lomefloxacin (*Maxaquin*), ofloxacin (*Floxin*), rufloxacin, sparfloxacin (*Zagam*), and temafloxacin.

➡ **Monitor.** Monitor patients maintained on theophylline for increased serum theophylline concentrations and signs of toxicity (eg, palpitations, tachycardia, nausea, tremor) during coadministration of ciprofloxacin.

REFERENCES:

1. Nix DE, et al. Effect of multiple dose oral ciprofloxacin on the pharmacokinetics of theophylline and indocyanine green. *J Antimicrob Chemother*. 1987;19:263.

2. Wijnands WJA, et al. The influence of quinolone derivatives on theophylline clearance. *Br J Clin Pharmacol*. 1986;22:677.

3. Schwartz J, et al. Impact of ciprofloxacin on theophylline clearance and steady-state concentrations in serum. *Antimicrob Agents Chemother*. 1988;32:75.

4. Bachmann KA, et al. Predicting the ciprofloxacin-theophylline interaction from single plasma theophylline measurements. *Br J Clin Pharmacol*. 1988;26:191.

5. Prince RA, et al. Effect of quinolone antimicrobials on theophylline pharmacokinetics. *J Clin Pharmacol*. 1989;29:650.

6. Karki SD, et al. Seizure with ciprofloxacin and theophylline combined therapy. *DICP, Ann Pharmacother*. 1990;24:595.

7. Wijnands WJA, et al. Steady-state kinetics of the quinolone derivatives ofloxacin, enoxacin, ciprofloxacin, and pefloxacin during maintenance treatment with theophylline. *Drugs*. 1987;34(Suppl. 1):159.

8. Loi CM, et al. Individual and combined effects of cimetidine and ciprofloxacin on theophylline metabolism in male nonsmokers. *Br J Clin Pharmacol*. 1993;36:195.

9. Bader MB. Role of ciprofloxacin in fatal seizures. *Chest*. 1992;101:883.

10. Batty KT, et al. The effect of ciprofloxacin on theophylline pharmacokinetics in healthy subjects. *Br J Clin Pharmacol*. 1995;39:305.

Ciprofloxacin (eg, *Cipro*)

Tizanidine (eg, *Zanaflex*)

SUMMARY: Ciprofloxacin markedly increases tizanidine concentrations; expect increased side effects.

RISK FACTORS: No specific risk factors are known.

MECHANISM: Ciprofloxacin inhibits the CYP1A2 metabolism of tizanidine.

CLINICAL EVALUATION: Ten healthy subjects were administered ciprofloxacin 500 mg or placebo twice daily for 3 days.[1] On day 3, a single dose of tizanidine 4 mg was administered. Ciprofloxacin increased the mean area under the concentration-time curve of tizanidine 10-fold. Peak tizanidine concentrations increased 7-fold. These changes in pharmacokinetics were accompanied by increased hypotensive and sedative effects. Given the severity of the interaction, consider the administration of ciprofloxacin (and all potent CYP1A2 inhibitors) as contraindicated with tizanidine.[2]

RELATED DRUGS: None known.

MANAGEMENT OPTIONS:

➡ *Use Alternative.* Use other fluoroquinolones with minimal effects on CYP1A2, including gatifloxacin (*Tequin*), levofloxacin (*Levaquin*), lomefloxacin (*Maxaquin*), moxifloxacin (*Avelox*), and ofloxacin (eg, *Floxin*), instead of ciprofloxacin in patients receiving tizanidine.

➡ *Monitor.* If the combination is used, monitor for hypotension and excessive CNS depression.

REFERENCES:

1. Granfors MT, et al. Ciprofloxacin greatly increases concentrations and hypotensive effect of tizanidine by inhibiting its cytochrome P450 1A2-mediated presystemic metabolism. *Clin Pharmacol Ther*. 2004;76:598-606.
2. *Cipro* [package insert]. West Haven, CT: Bayer Health Care; 2005.

Ciprofloxacin (*Cipro*)

Warfarin (eg, *Coumadin*)

SUMMARY: Several cases of enhanced hypoprothrombinemic responses to warfarin have been associated with ciprofloxacin administration, but prospective trials have not supported this observation.

RISK FACTORS:

➡ *Concurrent Diseases.* Fever may enhance the catabolism of clotting factors thus enhancing the oral anticoagulant effect.

MECHANISM: Not established. Ciprofloxacin is known to inhibit the metabolism of some drugs. Fever also may enhance the catabolism of clotting factors;[7] thus, the infection for which ciprofloxacin is used could theoretically enhance the effect of the oral anticoagulant. This effect should dissipate as ciprofloxacin lowers the fever.

CLINICAL EVALUATION: Several cases of possible ciprofloxacin-induced increases in warfarin response have been reported,[1-5,8] and additional unproved cases of marked increases in warfarin response associated with ciprofloxacin have been reported to the manufacturer of ciprofloxacin.[1] Conversely, ciprofloxacin 500 mg twice daily for 7 days did not affect the hypoprothrombinemic response in 9 men on low intensity chronic warfarin therapy,[6] nor did 10 days of ciprofloxacin change INR values in other patients.[9] Thus the evidence supporting an interaction between warfarin and ciprofloxacin is not consistent. Until further information is available, consider patients taking warfarin and ciprofloxacin at some increased risk of hypoprothrombinemia.

RELATED DRUGS: Norfloxacin (*Noroxin*) and ofloxacin (*Floxin*) have been noted to increase INRs in a few case reports.

MANAGEMENT OPTIONS:

➠ **Consider Alternative.** Consider using an antibiotic other than ciprofloxacin to avoid the potential interaction.

➠ **Monitor.** In patients receiving oral anticoagulants, monitor for altered hypoprothrombinemic response when ciprofloxacin is initiated or discontinued and adjust the anticoagulant dose as needed.

REFERENCES:

1. Kamada AK. Possible interaction between ciprofloxacin and warfarin. *DICP, Ann Pharmacother.* 1990;24:27.
2. Mott FE, et al. Ciprofloxacin and warfarin. *Ann Intern Med.* 1989;111:542.
3. Renzi R, et al. Ciprofloxacin interaction with sodium warfarin: a potentially dangerous side effect. *Am J Emerg Med.* 1991;9:551.
4. Dugoni-Kramer BM. Ciprofloxacin-warfarin interaction. *DICP, Ann Pharmacother.* 1991;25:1397.
5. Johnson KC, et al. Drug interaction. *J Fam Pract.* 1991;33:338.
6. Rindone JP, et al. Hypoprothrombinemic effect of warfarin not influenced by ciprofloxacin. *Clin Pharm.* 1991;10:136.
7. Loclinger EA, et al. The biological disappearance rate of prothrombin and factors VII, IX and X from plasma in hypothyroidism, hyperthyroidism and during fever. *Thromb Diath Haemorrh.* 1964;10:267.
8. Linville D, et al. Ciprofloxacin and warfarin interaction. *Am J Med.* 1991;90:765.

Ciprofloxacin (*Cipro*)

Zinc

SUMMARY: The administration of multivitamins with zinc may reduce the serum concentration of ciprofloxacin; however the clinical significance appears to be minimal.

RISK FACTORS: No specific risk factors are known.

MECHANISM: Zinc appears to inhibit the absorption of ciprofloxacin by binding to it in the GI tract.

CLINICAL EVALUATION: A single 500 mg dose of ciprofloxacin was administered alone and following the daily administration of 1 multivitamin tablet containing 23.9 mg of zinc (*Stresstabs 600 with Zinc*) for 7 days. The apparent oral absorption of ciprofloxacin was reduced 24% when it was taken following the multivitamin-zinc tablet.[1]

RELATED DRUGS: The absorption of other quinolones (eg, norfloxacin [*Noroxin*], enoxacin [*Penetrex*]) is likely to be reduced by zinc.

MANAGEMENT OPTIONS:

➡ *Circumvent/Minimize.* Patients taking ciprofloxacin, and probably other quinolone antibiotics, should avoid the coadministration of oral multivitamins containing zinc. If the drugs are used together, administer the ciprofloxacin 2 hours or mroe before the zinc.

➡ *Monitor.* Watch for antibiotic failure when zinc and a quinolone are coadministered.

REFERENCES:

1. Polk RE, et al. Effect of ferrous sulfate and multivitamins with zinc on absorption of ciprofloxacin in normal volunteers. *Antimicrob Agents Chemother.* 1989;33:1841.

Cisapride[†] (eg, *Propulsid*)

Clarithromycin (*Biaxin*)

SUMMARY: Clarithromycin may increase cisapride concentrations leading to toxicity including cardiac arrhythmias.

RISK FACTORS:

➡ *Concurrent Diseases.* Preexisting cardiovascular disease or an electrolyte imbalance may increase the risk of the interaction.

MECHANISM: Cisapride is metabolized by the hepatic enzyme CYP3A4. It appears that clarithromycin inhibits the metabolism of cisapride in vitro. This could increase cisapride's bioavailability and reduce its clearance resulting in higher serum cisapride concentrations.

CLINICAL EVALUATION: Several patients have developed QT prolongation and ventricular arrhythmias, including torsades de pointes, while receiving cisapride in combination with other drugs.[1] Details of these cases including drug dosages, underlying diseases, and concomitant drugs have not been released, but most were chronically ill and had additional risk factors for arrhythmias. The results of a study in healthy subjects indicate that ketoconazole can increase cisapride concentrations which may lead to prolonged QT intervals.[1] Clarithromycin appears to inhibit the metabolism of cisapride in vitro. The incidence and clinical significance of these effects are unknown.

RELATED DRUGS: Ketoconazole (eg, *Nizoral*) can increase cisapride concentrations. Troleandomycin (*TAO*) and erythromycin (eg, *E-Mycin*) also may inhibit cisapride metabolism. Azithromycin (*Zithromax*) and dirithromycin (*Dynabac*) would not be expected to inhibit cisapride metabolism.

MANAGEMENT OPTIONS:

➡ *Avoid Unless Benefit Outweighs Risk.* Patients who are receiving cisapride and require clarithromycin should have their cisapride temporarily discontinued. Metoclopramide (eg, *Reglan*) or an H_2-receptor antagonist could be considered as a substitute for cisapride.

➡ *Monitor.* If cisapride is used with clarithromycin, monitor patient for arrhythmias and prolonged QT intervals.

REFERENCES:

1. Product information. Cisapride (*Propulsid*). Janssen Pharmaceutica. 1995.

† Available only through an investigational limited access program.

5 Cisapride†

Digoxin (eg, *Lanoxin*)

SUMMARY: Cisapride administration has no significant effect on plasma digoxin concentrations.

RISK FACTORS: No specific risk factors are known.

MECHANISM: Cisapride increases GI motility which might reduce the time for digoxin absorption or alter its dissolution.

CLINICAL EVALUATION: Six healthy subjects received digoxin 0.5 mg twice daily orally for 3 days followed by 0.25 mg twice daily alone or with concomitant cisapride 10 mg 3 times daily.[1] No changes in digoxin pharmacokinetics were noted except for an insignificant decrease in the area under the concentration-time curve of digoxin (12%).

RELATED DRUGS: Metoclopramide (eg, *Reglan*) has been reported to reduce the bioavailability of digoxin tablets approximately 20%.[1,2]

MANAGEMENT OPTIONS: No interaction.

REFERENCES:

1. Kirch W, et al. Effect of cisapride and metoclopramide on digoxin bioavailability. *Eur J Drug Metab Pharmacokinet.* 1986;11:249.

2. Johnson BF, et al. Effect of metoclopramide on digoxin absorption from tablets and capsules. *Clin Pharmacol Ther.* 1984;36:724.

† Available only through an investigational limited access program.

4 Cisapride†

Disopyramide (eg, *Norpace*)

SUMMARY: Cisapride increases the gastric emptying in patients taking disopyramide.

RISK FACTORS: No specific risk factors are known.

MECHANISM: Disopyramide slows gastric emptying because of its anticholinergic effects. Cisapride is a prokinetic agent that increases gastric emptying by releasing acetylcholine from the myenteric plexus in the stomach.

CLINICAL EVALUATION: Twenty patients with arrhythmias who were taking disopyramide 100 mg 3 times daily were administered a gastric emptying test before and after cisapride 2.5 mg 3 times daily was administered with disopyramide for 7 days.[1] Gastric emptying was increased and the serum concentration of disopyramide 2 hours after a dose was significantly higher when coadministered with cisapride. The absorption rate constant of disopyramide nearly doubled following cisapride administration. Disopyramide area under the plasma concentration-time curve and half-life were not changed by cisapride administration.[1] This interaction may be beneficial in patients who suffer from delayed gastric emptying secondary to disopyramide.

RELATED DRUGS: Metoclopramide (eg, *Reglan*) may affect disopyramide in a similar manner.

MANAGEMENT OPTIONS: No specific action is required, but be alert for evidence of the interaction.

REFERENCES:

1. Kuroda T, et al. Effects of cisapride on gastrointestinal motor activity and gastric emptying of disopyramide. *J Pharmacobiodyn*. 1992;15:395.

† Available only through an investigational limited access program.

Cisapride† (eg, *Propulsid*)

Erythromycin (eg, *E-Mycin*)

SUMMARY: Erythromycin may increase cisapride concentrations leading to toxicity including cardiac arrhythmias.

RISK FACTORS:

➡ **Concurrent Diseases.** Preexisting cardiovascular disease or electrolyte imbalance may increase the risk of the interaction.

MECHANISM: Cisapride is metabolized by the hepatic enzyme CYP3A4. It appears that erythromycin inhibits the metabolism of cisapride in vitro. This could increase cisapride's bioavailability and reduce its clearance resulting in higher serum concentrations.

CLINICAL EVALUATION: Several patients have developed QT prolongation and ventricular arrhythmias, including torsades de pointes, while receiving cisapride in combination with other drugs.[1] Details of these cases including drug dosages, underlying diseases, and concomitant drugs have not been released, but most patients were chronically ill and had additional risk factors for arrhythmias. The results of a study in healthy subjects indicate that ketoconazole can increase cisapride concentrations, which may lead to prolonged QT intervals.[1] Erythromycin appears to inhibit the metabolism of cisapride in vitro. The incidence and clinical significance of these effects are unknown.

RELATED DRUGS: Ketoconazole (eg, *Nizoral*) can increase cisapride concentrations. Troleandomycin (*TAO*) and clarithromycin (*Biaxin*) also may inhibit cisapride metabolism.

MANAGEMENT OPTIONS:

➡ **Avoid Unless Benefit Outweighs Risk.** Patients who are receiving cisapride and require erythromycin should have their cisapride temporarily discontinued. Consider metoclopramide (eg, *Reglan*) or an H_2-receptor antagonist as a substitute for cisapride.

➡ **Monitor.** If cisapride is used with erythromycin, monitor patient for arrhythmias and prolonged QT intervals.

REFERENCES:

1. Product information. Cisapride (*Propulsid*). Janssen Pharmaceutica. 1998.

† Available only through an investigational limited access program.

Cisapride† (*Propulsid*)

Grapefruit Juice

SUMMARY: A single glass of grapefruit juice moderately increased cisapride plasma concentrations; although the risk of this combination is not known, grapefruit juice would be best avoided in patients on cisapride.

RISK FACTORS: No specific risk factors are known.

MECHANISM: Grapefruit juice probably reduces the metabolism of cisapride by CYP3A4 in the small intestine.

CLINICAL EVALUATION: In a randomized, crossover study, 12 healthy subjects received a single oral dose of cisapride 10 mg alone and with 250 mL grapefruit juice.[1] Grapefruit juice was associated with approximately 50% increase in the cisapride area under the plasma concentration-time curve, but electrocardiogram showed no increase in the QTc interval. However, note that multiple doses of grapefruit juice have been shown to have a substantially greater inhibitory effect on CYP3A4 than single doses. Thus, larger amounts of grapefruit juice may result in clinically important increases in cisapride plasma concentrations, with the possibility of ventricular arrhythmias (eg, torsades de pointes).

RELATED DRUGS: No information is available.

MANAGEMENT OPTIONS:

➡ ***Use Alternative.*** Orange juice is unlikely to interact with cisapride.

➡ ***Monitor.*** If grapefruit juice is used in a patient on cisapride, monitor for cardiac arrhythmias and prolonged QT intervals.

REFERENCES:
1. Offman EM, et al. Red wine-cisapride interaction: comparison with grapefruit juice. *Clin Pharmacol Ther.* 2001;70:17.

† Available only through an investigational limited access program.

 Cisapride† (eg, *Propulsid*)

Indinavir (*Crixivan*)

SUMMARY: Indinavir is likely to increase cisapride serum concentrations potentially resulting in adverse effects including cardiac arrhythmias. Until further information is available, avoid the concomitant use of indinavir and cisapride.

RISK FACTORS: No specific risk factors are known.

MECHANISM: Indinavir is known to inhibit the activity of CYP3A4, the enzyme responsible for the metabolism of cisapride. Cisapride accumulation can result in cardiac effects (prolonged QTc intervals) and arrhythmias.

CLINICAL EVALUATION: While no published data are available for evaluation, the manufacturer of cisapride has made available some information on this interaction. Indinavir is known to inhibit the metabolism of other CYP3A4 substrates and it is likely that cisapride would be similarly affected. Until specific studies defining the magnitude of this potential interaction are available, avoid the coadministration of cisapride and indinavir.[1]

RELATED DRUGS: Ritonavir (*Norvir*) would be likely to inhibit the metabolism of cisapride in a similar manner. Delavirdine (*Rescriptor*) is a CYP3A4 inhibitor and also may affect cisapride's metabolism. While no data are available, other antiviral agents such as saquinavir (*Fortovase*) or famciclovir (*Valtrex*) may be less likely to interact with cisapride. The metabolism of metoclopramide (eg, *Reglan*) would be unlikely to be affected by indinavir coadministration.

MANAGEMENT OPTIONS:

➡ *Use Alternative.* Avoid the combination of indinavir and cisapride because of the risk of a possibly serious arrhythmia. Nonintegrated alternatives are available and consider in patients requiring a prokinetic agent and an antiviral agent.

REFERENCES:

1. Product information. Cisapride (*Propulsid*). Janssen Pharmaceutica. 1998.

† Available only through an investigational limited access program.

Cisapride† (eg, *Propulsid*)

Itraconazole (*Sporanox*)

SUMMARY: Itraconazole may increase cisapride concentrations and lead to toxicity including arrhythmias.

RISK FACTORS:

➡ *Concurrent Diseases.* Preexisting cardiovascular disease or electrolyte imbalance may increase the risk of the interaction.

MECHANISM: Cisapride is metabolized by the hepatic enzyme CYP3A4. It appears that itraconazole inhibits the metabolism of cisapride in vitro. This could increase cisapride's bioavailability and reduce its clearance.

CLINICAL EVALUATION: Several patients have developed QT prolongation and ventricular arrhythmias, including torsades de pointes, while receiving cisapride in combination with other drugs.[1] Details of these cases including drug dosages, underlying diseases, and concomitant drugs have not been released, but most patients were chronically ill and had additional risk factors for arrhythmias. Itraconazole appears to inhibit the metabolism of cisapride in vitro. The incidence and clinical significance of these effects are unknown.

RELATED DRUGS: In vitro studies have shown ketoconazole (eg, *Nizoral*) and miconazole could interact with cisapride in a similar manner. Fluconazole (*Diflucan*) appears to produce less in vitro inhibition, but caution is warranted if this agent is administered (especially at high doses) with cisapride, particularly in patients with other risk factors for arrhythmias (eg, hypokalemia, cardiovascular disease, antiarrhythmic drug therapy). Itraconazole would not be expected to alter the elimination of metoclopramide (eg, *Reglan*).

MANAGEMENT OPTIONS:

➡ *Avoid Unless Benefit Outweighs Risk.* Patients who are receiving cisapride and require itraconazole should have their cisapride temporarily discontinued. The use of H_2-receptor antagonists or proton pump inhibitors is not recommended because they reduce the absorption of oral antifungal agents. Metoclopramide therapy could be considered as a substitute for cisapride.

➡ **Monitor.** Pending further information on this interaction, the manufacturer recommends avoiding the concomitant use of itraconazole and cisapride. If they are coadministered, monitor patients carefully for arrhythmias and prolonged QT intervals.

REFERENCES:

1. Product information. Cisapride (*Propulsid*). Janssen Pharmaceutica. 1998.

† Available only through an investigational limited access program.

 Cisapride†

Ketoconazole (eg, *Nizoral*)

SUMMARY: Ketoconazole increases cisapride concentrations and may lead to toxicity, including arrhythmias.

RISK FACTORS:

➡ **Concurrent Diseases.** Pre-existing cardiovascular disease or electrolyte imbalance may increase the risk of the interaction.

MECHANISM: Cisapride is metabolized by the hepatic enzyme CYP3A4. It appears that ketoconazole inhibits the metabolism of cisapride, probably increasing its bioavailability and reducing its clearance.

CLINICAL EVALUATION: Several patients developed QT prolongation and ventricular arrhythmias, including torsades de pointes, during cisapride and ketoconazole administration.[1] Details of these cases including drug dosages, underlying diseases, and concomitant drugs have not been published. The results of a study in healthy subjects indicate that ketoconazole can increase cisapride concentrations and may lead to prolonged QT intervals.[1] The effects of coadministration on cisapride's GI effects are unknown.

RELATED DRUGS: Other antifungal inhibitors of CYP3A4 (eg, itraconazole [*Sporanox*], fluconazole [*Diflucan*], miconazole) are likely to increase cisapride concentrations. Ketoconazole would not be expected to alter the elimination of metoclopramide (eg, *Reglan*).

MANAGEMENT OPTIONS:

➡ **Avoid Unless Benefit Outweighs Risk.** Until further information on this interaction is available, the manufacturer recommends avoiding the concomitant use of ketoconazole and cisapride. The use of H_2-receptor antagonists or proton pump inhibitors (omeprazole [*Prilosec*], lansoprazole [*Prevacid*]) is not recommended because they may reduce the absorption of some oral antifungal agents. Metoclopramide therapy could be considered as a substitute for cisapride.

➡ **Monitor.** Monitor patients who are receiving cisapride, particularly in patients with other risk factors for arrhythmias, and require ketoconazole for arrhythmias and prolonged QT intervals.

REFERENCES:

1. Product Information. Cisapride (*Propulsid*). Janssen Pharmaceutica. 1998.

† Available only through an investigational limited access program.

Cisapride†

Mibefradil (*Posicor*)

SUMMARY: Mibefradil is likely to increase cisapride serum concentrations, potentially resulting in adverse effects including cardiac arrhythmias. Pending further information on this interaction, avoid the concomitant use of mibefradil and cisapride.

RISK FACTORS: No specific risk factors are known.

MECHANISM: Mibefradil is known to inhibit the activity of CYP3A4, the enzyme responsible for the metabolism of cisapride. Cisapride accumulation can result in cardiac effects (prolonged QTc intervals) and arrhythmias.

CLINICAL EVALUATION: While no published data are available for evaluation, the manufacturer of mibefradil has made available some information on this interaction.[1] Mibefradil is known to inhibit the metabolism of other CYP3A4 substrates (eg, terfenadine) and it is likely that cisapride would be similarly affected. Until specific studies defining the magnitude of this potential interaction are available, avoid the coadministration of cisapride and mibefradil.

RELATED DRUGS: Other calcium channel blockers (eg, amlodipine [*Norvasc*], nifedipine [eg, *Procardia*], nicardipine [eg, *Cardene*]) would not be expected to change cisapride plasma concentrations. The metabolism of metoclopramide (eg, *Reglan*) would be unlikely to be affected by mibefradil coadministration.

MANAGEMENT OPTIONS:

➡ ***Use Alternative.*** Avoid the combination of mibefradil and cisapride because of a possibly serious arrhythmia. Noninteracting alternatives are available and consider in patients requiring a prokinetic agent and a calcium channel blocker.

REFERENCES:

1. Product information. Mibefradil (*Posicor*). Roche Laboratories, Inc. 1997.

† Available only through an investigational limited access program.

Cisapride†

Miconazole

SUMMARY: IV miconazole may increase cisapride concentrations and lead to toxicity including arrhythmias.

RISK FACTORS:

➡ ***Concurrent Diseases.*** Preexisting cardiovascular disease or electrolyte imbalance may increase the risk of the interaction.

MECHANISM: Cisapride is metabolized by the hepatic enzyme CYP3A4. It appears that miconazole inhibits the metabolism of cisapride in vitro. This could increase cisapride's bioavailability and reduce its clearance.

CLINICAL EVALUATION: Several patients have developed QT prolongation and ventricular arrhythmias, including torsades de pointes, while receiving cisapride in combination with other drugs.[1] Details of these cases including drug dosages, underlying diseases, and concomitant drugs have not been released, but most were chronically ill and had additional risk factors for arrhythmias. The results of a study in healthy subjects indicate that ketoconazole can increase cisapride concentrations which may lead to prolonged QT intervals.[1] Itraconazole appears to inhibit the metabolism of cisapride in vitro. The incidence and clinical significance of these effects are unknown.

RELATED DRUGS: Other antifungal agents that inhibit CYP3A4 (eg, ketoconazole [eg, *Nizoral*], itraconazole [*Sporanox*], fluconazole [*Diflucan*]) are likely to increase cisapride concentrations. Miconazole would not be expected to alter the elimination of metoclopramide (eg, *Reglan*).

MANAGEMENT OPTIONS:

➡ *Avoid Unless Benefit Outweighs Risk.* Until further information on this interaction is available, the manufacturer recommends avoiding the concomitant use of miconazole and cisapride. Patients who are receiving cisapride and require miconazole should have their cisapride temporarily discontinued. Metoclopramide therapy could be considered as a substitute for cisapride.

➡ *Monitor.* If a patient requires both cisapride and miconazole, monitor for cardiac arrhythmias and prolonged QT intervals.

REFERENCES:

1. Product information. Cisapride (*Propulsid*). Janssen Pharmaceutica. 1998.

† Available only through an investigational limited access program.

 Cisapride†

Nefazodone (*Serzone*)

SUMMARY: Nefazodone is likely to increase cisapride serum concentrations potentially resulting in adverse effects including cardiac arrhythmias. Until further information is available, avoid the concomitant use of nefazodone and cisapride.

RISK FACTORS: No specific risk factors are known.

MECHANISM: Nefazodone is known to inhibit the activity of CYP3A4, the enzyme responsible for the metabolism of cisapride. Cisapride accumulation can result in cardiac effects (prolonged QTc intervals) and arrhythmias.

CLINICAL EVALUATION: While no published data are available for evaluation, the manufacturer of cisapride has made available some information on this interaction. Nefazodone is known to inhibit the metabolism of other CYP3A4 substrates and it is likely that cisapride would be similarly affected. Until specific studies defining the magnitude of this potential interaction are available, avoid the coadministration of cisapride and nefazodone.[1]

RELATED DRUGS: While no data are available, other antidepressants including fluoxetine (*Prozac*), paroxetine (*Paxil*), and sertraline (*Zoloft*) would not be likely to affect the metabolism of cisapride. The metabolism of metoclopramide (eg, *Reglan*) would be unlikely to be affected by concomitant nefazodone administration.

MANAGEMENT OPTIONS:

➡ *Use Alternative.* Because of the risk of a possibly serious arrhythmia, avoid the combination of nefazodone and cisapride. Noninteracting alternatives are available and should be considered in patients requiring a prokinetic agent and an antidepressant.

REFERENCES:

1. Product information. Cisapride (*Propulsid*). Janssen Pharmaceutica. 1998.

† Available only through an investigational limited access program.

Cisapride†

Ritonavir (*Norvir*)

SUMMARY: Ritonavir is likely to increase cisapride serum concentrations, potentially resulting in adverse effects including cardiac arrhythmias. Until further information is available, avoid the concomitant use of ritonavir and cisapride.

RISK FACTORS: No specific risk factors are known.

MECHANISM: Ritonavir is known to inhibit the activity of CYP3A4, the enzyme responsible for the metabolism of cisapride. Cisapride accumulation can result in cardiac effects (prolonged QTc intervals) and arrhythmias.

CLINICAL EVALUATION: While no published data are available for evaluation, the manufacturer of cisapride has made available some information on this interaction. Ritonavir is known to inhibit the metabolism of other CYP3A4 substrates and it is likely that cisapride would be similarly affected. Until specific studies defining the magnitude of this potential interaction are available, avoid the coadministration of cisapride and ritonavir.[1]

RELATED DRUGS: Indinavir (*Crixivan*) may inhibit the metabolism of cisapride in a similar manner. Delavirdine (*Rescriptor*) is a CYP3A4 inhibitor and also may affect cisapride's metabolism. While no data are available, other antiviral agents such as saquinavir (eg, *Fortovase*) or famciclovir (*Valtrex*) may be less likely to interact with cisapride. The metabolism of metoclopramide (eg, *Reglan*) is unlikely to be affected by ritonavir coadministration.

MANAGEMENT OPTIONS:

➥ **Use Alternative.** Because of the risk of a possibly serious arrhythmia, avoid the combination of ritonavir and cisapride. Consider noninteracting alternatives in patients requiring a prokinetic agent and an antiviral agent.

REFERENCES:

1. *Propulsid* [package insert]. Titusville, NJ: Janssen Pharmaceutica; 1998.

† Available only through an investigational limited access program.

Cisapride†

Sertraline (*Zoloft*)

SUMMARY: Sertraline reduced cisapride plasma concentrations in healthy subjects; monitor for reduced cisapride response.

RISK FACTORS: No specific risk factors are known.

MECHANISM: Not established. It is possible that sertraline acts as a mild enzyme inducer and increases cisapride metabolism.

CLINICAL EVALUATION: In 15 healthy subjects given cisapride and sertraline concomitantly for about a month, sertraline was associated with about a 36% reduction in cisapride area under the plasma concentration-time curve.[1] The clinical importance of this interaction is not known, but theoretically it may reduce cisapride's efficacy.

RELATED DRUGS: Fluoxetine (eg, *Prozac*) 20 mg/day also has been reported to reduce cisapride plasma concentrations in healthy subjects.[2]

MANAGEMENT OPTIONS:

➡ *Monitor.* Monitor for reduced cisapride efficacy in patients who receive sertraline concomitantly.

REFERENCES:

1. Alderman J. Coadministration of sertraline with cisapride or pimozide: an open-label, nonrandomized examination of pharmacokinetics and corrected QT intervals in healthy adult volunteers. *Clin Ther.* 2005;27:1050-1063.

2. Zhao Q, et al. Influence of coadministration of fluoxetine on cisapride pharmacokinetics and QTc intervals in healthy volunteers. *Pharmacotherapy.* 2001;21:149-157.

† Available only through an investigational limited access program.

 Cisapride†

Simvastatin (*Zocor*)

SUMMARY: In healthy subjects, simvastatin slightly increased cisapride plasma concentrations and cisapride moderately decreased simvastatin acid plasma concentrations; the clinical importance of these changes is not established.

RISK FACTORS: No specific risk factors are known.

MECHANISM: Not established.

CLINICAL EVALUATION: Eleven healthy subjects were given cisapride 10 mg every 8 hours and simvastatin 20 mg every 12 hours alone and together, each regimen lasting 3 to 4 days.[1] Simvastatin slightly increased cisapride plasma concentrations 14%, and cisapride moderately decreased simvastatin acid plasma concentrations 33%. The clinical importance of the increase in cisapride concentration is probably minimal in most patients, but it is possible that a rare predisposed patient would have an adverse consequence. One of the subjects developed a 50% increase in cisapride plasma concentrations following simvastatin. The reduced simvastatin acid concentrations could decrease the cholesterol-lowering effects of simvastatin somewhat, but this likely could be counteracted by increases in the simvastatin dose or use of a statin that may be less likely to interact. Additional information from chronic administration of the 2 drugs is needed to determine the clinical importance of the interaction.

RELATED DRUGS: Theoretically, pravastatin (*Pravachol*) and fluvastatin (*Lescol*) are less likely to increase cisapride plasma concentrations, but clinical data are lacking. Lovastatin (eg, *Mevacor*) has drug interactions similar to simvastatin and can be expected to interact similarly with cisapride.

MANAGEMENT OPTIONS:

➡ *Consider Alternative.* Consider using an alternative to 1 of the drugs (see Related Drugs).

➡ *Monitor.* In patients receiving both drugs, monitor for a reduced cholesterol-lowering effect of simvastatin and for evidence of cisapride toxicity (eg, syncope, palpitations).

REFERENCES:

1. Simard C, et al. Study of the drug-drug interaction between simvastatin and cisapride in man. *Eur J Clin Pharmacol.* 2001;57:229-234.

† Available only through an investigational limited access program.

Cisapride†

Sparfloxacin (*Zagam*)

SUMMARY: Cisapride produced a small increase in the peak sparfloxacin concentration; however, no adverse effects were noted.

RISK FACTORS: No specific risk factors are known.

MECHANISM: Cisapride increases gastric motility, resulting in a more rapid delivery of sparfloxacin to the small bowel and an increase in the peak sparfloxacin plasma concentration.

CLINICAL EVALUATION: Fifteen healthy subjects received sparfloxacin 400 mg as a single oral dose alone and after 4 days of cisapride 10 mg 3 times daily.[1] Compared with sparfloxacin alone, administration with cisapride resulted in a 37% increase in the mean peak sparfloxacin concentration. The area under the plasma concentration-time curve, half-life, and clearance of sparfloxacin were not altered by cisapride. However, the mean time to peak sparfloxacin concentration was reduced from 4.1 to 1.9 hours after cisapride pretreatment. The electrocardiogram revealed that the QTc interval increased 7.7% during concurrent sparfloxacin and cisapride dosing compared with the QTc interval before any medications were given. No patient developed an arrhythmia. The effect of cisapride and sparfloxacin on the QTc when each drug was administered alone was not determined. Nevertheless, the small increase in QTc would not be likely to produce an arrhythmia in patients with normal cardiac conduction.

RELATED DRUGS: Metoclopramide (eg, *Reglan*) may produce a similar change in the absorption rate of sparfloxacin.

MANAGEMENT OPTIONS: No specific action is required, but be alert for evidence of the interaction.

REFERENCES:

1. Zix JA. Pharmacokinetics of sparfloxacin and interaction with cisapride and sucralfate. *Antimicrob Agents Chemother.* 1997;41:1668-1672.

† Available only through an investigational limited access program.

2   Cisapride[†]

Troleandomycin

SUMMARY: Troleandomycin may increase cisapride concentrations and lead to toxicity, including arrhythmias.

RISK FACTORS:

➡ **Concurrent Diseases.** Preexisting cardiovascular disease or electrolyte imbalance may increase the risk of the interaction.

MECHANISM: Cisapride is metabolized by the hepatic enzyme CYP3A4. Troleandomycin appears to inhibit the metabolism of cisapride in vitro. This could increase cisapride's bioavailability and reduce its clearance.

CLINICAL EVALUATION: Several patients developed QT prolongation and ventricular arrhythmias, including torsades de pointes, while receiving cisapride in combination with other drugs.[1] Details of these cases including drug dosages, underlying diseases, and concomitant drugs have not been released, but most patients were chronically ill and had risk factors for arrhythmias. The incidence and clinical significance of this interaction are unknown.

RELATED DRUGS: Erythromycin (eg, *Ery-Tab*) and clarithromycin (eg, *Biaxin*) also may inhibit cisapride metabolism.

MANAGEMENT OPTIONS:

➡ **Avoid Unless Benefit Outweighs Risk.** Temporarily discontinue cisapride in patients who are receiving cisapride and require troleandomycin. Consider metoclopramide (eg, *Reglan*) or an H_2-receptor antagonist as a substitute for cisapride. Azithromycin (eg, *Zithromax*) may be substituted for troleandomycin.

➡ **Monitor.** If cisapride is used with troleandomycin, monitor patients for arrhythmias and prolonged QT intervals.

REFERENCES:

1. *Propulsid* [package insert]. Titusville, NJ: Janssen Pharmaceutica; 1998.

† Available only through an investigational limited access program.

4   Cisapride[†]

Warfarin (eg, *Coumadin*)

SUMMARY: Isolated cases of an increased hypoprothrombinemic response to warfarin during cisapride therapy have been reported, but a causal relationship has not been established.

RISK FACTORS: No specific risk factors are known.

MECHANISM: Not established. The cytochrome P450 isozyme most important in the metabolism of S-warfarin is CYP2C9, but cisapride is not known to affect this enzyme.

CLINICAL EVALUATION: A 75-year-old man stabilized on warfarin 4 mg/day developed an increase in international normalized ratio (INR) from approximately 2.4 to 10.7 within 3 weeks after replacing metoclopramide therapy with cisapride.[1] It does not appear likely that discontinuation of the metoclopramide produced this effect, and other factors that may have affected the INR response were not present. The manufacturer of cisapride has received some case reports of increased oral antico-agulant response purportedly caused by cisapride, but details were not given.[2] Thus, the evidence to support an interaction between warfarin and cisapride is meager, but the possibility that an occasional patient is susceptible to an increased warfarin response cannot rule out.

RELATED DRUGS: The effect of cisapride on oral anticoagulants other than warfarin is not established.

MANAGEMENT OPTIONS: No specific action is required, but be alert for evidence of the interaction.

REFERENCES:

1. Darlington MR. Hypoprothrombinemia induced by warfarin sodium and cisapride. *Am J Health Syst Pharm.* 1997;54:320.

2. *Propulsid* [package insert]. Titusville, NJ: Janssen Pharmaceutica; 1998.

† Available only through an investigational limited access program.

Cisapride†

Wine

SUMMARY: A single glass of red wine had a minimal effect on cisapride plasma concentrations.

RISK FACTORS: No specific risk factors are known.

MECHANISM: Red wine may slightly reduce the metabolism of cisapride by CYP3A4 in the intestine.

CLINICAL EVALUATION: In a randomized, crossover study, 12 healthy subjects received a single oral dose of cisapride 10 mg alone and with 250 mL red wine (eg, cabernet sauvignon).[1] The wine was associated with a slight increase in the cisapride area under the plasma concentration-time curve (AUC), but the changes were not clinically significant. One person had a doubling of cisapride AUC with red wine, but it is not certain that the wine caused the change.

RELATED DRUGS: No information is available.

MANAGEMENT OPTIONS: No specific action is required, but be alert for evidence of the interaction.

REFERENCES:

1. Offman EM, et al. Red wine-cisapride interaction: comparison with grapefruit juice. *Clin Pharmacol Ther.* 2001;70:17-23.

† Available only through an investigational limited access program.

Cisplatin (eg, *Platinol-AQ*)

Diazoxide (*Hyperstat*)

SUMMARY: A patient developed nephrotoxicity following combined use of cisplatin and a potent combination of anti-hypertensive drugs, but a causal relationship was not established.

RISK FACTORS: No specific risk factors are known.

MECHANISM: Not established. Aggressive antihypertensive therapy may alter renal hemodynamics, resulting in increased nephrotoxic effect of cisplatin.

CLINICAL EVALUATION: A 58-year-old man with normal renal function developed severe hypertension 3 hours after receiving IV cisplatin 70 mg/m^2 body surface area.[1] The patient suffered severe nausea and vomiting, and his blood pressure increased to 248/140 mm Hg. Treatment with furosemide (eg, *Lasix*) 40 mg IV, hydralazine (eg, *Apresoline*) 10 mg IM, diazoxide 300 mg IV, and propranolol (eg, *Inderal*) 20 mg twice daily for 2 days decreased the blood pressure while maintaining a urine output of at least 150 mL/hr. At no time during treatment was the blood pressure less than 110/70 mm Hg. Nine days after this dose of cisplatin, the patient's renal function decreased, as evidenced by an elevated serum urea nitrogen. On 2 subsequent occasions, the use of cisplatin in the same dose again precipitated severe nausea, vomiting, and blood pressure elevation; however, antihypertensive therapy was not initiated and the renal function did not deteriorate. Although cisplatin or aggressive antihypertensive therapy can decrease renal function, this patient's renal dysfunction probably can be best explained by an interaction between these drugs. The renal function did not decrease after 2 subsequent cisplatin infusions, and the antihypertensive therapy did not result in excessive hypotension. Therefore, it is possible that aggressive antihypertensive treatment may have altered renal hemodynamics in a way that would promote cisplatin nephrotoxicity.

RELATED DRUGS: Theoretically, any potent hypotensive drug regimen could increase cisplatin or carboplatin nephrotoxicity.

MANAGEMENT OPTIONS:

➡ *Monitor.* Monitor renal function if potent antihypertensive drugs are used with cisplatin.

REFERENCES:

1. Markman M, et al. Nephrotoxicity with cisplatin and antihypertensive medications. *Ann Intern Med.* 1982;96:257.

 Cisplatin (eg, *Platinol-AQ*)

Ethacrynic Acid (*Edecrin*)

SUMMARY: Severe ototoxicity has been noted in animals given cisplatin and ethacrynic acid.

RISK FACTORS: No specific risk factors are known.

MECHANISM: Both cisplatin and ethacrynic acid can produce ototoxicity in humans when used alone. Additive ototoxicity may occur with combined use.

CLINICAL EVALUATION: Animal studies indicate that combined use of cisplatin and ethacrynic acid markedly enhances the likelihood of ototoxicity over either drug used alone.[1]

RELATED DRUGS: Furosemide (eg, *Lasix*) and bumetanide (eg, *Bumex*) appear to be less ototoxic than ethacrynic acid and might be less likely to cause ototoxicity when combined with cisplatin.

MANAGEMENT OPTIONS:

➡ *Avoid Unless Benefit Outweighs Risk.* Avoid concurrent use of ethacrynic acid and cisplatin if possible.

➡ **Monitor.** If any loop diuretic is used with cisplatin, monitor the patient carefully for ototoxicity.

REFERENCES:
1. Komune S, et al. Potentiating effects of cisplatin and ethacrynic acid in ototoxicity. *Arch Otolaryngol.* 1981;107:594-597.

Cisplatin (eg, *Platinol-AQ*)

Gentamicin (eg, *Garamycin*)

SUMMARY: Cisplatin may enhance the nephrotoxicity of aminoglycosides like gentamicin, but the clinical importance is not established.

RISK FACTORS:

➡ **Concurrent Diseases.** Renal dysfunction increases the risk of interaction.

MECHANISM: Not established.

CLINICAL EVALUATION: The combination of cisplatin and aminoglycosides may increase the risk of renal toxicity,[1] reduce the elimination of gentamicin,[2] or produce magnesium wasting.[3-5] However, a retrospective study failed to find an increase in nephrotoxicity in patients receiving cisplatin plus aminoglycosides compared with cisplatin alone.[6]

RELATED DRUGS: Other aminoglycosides may increase the risk of nephrotoxicity with cisplatin. Carboplatin may interact in a similar manner with aminoglycosides.

MANAGEMENT OPTIONS:

➡ **Consider Alternative.** Select an antibiotic other than an aminoglycoside.

➡ **Monitor.** Observe patients receiving the combination for renal dysfunction or hypomagnesemia.

REFERENCES:
1. Dentino M, et al. Long term effect of cis-diaminedichloride platinum (CDDP) on renal function and structure in man. *Cancer.* 1978;41:1274-1281.
2. Stewart CF, et al. The effect of cisplatin therapy on gentamicin pharmacokinetics. *Drug Intell Clin Pharm.* 1984;18:512.
3. Patel R, et al. Symptomatic hypomagnesemia associated with gentamicin therapy. *Nephron.* 1979;23:50-52.
4. Blachley JD, et al. Renal and electrolyte disturbances associated with cisplatin. *Ann Intern Med.* 1981;95:628-632.
5. Flombaum CD. Hypomagnesemia associated with cisplatin combination chemotherapy. *Ann Intern Med.* 1984;144:2336-2337.
6. Haas A, et al. The influence of aminoglycosides on nephrotoxicity of cis-diaminedichloroplatinum in cancer patients. *J Infect Dis.* 1983;147:363.

Cisplatin (eg, *Platinol-AQ*)

Lithium (eg, *Eskalith*)

SUMMARY: Cisplatin therapy may temporarily produce minor reductions in serum lithium concentrations; the clinical significance of this interaction is unknown but appears to be limited.

RISK FACTORS: No specific risk factors are known.

MECHANISM: Fluid loading and mannitol administration that coincides with cisplatin administration may result in a transient increase in lithium renal clearance. In addition, cisplatin-induced dysfunction of renal tubular reabsorption could lead to increased lithium excretion.

CLINICAL EVALUATION: A patient maintained on lithium 300 mg 4 times daily received cisplatin 100 mg/m², 25 g mannitol, and fluids on 2 separate occasions.[1] Her serum lithium concentrations fell from 0.8 to 1 mEq/L to 0.5 to 0.3 mEq/L over 24 to 36 hours following cisplatin administration and returned to near baseline by 48 to 72 hours. No change in clinical response to lithium therapy was noted. Another report noted no change in lithium concentrations following cisplatin 50 mg/m².[2]

RELATED DRUGS: No information is available.

MANAGEMENT OPTIONS: No specific action is required, but be alert for evidence of the interaction.

REFERENCES:
1. Pietruszka LJ, et al. Evaluation of cisplatin-lithium interaction. *Drug Intell Clin Pharm.* 1985;19:31-32.
2. Beijnen JH, et al. Effect of cisplatin-containing chemotherapy on lithium serum concentrations. *Ann Pharmacother.* 1992;26:488-490.

 Cisplatin (eg, *Platinol-AQ*)

Ondansetron (*Zofran*)

SUMMARY: Ondansetron was associated with small reductions in the plasma concentration of cisplatin in patients undergoing bone marrow transplantation, but the clinical importance of this effect is not established.

RISK FACTORS: No specific risk factors are known.

MECHANISM: Not established.

CLINICAL EVALUATION: In a group of patients undergoing bone marrow transplantation who all received high-dose cisplatin, cyclophosphamide (eg, *Cytoxan*) and carmustine (eg, *BiCNU*), 23 were give ondansetron as an antiemetic, and 129 received prochlorperazine (eg, *Compazine*).[1] In patients receiving ondansetron, the cisplatin and cyclophosphamide areas under the plasma concentration-time curves (AUCs) were 19% and 15% lower, respectively, than in patients receiving prochlorperazine. The AUC of carmustine was 20% lower with ondansetron vs prochlorperazine, but the difference was not statistically significant. The clinical importance of the changes in plasma concentrations of cisplatin and cyclophosphamide is not clear.

RELATED DRUGS: Ondansetron was also associated with a small reduction in cyclophosphamide plasma concentrations.

MANAGEMENT OPTIONS: No specific action is required, but be alert for evidence of the interaction.

REFERENCES:
1. Cagnoni PJ, et al. Modification of the pharmacokinetics of high-dose cyclophosphamide and cisplatin by antiemetics. *Bone Marrow Transplant.* 1999;24:1-4.

Cisplatin (eg, *Platinol-AQ*)

Phenytoin (eg, *Dilantin*)

SUMMARY: Phenytoin levels may be decreased by antineoplastic drugs like cisplatin, which may result in increased seizure activity or increased phenytoin dosage requirement.

RISK FACTORS: No specific risk factors are known.

MECHANISM: The mechanism for this interaction has not been fully established. It may be due in part to impaired oral absorption of phenytoin; however, this would not explain why patients receiving IV phenytoin have experienced declines in phenytoin levels. It most likely involves alterations in the metabolism of phenytoin.

CLINICAL EVALUATION: Several reports of decreased phenytoin levels following chemotherapy appear in the literature, including reports of seizures in patients who developed subtherapeutic phenytoin levels.[1-5,7] In the largest series, 14 of 19 patients (74%) receiving phenytoin while being treated with cisplatin and carmustine required phenytoin dosage increases to maintain therapeutic levels. Every patient who received 3 or more cycles of chemotherapy required dosage adjustment.[1] Decreases in phenytoin levels were noted as early as 2 days after initiation of chemotherapy. Based on information from cycles where patients received only 1 of the 2 agents, this interaction appeared to be caused by cisplatin and not carmustine; however, case reports suggest that a number of different chemotherapy agents may affect phenytoin levels. Decreased phenytoin levels and seizures developed in a 64-year-old man after receiving carboplatin.[5]

RELATED DRUGS: A 46-year-old man receiving chronic phenytoin experienced increased seizure activity associated with subtherapeutic phenytoin levels following chemotherapy with methotrexate, vinblastine, and carmustine.[2] In another case, a pharmacokinetic study of IV phenytoin was performed in a 10-year-old boy with acute lymphocytic leukemia being treated with prednisone, vincristine, methotrexate, leucovorin, and mercaptopurine. The clearance of phenytoin was more than doubled on the seventh day after starting chemotherapy. Plasma protein binding of phenytoin was unchanged.[6]

MANAGEMENT OPTIONS:

➡ *Circumvent/Minimize.* Case reports suggest that phenytoin levels will begin to return to normal 2 to 3 weeks following chemotherapy. If a patient had required a dosage increase to maintain a therapeutic level following chemotherapy, it would be important to anticipate this and reduce the dosage accordingly to prevent phenytoin toxicity from developing.

➡ *Monitor.* Monitor patient phenytoin levels 2 to 3 days after a dose of chemotherapy. If the phenytoin concentration has decreased significantly, adjust the phenytoin dosage and monitor phenytoin concentrations weekly.

REFERENCES:

1. Grossman SA, et al. Decreased phenytoin levels in patients receiving chemotherapy. *Am J Med.* 1989;87:505.
2. Bollini P, et al. Decreased phenytoin level during antineoplastic therapy: a case report. *Epilepsia.* 1983;24:75.
3. Neef C, et al. An interaction between cytostatic and anticonvulsant drugs. *Clin Pharmacol Ther.* 1988;43:372.

4. Sylvester RK, et al. Impaired phenytoin bioavailability secondary to cisplatinum, vinblastine, and bleomycin. *Ther Drug Monit.* 1984;6:302.

5. Dofferhoff ASM, et al. Decreased phenytoin level after carboplatin treatment. *Am J Med.* 1990;89:247.

6. Jarosinski PF, et al. Altered phenytoin clearance during intensive chemotherapy for acute lymphoblastic leukemia. *J Pediatr.* 1988;112:996.

7. Fincham RW, et al. Decreased phenytoin levels in antineoplastic therapy. *Ther Drug Monit.* 1979;1:277.

 Cisplatin

Valproic Acid (eg, *Depakene*)

SUMMARY: A patient on valproic acid developed decreased concentrations of valproic acid and seizures on several occasions after receiving cisplatin-containing chemotherapy.

RISK FACTORS: No specific risk factors are known.

MECHANISM: Not established.

CLINICAL EVALUATION: A 34-year-old man on valproic acid 1,200 mg daily developed reduced valproic acid serum concentrations and seizures several days after each of 7 cycles of chemotherapy with bleomycin-etoposide-cisplatin or paclitaxel-ifosfamide-cisplatin.[1] Because cisplatin was the only drug common to both regimens, it was considered the most likely cause for the reduced valproic acid concentrations. Although cisplatin does appear to be the most likely cause, the possibility that one of the noncisplatin chemotherapy agents in each regimen caused the interaction cannot be ruled out. Because the patient could feel the tonic-clonic seizures coming on, they were able to be stopped with intravenous phenytoin and diazepam.

RELATED DRUGS: No information is available.

MANAGEMENT OPTIONS:

➡ *Monitor.* Monitor patients on valproic acid who receive cisplatin-containing chemotherapy for reduced valproic acid serum concentrations. Based on these results, it may be possible to stop the seizures with acute administration of other anticonvulsants.

REFERENCES:

1. Ikeda H, et al. Pharmacokinetic interaction on valproic acid and recurrence of epileptic seizures during chemotherapy in an epileptic patient. *Br J Clin Pharmacol.* 2005;59(5):593-597.

 Citalopram (eg, *Celexa*)

Clozapine (eg, *Clozaril*)

SUMMARY: A patient developed evidence of clozapine toxicity after starting citalopram, but a causal relationship was not established.

RISK FACTORS: No specific risk factors are known.

MECHANISM: Not established.

CLINICAL EVALUATION: A 39-year-old man with schizoaffective disorder receiving clozapine 400 mg/day was started on citalopram 20 mg/day, increasing up to 40 mg/day.[1] One week after citalopram was increased to 40 mg/day, he developed sedation, fatigue, enuresis, hypersalivation, and confusion, and his clozapine and norclozapine serum concentrations were elevated. After the citalopram was reduced to 20 mg/day, the adverse reactions subsided within 2 weeks and clozapine serum concentrations decreased. Although the temporal relationship of this reaction is consistent with citalopram-induced clozapine toxicity, other evidence suggests that citalopram has only minor effects on CYP-450 isozymes. More study is needed to establish a causal relationship.

RELATED DRUGS: Fluvoxamine is a potent inhibitor of CYP1A2 and a moderate inhibitor of CYP3A4, which results in marked increases in clozapine serum concentrations.

MANAGEMENT OPTIONS: No specific action is required, but be alert for evidence of the interaction.

REFERENCES:
1. Borba CP, et al. Citalopram and clozapine: potential drug interaction. *J Clin Psychiatry*. 2000;61(4):301-302.

Citalopram (eg, *Celexa*)

Fentanyl (eg, *Actiq*)

SUMMARY: A patient developed evidence of serotonin toxicity after receiving citalopram and fentanyl.

RISK FACTORS: No specific risk factors known.

MECHANISM: Probably additive serotonergic effects.

CLINICAL EVALUATION: A 65-year-old woman on chronic citalopram developed serotonin toxicity (myoclonus, tremors, confusion, agitation) following administration of a fentanyl 25 mcg/hr patch.[1] Her symptoms clearly supported a diagnosis of serotonin toxicity.[2,3] The fentanyl was stopped, and her symptoms resolved over 24 to 36 hours.

RELATED DRUGS: Theoretically, other antidepressants that inhibit serotonin reuptake (clomipramine [eg, *Anafranil*], duloxetine [*Cymbalta*], escitalopram [*Lexapro*], fluoxetine [eg, *Prozac*], fluvoxamine, imipramine [eg, *Tofranil*], paroxetine [eg, *Paxil*], sertraline [eg, *Zoloft*], venlafaxine [*Effexor*]) may also increase the risk of serotonin toxicity when combined with fentanyl.

MANAGEMENT OPTIONS:

➥ *Monitor.* If the combination is used, monitor for symptoms of serotonin toxicity, including myoclonus, rigidity, tremor, hyperreflexia, seizures, confusion, agitation, hypomania, incoordination, fever, sweating, shivering, and coma.

REFERENCES:
1. Altman EM, Manos GH. Serotonin syndrome associated with citalopram and meperidine. *Psychosomatics*. 2007;48(4):361-363.

2. Isbister GK, et al. Serotonin toxicity: a practical approach to diagnosis and treatment. *Med J Aust*. 2007;187(6):361-365.

3. Boyer EW, Shannon M. The serotonin syndrome. *N Engl J Med*. 2005;352(11):1112-1120.

Citalopram (eg, *Celexa*)

Irinotecan (*Camptosar*)

SUMMARY: A patient developed rhabdomyolysis after receiving irinotecan and citalopram, but a causal relationship was not established.

RISK FACTORS: No specific risk factors are known.

MECHANISM: Not established.

CLINICAL EVALUATION: A 74-year-old man with gastric cancer developed rhabdomyolysis after concurrent therapy with irinotecan and citalopram.[1] Although the rhabdomyolysis may have been caused by the combination of citalopram and irinotecan, the relative contribution of irinotecan, citalopram, and his underlying conditions was not clear.

RELATED DRUGS: No information is available.

MANAGEMENT OPTIONS: No specific action is required, but be alert for evidence of the interaction.

REFERENCES:
1. Richards S, et al. Selective serotonin reuptake inhibitor-induced rhabdomyolysis associated with irinotecan. *South Med J*. 2003;96(10):1031-1033.

Citalopram (eg, *Celexa*)

Linezolid (*Zyvox*)

SUMMARY: Some cases of possible serotonin syndrome have been reported with concurrent linezolid and citalopram. Although the incidence of this reaction is not established, the linezolid prescribing information recommends careful monitoring if linezolid is used with drugs that inhibit serotonin uptake.

RISK FACTORS: No specific risk factors known.

MECHANISM: Linezolid is a weak nonselective monoamine oxidase inhibitor (MAOI), but in some patients it may increase the risk of serotonin syndrome when combined with serotonergic drugs such as citalopram.

CLINICAL EVALUATION: Several cases of serotonin syndrome have been reported in patients receiving linezolid and citalopram concomitantly.[1-5] Although it appears that most patients who receive linezolid and selective serotonin reuptake inhibitors (SSRIs) do not develop serotonin syndrome,[6] the manufacturer of linezolid states that serotonin reuptake inhibitors are contraindicated with linezolid unless the patient can be carefully observed for evidence of serotonin syndrome.[7]

RELATED DRUGS: Other SSRIs may interact similarly, including escitalopram (*Lexapro*), fluoxetine (eg, *Prozac*), fluvoxamine (eg, *Luvox*), and paroxetine (eg, *Paxil*). Selective serotonin/norepinephrine reuptake inhibitors may also interact, including clomipramine (eg, *Anafranil*), desvenlafaxine (*Pristiq*), duloxetine (*Cymbalta*), imipramine (eg, *Tofranil*), and venlafaxine (eg, *Effexor*).

MANAGEMENT OPTIONS:

➡ *Monitor.* Monitor for evidence of serotonin syndrome (eg, agitation, coma, confusion, fever, hyperreflexia, hypomania, incoordination, myoclonus, rigidity, seizures, shivering, sweating, tachycardia, tremor).

REFERENCES:

1. Bernard L, et al. Serotonin syndrome after concomitant treatment with linezolid and citalopram. *Clin Infect Dis.* 2003;36(9):1197.

2. Hachem RY, et al. Myelosuppression and serotonin syndrome associated with concurrent use of linezolid and selective serotonin reuptake inhibitors in bone marrow transplant patients. *Clin Infect Dis.* 2003;37(1):e8-e11.

3. Clark DB, et al. Drug interactions between linezolid and selective serotonin reuptake inhibitors: case report involving sertraline and review of the literature. *Pharmacotherapy.* 2006;26(2):269-276.

4. Tahir N. Serotonin syndrome as a consequence of drug-resistant infections: an interaction between linezolid and citalopram. *J Am Med Dir Assoc.* 2004;5(2):111-113.

5. Bergeron L, et al. Serotonin toxicity associated with concomitant use of linezolid. *Ann Pharmacother.* 2005;39(5):956-961.

6. Taylor JJ, et al. Linezolid and serotonergic drug interactions: a retrospective survey. *Clin Infect Dis.* 2006;43(2):180-187.

7. *Zyvox* [package insert]. New York, NY: Pfizer, Inc; 2008.

Citalopram (eg, *Celexa*)

Meperidine (eg, *Demerol*)

SUMMARY: A patient developed evidence of serotonin toxicity after receiving citalopram and meperidine.

RISK FACTORS: No specific risk factors are known.

MECHANISM: Probable additive serotonergic effects.

CLINICAL EVALUATION: A 44-year-old woman on citalopram 40 mg/day was given meperidine (230 mg over 8 hours).[1] Although her symptoms were not classic serotonin toxicity (no myoclonus, tremor, or rigidity),[2,3] both drugs are serotonergic, and it is possible that the reaction resulted from additive serotonergic effects.

RELATED DRUGS: Theoretically, other antidepressants that inhibit serotonin reuptake (eg, clomipramine [eg, *Anafranil*], duloxetine [*Cymbalta*], escitalopram [*Lexapro*], fluoxetine [eg, *Prozac*], fluvoxamine [eg, *Luvox*], imipramine [eg, *Tofranil*], paroxetine [eg, *Paxil*], sertraline [eg, *Zoloft*], venlafaxine [eg, *Effexor*]) may also increase the risk of serotonin toxicity when combined with meperidine.

MANAGEMENT OPTIONS:

➡ *Monitor.* If the combination is used, monitor for symptoms of serotonin toxicity (eg, agitation, coma, confusion, fever, hyperreflexia, hypomania, incoordination, myoclonus, rigidity, seizures, shivering, sweating, tremor).

REFERENCES:

1. Altman EM, et al. Serotonin syndrome associated with citalopram and meperidine. *Psychosomatics.* 2007;48(4):361-363.

2. Isbister GK, et al. Serotonin toxicity: a practical approach to diagnosis and treatment. *Med J Aust.* 2007;187(6):361-365.

3. Boyer EW, et al. The serotonin syndrome. *N Engl J Med.* 2005;352(11):1112-1120.

Citalopram (eg, *Celexa*)

AVOID **Methylene Blue (eg, *Urolene Blue*)**

SUMMARY: Giving methylene blue to patients taking citalopram or other serotonergic drugs may result in serotonin syndrome; the combination is best avoided.

RISK FACTORS: No specific risk factors are known.

MECHANISM: Methylene blue appears to be a strong inhibitor of monoamine oxidase type A (MAO-A) and a weak inhibitor of MAO-B.[1,2] Selective serotonin reuptake inhibitors (SSRIs), such as citalopram, and selective serotonin-norepinephrine reuptake inhibitors (SNRIs) may cause severe serotonin syndrome when combined with MAO inhibitors (MAOIs).

CLINICAL EVALUATION: A 55-year-old woman taking citalopram and bupropion was given methylene blue prior to parathyroid surgery. After the operation, she developed serotonin syndrome with agitation, confusion, sweating, hyperreflexia, and other symptoms.[3] A 65-year-old man taking citalopram was given methylene blue and soon developed agitation, disorientation, fever, sweating, shivering, and tachycardia.[4] A similar case was reported in a 44-year-old woman.[5] Virtually all cases of serotonin syndrome following methylene blue have occurred in patients receiving SSRIs or SNRIs, which is consistent with the view that a drug interaction is involved. (SSRIs and SNRIs given alone rarely produce serious serotonin toxicity, even when taken in overdose).

RELATED DRUGS: Methylene blue has been associated with serotonin syndrome in patients receiving other SSRIs, such as fluoxetine (eg, *Prozac*) and paroxetine (eg, *Paxil*), and also in patients receiving SNRIs, such as clomipramine (eg, *Anafranil*) and venlafaxine (eg, *Effexor*). Methylene blue is also likely to interact with other SSRIs, such as escitalopram (*Lexapro*), fluvoxamine (eg, *Luvox*), and sertraline (eg, *Zoloft*), and other SNRIs, such as desvenlafaxine (*Pristiq*), duloxetine (*Cymbalta*), and imipramine (eg, *Tofranil*).

MANAGEMENT OPTIONS:

➡ *AVOID COMBINATION.* Given that serotonin syndrome can be life-threatening, avoid the combination.[3] To minimize the risk of interactions, stop citalopram or other SSRIs or SNRIs for 2 weeks before administering methylene blue. In patients taking fluoxetine, allow 5 weeks to elapse before administering an MAOI, such as methylene blue. Available evidence suggests that the interaction cannot be avoided by decreasing the dose of methylene blue.[1,6]

REFERENCES:

1. Stanford SC, et al. Risk of severe serotonin toxicity following co-administration of methylene blue and serotonin reuptake inhibitors: an update on a case report of post-operative delirium [published online ahead of print May 7, 2009]. *J Psychopharmacol.* doi: 10.1177/0269881109105450.

2. Ramsay RR, et al. Methylene blue and serotonin toxicity: inhibition of monoamine oxidase A (MAO A) confirms a theoretical prediction. *Br J Pharmacol.* 2007;152(6):946-951.

3. Pollack G, et al. Parathyroid surgery and methylene blue: a review with guidelines for safe intraoperative use. *Laryngoscope.* 2009;119(10):1941-1946.

4. Mathew S, et al. Hyperpyrexia and prolonged postoperative disorientation following methylene blue infusion during parathyroidectomy. *Anaesthesia.* 2006;61(6):580-583.

5. Khavandi A, et al. Serotonin toxicity precipitated by concomitant use of citalopram and methylene blue. *Med J Aust.* 2008;189(9):534-535.

6. Schwiebert C, et al. Small doses of methylene blue, previously considered safe, can precipitate serotonin toxicity. *Anaesthesia.* 2009;64(8):924.

Citalopram (eg, *Celexa*)

Metoprolol (eg, *Lopressor*)

SUMMARY: Citalopram increases the plasma concentrations of metoprolol; however, little change in patient response is likely to be seen in most patients taking metoprolol.

RISK FACTORS:

➡ ***Pharmacogenetics.*** Only patients who are rapid CYP2D6 metabolizer genotypes are susceptible to the interaction.

MECHANISM: Citalopram inhibits CYP2D6, the enzyme responsible for the metabolism of metoprolol.

CLINICAL EVALUATION: The administration of citalopram 40 mg/day for 22 days resulted in a 2-fold increase in the plasma concentrations of metoprolol.[1] No further details are available regarding this interaction. Because of metoprolol's relatively wide therapeutic window, few patients should experience a significant change in their response to the beta-blocker.

RELATED DRUGS: Propranolol (eg, *Inderal*), timolol (eg, *Blocadren*), and carvedilol (eg, *Coreg*) are at least partially metabolized by CYP2D6 and, if coadministered with citalopram, their plasma concentrations would probably increase. Escitalopram (*Lexapro*) is known to inhibit the metabolism of metoprolol. Other antidepressants that inhibit CYP2D6 (eg, paroxetine [eg, *Paxil*], fluoxetine [eg, *Prozac*]) are expected to increase metoprolol plasma concentrations.

MANAGEMENT OPTIONS:

➡ ***Monitor.*** Monitor patients stabilized on metoprolol for any evidence of increased beta-blockade (eg, bradycardia, heart failure, hypotension) when citalopram is coadministered.

REFERENCES:

1. *Celexa* [package insert]. St. Louis, MO: Forest Laboratories; 2004.

Citalopram (eg, *Celexa*)

Moclobemide†

SUMMARY: Combined overdose of citalopram and moclobemide has resulted in fatal serotonin syndrome, but the danger of combining therapeutic doses of the 2 drugs is not known.

RISK FACTORS:

➡ ***Dosage Regimen.*** The observed reactions occurred in overdose situations.

MECHANISM: Citalopram is a selective serotonin reuptake inhibitor (SSRI) and moclobemide is a selective inhibitor of monoamine oxidase type A (MAO-A), the form of MAO that metabolizes serotonin. The combination may result in excessive serotonin effects, the serotonin syndrome.

CLINICAL EVALUATION: Three men (29, 34, and 41 years of age) died from serotonin syndrome (convulsions, hyperthermia, loss of consciousness) after taking overdoses of moclobemide and citalopram.[1] The authors suggest that the fatalities were caused by a combined effect of both drugs rather than either drug acting alone because: 1) the blood concentrations of citalopram were not markedly elevated, and 2) overdoses of moclobemide alone do not appear to be life-threatening. Note that combining an SSRI with nonselective MAO inhibitors (MAOIs), such as tranylcypromine (eg, *Parnate*) or phenelzine (*Nardil*), has resulted in fatalities, even at therapeutic doses.[2,3] Moclobemide might become a nonselective MAOI when given in overdose, but supporting evidence is lacking. Selegiline (eg, *Eldepryl*), a selective MAO-B inhibitor, can become nonselective at higher doses; it seems reasonable to suspect moclobemide could do the same. Thus, although it is not yet clear whether therapeutic doses of moclobemide and citalopram are dangerous, consider the possibility that they are until proven otherwise. Moreover, the therapeutic benefit of using the combination over either drug alone is not established.

RELATED DRUGS: In a preliminary report on the use of therapeutic moclobemide doses with another SSRI, fluoxetine (eg, *Prozac*), no unexpected adverse reaction occurred.[4] Little is known regarding the effect of moclobemide combined with SSRIs other than citalopram or fluoxetine.

MANAGEMENT OPTIONS:

➡ *Avoid Unless Benefit Outweighs Risk.* Although it is possible that the danger of concomitant use of citalopram and moclobemide is restricted to overdoses, the lack of safety data at therapeutic doses dictates extreme caution in using this combination.

➡ *Monitor.* Carefully monitor and use conservative dosing in patients given the combination.

REFERENCES:

1. Neuvonen PJ, et al. Five fatal cases of serotonin syndrome after moclobemide-citalopram or moclobemide-clomipramine overdoses. *Lancet*. 1993;342(8884):1419.
2. Beasley CM Jr, et al. Possible monoamine oxidase inhibitor-serotonin reuptake inhibitor interaction: fluoxetine clinical data and preclinical findings. *J Clin Psychopharmacol*. 1993;13(5):312-320.
3. Graber MA, et al. Sertraline-phenelzine drug interaction: a serotonin syndrome reaction. *Ann Pharmacother*. 1994;28(6):732-735.
4. Dingemanse J, et al. Pharmacodynamic and pharmacokinetic interactions between fluoxetine and moclobemide. *Clin Pharmacol Ther*. 1993;53:178.

† Not available in the United States.

Citalopram (eg, *Celexa*)

Quetiapine (*Seroquel*)

SUMMARY: A woman taking citalopram and quetiapine developed some symptoms of serotonin toxicity, but a causal relationship was not established.

RISK FACTORS: No specific risk factors are known.

MECHANISM: Not established.

CLINICAL EVALUATION: A 42-year-old woman on citalopram 40 mg/day and quetiapine 800 mg/day took an extra 200 mg of quetiapine one morning.[1] Within 12 hours, she developed agitation, delirium, and disorientation, and then developed hyperreflexia and muscle rigidity. Although her symptoms were indicative of serotonin toxicity, the lack of 2 of the classic signs of serotonin toxicity (myoclonus and tremor) made a definitive diagnosis of serotonin toxicity difficult.[2,3]

RELATED DRUGS: If this interaction proves to be valid, other antidepressants that inhibit serotonin reuptake (clomipramine [eg, *Anafranil*], duloxetine [*Cymbalta*], escitalopram [*Lexapro*], fluoxetine [eg, *Prozac*], fluvoxamine [eg, *Luvox CR*], imipramine [eg, *Tofranil*], paroxetine [eg, *Paxil*], sertraline [eg, *Zoloft*], venlafaxine [eg, *Effexor*]) may also interact with quetiapine.

MANAGEMENT OPTIONS:

➡ *Monitor.* If the combination is used, monitor for symptoms of serotonin toxicity (eg, agitation, coma, confusion, fever, hyperreflexia, hypomania, incoordination, myoclonus, rigidity, seizures, shivering, sweating, tremor).

REFERENCES:

1. Marlowe K, Schirgel D. Quetiapine and citalopram: aetiological significances in serotonin syndrome. *N Z Med J.* 2006;119(1237):U2058.

2. Isbister GK, et al. Serotonin toxicity: a practical approach to diagnosis and treatment. *Med J Aust.* 2007;187(6):361-365.

3. Boyer EW, Shannon M. The serotonin syndrome. *N Engl J Med.* 2005;352(11):1112-1120.

Citalopram (eg, *Celexa*)

Thiazides

SUMMARY: The combined use of citalopram and a thiazide diuretic increased the risk of hyponatremia and its associated symptoms (eg, confusion, disorientation, weakness).

RISK FACTORS:

➡ *Effects of Age.* Elderly patients appear to be at greater risk; lower body weight may play a role, as well as diseases and changes in kidney function, which may predispose patients to hyponatremia.

➡ *Gender.* The majority of case reports involve women, although it is not clear that female gender is an independent risk factor.

MECHANISM: Selective serotonin reuptake inhibitors (SSRIs) and selective serotonin-norepinephrine reuptake inhibitors (SNRIs) can produce syndrome of inappropriate antidiuretic hormone (SIADH), resulting in hyponatremia. The natriuretic effect of thiazide diuretics can result in additive hyponatremia.

CLINICAL EVALUATION: A 90-year-old woman with hypertension was taking an angiotensin-converting enzyme inhibitor, hydrochlorothiazide (eg, *HydroDIURIL*) 12.5 mg/day, and atorvastatin (*Lipitor*) 10 mg/day.[1] She was then placed on citalopram 10 mg/day, which was later increased to 20 mg/day. She subsequently developed disorientation and confusion and was found to have hyponatremia (serum sodium of 112 mg/dL). She responded to fluid restriction and discontinuation of the thiazide and citalopram. Citalopram alone has been associated with hyponatremia,[2,3,4] but it is likely that the thiazide diuretic contributed in this case. Numerous cases of hyponatremia have been reported with other combinations of SSRIs and diuretics.[5,6,7]

RELATED DRUGS: Most other SSRIs have also been associated with hyponatremia, including escitalopram (*Lexapro*), fluoxetine (eg, *Prozac*), fluvoxamine (eg, *Luvox CR*), paroxetine (eg, *Paxil*), and sertraline (eg, *Zoloft*). The following SNRIs may also interact: clomipramine (eg, *Anafranil*), duloxetine (*Cymbalta*), imipramine (eg, *Tofranil*), and venlafaxine (eg, *Effexor*).

MANAGEMENT OPTIONS:

➡ *Consider Alternative.* Mirtazapine (eg, *Remeron*) may be less likely to cause hyponatremia than SSRIs or SNRIs, and in one case of citalopram-induced hyponatremia, mirtazapine was substituted for citalopram without a recurrence of hyponatremia.[8] Mirtazapine, however, has been associated with hyponatremia in isolated case reports; use with caution.[2,9]

➡ *Monitor.* Hyponatremia usually occurs in the first 2 to 3 weeks of starting therapy with the second drug (SSRIs, SNRIs, or the diuretic). Monitor for the following symptoms of hyponatremia: anorexia, confusion, disorientation, fatigue, headache, muscle cramps, nausea, weakness; in severe cases, seizures, coma, and death can occur. In predisposed patients, such as elderly patients taking diuretics (especially women), measure serum sodium at baseline and repeat it 7 to 10 days after the second drug is started.

REFERENCES:

1. Wright SK, Schroeter S. Hyponatremia as a complication of selective serotonin reuptake inhibitors. *J Am Acad Nurse Pract*. 2008;20(1):47-51.
2. Bavbek N, et al. Recurrent hyponatremia associated with citalopram and mirtazapine. *Am J Kidney Dis*. 2006;48(4):e61-e62.
3. Romero S, et al. Syndrome of inappropriate secretion of antidiuretic hormone due to citalopram and venlafaxine. *Gen Hosp Psychiatry*. 2007;29(1):81-84.
4. Flores G, et al. Severe symptomatic hyponatremia during citalopram therapy—a case report. *BMC Nephrol*. 2004;5:2.
5. Rosner MH. Severe hyponatremia associated with the combined use of thiazide diuretics and selective serotonin reuptake inhibitors. *Am J Med Sci*. 2004;327(2):109-111.
6. Jacob S, et al. Hyponatremia associated with selective serotonin-reuptake inhibitors in older adults. *Ann Pharmacother*. 2006;40(9):1618-1622.
7. Fitzgerald MA. Hyponatremia associated with SSRI use in a 65-year-old woman. *Nurse Pract*. 2008;33(2):11-12.
8. Jagsch C, et al. Successful mirtazapine treatment of an 81-year-old patient with syndrome of inappropriate antidiuretic hormone secretion. *Pharmacopsychiatry*. 2007;40(3):129-131.
9. Ladino M, et al. Mirtazapine-induced hyponatremia in an elderly hospice patient. *J Palliat Med*. 2006;9(2):258-260.

Citalopram (eg, *Celexa*)

Tramadol (eg, *Ultram*)

SUMMARY: A patient developed serotonin toxicity after taking citalopram and tramadol; more data are needed to establish the incidence of this interaction.

RISK FACTORS: No specific risk factors are known.

MECHANISM: Probably additive serotonergic effects.

CLINICAL EVALUATION: A 70-year-old woman on chronic therapy with citalopram 10 mg/day started tramadol 50 mg/day and then developed confusion, fever, restlessness, tremors, and visual hallucinations.[1] A year later, she developed the same reaction when tramadol 20 mg/day was added to her citalopram therapy. Based on the standard diagnostic methods, the patient probably had serotonin toxicity.[2,3] Through genotyping, she was found to have lowered activity of both CYP2C9 and

CYP2D6, and lower than normal clearance of citalopram; therefore, she may have had higher than normal plasma concentrations of citalopram. Given that tramadol and citalopram are serotonergic, it seems likely that the combination was responsible for the serotonin toxicity.

RELATED DRUGS: Tramadol has produced serotonin toxicity when combined with several other selective serotonin reuptake inhibitors (SSRIs). Combining tramadol with meperidine (eg, *Demerol*) or fentanyl (eg, *Sublimaze*) may theoretically increase the risk of serotonin toxicity.

MANAGEMENT OPTIONS:

➡ *Consider Alternative.* In patients using SSRIs, consider using an analgesic other than tramadol, meperidine, or fentanyl.

➡ *Monitor.* If the combination is used, monitor for symptoms of serotonin toxicity (eg, agitation, coma, confusion, fever, hyperreflexia, hypomania, incoordination, myoclonus, rigidity, seizures, shivering, sweating, tremor).

REFERENCES:

1. Mahlberg R, et al. Serotonin syndrome with tramadol and citalopram. *Am J Psychiatry*. 2004;161(6):1129.
2. Isbister GK, et al. Serotonin toxicity: a practical approach to diagnosis and treatment. *Med J Aust.* 2007;187(6):361-365.
3. Boyer EW, et al. The serotonin syndrome. *N Engl J Med*. 2005;352(11):1112-1120.

Clarithromycin (eg, *Biaxin*)

Colchicine AVOID

SUMMARY: Severe colchicine toxicity can occur in patients concomitantly receiving clarithromycin; the combination is contraindicated.

RISK FACTORS:

➡ *Concurrent Diseases.* Patients with renal function impairment may be at higher risk from this interaction.

MECHANISM: Not established. Clarithromycin inhibits P-glycoprotein, and colchicine is a P-glycoprotein substrate. Thus, clarithromycin theoretically could affect the intestinal absorption, renal elimination, and biliary excretion of colchicine. It is possible that clarithromycin inhibition of CYP3A4 also is involved in the interaction.

CLINICAL EVALUATION: A patient with end-stage renal disease on continuous ambulatory peritoneal dialysis was taking colchicine 0.5 mg twice daily, erythropoietin, and calcium carbonate.[1] Four days after the addition of clarithromycin 500 mg twice daily, the patient developed fever, diarrhea, myalgia, and abdominal pain. Laboratory findings included anemia, thrombocytopenia, and leukopenia. The patient died as a result of pancytopenia and multiple organ failure. A second case was noted of a patient stabilized on colchicine 1.5 mg/day who developed fever, diarrhea, pancytopenia, renal failure, and pancreatitis beginning 3 days after the initiation of clarithromycin 1 g/day for the treatment of *Helicobacter pylori*.[2] Two additional cases of fatal agranulocytosis following use of clarithromycin and colchicine have been reported.[3] Additional evidence of an interaction comes from a retrospective case-control study of 116 patients who received colchicine and clarithromycin on the same admission.[4] Nine of 88 patients who received the drugs simultaneously died, while 1 of 28 patients who received the drugs sequentially died. Enough evidence exists to prohibit the concurrent use of colchicine and clarithromycin.

RELATED DRUGS: Erythromycin (eg, *Ery-Tab*) and josamycin[†] also have been reported to cause colchicine toxicity. Theoretically, troleandomycin[†] would interact similarly, but azithromycin (eg, *Zithromax*) and dirithromycin[†] would not. Any P-glycoprotein or CYP3A4 inhibitor would theoretically increase the risk of colchicine toxicity.

MANAGEMENT OPTIONS:

➡ *AVOID COMBINATION.* Avoid using colchicine and clarithromycin concurrently. Until more information is available, the same caution applies to other macrolides that can inhibit P-glycoprotein and/or CYP3A4.

REFERENCES:

1. Dogukan A, et al. Acute fatal colchicine intoxication in a patient on continuous ambulatory peritoneal dialysis (CAPD). Possible role of clarithromycin administration. *Clin Nephrol.* 2001;55(2):181-182.

2. Rollot F, et al. Acute colchicine intoxication during clarithromycin administration. *Ann Pharmacother.* 2004;38(12):2074-2077.

3. Cheng VC, et al. Two probable cases of serious drug interaction between clarithromycin and colchicine. *South Med J.* 2005;98(8):811-813.

4. Hung IF, et al. Fatal interaction between clarithromycin and colchicine in patients with renal insufficiency: a retrospective study. *Clin Infect Dis.* 2005;41(3):291-300.

† Not available in the United States.

Clarithromycin (*Biaxin*)

Cyclosporine (eg, *Neoral*)

SUMMARY: Cyclosporine concentrations are likely to be increased by clarithromycin coadministration; toxic cyclosporine concentrations and renal toxicity may result.

RISK FACTORS:

➡ *Concomitant Diseases.* Renal dysfunction can increase the risk of interaction.[1]

MECHANISM: Clarithromycin is a macrolide antibiotic that is known to inhibit the metabolism of other drugs that are metabolized in a manner similar to cyclosporine (CYP3A4), including carbamazepine (eg, *Tegretol*) and terfenadine.

CLINICAL EVALUATION: Three kidney transplant patients receiving cyclosporine experienced elevations of cyclosporine concentrations following the addition of clarithromycin.[2] Although cyclosporine concentrations were not obtained just before the administration of clarithromycin in any of the patients, cyclosporine concentrations in each were increased compared with values obtained in the weeks before clarithromycin administration. Serum creatinine concentrations were elevated during the increased cyclosporine concentrations. Prospective studies are needed to fully elucidate the potential magnitude of this interaction.

RELATED DRUGS: Erythromycin (eg, *E-Mycin*)[3] and, to a lesser extent, josamycin[4] and roxithromycin,[5] have been noted to increase cyclosporine concentrations; azithromycin (*Zithromax*) and dirithromycin (*Dynabac*) would be unlikely to inhibit cyclosporine metabolism. Tacrolimus (*Prograf*) is similarly affected by macrolide administration.

MANAGEMENT OPTIONS:

➡ *Monitor.* Carefully monitor cyclosporine concentrations in patients stabilized on cyclosporine and adjust doses as required during clarithromycin administration.

REFERENCES:

1. Neu HC. The development of macrolides: clarithromycin in perspective. *J Antimicrob Chemother.* 1991;27(suppl. A):1-9.

2. Ferrari SL, et al. The interaction between clarithromycin and cyclosporine in kidney transplant recipients. *Transplantation.* 1994;58:725-727.

3. Harnett JD, et al. Erythromycin-cyclosporine interaction in renal transplant recipients. *Transplantation.* 1987;43:316-318.

4. Kreft-Jais C, et al. Effect of josamycin on plasma cyclosporine levels. *Eur J Clin Pharmacol.* 1987;32:327-328.

5. Billaud EM, et al. Interaction between roxithromycin and cyclosporin in heart transplant patients. *Clin Pharmacokinet.* 1990;19:499-502.

Clarithromycin (eg, *Biaxin*)

Digoxin (eg, *Lanoxin*)

SUMMARY: Clarithromycin administration increases the plasma concentration of digoxin; digoxin toxicity including nausea, malaise, visual changes, and arrhythmias may occur.

RISK FACTORS: No specific risk factors are known.

MECHANISM: Clarithromycin may enhance the absorption of digoxin and/or reduce its renal and biliary elimination by inhibiting p-glycoprotein in the intestine, kidney, and liver.

CLINICAL EVALUATION: Clarithromycin has been reported in a number of case studies to increase the plasma concentration of digoxin.[1-5] Digoxin clearance may be reduced 60%, and plasma concentrations may increase 2-fold.

RELATED DRUGS: Digitoxin[†] would likely be affected in a similar manner by clarithromycin. Erythromycin also increases digoxin plasma concentrations. There is little data on the effect of other macrolides on digoxin.

MANAGEMENT OPTIONS:

➡ *Consider Alternative.* Select an antibiotic known to have no effect on digoxin concentrations in patients receiving chronic digoxin therapy. If azithromycin (*Zithromax*) or dirithromycin (*Dynabac*) are used, monitor for changes in digoxin concentrations.

➡ *Monitor.* In patients receiving digoxin, monitor for changes in digoxin concentrations when clarithromycin is added or removed from the drug regimen.

REFERENCES:

1. Xu H, et al. Clarithromycin-induced digoxin toxicity: a case report and review of the literature. *Conn Med.* 2001;65:527-529.

2. Zapater P, et al. A prospective study of the clarithromycin-digoxin interaction in elderly patients. *J Antimicrob Chemother.* 2002;50:601-606.

3. Tanaka H, et al. Effect of clarithromycin on steady-state digoxin concentrations. *Ann Pharmacother.* 2003;37:178-181.

4. Nordt SP, et al. Clarithromycin induced digoxin toxicity. *J Accid Emerg Med.* 1998;15:194-195.

5. Juurlink DN, et al. Drug-drug interactions among elderly patients hospitalized for drug toxicity. *JAMA.* 2003;289:1652-1658.

† Not available in the United States.

Clarithromycin (*Biaxin*)

Ergotamine (*Ergomar*)

SUMMARY: The coadministration of clarithromycin and ergotamine may result in ergotism, including hypertension and ischemia.

RISK FACTORS: No specific risk factors are known.

MECHANISM: Clarithromycin inhibits hepatic metabolism and appears to inhibit the metabolism of ergotamine.

CLINICAL EVALUATION: A 59-year-old woman was taking clarithromycin 500 mg twice daily for sinusitis.[1] She took 2 mg ergotamine tartrate for a migraine headache on the fifth day of clarithromycin administration. Two hours later she developed swelling in her neck and tongue, hypertension, and cyanotic fingers. Following treatment with nitroprusside, the cyanosis resolved. Prior use of ergotamine without clarithromycin did not produce any complications.

RELATED DRUGS: Erythromycin (eg, *E-Mycin*) also has been reported to cause ergotamine toxicity.[2] Although no data are available, azithromycin (*Zithromax*) or dirithromycin (*Dynabac*) would be unlikely to inhibit the metabolism of ergotamine.

MANAGEMENT OPTIONS:

➥ *Use Alternative.* The use of macrolides such as azithromycin or dirithromycin that do not inhibit drug metabolism is preferable in patients with migraine headaches who require ergotamine for acute migraine attacks.

REFERENCES:

1. Horowitz RS, et al. Clinical ergotism with lingual ischemia induced by clarithromycin-ergotamine interaction. *Arch Intern Med*. 1996;156:456-458.
2. Ghali R, et al. Erythromycin-associated ergotamine intoxication: arteriographic and electrophysiologic analysis of a rare cause of severe ischemia of the lower extremities and associated ischemic neuropathy. *Ann Vasc Surg*. 1993;7:291-296.

 Clarithromycin (eg, *Biaxin*)

Etravirine (*Intelence*)

SUMMARY: Clarithromycin administration will increase etravirine plasma concentrations, whereas etravirine reduces clarithromycin levels.

RISK FACTORS: No specific risk factors are known.

MECHANISM: Etravirine is partially metabolized by CYP3A4. Clarithromycin inhibits the activity of this enzyme, resulting in reduced etravirine metabolism. Etravirine induces CYP3A4, resulting in increased metabolism of clarithromycin.

CLINICAL EVALUATION: While specific data are limited, the manufacturer of etravirine notes that the coadministration of clarithromycin 500 mg twice daily prior to a dose of etravirine increased the mean area under the plasma concentration-time curve of etravirine approximately 42%.[1] Pending further data, observe patients receiving clarithromycin and etravirine for increased etravirine adverse reactions such as rash or nausea. Etravirine has been noted to reduce clarithromycin plasma concentrations approximately 40%. Some patients may experience a reduction in the antimicrobial efficacy of clarithromycin.

RELATED DRUGS: Erythromycin (eg, *Ery-Tab*) and telithromycin (*Ketek*) are likely to produce a similar interaction with etravirine.

MANAGEMENT OPTIONS:

➥ *Consider Alternative.* Azithromycin (eg, *Zithromax*) does not inhibit CYP3A4 and may be considered as an alternative to clarithromycin in patients receiving etravirine.

➥ *Monitor.* Monitor for etravirine adverse reactions (eg, skin rash, nausea) and reduced clarithromycin efficacy when the 2 agents are coadministered.

REFERENCES:

1. *Intelence* [package insert]. Raritan, NJ: Tibotec Therapeutics; 2008.

Clarithromycin (eg, *Biaxin*)

Fentanyl (eg, *Duragesic*)

SUMMARY: Fentanyl concentrations are likely to increase during clarithromycin administration; increased narcotic effects may occur.

RISK FACTORS: No specific risk factors are known.

MECHANISM: Clarithromycin is known to inhibit the enzyme (CYP3A4) responsible for the metabolism of fentanyl.

CLINICAL EVALUATION: While specific data are limited, the manufacturer of fentanyl notes that the coadministration of fentanyl and clarithromycin should be undertaken with caution.[1] Pending further data, observe patients receiving fentanyl and clarithromycin for evidence of increased fentanyl effect, including prolonged sedation and possible respiratory depression.

RELATED DRUGS: The metabolisms of alfentanil (eg, *Alfenta*) and sufentanil (eg, *Sufenta*) are likely to be reduced by clarithromycin administration. Erythromycin (eg, *Ery-Tab*) and troleandomycin[†] are likely to inhibit the metabolism of fentanyl in a similar manner to clarithromycin.

MANAGEMENT OPTIONS:

➥ *Consider Alternative.* Azithromycin (eg, *Zithromax*) does not inhibit CYP3A4 and may be considered as an alternative to clarithromycin in patients receiving fentanyl. Narcotics not metabolized by CYP3A4, such as morphine or oxycodone, may also be considered as alternatives.

➥ *Monitor.* Monitor patients for excess sedation and respiratory depression if fentanyl is coadministered with a CYP3A4 inhibitor.

REFERENCES:

1. *Duragesic* [package insert]. Titusville, NJ: Janssen LP; 2008.

† Not available in the United States.

4 Clarithromycin (eg, *Biaxin*)
Fluconazole (eg, *Diflucan*)

SUMMARY: Fluconazole administration produced a limited increase in clarithromycin concentrations; no adverse effect is expected.

RISK FACTORS: No specific risk factors are known.

MECHANISM: Not established. Fluconazole may inhibit the metabolism of clarithromycin.

CLINICAL EVALUATION: Clarithromycin 500 mg every 12 hours was taken by 20 healthy subjects for 8 days. On day 5, fluconazole 400 mg was taken, and on days 6 through 8, fluconazole 200 mg/day was administered with clarithromycin.[1] Clarithromycin concentrations were assessed on days 4 and 8. The coadministration of fluconazole resulted in a 33% and 18% increase in clarithromycin mean minimum plasma concentration and mean area under the concentration-time curve, respectively. It is unlikely that these increases in clarithromycin concentrations will alter patient response or produce clarithromycin toxicity. The potential influence of clarithromycin on fluconazole pharmacokinetics was not assessed.

RELATED DRUGS: The effects of other antifungal agents on clarithromycin plasma concentrations are unknown.

MANAGEMENT OPTIONS: No specific action is required, but be alert for evidence of the interaction.

REFERENCES:
1. Gustavson LE, et al. Drug interaction between clarithromycin and fluconazole in healthy subjects. *Clin Pharmacol Ther*. 1996;59:185.

3 Clarithromycin (eg, *Biaxin*)
Glyburide (eg, *DiaBeta*)

SUMMARY: Clarithromycin administration increases the plasma concentration of glyburide; some patients may experience enhanced hypoglycemic effects.

RISK FACTORS:

 Pharmacogenetics. Potentially, patients who are poor CYP2C9 metabolizers may be at greater risk; a larger portion of glyburide elimination may be dependent on P-glycoprotein activity.

MECHANISM: Clarithromycin inhibits P-glycoprotein, an efflux transporter that contributes to the elimination of glyburide.

CLINICAL EVALUATION: In a study of 12 healthy subjects, a single dose of glyburide 0.875 mg was administered following placebo or clarithromycin 250 mg twice daily for 2 days and on the morning of the third day.[1] The mean area under the plasma concentration-time curve of glyburide was increased approximately 35% following clarithromycin administration compared with placebo. No change in blood sugar was observed in the subjects who were treated with extra glucose during the study. Two cases of patients with diabetes who developed hypoglycemia following the addition of clarithromycin to a stable dose of glyburide have been reported.[2,3] In both cases, the dose of clarithromycin was 1,000 mg daily and the hypoglycemic episode occurred about 48 hours after the clarithromycin was initiated. The higher dose of clarithromycin in these cases may have contributed to the development of hypoglycemia.

RELATED DRUGS: Erythromycin (eg, *Ery-Tab*) may cause a similar increase in glyburide plasma concentrations. Oral hypoglycemic agents that are substrates for P-glycoprotein or CYP3A4 may have an increased effect when administered with clarithromycin.

MANAGEMENT OPTIONS:

➡ *Consider Alternative.* Glipizide (eg, *Glucotrol*) may be less affected by clarithromycin, but it has also been reported to interact with clarithromycin.[2] The hypoglycemic effect of some oral hypoglycemic agents (eg, chlorpropamide [eg, *Diabinese*], tolbutamide [eg, *Orinase*], rosiglitazone [*Avandia*], metformin [eg, *Glucophage*]) may not be affected by clarithromycin, but data are limited.

➡ *Monitor.* Monitor blood sugar in diabetic patients taking glyburide when clarithromycin is coadministered.

REFERENCES:

1. Lilja JJ, et al. Effects of clarithromycin and grapefruit juice on the pharmacokinetics of glibenclamide. *Br J Clin Pharmacol.* 2007;63(6):732-740.
2. Bussing R, et al. Severe hypoglycemia from clarithromycin-sulfonylurea drug interaction. *Diabetes Care.* 2002;25(9):1659-1661.
3. Leiba A, et al. An unusual case of hypoglycemia in a diabetic patient. *Ann Emerg Med.* 2004;44(4):427-428.

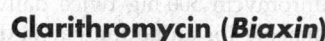

Clarithromycin (*Biaxin*)

Indinavir (*Crixivan*)

SUMMARY: Clarithromycin can increase indinavir serum concentrations, possibly resulting in toxicity. Indinavir increased clarithromycin concentrations; the clinical significance of these changes is unknown.

RISK FACTORS: No specific risk factors are known.

MECHANISM: Indinavir appears to inhibit the metabolism of clarithromycin and, to a lesser extent, clarithromycin inhibits the metabolism of indinavir.

CLINICAL EVALUATION: The administration of indinavir 800 mg every 8 hours with clarithromycin 500 mg every 12 hours for 1 week resulted in a 53% increase in clarithromycin area under the concentration-time curve (AUC).[1] The AUC of indinavir increased 29%. No additional details of the study are available. The increase in clarithromycin concentration is unlikely to cause adverse reactions, but indinavir may produce additional toxicity.

RELATED DRUGS: Clarithromycin produces a small increase in ritonavir (*Norvir*) serum concentrations that are unlikely to produce toxicity. Ritonavir significantly increased clarithromycin concentrations. Other macrolides (eg, erythromycin [eg, *Ery-Tab*], troleandomycin[+]) are likely to affect indinavir in a similar manner. Dirithromycin[+] and azithromycin (eg, *Zithromax*) are not likely to inhibit indinavir metabolism.

MANAGEMENT OPTIONS:

➡ *Circumvent/Minimize.* The dose of indinavir may require reduction during administration of clarithromycin or certain other macrolides.

➡ *Monitor.* Monitor patients for possible indinavir toxicity (eg, nausea, vomiting, headache).

REFERENCES:

1. *Crixivan* [package insert]. Whitehouse Station, NJ: Merck & Co, Inc; 1996.

† Not available in the United States.

Clarithromycin (eg, *Biaxin*)

Itraconazole (eg, *Sporanox*)

SUMMARY: Itraconazole concentrations are nearly doubled during clarithromycin coadministration; an increase in itraconazole adverse reactions is possible.

RISK FACTORS:

➡ *Route of Administration.* Oral administration of clarithromycin is likely to produce a greater effect on itraconazole concentrations than intravenous dosing.

MECHANISM: Not established. It is likely that clarithromycin inhibits the first-pass metabolism of itraconazole by inhibiting CYP3A4 or P-glycoprotein activity in the intestinal mucosa.

CLINICAL EVALUATION: Eight AIDS patients received itraconazole 200 mg/day for 14 days. Clarithromycin 500 mg twice daily was later administered in combination with itraconazole for an additional 14 days.[1] The mean area under the concentration-time curve and peak plasma concentration of itraconazole were both increased approximately 90% during clarithromycin coadministration. The potential effect of itraconazole on clarithromycin pharmacokinetics was not studied.

RELATED DRUGS: It is possible that other macrolide antibiotics (eg, erythromycin [eg, *Ery-Tab*]) could alter itraconazole pharmacokinetics in a similar manner. Macrolide antibiotics that have little effect on CYP3A4 activity include azithromycin (eg, *Zithromax*) or dirithromycin.†

MANAGEMENT OPTIONS:

➡ *Consider Alternative.* Consider macrolide antibiotics that have little effect on CYP3A4 activity (see Related Drugs) for patients taking itraconazole.

➡ *Monitor.* Observe patients receiving both drugs for increased itraconazole adverse reactions (eg, nausea, vomiting, headache) during the coadministration of clarithromycin.

REFERENCES:

1. Hardin TC, et al. Evaluation of the pharmacokinetic interaction between itraconazole and clarithromycin following chronic oral dosing in HIV-infected patients. *Pharmacotherapy.* 1997;17:52.

† Not available in the United States.

Clarithromycin (eg, *Biaxin*)

Lansoprazole (eg, *Prevacid*)

SUMMARY: Clarithromycin increases the plasma concentration of lansoprazole; some patients may experience an increase in adverse reactions.

RISK FACTORS: No significant risk factors are known.

MECHANISM: Clarithromycin inhibits the CYP3A4-mediated metabolism of lansoprazole.

CLINICAL EVALUATION: The mean plasma concentration of lansoprazole drawn 3 hours after the seventh daily dose was compared in 3 separate groups.[1] One group of 10 healthy subjects received lansoprazole 30 mg alone. Two other groups of 10 patients each were treated with lansoprazole 30 mg combined with clarithromycin 200 or 400 mg twice daily. Compared with the group not receiving clarithromycin, lansoprazole plasma concentrations were 80% and 145% higher during coadministration of clarithromycin 200 and 400 mg twice daily, respectively. In a second study, 18 healthy subjects received a single dose of lansoprazole 60 mg alone and following 6 days of clarithromycin 400 mg twice daily.[2] The mean area under the lansoprazole concentration-time curve was increased about 2-fold during clarithromycin administration. The increased lansoprazole concentrations may increase adverse reactions such as diarrhea.

RELATED DRUGS: Erythromycin is likely to increase lansoprazole plasma concentrations in a similar manner. The plasma concentrations of other proton pump inhibitors metabolized by CYP3A4, including omeprazole (eg, *Prilosec*), esomeprazole (*Nexium*), and pantoprazole (eg, *Protonix*), also have increased when coadministered with clarithromycin.

MANAGEMENT OPTIONS:

➥ *Consider Alternative.* Azithromycin (eg, *Zithromax*) is not expected to affect the plasma concentration of lansoprazole. Rabeprazole (*Aciphex*) pharmacokinetics do not appear to be affected by clarithromycin.

➥ *Monitor.* Observe patients taking lansoprazole for increased GI adverse reactions if clarithromycin is coadministered.

REFERENCES:

1. Ushiama H, et al. Dose-dependent inhibition of CYP3A activity by clarithromycin during *Helicobacter pylori* eradication therapy assessed by changes in plasma lansoprazole levels and partial cortisol clearance to 6β-hydroxycortisol. *Clin Pharmacol Ther.* 2002;72(1):33-43.
2. Miura M, et al. Effect of clarithromycin on enantioselective disposition of lansoprazole in relation to CYP2C19 genotypes. *Chirality.* 2005;17(6):338-344.

Clarithromycin (eg, *Biaxin*)

Midazolam

SUMMARY: Clarithromycin administration increases midazolam serum concentrations and accentuates its pharmacologic effects.

RISK FACTORS:

➡ ***Route of Administration.*** The oral administration of midazolam increases the risk of this interaction.

MECHANISM: Clarithromycin is known to inhibit CYP3A4, the enzyme responsible for midazolam's metabolism. This results in an increase in the bioavailability of orally administered midazolam and a reduction in its systemic clearance.

CLINICAL EVALUATION: Twelve healthy subjects ingested midazolam 15 mg alone and following 5 days of clarithromycin 250 mg twice daily.[1] The peak serum concentration of midazolam was increased 142%, and its area under the concentration-time curve was increased more than 250% following clarithromycin pretreatment. The half-life of midazolam increased from 3.4 to 7.4 hours. These pharmacokinetic changes were accompanied by a marked reduction in subject alertness. In another study, midazolam clearance following intravenous dosing was reduced 65% in subjects treated with clarithromycin 500 mg twice daily for 7 days.[2] Midazolam's bioavailability was increased from 0.31 to 0.75 after clarithromycin pretreatment.

RELATED DRUGS: Erythromycin (eg, *Ery-Tab*), troleandomycin,[†] and roxithromycin[†] have been reported to inhibit the metabolism of midazolam. Clarithromycin is likely to reduce the metabolism of other benzodiazepines, such as diazepam (eg, *Valium*), which are metabolized by CYP3A4. Other benzodiazepines (eg, lorazepam [eg, *Ativan*], oxazepam) that are not metabolized by CYP3A4 are unlikely to be affected by clarithromycin.

MANAGEMENT OPTIONS:

➡ ***Consider Alternative.*** Azithromycin (eg, *Zithromax*) and dirithromycin[†] do not inhibit CYP3A4 and are not expected to affect midazolam metabolism. Lorazepam (eg, *Ativan*) and oxazepam are benzodiazepines that are not expected to interact with clarithromycin.

➡ ***Monitor.*** Monitor for excess sedation in patients administered midazolam during therapy with clarithromycin.

REFERENCES:

1. Yeates RA, et al. Interaction between midazolam and clarithromycin: comparison with azithromycin. *Int J Clin Pharmacol Ther.* 1996;34(9):400-405.

2. Gorski JC, et al. The contribution of intestinal and hepatic CYP3A to the interaction between midazolam and clarithromycin. *Clin Pharmacol Ther.* 1998;64(2):133-143.

† Not available in the United States.

Clarithromycin (eg, *Biaxin*)
Nifedipine (eg, *Procardia*)

SUMMARY: Clarithromycin may increase the plasma concentration of nifedipine, increasing its hypotensive effects.

RISK FACTORS: No specific risk factors are known.

MECHANISM: Clarithromycin inhibits CYP3A4, the primary enzyme that metabolizes nifedipine.

CLINICAL EVALUATION: A 77-year-old patient with a history of diabetes, bronchitis, hypertension, renal dysfunction, and left ventricular dysfunction was taking doxazosin 8 mg daily, sustained-release nifedipine 60 mg daily, and captopril 25 mg daily.[1] After complaining of an upper respiratory tract infection, the patient was started on clarithromycin 500 mg every 12 hours. Two days later, following the discontinuation of captopril and the initiation of valsartan 80 mg every 12 hours, the patient developed dyspnea, hypotension, bradycardia, and abdominal pain. The patient was treated for hypotensive shock with discontinuation of hypotensive medications and erythromycin was substituted for clarithromycin. The patient was eventually restarted on nifedipine and clarithromycin without further problems. While this case is confounded by many variables, the administration of clarithromycin could have increased the nifedipine plasma concentrations, resulting in an interaction that was exacerbated by the presence of other classes of hypotensive drugs. A recent case-controlled study found a nearly 4-fold increase in risk of hypotension when clarithromycin was coadministered with calcium channel blockers, including nifedipine.[2]

RELATED DRUGS: Clarithromycin is expected to inhibit the metabolism of other calcium channel blockers. Erythromycin (eg, *Ery-Tab*) and telithromycin (*Ketek*) are likely to inhibit the metabolism of nifedipine in a similar manner.

MANAGEMENT OPTIONS:

➡ **Monitor.** Pending more data on this interaction, monitor patients stabilized on nifedipine for excess hypotensive response during clarithromycin coadministration.

REFERENCES:
1. Gerónimo-Pardo M, et al. Clarithromycin-nifedipine interaction as possible cause of vasodilatory shock. *Ann Pharmacother.* 2005;39(3):538-542.
2. Wright AJ, et al. The risk of hypotension following co-prescription of macrolide antibiotics and calcium-channel blockers. *CMAJ.* 2011;183(3):303-307.

Clarithromycin (eg, *Biaxin*) 4
Omeprazole (eg, *Prilosec*)

SUMMARY: Clarithromycin administration increased omeprazole concentrations. While toxicity is unlikely, increased omeprazole efficacy may result.

RISK FACTORS: No specific risk factors are known.

MECHANISM: Clarithromycin inhibits the CYP3A4 and perhaps the CYP2C19 metabolism of omeprazole.

CLINICAL EVALUATION: Twenty-one subjects were administered clarithromycin 400 mg or placebo twice daily for 3 days.[1] On the fourth day, each subject was administered a single dose of omeprazole 20 mg with a dose of clarithromycin 400 mg. Subjects were genotyped for CYP2C19 activity. Omeprazole is primarily metabolized by CYP2C19; CYP3A4 is a minor pathway in most patients. Six subjects were homozygous extensive metabolizers (EMs), 11 were heterozygous EMs, and 4 were CYP2C19 poor metabolizers (PMs). Omeprazole areas under the concentration-time curve (AUCs) when taken alone were 383, 1,001, and 5,589 ng/h/mL for the homozygous EMs, heterozygous EMs, and PMs, respectively. The coadministration of clarithromycin increased these AUCs 117%, 110%, and 134%, respectively. This clarithromycin-induced increase in omeprazole concentrations probably contributes to omeprazole's efficacy when combined with clarithromycin for the treatment of *Helicobacter pylori* infections.

RELATED DRUGS: Erythromycin (eg, *Ery-Tab*) and troleandomycin[†] are likely to produce similar changes in omeprazole concentrations. While other proton pump inhibitors undergo some CYP3A4 metabolism, the effect of clarithromycin on plasma concentration is unreported.

MANAGEMENT OPTIONS:

➡ *Monitor.* No specific action is required, but be alert for evidence of an interaction.

REFERENCES:
1. Furuta T, et al. Effects of clarithromycin on the metabolism of omeprazole in relation to CYP2C19 genotype status in humans. *Clin Pharmacol Ther.* 1999;66(3):265-274.

† Not available in the United States.

Clarithromycin (eg, *Biaxin*)

Oxycodone (eg, *Oxycontin*)

SUMMARY: Clarithromycin administration increases oxycodone and oxymorphone plasma concentrations; some patients may experience enhanced opioid effects.

RISK FACTORS: No specific risk factors are known.

MECHANISM: Clarithromycin inhibits the metabolism of oxycodone to noroxycodone; this enables more oxycodone to be metabolized by CYP2D6 to oxymorphone.

CLINICAL EVALUATION: Ten young and ten elderly subjects took a single dose of oral oxycodone 10 mg on day 4 of a 5-day course of clarithromycin 500 mg twice daily or placebo.[1] The administration of clarithromycin reduced the oral clearance of oxycodone approximately 50%, resulting in a mean increase in the area under the plasma concentration-time curve of oxycodone of approximately 200%. The half-life of oxycodone was increased from 4.4 to 5.8 hours and from 5.9 to 7 hours in the young and elderly subjects, respectively. The concentration of noroxycodone was reduced following clarithromycin dosing while the concentration of the active metabolite oxymorphone was increased more than 300% in both subject groups.

RELATED DRUGS: Other opioids that are substrates for CYP3A4 (eg, fentanyl [eg, *Fentora*], alfentanil [eg, *Alfenta*]) are expected to interact in a similar manner. Erythromycin (eg, *Ery-Tab*) is likely to produce a similar reduction in the clearance of oxycodone.

MANAGEMENT OPTIONS:

➥ *Consider Alternative.* Azithromycin (eg, *Zithromax*) does not inhibit CYP3A4 and could be considered as an alternative to clarithromycin in patients receiving oxycodone.

➥ *Monitor.* Observe patients receiving oxycodone and clarithromycin for increased opioid effects, including nausea, vomiting, sedation, and respiratory depression; oxycodone dose reduction may be needed to avoid toxicity.

REFERENCES:

1. Liukas A, et al. Inhibition of cytochrome P450 3A by clarithromycin uniformly affects the pharmacokinetics and pharmacodynamics of oxycodone in young and elderly volunteers. *J Clin Psychopharmacol.* 2011;31(3):302-308.

Clarithromycin (eg, *Biaxin*)

Pimozide (*Orap*)

SUMMARY: Elevated pimozide concentrations and cardiac arrhythmias may occur if pimozide and clarithromycin are coadministered.

RISK FACTORS: No specific risk factors are known.

MECHANISM: Clarithromycin inhibits the CYP3A4 metabolism of pimozide. Both drugs can produce a prolongation of the QTc interval. The coadministration of pimozide and clarithromycin may lead to a pharmacokinetic and pharmacodynamic interaction, potentially producing ventricular arrhythmias including torsades de pointes.

CLINICAL EVALUATION: Nine subjects were administered a single dose of pimozide 6 mg following a 5-day regimen of clarithromycin 500 mg twice daily or placebo.[1] Compared with placebo, clarithromycin pretreatment reduced the clearance of pimozide an average of 46%. The mean QTc was prolonged 13.3 and 15.7 seconds during pimozide alone and pimozide plus clarithromycin, respectively. The manufacturer of pimozide contraindicates the use of azithromycin (eg, *Zithromax*) and dirithromycin[+] with pimozide.[2] However, azithromycin has been shown to have no effect on the in vitro metabolism of pimozide and is unlikely to affect its CYP3A4 metabolism in vivo.[3] The administration of clarithromycin and pimozide has been associated with sudden cardiac death in at least 1 patient.[4] Patients with bradycardia, hypokalemia, or hypomagnesemia may be at increased risk of torsades de pointes.

RELATED DRUGS: Erythromycin (eg, *Ery-Tab*) and troleandomycin[+] are likely to produce similar increases in pimozide plasma concentrations. Azithromycin and dirithromycin do not inhibit CYP3A4 activity and are not expected to reduce pimozide metabolism.

MANAGEMENT OPTIONS:

➥ *Use Alternative.* Do not administer clarithromycin or erythromycin to patients receiving pimozide. Azithromycin or dirithromycin are suitable alternatives.

➥ **Monitor.** If clarithromycin, troleandomycin, or erythromycin is coadministered with pimozide, monitor the electrocardiogram for evidence of QTc prolongation.

REFERENCES:

1. Desta Z, et al. Effect of clarithromycin on the pharmacokinetics and pharmacodynamics of pimozide in healthy poor and extensive metabolizers of cytochrome P450 2D6 (CYP2D6). *Clin Pharmacol Ther.* 1999;65(1):10-20.

2. *Orap* [package insert]. North Wales, PA: Gate Pharmaceuticals; 1999.

3. Desta Z, et al. In vitro inhibition of pimozide N-dealkylation by selective serotonin reuptake inhibitors and azithromycin. *J Clin Psychopharmacol.* 2002;22(2):162-168.

4. Flockhart DA, et al. Studies on the mechanism of a fatal clarithromycin-pimozide interaction in a patient with Tourette syndrome. *J Clin Psychopharmacol.* 2000;20(3):317-324.

† Not available in the United States.

Clarithromycin (eg, *Biaxin*)

Prednisone

SUMMARY: The coadministration of clarithromycin and prednisone may lead to elevated prednisone concentrations and altered mental function.

RISK FACTORS: No specific risk factors are known.

MECHANISM: Clarithromycin may inhibit the metabolism (CYP3A4) of prednisone or its metabolite prednisolone, leading to toxic steroid concentrations and altered mental status.

CLINICAL EVALUATION: Two cases of acutely altered mental status have been reported during the coadministration of prednisone and clarithromycin.[1,2] In both cases, the mental changes occurred within a few days of the initiation of clarithromycin and prednisone. One patient had been taking prednisone 20 mg/day for 1 month prior to the addition of clarithromycin without adverse reaction. In the other patient, prednisone was begun simultaneously with clarithromycin. Although the possibility exists that the prednisone alone accounted for the mental status changes, an interaction seems likely.

RELATED DRUGS: Erythromycin (eg, *Ery-Tab*) and troleandomycin† are likely to inhibit the metabolism of prednisone and prednisolone (eg, *Orapred*). Methylprednisolone (eg, *Medrol*) is also a substrate for CYP3A4 and may interact with these macrolides in a similar manner. Azithromycin (eg, *Zithromax*) and dirithromycin† do not inhibit CYP3A4 activity and are not expected to interact with corticosteroids.

MANAGEMENT OPTIONS:

➥ **Consider Alternative.** Consider azithromycin or dirithromycin for patients taking corticosteroids who require macrolide antibiotics.

➥ **Monitor.** Observe patients receiving prednisone and CYP3A4-inhibiting macrolides for evidence of excessive steroid effects, including changing mental function, glucose intolerance, and muscle weakness.

REFERENCES:

1. Finkenbine R, et al. Case of mania due to prednisone-clarithromycin interaction. *Can J Psychiatry.* 1997;42(7):778.

2. Finkenbine RD, et al. Case of psychosis due to prednisone-clarithromycin interaction. *Gen Hosp Psychiatry.* 1998;20(5):325-326.

† Not available in the United States.

Clarithromycin (eg, *Biaxin*)

Repaglinide (*Prandin*)

SUMMARY: Clarithromycin increases repaglinide serum concentrations and the insulin response to repaglinide. The effect on glycemic control in patients with diabetes is unknown.

RISK FACTORS: No specific risk factors are known.

MECHANISM: Clarithromycin inhibits the CYP3A4 pathway of repaglinide metabolism.

CLINICAL EVALUATION: Nine subjects received placebo or clarithromycin 250 mg twice daily for 4 days.[1] On day 5, they were administered a single dose of clarithromycin and repaglinide 0.25 mg. Compared with placebo, clarithromycin increased the mean area under the concentration-time curve of repaglinide 40% and the mean peak repaglinide concentration 67%. The half-life of repaglinide was significantly increased from 1.4 to 1.7 hours following clarithromycin administration. The serum insulin response to repaglinide was also increased following clarithromycin administration. Larger doses of clarithromycin are expected to produce a greater effect on repaglinide pharmacokinetics. The effect of these changes in repaglinide serum concentrations in patients with diabetes is unknown, but some may have enhanced hypoglycemic response during clarithromycin and repaglinide coadministration.

RELATED DRUGS: Erythromycin (eg, *E-Mycin*) and troleandomycin (*TAO*) also inhibit CYP3A4 and would be expected to affect repaglinide in a manner similar to that seen with clarithromycin.

MANAGEMENT OPTIONS:

➡ **Consider Alternative.** Azithromycin (*Zithromax*) and dirithromycin (*Dynabac*) do not inhibit CYP3A4 and would not be expected to alter repaglinide serum concentrations.

➡ **Monitor.** Monitor patients requiring clarithromycin and repaglinide for symptoms of hypoglycemia, including tachycardia, tremor, and sweating.

REFERENCES:
1. Niemi M, et al. The cytochrome P4503A4 inhibitor clarithromycin increases the plasma concentrations and effects of repaglinide. *Clin Pharmacol Ther*. 2001;70:58-65.

Clarithromycin (eg, *Biaxin*)

Rifabutin (*Mycobutin*) AVOID

SUMMARY: Clarithromycin increases the plasma concentrations of rifabutin and increases its toxicity. Rifabutin reduces the concentration of clarithromycin and may result in a loss of efficacy. Avoid the combination.

RISK FACTORS: No specific risk factors are known.

MECHANISM: Clarithromycin inhibits the metabolism (CYP3A4) of rifabutin. Rifabutin increases the metabolism of clarithromycin.

CLINICAL EVALUATION: The coadministration of clarithromycin 500 mg and rifabutin 300 mg daily for 7 days increased the mean area under the plasma concentration-time curve (AUC) of rifabutin 76% compared with the AUC of rifabutin administered alone to patients with HIV.[1] In another study of clarithromycin 500 mg twice daily coadministered with rifabutin 300 mg daily for several weeks, mean rifabutin AUC was increased 99%.[2] Healthy subjects taking clarithromycin 500 mg twice daily and rifabutin 300 mg daily had rifabutin plasma concentrations about 4 times higher than subjects taking only rifabutin.[3] Side effects, including uveitis, GI upset, myalgia, and neutropenia were observed in these trials and in patients receiving combination therapy with clarithromycin and rifabutin.[4,5,6] Avoid the combination of clarithromycin and rifabutin.

Rifabutin 300 mg daily reduced the AUC of clarithromycin 44%,[2] while the administration of rifabutin 600 mg daily reduced the mean clarithromycin concentration 63%.[7] This magnitude of reduction in clarithromycin plasma concentration will reduce the antibacterial efficacy of clarithromycin.

RELATED DRUGS: Troleandomycin and erythromycin would be expected to interact in a similar manner with rifabutin. Azithromycin (*Zithromax*) does not increase rifabutin concentrations, but increased adverse effects have been reported during coadministration of rifabutin and azithromycin.[8] The effect of the coadministration of dirithromycin (*Dynabac*) and rifabutin is unknown but should be avoided pending trial outcomes. Rifampin also induces the metabolism of clarithromycin.

MANAGEMENT OPTIONS:

➡ *AVOID COMBINATION.* Because of the risk of increased toxicity and potential loss of efficacy, avoid the combination of clarithromycin and rifabutin.

REFERENCES:

1. Jordan MK, et al. Effects of fluconazole and clarithromycin on rifabutin and 25-O-desacetylrifabutin pharmacokinetics. *Antimicrob Agents Chemother.* 2000;44:2170-2172.
2. Hafner R, et al. Tolerance and pharmacokinetic interactions of rifabutin and clarithromycin in human immunodeficiency virus-infected volunteers. *Antimicrob Agents Chemother.* 1998;42:631-639.
3. Apseloff G, et al. Comparison of azithromycin and clarithromycin in their interactions with rifabutin in healthy volunteers. *J Clin Pharmacol.* 1998;38:830-835.
4. Griffith DE, et al. Adverse events associated with high-dose rifabutin in macrolide-containing regimens for the treatment of *Mycobacterium avium* complex lung disease. *Clin Infect Dis.* 1995;21:594-598.
5. Benson CA, et al. Clarithromycin or rifabutin alone or in combination for primary prophylaxis of *Mycobacterium avium* complex disease in patients with AIDS: a randomized, double-blind, placebo-controlled trial. *J Infect Dis.* 2000;181:1289-1297.
6. Lowe SH, et al. Uveitis during treatment of disseminated *Mycobacterium avium*-intracellulare complex infection with the combination of rifabutin, clarithromycin and ethambutol. *Neth J Med.* 1996;48:211-215.
7. Wallace RJ, et al. Reduced serum levels of clarithromycin in patients treated with multidrug regimens including rifampin or rifabutin for *Mycobacterium avium-M. intracellulare* infection. *J Infect Dis.* 1995;171:747-750.
8. Hafner R, et al. Tolerance and pharmacokinetic interactions of rifabutin and azithromycin. *Antimicrob Agents Chemother.* 2001;45:1572-1577.

Clarithromycin (eg, *Biaxin*)

Rifampin (eg, *Rifadin*)

SUMMARY: Rifampin reduces the plasma concentrations of clarithromycin. Loss of antimicrobial activity may result.

RISK FACTORS: No specific risk factors are known.

MECHANISM: Rifampin induces the activity of CYP3A4, the enzyme responsible for the metabolism of clarithromycin.

CLINICAL EVALUATION: Nine patients with *Mycobacterium avium* received clarithromycin 500 mg twice daily alone and with rifampin 600 mg/day.[1] The plasma concentration of clarithromycin was reduced by 87% during rifampin coadministration. This degree of reduction in clarithromycin concentration is likely to markedly reduce its antimicrobial activity.

RELATED DRUGS: Erythromycin may be affected in a similar manner by rifampin coadministration. Rifabutin also increases the metabolism of clarithromycin.

MANAGEMENT OPTIONS:

➡ *Consider Alternative.* Azithromycin (eg, *Zithromax*) is not metabolized by CYP3A4 and may offer an alternative to clarithromycin in patients receiving rifampin.

➡ *Monitor.* If rifampin is coadministered to patients taking clarithromycin or erythromycin, monitor for the potential loss of antibiotic efficacy.

REFERENCES:

1. Wallace RJ Jr, et al. Reduced serum levels of clarithromycin in patients treated with multidrug regimens including rifampin or rifabutin for *Mycobacterium avium-M. intracellulare* infection. *J Infect Dis.* 1995;171:747-750.

Clarithromycin (eg, *Biaxin*)

Ritonavir (*Norvir*)

SUMMARY: Clarithromycin produces a small increase in ritonavir serum concentrations that is unlikely to produce toxicity. Ritonavir significantly increased clarithromycin concentrations; the clinical significance of this change is unknown.

RISK FACTORS: No specific risk factors are known.

MECHANISM: Ritonavir appears to inhibit the metabolism of clarithromycin and, to a lesser extent, clarithromycin inhibits the metabolism of ritonavir.

CLINICAL EVALUATION: Ritonavir 200 mg every 8 hours and clarithromycin 500 mg every 12 hours were each administered orally for 4 days alone and in combination to 22 healthy subjects.[1] The administration of clarithromycin with ritonavir increased the area under the concentration-time curve (AUC) of ritonavir by a small amount (13%). This change is not likely to alter a patient's response to ritonavir. Ritonavir administration increased the mean AUC of clarithromycin 77% compared with the AUC of clarithromycin after its administration alone. The mean half-life of clarithromycin increased from a baseline of 5 hours to 14 hours following ritonavir coadministration. The significance of this increase in clarithromycin serum concentration is unknown but could result in increased GI intolerance.

RELATED DRUGS: A similar interaction was seen between clarithromycin and indinavir (*Crixivan*). Other macrolides (eg, erythromycin [eg, *Ery-Tab*]) are likely to affect ritonavir in a similar manner. Dirithromycin (*Dynabac*) and azithromycin (eg, *Zithromax*) are unlikely to inhibit ritonavir metabolism.

MANAGEMENT OPTIONS: No specific action is required, but be alert for evidence of the interaction.

REFERENCES:

1. Ouellet D, et al. Assessment of the pharmacokinetic interaction between ritonavir and clarithromycin. *Clin Pharmacol Ther.* 1996;59:143.

Clarithromycin (eg, *Biaxin*)

Sildenafil (eg, *Viagra*)

SUMMARY: Clarithromycin administration increases sildenafil plasma concentrations; increased sildenafil adverse reactions are likely to occur.

RISK FACTORS: No specific risk factors are known.

MECHANISM: Clarithromycin appears to inhibit the metabolism of sildenafil, probably via the CYP3A4 pathway.

CLINICAL EVALUATION: Twelve healthy men received sildenafil 50 mg alone or 2 hours after taking a single dose of clarithromycin 500 mg.[1] The mean area under the plasma concentration-time curve of sildenafil was increased 128% by the coadministration of clarithromycin. Peak sildenafil concentrations increased 142%. Sildenafil's half-life increased from 2.5 to 3 hours with concurrent clarithromycin administration. The effect of multiple doses of clarithromycin on sildenafil plasma concentrations is likely to be even greater.

RELATED DRUGS: Erythromycin (eg, *Ery-Tab*) would be likely to inhibit the metabolism of sildenafil in a similar manner. Clarithromycin may increase the plasma concentrations of vardenafil (*Levitra*) and tadalafil (*Cialis*).

MANAGEMENT OPTIONS:

➡ *Consider Alternative.* Azithromycin (eg, *Zithromax*) does not inhibit CYP3A4 and could be considered as an alternative to clarithromycin in patients receiving sildenafil.

➡ *Monitor.* Patients using sildenafil should be alert for adverse reactions (dizziness, headache, hypotension) if clarithromycin is coadministered.

REFERENCES:

1. Hedaya MA, et al. The effect of ciprofloxacin and clarithromycin on sildenafil oral bioavailability in human volunteers. *Biopharm Drug Dispos.* 2006;27:103-110.

Clarithromycin (eg, *Biaxin*)

Simvastatin (eg, *Zocor*)

SUMMARY: Clarithromycin administration can increase simvastatin concentrations; myalgia and rhabdomyolysis may result.

RISK FACTORS: No specific risk factors are known.

MECHANISM: Clarithromycin inhibits the first-pass and systemic metabolism of simvastatin by inhibiting the activity of CYP3A4 in the small intestine and the liver. The dual site of CYP3A4 inhibition by clarithromycin may result in a marked increase in simvastatin plasma concentrations.

CLINICAL EVALUATION: A patient with several disease states, including diabetes mellitus, dyslipidemia, hypertension, and renal dysfunction, was taking a number of medications, including simvastatin 80 mg daily. The patient was stabilized on simvastatin for 6 months prior to the administration of clarithromycin 500 mg twice daily for 21 days.[1] Progressive muscle weakness and darkened urine with decreased urinary output and elevated creatine phosphokinase developed. The patient was admitted to the hospital with a diagnosis of rhabdomyolysis and subsequently died from complications. Controlled studies are needed to define the magnitude of clarithromycin-induced inhibition of simvastatin metabolism.

RELATED DRUGS: Erythromycin (eg, *Ery-Tab*) is expected to affect simvastatin metabolism in a similar manner. Lovastatin (eg, *Mevacor*) also appears to be very sensitive to CYP3A4 inhibitors. Atorvastatin (*Lipitor*) is metabolized by CYP3A4 as well.

MANAGEMENT OPTIONS:

➠ *Use Alternative.* A macrolide that does not inhibit CYP3A4, such as azithromycin (eg, *Zithromax*), is preferred in patients taking HMG-CoA reductase inhibitors. Pravastatin (eg, *Pravachol*) and fluvastatin (*Lescol*) are not metabolized by CYP3A4 and are safer alternatives for patients requiring drugs that inhibit the enzyme.

➠ *Circumvent/Minimize.* If the course of clarithromycin therapy is short, discontinue simvastatin during clarithromycin therapy. Simvastatin may be restarted several days after completion of the clarithromycin therapy.

➠ *Monitor.* Monitor patients taking HMG-CoA reductase inhibitors for muscle pain or weakness.

REFERENCES:

1. Lee AJ, et al. Rhabdomyolysis secondary to a drug interaction between simvastatin and clarithromycin. *Ann Pharmacother*. 2001;35:26-31.

Clarithromycin (eg, *Biaxin*)

Sirolimus (*Rapamune*)

SUMMARY: Clarithromycin administration increased sirolimus plasma concentrations; some patients may experience sirolimus toxicity.

RISK FACTORS: No specific risk factors are known.

MECHANISM: Clarithromycin appears to affect the metabolism of sirolimus by CYP3A4 and to inhibit the efflux of sirolimus by the transporter P-glycoprotein.

CLINICAL EVALUATION: About one year following a cadaver-donor kidney transplant, a patient taking sirolimus 2 mg/day was treated with clarithromycin 250 mg twice a day for a week for pneumonia.[1] During the course of clarithromycin, the patient's sirolimus plasma concentration increased from 6.2 to 52.2 ng/mL and was accompanied by a rise in the serum creatinine levels. Sirolimus concentrations declined after stopping both drugs and restabilized at 6.5 ng/mL 6 days after restarting sirolimus at 1.5 mg/day. Kidney function improved with the normalization of sirolimus concentrations.

RELATED DRUGS: Tacrolimus (*Prograf*) and cyclosporine (eg, *Neoral*) are also known to interact with clarithromycin. Everolimus may also interact in a similar manner with clarithromycin. Erythromycin (eg, *Ery-Tab*) and troleandomycin[†] are likely to reduce the elimination of sirolimus.

MANAGEMENT OPTIONS:

➥ **Consider Alternative.** Azithromycin (eg, *Zithromax*) does not inhibit CYP3A4 and may be considered as an alternative to clarithromycin in patients receiving sirolimus.

➥ **Monitor.** Be alert for signs of sirolimus toxicity (eg, thrombocytopenia and hyperlipidemia) if clarithromycin or other CYP3A4 or P-glycoprotein inhibitors are coadministered.

REFERENCES:

1. Capone D, et al. A pharmacokinetic interaction between clarithromycin and sirolimus in kidney transplant recipient. *Curr Drug Metab.* 2007;8(4):379-381.

† Not available in the United States.

 Clarithromycin (eg, *Biaxin*)

Tacrolimus (*Prograf*)

SUMMARY: Tacrolimus concentrations may increase during clarithromycin administration; nephrotoxicity could result.

RISK FACTORS: No specific risk factors are known.

MECHANISM: Clarithromycin is known to inhibit CYP3A4, the enzyme that metabolizes tacrolimus. Thus, it may inhibit the metabolism of tacrolimus, resulting in elevated plasma concentrations.

CLINICAL EVALUATION: A case report noted that tacrolimus concentrations increased after 6 days of clarithromycin therapy, and serum creatinine increased with the tacrolimus concentrations.[1] Tacrolimus was withheld and renal function returned to baseline. Thirty days later, tacrolimus dose requirements were markedly less than the pre-clarithromycin therapy. Clarithromycin is not expected to continue to affect the pharmacokinetics of tacrolimus for several weeks after its administration is discontinued.

RELATED DRUGS: Erythromycin (eg, *Ery-Tab*) also has been reported to increase tacrolimus concentrations.[2] Azithromycin (eg, *Zithromax*) is unlikely to increase tacrolimus concentrations. Clarithromycin is expected to affect cyclosporine (eg, *Neoral*) in a similar manner.

MANAGEMENT OPTIONS:

➥ **Monitor.** Until more information is available, monitor tacrolimus patients for decreasing renal function and increasing tacrolimus serum concentrations following the addition of clarithromycin.

REFERENCES:

1. Wolter K, et al. Interaction between FK 506 and clarithromycin in a renal transplant patient. *Eur J Clin Pharmacol.* 1994;47(2):207-208.
2. Shaeffer MS, et al. Interaction between FK506 and erythromycin. *Ann Pharmacother.* 1994;28(2):280-281.

Clarithromycin (eg, *Biaxin*)

Terfenadine[†]

SUMMARY: Clarithromycin appears to increase terfenadine and terfenadine carboxylate plasma concentrations. Cardiac arrhythmias could result from elevated terfenadine concentrations.

RISK FACTORS: No specific risk factors are known.

MECHANISM: Clarithromycin appears to inhibit the hepatic metabolism of terfenadine and its metabolite, probably by inhibiting the CYP3A4 enzyme.

CLINICAL EVALUATION: The area under the plasma concentration-time curve of terfenadine carboxylate, terfenadine's active metabolite, increased 156% during clarithromycin administration.[1] Terfenadine was not detectable in the plasma of any subject during terfenadine administration alone; 4 of the 6 subjects had terfenadine in their plasma during the terfenadine-clarithromycin phase of the study. The administration of clarithromycin and terfenadine resulted in a prolongation of the QT interval. These changes could result in arrhythmias in some patients.

RELATED DRUGS: Erythromycin (eg, *Ery-Tab*) and troleandomycin[†] have been reported to inhibit the metabolism of terfenadine. Azithromycin (eg, *Zithromax*) and dirithromycin are unlikely to increase terfenadine concentrations. Astemizole is likely to be similarly affected by clarithromycin.

MANAGEMENT OPTIONS:

➡ ***Use Alternative.*** Astemizole may not be a safe alternative to terfenadine because it has been associated with arrhythmias when administered with drugs that inhibit its metabolism. The use of sedating antihistamines, such as loratadine (eg, *Claritin*), fexofenadine (eg, *Allegra*), or cetirizine (eg, *Zyrtec*), may be preferable in patients who require antihistamine therapy during clarithromycin treatment. Azithromycin may be substituted for clarithromycin in some cases.

➡ ***Monitor.*** Monitor patients taking clarithromycin and terfenadine for changes in cardiac conduction.

REFERENCES:

1. Honig PK, et al. Comparison of the effect of the macrolide antibiotics erythromycin, clarithromycin and azithromycin on terfenadine steady-state pharmacokinetics and electrocardiographic parameters. *Drug Invest*. 1994;7:148-156.

† Not available in the US.

Clarithromycin (eg, *Biaxin*)

Theophylline (eg, *Theochron*)

SUMMARY: Clarithromycin produces a small increase in theophylline serum concentrations; toxicity is not likely to result.

RISK FACTORS: No specific risk factors are known.

MECHANISM: Clarithromycin is a relatively weak inhibitor of theophylline metabolism.

CLINICAL EVALUATION: The manufacturer of clarithromycin notes a 20% increase in theophylline concentrations following clarithromycin 250 or 500 mg twice daily.[1] No further details are provided. Five subjects received a single dose of theophylline alone and on the sixth day of clarithromycin 500 mg twice daily for 7 days.[2] The mean area under the concentration-time curve of theophylline was increased 8% and the theophylline half-life increased from 9.8 to 10.5 hours during the clarithromycin phase. Neither of these changes was statistically significant nor is likely to produce adverse clinical effects. An abstract noted no change in theophylline concentrations during coadministration of clarithromycin 500 mg twice daily for 5 days.[3] It appears that clarithromycin has a minimal effect on the metabolism of theophylline, and the coadministration of the 2 drugs should be well tolerated by most patients.

RELATED DRUGS: Erythromycin (eg, *Ery-Tab*) and troleandomycin[†] are more potent inhibitors of theophylline metabolism. Dirithromycin and azithromycin (eg, *Zithromax*) do not inhibit theophylline metabolism.

MANAGEMENT OPTIONS: No specific action is required, but be alert for evidence of the interaction.

REFERENCES:
1. *Biaxin* [package insert]. Abbott Park, IL: Abbott Laboratories; 1992.
2. Gillum JG, et al. Effect of combination therapy with ciprofloxacin and clarithromycin on theophylline pharmacokinetics in healthy volunteers. *Antimicrob Agents Chemother*. 1996;40(7):1715-1716.
3. Ruff F, et al. Effect of multiple doses of clarithromycin on the pharmacokinetics of theophylline [abstract]. In: Program and Abstracts of the 30th Interscience Conference on Antimicrobial Agents and Chemotherapy; October 21–24, 1990; Atlanta, GA. Abstract 761.

† Not available in the US.

Clarithromycin (eg, *Biaxin*)

Tipranavir (*Aptivus*)

SUMMARY: During the coadministration of clarithromycin and tipranavir, the mean area under the plasma concentration-time curves (AUCs) of tipranavir and clarithromycin were increased; an increase in tipranavir adverse reactions may occur in some patients.

RISK FACTORS: No specific risk factors are known.

MECHANISM: Tipranavir/ritonavir appears to inhibit the metabolism of clarithromycin, while clarithromycin inhibits the metabolism of tipranavir. Both effects are likely caused by the inhibition CYP3A4.

CLINICAL EVALUATION: While specific data are limited, the manufacturer of tipranavir notes that clarithromycin 500 mg twice daily for 12 days increased the mean AUC of tipranavir 66%.[1] Some patients may experience an increase in tipranavir toxicity. Tipranavir 500 mg twice daily plus ritonavir 200 mg twice daily coadministered with clarithromycin increased the clarithromycin mean AUC 19%.

RELATED DRUGS: Erythromycin (eg, *Ery-Tab*) and troleandomycin are expected to affect tipranavir in a similar manner.

MANAGEMENT OPTIONS:

➡ *Consider Alternative.* Azithromycin (eg, *Zithromax*) does not inhibit CYP3A4 and could be considered as an alternative to clarithromycin in patients receiving tipranavir.

➡ **Monitor.** If agents that inhibit CYP3A4 are coadministered with tipranavir, watch for signs of tipranavir toxicity (eg, hepatic function impairment, bleeding).

REFERENCES:

1. *Aptivus* [package insert]. Ridgefield, CT: Boehringer Ingelheim Pharmaceuticals, Inc; 2007.

Clarithromycin (eg, *Biaxin*)

Triazolam (eg, *Halcion*)

SUMMARY: Clarithromycin administration can increase triazolam plasma concentrations and pharmacologic effects.

RISK FACTORS: No specific risk factors are known.

MECHANISM: Clarithromycin inhibits the metabolism (CYP3A4) of triazolam in the small intestine and liver. A reduction in first-pass and systemic clearance of triazolam is likely to occur.

CLINICAL EVALUATION: Twelve subjects received clarithromycin 500 mg twice daily for 2 days.[1] Following the third dose of clarithromycin, a single oral dose of triazolam 0.125 mg was administered. The peak plasma concentration and area under the concentration-time curve of triazolam were increased 2- and 5.25-fold, respectively. Triazolam half-life increased from 2.7 to 8.3 hours following clarithromycin administration. The pharmacologic response (eg, sedation, fatigue, decreased mental ability) to triazolam increased following clarithromycin. The effects of a longer duration of clarithromycin administration are unknown; however, it is possible that a larger effect on triazolam pharmacokinetics might be noted.

RELATED DRUGS: Erythromycin (eg, *Ery-Tab*) and troleandomycin† are known to inhibit triazolam metabolism. Azithromycin (eg, *Zithromax*) does not alter triazolam metabolism.

MANAGEMENT OPTIONS:

➡ **Consider Alternative.** Consider azithromycin as an alternative for patients taking triazolam. A benzodiazepine that is not metabolized by CYP3A4 (eg, temazepam [eg, *Restoril*], lorazepam [eg, *Ativan*]) can be considered for administration when patients are taking clarithromycin.

➡ **Monitor.** If clarithromycin is administered to patients taking triazolam, monitor for increased CNS effects.

REFERENCES:

1. Greenblatt DJ, et al. Inhibition of triazolam clearance by macrolide antimicrobial agents: in vitro correlates and dynamic consequences. *Clin Pharmacol Ther.* 1998;64(3):278-285.

† Not available in the US.

Clarithromycin (eg, *Biaxin*)

Verapamil (eg, *Isoptin*)

SUMMARY: The combination of verapamil and clarithromycin has been reported to lead to hypotension and bradycardia.

RISK FACTORS: No specific risk factors are known.

MECHANISM: Clarithromycin is known to inhibit CYP3A4 and P-glycoprotein, both of which contribute to the elimination of verapamil.

CLINICAL EVALUATION: A patient with chronic renal failure, intermittent atrial fibrillation, and chronic obstructive pulmonary disease was being treated with digoxin 0.125 mg 3 times weekly.[1] Because of an increase in pulmonary symptoms and atrial fibrillation, clarithromycin 250 mg twice daily and verapamil 120 mg were initiated. Within 2 days the patient's blood pressure was 89/39 mm Hg and her pulse was 50 beats per minute (no electrocardiogram recorded). Verapamil was discontinued and her hemodynamic status normalized. Digoxin concentration was 0.8 ng/mL prior to the institution of verapamil and clarithromycin; no levels were determined during the hypotensive episode. The hypotension and bradycardia could be related to the combination of verapamil and clarithromycin. However, it is not possible to rule out some contribution of digoxin to the cardiac adverse reactions observed in this patient because both verapamil and clarithromycin can increase digoxin concentrations. A recent case-controlled study found a nearly 4-fold increase in risk of hypotension when clarithromycin was coadministered with calcium channel blockers, including verapamil.[2]

RELATED DRUGS: Clarithromycin is expected to inhibit the metabolism of other calcium channel blockers. Erythromycin (eg, *Ery-Tab*) is known to increase verapamil concentrations. Azithromycin (eg, *Zithromax*), because of its weak P-glycoprotein inhibition, may potentially reduce verapamil elimination. However, no data are available.

MANAGEMENT OPTIONS:

➡ *Consider Alternative.* As noted, azithromycin may have a lower potential to produce an adverse reaction with verapamil because it does not inhibit CYP3A4 and has a modest effect on P-glycoprotein.

➡ *Monitor.* Monitor patients taking verapamil for bradycardia, heart block, and hypotension if clarithromycin is coadministered.

REFERENCES:

1. Kaeser YA, et al. Severe hypotension and bradycardia associated with verapamil and clarithromycin. *Am J Health Syst Pharm.* 1998;55(22):2417-2418.
2. Wright AJ, et al. The risk of hypotension following co-prescription of macrolide antibiotics and calcium-channel blockers. *CMAJ.* 2011;183(3):303-307.

 Clarithromycin (eg, *Biaxin*)

Vinorelbine (eg, *Navelbine*)

SUMMARY: The coadministration of clarithromycin is associated with an increased risk of neutropenia in patients being treated with vinorelbine.

RISK FACTORS: No specific risk factors are known.

MECHANISM: Clarithromycin is known to inhibit the activity of CYP3A4, the enzyme responsible for the metabolism of vinorelbine. Clarithromycin-induced reduction in P-glycoprotein activity may also contribute to reduced clearance of vinorelbine.

CLINICAL EVALUATION: A retrospective cohort study was undertaken of patients treated with vinorelbine for non–small cell lung cancer.[1] Patients were categorized based on their exposure to clarithromycin during vinorelbine administration. The use of other drugs that might inhibit CYP3A4 or contribute to cytotoxicity was noted. The severity of neutropenia during vinorelbine administration was correlated to the dose of vinorelbine, female gender, and concurrent clarithromycin exposure. Four of 12 patients receiving vinorelbine and clarithromycin also received vinorelbine without clarithromycin. In each of these patients, neutrophil counts were lower during concurrent clarithromycin dosing. Clarithromycin administration is likely to increase vinorelbine plasma concentration and produce adverse reactions.

RELATED DRUGS: Erythromycin (eg, *Ery-Tab*) and troleandomycin[†] are likely to inhibit the metabolism of vinorelbine in a similar manner. Vinblastine and vincristine (eg, *Vincasar*) are also CYP3A4 substrates and are likely to interact with clarithromycin.

MANAGEMENT OPTIONS:

➡ **Use Alternative.** Azithromycin (eg, *Zithromax*) does not appear to inhibit CYP3A4 and can be considered as an alternative to clarithromycin in patients receiving vinorelbine.

➡ **Monitor.** Carefully monitor patients for any evidence of neurotoxicity if clarithromycin is coadministered with vinorelbine.

REFERENCES:

1. Yano R, et al. Evaluation of potential interaction between vinorelbine and clarithromycin. *Ann Pharmacother.* 2009;43(3):453-458.

† Not available in the United States.

Clarithromycin (eg, *Biaxin*)

Warfarin (eg, *Coumadin*)

SUMMARY: Clarithromycin appears to increase the anticoagulant effect of warfarin.

RISK FACTORS: No specific risk factors are known.

MECHANISM: Unknown. Clarithromycin is known to inhibit CYP3A4, an enzyme partially responsible for the metabolism of warfarin.

CLINICAL EVALUATION: Two published case reports noted 3 patients who developed an increased international normalized ratio (INR) following the addition of clarithromycin to stable doses of warfarin.[1,2] Clarithromycin dosage was 500 mg twice daily for 10 to 14 days. All patients experienced elevated INR during treatment with clarithromycin. INR returned to baseline values after the discontinuation of clarithromycin and warfarin and the administration of vitamin K. Evaluation of causation in these cases is complicated by the presence of other factors that may alter warfarin metabolism including concomitant drug therapy and infectious diseases.

Prospective studies on the effect of clarithromycin on warfarin metabolism and INR response are needed to substantiate this interaction.

RELATED DRUGS: Erythromycin (eg, *Ery-Tab*) has been reported to reduce the metabolism of warfarin. The metabolism of acenocoumarol also appears to be inhibited by clarithromycin administration.

MANAGEMENT OPTIONS:

➡ **Consider Alternative.** Consider a macrolide antibiotic that does not inhibit metabolism (eg, azithromycin [eg, *Zithromax*]). Note that while cases of azithromycin-induced enhanced warfarin response have been noted, no definitive studies have confirmed this effect.

➡ **Monitor.** Monitor INR in patients stabilized on warfarin therapy during clarithromycin therapy. Check the INR after 3 to 5 days of clarithromycin administration for evidence of increased response.

REFERENCES:

1. Recker MW, et al. Potential interaction between clarithromycin and warfarin. *Ann Pharmacother.* 1997;31(9):996-998.

2. Oberg KC. Delayed elevation of international normalized ratio with concurrent clarithromycin and warfarin therapy. *Pharmacotherapy.* 1998;18(2):386-391.

Clarithromycin (eg, *Biaxin*)

Zidovudine (*Retrovir*)

SUMMARY: Clarithromycin produces minimal changes in zidovudine concentrations; the clinical significance of these changes is unknown.

RISK FACTORS: No specific risk factors are known.

MECHANISM: Clarithromycin may inhibit the absorption of zidovudine.

CLINICAL EVALUATION: The mean area under the plasma concentration-time curve (AUC) of zidovudine in 4 patients with HIV was reduced 27% by clarithromycin 4 g/day. Mean peak zidovudine concentrations were reduced 25% to 45%, although statistical significance was not achieved.[1] Zidovudine administration did not affect the plasma concentrations of clarithromycin. In another study, clarithromycin 1 g twice daily for 3 days increased zidovudine peak concentrations 54% but did not significantly alter the AUC of zidovudine.[2] The clinical effects of clarithromycin-induced changes in zidovudine concentrations are probably limited.

RELATED DRUGS: Azithromycin (*Zithromax*) does not appear to affect zidovudine.

MANAGEMENT OPTIONS: No specific action is required, but be alert for evidence of the interaction.

REFERENCES:

1. Gustavson LE, et al. Drug interaction between clarithromycin and oral zidovudine in HIV-1 infected patients. *Clin Pharmacol Ther.* 1993;53:163.

2. Vance E, et al. Pharmacokinetics of clarithromycin and zidovudine in patients with AIDS. *Antimicrob Agents Chemother.* 1995;39:1355-1360.

Clinafloxacin†

Theophylline (eg, *Theolair*)

SUMMARY: A case report noted an apparent increase in theophylline concentration following the addition of clinafloxacin therapy.

RISK FACTORS: No specific risk factors are known.

MECHANISM: Not established. Clinafloxacin may inhibit the metabolism of theophylline.

CLINICAL EVALUATION: A 78-year-old man with chronic obstructive pulmonary disease had his dose of extended-release theophylline increased from 400 mg twice daily to 300 mg every 8 hours.[1] His plasma theophylline concentration was between 65 and 75 µmol/L (12.9 and 14.9 mg/L) 2 days later. Six days later he was started on clinafloxacin 200 mg IV every 12 hours. Five days after starting clinafloxacin, his theophylline concentration was noted to be 156 µmol/L (30.9 mg/L), but no symptoms of theophylline toxicity were noted. The theophylline dose was reduced to 200 mg every 8 hours and 3 days later the theophylline concentration was 80 µmol/L (15.8 mg/L). No dechallenge was attempted and the patient expired before more data could be obtained. Based upon this report, causation cannot be established. However, clinafloxacin, like other quinolones, may inhibit the metabolism of theophylline and could result in theophylline toxicity.

RELATED DRUGS: Other quinolones known to inhibit the metabolism of theophylline include ciprofloxacin (*Cipro*), enoxacin (*Penetrex*), norfloxacin (*Noroxin*), pipemidic acid, and pefloxacin. Quinolones reported to produce no or minor changes in theophylline pharmacokinetics include fleroxacin, flosequinan, lomefloxacin (*Maxaquin*), ofloxacin (*Floxin*), rufloxacin, sparfloxacin (*Zagam*), and temafloxacin. (Also, see Ciprofloxacin/Theophylline; Enoxacin/Theophylline; Norfloxacin/Theophylline; Pefloxacin/Theophylline monographs.)

MANAGEMENT OPTIONS:

➡ ***Consider Alternative.*** Consider using a quinolone reported to produce no or minor changes in theophylline pharmacokinetics (eg, fleroxacin, flosequinan, lomefloxacin, ofloxacin, rufloxacin, sparfloxacin, temafloxacin).

➡ ***Monitor.*** Monitor patients maintained on theophylline for increased serum theophylline concentrations and signs of toxicity (eg, palpitations, tachycardia, nausea, tremor) during coadministration of clinafloxacin.

REFERENCES:

1. Matuschka PR, et al. Clinafloxacin-theophylline drug interaction. *Ann Pharmacother*. 1995;29:378-380.

† Not available in the US.

Clindamycin (eg, *Cleocin*)

Gentamicin (eg, *Garamycin*)

SUMMARY: Preliminary data suggest that clindamycin may increase the risk of renal toxicity following gentamicin administration.

RISK FACTORS: No specific risk factors are known.

MECHANISM: Not established.

CLINICAL EVALUATION: Three patients have been described in whom the administration of clindamycin appeared to predispose to gentamicin nephrotoxicity.[1] All had normal renal function before therapy and improved rapidly when the antibiotics were discontinued. Causation was not established and confirmation of these preliminary results is needed.

RELATED DRUGS: Clindamycin may increase nephrotoxicity associated with other aminoglycosides as well.

MANAGEMENT OPTIONS: No specific action is required, but be alert for evidence of the interaction.

REFERENCES:

1. Butkus DE, et al. Renal failure following gentamicin in combination with clindamycin. *Nephron*. 1976;17:307-313.

Clobazam (*Frisium*)

Phenytoin (eg, *Dilantin*)

SUMMARY: Case reports suggest that clobazam addition to phenytoin can lead to clinically obvious phenytoin toxicity in patients who have been taking maximum tolerated phenytoin doses.

RISK FACTORS: No specific risk factors are known.

MECHANISM: Not established, but clobazam may inhibit the metabolism of phenytoin.

CLINICAL EVALUATION: In case reports of 3 patients who previously were maintained at high steady-state plasma phenytoin concentrations, 2 to 3 weeks after clobazam therapy was initiated, the patients became clinically toxic (drowsiness, ataxia, incoordination, lethargy). In the 2 patients where laboratory data were available, phenytoin concentrations had increased 25% and 72%.[1]

RELATED DRUGS: No information is available.

MANAGEMENT OPTIONS:

➡ *Monitor.* Be alert for signs of increased phenytoin concentrations when clobazam is initiated, especially in patients maintained at high therapeutic phenytoin concentrations.

REFERENCES:

    1. Zifkin, et al. Phenytoin toxicity due to interaction with clobazam. *Neurology.* 1991;41:313.

Clofibrate (*Atromid-S*)

Contraceptives, Oral (eg, *Ortho-Novum*)

SUMMARY: Some clinical information indicates that oral contraceptives may inhibit the response to clofibrate, but more study is needed.

RISK FACTORS: No specific risk factors are known.

MECHANISM: Oral contraceptives probably enhance the glucuronide conjugation of clofibric acid, the active form of clofibrate. Such a mechanism is consistent with the ability of oral contraceptives to enhance the glucuronide conjugation of other drugs such as benzodiazepines. Oral contraceptives also may have significant intrinsic hyperlipidemic effects in some patients.

CLINICAL EVALUATION: Oral contraceptives appeared to enhance the metabolism of clofibric acid in 1 study comparing 8 women on oral contraceptives with 8 nonusers.[2] Also, serum cholesterol and triglyceride concentrations that previously had been controlled with clofibrate rose in a patient with type IV hyperlipoproteinemia who took an oral contraceptive.[1] Although the study[2] and the case report[1] both indicate that oral contraceptives may reduce clofibrate effect, more evidence is needed to substantiate this interaction. The effect of oral contraceptives on other hypolipidemic drugs is not established.

RELATED DRUGS: The effect of oral contraceptives on other hypolipidemic drugs is not established.

MANAGEMENT OPTIONS: No specific action is required, but be alert for evidence of the interaction.

REFERENCES:

1. Robertson-Rintoul J. Raised serum-lipids and oral contraceptives. *Lancet*. 1972;2:1320.

2. Miners JO, et al. Gender and oral contraceptive steroids as determinants of drug glucuronidation: effects on clofibric acid elimination. *Br J Clin Pharmacol*. 1984;18:240.

Clofibrate (*Atromid-S*)

Furosemide (eg, *Lasix*)

SUMMARY: Furosemide and clofibrate effects may be enhanced in patients with hypoalbuminemia who receive both agents.

RISK FACTORS:

➡ **Concurrent Diseases.** Risk appears higher in nephrotic syndrome or other disorders resulting in hypoalbuminemia.

MECHANISM: Furosemide and clofibrate may compete for plasma albumin-binding sites. Experimental evidence indicates that at plasma albumin concentrations less than 2 g/dL, the unbound fraction of furosemide increases considerably,[2] lending support to a mechanism of protein-binding competition in the patients described below.

CLINICAL EVALUATION: In several patients with nephrotic syndrome, hypoalbuminemia, and hyperlipoproteinemia, combined treatment with furosemide and clofibrate resulted in muscular symptoms (eg, pain, stiffness) as well as a marked diuresis.[1] It seems likely that the competition for albumin binding between the 2 drugs and the hypoalbuminemia resulted in higher free concentrations of both drugs, causing the muscular syndrome and the pronounced diuresis. However, additional study will be required to establish conclusively that the interaction was responsible for the effects.

RELATED DRUGS: It is not known whether other fibric acids such as gemfibrozil (eg, *Lopid*) would interact with furosemide, nor is it known whether loop diuretics other than furosemide would interact with clofibrate.

MANAGEMENT OPTIONS:

➡ **Consider Alternative.** In patients with hypoalbuminemia who are receiving furosemide, consider using hypolipidemic agents other than clofibrate.

➡ **Circumvent/Minimize.** If furosemide and clofibrate are used concurrently in patients with hypoalbuminemia, consider using conservative doses of 1 or both drugs until patient response is determined.

➡ **Monitor.** If furosemide and clofibrate are used concurrently in patients with hypoalbuminemia, monitor for evidence of myopathy (eg, muscle pain, weakness) and for excessive diuretic effect.

REFERENCES:

1. Bridgman JF, et al. Complications during clofibrate treatment of nephrotic-syndrome hyperlipoproteinemia. *Lancet*. 1972,2:506.

2. Prandota J, et al. Furosemide binding to human albumin and plasma of nephrotic children. *Clin Pharmacol Ther*. 1975;17:159.

Clofibrate (*Atromid-S*)

Rifampin (eg, *Rifadin*)

SUMMARY: Clofibrate serum concentrations can be reduced by rifampin.

RISK FACTORS: No specific risk factors are known.

MECHANISM: Rifampin appears to enhance the hepatic metabolism of clofibrate.

CLINICAL EVALUATION: In 5 healthy subjects, rifampin 600 mg/day for 7 days reduced the steady-state plasma concentrations of the active metabolite of clofibrate 40%.[1] The degree to which this reduces the long-term therapeutic effect of clofibrate has not been established, but in the short term, rifampin probably reduces the therapeutic response to clofibrate.

RELATED DRUGS: No information is available.

MANAGEMENT OPTIONS:

➥ *Circumvent/Minimize.* An increased dose of clofibrate may be necessary during rifampin coadministration.

➥ *Monitor.* When rifampin therapy is prolonged in patients on clofibrate, monitor serum lipid levels to detect inhibition of clofibrate effect.

REFERENCES:

1. Houin G, et al. Clofibrate and enzymatic induction in man. *Int J Clin Pharmacol*. 1978;16:150.

 Clofibrate (*Atromid-S*)

Warfarin (eg, *Coumadin*)

SUMMARY: Clofibrate increases the hypoprothrombinemic effect of warfarin and probably other oral anticoagulants; serious bleeding episodes have occurred in some patients receiving warfarin and clofibrate.

RISK FACTORS: No specific risk factors are known.

MECHANISM: Not established. Clofibrate may enhance warfarin's effect on the synthesis of vitamin K-dependent clotting factors or affect the turnover of vitamin K. Clofibrate also may displace warfarin from plasma protein binding sites,[12] but it does not appear to affect warfarin metabolism.[14]

CLINICAL EVALUATION: Clofibrate has been shown to increase the hypoprothrombinemic response to warfarin and other oral anticoagulants.[1-11,13] At least 1 death from massive hemorrhage has been attributed to this interaction.[3] Some people appear more likely to develop the interaction than others,[1,2] but the risk factors are not established.

RELATED DRUGS: Gemfibrozil (eg, *Lopid*), lovastatin (*Mevacor*), and simvastatin (*Zocor*) may increase the effect of oral anticoagulants while cholestyramine (eg, *Questran*) and colestipol (*Colestid*) may reduce their effect.

MANAGEMENT OPTIONS:

➥ *Avoid Unless Benefit Outweighs Risk.* Avoid concomitant therapy with clofibrate and oral anticoagulants if possible. If oral anticoagulant therapy is begun in a patient receiving clofibrate, anticoagulant doses probably should be conservative until the maintenance dose is established.

➡ **Monitor.** Monitor for altered oral anticoagulant effect if clofibrate is initiated, discontinued, or changed in dosage.

REFERENCES:

1. Starr KJ, et al. Drug interactions in patients on long term oral anticoagulant and antihypertensive adrenergic neuron-blocking drugs. *BMJ.* 1972;4:133.
2. Udall JA. Drug interference with warfarin therapy. *Clin Med.* 1970;77:20.
3. Solomon RB, et al. Massive hemorrhage and death during treatment with clofibrate and warfarin. *NY State J Med.* 1973;73:2002.
4. Eastham RD. Warfarin dosage influenced by clofibrate plus age. *Lancet.* 1973;1:1450.
5. Oliver MF, et al. Effect of Atromid and ethyl chlorophenoxyisobutyrate on anticoagulant requirements. *Lancet.* 1963;1:143.
6. Schrogie JJ, et al. The anticoagulant response to bishydroxycoumarin II: the effect of D-thyroxine, clofibrate, and norethandrolone. *Clin Pharmacol Ther.* 1967;8:70.
7. Hunninghake DB, et al. Drug interactions with warfarin. *Arch Intern Med.* 1968;121:349.
8. Pond SM, et al. The effects of allopurinol and clofibrate on the elimination of coumarin anticoagulants in man. *Aust NZ J Med.* 1975;5:324.
9. Corrigan JJ, et al. Coagulopathy associated with vitamin E ingestion. *JAMA.* 1974;230:1300.
10. Williams JRB, et al. Effect of concomitantly administered drugs on the control of long term anticoagulant therapy. *Q J Med.* 1976;45:63.
11. Bjornsson TD, et al. Interaction of clofibrate with warfarin: studies using radiolabeled vitamin K. *Clin Pharmacol Ther.* 1977;21:99.
12. Bjornsson TD, et al. Clofibrate displaces warfarin from plasma proteins in man: an example of a pure displacement interaction. *J Pharmacol Exp Ther.* 1979;210:316.
13. Roberts SD, et al. Effect of Atromid on requirements of warfarin. *J Atheroscler Res.* 1963;3:655.
14. Bjornsson TD, et al. Interaction of clofibrate with warfarin: effect of clofibrate on the disposition of the optical enantiomorphs of warfarin. *J Pharmacokinet Biopharm.* 1977;5:495.

Clomipramine (eg, *Anafranil*)

Fluvoxamine (*Luvox*)

SUMMARY: Fluvoxamine substantially increased clomipramine serum concentrations in 1 patient, probably by inhibition of clomipramine metabolism; adjustments in clomipramine dosage may be needed.

RISK FACTORS: No specific risk factors are known.

MECHANISM: The demethylation of clomipramine to desmethylclomipramine appears to be mediated by the cytochrome P450 isozymes, CYP1A2 and CYP3A4. Fluvoxamine is known to inhibit both of these isozymes (especially CYP1A2).

CLINICAL EVALUATION: A 15-year-old autistic boy was given clomipramine up to 50 mg 3 times daily for 8 weeks with minimal response.[1] The addition of fluvoxamine 25 mg/day resulted in a 3-fold increase in trough serum concentrations of both clomipramine and a major metabolite, desmethylclomipramine (DCMI). An adequate clinical response was still not obtained. Although the clinical importance of this interaction is not established, the magnitude of the increases in clomipramine serum concentrations appears sufficient to increase the risk of clomipramine adverse effects. Moreover, some evidence suggests a negative correlation between DCMI levels and clinical improvement in obsessive compulsive symptoms. Thus, elevated DCMI levels theoretically would reduce the clinical response.

RELATED DRUGS: Other combinations of tricyclic antidepressants and selective serotonin reuptake inhibitors also may interact (see Desipramine-Fluoxetine monograph and Index).

MANAGEMENT OPTIONS:

➡ *Monitor.* Monitor for evidence of excessive clomipramine effect if fluvoxamine is given concurrently; adjust the clomipramine dosage as needed.

REFERENCES:

1. Oesterheld J, et al. Grapefruit juice and clomipramine: shifting metabolic ratios. *J Clin Psychopharmacol.* 1997;17:62.

 Clomipramine (eg, *Anafranil*)

Grapefruit Juice

SUMMARY: Grapefruit juice increased clomipramine serum concentrations in 2 patients, probably by inhibition of clomipramine metabolism; adjustments in clomipramine dosage may be needed.

RISK FACTORS: No specific risk factors are known.

MECHANISM: The demethylation of clomipramine to desmethylclomipramine appears to be at least partly mediated by cytochrome P4503A4. Grapefruit juice is known to inhibit CYP3A4, and thus may reduce the metabolism of clomipramine.

CLINICAL EVALUATION: An 8-year-old boy with Tourette's syndrome and obsessive compulsive disorder had minimal improvement with clomipramine 25 mg 3 times daily for 3 months. After 3 days of giving each dose of clomipramine with 250 ml grapefruit juice, his clomipramine serum concentrations almost tripled, and he subsequently developed sustained clinical improvement.[1] Another patient, a 13-year-old girl with autistic disorder who was not responding to clomipramine, developed an approximately 50% increase in clomipramine serum concentrations after 3 days of giving the clomipramine with grapefruit juice. Nonetheless, clinical improvement did not occur. Although the clinical importance of this interaction is not established, the magnitude of the increases in clomipramine serum concentrations may be sufficient to increase the risk of clomipramine adverse effects in some patients.

RELATED DRUGS: The effect of grapefruit juice on other tricyclic antidepressants is not established.

MANAGEMENT OPTIONS:

➡ *Monitor.* Monitor for evidence of excessive clomipramine effect if it is taken with grapefruit juice; adjust the clomipramine dosage as needed.

REFERENCES:

1. Oesterheld J, et al. Grapefruit juice and clomipramine: shifting metabolic ratios. *J Clin Psychopharmacol.* 1997;17:62.

 Clomipramine (eg, *Anafranil*)

Ibuprofen (eg, *Motrin*)

SUMMARY: The combined use of clomipramine with ibuprofen (or other nonsteroidal anti-inflammatory drugs [NSAIDs]) appears to increase the risk of upper GI bleeding.

RISK FACTORS: No specific risk factors are known.

MECHANISM: NSAIDs impair the defenses of the gastric mucosa, which can lead to gastric erosions and bleeding. Also, both NSAIDs and clomipramine can impair platelet function. Serotonin appears to play a role in platelet function, but platelets do not synthesize serotonin. Clomipramine is a potent inhibitor of serotonin reuptake, and, like selective serotonin reuptake inhibitors (SSRIs), probably inhibits the uptake of serotonin by platelets. This may add to the antiplatelet effects of NSAIDs.

CLINICAL EVALUATION: In a population-based cohort study of 26,005 antidepressant users, clomipramine or other SSRIs without an NSAID increased the risk of serious GI bleeding by 3.6-fold, but patients on both an SSRI and NSAID had more than a 12-fold increase in risk.[1] The increase in GI bleeding risk appeared to correlate with the potency of the antidepressant as a serotonin reuptake inhibitor. Antidepressants with less serotonergic effect than SSRIs, such as imipramine (eg, *Tofranil*), amitriptyline, and doxepin (eg, *Sinequan*), appeared somewhat less likely to be associated with GI bleeding than clomipramine or SSRIs, although the risk was increased. Antidepressants with minimal serotonergic effects, such as desipramine (eg, *Norpramin*), trimipramine (*Surmontil*), nortriptyline (eg, *Aventyl*), maprotiline, and mianserin,[+] did not appear to increase the risk of GI bleeding.[1] In another report of a 5-year case-control study of 1,651 cases of serious GI bleeding compared with 10,000 matched controls, there was a 3-fold increase in GI bleeding in users of SSRIs (without NSAIDs) compared with nonusers.[2] Patients receiving both an SSRI and an NSAID had an almost 16-fold increase of GI bleeding.

Given the plausible biological mechanism (see Mechanism) and the consistent findings from 2 studies, assume that the combination of clomipramine or SSRIs with NSAIDs substantially increases the relative risk of upper GI bleeding. Nonetheless, note that the absolute risk of GI bleeding was not high; GI bleeding occurred in only 17 of 4,107 patients receiving clomipramine or SSRIs with NSAIDs.[1] Given the low absolute risk, there may be situations in which the benefit of the combination outweighs the risk.

RELATED DRUGS: Assume that all other drugs that inhibit serotonin reuptake (eg, citalopram [eg, *Celexa*], fluoxetine [eg, *Prozac*], fluvoxamine [eg, *Luvox*], nefazodone, paroxetine [eg, *Paxil*], sertraline [eg, *Zoloft*], venlafaxine [eg, *Effexor*]) would interact with all NSAIDs (eg, diclofenac [eg, *Voltaren*], diflunisal, etodolac, fenoprofen [eg, *Nalfon*], flurbiprofen [eg, *Ansaid*], ibuprofen [eg, *Motrin*], indomethacin [eg, *Indocin*], ketoprofen, ketorolac, meclofenamate, mefenamic acid [eg, *Ponstel*], meloxicam [eg, *Mobic*], nabumetone, naproxen [eg, *Aleve*], oxaprozin [eg, *Daypro*], piroxicam [eg, *Feldene*], sulindac [eg, *Clinoril*], tolmetin).

MANAGEMENT OPTIONS:

➡ *Consider Alternative.* Consider using a non-NSAID analgesic, such as acetaminophen (eg, *Tylenol*). If an NSAID is needed, consider a nonacetylated salicylate, such as choline magnesium trisalicylate, salsalate (eg, *Amigesic*), or magnesium salicylate (eg, *Doan's*), because these products have minimal effects on platelets and the gastric mucosa. It is not known whether COX-2 inhibitors such as celecoxib (*Celebrex*) or valdecoxib[+] are less likely to cause GI bleeding with clomipramine. Antidepressants with less effect on serotonin (see Clinical Evaluation) may reduce the risk of GI bleeding when combined with NSAIDs.

➡ **Monitor.** Patients receiving both clomipramine and an NSAID should be alert for evidence of GI bleeding.

REFERENCES:

1. Dalton SO, et al. Use of selective serotonin reuptake inhibitors and risk of upper gastrointestinal tract bleeding: a population-based cohort study. *Arch Intern Med.* 2003;163(1):59-64.

2. de Abajo FJ, et al. Association between selective serotonin reuptake inhibitors and upper gastrointestinal bleeding: population based case-control study. *BMJ.* 1999;319(7217):1106-1109.

† Not available in the United States.

 Clomipramine (eg, *Anafranil*)

AVOID **Methylene Blue (eg, *Urolene Blue*)**

SUMMARY: Giving methylene blue to patients receiving clomipramine or other serotonergic drugs may result in serotonin syndrome; the combination is best avoided.

RISK FACTORS: No specific risk factors are known.

MECHANISM: Methylene blue appears to be a strong inhibitor of monoamine oxidase type A (MAO-A) and a weak inhibitor of MAO-B.[1,2] Selective serotonin-norepinephrine reuptake inhibitors (SNRIs), such as clomipramine, and selective serotonin reuptake inhibitors (SSRIs) may cause severe serotonin syndrome when combined with MAO inhibitors (MAOIs).

CLINICAL EVALUATION: A 66-year-old woman on long-term clomipramine who was given methylene blue during a parathyroidectomy developed evidence of serotonin syndrome after surgery (eg, agitation, confusion, jerking movements of limbs).[3] Virtually all cases of serotonin syndrome following methylene blue have occurred in patients receiving SNRIs or SSRIs, which is consistent with the view that a drug interaction is involved. (SNRIs or SSRIs given alone rarely produce serious serotonin toxicity, even when taken in overdose.)

RELATED DRUGS: Methylene blue has been associated with serotonin syndrome in patients receiving other SSRIs, such as citalopram (eg, *Celexa*), fluoxetine (eg, *Prozac*), and paroxetine (eg, *Paxil*), and also in patients receiving SNRIs, such as venlafaxine (eg, *Effexor*). Methylene blue is likely to also interact with other SSRIs, such as escitalopram (*Lexapro*), fluvoxamine (eg, *Luvox*), and sertraline (eg, *Zoloft*), and other SNRIs, such as desvenlafaxine (*Pristiq*), duloxetine (*Cymbalta*), and imipramine (eg, *Tofranil*).

MANAGEMENT OPTIONS:

➡ **AVOID COMBINATION.** Given that serotonin syndrome can be life-threatening, it is prudent to avoid the combination.[4] Stopping clomipramine or other SSRIs or SNRIs for 2 weeks before using methylene blue would minimize the risk, except for fluoxetine, where 5 weeks should elapse before using an MAOI, such as methylene blue. Available evidence suggests that the interaction cannot be avoided by decreasing the dose of methylene blue.[1,5]

REFERENCES:

1. Stanford SC, et al. Risk of severe serotonin toxicity following co-administration of methylene blue and serotonin reuptake inhibitors: an update on a case report of post-operative delirium [published online ahead of print May 7, 2009]. *J Psychopharmacol.* doi: 10.1177/0269881109105450.

2. Ramsay RR, et al. Methylene blue and serotonin toxicity: inhibition of monoamine oxidase A (MAO A) confirms a theoretical prediction. *Br J Pharmacol.* 2007;152(6):946-951.

3. Khan MA, et al. Prolonged postoperative altered mental status after methylene blue infusion during parathyroidectomy: a case report and review of the literature. *Ann R Coll Surg Engl.* 2007;89(2):W9-W11.

4. Pollack G, et al. Parathyroid surgery and methylene blue: a review with guidelines for safe intraoperative use [published online ahead of print May 13, 2009]. *Laryngoscope.* doi: 10.1002/lary.20581.

5. Schwiebert C, et al. Small doses of methylene blue, previously considered safe, can precipitate serotonin toxicity. *Anaesthesia.* 2009;64(8):924.

Clomipramine (eg, *Anafranil*)

Moclobemide†

SUMMARY: The combination of moclobemide and clomipramine (in overdose) has been associated with fatal serotonin syndrome and (in therapeutic doses) with nonfatal serotonin syndrome. Moclobemide generally should not be given with clomipramine or with other tricyclic antidepressants (TCAs) that inhibit serotonin reuptake (eg, amitriptyline, imipramine, trazodone), or with selective serotonin reuptake inhibitors (SSRIs).

RISK FACTORS: No specific risk factors are known.

MECHANISM: Clomipramine, a potent inhibitor of serotonin uptake, and other TCAs are dangerous when combined with nonselective monoamine oxidase inhibitors (MAOIs), such as phenelzine (*Nardil*) and tranylcypromine (eg, *Parnate*). Moclobemide is a selective inhibitor of MAO-A, the form of MAO that metabolizes serotonin.

CLINICAL EVALUATION: A 23-year-old man and a 19-year-old woman each took moclobemide 1,000 to 1,500 mg along with clomipramine 225 to 500 mg. Although they were euphoric 2 to 3 hours after ingestion, they soon developed extreme tremor, convulsions, and hyperthermia; both died within 10 hours of taking the drugs.[1] Blood concentrations of both drugs on admission and at necropsy showed moderate overdose. Another patient developed nonfatal serotonin syndrome with therapeutic doses of the drugs after being switched from clomipramine 50 mg/day to moclobemide 300 mg/day. Thus, although data are limited, assume that therapeutic doses of the combination also may be dangerous.

RELATED DRUGS: Other antidepressants that inhibit serotonin reuptake such as SSRIs, amitriptyline, imipramine (eg, *Tofranil*), and trazodone also are expected to interact adversely with moclobemide.

MANAGEMENT OPTIONS:

➡ *Avoid Unless Benefit Outweighs Risk.* Avoid combined use of moclobemide and clomipramine. Also avoid other TCAs that can inhibit serotonin uptake (eg, amitriptyline, imipramine, trazodone) in patients taking moclobemide unless additional data prove that they are safe. SSRIs probably also should be avoided with moclobemide, although some combinations may be safe. If severe serotonin syndrome develops from one of these interactions, intensive supportive therapy is needed to treat convulsions, hyperthermia, and cardiorespiratory problems. The use of methysergide (a serotonin antagonist) and dantrolene (for muscle rigidity and hyperpyrexia) also has been recommended.[2]

➡ *Monitor.* If the combination is used, be alert for evidence of serotonin syndrome (eg, coma, dizziness, incoordination, myoclonus, rigidity, seizures, tremor), psychiatric symptoms (eg, agitation, confusion, hypomania), and disorders of temperature regulation (eg, fever, shivering, sweating); severe cases can be fatal.

REFERENCES:

1. Spigset O, et al. Serotonin syndrome caused by a moclobemide-clomipramine interaction. *BMJ.* 1993;306(6872):248.

2. Neuvonen PJ, et al. Five fatal cases of serotonin syndrome after moclobemide-citalopram or moclobemide-clomipramine overdoses. *Lancet.* 1993;342(8884):1419.

† Not available in the United States.

Clomipramine (eg, *Anafranil*)

Olanzapine (*Zyprexa*)

SUMMARY: A patient on olanzapine and clomipramine developed serotonin toxicity, but a causal relationship was not established.

RISK FACTORS: No specific risk factors are known.

MECHANISM: Not established.

CLINICAL EVALUATION: A patient taking olanzapine and clomipramine developed myoclonus, hyperreflexia, diaphoresis, fever, disorientation, diarrhea, and coma.[1] The symptoms clearly supported a diagnosis of serotonin toxicity,[2,3] but the serotonergic effect of olanzapine is not well established (although clomipramine is a well-known serotonergic agent).

RELATED DRUGS: No information available.

MANAGEMENT OPTIONS:

➥ *Monitor.* Although the interaction is not well documented, if the combination is used, monitor for symptoms of serotonin toxicity, including myoclonus, rigidity, tremor, hyperreflexia, seizures, confusion, agitation, hypomania, incoordination, fever, sweating, shivering, and coma.

REFERENCES:

1. Verre M, et al. Serotonin syndrome caused by olanzapine and clomipramine. *Minerva Anestesiol.* 2008;74(1-2):41-45.

2. Isbister GK, et al. Serotonin toxicity: a practical approach to diagnosis and treatment. *Med J Aust.* 2007;187(6):361-365.

3. Boyer EW, et al. The serotonin syndrome. *N Engl J Med.* 2005;352(11):1112-1120.

4   Clomipramine (eg, *Anafranil*)

Oxybutynin (eg, *Ditropan*)

SUMMARY: A patient developed decreased clomipramine plasma concentrations after starting oxybutynin, but a causal relationship was not established.

RISK FACTORS: No specific risk factors are known.

MECHANISM: Not established. It is possible that oxybutynin induces the CYP3A4 metabolism of clomipramine, but little information is available.

CLINICAL EVALUATION: A 72-year-old woman receiving clomipramine developed substantial reductions in clomipramine and desmethylclomipramine plasma concentrations after starting oxybutynin therapy.[1] More data are needed to establish a causal relationship.

RELATED DRUGS: No information is available.

MANAGEMENT OPTIONS: No specific action is required, but be alert for evidence of the interaction.

REFERENCES:

1. Grözinger M, et al. Oxybutynin enhances the metabolism of clomipramine and dextrorphan possibly by induction of a cytochrome P450 isozyme. *J Clin Psychopharmacol.* 1999;19(3):287-289.

Clomipramine (eg, *Anafranil*)

Phenelzine (*Nardil*) AVOID

SUMMARY: Avoid clomipramine and imipramine in patients receiving phenelzine or other nonselective monoamine oxidase inhibitors (MAOIs).

RISK FACTORS: No specific risk factors are known.

MECHANISM: The mechanism of this interaction has not been established, but it may be related to the combined inhibition of serotonin reuptake by tricyclic antidepressants (TCAs) and interference with serotonin metabolism by MAOIs.

CLINICAL EVALUATION: Three patients died, likely as a result of an interaction between clomipramine and a nonselective MAOI. Two of these patients were receiving therapeutic doses of both drugs.[1] Imipramine (eg, *Tofranil*) also has been associated with severe reactions, probably resulting from serotonin syndrome. Symptoms of serotonin syndrome can include neurologic symptoms (dizziness, incoordination, myoclonus, rigidity, seizures, tremor), disorders of temperature regulation (fever, shivering, sweating), and psychiatric effects (agitation, confusion, hypomania). Fatalities have occurred. Still, there is convincing evidence[2-9] that an MAOI and a TCA can be used together safely by experienced clinicians.

RELATED DRUGS: Other antidepressants that inhibit serotonin reuptake such as amitriptyline, imipramine, and trazodone are expected to interact adversely with nonselective MAOIs, including tranylcypromine (eg, *Parnate*) and isocarboxazid. Other TCAs also may interact with MAOIs, but some TCAs and nonselective MAOIs can be given together safely if the following precautions are observed: 1) avoid large doses, 2) give the drugs orally, 3) avoid clomipramine and imipramine, and 4) monitor patients closely.[1-11]

MANAGEMENT OPTIONS:

➡ *AVOID COMBINATION.* Avoid combined use of clomipramine or imipramine with nonselective MAOIs.

REFERENCES:

1. Beaumont G. Drug interactions with clomipramine (*Anafranil*). *J Int Med Res.* 1973;1:480-484.

2. Kline NS. Experimental use of monoamine oxidase inhibitors with tricyclic antidepressants (Questions and Answers). *JAMA.* 1974;227:807.

3. Winston F. Combined antidepressant therapy. *Br J Psychiatry.* 1971;118(544):301-304.

4. Schuckit M, et al. Tricyclic antidepressants and monoamine oxidase inhibitors. *Arch Gen Psychiatry.* 1971;24(6):509 514.

5. Spiker DG, et al. Combining tricyclic and monoamine oxidase inhibitor antidepressants. *Arch Gen Psychiatry.* 1976;33(7):828-830.

6. Ananth J, et al. A review of combined tricyclic and MAOI therapy. *Compr Psychiatry.* 1977;18(3):221-230.

7. White K. Tricyclic overdose in a patient given combined tricyclic-MAOI treatment. *Am J Psychiatry.* 1978;135(11):1411.

8. Young JP, et al. Controlled trial of trimipramine, monoamine oxidase inhibitors, and combined treatment in depressed outpatients. *Br Med J.* 1979;2(6201):1315-1317.

9. White K. Combined tricyclic and monoamine-oxidase inhibitor antidepressant treatment. *West J Med.* 1983;138(3):406-407.

10. de la Fuente JR, et al. Mania induced by tricyclic-MAOI combination therapy in bipolar treatment-resistant disorder: case reports. *J Clin Psychiatry.* 1986;47(1):40-41.

11. White K, et al. The combined use of MAOIs and tricyclics. *J Clin Psychiatry.* 1984;45(7 pt 2):67-69.

 Clomipramine (eg, *Anafranil*)

Rasagiline (*Azilect*)

SUMMARY: Theoretically, the concomitant use of rasagiline and serotonergic tricyclic antidepressants (TCAs) such as clomipramine could increase the risk of serotonin syndrome.

RISK FACTORS: No specific risk factors are known.

MECHANISM: The combination may have additive serotonergic effects.

CLINICAL EVALUATION: Severe serotonin syndrome-like reactions (including fatalities) have occurred when serotonergic TCAs were used in patients on nonselective MAO inhibitors or selegiline. Because it cannot be ruled out that rasagiline produces nonselective MAO inhibition in some patients, combining rasagiline with TCAs could theoretically increase the risk of serotonin syndrome.[1,2] The serotonergic effect of TCAs varies, with clomipramine and imipramine (eg, *Tofranil*) having the greatest effect, and amitriptyline and doxepin (eg, *Sinequan*) having some effect. Nonetheless, over 100 patients in rasagiline clinical trials received TCAs, apparently without evidence of serotonin syndrome.[2] Thus, it is likely that most patients receiving rasagiline and TCAs concurrently would not develop a severe adverse drug interaction.

RELATED DRUGS: The other TCAs most likely to interact with rasagiline include imipramine and possibly amitriptyline and doxepin. Any interaction between rasagiline and TCAs is likely to be similar with selegiline and TCAs.

MANAGEMENT OPTIONS:

➡ ***Avoid Unless Benefit Outweighs Risk.*** Although it is difficult to assess the risk of this interaction given current data, consider the severity of the interaction should it occur. Rasagiline product information recommends avoiding TCAs concurrently or within 2 weeks of stopping rasagiline.

➡ ***Use Alternative.*** If a TCA is used, avoid agents with the largest serotonergic effects (eg, clomipramine, imipramine).

➡ ***Monitor.*** If TCAs are used with rasagiline, monitor for symptoms of serotonin syndrome such as agitation, coma, confusion, fever, hyperreflexia, hypomania, incoordination, myoclonus, rigidity, seizures, shivering, sweating, and tremor.

REFERENCES:

1. Chen JJ, et al. Rasagiline: A second-generation monoamine oxidase type-B inhibitor for the treatment of Parkinson disease. *Am J Health Syst Pharm.* 2006;63:915-928.

2. *Azilect* [package insert]. North Wales, PA: Teva Neuroscience, Inc.; 2006.

Clonazepam (eg, *Klonopin*) 4

Clozapine (eg, *Clozaril*)

SUMMARY: A patient on clonazepam developed delirium after starting clozapine therapy, but a causal relationship was not established.

RISK FACTORS: No specific risk factors are known.

MECHANISM: Not established.

CLINICAL EVALUATION: A 42-year-old woman on chronic clonazepam 2 mg/day was started on clozapine 150 mg/day. A week later she developed somnolence, confusion, disorientation, ataxia, slurred speech, and profuse salivation.[1] The clonazepam was discontinued and the delirium cleared over the next week. Since the patient was not rechallenged or given clonazepam in the absence of clozapine, it was not possible to establish a causal relationship. Nonetheless, delirium has been reported in patients receiving clozapine and lorazepam, so it is possible that the reaction observed in this patient resulted from a drug interaction.

RELATED DRUGS: Delirium has been reported in patients treated with the combination of clozapine and another benzodiazepine, lorazepam (eg, *Ativan*), but little is known regarding other benzodiazepines.

MANAGEMENT OPTIONS: No specific action is required, but be alert for evidence of the interaction.

REFERENCES:
1. Jackson CW. Delirium associated with clozapine and benzodiazepine combinations. *Ann Clin Psychiatry.* 1995;7:139.

Clonazepam (eg, *Klonopin*) 5

Fluoxetine (*Prozac*)

SUMMARY: Study in healthy subjects suggests that fluoxetine does not affect the pharmacokinetics of clonazepam.

RISK FACTORS: No specific risk factors are known.

MECHANISM: No interaction.

CLINICAL EVALUATION: Twelve healthy subjects received a single oral 1 mg dose of clonazepam with and without fluoxetine 40 mg/day for 3 to 7 days.[1] Fluoxetine had no effect on clonazepam clearance, half-life, or area under the plasma concentration-time curve. However, 8 days of fluoxetine does not rule out the possibility of an interaction with clonazepam. For example, the ability of fluoxetine to increase carbamazepine (eg, *Tegretol*) serum concentrations may take at least 10 days.

RELATED DRUGS: The effect of selective serotonin reuptake inhibitors other than fluoxetine on clonazepam is not established.

MANAGEMENT OPTIONS: No interaction.

REFERENCES:
1. Greenblatt DG, et al. Fluoxetine impairs clearance of alprazolam but not of clonazepam. *Clin Pharmacol Ther.* 1992;52:479.

Clonazepam (eg, *Klonopin*)

Phenobarbital

SUMMARY: Phenobarbital slightly enhances the elimination of clonazepam, but the effect is unlikely to be clinically significant. Clonazepam does not appear to affect barbiturate serum concentrations.

RISK FACTORS: No specific risk factors are known.

MECHANISM: Phenobarbital probably increases the hepatic metabolism of clonazepam.

CLINICAL EVALUATION: Eight healthy subjects were given a single oral dose of clonazepam 0.03 mg/kg before and after 19 days of phenobarbital 1.4 mg/kg/day.[2] Clonazepam clearance was increased approximately 20%, but it is unlikely that this effect would be clinically important. The additive anticonvulsant effect of the 2 drugs may offset the small reduction in clonazepam serum concentrations. Clonazepam does not affect barbiturate serum concentrations.[1]

RELATED DRUGS: Little is known regarding the effect of barbiturates other than phenobarbital on clonazepam, but they probably also reduce clonazepam serum concentrations. Theoretically, administration of a barbiturate in doses capable of inducing enzymes but not sufficient to exert significant anticonvulsant effect (eg, a nightly hypnotic barbiturate) might be more likely to interfere with the anticonvulsant effect of clonazepam. However, this has not been studied clinically.

MANAGEMENT OPTIONS: No specific action is required, but be alert for evidence of the interaction.

REFERENCES:
1. Johannessen SI, et al. Lack of effect of clonazepam on serum levels of diphenylhydantoin, phenobarbital and carbamazepine. *Acta Neurol Scand.* 1977;55:506.
2. Khoo KC, et al. Influence of phenytoin and phenobarbital on the disposition of a single oral dose of clonazepam. *Clin Pharmacol Ther.* 1980;28:368.

4 **Clonazepam (eg, *Klonopin*)**

Phenytoin (eg, *Dilantin*)

SUMMARY: Phenytoin lowers plasma clonazepam concentrations, but the clinical importance of this effect is probably minimal.

RISK FACTORS: No specific risk factors are known.

MECHANISM: Phenytoin probably enhances the hepatic metabolism of clonazepam.

CLINICAL EVALUATION: Eight healthy subjects were given an oral dose of clonazepam 0.03 mg/kg before and after 19 days of phenytoin 4.3 mg/kg/day.[3] Although clonazepam clearance was increased approximately 50%, the clinical importance of this effect is questionable because the additive anticonvulsant effect could compensate for the decrease in the plasma concentration of clonazepam. Clonazepam does not affect phenytoin serum concentrations.[1] In another study, short-term therapy with clonazepam and valproate reportedly was associated with increased phenytoin concentrations,[2] but it does not seem likely that clonazepam was responsible.

RELATED DRUGS: No information is available.

MANAGEMENT OPTIONS: No specific action is required, but be alert for evidence of the interaction.

REFERENCES:

1. Johannessen SI, et al. Lack of effect of clonazepam on serum levels of diphenylhydantoin, phenobarbital and carbamazepine. *Acta Neurol Scand.* 1977;55:506.
2. Windorfer A. Drug interaction during anticonvulsive therapy. *Int J Clin Pharmacol.* 1976;14:236.
3. Khoo KC, et al. Influence of phenytoin and phenobarbital on the disposition of a single oral dose of clonazepam. *Clin Pharmacol Ther.* 1980;28:368.

Clonazepam (eg, *Klonopin*)

Primidone (eg, *Mysoline*)

SUMMARY: Primidone may decrease plasma clonazepam concentrations slightly, but the clinical importance of this effect is probably minimal.

RISK FACTORS: No specific risk factors are known.

MECHANISM: The phenobarbital produced from primidone metabolism may enhance the hepatic metabolism of clonazepam.

CLINICAL EVALUATION: Some primidone is metabolized to phenobarbital which lowers plasma clonazepam concentrations. The interaction is unlikely to be clinically important. Clonazepam has been associated with increased serum concentrations of primidone in epileptic patients,[1] but no details were given.

RELATED DRUGS: Phenobarbital and other barbiturates would also be expected to enhance clonazepam metabolism.

MANAGEMENT OPTIONS: No specific action is required, but be alert for evidence of the interaction.

REFERENCES:

1. Windorfer A. Drug interaction during anticonvulsive therapy. *Int J Clin Pharmacol.* 1976;14:236.

Clonazepam (eg, *Klonopin*)

Valproic Acid (eg, *Depakene*)

SUMMARY: Absence seizures have been reported in patients receiving valproic acid and clonazepam, but a causal relationship has not been established.

RISK FACTORS: No specific risk factors are known.

MECHANISM: Not established.

CLINICAL EVALUATION: The combined use of clonazepam and valproic acid has been associated with absence seizures,[1,2] although the role of a drug interaction between clonazepam and valproic acid in this phenomenon is not established.

RELATED DRUGS: No information is available.

MANAGEMENT OPTIONS:

➥ *Monitor.* If absence seizures increase with combined clonazepam and valproic acid, consider an alternative anticonvulsant regimen.

REFERENCES:

1. Jeavons PM, et al. Treatment of generalized epilepsies of childhood and adolescence with sodium valproate ("epilim"). *Dev Med Child Neurol.* 1977;19:9.

2. Browne TR. Interaction between clonazepam and sodium valproate. *N Engl J Med.* 1979;300:678.

Clonidine (eg, *Catapres*)

Cyclosporine (eg, *Neoral*)

SUMMARY: Limited clinical evidence suggests that clonidine increases cyclosporine blood concentrations; more study is needed to establish the incidence and magnitude of this interaction.

RISK FACTORS: No specific risk factors are known.

MECHANISM: None known.

CLINICAL EVALUATION: A 3-year-old boy developed elevated blood pressure after a renal transplant that was resistant to a combination of propranolol, hydralazine, furosemide, and nifedipine.[1] The addition of minoxidil controlled his blood pressure, but adverse effects resulted in the substitution of clonidine for minoxidil. Whole blood cyclosporine concentrations increased markedly, reaching a peak of 927 mcg/L despite a reduction in cyclosporine dose. The cyclosporine blood concentration fell rapidly when the clonidine was withdrawn. Although the temporal relationship between clonidine administration and cyclosporine blood concentrations suggests that an interaction occurred, additional study is needed to prove that the interaction occurs. A previous study in bone marrow transplant recipients supports the existence of an interaction; the study found increased cyclosporine blood concentrations in the presence of transdermal clonidine.[2]

RELATED DRUGS: The effect of clonidine on tacrolimus (*Prograf*) is not established, but the drug interactions of cyclosporine and tacrolimus tend to be similar.

MANAGEMENT OPTIONS:

➥ *Monitor.* Monitor for altered cyclosporine blood concentrations if clonidine is initiated, discontinued, or changed in dosage; adjust cyclosporine dose as needed.

REFERENCES:

1. Gilbert RD, et al. Interaction between clonidine and cyclosporine A. *Nephron.* 1995;71:105.

2. Luke J, et al. Prevention of cyclosporine-induced nephrotoxicity with transdermal clonidine. *Clin Pharmacol.* 1990;9:49.

Clonidine (eg, *Catapres*)

Desipramine (eg, *Norpramin*)

SUMMARY: Tricyclic antidepressants (TCAs) such as desipramine can inhibit the antihypertensive response to clonidine; preliminary evidence indicates that TCAs also may enhance the hypertensive response to abrupt clonidine withdrawal.

RISK FACTORS:

➡ ***Dosage Regimen.*** Abrupt withdrawal of clonidine in the presence of a TCA may lead to an exaggerated hypertensive response.

MECHANISM: The mechanism for inhibition of clonidine antihypertensive response by TCAs is not established.[1] Tricyclic antidepressants markedly enhance the pressor response to catecholamines, such as norepinephrine and epinephrine, which may account for the proposed increased hypertensive response to clonidine withdrawal.

CLINICAL EVALUATION: Four of five hypertensive patients on chronic clonidine therapy developed a 22/15 mmHg rise in mean supine blood pressure during therapy with desipramine 75 mg/day for 2 weeks.[2] Although the increases in blood pressure usually occurred in the second week of desipramine treatment, 1 patient developed a considerable increase in blood pressure, along with headache and sweating, 24 hours after desipramine was ingested. A hypertensive crisis also occurred 2 days after starting 50 mg/day of imipramine (eg, *Tofranil*) in a 77-year-old woman stabilized on clonidine 0.4 mg/day.[3] Some evidence suggests that TCAs enhance the rebound hypertensive reactions following clonidine withdrawal. A patient on chronic therapy with amitriptyline (eg, *Elavil*) 100 mg/day and clonidine 0.2 mg/day developed hypertension, tachycardia, and anxiety after drugs were discontinued.[4] This reaction may have resulted from amitriptyline-induced potentiation of the catecholamines released in response to the withdrawal of clonidine.

RELATED DRUGS: Little is known regarding the effect of other TCAs on clonidine response; assume that they interact until proven otherwise. Trazodone (eg, *Desyrel*) reportedly inhibits the hypotensive response to clonidine, but more evidence is needed.[5] Theoretically, maprotiline (eg, *Ludiomil*) would be less likely to interact with clonidine than other TCAs, but clinical studies are lacking. The tetracyclic drug mianserin has minimal effects on clonidine response in both healthy subjects and patients with essential hypertension.[6-8] Clonidine-like drugs such as guanabenz (eg, *Wytensin*) and guanfacine (*Tenex*) theoretically also would interact with TCAs.

MANAGEMENT OPTIONS:

➡ ***Avoid Unless Benefit Outweighs Risk.*** If possible, avoid concomitant use of clonidine and tricyclic antidepressants. Since TCAs also appear to interact with guanethidine (*Ismelin*), bethanidine, and debrisoquin, these drugs would not be suitable alternatives. Methyldopa (eg, *Aldomet*) apparently can be used safely with TCAs, but methyldopa has other disadvantages. In any case, blood monitor pressure if TCAs are initiated, discontinued, or changed in dosage in a patient on antihypertensive drugs.

➡ **Monitor.** If TCAs and clonidine are used concurrently, monitor blood pressure carefully when the TCA is started and also if the clonidine is withdrawn. Gradual tapering of the clonidine dosage may be helpful in reducing the likelihood of severe rebound hypertension.

REFERENCES:

1. Gutkind JS, et al. Differential pharmacological interaction of clonidine and guanabenz with antidepressive drugs. *Clin Exp Hypertens.* 1987;A9:1531.

2. Briant RH, et al. Interaction between clonidine and desipramine in man. *BMJ.* 1973;1:522.

3. Hui KK. Hypertensive crisis induced by interaction of clonidine with imipramine. *J Am Geriatr Soc.* 1983;31:164.

4. Stiff JL, et al. Clonidine withdrawal complicated by amitriptyline therapy. *Anesthesiology.* 1983;59:73.

5. Barnes JS, et al. Lack of interaction between tricyclic antidepressants and clonidine at the alpha-2-adrenoceptor on human platelets. *Clin Pharmacol Ther.* 1982;32:744.

6. Elliott HL, et al. Pharmacodynamics studies on mianserin and its interaction with clonidine. *Eur J Clin Pharmacol.* 1981;21:97.

7. Elliot HL, et al. Absence of an effect of mianserin on the actions of clonidine or methyldopa in hypertensive patients. *Eur J Clin Pharmacol.* 1983;24:15.

8. Elliot HL, et al. Assessment of the interaction between mianserin and centrally-acting antihypertensive drugs. *Br J Clin Pharmacol.* 1983;15:323S.

Clonidine (eg, *Catapres*)

Insulin

SUMMARY: Clonidine may diminish the symptoms of hypoglycemia.

RISK FACTORS: No specific risk factors are known.

MECHANISM: The increased production of catecholamines in response to insulin-induced hypoglycemia is inhibited by pretreatment with clonidine.

CLINICAL EVALUATION: A group of hypertensive and normal subjects were given a single dose of insulin before and during treatment with clonidine.[1] Clonidine suppressed the marked increase in catecholamine production that normally follows insulin hypoglycemia and also reduced the signs and symptoms of hypoglycemia without affecting the ability to recover from hypoglycemia. Similar results were obtained when transdermal clonidine 0.1 mg/day was applied to subjects before insulin 0.1 units/kg.[2]

RELATED DRUGS: Guanfacine (*Tenex*) and guanabenz (eg, *Wytensin*) theoretically would produce a similar effect during hypoglycemic episodes.

MANAGEMENT OPTIONS:

➡ **Monitor.** Patients receiving antidiabetic drugs and clonidine should be aware that clonidine may suppress the signs and symptoms of hypoglycemia.

REFERENCES:

1. Hedeland H, et al. The effect of insulin-induced hypoglycaemia on plasma renin activity and urinary catecholamines before and following clonidine (*Catapres*) in man. *Acta Endocrinol.* 1972;71:321.

2. Guthrie GP, et al. Effect of transdermal clonidine on the endocrine responses to insulin-induced hypoglycemia in essential hypertension. *Clin Pharmacol Ther.* 1989;45:417.

Clonidine (eg, *Catapres*) 4

Levodopa (eg, *Larodopa*)

SUMMARY: Clonidine appeared to inhibit the antiparkinsonian effect of levodopa in one study but not in another; more study is needed.

RISK FACTORS: No specific risk factors are known.

MECHANISM: Clonidine may inhibit the antiparkinsonian activity of levodopa by stimulating central alpha-adrenergic receptors.

CLINICAL EVALUATION: In 7 patients with parkinsonism (5 on piribedil, 2 on levodopa plus carbidopa), clonidine administration was associated with an exacerbation of the parkinsonism.[1] Patients who were receiving anticholinergics in addition to the levodopa or piribedil seemed to be less affected by clonidine. The interaction was not confirmed in another study of 10 patients receiving levodopa.[2]

RELATED DRUGS: Although little is known regarding the effect of centrally acting alpha-agonists other than clonidine such as guanabenz (eg, *Wytensin*) and guanfacine (*Tenex*), consider the possibility that they interact with levodopa until clinical information is available.

MANAGEMENT OPTIONS: No specific action is required, but be alert for the evidence of the interaction.

REFERENCES:

1. Shoulson I, et al. Clonidine and the anti-parkinsonian response to L-dopa or piribedil. *Neuropharmacology.* 1976;15:25.
2. Tarsy D, et al. Clonidine in parkinson disease. *Arch Neurol.* 1975;32:134.

Clonidine (eg, *Catapres*)

Milnacipran (eg, *Savella*)

SUMMARY: Theoretically, combining milnacipran with clonidine may inhibit the antihypertensive effect of clonidine.

RISK FACTORS: No specific risk factors are known.

MECHANISM: Milnacipran inhibits the reuptake of both serotonin and norepinephrine; other norepinephrine reuptake inhibitors, such as tricyclic antidepressants, have been shown to markedly reduce the antihypertensive effects of clonidine.

CLINICAL EVALUATION: This interaction is based largely on theoretical considerations, and it is not known how often adverse outcomes would be observed. The manufacturer lists this interaction as clinically important.[1]

RELATED DRUGS: Theoretically, milnacipran also impairs the antihypertensive effect of drugs with a mechanism of action similar to clonidine, such as guanabenz and guanfacine (eg, *Tenex*).

MANAGEMENT OPTIONS:

➥ *Consider Alternative.* If possible, use an alternative to one of the drugs.

➥ *Monitor.* If the combination is used, monitor the antihypertensive response to clonidine if milnacipran therapy is initiated or discontinued.

REFERENCES:

1. *Savella* [package insert]. St. Louis, MO: Forest Pharmaceuticals; 2010.

 Clonidine (eg, *Duraclon*)

Mirtazapine (eg, *Remeron*)

SUMMARY: A man with well-controlled hypertension developed a severe hypertensive reaction after mirtazapine was added to his therapy.

RISK FACTORS: No specific risk factors are known.

MECHANISM: The antihypertensive effect of clonidine is related to stimulation of central alpha-2 receptors; mirtazapine inhibits these same receptors. This may explain the observed loss of clonidine antihypertensive effect.

CLINICAL EVALUATION: A 20-year-old man whose hypertension had been well controlled (usually 140 to 150/80 to 85 mm Hg) on metoprolol (eg, *Lopressor*), losartan (eg, *Cozaar*), and clonidine started mirtazapine 15 mg/day.[1] Within a few days, his blood pressure began to rise, and after 2 weeks, he was admitted with shortness of breath and blood pressures ranging from 187 to 208/113 to 131 mm Hg. The hypertension was refractory to treatment, but eventually responded to a nitro-prusside infusion and emergency dialysis in the intensive care unit. After stopping the mirtazapine, he was again controlled by the same antihypertensive regimen he was on prior to the mirtazapine.

RELATED DRUGS: Tricyclic antidepressants (TCAs) also antagonize the antihypertensive response to clonidine, and they are not appropriate substitutes for mirtazapine in a patient on clonidine. Trazodone (eg, *Desyrel*) reportedly inhibits the hypotensive response to clonidine, but more evidence is needed.[2] Mianserin[†] has minimal effects on clonidine response in healthy subjects and hypertensive patients.[3,4] Antihypertensive drugs, such as guanabenz and guanfacine (eg, *Tenex*), stimulate central alpha-2 receptors, and theoretically would interact with mirtazapine or TCAs in the same manner as clonidine.

MANAGEMENT OPTIONS:

➥ *Use Alternative.* In patients on clonidine, use antidepressants other than mirtazapine or TCAs (see Related Drugs).

REFERENCES:

1. Abo-Zena RA, et al. Hypertensive urgency induced by an interaction of mirtazapine and clonidine. *Pharmacotherapy*. 2000;20(4):476-478.

2. Barnes JS, et al. Lack of interaction between tricyclic antidepressants and clonidine at the alpha 2-adrenoceptor on human platelets. *Clin Pharmacol Ther*. 1982;32(6):744-748.

3. Elliott HL, et al. Pharmacodynamic studies on mianserin and its interaction with clonidine. *Eur J Clin Pharmacol*. 1981;21(2):97-102.

4. Elliott HL, et al. Absence of an effect of mianserin on the actions of clonidine or methyldopa in hyper-tensive patients. *Eur J Clin Pharmacol*. 1983;24(1):15-19.

† Not available in the United States.

Clonidine (eg, *Catapres*)

Nitroprusside

SUMMARY: Cases of severe hypotensive reactions with the combined use of clonidine and nitroprusside have been reported.

RISK FACTORS: No specific risk factors are known.

MECHANISM: Clonidine and nitroprusside appear to have additive hypotensive effects.

CLINICAL EVALUATION: Three patients have been described in whom simultaneous discontinuation of nitroprusside and initiation of clonidine were associated with severe hypotensive reactions.[1] More study is needed to better define the consequences of an interaction between these drugs.

RELATED DRUGS: Although little is known regarding the effect of centrally acting alpha-agonists other than clonidine, such as guanabenz (eg, *Wytensin*) and guanfacine (*Tenex*), consider the possibility that they interact with nitroprusside until clinical information is available.

MANAGEMENT OPTIONS:

➥ *Monitor.* Monitor for excessive hypotensive effects when clonidine is used in patients who are receiving nitroprusside or who have recently received it.

REFERENCES:

1. Cohen IM, et al. Danger in nitroprusside therapy. *Ann Intern Med*. 1976;85:205.

Clonidine (eg, *Catapres*)

Piribedil

SUMMARY: Preliminary evidence indicates that clonidine inhibits the antiparkinsonian effect of piribedil.

RISK FACTORS: No specific risk factors are known.

MECHANISM: Clonidine may inhibit the antiparkinsonian activity of piribedil by stimulating central alpha-adrenergic receptors.

CLINICAL EVALUATION: In 5 patients with parkinsonism receiving piribedil, clonidine administration was associated with an exacerbation of the parkinsonism.[1] Patients who were receiving anticholinergics in addition to the piribedil seemed to be less affected by the clonidine.

RELATED DRUGS: Although little is known regarding the effect of centrally acting alpha-agonists other than clonidine, such as guanabenz (eg, *Wystensin*) and guanfacine (*Tenex*), consider the possibility that they interact with piribedil until clinical information is available.

MANAGEMENT OPTIONS: No specific action is required, but be alert for evidence of the interaction.

REFERENCES:

1. Shoulson I, et al. Clonidine and the anti-parkinsonian response to L-dopa or piribedil. *Neuropharmacology*. 1976;15:25.

Clonidine (eg, *Catapres*)

Propranolol (eg, *Inderal*)

SUMMARY: Hypertension occurring upon withdrawal of clonidine may be exacerbated by noncardioselective (eg, propranolol, nadolol [eg, *Corgard*]) beta blocker therapy.

RISK FACTORS:

➡ *Order of Drug Administration.* Withdrawal of clonidine during noncardioselective beta blocker therapy.

MECHANISM: The hypertension that may accompany rapid clonidine withdrawal is thought to result from increased circulating catecholamine levels. If the patient is receiving a beta blocker during withdrawal from clonidine, the β-(vasodilator) response of epinephrine would be blocked, resulting in an exaggerated α-(vasoconstrictor) response and, possibly, hypertension. Theoretically, cardioselective beta blockers would not produce this effect, because they do not appear to enhance the pressor response to epinephrine.

CLINICAL EVALUATION: In several patients, beta blockers appeared to enhance the hypertensive response following clonidine withdrawal.[1-5] Even gradual withdrawal of clonidine has been associated with hypertensive reactions in the presence of beta blockade.[2,4] A paradoxical hypertensive response also has been reported in patients on continued clonidine therapy who also receive propranolol[6] or sotalol (eg, *Betapace*).[9] However, neither propranolol nor sotalol increased blood pressure in 12 clonidine-treated patients, and the significance of the hypertensive effect of continued combination therapy remains to be established.[7]

RELATED DRUGS: Centrally acting alpha-agonists other than clonidine, such as guanabenz (eg, *Wystensin*) and guanfacine (*Tenex*), can produce rebound hypertension when discontinued; thus, assume that beta-adrenergic blockers can enhance this hypertensive reaction until proven otherwise.

MANAGEMENT OPTIONS:

➡ *Consider Alternative.* The use of labetalol (*Normodyne*) (which has both alpha- and beta-blocking activity) may prove useful in preventing rebound hypertension following clonidine withdrawal.[8] Cardioselective beta blockers (eg, atenolol [eg, *Tenormin*], metoprolol [eg, *Lopressor*]) would be less likely to produce rebound hypertension.

➡ *Circumvent/Minimize.* In patients receiving both nonselective beta-adrenergic blockers and clonidine, the beta blocker could be withdrawn before the clonidine to reduce the danger of rebound hypertension.

➡ *Monitor.* If clonidine is withdrawn while the patient remains on a beta-adrenergic blocker, monitor the patient very carefully for a hypertensive response.

REFERENCES:

1. Harris AL. Clonidine withdrawal and blockade. *Lancet.* 1976;1:596.
2. Cairns SA, et al. Clonidine withdrawal. *Lancet.* 1976;1:368.
3. Bailey RR, et al. Rapid clonidine withdrawal with blood pressure overshoot exaggerated by beta blockade. *BMJ.* 1976;2:942.
4. Strauss FG, et al. Withdrawal of antihypertensive therapy. *JAMA.* 1977;238:1734.
5. Vernon C, et al. Fatal rebound hypertension after abrupt withdrawal of clonidine and propranolol. *Br J Clin Pract.* 1979;33:112.

6. Warren SE, et al. Clonidine and propranolol paradoxical hypertension. *Arch Intern Med.* 1979;139:253.

7. Lilja M, et al. Interaction of clonidine and beta blockers. *Acta Med Scand.* 1980;207:173.

8. Rosenthal T, et al. Use of labetalol in hypertensive patients during discontinuation of clonidine therapy. *Eur J Clin Pharmacol.* 1981;20:237.

9. Saarimaa H. Combination of clonidine and sotalol in hypertension. *BMJ.* 1976;1:810.

Clonidine (eg, *Catapres*)

Verapamil (eg, *Calan*)

SUMMARY: The combined use of verapamil and clonidine was associated with arrhythmias in 2 patients, but a causal relationship was not established.

RISK FACTORS: No specific risk factors are known.

MECHANISM: Not established.

CLINICAL EVALUATION: Two hypertensive patients developed atrioventricular nodal rhythms following the addition of clonidine 0.15 mg twice daily to chronic verapamil therapy.[1] In both cases, the arrhythmia occurred within 1 day after clonidine was started and was accompanied by a fall in blood pressure. Causation was not established in either case.

RELATED DRUGS: No information is available.

MANAGEMENT OPTIONS: No specific action is required, but be alert for evidence of the interaction.

REFERENCES:

1. Jaffe, et al. Adverse interaction between clonidine and verapamil. *Annals Pharmacother.* 1994;28:881.

Clopidogrel (eg, *Plavix*)

Itraconazole (eg, *Sporanox*)

SUMMARY: Itraconazole inhibits the conversion of clopidogrel to its active metabolite and may reduce its antiplatelet activity in some patients.

RISK FACTORS:

➡ ***Pharmacogenetics.*** Patients without CYP3A5 activity will not be able to convert clopidogrel to its active metabolite in the presence of itraconazole.

MECHANISM: Itraconazole inhibits one of the pathways (CYP3A4) responsible for the conversion of clopidogrel to its active metabolite.

CLINICAL EVALUATION: Thirty-two subjects received a loading dose of clopidogrel 300 mg followed by 75 mg daily for 6 days with and without a pretreatment of itraconazole 200 mg for 4 days.[1] Half of the subjects were known to be genetically deficient in the enzyme CYP3A5. Itraconazole pretreatment inhibited the antiplatelet aggregation activity of clopidogrel in the patients deficient in CYP3A5 but had less effect on clopidogrel's activity in patients with the enzyme. Clopidogrel requires conversion to an active metabolite by CYP3A4 or CYP3A5 to exert its antiplatelet action. Patients without CYP3A5 had similar antiplatelet activity following clopidogrel alone as those with the CYP3A5 enzyme.

RELATED DRUGS: Other antifungal agents that inhibit CYP3A4 (eg, ketoconazole [eg, *Nizoral*], voriconazole [*Vfend*], posaconazole [*Noxafil*], fluconazole [eg, *Diflucan*]) are expected to affect clopidogrel in a similar manner.

MANAGEMENT OPTIONS:

➡ *Consider Alternative.* Terbinafine (eg, *Lamisil*) may be considered as an alternative antifungal agent because it does not affect CYP3A4 activity. Aspirin's antiplatelet activity is not affected by itraconazole.

➡ *Monitor.* Monitor patients receiving clopidogrel and itraconazole for possible reduction in antiplatelet activity.

REFERENCES:

1. Suh JW, et al. Increased risk of atherothrombotic events associated with cytochrome P450 3A5 polymorphism in patients taking clopidogrel. *CMAJ.* 2006;174(12):1715-1722.

Clopidogrel (eg, *Plavix*)

Ketoconazole (eg, *Nizoral*)

SUMMARY: Ketoconazole administration produces a modest reduction in the plasma concentration of clopidogrel's active metabolite; some patients may have reduced antiplatelet activity.

RISK FACTORS: No specific risk factors are known.

MECHANISM: Ketoconazole is known to inhibit the activity of CYP3A4, an enzyme partially responsible for the conversion of clopidogrel to its active metabolite.

CLINICAL EVALUATION: Eighteen subjects received a loading dose of clopidogrel 300 mg followed by 75 mg daily for 5 days, either alone or with ketoconazole 400 mg daily beginning 3 days prior to starting the clopidogrel regimen and continued until 1 day after the last dose of clopidogrel.[1] The coadministration of ketoconazole resulted in a reduction of 14% and 22% in the mean area under the concentration-time curve (AUC) of the active metabolite of clopidogrel after the single and multiple dose periods, respectively.

RELATED DRUGS: Fluconazole (eg, *Diflucan*), itraconazole (eg, *Sporanox*), posaconazole (*Noxafil*), and voriconazole (*Vfend*) also inhibit the activity of CYP3A4 and are expected to decrease the plasma concentrations of clopidogrel's active metabolite. Ketoconazole administration with prasugrel (*Effient*) produced a reduction in its peak concentration but not its AUC or antiplatelet activity.[1]

MANAGEMENT OPTIONS:

➡ *Consider Alternative.* Terbinafine (eg, *Lamisil*) may be considered as an alternative antifungal agent because it does not affect CYP3A4 activity. Amphotericin, caspofungin (*Cancidas*), and anidulafungin (*Eraxis*) do not appear to inhibit CYP3A4. Based on limited data, the activity of prasugrel may be less affected by ketoconazole coadministration.

➡ *Monitor.* While platelet activity can be tested, it will not be practical for all patients. Consider using aspirin (unless contraindicated) with clopidogrel to provide an alternative antiplatelet therapy.

REFERENCES:

1. Farid NA, et al. Cytochrome P450 3A inhibition by ketoconazole affects prasugrel and clopidogrel pharmacokinetics and pharmacodynamics differently. *Clin Pharmacol Ther.* 2007;81(5):735-741.

Clopidogrel (eg, *Plavix*)

Omeprazole (eg, *Prilosec*)

SUMMARY: Some reports have noted an association between omeprazole administration and reduced antiplatelet effect of clopidogrel. Carefully controlled studies are necessary to establish the extent of this interaction and its clinical significance.

RISK FACTORS: There are a number of potential risk factors, including genetically determined P-glycoprotein, CYP2C19, and CYP3A5 activity, concurrent disease states, and moderating effects of other drugs such as aspirin.

MECHANISM: Clopidogrel requires metabolism by CYP3A4/5 and CYP2C19 (and possibly other enzymes) to an active metabolite. Omeprazole is an inhibitor of CYP2C19 and may reduce the formation of clopidogrel's active metabolite in some patients.

CLINICAL EVALUATION: A number of studies have suggested a reduced efficacy of clopidogrel in patients taking proton pump inhibitors in general or omeprazole specifically.[1-3] These are observational or case-controlled studies that raise questions about association but do not provide adequate controls to positively define the causal relationship that might exist between proton pump inhibitors and clopidogrel activity. Because clopidogrel is metabolized by multiple pathways, including at least 2 (CYP3A5 and CYP2C19) that are genetically determined, and is a substrate for P-glycoprotein, whose activity is also genetically determined, very careful subject selection and study design will be necessary to establish the exact nature of an interaction between clopidogrel and proton pump inhibitors. The potential clinical effect of the interaction will also require carefully controlled studies.

RELATED DRUGS: While esomeprazole (*Nexium*) is known to inhibit CYP2C19, the potential for other proton pump inhibitors to interact has not been adequately studied.

MANAGEMENT OPTIONS:

➡ **Consider Alternative.** Pending further data, for patients treated with clopidogrel who require acid suppression, consider using proton pump inhibitors other than omeprazole or esomeprazole, or H$_2$-receptor antagonists except cimetidine, which appears to inhibit suggested pathways of clopidogrel metabolism.

➡ **Monitor.** While platelet activity can be tested, it will not be practical for all patients. Consider using aspirin (unless contraindicated) with clopidogrel to provide an alternative antiplatelet therapy.

REFERENCES:

1. Gilard M, et al. Influence of omeprazole on the antiplatelet action of clopidogrel associated with aspirin: the randomized, double-blind OCLA (Omeprazole Clopidogrel Aspirin) study. *J Am Coll Cardiol.* 2008;51(3):256-260.

2. Pezalla E, et al. Initial assessment of clinical impact of a drug interaction between clopidogrel and proton pump inhibitors. *J Am Coll Cardiol.* 2008;52(12):1038-1039.

3. Juurlink DN, et al. A population-based study of the drug interaction between proton pump inhibitors and clopidogrel. [published online ahead of print]. *CMAJ.* 2009;180(7). doi:10.1503/cmaj.082001.

Clopidogrel (eg, *Plavix*)

Rifampin (eg, *Rifadin*)

SUMMARY: Rifampin appears to enhance the antiplatelet effects of clopidogrel, but the clinical importance of this effect is not established.

RISK FACTORS: No specific risk factors are known.

MECHANISM: Clopidogrel is a prodrug, and CYP3A4 appears to be the primary isozyme involved in formation of the active metabolite.[1] Rifampin is a potent CYP3A4 inducer and probably increases the conversion of clopidogrel to its active metabolite.

CLINICAL EVALUATION: Ten healthy subjects were given clopidogrel 75 mg/day for 6 days alone and with rifampin 300 mg twice daily.[2] Rifampin was associated with an increase in the ability of clopidogrel to inhibit platelet aggregation. With clopidogrel alone, platelet aggregation was 56%, but with concurrent rifampin, platelet aggregation increased to 33% of control. It is not know if this effect increases the risk of bleeding in patients taking clopidogrel.

RELATED DRUGS: Although clinical information is not available, other CYP3A4 inducers also are expected to increase clopidogrel effect.

MANAGEMENT OPTIONS:

➥ **Monitor.** Consider monitoring platelet function if rifampin is initiated, discontinued, or changed in dosage. Adjustments in clopidogrel dose may be needed.

REFERENCES:

1. Clarke TA, et al. The metabolism of clopidogrel is catalyzed by human cytochrome P450 3A and is inhibited by atorvastatin. *Drug Metab Dispos.* 2003;31(1):53-59.
2. Lau WC, et al. Atorvastatin reduces the ability of clopidogrel to inhibit platelet aggregation: a new drug-drug interaction. *Circulation.* 2003;107(1):32-37.

Clorazepate (eg, *Tranxene*)

Omeprazole (eg, *Prilosec*)

SUMMARY: A patient became comatose after taking clorazepate and omeprazole concurrently, but a causal relationship was not established.

RISK FACTORS: No specific risk factors are known.

MECHANISM: Not established. Omeprazole is a known inhibitor of CYP2C19, and it was proposed that omeprazole inhibited the CYP2C19 metabolism of desmethyldiazepam, the major active metabolite of clorazepate.

CLINICAL EVALUATION: A 60-year-old alcoholic man became comatose after receiving large doses of clorazepate to treat acute alcohol withdrawal.[1] The unconsciousness resolved slowly, and he required treatment in the intensive care unit for almost 2 weeks. Although it is not possible to rule out the possibility that the unconsciousness was caused by clorazepate alone, the severity and duration of the reaction are consistent with reduced desmethyldiazepam metabolism.

RELATED DRUGS: Other proton pump inhibitors, such as lansoprazole (eg, *Prevacid*), pantoprazole (eg, *Protonix*), and rabeprazole (*Aciphex*), are unlikely to inhibit CYP2C19, and theoretically are less likely to interact with clorazepate.

MANAGEMENT OPTIONS: No specific action is required, but be alert for evidence of the interaction.

REFERENCES:
1. Konrad A. Protracted episode of reduced consciousness following co-medication with omeprazole and clorazepate. *Clin Drug Invest.* 2000;19:307-311.

Clorazepate (eg, *Tranxene*)

Primidone (eg, *Mysoline*)

SUMMARY: The combined use of primidone and clorazepate may result in mental changes, but data are limited.

RISK FACTORS: No specific risk factors are known.

MECHANISM: Not established.

CLINICAL EVALUATION: Several patients receiving primidone and clorazepate developed personality changes, including aggressive behavior, depression, and irritability.[1] A drug interaction between primidone and clorazepate was proposed to explain these findings, but little supporting evidence was given.

RELATED DRUGS: No information is available.

MANAGEMENT OPTIONS: No specific action is required, but be alert for evidence of the interaction.

REFERENCES:
1. Feldman RG. Chlorazepate in temporal lobe epilepsy. *JAMA.* 1976;236(23):2603.

Clotrimazole (eg, *Mycelex*)

Midazolam

SUMMARY: Clotrimazole increases the concentration of orally administered midazolam; increased sedation may occur in some patients.

RISK FACTORS: No specific risk factors are known.

MECHANISM: Clotrimazole inhibits CYP3A4, the enzyme responsible for midazolam metabolism. It appears that only enterocyte CYP3A4 is inhibited by oral clotrimazole.

CLINICAL EVALUATION: Ten healthy subjects received midazolam 2 mg orally or 0.025 mg/kg intravenously (IV) alone and following clotrimazole troches 10 mg 3 times a day for 5 days.[1] Compared with midazolam alone, the pretreatment with clotrimazole increased the mean area under the concentration-time curve of midazolam more than 60%. Midazolam half-life was not changed. Clotrimazole did not affect the pharmacokinetics of midazolam administered IV.

RELATED DRUGS: Ketoconazole (eg, *Nizoral*), fluconazole (eg, *Diflucan*), itraconazole (eg, *Sporanox*), posaconazole (*Noxafil*), and voriconazole (*Vfend*) also inhibit the activity of CYP3A4 and are expected to increase the plasma concentrations of midazolam. The first-pass metabolism of benzodiazepines that are metabolized by CYP3A4, such as alprazolam (eg, *Xanax*), flurazepam, or triazolam (eg, *Halcion*), might also be reduced by clotrimazole.

MANAGEMENT OPTIONS:

➡ *Consider Alternative.* Nystatin suspension may be considered in patients taking oral drugs that are CYP3A4 substrates. Other benzodiazepines (eg, lorazepam [eg, *Ativan*], oxazepam) that are not metabolized by CYP3A4 are unlikely to be affected by clotrimazole.

➡ *Monitor.* If clotrimazole is administered to patients receiving oral midazolam, monitor for excess sedation.

REFERENCES:

   1. Shord SS, et al. Effects of oral clotrimazole troches on the pharmacokinetics of oral and intravenous midazolam. *Br J Clin Pharmacol.* 2010;69:160-166.

Clotrimazole (eg, *Mycelex*)

Tacrolimus (*Prograf*)

SUMMARY: The administration of oral clotrimazole troches results in an increase in tacrolimus plasma concentrations.

RISK FACTORS: No specific risk factors are known.

MECHANISM: Clotrimazole is an inhibitor of CYP3A4, the primary metabolic pathway for tacrolimus, and inhibits P-glycoprotein, which is known to transport tacrolimus. Both of these effects are expected to increase the bioavailability of tacrolimus and its plasma concentrations.

CLINICAL EVALUATION: Tacrolimus plasma concentrations were measured in 6 renal transplant patients taking maintenance tacrolimus before and following 5 days of oral clotrimazole troche 3 times daily.[1] The mean area under the plasma concentration-time curve (AUC) of tacrolimus increased about 150% when clotrimazole was administered. Tacrolimus sampling time was insufficient to calculate its half-life. In a case report, a patient receiving tacrolimus, prednisone, and clotrimazole troches developed elevated tacrolimus concentrations, serum creatinine, and hepatic function tests.[2] The AUC of tacrolimus was reduced 45% following the discontinuation of clotrimazole. Some patients stabilized on tacrolimus may require a dose adjustment when clotrimazole is added to or deleted from the dosage regimen.

RELATED DRUGS: Other antifungal agents that inhibit CYP3A4 (eg, fluconazole [eg, *Diflucan*], itraconazole [eg, *Sporanox*], voriconazole [*Vfend*]) have been reported to affect tacrolimus similarly. Sirolimus (*Rapamune*) and cyclosporine (eg, *Neoral*) are also substrates for CYP3A4 and would likely be similarly affected by clotrimazole.

MANAGEMENT OPTIONS:

➡ *Consider Alternative.* Consider terbinafine (eg, *Lamisil*) as an alternative antifungal agent because it does not affect CYP3A4 activity.

➡ *Monitor.* Monitor patients for altered tacrolimus plasma concentrations whenever clotrimazole is added to or removed from drug regimens.

REFERENCES:

   1. Vasquez EM, et al. Concomitant clotrimazole therapy more than doubles the relative oral bioavailability of tacrolimus. *Ther Drug Monit.* 2005;27(5):587-591.

2. Mieles L, et al. Interaction between FK506 and clotrimazole in a liver transplant recipient. *Transplantation*. 1991;52(6):1086-1087.

Clozapine (eg, *Clozaril*)

Cigarette Smoking

SUMMARY: Serious clozapine toxicity has occurred following smoking cessation; monitor clozapine concentrations carefully and reduce clozapine dosage as needed.

RISK FACTORS: No specific risk factors are known.

MECHANISM: Cigarette smoking induces the metabolism of clozapine by CYP1A2; discontinuation of smoking results in reduction in CYP1A2 activity and increased clozapine serum concentrations. The reduction in CYP1A2 activity following cessation of smoking appears quickly, with a half-life decrease in CYP1A2 activity of about 40 hours in 1 study.[1]

CLINICAL EVALUATION: In 11 patients stabilized on clozapine who stopped smoking, the clozapine serum concentrations increased a mean of 72% over the next 18 to 47 days.[2] One patient manifested a 261% increase in clozapine concentrations (to 3,066 ng/mL) and developed aspiration pneumonia. Other cases of clozapine toxicity have been reported after smoking cessation, with findings such as generalized tonic-clonic seizures, stupor, coma, myoclonus, and confusion.[3-5] The magnitude of the changes in clozapine concentrations and the severity of the adverse outcomes suggest that smoking activity has a substantial effect on clozapine response.

RELATED DRUGS: Smoking may also reduce concentrations of another CYP1A2 substrate, olanzapine (*Zyprexa*), and possibly also thioridazine and chlorpromazine (eg, *Thorazine*).

MANAGEMENT OPTIONS:

➡ *Monitor.* Carefully monitor patients receiving clozapine for elevated clozapine concentrations if they stop smoking cigarettes. Patients on clozapine who start smoking (or who substantially increase the number of cigarettes smoked per day) are likely to need an increase in clozapine dosage. Any change in cigarette smoking may affect clozapine dosage requirements, and patients must be monitored accordingly.

REFERENCES:

1. Faber MS, Fuhr U. Time response of cytochrome P450 1A2 activity on cessation of heavy smoking. *Clin Pharmacol Ther*. 2004;76:178-184.
2. Meyer JM. Individual changes in clozapine levels after smoking cessation: results and a predictive model. *J Clin Psychopharmacol*. 2001;21:569-574.
3. McCarthy RH. Seizures following smoking cessation in a clozapine responder. *Pharmacopsychiatry*. 1994;27:210-211.
4. Skogh E, et al. Could discontinuing smoking be hazardous for patients administered clozapine medication? A case report. *Ther Drug Monit*. 1999;21.580-582.
5. Zullino DF, et al. Tobacco and cannabis smoking cessation can lead to intoxication with clozapine or olanzapine. *Int Clin Psychopharmacol*. 2002;17:141-143.

Clozapine (eg, *Clozaril*)

Diazepam (eg, *Valium*)

SUMMARY: Isolated cases of cardiorespiratory collapse have been reported in patients receiving diazepam and clozapine, but a causal relationship has not been established.

RISK FACTORS: No specific risk factors are known.

MECHANISM: Not established. It is possible that clozapine and diazepam have additive pharmacodynamic effects on the cardiovascular and respiratory systems.

CLINICAL EVALUATION: A 51-year-old man with schizophrenia who was receiving diazepam 20 mg/day developed loss of consciousness, no visible respiration, and unmeasurable blood pressure after receiving clozapine 25 mg.[1] A 36-year-old schizophrenic man receiving diazepam 5 mg/day developed delirium and cardiorespiratory collapse after receiving clozapine 12.5 mg.[1] This second patient also received flurazepam (eg, *Dalmane*) 30 mg the day before collapse. Because a drug interaction between the benzodiazepines and clozapine was suspected, a retrospective review was conducted of patients who had received clozapine with and without concurrent benzodiazepines. Of the 39 patients reviewed, 3 collapsed with clozapine plus benzodiazepines, while 1 collapsed with clozapine alone. Dizziness and sedation also were found more often with the combination than with clozapine monotherapy. However, firm conclusions cannot be drawn given the number of subjects studied. Although one cannot rule out the possibility that a drug interaction contributed to the reactions, a causal relationship was not established. Clozapine in the absence of benzodiazepine therapy has been associated with isolated cases of respiratory arrest and orthostatic hypotension with syncope.[2] Moreover, many patients have received clozapine and benzodiazepines concurrently without manifesting such reactions.[3] Nonetheless, the possibility that in certain predisposed patients diazepam can increase the risk of cardiorespiratory collapse caused by clozapine cannot be ruled out.

RELATED DRUGS: Lorazepam (eg, *Ativan*) has also been associated with similar reactions when combined with clozapine, but a causal relationship has not been established.

MANAGEMENT OPTIONS:

➡ ***Monitor.*** Although a causal relationship has not been established for this interaction, the severity of the reaction dictates that patients receiving clozapine and diazepam be monitored closely for evidence of respiratory depression and hypotension, especially during the first few weeks of therapy and after an increase in the dose of either drug. Until more information is available, the same precautions should pertain to the use of clozapine concurrently with benzodiazepines other than diazepam.

REFERENCES:

1. Sassim N, et al. Adverse drug reactions with clozapine and simultaneous application of benzodiazepines. *Pharmacopsychiatry.* 1988;21:306-307.
2. Finkel M, et al. Clozapine—a novel antipsychotic agent. *N Engl J Med.* 1991;325:518.
3. Frankenburg F, et al. Clozapine—a novel antipsychotic agent. *N Engl J Med.* 1991;325:518.

Clozapine (eg, *Clozaril*)

Erythromycin (eg, *E-Mycin*)

SUMMARY: A patient receiving clozapine developed elevated plasma concentrations and a seizure following the addition of erythromycin therapy.

RISK FACTORS: No specific risk factors are known.

MECHANISM: Not established. It is probable that erythromycin inhibits the metabolism of clozapine.

CLINICAL EVALUATION: A patient receiving clozapine had elevated clozapine concentrations and a tonic-clonic seizure 7 days after starting erythromycin.[1] Erythromycin was discontinued, the clozapine dose was reduced, and no further seizures occurred. The temporal relationship between the administration of erythromycin and the toxicity make it likely that erythromycin was responsible for the elevated clozapine concentration and apparent clozapine-induced seizure. More study is needed to determine the frequency with which this interaction would result in adverse patient outcomes.

RELATED DRUGS: Troleandomycin (*TAO*) or clarithromycin (*Biaxin*) may inhibit the metabolism of clozapine. Azithromycin (*Zithromax*) and dirithromycin (*Dynabac*) would be unlikely to inhibit the metabolism of clozapine.

MANAGEMENT OPTIONS:

➡ **Use Alternative.** Noninteracting antibiotics (eg, azithromycin, dirithromycin) are preferable in patients receiving clozapine.

REFERENCES:
1. Funderburg LG, et al. Seizure following the addition of erythromycin to clozapine treatment. *Am J Psychiatry*. 1994;151:1840.

Clozapine (eg, *Clozaril*)

Fluvoxamine (*Luvox*)

SUMMARY: Fluvoxamine can markedly increase clozapine plasma concentrations; dosage adjustments are likely to be needed.

RISK FACTORS: No specific risk factors are known.

MECHANISM: Fluvoxamine is a potent inhibitor of cytochrome P4501A2, an enzyme that appears to be important in the metabolism of clozapine.

CLINICAL EVALUATION: A 36-year-old schizophrenic woman receiving clozapine 400 mg/day was started on fluvoxamine 100 mg/day. Four and 7 days after starting fluvoxamine, the clozapine serum concentration increased from 267 to 2166 and 3151 ng/mL, respectively (a 7- to 11-fold increase). She subsequently was stabilized on reduced doses of clozapine 200 mg/day and fluvoxamine 50 mg/day. Two other patients, a 22-year-old man and a 41-year-old woman, also manifested extremely high clozapine plasma concentrations while taking fluvoxamine concurrently.[1] In another study, data from a therapeutic drug monitoring service were used to determine the effect of other drugs on clozapine serum concentrations.[2] In 3 to 4 patients on combined clozapine-fluvoxamine therapy, the ratio of clozapine plasma concentration to dose (C/D ratio) was markedly higher than in patients receiving clozapine without fluvoxamine. In 2 of the patients who had clozapine levels determined with and without fluvoxamine, the C/D ratio increased 5- to 10-fold. One of the patients developed marked sedation and urinary incontinence when fluvoxamine 150 mg/day was added to clozapine 550 mg/day; his clozapine plasma concentration had increased approximately 8-fold.

RELATED DRUGS: The effect of selective serotonin reuptake inhibitors (SSRIs) other than fluvoxamine on clozapine is not established, but fluoxetine (*Prozac*), paroxetine (*Paxil*), and sertraline (*Zoloft*) appear to have little effect on cytochrome P4501A2.

MANAGEMENT OPTIONS:

➡ *Use Alternative.* Given the large magnitude of the increases in clozapine plasma concentrations because of fluvoxamine, an SSRI other than fluvoxamine generally would be preferable. If fluvoxamine is used, adjustments in clozapine dosage are likely to be needed. Monitor for altered clozapine response if fluvoxamine therapy is initiated, discontinued, or changed in dosage.

REFERENCES:

1. Hiemke C, et al. Elevated levels of clozapine in serum after addition of fluvoxamine. *J Clin Psychopharmacol.* 1994;14:279.

2. Jerling M, et al. Fluvoxamine inhibition and carbamazepine induction of the metabolism of clozapine: evidence from a therapeutic drug monitoring service. *Ther Drug Monit.* 1994;16:368.

Clozapine (*Clozaril*)

Haloperidol (*Haldol*)

SUMMARY: A patient on clozapine developed symptoms consistent with neuroleptic malignant syndrome (NMS) after haloperidol was added to his therapy, but a causal relationship was not established.

RISK FACTORS: No specific risk factors are known.

MECHANISM: Not established. It is possible that the reaction resulted from additive pharmacodynamic effects of clozapine and haloperidol. Both drugs have been associated with NMS when given alone.

CLINICAL EVALUATION: A 68-year-old man on clozapine 600 mg/day and venlafaxine 150 mg/day was given haloperidol 4 mg/day.[1] About 4 weeks after starting the haloperidol, he was found slumped over a table with clammy skin and was brought to an emergency department. He was noted to have fever, tachycardia, diaphoresis, delirium, and unintelligible speech. A diagnosis of neuroleptic malignant syndrome caused by combined effects of clozapine and haloperidol was made. Nonetheless, one cannot rule out the possibility that the reaction was from the haloperidol alone.

RELATED DRUGS: No information is available.

MANAGEMENT OPTIONS: No specific action is required, but be alert for evidence of the interaction.

REFERENCES:

1. Garcia G, et al. Neuroleptic malignant syndrome with antidepressant/antipsychotic drug combination. *Ann Pharmacother.* 2001;35:784.

Clozapine (eg, *Clozaril*)

Lithium (eg, *Eskalith*)

SUMMARY: Patients on clozapine and lithium have developed diabetic ketoacidosis, but a causal relationship was not established.

RISK FACTORS: No specific risk factors are known.

MECHANISM: Not established.

CLINICAL EVALUATION: Isolated cases of diabetic ketoacidosis have been reported in patients receiving clozapine and lithium.[1,2] More study is needed to establish whether or not the ketoacidosis resulted from combined effects of clozapine and lithium.

RELATED DRUGS: No information is available.

MANAGEMENT OPTIONS: No specific action is required, but be alert for evidence of the interaction.

REFERENCES:

1. Peterson GA, et al. Diabetic ketoacidosis from clozapine and lithium cotreatment. *Am J Psychiatry.* 1996;153:737.

2. Koval MS, et al. Diabetic ketoacidosis associated with clozapine treatment. *Am J Psychiatry.* 1994;151:1520.

Clozapine (*Clozaril*) 4

Loperamide (eg, *Imodium*)

SUMMARY: A patient on clozapine and loperamide developed fatal gastroenteritis, but a causal relationship was not established.

RISK FACTORS: No specific risk factors are known.

MECHANISM: It was proposed that the anticholinergic effect of clozapine added to the antimotility effects of loperamide, leading to toxic megacolon.

CLINICAL EVALUATION: A 36-year-old man receiving clozapine developed fatal toxic megacolon after starting loperamide therapy for diarrhea.[1] It is possible that the fatal reaction resulted from the combined use of clozapine and loperamide, but one cannot rule out that loperamide alone was responsible.

RELATED DRUGS: No information is available.

MANAGEMENT OPTIONS: No specific action is required, but be alert for evidence of the interaction.

REFERENCES:

1. Eronen M, et al. Lethal gastroenteritis associated with clozapine and loperamide. *Am J Psychiatry.* 2003;160.2242-2243.

Clozapine (eg, *Clozaril*)

Lorazepam (eg, *Ativan*)

SUMMARY: Isolated cases of cardiovascular or respiratory collapse have been reported in patients receiving lorazepam and clozapine, but a causal relationship has not been established.

RISK FACTORS: No specific risk factors are known.

MECHANISM: Not established. It is possible that clozapine and lorazepam have additive pharmacodynamic effects on the cardiovascular and respiratory systems.

CLINICAL EVALUATION: A 47-year-old woman with schizophrenia who was admitted with an acute exacerbation was given lorazepam and clozapine (daily doses not stated).[1] After 7 days of combined therapy, she developed cardiorespiratory collapse with cyanosis and apnea 90 minutes after taking a 25-mg dose of clozapine (the dose and timing of lorazepam was not stated). She responded to cardiopulmonary resuscitation. Given that cardiovascular collapse had been reported in patients receiving clozapine and diazepam,[2] the authors proposed that this patient's reaction may have been caused by a drug interaction. Another report described a 43-year-old man who was receiving clozapine in increasing doses up to 400 mg/day along with lorazepam 1 mg 3 times daily and flunitrazepam 2 mg/day.[3] He refused to take the clozapine on the seventeenth day of therapy and was given 3 IV doses of lorazepam over 9 hours at 8:00, 1:00, and 5:00. He was found dead in bed at 5:00 the next morning, presumably because of respiratory arrest during sleep. Given the delayed nature of the reaction, it is not clear what role the combined effects of clozapine and lorazepam played in the fatal episode. Although one cannot rule out the possibility that a drug interaction contributed to the above reactions, a causal relationship was not established. Clozapine in the absence of benzodiazepine therapy has been associated with isolated cases of respiratory arrest and orthostatic hypotension with syncope.[4] Moreover, many patients have received clozapine and benzodiazepines concurrently without manifesting such reactions.[4] Nonetheless, one cannot rule out the possibility that lorazepam might increase the risk of cardiorespiratory collapse in certain predisposed patients receiving clozapine.

RELATED DRUGS: Diazepam (eg, *Valium*) also has been associated with similar reactions when combined with clozapine, but a causal relationship has not been established.

MANAGEMENT OPTIONS:

➡ ***Monitor.*** Although a causal relationship has not been established for this interaction, the severity of the reaction dictates that patients receiving clozapine and lorazepam be monitored closely for evidence of respiratory depression and hypotension, especially during the first few weeks of therapy and after an increase in the dose of either drug. Until more information is available, the same precautions also pertain to the use of clozapine concurrently with benzodiazepines other than lorazepam.

REFERENCES:

1. Friedman LJ, et al. Clozapine–a novel antipsychotic agent. *N Engl J Med.* 1991;325:518-519.
2. Sassim N, et al. Adverse drug reactions with clozapine and simultaneous application of benzodiazepines. *Pharmacopsychiatry.* 1988;21:306-307.
3. Klimke A, et al. Sudden death after intravenous application of lorazepam in a patient treated with clozapine. *Am J Psychiatry.* 1994;151:780.
4. Finkel M, et al. Clozapine–a novel antipsychotic agent. *N Engl J Med.* 1991;325:518.

Clozapine (eg, *Clozaril*)

Modafinil (*Provigil*)

SUMMARY: A patient on clozapine developed evidence of clozapine toxicity after starting modafinil, but a causal relationship was not established.

RISK FACTORS: No specific risk factors are known.

MECHANISM: Not established. It was proposed that modafinil inhibits the hepatic metabolism of clozapine by CYP2C19.

CLINICAL EVALUATION: A 42-year-old schizophrenic man on clozapine 450 mg/day developed evidence of clozapine toxicity and an elevated clozapine serum concentration after starting modafinil 300 mg/day.[1] More clinical study is needed to establish whether modafinil interacts with clozapine.

RELATED DRUGS: No information is available.

MANAGEMENT OPTIONS: No specific action is required, but be alert for evidence of the interaction.

REFERENCES:

1. Dequardo JR. Modafinil-associated clozapine toxicity. *Am J Psychiatry*. 2002;159:1243-1244.

Clozapine (eg, *Clozaril*)

Nefazodone

SUMMARY: A case of possible clozapine toxicity occurred following addition of nefazodone, but a causal relationship was not established. Pharmacokinetic data suggest a minimal interaction between clozapine and nefazodone.

RISK FACTORS: No specific risk factors are known.

MECHANISM: Not established. Some evidence suggests that clozapine is partially metabolized by CYP3A4, and nefazodone is a known CYP3A4 inhibitor.

CLINICAL EVALUATION: A 40-year-old schizophrenic man on clozapine and risperidone was started on nefazodone 200 mg/day for 7 days, then 300 mg/day.[1] After 7 days on the higher dose, he developed dizziness, hypotension, and increased anxiety. His clozapine and norclozapine plasma concentrations were 75% and 89% higher, respectively, than before he started nefazodone. When the nefazodone dose was decreased to 200 mg/day, the hypotension and symptoms resolved within 7 days, and the serum concentrations of clozapine and norclozapine declined. Conversely, in a study of 6 patients, nefazodone 100 mg twice daily for 1 week, then 200 mg twice daily for 2 weeks had negligible effects on clozapine plasma concentrations.[2] Although CYP3A4 does not appear to be an important isozyme in the metabolism of clozapine, it is possible that CYP3A4 inhibitors such as nefazodone may increase clozapine plasma concentrations in certain predisposed patients.

RELATED DRUGS: The selective serotonin reuptake inhibitor fluvoxamine is a potent inhibitor of CYP1A2 and can substantially increase clozapine plasma concentrations.

MANAGEMENT OPTIONS: No specific action is required, but be alert for evidence of the interaction.

REFERENCES:

1. Khan AY, et al. Increase in plasma levels of clozapine and norclozapine after administration of nefazodone. *J Clin Psychiatry.* 2001;62:375-376.

2. Taylor D, et al. The effect of nefazodone on clozapine plasma concentrations. *Int Clin Psychopharmacol.* 1999;14:185-187.

4   Clozapine (eg, *Clozaril*)

Omeprazole (eg, *Prilosec*)

SUMMARY: Two patients developed reduced clozapine concentrations with concomitant omeprazole, but a causal relationship was not established.

RISK FACTORS: No specific risk factors are known.

MECHANISM: Not established.

CLINICAL EVALUATION: In 2 patients stabilized on clozapine, the addition of omeprazole therapy was associated with an over 40% reduction in clozapine plasma concentrations.[1] More study is needed to establish a causal relationship and to determine if the interaction reduces the efficacy of clozapine.

RELATED DRUGS: The effect of other proton pump inhibitors on clozapine is not established.

MANAGEMENT OPTIONS: No specific action is required, but be alert for evidence of the interaction.

REFERENCES:

1. Frick A, et al. Omeprazole reduces clozapine plasma concentrations. A case report. *Pharmacopsychiatry.* 2003;36:121-123.

4   Clozapine (eg, *Clozaril*)

Risperidone (eg, *Risperdal*)

SUMMARY: Although isolated case reports suggest that risperidone may increase clozapine serum concentrations, a study in 18 patients found no effect.

RISK FACTORS: No specific risk factors are known.

MECHANISM: Not established. It is possible that risperidone inhibits the hepatic metabolism of clozapine.

CLINICAL EVALUATION: A 32-year-old man with schizoaffective disorder was started on clozapine following failure to respond to haloperidol (eg, *Haldol*), thioridazine, and thiothixene (eg, *Navane*).[1] He responded partially to clozapine titrated to 300 mg twice daily, and risperidone was added. After 2 weeks of risperidone 1 mg twice daily, the clozapine plasma concentration was 74% higher than when clozapine was given alone. The increase in clozapine concentrations was associated with improved antipsychotic effect and no adverse effects. Nonetheless, a study in 18 patients who received clozapine with and without concurrent risperidone therapy found no effect on risperidone and clozapine serum concentrations.[2]

RELATED DRUGS: No information is available.

MANAGEMENT OPTIONS: No specific action is required, but be alert for evidence of the interaction.

REFERENCES:

1. Tyson SC, et al. Pharmacokinetic interaction between risperidone and clozapine. *Am J Psychiatry.* 1995;152:1401-1402.
2. Raaska K, et al. Therapeutic drug monitoring data: risperidone does not increase serum clozapine concentration. *Eur J Clin Pharmacol.* 2002;58:587-591.

Clozapine (eg, *Clozaril*)

Sertraline (*Zoloft*)

SUMMARY: A man on clozapine and sertraline died of an apparent cardiac arrhythmia, but a causal relationship was not established.

RISK FACTORS: No specific risk factors are known.

MECHANISM: Not established.

CLINICAL EVALUATION: A 26-year-old man with schizophrenia, obsessive-compulsive disorder, and depression was found dead at his home, presumably of an acute cardiac arrhythmia.[1] He had been taking clozapine 100 mg twice daily, sertraline 200 mg once daily, and atenolol 50 mg twice daily. It was not clear if any of his medications played a role in his death, but the combination of clozapine and sertraline might have contributed to sudden cardiac death.

RELATED DRUGS: No information is available.

MANAGEMENT OPTIONS: No specific action is required, but be alert for evidence of the interaction.

REFERENCES:

1. Hoehns JD, et al. Sudden cardiac death with clozapine and sertraline combination. *Ann Pharmacother.* 2001;35:862-866.

Clozapine (eg, *Clozaril*)

Valproic Acid (eg, *Depakene*)

SUMMARY: Several patients stabilized on clozapine developed substantial reductions in clozapine total serum concentrations after valproic acid was started, but clozapine therapeutic response was not affected.

RISK FACTORS: No specific risk factors are known.

MECHANISM: Not established. The observed effects are consistent with valproic acid-induced displacement of clozapine from plasma protein binding sites, but binding studies have not been performed.

CLINICAL EVALUATION: Four schizophrenic subjects stabilized on large doses of clozapine 550 to 650 mg/day were started on valproic acid and titrated up to a valproic acid serum concentration in the therapeutic range (50 to 100 mcg/mL).[1] Total clozapine serum concentrations decreased gradually over 3 weeks (average decrease, 41% at 3 weeks). However, the reduced total clozapine serum concentrations were not associated with inhibition in the antipsychotic effect of clozapine. A possible reason for this apparent discrepancy is that valproic acid displaces clozapine from plasma protein binding, thus reducing total but not unbound clozapine in the serum. This presents the theoretical danger of a clinician increasing clozapine dosage in response to low total clozapine serum concentrations. Nonetheless, more study is needed to establish the mechanism and clinical importance of this interaction.

RELATED DRUGS: No information is available.

MANAGEMENT OPTIONS:

➡ **Monitor.** Until more data are available, monitor for altered clozapine response if valproic acid therapy is initiated, discontinued, or changed in dosage. When interpreting clozapine serum concentrations, keep in mind that if displacement of clozapine from plasma protein binding is involved, subtherapeutic total clozapine levels may not indicate subtherapeutic unbound levels.

REFERENCES:

1. Finley P, et al. Potential impact of valproic acid therapy on clozapine disposition. *Biol Psychiatry.* 1994;36:487-488.

Cocaine

Disulfiram (*Antabuse*)

SUMMARY: Disulfiram may substantially increase cocaine plasma concentrations and cardiovascular effects, but the clinical importance of this effect is not established.

RISK FACTORS: No specific risk factors are known.

MECHANISM: Not established. Disulfiram may inhibit the metabolism of cocaine by plasma and microsomal carboxylesterases and plasma cholinesterase.[1]

CLINICAL EVALUATION: In a randomized, double-blind, placebo-controlled study, 7 cocaine abusers were given intranasal cocaine 1 or 2 mg/kg with disulfiram 250 and 500 mg/day.[1] Disulfiram increased cocaine area under the plasma concentration-time curve 3- to 6-fold, and also increased the cardiovascular effects of cocaine, particularly the heart rate. However, subjects' behavioral responses to cocaine were not affected. The extent to which this interaction increases the risk of adverse cardiovascular effects of cocaine in patients receiving disulfiram as treatment for cocaine-alcohol abuse is not established.

RELATED DRUGS: No information is available.

MANAGEMENT OPTIONS:

➡ **Circumvent/Minimize.** Inform patients receiving disulfiram that cocaine may have greater toxicity.

REFERENCES:

1. McCance-Katz EF, et al. Disulfiram effects on acute cocaine administration. *Drug Alcohol Depend.* 1998;52:27-39.

Cocaine **3**

Propranolol (eg, *Inderal*)

SUMMARY: Propranolol increases the angina-inducing potential of cocaine; other beta-adrenergic blockers would be expected to have similar effects.

RISK FACTORS: No specific risk factors are known.

MECHANISM: Cocaine-induced coronary vasoconstriction is potentiated by beta-adrenergic blockers, resulting in a reduction in coronary blood flow.

CLINICAL EVALUATION: Thirty patients being evaluated for chest pain underwent cardiac catheterization.[1] One-half of the patients received intranasal saline while the other half received 2 mg/kg of an intranasal cocaine solution. Intracoronary propranolol 2 mg was administered 15 minutes after the cocaine or saline administration. Cocaine increased blood pressure and myocardial oxygen demand while decreasing coronary blood flow. Saline and propranolol alone had no effect. The administration of propranolol following cocaine produced a greater reduction in coronary blood flow and increased coronary vascular resistance. One patient developed symptoms of angina following propranolol and cocaine administration. The significance of this interaction in patients using therapeutic or recreational doses of cocaine is unknown, but it is likely to heighten as the cocaine dose increases. Beta blockers with vasodilating properties (eg, labetalol) theoretically would be less likely to potentiate the vasoconstricting effects of cocaine.

RELATED DRUGS: Other beta blockers are likely to produce a similar reaction.

MANAGEMENT OPTIONS:

➡ *Consider Alternative.* The use of cocaine for local anesthesia might pose an increased risk to patients taking beta blockers. Consider other local anesthetics for use.

➡ *Monitor.* Caution patients, particularly those with coronary artery disease, taking beta-adrenergic blockers regarding the potential for angina during cocaine use.

REFERENCES:

1. Lange RA, et al. Potentiation of cocaine-induced coronary vasoconstriction by beta-adrenergic blockade. *Ann Intern Med.* 1990;112:897.

Codeine **4**

Fluoxetine (*Prozac*)

SUMMARY: Fluoxetine inhibits CYP2D6, and theoretically would interfere with the bioactivation of codeine to morphine, but the extent to which it inhibits the analgesic effect of codeine is not established.

RISK FACTORS:

➡ *Pharmacogenetics.* Only patients with the extensive metabolizer CYP2D6 phenotype (EMs) would be expected to experience this interaction. Poor metabolizers (PMs) do not have the gene for production of CYP2D6, so there would be no CYP2D6 for the fluoxetine to inhibit. Approximately 8% of whites are deficient in CYP2D6, but the deficiency is rare in Asians, usually 2% or less.

MECHANISM: Codeine exerts its analgesic effects (and probably also its side effects) primarily through its metabolic conversion to morphine by the isozyme, CYP2D6.[1,2]

Thus, patients genetically deficient in CYP2D6 or receiving CYP2D6 inhibitors such as fluoxetine are likely to produce little or no morphine during codeine administration.

CLINICAL EVALUATION: Fluoxetine is a potent inhibitor of CYP2D6. Because several studies have shown that another CYP2D6 inhibitor, quinidine (eg, *Quinora*), inhibits the analgesic effect of codeine,[3-6] fluoxetine might be expected to inhibit codeine analgesia as well. Nonetheless, clinical studies are needed to determine the clinical importance of this potential interaction.

RELATED DRUGS: The analgesic effect of dihydrocodeine (eg, *Synalgos-DC*) and hydrocodone (eg, *Vicodin*) may be dependent on conversion to morphine-like active metabolites, and early evidence suggests that CYP2D6 inhibitors can reduce their analgesic efficacy. Whether fluoxetine affects these drugs is not known. Tramadol (*Ultram*) appears to be partially dependent upon CYP2D6 for analgesic activity, but theoretically would be less affected than codeine by fluoxetine. Early pharmacodynamic evidence suggests that oxycodone (eg, *Percodan*) does not require conversion by CYP2D6 to an active metabolite. Theoretically, oxycodone would not be affected by fluoxetine, but more study is needed.

MANAGEMENT OPTIONS: No specific action is required, but be alert for evidence of the interaction.

REFERENCES:

1. Sindrup SH, et al. Codeine increases pain thresholds to copper vapor laser stimuli in extensive but not poor metabolizers of sparteine. *Clin Pharmacol Ther*. 1990;48:686.
2. Poulsen L, et al. Codeine and morphine in extensive and poor metabolizers of sparteine: pharmacokinetics, analgesic effect and side effects. *Eur J Clin Pharmacol*. 1996;51:289.
3. Desmeules J, et al. Impact of environmental and genetic factors on codeine analgesia. *Eur J Clin Pharmacol*. 1991;41:23.
4. Sindrup SH, et al. The effect of quinidine on the analgesic effect of codeine. *Eur J Clin Pharmacol*. 1992;42:587.
5. Sindrup SH, et al. Impact of quinidine on plasma and cerebrospinal fluid concentrations of codeine and morphine after codeine intake. *Eur J Clin Pharmacol*. 1996;49:503.
6. Caraco Y, et al. Pharmacogenetic determination of the effects of codeine and prediction of drug interactions. *J Pharmacol Exp Ther*. 1996;278:1165.

4   Codeine

Haloperidol (*Haldol*)

SUMMARY: Haloperidol inhibits the bioactivation of codeine to morphine in vitro, but the extent to which haloperidol inhibits the analgesic effect of codeine is not established.

RISK FACTORS:

➡ **Pharmacogenetics.** Only patients with the extensive metabolizer CYP2D6 phenotype (EMs) would be expected to experience this interaction. Poor metabolizers (PMs) do not have the gene for production of CYP2D6, so there would be no CYP2D6 for the haloperidol to inhibit. Approximately 8% of whites are deficient in CYP2D6, but the deficiency is rare in Asians, usually 2% or less.

MECHANISM: Codeine exerts its analgesic effects (and probably also its side effects) primarily through its metabolic conversion to morphine by the isozyme, CYP2D6.[1,2] Thus, patients genetically deficient in CYP2D6 or receiving CYP2D6 inhibitors such as haloperidol produce little or no morphine during codeine administration.

CLINICAL EVALUATION: Using hepatic microsomes from an extensive metabolizer, haloperidol was found to inhibit the conversion of codeine to morphine *in vitro*.[3] Several studies have shown that the CYP2D6 inhibitor, quinidine (eg, *Quinora*), inhibits the analgesic effect of codeine.[4-7] Thus, haloperidol, a known CYP2D6 inhibitor, might be expected to inhibit codeine analgesia as well. Nonetheless, clinical studies are needed to determine the clinical importance of this potential interaction.

RELATED DRUGS: The analgesic effect of dihydrocodeine (eg, *Synalgos-DC*) and hydrocodone (eg, *Vicodin*) may be dependent on conversion to morphine-like active metabolites, and early evidence suggests that CYP2D6 inhibitors can reduce their analgesic efficacy. Whether haloperidol affects these drugs is unknown. Tramadol (*Ultram*) appears to be partially dependent upon CYP2D6 for analgesic activity, but theoretically would be less affected than codeine by haloperidol. Early pharmacodynamic evidence suggests that oxycodone (eg, *Percodan*) does not require conversion by CYP2D6 to an active metabolite. Theoretically, oxycodone would not be affected by haloperidol, but more study is needed.

MANAGEMENT OPTIONS: No specific action is required, but be alert for evidence of the interaction.

REFERENCES:

1. Sindrup SH, et al. Codeine increases pain thresholds to copper vapor laser stimuli in extensive but not poor metabolizers of sparteine. *Clin Pharmacol Ther.* 1990;48:686.
2. Poulsen L, et al. Codeine and morphine in extensive and poor metabolizers of sparteine: pharmacokinetics, analgesic effect and side effects.*Eur J Clin Pharmacol.* 1996;51:289.
3. Dayer P, et al. *In vitro* forecasting of drugs that may interfere with codeine bioactivation. *Eur J Drug Metab Pharmacokinet.* 1992;17:115.
4. Desmeules J, et al. Impact of environmental and genetic factors on codeine analgesia. *Eur J Clin Pharmacol.* 1991;41:23.
5. Sindrup SH, et al. The effect of quinidine on the analgesic effect of codeine. *Eur J Clin Pharmacol.* 1992;42:587.
6. Sindrup SH, et al. Impact of quinidine on plasma and cerebrospinal fluid concentrations of codeine and morphine after codeine intake. *Eur J Clin Pharmacol.* 1996;49:503.
7. Caraco Y, et al. Pharmacogenetic determination of the effects of codeine and prediction of drug interactions. *J Pharmacol Exp Ther.* 1996;278:1165.

Codeine **4**

Mibefradil

SUMMARY: Mibefradil inhibits CYP2D6, and theoretically would interfere with the bioactivation of codeine to morphine, but the extent to which it inhibits the analgesic effect of codeine is not established.

RISK FACTORS:

➡ **Pharmacogenetics.** Only patients with the extensive metabolizer CYP2D6 phenotype (EMs) would be expected to experience this interaction. Poor metabolizers (PMs) do not have the gene for production of CYP2D6, so there would be no CYP2D6 for the mibefradil to inhibit. Approximately 8% of whites are deficient in CYP2D6, but the deficiency is rare in Asians, usually 2% or less.

MECHANISM: Codeine exerts its analgesic effects (and probably also its side effects) primarily through its metabolic conversion to morphine by the isozyme, CYP2D6.[1,2] Thus, patients genetically deficient in CYP2D6 or receiving CYP2D6 inhibitors such as mibefradil are likely to produce little or no morphine during codeine administration.

CLINICAL EVALUATION: Mibefradil is known to inhibit CYP2D6. Because several studies have shown that another CYP2D6 inhibitor, quinidine (eg, *Quinora*), inhibits the analgesic effect of codeine,[3-6] mibefradil might be expected to inhibit codeine analgesia as well. Nonetheless, clinical studies are needed to determine the clinical importance of this potential interaction.

RELATED DRUGS: The analgesic effect of dihydrocodeine (eg, *Synalgos-DC*) and hydrocodone (eg, *Vicodin*) may be dependent on conversion to morphine-like active metabolites, and early evidence suggests that CYP2D6 inhibitors can reduce their analgesic efficacy. Whether mibefradil affects these drugs is unknown. Tramadol (*Ultram*) appears to be partially dependent upon CYP2D6 for analgesic activity, but theoretically would be less affected than codeine by mibefradil. Early pharmacodynamic evidence suggests that oxycodone (eg, *Percodan*) does not require conversion by CYP2D6 to an active metabolite. Theoretically, oxycodone would not be affected by mibefradil, but more study is needed.

MANAGEMENT OPTIONS: No specific action is required, but be alert for evidence of the interaction.

REFERENCES:
1. Sindrup SH, et al. Codeine increases pain thresholds to copper vapor laser stimuli in extensive but not poor metabolizers of sparteine. *Clin Pharmacol Ther*. 1990;48:686.
2. Poulsen L, et al. Codeine and morphine in extensive and poor metabolizers of sparteine: pharmacokinetics, analgesic effect and side effects.*Eur J Clin Pharmacol*. 1996;51:289.
3. Desmeules J, et al. Impact of environmental and genetic factors on codeine analgesia. *Eur J Clin Pharmacol*. 1991;41:23.
4. Sindrup SH, et al. The effect of quinidine on the analgesic effect of codeine. *Eur J Clin Pharmacol*. 1992;42:587.
5. Sindrup SH, et al. Impact of quinidine on plasma and cerebrospinal fluid concentrations of codeine and morphine after codeine intake. *Eur J Clin Pharmacol*. 1996;49:503.
6. Caraco Y, et al. Pharmacogenetic determination of the effects of codeine and prediction of drug interactions. *J Pharmacol Exp Ther*. 1996;278:1165.

 4   Codeine

Paroxetine (*Paxil*)

SUMMARY: Paroxetine inhibits CYP2D6, and theoretically would interfere with the bioactivation of codeine to morphine, but the extent to which it inhibits the analgesic effect of codeine is not established.

RISK FACTORS:

➡ **Pharmacogenetics.** Only patients with the extensive metabolizer CYP2D6 phenotype (EMs) would be expected to experience this interaction. Poor metabolizers (PMs) do not have the gene for production of CYP2D6, so there would be no CYP2D6 for the paroxetine to inhibit. Approximately 8% of whites are deficient in CYP2D6, but the deficiency is rare in Asians, usually 2% or less.

MECHANISM: Codeine exerts its analgesic effects (and probably also its side effects) primarily through its metabolic conversion to morphine by the isozyme, CYP2D6.[1,2] Thus, patients genetically deficient in CYP2D6 or receiving CYP2D6 inhibitors such as paroxetine are likely to produce little or no morphine during codeine administration.

CLINICAL EVALUATION: Paroxetine is a potent inhibitor of CYP2D6. Because several studies have shown that another CYP2D6 inhibitor, quinidine (eg, *Quinora*), inhibits the analgesic effect of codeine,[3-6] paroxetine might be expected to inhibit codeine analgesia as well. Nonetheless, clinical studies are needed to determine the clinical importance of this potential interaction.

RELATED DRUGS: The analgesic effect of dihydrocodeine (eg, *Synalgos-DC*) and hydrocodone (eg, *Vicodin*) may be dependent on conversion to morphine-like active metabolites, and early evidence suggests that CYP2D6 inhibitors can reduce their analgesic efficacy. Whether paroxetine affects these drugs is unknown. Tramadol (*Ultram*) appears to be partially dependent upon CYP2D6 for analgesic activity, but theoretically would be less affected than codeine by paroxetine. Early pharmacodynamic evidence suggests that oxycodone (eg, *Percodan*) does not require conversion by CYP2D6 to an active metabolite. Theoretically, oxycodone would not be affected by paroxetine, but more study is needed.

MANAGEMENT OPTIONS: No specific action is required, but be alert for evidence of the interaction.

REFERENCES:

1. Sindrup SH, et al. Codeine increases pain thresholds to copper vapor laser stimuli in extensive but not poor metabolizers of sparteine. *Clin Pharmacol Ther.* 1990;48:686.

2. Poulsen L, et al. Codeine and morphine in extensive and poor metabolizers of sparteine: pharmacokinetics, analgesic effect and side effects. *Eur J Clin Pharmacol.* 1996;51:289.

3. Desmeules J, et al. Impact of environmental and genetic factors on codeine analgesia. *Eur J Clin Pharmacol.* 1991;41:23.

4. Sindrup SH, et al. The effect of quinidine on the analgesic effect of codeine. *Eur J Clin Pharmacol.* 1992;42:587.

5. Sindrup SH, et al. Impact of quinidine on plasma and cerebrospinal fluid concentrations of codeine and morphine after codeine intake. *Eur J Clin Pharmacol.* 1996;49:503.

6. Caraco Y, et al. Pharmacogenetic determination of the effects of codeine and prediction of drug interactions. *J Pharmacol Exp Ther.* 1996;278:1165.

Codeine 4

Perphenazine (*Trilafon*)

SUMMARY: Perphenazine inhibits CYP2D6, and theoretically would interfere with the bioactivation of codeine to morphine, but the extent to which it inhibits the analgesic effect of codeine is not established.

RISK FACTORS:

➡ ***Pharmacogenetics.*** Only patients with the extensive metabolizer CYP2D6 phenotype (EMs) would be expected to experience this interaction. Poor metabolizers (PMs) do not have the gene for production of CYP2D6, so there would be no CYP2D6 for the perphenazine to inhibit. Approximately 8% of whites are deficient in CYP2D6, but the deficiency is rare in Asians, usually 2% or less.

MECHANISM: Codeine exerts its analgesic effects (and probably also its side effects) primarily through its metabolic conversion to morphine by the isozyme, CYP2D6.[1,2] Thus, patients genetically deficient in CYP2D6 or receiving CYP2D6 inhibitors such as perphenazine are likely to produce little or no morphine during codeine administration.

CLINICAL EVALUATION: Perphenazine is known to inhibit CYP2D6. Because several studies have shown that another CYP2D6 inhibitor, quinidine (eg, *Quinora*), inhibits the analgesic effect of codeine,[3-6] perphenazine might be expected to inhibit codeine analgesia as well. Nonetheless, clinical studies are needed to determine the clinical importance of this potential interaction.

RELATED DRUGS: The analgesic effect of dihydrocodeine (eg, *Synalgos-DC*) and hydrocodone (eg, *Vicodin*) may be dependent on conversion to morphine-like active metabolites, and early evidence suggests that CYP2D6 inhibitors can reduce their analgesic efficacy. Whether perphenazine affects these drugs is unknown. Tramadol (*Ultram*) appears to be partially dependent upon CYP2D6 for analgesic activity, but theoretically would be less affected than codeine by perphenazine. Early pharmacodynamic evidence suggests that oxycodone (eg, *Percodan*) does not require conversion by CYP2D6 to an active metabolite. Theoretically, oxycodone would not be affected by perphenazine, but more study is needed.

MANAGEMENT OPTIONS: No specific action is required, but be alert for evidence of the interaction.

REFERENCES:

1. Sindrup SH, et al. Codeine increases pain thresholds to copper vapor laser stimuli in extensive but not poor metabolizers of sparteine. *Clin Pharmacol Ther.* 1990;48:686.
2. Poulsen L, et al. Codeine and morphine in extensive and poor metabolizers of sparteine: pharmacokinetics, analgesic effect and side effects.*Eur J Clin Pharmacol.* 1996;51:289.
3. Desmeules J, et al. Impact of environmental and genetic factors on codeine analgesia. *Eur J Clin Pharmacol.* 1991;41:23.
4. Sindrup SH, et al. The effect of quinidine on the analgesic effect of codeine. *Eur J Clin Pharmacol.* 1992;42:587.
5. Sindrup SH, et al. Impact of quinidine on plasma and cerebrospinal fluid concentrations of codeine and morphine after codeine intake. *Eur J Clin Pharmacol.* 1996;49:503.
6. Caraco Y, et al. Pharmacogenetic determination of the effects of codeine and prediction of drug interactions. *J Pharmacol Exp Ther.* 1996;278:1165.

4   Codeine

Propafenone (*Rythmol*)

SUMMARY: Propafenone inhibits CYP2D6, and theoretically would interfere with the bioactivation of codeine to morphine, but the extent to which it inhibits the analgesic effect of codeine is not established.

RISK FACTORS:

➡ **Pharmacogenetics.** Only patients with the extensive metabolizer CYP2D6 phenotype (EMs) would be expected to experience this interaction. Poor metabolizers (PMs) do not have the gene for production of CYP2D6, so there would be no CYP2D6 for the propafenone to inhibit. Approximately 8% of whites are deficient in CYP2D6, but the deficiency is rare in Asians, usually 2% or less.

MECHANISM: Codeine exerts its analgesic effects (and probably also its side effects) primarily through its metabolic conversion to morphine by the isozyme, CYP2D6.[1,2] Thus, patients genetically deficient in CYP2D6 or receiving CYP2D6 inhibitors such as propafenone are likely to produce little or no morphine during codeine administration.

CLINICAL EVALUATION: Propafenone is known to inhibit CYP2D6. Because several studies have shown that another CYP2D6 inhibitor, quinidine (eg, *Quinora*), inhibits the analgesic effect of codeine,[3-6] propafenone might be expected to inhibit codeine analgesia as well. Nonetheless, clinical studies are needed to determine the clinical importance of this potential interaction.

RELATED DRUGS: The analgesic effect of dihydrocodeine (eg, *Synalgos-DC*) and hydrocodone (eg, *Vicodin*) may be dependent on conversion to morphine-like active metabolites, and early evidence suggests that CYP2D6 inhibitors can reduce their analgesic efficacy. Whether propafenone affects these drugs is unknown. Tramadol (*Ultram*) appears to be partially dependent upon CYP2D6 for analgesic activity, but theoretically would be less affected than codeine by propafenone. Early pharmacodynamic evidence suggests that oxycodone (eg, *Percodan*) does not require conversion by CYP2D6 to an active metabolite. Theoretically, oxycodone would not be affected by propafenone, but more study is needed.

MANAGEMENT OPTIONS: No specific action is required, but be alert for evidence of the interaction.

REFERENCES:

1. Sindrup SH, et al. Codeine increases pain thresholds to copper vapor laser stimuli in extensive but not poor metabolizers of sparteine. *Clin Pharmacol Ther.* 1990;48:686.

2. Poulsen L, et al. Codeine and morphine in extensive and poor metabolizers of sparteine: pharmacokinetics, analgesic effect and side effects. *Eur J Clin Pharmacol.* 1996;51:289.

3. Desmeules J, et al. Impact of environmental and genetic factors on codeine analgesia. *Eur J Clin Pharmacol.* 1991;41:23.

4. Sindrup SH, et al. The effect of quinidine on the analgesic effect of codeine. *Eur J Clin Pharmacol.* 1992;42:587.

5. Sindrup SH, et al. Impact of quinidine on plasma and cerebrospinal fluid concentrations of codeine and morphine after codeine intake. *Eur J Clin Pharmacol.* 1996;49:503.

6. Caraco Y, et al. Pharmacogenetic determination of the effects of codeine and prediction of drug interactions. *J Pharmacol Exp Ther.* 1996;278:1165.

Codeine

Propoxyphene (eg, *Darvocet-N*)

SUMMARY: Propoxyphene inhibits CYP2D6, and theoretically would interfere with the bioactivation of codeine to morphine, but the extent to which it inhibits the analgesic effect of codeine is not established.

RISK FACTORS:

➡ ***Pharmacogenetics.*** Only patients with the extensive metabolizer CYP2D6 phenotype (EMs) would be expected to experience this interaction. Poor metabolizers (PMs) do not have the gene for production of CYP2D6, so there would be no CYP2D6 for the propoxyphene to inhibit. Approximately 8% of whites are deficient in CYP2D6, but the deficiency is rare in Asians, usually 2% or less.

MECHANISM: Codeine exerts its analgesic effects (and probably also its side effects) primarily through its metabolic conversion to morphine by the isozyme, CYP2D6.[1,2] Thus, patients genetically deficient in CYP2D6 or receiving CYP2D6 inhibitors such as propoxyphene are likely to produce little or no morphine during codeine administration.

CLINICAL EVALUATION: Propoxyphene is known to inhibit CYP2D6. Because several studies have shown that another CYP2D6 inhibitor, quinidine (eg, *Quinora*) inhibits the analgesic effect of codeine,[3-6] propoxyphene might be expected to inhibit codeine analgesia as well. Nonetheless, clinical studies are needed to determine the clinical importance of this potential interaction. Because propoxyphene is a relatively weak analgesic, it is possible that the inhibitory effect of propoxyphene on the analgesic effect of codeine (or related opiates) would outweigh any intrinsic analgesic effects of the propoxyphene.

RELATED DRUGS: The analgesic effect of dihydrocodeine (eg, *Synalgos-DC*) and hydrocodone (eg, *Vicodin*) may be dependent on conversion to morphine-like active metabolites, and early evidence suggests that CYP2D6 inhibitors can reduce their analgesic efficacy. Whether propoxyphene affects these drugs is unknown. Tramadol (*Ultram*) appears to be partially dependent upon CYP2D6 for analgesic activity, but theoretically would be less affected than codeine by propoxyphene. Early pharmacodynamic evidence suggests that oxycodone (eg, *Percodan*) does not require conversion by CYP2D6 to an active metabolite. Theoretically, oxycodone would not be affected by propoxyphene, but more study is needed.

MANAGEMENT OPTIONS: No specific action is required, but be alert for evidence of the interaction.

REFERENCES:
1. Sindrup SH, et al. Codeine increases pain thresholds to copper vapor laser stimuli in extensive but not poor metabolizers of sparteine. *Clin Pharmacol Ther*. 1990;48:686.
2. Poulsen L, et al. Codeine and morphine in extensive and poor metabolizers of sparteine: pharmacokinetics, analgesic effect and side effects. *Eur J Clin Pharmacol*. 1996;51:289.
3. Desmeules J, et al. Impact of environmental and genetic factors on codeine analgesia. *Eur J Clin Pharmacol*. 1991;41:23.
4. Sindrup SH, et al. The effect of quinidine on the analgesic effect of codeine. *Eur J Clin Pharmacol*. 1992;42:587.
5. Sindrup SH, et al. Impact of quinidine on plasma and cerebrospinal fluid concentrations of codeine and morphine after codeine intake. *Eur J Clin Pharmacol*. 1996;49:503.
6. Caraco Y, et al. Pharmacogenetic determination of the effects of codeine and prediction of drug interactions. *J Pharmacol Exp Ther*. 1996;278:1165.

4   Codeine

Quinacrine

SUMMARY: Quinacrine inhibits CYP2D6, and theoretically would interfere with the bioactivation of codeine to morphine, but the extent to which it inhibits the analgesic effect of codeine is not established.

RISK FACTORS:

➡ ***Pharmacogenetics.*** Only patients with the extensive metabolizer CYP2D6 phenotype (EMs) would be expected to experience this interaction. Poor metabolizers (PMs) do not have the gene for production of CYP2D6, so there would be no CYP2D6 for the quinacrine to inhibit. Approximately 8% of whites are deficient in CYP2D6, but the deficiency is rare in Asians, usually 2% or less.

MECHANISM: Codeine exerts its analgesic effects (and probably also its side effects) primarily through its metabolic conversion to morphine by the isozyme, CYP2D6.[1,2] Thus, patients genetically deficient in CYP2D6 or receiving CYP2D6 inhibitors such as quinacrine are likely to produce little or no morphine during codeine administration.

CLINICAL EVALUATION: Quinacrine is know to inhibit CYP2D6. Because several studies have shown that another CYP2D6 inhibitor, quinidine (eg, *Quinora*), inhibits the analgesic effect of codeine,[3-6] quinacrine might be expected to inhibit codeine analgesia as well. Nonetheless, clinical studies are needed to determine the clinical importance of this potential interaction.

RELATED DRUGS: The analgesic effect of dihydrocodeine (*Synalgos-DC*) and hydrocodone (eg, *Vicodin*) may be dependent on conversion to morphine-like active metabolites, and early evidence suggests that CYP2D6 inhibitors can reduce their analgesic efficacy. Whether quinacrine affects these drugs is unknown. Tramadol (*Ultram*) appears to be partially dependent upon CYP2D6 for analgesic activity, but theoretically would be less affected than codeine by quinacrine. Early pharmacodynamic evidence suggests that oxycodone (eg, *Percodan*) does not require conversion by CYP2D6 to an active metabolite. Theoretically, oxycodone would not be affect by quinacrine, but more study is needed.

MANAGEMENT OPTIONS: No specific action is required, but be alert for evidence of the interaction.

REFERENCES:

1. Sindrup SH, et al. Codeine increases pain thresholds to copper vapor laser stimuli in extensive but not poor metabolizers of sparteine. *Clin Pharmacol Ther.* 1990;48;686.

2. Poulsen L, et al. Codeine and morphine in extensive and poor metabolizers of sparteine: pharmacokinetics, analgesic effect and side effects. *Eur J Clin Pharmacol.* 1996;51;289.

3. Desmeules J, et al. Impact of environmental and genetic factors on codeine analgesia. *Eur J Clin Pharmacol.* 1991;41;23.

4. Sindrup SH, et al. The effect of quinidine on the analgesic effect of codeine. *Eur J Clin Pharmacol.* 1992;42;587.

5. Sindrup SH, et al. Impact of quinidine on plasma and cerebrospinal fluid concentrations of codeine and morphine after codeine intake. *Eur J Clin Pharmacol.* 1996;49;503.

6. Caraco Y, et al. Pharmacogenetic determination of the effects of codeine and prediction of drug interactions. *J Pharmacol Exp Ther.* 1996;278;1165.

Codeine

Quinidine (eg, *Quinora*)

SUMMARY: Quinidine inhibits the bioactivation of codeine to morphine, thus reducing the analgesic effect of codeine.

RISK FACTORS:

➥ *Pharmacogenetics.* Only patients with the extensive metabolizer CYP2D6 phenotype (EMs) would be expected to experience this interaction. Poor metabolizers (PMs) do not have the gene for production of CYP2D6, so there would be no CYP2D6 for the quinidine to inhibit. Approximately 8% of whites are deficient in CYP2D6, but the deficiency is rare in Asians, usually 2% or less.[1,2]

MECHANISM: Codeine exerts its analgesic effects (and probably also its side effects) primarily through its metabolic conversion to morphine by the isozyme, CYP2D6.[3,4] Thus, patients genetically deficient in CYP2D6 or receiving a potent CYP2D6 inhibitor such as quinidine produce little or no morphine during codeine administration.

CLINICAL EVALUATION: Several clinical studies have shown that quinidine markedly reduces morphine plasma concentrations in patients receiving codeine, accompanied by reduction in the analgesic effect of codeine.[5-8] The effect of quinidine on the antitussive effect of codeine is not established, but it seems likely that it too would be inhibited. Codeine slows GI motility in EMs but not in PMs, suggesting that this side effect of codeine is more likely because of the morphine produced than codeine itself.[9]

RELATED DRUGS: The analgesic effect of dihydrocodeine (eg, *Synalgos-DC*) and hydrocodone (eg, *Vicodin*) also may be dependent on conversion to morphine-like active metabolites, and early evidence suggests that quinidine can reduce their analgesic efficacy.[10-12] Tramadol (*Ultram*) appears to be partially dependent upon CYP2D6 for analgesic activity, but theoretically would be less affected than codeine by quinidine therapy.[13] Early pharmacodynamic evidence suggest that oxycodone (eg, *Percodan*) does not require conversion by CYP2D6 to an active metabolite.[14-15] Theoretically, oxycodone would not be affected by quinidine, but more study is needed.

MANAGEMENT OPTIONS:

➡ *Consider Alternative.* Consider use of an analgesic other than codeine, dihydrocodeine, hydrocodone, or tramadol. (See Related Drugs.)

➡ *Monitor.* If codeine and quinidine are used together, monitor for reduced analgesic effect.

REFERENCES:

1. Tseng C-Y, et al. Formation of morphine from codeine in Chinese subjects of different CYP2D6 genotypes. Clin Pharmacol Ther. 1996;60:177.

2. Straka RJ, et al. Comparison of the prevalence of the poor metabolizer phenotype for CYP2D6 between 203 Hmong subjects and 280 white subjects residing in Minnesota. Clin Pharmacol Ther. 1995;58:29.

3. Sindrup SH, et al. Codeine increases pain thresholds to copper vapor laser stimuli in extensive but not poor metabolizers of sparteine. Clin Pharmacol Ther. 1990;48:686.

4. Poulsen L, et al. Codeine and morphine in extensive and poor metabolizers of sparteine: pharmacokinetics, analgesic effect and side effects. Eur J Clin Pharmacol. 1996;51:289.

5. Desmeules J, et al. Impact of genetic and environmental factors on codeine analgesia. Clin Pharmacol Ther. 1989;45:122.

6. Sindrup SH, et al. The effect of quinidine on the analgesic effect of codeine. Eur J Clin Pharmacol. 1992;42:587.

7. Sindrup SH, et al. Impact of quinidine on plasma and cerebrospinal fluid concentrations of codeine and morphine after codeine intake. Eur J Clin Pharmacol. 1996;49:503.

8. Caraco Y, et al. Pharmacogenetic determination of the effects of codeine and prediction of drug interactions. J Pharmacol Exp Ther. 1996;278:1165.

9. Mikus G, et al. Effect of codeine on gastrointestinal motility in relation to CYP2D6 phenotype. Clin Pharmacol Ther. 1997;61:459.

10. Fromm MF, et al. Dihydrocodeine: a new opioid substrate for the polymorphic CYP2D6 in humans. Clin Pharmacol Ther. 1995;58:374.

11. Hufschmid E, et al. Exploration of the metabolism of dihydrocodeine via determination of its metabolites in human urine using micellar electrokinetic capillary chromatography. J Chromatogr B Biome Appl. 1995;668:159.

12. Otton SV, et al. CYP2D6 phenotype determines the metabolic conversion of hydrocodone to hydromorphone. Clin Pharmacol Ther. 1993;54:463.

13. Poulsen L, et al. The hypoalgesic effect of tramadol in relation to CYP2D6. Clin Pharmacol Ther. 1996;60:636.

14. Poyhia R, et al. A review of oxycodone's clinical pharmacokinetics and pharmacodynamics. J Pain Symptom Manage. 1993;8:63.

15. Kaiko RF, et al. Phamacokinetic-phamacodynamic relationships of controlled-release oxycodone. Clin Pharmacol Ther. 1996;59:52.

Codeine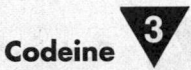

Rifampin (eg, *Rifadin*)

SUMMARY: Rifampin reduces the conversion of codeine to morphine, and may inhibit the analgesic effect of codeine.

RISK FACTORS:

➥ *Pharmacogenetics.* This interaction was shown to occur only in people with normal CYP2D6 activity.

MECHANISM: Rifampin appears to enhance the metabolism of codeine to inactive metabolites (probably by CYP3A4), thus reducing the amount of codeine converted by CYP2D6 to its active metabolite, morphine.

CLINICAL EVALUATION: Fifteen healthy subjects were given a single dose of codeine 120 mg with and without pretreatment with rifampin (600 mg/day for 3 weeks).[1] In the 9 extensive metabolizers (EMs) (those with normal CYP2D6 activity), rifampin reduced plasma morphine concentrations, and attenuated the respiratory and psychomotor effects of codeine. In the 6 poor metabolizers (PMs) (those deficient in CYP2D6), rifampin had no effect on the respiratory or psychomotor effects of codeine. Rifampin is expected to reduce the analgesic effects of codeine in EMs, but clinical studies are needed for confirmation. PMs do not respond well to codeine regardless of coadministration with enzymes inducers such as rifampin.

RELATED DRUGS: Theoretically, other enzyme inducers may also impair codeine effect, such as barbiturates, carbamazepine (eg, *Tegretol*), efavirenz (*Sustiva*), nafcillin, nevirapine (*Viramune*), oxcarbazepine (eg, *Trileptal*), phenytoin (eg, *Dilantin*), primidone (eg, *Mysoline*), rifabutin (*Mycobutin*), rifapentine (*Priftin*), and St. John's wort. However, most of these inducers are less potent than rifampin. Rifampin may also impair the efficacy of other opioid analgesics, such as alfentanil (eg, *Alfenta*), fentanyl (eg, *Sublimaze*), methadone (eg, *Dolophine*), morphine (eg, *Oramorph*), oxycodone (eg, *OxyContin*), and sufentanil (eg, *Sufenta*).

MANAGEMENT OPTIONS:

➥ *Monitor.* Monitor for reduced analgesic effect of codeine if rifampin or other enzyme inducers are given concomitantly.

REFERENCES:

1. Caraco Y, et al. Pharmacogenetic determinants of codeine induction by rifampin: the impact on codeine's respiratory, psychomotor and miotic effects. *J Pharmacol Exp Ther.* 1997;281(1):330-336.

4   Codeine

Thioridazine

SUMMARY: Thioridazine inhibits the bioactivation of codeine to morphine in vitro, but the extent to which it inhibits the analgesic effect of codeine is not established.

RISK FACTORS:

➡ ***Pharmacogenetics.*** Only patients with the extensive metabolizer CYP2D6 phenotype (EMs) can be expected to experience this interaction. Poor metabolizers do not have the gene for production of CYP2D6, so there is no CYP2D6 for the thioridazine to inhibit in these patients. Approximately 8% of white patients are deficient in CYP2D6, but the deficiency is rare in Asian patients, usually up to 2%.

MECHANISM: Codeine exerts its analgesic effects (and probably also its adverse reactions) primarily through its metabolic conversion to morphine by the isozyme CYP2D6.[1,2] Thus, patients genetically deficient in CYP2D6 or receiving CYP2D6 inhibitors such as thioridazine produce little or no morphine during codeine administration.

CLINICAL EVALUATION: Using hepatic microsomes from an extensive metabolizer, thioridazine inhibited the conversion of codeine to morphine in vitro.[3] Several studies have shown that the CYP2D6 inhibitor quinidine reduces the analgesic effect of codeine.[4,5,6,7] Thus, thioridazine, a known CYP2D6 inhibitor, might be expected to inhibit codeine analgesia as well. Nonetheless, studies are needed to determine the clinical importance of this potential interaction.

RELATED DRUGS: The analgesic effect of dihydrocodeine and hydrocodone (eg, *Vicodin*) may be dependent on conversion to morphine-like active metabolites; early evidence suggests that CYP2D6 inhibitors can reduce their analgesic efficacy. Whether thioridazine affects these drugs is unknown. Tramadol (eg, *Ultram*) appears to be partially dependent upon CYP2D6 for analgesic activity, but theoretically would be less affected than codeine by thioridazine. Early pharmacodynamic evidence suggests that oxycodone (eg, *Percocet*) does not require conversion by CYP2D6 to an active metabolite. Theoretically, oxycodone would not be affected by thioridazine, but more study is needed.

MANAGEMENT OPTIONS: No specific action is required, but be alert for evidence of the interaction.

REFERENCES:

1. Sindrup SH, et al. Codeine increases pain thresholds to copper vapor laser stimuli in extensive but not poor metabolizers of sparteine. *Clin Pharmacol Ther*. 1990;48(6):686-693.
2. Poulsen L, et al. Codeine and morphine in extensive and poor metabolizers of sparteine: pharmacokinetics, analgesic effect and side effects. *Eur J Clin Pharmacol*. 1996;51(3-4):289-295.
3. Dayer P, et al. In vitro forecasting of drugs that may interfere with codeine bioactivation. *Eur J Drug Metab Pharmacokinet*. 1992;17(2):115-120.
4. Desmeules J, et al. Impact of environmental and genetic factors on codeine analgesia. *Eur J Clin Pharmacol*. 1991;41(1):23-26.
5. Sindrup SH, et al. The effect of quinidine on the analgesic effect of codeine. *Eur J Clin Pharmacol*. 1992;42(6):587-591.
6. Sindrup SH, et al. Impact of quinidine on plasma and cerebrospinal fluid concentrations of codeine and morphine after codeine intake. *Eur J Clin Pharmacol*. 1996;49(6):503-509.
7. Caraco Y, et al. Pharmacogenetic determination of the effects of codeine and prediction of drug interactions. *J Pharmacol Exp Ther*. 1996;278(3):1165-1174.

Colchicine (eg, *Colcrys*)

Atorvastatin (*Lipitor*)

SUMMARY: The combination of colchicine and atorvastatin may increase the risk of myopathy; if the combination is necessary, monitor for evidence of myopathy.

RISK FACTORS:

➡ **Concurrent Diseases.** Based on case reports, renal impairment appears to be an important risk factor for toxicity from colchicine drug interactions; all of the patients who developed myopathy during colchicine and atorvastatin had renal impairment.[1-4] Theoretically, hepatic disease may also increase the risk of colchicine toxicity.

MECHANISM: Colchicine and atorvastatin have both been associated with myopathy when given alone, and it is proposed that the combination may produce additive damage to muscle cells.[5] Clinical evidence suggests that atorvastatin may be a weak P-glycoprotein inhibitor, which may contribute somewhat to the interaction.[6]

CLINICAL EVALUATION: Several case reports of myopathy have been reported in patients taking colchicine who were started on atorvastatin.[1-4] Three cases were rated as probable on the Drug Interaction Probability Scale (DIPS) and one case was rated possible.[7] (He was also taking cyclosporine, which also interacts with colchicine to produce myopathy.[3]) All patients developed evidence of myopathy (muscle weakness with or without myalgia and dark urine), and one proceeded to rhabdomyolysis, renal failure, and death from pneumonia.[1] The onset of myopathy symptoms after starting atorvastatin ranged from 2 weeks to 2 months, and all patients had elevated creatine kinase concentrations.

RELATED DRUGS: Myopathy has been reported in patients receiving colchicine with simvastatin (eg, *Zocor*), lovastatin (eg, *Mevacor*), fluvastatin (eg, *Lescol*), and pravastatin (eg, *Pravachol*), although the fluvastatin and pravastatin cases were not convincing. Nonetheless, all statins should be considered capable of increasing the risk of myopathy if combined with colchicine.

MANAGEMENT OPTIONS:

➡ **Consider Alternative.** Given the potential for severe myopathy in at least some patients, avoid combining colchicine and atorvastatin if possible. Theoretically, pravastatin might be less likely to interact with colchicine than atorvastatin.

➡ **Circumvent/Minimize.** If the combination is needed, use the lowest effective dose of atorvastatin or other statins. (Statin-induced myopathy is known to be dose-related.)

➡ **Monitor.** In patients receiving colchicine with atorvastatin or other statins, monitor for evidence of myopathy (eg, muscle weakness, myalgia, dark urine, paresthesia). Advise patients to stop both drugs immediately and contact their health care provider if they experience any of these symptoms.

REFERENCES:

1. Tufan A, et al. Rhabdomyolysis in a patient treated with colchicine and atorvastatin. *Ann Pharmacother*. 2006;40:(7-8)1466-1469.
2. Sahin G, et al. Which statin should be used together with colchicine? Clinical experience in three patients with nephrotic syndrome due to AA type amyloidosis. *Rheumatol Int*. 2008;28(3):289-291.

3. Phanish MK, et al. Colchicine-induced rhabdomyolysis. *Am J Med*. 2003;114(2):166-167.

4. Vasudevan AR, et al. Colchicine-induced rhabdomyolysis: the whole is greater than the sum of its parts! *Am J Med*. 2003;115(3):249.

5. Wilbur K, Makowsky M. Colchicine myotoxicity: case reports and literature review. *Pharmacotherapy*. 2004;24(12):1784-1792.

6. Boyd RA, et al. Atorvastatin coadministration may increase digoxin concentrations by inhibition of intestinal P-glycoprotein-mediated secretion. *J Clin Pharmacol*. 2000;40(1):91-98.

7. Horn JR, et al. Proposal for a new tool to evaluate drug interaction cases. *Ann Pharmacother*. 2007;41(4):674-680.

Colchicine (eg, *Colcrys*)

Cyclosporine (eg, *Neoral*)

SUMMARY: Cyclosporine blood concentrations increased and nephrotoxicity developed after administration of colchicine in renal transplant patients.

RISK FACTORS: No specific risk factors are known.

MECHANISM: Not established.

CLINICAL EVALUATION: In 4 renal transplant patients receiving prophylactic colchicine, an attempt was made to convert them from azathioprine (eg, *Imuran*) therapy to cyclosporine therapy. All 4 patients developed severe adverse reactions after starting cyclosporine, including diarrhea, and elevated lactate dehydrogenase, ALT, and bilirubin; 2 had elevated serum creatinine and 1 was hospitalized with severe muscle pain and weakness.[1] The reactions were reversible. In another report, a 45-year-old renal transplant recipient receiving cyclosporine 3 mg/kg/day developed marked increases in blood cyclosporine concentrations (to 1,519 ng/mL) and acute impairment of renal function within 2 days after receiving 1 day of colchicine 2 mg twice daily.[2] Renal biopsy excluded a rejection episode. Authors could not find other potential causes for the reduced renal function or elevated cyclosporine concentrations. The temporal relationship of the reaction with colchicine administration and the lack of other identifiable causes suggest colchicine may have caused the nephrotoxicity through an increase in blood cyclosporine concentrations. One case of multiple organ failure has been reported in a renal transplant patient when colchicine was added to his cyclosporine therapy.[3] However, cyclosporine concentrations were not elevated and it was proposed that cyclosporine may have increased intracellular colchicine concentrations.

RELATED DRUGS: Tacrolimus (eg, *Prograf*) and cyclosporine tend to have similar interactions, but it is unknown if tacrolimus interacts with colchicine.

MANAGEMENT OPTIONS:

➡ **Monitor.** Monitor for altered cyclosporine blood concentrations and renal function if colchicine is initiated, discontinued, or changed in dosage. Note: Cyclosporine commonly induces hyperuricemia by decreasing urate clearance.[4] Colchicine must be used with caution in patients with decreased renal function because they are at increased risk for neuromuscular toxicity and bone marrow dysplasia.[5]

REFERENCES:

1. Yussim A, et al. Gastrointestinal, hepatorenal, and neuromuscular toxicity caused by cyclosporine-colchicine interaction in renal transplantation. *Transplant Proc*. 1994;26(5):2825-2826.

2. Menta R, et al. Reversible acute cyclosporin nephrotoxicity induced by colchicine administration. *Nephrol Dial Transplant*. 1987;2(5):380-381.

3. Minetti EE, Minetti L. Multiple organ failure in a kidney transplant patient receiving both colchicine and cyclosporine. *J Nephrol*. 2003;16(3):421-425.

4. Lin HY, et al. Cyclosporine-induced hyperuricemia and gout. *N Engl J Med*. 1989;321(5):287-292.

5. Kuncl RW, et al. Colchicine myopathy and neuropathy. *N Engl J Med*. 1987;316(25):1562-1568.

Colchicine (eg, *Colcrys*)

Diltiazem (eg, *Cardizem*)

SUMMARY: Diltiazem increases colchicine plasma concentrations and the risk of serious colchicine toxicity; the combination should generally be avoided.

RISK FACTORS:

➡ *Concurrent Diseases.* Based on case reports, renal impairment appears to be an important risk factor for toxicity from colchicine drug interactions. Theoretically, hepatic disease may also increase the risk of colchicine toxicity.

MECHANISM: Colchicine is a substrate for CYP3A4 in the gut wall and liver, and a substrate for P-glycoprotein (P-gp) in the gut wall, liver, and renal tubules. Because diltiazem inhibits both CYP3A4 and P-gp, it may increase colchicine bioavailability, inhibit systemic colchicine metabolism, and reduce biliary and renal tubular secretion of colchicine.

CLINICAL EVALUATION: Twenty healthy subjects were given a single dose of colchicine 0.6 mg with and without pretreatment with diltiazem 240 mg daily for 7 days.[1,2] The colchicine area under the plasma concentration-time curve increased 93%, but the range was large (30% decrease to a 339% increase). Diltiazem increased colchicine half-life from approximately 6 hours to approximately 12 hours. The *Colcrys* product information suggests that in the presence of diltiazem therapy, the colchicine dose for gout should be cut in half. Nonetheless, given the marked intersubject variability observed in the healthy volunteers (variability would probably be higher in actual patients), a 50% reduction in dosage is likely to be too small or too large for many patients. Given that colchicine toxicity can be fatal, it would be preferable to avoid giving diltiazem (or verapamil) to patients on colchicine.

RELATED DRUGS: Verapamil (eg, *Calan*) also inhibits the activity of CYP3A4 and P-gp and has been shown to increase colchicine plasma concentrations. There is some evidence that nicardipine can inhibit P-gp, so theoretically it could increase the plasma concentrations of colchicine. Most other calcium channel blockers appear to have little inhibitory effect on CYP3A4 (and probably P-gp) and are unlikely to interact with colchicine.

MANAGEMENT OPTIONS:

➡ *Use Alternative.* Given the potential for life-threatening colchicine toxicity with concurrent diltiazem or verapamil, it should be rare for the benefit of the combination to outweigh the risks. Consider using a calcium channel blocker other than diltiazem or verapamil. If diltiazem or verapamil is absolutely necessary, consider stopping colchicine during calcium channel blocker therapy and using an alternative treatment for gout.

➡ *Monitor.* If diltiazem or verapamil is given with colchicine, reduce the colchicine dose by at least 75%, and monitor the patient carefully for evidence of colchicine toxicity. Colchicine can produce diarrhea, vomiting, abdominal pain, fever, bleeding, and myopathy (muscle pain, weakness, dark urine, paresthesia); severe cases can result in multiorgan failure and death. Based on patient response, increase the colchicine dose very gradually as needed with continued monitoring for colchicine toxicity. Because of the long half-life of colchicine in the presence of inhibitors of CYP3A4 and/or P-gp, it may take several days or up to 1 week to achieve a new steady state after changes in colchicine dosage.

REFERENCES:

1. Terkeltaub RA, et al. Novel evidence-based colchicine dose-reduction algorithm to predict and prevent colchicine toxicity in the presence of cytochrome P450 3A4/P-glycoprotein inhibitors. *Arthritis Rheum.* 2011;63(8):2226-2237.

2. *Colcrys* [package insert]. Philadelphia, PA: Mutual Pharmaceutical Company, Inc; 2010.

4   Colchicine (eg, *Colcrys*)

Disulfiram (eg, *Antabuse*)

SUMMARY: A patient taking colchicine and disulfiram developed a severe skin eruption, but a causal relationship is doubtful.

RISK FACTORS: No specific risk factors are known.

MECHANISM: Preliminary evidence (primarily in vitro) suggests that disulfiram may inhibit P-glycoprotein (P-gp), which theoretically could increase the risk of colchicine toxicity.[1,2] More evidence is needed to establish that disulfiram inhibits P-gp.

CLINICAL EVALUATION: A 44-year-old man taking colchicine 1 mg/day was given 1 dose of disulfiram 200 mg, and developed a severe erythematous skin eruption 12 hours later.[3] The authors propose that the reaction was caused by elevated colchicine plasma concentrations from disulfiram-induced inhibition of P-gp and CYP3A4. It seems unlikely, however, that a single dose of a P-gp inhibitor could cause such a reaction, and it is not clear that elevated colchicine concentrations would produce a skin eruption of this type. Nonetheless, it is possible that disulfiram could increase colchicine plasma concentrations, if disulfiram actually inhibits P-gp clinically and not just in vitro. More data are needed to determine if disulfiram increases the risk of colchicine toxicity. The case was rated as doubtful on the Drug Interaction Probability Scale (DIPS).[4]

RELATED DRUGS: No information is available.

MANAGEMENT OPTIONS:

➠ *Monitor.* In patients receiving concurrent colchicine and disulfiram, monitor for colchicine toxicity (eg, diarrhea, vomiting, abdominal pain, fever, bleeding, myopathy [muscle pain, weakness, dark urine, paresthesia]); severe cases can result in multiorgan failure and death.

REFERENCES:

1. Sauna ZE, et al. The molecular basis of the action of disulfiram as a modulator of the multidrug resistance-linked ATP binding cassette transporters MDR1 (ABCB1) and MRP1 (ABCC1). *Mol Pharmacol.* 2004;65(3):675-684.

2. Loo TW, et al. Disulfiram metabolites permanently inactivate the human multidrug resistance P-glycoprotein. *Mol Pharm.* 2004;1(6):426-433.

3. Chen SC, et al. Potentially fatal interaction between colchicine and disulfiram. *Prog Neuropsychopharmacol Biol Psychiatry.* 2009;33(7):1281.

4. Horn JR, et al. Proposal for a new tool to evaluate drug interaction cases. *Ann Pharmacother.* 2007;41(4):674-680.

Colchicine (eg, *Colcrys*)

Erythromycin (eg, *Ery-Tab*) AVOID

SUMMARY: A patient developed severe colchicine toxicity following 2 weeks of erythromycin coadministration; given several fatal case reports of colchicine and clarithromycin (eg, *Biaxin*) coadministration, clarithromycin and erythromycin are contraindicated with colchicine.

RISK FACTORS:

➡ ***Concurrent Diseases.*** Patients with impaired renal function may be at higher risk of this interaction.

MECHANISM: Not established. Erythromycin inhibits P-glycoprotein (P-gp) and CYP3A4, and colchicine appears to be a substrate for both. Thus, erythromycin theoretically could affect the absorption, metabolism, and biliary elimination of colchicine.

CLINICAL EVALUATION: A patient with familial Mediterranean fever and renal amyloidosis with chronic renal failure was receiving colchicine 1 mg/day.[1] She was administered erythromycin 2 g/day and 2 weeks later was admitted with fever, pancytopenia, abdominal pain, myalgia, vomiting, and elevated hepatic enzymes. This case does not establish causation for an interaction between colchicine and erythromycin. Nevertheless, given the strong evidence that clarithromycin can cause serious, even fatal, colchicine toxicity, erythromycin (which has similar effects on P-gp and CYP3A4) also should be considered as contraindicated.

RELATED DRUGS: Clarithromycin (eg, *Biaxin*) and josamycin[+] also have been reported to cause colchicine toxicity. Theoretically, troleandomycin[+] would interact similarly, but azithromycin (eg, *Zithromax*) and dirithromycin[+] would not. Any P-gp inhibitor or CYP3A4 inhibitor would theoretically increase the risk of colchicine toxicity.

MANAGEMENT OPTIONS:

➡ ***AVOID COMBINATION.*** Avoid using colchicine and erythromycin concurrently. Until more information is available, the same caution applies to other macrolides that can inhibit P-gp and/or CYP3A4.

REFERENCES:

1. Caraco Y, et al. Acute colchicine intoxication—possible role of erythromycin administration. *J Rheumatol.* 1992;19(3):494-496.

† Not available in the United States.

Colchicine (eg, *Colcrys*)

Fluvastatin (*Lescol*)

SUMMARY: The combination of colchicine and fluvastatin may increase the risk of myopathy; if the combination is necessary, monitor for evidence of myopathy.

RISK FACTORS:

➡ ***Concurrent Diseases.*** Based on case reports, renal impairment appears to be an important risk factor for toxicity from colchicine drug interactions. Theoretically, hepatic disease may also increase the risk of colchicine toxicity.

MECHANISM: Colchicine and fluvastatin have both been associated with myopathy when given alone, and it is proposed that the combination may produce additive damage to muscle cells.[1]

CLINICAL EVALUATION: Two men aged 70 and 77 years developed rhabdomyolysis with muscle weakness and myalgia following addition of colchicine to long-term fluvastatin 80 mg/day.[2,3] Both cases were rated as possible on the Drug Interaction Probability Scale (DIPS).[4] As with other statin-colchicine case reports of myopathy, it is usually not possible to strictly rule out that the muscle damage was only due to the second drug added to the regimen (in these 2 cases, colchicine).

RELATED DRUGS: Myopathy has been reported in patients receiving colchicine with atorvastatin (*Lipitor*), simvastatin (eg, *Zocor*), lovastatin (eg, *Mevacor*), and pravastatin (eg, *Pravachol*), although the fluvastatin and pravastatin cases were not convincing. Nonetheless, consider all statins capable of increasing the risk of myopathy if combined with colchicine.

MANAGEMENT OPTIONS:

➡ *Consider Alternative.* Given the potential for severe myopathy in at least some patients, avoid combining colchicine and fluvastatin if possible. Theoretically, pravastatin might be less likely to interact with colchicine than atorvastatin.

➡ *Circumvent/Minimize.* If the combination is needed, use the lowest effective dose of fluvastatin or other statin. (Statin-induced myopathy is known to be dose-related.)

➡ *Monitor.* In patients receiving colchicine with fluvastatin or other statins, monitor for evidence of myopathy (muscle weakness, myalgia, dark urine, paresthesia). Advise patients to stop both drugs immediately and contact their health care provider if they experience any of these symptoms.

REFERENCES:

1. Wilbur K, Makowsky M. Colchicine myotoxicity: case reports and literature review. *Pharmacotherapy.* 2004;24(12):1784-1792.
2. Atasoyu EM, et al. Possible colchicine rhabdomyolysis in a fluvastatin-treated patient. *Ann Pharmacother.* 2005;39(7-8):1368-1369 .
3. Sarullo FM, et al. Rhabdomyolysis induced by co-administration of fluvastatin and colchicine. *Monaldi Arch Chest Dis.* 2010;74(3):147-149.
4. Horn JR, et al. Proposal for a new tool to evaluate drug interaction cases. *Ann Pharmacother.* 2007;41(4):674-680.

4   Colchicine (eg, *Colcrys*)

Gemfibrozil (eg, *Lopid*)

SUMMARY: The combination of colchicine and gemfibrozil may increase the risk of myopathy; if the combination is necessary, monitor for evidence of myopathy.

RISK FACTORS:

➡ *Concurrent diseases.* Based on case reports, renal impairment appears to be an important risk factor for toxicity from colchicine drug interactions. Theoretically, hepatic disease may also increase the risk of colchicine toxicity.

MECHANISM: Colchicine and gemfibrozil have both been associated with myopathy when given alone, and it is proposed that the combination may produce additive damage to muscle cells.[1]

CLINICAL EVALUATION: A 40-year-old man with amyloidosis, nephrotic syndrome, and chronic liver disease developed rhabdomyolysis after gemfibrozil 1,200 mg/day was added to his long-term colchicine therapy (1.5 mg/day).[2] He developed myalgia and dark brown urine (without muscle weakness), and an elevation in creatine kinase and other muscle enzymes. After the myopathy resolved, he was restarted on colchicine 1 mg/day without gemfibrozil with no recurrence of myopathy. Because gemfibrozil alone has been reported to cause muscle toxicity, it is not possible to rule out the possibility that the myopathy was caused by gemfibrozil. Nonetheless, because both gemfibrozil and colchicine can cause myopathy, it is plausible that the reaction resulted from an additive myotoxic effect. The case was rated as possible on the Drug Interaction Probability Scale (DIPS).[3]

RELATED DRUGS: Theoretically, other fibrates, such as fenofibrate (eg, *Tricor*), may also have additive toxic effects on skeletal muscle when combined with colchicine, but clinical evidence is lacking.

MANAGEMENT OPTIONS:

➡ *Monitor.* In patients receiving colchicine with gemfibrozil or other fibrates, monitor for evidence of myopathy (muscle weakness, myalgia, dark urine, paresthesia). Advise patients to stop both drugs immediately and contact their health care provider if they experience any of these symptoms.

REFERENCES:

1. Wilbur K, Makowsky M. Colchicine myotoxicity: case reports and literature review. *Pharmacotherapy*. 2004;24(12):1784-1792.

2. Atmaca H, et al. Rhabdomyolysis associated with gemfibrozil-colchicine therapy. *Ann Pharmacother*. 2002;36(11):1719-1721.

3. Horn JR, et al. Proposal for a new tool to evaluate drug interaction cases. *Ann Pharmacother*. 2007;41(4):674-680.

Colchicine (eg, *Colcrys*)

Grapefruit AVOID

SUMMARY: Grapefruit juice may increase colchicine plasma concentrations and the risk of colchicine toxicity; avoid the combination.

RISK FACTORS:

➡ *Concurrent Diseases.* Based on case reports, renal impairment appears to be an important risk factor for toxicity from colchicine drug interactions. Theoretically, hepatic disease may also increase the risk of colchicine toxicity.

MECHANISM: Colchicine is a substrate for CYP3A4 and P-glycoprotein, both of which are inhibited by grapefruit juice.

CLINICAL EVALUATION: An 8-year-old girl with familial Mediterranean fever taking colchicine 2 mg/day developed a nearly fatal episode of colchicine toxicity approximately 2 months after starting to drink approximately 1 L of grapefruit juice per day.[1] She presented with fever, vomiting, severe abdominal pain, and a sore throat and soon developed circulatory shock and pancytopenia. The *Colcrys* product information describes a study of 21 healthy subjects who received a single dose of colchicine 0.6 mg with and without pretreatment with grapefruit juice 240 mL twice daily for 4 days.[2] Although they did not detect any effect of grapefruit juice on colchicine plasma concentrations, the type of grapefruit juice used may not have contained a high enough concentration of the inhibitor. Given that colchicine toxicity can be fatal, avoid giving any type of grapefruit juice to patients taking colchicine when possible.

RELATED DRUGS: Orange juice does not appear to affect CYP3A4 or P-glycoprotein, and is unlikely to affect colchicine.

MANAGEMENT OPTIONS:

➥ **Use Alternative.** Given the potential for life-threatening colchicine toxicity, advise patients to avoid grapefruit juice. Orange juice does not affect the pharmacokinetics of CYP3A4 substrates.

➥ **Monitor.** If a patient does drink grapefruit juice with colchicine, monitor carefully for evidence of colchicine toxicity (eg, diarrhea, vomiting, abdominal pain, fever, bleeding, myopathy [muscle pain, weakness, dark urine, paresthesia]); severe cases can result in multiorgan failure and death.

REFERENCES:

1. Goldbart A, et al. Near fatal acute colchicine intoxication in a child. A case report. *Eur J Pediatr.* 2000;159(12):895-897.
2. *Colcrys* [package insert]. Philadelphia, PA: Mutual Pharmaceutical Company, Inc; 2010.

Colchicine (eg, *Colcrys*)

Hydroxychloroquine (eg, *Plaquenil*)

SUMMARY: Limited evidence suggests that the combination of colchicine and hydroxychloroquine may increase the risk of myopathy; if the combination is necessary, monitor for evidence of myopathy.

RISK FACTORS:

➥ **Concurrent Diseases.** Based on case reports, renal impairment appears to be an important risk factor for toxicity from colchicine drug interactions. Theoretically, hepatic disease may also increase the risk of colchicine toxicity.

MECHANISM: Hydroxychloroquine alone is known to produce myotoxicity and could theoretically increase the risk of colchicine-induced muscle damage through additive myotoxic effects.[1-3] It is also possible that hydroxychloroquine inhibits P-glycoprotein, given a possible interaction of hydroxychloroquine with digoxin.[4] Digoxin, like colchicine, is a P-glycoprotein substrate, but more data are needed to establish this as a possible mechanism for a hydroxychloroquine-colchicine drug interaction.

CLINICAL EVALUATION: A 66-year-old woman on long-term hydroxychloroquine therapy (200 mg/day) was started on colchicine therapy for gout, and 4 weeks later she developed severe muscle weakness and muscle biopsy findings consistent with both colchicine- and hydroxychloroquine-induced myopathy.[5] Because both hydroxychloroquine and colchicine can cause myopathy, it is plausible that the reaction resulted from an additive myotoxic effect. The case was rated as possible on the Drug Interaction Probability Scale (DIPS).[6]

RELATED DRUGS: No information is available.

MANAGEMENT OPTIONS:

➥ **Monitor.** In patients receiving colchicine with hydroxychloroquine, monitor for evidence of myopathy (muscle weakness, myalgia, dark urine, paresthesia). Advise patients to stop both drugs immediately and contact their health care provider if they experience any of these symptoms.

REFERENCES:

1. Wilbur K, Makowsky M. Colchicine myotoxicity: case reports and literature review. *Pharmacotherapy.* 2004;24(12):1784-1792.

2. Kwon JB, et al. Hydroxychloroquine-induced myopathy. *J Clin Rheumatol.* 2010;16(1):28-31.

3. Abdel-Hamid H, et al. Severe hydroxychloroquine myopathy. *Muscle Nerve.* 2008;38(3):1206-1210.

4. Leden I. Digoxin-hydroxychloroquine interaction? *Acta Med Scand.* 1982;211(5):411-412.

5. Lonesky TA, et al. Hydroxychloroquine and colchicine induced myopathy. *J Rheumatol.* 2009;36(11):2617-2618.

6. Horn JR, et al. Proposal for a new tool to evaluate drug interaction cases. *Ann Pharmacother.* 2007;41(4):674-680.

Colchicine (eg, *Colcrys*)

Ketoconazole (eg, *Nizoral*)

SUMMARY: Ketoconazole increases colchicine plasma concentrations and the risk of serious colchicine toxicity; generally avoid the combination.

RISK FACTORS:

➡ **Concurrent Diseases.** Based on case reports, renal impairment appears to be an important risk factor for toxicity from colchicine drug interactions. Theoretically, hepatic disease may also increase the risk of colchicine toxicity.

MECHANISM: Colchicine is a substrate for CYP3A4 in the gut wall and liver, and a substrate for P-glycoprotein (P-gp) in the gut wall, liver, and renal tubules. Because ketoconazole inhibits both CYP3A4 and P-gp, it may increase colchicine bioavailability, inhibit systemic colchicine metabolism, and reduce biliary and renal tubular secretion of colchicine.

CLINICAL EVALUATION: Twenty-four healthy subjects were given a single dose of colchicine 0.6 mg with and without pretreatment with ketoconazole 200 mg twice daily for 5 days.[1,2] Colchicine area under the plasma concentration-time curve increased by a mean of 212%, but the range was large (77% to 420%). Ketoconazole increased colchicine half-life from approximately 6.3 to 26 hours. The *Colcrys* product information suggests that in the presence of ketoconazole therapy, the colchicine dose for gout should be cut in half. Nonetheless, given the high intersubject variability observed in healthy volunteers (variability is likely to be higher in actual patients), a 50% reduction in dosage is likely to be too small or too large for many patients. Given that colchicine toxicity can be fatal, avoid giving azole antifungals to patients taking colchicine when possible.

RELATED DRUGS: Like ketoconazole, itraconazole (eg, *Sporanox*) and posaconazole (*Noxafil*) inhibit both CYP3A4 and P-gp, and are expected to interact with colchicine. Fluconazole (eg, *Diflucan*) and voriconazole (eg, *Vfend*) inhibit the activity of CYP3A4 and are expected to increase colchicine plasma concentrations, although the magnitude of the interaction may be less than with other azoles.

MANAGEMENT OPTIONS:

➡ **Use Alternative.** Given the potential for life-threatening colchicine toxicity with concurrent ketoconazole (or other azole antifungals that inhibit CYP3A4), it should be rare for the benefit of the combination to outweigh the risks. Consider terbinafine (eg, *Lamisil*) as an alternative antifungal agent because it does not affect CYP3A4 activity. Amphotericin (eg, *Amphotec*), caspofungin (*Cancidas*), and anidulafungin (*Eraxis*) do not appear to inhibit CYP3A4. If an azole antifungal agent is absolutely necessary, consider stopping colchicine treatment during therapy with the antifungal and using an alternative treatment for gout.

➥ *Monitor.* If it is absolutely necessary to use ketoconazole or other azole antifungal agents with colchicine, reduce the colchicine dose by at least 75%, and monitor the patient carefully for evidence of colchicine toxicity. Colchicine can produce diarrhea, vomiting, abdominal pain, fever, bleeding, myopathy (muscle pain, weakness, dark urine, paresthesia); severe cases can result in multiorgan failure and death. Based on patient response, increase the colchicine dose very gradually as needed with continued monitoring for colchicine toxicity. Because of the long half-life of colchicine in the presence of ketoconazole, it may take several days or 1 week or more to achieve a new steady state after changes in colchicine dosage.

REFERENCES:
1. Terkeltaub RA, et al. Novel evidence-based colchicine dose-reduction algorithm to predict and prevent colchicine toxicity in the presence of cytochrome P450 3A4/P-glycoprotein inhibitors. *Arthritis Rheum.* 2011;63(8):2226-2237.

2. *Colcrys* [package insert]. Philadelphia, PA: Mutual Pharmaceutical Company, Inc; 2010.

Colchicine (eg, *Colcrys*)

Lovastatin (eg, *Mevacor*)

SUMMARY: The combination of colchicine and lovastatin may increase the risk of myopathy; if the combination is necessary, monitor for evidence of myopathy.

RISK FACTORS:

➥ *Concurrent Diseases.* Based on case reports, renal impairment appears to be an important risk factor for toxicity from colchicine drug interactions.[1] Theoretically, hepatic disease may also increase the risk of colchicine toxicity.

MECHANISM: Colchicine and lovastatin have both been associated with myopathy when given alone, and it is proposed that the combination may produce additive damage to muscle cells.[2]

CLINICAL EVALUATION: A 79-year-old man taking colchicine developed weakness and elevated creatine kinase 2 weeks after starting lovastatin. The case was rated as possible on the Drug Interaction Probability Scale (DIPS).[3] Although there is little clinical evidence for an interaction between colchicine and lovastatin, the interactive properties of lovastatin are almost identical to those of simvastatin, a drug for which there is considerably more evidence for an interaction with colchicine.

RELATED DRUGS: Myopathy has been reported in patients receiving colchicine with atorvastatin (*Lipitor*), simvastatin (eg, *Zocor*), fluvastatin (*Lescol*), and pravastatin (eg, *Pravachol*), although the fluvastatin and pravastatin cases were not convincing. Nonetheless, consider all statins capable of increasing the risk of myopathy if combined with colchicine.

MANAGEMENT OPTIONS:

➡ *Consider Alternative.* Given the potential for severe myopathy in at least some patients, avoid combining colchicine and lovastatin if possible. Theoretically, pravastatin might be less likely to interact with colchicine than atorvastatin.

➡ *Circumvent/Minimize.* If the combination is needed, use the lowest effective dose of lovastatin or other statin. (Statin-induced myopathy is known to be dose-related.)

➡ *Monitor.* In patients receiving colchicine with lovastatin or other statins, monitor for evidence of myopathy (muscle weakness, myalgia, dark urine, paresthesia). Advise patients to stop both drugs immediately and contact their health care provider if they experience any of these symptoms.

REFERENCES:

1. Torgovnick J, et al. Colchicine and HMG Co-A reductase inhibitors induced myopathy—a case report. *Neurotoxicology.* 2006;27(6):1126-1127.
2. Wilbur K, Makowsky M. Colchicine myotoxicity: case reports and literature review. *Pharmacotherapy.* 2004;24(12):1784-1792.
3. Horn JR, et al. Proposal for a new tool to evaluate drug interaction cases. *Ann Pharmacother.* 2007;41(4):674-680.

Colchicine (eg, *Colcrys*)

Pravastatin (eg, *Pravachol*)

SUMMARY: The combination of colchicine and pravastatin may increase the risk of myopathy; if the combination is necessary, monitor for evidence of myopathy.

RISK FACTORS:

➡ *Concurrent Diseases.* Based on case reports, renal impairment appears to be an important risk factor for toxicity from colchicine drug interactions. Theoretically, hepatic disease may also increase the risk of colchicine toxicity.

MECHANISM: Colchicine and pravastatin have both been associated with myopathy when given alone, and it is proposed that the combination may produce additive damage to muscle cells.[1]

CLINICAL EVALUATION: A 65-year-old woman on long-term pravastatin therapy (20 mg/day) developed muscle weakness and marked elevations of creatine kinase after starting colchicine.[2] Seven days after both drugs were discontinued, the muscle weakness improved, and the abnormal muscle enzymes returned to normal. Colchicine was subsequently restarted at 1 mg/day without incident. Another case of rhabdomyolysis was reported following initiation of colchicine in a patient receiving pravastatin 20 mg/day and cyclosporine, but the myotoxicity was much more likely to be due to the patient's combination of colchicine with cyclosporine.[3] The ability of cyclosporine to increase plasma concentrations of both colchicine and pravastatin is well documented, while the pravastatin-colchicine interaction is not. The first case was rated as possible on the Drug Interaction Probability Scale (DIPS), and the second case was rated as doubtful.[4]

RELATED DRUGS: Myopathy has been reported in patients receiving colchicine with atorvastatin (*Lipitor*), simvastatin (eg, *Zocor*), lovastatin (eg, *Mevacor*), fluvastatin (eg, *Lescol*), and pravastatin (eg, *Pravachol*), although the fluvastatin and pravastatin cases were not convincing. Nonetheless, consider all statins capable of increasing the risk of myopathy if combined with colchicine.

MANAGEMENT OPTIONS:

➡ **Consider Alternative.** An alternative to colchicine could be considered, but using a statin other than pravastatin may actually increase the risk. Theoretically, pravastatin may be less likely to interact with colchicine than other statins.

➡ **Circumvent/Minimize.** If the combination is needed, use the lowest effective dose of pravastatin or other statin.

➡ **Monitor.** In patients receiving colchicine with pravastatin or other statins, monitor for evidence of myopathy (muscle weakness, myalgia, dark urine, paresthesia). Advise patients to stop both drugs immediately and contact their health care provider if they experience any of these symptoms.

REFERENCES:

1. Wilbur K, Makowsky M. Colchicine myotoxicity: case reports and literature review. *Pharmacotherapy.* 2004;24(12):1784-1792.

2. Alayi G, et al. Acute myopathy in a patient with concomitant use of pravastatin and colchicine. *Ann Pharmacother.* 2005;39(7-8):1358-1361.

3. Bouquié R, et al. Colchicine-induced rhabdomyolysis in a heart/lung transplant patient with concurrent use of cyclosporine, pravastatin, and azithromycin. *J Clin Rheumatol.* 2011;17(1):28-30.

4. Horn JR, et al. Proposal for a new tool to evaluate drug interaction cases. *Ann Pharmacother.* 2007;41(4):674-680.

 Colchicine (eg, *Colcrys*)

Ritonavir (*Norvir*)

SUMMARY: Ritonavir increases colchicine plasma concentrations and the risk of serious colchicine toxicity; generally avoid the combination.

RISK FACTORS:

➡ **Concurrent Diseases.** Based on case reports, renal impairment appears to be an important risk factor for toxicity from colchicine drug interactions. Theoretically, hepatic disease may also increase the risk of colchicine toxicity.

➡ **Order of Drug Administration.** Clinical evidence suggests that ritonavir initially acts as a CYP3A4 inhibitor, but long-term administration may actually induce CYP3A4. For example, a single dose of ritonavir increased telaprevir plasma concentrations by approximately 2–fold, while ritonavir for 14 days reduced telaprevir levels 25%.[1] Thus, starting ritonavir therapy in a patient on long-term colchicine therapy is likely to increase colchicine concentrations, while starting colchicine in the presence of long-term ritonavir therapy may result in lower than expected colchicine levels.

MECHANISM: Colchicine is a substrate for CYP3A4 in the gut wall and liver, and a substrate for P-glycoprotein (P-gp) in the gut wall, liver, and renal tubules. Because ritonavir inhibits both CYP3A4 and P-gp, short-term ritonavir may increase colchicine bioavailability, inhibit systemic colchicine metabolism, and reduce biliary and renal tubular secretion of colchicine.

CLINICAL EVALUATION: Eighteen healthy subjects were given a single dose of colchicine 0.6 mg with and without pretreatment with ritonavir 100 mg twice daily for 5 days.[2,3] The colchicine area under the plasma concentration-time curve increased

296%, but the range was large (54% to 924%). Ritonavir increased colchicine half-life from approximately 5 to 17 hours. The *Colcrys* product information suggests that in the presence of ritonavir therapy, the colchicine dose for gout should be cut in half. Nonetheless, given the marked intersubject variability observed in healthy volunteers (variability would probably be higher in actual patients), a 50% reduction in dosage is likely to be too small or too large for many patients. Given that colchicine toxicity can be fatal, avoid concurrent use of ritonavir and colchicine when possible.

RELATED DRUGS: Atazanavir (*Reyataz*), darunavir (*Prezista*), delavirdine (*Rescriptor*), fosamprenavir (*Lexiva*), indinavir (*Crixivan*), nelfinavir (*Viracept*), and saquinavir (*Invirase*) also inhibit the activity of CYP3A4 (some also inhibit P-gp and are expected to increase the plasma concentrations of colchicine).

MANAGEMENT OPTIONS:

➡ *Use Alternative.* Given the potential for life-threatening colchicine toxicity with concurrent ritonavir (or other protease inhibitors that inhibit CYP3A4 or P-gp), it should be rare for the benefit of the combination to outweigh the risks. If ritonavir is absolutely necessary, consider stopping colchicine treatment during ritonavir therapy and using alternative gout therapy.

➡ *Monitor.* If it is absolutely necessary to use ritonavir with colchicine, reduce the colchicine dose by at least 75% and monitor the patient carefully for evidence of colchicine toxicity. Colchicine can produce diarrhea, vomiting, abdominal pain, fever, bleeding, myopathy (muscle pain, weakness, dark urine, paresthesia); severe cases can result in multiorgan failure and death. Based on the patient's response, increase the colchicine dose very gradually as needed with continued monitoring for colchicine toxicity. Because of the long half-life of colchicine in the presence of ritonavir, it may take several days or 1 week or more in some patients to achieve a new steady state after changes in colchicine dosage.

REFERENCES:

1. *Incivek* [package insert]. Cambridge, MA: Vertex Pharmaceuticals Inc; 2011.
2. Terkeltaub RA, et al. Novel evidence-based colchicine dose-reduction algorithm to predict and prevent colchicine toxicity in the presence of cytochrome P450 3A4/P-glycoprotein inhibitors. *Arthritis Rheum.* 2011;63(8):2226-2237.
3. *Colcrys* [package insert]. Philadelphia, PA: Mutual Pharmaceutical Company Inc; 2010.

Colchicine (eg, *Colcrys*)

Simvastatin (eg, *Zocor*)

SUMMARY: The combination of colchicine and simvastatin may increase the risk of myopathy; if the combination is necessary, monitor for evidence of myopathy.

RISK FACTORS:

➡ *Concurrent Diseases.* Based on case reports, renal impairment appears to be an important risk factor for toxicity from colchicine drug interactions; almost all of the patients who developed myopathy during treatment with colchicine and simvastatin had renal impairment.[1-6] Theoretically, hepatic disease may also increase the risk of colchicine toxicity.

MECHANISM: Colchicine and simvastatin have both been associated with myopathy when given alone, and it is proposed that the combination may produce additive damage to muscle cells.[5]

CLINICAL EVALUATION: Several case reports of myopathy have been reported in patients taking colchicine who were started on simvastatin.[1-5] Four cases were rated as probable on the Drug Interaction Probability Scale (DIPS) and the one fatal case was rated possible.[7] (He was also taking cyclosporine and propofol, which may have contributed to the myopathy.[3]) All patients developed evidence of myopathy (muscle weakness with or without myalgia) and elevated creatine kinase. The onset of myopathy symptoms after starting simvastatin was usually 1 to 3 weeks.

RELATED DRUGS: Myopathy has been reported in patients receiving colchicine with atorvastatin (*Lipitor*), lovastatin (eg, *Mevacor*), fluvastatin (*Lescol*), and pravastatin (eg, *Pravachol*), although the fluvastatin and pravastatin cases were not convincing. Nonetheless, consider all statins capable of increasing the risk of myopathy if combined with colchicine.

MANAGEMENT OPTIONS:

➡ *Consider Alternative.* Given the potential for severe myopathy in at least some patients, avoid combining colchicine and simvastatin if possible. Theoretically, pravastatin might be less likely to interact with colchicine than atorvastatin.

➡ *Circumvent/Minimize.* If the combination is needed, use the lowest effective dose of simvastatin or other statin. (Simvastatin-induced myopathy is known to be dose-related.)

➡ *Monitor.* In patients receiving colchicine with simvastatin or other statins, monitor for evidence of myopathy (muscle weakness, myalgia, dark urine, paresthesia). Advise patients to stop both drugs immediately and contact their health care provider if they experience any of these symptoms.

REFERENCES:

1. Hsu WC, et al. Colchicine-induced acute myopathy in a patient with concomitant use of simvastatin. *Clin Neuropharmacol.* 2002;25(5):266-268.
2. Baker SK, et al. Cytoskeletal myotoxicity from simvastatin and colchicine. *Muscle Nerve.* 2004;30(6):799-802.
3. Justiniano M, et al. Rapid onset of muscle weakness (rhabdomyolysis) associated with the combined use of simvastatin and colchicine. *J Clin Rheumatol.* 2007;13(5):266-268.
4. Sahin G, et al. Which statin should be used together with colchicine? Clinical experience in three patients with nephrotic syndrome due to AA type amyloidosis. *Rheumatol Int.* 2008;28(3):289-291.
5. Francis L, et al. Fatal toxic myopathy attributed to propofol, methylprednisolone, and cyclosporine after prior exposure to colchicine and simvastatin. *Clin Rheumatol.* 2008;27(1):129-131.
6. Wilbur K, Makowsky M. Colchicine myotoxicity: case reports and literature review. *Pharmacotherapy.* 2004;24(12):1784-1792.
7. Horn JR, et al. Proposal for a new tool to evaluate drug interaction cases. *Ann Pharmacother.* 2007;41(4):674-680.

2 Colchicine (eg, *Colcrys*)

Telaprevir (*Incivek*)

SUMMARY: The coadministration of telaprevir is expected to markedly increase the plasma concentration of colchicine; adverse reactions, including GI and hematologic toxicity, may be more likely to occur.

RISK FACTORS: No specific risk factors are known.

MECHANISM: Telaprevir inhibits the CYP3A4-mediated metabolism and P-glycoprotein elimination of colchicine.

CLINICAL EVALUATION: While specific data are limited, the manufacturer of telaprevir notes that the coadministration of telaprevir and colchicine should be avoided if possible.[1] Pending further data, carefully observe patients receiving telaprevir and colchicine for colchicine adverse reactions.

RELATED DRUGS: Atazanavir (*Reyataz*), darunavir (*Prezista*), fosamprenavir (*Lexiva*), indinavir (*Crixivan*), nelfinavir (*Viracept*), and saquinavir (*Invirase*) also inhibit the activity of CYP3A4 and are expected to increase the plasma concentrations of colchicine.

MANAGEMENT OPTIONS:

➡ *Avoid Unless Benefit Outweighs Risk.* Avoid the coadministration of telaprevir and colchicine when possible.

➡ *Monitor.* Monitor patients stabilized on telaprevir for adverse reactions if colchicine is coadministered. Colchicine can produce diarrhea, vomiting, abdominal pain, fever, bleeding, myopathy (muscle pain, weakness, dark urine, paresthesia); severe cases can result in multiorgan failure and death. The telaprevir package insert recommends limiting the dose of colchicine for patients taking telaprevir; however, no data are provided to support the recommendation.

REFERENCES:

1. *Incivek* [package insert]. Cambridge, MA: Vertex Pharmaceuticals Inc; 2011.

Colesevelam (*Welchol*)
Contraceptives, Oral

SUMMARY: Colesevelam modestly reduces ethinyl estradiol bioavailability; separate doses appropriately to minimize the interaction.

RISK FACTORS: No specific risk factors are known.

MECHANISM: Colesevelam appears to bind with ethinyl estradiol in the GI tract, thus reducing its absorption.

CLINICAL EVALUATION: Healthy subjects were given an oral contraceptive (norethindrone 1 mg plus ethinyl estradiol 0.035 mg) in the following 4 different ways: (a) alone, (b) simultaneously with colesevelam 3.75 g, (c) 1 hour before colesevelam, (d) 4 hours before colesevelam.[1] The ethinyl estradiol area under the concentration-time curve (AUC) was somewhat lower when given simultaneously with colesevelam and with the oral contraceptive given 1 hour before, but no interaction was observed with the contraceptive given 4 hours before the colesevelam. Norethindrone AUC was not significantly affected by colesevelam.

RELATED DRUGS: Other bile acid sequestrants, such as cholestyramine (eg, *Questran*) and colestipol (eg, *Colestid*), may also interfere with the absorption of ethinyl estradiol. The effect of colesevelam on estrogens other than ethinyl estradiol is not established, but assume that they interact until proven otherwise. The effect of colesevelam on the bioavailability of progestins other than norethindrone is not established.

MANAGEMENT OPTIONS:

➡ *Circumvent/Minimize.* Give oral contraceptives containing ethinyl estradiol (or other estrogens) at least 4 hours before colesevelam.[2]

➡ *Monitor.* If the combination is used, spotting or breakthrough bleeding could be an indication that colesevelam is reducing the plasma estrogen concentrations, but lack of breakthrough bleeding does not ensure contraceptive protection.

REFERENCES:

1. Brown KS, et al. Effect of the bile acid sequestrant colesevelam on the pharmacokinetics of pioglitazone, repaglinide, estrogen estradiol, norethindrone, levothyroxine, and glyburide. *J Clin Pharmacol.* 2010;50(5):554-565.

2. *Welchol* [package insert]. Parsippany, NJ: Daiichi Sankyo Inc; 2010.

Colesevelam (*Welchol*)

Cyclosporine (eg, *Neoral*)

SUMMARY: Colesevelam reduces cyclosporine bioavailability; separate doses appropriately to minimize the interaction.

RISK FACTORS: No specific risk factors are known.

MECHANISM: Colesevelam appears to bind with cyclosporine in the GI tract, thus reducing its absorption.

CLINICAL EVALUATION: Administration of cyclosporine 200 mg with colesevelam 3.75 g reduced cyclosporine area under the plasma concentration-time curve 34%.[1] No details of the study were given; until more data are available, assume that colesevelam can reduce cyclosporine efficacy.

RELATED DRUGS: Other bile acid sequestrants, such as cholestyramine (eg, *Questran*) and colestipol (eg, *Colestid*), may also interfere with the absorption of cyclosporine. The effect of colesevelam on other immunosuppressants, such as sirolimus (*Rapamune*) and tacrolimus (eg, *Prograf*), is not established, but assume that they interact until proven otherwise.

MANAGEMENT OPTIONS:

➡ *Circumvent/Minimize.* Give cyclosporine at least 4 hours before colesevelam.[1] It is advised to keep the dosing interval between the drugs as consistent as possible from day to day.

➡ *Monitor.* If the combination is used, monitor for reduced cyclosporine effect if colesevelam is started or stopped, or if the dosing interval between the 2 drugs changes.

REFERENCES:

1. *Welchol* [package insert]. Parsippany, NJ: Daiichi Sankyo Inc; 2010.

Colesevelam (*Welchol*)

Glyburide (eg, *DiaBeta*)

SUMMARY: Colesevelam reduces glyburide plasma concentrations; some loss of hypoglycemic effect may occur.

RISK FACTORS: No specific risk factors are known.

MECHANISM: Colesevelam appears to interfere with the GI absorption of glyburide.

CLINICAL EVALUATION: Subjects were administered a single dose of glyburide 3 mg in 4 different ways: a) alone, b) simultaneously with colesevelam 3,750 mg, c) 1 hour before colesevelam, d) 4 hours before colesevelam.[1] The area under the concentration-time curve of glyburide was reduced 32%, 20%, and 8%, when administered concurrently, 1 hour, and 4 hours before the colesevelam, respectively. Glyburide doses should be administered several hours before colesevelam to minimize the magnitude of the interaction.

RELATED DRUGS: None known.

MANAGEMENT OPTIONS:

➡ *Monitor.* Avoid coadministration of glyburide and colesevelam. Give glyburide 2 to 4 hours prior to a dose of colesevelam to minimize any loss of hypoglycemic efficacy.

REFERENCES:

1. Brown KS, et al. Effect of the bile acid sequestrant colesevelam on the pharmacokinetics of pioglitazone, repaglinide, estrogen estradiol, norethindrone, levothyroxine, and glyburide. *J Clin Pharmacol.* 2010;50(5):554-565.

Colesevelam (*Welchol*)

Levothyroxine (eg, Synthroid)

SUMMARY: Colesevelam can markedly reduce levothyroxine bioavailability; separate doses appropriately to minimize the interaction.

RISK FACTORS: No specific risk factors are known.

MECHANISM: Colesevelam appears to bind with levothyroxine in the GI tract, thus reducing its absorption.

CLINICAL EVALUATION: Six healthy subjects were given oral levothyroxine 1 mg with and without concurrent colesevelam 3.75 g.[1] The thyroxine area under the serum concentration-time curve (AUC) was reduced by 96% in the presence of colesevelam. In another study, subjects were administered a single dose of levothyroxine 0.6 mg alone and with colcsevelam 3.75 g simultaneously, 1 hour, and 4 hours after levothyroxine.[2] The thyroxine AUC was markedly lower when given simultaneously with colesevelam, only slightly lower with colesevelam 1 hour after levothyroxine, and no interaction was observed with the colesevelam given 4 hours later.

RELATED DRUGS: Other bile acid sequestrants, such as cholestyramine (eg, *Questran*) and colestipol (eg, *Colestid*), may also interfere with the absorption of levothyroxine.

MANAGEMENT OPTIONS:

➡ *Circumvent/Minimize.* Give levothyroxine or other thyroid replacement products 4 hours before colesevelam.[3] It is advised to keep the dosing interval between levothyroxine and colescvelam as consistent as possible from day to day.

➥ **Monitor.** Even if the doses are separated, monitor for altered thyroid function if colesevelam is started, stopped, or changed in dosage, or if the interval between the colesevelam and the levothyroxine is changed.

REFERENCES:

1. Weitzman SP, et al. Colesevelam hydrochloride and lanthanum carbonate interfere with the absorption of levothyroxine. *Thyroid.* 2009;19(1):77-79.

2. Brown KS, et al. Effect of the bile acid sequestrants colesevelam on the pharmacokinetics of pioglitazone, repaglinide, estrogen estradiol, norethindrone, levothyroxine, and glyburide. *J Clin Pharmacol.* 2010;50(5):554-565.

3. *Welchol* [package insert]. Parsippany, NJ: Daiichi Sankyo Inc; 2010.

Colesevelam (*Welchol*)

Phenytoin (eg, *Dilantin*)

SUMMARY: There have been isolated reports of reduced phenytoin response due to concurrent colesevelam, but a causal relationship has not been established.

RISK FACTORS: No specific risk factors are known.

MECHANISM: Not established. Theoretically, colesevelam may bind with phenytoin in the GI tract, thus reducing its absorption.

CLINICAL EVALUATION: The manufacturer of *Welchol* received reports of increased seizure activity and reduced phenytoin plasma concentrations in patients given colesevelam and phenytoin.[1] No details were given; thus, it is not possible to assess the validity of these reports.

RELATED DRUGS: Theoretically, other bile acid sequestrants, such as cholestyramine (eg, *Questran*) and colestipol (eg, *Colestid*), may also interfere with the absorption of phenytoin.

MANAGEMENT OPTIONS:

➥ **Circumvent/Minimize.** Give phenytoin at least 4 hours before colesevelam.

➥ **Monitor.** If the combination is used, monitor for altered phenytoin response if colesevelam is started or stopped, or if the dosing interval between the two drugs changes.

REFERENCES:

1. *Welchol* [package insert]. Parsippany, NJ: Daiichi Sankyo Inc; 2010.

Colesevelam (*Welchol*)

Verapamil (eg, *Calan*)

SUMMARY: Colesevelam may reduce verapamil bioavailability; separate doses appropriately to minimize the interaction.

RISK FACTORS: No specific risk factors are known.

MECHANISM: Colesevelam probably binds with verapamil in the GI tract, thus reducing its absorption.

CLINICAL EVALUATION: Giving sustained-release verapamil 240 mg with colesevelam 4.5 g reduced verapamil area under the plasma concentration-time curve 31%.[1] No details of the study were given, but until more data are available it should be assumed that colesevelam can reduce verapamil efficacy.

RELATED DRUGS: Theoretically, other bile acid sequestrants, such as cholestyramine (eg, *Questran*) and colestipol (eg, *Colestid*), may also interfere with the absorption of verapamil.

MANAGEMENT OPTIONS:

➥ *Circumvent/Minimize.* Give verapamil at least 4 hours before colesevelam.

➥ *Monitor.* If the combination is used, monitor for altered verapamil response if colesevelam is started or stopped, or if the dosing interval between the two drugs changes.

REFERENCES:

1. *Welchol* [package insert]. Parsippany, NJ: Daiichi Sankyo Inc; 2010.

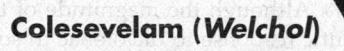

Colesevelam (*Welchol*)

Warfarin (eg, *Coumadin*)

SUMMARY: There have been isolated reports of reduced international normalized ration (INR) response to warfarin following colesevelam therapy, but a causal relationship has not been established.

RISK FACTORS: No specific risk factors are known.

MECHANISM: Not established. Theoretically, colesevelam may bind with warfarin in the GI tract, thus reducing its absorption.

CLINICAL EVALUATION: There are case reports of decreased INR in patients on warfarin during colesevelam therapy.[1] No details were given; thus, it is not possible to assess the validity of these reports. Moreover, the manufacturer found no effect of colesevelam on warfarin plasma concentrations in healthy subjects.[1] Taken together, the evidence for an interaction between warfarin and colesevelam is minimal, but it cannot be ruled out that some patients would be affected.

RELATED DRUGS: Cholestyramine (eg, *Questran*) has been reported to interfere with the absorption of warfarin, but colestipol (eg, *Colestid*) may be less likely to do so.

MANAGEMENT OPTIONS:

➥ *Circumvent/Minimize.* It is advised to give warfarin at least 4 hours before colesevelam, and probably more important to keep the interval between the doses of warfarin and colesevelam as consistent as possible.

➥ *Monitor.* If the combination is used, monitor for altered INR response if colesevelam is started, stopped, changed in dosage, or if the interval between the doses of the two drugs changes.

REFERENCES:

1. *Welchol* [package insert]. Parsippany, NJ: Daiichi Sankyo Inc; 2010.

Colestipol (*Colestid*)

Diclofenac (eg, *Voltaren*)

SUMMARY: Single dose studies suggest that colestipol moderately reduces the bioavailability of diclofenac; the clinical importance of this effect is not established, but reduced diclofenac effect may occur.

RISK FACTORS: No specific risk factors are known.

MECHANISM: Colestipol probably binds with diclofenac in the GI tract, thus inhibiting diclofenac absorption. Colestipol also may interfere with the enterohepatic circulation of diclofenac.

CLINICAL EVALUATION: Six healthy subjects took oral diclofenac 100 mg alone and with cholestyramine 8 g or colestipol 10 g in a randomized 3-way crossover study.[1] Colestipol reduced the diclofenac area under the plasma concentration-time curve 33%. Although the magnitude of this effect may be sufficient to reduce the therapeutic response to diclofenac in some patients, chronic dosing studies are needed to establish the clinical importance of this interaction.

RELATED DRUGS: Cholestyramine (eg, *Questran*) also appears to inhibit the absorption of diclofenac, and to a greater extent than colestipol.

MANAGEMENT OPTIONS:

➡ ***Circumvent/Minimize.*** Give the diclofenac 2 hours before or 6 hours after the colestipol to optimize the absorption of the diclofenac. However, because diclofenac undergoes enterohepatic circulation, reduced diclofenac plasma concentrations may occur even if the doses are separated.

➡ ***Monitor.*** Monitor for reduced diclofenac effect, regardless of how far apart the doses are separated.

REFERENCES:
1. Al-balla SR, et al. The effects of cholestyramine and colestipol on the absorption of diclofenac in man. *Int J Clin Pharmacol Ther*. 1994;32:441.

 Colestipol (*Colestid*)

Digitoxin[†]

SUMMARY: Colestipol may reduce the serum concentration of digitoxin, but this has not been a consistent finding.

RISK FACTORS: No specific risk factors are known.

MECHANISM: Colestipol appears to bind digitoxin in the GI tract, thus impairing its initial absorption and enterohepatic circulation.

CLINICAL EVALUATION: In 4 patients with digitoxin intoxication, colestipol appeared to reduce plasma digitoxin concentrations, presumably by interrupting enterohepatic circulation.[1] A similar effect was seen in 1 patient with digoxin (eg, *Lanoxin*) intoxication, but one would expect digoxin to be less affected, because it undergoes less enterohepatic circulation. However, neither colestipol 10 g as a single dose[3] nor 5 g 4 times daily[2] altered the pharmacokinetics of digoxin or digitoxin, respectively, in nontoxic subjects. Studies in patients receiving therapeutic doses of digitalis glycosides are needed to evaluate the clinical importance of the interaction between colestipol and digitalis glycosides.

RELATED DRUGS: Cholestyramine (eg, *Questran*) also may reduce digitoxin concentrations.

MANAGEMENT OPTIONS: No specific action is required, but be alert for evidence of the interaction.

REFERENCES:

1. Bazzano G, et al. Digitalis intoxication: treatment with a new steroidbinding resin. *JAMA.* 1972;220:828.

2. van Bever RJ, et al. The effect of colesripol on digitoxin plasma levels. *Arzneimittelforschung.* 1976;26:1891.

3. Neuvonen PJ, et al. Effects of resins and activated charcoal on the absorption of digoxin, carbamazepine and furosemide. *Br J Clin Pharmacol.* 1988;25:229.

† Not available in the US.

Colestipol (*Colestid*)   4

Digoxin (eg, *Lanoxin*)

SUMMARY: Colestipol may reduce the serum concentrations of digitalis glycosides, but this has not been a consistent finding.

RISK FACTORS: No specific risk factors are known.

MECHANISM: Colestipol appears to bind digitalis glycosides in the GI tract, thus impairing their initial absorption and enterohepatic circulation.

CLINICAL EVALUATION: In 4 patients with digitoxin intoxication, colestipol appeared to reduce plasma digitoxin concentrations, presumably by interrupting enterohepatic circulation.[1] A similar effect was seen in 1 patient with digoxin intoxication, but one would expect digoxin to be less affected, since it undergoes less enterohepatic circulation. However, neither colestipol 10 g as a single dose[3] nor 5 g 4 times daily[2] altered the pharmacokinetics of digoxin or digitoxin (*Crystodigin*), respectively, in nontoxic subjects. Studies in patients receiving therapeutic doses of digitalis glycosides are needed to evaluate the clinical importance of the interaction between colestipol and digitalis glycosides.

RELATED DRUGS: Cholestyramine (eg, *Questran*) also may reduce digitalis glycoside concentrations.

MANAGEMENT OPTIONS: No specific action is required, but be alert for evidence of the interaction.

REFERENCES:

1. Bazzano G, et al. Digitalis intoxication: treatment with a new steroidbinding resin. *JAMA.* 1972;220:828.

2. van Bever RJ, et al. The effect of colestripol on digitoxin plasma levels. *Arzneimittelforschung.* 1976;26:1891.

3. Neuvonen PJ, et al. Effects of resins and activated charcoal on the absorption of digoxin, carbamazepine and furosemide. *Br J Clin Pharmacol.* 1988;25:229.

Colestipol (*Colestid*)

Furosemide (eg, *Lasix*)

SUMMARY: Study in healthy subjects suggests that colestipol considerably reduces the bioavailability and diuretic response of furosemide.

RISK FACTORS: No specific risk factors are known.

MECHANISM: Colestipol probably binds with furosemide in the GI tract, thus reducing its bioavailability.

CLINICAL EVALUATION: Six healthy subjects received a single oral 40 mg dose of furosemide with and without coadministration of 10 g of colestipol.[1] The bioavailability of furosemide, as measured by the area under the plasma concentration-time curve and total urinary elimination, was reduced 80% by colestipol. The reduction in furosemide bioavailability was accompanied by a 58% reduction in furosemide diuretic response. Thus, it appears that colestipol can reduce furosemide response considerably.

RELATED DRUGS: Cholestyramine (eg, *Questran*) also substantially reduces the bioavailability of furosemide.

MANAGEMENT OPTIONS:

➡ *Circumvent/Minimize.* Although the ability to circumvent the interaction by separating doses of furosemide from colestipol has not been studied systematically, giving furosemide 2 hours before or 6 hours after the colestipol would be expected to minimize the interaction.

➡ *Monitor.* Monitor for altered furosemide response if colestipol therapy is initiated, discontinued, changed in dosage, or if the interval between doses of the 2 drugs is changed.

REFERENCES:

    1. Neuvonen PJ, et al. Effects of resins and activated charcoal on the absorption of digoxin, carbamazepine and furosemide. *Br J Clin Pharmacol.* 1988;25:229.

Colestipol (eg, *Colestid*)

Gemfibrozil (eg, *Lopid*)

SUMMARY: Colestipol appears to reduce the bioavailability of gemfibrozil if the drugs are given concurrently but not if the doses are separated by at least 2 hours.

RISK FACTORS: No specific risk factors are known.

MECHANISM: Although the mechanism has not been studied, colestipol probably binds with gemfibrozil in the GI tract, thus reducing gemfibrozil bioavailability.

CLINICAL EVALUATION: Ten patients with hyperlipidemia were randomly given gemfibrozil 600 mg under 4 conditions: alone, with colestipol 5 g, 2 hours before colestipol, and 2 hours after colestipol.[1] Coadministration resulted in a 30% reduction in gemfibrozil absorption as measured by the area under the plasma concentration-time curve; administration of gemfibrozil 2 hours before or after colestipol did not affect gemfibrozil bioavailability. Although the clinical significance of a 30% reduction in the bioavailability of gemfibrozil is not established, a decreased gemfibrozil response in at least some patients is expected.

RELATED DRUGS: Cholestyramine (eg, *Questran*) probably inhibits the absorption of gemfibrozil.

MANAGEMENT OPTIONS:

➡ *Circumvent/Minimize.* Until more is known about this interaction, it would be prudent to separate doses of gemfibrozil and colestipol (or cholestyramine) by at least 2 hours.

➡ *Monitor.* Monitor for reduced gemfibrozil response if colestipol or cholestyramine is also given.

REFERENCES:

1. Forland SC, et al. Apparent reduced absorption of gemfibrozil when given with colestipol. *J Clin Pharmacol*. 1990;30:29-32.

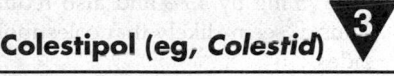

Colestipol (eg, *Colestid*)

Tetracycline (eg, *Sumycin*)

SUMMARY: Colestipol reduces the bioavailability of tetracycline; however, the clinical importance of this interaction is not established.

RISK FACTORS: No specific risk factors are known.

MECHANISM: Colestipol appears to bind tetracycline in the intestinal tract, inhibiting its absorption.

CLINICAL EVALUATION: Colestipol 30 g reduced tetracycline absorption more than 50%.[1] No information is available regarding the magnitude of this interaction when colestipol is given in daily divided doses (5 to 10 g) or when the doses of colestipol and tetracycline are given at separate times.

RELATED DRUGS: Cholestyramine (eg, *Questran*) might reduce absorption of tetracycline as well.

MANAGEMENT OPTIONS:

➡ *Circumvent/Minimize.* Until further information is available, patients receiving colestipol and tetracycline should separate the doses in an attempt to minimize the effect of colestipol on tetracycline absorption. Administer tetracycline 2 hours before or at least 3 hours after colestipol.

➡ *Monitor.* If doses of tetracycline and bile acid binding resin must be administered together, monitor patients for reduced antibiotic effect.

REFERENCES:

1. Friedman H, et al. Impaired absorption of tetracycline by colestipol is not reversed by orange juice. *J Clin Pharmacol*. 1989;29:748-751.

Colestipol (eg, *Colestid*)

Thiazides

SUMMARY: Colestipol has been reported to reduce the serum concentrations of thiazides and may lessen their diuretic effect.

RISK FACTORS: No specific risk factors are known.

MECHANISM: Colestipol appears to inhibit the GI absorption of thiazides such as chlorothiazide (eg, *Diuril*).

CLINICAL EVALUATION: In 10 patients with hyperlipoproteinemia, colestipol given at the same time or 1 hour after chlorothiazide decreased chlorothiazide absorption considerably as measured by cumulative urinary excretion.[1] In 6 healthy subjects, colestipol 10 g reduced total urinary excretion of a single dose of hydrochlorothiazide 75 mg by 43% and also reduced the plasma concentrations of the diuretic.[2] Thus, it seems likely that colestipol would inhibit the therapeutic response to thiazides.

RELATED DRUGS: Assume that all thiazides interact with colestipol until proved otherwise. Cholestyramine (eg, *Questran*) also inhibits thiazide diuretic absorption.

MANAGEMENT OPTIONS:

➡ *Circumvent/Minimize.* Administer thiazides at least 2 hours before or 6 hours after colestipol, and try to maintain a relatively constant interval and sequence of administration of the 2 drugs.

➡ *Monitor.* Monitor for altered thiazide response if colestipol therapy is initiated, discontinued, changed in dosage, or if the interval between doses of the 2 drugs is changed.

REFERENCES:

1. Kauffman RE, et al. Effect of colestipol on gastrointestinal absorption of chlorothiazide in man. *Clin Pharmacol Ther.* 1973;14:886-890.
2. Hunninghake DB, et al. The effect of cholestyramine and colestipol on the absorption of hydrochlorothiazide. *Int J Clin Pharmacol Ther Toxicol.* 1982;20:151-154.

Conivaptan (*Vaprisol*)

Amlodipine (eg, *Norvasc*)

SUMMARY: Conivaptan is likely to increase amlodipine plasma concentrations.

RISK FACTORS: No specific risk factors are known.

MECHANISM: Conivaptan is a CYP3A4 inhibitor and is likely to inhibit the intestinal and hepatic metabolism of amlodipine.

CLINICAL EVALUATION: The development of an oral formulation of conivaptan was discontinued because of its ability to inhibit CYP3A4 and the resultant risk of drug interactions.[1] The manufacturer reported that conivaptan 40 mg/day intravenous resulted in a 2-fold increase in amlodipine area under the plasma concentration-time curve.[2] The extent to which an interaction of this magnitude increases amlodipine toxicity is not clear, but the risk is probably small.

RELATED DRUGS: Theoretically, conivaptan increases the plasma concentrations of other calcium-channel blockers, which are also metabolized by CYP3A4.

MANAGEMENT OPTIONS: No specific action is required, but be alert for evidence of the interaction.

REFERENCES:
1. Ali F, et al. Therapeutic potential of vasopressin receptor antagonists. *Drugs.* 2007;67:847-858.
2. *Vaprisol* [package insert]. Deerfield, IL: Astellas Pharma US Inc.; 2007.

Conivaptan (*Vaprisol*)

Atorvastatin (*Lipitor*)

SUMMARY: Conivaptan is likely to increase atorvastatin plasma concentrations; the combination should generally be avoided.

RISK FACTORS: No specific risk factors are known.

MECHANISM: Conivaptan is a CYP3A4 inhibitor and is likely to inhibit the intestinal and hepatic metabolism of atorvastatin.

CLINICAL EVALUATION: The development of an oral formulation of conivaptan was discontinued because of its ability to inhibit CYP3A4 and the resultant risk of drug interactions.[1] The manufacturer reported that 2 cases of rhabdomyolysis were reported when conivaptan was used concurrently with CYP3A4-metabolized statins, although the specific statins involved were not stated.[2] Even though little clinical evidence of an interaction is available, the use of conivaptan with atorvastatin should generally be avoided.

RELATED DRUGS: Conivaptan is likely to produce even greater increases in plasma concentrations of lovastatin (eg, *Mevacor*) and simvastatin (eg, *Zocor*) than of atorvastatin. Pravastatin (eg, *Pravachol*), fluvastatin (*Lescol*), and rosuvastatin (*Crestor*) are not metabolized by CYP3A4, and theoretically are unlikely to interact with conivaptan.

MANAGEMENT OPTIONS:

➥ *Consider Alternative.* Pravastatin, fluvastatin, and rosuvastatin are less likely to interact with conivaptan than atorvastatin.

➥ *Circumvent/Minimize.* In patients receiving atorvastatin, consider discontinuing atorvastatin during short-term conivaptan therapy.

➥ *Monitor.* If conivaptan is used with atorvastatin, monitor for evidence of rhabdomyolysis (eg, muscle pain, weakness, dark urine).

REFERENCES:
1. Ali F, et al. Therapeutic potential of vasopressin receptor antagonists. *Drugs.* 2007;67:847-858.
2. *Vaprisol* [package insert]. Deerfield, IL: Astellas Pharma US Inc.; 2007.

Conivaptan (*Vaprisol*)

Clarithromycin (eg, *Biaxin*)

SUMMARY: Conivaptan is listed as contraindicated with CYP3A4 inhibitors such as clarithromycin, but the contraindication is based on lack of information on conivaptan toxicity.

RISK FACTORS: No specific risk factors are known.

MECHANISM: Clarithromycin is likely to inhibit the CYP3A4 metabolism of conivaptan.

CLINICAL EVALUATION: The manufacturer reports that the CYP3A4 inhibitor ketoconazole resulted in a marked increase in plasma concentrations of oral conivaptan.[1] Based on these data, the product information for conivaptan states that conivaptan is contraindicated with potent inhibitors of CYP3A4 such as clarithromycin because the clinical consequences of elevated conivaptan concentrations are unknown. But because the risk of elevated conivaptan concentrations has not been established, it is possible that the benefit of combined therapy could outweigh the risk in some patients.

RELATED DRUGS: Erythromycin (eg, *Ery-Tab*) and troleandomycin[†] are not mentioned in the conivaptan product information but they can also inhibit CYP3A4 and are expected to interact with conivaptan.

MANAGEMENT OPTIONS:

➥ *Avoid Unless Benefit Outweighs Risk.* Although the risk of elevated conivaptan concentrations has not been established, one should generally avoid concurrent use with clarithromycin, erythromycin, or troleandomycin[†]. If concurrent use is deemed necessary, monitor the patient closely.

➥ *Use Alternative.* Azithromycin (*Zithromax*) and dirithromycin[†] do not appear to inhibit CYP3A4, and theoretically are not expected to interact with conivaptan.

REFERENCES:

    1. *Vaprisol* [package insert]. Deerfield, IL: Astellas Pharma US Inc.; 2007.

    † Not available in the United States.

2 **Conivaptan (*Vaprisol*)**

Colchicine

SUMMARY: Based on the interactive properties of the 2 drugs, it is likely that conivaptan substantially increases colchicine plasma concentrations. Avoid the combination when possible.

RISK FACTORS: No specific risk factors are known.

MECHANISM: Colchicine is a P-glycoprotein and CYP3A4 substrate, and conivaptan inhibits both P-glycoprotein and CYP3A4; colchicine plasma concentrations are likely to increase.[1]

CLINICAL EVALUATION: Although the interaction is based primarily on theoretical considerations, it is likely that conivaptan would increase the risk of colchicine toxicity. Given that colchicine toxicity can be fatal, even a theoretical interaction warrants close attention.

RELATED DRUGS: No information available.

MANAGEMENT OPTIONS:

➡ *Avoid Unless Benefit Outweighs Risk.* Given that colchicine toxicity can be life-threatening, use conivaptan only if it is likely to provide therapeutic benefits that cannot be achieved with noninteracting alternatives.

➡ *Use Alternative.* If possible, use a therapeutic alternative to conivaptan that does not inhibit P-glycoprotein, or use an alternative to colchicine.

➡ *Monitor.* If the combination must be used, monitor carefully for colchicine toxicity (eg, diarrhea, vomiting, fever, abdominal pain, muscle pains). Advise the patient to immediately contact a health care provider if any of these symptoms occur. Colchicine-induced pancytopenia can result in infections, bleeding, and anemia, and is often the cause of death in fatal cases.

REFERENCES:

1. Rautio J, et al. In vitro p-glycoprotein inhibition assays for assessment of clinical drug interaction potential of new drug candidates: a recommendation for probe substrates. *Drug Metab Dispos.* 2006;34(5):786-792.

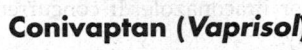

Conivaptan (*Vaprisol*)

Digoxin (eg, *Lanoxin*)

SUMMARY: Conivaptan may increase the risk of digoxin toxicity.

RISK FACTORS: No specific risk factors are known.

MECHANISM: Not established. Conivaptan may inhibit P-glycoprotein, thus increasing digoxin absorption and impairing its elimination.

CLINICAL EVALUATION: The manufacturer stated that oral conivaptan (40 mg twice daily) increased digoxin area under the plasma concentration-time curve by 43%, but details of the study were not given.[1] Intravenous conivaptan was not studied, but it may also interact with digoxin.

RELATED DRUGS: No information is available.

MANAGEMENT OPTIONS:

➡ *Monitor.* If conivaptan is given concurrently with digoxin, monitor for excessive digoxin effect and digoxin toxicity.

REFERENCES:

1. *Vaprisol* [package insert]. Deerfield, IL: Astellas Pharma US Inc.; 2007.

Conivaptan (*Vaprisol*)

Ketoconazole (eg, *Nizoral*)

SUMMARY: Potent CYP3A4 inhibitors such as ketoconazole are listed as contraindicated with conivaptan, but the contraindication is based on lack of information on conivaptan toxicity.

RISK FACTORS: No specific risk factors are known.

MECHANISM: Ketoconazole is likely to inhibit the CYP3A4 metabolism of conivaptan.

CLINICAL EVALUATION: The manufacturer reported that concurrent use of ketoconazole with oral conivaptan resulted in an 11-fold increase in conivaptan area under the plasma concentration-time curve.[1] No details of the study were given. Intravenous conivaptan is expected to interact with ketoconazole to a lesser degree. The product information for conivaptan states that concurrent use with ketoconazole is contraindicated because the clinical consequences of elevated conivaptan concentrations have not been established. Based on this, the combination should be avoided, but because the risk of elevated conivaptan concentrations is not established, it is possible that the benefit of combined therapy could outweigh the risk in some patients.

RELATED DRUGS: Itraconazole (eg, *Sporanox*) is also contraindicated with conivaptan in the product information. Voriconazole (*Vfend*), posaconazole (*Noxafil*), and fluconazole (eg, *Diflucan*) are not mentioned in the conivaptan product information; however, they can also inhibit CYP3A4 and are expected to interact with conivaptan, but to a lesser extent than itraconazole or ketoconazole.

MANAGEMENT OPTIONS:

➡ *Avoid Unless Benefit Outweighs Risk.* Although the risk of elevated conivaptan concentrations has not been established, generally avoid concurrent use with ketoconazole or itraconazole. If concurrent use is deemed necessary, monitor the patient closely.

REFERENCES:

1. *Vaprisol* [package insert]. Deerfield, IL: Astellas Pharma US Inc.; 2007.

 Conivaptan (*Vaprisol*)

Lovastatin (eg, *Mevacor*)

SUMMARY: Conivaptan is likely to markedly increase lovastatin plasma concentrations; the combination should generally be avoided.

RISK FACTORS: No specific risk factors are known.

MECHANISM: Conivaptan is a CYP3A4 inhibitor and is likely to inhibit the intestinal and hepatic metabolism of lovastatin.

CLINICAL EVALUATION: The development of an oral formulation of conivaptan was discontinued because of its ability to inhibit CYP3A4 and the resultant risk of drug interactions.[1] The manufacturer reported that 2 cases of rhabdomyolysis were reported when conivaptan was used concurrently with CYP3A4-metabolized statins, although the specific statins involved were not stated.[2] Even though little clinical evidence of an interaction is available, the use of a strong CYP3A4 inhibitor with lovastatin should generally be avoided.

RELATED DRUGS: Conivaptan is also likely to inhibit the CYP3A4 metabolism of simvastatin (eg, *Zocor*) and, to a lesser extent, atorvastatin (*Lipitor*). Pravastatin (*Pravachol*), fluvastatin (*Lescol*), and rosuvastatin (*Crestor*) are not metabolized by CYP3A4, and theoretically are unlikely to interact with conivaptan.

MANAGEMENT OPTIONS:

➡ *Use Alternative.* Pravastatin, fluvastatin, and rosuvastatin are theoretically less likely to interact with conivaptan than lovastatin.

➡ *Circumvent/Minimize.* In patients receiving lovastatin, consider discontinuing the lovastatin during short-term conivaptan therapy.

➡ **Monitor.** If conivaptan is used with lovastatin, monitor for evidence of rhabdomyolysis (eg, muscle pain, weakness, dark urine).

REFERENCES:

1. Ali F, et al. Therapeutic potential of vasopressin receptor antagonists. *Drugs.* 2007;67:847-858.

2. *Vaprisol* [package insert]. Deerfield, IL: Astellas Pharma US Inc.; 2007.

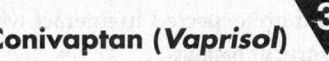

Conivaptan (*Vaprisol*)

Midazolam

SUMMARY: Conivaptan is likely to increase midazolam plasma concentrations.

RISK FACTORS: No specific risk factors are known.

MECHANISM: Conivaptan is a CYP3A4 inhibitor and is likely to inhibit the intestinal and hepatic metabolism of midazolam.

CLINICAL EVALUATION: The development of an oral formulation of conivaptan was discontinued because of its ability to inhibit CYP3A4 and the resultant risk of drug interactions.[1] The manufacturer reports that intravenous conivaptan (40 mg/day) resulted in a 2-fold increase in intravenous midazolam area under the concentration-time curve (AUC) and a 3-fold increase in oral midazolam AUC.[2] The magnitude of the interaction is likely to result in enhanced CNS depression with midazolam.

RELATED DRUGS: Conivaptan is likely to increase the plasma concentrations of other CYP3A4-metabolized benzodiazepines such as alprazolam (eg, *Xanax*) and triazolam (eg, *Halcion*).

MANAGEMENT OPTIONS:

➡ **Monitor.** Monitor for excessive CNS depression in patients who receive concurrent therapy with conivaptan and midazolam. It may be necessary to reduce the dose of midazolam.

REFERENCES:

1. Ali F, et al. Therapeutic potential of vasopressin receptor antagonists. *Drugs.* 2007;67:847-858.

2. *Vaprisol* [package insert]. Deerfield, IL: Astellas Pharma US Inc.; 2007.

Conivaptan (*Vaprisol*)

Ritonavir (*Norvir*)

SUMMARY: Potent CYP3A4 inhibitors such as ritonavir are listed as contraindicated with conivaptan, but the contraindication is based on lack of information on conivaptan toxicity.

RISK FACTORS: No specific risk factors are known.

MECHANISM: Ritonavir is likely to inhibit the CYP3A4 metabolism of conivaptan.

CLINICAL EVALUATION: The manufacturer reported that the CYP3A4 inhibitor ketoconazole resulted in a marked increase in plasma concentrations of oral conivaptan.[1] Based on these data, the product information for conivaptan states that conivaptan is contraindicated with potent inhibitors of CYP3A4 such as ritonavir because the clinical consequences of elevated conivaptan concentrations are unknown. But because the risk of elevated conivaptan concentrations has not been established, it is possible that the benefit of combined therapy could outweigh the risk in some patients.

RELATED DRUGS: Indinavir (*Crixivan*) is also contraindicated with conivaptan in the product information. Amprenavir (*Agenerase*), atazanavir (*Reyataz*), darunavir (*Prezista*), delavirdine (*Rescriptor*), nelfinavir (*Viracept*), and saquinavir (*Invirase*) are not mentioned in the conivaptan product information, but they can also inhibit CYP3A4 and are expected to interact with conivaptan.

MANAGEMENT OPTIONS:

➡ *Avoid Unless Benefit Outweighs Risk.* Although the risk of elevated conivaptan concentrations is not established, generally avoid concurrent use with ritonavir, indinavir, and other CYP3A4 inhibitors. If concurrent use is deemed necessary, monitor the patient closely.

REFERENCES:

1. *Vaprisol* [package insert]. Deerfield, IL: Astellas Pharma US Inc.; 2007.

 Conivaptan (*Vaprisol*)

Simvastatin (eg, *Zocor*)

SUMMARY: Conivaptan is likely to markedly increase simvastatin plasma concentrations; the combination should generally be avoided.

RISK FACTORS: No specific risk factors are known.

MECHANISM: Conivaptan is a CYP3A4 inhibitor and is likely to inhibit the intestinal and hepatic metabolism of simvastatin.

CLINICAL EVALUATION: The development of an oral formulation of conivaptan was discontinued because of its ability to inhibit CYP3A4 and the resultant risk of drug interactions.[1] The manufacturer cites a study in which intravenous conivaptan (30 mg/day) produced a 3-fold increase in simvastatin area under the plasma concentration-time curve.[2] The manufacturer also stated that 2 cases of rhabdomyolysis were reported when conivaptan was used concurrently with CYP3A4-metabolized statins, although the specific statins involved were not stated. Even though little clinical evidence of an interaction is available, the use conivaptan with simvastatin should generally be avoided.

RELATED DRUGS: Conivaptan is also likely to inhibit the CYP3A4 metabolism of lovastatin (eg, *Mevacor*) and to a lesser extent atorvastatin (*Lipitor*). Pravastatin (eg, *Pravachol*), fluvastatin (*Lescol*), and rosuvastatin (*Crestor*) are not metabolized by CYP3A4, and theoretically are unlikely to interact with conivaptan.

MANAGEMENT OPTIONS:

➡ *Use Alternative.* Pravastatin, fluvastatin, and rosuvastatin are less likely to interact with conivaptan than simvastatin.

➡ *Circumvent/Minimize.* In patients receiving simvastatin, consider discontinuing the simvastatin during short-term conivaptan therapy.

➡ *Monitor.* If conivaptan is used with simvastatin, monitor for evidence of rhabdomyolysis (eg, muscle pain, weakness, dark urine).

REFERENCES:

1. Ali F, et al. Therapeutic potential of vasopressin receptor antagonists. *Drugs.* 2007;67:847-858.
2. *Vaprisol* [package insert]. Deerfield, IL: Astellas Pharma US Inc.; 2007.

Conivaptan (*Vaprisol*) 5

Warfarin (eg, *Coumadin*)

SUMMARY: Conivaptan does not appear to interact with warfarin.

RISK FACTORS: None (no interaction).

MECHANISM: None (no interaction).

CLINICAL EVALUATION: The manufacturer stated that oral conivaptan (40 mg twice daily for 10 days) did not affect the pharmacokinetics or pharmacodynamics of warfarin.[1] Intravenous conivaptan was not studied, but there is no reason to believe that it interacts with warfarin if oral conivaptan does not.

RELATED DRUGS: No information is available.

MANAGEMENT OPTIONS: No interaction.

REFERENCES:

1. *Vaprisol* [package insert]. Deerfield, IL: Astellas Pharma US Inc.; 2007.

Contraceptives, Oral (eg, *Ortho-Novum*)

Felbamate (*Felbatol*)

SUMMARY: Felbamate substantially reduced plasma gestodene concentrations and slightly reduced plasma ethinyl estradiol concentrations in women on an oral contraceptive containing ethinyl estradiol and gestodene, but the extent to which felbamate reduces oral contraceptive efficacy has not been established.

RISK FACTORS: No specific risk factors are known.

MECHANISM: Not established. It is possible that felbamate enhances the metabolism of gestodene and ethinyl estradiol.

CLINICAL EVALUATION: In a randomized, double-blind, parallel study, 31 women taking chronic oral contraceptives (ethinyl estradiol 30 mcg plus gestodene 75 mcg) received placebo (n = 11) or felbamate 2,400 mg/day (n = 21) from the midcycle of 1 month to the midcycle of the next month for 2 consecutive cycles.[1] Felbamate was associated with a 42% decrease in gestodene area under the plasma concentration-time curve (AUC), but ethinyl estradiol AUC was decreased only 13%. Ovulation was not detected in either group based on determinations of plasma hormone concentrations. Nonetheless, one patient on felbamate developed breakthrough bleeding, which is consistent with reduced circulating hormone levels in women receiving oral contraceptives. Thus, while it is not known whether felbamate can decrease the efficacy of oral contraceptives, consider that it may occur.[2]

RELATED DRUGS: The effect of felbamate on progestins other than gestodene or estrogens other than ethinyl estradiol has not been established, but an interaction could occur.[2]

MANAGEMENT OPTIONS:

➡ *Consider Alternative.* Consider adding other means of contraception to the oral contraceptive, especially during the first 2 to 3 months of combined therapy with felbamate. Alternatively, some studies have recommended using a higher-dose oral contraceptive to maintain adequate hormonal concentrations. This appears to be a reasonable recommendation, but the magnitude of the required dosage increase is likely to vary considerably from one patient to another.

➠ **Monitor.** Spotting or breakthrough bleeding in patients taking oral contraceptives and felbamate could indicate that the drugs are interacting, although lack of breakthrough bleeding does not ensure contraceptive protection.

REFERENCES:

1. Saano V, et al. Effects of felbamate on the pharmacokinetics of a low-dose combination oral contraceptive. *Clin Pharmacol Ther.* 1995;58:523-531.

2. Wilbur K, et al. Pharmacokinetic drug interactions between oral contraceptives and second-generation anticonvulsants. *Clin Pharmacokinet.* 2000;38:355-365.

5 Contraceptives, Oral (eg, *Ortho-Novum*)

Gabapentin (eg, *Neurontin*)

SUMMARY: Gabapentin does not appear to affect the pharmacokinetics of an oral contraceptive containing ethinyl estradiol and norethindrone.

RISK FACTORS: No specific risk factors are known.

MECHANISM: No interaction.

CLINICAL EVALUATION: Gabapentin 1,200 mg/day was given to 13 healthy women on an oral contraceptive containing ethinyl estradiol 50 mcg plus norethindrone 2.5 mg.[1] Gabapentin had no effect on the pharmacokinetics of ethinyl estradiol. This lack of interaction is consistent with the fact that gabapentin is not metabolized and is unlikely to be involved in metabolic interactions.

RELATED DRUGS: No information is available.

MANAGEMENT OPTIONS: No interaction.

REFERENCES:

1. Eldon MA, et al. Gabapentin does not interact with a contraceptive regimen of norethindrone acetate and ethinyl estradiol. *Neurology.* 1998;50:1146-1148.

Contraceptives, Oral (eg, *Ortho-Novum*)

Lamotrigine (*Lamictal*)

SUMMARY: Preliminary evidence suggests that lamotrigine has little or no effect on the pharmacokinetics of ethinyl estradiol or levonorgestrel.

RISK FACTORS: No specific risk factors are known.

MECHANISM: No interaction.

CLINICAL EVALUATION: Although earlier reports suggested little or no interaction between lamotrigine and oral contraceptives,[1,2] 2 subsequent studies found reduced lamotrigine plasma concentrations.[3,4] In 1 study, lamotrigine serum concentrations were compared in 3 groups: women on no hormonal contraception; women on oral contraceptives with ethinyl estradiol; and women on progestin-only contraception.[3] Lamotrigine serum concentration-to-dose ratio was 41% lower in women on ethinyl estradiol compared with those not on hormonal contraception. There was no significant difference in lamotrigine concentrations in women on progestin-only contraception compared with those not on hormonal contraception. Another study found lamotrigine AUC was 21% lower in women taking ethinyl estradiol-containing contraception compared with these same women when not taking hormonal contraception.[4] Decreases in ethinyl estradiol and levonorgestrel plasma concentrations have been reported following lamotrigine administration,[1,4] but the effect has generally been small. Nonetheless, the possibility that a rare patient may have reduced oral contraceptive efficacy because of lamotrigine cannot be ruled out.

RELATED DRUGS: No information is available.

MANAGEMENT OPTIONS:

➡ **Monitor.** Monitor for reduced lamotrigine effect if oral contraceptives are used concurrently. Although lamotrigine appears to have only a small effect on plasma concentrations of ethinyl estradiol or levonorgestrel, monitor for evidence of inadequate contraceptive efficacy, such as menstrual irregularities (eg, spotting, breakthrough bleeding).

REFERENCES:

1. Holdich T, et al. Effect of lamotrigine on the pharmacology of the combine oral contraceptive pill. *Epilepsia*. 1991;32:(suppl):96.

2. Hussein Z, et al. Population pharmacokinetics of lamotrigine monotherapy in patients with epilepsy: retrospective analysis of routine monitoring data. *Br J Clin Pharmacol*. 1997;43:457-465.

3. Reimers A, et al. Ethinyl estradiol, not progestogens, reduces lamotrigine serum concentrations. *Epilepsia*. 2005;46:1414-1417.

4. Sidhu J, et al. The pharmacokinetic and pharmacodynamic consequences of the coadministration of lamotrigine and a combined oral contraceptive in healthy female subjects. *Br J Clin Pharmacol*. 2006;61:191-199.

Contraceptives, Oral (eg, *Ortho-Novum*)

Nefazodone

SUMMARY: A woman taking a low-dose oral contraceptive developed symptoms of excessive estrogen effect after starting nefazodone, but the clinical importance of this effect is not established.

RISK FACTORS: No specific risk factors are known.

MECHANISM: Not established. Nefazodone is a potent inhibitor of CYP3A4, and ethinyl estradiol is metabolized by this isozyme. Thus, nefazodone may inhibit ethinyl estradiol metabolism, resulting in increased estrogenic effect.

CLINICAL EVALUATION: A 27-year-old woman on a low-dose oral contraceptive (ethinyl estradiol 20 mcg plus desogestrel 0.15 mg) developed evidence of excessive estrogen effect (eg, breast tenderness, bloating, weight gain) after nefazodone 100 to 150 mg/day was started.[1] The adverse effects resolved after nefazodone was discontinued. Nefazodone appeared to interact with the estrogen in this patient, but the incidence and magnitude of this interaction is not established.

RELATED DRUGS: Fluvoxamine also inhibits CYP3A4, but it is probably less potent than nefazodone. Fluoxetine (eg, *Prozac*) is a weak inhibitor of CYP3A4, but citalopram (eg, *Celexa*), paroxetine (eg, *Paxil*), sertraline (*Zoloft*), and venlafaxine (*Effexor*) appear to have minimal effects on CYP3A4.

MANAGEMENT OPTIONS: No specific action is required, but be alert for evidence of the interaction.

REFERENCES:

1. Adson DE, et al. A probable interaction between a very low-dose oral contraceptive and the antidepressant nefazodone: a case report. *J Clin Psychopharmacol.* 2001;21:618-619.

Contraceptives, Oral (eg, *Nordette-28*)

Oxcarbazepine (*Trileptal*)

SUMMARY: Two studies suggest that oxcarbazepine reduces the plasma concentrations of ethinyl estradiol and levonorgestrel, and may reduce the efficacy of oral contraceptives.

RISK FACTORS: No specific risk factors are known.

MECHANISM: Not established. Oxcarbazepine probably increases the first-pass metabolism of ethinyl estradiol and levonorgestrel.

CLINICAL EVALUATION: In a randomized, crossover study, 16 healthy women took a combination oral contraceptive (ethinyl estradiol 50 mcg and levonorgestrel 250 mcg) with and without concurrent oxcarbazepine (1,200 mg/day).[1] Oxcarbazepine was associated with a 47% reduction in the area under the plasma concentration-time curve (AUC) for both hormones. These results were consistent with an earlier report of reduced AUC for ethinyl estradiol and levonorgestrel in 13 healthy women given oxcarbazepine with a triphasic oral contraceptive.[2] Oxcarbazepine was associated with menstrual irregularities in both studies. These results suggest that oxcarbazepine may reduce the efficacy of oral contraceptives.

RELATED DRUGS: The effect of oxcarbazepine on progestins other than levonorgestrel or estrogens other than ethinyl estradiol is not established, but an interaction could occur.

MANAGEMENT OPTIONS:

➡ *Consider Alternative.* Consider adding other means of contraception to oral contraceptives, especially during the first 2 to 3 months of combined therapy with oxcarbazepine. Alternatively, some studies have recommended using a higher-dose oral contraceptive to maintain adequate hormonal concentrations. This appears to be a reasonable recommendation, but the magnitude of the required dosage increase is likely to vary considerably from 1 patient to another.

➡ *Monitor.* Spotting or breakthrough bleeding in patients taking oral contraceptives and oxcarbazepine could indicate that the drugs are interacting, although lack of breakthrough bleeding does not ensure contraceptive protection.

REFERENCES:

1. Fattore C, et al. Induction of ethinylestradiol and levonorgestrel metabolism by oxycarbazepine in healthy women. *Epilepsia.* 1999;40:783-787.
2. Klosterskov Jensen P, et al. Possible interaction between oxcarbazepine and an oral contraceptive. *Epilepsia.* 1992;33:1149-1152.

Contraceptives, Oral (eg, *Ortho-Novum*) `5`

Oxybutynin (eg, *Ditropan*)

SUMMARY: Available evidence suggests that oral contraceptives do not affect oxybutynin plasma concentrations.

RISK FACTORS: No specific risk factors are known.

MECHANISM: None (no interaction).

CLINICAL EVALUATION: A study in 24 women (13 on oral contraceptives) found no difference in oxybutynin pharmacokinetics in women taking oral contraceptives versus those not on oral contraceptives.[1]

RELATED DRUGS: No information is available.

MANAGEMENT OPTIONS: No interaction.

REFERENCES:
1. Lukkari E, et al. The pharmacokinetics of oxybutynin is unaffected by gender and contraceptive steroids. *Eur J Clin Pharmacol.* 1998;53:351-354.

Contraceptives, Oral (eg, *Ortho-Novum*)

Phenobarbital (eg, *Solfoton*)

SUMMARY: Phenobarbital may reduce the efficacy of oral contraceptives; menstrual irregularities and unintended pregnancies may occur.

RISK FACTORS:

➡ **Dosage Regimen.** It is likely that patients taking low-dose oral contraceptives containing the lowest doses of steroids are most susceptible to this interaction.

MECHANISM: Barbiturates probably enhance the hepatic metabolism of estrogens.

CLINICAL EVALUATION: There are many case reports of patients with seizure disorders who have become pregnant while taking oral contraceptives in combination with anticonvulsants, including phenobarbital.[1-4]

RELATED DRUGS: All barbiturates are likely to enhance estrogen metabolism.

MANAGEMENT OPTIONS:

➡ **Circumvent/Minimize.** Patients receiving chronic barbiturate therapy may require oral contraceptives with a higher estrogen content. If barbiturate use is short-term, use alternative methods of contraception (in addition to the oral contraceptives) during, and for at least several weeks after, barbiturate therapy has been discontinued.

➡ **Monitor.** Spotting or breakthrough bleeding may be an indication that significant enzyme induction is occurring, but a lack of menstrual irregularities does not ensure that the interaction has not occurred.

REFERENCES:
1. Janz D, et al. Letter: Anti-epileptic drugs and failure of oral contraceptives. *Lancet.* 1974;1:1113.
2. Conney AH. Pharmacological implications of microsomal enzyme induction. *Pharmacol Rev.* 1967;19:317-366.
3. Robertson YR, et al. Interactions between oral contraceptives and other drugs: a review. *Curr Med Res Opin.* 1976;3:647.
4. Hempel E, et al. Drug stimulated biotransformation of hormonal steroid contraceptives: clinical implications. *Drugs.* 1976;12:442-448.

Contraceptives, Oral (eg, *Ortho-Novum*)

Phenytoin (eg, *Dilantin*)

SUMMARY: Phenytoin and other enzyme-inducing anticonvulsants, such as barbiturates, carbamazepine, and primidone, may inhibit the effect of oral contraceptives resulting in menstrual irregularities and unplanned pregnancies.

RISK FACTORS: No specific risk factors are known.

MECHANISM: Anticonvulsant-induced enzyme induction may enhance the metabolism of oral contraceptives.[3,9] Conversely, estrogens may inhibit phenytoin metabolism.[2] The suggestion that contraceptive steroids may affect plasma protein binding of anticonvulsants[4] was not confirmed in a study of oral contraceptives on the plasma protein binding of phenytoin.[1]

CLINICAL EVALUATION: A number of unplanned pregnancies have occurred in women taking phenytoin or other anticonvulsants and oral contraceptives concurrently.[6-8] In a retrospective study, 3 of 41 women developed unplanned pregnancies while on oral contraceptives and anticonvulsants; none of the women with seizure disorders on oral contraceptives alone became pregnant.[10] Phenytoin and other anticonvulsants have also been associated with unplanned pregnancies and low norgestrel plasma concentrations in women receiving norgestrel (progestin-only contraception) subdermal capsules.[12] Single-dose pharmacokinetics of oral doses of ethinyl estradiol and levonorgestrel were studied in women before and 8 to 12 weeks after initiating phenytoin (n = 6). Phenytoin decreased the area under the concentration-time curve (AUC) of ethinyl estradiol 49% and levonorgestrel 40%. Although oral contraceptives purportedly can induce seizures,[5] a study of 20 patients with seizure disorders failed to show an effect of oral contraceptives on seizure frequency compared with placebo.[4] Rare clinical cases of estrogen-induced inhibition of phenytoin metabolism have been reported, but the incidence and magnitude of this effect cannot be determined from the data presented.[2]

RELATED DRUGS: Valproic acid (eg, *Depakene*) does not appear to affect the pharmacokinetics of oral contraceptives;[11] clinical evidence and theoretical considerations suggest that benzodiazepine anticonvulsants are unlikely to affect oral contraceptive efficacy. Carbamazepine (eg, *Tegretol*) and primidone (eg, *Mysoline*) may inhibit the effect of oral contraceptives resulting in menstrual irregularities and unplanned pregnancies.

MANAGEMENT OPTIONS:

➡ *Consider Alternative.* When pregnancy is to be avoided in women receiving enzyme-inducing anticonvulsants such as carbamazepine, phenobarbital, phenytoin, and primidone, use a means of contraception other than oral contraceptives. Alternatively, some studies have recommended using a higher estrogen content oral contraceptive for women being treated with an enzyme reducing drug. This method would work best for women on a relatively stable anticonvulsant regimen.

➡ *Monitor.* Individualize this method based on patient response (eg, lack of breakthrough bleeding). Spotting or breakthrough bleeding in patients who are taking oral contraceptives and enzyme-inducing anticonvulsants could indicate that the drugs are interacting, although lack of breakthrough bleeding does not ensure contraceptive protection.[13] Also be alert for evidence of increased phenytoin effect in patients taking oral contraceptives.

REFERENCES:

1. Hooper WD, et al. Plasma protein binding of diphenylhydantoin. Effects of sex hormones, renal and hepatic disease. *Clin Pharmacol Ther.* 1974; 15:276.

2. Kutt H, et al. Management of epilepsy with diphenylhydantoin sodium. *JAMA.* 1968;203:969.

3. Kutt H, et al. Metabolism of diphenylhydantoin by rat liver microsomes. I. Characteristics of the reaction. *Biochem Pharmacol.* 1970;19:675.

4. Espir M, et al. Epilepsy and oral contraception. *BMJ.* 1969;1:294.

5. McArthur J. Oral contraceptives and epilepsy (Notes and Comments). *BMJ.* 1967;3:162.

6. Kenyon IE. Unplanned pregnancy in an epileptic. *BMJ.* 1972;1:686.

7. Janz D, et al. Anti-epileptic drugs and failure of oral contraceptives. *Lancet.* 1974;1:113.

8. Laengner H, et al. Antiepileptic drugs and failure of oral contraceptives. *Lancet.* 1974;2:600.

9. Robertson YR, et al. Interactions between oral contraceptives and other drugs:a review. *Curr Med Res Opin.* 1976;3:647.

10. Coulam CB, et al. Do anticonvulsants reduce the efficacy of oral contraceptives? *Epilepsia.* 1979;20:519.

11. Crawford P, et al. The lack of effect of sodium valproate on the pharmacokinetics or oral contraceptive steroids. *Contraception.* 1986;33:23.

12. Haukkamaa M. Contraception by Norplant subdermal capsules is not reliable in epileptic patients on anticonvulsant treatment. *Contraception.* 1986;33:559.

13. Mattson RH, et al. Use of oral contraceptives by women with epilepsy. *JAMA.* 1986;256:238.

Contraceptives, Oral (eg, *Ortho-Novum*)

Prednisolone (eg, *Prelone*)

SUMMARY: Oral contraceptives and estrogens may enhance the effect of hydrocortisone, prednisolone, and possibly other corticosteroids; adjustments in corticosteroid dosage may be required.

RISK FACTORS: No specific risk factors are known.

MECHANISM: Not established. It is possible that the estrogen-induced increase in serum cortisol-binding globulin retards the metabolism of corticosteroids.

CLINICAL EVALUATION: Women taking oral contraceptives may have a lower metabolic clearance rate for prednisolone than subjects who are not receiving oral contraceptives.[3] The pharmacokinetics of prednisolone 40 mg IV were compared in 8 women receiving oral contraceptives, 5 healthy women who were not taking oral contraceptives, and 8 healthy men.[4] In women taking oral contraceptives, the total plasma clearance of prednisolone was approximately 50% less than that seen in the other 2 groups, and the area under the plasma concentration-time curve for unbound prednisolone was approximately twice that of the other 2 groups. Thus, there is substantial evidence that estrogens and oral contraceptives can enhance the effect of corticosteroids. Estrogen enhances the anti-inflammatory effect of hydrocortisone in patients with chronic inflammatory skin diseases.[2] When estrogen was added, a 3- to 20-fold reduction in the dose of corticosteroid was possible. In another study, estrogen consistently enhanced the glucosuric effect of hydrocortisone administered to 9 diabetic subjects; however, the glucosuric effect of prednisone (eg, *Deltasone*), prednisolone, dexamethasone (eg, *Decadron*), and methylprednisolone (eg, *Medrol*) was not affected consistently by estrogen.[1]

RELATED DRUGS: Most combinations of oral contraceptives and corticosteroids probably interact. (See Clinical Evaluation.)

MANAGEMENT OPTIONS:

➡ *Monitor.* In patients receiving both corticosteroids and oral contraceptives estrogen, watch for evidence of excessive corticosteroid effects. It may be necessary to reduce the dose of the corticosteroid.

REFERENCES:

1. Nelson DH, et al. Potentiation of the biologic effect of administered cortisol by estrogen treatment. *J Clin Endocrinol Metab.* 1963;23:261.

2. Spangler AS, et al. Enhancement of the anti-inflammatory action of hydrocortisone by estrogen. *J Clin Endocrinol.* 1969;29:650.

3. Kozower M, et al. Decreased clearance of prednisolone, a factor in the development of corticosteroid side effects. *J Clin Endocrinol Metab.* 1974;38:407.

4. Boekenoogen SJ, et al. Prednisolone disposition and protein binding in oral contraceptive users. *J Clin Endocrinol Metab.* 1983;56:702.

Contraceptives, Oral (eg, *Ortho-Novum*)

Prochlorperazine (*Compazine*)

SUMMARY: Preliminary evidence indicates that estrogens increase the serum concentrations of some phenothiazines; however, more study is needed.

RISK FACTORS: No specific risk factors are known.

MECHANISM: Not established. Estrogens may decrease the elimination rate of prochlorperazine and butaperazine.

CLINICAL EVALUATION: A dystonic reaction to prochlorperazine was observed in a patient with morning sickness (and presumably high estrogen concentrations). Based on this observation, the effect of conjugated estrogens (*Premarin*) on butaperazine blood concentrations was measured in 4 postmenopausal schizophrenic patients.[1] The plasma concentrations of butaperazine were increased following estrogen treatment as was the area under the plasma concentration-time curve. However, these are preliminary results, and further study is needed to assess the clinical significance of this interaction.

RELATED DRUGS: Butaperazine may interact similarly. The effect of estrogens on other phenothiazines is not established.

MANAGEMENT OPTIONS: No specific action is required, but be alert for evidence of the interaction.

REFERENCES:

1. El-Yousef MK, et al. Estrogen effects on phenothiazine derivative blood levels. *JAMA.* 1974;228:827.

Contraceptives, Oral (eg, *Ortho-Novum*)

Rifabutin (*Mycobutin*)

SUMMARY: Rifabutin can reduce the plasma concentrations of ethinyl estradiol and norethindrone and may reduce oral contraceptive effectiveness; unintended pregnancy may result.

RISK FACTORS: No specific risk factors are known.

MECHANISM: Rifabutin increases the metabolism of ethinyl estradiol and norethindrone, probably by induction of the CYP3A4 enzyme.

CLINICAL EVALUATION: Twenty-two healthy women took an oral contraceptive containing 35 mcg ethinyl estradiol and 1 mg of norethindrone for 21 days.[1] Following baseline pharmacokinetic studies, they resumed the oral contraceptive with the coadministration of rifabutin 300 mg/day for 10 days starting on day 1 of their cycle. Pharmacokinetic studies were repeated on day 10 of rifabutin dosing. The mean area under the concentration-time curve (AUC) of ethinyl estradiol and the peak ethinyl estradiol concentration were reduced 64% and 42%, respectively, by rifabutin treatment. Similar results were noted in a study involving 12 subjects who were given an oral contraceptive with and without rifabutin (300 mg/day).[2] Side effects of reduced ethinyl estradiol, such as spotting, were increased during rifabutin administration. Norethindrone AUC was reduced 20%[1] and 13%[2] during rifabutin administration in the studies.

RELATED DRUGS: All oral contraceptives would be expected to interact in a similar manner with rifabutin. Rifampin is also known to reduce the plasma concentrations of estrogens.

MANAGEMENT OPTIONS:

➡ **Consider Alternative.** Patients receiving rifabutin should use contraceptive methods other than oral contraceptives or use additional contraceptive methods during and for at least 1 cycle after rifabutin is discontinued.

➡ **Monitor.** Watch for evidence of reduced estrogen effect, including menstrual irregularities, as evidence of reduced estrogen concentrations. Counsel patients taking oral contraceptives on the risk of pregnancy during rifabutin administration.

REFERENCES:
1. LeBel M, et al. Effects of rifabutin and rifampicin on the pharmacokinetics of ethinylestradiol and norethindrone. *J Clin Pharmacol.* 1998;38:1042-1050.
2. Barditch-Crovo P, et al. The effects of rifampin and rifabutin on the pharmacokinetics and pharmacodynamics of a combination oral contraceptive. *Clin Pharmacol Ther.* 1999;65:428-438.

Contraceptives, Oral (eg, *Ortho-Novum*)

Rifampin (eg, *Rifadin*)

SUMMARY: Rifampin can reduce the plasma concentrations of ethinyl estradiol and norethindrone and may reduce oral contraceptive effectiveness; unintended pregnancy may result.

RISK FACTORS: No specific risk factors are known.

MECHANISM: Rifampin increases the metabolism of ethinyl estradiol and norethindrone, probably by induction of the CYP3A4 enzyme.

CLINICAL EVALUATION: Twenty-two healthy women took an oral contraceptive containing 35 mcg ethinyl estradiol and 1 mg of norethindrone for 21 days.[1] Following baseline pharmacokinetic studies, they resumed the oral contraceptive with the concurrent administration of rifampin 300 mg/day for 10 days starting on day 1 of their cycle. Pharmacokinetic studies were repeated on day 10 of rifampin dosing. The mean area under the concentration-time curve (AUC) of ethinyl estradiol and the peak ethinyl estradiol concentration were reduced 64% and 42%, respectively, by rifampin treatment. Side effects of reduced ethinyl estradiol, such as spotting, were increased during rifampin administration. Similar results were noted in a study involving 12 subjects who were given an oral contraceptive with and without rifampin (600 mg/day).[2] A reduction in ethinyl estradiol concentrations was also reported during rifampin coadministration.[3] Case reports have noted menstrual irregularities and an increased prevalence of unplanned pregnancies when rifampin is administered with oral contraceptives.[4] An elevation of progesterone, indicating ovulation, has also been noted in women taking oral contraceptives and rifampin.[5] Norethindrone AUC was reduced 60%[1] and 51%[2] during rifampin administration in the studies noted above.

RELATED DRUGS: All oral contraceptives would be expected to interact in a similar manner with rifampin. Rifabutin is also known to reduce the plasma concentrations of estrogens.

MANAGEMENT OPTIONS:

➡ *Consider Alternative.* Patients receiving rifampin should use contraceptive methods other than oral contraceptives or use additional contraceptive methods during and for at least 1 cycle after rifampin is discontinued.

➡ *Monitor.* Watch for evidence of reduced estrogen effect, including menstrual irregularities, as evidence of reduced estrogen concentrations. Counsel patients taking oral contraceptives on the risk of pregnancy during rifampin administration.

REFERENCES:
1. LeBel M, et al. Effects of rifabutin and rifampicin on the pharmacokinetics of ethinylestradiol and norethindrone. *J Clin Pharmacol*. 1998;38:1042-1050.
2. Barditch-Crovo P, et al. The effects of rifampin and rifabutin on the pharmacokinetics and pharmacodynamics of a combination oral contraceptive. *Clin Pharmacol Ther*. 1999;65:428-438.
3. Back DJ, et al. The effect of rifampicin on the pharmacokinetics of ethynylestradiol in women. *Contraception*. 1980;21:135-143.
4. Skolnick JL, et al. Rifampin, oral contraceptives, and pregnancy. *JAMA*. 1976;236:1382.
5. Meyer B, et al. A model to detect interactions between roxithromycin and oral contraceptives. *Clin Pharmacol Ther*. 1990;47:671-674.

 3

Contraceptives, Oral (eg, *Ortho-Novum*)

Ritonavir (*Norvir*)

SUMMARY: Ritonavir is reported to reduce ethinyl estradiol concentrations. Loss of contraceptive activity could occur.

RISK FACTORS: No specific risk factors are known.

MECHANISM: Not established. Ritonavir may increase the activity of glucuronyl transferases or other enzymes responsible for ethinyl estradiol metabolism. The oral bioavailability of ethinyl estradiol is 40% to 50%.[1] Approximately 60% of the first-pass metabolism is by conjugation with sulfate and the remainder of the first-pass metabolism is probably via CYP3A4 hydroxylation or glucuronidation. Ethinyl estradiol that reaches the systemic circulation is hydroxylated by CYP3A4 or conjugated with glucuronide. The glucuronides are secreted into the liver bile and may be hydrolyzed by gut bacteria back to ethinyl estradiol that can then be reabsorbed. An increase in glucuronidation or a reduction in the bacterial hydrolysis of glucuronide metabolites could result in reduced ethinyl estradiol plasma concentrations. It is also thought that ritonavir induces CYP3A4 and then inhibits the metabolism of other drugs that are metabolized by CYP3A4. Thus, one would assume that ritonavir also would reduce the metabolism of ethinyl estradiol, resulting in an increase in estradiol concentrations. While the manufacturer suggests that this interaction is the result of enhanced glucuronidation, the mechanism of this interaction awaits further study.

CLINICAL EVALUATION: While no published data are available for evaluation, the manufacturer of ritonavir has made available some data on this interaction. The pharmacokinetics of an oral contraceptive containing 50 mcg ethinyl estradiol were compared in a noncrossover trial involving 23 subjects.[2] The administration of ritonavir 500 mg every 12 hours for 16 days resulted in a 40% reduction in the area under the concentration-time curve (AUC) of ethinyl estradiol compared with the AUC measured in subjects receiving only ethinyl estradiol. The half-life of ethinyl estradiol averaged 32% shorter in women taking concomitant ritonavir. These changes suggest an increase in the metabolism of ethinyl estradiol, a reduction in its bioavailability, a reduction in its tissue binding, or some combination of the three. A reduction in contraceptive efficacy is possible.

RELATED DRUGS: Indinavir (*Crixivan*) has been noted to increase ethinyl estradiol concentrations 24%.[3] The effect of ritonavir on other estrogens is unknown. While no data are available, saquinavir (*Fortovase*) and nelfinavir (*Viracept*) would be less likely to interact with ethinyl estradiol.

MANAGEMENT OPTIONS:

➡ *Consider Alternative.* Patients receiving ritonavir and oral contraceptives should utilize an alternative method of birth control during ritonavir administration and for at least 1 cycle following its discontinuation. Indinavir does not appear to reduce oral contraceptive concentrations and could be considered as an alternative antiviral agent.

➡ *Monitor.* Monitor patients for signs that may indicate insufficient estrogen concentrations such as breakthrough bleeding.

REFERENCES:

1. Shenfield GM. Oral contraceptives. Are drug interactions of clinical significance? *Drug Saf.* 1993;9:21-37.

2. Product information. Ritonavir (*Norvir*). Abbott Laboratories. 1996.

3. Product information. Indinavir (*Crixivan*). Merck and Company, Inc. 1996.

Contraceptives, Oral (eg, *Ortho-Novum*)

Selegiline (eg, *Eldepryl*)

SUMMARY: Women on oral contraceptives appear to have considerably higher serum concentrations of selegiline, but the extent to which this increases the risk of selegiline drug interactions or adverse effects is not established.

RISK FACTORS: No specific risk factors are known.

MECHANISM: Not established. It is possible that oral contraceptives inhibit the N-demethylation of selegiline.

CLINICAL EVALUATION: Eight women (4 taking oral contraceptives) were given 4 different doses of selegiline (5, 10, 20, and 40 mg) in a 4-period randomized study.[1] The serum concentrations of selegiline in the 4 women taking oral contraceptives were approximately 20-fold higher than in the women not taking oral contraceptives.

This is of potential clinical concern because at higher serum concentrations selegiline can lose its MAO-B selectivity and can become a nonselective MAO inhibitor. This, in turn, can increase the risk of serious drug-drug and drug-food interactions, resulting in acute hypertensive reactions or serotonin syndrome.

RELATED DRUGS: No information is available.

MANAGEMENT OPTIONS:

➡ *Consider Alternative.* In patients receiving selegiline, consider advising use of contraceptive methods other than oral contraceptives. When selegiline is being used for parkinsonism, most patients would not be of an age to need contraception, but selegiline is occasionally used for disorders other than parkinsonism.

➡ *Monitor.* When selegiline is used in women taking oral contraceptives, watch for evidence of nonselective MAO inhibition (eg, hypertensive reactions to tyramine or sympathomimetics, serotonin syndrome when combined with other serotonergic drugs).

REFERENCES:

1. Laine K, et al. Dose linearity study of selegiline pharmacokinetics after oral administration: evidence for strong drug interaction with female sex steroids. *Br J Clin Pharmacol.* 1999;47:249-254.

Contraceptives, Oral (eg, *Ortho-Novum*)

St. John's Wort

SUMMARY: Several cases of menstrual breakthrough bleeding and at least 1 unintended pregnancy have been reported in association with use of St. John's wort in patients taking oral contraceptives. Although a causal relationship has not been established, patients on oral contraceptives should avoid St. John's wort or consider using additional contraceptive methods.

RISK FACTORS: No specific risk factors are known.

MECHANISM: Not established. Other clinical evidence suggest St. John's wort enhances CYP3A4 activity, and estrogens are metabolized by this isozyme. Therefore, it is possible that St. John's wort enhances the hepatic metabolism of the estrogens (and possibly the progestins) in oral contraceptives.

CLINICAL EVALUATION: The Swedish Medical Products Agency has received several case reports of breakthrough menstrual bleeding following the use of St. John's wort in patients taking long-term oral contraceptives.[1] Menstrual irregularities can be a sign of inadequate circulating contraceptive hormone concentrations. Although only a few cases of breakthrough bleeding were reported and few details were presented, the findings are consistent with other reports of St. John's wort reducing the plasma concentrations of drugs that are substrates for CYP3A4 or p-glycoprotein.[2-4] Unintended pregnancy has been reported in women on oral contraceptives who took St. John's wort.[5] It is not possible to establish a causal relationship in such anecdotal cases, but it is consistent with the menstrual irregularities described above.

RELATED DRUGS: No information is available.

MANAGEMENT OPTIONS:

➡ *Consider Alternative.* In patients receiving oral contraceptives, consider using alternative antidepressants. Selective serotonin reuptake inhibitors (SSRIs) are not known to induce CYP3A4. SSRIs include fluoxetine (*Prozac*), paroxetine (*Paxil*), sertraline (*Zoloft*), and citalopram (*Celexa*).

➥ **Circumvent/Minimize.** Consider the use of additional forms of contraception if St. John's wort is used with oral contraceptives.

➥ **Monitor.** Menstrual irregularities, such as breakthrough bleeding, may be signs of reduced oral contraceptive efficacy, but the absence of menstrual irregularities does not ensure adequate contraception.

REFERENCES:
1. Yue QY, et al. Safety of St. John's wort. *Lancet*. 2000;355:576-577.
2. Ruschitzka F, et al. Acute heart transplant rejection due to Saint John's wort. *Lancet*. 2000;355:548-549.
3. Piscitelli SC, et al. Indinavir concentrations and St. John's wort. *Lancet*. 2000;355:547-548.
4. Johne A, et al. Pharmacokinetic interaction of digoxin with an herbal extract from St. John's wort (*hypericum perforatum*). *Clin Pharmacol Ther*. 1999;66:338-345.
5. Schwarz UI, et al. Unwanted pregnancy on self-medication with St. John's wort despite hormonal contraception. *Br J Clin Pharmacol*. 2003;55:112-113.

Contraceptives, Oral (eg, *Ortho-Novum*)

Tetracycline (eg, *Sumycin*)

SUMMARY: Case reports suggest that tetracycline can reduce the effectiveness of oral contraceptives; a prospective study failed to demonstrate an effect in a small number of women.

RISK FACTORS: No specific risk factors are known.

MECHANISM: Not established. Tetracycline may interfere with the enterohepatic circulation of estrogens by reducing bacterial hydrolysis of conjugated estrogens in the intestine.

CLINICAL EVALUATION: Several cases of unintended pregnancy and menstrual irregularities have been reported following concurrent use of tetracyclines and oral contraceptives.[1-4] Tetracycline 500 mg every 6 hours had no effect on plasma ethinyl estradiol or norethindrone concentrations in 7 healthy subjects taking an oral contraceptive.[5] Likewise, doxycycline (eg, *Vibramycin*) had no effect on ethinyl estradiol or norethindrone concentrations.[6] Interactions with antibiotics may be rare and, therefore, difficult to detect in small, prospective studies.

RELATED DRUGS: Other oral antibiotics have been associated with oral contraceptive failure.

MANAGEMENT OPTIONS:

➥ **Monitor.** Although evidence of interaction between tetracyclines and oral contraceptives is limited, counsel women taking oral contraceptives to use additional forms of contraception during tetracycline therapy.

REFERENCES:
1. Orme ML. The clinical pharmacology of oral contraceptive steroids. *Br J Clin Pharmacol*. 1982;14:31-42.
2. Bacon JF, et al. Pregnancy attributable to interaction between tetracycline and oral contraceptives. *Br Med J*. 1980;280:293.
3. DeSano EA, et al. Possible interactions of antihistamines and antibiotics with oral contraceptive effectiveness. *Fertil Steril*. 1982;37:853-854.

4. Back DJ, et al. Evaluation of Committee on Safety of Medicines yellow card reports on oral contraceptive-drug interactions with anticonvulsants and antibiotics. *Br J Clin Pharmacol.* 1988;25:527-532.

5. Murphy AA, et al. The effect of tetracycline on levels of oral contraceptives. *Am J Obstet Gynecol.* 1991;164:28-33.

6. Neely JL, et al. The effect of doxycycline on serum levels of ethinyl estradiol, norethindrone, and endogenous progesterone. *Obstet Gynecol.* 1991;77:416-420.

5   Contraceptives, Oral (eg, *Ortho-Novum*)

Thalidomide (*Thalomid*)

SUMMARY: Thalidomide does not appear to affect the pharmacokinetics of ethinyl estradiol or norethindrone.

RISK FACTORS: No specific risk factors are known.

MECHANISM: No interaction.

CLINICAL EVALUATION: Ten healthy women were given single oral doses of ethinyl estradiol 0.07 mg plus norethindrone 2 mg with and without pretreatment with 3 weeks of thalidomide 200 mg/day.[1] Thalidomide did not affect any of the pharmacokinetic measurements for ethinyl estradiol or norethindrone (maximal plasma concentrations, area under the concentration-time curve, half-life, oral clearance). This suggests that thalidomide is not likely to impair the efficacy of oral contraceptives containing these 2 hormones. Nonetheless, these results do not rule out the possibility of an interaction between thalidomide and other estrogens or progestins, nor do they rule out the possibility of a nonpharmacokinetic interaction between thalidomide and ethinyl estradiol or norethindrone. These possibilities appear unlikely, but given the danger of a pregnancy during thalidomide therapy, it is important to rigorously rule out the possibility of interactions.

RELATED DRUGS: The effect of thalidomide on other estrogens and progestins has not been established. Interactions appear unlikely, but studies are needed to establish this with certainty.

MANAGEMENT OPTIONS: No interaction.

REFERENCES:
1. Trapnell CB, et al. Thalidomide does not alter the pharmacokinetics of ethinyl estradiol and norethindrone. *Clin Pharmacol Ther.* 1998;64:597-602.

4   Contraceptives, Oral (eg, *Ortho-Novum*)

Theophylline (eg, *Theochron*)

SUMMARY: Oral contraceptives have been reported to increase serum theophylline concentrations. The effect may be greater when theophylline is given orally rather than intravenously (IV) and when oral contraceptives containing more than estrogen 35 mcg are used. More study is needed.

RISK FACTORS: No specific risk factors are known.

MECHANISM: Oral contraceptives appear to inhibit the hepatic metabolism of theophylline.[1]

CLINICAL EVALUATION: Aminophylline oral 4 mg/kg solution was given to 8 healthy women on long-term treatment with an oral contraceptive (norgestrel 0.5 mg with ethinyl estradiol 50 mcg). Aminophylline clearances were compared with those of

8 matched control patients who were not taking oral contraceptives.[2] Those taking oral contraceptives had a 34% lower plasma clearance of theophylline than controls. In another study of 22 women, those taking an oral contraceptive (norgestrel 0.5 mg with ethinyl estradiol 50 mcg) had a lower theophylline clearance than women who were not taking oral contraceptives.[2] The inhibitory effect of oral contraceptives on theophylline clearance was more notably offset if the subject was also a smoker. Inhibition of theophylline elimination associated with oral contraceptives was found in another study of women taking oral contraceptives (estrogen dose not stated) who received oral theophylline.[3] Conversely, a subsequent study of 10 adolescent girls taking oral contraceptives (containing estrogen 35 mcg) found no difference in the pharmacokinetics of IV theophylline (given as aminophylline 7.6 mg/kg) when compared with 10 matched control subjects.[4] Although the reasons for the conflicting results are not clear, compared with the positive studies,[1-3] the negative study[4] involved IV instead of oral theophylline, low-dose oral contraceptives, shorter-term use of oral contraceptives, and younger subjects. It is possible the oral contraceptive–induced inhibition of theophylline elimination is most likely to occur with oral administration of theophylline and with oral contraceptives containing more than 35 mcg of estrogen, but additional study is needed to confirm this possibility.

RELATED DRUGS: No information is available.

MANAGEMENT OPTIONS: No specific action is required, but be alert for evidence of the interaction.

REFERENCES:
1. Gardner MJ, et al. Effects of oral contraceptives and tobacco use on the metabolic pathways of theophylline. *Int J Pharmaceut.* 1986;33:55.
2. Tornatore KM, et al. Effect of chronic oral contraceptive steroids on theophylline disposition. *Eur J Clin Pharmacol.* 1982;23:129-134.
3. Roberts RK, et al. Oral contraceptive steroids impair the elimination of theophylline. *J Lab Clin Med.* 1983;101:821-825.
4. Koren G, et al. Theophylline pharmacokinetics in adolescent females following coadministration of oral contraceptives. *Clin Invest Med.* 1985;8:222-226.

Contraceptives, Oral (eg, *Ortho-Novum*)

Thyroid

SUMMARY: Theoretically, oral contraceptives or estrogen therapy lower unbound (pharmacologically active) thyroxine concentrations in patients who depend upon exogenous thyroid to maintain a euthyroid state.

RISK FACTORS: No specific risk factors are known.

MECHANISM: Estrogens increase serum thyroxine-binding globulin (TBG), which would tend to decrease "free" or unbound thyroxine concentrations. A patient with normal thyroid function will compensate by increasing thyroxine synthesis. In contrast, a hypothyroid patient who must depend on exogenous thyroid replacement therapy will be unable to compensate for decreased concentrations of the free or active form of thyroxine. Thus, the response to exogenous thyroid replacement therapy may decrease, and dose requirements may increase. Patients without a functioning thyroid gland who are on thyroid replacement therapy may require higher thyroid replacement doses if estrogens or oral contraceptives are started.

CLINICAL EVALUATION: The ability of oral contraceptives and estrogens to increase serum TBG is well established, but the effect of this increase on patients receiving thyroid replacement therapy is based largely on theoretical considerations rather than clinical evidence.[1,2]

RELATED DRUGS: No information is available.

MANAGEMENT OPTIONS: No specific action is required, but be alert for evidence of the interaction.

REFERENCES:
1. Margulis RR, et al. Effect of oral contraceptives on thyroid function (Questions and Answers). *JAMA.* 1968;206:2326.
2. Wiener JD. Thyroid hormones and protein-bound iodine. *JAMA.* 1969;207:1717.

Contraceptives, Oral (eg, *Ortho-Novum*)

Tizanidine (eg, *Zanaflex*)

SUMMARY: Women taking oral contraceptives (OCs) may have higher than expected tizanidine plasma concentrations; tizanidine dosage adjustments may be needed.

RISK FACTORS: No specific risk factors are known.

MECHANISM: Not established. Oral contraceptives may inhibit the metabolism of tizanidine by CYP1A2.

CLINICAL EVALUATION: In a parallel-group study of tizanidine pharmacokinetics and pharmacodynamics in 15 healthy women using OCs compared with 15 healthy women not taking OCs, the women on OCs had an almost 4-fold higher area under the tizanidine plasma concentration-time curve and increased hypotensive effect.[1] Theoretically, this could increase the risk of tizanidine toxicity (eg, hypotension, bradycardia, CNS depression).

RELATED DRUGS: No information is available.

MANAGEMENT OPTIONS: No specific action is required, but be alert for evidence of the interaction.

REFERENCES:
1. Granfors MT, et al. Oral contraceptives containing ethinyl estradiol and gestodene markedly increase plasma concentrations and effects of tizanidine by inhibiting cytochrome P450 1A2. *Clin Pharmacol Ther.* 2005;78:400-411.

Contraceptives, Oral (eg, *Ortho-Novum*)

Topiramate (*Topamax*)

SUMMARY: Topiramate can moderately reduce serum concentrations of ethinyl estradiol, but the degree to which this would increase the risk of contraceptive failure is not established.

RISK FACTORS: No specific risk factors are known.

MECHANISM: Not established. It is possible that topiramate enhances the metabolism of estrogens.

CLINICAL EVALUATION: Twelve healthy women taking valproic acid (eg, *Depakene*) were given a combination oral contraceptive (norethindrone 1 mg plus ethinyl estradiol 35 mcg) for 1 cycle (baseline).[1] Topiramate was then added in increasing doses (up to 400 mg twice daily) for the next 3 cycles. All topiramate doses were associated with a decrease in ethinyl estradiol area under the concentration-time curve, with the largest topiramate dose producing a moderate 30% decreases. It is not known whether the magnitude of this effect would be sufficient to reduce the efficacy of oral contraceptives, but it seems likely that at least an occasional patient would be affected.

RELATED DRUGS: The effect of topiramate on estrogens other than ethinyl estradiol is not established, but an interaction could occur.

MANAGEMENT OPTIONS:

➡ *Consider Alternative.* Consider adding other means of contraception to the oral contraceptive, especially during the first 2 to 3 months of combined therapy with topiramate. Alternatively, some have recommended using a higher-dose oral contraceptive to maintain adequate hormonal concentrations. This appears to be a reasonable recommendation, but the magnitude of the required dosage increase is likely to vary considerably from one patient to another.

➡ *Monitor.* Spotting or breakthrough bleeding in patients taking oral contraceptives and topiramate could indicate that the drugs are interacting, although lack of breakthrough bleeding does not ensure contraceptive protection.

REFERENCES:

1. Rosenfeld WE, et al. Effect of topiramate on the pharmacokinetics of an oral contraceptive containing norethindrone and ethinyl estradiol in patients with epilepsy. *Epilepsia.* 1997;38(3):317-23.

Contraceptives, Oral (eg, *Nordette-28*)

Vigabatrin (*Sabril;* investigational)

SUMMARY: Vigabatrin does not appear to affect the pharmacokinetics of ethinyl estradiol or levonorgestrel.

RISK FACTORS: No specific risk factors are known.

MECHANISM: No interaction.

CLINICAL EVALUATION: In 13 healthy women, vigabatrin 3 g/day for 4 weeks had no effect on the pharmacokinetics of ethinyl estradiol or levonorgestrel.[1]

RELATED DRUGS: No information is available.

MANAGEMENT OPTIONS: No interaction.

REFERENCES:

1. Bartoli A, et al. A double-blind, placebo-controlled study on the effect of vigabatrin on in vivo parameters of hepatic microsomal enzyme induction and on the kinetics of steroid oral contraceptives in healthy female volunteers. *Epilepsia.* 1997;38:702-707.

2   Contraceptives, Oral (eg, *Ortho-Novum*)

Warfarin (eg, *Coumadin*)

SUMMARY: Oral contraceptives have been reported to increase and decrease anticoagulant response, depending upon the oral anticoagulant. Most patients requiring oral anticoagulants should avoid oral contraceptives because they may increase the risk of thromboembolic disorders.

RISK FACTORS: No specific risk factors are known.

MECHANISM: Oral contraceptives may increase the activity of certain clotting factors in the blood. The ability of oral contraceptives to increase the clearance of phenprocoumon[†] may be related to enhanced phenprocoumon metabolism. Phenprocoumon undergoes glucuronide conjugation, a process that is increased by oral contraceptives. However, oral contraceptives also have been shown to inhibit oxidative drug metabolism; thus, it cannot be assumed that the clearance of oral anticoagulants other than phenprocoumon would be increased.

CLINICAL EVALUATION: Because oral contraceptives should be avoided in patients with thromboembolic disorders, the combined use of oral contraceptives and oral anticoagulants should be uncommon. Nonetheless, some reports have described the effect of oral contraceptives on oral anticoagulants. Seven women on various oral contraceptives (containing 30 to 50 mcg estrogen) were given a single oral dose of phenprocoumon 0.22 mg/kg.[1] The clearance of phenprocoumon was 25% higher in these women than in 7 matched controls not receiving oral contraceptives. Similarly, oral contraceptives have been shown clinically to decrease the anticoagulant response to dicumarol.[2] However, a subsequent study found that the response to acenocoumarol was enhanced in the presence of oral contraceptives.[3] Limited data are available concerning the effect of oral contraceptives on the response to warfarin.

RELATED DRUGS: No information is available.

MANAGEMENT OPTIONS:

➡ *Avoid Unless Benefit Outweighs Risk.* Patients on oral anticoagulants should avoid oral contraceptives because the contraceptives may increase the risk of thromboembolic disorders.

➡ *Monitor.* If an oral contraceptive must be used in a patient receiving an oral anticoagulant, monitor for altered hypoprothrombinemic response when the oral contraceptive is initiated, or discontinued, or if its hormone content is changed.

REFERENCES:

1. Monig H, et al. Effect of oral contraceptive steroids on the pharmacokinetics of phenprocoumon. *Br J Clin Pharmacol*. 1990;30:115-118.
2. Schrogie JJ, et al. Effect of oral contraceptives on vitamin K-dependent clotting activity. *Clin Pharmacol Ther*. 1967;8:670-675.
3. de Teresa E, et al. Interaction between anticoagulants and contraceptives: an unsuspected finding. *Br Med J*. 1979;2:1260-1261.

† Not available in the United States.

Contrast Media

Propranolol (eg, *Inderal*)

SUMMARY: Patients taking beta-blockers, such as propranolol, are at increased risk for anaphylaxis following the administration of IV contrast media.

RISK FACTORS:

➡ ***Concurrent Diseases.*** Patients with a prior history of anaphylactoid reactions may be at particular risk.

MECHANISM: Not established.

CLINICAL EVALUATION: Forty-nine patients who developed anaphylactoid reactions after receiving IV contrast media were compared with 83 case-control patients.[1] The risk of developing anaphylaxis was 3 times higher (0.12% versus 0.38%) among patients taking beta-blockers compared with those who were not. Additionally, the risk of hospitalization following the anaphylactic reaction was 9 times higher in the group taking beta-blockers. No class of beta-blockers (eg, $beta_1$-selective agents) appears to offer a reduced risk. Note that beta-blockers can inhibit the pressor and bronchodilator response of epinephrine in patients who develop anaphylaxis.[2,3]

RELATED DRUGS: All beta-blockers may increase the risk of anaphylaxis following contrast media.

MANAGEMENT OPTIONS:

➡ ***Circumvent/Minimize.*** While the overall incidence of anaphylaxis is low following contrast media, the use of lower-osmolality contrast agents or pretreatment with antihistamines and corticosteroids might be considered for patients taking beta-blockers.

➡ ***Monitor.*** Watch for an increased incidence of anaphylaxis in patients taking beta-blockers who receive contrast media.

REFERENCES:

1. Lang DM, et al. Increased risk for anaphylactoid reaction from contrast media in patients on beta-adrenergic blockers or with asthma. *Ann Intern Med*. 1991;115:270-276.
2. Jacobs RL, et al. Potentiated anaphylaxis in patients with drug-induced beta-adrenergic blockade. *J Allergy Clin Immunol*. 1981;68:125-127.
3. Hannaway PJ, et al. Severe anaphylaxis and drug-induced beta-blockade. *N Engl J Med*. 1983;308:1536.

Cranberry Juice **4**

Warfarin (eg, *Coumadin*)

SUMMARY: A man on warfarin developed an excessive hypoprothrombinemic response and fatal bleeding after extensive ingestion of cranberry juice, but a causal relationship was not established.

RISK FACTORS: No specific risk factors are known.

MECHANISM: Not established. Study in healthy subjects suggests that cranberry juice does not inhibit CYP2C9, so if an interaction exists it may be because of a mechanism other than inhibition of the CYP2C9 metabolism of warfarin.[1]

CLINICAL EVALUATION: A man on chronic warfarin developed an international normalized ratio (INR) over 50 and fatal hemorrhage after ingesting large amounts of cranberry juice.[2] He also ate very little during this time, and it is not possible to determine whether cranberry juice played a role in the excessive hypoprothrombinemia. In another case, a 69-year-old man on warfarin developed marked elevation in INR after ingesting cranberry juice (about 2 L/day) for prevention of urinary tract infections.[3] Although a causal relationship was not established in these 2 cases, it is possible that large amounts of cranberry juice increased warfarin response.

RELATED DRUGS: No information is available.

MANAGEMENT OPTIONS: No specific action is required, but be alert for evidence of the interaction.

REFERENCES:

1. Greenblatt DJ, et al. Interaction of flurbiprofen with cranberry juice, grape juice, tea, and fluconazole: in vitro and clinical studies. *Clin Pharmacol Ther*. 2006;79:125-133.
2. Suvarna R, et al. Possible interaction between warfarin and cranberry juice. *BMJ*. 2003;327:1454.
3. Grant P. Warfarin and cranberry juice: an interaction? *J Heart Valve Dis*. 2004;13:25-26.

Cromolyn (eg, *Intal*)

Dexamethasone (eg, *Decadron*)

SUMMARY: The small effect of cromolyn on dexamethasone disposition is unlikely to be clinically important.

RISK FACTORS: No specific risk factors are known.

MECHANISM: Not established.

CLINICAL EVALUATION: Cromolyn therapy produced a slight decrease in the clearance of dexamethasone in 4 asthmatic patients,[1] but the magnitude of the change seems insufficient to affect dexamethasone response.

RELATED DRUGS: No information is available.

MANAGEMENT OPTIONS: No specific action is required, but be alert for evidence of the interaction.

REFERENCES:

1. Brooks SM, et al. The effects of disodium cromoglycate on dexamethasone metabolism. *Am Rev Respir Dis*. 1976;114(6):1191-1194.

5 Cromolyn (eg, *Intal*)

Ethanol (Ethyl Alcohol)

SUMMARY: Cromolyn does not appear to interact with ethanol.

RISK FACTORS: No specific risk factors are known.

MECHANISM: No interaction.

CLINICAL EVALUATION: Results of psychomotor tests in subjects receiving cromolyn and ethanol failed to reveal evidence of a clinically significant interaction.[1]

RELATED DRUGS: No information is available.

MANAGEMENT OPTIONS: No interaction.

REFERENCES:
1. Crawford WA, et al. The effect of disodium cromoglycate on human performance, alone and in combination with ethanol. *Med J Aust.* 1976;1(26):997-999.

Cyclizine (eg, *Marezine*)

Donepezil (eg, *Aricept*)

SUMMARY: Cyclizine is an anticholinergic drug and may inhibit the therapeutic effect of donepezil in Alzheimer disease.

RISK FACTORS: No specific risk factors are known.

MECHANISM: Donepezil is a cholinesterase inhibitor and thus increases cholinergic activity; its efficacy is likely to be inhibited by anticholinergic drugs such as cyclizine.[1]

CLINICAL EVALUATION: In a preliminary study of 69 patients with Alzheimer disease receiving donepezil 10 mg/day and followed for 2 years, 16 patients received concurrent therapy with anticholinergic drugs and 53 patients did not.[2] Mental functioning, as measured by the Mini-Mental State Exam (MMSE), was significantly lower in the patients receiving concomitant anticholinergic drugs. Also, the French Pharmacovigilance Database received 118 spontaneous reports of adverse reactions in patients receiving anticholinergic drugs with cholinesterase inhibitors (eg, donepezil, galantamine, rivastigmine). After evaluation by clinical pharmacologists, 24 were thought to be adverse drug interactions.[3] Although additional study is needed to establish the clinical importance of these interactions, the evidence is consistent with the known pharmacological effects of the drugs. Short-term use of an anticholinergic antiemetic may not cause significant interaction.

RELATED DRUGS: All cholinesterase inhibitors used to treat Alzheimer disease (donepezil, galantamine [eg, *Razadyne*], rivastigmine [eg, *Exelon*]) are expected to interact similarly with cyclizine and other anticholinergic antiemetics, such as dimenhydrinate (eg, *Dramamine*), meclizine (eg, *Antivert*), prochlorperazine (eg, *Compro*), and scopolamine (eg, *Scopace*).

MANAGEMENT OPTIONS:

➡ ***Consider Alternative.*** If possible, use an alternative to cyclizine or other anticholinergic antiemetic drugs (see Related Drugs).

➡ ***Monitor.*** If cyclizine or other anticholinergic antiemetic drugs are used with donepezil or another cholinesterase inhibitor, be alert for evidence of reduced mental functioning.

REFERENCES:
1. *Aricept* [package insert]. New York, NY: Pfizer; 2011.
2. Lu CJ, Tune LE. Chronic exposure to anticholinergic medications adversely affects the course of Alzheimer disease. *Am J Geriatr Psychiatry.* 2003;11(4):458-461.
3. Tavassoli N, et al. Drug interactions with cholinesterase inhibitors: an analysis of the French Pharmacovigilance Database and a comparison of two national drug formularies (Vidal, British National Formulary). *Drug Saf.* 2007;30(11):1063-1071.

Cyclobenzaprine (eg, *Flexeril*)

Donepezil (eg, *Aricept*)

SUMMARY: Cyclobenzaprine has anticholinergic properties and may inhibit the therapeutic effect of donepezil in Alzheimer disease.

RISK FACTORS: No specific risk factors are known.

MECHANISM: Donepezil is a cholinesterase inhibitor and thus increases cholinergic activity; its efficacy is likely to be inhibited by anticholinergic drugs such as cyclobenzaprine.[1]

CLINICAL EVALUATION: In a preliminary study of 69 patients with Alzheimer disease receiving donepezil 10 mg/day and followed for 2 years, 16 patients received concurrent therapy with anticholinergic drugs and 53 patients did not.[2] Mental functioning, as measured by the Mini-Mental State Exam (MMSE), was significantly lower in the patients receiving concomitant anticholinergic drugs. Also, the French Pharmacovigilance Database received 118 spontaneous reports of adverse reactions in patients receiving anticholinergic drugs with cholinesterase inhibitors (eg, donepezil, galantamine, rivastigmine). After evaluation by clinical pharmacologists, 24 were thought to be adverse drug interactions.[3] Although additional study is needed to establish the clinical importance of these interactions, the evidence is consistent with the known pharmacological effects of the drugs. Short-term use of an anticholinergic muscle relaxant may not cause significant interaction.

RELATED DRUGS: All cholinesterase inhibitors used to treat Alzheimer disease (donepezil, galantamine [eg, *Razadyne*], rivastigmine [eg, *Exelon*]) are expected to interact similarly with cyclobenzaprine or other muscle relaxants with anticholinergic properties, such as methocarbamol (eg, *Robaxin*) and orphenadrine (eg, *Norflex*).

MANAGEMENT OPTIONS:

➡ **Consider Alternative.** If possible, use an alternative to cyclobenzaprine or other anticholinergic muscle relaxants (see Related Drugs).

➡ **Monitor.** If cyclobenzaprine or other anticholinergic muscle relaxants are used with donepezil or another cholinesterase inhibitor, be alert for evidence of reduced mental functioning.

REFERENCES:

1. *Aricept* [package insert]. New York, NY: Pfizer; 2011.
2. Lu CJ, Tune LE. Chronic exposure to anticholinergic medications adversely affects the course of Alzheimer disease. *Am J Geriatr Psychiatry.* 2003;11(4):458-461.
3. Tavassoli N, et al. Drug interactions with cholinesterase inhibitors: an analysis of the French Pharmacovigilance Database and a comparison of two national drug formularies (Vidal, British National Formulary). *Drug Saf.* 2007;30(11):1063-1071.

Cyclobenzaprine (eg, *Flexeril*)

Droperidol (eg, *Inapsine*)

SUMMARY: A patient receiving cyclobenzaprine and fluoxetine (eg, *Prozac*) developed ventricular tachycardia and fibrillation after droperidol was added, but the relative contribution of each drug to the adverse reaction is not clear.

RISK FACTORS: No specific risk factors are known.

MECHANISM: It was proposed that droperidol and cyclobenzaprine had additive effects in prolonging the QT interval and contributing to the arrhythmia. Fluoxetine also may inhibit cyclobenzaprine metabolism, with resulting increased cyclobenzaprine serum concentrations contributing to the reaction. Nonetheless, the ability of fluoxetine to inhibit cyclobenzaprine metabolism and the ability of cyclobenzaprine to prolong the QT interval are based primarily on theoretical considerations rather than clinical evidence.

CLINICAL EVALUATION: A 59-year-old woman on long-term therapy with cyclobenzaprine 10 mg/day and fluoxetine 30 mg/day was noted on electrocardiogram (ECG) to have a prolonged QTc interval.[1] Prior to surgery to repair her Achilles tendon, she received droperidol 0.625 mg intravenous and metoclopramide (eg, *Reglan*) 10 mg IV. During surgery she developed polymorphic ventricular tachycardia (torsades de pointes), which progressed into ventricular fibrillation. She was successfully defibrillated. While it is reasonable to assume that the droperidol contributed to the arrhythmia, the role of the cyclobenzaprine and fluoxetine is not clear. Although the case for a causal relationship is weak, the severity of the adverse reaction warrants monitoring.

RELATED DRUGS: Theoretically, antipsychotic drugs other than droperidol that also prolong the QT interval could produce similar effects.

MANAGEMENT OPTIONS:

➡ **Monitor.** Monitor for evidence of polymorphic ventricular tachycardia (eg, fainting, light-headedness). Monitor the ECG for excessive prolongation of the QTc interval.

REFERENCES:

1. Michalets EL, et al. Torsade de pointes resulting from the addition of droperidol to an existing cytochrome P450 drug interaction. *Ann Pharmacother.* 1998;32(7-8):761-765.

Cyclobenzaprine (eg, *Flexeril*)

Duloxetine (*Cymbalta*)

SUMMARY: A patient developed serotonin toxicity after receiving concurrent cyclobenzaprine and duloxetine.

RISK FACTORS: No specific risk factors are known.

MECHANISM: Probably additive serotonergic effects.

CLINICAL EVALUATION: A 53-year-old man on duloxetine 60 mg/day developed symptoms of serotonin toxicity after starting cyclobenzaprine 10 mg 3 times daily.[1] After starting cyclobenzaprine, he developed diaphoresis, confusion, hallucinations, and agitation, as well as tremors and myoclonus. The symptoms clearly supported a diagnosis of serotonin toxicity.[2,3]

RELATED DRUGS: Theoretically, other antidepressants that inhibit serotonin reuptake (eg, citalopram [eg, *Celexa*], clomipramine [eg, *Anafranil*], escitalopram [*Lexapro*], fluoxetine [eg, *Prozac*], fluvoxamine, imipramine [eg, *Tofranil*], paroxetine [eg, *Paxil*], sertraline [eg, *Zoloft*], venlafaxine [*Effexor*]) might interact similarly with cyclobenzaprine.

MANAGEMENT OPTIONS:

➡ *Avoid Unless Benefit Outweighs Risk.* Given the severity of the adverse outcome, avoid the combination when possible. If the combination is used, monitor for symptoms of serotonin toxicity, including myoclonus, tremor, hyperreflexia, muscle rigidity, fever, sweating, agitation, confusion, hypomania, incoordination, seizures, and coma.

REFERENCES:

1. Keegan MT, et al. Serotonin syndrome from the interaction of cyclobenzaprine with other serotoninergic drugs. *Anesth Analg.* 2006;103(6):1466-1468.
2. Isbister GK, et al. Serotonin toxicity: a practical approach to diagnosis and treatment. *Med J Aust.* 2007;187(6):361-365.
3. Boyer EW, Shannon M. The serotonin syndrome. *N Engl J Med.* 2005;352(11):1112-1120.

Cyclobenzaprine (eg, *Flexeril*)

Fluoxetine (eg, *Prozac*)

SUMMARY: A patient receiving cyclobenzaprine and fluoxetine developed ventricular tachycardia and fibrillation after droperidol was added, but the relative contribution of each drug to the adverse reaction is not clear.

RISK FACTORS: No specific risk factors are known.

MECHANISM: It was proposed that fluoxetine inhibited cyclobenzaprine metabolism, and the resulting increased cyclobenzaprine serum concentrations combined with droperidol (eg, *Inapsine*) prolonged the QT interval and produced the ventricular arrhythmia. Nonetheless, the ability of fluoxetine to inhibit cyclobenzaprine metabolism and the ability of cyclobenzaprine to prolong the QT interval are based primarily on theoretical considerations rather than clinical evidence.

CLINICAL EVALUATION: A 59-year-old woman on long-term therapy with cyclobenzaprine 10 mg/day and fluoxetine 30 mg/day was noted on electrocardiogram (ECG) to have a prolonged QTc interval.[1] Prior to surgery to repair her Achilles tendon, she received droperidol 0.625 mg intravenously (IV) and metoclopramide (eg, *Reglan*) 10 mg IV. During surgery she developed polymorphic ventricular tachycardia (torsades de pointes), which progressed into ventricular fibrillation. She was successfully defibrillated. While it is reasonable to assume that the droperidol contributed to the arrhythmia, the role of the cyclobenzaprine and fluoxetine is not clear. Although the case for a causal relationship is weak, the severity of the adverse reaction warrants monitoring of the patient.

RELATED DRUGS: No information is available.

MANAGEMENT OPTIONS:

➡ *Monitor.* Monitor for evidence of polymorphic ventricular tachycardia (eg, fainting, light-headedness). Monitor the ECG for excessive prolongation of the QTc interval.

REFERENCES:

1. Michalets EL, et al. Torsade de pointes resulting from the addition of droperidol to an existing cytochrome P450 drug interaction. *Ann Pharmacother.* 1998;32(7-8):761-765.

Cyclobenzaprine (eg, *Flexeril*)

Phenelzine (*Nardil*)

SUMMARY: A patient on phenelzine developed serotonin toxicity after starting cyclobenzaprine; avoid this combination if possible.

RISK FACTORS: No specific risk factors are known.

MECHANISM: Probably additive serotonergic effects.

CLINICAL EVALUATION: A 70-year-old woman on phenelzine 60 mg/day developed symptoms of serotonin toxicity after starting cyclobenzaprine 10 mg 3 times daily.[1] After 3 doses of cyclobenzaprine, she started to develop symptoms of serotonin toxicity, and eventually manifested myoclonus, tremors, fever, diaphoresis, confusion, and tachycardia. The symptoms clearly supported a diagnosis of serotonin toxicity.[2,3]

RELATED DRUGS: Other nonselective monoamine oxidase inhibitors such as tranylcypromine (eg, *Parnate*) are expected to interact similarly with cyclobenzaprine.

MANAGEMENT OPTIONS:

➡ *Avoid Unless Benefit Outweighs Risk.* Given the severity of the adverse outcome, it would be wise to avoid the combination. If the combination is used, monitor for symptoms of serotonin toxicity, including myoclonus, tremor, hyperreflexia, muscle rigidity, fever, sweating, agitation, confusion, hypomania, incoordination, seizures, and coma.

REFERENCES:

1. Keegan MT, et al. Serotonin syndrome from the interaction of cyclobenzaprine with other serotoninergic drugs. *Anesth Analg.* 2006;103(6):1466-1468.

2. Isbister GK, et al. Serotonin toxicity: a practical approach to diagnosis and treatment. *Med J Aust.* 2007;187(6):361-365.

3. Boyer EW, et al. The serotonin syndrome. *N Engl J Med.* 2005;352(11):1112-1120.

Cyclobenzaprine (eg, *Flexeril*)

Rasagiline (*Azilect*)

SUMMARY: Generally avoid concomitant use of rasagiline and cyclobenzaprine.

RISK FACTORS: No specific risk factors are known.

MECHANISM: Not established. The combination may have additive serotonergic effects.

CLINICAL EVALUATION: Because of its structural similarity to tricyclic antidepressants, cyclobenzaprine is contraindicated with monoamine oxidase inhibitors (MAOIs). The risk of using cyclobenzaprine with rasagiline or even nonselective MAOIs is not clear. Nonetheless, the combination is contraindicated in the rasagiline product information.[1]

RELATED DRUGS: Any interaction between cyclobenzaprine and rasagiline is likely to be similar to that of cyclobenzaprine and selegiline (eg, *Eldepryl*).

MANAGEMENT OPTIONS:

➡ ***AVOID COMBINATION.*** Generally, do not use cyclobenzaprine concurrently with rasagiline or within 2 weeks of the discontinuation of rasagiline.

REFERENCES:

1. *Azilect* [package insert]. North Wales, PA: Teva Neuroscience, Inc; 2006.

Cyclophosphamide (eg, *Cytoxan*)

Digoxin (eg, *Lanoxin*)

SUMMARY: Patients receiving cancer chemotherapy may have impaired absorption of digoxin tablets; the magnitude of the reduction appears sufficient to reduce the therapeutic effect of digoxin in some patients. The absorption of digoxin capsules does not appear to be affected by cytotoxic drugs.

RISK FACTORS: No specific risk factors are known.

MECHANISM: Cytotoxic drugs appear to affect the intestinal mucosa, resulting in malabsorption of digoxin.

CLINICAL EVALUATION: Six patients with lymphoma were given a single dose of beta-acetyldigoxin 0.8 mg (a digitalis glycoside similar to digoxin) before and 25 hours after therapy with a variety of cytotoxic agents alone or in combination (cyclophosphamide, prednisone [eg, *Sterapred*], procarbazine [*Matulane*]).[1] Several plasma digitalis glycoside concentrations measured 0 to 8 hours thereafter indicated that the rate of absorption was delayed, and the extent of absorption may have been decreased. Mean steady-state digoxin concentrations after similar chemotherapy in 15 cancer patients were 50% lower than those before chemotherapy. Digoxin concentrations began to fall 24 hours after therapy and reached their nadir at 48 hours. Digoxin concentrations returned to original values 8 days after the last dose of cytotoxic agents. The renal excretion of digoxin also was decreased. In another study of 13 patients, cancer chemotherapy reduced the absorption of digoxin tablets but not digoxin capsules.[2]

RELATED DRUGS: Other cytotoxic drugs also may inhibit the absorption of digoxin. Unlike digoxin, digitoxin[†] absorption does not appear to be reduced by cytotoxic drugs.[3]

MANAGEMENT OPTIONS:

➡ ***Consider Alternative.*** Digoxin capsules appear less likely to interact with cytotoxic drugs.

➡ ***Monitor.*** Be alert for evidence of reduced digoxin response during cytotoxic drug therapy. If oral doses of digoxin are increased to compensate for this effect, reductions in digoxin dosage will probably be required if the cytotoxic drugs are stopped for more than a few days.

REFERENCES:

1. Kuhlmann J, et al. Effects of cytostatic drugs on plasma level and renal excretion of beta-acetyldigoxin. *Clin Pharmacol Ther.* 1981;30(4):518-527.

2. Bjornsson TD, et al. Effects of high-dose cancer chemotherapy on the absorption of digoxin in two different formulations. *Clin Pharmacol Ther.* 1986;39(1):25-28.

3. Kuhlmann J, et al. Cytostatic drugs are without significant effect on digitoxin plasma level and renal excretion. *Clin Pharmacol Ther.* 1982;32(5):646-651.

† Not available in the United States.

Cyclophosphamide (eg, *Cytoxan*)

Ondansetron (eg, *Zofran*)

SUMMARY: Ondansetron was associated with small reductions in the plasma concentration of cyclophosphamide in patients undergoing bone marrow transplantation, but the clinical importance of this effect is not established.

RISK FACTORS: No specific risk factors are known.

MECHANISM: Not established.

CLINICAL EVALUATION: A group of patients undergoing bone marrow transplantation received high-dose cyclophosphamide, cisplatin, and carmustine (eg, *BiCNU*). Twenty-three patients were given ondansetron and 129 patients received prochlorperazine (eg, *Compazine*) as an antiemetic regimen.[1] In the patients receiving ondansetron, the cyclophosphamide and cisplatin areas under the plasma concentration-time curve (AUCs) were 15% and 19% lower, respectively, than in the patients receiving prochlorperazine. The AUC of carmustine was 20% lower with ondansetron versus prochlorperazine, but the difference was not statistically significant. The clinical importance of the changes in plasma concentrations of cyclophosphamide and cisplatin is not clear.

RELATED DRUGS: Ondansetron was also associated with a small reduction in cisplatin plasma concentrations.

MANAGEMENT OPTIONS: No specific action is required, but be alert for evidence of the interaction.

REFERENCES:
1. Cagnoni PJ, et al. Modification of the pharmacokinetics of high-dose cyclophosphamide and cisplatin by antiemetics. *Bone Marrow Transplant.* 1999;24(1):1-4.

Cyclophosphamide (eg, *Cytoxan*)

Phenobarbital

SUMMARY: Barbiturates like phenobarbital may affect the metabolism of cyclophosphamide, but reports of adverse clinical effects from this interaction are lacking.

RISK FACTORS: No specific risk factors are known.

MECHANISM: Barbiturates may promote the conversion of cyclophosphamide to active alkylating metabolites, but the inactivation of these metabolites also may be enhanced.

CLINICAL EVALUATION: In a group of patients receiving cyclophosphamide, those receiving enzyme-inducing agents such as barbiturates not only developed higher peak plasma concentrations of alkylating metabolites of cyclophosphamide, but also showed a more rapid decline in plasma concentrations of these metabolites than did those not receiving enzyme inducers. Thus, although it appears that barbiturates may alter cyclophosphamide disposition, the clinical effect of such altered disposition is not clear.[1,2]

RELATED DRUGS: No information is available.

MANAGEMENT OPTIONS: No specific action is required, but be alert for evidence of the interaction.

REFERENCES:
1. Bagley CM Jr, et al. Clinical pharmacology of cyclophosphamide. *Cancer Res.* 1973;33:226.
2. Kaplan SR, et al. Immunosuppressive agents (first of two parts). *N Engl J Med.* 1973;289:952.

 Cyclophosphamide (eg, *Cytoxan*)

Phenytoin (eg, *Dilantin*)

SUMMARY: Although phenytoin may affect the metabolism of cyclophosphamide, the clinical importance of this effect is not established.

RISK FACTORS: No specific risk factors are known.

MECHANISM: Enzyme-inducing agents such as phenytoin theoretically could enhance the formation of alkylating metabolites of cyclophosphamide.

CLINICAL EVALUATION: Although some limited clinical evidence indicates that enzyme inducers may increase peak plasma concentrations of alkylating metabolites of cyclophosphamide, this might be counteracted by a more rapid disposition of such metabolites.[1] Thus, the clinical significance of the concomitant use of phenytoin and cyclophosphamide remains unknown.

RELATED DRUGS: No information is available.

MANAGEMENT OPTIONS: No specific action is required, but be alert for evidence of the interaction.

REFERENCES:
1. Bagley CM, et al. Clinical pharmacology of cyclophosphamide. *Cancer Res.* 1973;33:226.

4 Cyclophosphamide (eg, *Cytoxan*)

Prednisone (eg, *Deltasone*)

SUMMARY: Corticosteroids like prednisone reportedly may alter cyclophosphamide effect, but the clinical importance of this interaction is not clear.

RISK FACTORS: No specific risk factors are known.

MECHANISM: It has been proposed that corticosteroids may inhibit the hepatic microsomal enzymes that activate cyclophosphamide to its alkylating metabolites.[1]

CLINICAL EVALUATION: Some have indicated that reduction of corticosteroid dosage in a patient also receiving cyclophosphamide may result in excessive cyclophosphamide effect,[2] but this has been refuted by others.[3] In 1 study, massive single doses of prednisolone (eg, *Prelone*) did not appear to affect cyclophosphamide metabolism in several patients. Thus, more study is needed to resolve the clinical significance of this purported interaction.

RELATED DRUGS: No information is available.

MANAGEMENT OPTIONS: No specific action is required, but be alert for evidence of the interaction.

REFERENCES:

1. Bagley CM Jr, et al. Clinical pharmacology of cyclophosphamide. *Cancer Res.* 1973;33:226.
2. Kaplan SR, et al. Immunosuppressive agents (first two parts). *N Engl J Med.* 1973;289:952.
3. Faber OK, et al. Cyclophosphamide activation and corticosteroids. *N Engl J Med.* 1974;291:211.

Cyclophosphamide (eg, *Cytoxan*)

Succinylcholine (eg, *Anectine*)

SUMMARY: Cyclophosphamide may prolong the neuromuscular blocking effect of succinylcholine.

RISK FACTORS: No specific risk factors are known.

MECHANISM: Cyclophosphamide may decrease plasma levels of pseudocholinesterase, which metabolizes succinylcholine.

CLINICAL EVALUATION: Evidence from limited clinical observations and in vitro studies indicates that prolonged apnea might occur following succinylcholine administration in some patients who also receive cyclophosphamide.[1-5] The possibility may be higher in very ill patients who are receiving large IV doses of cyclophosphamide.

RELATED DRUGS: No information is available.

MANAGEMENT OPTIONS:

➡ **Monitor.** Monitor patients for prolonged succinylcholine effect in patients also receiving cyclophosphamide (and probably other antineoplastics). Plasma pseudocholinesterase determinations may be desirable prior to succinylcholine administration. Avoidance of succinylcholine or cyclophosphamide has been recommended if the patient has significantly depressed pseudocholinesterase levels.[1]

REFERENCES:

1. Walker IR, et al. Cyclophosphamide, cholinesterase and anaesthesia. *Aust NZ J Med.* 1972;2:247.
2. Mone JG, et al. Qualitative and quantitative defects of pseudocholinesterase activity. *Anaesthesia.* 1967;22:55.
3. Smith RM Jr, et al. Succinylcholine-pantothenyl alcohol: a reappraisal. *Anesth Analg Curr Res.* 1969;48:205.
4. Zsigmond EK, et al. The effect of a series of anticancer drugs on plasma cholinesterase activity. *Can Anaesth Soc J.* 1972;19:75.
5. Wolff H. Die Hemmung der Serumcholinesterase durch Cyclophosphamid (*Endoxan*). *Klin Wochenschr.* 1965;43:819.

Cyclophosphamide (eg, *Cytoxan*)

Warfarin (eg, *Coumadin*)

SUMMARY: Cyclophosphamide appeared to inhibit the hypoprothrombinemic response to warfarin in one patient; more study is needed.

RISK FACTORS: No specific risk factors are known.

MECHANISM: Not established.

CLINICAL EVALUATION: A patient on warfarin and cyclophosphamide 450 mg/day developed a marked increase in prothrombin time when cyclophosphamide was discontinued.[1] Although the cyclophosphamide may have been responsible for the reduced warfarin effect in this patient, confirmation is needed.

RELATED DRUGS: The effect of cyclophosphamide on oral anticoagulants other than warfarin is not established, but be alert for the possibility. Several other cytotoxic drugs have been reported to affect warfarin response.

MANAGEMENT OPTIONS:

➡ *Monitor.* Watch for an alteration in the hypoprothrombinemic response to oral anticoagulants if cyclophosphamide is initiated, discontinued, or changed in dosage; adjust oral anticoagulant dosage as needed.

REFERENCES:
  1. Tashima CK. Cyclophosphamide effect on coumarin anticoagulation. *South Med J.* 1979;72:633.

Cycloserine (*Seromycin*)

Isoniazid (INH)

SUMMARY: The combined use of cycloserine and INH may result in increased central nervous system (CNS) toxicity.

RISK FACTORS: No specific risk factors are known.

MECHANISM: It is proposed that cycloserine and isoniazid have a combined toxic action on the CNS.

CLINICAL EVALUATION: In a study of 11 subjects given cycloserine with and without isoniazid, CNS effects occurred in 9 of 11 on combined therapy.[1] With cycloserine alone only 1 of the 11 subjects developed such symptoms. The frequency and severity of these effects is unclear.

RELATED DRUGS: No information is available.

MANAGEMENT OPTIONS:

➡ *Monitor.* Monitor patients receiving cycloserine and INH more closely for signs of CNS toxicity including dizziness or drowsiness.

REFERENCES:
  1. Mattila MJ, et al. Serum levels, urinary excretion, and side-effects of cycloserine in the presence of isoniazid and p-aminosalicylic acid. *Scand J Respir Dis.* 1969;50:291.

Cyclosporine (eg, *Neoral*)

Contraceptives, Oral (eg, *Ortho-Novum*)

SUMMARY: Isolated cases of elevated plasma cyclosporine concentrations have been observed following oral contraceptive use.

RISK FACTORS: No specific risk factors are known.

MECHANISM: Not established. Oral contraceptives are known to inhibit hepatic microsomal drug metabolism,[1-3] and it is possible that they also inhibit the metabolism of cyclosporine.

CLINICAL EVALUATION: Cyclosporine concentrations increased following initiation of an oral contraceptive containing levonorgestrel 150 mcg and ethinyl estradiol 30 mcg, in a 32-year-old woman receiving cyclosporine 5 mg/kg/day.[4] The plasma cyclosporine concentrations declined after the oral contraceptive was stopped; similar changes in plasma cyclosporine concentrations were observed when the contraceptive was later started and stopped. The fact that the serum cyclosporine concentrations increased when the contraceptive was started and decreased when the contraceptive was stopped on 2 separate occasions suggests that a drug interaction occurred in this patient. Moreover, another case of oral contraceptive-induced increase in cyclosporine concentrations and toxicity had been reported earlier.[5] Nevertheless, it is not clear how often this effect would be observed in other patients receiving the combination.

RELATED DRUGS: The effect of replacement estrogen therapy on cyclosporine is not established; given the lower doses of estrogen used in replacement therapy, an interaction seems less likely.

MANAGEMENT OPTIONS:

➥ *Consider Alternative.* Although this interaction is not well documented, consider using contraception other than oral contraceptives in patients receiving cyclosporine, because the consequences are potentially severe.

➥ *Monitor.* If oral contraceptives are used, monitor the patient's clinical response and cyclosporine serum concentrations. When cyclosporine therapy is started in a patient who is already taking oral contraceptives, anticipate the possibility that cyclosporine dosage requirements may be lower than expected. In a patient stabilized on both cyclosporine and an oral contraceptive, discontinuation of the contraceptive may cause a fall in cyclosporine blood concentrations. In both situations, carefully monitor the clinical response of the patient and adjust the cyclosporine dose as necessary. Based on the case reported and theoretical considerations, the changes in cyclosporine concentrations caused by hormone therapy probably occur gradually over several weeks. Keep this in mind when monitoring patients for this interaction.

REFERENCES:

1. Chambers DM, et al. Antipyrine elimination in saliva after low-dose combined or progestogen only oral contraceptive steroids. *Br J Clin Phamacol.* 1982;13:229.

2. Abernethy DR, et al. Impairment of antipyrine metabolism by low-dose oral contraceptive steroids. *Clin Pharmacol Ther.* 1981;29:106.

3. O'Malley K, et al. Increased antipyrine half-life in women taking oral contraceptives. *Scot Med J.* 1970;15:454.

4. Deray G. Oral contraceptive interaction with cyclosporine. *Lancet.* 1987;1:158.

5. Maurer G. Metabolism of cyclosporine. *Transplant Proc.* 1985;17(Suppl. 1):19.

Cyclosporine (eg, *Neoral*)

Danazol (eg, *Danocrine*)

SUMMARY: Preliminary case reports suggest that danazol and other androgens can increase serum cyclosporine concentrations and may result in cyclosporine toxicity.

RISK FACTORS: No specific risk factors are known.

MECHANISM: Not established. Danazol and other androgens can inhibit the metabolism of other drugs,[1,2] and cyclosporine perhaps is susceptible to such inhibition.

CLINICAL EVALUATION: A 15-year-old girl with a cadaver kidney graft 15 months earlier was well maintained on a stable dose of cyclosporine and prednisone.[4] Her cyclosporine dose, cyclosporine blood concentrations, and serum creatinine levels were all stable. Her blood cyclosporine concentrations and serum creatinine levels increased following initiation of danazol for menorrhagia; this persisted even after the cyclosporine dose was reduced. When the danazol was replaced with a progestin (norethindrone) in a dose of 5 mg 3 times daily, blood cyclosporine concentrations fell only slightly. When norethindrone was discontinued, the blood cyclosporine concentrations fell substantially. In another report, a 59-year-old man with a cadaver kidney transplant who was receiving azathioprine (eg, *Imuran*) and prednisone (eg, *Deltasone*) was started on methyltestosterone for hypogonadism and osteoporosis.[3] Cyclosporine 15 mg/kg/day then was started while the azathioprine dosage was halved to 0.75 mg/kg/day. Blood cyclosporine concentrations were excessive (more than 2000 ng/ml), and the half-life was several times longer than normal. Laboratory evidence of cyclosporine toxicity normalized after the cyclosporine and methyltestosterone were discontinued. Thus, androgens (and possibly progestins) appear to have increased cyclosporine levels in these patients, but the predictability of the interaction is unknown.

RELATED DRUGS: Tacrolimus (*Prograf*), like cyclosporine, is metabolized by CYP3A4, and its effect also appears to be increased by danazol.[5] Other androgens appear to interact similarly.

MANAGEMENT OPTIONS:

➡ *Avoid Unless Benefit Outweighs Risk.* Although this interaction is based upon isolated cases, the potentially severe consequences warrant avoiding the use of anabolic steroids in patients receiving cyclosporine.

➡ *Monitor.* If anabolic steroids are started in a patient receiving cyclosporine, monitor the patient's cyclosporine response and serum concentrations carefully. When cyclosporine therapy is started in a patient who is already taking anabolic steroids, the cyclosporine dose requirements may be lower than expected. In a patient stabilized on both cyclosporine and anabolic steroids, stopping the hormone may cause a fall in cyclosporine blood concentrations; monitor the clinical response of the patient carefully and increase the cyclosporine dose as necessary. Based upon the cases reported as well as theoretical considerations, the changes in cyclosporine concentrations caused by such hormones probably occur gradually over several weeks; keep this in mind when monitoring for this interaction.

REFERENCES:

1. Kramer G, et al. Carbamazepine-danazol drug interaction: its mechanism examined by a stable isotope technique. *Ther Drug Monit.* 1986;8:387.

2. Hvidberg EF, et al. Studies of the interaction of phenylbutazone, oxyphenbutazone and methandrostenolone in man. *Proc Soc Exp Biol Med.* 1968;129:438.

3. Moller BB, et al. Toxicity of cyclosporine during treatment with androgens. *N Engl J Med.* 1985;313:1416.

4. Ross WB, et al. Cyclosporine interaction with danazol and noresthisterone. *Lancet.* 1986;1:330.

5. Shapiro R, et al. FK 506 interaction with danazol. *Lancet.* 1993;341:1344.

Cyclosporine (eg, *Neoral*)

Diclofenac (eg, *Voltaren*)

SUMMARY: Diclofenac has been associated with increased serum concentrations of creatinine and potassium as well as increased blood pressure in a number of patients receiving cyclosporine.

RISK FACTORS: No specific risk factors are known.

MECHANISM: Not established. It has been proposed that nonsteroidal anti-inflammatory drugs (NSAIDs) such as diclofenac may inhibit the protective effect of prostaglandins against cyclosporine nephrotoxicity.

CLINICAL EVALUATION: Of 20 patients with rheumatoid arthritis who were treated with cyclosporine 2.5 to 5 mg/kg/day and diclofenac, 7 were considered to have a "high probability" of interaction, as evidenced by elevated plasma creatinine and serum potassium concentrations or an increase in blood pressure that normalized following discontinuation of only diclofenac.[1] Nine of the patients had a "possible" interaction; in these patients there was no "dechallenge" (ie, diclofenac was not discontinued while continuing with cyclosporine therapy). Diclofenac did not appear to affect blood cyclosporine concentrations. Another patient receiving cyclosporine for idiopathic uveitis developed a marked increase in serum creatinine 48 hours after starting diclofenac;[2] plasma cyclosporine concentrations were not elevated during this period.

RELATED DRUGS: Sulindac (eg, *Clinoril*) was associated with increased serum cyclosporine and serum creatinine concentrations in 1 patient.[3] On the other hand, indomethacin (*Indocin*) and ketoprofen (eg, *Orudis*) appeared *less* likely than diclofenac to interact with cyclosporine in another patient.[1] Given the paucity of data, the relative likelihood of various NSAIDs to increase cyclosporine-induced nephrotoxicity cannot be determined. Assume that all NSAIDs are capable of interacting with cyclosporine until evidence to the contrary is available.

MANAGEMENT OPTIONS:

➡ **Consider Alternative.** Until the clinical importance of this potential interaction is better defined, patients taking cyclosporine should use diclofenac or other NSAIDs only when the expected benefit clearly outweighs the risk of nephrotoxicity.

➡ **Monitor.** If the combination is used, monitor the patient's renal function carefully and be prepared to discontinue one or both drugs.

REFERENCES:

1. Branthwaite JP, et al. Cyclosporin and diclofenac interaction in rheumatoid arthritis. *Lancet*. 1991;337:252.
2. Deray G, et al. Enhancement of cyclosporine A nephrotoxicity of diclofenac. *Clin Nephrol*. 1987;27:213.
3. Sesin GP, et al. Sulindac-induced elevation of serum cyclosporine concentration. *Clin Pharm*. 1989;8:445.

Cyclosporine (eg, *Neoral*)

Digoxin (eg, *Lanoxin*)

SUMMARY: The administration of cyclosporine to patients stabilized on digoxin may result in increased digoxin serum concentrations and digoxin toxicity.

RISK FACTORS: No specific risk factors are known.

MECHANISM: The mechanism of this interaction is not known, but cyclosporine may decrease the clearance or renal tubular secretion of digoxin.[3] A reduction in creatinine clearance noted with the administration of cyclosporine also could contribute to the changes observed.

CLINICAL EVALUATION: Several case studies have noted an average reduction in digoxin clearance (approximately 50%) and an increase in digoxin concentrations following the coadministration of cyclosporine.[1] Cyclosporine administration also reduced the patient's creatinine clearances approximately 60%; this would reduce digoxin clearance and volume of distribution. The pharmacokinetics of a single dose of digoxin 0.25 or 0.5 mg IV were studied in 7 cardiac transplant patients before and after transplantation while they received chronic cyclosporine therapy.[2] Digoxin volume of distribution and half-life were increased, but renal clearance did not change.

RELATED DRUGS: Tacrolimus (*Prograf*) may produce a similar interaction with digoxin, but data are not available.

MANAGEMENT OPTIONS:

➥ *Circumvent/Minimize.* A reduction in the digoxin dosage may be required. With the discontinuation of cyclosporine, patients may require increased digoxin dosages.

➥ *Monitor.* Until more data regarding this interaction are available, monitor patients maintained on digoxin carefully for digitalis toxicity if cyclosporine is added to their regimen.

REFERENCES:

1. Dorian P, et al. Digoxin-cyclosporine interaction: severe digitalis toxicity after cyclosporine treatment. *Clin Invest Med.* 1988;11:108.
2. Robieux LC, et al. The effect of cardiac transplantation and cyclosporin therapy on digoxin pharmacokinetics. *J Clin Pharmacol.* 1992;32:338.
3. Okamura N, et al. Digoxin-cyclosporin A interaction: modulation of the multidrug transporter P-glycoprotein in the kidney. *J Pharmacol Exp Ther.* 1993;266:1614.

Cyclosporine (eg, *Neoral*)

Diltiazem (eg, *Cardizem*)

SUMMARY: Cyclosporine blood concentrations are increased by diltiazem; renal toxicity has been reported with the elevated cyclosporine concentrations.

RISK FACTORS: No specific risk factors are known.

MECHANISM: Diltiazem appears to inhibit the metabolism (CYP3A4) and may increase the bioavailability of cyclosporine.

CLINICAL EVALUATION: The coadministration of diltiazem and cyclosporine has been associated with increased cyclosporine concentrations and renal toxicity.[1] Several days were required for cyclosporine concentrations to decline to baseline after the diltiazem was discontinued. Diltiazem reduced cyclosporine clearance 30% to 70%.[2,4,5] The resulting cyclosporine dose reduction may result in a cost savings.[2-4,7,8] A single 90 mg dose of diltiazem did not alter the pharmacokinetics of cyclosporine.[6]

RELATED DRUGS: Nicardipine (eg, *Cardene*) and verapamil (eg, *Calan*) inhibit cyclosporine metabolism while isradipine (*DynaCirc*), nifedipine (eg, *Procardia*), amlodipine (*Norvasc*), and nitrendipine have minimal effect. Diltiazem may affect tacrolimus (*Prograf*) in a similar manner.

MANAGEMENT OPTIONS:

➡ *Consider Alternative.* Calcium channel blockers that do not appear to alter cyclosporine pharmacokinetics include isradipine,[9] nitrendipine,[10] and amlodipine.[11]

➡ *Circumvent/Minimize.* Reduce cyclosporine dosage and monitor blood concentrations when diltiazem is coadministered.

➡ *Monitor.* Observe patients receiving both drugs for increased cyclosporine concentrations and decreasing renal function.

REFERENCES:

1. Pochet JM, et al. Cyclosporine-diltiazem interactions. *Lancet.* 1986;1:979.
2. Smith CL, et al. Clinical and medicoeconomic impact of the cyclosporine-diltiazem interaction in renal transplant recipients. *Pharmacotherapy.* 1994;14:471.
3. Chrysostomou A, et al. Diltiazem in renal allograft recipients receiving cyclosporine. *Transplantation.* 1993;55:300.
4. Wagner K, et al. Interaction of cyclosporin and calcium antagonists. *Transplant Proc.* 1989;21:1453.
5. Sabate I, et al. Cyclosporin-diltiazem interaction: comparison of cyclosporin levels measured with two monoclonal antibodies. *Transplant Proc.* 1989;21:1460.
6. Roy LF, et al. Short-term effects of calcium antagonists on hemodynamics and cyclosporine pharmacokinetics in heart-transplant and kidney-transplant patients. *Clin Pharmacol Ther.* 1989;46:657.
7. Campistol JM, et al. Interactions between cyclosporine and diltiazem in renal transplant patients. *Nephron.* 1991;57:241.
8. Bourge RC, et al. Diltiazem-cyclosporine interaction in cardiac transplant recipients: impact on cyclosporine dose and medication costs. *Am J Med.* 1991;90:402.
9. Martinez F, et al. No clinically significant interaction between cyclosporin and isradipine. *Nephron.* 1991;59:658.
10. Copur MS, et al. Effects of nitrendipine on blood pressure and blood cyclosporine A level in patients with posttransplant hypertension. *Nephron.* 1989;52:227.
11. Toupance O, et al. Antihypertensive effect of amlodipine and lack of interference with cyclosporine metabolism in renal transplant recipients. *Hypertension.* 1994;24:297.

Cyclosporine (eg, *Neoral*)

Doxorubicin (eg, *Adriamycin*)

SUMMARY: A patient receiving cyclosporine and doxorubicin developed CNS toxicity including coma and seizures; causation has not been established.

RISK FACTORS: No specific risk factors are known.

MECHANISM: Not established.

CLINICAL EVALUATION: A 49-year-old patient taking cyclosporine 2 mg/kg/day for immunosuppression following a heart transplantation developed Burkitt's lymphoma.[1] Cyclosporine was discontinued and chemotherapy consisting of doxorubicin 60 mg, vincristine 2 mg, cyclophosphamide 600 mg, and prednisone 80 mg was administered. Eight hours later, the patient developed a coma that resolved after 12 hours. A second course of chemotherapy 1 week later resulted in coma and tonic clonic seizures shortly after doxorubicin and vincristine administration. Causation was not demonstrated by this case report; however, animal toxicity studies suggest cyclosporine increases the neurological toxicity of doxorubicin.

RELATED DRUGS: The effect of tacrolimus (*Prograf*) on doxorubicin is not established.

MANAGEMENT OPTIONS:

➡ **Monitor.** Until further information is available, carefully observe patients taking cyclosporine for changing mental status and CNS toxicity if they receive doxorubicin.

REFERENCES:

　　1.　Barbui T, et al. Neurological symptoms and coma associated with doxorubicin administration during chronic cyclosporine therapy. *Lancet*. 1992;339:1421.

 Cyclosporine (eg, *Neoral*)

Enalapril (*Vasotec*)

SUMMARY: Initiation of enalapril therapy in 2 renal transplant patients receiving cyclosporine was associated with acute renal failure; more study is needed to assess the clinical importance of this purported interaction.

RISK FACTORS:

➡ **Other Drugs.** Diuretic-induced hypovolemia is a possible risk factor.

MECHANISM: The mechanism is not established, but the following sequence of events has been proposed.[1] Cyclosporine results in renal afferent vasoconstriction and glomerular hypoperfusion. In this situation, intrarenal angiotensin II is needed to maintain an adequate glomerular filtration rate; therefore, subsequent inhibition of angiotensin-converting enzyme (ACE) could reduce renal function acutely.

CLINICAL EVALUATION: Two renal transplant patients receiving cyclosporine experienced acute deterioration of renal function after initiation of enalapril therapy.[1] In 1 case, renal failure was detected 10 days after initiating enalapril; in the other case, renal function gradually declined over 6 weeks. Renal biopsy showed no evidence of rejection. Concomitant furosemide therapy in both patients could have contributed to the decreased renal function, because the use of ACE inhibitors in the presence of diuretic-induced hypovolemia has been associated with acute renal failure.[2] Although the renal failure could have been caused by cyclosporine alone, that appears unlikely because in 1 patient the renal function improved after the discontinuation of enalapril despite continued cyclosporine treatment. Furthermore, cyclosporine was restarted with no renal impairment in the other patient. Since enalapril was associated with acute renal failure in only 2 patients receiving cyclosporine, additional evidence will be needed to establish a causal relationship.

RELATED DRUGS: Based on the proposed mechanism, expect other ACE inhibitors to interact with cyclosporine in a similar manner.

MANAGEMENT OPTIONS:

➡ *Monitor.* Until further information is available, initiate ACE inhibitors cautiously in patients receiving cyclosporine; monitor renal function carefully.

REFERENCES:

1. Murray BM, et al. Enalapril-associated acute renal failure in renal transplants: possible role of cyclosporine. *Am J Kidney Dis.* 1990;16:66.

2. Funck-Brentano C, et al. Reversible renal failure after combined treatment with enalapril and furosemide in a patient with congestive heart failure. *Br Heart J.* 1986;55:596.

Cyclosporine (eg, *Neoral*)

Erythromycin (eg, *E-Mycin*)

SUMMARY: The combination of cyclosporine and erythromycin should be used with caution because of the potential for elevated cyclosporine concentrations and nephrotoxicity.

RISK FACTORS: No specific risk factors are known.

MECHANISM: Erythromycin appears to inhibit the metabolism of cyclosporine.

CLINICAL EVALUATION: The administration of erythromycin reduces cyclosporine clearance by one-half and may more than double the maximum cyclosporine concentration.[3] A patient receiving 19 mg/kg/day of cyclosporine following a renal transplantation was reported to have a trough cyclosporine concentration of 122 ng/ml.[1] Several days may be required to observe the maximum effect of erythromycin on cyclosporine concentrations. Other reports have noted similar increases in cyclosporine concentrations after erythromycin administration, and some patients experienced nephrotoxicity because of the increased cyclosporine concentrations.[2,4-11]

RELATED DRUGS: Troleandomycin (*TAO*) or clarithromycin (*Biaxin*) also may inhibit the metabolism of cyclosporine. Tacrolimus (*Prograf*) is affected similarly by erythromycin administration. Azithromycin (*Zithromax*) does not appear to affect cyclosporine.

MANAGEMENT OPTIONS:

➡ *Circumvent/Minimize.* Cyclosporine doses may require reduction during erythromycin administration.

➡ *Monitor.* Monitor renal function and cyclosporine concentrations when erythromycin is added to or deleted from the regimen of patients receiving cyclosporine.

REFERENCES:

1. Ptachcinski RJ, et al. Effect of erythromycin on cyclosporine levels. *N Engl J Med.* 1985;313:1416.

2. Kohan DE. Possible interaction between cyclosporine and erythromycin. *N Engl J Med.* 1986;314:448.

3. Freeman DJ, et al. Cyclosporin-erythromycin interaction in normal subjects. *Br J Clin Pharmacol.* 1987;23:776.

4. Godin JRP, et al. Erythromycin-cyclosporin interaction. *Drug Intell Clin Pharm.* 1986;20:504.

5. Hourmant M, et al. Co-administration of erythromycin results in an increase of blood cyclosporine to toxic levels. *Transplant Proc.* 1985;17:2723.

6. Kessler M, et al. Interaction between cyclosporine and erythromycin in a kidney transplant patient. *Eur J Clin Pharmacol.* 1986;30:633.

7. Grino JM, et al. Erythromycin and cyclosporine. *Ann Intern Med.* 1986;105:467.

8. Jensen CWB, et al. Exacerbation of cyclosporine toxicity of concomitant administration of erythromycin. *Transplantation.* 1987;43:263.

9. Wadhwa NK, et al. Interaction between erythromycin and cyclosporine in a kidney and pancreas allograft recipient. *Ther Drug Monit*. 1987;9:123.

10. Gupta SK, et al. Cyclosporin-erythromycin interaction in renal transplant patients. *Br J Clin Pharmacol*. 1989;27:475.

11. Koselj M, et al. Drug interaction between cyclosporine and rifampicin, erythromycin, and azoles in kidney recipients with opportunistic infections. *Transplant Proc*. 1994;26:2823.

 4 ## Cyclosporine (eg, *Neoral*)

Ethanol (Ethyl Alcohol)

SUMMARY: Acute ethanol intoxication was associated with increased serum cyclosporine concentrations in one patient, but additional study involving smaller amounts of ethanol (equal to a few drinks) showed no effect.

RISK FACTORS:

➡ **Dosage Regimen.** If this interaction occurs, it may occur only with acute overdoses of alcohol.

MECHANISM: Not established. Acute ethanol intoxication is known to inhibit the ability of the liver to metabolize drugs, and it is possible that cyclosporine is similarly affected.

CLINICAL EVALUATION: A 51-year-old renal transplant recipient developed an approximately 2-fold increase in his serum cyclosporine concentrations following an alcohol binge.[1] In a subsequent crossover study in 8 male renal transplant recipients, acute intake of 50 ml of 100% ethanol (equivalent to approximately 4 oz of whiskey) did not affect serum cyclosporine concentrations.

RELATED DRUGS: The effect of ethanol on tacrolimus (*Prograf*) is not established; given the similarity of its metabolism to cyclosporine, interactions with alcohol may be similar.

MANAGEMENT OPTIONS: No specific action is required, but be alert for evidence of the interaction.

REFERENCES:

1. Paul MD, et al. The effect of ethanol on serum cyclosporine A levels in renal transplant recipients. *Am J Kidney Dis*. 1987;10:133.

 3 ## Cyclosporine (eg, *Neoral*)

Etoposide (eg, *VePesid*)

SUMMARY: High-dose cyclosporine may improve tumor response to etoposide, but also increases toxicity; adjustments to etoposide dose may be necessary.

RISK FACTORS: No specific risk factors are known.

MECHANISM: Not established.

CLINICAL EVALUATION: Eighteen children with refractory solid tumors (who had previously received etoposide) were given etoposide plus high-dose cyclosporine in an effort to enhance tumor sensitivity.[1] Cyclosporine substantially increased etoposide plasma concentrations, and resulted in a 24% tumor response rate. But acute toxicity was also increased; hypersensitivity reactions were common, and in some cases were severe.

RELATED DRUGS: No information is available.

MANAGEMENT OPTIONS:

➥ *Circumvent/Minimize.* The authors recommend halving the etoposide dose if high-dose cyclosporine is used concurrently.[1]

➥ *Monitor.* Closely monitor patients on this combination, especially for hypersensitivity reactions such as rash, fever, and bronchospasm.

REFERENCES:

1. Bisogno G, et al. High-dose cyclosporin with etoposide—toxicity and pharmacokinetic interaction in children with solid tumors. *Br J Cancer.* 1998;77:2304.

Cyclosporine (eg, *Neoral*)

Felodipine (*Plendil*)

SUMMARY: When cyclosporine and felodipine are coadministered, cyclosporine markedly increases felodipine concentrations while the concentrations of cyclosporine are minimally increased.

RISK FACTORS:

➥ *Route of Administration.* The administration of oral cyclosporine would be expected to produce a greater effect on felodipine concentrations than IV cyclosporine.

MECHANISM: Cyclosporine and felodipine are subject to intestinal wall first-pass metabolism by CYP3A4. Because the molar concentration of cyclosporine is much larger than that of felodipine, cyclosporine may competitively inhibit the first-pass metabolism of felodipine resulting in an increased bioavailability of felodipine. Additionally, the affinity of cyclosporine for the enzyme may be greater than felodipine. This may explain the larger effect of cyclosporine on felodipine than the effect of felodipine on cyclosporine concentrations.

CLINICAL EVALUATION: Twelve healthy subjects were administered single oral doses of felodipine extended-release 10 mg, cyclosporine 5 mg/kg, and the combination of both felodipine and cyclosporine.[1] Felodipine increased the peak blood concentration of cyclosporine (16%) but did not affect its area under the concentration-time curve (AUC). The coadministration of cyclosporine and felodipine significantly increased the peak plasma concentration (151%) and AUC (58%) of felodipine. The combination treatment resulted in a greater decrease in mean diastolic blood pressure over 24 hours than either drug given alone. The chronic administration of felodipine with cyclosporine could produce increased hypotensive effects.

RELATED DRUGS: It is possible that other dihydropyridines that have a large first-pass clearance (eg, nitrendipine) may be similarly affected by cyclosporine coadministration. Dihydropyridines that have less first-pass metabolism include amlodipine (*Norvasc*).

MANAGEMENT OPTIONS:

➥ *Consider Alternative.* Patients receiving cyclosporine could be treated with a dihydropyridine that has less first-pass metabolism than felodipine (see Related Drugs) or a different class of antihypertensive could be selected.

➥ *Circumvent/Minimize.* Avoid taking felodipine with cyclosporine. Separate the doses by at least 2 hours.

➥ **Monitor.** If felodipine and cyclosporine are administered together, watch for excessive hypotensive effects.

REFERENCES:
1. Madsen JK, et al. Pharmacokinetic interaction between cyclosporine and the dihydropyridine calcium antagonist felodipine. *Eur J Clin Pharmacol.* 1996;50:203.

Cyclosporine (eg, *Neoral*)

Fluconazole (eg, *Diflucan*)

SUMMARY: Fluconazole appears to increase cyclosporine plasma concentrations, particularly at higher fluconazole doses; cyclosporine toxicity could result in some patients.

RISK FACTORS:

➥ **Dosage Regimen.** Fluconazole doses higher than 100 mg/day might increase the likelihood of the interaction.

MECHANISM: It appears that fluconazole inhibits the metabolism (CYP3A4) of cyclosporine.[1]

CLINICAL EVALUATION: In several case reports, elevated cyclosporine concentrations or rising serum creatinine concentrations have been noted following the addition of fluconazole therapy.[2-4] Details of these cases are limited, and causation is difficult to establish. The average cyclosporine clearance after oral administration decreased 55% following fluconazole 200 mg/day for 14 days.[5] Trough cyclosporine concentrations increased from 27 to 58 ng/mL; however, adverse effects were not observed. Other patients taking fluconazole 100 mg/day[6-8] or 200 mg/day[9] displayed no changes in their cyclosporine concentrations. A well-designed trial is needed to resolve the clinical significance of this interaction.

RELATED DRUGS: Fluconazole inhibits tacrolimus (*Prograf*) metabolism. Ketoconazole (eg, *Nizoral*), miconazole (eg, *Micatin*), and itraconazole (*Sporanox*) are also inhibitors of cyclosporine metabolism.

MANAGEMENT OPTIONS:

➥ **Monitor.** Until more studies have been done, monitor cyclosporine plasma concentrations and renal function when fluconazole is administered. Cyclosporine dosage adjustments may be required in some patients.

REFERENCES:
1. Back DJ, et al. Comparative effects of the antimycotic drugs ketoconazole, fluconazole, itraconazole and terbinafine on the metabolism of cyclosporin by human liver microsomes. *Br J Clin Pharmacol.* 1991;32:624-626.
2. Lopez-Gil JA. Fluconazole-cyclosporine interaction: a dose-dependent effect? *Ann Pharmacother.* 1993;27:427-430.
3. Collingnon P, et al. Interaction of fluconazole with cyclosporin. *Lancet.* 1989;1:1262.
4. Torregrosa V, et al. Interaction of fluconazole with ciclosporin A. *Nephron.* 1992;60:125-126.
5. Canafax DM, et al. Increased cyclosporine levels as a result of simultaneous fluconazole and cyclosporine therapy in renal transplant recipients: a double-blind, randomized pharmacokinetic and safety study. *Transplant Proc.* 1991;23(1 pt 2):1041-1042.
6. Kruger HU, et al. No severe interactions between fluconazole, a triazole antifungal agent, with cyclosporin. *Bone Marrow Transplant.* 1988;3:271.
7. Lazar JD, et al. Drug interactions with fluconazole. *Rev Infect Dis.* 1990;12(suppl 3):S327-S333.

8. Kruger HU, et al. Absence of significant interaction of fluconazole with cyclosporin. *J Antimicrob Chemother*. 1989;24:781-786.

9. Ehninger G, et al. Interaction of fluconazole with cyclosporin. *Lancet*. 1989;2:104-105.

Cyclosporine (eg, *Neoral*)

Fluvastatin (*Lescol*)

SUMMARY: Cyclosporine increases plasma fluvastatin concentrations, but the clinical importance of this effect is not established.

RISK FACTORS: No specific risk factors are known.

MECHANISM: Not established. Cyclosporine may inhibit the hepatic uptake of fluvastatin by transporters such as OATP-C.

CLINICAL EVALUATION: In transplant patients, those receiving cyclosporine developed higher serum fluvastatin concentrations than similar patients not receiving cyclosporine.[1] The degree to which this pharmacokinetic interaction increases the risk of fluvastatin-induced myopathy is not established, but available evidence suggests that the risk is not large. A study in 16 stable renal transplant patients found no effect of fluvastatin on mean trough cyclosporine flood concentrations.[2]

RELATED DRUGS: Cyclosporine can also increase the serum concentrations of lovastatin (eg, *Mevacor*), simvastatin (*Zocor*), atorvastatin (*Lipitor*), rosuvastatin (*Crestor*), and pravastatin (*Pravachol*), although the risk of adverse consequences appears to differ depending on the statin. Pravastatin, for example, is frequently used in transplant patients without evidence of adverse drug interactions.

MANAGEMENT OPTIONS: No specific action is required, but be alert for evidence of the interaction.

REFERENCES:

1. Park JW, et al. Pharmacokinetics and pharmacodynamics of fluvastatin in heart transplant recipients taking cyclosporine A. *J Cardiovasc Pharmacol Ther*. 2001;6:351-361.

2. Li PK, et al. The interaction of fluvastatin and cyclosprin A in renal transplant patients. *Int J Clin Pharmacol Ther*. 1995;33:246-248.

Cyclosporine (eg, *Neoral*)

Gentamicin (eg, *Garamycin*)

SUMMARY: Cyclosporine and gentamicin are nephrotoxic and produce additive renal damage when administered together.

RISK FACTORS: No specific risk factors are known.

MECHANISM: Both drugs appear to injure the renal tubule.

CLINICAL EVALUATION: The combined use of gentamicin and cyclosporine in renal transplant patients increased the incidence of acute tubular necrosis to 67% compared with 5% to 10% when gentamicin was used alone or when cyclosporine was used with another antibiotic (ampicillin [eg, *Principen*]).[1] Animal studies have demonstrated additive renal toxicity when cyclosporine and gentamicin are coadministered.[2]

RELATED DRUGS: Other aminoglycosides may produce additive nephrotoxicity with cyclosporine. The effect of aminoglycosides on tacrolimus (*Prograf*) nephrotoxicity is unknown.

MANAGEMENT OPTIONS:

➡ *Consider Alternative.* If possible, avoid the administration of aminoglycosides in patients receiving cyclosporine for immunosuppression after renal transplantation.

➡ *Monitor.* Monitor patients receiving the combination for reduced renal function.

REFERENCES:

1. Termeer A, et al. Severe nephrotoxicity caused by the combined use of gentamicin and cyclosporine in renal allograft recipients. *Transplantation.* 1986;42:220-221.

2. Whiting PH, et al. The enhancement of cyclosporin A-induced nephrotoxicity by gentamicin. *Biochem Pharmacol.* 1983;32:2025-2028.

Cyclosporine (eg, *Neoral*)

Glipizide (eg, *Glucotrol*)

SUMMARY: Glipizide administration appears to increase cyclosporine concentrations; nephrotoxicity could occur.

RISK FACTORS: No specific risk factors are known.

MECHANISM: Not established. Glipizide may reduce the first-pass or systemic clearance of cyclosporine.

CLINICAL EVALUATION: Two cases of increased cyclosporine concentrations following the addition of glipizide 10 mg/day to renal transplant patients have been noted.[1] In both cases, increased cyclosporine concentrations were accompanied by elevated serum creatinine concentrations. Cyclosporine dosage reductions of 20% to 30% were required after the addition of glipizide. Causation was not established in either case.

RELATED DRUGS: Other sulfonylureas may affect cyclosporine in a similar manner. It is possible that tacrolimus (*Prograf*) interacts with glipizide.

MANAGEMENT OPTIONS:

➡ *Circumvent/Minimize.* Cyclosporine doses may require adjustment to avoid cyclosporine-induced renal toxicity.

➡ *Monitor.* Until further information is available, monitor patients stabilized on cyclosporine for increased cyclosporine concentrations following the addition of glipizide.

REFERENCES:

1. Chidester PD, et al. Interaction between glipizide and cyclosporine: report of two cases. *Transplant Proc.* 1993;25:2136-2137.

Cyclosporine (eg, *Neoral*)

Grapefruit Juice

SUMMARY: Grapefruit juice can increase cyclosporine blood concentrations; adjustments in cyclosporine dosage may be necessary.

RISK FACTORS: No specific risk factors are known.

MECHANISM: Grapefruit juice inhibits the presystemic metabolism of cyclosporine by intestinal CYP3A4.

CLINICAL EVALUATION: Studies in both healthy subjects[1] and renal transplant patients[2-5] have shown that grapefruit juice can increase cyclosporine blood concentrations. In multiple-dose trials (grapefruit juice given daily for several days with cyclosporine) the mean increase in cyclosporine blood concentrations is usually approximately 30% to 40%,[1,2] although 1 study found a larger effect.[3] Only small increases in cyclosporine blood concentrations have been noted in single-dose studies[4] and when the grapefruit juice was separated from the cyclosporine 90 minutes or more.[5] Thus, it is clear that grapefruit juice (and probably other forms of grapefruit) can increase cyclosporine blood concentrations. The intentional use of grapefruit juice with cyclosporine to reduce the cost of cyclosporine therapy has been proposed, but studies are needed to assess the safety of this proposal.

RELATED DRUGS: Like cyclosporine, tacrolimus (*Prograf*) also undergoes first-pass metabolism by CYP3A4. Thus, grapefruit juice probably also increases tacrolimus blood concentrations.

MANAGEMENT OPTIONS:

➡ *Consider Alternative.* Orange juice does not appear to interact with cyclosporine.

➡ *Circumvent/Minimize.* Advise patients on cyclosporine to avoid grapefruit juice (unless the combination is being used intentionally to elevate cyclosporine blood levels). Separating doses of grapefruit juice from cyclosporine may not eliminate the interaction completely, since the inhibitory effect of grapefruit juice on CYP3A4 can last for several hours.

➡ *Monitor.* If grapefruit juice is taken concurrently with cyclosporine, carefully monitor the patient's response to cyclosporine, especially if grapefruit juice is initiated, discontinued, or if the interval between the cyclosporine and grapefruit juice is changed.

REFERENCES:

1. Yee G, et al. Effect of grapefruit juice on blood cyclosporin concentration. *Lancet.* 1995;345:955.
2. Ducharme MP, et al. Trough concentrations of cyclosporine in blood following administration with grapefruit juice. *Br J Clin Pharmacol.* 1993;36:457.
3. Proppe DG, et al. Influence of chronic ingestion of grapefruit juice on steady-state blood concentrations of cyclosporine A in renal transplant patients with stable graft function. *Br J Clin Pharmacol.* 1995;39:337.
4. Herlitz H, et al. Grapefruit juice: a possible source of variability in blood concentration of cyclosporin A. *Nephrol Dial Transplant.* 1993;8:375.
5. Hollander AAMJ, et al. The effect of grapefruit juice on cyclosporine and prednisone metabolism in transplant patients. *Clin Pharmacol Ther.* 1995;57:318.

Cyclosporine (eg, *Neoral*)

Griseofulvin (eg, *Grisactin*)

SUMMARY: Griseofulvin administration decreased the blood concentrations of cyclosporine in 1 patient; cyclosporine efficacy could be reduced during griseofulvin administration.

RISK FACTORS: No specific risk factors are known.

MECHANISM: Not established. Griseofulvin appears to increase the metabolism or decrease the absorption of cyclosporine.

CLINICAL EVALUATION: A renal transplant patient was receiving cyclosporine, azathioprine, prednisone, nifedipine, and isoniazid.[1] Cyclosporine concentrations were 90 ng/ml before the addition of griseofulvin. Two weeks after griseofulvin 500 mg/day was added, cyclosporine concentrations had fallen to 50 ng/ml. During this period the cyclosporine dose had been increased from 2.8 to 4.8 mg/kg. Four months later griseofulvin was discontinued and blood cyclosporine concentrations increased to over 200 ng/ml. While methylprednisolone has been reported to increase cyclosporine concentrations,[2] the contribution of prednisolone or other drugs taken by this patient to this case report is unknown.

RELATED DRUGS: Griseofulvin may affect tacrolimus (*Prograf*) similarly. Other antifungal agents (eg, ketoconazole [eg, *Nizoral*]) may reduce cyclosporine metabolism.

MANAGEMENT OPTIONS:

➡ *Circumvent/Minimize.* Cyclosporine doses may have to be increased during griseofulvin therapy and decreased when griseofulvin is discontinued.

➡ *Monitor.* Monitor cyclosporine concentrations and signs of transplant rejection when griseofulvin is added to or removed from the therapy of a patient receiving cyclosporine.

REFERENCES:
1. Abu-Romeh SH, et al. Cyclosporin A and griseofulvin: another drug interaction. *Nephron.* 1991;58:237.
2. Klintmalm G, et al. High dose methylprednisolone increases plasma cyclosporin levels in renal transplant recipients. *Lancet.* 1984;1:731.

 Cyclosporine (eg, *Neoral*)

Imipenem (*Primaxin*)

SUMMARY: Taking imipenem with cyclosporine resulted in acute CNS toxicity in 1 patient.

RISK FACTORS: No specific risk factors are known.

MECHANISM: The interaction between imipenem and cyclosporine may be caused by a summation of CNS side effects, an imipenem-induced increase in cyclosporine concentrations, or both.

CLINICAL EVALUATION: A 62-year-old patient who was receiving cyclosporine after a renal transplant was treated with the combination imipenem/cilastatin IV 500 mg every 12 hours.[1] Twenty minutes after the second dose of imipenem, the patient developed neurologic side effects, including disorientation, motor aphasia, agitation, and tremor. The imipenem was discontinued; within 7 days the mental changes cleared, but the tremor remained. The patient's cyclosporine blood concentration increased from 400 ng/ml before the imipenem to 1000 ng/ml 4 days after imipenem. Cross-reactivity of imipenem with the cyclosporine radioimmunoassay was not ruled out.

RELATED DRUGS: A similar interaction with tacrolimus (*Prograf*) and imipenem may occur, but data are not available.

MANAGEMENT OPTIONS:

➡ *Monitor.* Until more information about this is available, carefully observe patients receiving both drugs for CNS toxic symptoms and altered cyclosporine serum concentrations.

REFERENCES:

1. Zazgornik J, et al. Potentiation of neurotoxic side effects by co-administration of imipenem to cyclosporine therapy in a kidney transplant recipient—synergism of side effects or drug interaction? *Clin Nephrol.* 1986;26:265.

Cyclosporine (eg, *Neoral*)

Indomethacin (eg, *Indocin*)

SUMMARY: Some nonsteroidal anti-inflammatory drugs (NSAIDs) may increase the risk of cyclosporine nephrotoxicity, but little clinical information is available for indomethacin.

RISK FACTORS: No specific risk factors are known.

MECHANISM: Not established.

CLINICAL EVALUATION: Although animal studies suggest that indomethacin may enhance the nephrotoxicity of cyclosporine,[1] clinical evidence is limited. In 1 patient, indomethacin did not appear to affect cyclosporine response significantly, but few details were given.[2]

RELATED DRUGS: Another NSAID, diclofenac (eg, *Voltaren*), has been associated with impaired renal function in a number of patients receiving cyclosporine;[2,3] and sulindac (eg, *Clinoril*) was associated with increased serum cyclosporine and serum creatinine concentrations in 1 patient.[4] However, because little is known regarding the effect of other NSAIDs on cyclosporine response, assume that all NSAIDs are capable of interacting with cyclosporine until evidence to the contrary is available.

MANAGEMENT OPTIONS:

➡ *Consider Alternative.* Even though there is little clinical information available regarding the effect of indomethacin on the response to cyclosporine, use all NSAIDs cautiously in patients taking cyclosporine.

➡ *Monitor.* If the combination is used, monitor the patient's renal function carefully and be prepared to discontinue one or both drugs.

REFERENCES:

1. Whiting PM, et al. Drug interactions with cyclosporine; implications from animal studies. *Transplant Proc.* 1986;18(Suppl. 5):56.

2. Branthwaite JP, et al. Cyclosporin and diclofenac interaction in rheumatoid arthritis. *Lancet.* 1991;337:252.

3. Deray G, et al. Enhancement of cyclosporine A nephrotoxicity of diclofenac. *Clin Nephrol.* 1987;27:213.

4. Sesin GP, et al. Sulindac-induced elevation of serum cyclosporine concentration. *Clin Pharm.* 1989;8:445.

4 Cyclosporine (eg, *Neoral*)

Isotretinoin (*Accutane*)

SUMMARY: Limited clinical data suggest that isotretinoin does not affect cyclosporine blood concentrations.

RISK FACTORS: No specific risk factors are known.

MECHANISM: Not established.

CLINICAL EVALUATION: In at least 2 heart transplant patients with severe acne, isotretinoin has been used concurrently with cyclosporine without any apparent alteration in blood cyclosporine concentrations or other difficulties caused by drug interaction.[1,2] Although this suggests that isotretinoin does not affect cyclosporine response, confirmation is needed. Since both cyclosporine and isotretinoin have been associated with elevated serum lipids, it has been suggested that patients receiving both drugs should be monitored for increased cholesterol and triglyceride levels.[3]

RELATED DRUGS: No information is available.

MANAGEMENT OPTIONS: No specific action is required, but be alert for evidence of the interaction.

REFERENCES:

1. O'Connell BM, et al. Dermatological complications following cardiac transplantation. *Heart Transplant.* 1986;5:430.

2. Bunker CB, et al. Isotretinoin treatment of severe acne in post-transplant patients taking cyclosporine. *J Am Acad Dermatol.* 1990;22:693.

3. Abel EA. Isotretinoin treatment of severe cystic acne in a heart transplant patient receiving cyclosporine: consideration of drug interactions. *J Am Acad Dermatol.* 1991;24:511.

3 Cyclosporine (eg, *Neoral*)

Itraconazole (*Sporanox*)

SUMMARY: Itraconazole may increase cyclosporine serum concentrations; nephrotoxicity may result.

RISK FACTORS: No specific risk factors are known.

MECHANISM: Itraconazole appears to inhibit the metabolism (CYP3A4) of cyclosporine.[5,6]

CLINICAL EVALUATION: Cyclosporine blood concentrations increased from 367 to 850 ng/ml after the addition of itraconazole and decreased to 396 ng/ml after itraconazole was withdrawn. A decrease in creatinine clearance was noted while cyclosporine concentrations were elevated.[1] In a second case report, dose-adjusted (concentration/dose) cyclosporine concentrations increased 3-fold during itraconazole administration and remained elevated for 4 weeks after itraconazole was discontinued. This may have been because of very slow elimination of the metabolites.[2] Seven transplant patients required an average cyclosporine dose reduction of 56% following itraconazole administration.[4] In an uncontrolled study 13 patients receiving itraconazole 100 mg twice daily for 4 to 7 weeks had cyclosporine concentrations similar to 210 other patients receiving cyclosporine without itraconazole.[3] Because of the design of this study, interpret these results with caution.

RELATED DRUGS: Ketoconazole (eg, *Nizoral*), miconazole, and fluconazole (*Diflucan*) are also inhibitors of cyclosporine metabolism. Itraconazole may affect tacrolimus (*Prograf*) similarly.

MANAGEMENT OPTIONS:

➧ *Monitor.* Monitor cyclosporine concentrations and renal function when itraconazole is added to or removed from the therapy of patients taking cyclosporine.

REFERENCES:

1. Kwan JTC, et al. Interaction of cyclosporine and itraconazole. *Lancet.* 1987;2:282.
2. Trenk D, et al. Time course of cyclosporin/itraconazole interaction. *Lancet.* 1987;2:1335.
3. Novakova I, et al. Itraconazole and cyclosporin nephrotoxicity. *Lancet.* 1987;2:920.
4. Kramer MR, et al. Cyclosporin and itraconazole interaction in heart and lung transplant recipients. *Ann Intern Med.* 1990;113:327.
5. Back DJ, et al. Comparative effects of the antimycotic drugs ketoconazole, fluconazole, itraconazole, and terbinafine on the metabolism of cyclosporin by human liver microsomes. *Br J Clin Pharmacol.* 1991;32:624.
6. Berenguer J, et al. Itraconazole for experimental pulmonary aspergillosis: comparison with amphotericin B, interaction with cyclosporine A, and correlation between therapeutic response and itraconazole concentrations in plasma. *Antimicrob Agents Chemother.* 1994;38:1303.

Cyclosporine (eg, *Neoral*)

Josamycin

SUMMARY: Josamycin, a macrolide antibiotic, appears to increase cyclosporine plasma concentrations, but additional study is needed to assess the incidence and magnitude of this effect.

RISK FACTORS: No specific risk factors are known.

MECHANISM: Not established; however, josamycin is a macrolide antibiotic related to erythromycin (eg, *E-Mycin*) and may inhibit cyclosporine metabolism.

CLINICAL EVALUATION: A renal transplant patient's cyclosporine concentration increased following 5 days of josamycin 2 g/day. A second case report noted that a cyclosporine dose was reduced from 300 to 100 mg/day during treatment with josamycin 2 g/day.[1] Another report noted a rise in cyclosporine concentrations within 2 to 4 days after starting josamycin in several patients.[2,3]

RELATED DRUGS: Tacrolimus (*Prograf*) is likely to be affected similarly by josamycin administration. Other macrolides (eg, erythromycin, troleandomycin [*TAO*], clarithromycin [*Biaxin*]) are known to inhibit cyclosporine metabolism. Azithromycin (*Zithromax*) and dirithromycin (*Dynabac*) would be unlikely to inhibit cyclosporine metabolism.

MANAGEMENT OPTIONS:

➧ *Monitor.* Monitor patients receiving cyclosporine for elevated cyclosporine concentrations and nephrotoxicity if josamycin is administered. Cyclosporine concentrations may decline following discontinuation of josamycin dosing.

REFERENCES:

1. Kreft-Jais C, et al. Effect of josamycin on plasma cyclosporine levels. *Eur J Clin Pharmacol.* 1987;32:327.
2. Azana J, et al. Possible interaction between cyclosporine and josamycin: a description of three cases. *Clin Pharmacol Ther.* 1992;51:572.
3. Torregrosa JV, et al. Interaction of josamycin with cyclosporin A. *Nephron.* 1993;65:476.

Cyclosporine (eg, Neoral)

Ketoconazole (eg, Nizoral)

SUMMARY: Ketoconazole appears to increase the serum concentration of cyclosporine, thereby increasing the risk of cyclosporine-induced renal toxicity.

RISK FACTORS: No specific risk factors are known.

MECHANISM: Ketoconazole inhibits the metabolism (CYP3A4) and increases the bioavailability of cyclosporine.[7]

CLINICAL EVALUATION: Both clinical studies and numerous case reports have identified ketoconazole-induced reduction in cyclosporine metabolism.[2,3] Cyclosporine clearance has been reduced by up to 85%[1,5,8] and its bioavailability increased from approximately 20% to 56%.[8] Renal toxicity has been noted to accompany the increased cyclosporine concentrations.[4-6] The large dose reductions (60% to 80%) necessitated by the ketoconazole-induced decrease in cyclosporine clearance have been advocated as a method to reduce the cost of immunosuppressant therapy.[4,5]

RELATED DRUGS: Other antifungal agents (eg, miconazole, itraconazole [*Sporanox*], fluconazole [*Diflucan*]) are likely to increase cyclosporine concentrations. It is likely that tacrolimus (*Prograf*) concentrations will be increased by ketoconazole and other antifungal agents.

MANAGEMENT OPTIONS:

➡ *Circumvent/Minimize.* Cyclosporine dose reduction is usually necessary when administered with ketoconazole.

➡ *Monitor.* Monitor cyclosporine concentrations and renal function when ketoconazole is prescribed during cyclosporine therapy. In patients stabilized on both drugs, large reductions in cyclosporine concentrations may occur when ketoconazole is discontinued.

REFERENCES:

1. First MR, et al. Cyclosporine-ketoconazole interaction. *Transplantation.* 1993;55:1000.
2. Sorenson AL, et al. Effects of ketoconazole on cyclosporine metabolism in renal allograft recipients. *Transplant Proc.* 1994;26:2822.
3. Shepard JH, et al. Cyclosporine-ketoconazole: a potentially dangerous drug-drug interaction. *Clin Pharm.* 1986;5:648.
4. Nolan PE, et al. Potentially favorable pharmacokinetic interaction between cyclosporine and ketoconazole in cardiac transplant recipients. *Pharmacotherapy.* 1989;9:192.
5. First MR, et al. Concomitant administration of cyclosporin and ketoconazole in renal transplant recipients. *Lancet.* 1989;2:1198.
6. Charles BG, et al. The ketoconazole-cyclosporin interaction in an elderly renal transplant patient. *Aust N Z J Med.* 1989;19:292.
7. Back DJ, et al. Comparative effects of the antimycotic drugs ketoconazole, fluconazole, itraconazole, and terbinafine on the metabolism of cyclosporin by human liver microsomes. *Br J Clin Pharmacol.* 1991;32:624.
8. Gomez DY, et al. The effects of ketoconazole on the intestinal metabolism and bioavailability of cyclosporine. *Clin Pharmacol Ther.* 1995;58:15.

Cyclosporine (eg, *Neoral*)

Ketoprofen (eg, *Oruvail*)

SUMMARY: Although some nonsteroidal anti-inflammatory drugs (NSAIDs) may increase the risk of cyclosporine nephrotoxicity, little clinical information is available for ketoprofen.

RISK FACTORS: No specific risk factors are known.

MECHANISM: Not established.

CLINICAL EVALUATION: Ketoprofen and cyclosporine were given concurrently in 1 patient without apparent interaction, but few details were given.[1]

RELATED DRUGS: Another NSAID, diclofenac (eg, *Voltaren*), has been associated with impaired renal function in a number of patients receiving cyclosporine[1,2]; sulindac (eg, *Clinoril*) was associated with increased serum cyclosporine and serum creatinine concentrations in 1 patient.[3] However, because little is known regarding the effect of other NSAIDs on cyclosporine response, assume that all NSAIDs are capable of interacting with cyclosporine until evidence to the contrary is available.

MANAGEMENT OPTIONS:

➥ **Consider Alternative.** Although little clinical information is available regarding the effect of ketoprofen on the response to cyclosporine, use all NSAIDs cautiously in patients receiving cyclosporine.

➥ **Monitor.** If the combination is used, monitor renal function carefully and be prepared to discontinue 1 or both drugs.

REFERENCES:

1. Branthwaite JP, et al. Cyclosporin and diclofenac interaction in rheumatoid arthritis. *Lancet.* 1991;337:252.
2. Deray G, et al. Enhancement of cyclosporine A nephrotoxicity of diclofenac. *Clin Nephrol.* 1987;27:213-214.
3. Sesin GP, et al. Sulindac-induced elevation of serum cyclosporine concentration. *Clin Pharm.* 1989;8:445-446.

Cyclosporine (eg, *Neoral*)

Levofloxacin (*Levaquin*)

SUMMARY: Levofloxacin does not appear to affect cyclosporine plasma concentrations.

RISK FACTORS: No specific risk factors are known.

MECHANISM: No interaction.

CLINICAL EVALUATION: Levofloxacin 500 mg 3 times daily for 6 days did not affect the pharmacokinetics of a single oral dose of cyclosporine 10 mg in 12 healthy subjects.[1]

RELATED DRUGS: Ofloxacin (eg, *Floxin*) does not affect cyclosporine pharmacokinetics. Norfloxacin (*Noroxin*) has been reported to affect cyclosporine concentrations in some patients, but other investigators found no changes.

MANAGEMENT OPTIONS: No interaction.

REFERENCES:

1. Doose DR, et al. Levofloxacin does not alter cyclosporine disposition. *J Clin Pharmacol.* 1998;38:90-93.

Cyclosporine (eg, *Neoral*)

Levothyroxine (eg, *Levoxyl*)

SUMMARY: Patients on chronic levothyroxine therapy may have decreased cyclosporine blood concentrations.

RISK FACTORS: No specific risk factors are known.

MECHANISM: Some clinical and animal data suggest that levothyroxine induces P-glycoprotein; it is possible that levothyroxine reduces cyclosporine bioavailability by inducing intestinal P-glycoprotein.

CLINICAL EVALUATION: Trough cyclosporine blood concentrations were measured in 40 patients, 10 of whom were on chronic therapy with levothyroxine.[1] Patients on levothyroxine had lower cyclosporine blood concentrations than those not taking levothyroxine. Subsequent study in rats also found lower cyclosporine blood concentrations in the presence of levothyroxine. More study is needed to establish the magnitude and clinical importance of this interaction.

RELATED DRUGS: No information is available.

MANAGEMENT OPTIONS:

➥ *Monitor.* Monitor for reduced cyclosporine blood concentrations if levothyroxine is given concurrently.

REFERENCES:

1. Jin M, et al. Long-term levothyroxine treatment decreases the oral bioavailability of cyclosporine A by inducing P-glycoprotein in small intestine. *Drug Metab Pharmacokinet.* 2005;20:324-330.

Cyclosporine (eg, *Neoral*)

Lovastatin (eg, *Mevacor*)

SUMMARY: Cyclosporine substantially increases plasma lovastatin concentrations, and the combination may increase the risk of skeletal muscle damage.

RISK FACTORS: No specific risk factors are known.

MECHANISM: Not established. Cyclosporine may inhibit the hepatic uptake of lovastatin by transporters such as OATP-C and also may inhibit the metabolism of lovastatin by CYP3A4.

CLINICAL EVALUATION: Kidney transplant patients receiving cyclosporine appear to develop serum lovastatin concentrations that are up to 20-fold higher than in patients not receiving cyclosporine.[1] Some transplant recipients taking cyclosporine and lovastatin have developed rhabdomyolysis; it is reasonable to assume that the observed pharmacokinetic interaction contributes to these adverse reactions.[2]

RELATED DRUGS: Cyclosporine also can increase the serum concentrations of simvastatin (*Zocor*), atorvastatin (*Lipitor*), fluvastatin (*Lescol*), rosuvastatin (*Crestor*), and pravastatin (*Pravachol*), although the risk of adverse consequences appears to differ depending on the statin. Pravastatin, for example, is frequently used in transplant patients without evidence of adverse drug interactions.

MANAGEMENT OPTIONS:

➡ *Circumvent/Minimize.* For patients receiving cyclosporine, the product information for lovastatin states that the dose of lovastatin should not exceed 20 mg/day. While many cyclosporine-treated patients have received larger doses of lovastatin without harm, exceeding this dosage recommendation could present medico-legal problems if the patient develops myopathy.

➡ *Monitor.* Be alert for evidence of myopathy (eg, darkened urine, muscle pain, muscle weakness) in patients receiving cyclosporine and lovastatin (or any other statin).

REFERENCES:

1. Olbricht C, et al. Accumulation of lovastatin, but not pravastatin, in the blood of cyclosporine-treated kidney graft patients after multiple doses. *Clin Pharmacol Ther*. 1997;62:311-321.
2. Asberg A. Interactions between cyclosporin and lipid-lowering drugs: implications for organ transplant recipients. *Drugs*. 2003;63:367-378.

Cyclosporine (eg, *Neoral*)
Mefenamic Acid (*Ponstel*)

SUMMARY: A renal transplant patient rapidly developed nephrotoxicity and an increase in plasma cyclosporine concentrations following the use of mefenamic acid, but the clinical importance is not established.

RISK FACTORS: No specific risk factors are known.

MECHANISM: Not established.

CLINICAL EVALUATION: A 36-year-old renal transplant patient stabilized on cyclosporine developed an increase in serum creatinine from 113 µmol/L (normal 50 to 110 mcmol/L) 1 day after starting mefenamic acid for dysmenorrhea.[1] Her plasma cyclosporine concentration abruptly rose to approximately twice the previous value. When the mefenamic acid was discontinued, the serum creatinine and cyclosporine concentrations fell to previous levels within approximately 1 week. The temporal relationship between the initiation and discontinuation of mefenamic acid therapy and the changes in cyclosporine plasma concentrations and renal function suggest that mefenamic acid interacts with cyclosporine. Moreover, some other nonsteroidal anti-inflammatory drugs (NSAIDs) have been shown to increase plasma cyclosporine concentrations or increase cyclosporine nephrotoxicity. Nonetheless, more information is needed to establish the incidence and magnitude of this interaction.

RELATED DRUGS: Several NSAIDs (eg, diclofenac [eg, *Voltaren*], sulindac [eg, *Clinoril*]) have been associated with impaired renal function or increased cyclosporine blood concentrations. The relative likelihood of various NSAIDs increasing cyclosporine-induced nephrotoxicity is not established but assume that all NSAIDs are capable of interacting with cyclosporine until evidence to the contrary is available.

MANAGEMENT OPTIONS:

➡ *Consider Alternative.* Until the clinical importance of this potential interaction is better defined, use mefenamic acid (or other NSAIDs) in patients receiving cyclosporine only when the expected benefit clearly outweighs the risk of excessive cyclosporine response and nephrotoxicity.

➡ **Monitor.** If the combination is used, monitor the patient's renal function and cyclosporine concentrations carefully, and be prepared to discontinue one or both drugs.

REFERENCES:

1. Agar JW. Cyclosporin A and mefenamic acid in a renal transplant patient. *Aust N Z J Med.* 1991;21:784-785.

Cyclosporine (eg, *Neoral*)

Melphalan (*Alkeran*)

SUMMARY: Preliminary evidence indicates that melphalan may increase the likelihood of nephrotoxicity in patients receiving cyclosporine.

RISK FACTORS: No specific risk factors are known.

MECHANISM: Not established.

CLINICAL EVALUATION: In 1 clinical study, renal failure occurred in 13 of 17 patients who received cyclosporine 12.5 mg/kg/day and melphalan 140 to 250 mg/m^2 as a single dose; the authors concluded the reactions resulted from a drug interaction between cyclosporine and melphalan.[1] Similar doses of melphalan in 7 patients without cyclosporine therapy did not cause nephrotoxicity.

RELATED DRUGS: No information is available.

MANAGEMENT OPTIONS:

➡ **Monitor.** Monitor renal function carefully in patients receiving concurrent therapy with cyclosporine and melphalan.

REFERENCES:

1. Morgenstern GR, et al. Cyclosporin interaction with ketoconazole and melphalan. *Lancet.* 1982;2:1342.

Cyclosporine (eg, *Neoral*)

Methotrexate

SUMMARY: The combination of methotrexate and cyclosporine in the treatment of psoriasis appears to increase toxicity.

RISK FACTORS: No specific risk factors are known.

MECHANISM: Not established. Methotrexate may inhibit the clearance of cyclosporine or its metabolites; cyclosporine may inhibit methotrexate elimination.

CLINICAL EVALUATION: Thirteen patients with psoriasis were treated with cyclosporine for an average of 2.5 years.[1] Seven of the patients had previously received methotrexate, 6 had not. Patients receiving cyclosporine after methotrexate had higher cyclosporine plus metabolite plasma concentrations (626 vs 296 ng/ml) and developed increased serum creatinine concentrations and hypertension more frequently than patients taking only cyclosporine. Another report of 4 patients with psoriasis described elevations in hepatic enzymes and serum creatinine, nausea, vomiting, and oral mucosal ulcers following combination therapy with cyclosporine 2.5 to 5 mg/kg/day and methotrexate 2.5 mg twice daily for 3 doses per week.[2] The data presented do not indicate whether cyclosporine concentrations (range, 135 to 325 ng/mL) changed following methotrexate administration. The side effects resolved following discontinuation of both drugs.

RELATED DRUGS: No information is available.

MANAGEMENT OPTIONS:

➥ *Monitor.* Carefully monitor patients receiving methotrexate and cyclosporine for toxicity from both agents. Monitor cyclosporine and methotrexate concentrations; the dosage of either drug may require adjustment.

REFERENCES:

1. Powles AV, et al. Cyclosporin toxicity. *Lancet.* 1990;335:610.
2. Korstanje MJ, et al. Cyclosporine and methotrexate: a dangerous combination. *J Am Acad Derm.* 1990;23:320.

Cyclosporine (eg, *Neoral*)

Methylphenidate (eg, *Ritalin*)

SUMMARY: A boy receiving cyclosporine following a heart transplant developed an increase in cyclosporine concentrations during methylphenidate administration, but a causal relationship was not established.

RISK FACTORS: No specific risk factors are known.

MECHANISM: Not established.

CLINICAL EVALUATION: A 10-year-old boy on cyclosporine following a heart transplant developed a substantial increase in cyclosporine blood concentrations after starting methylphenidate 5 mg twice daily.[1] It was not possible to be certain that the patient adhered to the cyclosporine dosing schedule, so a causal relationship was not established.

RELATED DRUGS: No information is available.

MANAGEMENT OPTIONS: No specific action is required, but be alert for evidence of the interaction.

REFERENCES:

1. Lewis BR, et al. Pharmacokinetic interactions between cyclosporine and bupropion or methylphenidate. *J Child Adolesc Psychopharmacol.* 2001;11:193-198.

Cyclosporine (eg, *Neoral*)

Metoclopramide (eg, *Reglan*)

SUMMARY: Metoclopramide increases the bioavailability and serum concentrations of single-dose cyclosporine, probably by increasing gastric emptying; nevertheless, it is not known how often this effect would cause clinical difficulties.

RISK FACTORS: No specific risk factors are known.

MECHANISM: Not established. Cyclosporine is variably and poorly absorbed, probably because of one or more of the following factors: degradation within the GI tract, first-pass metabolism, and carrier-mediated absorption.[1] Metoclopramide-induced increases in GI motility and gastric emptying could reduce degradation of cyclosporine within the GI tract by transporting the cyclosporine to sites of absorption more rapidly. Theoretically, this more rapid absorption also could reduce first-pass metabolism of cyclosporine, but this has not been studied.

CLINICAL EVALUATION: The effect of single 20 mg oral doses of metoclopramide on the absorption of cyclosporine was studied in 14 renal transplant patients (cyclosporine doses were 4 to 10 mg/kg/day in 2 divided doses).[2] Metoclopramide increased the mean bioavailability of cyclosporine approximately 30%, but much larger increases were seen in a few patients. It is not known whether the increase in cyclosporine bioavailability would be sustained with multiple doses of metoclopramide. If so, it is likely that some patients would develop excessive cyclosporine effects with this combination.

RELATED DRUGS: The effect of cisapride on cyclosporine is not established, but caution is in order as both are metabolized by CYP3A4. Competition for metabolism is theoretically possible.

MANAGEMENT OPTIONS:

➡ **Monitor.** Until multiple-dose studies are performed, monitor cyclosporine serum concentrations and responses carefully when metoclopramide is given concurrently. It may be necessary to reduce the cyclosporine dose in some patients.

REFERENCES:

1. Yee GC, et al. Cyclosporine. In: Evans WE, et al, eds. *Applied Pharmacokinetics: Principles of Therapeutic Drug Monitoring.* 3rd ed. Vancouver: Applied Therapeutics, Inc.; 1992.

2. Wadhwa NK, et al. The effect of oral metoclopramide on the absorption of cyclosporine. *Transplantation.* 1987;43:211-213.

4 Cyclosporine (eg, *Neoral*)

Metronidazole (eg, *Flagyl*)

SUMMARY: Metronidazole appeared to increase blood cyclosporine concentrations in 1 patient, but a causal relationship was not established.

RISK FACTORS: No specific risk factors are known.

MECHANISM: Not established. Metronidazole can inhibit hepatic drug metabolism, and it is possible that cyclosporine metabolism is affected similarly.

CLINICAL EVALUATION: A renal transplant patient developed more than a 2-fold increase in her blood cyclosporine concentrations over about 2 weeks after metronidazole 2250 mg/day and cimetidine (eg, *Tagamet*) 800 mg/day were started simultaneously.[1] When the metronidazole dosage was reduced to 1200 mg/day (at the same time that the cimetidine was discontinued), the cyclosporine concentrations fell to approximately 50% of baseline levels and then returned to baseline after the metronidazole was discontinued. Although the presence of cimetidine therapy complicates evaluation of metronidazole's role in the altered cyclosporine concentrations, limited evidence suggests that cimetidine does not affect cyclosporine blood concentrations.[2] Nonetheless, additional study under more controlled conditions is needed to determine whether metronidazole affects cyclosporine disposition.

RELATED DRUGS: If this interaction is substantiated, tacrolimus (*Prograf*) is likely to be affected similarly.

MANAGEMENT OPTIONS: No specific action is required, but be alert for evidence of the interaction.

REFERENCES:

1. Zylber-Katz E, et al. Cyclosporine interactions with metronidazole and cimetidine. *Drug Intell Clin Pharm.* 1988;22:504-505.

2. Pachon J, et al. Effects of H$_2$-receptor antagonists on renal function in cyclosporine-treated renal transplant patients. *Transplantation.* 1989;47:254-259.

Cyclosporine (eg, *Neoral*)

Miconazole (eg, *Monistat*)

SUMMARY: Miconazole administration to a patient receiving cyclosporine appears to increase cyclosporine concentrations; the clinical significance of this increase is unknown.

RISK FACTORS: No specific risk factors are known.

MECHANISM: Not established. Miconazole-induced reduction in cyclosporine (CYP3A4) metabolism may be responsible for the increased cyclosporine concentrations observed in this patient.

CLINICAL EVALUATION: A heart transplant patient was receiving several different antimycotic drugs including ketoconazole (eg, *Nizoral*), fluconazole (*Diflucan*), and miconazole during his hospitalization.[1] Miconazole 1 g IV every 8 hours was initiated while the patient was taking cyclosporine 220 mg/day. The cyclosporine plasma concentration increased from 227 to 376 ng/mL 3 days after starting miconazole. The miconazole was discontinued after 13 days but was restarted 4 days later. Cyclosporine concentrations again increased following miconazole administration, although the cyclosporine dose had been increased just before adding the miconazole. The second time miconazole was discontinued, the initiation of another antimycotic agent (SCH 39304) also appeared to increase cyclosporine concentrations. Fluconazole did not appear to affect cyclosporine concentrations in this patient, although it has been reported to increase cyclosporine concentrations in other studies.[2]

RELATED DRUGS: Other antifungal agents (ketoconazole, itraconazole [eg, *Sporanox*], fluconazole) are likely to increase cyclosporine concentrations. Miconazole may produce a similar reaction with tacrolimus (eg, *Prograf*).

MANAGEMENT OPTIONS:

➡ **Monitor.** Until further studies of this interaction are available, closely monitor patients stabilized on cyclosporine for increased concentrations of cyclosporine when miconazole is administered.

REFERENCES:

1. Horton CM, et al. Cyclosporine interactions with miconazole and other azole-antimycotics: a case report and review of the literature. *J Heart Lung Transplant.* 1992;11:1127-1132.

2. Canafax DM, et al. Increased cyclosporine levels as a result of simultaneous fluconazole and cyclosporine therapy in renal transplant recipients: a double-blind, randomized pharmacokinetic and safety study. *Transplant Proc.* 1991;23:1041-1042.

Cyclosporine (eg, *Sandimmune*)

Modafinil (*Provigil*)

SUMMARY: Limited clinical evidence and theoretical considerations suggest that modafinil can reduce cyclosporine blood concentrations; monitor patients carefully.

RISK FACTORS: No specific risk factors are known.

MECHANISM: Modafinil is known to induce intestinal CYP3A4, and it probably reduces cyclosporine bioavailability through increased presystemic metabolism.

CLINICAL EVALUATION: A 41-year-old woman on cyclosporine developed a 50% reduction in cyclosporine blood concentrations after taking modafinil (200 mg/day for 1 month).[1] This effect is consistent with another study finding that modafinil produced a 59% reduction in triazolam area under the concentration-time curve. Cyclosporine and triazolam undergo extensive first-pass metabolism by intestinal CYP3A4.

RELATED DRUGS: No information is available.

MANAGEMENT OPTIONS:

➡ *Circumvent/Minimize.* Given the importance of maintaining adequate cyclosporine blood concentrations in transplant patients, avoid concurrent use of modafinil and cyclosporine if possible.

➡ *Monitor.* If modafinil is used concurrently with cyclosporine, monitor cyclosporine blood concentrations carefully when modafinil is initiated, discontinued, or changed in dosage. Note that the onset and offset of enzyme induction can be gradual, so continue cyclosporine monitoring until it is clear that blood concentrations are stable.

REFERENCES:

1. Product information. Modafinil (*Provigil*). Cephalon, Inc. 2002.
2. Robertson P, et al. Effect of modafinil on the pharmacokinetics of ethinyl estradiol and triazolam in healthy volunteers. *Clin Pharmacol Ther.* 2002;71:46-56.

Cyclosporine (eg, *Neoral*)

Nafcillin

SUMMARY: Nafcillin therapy reduced cyclosporine blood concentrations during coadministration; the clinical significance of this interaction is unknown, but a reduction in cyclosporine activity may be anticipated.

RISK FACTORS: No specific risk factors are known.

MECHANISM: Not established. Nafcillin appears to increase the metabolism or reduce the bioavailability of cyclosporine.

CLINICAL EVALUATION: The cyclosporine concentration in a 34-year-old woman taking cyclosporine 400 mg/day declined more than 50% when nafcillin was administered on 2 separate occasions.[1] No deterioration in graft function was noted during the periods of low cyclosporine concentrations. While the temporal relationship between the repeated administration of nafcillin and the changes in cyclosporine concentration indicate an interaction is likely, more study is needed to establish a causal relationship.

RELATED DRUGS: If this interaction is substantiated, tacrolimus (*Prograf*) is likely to be affected similarly.

MANAGEMENT OPTIONS:

➡ *Monitor.* Monitor patients receiving cyclosporine for reduced blood concentrations of cyclosporine and evidence of organ rejection during nafcillin administration.

REFERENCES:

1. Veremis SA, et al. Subtherapeutic cyclosporine concentrations during nafcillin therapy. *Transplantation.* 1987;43:913.

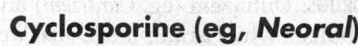

Cyclosporine (eg, *Neoral*)

Naproxen (eg, *Naprosyn*)

SUMMARY: Impaired renal function appears to be greater with naproxen plus cyclosporine than with either drug alone.

RISK FACTORS: No specific risk factors are known.

MECHANISM: Not established.

CLINICAL EVALUATION: Eleven patients with rheumatoid arthritis were treated with cyclosporine and nonsteroidal anti-inflammatory drugs (NSAIDs) (sulindac [eg, *Clinoril*] or naproxen), alone and in combination. Impairment of renal function was greater with cyclosporine plus an NSAID than with either drug alone.[4] The effect was reversible.

RELATED DRUGS: In patients receiving cyclosporine, several NSAIDs have been associated with impaired renal function or increased cyclosporine blood concentrations.[1-4] The relative likelihood of various NSAIDs to increase cyclosporine-induced nephrotoxicity is not established, but assume that all NSAIDs are capable of interacting with cyclosporine until evidence to the contrary is available.

MANAGEMENT OPTIONS:

➡ *Consider Alternative.* Until the clinical importance of this potential interaction is better defined, use naproxen (or other NSAIDs) in patients receiving cyclosporine only when the expected benefit clearly outweighs the risk of excessive cyclosporine response and nephrotoxicity.

➡ *Monitor.* If the combination is used, monitor the patient's renal function carefully and be prepared to discontinue one or both drugs.

REFERENCES:

1. Sesin GP, et al. Sulindac-induced elevation of serum cyclosporine concentrations. *Clin Pharm.* 1989;8:445.

2. Branthwaite JP, et al. Cyclosporin and diclofenac interaction in rheumatoid arthritis. *Lancet.* 1991;337:252.

3. Deray G, et al. Enhancement of cyclosporine A nephrotoxicity by diclofenac. *Clin Nephrol.* 1987;27:213.

4. Altman RD, et al. Interaction of cyclosporine A and nonsteroidal antiinflammatory drugs on renal function in patients with rheumatoid arthritis. *Am J Med.* 1992;93:396.

Cyclosporine (*Neoral*)

Nicardipine (eg, *Cardene*)

SUMMARY: Cyclosporine blood concentrations are increased by nicardipine; cyclosporine toxicity could result.

RISK FACTORS: No specific risk factors are known.

MECHANISM: Nicardipine appears to inhibit the metabolism of cyclosporine.

CLINICAL EVALUATION: An increase in cyclosporine concentrations more than 100% has been noted during coadministration of nicardipine 60 to 120 mg/day.[1-3] This degree of increase could result in cyclosporine-induced nephrotoxicity.

RELATED DRUGS: Diltiazem (eg, *Cardizem*) and verapamil (eg, *Calan*) inhibit cyclosporine metabolism while isradipine (*DynaCirc*), nifedipine (eg, *Procardia*), amlodipine (*Norvasc*) and nitrendipine have minimal effect. Nicardipine may affect tacrolimus (*Prograf*) in a similar manner.

MANAGEMENT OPTIONS:

➡ *Consider Alternative.* Calcium channel blockers that do not appear to alter cyclosporine pharmacokinetics include isradipine,[4] nitrendipine,[5] and amlodipine.[6]

➡ *Circumvent/Minimize.* Reduce cyclosporine dosage and monitor blood concentrations when nicardipine is coadministered.

➡ *Monitor.* Observe patients receiving both drugs for increased cyclosporine concentrations and decreasing renal function.

REFERENCES:

1. Bourbigot B, et al. Nicardipine increases cyclosporine blood levels. *Lancet.* 1986;1:1447.
2. Cantarovich M, et al. Confirmation of the interaction between cyclosporine and the calcium channel blocker nicardipine in renal transplant patients. *Clin Nephrol.* 1987;29:190.
3. Todd P, et al. Nicardipine interacts with cyclosporin. *Br J Dermatol.* 1989;121:820.
4. Martinez F, et al. No clinically significant interaction between cyclosporin and isradipine. *Nephron.* 1991;59:658.
5. Coupur MS, et al. Effects of nitrendipine on blood pressure and blood cyclosporine A level in patients with posttransplant hypertension. *Nephron.* 1989;52:227.
6. Toupance O, et al. Antihypertensive effect of amlodipine and lack of interference with cyclosporine metabolism in renal transplant recipients. *Hypertension.* 1994;24:297.

Cyclosporine (eg, *Neoral*)

Nifedipine (eg, *Procardia*)

SUMMARY: Nifedipine does not appear to affect cyclosporine concentrations, but cyclosporine may increase nifedipine concentrations.

RISK FACTORS: No specific risk factors are known.

MECHANISM: Cyclosporine may inhibit the renal elimination of a nifedipine metabolite.

CLINICAL EVALUATION: Nifedipine has little or no effect on cyclosporine concentrations.[1,3-6] In a preliminary report in 8 patients, cyclosporine 3 to 4 mg/kg/day reduced the urinary excretion of a nifedipine metabolite.[2] The significance of these changes is probably limited.

RELATED DRUGS: Diltiazem (eg, *Cardizem*), nicardipine (eg, *Cardene*) and verapamil (eg, *Calan*) inhibit cyclosporine metabolism while isradipine (*DynaCirc*) and nitrendipine have minimal effect. While no data exist, nifedipine would be expected to have minimal effect on tacrolimus (*Prograf*) metabolism.

MANAGEMENT OPTIONS: No specific action is required, but be alert for evidence of an interaction.

REFERENCES:

1. Robson RA, et al. Cyclosporin-verapamil interaction. *Br J Clin Pharmacol.* 1988;25:402.
2. McFadden JP, et al. Cyclosporin decreases nifedipine metabolism. *BMJ.* 1989;299:1224.
3. Wagner K, et al. Interaction of cyclosporin and calcium antagonists. *Transplant Proc.* 1989;21:1453.
4. Wagner K, et al. Interaction of calcium blockers and cyclosporine. *Transplant Proc.* 1988;20(Suppl. 2):561.
5. Roy LF, et al. Short-term effects of calcium antagonists on hemodynamics and cyclosporine pharmacokinetics in heart-transplant and kidney-transplant patients. *Clin Pharmacol Ther.* 1989;46:657.
6. Howard RL, et al. The effect of calcium channel blockers on the cyclosporine dose requirement in renal transplant recipients. *Ren Fail.* 1990;12:89.

Cyclosporine (eg, *Neoral*)

Norfloxacin (*Noroxin*)

SUMMARY: Norfloxacin may increase cyclosporine concentrations, but the frequency and magnitude of the effect is unknown.

RISK FACTORS: No specific risk factors are known.

MECHANISM: Not established.

CLINICAL EVALUATION: A cardiac transplant patient developed a sudden increase in serum cyclosporine concentrations following the addition of norfloxacin 400 mg twice daily for 5 days.[1] However, in 6 renal transplant patients, norfloxacin 400 mg twice daily for an average of 9 days had no effect on serum cyclosporine concentrations.[2] Additional study is required to define the significance of this potential interaction.

RELATED DRUGS: Ciprofloxacin (*Cipro*) has been reported to cause nephrotoxicity when administered with cyclosporine. Ofloxacin (eg, *Floxin*) and pefloxacin have been shown to produce no change in cyclosporine concentration or toxicity. Norfloxacin may produce a similar effect on tacrolimus (*Prograf*).

MANAGEMENT OPTIONS: No specific action is required, but be alert for evidence of the interaction.

REFERENCES:

1. Thomson DJ, et al. Norfloxacin-cyclosporine interaction. *Transplantation.* 1988;46:312-313.
2. Jadoul M, et al. Norfloxacin and cyclosporine—a safe combination. *Transplantation.* 1989;47:747-748.

Cyclosporine (eg, *Neoral*) 5

Ofloxacin (eg, *Floxin*)

SUMMARY: Limited evidence suggests there is no interaction between cyclosporine and ofloxacin.

RISK FACTORS: No specific risk factors are known.

MECHANISM: No interaction.

CLINICAL EVALUATION: Thirty-nine renal transplant recipients taking cyclosporine were treated with ofloxacin at varying dosages for urinary tract infections.[1] Cyclosporine blood concentrations and serum creatinine levels were not affected.

RELATED DRUGS: Ciprofloxacin (*Cipro*) may increase cyclosporine concentrations. Pefloxacin does not appear to affect cyclosporine metabolism. Ofloxacin would be unlikely to affect tacrolimus (*Prograf*) metabolism.

MANAGEMENT OPTIONS: No interaction.

REFERENCES:
1. Vogt P, et al. Ofloxacin in the treatment of urinary tract infection in renal transplant recipients. *Infection.* 1988;16:175-178.

Cyclosporine (eg, *Neoral*)

Omeprazole (eg, *Prilosec*)

SUMMARY: One patient appeared to develop reduced cyclosporine concentrations with omeprazole; subsequent study has not confirmed this effect.

RISK FACTORS: No specific risk factors are known.

MECHANISM: Not established.

CLINICAL EVALUATION: Although omeprazole appeared to inhibit cyclosporine metabolism in 1 case,[1] subsequent reports in 11 patients[2,3] failed to confirm an effect of omeprazole 20 mg/day on cyclosporine blood concentrations. Nonetheless, the ability of omeprazole to inhibit hepatic drug metabolism is known to be dose-related, and it is possible that an effect on cyclosporine metabolism would occur with omeprazole doses of more than 20 mg/day.

RELATED DRUGS: Ranitidine (eg, *Zantac*), and probably cimetidine (eg, *Tagamet*), appears unlikely to affect cyclosporine blood concentrations (see Index). Theoretically, lansoprazole (*Prevacid*) would be unlikely to interact with cyclosporine, but little information is available.

MANAGEMENT OPTIONS: No specific action is required, but be alert for evidence of the interaction.

REFERENCES:
1. Schouler L, et al. Omeprazole-cyclosporine interaction. *Am J Gastroenterol.* 1991;86:1097.
2. Blohme I, et al. A study of the interaction between omeprazole and cyclosporine in renal transplant patients. *Br J Clin Pharmacol.* 1993;35:156-160.
3. Castellote E, et al. Does interaction between omeprazole and cyclosporin exist? *Nephron.* 1993;65:478.

Cyclosporine (eg, *Neoral*)

Oxybutynin (eg, *Ditropan*)

SUMMARY: Limited clinical evidence suggests that oxybutynin does not interact with cyclosporine.

RISK FACTORS: No specific risk factors are known.

MECHANISM: None (no interaction).

CLINICAL EVALUATION: Two children received cyclosporine with and without concurrent oxybutynin therapy, and there was no change in the trough blood cyclosporine concentrations.[1] Additional study is needed to establish that oxybutynin does not interact with cyclosporine.

RELATED DRUGS: No information is available.

MANAGEMENT OPTIONS: No interaction.

REFERENCES:

1. Springate JE. Oxybutynin does not affect cyclosporine blood levels. *Ther Drug Monit.* 2001;23:155-156.

Cyclosporine (eg, *Neoral*)

Pefloxacin†

SUMMARY: Limited evidence suggests there is no interaction between cyclosporine and pefloxacin.

RISK FACTORS: No specific risk factors are known.

MECHANISM: No interaction.

CLINICAL EVALUATION: Pefloxacin 400 mg every 12 hours had no effect on the pharmacokinetics of chronically administered cyclosporine in renal transplant patients.[1]

RELATED DRUGS: Ciprofloxacin (*Cipro*) has been reported to inhibit cyclosporine metabolism. Ofloxacin (eg, *Floxin*) would be unlikely to affect cyclosporine metabolism.

MANAGEMENT OPTIONS: No interaction.

REFERENCES:

1. Lang J, et al. Absence of pharmacokinetic interaction between pefloxacin and cyclosporin A in patients with renal transplants. *Rev Infect Dis.* 1989;11(suppl 5): S1094.

† Not available in the United States.

Cyclosporine (eg, *Neoral*)

Phenobarbital (eg, *Solfoton*)

SUMMARY: Phenobarbital (and probably other barbiturates) can reduce the effect of cyclosporine; adjustments in the cyclosporine dose may be needed.

RISK FACTORS: No specific risk factors are known.

MECHANISM: Barbiturates are likely to enhance the hepatic microsomal metabolism of cyclosporine.[1]

CLINICAL EVALUATION: Those involved in the clinical use of cyclosporine have observed that enzyme inducers such as phenobarbital may lower serum cyclosporine concentrations,[2,3] although little specific evidence has been presented. A 4-year-old girl on long-term phenobarbital 100 mg/day therapy received cyclosporine 25 mg/kg for 4 days, then 12.5 mg/kg. Trough serum cyclosporine concentrations were undetectable during this dosage of phenobarbital, but increased gradually as the phenobarbital dosage was reduced to 50 mg/day and then to 25 mg/day.[4] Although this interaction requires further study, the well-documented ability of another enzyme inducer, rifampin (eg, *Rifadin*), to stimulate cyclosporine metabolism[5] supports the suggestion that phenobarbital acts in a similar way.

RELATED DRUGS: Expect other barbiturates to reduce cyclosporine response until evidence to the contrary becomes available.

MANAGEMENT OPTIONS:

➡ **Consider Alternative.** If the barbiturate is being used as a sedative-hypnotic, consider using a benzodiazepine in place of the barbiturate.

➡ **Monitor.** In a patient stabilized on cyclosporine, monitor for altered cyclosporine response if barbiturate therapy is started or stopped or if the barbiturate dose is changed. Note that the enzyme-inducing effects of barbiturates tend to have a gradual onset and offset (at least 1 to 2 weeks, depending on the barbiturate). When initiating cyclosporine therapy in a patient receiving a barbiturate, be aware that the cyclosporine dosage requirements may be higher than anticipated.

REFERENCES:

1. Cockburn IT, et al. An appraisal of drug interactions with *Sandimmun. Transplant Proc.* 1989;21(5):3845-3850.
2. Burkle WS. Usefulness of cyclosporine monitoring questioned. *Clin Pharm.* 1984;3(3):239, 243.
3. Kerr LE. Drug interactions with cyclosporine. *Clin Pharm.* 1984;3(4):346, 348.
4. Carstensen H, et al. Interaction between cyclosporine A and phenobarbitone. *Br J Clin Pharmacol.* 1986;21(5):550-551.
5. Offermann G, et al. Low cyclosporin A blood levels and acute graft rejection in a renal transplant recipient during rifampin treatment. *Am J Nephrol.* 1985;5(5):385-387.

Cyclosporine (eg, *Neoral*)

Phenytoin (eg, *Dilantin*)

SUMMARY: Phenytoin markedly reduces serum cyclosporine concentrations and is likely to increase cyclosporine dosage requirements.

RISK FACTORS: No specific risk factors are known.

MECHANISM: Phenytoin is a known enzyme inducer of hepatic microsomal enzymes, and enzyme induction is probably responsible for at least part of the reduction in cyclosporine serum concentrations. Nevertheless, the rapid onset and offset of the interaction noted in one study (a few days) suggests that additional mechanisms may be involved. Indeed, some of the data suggest that phenytoin inhibits the absorption of cyclosporine.[1]

CLINICAL EVALUATION: Five patients receiving oral cyclosporine following renal transplantation developed reductions in trough cyclosporine serum concentrations within a few days of starting phenytoin therapy; the interaction dissipated within 3 days after discontinuing phenytoin.[2] The area under the intravenous cyclosporine concentration-time curve decreased 50% in the presence of phenytoin therapy. In 2 subsequent studies involving healthy subjects[3] and transplant patients,[4] phenytoin was associated with marked reductions in cyclosporine serum concentrations. The magnitude of the interaction observed in these studies is expected to result in insufficient serum cyclosporine concentrations if the cyclosporine dosages are not adjusted.

RELATED DRUGS: Other enzyme-inducing anticonvulsants also appear to reduce blood cyclosporine concentrations. Tacrolimus (*Prograf*) is likely affected similarly by enzyme inducers.

MANAGEMENT OPTIONS:

➥ *Circumvent/Minimize.* When initiating cyclosporine therapy in a patient receiving phenytoin, be aware that the cyclosporine dosage requirements may be higher than anticipated.

➥ *Monitor.* In a patient stabilized on cyclosporine, monitor for altered cyclosporine response if phenytoin therapy is started or stopped or if the dose is changed. Starting phenytoin therapy may increase the risk of rejection in patients taking cyclosporine.

REFERENCES:

1. Rowland M, et al. Cyclosporin-phenytoin interaction: re-evaluation using metabolite data. *Br J Clin Pharmacol.* 1987;24(3):329-334.

2. Keown PA, et al. The effects and side effects of cyclosporine: relationship to drug pharmacokinetics. *Transplant Proc.* 1982;14(4):659-661.

3. Freeman DJ, et al. Evaluation on cyclosporin-phenytoin interaction with observations of cyclosporin metabolites. *Br J Clin Pharmacol.* 1984;18(6):887-893.

4. Keown PA, et al. Interaction between phenytoin and cyclosporine following organ transplantation. *Transplantation.* 1984;38(3):304-306.

Cyclosporine (eg, *Neoral*)

Pitavastatin (*Livalo*)

SUMMARY: Cyclosporine has been reported to increase the concentrations of pitavastatin; increased adverse reactions may occur in some patients.

RISK FACTORS: No specific risk factors are known.

MECHANISM: Unknown. Pitavastatin is a substrate for the organic anion-transporting polypeptide (OATP), and cyclosporine is known to inhibit this transporter. Inhibition of OATP would reduce the uptake of pitavastatin into hepatocytes where it is metabolized.

CLINICAL EVALUATION: While specific data are limited, the manufacturer of pitavastatin notes that the coadministration of pitavastatin 2 mg daily for 6 days with cyclosporine 2 mg/kg on day 6 increased the mean area under the plasma concentration-time curve of pitavastatin approximately 4.6-fold.[1] Pending further data, observe patients receiving pitavastatin and cyclosporine for increased pitavastatin effect. Pitavastatin labeling contraindicates the administration of pitavastatin with cyclosporine.

RELATED DRUGS: No information is available.

MANAGEMENT OPTIONS:

➥ *Avoid Unless Benefit Outweighs Risk.* The use of an alternate statin, such as pravastatin (eg, *Pravachol*), is suggested for patients taking cyclosporine. Note that pravastatin concentrations are increased by cyclosporine; start with a low dose of pravastatin when possible.

➥ *Monitor.* Carefully monitor patients receiving pitavastatin who require cyclosporine for signs of pitavastatin toxicity, including hepatotoxicity, muscle weakness, and myalgia.

REFERENCES:

1. *Livalo* [package insert]. Montgomery, AL: Kowa Pharmaceuticals America Inc; 2009.

Cyclosporine (eg, *Neoral*)

Posaconazole (*Noxafil*)

SUMMARY: Posaconazole administration results in elevated cyclosporine plasma concentrations; cyclosporine toxicity may result.

RISK FACTORS: No specific risk factors are known.

MECHANISM: Posaconazole is known to inhibit CYP3A4, the primary metabolic pathway for cyclosporine.

CLINICAL EVALUATION: Four patients taking cyclosporine for immunosuppression received concomitant posaconazole 200 mg daily for 10 days.[1] Cyclosporine dosages were adjusted if trough concentrations were altered. The apparent clearance of cyclosporine was reduced approximately 25% during posaconazole administration. Cyclosporine dose reductions ranged from 14% to 29% in these patients. Larger doses of posaconazole are expected to produce a greater increase in cyclosporine plasma concentrations.

RELATED DRUGS: Ketoconazole (eg, *Nizoral*), fluconazole (eg, *Diflucan*), itraconazole (eg, *Sporanox*), and voriconazole (*Vfend*) also inhibit the activity of CYP3A4 and are expected to increase the plasma concentrations of cyclosporine. Posaconazole also reduced the clearance of tacrolimus (*Prograf*) and is expected to affect sirolimus (*Rapamune*) in a similar manner.

MANAGEMENT OPTIONS:

➡ ***Consider Alternative.*** Terbinafine (eg, *Lamisil*) may be an alternative antifungal agent because it does not affect CYP3A4 activity. Amphotericin, caspofungin (*Cansidas*), and anidulafungin (*Eraxis*) do not appear to inhibit CYP3A4.

➡ ***Monitor.*** Monitor patients stabilized on cyclosporine for altered cyclosporine dose requirements if posaconazole is added to or discontinued from their drug regimen.

REFERENCES:

1. Sansone-Parsons A, et al. Effect of oral posaconazole on the pharmacokinetics of cyclosporine and tacrolimus. *Pharmacotherapy.* 2007;27(6):825-834.

 Cyclosporine (eg, *Neoral*)

Pravastatin (*Pravachol*)

SUMMARY: Clinical trials in patients with renal or cardiac transplants have found no evidence that pravastatin results in myopathy when combined with cyclosporine, but 1 preliminary report suggests that pravastatin may increase serum cyclosporine concentrations.

RISK FACTORS: No specific risk factors are known.

MECHANISM: Not established.

CLINICAL EVALUATION: In 24 renal transplant recipients taking cyclosporine (mean dose, 2.7 mg/kg/day), azathioprine, and prednisolone, the addition of pravastatin 10 mg/day did not result in symptoms of myopathy, an elevated creatine kinase (CK) level or impaired renal function.[1] Similar results were found in a preliminary report of 21 cyclosporine-treated heart transplant patients (6 months or longer postoperative); the addition of pravastatin 10 mg/day for a mean of 119 days did not result in myalgia, nor did it affect CK or cyclosporine concentrations.[2] In another preliminary report, 33 post-cardiac transplant patients on cyclosporine were given pravastatin 20 mg/day for 3 months.[3] The use of pravastatin appeared to be safe and effective in these patients; serum CK levels were not affected. However, 17 of the 19 patients on a stable cyclosporine dose developed a 74% increase in plasma cyclosporine concentrations. The reason for the finding of increased cyclosporine concentrations in one study[3] but not another[2] is not clear; the dose of the pravastatin (20 vs 10 mg/day) may be one reason. More study is needed to determine whether pravastatin (or other hepatic hydroxymethylglutaryl coenzyme A reductase inhibitors) affects cyclosporine serum concentrations.

RELATED DRUGS: Available evidence suggests that pravastatin and fluvastatin (*Lescol*) are safer than lovastatin (*Mevacor*) in patients receiving cyclosporine. Since little is known regarding the effect of combined cyclosporine-simvastatin (*Zocor*) therapy, pravastatin is probably preferable to this agent as well.

MANAGEMENT OPTIONS: No specific action is required, but be alert for evidence of the interaction.

REFERENCES:

1. Yoshimura N, et al. The effects of pravastatin on hyperlipidemia in renal transplant recipients. *Transplantation.* 1992;53:94.

2. Davies RA. Safety and efficacy of pravastatin after heart transplantation: preliminary patient studies. XI International Symposium on Drugs Affecting Lipid Metabolism. Florence, Italy: 1992 May. Abstract Book: 18.

3. Brownfield ED, et al. Pravastatin safely lowers cholesterol after cardiac transplant and may allow reduction of cyclosporine. American Heart Association, 65th Scientific Sessions. New Orleans, LA: 1992 November.

Cyclosporine (eg, *Neoral*)

Prednisolone (eg, *Prelone*)

SUMMARY: The concurrent use of cyclosporine and methylprednisolone may increase the plasma concentrations of both drugs; isolated case reports indicate that the combination may result in seizures. The clinical importance of these findings is unclear.

RISK FACTORS: No specific risk factors are known.

MECHANISM: Not established. Both cyclosporine and corticosteroids are metabolized by CYP3A4, and it is possible that they compete for CYP3A4 metabolism.

CLINICAL EVALUATION: Cyclosporine reduced the plasma clearance of prednisolone in renal transplant patients and thus may increase prednisolone effects.[3] In another preliminary study, plasma cyclosporine levels were increased in the presence of methylprednisolone.[4] Nonetheless, in patients whose drug response is being carefully monitored, one would not expect these changes to result in adverse effects. Several patients receiving concurrent cyclosporine and high-dose methylprednisolone developed seizures, but a causal relationship was not established.[1,2]

RELATED DRUGS: There is little evidence of drug interactions when combining cyclosporine with other corticosteroids, but it is possible that they interact as well. Tacrolimus (*Prograf*) may interact with corticosteroids, but little information is available.

MANAGEMENT OPTIONS:

➡ **Monitor.** Although cyclosporine and corticosteroids commonly are used concurrently, be alert for evidence of increased response to both drugs.

REFERENCES:

1. Durrant S, et al. Cyclosporin A, methylprednisolone, and convulsions. *Lancet.* 1982;2:829.
2. Boogaerts MA, et al. Cyclosporin, methylprednisolone, and convulsions. *Lancet.* 1982;2:1216.
3. Ost L. Effects of cyclosporin on prednisolone metabolism. *Lancet.* 1984;1:451.
4. Klintmalm G, et al. High dose methylprednisolone increases plasma cyclosporin levels in renal transplant recipients. *Lancet.* 1984;1:731.

Cyclosporine (eg, *Neoral*)

Probucol

SUMMARY: A preliminary report suggests that probucol slightly reduces blood cyclosporine concentrations, but the clinical importance of this effect is unknown.

RISK FACTORS: No specific risk factors are known.

MECHANISM: Not established. Probucol might decrease the GI absorption of cyclosporine.

CLINICAL EVALUATION: Several studies in heart and renal transplant patients have found that probucol reduces cyclosporine blood concentrations. Although the reductions in blood cyclosporine are usually modest, the effect is substantial in some patients.[1-4] Probucol does not appear to affect the half-life of cyclosporine.[2]

RELATED DRUGS: No information is available.

MANAGEMENT OPTIONS:

➡ **Monitor.** Although the interaction is not well documented, it would be prudent to monitor patients for altered cyclosporine blood levels and response if probucol is initiated or discontinued.

REFERENCES:

1. Chen P, et al. Clinical pharmacokinetic interaction of cyclosporine and probucol studied using a HPLC assay procedure. *Pharm Res.* 1990;7:S-254.
2. Corder CN, et al. Interference with steady state cyclosporine levels by probucol. *Clin Pharmacol Ther.* 1990;47:204.
3. Gallego C, et al. Interaction between probucol and cyclosporine in renal transplant patients. *Ann Pharmacother.* 1994;28:940.
4. Sundararajan V, et al. Interaction of cyclosporine and probucol in heart transplant patients. *Transplant Proc.* 1991;23:2028.

4   Cyclosporine (eg, *Neoral*)

Propafenone (*Rythmol*)

SUMMARY: Propafenone administration may increase blood cyclosporine concentrations; the clinical importance of this interaction is not defined.

RISK FACTORS: No specific risk factors are known.

MECHANISM: Not established. Propafenone may increase the bioavailability of cyclosporine or inhibit its metabolism.

CLINICAL EVALUATION: A cardiac transplant patient who was maintained on cyclosporine 240 mg/day had whole blood concentrations of approximately 450 ng/ml.[1] Propafenone 750 mg/day was added to his therapy, and cyclosporine concentrations increased to approximately 750 ng/ml over 5 days. The propafenone dose was reduced to 600 mg/day and cyclosporine reduced to 200 mg/day; cyclosporine concentrations fell to 400 to 450 ng/ml. No dechallenge or rechallenge was attempted. More study of this interaction is needed to assess its clinical significance.

RELATED DRUGS: Tacrolimus (*Prograf*) may be affected similarly.

MANAGEMENT OPTIONS: No specific action is required, but be alert for evidence of the interaction.

REFERENCES:

1. Spes CH, et al. Ciclosporin-Propafenone interaction. *Klin Wochenschr*. 1990;68:872.

Cyclosporine (eg, *Neoral*)

Pyrazinamide

SUMMARY: The administration of pyrazinamide to a patient receiving cyclosporine resulted in a need to increase cyclosporine doses to maintain therapeutic plasma concentrations of cyclosporine.

RISK FACTORS: No specific risk factors are known.

MECHANISM: Not established. Pyrazinamide appears to increase the clearance of cyclosporine or reduce its absorption.

CLINICAL EVALUATION: A 28-year-old renal transplant patient was receiving cyclosporine, prednisone, isoniazid, rifampicin, and ethambutol.[1] Pyrazinamide 15 mg/kg was added to his therapy, and 2 days later the cyclosporine concentration was reduced 40%. The cyclosporine dose was increased to 9.3 mg/kg with a rise in cyclosporine concentration to 94 ng/ml 3 days later. The pyrazinamide dose was increased to 30 mg/kg/day. The cyclosporine dose again was increased to 11.5 mg/kg/day, resulting in a cyclosporine concentration of 175 ng/ml. After the pyrazinamide was discontinued, cyclosporine dosage was reduced. While this case does not prove causation, it would appear that the coadministration of pyrazinamide with cyclosporine results in lower cyclosporine concentrations.

RELATED DRUGS: If this interaction is substantiated, tacrolimus (*Prograf*) is likely to be affected similarly.

MANAGEMENT OPTIONS:

➡ *Circumvent/Minimize.* Cyclosporine dosages may need to be increased during the coadministration of pyrazinamide to maintain therapeutic concentrations.

➡ *Monitor.* Until further information regarding this interaction is available, monitor patients stabilized on cyclosporine for reduced concentrations if pyrazinamide therapy is initiated.

REFERENCES:

1. del Cerro LAJ, et al. Effect of pyrazinamide on cyclosporine levels. *Nephron*. 1992;62:113.

Cyclosporine (eg, *Neoral*)

Quinupristin/Dalfopristin (*Synercid*)

SUMMARY: The blood concentration of cyclosporine was increased by coadministration of quinupristin/dalfopristin; reduced doses of cyclosporine may be necessary.

RISK FACTORS: No specific risk factors are known.

MECHANISM: The metabolism of cyclosporine (CYP3A4) is inhibited by quinupristin/dalfopristin.

CLINICAL EVALUATION: Although published data are lacking, the manufacturer of quinupristin/dalfopristin reported on 24 subjects who received a single 300 mg dose of cyclosporine following placebo or quinupristin/dalfopristin 7.5 mg/kg every 8 hours for 2 days.[1] The administration of quinupristin/dalfopristin produced a 63% increase in the area under the concentration-time curve and a 34% reduction in the clearance of cyclosporine. The half-life of cyclosporine increased 77%. The magnitude of the increase in cyclosporine concentration is greater in patients taking oral cyclosporine than in those receiving IV cyclosporine. An increased risk of cyclosporine toxicity would be expected from this combination.

RELATED DRUGS: Tacrolimus (*Prograf*) would probably be affected by quinupristin/dalfopristin in a similar manner.

MANAGEMENT OPTIONS:

➥ *Monitor.* Carefully monitor patients stabilized on cyclosporine for increasing cyclosporine concentrations when quinupristin/dalfopristin is added. Cyclosporine dosages may need to be reduced during coadministration with quinupristin/dalfopristin.

REFERENCES:
1. Product information. Quinupristin/dalfopristin (*Synercid*). Rhône-Poulenc Rorer. 1999.

 Cyclosporine (eg, *Neoral*)

Ranitidine (eg, *Zantac*)

SUMMARY: Ranitidine does not appear to affect blood cyclosporine concentrations.

RISK FACTORS: No specific risk factors are known.

MECHANISM: Ranitidine does not appear to affect cyclosporine metabolism.

CLINICAL EVALUATION: Ranitidine appears to have minimal effects on serum creatinine, creatinine clearance, and inulin clearance in patients receiving cyclosporine.[1,2] Moreover, 3 studies in renal transplant patients have shown that ranitidine does not affect blood cyclosporine concentrations.[1-3] In one study, ranitidine was reported to increase serum creatinine concentrations in kidney and heart transplant patients receiving cyclosporine;[4] however, the data from patients receiving ranitidine was mixed with patients receiving cimetidine, and it is not likely that ranitidine contributed to the effect.

RELATED DRUGS: Ranitidine appears to have less effect on serum creatinine than does cimetidine (eg, *Tagamet*), and its lack of effect on blood cyclosporine concentrations is better documented. Thus, it may be preferable to cimetidine in patients on cyclosporine. Other H_2-receptor antagonists, such as famotidine (eg, *Pepcid*) and nizatidine (*Axid*), are probably similar to ranitidine when combined with cyclosporine, but little information is available.

MANAGEMENT OPTIONS: No interaction.

REFERENCES:

1. Pachon J, et al. Creatinine serum concentrations and H_2-receptor antagonists. *Clin Nephrol.* 1984;22:214.
2. Jadoul M, et al. Ranitidine and the cyclosporine-treated patient. *Transplantation.* 1989;48:359.
3. Zazgornik J, et al. Ranitidine does not influence the blood cyclosporin levels in renal transplant patients. *Kidney Int.* 1985;28:401.
4. Jarowenko MV, et al. Ranitidine, Cimetidine, and the Cyclosporinetreated recipient. *Transplantation.* 1986;42:311.

Cyclosporine (eg, *Neoral*)

Repaglinide (*Prandin*)

SUMMARY: Cyclosporine administration increases the plasma concentrations of repaglinide (CYP3A4) and its hypoglycemic activity.

RISK FACTORS: No specific risk factors are known.

MECHANISM: Cyclosporine appears to inhibit the metabolism of repaglinide (CYP3A4) and its uptake into the liver (via OATP1B1 inhibition), where it also is metabolized by CYP2C8.

CLINICAL EVALUATION: Twelve healthy subjects received 2 consecutive daily doses of oral cyclosporine 100 mg or placebo.[1] On the second day, they also received a single oral dose of repaglinide 0.25 mg. The mean area under the plasma concentration-time curve of repaglinide was increased 244% (range 119% to 533%) by cyclosporine compared with placebo. Repaglinide half-life did not change when administered with cyclosporine. The blood glucose-lowering effect of repaglinide is concentration dependent; patients may experience hypoglycemic episodes if the 2 drugs are coadministered without adequate monitoring.

RELATED DRUGS: Pioglitazone (*Actos*) is also partially metabolized by CYP3A4 and may be affected by cyclosporine.

MANAGEMENT OPTIONS:

➡ *Consider Alternative.* An oral hypoglycemic agent that is not metabolized by CYP3A4 (eg, glipizide [eg, *Glucotrol*] or glyburide [eg, *Diabeta*]) may be preferable in patients taking cyclosporine.

➡ *Monitor.* Caution patients taking repaglinide to carefully monitor blood sugar when cyclosporine is added or removed from the drug regimen.

REFERENCES:

1. Kajosaari LI, et al. Cyclosporine markedly raises the plasma concentrations of repaglinide. *Clin Pharmacol Ther.* 2005;78:388-399.

Cyclosporine (eg, *Neoral*)

Rifampin (eg, *Rifadin*)

SUMMARY: Rifampin may reduce cyclosporine concentrations and cause therapeutic failure.

RISK FACTORS: No specific risk factors are known.

MECHANISM: Rifampin increases the hepatic and gut metabolism (CYP3A4) of cyclosporine and appears to reduce its bioavailability.[1-3]

CLINICAL EVALUATION: Cyclosporine serum or blood concentrations are reduced after the coadministration of rifampin.[1,4-9] In 1 case, rifampin reduced the area under the concentration-time curve of cyclosporine nearly 60% and shortened its half-life from 4.1 to 1.85 hours.[8] It appears that the interaction between rifampin and cyclosporine predictably reduces the blood concentration of cyclosporine and may result in a loss of cyclosporine efficacy. As with other enzyme inducers, rifampin requires several days to 2 weeks to produce its maximal effect.

RELATED DRUGS: Tacrolimus (*Prograf*) is likely to be affected similarly by rifampin administration.

MANAGEMENT OPTIONS:

➡ ***Avoid Unless Benefit Outweighs Risk.*** Coadminister rifampin and cyclosporine only with careful monitoring of cyclosporine concentrations.

➡ ***Monitor.*** Monitor cyclosporine blood concentrations when cyclosporine and rifampin are used simultaneously. The addition of rifampin to cyclosporine regimens may require a 2- to 4-fold increase in cyclosporine dosages to maintain therapeutic blood concentrations. The discontinuation of rifampin may cause cyclosporine concentrations to increase over 5 to 10 days, possibly resulting in toxicity. Dosage reduction will most likely be required, particularly in patients who have had their dosage increased as a result of rifampin administration.

REFERENCES:

1. Hebert MF, et al. Bioavailability of cyclosporine with concomitant rifampin administration is markedly less than predicted by hepatic enzyme induction. *Clin Pharmacol Ther.* 1992;52:453-457.

2. Combalbert J, et al. Metabolism of cyclosporin A. IV. Purification and identification of the rifampicin-inducible human liver cytochrome P450 (cyclosporin A oxidase) as a product of P450IIIA gene subfamily. *Drug Metab Dispos.* 1989;17:197-207.

3. Hebert MF, et al. Clinical evidence of metabolic differences between intestinal and hepatic cytochrome P450. *Clin Pharmacol Ther.* 1993;53:190.

4. Modry DL, et al. Acute rejection and massive cyclosporine requirements in heart transplant recipients treated with rifampin. *Transplantation.* 1985;39:313-314.

5. Howard P, et al. Cyclosporine-rifampin drug interaction. *Drug Intell Clin Pharm.* 1985;19:763-764.

6. Cassidy MJ, et al. Effect of rifampicin on cyclosporin A blood levels in a renal transplant recipient. *Nephron.* 1985;41:207-208.

7. Van Buren D, et al. The antagonistic effect of rifampin upon cyclosporine bioavailability. *Transplant Proc.* 1984;16:1642-1645.

8. Offermann G, et al. Low cyclosporin A blood levels and acute graft rejection in a renal transplant recipient during rifampin treatment. *Am J Nephrol.* 1985;5:385-387.

9. Koselj M, et al. Drug interactions between cyclosporine and rifampicin, erythromycin, and azoles in kidney recipients with opportunistic infections. *Transplant Proc.* 1994;26:2823-2824.

Cyclosporine (eg, *Neoral*)

Rosuvastatin (*Crestor*)

SUMMARY: Cyclosporine substantially increases plasma rosuvastatin concentrations, but the clinical importance of this effect is not established.

RISK FACTORS: No specific risk factors are known.

MECHANISM: Not established. Cyclosporine may inhibit the hepatic uptake of rosuvastatin by the transporter OATP-C.

CLINICAL EVALUATION: In transplant recipients taking cyclosporine who were given rosuvastatin 10 mg/day for 10 days, plasma concentrations of rosuvastatin were more than 7-fold higher than historical controls.[1] Although the combination was well-tolerated, statin-induced skeletal muscle damage usually occurs only after 2 or more weeks of elevated plasma statin concentrations. Until more data are available on this interaction, it should be assumed that cyclosporine could increase the risk of rosuvastatin toxicity.

RELATED DRUGS: Cyclosporine also can increase the serum concentrations of lovastatin (eg, *Mevacor*), simvastatin (*Zocor*), atorvastatin (*Lipitor*), fluvastatin (*Lescol*), and pravastatin (*Pravachol*), although the risk of adverse consequences appears to differ depending on the statin. Pravastatin, for example, is frequently used in transplant patients without evidence of adverse drug interactions.

MANAGEMENT OPTIONS: No specific action is required, but be alert for evidence of the interaction.

REFERENCES:
1. Simonson SG, et al. Rosuvastatin pharmacokinetics in heart transplant recipients administered an antirejection regimen including cyclosporine. *Clin Pharmacol Ther.* 2004;76:167-177.

Cyclosporine (eg, *Neoral*) ▼³

Roxithromycin†

SUMMARY: Roxithromycin administration appears to increase cyclosporine concentrations; and cyclosporine appears to increase the concentration of roxithromycin. The clinical significance of these effects is not established.

RISK FACTORS: No specific risk factors are known.

MECHANISM: Roxithromycin may inhibit the metabolism of cyclosporine; cyclosporine appears to inhibit roxithromycin elimination.

CLINICAL EVALUATION: Eight heart transplant patients stabilized on cyclosporine received roxithromycin 150 mg twice daily for 11 days.[1] Cyclosporine concentrations rose between 25% and 40% during roxithromycin dosing and returned to baseline over 2 weeks following the discontinuation of roxithromycin. Serum creatinine concentrations did not change. In another study, 6 healthy subjects, 9 renal transplant patients taking cyclosporine, and 10 transplant patients taking azathioprine (eg, *Imuran*) were given roxithromycin 300 mg.[2] Compared with controls, the patients taking cyclosporine had roxithromycin clearances that were 57% lower; their roxithromycin half-lives were twice as long. The clinical significance of these interactions is not known.

RELATED DRUGS: Other macrolide antibiotics including erythromycin (eg, *Ery-Tab*), troleandomycin†, and clarithromycin (eg, *Biaxin*) may inhibit the metabolism of cyclosporine. Azithromycin (eg, *Zithromax*) would not interact with cyclosporine. Roxithromycin may have a similar effect on tacrolimus (*Prograf*) elimination.

MANAGEMENT OPTIONS:

➡ *Monitor.* Until more studies of these interactions are available, monitor patients stabilized on cyclosporine for changing cyclosporine concentrations when roxithromycin is added to or deleted from dosage regimens.

REFERENCES:
1. Billaud EM, et al. Interaction between roxithromycin and cyclosporin in heart transplant patients. *Clin Pharmacokinet.* 1990;19:499-502.

2. Moravek J, et al. Pharmacokinetics of roxithromycin in kidney grafted patients under cyclosporin A or azathioprine immunosuppression and in healthy volunteers. *Int J Clin Pharmacol Ther Toxicol.* 1990;28:262-267.

† Not available in the United States.

4 Cyclosporine (eg, *Neoral*)

Sertraline (*Zoloft*)

SUMMARY: A patient on cyclosporine developed serotonin syndrome after sertraline therapy was started, but a causal relationship was not established.

RISK FACTORS: No specific risk factors are known.

MECHANISM: Not established. The authors propose an additive serotonergic effect of cyclosporine and sertraline in the CNS, but it is not known if cyclosporine is serotonergic in humans. Sertraline is partially metabolized by CYP3A4, and it is possible that cyclosporine, a known inhibitor of CYP3A4, increased sertraline serum concentrations.

CLINICAL EVALUATION: A 53-year-old man on cyclosporine 100 mg twice daily following a renal transplant was started on sertraline 50 mg/day. Five days later, he developed a generalized tremor, profuse sweating, fever, tachycardia, elevated blood pressure, ankle clonus, and hyperreflexia. This constellation of findings strongly suggest serotonin syndrome.[1]

RELATED DRUGS: No information is available.

MANAGEMENT OPTIONS: No specific action is required, but be alert for evidence of the interaction.

REFERENCES:
1. Wong EH, et al. Serotonin syndrome in a renal transplant patient. *J R Soc Med.* 2002;95:304-305.

3 Cyclosporine (eg, *Neoral*)

Simvastatin (*Zocor*)

SUMMARY: Cyclosporine increases plasma simvastatin concentrations; some evidence suggests that the combination may increase the risk of skeletal muscle damage.

RISK FACTORS: No specific risk factors are known.

MECHANISM: Not established. Cyclosporine may inhibit the hepatic uptake of simvastatin by transporters such as OATP-C, and may also inhibit the metabolism of simvastatin by CYP3A4.

CLINICAL EVALUATION: In a small study of kidney transplant patients, those receiving cyclosporine developed higher serum simvastatin concentrations than similar patients not receiving cyclosporine.[1] Some transplant recipients taking cyclosporine with simvastatin or lovastatin have developed rhabdomyolysis, and it is reasonable to assume that a pharmacokinetic interaction contributes to these adverse reactions.[2]

RELATED DRUGS: Cyclosporine can also increase the serum concentrations of lovastatin (eg, *Mevacor*), atorvastatin (*Lipitor*), fluvastatin (*Lescol*), rosuvastatin (*Crestor*), and pravastatin (*Pravachol*), although the risk of adverse consequences appears to differ depending on the statin. Pravastatin, for example, is frequently used in transplant patients without evidence of adverse drug interactions.

MANAGEMENT OPTIONS:

➡ *Circumvent/Minimize.* In patients receiving cyclosporine, the product information for simvastatin states that the dose of simvastatin should not exceed 10 mg/day. While many cyclosporine-treated patients have received larger doses of simvastatin without harm, exceeding this dosage recommendation could present medico-legal problems if the patient develops myopathy.

➡ *Monitor.* Be alert for evidence of myopathy (eg, muscle pain, muscle weakness, darkened urine) in patients receiving cyclosporine and simvastatin (or any other statin).

REFERENCES:

1. Arnadottir M, et al. Plasma concentration profiles of simvastatin 3-hydroxy 3-methyl-glutaryl-coenzyme A reductase inhibitory activity in kidney transplant recipients with and without ciclosporin. *Nephron.* 1993;65:410-413.

2. Asberg A. Interactions between cyclosporin and lipid-lowering drugs: implications for organ transplant recipients. *Drugs.* 2003;63:367-378.

Cyclosporine (eg, *Neoral*)

St. John's Wort

SUMMARY: Two heart transplant patients receiving cyclosporine developed acute rejection reactions after starting therapy with St. John's wort; monitor patients for altered cyclosporine effect if St. John's wort is used concurrently.

RISK FACTORS: No specific risk factors are known.

MECHANISM: Not established. Other clinical evidence suggests that St. John's wort may enhance the activity of CYP3A4 or p-glycoprotein. Therefore, it is possible that St. John's wort reduces cyclosporine's bioavailability or enhances its hepatic metabolism.

CLINICAL EVALUATION: Two heart transplant patients (61 and 63 years of age) developed acute rejection episodes 3 weeks after starting St. John's wort extract 300 mg 3 times daily.[1] In both cases, the acute rejection was accompanied by dramatic reductions in cyclosporine plasma concentrations. Although only 2 cases were reported, the findings are consistent with other reports of St. John's wort reducing the plasma concentrations of drugs that are substrates for CYP3A4 or p-glycoprotein.[2-4]

RELATED DRUGS: Theoretically, St. John's wort would also reduce the serum plasma concentrations of related immunosuppressants that are metabolized by CYP3A4 and may be transported by p-glycoprotein, examples include tacrolimus (*Prograf*) and sirolimus (*Rapamune*).

MANAGEMENT OPTIONS:

➡ *Use Alternative.* The use of antidepressants other than St. John's wort in patients receiving cyclosporine (and perhaps also tacrolimus or sirolimus) is preferable. Selective serotonin reuptake inhibitors and related antidepressants (eg, paroxetine [eg, *Paxil*], sertraline [*Zoloft*], citalopram [eg, *Celexa*], venlafaxine [*Effexor*]) are not known to induce or inhibit CYP3A4 to a clinically important extent. Fluoxetine (eg, *Prozac*) appears to be a weak inhibitor of CYP3A4, fluvoxamine is a moderate CYP3A4 inhibitor, and nefazodone is a potent inhibitor of CYP3A4.

➡ *Monitor.* If St. John's wort is used with cyclosporine, tacrolimus, or sirolimus, monitor the patient for reduced immunosuppressant effect.

REFERENCES:

1. Ruschitzka F, et al. Acute heart transplant rejection due to Saint John's wort. *Lancet.* 2000;355:548-549.
2. Yue QY, et al. Safety of St. John's wort (*Hypericum perforatum*). *Lancet.* 2000;355:576-577.
3. Piscitelli SC, et al. Indinavir concentrations and St. John's wort. *Lancet.* 2000;355:547-548. Erratum in: *Lancet.* 2001;357:1210.
4. Johne A, et al. Pharmacokinetic interaction of digoxin with an herbal extract from St. John's wort (*Hypericum perforatum*). *Clin Pharmacol Ther.* 1999;66:338-345.

Cyclosporine (eg, *Neoral*)

Sulindac (eg, *Clinoril*)

SUMMARY: Impaired renal function appears to be greater with sulindac plus cyclosporine than with either drug alone; sulindac has also been reported to increase serum cyclosporine concentrations.

RISK FACTORS: No specific risk factors are known.

MECHANISM: Not established.

CLINICAL EVALUATION: Eleven patients with rheumatoid arthritis were treated with cyclosporine and nonsteroidal anti-inflammatory drugs (NSAIDs) (sulindac or naproxen [eg, *Naprosyn*]), alone and in combination. Impairment of renal function was greater with cyclosporine plus an NSAID than with either drug alone.[1] The effect was reversible. A 47-year-old woman receiving cyclosporine 400 mg/day following a cadaver kidney transplant had stable trough serum cyclosporine concentrations (450 to 525 ng/mL) and stable serum creatinine concentrations.[2] Three days after starting sulindac 150 mg twice daily, cyclosporine concentrations had increased to 1,218 ng/mL, and there were slight increases in serum creatinine and blood urea nitrogen. The patient had been receiving trimethoprim/sulfamethoxazole (eg, *Bactrim*), which was discontinued 1 week before the sulindac was started. However, because previous trimethoprim/sulfamethoxazole therapy had not affected serum cyclosporine concentrations, the authors concluded that discontinuation of trimethoprim/sulfamethoxazole was not involved in the increase in serum cyclosporine concentrations.

RELATED DRUGS: In patients receiving cyclosporine, several NSAIDs have been associated with impaired renal function or increased cyclosporine blood concentrations.[1,3,4] The relative likelihood of various NSAIDs to increase cyclosporine-induced nephrotoxicity is not established, but assume that all NSAIDs are capable of interacting with cyclosporine until more evidence is available.

MANAGEMENT OPTIONS:

➠ *Consider Alternative.* Until the clinical importance of this potential interaction is better defined, use sulindac (or other NSAIDs) in patients receiving cyclosporine only when the expected benefit clearly outweighs the risk of excessive cyclosporine response and nephrotoxicity.

➠ *Monitor.* If the combination is used, monitor the patient's renal function carefully and be prepared to discontinue one or both drugs.

REFERENCES:

1. Altman RD, et al. Interaction of cyclosporine A and nonsteroidal anti-inflammatory drugs on renal function in patients with rheumatoid arthritis. *Am J Med.* 1992;93(4):396-402.
2. Sesin GP, et al. Sulindac-induced elevation of serum cyclosporine concentration. *Clin Pharm.* 1989;8(6):445-446.
3. Branthwaite JP, Nicholls A. Cyclosporin and diclofenac interaction in rheumatoid arthritis. *Lancet.* 1991;337(8735):252.
4. Deray G, et al. Enhancement of cyclosporine A nephrotoxicity by diclofenac. *Clin Nephrol.* 1987;27(4):213-214.

Cyclosporine (eg, *Neoral*)

Sulphadimidine†

SUMMARY: Some sulfonamides can reduce the plasma concentration of cyclosporine, potentially reducing its efficacy.

RISK FACTORS:

➠ *Dosage Regimen.* Intravenous (IV) administration of sulphadimidine is a probable risk factor.

MECHANISM: Not established. Sulfonamides may increase the hepatic metabolism of cyclosporine.

CLINICAL EVALUATION: Five cardiac transplant patients receiving cyclosporine were treated with IV sulphadimidine and trimethoprim (eg, *Primsol*).[1] Serum cyclosporine concentrations in all 5 patients were more than 100 ng/mL before sulphadimidine treatment; however, the cyclosporine concentrations fell to unmeasurable values in 4 patients and to 40 ng/mL in the other patient within 4 days after antibiotic therapy was started. These decreases in cyclosporine concentrations were followed by transplant rejection episodes in 2 of the patients. After 4 to 24 days patients were switched from IV antibiotics to oral trimethoprim/sulfamethoxazole (eg, *Bactrim*). No suppression of cyclosporine concentrations was noted during the oral antibiotic therapy. Other cases describing sulfadimidine- and sulfadiazine-induced reduction in cyclosporine concentration have also been reported.[2,3]

RELATED DRUGS: Tacrolimus (eg, *Prograf*) concentrations may be reduced in a similar manner.

MANAGEMENT OPTIONS:

➥ *Circumvent/Minimize.* Oral trimethoprim/sulfamethoxazole did not affect cyclosporine plasma concentrations.

➥ *Monitor.* During the administration of sulfadimidine to patients receiving cyclosporine, monitor plasma cyclosporine concentrations.

REFERENCES:

1. Jones DK, et al. Serious interaction between cyclosporine A and sulphadimidine. *Br Med J (Clin Red Ed).* 1986;292(6522):728-729.

2. Wallwork H, et al. Cyclosporin and intravenous sulphadimidine and trimethoprim therapy. *Lancet.* 1983;1(8320):366-367.

3. Spes CH, et al. Sulfadiazine therapy for toxoplasmosis in heart transplant recipients decreases cyclosporine concentration. *Clin Investig.* 1992;70(9):752-754.

† Not available in the United States.

Cyclosporine (eg, *Neoral*)

Telaprevir (*Incivek*)

SUMMARY: The coadministration of telaprevir increases the plasma concentration of cyclosporine; adverse reactions, including renal dysfunction, may be more likely to occur.

RISK FACTORS: No specific risk factors are known.

MECHANISM: Telaprevir inhibits the CYP3A4-mediated metabolism and P-glycoprotein elimination of cyclosporine.

CLINICAL EVALUATION: While specific data are limited, the manufacturer of telaprevir notes that the coadministration of telaprevir 750 mg every 8 hours for 11 days increased the mean area under the plasma concentration-time curve of cyclosporine approximately 5-fold.[1] Pending further data, observe patients receiving telaprevir and cyclosporine for increased cyclosporine plasma concentrations and adverse reactions.

RELATED DRUGS: Atazanavir (*Reyataz*), darunavir (*Prezista*), fosamprenavir (*Lexiva*), indinavir (*Crixivan*), nelfinavir (*Viracept*), and saquinavir (*Invirase*) also inhibit the activity of CYP3A4 and are expected to increase the plasma concentration of cyclosporine. Telaprevir markedly increases the plasma concentration of tacrolimus (eg, *Prograf*); sirolimus (*Rapammune*) may be affected in a similar manner.

MANAGEMENT OPTIONS:

➥ *Avoid Unless Benefit Outweighs Risk.* Generally avoid the coadministration of cyclosporine and telaprevir.

➥ *Monitor.* Monitor patients stabilized on cyclosporine for adverse reactions if telaprevir is coadministered.

REFERENCES:

1. *Incivek* [package insert]. Cambridge, MA: Vertex Pharmaceuticals Inc; 2011.

Cyclosporine (eg, *Neoral*)

Ticlopidine

SUMMARY: A patient with nephrotic syndrome developed a marked reduction in blood cyclosporine concentrations during ticlopidine therapy; a causal relationship was likely in this patient, but more study is needed to assess the clinical importance.

RISK FACTORS: No specific risk factors are known.

MECHANISM: Not established.

CLINICAL EVALUATION: In an 18-year-old man receiving cyclosporine 5.6 mg/kg/day for nephrotic syndrome, blood cyclosporine concentrations fell more than 50% after ticlopidine 500 mg/day was added.[1] When ticlopidine was stopped, blood cyclosporine concentrations increased substantially and proteinuria subsided. Several months later while he was receiving cyclosporine 6.7 mg/kg/day, initiation of ticlopidine again reduced the blood cyclosporine concentrations approximately 50%, and blood concentrations returned to the previous value when the ticlopidine was stopped. Given the temporal relationship between the cyclosporine blood concentrations and the starting and stopping of ticlopidine, it is highly likely that ticlopidine was responsible for the changes. Moreover, there was evidence of reduced cyclosporine effect (in the form of proteinuria) while the ticlopidine was given. The possibility that ticlopidine might have interfered with the cyclosporine assays apparently was not ruled out, but that does not appear likely.

RELATED DRUGS: No information is available.

MANAGEMENT OPTIONS:

➡ **Monitor.** Until more information is available, monitor cyclosporine blood concentrations and therapeutic response carefully if ticlopidine is initiated or discontinued in patients taking cyclosporine.

REFERENCES:

1. Birmelé B, et al. Interaction of cyclosporin and ticlopidine. *Nephrol Dial Transplant.* 1991;6(2):150-151.

Cyclosporine (eg, *Neoral*)

Trimethoprim/Sulfamethoxazole (eg, *Bactrim*)

SUMMARY: Trimethoprim/sulfamethoxazole may produce additive nephrotoxicity with cyclosporine.

RISK FACTORS:

➡ **Dosage Regimen.** Intravenous (IV) trimethoprim/sulfamethoxazole administration increases the potential for cyclosporine nephrotoxicity.

MECHANISM: Not established. Trimethoprim/sulfamethoxazole may increase the nephrotoxicity of cyclosporine.

CLINICAL EVALUATION: In one report, IV trimethoprim/sulfamethoxazole increased the potential for cyclosporine nephrotoxicity.[1] It is not clear whether this interaction resulted from altered cyclosporine pharmacokinetics or from combined nephrotoxicity. The oral administration of trimethoprim/sulfamethoxazole has not been reported to increase the nephrotoxicity of cyclosporine.

RELATED DRUGS: Trimethoprim/sulfamethoxazole may produce a similar effect when administered with tacrolimus (eg, *Prograf*).

MANAGEMENT OPTIONS: No specific action is required, but be alert for evidence of the interaction.

REFERENCES:

1. Ringdén O, et al. Nephrotoxicity by co-trimoxazole and cyclosporin in transplanted patients. *Lancet*. 1984;1(8384):1016-1017.

Cyclosporine (eg, *Neoral*)

Verapamil (eg, *Calan*)

SUMMARY: Cyclosporine blood concentrations are increased by verapamil; cyclosporine toxicity could result.

RISK FACTORS: No specific risk factors are known.

MECHANISM: Verapamil appears to inhibit the metabolism of cyclosporine.

CLINICAL EVALUATION: Verapamil 120 to 360 mg/day for 7 days has been associated with 2- to 4-fold increases in cyclosporine concentrations.[1-5] Changes in cyclosporine concentrations of this magnitude are expected to increase cyclosporine toxicity. The clinical significance of these changes requires further study.

RELATED DRUGS: Diltiazem (eg, *Cardizem*) and nicardipine (eg, *Cardene*) inhibit cyclosporine metabolism, while isradipine (eg, *DynaCirc*), nifedipine (eg, *Procardia*), amlodipine (eg, *Norvasc*), and nitrendipine have minimal effect. Verapamil may affect tacrolimus (eg, *Prograf*) in a similar manner.

MANAGEMENT OPTIONS:

➥ ***Consider Alternative.*** Calcium channel blockers that do not appear to alter cyclosporine pharmacokinetics include isradipine,[6] nitrendipine,[7] and amlodipine.[8]

➥ ***Circumvent/Minimize.*** Reduce cyclosporine dosage and monitor blood concentrations when verapamil is coadministered.

➥ ***Monitor.*** Observe patients receiving both drugs for increased cyclosporine concentrations and decreased renal function.

REFERENCES:

1. Lindholm A, Henricsson S. Verapamil inhibits cyclosporin metabolism. *Lancet*. 1987;1(8544):1262-1263.
2. Maggio TG, Bartels DW. Increased cyclosporine blood concentrations due to verapamil administration. *Drug Intell Clin Pharm*. 1988;22(9):705-707.
3. Robson RA, et al. Cyclosporin-verapamil interaction. *Br J Clin Pharmacol*. 1988;25(3):402-403.
4. Sabaté I, et al. Evaluation of cyclosporin-verapamil interaction, with observations on patient cyclosporin and metabolites. *Clin Chem*. 1988;34(10):2151.
5. Howard RL, et al. The effect of calcium channel blockers on the cyclosporine dose requirement in renal transplant patients. *Ren Fail*. 1990;12(2):89-92.
6. Martinez F, et al. No clinically significant interaction between ciclosporin and isradipine. *Nephron*. 1991;59(4):658-659.
7. Copur MS, et al. Effects of nitrendipine on blood pressure and blood ciclosporin A level in patients with posttransplant hypertension. *Nephron*. 1989;52(3):227-230.
8. Toupance O, et al. Antihypertensive effect of amlodipine and lack of interference with cyclosporine metabolism in renal transplant recipients. *Hypertension*. 1994;24(3):297-300.

Cyclosporine (eg, *Neoral*)

Voriconazole (*Vfend*)

SUMMARY: Cyclosporine blood concentrations are increased by concurrent voriconazole administration.

RISK FACTORS:

➥ ***Pharmacogenetics.*** Patients who are poor metabolizers for CYP2C19 will have higher voriconazole concentrations and thus are likely to have an interaction of larger magnitude.

MECHANISM: Voriconazole diminishes the metabolism of cyclosporine by inhibiting the activity of cytochrome P4503A4.

CLINICAL EVALUATION: Seven renal transplant patients received cyclosporine doses of 150 to 375 mg/day with voriconazole 200 mg every 12 hours or placebo for 8 days.[1] The coadministration of voriconazole with cyclosporine resulted in a mean 1.7-fold increase in the area under the concentration-time curve of cyclosporine compared with placebo. Mean peak cyclosporine blood concentration increased 13% during voriconazole administration. Patients experienced more adverse effects (eg, elevated cyclosporine or creatinine concentrations, dyspnea, lower limb edema) during the coadministration of voriconazole and cyclosporine.

RELATED DRUGS: Tacrolimus (eg, *Prograf*) is similarly affected by voriconazole administration. Sirolimus (*Rapamune*) concentrations are increased to a greater extent than cyclosporine by voriconazole. The metabolism of other immunosuppressants such as everolimus (*Certican*) is likely to be decreased by voriconazole. Other azole antifungal agents including ketoconazole (eg, *Nizoral*), fluconazole (*Diflucan*), and itraconazole (eg, *Sporanox*) are known to reduce the metabolism of cyclosporine.

MANAGEMENT OPTIONS:

➥ ***Circumvent/Minimize.*** A reduction in cyclosporine dose may be required during treatment with voriconazole.

➥ ***Monitor.*** Carefully monitor patients for elevated cyclosporine concentrations or evidence of cyclosporine toxicity (eg, increased serum creatinine) during voriconazole coadministration. When voriconazole is discontinued, monitor for decreasing cyclosporine concentrations

REFERENCES:

1. Romero AJ et al. Effect of voriconazole on the pharmacokinetics of cyclosporine in renal transplant patients. *Clin Pharmacol Ther*. 2002;71:226-234.

Cyclosporine (eg, *Neoral*)

Warfarin (eg, *Coumadin*)

SUMMARY: In 1 patient concurrent therapy with warfarin and cyclosporine was associated with a reduced effect of both drugs, but increased effects of both drugs were observed in another patient receiving cyclosporine and acenocoumarol; more study is needed.

RISK FACTORS: No specific risk factors are known.

MECHANISM: Not established.

CLINICAL EVALUATION: In a patient with pure erythrocyte aplasia receiving chronic therapy with cyclosporine, the cyclosporine blood concentration dropped and erythrocyte aplasia worsened following initiation of warfarin for deep vein thrombosis.[1] When the cyclosporine dose was increased from 3 to 7 mg/kg, the hypoprothrombinemic response to warfarin declined and the dose of warfarin had to be increased. Although the temporal relationship suggests a mutual reduction in drug response, the findings are not consistent with the known properties of the 2 drugs. Note that the patient also was receiving chronic phenobarbital therapy. Because phenobarbital is capable of stimulating the metabolism of cyclosporine[2] and warfarin,[3] the reduced effects of these drugs may have been caused by phenobarbital. Although this interaction is not well established, monitor patients receiving cyclosporine and oral anticoagulants for an altered response to both drugs if either drug is initiated, discontinued, or changed in dosage.

RELATED DRUGS: In 1 patient anticoagulated with acenocoumarol, the addition of cyclosporine was associated with an increase in the effect of both drugs.[4] Although it is possible that cyclosporine interacts differently with warfarin and acenocoumarol, study under more controlled conditions will be necessary to establish whether or not oral anticoagulants and cyclosporine interact with each other.

MANAGEMENT OPTIONS: No specific action is required, but be alert for evidence of the interaction.

REFERENCES:

1. Snyder DS. Interaction between cyclosporine and warfarin. *Ann Intern Med*. 1988;108:311.
2. Carstensen H, et al. Interaction between cyclosporin A and phenobarbitone. *Br J Clin Pharmacol*. 1986;21:550.
3. Levy G, et al. Pharmacokinetic analysis of the effect of barbiturate on the anticoagulant action of warfarin in man. *Clin Pharmacol Ther*. 1970;11:372.
4. Campistol JM, et al. Interaction between cyclosporine A and Sintrom. *Nephron*. 1989;53:291.

Cyclosporine (eg, *Sandimmune*)

Wine, Red

SUMMARY: Red wine moderately reduced cyclosporine blood concentrations following use of *Sandimmune*; the effect of red wine on *Neoral* is not established.

RISK FACTORS:

➡ **Pharmacogenetics.** Although data are limited (9 Caucasians and 3 Asians), the Asians experienced a smaller decrease (14%) than the Caucasians (35%). More study is needed to determine whether this difference is real.

MECHANISM: Because serum concentrations of cyclosporine declined, but the half-life was not affected, the red wine probably reduced cyclosporine bioavailability. The mechanism by which the wine produces this effect is not known.

CLINICAL EVALUATION: In a randomized crossover study, 12 healthy subjects were given a single oral 8 mg/kg dose of cyclosporine (eg, *Sandimmune*) with and without coadministration of 360 mL red wine (Blackstone Merlot, 1996).[1] The red wine was associated with a 29% reduction in cyclosporine area under the blood concentration-time curve. Although the average effect was not large, there was considerable variability between subjects-decreases ranged from 1.5% to 56%. It seems likely that at least some patients would have a clinically significant reduction in cyclosporine effect with red wine.

RELATED DRUGS: The microemulsion form of cyclosporine (*Neoral*) is better absorbed than the standard formulation used in this study (*Sandimmune*). Thus, these results do not necessarily apply to patients taking *Neoral*. Theoretically, *Neoral* would be less likely to be affected than *Sandimmune*. The effect of other red wines on cyclosporine is not known, but it is likely that some would have a greater effect on cyclosporine, and some would have less. Preliminary results from the same authors suggest that white wine may not affect cyclosporine bioavailability.[1]

MANAGEMENT OPTIONS:

➡ *Consider Alternative.* Preliminary evidence suggests that white wine may be less likely to interact. Theoretically, the microemulsion form of cyclosporine would be less likely to interact.

➡ *Circumvent/Minimize.* In patients receiving the standard cyclosporine formulation (eg, *Sandimmune*) it may be prudent for them to avoid red wine. The effect of separating doses of *Sandimmune* from red wine is not known.

➡ *Monitor.* Be alert for altered cyclosporine blood concentrations if patients ingest red wine.

REFERENCES:

1. Tsunoda SM, et al. Red wine decreases cyclosporine bioavailability. *Clin Pharmacol Ther.* 2001;70:462-467.

Cyproheptadine (*Periactin*)

Fluoxetine (eg, *Prozac*)

SUMMARY: Some patients on fluoxetine have developed a worsening of depression when cyproheptadine was added, but this has not been a consistent finding; more study is needed.

RISK FACTORS: No specific risk factors are known.

MECHANISM: Cyproheptadine is a serotonin antagonist, which theoretically could inhibit the effects of serotonin reuptake inhibitors such as fluoxetine.

CLINICAL EVALUATION: Three men taking fluoxetine developed a return of depressive symptoms after starting cyproheptadine 2 to 6 mg/day to treat their ejaculatory disturbances.[1] In 2 of the patients, the dysphoria was noted within 3 to 4 hours after taking a dose of cyproheptadine; the other patient noticed the return of depression after 2 days. Two other patients taking fluoxetine did not experience an exacerbation of depression after successfully using cyproheptadine for ejaculatory problems.[2] One patient took single 8 mg doses of cyproheptadine, while the other took cyproheptadine chronically in doses up to 16 mg/day. The reason for the conflicting results is unclear.

RELATED DRUGS: Theoretically, other selective serotonin reuptake inhibitors would interact similarly with cyproheptadine.

MANAGEMENT OPTIONS:

➥ *Monitor.* Until more information is available, monitor for reduced antidepressant response to fluoxetine if cyproheptadine is started.

REFERENCES:

1. Feder R. Reversal of antidepressant activity of fluoxetine by cyproheptadine in three patients. *J Clin Psychiatry.* 1991;52:163.

2. McCormick S, et al. Reversal of fluoxetine-induced anorgasmia by cyproheptadine in two patients. *J Clin Psychiatry.* 1990;51:383.

4   Cyproheptadine (*Periactin*)

Phenelzine (*Nardil*)

SUMMARY: A case report noted visual hallucinations in a patient treated with cyproheptadine and phenelzine; but a causal relationship was not established.

RISK FACTORS: No specific risk factors are known.

MECHANISM: Not established.

CLINICAL EVALUATION: A patient treated with phenelzine 30 mg/day was given cyproheptadine 2 mg/day to treat phenelzine-induced anorgasmia.[1] After 2 months of combination therapy, she became irritable and developed visual hallucinations. All medications were discontinued, and the hallucinations resolved over 48 hours. No rechallenge was attempted, so it is difficult to determine whether an interaction between the 2 drugs caused the reaction.

RELATED DRUGS: The effect of combined use of cyproheptadine with other monoamine oxidize inhibitors such as isocarboxazid (*Marplan*) and tranylcypromine (*Parnate*) is not established.

MANAGEMENT OPTIONS: No specific action is required, but be alert for evidence of the interaction.

REFERENCES:

1. Kahn DA. Possible toxic interaction between cyproheptadine and phenelzine. *Am J Psych.* 1987;144:1242.

Danazol (eg, *Danocrine*)

Lovastatin (*Mevacor*)

SUMMARY: A patient developed myositis with rhabdomyolysis after danazol was added to his lovastatin therapy; although a causal relationship was not proved, the reaction is consistent with the known interactive properties of the drugs.

RISK FACTORS: No specific risk factors are known.

MECHANISM: Evidence from in vitro studies using human hepatic microsomes suggests that lovastatin is metabolized by cytochrome P4503A4 (CYP3A4). Other drugs known to inhibit CYP3A4 (eg, cyclosporine, erythromycin) have been reported to increase the risk of lovastatin myopathy. Therefore, it is possible that danazol inhibits the metabolism of lovastatin by CYP3A4, thereby increasing lovastatin serum concentrations and the risk of lovastatin-induced myopathy.

CLINICAL EVALUATION: A 72-year-old man receiving lovastatin 20 mg twice daily was started on danazol 200 mg 3 times/day and prednisone 10 mg twice daily.[1] About 2 months later he developed myositis, which progressed to rhabdomyolysis and myoglobinuria. The lovastatin and danazol were discontinued, and the syndrome resolved over the next 2 weeks. At the onset of the myositis, he also was receiving atenolol (eg, *Tonormin*), aspirin, dipyridamole (eg, *Persantine*), and doxycycline (eg, *Vibramycin*), but it is not known if they had any role in the reaction; based upon current evidence, it does not seem likely. Given the known ability of danazol to inhibit hepatic drug metabolism, the most plausible explanation is a danazol-lovastatin interaction. Nonetheless, do not rule out the possibility that the myositis was caused by lovastatin alone.

RELATED DRUGS: It is not known whether androgens other than danazol interact with lovastatin, but consider the possibility. The effect of danazol on other hepatic hydroxymethylglutaryl coenzyme A reductase inhibitors is not established. Because pravastatin (*Pravachol*) and fluvastatin (*Lescol*) appear less likely to interact with cyclosporine than lovastatin, they also may be less likely to interact with danazol.

MANAGEMENT OPTIONS:

➥ *Consider Alternative.* See Related Drugs.

➥ *Monitor.* If the combination is used, monitor the patient for evidence of myositis. Advise patients to contact health care provider if developing unexpected muscle pain or weakness.

REFERENCES:
1. Dallaire M, et al. Severe rhabdomyolysis in a patient receiving lovastatin, danazol, and doxycycline [in French]. *CMAJ.* 1994;150:1991.

Danazol (eg, *Danocrine*)

Warfarin (eg, *Coumadin*)

SUMMARY: Several cases of enhanced hypoprothrombinemic response to warfarin following danazol therapy have been reported.

RISK FACTORS: No specific risk factors are known.

MECHANISM: Not established. Danazol may increase the endogenous anticoagulants, antithrombin III and protein C, thereby enhancing the hypoprothrombinemic response to oral anticoagulants.[3] Danazol also may increase fibrinolytic activity, thus increasing the bleeding risk.

CLINICAL EVALUATION: Danazol therapy was associated with excessive hypoprothrombinemia and bleeding in several women on chronic warfarin therapy. One woman on warfarin developed hematemesis and a prothrombin time of 168 seconds 3 weeks after starting danazol 400 mg/day.[1] Another woman receiving warfarin developed excessive hypoprothrombinemia 2 days after starting danazol 800 mg/day;[2] this woman subsequently had a severe bleeding episode even though the warfarin was discontinued. A 47-year-old woman on chronic warfarin therapy developed gross hematuria, back pain, and a prothrombin time of 56 seconds 1 month after starting danazol 400 mg/day; there was a positive rechallenge with danazol 1 month later.[3] A 28-year-old woman on chronic warfarin developed hemarthrosis of the knee and a prothrombin time of 39 seconds 3 weeks after starting danazol 600 mg/day.[3]

RELATED DRUGS: Anabolic steroids other than danazol are known to increase the hypoprothrombinemic response to oral anticoagulants. Oral anticoagulants other than warfarin also are likely to interact with danazol.

MANAGEMENT OPTIONS:

➡ *Avoid Unless Benefit Outweighs Risk.* Avoid concomitant therapy with oral anticoagulants and danazol if possible.

➡ *Monitor.* If the combination is used, watch for an alteration in the hypoprothrombinemic response to oral anticoagulants if danazol is initiated, discontinued, or changed in dosage; adjust oral anticoagulant dosage as needed. It is possible that danazol, by increasing fibrinolytic activity, increases the bleeding risk in anticoagulated patients even when the warfarin dose has been adjusted to achieve the desired hypoprothrombinemic response. Thus, give careful attention to early detection of bleeding.

REFERENCES:

1. Goulbourne IA, et al. An interaction between danazol and warfarin: case report. *Br J Obstet Gynaecol.* 1981;88:950.

2. Small M, et al. Danazol and oral anticoagulants. *Scott Med J.* 1982;27:331.

3. Meeks ML, et al. Danazol increases the anticoagulant effect of warfarin. *Ann Pharmacother.* 1992;26:641.

Danshen

Warfarin (eg, *Coumadin*)

SUMMARY: Danshen has been reported to increase the bleeding risk in patients on warfarin, but more study is needed to establish the clinical importance of this interaction.

RISK FACTORS: No specific risk factors are known.

MECHANISM: Animal and in vitro studies suggest that danshen may impair hemostasis (eg, inhibition of platelet function, increased fibrinolysis) and also may inhibit the elimination of warfarin.

CLINICAL EVALUATION: Isolated cases of excessive hypoprothrombinemia and bleeding have been reported in patients on warfarin who took danshen.[1] Although more information is needed to establish a causal relationship, until proven otherwise assume that danshen may increase the bleeding risk in patients on warfarin or other oral anticoagulants.

RELATED DRUGS: Theoretically, danshen could increase the bleeding risk in patients on other oral anticoagulants such as acenocoumarol and phenprocoumon.

MANAGEMENT OPTIONS:

➡ *Consider Alternative.* In patients receiving warfarin or other oral anticoagulants, consider using an alternative to danshen.

➡ *Monitor.* In patients receiving warfarin or other oral anticoagulants, monitor the INR when danshen is started, stopped, or changed in dosage. Note that some of the purported mechanisms (eg, platelet inhibition) would not be reflected in an increased INR, so an INR in the desired range does not ensure that there is not an increased risk of bleeding.

REFERENCES:

1. Chan TK. Interaction between warfarin and danshen (*Salvia miltiorrhiza*). *Ann Pharmacother.* 2001;35:501.

Dantrolene (*Dantrium*)
Verapamil (eg, *Calan*)

SUMMARY: A patient developed hyperkalemia and cardiovascular depression following verapamil and dantrolene administration.

RISK FACTORS: No specific risk factors are known.

MECHANISM: Not established.

CLINICAL EVALUATION: A diabetic patient undergoing a hemicolectomy received dantrolene 2.4 mg IV prophylactically because of a history of malignant hyperthermia.[1] The patient was being treated with verapamil 80 mg 3 times/day, insulin, and transdermal nitroglycerin (eg, *Nitro-Dur*). When dantrolene was administered 2 hours after an oral dose of verapamil, the patient was noted to be hyperkalemic and hyperglycemic 2 hours later. The hyperkalemia was accompanied by decreased cardiac output, metabolic acidosis, and elevated pulmonary artery pressures. Six months later, the same patient received dantrolene 2.4 mg IV preoperatively; however, metabolic changes were not noted, possibly because the patient no longer was treated with verapamil but with nifedipine 10 mg 3 times/day.

RELATED DRUGS: Based on this case report, nifedipine (eg, *Procardia*) does not interact with dantrolene. No data are available regarding other calcium channel blockers.

MANAGEMENT OPTIONS: No specific action is required, but be alert for evidence of the interaction.

REFERENCES:

1. Rubin AS, et al. Hyperkalemia, verapamil, and dantrolene. *Anesthesiology.* 1987;66:246.

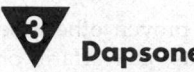 **Dapsone**

Didanosine (*Videx*)

SUMMARY: Dapsone failed to prevent pneumocystis infections in patients being treated with didanosine for human immunodeficiency virus (HIV).

RISK FACTORS: No specific risk factors are known.

MECHANISM: Not established. It is possible that the citrate-phosphate buffer in the didanosine formulation inhibited the dissolution of dapsone in the stomach.

CLINICAL EVALUATION: In a study of patients with HIV being treated with didanosine, dapsone prophylaxis for pneumocystis infection failed in approximately 35% of the cases.[1] This is a much higher failure rate than expected. Pending prospective studies, this interaction may reduce the efficacy of didanosine.

RELATED DRUGS: No information is available.

MANAGEMENT OPTIONS:

➡ *Circumvent/Minimize.* Administer dapsone 2 to 3 hours before didanosine to avoid a reduction in dapsone absorption.

➡ *Monitor.* Watch patients receiving the combination for reduced dapsone efficacy.

REFERENCES:

1. Metroka CE, et al. Failure of prophylaxis with dapsone in patients taking dideoxyinosine. *N Engl J Med*. 1991;325:737.

 Dapsone

Probenecid

SUMMARY: Probenecid may increase serum dapsone concentrations, but the clinical importance of this effect is not established.

RISK FACTORS: No specific risk factors are known.

MECHANISM: Probenecid appears to inhibit the renal excretion of dapsone.

CLINICAL EVALUATION: In one preliminary study, dapsone serum concentrations were increased approximately 50% after 4 hours and 25% after 8 hours when probenecid was given at the same time as dapsone.[1] The increased serum dapsone concentrations may increase dapsone toxicity, but this has not been studied.

RELATED DRUGS: No information is available.

MANAGEMENT OPTIONS:

➡ *Circumvent/Minimize.* The dapsone dose may need to be reduced in some patients taking concomitant probenecid.

➡ *Monitor.* Monitor patients taking dapsone and probenecid for evidence of increased dapsone serum concentrations including hemolytic anemia, methemoglobinemia, and peripheral neuropathy with muscle weakness.

REFERENCES:

1. Goodwin CS, et al. Inhibition of dapsone excretion by probenecid. *Lancet*. 1969;2:884.

Dapsone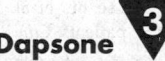

Rifampin (eg, *Rifadin*)

SUMMARY: Rifampin reduces dapsone serum concentrations; methemoglobin concentrations were increased.

RISK FACTORS: No specific risk factors are known.

MECHANISM: Rifampin appears to induce the metabolism of dapsone resulting in lower serum concentrations.[5]

CLINICAL EVALUATION: Dapsone half-life was reduced 37% 3 days after a single 600 mg dose of rifampin.[1] During 15 days of rifampin administration, plasma dapsone concentrations decreased 35% to 70%.[2] Dapsone clearance increased 250% and methemoglobin increased 68%.[6] The risk of methemoglobin toxicity appears to be increased by this combination. These studies confirm earlier reports of rifampin-induced reductions in dapsone serum concentrations.[3,4] However, dapsone concentrations remained well above minimum inhibitory concentrations for *M. leprae*. Dapsone is less active against *P. carinii* than *M. leprae*; rifampin coadministration may reduce the efficacy of dapsone when used for *P. carinii* infections.

RELATED DRUGS: No information is available.

MANAGEMENT OPTIONS:

➥ *Circumvent/Minimize.* Dapsone doses may need to be increased during rifampin administration.

➥ *Monitor.* Monitor patients for methemoglobin accumulation during rifampin coadministration. Observe patients being treated for pneumocystis for reduced efficacy.

REFERENCES:

1. Pieters FAJM, et al. Influence of once-monthly rifampicin and daily clofazimine on the pharmacokinetics of dapsone in leprosy patients in Nigeria. *Eur J Clin Pharmacol.* 1988;34:73.
2. George J, et al. Drug interaction during multidrug regimens for treatment of leprosy. *Indian J Med Res.* 1988;87:151.
3. Balakrishnan S, et al. Drug interactions. The influence of rifampicin and clofazimine on the urinary excretion of DDS. *Lepr India.* 1981;53:17.
4. Balakrishnan S, et al. Influence of rifampicin on DDS excretion in urine. *Lepr India.* 1979;51:54.
5. Horowitz HW, et al. Drug interactions in use of dapsone for Pneumocystis carinii prophylaxis. *Lancet.* 1992;339:747.
6. Occhipinti DJ, et al. Influence of rifampin and clarithromycin on dapsone disposition and methemoglobin concentrations. *Clin Pharmacol Ther.* 1995;57:163.

Dapsone

Trimethoprim (eg, *Proloprim*)

SUMMARY: Trimethoprim appears to increase dapsone serum concentrations and effects; dapsone increases trimethoprim concentrations.

RISK FACTORS: No specific risk factors are known.

MECHANISM: Trimethoprim may reduce the elimination of dapsone; dapsone appears to reduce the elimination of trimethoprim.

CLINICAL EVALUATION: Dapsone serum concentrations were noted to be 40% higher in subjects taking dapsone plus trimethoprim.[1] Dapsone toxicity (methemoglobinemia) and efficacy were greater in the patients receiving trimethoprim plus dapsone. Trimethoprim concentrations were 48% greater in the patients receiving dapsone concomitantly compared with those receiving trimethoprim plus sulfamethoxazole (*Gantanol*) although no additional toxicity was noted.

RELATED DRUGS: Trimethoprim-sulfamethoxazole (eg, *Bactrim*) also may produce similar effects.

MANAGEMENT OPTIONS:

➡ *Monitor.* Monitor methemoglobin levels of patients receiving dapsone plus trimethoprim for increased dapsone toxicity.

REFERENCES:

1. Lee BL, et al. Dapsone, trimethoprim, and sulfamethoxazole plasma levels during treatment of pneumocystis pneumonia in patients with the acquired immunodeficiency syndrome (AIDS). *Ann Intern Med.* 1989;110:606.

4   Dapsone

Zalcitabine†

SUMMARY: Dapsone did not alter the serum concentrations of zalcitabine. Zalcitabine caused a small increase in dapsone concentrations, which is not likely to produce a clinically significant change in dapsone response.

RISK FACTORS: No specific risk factors are known.

MECHANISM: Not established.

CLINICAL EVALUATION: Twelve HIV-infected patients received 3 drug regimens: dapsone 100 mg orally, zalcitabine 1.5 mg orally 3 times a day, and the combination of dapsone and zalcitabine.[1] The administration of dapsone with zalcitabine did not significantly alter the pharmacokinetics of zalcitabine compared with its administration alone; however, the peak dapsone concentration increased 19% and the clearance of dapsone after oral administration fell approximately 20%. The clinical significance of these changes is likely to be limited.

RELATED DRUGS: No information is available.

MANAGEMENT OPTIONS: No specific action is required, but be alert for evidence of the interaction.

REFERENCES:

1. Lee BL, et al. Zalcitabine (DDC) and dapsone (DAP) pharmacokinetic interaction in HIV-infected patients. *Clin Pharmacol Ther.* 1995;57(2):186.

† Not available in the United States.

5   Dapsone

Zidovudine (eg, *Retrovir*)

SUMMARY: No interaction.

RISK FACTORS: No specific risk factors are known.

MECHANISM: No interaction.

CLINICAL EVALUATION: Eight HIV-infected men received a single oral dose of zidovudine 200 mg and another single dose of zidovudine after 5 days of dapsone 100 mg/day.[1] Dapsone administration had no effect on the serum concentrations of zidovudine.

RELATED DRUGS: No information is available.

MANAGEMENT OPTIONS: No interaction.

REFERENCES:
1. Lee BL, et al. Zidovudine, trimethoprim, and dapsone pharmacokinetic interactions in patients with human immunodeficiency virus infection. *Antimicrob Agents Chemother.* 1996;40(5):1231-1236.

Darunavir (*Prezista*)

Etravirine (*Intelence*)

SUMMARY: Darunavir administration appears to reduce etravirine plasma concentrations; further study is needed to establish the clinical relevance of this interaction.

RISK FACTORS: No specific risk factors are known.

MECHANISM: Unknown.

CLINICAL EVALUATION: While specific data are limited, the manufacturer of etravirine notes that the coadministration of darunavir 600 mg plus ritonavir (*Norvir*) 100 mg twice daily with etravirine reduced the mean area under the plasma concentration-time curve (AUC) of etravirine by approximately 30%.[1] This data appears to reflect a study done in HIV-infected patients in which plasma concentrations of etravirine obtained during darunavir/ritonavir coadministration were compared with historic controls.[2] In a study of 32 healthy subjects, etravirine 100 or 200 mg twice daily was administered alone or for the last 7 days of a 16-day regimen of darunavir 600 mg/ritonavir 100 mg twice daily.[3] The coadministration of darunavir/ritonavir decreased the mean AUC of etravirine 37%. It was also noted that ritonavir 600 mg twice daily reduced etravirine AUC by approximately 50%. Some patients may have a reduction in antiviral efficacy; however, more data are needed to establish clinical significance.

RELATED DRUGS: Ritonavir, saquinavir (*Invirase*), and tipranavir (*Aptivus*) have also been noted to reduce etravirine plasma concentrations.

MANAGEMENT OPTIONS:

➡ ***Monitor.*** Monitor for reduced etravirine antiviral efficacy when it is coadministered with darunavir.

REFERENCES:
1. *Intelence* [package insert]. Raritan, NJ: Tibotec Therapeutics; 2008.
2. Boffito M, et al. Pharmacokinetic and antiretroviral response to darunavir/ritonavir and etravirine combination in patients with high-level viral resistance. *AIDS.* 2007;21(11):1449-1455.
3. Schöller-Gyüre M, et al. Pharmacokinetics of darunavir/ritonavir and TMC125 alone and coadministered in HIV-negative volunteers. *Antivir Ther.* 2007;12(5):789-796.

Darunavir (*Prezista*)/Ritonavir (*Norvir*)

Ketoconazole

SUMMARY: The coadministration of darunavir/ritonavir and ketoconazole results in an increase in the plasma concentrations of both ketoconazole and darunavir.

RISK FACTORS: No specific risk factors are known.

MECHANISM: The ritonavir component of darunavir/ritonavir appears to inhibit the elimination of ketoconazole, while ketoconazole inhibits the elimination of darunavir. The CYP3A4 enzyme is probably involved in both interactions.

CLINICAL EVALUATION: While specific data are limited, it has been noted that the coadministration of darunavir 400 mg/ritonavir 100 mg twice daily with ketoconazole 200 mg twice daily increased the mean area under the plasma concentration-time curve (AUC) of darunavir approximately 40%.[1] The mean AUC of ketoconazole was increased over 3-fold during darunavir/ritonavir coadministration. Pending further data, patients receiving darunavir/ritonavir and ketoconazole should be observed for increased effects of both drugs.

RELATED DRUGS: Other antifungal agents that inhibit CYP3A4 (eg, itraconazole [eg, *Sporanox*], voriconazole [*Vfend*], posaconazole [*Noxafil*], and fluconazole [eg, *Diflucan*]) are expected to affect darunavir in a similar manner. Atazanavir (*Reyataz*), indinavir (*Crixivan*), nelfinavir (*Viracept*), saquinavir (*Invirase*), and ritonavir (*Norvir*) also inhibit the activity of CYP3A4 and would be expected to increase the plasma concentrations of ketoconazole.

MANAGEMENT OPTIONS:

➡ *Consider Alternative.* Consider terbinafine (eg, *Lamisil*) as an alternative antifungal agent because it does not affect CYP3A4 activity. Amphotericin, caspofungin (*Cancidas*), and anidulafungin (*Eraxis*) do not appear to inhibit CYP3A4.

➡ *Monitor.* An excessive response to darunavir/ritonavir (eg, glucose intolerance, hepatotoxicity, skin rashes) may occur if ketoconazole is coadministered.

REFERENCES:

1. *Prezista* [package insert]. Raritan, NJ: Tibotec Therapeutics; 2008.

 Dasatinib (*Sprycel*)

Famotidine (eg, *Pepcid*)

SUMMARY: Famotidine reduces dasatinib plasma concentrations; some loss of efficacy is likely to occur.

RISK FACTORS: No specific risk factors are known.

MECHANISM: Dasatinib is known to require an acidic pH to complete dissolution. Drugs that increase gastric acidity may reduce its dissolution and, thus, its absorption.

CLINICAL EVALUATION: Twenty-one healthy subjects received 2 doses of dasatinib 50 mg separated by 12 hours.[1] The same regimen was repeated with a single dose of famotidine 40 mg administered 2 hours after the first dose of dasatinib. Pretreatment with famotidine reduced the 12-hour area under the concentration-time curve (AUC) and maximum concentration of dasatinib by more than 60% compared with dasatinib administered alone. No pH monitoring was done. The coadministration of antacid (aluminum/magnesium hydroxide 30 mL) reduced the AUC of dasatinib by about 50%. Giving the antacid 2 hours prior to the dasatinib had no effect on dasatinib pharmacokinetics. Repeated doses of famotidine or the use of more potent acid-suppressing drugs (eg, proton pump inhibitors) would be expected to produce a greater effect. Doses of dasatinib may require adjustment to maintain adequate antineoplastic activity.

RELATED DRUGS: Imatinib (*Gleevec*) does not appear to be affected by antacid administration.[2] Other H_2-receptor antagonists (cimetidine [eg, *Tagamet*], nizatidine [eg, *Axid*], and ranitidine [eg, *Zantac*]), antacids, and proton pump inhibitors (esomeprazole [*Nexium*], lansoprazole [*Prevacid*], omeprazole [eg, *Prilosec*], pantoprazole [eg, *Protonix*], and rabeprazole [*AcipHex*]) may also reduce the absorption of dasatinib.

MANAGEMENT OPTIONS:

➡ **Monitor.** Carefully monitor patients taking dasatinib if drugs that reduce gastric acidity are coadministered. Separating antacids and dasatinib should avoid the interaction; administration of dasatinib 2 to 3 hours prior to the antacid would be reasonable.

REFERENCES:

1. Eley T, et al. Phase I study of the effect of gastric acid pH modulators on the bioavailability of oral dasatinib in healthy subjects. *J Clin Pharmacol.* 2009;49(6):700-709.

2. Sparano BA, et al. Effect of antacid on imatinib absorption. *Cancer Chemother Pharmacol.* 2009;63(3):525-528.

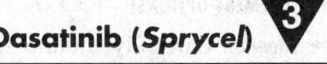

Dasatinib (*Sprycel*)

Ketoconazole (eg, *Nizoral*)

SUMMARY: The administration of ketoconazole to patients stabilized on dasatinib results in a marked increase in dasatinib plasma concentrations; increased adverse effects are likely to occur.

RISK FACTORS: No specific risk factors are known.

MECHANISM: Ketoconazole appears to inhibit the CYP3A4 metabolism of dasatinib, resulting in elevated dasatinib plasma concentrations.

CLINICAL EVALUATION: While specific data are limited, the manufacturer of dasatinib notes that the coadministration of ketoconazole 200 mg twice a day with dasatinib 20 mg daily in patients with tumors increased the mean area under the plasma concentration-time curve of dasatinib by about 5-fold.[1] Pending further data, patients receiving dasatinib and ketoconazole should be observed for increased dasatinib adverse effects, such as myelosuppression.

RELATED DRUGS: Fluconazole (eg, *Diflucan*), itraconazole (eg, *Sporanox*), posaconazole (*Noxafil*), and voriconazole (*Vfend*) also inhibit the activity of CYP3A4 and would be expected to increase the plasma concentration of dasatinib.

MANAGEMENT OPTIONS:

➡ **Consider Alternative.** Terbinafine (eg, *Lamisil*) may be considered as an alternative antifungal agent because it does not affect CYP3A4 activity. Amphotericin, caspofungin (*Cancidas*), and anidulafungin (*Eraxis*) do not appear to inhibit CYP3A4.

➡ *Monitor.* Carefully monitor patients taking dasatinib for altered response if keto-conazole is initiated or discontinued from their regimen.

REFERENCES:
1. *Sprycel* [package insert]. Princeton, NJ: Bristol-Myers Squibb Company; 2009.

 Dasatinib (*Sprycel*)

Rifampin (eg, *Rifadin*)

SUMMARY: The administration of rifampin to patients stabilized on dasatinib results in a marked decrease in dasatinib plasma concentrations; reduction in efficacy is likely to occur.

RISK FACTORS: No specific risk factors are known.

MECHANISM: Rifampin appears to induce the CYP3A4 metabolism of dasatinib, result-ing in decreased dasatinib plasma concentrations.

CLINICAL EVALUATION: While specific data are limited, the manufacturer of dasatinib notes that the coadministration of rifampin 600 mg daily for 8 days reduced the area under the plasma concentration-time curve of a single dose of dasatinib by 82%.[1] Pending further data, patients receiving dasatinib and rifampin should be observed for loss of dasatinib efficacy.

RELATED DRUGS: Rifabutin (*Mycobutin*) and rifapentine (*Priftin*) are known to induce CYP3A4 and would likely affect dasatinib in a similar manner.

MANAGEMENT OPTIONS:

➡ *Monitor.* Carefully monitor patients taking dasatinib for alteration of response if rifampin is initiated or discontinued from their regimen. Dasatinib will likely require an increase in dose if it is coadministered with rifampin.

REFERENCES:
1. *Sprycel* [package insert]. Princeton, NJ: Bristol-Myers Squibb Company; 2009.

 Debrisoquin†

Desipramine (eg, *Norpramin*)

SUMMARY: Desipramine and other tricyclic antidepressants (TCAs) appear to inhibit the antihypertensive response to debrisoquin.

RISK FACTORS: No specific risk factors are known.

MECHANISM: TCAs probably inhibit the adrenergic neuronal uptake of debrisoquin.

CLINICAL EVALUATION: In 2 patients receiving debrisoquin, the antihypertensive effect was reversed when desipramine was given.[1] In another patient, amitriptyline reduced the antihypertensive response to debrisoquin.[2] These reports, combined with theo-retical considerations, indicate that the interaction between debrisoquin and these TCAs probably exists.

RELATED DRUGS: Amitriptyline reduced antihypertensive response to debrisoquin. The effect of other TCAs on the response to debrisoquin is not known, but assume that they interact until proven otherwise.

MANAGEMENT OPTIONS:

➡ *Consider Alternative.* Although limited clinical evidence is available, avoid the use of TCAs in patients receiving debrisoquin.

➡ *Monitor.* If the combination is used, monitor for altered debrisoquin effect if TCAs are initiated, discontinued, or changed in dosage; adjust the debrisoquin dose as needed.

REFERENCES:

1. Mitchell JR, et al. Guanethidine and related agents. 3. Antagonism by drugs which inhibit the norepinephrine pump in man. *J Clin Invest.* 1970;49(8):1596-1604.

2. Skinner C, et al. Antagonism of the hypotensive action of bethanidine and debrisoquine by tricyclic antidepressants. *Lancet.* 1969;2(7620):564-566.

† Not available in the United States.

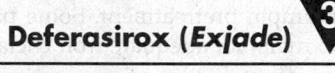

Deferasirox (*Exjade*)

Repaglinide (*Prandin*)

SUMMARY: Deferasirox administration increases the plasma concentration of repaglinide; increased hypoglycemic response may occur.

RISK FACTORS: No specific risk factors are known.

MECHANISM: Deferasirox inhibits the activity of CYP2C8, an enzyme partially responsible for the metabolism of repaglinide.

CLINICAL EVALUATION: Thirty-four subjects were administered placebo or deferasirox 30 mg/kg orally once daily for 3 days.[1] On the last day of deferasirox administration, a single dose of repaglinide 0.5 mg was administered 1 hour after the deferasirox dose. The mean area under the concentration-time curve and peak concentration of repaglinide were each increased approximately 2.3-fold after deferasirox compared with placebo. Serum glucose concentrations were lower during deferasirox plus repaglinide administration. It is likely that some patients with diabetes could experience hypoglycemia during the coadministration of deferasirox and repaglinide.

RELATED DRUGS: Pioglitazone (*Actos*) and rosiglitazone (*Avandia*) are also substrates for CYP2C8 and could be affected in a similar manner by deferasirox.

MANAGEMENT OPTIONS:

➡ *Consider Alternative.* Consider the use of oral hypoglycemic agents that are not substrates of CYP2C8, such as glipizide (eg, *Glucotrol*) or metformin (eg, *Glucophage*), in patients requiring deferasirox.

➡ *Monitor.* Monitor patients receiving repaglinide for increased hypoglycemic response during coadministration of deferasirox.

REFERENCES:

1. Skerjanec A, et al. Investigation of the pharmacokinetic interactions of deferasirox, a once-daily oral iron chelator, with midazolam, rifampin, and repaglinide in healthy volunteers. *J Clin Pharmacol.* 2010;50(2):205-213.

Deferasirox (*Exjade*)

Rifampin (eg, *Rifadin*)

SUMMARY: Rifampin reduces the plasma concentration of deferasirox; some loss of efficacy may occur.

RISK FACTORS: No specific risk factors are known.

MECHANISM: Rifampin appears to induce the glucuronidation-based metabolism of deferasirox.

CLINICAL EVALUATION: Twenty subjects received a single oral dose of deferasirox 30 mg/kg alone or on day 13 of a 15-day regimen of rifampin 300 mg daily.[1] The mean area under the concentration-time curve of deferasirox was reduced by 44% following pretreatment with rifampin. The mean half-life of deferasirox was reduced with rifampin pretreatment. Some patients may require an increased deferasirox dose to maintain adequate iron chelation efficacy.

RELATED DRUGS: Rifabutin (*Mycobutin*) may also induce the glucuronidation of deferasirox.

MANAGEMENT OPTIONS:

➡ **Monitor.** Monitor patients taking deferasirox for iron chelation for appropriate response if rifampin is added to or removed from their drug regimen.

REFERENCES:
1. Skerjanec A, et al. Investigation of the pharmacokinetic interactions of deferasirox, a once-daily oral iron chelator, with midazolam, rifampin, and repaglinide in healthy volunteers. *J Clin Pharmacol.* 2010;50(2):205-213.

Delavirdine (*Rescriptor*)

Omeprazole (eg, *Prilosec*)

SUMMARY: The absorption of delavirdine is reduced when gastric pH is increased; a reduction in antiviral efficacy may result.

RISK FACTORS: No specific risk factors are known.

MECHANISM: The absorption of delavirdine appears to be reduced as the pH of the gastric contents is increased. Delavirdine may require an acidic gastric pH for dissolution.

CLINICAL EVALUATION: Eight patients with HIV and gastric hypoacidity were treated with delavirdine 400 mg 3 times daily with and without concurrent glutamic acid 1,360 mg 3 times daily.[1] The minimum gastric pH in the patients without glutamic acid administration averaged 3.6. Under these conditions, the mean area under the concentration-time curve (AUC) over 8 hours following a dose of delavirdine was 46 mcmol/h. The administration of glutamic acid resulted in a mean minimum gastric pH of 1.5. Under these conditions, the AUC of delavirdine was increased 50% compared with the baseline value. Although no detail is provided, the manufacturer of delavirdine notes that the simultaneous administration of antacids reduces the AUC approximately 40%.[2] While additional study is indicated, it appears that the absorption of delavirdine is reduced in patients with increased gastric pH. Potent inhibitors of gastric acid secretion such as proton pump inhibitors or high doses of H_2-receptor antagonists would be expected to affect the absorption of delavirdine.

RELATED DRUGS: Other proton pump inhibitors (eg, lansoprazole [*Prevacid*], rabeprazole [*Aciphex*], pantoprazole [eg, *Protonix*]) or H_2-receptor antagonists (eg, cimetidine [eg, *Tagamet*], ranitidine [eg, *Zantac*], famotidine [eg, *Pepcid*], nizatidine [eg, *Axid*]) may also reduce the absorption of delavirdine.

MANAGEMENT OPTIONS:

➡ *Circumvent/Minimize.* Pending further study of this potential interaction, patients receiving delavirdine should avoid drugs that produce reduced gastric acidity at the time of delavirdine administration. The separation of the administration of antacids by 3 to 4 hours from the administration of delavirdine may reduce their effect on delavirdine absorption.

➡ *Monitor.* Monitor patients taking delavirdine and acid-suppressing drugs for a reduced antiviral effect.

REFERENCES:

1. Morse GD, et al. Gastric acidification increases delavirdine (DLV) mesylate exposure in HIV + subjects with gastric hypoacidity. *Clin Pharmacol Ther*. 1996;59:141.
2. *Rescriptor* [package insert]. Kalamazoo, MI: Pharmacia & Upjohn; 1999.

Delavirdine (*Rescriptor*)

Paclitaxel (eg, *Taxol*)

SUMMARY: Two patients on combined therapy with delavirdine and saquinavir (*Invirase*) developed unexpectedly severe paclitaxel toxicity, but a causal relationship was not established.

RISK FACTORS: No specific risk factors are known.

MECHANISM: Not established. Delavirdine and saquinavir may inhibit the metabolism of paclitaxel by CYP3A4.

CLINICAL EVALUATION: Two patients on combination antiretroviral therapy with delavirdine, saquinavir, and didanosine (eg, *Videx*) developed severe paclitaxel toxicity (mucositis, neutropenia, alopecia).[1] One of the patients also received fluconazole (eg, *Diflucan*), a known CYP3A4 inhibitor. Both patients had tolerated numerous previous cycles of paclitaxel therapy with only relatively mild toxicity (eg, nausea, alopecia). During these paclitaxel courses, the patients received various combinations of antiretroviral drugs, such as zidovudine (eg, *Retrovir*), zalcitabine,[†] lamivudine (*Epivir*), stavudine (*Zerit*), and indinavir (*Crixivan*). Although the findings in these patients are consistent with an interaction between paclitaxel and delavirdine/saquinavir, a causal relationship was not established. Additional study is needed for confirmation.

RELATED DRUGS: Little is known about the effect of other antiretroviral agents on paclitaxel toxicity. Theoretically, any antiretroviral agent that inhibits CYP3A4, including ritonavir (*Norvir*), indinavir, and nelfinavir (*Viracept*), may be expected to increase paclitaxel serum concentrations.

MANAGEMENT OPTIONS:

➥ *Monitor.* Monitor patients on delavirdine or other antiretroviral agents that inhibit CYP3A4 for excessive paclitaxel toxicity; reduce paclitaxel doses if necessary.

REFERENCES:

1. Schwartz JD, et al. Potential interaction of antiretroviral therapy with paclitaxel in patients with AIDS-related Kaposi's sarcoma. *AIDS.* 1999; 13(2):283-284.

† Not available in the United States.

Delavirdine (*Rescriptor*)

Rifabutin (*Mycobutin*)

SUMMARY: Rifabutin significantly reduces the plasma concentration of delavirdine; if coadministration cannot be avoided, delavirdine doses may need to be increased.

RISK FACTORS: No specific risk factors are known.

MECHANISM: Rifabutin appears to induce the first-pass or systemic metabolism (CYP3A4) of delavirdine.

CLINICAL EVALUATION: Twelve HIV-positive patients received delavirdine 400 mg orally 3 times a day for 29 days and a single dose on day 30.[1] Seven of the patients also received rifabutin 300 mg/day on days 16 to 30. The oral clearance of delavirdine increased from 4.4 L/hr on day 15 to 24 L/hr after 15 days of rifabutin coadministration. Delavirdine half-life was reduced from 4.8 hours to 2.1 hours following rifabutin administration. These changes are likely to reduce the antiviral efficacy of delavirdine. Rifabutin oral clearance was reduced 20% during delavirdine dosing but this change was not statistically significant, nor is it likely to be of clinical significance.

RELATED DRUGS: Rifampin (eg, *Rifadin*) is known to be an inducer of CYP3A4 and is likely to reduce the plasma concentration of delavirdine.

MANAGEMENT OPTIONS:

➥ *Circumvent/Minimize.* The dose of delavirdine may need to be increased during coadministration with rifabutin.

➥ *Monitor.* Monitor patients receiving rifabutin and delavirdine for reduced antiviral effect.

REFERENCES:

1. Borin MT, et al. Pharmacokinetic study of the interaction between rifabutin and delavirdine mesylate in HIV-1 infected patients. *Antiviral Res.* 1997;35:53.

Delavirdine (*Rescriptor*)

Rifampin (eg, *Rifadin*)

SUMMARY: Rifampin administration reduces the plasma concentrations of delavirdine; a loss of antiviral efficacy is likely to result.

RISK FACTORS: No specific risk factors are known.

MECHANISM: Rifampin increases the activity of CYP3A, the isozyme responsible for the metabolism of delavirdine. This probably leads to a reduction in delavirdine bio-availability and an increase in its clearance.

CLINICAL EVALUATION: Twelve patients with human immunodeficiency virus (HIV) were treated with delavirdine 400 mg every 8 hours for 30 days.[1] Seven of the 12 patients received rifampin 600 mg/day on days 16 through 30 of delavirdine administration. The pharmacokinetics of delavirdine in the 5 patients taking only delavirdine were compared with its pharmacokinetics in the 7 patients taking both rifampin and delavirdine. Delavirdine oral clearance was increased from 7.7 L/hr to 205 L/hr following 15 days of rifampin therapy. Steady-state delavirdine concentrations fell from 23 mcmol/L to 0.56 mcmol/L, and delavirdine's half-life was reduced from over 4 hours to 1.7 hours. The coadministration of rifampin would likely inhibit the antiviral activity of delavirdine.

RELATED DRUGS: Rifabutin (*Mycobutin*) also increases the clearance of delavirdine but to a somewhat lesser (5-fold increase) extent.[2]

MANAGEMENT OPTIONS:

➡ **Consider Alternative.** In view of the magnitude of this interaction, avoiding the use of rifampin in patients taking delavirdine seems prudent.

➡ **Monitor.** Monitor patients receiving delavirdine for loss of efficacy if rifampin or rifabutin are administered.

REFERENCES:

1. Borin MT, et al. Pharmacokinetic study of the interaction between rifampin and delavirdine mesylate. *Clin Pharmacol Ther.* 1997;61:544–53.
2. Borin MT, et al. Effect of rifabutin on delavirdine pharmacokinetics in HIV positive patients. Presented at the 34th Interscience Conference on Antimicrobial Agents and Chemotherapy, Orlando, Florida, 1994.

Desflurane (*Suprane*) 4

Dobutamine (eg, *Dobutrex*)

SUMMARY: Four patients died from cardiac ischemic events after receiving dobutamine or dopamine (eg, *Intropin*) following desflurane anesthesia, but it was not proven that the events were a result of the combined use of these agents.

RISK FACTORS: No specific risk factors are known.

MECHANISM: Not established.

CLINICAL EVALUATION: Twenty-one consecutive patients undergoing advanced head and neck reconstructive surgery under desflurane anesthesia received low-dose dopamine or dobutamine.[1,2] Four of the patients (all with a history of coronary artery disease) developed cardiac ischemia and died. Two had received dobutamine, and 2 had received dopamine. The combined use of desflurane with dobutamine or dopamine may have contributed to these reactions; a causal relationship was not established.

RELATED DRUGS: Dopamine was involved in 2 of the 4 deaths.

MANAGEMENT OPTIONS: No specific action is required, but be alert for evidence of the interaction.

REFERENCES:

1. Murray JM, et al. Fatal cardiac ischaemia associated with prolonged desflurane anaesthesia and administration of exogenous catecholamines. *Can J Anaesth.* 1998;45:1200–2.

2. Moir CL. Cardiac ischemia and desflurane. *Can J Anaesth.* 1999;46:810.

Desflurane (*Suprane*)

Dopamine (eg, *Intropin*)

SUMMARY: Four patients died from cardiac ischemic events after receiving dopamine or dobutamine following desflurane anesthesia, but it was not proven that the events were a result of the combined use of these agents.

RISK FACTORS: No specific risk factors are known.

MECHANISM: Not established.

CLINICAL EVALUATION: Twenty-one consecutive patients undergoing advanced head and neck reconstructive surgery under desflurane anesthesia received low-dose dopamine or dobutamine (eg, *Dobutrex*).[1,2] Four of the patients (all with a history of coronary artery disease) developed cardiac ischemia and died. Two had received dopamine, and 2 had received dobutamine. It is possible that the combined use of desflurane with dopamine or dobutamine contributed to these reactions, but a causal relationship was not established.

RELATED DRUGS: Dobutamine was involved in 2 of the 4 deaths.

MANAGEMENT OPTIONS: No specific action is required, but be alert for evidence of the interaction.

REFERENCES:

1. Murray JM, et al. Fatal cardiac ischaemia associated with prolonged desflurane anaesthesia and administration of exogenous catecholamines. *Can J Anaesth.* 1998;45:1200–2.

2. Moir CL. Cardiac ischemia and desflurane. *Can J Anaesth.* 1999;46:810.

Desipramine (eg, *Norpramin*)

Fluoxetine (*Prozac*)

SUMMARY: Patients receiving desipramine or other tricyclic antidepressants (TCAs) may manifest marked increases in their antidepressant plasma concentration when fluoxetine is added; some may develop symptoms of antidepressant toxicity.

RISK FACTORS: No specific risk factors are known.

MECHANISM: Fluoxetine (*Prozac*) markedly inhibits cytochrome P4502D6, an enzyme involved in the hepatic metabolism of a number of TCAs.[5,7]

CLINICAL EVALUATION: Six healthy subjects were given single 50 mg doses of desipramine on 3 occasions: alone, after a single 60 mg dose of fluoxetine, and after 8 days of fluoxetine 60 mg/day. Plasma desipramine concentrations were approximately 10 times higher after 8 days of fluoxetine. Even the single dose of fluoxetine increased plasma desipramine levels and reduced desipramine clearance by more than half. Imipramine (eg, *Tofranil*) plasma concentrations also were increased markedly by fluoxetine, but not to the same degree as desipramine. Numerous case reports have appeared describing TCA toxicity with concurrent fluoxetine.[1-4] A 75-year-old woman had been receiving desipramine 300 mg and tryptophan 2 g at bedtime with plasma desipramine concentrations averaging 130 ng/mL.[1] Because this regimen only partially relieved her depressive symptoms, fluoxetine was added (20 mg/day for 8 days, then 40 mg/day). The plasma desipramine concentration had increased to 212 ng/mL by day 5 of fluoxetine therapy and to 419 ng/mL by day 12. This was accompanied by a marked increase in her depressive symptoms (severe lethargy, fatigue, hopelessness). The patient improved to her baseline status after fluoxetine was stopped and the desipramine dose was reduced. Whether an interaction between fluoxetine and tryptophan contributed to this reaction is not known. caused by the long half-life of fluoxetine (2 or 3 days) and its active metabolite, norfluoxetine (7 to 9 days), fluoxetine interactions theoretically could occur for weeks after its discontinuation. Indeed, 1 patient appeared to manifest markedly increased plasma concentrations of amitriptyline (eg, *Elavil*) and nortriptyline (eg, *Pamelor*) with anticholinergic toxicity even though her fluoxetine had already been discontinued.[6]

RELATED DRUGS: Five patients receiving antidepressants including desipramine, imipramine, nortriptyline, and trazodone (eg, *Desyrel*) developed marked increases in their plasma antidepressant concentrations after the addition of fluoxetine.[2] Within 1 or 2 weeks of starting fluoxetine, 3 of the patients developed adverse effects characteristic of the antidepressant they were receiving (eg, anticholinergic symptoms, sedation). Three other patients developed elevated plasma cyclic concentrations and cyclic toxicity such as seizures and delirium after fluoxetine was added to TCA (desipramine, imipramine, or doxepin [eg, *Sinequan*]) therapy.[3] In 8 depressed patients given fluoxetine plus trazodone, 3 had a good response but 5 experienced intolerable side effects (eg, headaches, dizziness, sedation, fatigue) or did not respond.[8] Paroxetine (*Paxil*) is also a potent inhibitor of CYP2D6 and can increase serum desipramine concentrations substantially.

MANAGEMENT OPTIONS:

➥ *Monitor.* Monitor patients for increased antidepressant plasma levels and toxicity when fluoxetine is used concurrently; adjustment of the antidepressant dosage is likely to be required. Because of the slow elimination of fluoxetine and its active metabolite, its effect on the metabolism of other antidepressants is likely to dissipate gradually over 2 to 4 weeks.

REFERENCES:

1. Bell IR, et al. Fluoxetine induces elevation of desipramine level and exacerbation of geriatric nonpsychotic depression. *J Clin Psychopharmacol.* 1988;8:447.

2. Aranow RB, et al. Elevated antidepressant plasma levels after addition of fluoxetine. *Am J Psychiatry.* 1989;146:911.

3. Preskorn SH, et al. Serious adverse effects of combining fluoxetine and tricyclic antidepressants. *Am J Psychiatry.* 1990;147:532.

4. Kahn DG, et al. Increased plasma nortriptyline concentration in a patient cotreated with fluoxetine. *J Clin Psychiatry.* 1990;51:36.

5. Brosen K, et al. Fluoxetine and norfluoxetine are potent inhibitors of P450IID6: the source of sparteine/debrisoquine oxidation polymorphism. *Br J Clin Pharmacol.* 1991;32:136.

6. Muller N, et al. Extremely long plasma half-life of amitriptyline in a woman with the cytochrome P450IID6 29/ 29-Kilobase Wild-Type Allele: a slowly reversible interaction with fluoxetine. *Ther Drug Monit.* 1991;13:533.

7. Bergstrom RF, et al. Quantification and mechanism of the fluoxetine and tricyclic antidepressant interaction. *Clin Pharmacol Ther.* 1992;51:239.

8. Nierenberg AA, et al. Possible trazodone potentiation of fluoxetine:a case series. *J Clin Psychiatry.* 1992;53:83.

Desipramine (eg, *Norpramin*)

Guanethidine (*Ismelin*)

SUMMARY: Tricyclic antidepressants (TCAs) consistently inhibit the antihypertensive response to guanethidine.

RISK FACTORS: No specific risk factors are known.

MECHANISM: TCAs inhibit the uptake of guanethidine into the adrenergic neuron, resulting in an inhibition of guanethidine's antihypertensive effect.[3,4,14] The ability of TCAs to inhibit the neuronal uptake of norepinephrine may also be involved.

CLINICAL EVALUATION: The interaction between TCAs and guanethidine is well documented.[2,5-11,13] It is especially important in patients with moderate-to-severe hypertension, the group most likely to receive guanethidine. Although increasing the guanethidine dose may overcome the interaction, subsequent discontinuation of the TCA in a patient on high doses may result in severe hypotensive reactions. Preliminary reports indicate that 300 mg/day of doxepin (eg, *Sinequan*) is less potent as an antagonist to the antihypertensive effect of guanethidine than other TCAs, and 200 mg/day or less probably has minimal effect.[1]

RELATED DRUGS: In one case report, an interaction between guanethidine and imipramine (eg, *Tofranil*) was implicated in producing cardiac standstill and death.[12] However, a causal relationship was not established. Limited clinical evidence indicates that guanethidine's antihypertensive response is unaffected by mianserin[15,18] and is only occasionally affected by maprotiline (eg, *Ludiomil*).[16,17] Guanadrel (*Hylorel*) is pharmacologically similar to guanethidine and also may be inhibited by TCAs. Methyldopa (eg, *Aldomet*) may be less likely to interact with tricyclic antidepressants than guanethidine, but more information is needed.

MANAGEMENT OPTIONS:

➡ *Consider Alternative.* Although satisfactory control of hypertension can sometimes be achieved by alteration in guanethidine dosage, it is preferable to avoid the combination when possible. Maprotiline may be less likely to interact with guanethidine than tricyclic antidepressants.

➡ *Monitor.* If the combination is used, monitor patients for rising blood pressures when TCAs are started and for hypotension when cyclics are stopped.

REFERENCES:

1. Oates JA, et al. Effect of doxepin on the norepinephrine pump. A preliminary report. *Psychosomatics.* 1969;10:12.

2. Mitchell JR, et al. Antagonism of the antihypertensive action of guanethidine sulfate by desipramine hydrochloride. *JAMA.* 1967;202:973.

3. Feagin OT, et al. Uptake and release of guanethidine and bethanidine by the adrenergic neuron. *J Clin Invest.* 1969;48:23a.

4. Mitchell JR, et al. Guanethidine and related agents. III. Antagonism by drugs which inhibit the norepinephrine pump in man. *J Clin Invest.* 1970;49:1596.

5. Ober KF, et al. Drug interactions with guanethidine. *Clin Pharmacol Ther.* 1973;14:190.

6. Gulati OD, et al. Antagonism of adrenergic neuron blockade in hypertensive subjects. *Clin Pharmacol Ther.* 1966;7:510.

7. Stone CA, et al. Antagonism of certain effects of catecholamine depleting agents by antidepressant and related drugs. *J Pharmacol Exp Ther.* 1964;144:196.

8. Leishman AWD, et al. Antagonism of guanethidine by imipramine. *Lancet.* 1963;1:112.

9. Pitts NE. The clinical evaluation of doxepin. A new psychotherapeutic agent. *Psychosomatics.* 1969;10:164.

10. Meyer JF, et al. Insidious and prolonged antagonism of guanethidine by amitriptyline. *JAMA.* 1970;213:1487.

11. Lahti RA, et al. The tricyclic antidepressants: inhibition of norepinephrine uptake as related to potentiation of norepinephrine and clinical efficacy. *Biochem Pharmacol.* 1971;20:482.

12. Williams RB Jr, et al. Cardiac complications of tricyclic antidepressant therapy. *Ann Intern Med.* 1971;74:395.

13. Boston Collaborative Drug Surveillance Program. Adverse reactions to the tricyclic antidepressant drugs. *Lancet.* 1972;1:529.

14. Mitchell JR, et al. Guanethidine and related agents. I. Mechanism of the selective blockade of adrenergic neurons and its antagonism by drugs. *J Pharmacol Exp Ther.* 1970;172:100.

15. Ghose K, et al. Autonomic actions and interactions of mianserin hydrochloride (org. GB 94) and amitriptyline in patients with depressive illness. *Psychopharmacology.* 1976;49:201.

16. Smith AJ, et al. Interaction between postganglionic sympathetic blocking drugs and antidepressants. *J Int Med Res.* 1975;3(Suppl. 2):55.

17. Briant RH, et al. The assessment of potential drug interaction with a new tricyclic antidepressant drug. *Br J Clin Pharmacol.* 1974;1:113.

18. Burgess CD, et al. Cardiovascular responses to mianserin hydrochloride: A comparison with tricyclic antidepressant drugs. *Br J Clin Pharmacol.* 1978;5:215.

Desipramine (eg, *Norpramin*) 4

Ibuprofen (eg, *Motrin*)

SUMMARY: A patient developed desipramine toxicity after starting ibuprofen, but a causal relationship was not established.

RISK FACTORS: No specific risk factors are known.

MECHANISM: Not established.

CLINICAL EVALUATION: A 15-year-old boy with attention deficit disorder (ADD) and major depression was taking desipramine 300 mg/day, which was increased to 375 mg/day.[1] One week after the increased dosage, he developed symptoms consistent with chest wall pain, which was treated with ibuprofen 600 mg 3 times a day. One week later he developed blurred vision, clouding of consciousness, tachycardia, and a grand mal seizure. His sensorium cleared after administration of 2 mg physostigmine IV (*Antilirium*). His desipramine serum concentration was in the toxic range (657 ng/mL). The desipramine toxicity was attributed to the ibuprofen, but the increase in desipramine dose cannot be ruled out as the primary factor.

RELATED DRUGS: No information is available.

MANAGEMENT OPTIONS: No specific action is required, but be alert for evidence of the interaction.

REFERENCES:

1. Gillette DW. Desipramine and ibuprofen. *J Am Acad Child Adolesc Psychiatry.* 1998;37:1129.

5　Desipramine (eg, *Norpramin*)

Ketoconazole (eg, *Nizoral*)

SUMMARY: Ketoconazole does not affect desipramine concentrations.

RISK FACTORS: No specific risk factors are known.

MECHANISM: No interaction.

CLINICAL EVALUATION: Six healthy subjects received a single dose of desipramine 100 mg alone and on day 10 of a 14-day regimen of ketoconazole 200 mg/day.[1] Pretreatment with ketoconazole resulted in no significant changes in desipramine plasma concentrations.

RELATED DRUGS: Ketoconazole produces a small increase in the plasma concentration of imipramine (eg, *Tofranil*).

MANAGEMENT OPTIONS: No interaction.

REFERENCES:
1. Spina E, et al. Effect of ketoconazole on the pharmacokinetics of imipramine and desipramine in healthy subjects. *Br J Clin Pharmacol.* 1997;43(3):315–18.

4　Desipramine (eg, *Norpramin*)

Phenylbutazone

SUMMARY: Desipramine may delay the absorption of phenylbutazone, but the effect is not likely to be clinically important since the bioavailability of phenylbutazone was not affected.

RISK FACTORS: No specific risk factors are known.

MECHANISM: Desipramine appears to inhibit the rate of gastrointestinal (GI) absorption of phenylbutazone, possibly caused by slowed GI motility from the anticholinergic effect of the desipramine.

CLINICAL EVALUATION: In a study of 4 subjects, the time required to reach peak plasma phenylbutazone concentrations was delayed considerably by the prior administration of desipramine.[1] However, total phenylbutazone absorption (based on urinary excretion of oxyphenbutazone) did not appear to be affected. Thus, under the conditions of multiple dosing of phenylbutazone, this interaction would not be expected to impair phenylbutazone effect.

RELATED DRUGS: The effect of other tricyclic antidepressants on phenylbutazone is not established.

MANAGEMENT OPTIONS: No specific action is required, but be alert for evidence of the interaction.

REFERENCES:
1. Consolo S, et al. Delayed absorption of phenylbutazone caused by desmethylimipramine in humans. *Eur J Pharmacol.* 1970;10:239.

Desipramine (eg, *Norpramin*)

Ritonavir (*Norvir*)

SUMMARY: Desipramine concentrations are markedly increased by ritonavir administration; toxicity could result.

RISK FACTORS: No specific risk factors are known.

MECHANISM: Ritonavir (*Norvir*) appears to inhibit the metabolism (CYP3A4) of desipramine.

CLINICAL EVALUATION: A single dose of desipramine 100 mg was administered alone and following the administration of ritonavir 500 mg every 12 hours to 14 patients.[1] Although details of the study were not provided, the area under the concentration time curve of desipramine increased by 145% when it was administered after ritonavir. This degree of increase is likely to produce toxicity in patients maintained on chronic desipramine.

RELATED DRUGS: Other tricyclic antidepressants may be similarly affected by ritonavir. Indinavir (*Crixivan*) may inhibit the metabolism of tricyclic antidepressants; the magnitude of any inhibition is unknown.

MANAGEMENT OPTIONS:

➡ **Circumvent/Minimize.** Dosage of desipramine may require reduction.

➡ **Monitor.** Monitor patients stabilized on desipramine and other tricyclic antidepressants for cardiac, central nervous system, and anticholinergic side effects.

REFERENCES:
1. Product information. Ritonavir (*Norvir*). Abbott Laboratories. 1996.

Desipramine (eg, *Norpramin*)

Venlafaxine (eg, *Effexor*)

SUMMARY: Study in healthy subjects suggests that venlafaxine increases desipramine serum concentrations, but the extent to which this increases the risk of desipramine toxicity is not established.

RISK FACTORS:

➡ **Pharmacogenetics.** Only patients who have CYP2D6 would be expected to experience this interaction.

MECHANISM: Desipramine is metabolized primarily by CYP2D6, and venlafaxine probably inhibits its CYP2D6 metabolism.

CLINICAL EVALUATION: Six subjects took a single oral dose of imipramine 100 mg with and without pretreatment with venlafaxine 50 mg 3 times daily for 3 days.[1] Venlafaxine modestly increased imipramine area under the plasma concentration-time curve (AUC), but the AUC of desipramine (an active metabolite of imipramine) was increased 40%. It is not known how often this interaction would produce consequences.

RELATED DRUGS: Theoretically, other tricyclic antidepressants that are metabolized by CYP2D6 such as amitriptyline (eg, *Elavil*) would be similarly affected.

MANAGEMENT OPTIONS:

➥ *Monitor.* Monitor for altered desipramine effect if venlafaxine is initiated, discontinued, or changed in dosage.

REFERENCES:

1. Albers LJ, et al. Effect of venlafaxine on imipramine metabolism. *Psychiatry Res.* 2000;96:235-243.

 Dexamethasone (eg, *Decadron*)

Ephedrine

SUMMARY: Ephedrine may enhance the elimination of dexamethasone, but the clinical importance of this effect is not established.

RISK FACTORS: No specific risk factors are known.

MECHANISM: Not established.

CLINICAL EVALUATION: Nine patients with asthma were given dexamethasone before and after ephedrine 100 mg/day for 3 weeks.[1] Ephedrine therapy was associated with a 36% decrease in dexamethasone half-life and a 42% increase in the metabolic clearance of dexamethasone. In the same study, theophylline (eg, *Theolair*) did not appear to affect dexamethasone disposition in 7 patients.

RELATED DRUGS: The effect of ephedrine on the disposition of other corticosteroids is unknown.

MANAGEMENT OPTIONS: No specific action is required, but be alert for evidence of the interaction.

REFERENCES:

1. Brooks SM, et al. The effects of ephedrine and theophylline on dexamethasone metabolism in bronchial asthma. *J Clin Pharmacol.* 1977;17:308.

 Dexfenfluramine

Fluoxetine (*Prozac*)

SUMMARY: Cotherapy with dexfenfluramine and selective serotonin reuptake inhibitors (SSRIs) such as fluoxetine theoretically could result in serotonin syndrome.

RISK FACTORS: No specific risk factors are known.

MECHANISM: Dexfenfluramine releases serotonin and inhibits its uptake. Since SSRIs are also serotonergic, combined use theoretically increases the risk of serotonin syndrome. Also, fluoxetine and paroxetine (*Paxil*) are potent inhibitors of CYP2D6, an isozyme important in the metabolism of dexfenfluramine. Sertraline (*Zoloft*) and fluvoxamine (*Luvox*) are much weaker inhibitors of CYP2D6.

CLINICAL EVALUATION: Although this interaction is based primarily on theoretical considerations, the potential outcome is serious. Serotonin syndrome has occurred when SSRIs such as fluoxetine have been combined with other serotonergic agents such as nonselective monoamine oxidase inhibitors. Serotonin syndrome can result in severe toxicity; fatalities have occurred. Given the potential severity of the reaction, the product information states that dexfenfluramine should not be used with SSRIs or any other serotonergic agent.[2] Anecdotal evidence suggests that many patients have received dexfenfluramine with SSRIs without manifesting serious adverse consequences, but such evidence does not rule out an occasional serious reaction. Dexfenfluramine serum concentrations are likely to be higher in a) patients who are genetically deficient in CYP2D6 (deficiency occurs in about 5% to 10% of Caucasians and blacks, 1% or fewer of Asians);[1] b) patients who are taking potent inhibitors of CYP2D6 such as fluoxetine or paroxetine; or c) patients whose urinary pH is more alkaline. It is not known, however, whether patients with higher levels of dexfenfluramine are more likely to manifest an adverse drug interaction with SSRIs.

RELATED DRUGS: Avoid dexfenfluramine in combinations with other SSRIs such as paroxetine, sertraline, and fluvoxamine. Dexfenfluramine is the S-enantiomer of the racemate fenfluramine, so the 2 drugs probably interact in a similar way with SSRIs.

MANAGEMENT OPTIONS:

➡ *Avoid Unless Benefit Outweighs Risk.* Patients should avoid the use of SSRIs with either dexfenfluramine or fenfluramine, unless the combinations are found to be safe in well controlled clinical trials. There is also a medicolegal risk in using the combinations, since the manufacturer's information states that cotherapy should be avoided.

➡ *Monitor.* If the combination is used, be alert for evidence of serotonin syndrome which can result in neurotoxicity (eg, myoclonus, tremors, rigidity, incoordination, restlessness, hyperreflexia, seizures, coma); psychiatric symptoms (eg, agitation, confusion, hypomania); and temperature regulation abnormalities (eg, fever, sweating).

REFERENCES:

1. Gross AS, et al. The influence of the sparteine/debrisoquine genetic polymorphism on the disposition of dexfenfluramine. *Br J Clin Pharmacol.* 1996;41:311.
2. Product Information. Dexfenfluramine (*Redux*). Wyeth-Ayerst Laboratories. 1996.

Dexfenfluramine
Phenelzine (*Nardil*) AVOID

SUMMARY: Cotherapy with dexfenfluramine and nonselective monoamine oxidase inhibitors (MAOIs) such as phenelzine theoretically could result in serotonin syndrome.

RISK FACTORS: No specific risk factors are known.

MECHANISM: Dexfenfluramine releases serotonin and inhibits its uptake. Since nonselective MAOIs are also serotonergic, combined use theoretically increases the risk of serotonin syndrome.

CLINICAL EVALUATION: Although this interaction is based primarily on theoretical considerations, the potential outcome is serious. Serotonin syndrome has occurred when nonselective MAOIs such as phenelzine and tranylcypromine (*Parnate*) have been combined with other serotonergic agents. Serotonin syndrome can result in neurotoxicity (eg, myoclonus, tremors, rigidity, incoordination, restlessness, hyperreflexia, seizures, coma); psychiatric symptoms (eg, agitation, confusion, hypomania); and temperature regulation abnormalities (eg, fever, sweating). Fatalities have occurred. Given the potential severity of the reaction, the product information states that combined use of dexfenfluramine and MAOIs is contraindicated.[2] Dexfenfluramine serum concentrations are likely to be higher in patients who are genetically deficient in CYP2D6 (deficiency occurs in approximately 5% to 10% of Caucasians and blacks, 1% or fewer of Asians),[1] and also in patients whose urinary pH is more alkaline. It is not known, however, whether patients with higher levels of dexfenfluramine are more likely to manifest an adverse drug interaction with nonselective MAOIs.

RELATED DRUGS: Dexfenfluramine also is contraindicated with other nonselective MAOIs such as tranylcypromine and isocarboxazid (*Marplan*). Given that selegiline (eg, *Eldepryl*) can sometimes act as a nonselective MAOI (especially if given in large doses), it also might interact adversely with dexfenfluramine. Dexfenfluramine is the S-enantiomer of the racemate fenfluramine, so the 2 drugs probably interact in a similar way with nonselective MAOIs.

MANAGEMENT OPTIONS:

➡ *AVOID COMBINATION.* Patients should avoid any combination of a nonselective MAOI with either dexfenfluramine or fenfluramine.

REFERENCES:

1. Gross AS, et al. The influence of the sparteine/debrisoquine genetic polymorphism on the disposition of dexfenfluramine. *Br J Clin Pharmacol.* 1996;41:311.

2. Product information. Dexfenfluramine (*Redux*). Wyeth-Ayerst Laboratories. 1996.

Dextroamphetamine (eg, *Dexedrine*)

Furazolidone (*Furoxone*)

SUMMARY: Amphetamines may induce a hypertensive response in patients taking furazolidone.

RISK FACTORS: No specific risk factors are known.

MECHANISM: Furazolidone appears to inhibit monoamine oxidase, thus increasing the pressor effect of indirect-acting sympathomimetics such as amphetamines.

CLINICAL EVALUATION: The pressor response to dextroamphetamine was increased in 9 hypertensive patients after administration of furazolidone 400 to 800 mg/day.[1] The effect apparently was seen only after several days of furazolidone administration.

RELATED DRUGS: One would expect an enhanced response to other sympathomimetics with indirect activity (eg, ephedrine), but this apparently has not been studied.

MANAGEMENT OPTIONS:

➡ *Consider Alternative.* Patients receiving furazolidone probably should avoid taking amphetamines.

➡ *Monitor.* Watch for increased blood pressure if amphetamine and furazolidone are coadministered.

REFERENCES:

1. Pettinger WA, et al. Inhibition of monoamine oxidase in man by furazolidone. *Clin Pharmacol Ther.* 1968;9:442-447.

Dextroamphetamine (eg, *Dexedrine*)

Guanethidine (*Ismelin*)

SUMMARY: Amphetamines, and probably related sympathomimetics, inhibit the antihypertensive response to guanethidine.

RISK FACTORS: No specific risk factors are known.

MECHANISM: Amphetamines antagonize the adrenergic neuron blockage produced by guanethidine, probably by displacing guanethidine from adrenergic neurons and inhibiting its uptake by adrenergic neurons. Also, amphetamines may have a direct effect on vasoconstrictor receptors.[1]

CLINICAL EVALUATION: An interaction between amphetamines and guanethidine has been described in several hypertensive patients and is likely to be clinically significant.[2-5] The effect has been noted with both dextroamphetamine and methamphetamine and is pronounced enough to interfere considerably with hypertensive control.

RELATED DRUGS: Although little is known regarding other sympathomimetics, their pharmacologic similarity to amphetamines suggests that they are likely to inhibit guanethidine's effect as well. Guanadrel (*Hylorel*) is similar to guanethidine and also may be inhibited by amphetamines.

MANAGEMENT OPTIONS:

➡ ***Consider Alternative.*** Consider using an alternative to amphetamine or guanethidine.

➡ ***Monitor.*** If the combination is used, monitor for inhibition of antihypertensive response to guanethidine or guanadrel.

REFERENCES:

1. Ober KF, et al. Drug interactions with guanethidine. *Clin Pharmacol Ther*. 1973;14:190-195.
2. Feagin OT, et al. Uptake and release of guanethidine and bethanidine by the adrenergic neuron. *J Clin Invest*. 1969;48:23a.
3. Day MD, et al. Antagonism of guanethidine and bretylium by various agents. *Lancet*. 1962;2:1282.
4. Gulati OD, et al. Antagonism of adrenergic neuron blockade in hypertensive subjects. *Clin Pharmacol Ther*. 1966;7:510 514.
5. Starke K. Interactions of guanethidine and indirect-acting sympathomimetic amines. *Arch Int Pharmacodyn Ther*. 1972;195:309-314.

Dextroamphetamine (eg, *Dexedrine*)

Imipramine (eg, *Tofranil*)

SUMMARY: Theoretically, tricyclic antidepressants (TCAs) such as imipramine would increase the effect of amphetamines, but clinical evidence is lacking.

RISK FACTORS: No specific risk factors are known.

MECHANISM: Not established. However, in view of the effect of norepinephrine in patients receiving TCAs, it seems likely that amphetamines would have an enhanced effect in patients on cyclic antidepressants caused by the release of norepinephrine.

CLINICAL EVALUATION: Amphetamine abuse in patients receiving TCAs purportedly may be fatal, but case reports of such an effect are lacking.[1,2]

RELATED DRUGS: Other amphetamines may be similarly affected.

MANAGEMENT OPTIONS:

➡ *Circumvent/Minimize.* Patients receiving tricyclic antidepressants should avoid recreational use of amphetamines. The risk of therapeutic use of amphetamines with tricyclic antidepressants is not established.

➡ *Monitor.* Monitor for adverse cardiovascular effects in patients on the combination.

REFERENCES:

1. Raisfeld IH. Cardiovascular complications of antidepressant therapy. *Am Heart J.* 1972;83:129-133.
2. Beaumont G. Drug interactions with clomipramine (*Anafranil*). *J Int Med Res.* 1973;1:480.

Dextroamphetamine (eg, *Dexedrine*)

Norepinephrine (*Levophed*)

SUMMARY: Amphetamine abuse may enhance the pressor response to norepinephrine.

RISK FACTORS: No specific risk factors are known.

MECHANISM: Not established.

CLINICAL EVALUATION: After large oral amphetamine doses for several days, amphetamine IV considerably enhanced the pressor response to norepinephrine IV in 6 patients with histories of amphetamine abuse.[1]

RELATED DRUGS: Other amphetamines may be affected similarly.

MANAGEMENT OPTIONS: No specific action is required, but be alert for evidence of the interaction.

REFERENCES:

1. Cavanaugh JH, et al. Effect of amphetamine on the pressor response to tyramine: formation of p-hydroxynorephedrine from amphetamine in man. *Clin Pharmacol Ther.* 1970;11:656-664.

Dextroamphetamine (eg, *Dexedrine*)

AVOID Tranylcypromine (*Parnate*)

SUMMARY: Severe hypertensive reactions have occurred when amphetamines were ingested by patients taking monoamine oxidase inhibitors (MAOIs).

RISK FACTORS: No specific risk factors are known.

MECHANISM: MAOIs tend to increase the amount of norepinephrine present in storage sites of the adrenergic neuron; the subsequent administration of agents that cause catecholamine release (eg, amphetamines) results in the liberation of large amounts of norepinephrine to react with the receptor. MAOIs with intrinsic amphetamine-like activity (eg, phenelzine [*Nardil*], tranylcypromine) may be more dangerous in combination with amphetamines than pargyline and nialamide, which do not have amphetamine-like pharmacologic actions.

CLINICAL EVALUATION: Fatalities and near-fatalities have occurred in patients receiving amphetamines and an MAOI concomitantly. Tranylcypromine appears to have the greatest risk in this regard. Hyperpyrexia, headache, hypertension, and cerebral hemorrhage have occurred following MAOI plus amphetamine administration.[1-3,8] Cardiac arrhythmias, flushing, vomiting, and seizures have also been reported.

RELATED DRUGS: Although methylphenidate (eg, *Ritalin*) has amphetamine-like pharmacologic activity, some evidence indicates that the reactions it causes when used with MAOIs are less severe than those caused by amphetamines. Nevertheless, use methylphenidate cautiously in combination with MAOIs.[5,9] All nonselective MAOIs probably interact similarly with amphetamines: isocarboxazid (*Marplan*), phenelzine, tranylcypromine. Furazolidone (*Furoxone*), another MAOI, has been shown to increase pressor sensitivity to amphetamines.[6,7] Selegiline (eg, *Eldepryl*) has been reported to enhance the pressor effect of tyramine, particularly following doses greater than 10 mg/day; it could theoretically interact with amphetamines as well.[10] Type B MAOIs (eg, selegiline) should be less likely than the type A MAOIs (eg, moclobemide[†]) to interact with drugs that release catecholamines (eg, amphetamines). Nevertheless, little is known regarding drug interactions with type B MAOIs. Use cautiously until more data are available.

MANAGEMENT OPTIONS:

➡ *AVOID COMBINATION.* Amphetamines should not be given to patients receiving a nonselective MAOI. Phentolamine (*Regitine*) appears to be the logical therapy for severe hypertension resulting from this interaction, since it blocks the alpha effects of the released norepinephrine.[4] Remember that the effects of nonselective MAOIs should be assumed to persist for 2 weeks after they are discontinued.

REFERENCES:

1. Zeck P. The dangers of some antidepressant drugs. *Med J Aust.* 1961;2:607.
2. Krisko I, et al. Severe hyperpyrexia due to tranylcypromineamphetamine toxicity. *Ann Intern Med.* 1969;70:559.
3. Brownlee G, et al. Potentiation of amphetamine and pethidine by monoamine oxidase inhibitors. *Lancet.* 1963;1:669.
4. Goldberg LI. Monoamine oxidase inhibitors. Adverse reactions and possible mechanisms. *JAMA.* 1964;190:456.
5. Sjoqvist F. Psychotropic drugs (2). Interaction between monoamine oxidase (MAO) inhibitors and other substances. *Proc R Soc Med.* 1965;58:967.
6. Pettinger WA, et al. Inhibition of monoamine oxidase in man by furazolidone. *Clin Pharmacol Ther.* 1968;9:442.
7. Pettinger WA, et al. Supersensitivity to tyramine during monoamine oxidase inhibition in man. Mechanism at the level of the adrenergic neuron. *Clin Pharmacol Ther.* 1968;9:341.
8. Lloyd JTA, et al. Death after combined dexamphetamine and phenelzine. *BMJ.* 1965;2:168.
9. Product information. Dextroamphetamine (*Dexedrine*). 1990.
10. Schulz R, et al. Tyramine kinetics and pressor sensitivity during monoamine oxidase inhibition by selegiline. *Clin Pharmacol Ther.* 1989;46:528.

† Not available in the United States.

Dextromethorphan (eg, *Robitussin-DM*)

Fluoxetine (*Prozac*)

SUMMARY: A patient receiving fluoxetine developed visual hallucinations when she began to take dextromethorphan for her cough. A causal relationship was not established, but theoretical considerations suggest that an interaction may have occurred.

RISK FACTORS: No specific risk factors are known.

MECHANISM: Dextromethorphan is metabolized by cytochrome P4502D6 (CYP2D6), and fluoxetine is known to be a potent inhibitor of this enzyme.[2] Thus, it is likely that fluoxetine inhibits the hepatic metabolism of dextromethorphan. It is also possible that dextromethorphan adds to the serotonergic effect of fluoxetine, based on the fact that dextromethorphan can cause serotonin syndrome when combined with nonselective monoamine oxidase inhibitors.

CLINICAL EVALUATION: A 32-year-old woman on fluoxetine 20 mg/day developed a cold and cough for which she took 2 teaspoonfuls of a dextromethorphan-containing cough syrup on 1 day and 2 more teaspoonfuls the next morning.[1] Two hours later she developed vivid visual hallucinations with bright colors and distorted shapes. The hallucinations, which lasted for 6 to 8 hours, were similar to those she had experienced with LSD 12 years earlier. She had previously taken dextromethorphan in the absence of fluoxetine without any adverse effects. Nonetheless, it is likely that large numbers of patients receiving fluoxetine have taken dextromethorphan without serious adverse consequences. This suggests that, if an adverse interaction occurs, it may occur only in certain predisposed individuals.

RELATED DRUGS: A patient on paroxetine (*Paxil*) developed symptoms of serotonin syndrome after taking dextromethorphan, but a causal relationship was not established. Sertraline (*Zoloft*) and fluvoxamine (*Luvox*) appear to have less effect on CYP2D6 than fluoxetine and paroxetine, but little is known regarding their use with dextromethorphan. When considering codeine as an alternative to dextromethorphan, keep in mind that inhibitors of CYP2D6 may reduce the analgesic effect of codeine by inhibiting its conversion to morphine. The extent to which the antitussive effect of codeine is affected by inhibitors of CYP2D6 is not established.

MANAGEMENT OPTIONS:

➡ *Consider Alternative.* Although clinical data are very limited, there are theoretical reasons for limiting the use of dextromethorphan in patients taking fluoxetine (or other selective serotonin reuptake inhibitors). Moreover, the limited therapeutic usefulness of dextromethorphan in many patients is another reason for avoiding it in patients receiving fluoxetine, even though the risk of the combination is not established.

➡ *Monitor.* If the combination is used, monitor for evidence of serotonin syndrome which can result in neurologic findings (eg, dizziness, tremor, myoclonus, rigidity, seizures, incoordination, and coma), psychiatric symptoms (eg, agitation, confusion, hypomania), and disorders of temperature regulation (eg, fever, sweating, shivering); severe cases can be fatal.

REFERENCES:
   1. Achamallah NS. Visual hallucinations after combining fluoxetine and dextromethorphan. *Am J Med.* 1992;149:1406.

2. Crewe HK, et al. The effect of selective serotonin re-uptake inhibitors on cytochrome P4052D6 (CYP2D6) activity in human liver microsomes. *Br J Clin Pharmacol.* 1992; 34:262.

Dextromethorphan (eg, *Robitussin*)

Linezolid (*Zyvox*)

SUMMARY: Linezolid reduces the conversion of dextromethorphan to dextrorphan. Alteration in patient response does not appear likely.

RISK FACTORS: No specific risk factors are known.

MECHANISM: Linezolid appears to reduce the metabolism of dextromethorphan to dextrorphan; however, the mechanism is unclear. In this study, there was no evidence of linezolid's modest monoamine oxidase inhibition inhibiting the metabolism of serotonin.

CLINICAL EVALUATION: Two 20 mg doses of dextromethorphan or placebo were administered to 14 healthy subjects 4 hours apart before and following 2 days of linezolid 600 mg daily.[1] Because dextromethorphan plasma concentrations are very low, the concentration of its major metabolite, dextrorphan, was determined. Linezolid administration resulted in a mean decrease in the dextrorphan area under the plasma concentration-time curve (AUC) of 30%. No change was noted in systolic or diastolic blood pressure during linezolid and dextromethorphan compared with the drugs administered alone. Dextromethorphan did not affect the AUC of linezolid compared with placebo. No changes in autonomic responses (eg, temperature, heart rate, blood pressure, sedation) were noted.

RELATED DRUGS: The effect of linezolid on the pharmacokinetics of other selective serotonin reuptake inhibitors (SSRIs) (eg, fluoxetine [eg, *Prozac*], paroxetine [eg, *Paxil*]) is unknown, but case reports of serotonin syndrome in patients taking an SSRI and linezolid have appeared.

MANAGEMENT OPTIONS:

➥ **Monitor.** Pending further studies, monitor patients taking SSRIs for autonomic adverse reactions if linezolid is coadministered.

REFERENCES:
1. Hendershot PE, et al. Linezolid: pharmacokinetic and pharmacodynamic evaluation of coadministration with pseudoephedrine HCl, phenylpropanolamine HCl, and dextromethorphan HBr. *J Clin Pharmacol.* 2001;41(5):563-572.

Dextromethorphan (eg, *Robitussin*)

Moclobemide† AVOID

SUMMARY: Because dextromethorphan can cause serotonin syndrome when administered with nonselective monoamine oxidase inhibitors (MAOIs), cotherapy of dextromethorphan with moclobemide or other MAO-A inhibitors would theoretically produce the same effect.

RISK FACTORS: No specific risk factors are known.

MECHANISM: Dextromethorphan appears to block the neuronal uptake of serotonin. The combination of dextromethorphan and MAOIs that inhibit MAO-A may result in accumulation of CNS serotonin, resulting in serotonin syndrome.

CLINICAL EVALUATION: Dextromethorphan can produce serotonin syndrome (agitation, coma, confusion, hyperreflexia, hypomania, incoordination, myoclonus, rigidity, seizures, shivering, sweating, tremor) in patients taking nonselective MAOIs.[1-3] Because moclobemide inhibits MAO-A (which metabolizes serotonin), it theoretically would produce the same effect.[4]

RELATED DRUGS: Because serotonin is metabolized by MAO-A, all MAO-A inhibitors are expected to interact with dextromethorphan.

MANAGEMENT OPTIONS:

➡ *AVOID COMBINATION.* Dextromethorphan is contraindicated in patients receiving nonselective MAOIs or MAO-A inhibitors.

REFERENCES:

1. Rivers N, et al. Possible lethal reaction between *Nardil* and dextromethorphan. *Can Med Assoc J.* 1970;103(1):85.

2. Sovner R, et al. Interaction between dextromethorphan and monoamine oxidase inhibitor therapy with isocarboxazid. *N Engl J Med.* 1988;319(25):1671.

3. Nierenberg DW, et al. The central nervous system serotonin syndrome. *Clin Pharmacol Ther.* 1993;53(1):84-88.

4. Amrein R, et al. Interactions of moclobemide with concomitantly administered medication: evidence from pharmacological and clinical studies. *Psychopharmacology.* 1992;106(suppl):S24-S31.

† Not available in the United States.

 Dextromethorphan (eg, *Robitussin*)

AVOID **Phenelzine (*Nardil*)**

SUMMARY: Dextromethorphan may cause serotonin syndrome (agitation, coma, confusion, hyperreflexia, hypomania, incoordination, myoclonus, rigidity, seizures, shivering, sweating, tremor) when administered with monoamine oxidase inhibitors (MAOIs).

RISK FACTORS: No specific risk factors are known.

MECHANISM: Dextromethorphan appears to block the neuronal uptake of serotonin. The combination of dextromethorphan and MAOIs may result in accumulation of CNS serotonin, leading to the serotonin syndrome.

CLINICAL EVALUATION: A patient receiving phenelzine developed nausea, coma, hypotension, and hyperpyrexia following ingestion of 2 oz of a cough syrup containing dextromethorphan.[1] Subsequent death may have been caused by the combination of hyperpyrexia and cerebral hypoxia. Another patient on phenelzine 45 mg/day developed dizziness, headache, and nausea an hour after taking a dose of dextromethorphan. She subsequently became unresponsive and developed apnea, myoclonus, and rigidity; she recovered after 2 days in the intensive care unit.[2]

RELATED DRUGS: In one case, a patient taking isocarboxazid (*Marplan*) 30 mg/day developed dizziness, muscle tremor, and urinary retention within 1 hour of ingesting dextromethorphan 15 mg.[3] Assume tranylcypromine (eg, *Parnate*) produces serotonin syndrome with dextromethorphan.

MANAGEMENT OPTIONS:

➡ *AVOID COMBINATION.* Dextromethorphan is contraindicated in patients receiving nonselective MAOIs. The effects of nonselective MAOIs can persist for 2 weeks after discontinuation.

REFERENCES:

1. Rivers N, et al. Possible lethal reaction between *Nardil* and dextromethorphan. *Can Med Assoc J.* 1970;103(1):85.

2. Nierenberg DW, et al. The central nervous system serotonin syndrome. *Clin Pharmacol Ther.* 1993;53(1):84-88.

3. Sovner R, et al. Interaction between dextromethorphan and monoamine oxidase inhibitor therapy with isocarboxazid. *N Engl J Med.* 1988;319(25):1671.

Dextromethorphan (eg, *Robitussin*)

Propoxyphene (eg, *Darvocet-N*)

SUMMARY: A patient developed psychosis after taking dextromethorphan, propoxyphene, and hydrocodone, but it was not established that the reaction resulted from a drug interaction.

RISK FACTORS: No specific risk factors are known.

MECHANISM: Propoxyphene is likely to inhibit the CYP2D6 metabolism of dextromethorphan, and both drugs can have serotonergic effects. It is also possible that propoxyphene inhibited the CYP2D6 metabolism of hydrocodone. Nonetheless, it is not clear that any of these mechanisms were the cause of the reaction in this patient.

CLINICAL EVALUATION: A 60-year-old woman taking propoxyphene and hydrocodone developed a psychotic reaction after taking larger than recommended doses of dextromethorphan.[1] It is possible that the psychosis resulted from an interaction among these medications, but a causal relationship was not established. This case is rated "possible" using the Drug Interaction Probability Scale (DIPS).[2] The patient had some evidence of prior psychiatric disease, and had a urinary tract infection at the time of the reaction, both of which could have predisposed her to the psychosis.

RELATED DRUGS: No information is available.

MANAGEMENT OPTIONS: No specific action is required, but be alert for evidence of the interaction.

REFERENCES:

1. Jamison SC, et al. A 60-year-old woman with agitation and psychosis following ingestion of dextromethorphan and opioid analgesics. *J Psychopharmacol.* 2009;23(8):989-991.

2. Horn JR, et al. Proposal for a new tool to evaluate drug interaction cases. *Ann Pharmacother.* 2007;41(4):674-680.

Dextromethorphan (eg, *Robitussin*)

Quinidine

SUMMARY: Dextromethorphan concentrations may be increased to toxic levels during quinidine coadministration.

RISK FACTORS:

➡ ***Pharmacogenetics.*** Rapid metabolizers of dextromethorphan are at risk.

MECHANISM: Quinidine inhibits the hepatic metabolism of dextromethorphan by CYP2D6, resulting in reduced first-pass metabolism and intrinsic clearance.

CLINICAL EVALUATION: Six patients with amyotrophic lateral sclerosis received dextromethorphan 60 mg twice daily.[1] All patients were rapid metabolizers; trough dextromethorphan concentrations averaged 12 ng/mL. The same patients received a single dose of dextromethorphan 60 mg after quinidine 75 mg twice daily had been given for 1 week. Average trough dextromethorphan concentrations increased to 38 ng/mL. This degree of inhibition in dextromethorphan metabolism may result in toxic symptoms (eg, confusion, headache, insomnia, nausea, nervousness, tremors).

RELATED DRUGS: No information is available.

MANAGEMENT OPTIONS:

➡ ***Circumvent/Minimize.*** Patients taking quinidine should avoid dextromethorphan-containing medications. Consider dextromethorphan dosage reduction if administered with quinidine. Codeine may not be a suitable alternative because quinidine inhibits its conversion to morphine and may limit its antitussive effects.

➡ ***Monitor.*** If dextromethorphan is administered with quinidine, monitor for adverse reactions (eg, confusion, headache, insomnia, nausea, nervousness, tremors).

REFERENCES:

1. Zhang Y, et al. Dextromethorphan: enhancing its systemic availability by way of low-dose quinidine-mediated inhibition of cytochrome P4502D6. *Clin Pharmacol Ther*. 1992;51(6):647-655.

 Dextromethorphan (eg, *Robitussin*)

Rasagiline (*Azilect*)

SUMMARY: Generally avoid concomitant use of rasagiline and dextromethorphan.

RISK FACTORS: No specific risk factors are known.

MECHANISM: Not established. The combination may have additive serotonergic effects.

CLINICAL EVALUATION: Isolated cases of severe serotonin syndrome have been reported following the use of dextromethorphan with nonselective monoamine oxidase inhibitors (MAOIs). Because rasagiline may become a nonselective MAOI in some patients, generally avoid the use of dextromethorphan.[1]

RELATED DRUGS: Theoretically, codeine is not expected to interact with rasagiline, but clinical data are lacking. Any interaction between rasagiline and dextromethorphan is likely to be similar to that of selegiline and dextromethorphan.

MANAGEMENT OPTIONS:

➡ *Avoid Unless Benefit Outweighs Risk.* Do not use dextromethorphan concomitantly with rasagiline or within 2 weeks of discontinuing rasagiline. Caution patients taking rasagiline that many nonprescription cough and cold products contain dextromethorphan.

REFERENCES:

1. *Azilect* [package insert]. Kansas City, MO: Teva Neuroscience Inc; 2006.

Dextromethorphan (eg, *Robitussin*)

Selegiline (eg, *Eldepryl*)

SUMMARY: Because dextromethorphan can cause serotonin syndrome when administered with nonselective monoamine oxidase inhibitors (MAOIs), selegiline (especially in large doses) theoretically could produce the same effect.

RISK FACTORS:

➡ *Dosage Regimen.* Selegiline doses of 10 mg/day can have some inhibitory effect on MAO type A (MAO-A), and this effect increases as the daily dose is increased.

MECHANISM: Dextromethorphan appears to block the neuronal uptake of serotonin. The combination of dextromethorphan and MAOIs may result in accumulation of central nervous system serotonin, resulting in serotonin syndrome.

CLINICAL EVALUATION: Dextromethorphan can produce serotonin syndrome in patients taking nonselective MAOIs.[1-3] Because selegiline can have nonselective MAO inhibitory activity, it could theoretically produce the same effect. The combination of selegiline and meperidine (eg, *Demerol*) has been reported to produce serotonin syndrome,[4] lending support to the possibility that selegiline can contribute to this syndrome.

RELATED DRUGS: Meperidine and other nonselective MAOIs interact similarly with selegiline.

MANAGEMENT OPTIONS:

➡ *Avoid Unless Benefit Outweighs Risk.* Although dextromethorphan is contraindicated in patients receiving nonselective MAOIs or MAO-A inhibitors, little is known about the use of type B MAO inhibitors such as selegiline with dextromethorphan. Nonetheless, avoid concomitant use until more data are available.

➡ *Monitor.* If the combination is used, monitor for evidence of serotonin syndrome (eg, agitation, coma, confusion, hyperreflexia, hypomania, incoordination, myoclonus, rigidity, seizures, shivering, sweating, tremor).

REFERENCES:

1. Rivers N, et al. Possible lethal reaction between *Nardil* and dextromethorphan. *Can Med Assoc J.* 1970;103:85.
2. Sovner R, et al. Interaction between dextromethorphan and monoamine oxidase inhibitor therapy with isocarboxazid. *N Engl J Med.* 1988;319:1671.
3. Nierenberg DW, et al. The central nervous system serotonin syndrome. *Clin Pharmacol Ther.* 1993;53:84-88.
4. Zornberg GL, et al. Severe adverse interaction between pethidine and selegiline. *Lancet* 1991;337:246.

Dextromethorphan (eg, _Robitussin_)

Sibutramine (_Meridia_)

SUMMARY: The risk of serotonin syndrome would theoretically increase when sibutramine is combined with other serotonergic drugs such as dextromethorphan.

RISK FACTORS: No specific risk factors are known.

MECHANISM: Sibutramine inhibits serotonin reuptake; additive serotonergic effects may occur with dextromethorphan.

CLINICAL EVALUATION: While no published data are available for evaluation, the manufacturer of sibutramine has made some data on this interaction available.[1] Because sibutramine has serotonergic effects, its concurrent use with other serotonergic drugs (eg, dextromethorphan) may increase the risk of serotonin syndrome.[2] Although the actual risk of combining sibutramine with serotonergic drugs is unknown, the fact that serotonin syndrome can result in serious or fatal reactions must be considered.

RELATED DRUGS: No information is available.

MANAGEMENT OPTIONS:

➥ **Avoid Unless Benefit Outweighs Risk.** Do not use sibutramine with meperidine (eg, _Demerol_) until more information is available.

➥ **Monitor.** Serotonin syndrome can result in neurotoxicity (eg, coma, hyperreflexia, incoordination, myoclonus, restlessness, rigidity, seizures, tremors), psychiatric symptoms (eg, agitation, confusion, hypomania), and temperature regulation abnormalities (eg, fever, sweating). Note that mild forms of serotonin syndrome have also been reported, so consider any combination of symptoms as possibly related to excessive serotonin activity.

REFERENCES:

1. _Meridia_ [package insert]. North Chicago, Il: Abbott Laboratories; 1997.
2. Mills KC. Serotonin syndrome. A clinical update. _Crit Care Clin._ 1997;13:763-783.

 Dextromethorphan (eg, _Robitussin_)

Terbinafine (_Lamisil_)

SUMMARY: Terbinafine increases the concentration of dextromethorphan, a marker drug for CYP2D6 activity; the clearance of other CYP2D6 substrates is also likely to be reduced by terbinafine.

RISK FACTORS: Patients who are extensive CYP2D6 metabolizers (about 93% of the US population) will exhibit a greater reduction in metabolic activity following terbinafine administration compared with poor CYP2D6 metabolizers.

MECHANISM: Terbinafine inhibits the metabolic activity of CYP2D6 and reduces the clearance of CYP2D6 substrates such as dextromethorphan.

CLINICAL EVALUATION: Terbinafine 250 mg/day was administered for 14 days to 9 healthy subjects.[1] Dextromethorphan metabolism was evaluated 3 times before terbinafine administration, at the end of the 14-day terbinafine dosage regimen, and monthly thereafter for 6 months. Terbinafine markedly reduced CYP2D6 activity in rapid metabolizers. While this effect is of limited clinical significance with dextromethorphan, a number of other drugs are metabolized by CYP2D6 (see Related Drugs); terbinafine administration would also reduce the clearance of these drugs.

RELATED DRUGS: Other drugs metabolized by CYP2D6 include amitriptyline, carvedilol (*Coreg*), codeine, haloperidol (eg, *Haldol*), metoprolol (eg, *Lopressor*), nortriptyline (eg, *Pamelor*), and timolol (eg, *Blocadren*). The magnitude of terbinafine's effect of on these drugs awaits further study.

MANAGEMENT OPTIONS:

➥ *Monitor.* Pending data on the effect of terbinafine on other CYP2D6 substrates, monitor carefully for altered effect if terbinafine is added to or discontinued from a drug regimen.

REFERENCES:

1. Abdel-Rahman SM, et al. Investigation of terbinafine as a CYP2D6 inhibitor in vivo. *Clin Pharmacol Ther.* 1999;65:465-472.

Dextrothyroxine†

Warfarin (eg, *Coumadin*)

SUMMARY: Dextrothyroxine consistently increases the hypoprothrombinemic response to warfarin and probably other oral anticoagulants. Adjustments in oral anticoagulant dosage are likely to be necessary when dextrothyroxine therapy is initiated or discontinued.

RISK FACTORS: No specific risk factors are known.

MECHANISM: Not established. In animals, dextrothyroxine enhances the rate of degradation of factor II. This is consistent with the finding that increased circulating concentrations of thyroid hormones increase the catabolism of vitamin K–dependent clotting factors in humans.[1-5]

CLINICAL EVALUATION: Increases in the hypoprothrombinemic response to oral anticoagulants when dextrothyroxine is coadministered are well documented; some patients have developed bleeding episodes. Although most published information on this interaction involves warfarin, other oral anticoagulants also are likely to interact with dextrothyroxine.

RELATED DRUGS: All combinations of thyroid and oral anticoagulants are likely to interact.

MANAGEMENT OPTIONS:

➥ *Avoid Unless Benefit Outweighs Risk.* Avoid concomitant therapy with dextrothyroxine and oral anticoagulants if possible. If oral anticoagulant therapy is begun in a patient receiving dextrothyroxine, use conservative doses until the maintenance dose is established.

➥ *Monitor.* Initiation or discontinuation of dextrothyroxine therapy in a patient stabilized on an oral anticoagulant is likely to necessitate a change in the anticoagulant maintenance dose.

REFERENCES:

1. Weintraub M, et al. The effects of dextrothyroxine on the kinetics of prothrombin activity: proposed mechanism of the potentiation of warfarin by D-thyroxine. *J Lab Clin Med.* 1973;81:273-279.
2. Loeliger EA, et al. The biological disappearance rate of prothrombin, factors VII, IX and X from plasma in hypothyroidism, hyperthyroidism, and during fever. *Thromb Dia Haemorrh.* 1964;10:267-277.

3. Schrogie JJ, et al. The anticoagulant response to bishydroxycoumarin II. The effect of D-thyroxine, clofibrate, and norethandrolone. *Clin Pharmacol Ther*. 1967;8:70-77.

4. Solomon HM, et al. Change in receptor site affinity: a proposed explanation for the potentiating effect of D-thyroxine on the anticoagulant response to warfarin. *Clin Pharmacol Ther*. 1967;8:797-799.

5. Owens JC, et al. Effect of sodium dextrothyroxine in patients receiving anticoagulants. *N Engl J Med*. 1962;266:76-79.

† Not available in the United States.

 DHEA

Triazolam (eg, *Halcion*)

SUMMARY: Preliminary evidence suggests that DHEA increases triazolam plasma concentrations, but the clinical importance of this effect is not established.

RISK FACTORS: No specific risk factors are known.

MECHANISM: Not established. DHEA might inhibit CYP3A4-mediated metabolism of triazolam.

CLINICAL EVALUATION: In a preliminary study, 13 elderly subjects received a single oral dose of triazolam 0.25 mg with and without pretreatment with DHEA 200 mg/day for 2 weeks.[1] DHEA was associated with a 28% reduction in triazolam oral clearance, with a range of 0.6% to 42%. It is not clear how often this interaction would result in adverse outcomes, but one would expect a greater CNS-depressant effect of triazolam in at least some patients.

RELATED DRUGS: The effect of DHEA on other benzodiazepines is not established, but theoretically it would inhibit the metabolism of other CYP3A4-metabolized agents such as alprazolam (eg, *Xanax*) and midazolam (eg, *Versed*).

MANAGEMENT OPTIONS: No specific action is required, but be alert for evidence of the interaction.

REFERENCES:
1. Frye RF, et al. Effect of DHEA on CYP3A4-mediated metabolism of triazolam. *Clin Pharmacol Ther*. 2000;67:109.

4 **Diazepam (eg, *Valium*)**

Digoxin (eg, *Lanoxin*)

SUMMARY: Diazepam has been reported to increase digoxin concentrations.

RISK FACTORS: No specific risk factors are known.

MECHANISM: Not established.

CLINICAL EVALUATION: Preliminary results in a study of 7 subjects indicated that diazepam increased digoxin half-life and reduced urinary digoxin excretion.[1] The significance of these findings is unknown.

RELATED DRUGS: No information is available.

MANAGEMENT OPTIONS: No specific action is required, but be alert for evidence of the interaction.

REFERENCES:
1. Castillo-Ferrando JR, et al. Digoxin levels and diazepam. *Lancet*. 1980;2:368.

Diazepam (eg, *Valium*) 4

Diltiazem (eg, *Cardizem*)

SUMMARY: Diltiazem administration can produce a modest increase in diazepam concentrations; an increase in benzodiazepine effect may occur in some patients.

RISK FACTORS: No specific risk factors are known.

MECHANISM: Diazepam is metabolized by CYP2C19 and CYP3A4. Diltiazem is an inhibitor of CYP3A4 and increases diazepam serum concentrations.

CLINICAL EVALUATION: Thirteen volunteers, 8 extensive metabolizers (EMs) and 5 poor metabolizers (PMs) for CYP2C19, were administered diltiazem 200 mg or placebo daily for 3 days before and for 7 days after an oral, 2 mg dose of diazepam.[1] Both the EMs and PMs for CYP2C19 experienced about a 25% increase in the mean diazepam area under the concentration-time curve following diltiazem treatment. In the EMs, mean diazepam half-life was increased from 45 to 65 hours; in the PMs, the mean half-life increased from 77 to 104 hours. No pharmacodynamic response was noted in this study, but the dose of diazepam was small. The effect of an interaction between diltiazem and other benzodiazepines not cometabolized by CYP2C19 (see below) may be of larger magnitude.

RELATED DRUGS: Verapamil (eg, *Calan*) is also a known inhibitor of CYP3A4 and would be expected to interact with diazepam in a similar manner. Diltiazem increased triazolam (eg, *Halcion*) serum concentrations[2] and would be expected to interact with other benzodiazepines that are metabolized by CYP3A4 such as alprazolam (eg, *Xanax*), midazolam (eg, *Versed*), or halazepam.

MANAGEMENT OPTIONS:

➡ *Monitor.* Observe patients maintained on diazepam for increased effect (sedation, ataxia) if diltiazem is added to the regimen.

REFERENCES:

1. Kosuge K, Jun Y, Watanabe H, et al. Effects of CYP3A4 inhibition by diltiazem on pharmacokinetics and dynamics of diazepam in relation to CYP2C19 genotype status. *Drug Metab Dispos.* 2001;29:1284-1289.
2. Kosuge K, Nishimoto M, Kimura M, Umemura K, Nakashima M, Ohashi K. Enhanced effect of triazolam with diltiazem. *Br J Clin Pharmacol.* 1997;43:367-372.

Diazepam (eg, *Valium*)

Disulfiram (*Antabuse*)

SUMMARY: Disulfiram may increase serum concentrations of diazepam and benzodiazepines that undergo oxidative metabolism, but the frequency of excessive benzodiazepine response is unknown.

RISK FACTORS: No specific risk factors are known.

MECHANISM: Disulfiram inhibits the hepatic metabolism of some benzodiazepines.

CLINICAL EVALUATION: Disulfiram 500 mg/day for approximately 2 weeks reduced the clearance and prolonged the half-life of chlordiazepoxide (eg, *Librium*) and diazepam.[1] The magnitude of these changes appears sufficient to enhance the pharmacologic response of the benzodiazepines, but this was not assessed.

RELATED DRUGS: Other benzodiazepines that undergo oxidative metabolism (eg, clonazepam [eg, *Klonopin*], clorazepate [eg, *Tranxene*], flurazepam [eg, *Dalmane*], halazepam [*Paxipam*], prazepam†, and triazolam [eg, *Halcion*]) also might be affected by disulfiram treatment, but studies are not available. In 11 alcoholic patients undergoing withdrawal, disulfiram 0.5 g/day for 14 days did not appear to affect the pharmacokinetics of alprazolam (eg, *Xanax*);[2] however, poor compliance with the disulfiram therapy and the alcohol withdrawal process may have affected the results of this study. Oxazepam (eg, *Serax*) and lorazepam (eg, *Ativan*) are converted to inactive glucuronides, a process that does not appear to be affected by disulfiram.[1,3] Temazepam (eg, *Restoril*) also undergoes glucuronide conjugation and would not be expected to be affected by disulfiram.

MANAGEMENT OPTIONS:

➡ *Monitor.* Be alert for evidence of enhanced benzodiazepine response in patients receiving disulfiram. Some patients may require a reduction in benzodiazepine dosage during concurrent disulfiram use.

REFERENCES:

1. MacLeod SM, Sellers EM, Giles HG, et al. Interaction of disulfiram with benzodiazepines. *Clin Pharmacol Ther.* 1978;24:583-589.
2. Diquet B, Gujadhur L, Lamiable D, Warot D, Hayoun H, Choisy H. Lack of interaction between disulfiram and alprazolam in alcoholic patients. *Eur J Clin Pharmacol.* 1990;38:157.
3. Sellers EM, Giles HG, Greenblatt DJ, Naranjo CA. Differential effects of benzodiazepine disposition by disulfiram and ethanol. *Arzneimittelforschung.* 1980;30:882-886.

† Not available in the United States.

Diazepam (eg, *Valium*)

Ethanol (*ethyl alcohol*)

SUMMARY: Ethanol may enhance the adverse psychomotor effects of benzodiazepines such as diazepam; combined use may be dangerous in patients performing tasks requiring alertness.

RISK FACTORS: No specific risk factors are known.

MECHANISM: Ethanol and benzodiazepines are likely to have additive CNS depressant activity. Ethanol may increase the absorption of diazepam[1,2] and reduce its hepatic metabolism.[3,4] Patients with alcoholic liver disease may eliminate benzodiazepines more slowly than those with normal liver function.[5]

CLINICAL EVALUATION: Studies have demonstrated that benzodiazepines enhance the detrimental effects of ethanol on psychomotor skills and simulated driving.[2,6-14] Most of these studies have involved ethanol plus diazepam. Many ethanol and benzodiazepines interaction studies have differed with regard to degree of interaction. This is largely because of the many variables, including doses of drug and alcohol, type of test used, interval between drugs and testing, age of the subjects, trial design, and chronic versus acute administration of drugs or ethanol.

RELATED DRUGS: Nitrazepam,† bromazepam,† and lorazepam (eg, *Ativan*)[15,16] appear to have a similar effect when given with ethanol. Chlordiazepoxide (eg, *Librium*) may be less likely and diazepam more likely to enhance the adverse psychomotor effects of alcohol.[17-23] Ethanol seems less likely to affect the hepatic metabolism of oxazepam than diazepam,[4] but additive CNS depression is expected in either case. Expect all benzodiazepines to result in additive CNS depression with alcohol.[24]

MANAGEMENT OPTIONS:

➥ *Circumvent/Minimize.* Warn patients receiving benzodiazepines against moderate to large amounts of ethanol ingestion. Occasional ingestion of small amounts of ethanol (especially if taken with food) probably causes little difficulty unless alertness is required (eg, driving) or there is a disease or condition that makes the patient sensitive to CNS depression.

➥ *Monitor.* Monitor for excessive CNS depression if the combination is used.

REFERENCES:

1. Hayes SL, et al. Ethanol and oral diazepam absorption. *N Engl J Med.* 1977;296(4):186-189.
2. MacLeod SM, et al. Diazepam actions and plasma concentrations following ethanol ingestion. *Eur J Clin Pharmacol.* 1977;11(5):345-349.
3. Sellers EM, et al. Intravenous diazepam and oral ethanol interaction. *Clin Pharmacol Ther.* 1980;28(5):645.
4. Sellers EM, et al. Different effects on benzodiazepine disposition by disulfiram and ethanol. *Arzneimittelforschung.* 1980;30(5a):882-886.
5. Juhl RP, et al. Alprazolam pharmacokinetics in alcoholic liver disease. *J Clin Pharmacol.* 1984;24(2-3):113-119.
6. Linnoila M, Häkkinen S. Effects of diazepam and codeine, alone and in combination with alcohol, on simulated driving. *Clin Pharmacol Ther.* 1974;15(4):368-373.
7. Saarrio I, et al. Interaction of drugs with alcohol on human psychomotor skills related to driving: effect of sleep deprivation or two weeks' treatment with hypnotics. *J Clin Pharmacol.* 1975;15:52-59.
8. Saario I. Psychomotor skills during subacute treatment with thioridazine and bromazepam, and their combined effects with alcohol. *Ann Clin Res.* 1976;8(2):117-123.
9. Linnoila M. Effects of diazepam, chlordiazepoxide, thioridazine, haloperidol, flupenthixole and alcohol on psychomotor skills related to driving. *Ann Med Exp Biol Fenn.* 1973;51(3):125-132.
10. Linnoila M. Drug interaction on psychomotor skills related to driving: hypnotics and alcohol. *Ann Med Exp Biol Fenn.* 1973;51(3):118-124.
11. Linnoila M, et al. Drug interaction on psychomotor skills related to driving: diazepam and alcohol. *Eur J Clin Pharmacol.* 1973;5:186-194.
12. Morland J, et al. Combined effects of diazepam and ethanol on mental and psychomotor functions. *Acta Pharmacol Toxicol.* 1974;34(1):5-15.
13. Linnoila M, et al. Effect of treatment with diazepam or lithium and alcohol on psychomotor skills related to driving. *Eur J Clin Pharmacol.* 1974;7(5):337-342.
14. van Steveninck AL, et al. Pharmacodynamic interactions of diazepam and intravenous alcohol at pseudo steady state. *Psychopharmacology.* 1993;110(4):471-478.
15. Mattila MJ, et al. Acute effects of buspirone and alcohol on psychomotor skills. *J Clin Psychiatry.* 1982;43(12, Pt 2):56-61.
16. Linnoila M, et al. Effect of adinazolam and diazepam, alone and in combination with ethanol, on psychomotor and cognitive performance and on autonomic nervous system reactivity in healthy volunteers. *Eur J Clin Pharmacol.* 1990;38(4):371-377.
17. Reggiani G, et al. Some aspects of the experimental and clinical toxicology of chlordiazepoxide. In: Toxicity and Side-Effects of Psychotropic Drugs. Amsterdam: Excerpta Medica Foundation; 1968:79-97.
18. Hughes FW, et al. Comparative effect in human subjects of chlordiazepoxide, diazepam, and placebo on mental and physical performance. *Clin Pharmacol Ther.* 1965;6:139-145.
19. Hoffer A. Lack of potentiation by chlordiazepoxide (*Librium*) of depression or excitation due to alcohol. *Can Med Assoc J.* 1962;87:920-921.
20. Betts TA, et al. Effect of four commonly-used tranquilizers on low-speed driving performance tests. *Br Med J.* 1972;4(5840):580-584.
21. Dundee JW, et al. Alcohol and the benzodiazepines. The interaction between intravenous ethanol and chlordiazepoxide and diazepam. *Q J Stud Alcohol.* 1971;32(4):960-968.

22. Goldberg L. Behavioral and physiological effects of alcohol on man. *Psychosom Med*. 1966;28:570-595.

23. Miller AI, et al. Effects of combined chlordiazepoxide and alcohol in man. *Q J Stud Alcohol*. 1963;24:9.

24. Rosinga WM. Interaction of drugs and alcohol in relation to traffic safety. In: Meyer L, Peck HM, eds. *Drug Induced Disease*. Vol. 3. Amsterdam: Excerpta Medica Foundation; 1968:295-306.

† Not available in the United States.

5   Diazepam (eg, *Valium*)

Felodipine

SUMMARY: Felodipine appears to have little effect on the pharmacokinetics of diazepam.

RISK FACTORS: No specific risk factors are known.

MECHANISM: No interaction.

CLINICAL EVALUATION: Twelve healthy subjects received either a placebo or felodipine 10 mg extended-release tablets daily for 12 days.[1] On the sixth day of each 12-day period, subjects received diazepam 10 mg intravenous over 2 minutes, 30 minutes after the placebo or felodipine dose. No significant changes in diazepam pharmacokinetics were observed following felodipine administration. The area under the desmethyldiazepam concentration-time curve tended to be larger (14%) during felodipine administration. The clinical significance of this interaction appears limited.

RELATED DRUGS: Diazepam 10 mg/day had no effect on the pharmacokinetics of nimodipine (eg, *Nimotop*) administered 30 mg 3 times a day to 24 healthy elderly subjects.[2]

MANAGEMENT OPTIONS: No interaction.

REFERENCES:

1. Meyer BH, et al. The effects of felodipine on the pharmacokinetics of diazepam. *Int J Clin Pharmacol Ther Toxicol*. 1992;30(4):117-121.

2. Heine PR, et al. Lack of interaction between diazepam and nimodipine during chronic oral administration to healthy elderly subjects. *Br J Clin Pharmacol*. 1994;38(1):39-43.

3   Diazepam (eg, *Valium*)

Fluconazole (eg, *Diflucan*)

SUMMARY: Fluconazole increases the plasma concentration of diazepam; anticipate increased adverse reactions, including sedation and ataxia.

RISK FACTORS:

 Pharmacogenetics. Patients who are rapid metabolizers of CYP2C19 may be at risk to demonstrate a larger effect of fluconazole on diazepam metabolism.

MECHANISM: Fluconazole inhibits both of the primary pathways of diazepam metabolism, CYP2C19 and CYP3A4.

CLINICAL EVALUATION: Twelve healthy subjects received a single oral dose of diazepam 5 mg alone and following fluconazole 400 mg on the first day and 200 mg on the second day.[1] The mean area under the concentration-time curve of diazepam was increased 2.5-fold during fluconazole dosing. Diazepam half-life increased from 31 to 73 hours during fluconazole coadministration. Because this study used only

2 days of fluconazole dosing, the magnitude of this interaction may differ with long-term fluconazole dosing. All of the subjects were either homozygous (n = 8) or heterozygous extensive metabolizers for CYP2C19, so no conclusions could be drawn on the possible role of CYP2C19 polymorphism in the magnitude of the interaction.

RELATED DRUGS: The metabolism of other benzodiazepines metabolized by CYP3A4 (eg, alprazolam [eg, *Xanax*], midazolam, triazolam [eg, *Halcion*]) is also likely to be inhibited by fluconazole.

MANAGEMENT OPTIONS:

➡ *Consider Alternative.* Benzodiazepines (eg, lorazepam [eg, *Ativan*], oxazepam) that are not metabolized by CYP3A4 are unlikely to be affected by fluconazole. Consider using an antifungal that does not affect CYP3A4 or CYP2C19, such as terbinafine (eg, *Lamisil*).

➡ *Monitor.* Monitor patients receiving diazepam and fluconazole for evidence of increased diazepam effects.

REFERENCES:

1. Saari TI, et al. Voriconazole and fluconazole increase the exposure to oral diazepam. *Eur J Clin Pharmacol.* 2007;63(10):941-949.

Diazepam (eg, *Valium*)

Fluoxetine (eg, *Prozac*)

SUMMARY: A study in healthy subjects suggests that fluoxetine increases plasma diazepam concentrations and reduces the plasma concentration of its active metabolite, desmethyldiazepam. Fluoxetine may increase modestly the psychomotor impairment produced by diazepam in some patients, but the clinical importance of this effect is not established.

RISK FACTORS:

➡ *Effects of Age.* Elderly patients are known to be more sensitive to diazepam and may be more sensitive to this interaction.

MECHANISM: Not established. The results are consistent with fluoxetine-induced inhibition of the conversion of diazepam to desmethyldiazepam.

CLINICAL EVALUATION: Six healthy subjects received single oral doses of diazepam 10 mg under 3 conditions: alone, with a single dose of fluoxetine 60 mg, and with fluoxetine pretreatment (60 mg/day for 8 days).[1] Both single and multiple doses of fluoxetine increased the area under the diazepam plasma concentration-time curve and reduced diazepam clearance, but this was offset by a decrease in the plasma concentrations of desmethyldiazepam, the active metabolite of diazepam. Fluoxetine did not affect the psychomotor impairment produced by diazepam. In another study, healthy subjects received diazepam 5 mg with and without concurrent fluoxetine 60 mg.[2] Although fluoxetine alone did not affect psychomotor performance, it did increase diazepam-induced impairment of some psychomotor function tests. Thus, it is possible that patients who are more sensitive to benzodiazepines (ie, elderly patients) may have a clinically important interaction with combined use of fluoxetine and diazepam.

RELATED DRUGS: Preliminary evidence suggests that sertraline (eg, *Zoloft*) slightly reduces diazepam elimination. The effect of selective serotonin reuptake inhibitors other than fluoxetine on diazepam is not established, but fluvoxamine (eg, *Luvox*) is known to inhibit CYP3A4, an isozyme important in the metabolism of diazepam. Fluoxetine also inhibits the metabolism of alprazolam (eg, *Xanax*).

MANAGEMENT OPTIONS:

➥ *Circumvent/Minimize.* Use conservative doses of diazepam in the presence of fluoxetine until patient response is assessed. Advise patients receiving combined therapy to watch for excessive sedation.

➥ *Monitor.* Monitor for altered diazepam effect if fluoxetine is initiated, discontinued, or changed in dosage; adjust diazepam dose as needed.

REFERENCES:

1. Lemberger L, et al. The effect of fluoxetine on the pharmacokinetics and psychomotor responses of diazepam. *Clin Pharmacol Ther.* 1988;43(4):412-419.
2. Moskowitz H, Burns M. The effects on performance of two antidepressants, alone and in combination with diazepam. *Prog Neuropsychopharmacol Biol Psychiatry.* 1988;12(5):783-792.

Diazepam (eg, *Valium*)

Gallamine

SUMMARY: Diazepam reportedly prolongs gallamine effect, but this has not been a consistent finding.

RISK FACTORS: No specific risk factors are known.

MECHANISM: Not established. Study in normal volunteers given diazepam indicates that the drug may inhibit the contractile mechanism of skeletal muscle directly.[4]

CLINICAL EVALUATION: In a preliminary clinical study, diazepam increased the duration of action of gallamine and decreased the duration of succinylcholine activity.[1] Subsequent studies[2,3] did not substantiate these findings, and diazepam itself probably does not significantly affect the response to neuromuscular blockers. When the injectable form of diazepam was given intra-arterially, neuromuscular blockade was inhibited presumably by the preservatives or solvents in this formulation. The effect of IV or IM doses of diazepam on the response to neuromuscular blockers under clinical conditions remains to be determined.

RELATED DRUGS: No information is available.

MANAGEMENT OPTIONS: No specific action is required, but be alert for evidence of the interaction.

REFERENCES:

1. Feldman SA, et al. Interaction of diazepam with the muscle-relaxant drugs. *BMJ.* 1970;2:336.
2. Dretchen K, et al. The interaction of diazepam with myoneural blocking agents. *Anesthesiology.* 1971;34:463.
3. Webb SN, et al. Diazepam and neuromuscular blocking drugs. *BMJ.* 1971;3:640.
4. Ludin HP, et al. Action of diazepam on muscular contraction in man. *Z Neurol.* 1971;199:30.

Diazepam (eg, *Valium*)

Haloperidol (eg, *Haldol*)

SUMMARY: Diazepam may increase haloperidol-induced increases in serum prolactin, but the clinical importance is unknown.

RISK FACTORS: No specific risk factors are known.

MECHANISM: Not established.

CLINICAL EVALUATION: In a single-dose study, diazepam 10 mg IM produced about a two-fold increase in the ability of haloperidol 5 mg IM to elevate serum prolactin concentrations, but the clinical importance of this finding is not established.[1]

RELATED DRUGS: No information is available.

MANAGEMENT OPTIONS: No specific action is required, but be alert for evidence of the interaction.

REFERENCES:

   1. Aratao M. Promethazine and diazepam potentiate the haloperidol induced prolactin responses. *Commun Psychopharmacol.* 1980;4:317.

Diazepam (eg, *Valium*)

Isoniazid (INH; eg, *Nydrazid*)

SUMMARY: Isoniazid may increase diazepam serum concentrations; the clinical significance is not known.

RISK FACTORS: No specific risk factors are known.

MECHANISM: INH probably inhibits the hepatic metabolism of some benzodiazepines.

CLINICAL EVALUATION: In 9 healthy subjects, single 5 or 7.5 mg IV doses of diazepam were given with and without pretreatment with INH 180 mg/day.[1] INH prolonged the diazepam plasma half-life from 34 hours to 45 hours and reduced diazepam clearance from 0.54 mL/min/kg to 0.40 mL/min/kg body weight. It is likely that the typical doses of INH (300 mg/day) would increase the magnitude of this interaction.

RELATED DRUGS: The effect of isoniazid on other benzodiazepines is unknown. Isoniazid may affect other benzodiazepines (eg, triazolam [eg, *Halcion*]) in a similar manner.

MANAGEMENT OPTIONS:

➠ *Monitor.* Watch for evidence of altered diazepam effects when isoniazid is initiated or discontinued.

REFERENCES:

   1. Ochs HR, et al. Diazepam interaction with antituberculosis drugs. *Clin Pharmacol Ther.* 1981;29:671.

Diazepam (eg, *Valium*)

Itraconazole (*Sporanox*)

SUMMARY: Itraconazole administration increases the serum concentration of diazepam; diazepam toxicity could result.

RISK FACTORS: No specific risk factors are known.

MECHANISM: Itraconazole inhibits the metabolism of diazepam to temazepam via the CYP3A4 enzyme pathway. Even though CYP3A4 metabolism of diazepam to N-desmethyl-diazepam probably is inhibited by itraconazole, the concentrations of this enzyme are not altered. This is mostly explained by the fact that CYP2C19, an enzyme that is not inhibited by itraconazole, also converts diazepam to N-desmethyl-diazepam. Therefore, during itraconazole administration, diazepam metabolism continues via CYP2C19 limiting the magnitude of the interaction.

CLINICAL EVALUATION: Ten healthy subjects were given either placebo or itraconazole 200 mg/day for 4 days.[1] A single dose of 5 mg diazepam orally was given on the fourth day of treatment with either placebo or itraconazole. The diazepam area under the concentration-time curve was increased 31% and half-life prolonged by 34% following itraconazole pretreatment. The concentration of N-desmethyl-diazepam was not altered by itraconazole pretreatment. Measures of diazepam pharmacodynamic effects were similar following placebo and itraconazole.

RELATED DRUGS: Itraconazole is known to inhibit triazolam (eg, *Halcion*) and temazepam (eg, *Restoril*) metabolism. It also is likely to reduce the metabolism of chlordiazepoxide (eg, *Librium*) and midazolam (*Versed*). Lorazepam (eg, *Ativan*), a benzodiazepine not metabolized by CYP3A4, may be less likely to interact. Other antifungal agents such as ketoconazole (eg, *Nizoral*) and fluconazole (*Diflucan*) would be likely to inhibit the metabolism of diazepam.

MANAGEMENT OPTIONS:

➥ *Consider Alternative.* A benzodiazepine such as lorazepam that is not metabolized by CYP3A4 would be a potential alternative anxiolytic agent.

➥ *Monitor.* Monitor for increased diazepam effects (eg, sedation, ataxia, mental confusion) when itraconazole is coadministered with diazepam.

REFERENCES:
1. Ahonen J, et al. The effects of the antimycotic itraconazole on the pharmacokinetics and pharmacodynamics of diazepam. *Fundam Clin Pharmacol.* 1996;10:314.

Diazepam (eg, *Valium*)

Levodopa (eg, *Larodopa*)

SUMMARY: Diazepam appeared to exacerbate parkinsonism in a few patients receiving levodopa, but a causal relationship was not established.

RISK FACTORS: No specific risk factors are known.

MECHANISM: Not established.

CLINICAL EVALUATION: Case reports have described several levodopa-treated patients who developed deterioration of their parkinsonism when diazepam was initiated.[1,2]

RELATED DRUGS: Another patient well controlled on levodopa, benztropine (eg, *Cogentin*), and diphenhydramine (eg, *Antivert*) developed an acute exacerbation of parkinsonism following administration of chlordiazepoxide (eg, *Librium*); control returned 5 days after the chlordiazepoxide was discontinued.[3] These case reports suggest that benzodiazepines are capable of inhibiting the antiparkinsonian effects of levodopa, but little is known regarding the incidence of the interaction between these drugs or the factors that make it more likely to occur. The effect of other benzodiazepines on levodopa is not established.

MANAGEMENT OPTIONS:

➡ *Monitor.* Monitor for evidence of a reduced antiparkinsonian effect of levodopa in the presence of benzodiazepine therapy. If this suspected interaction may be occurring, discontinue benzodiazepine and monitor the patient to determine whether improvement occurs.

REFERENCES:

1. Wodak J, et al. Review of 12 months' treatment with L-DOPA in Parkinson's disease, with remarks on unusual side effects. *Med J Aust.* 1972;2:1277.
2. Hunter KR, et al. Use of levodopa with other drugs. *Lancet.* 1970;2:1283.
3. Yosselson-Superstine S, et al. Chlordiazepoxide interaction with levodopa. *Ann Intern Med.* 1982;96:259.

Diazepam (eg, *Valium*)

Lithium (eg, *Eskalith*)

SUMMARY: The combination of lithium and diazepam appeared to result in hypothermia in 1 patient, but the incidence of this interaction is unknown.

RISK FACTORS: No specific risk factors are known.

MECHANISM: Not established.

CLINICAL EVALUATION: A patient repeatedly became hypothermic while taking lithium and diazepam but did not manifest hypothermia when taking either drug alone.[1] The drug combination was probably responsible for the reaction in this patient, but it is unknown whether it is an idiosyncratic reaction or one that may be expected in a significant number of other patients treated with lithium and diazepam concurrently.

RELATED DRUGS: No information is available.

MANAGEMENT OPTIONS: No specific action is required, but be alert for evidence of the interaction.

REFERENCES:

1. Naylor GJ, et al. Profound hypothermia on combined lithium carbonate and diazepam treatment. *BMJ.* 1977;3:22.

Diazepam (eg, *Valium*)

Metoprolol (eg, *Lopressor*)

SUMMARY: Metoprolol may slightly reduce the metabolism of diazepam, but it does not affect the metabolism of lorazepam (eg, *Ativan*) or alprazolam (eg, *Xanax*). Metoprolol may increase the pharmacodynamic effects of some benzodiazepines.

RISK FACTORS: No specific risk factors are known.

MECHANISM: Metoprolol appears to reduce the oxidative N-demethylation of diazepam. The glucuronidation of lorazepam was unaffected by metoprolol.[1]

CLINICAL EVALUATION: The area under the diazepam serum concentration-time curve (AUC) was increased significantly (19%) by metoprolol 50 mg twice daily.[2] The pharmacodynamics of diazepam (as measured by visual acuity testing) were significantly impaired by the combination of metoprolol and diazepam compared with diazepam alone.

RELATED DRUGS: Atenolol (eg, *Tenormin*) had no effect on diazepam pharmacokinetics or pharmacodynamics.[2] Propranolol (eg, *Inderal*) and labetalol (eg, *Normodyne*) increased the pharmacodynamic effects of oxazepam (eg, *Serax*) without affecting its pharmacokinetics.[3] Propranolol produces a small reduction in diazepam clearance. Metoprolol increased bromazepam† AUC 35%.[1] Lorazepam (eg, *Ativan*) and alprazolam (eg, *Xanax*) metabolisms are unaffected by metoprolol.

MANAGEMENT OPTIONS:

➥ *Monitor.* Monitor patients receiving diazepam and metoprolol or propranolol for increased central nervous system depression.

REFERENCES:

1. Scott AK, et al. Interaction of metoprolol with lorazepam and bromazepam. *Eur J Clin Pharmacol.* 1991;40:405.

2. Hawksorth G, et al. Diazepam/beta-adrenoceptor antagonist interactions. *Br J Clin Pharmacol.* 1984;17:69S.

3. Sonne J, et al. Single dose pharmacokinetics and pharmacodynamics of oral oxazepam during concomitant administration of propranolol and labetalol. *Br J Clin Pharmacol.* 1990;29:33.

† Not available in the United States.

5   Diazepam (eg, *Valium*)

Naproxen (eg, *Naprosyn*)

SUMMARY: Diazepam and naproxen did not interact in a single-dose study.

RISK FACTORS: No specific risk factors are known.

MECHANISM: No interaction.

CLINICAL EVALUATION: A double-blind crossover study in 24 healthy subjects indicated that diazepam and naproxen do not interact as measured by various psychological tests.[1] However, the results of this single-dose study do not apply necessarily to clinical situations where one or both drugs are used chronically.

RELATED DRUGS: No information is available.

MANAGEMENT OPTIONS: No interaction.
REFERENCES:
1. Stitt FW, et al. A clinical study of naproxen-diazepam drug interaction on tests of mood and attention. *Curr Ther Res.* 1977;21:149.

Diazepam (eg, *Valium*)

Omeprazole (*Prilosec*)

SUMMARY: Omeprazole increases plasma diazepam concentrations considerably after single doses of diazepam in healthy subjects; the effect of this interaction on diazepam response is not established.

RISK FACTORS: No specific risk factors are known.

MECHANISM: Omeprazole probably inhibits the hepatic metabolism of diazepam. Studies of omeprazole with aminopyrine and antipyrine, as well as studies with human liver microsomes, suggest that omeprazole inhibits cytochrome P450 monooxygenases.[1,2]

CLINICAL EVALUATION: Eight healthy subjects were given a single IV dose of diazepam 0.1 mg/kg before and after omeprazole 40 mg/day for 7 days.[3] Omeprazole reduced the plasma clearance of diazepam by 54%. Plasma concentrations of desmethyldiazepam, the major metabolite of diazepam, increased more slowly after omeprazole; plasma concentrations of desmethyldiazepam on day 3 were 34% lower than when diazepam was given alone. Taken together, one would expect that these pharmacokinetic changes would increase the activity of diazepam. However, since the pharmacodynamic response to diazepam with and without omeprazole was not studied, the clinical importance of these findings remains to be determined. Furthermore, the effect of multiple doses of both diazepam and omeprazole must be studied to establish that the interaction occurs under more typical clinical conditions. Omeprazole in a dose of 20 mg/day would be expected to interact with diazepam to a lesser degree.

RELATED DRUGS: The effect of omeprazole on other benzodiazepines is unknown, but it would be most likely to affect benzodiazepines that undergo phase I metabolism (eg, agents *other than* lorazepam [eg, *Ativan*], oxazepam [eg, *Serax*], and temazepam [eg, *Restoril*]). The effect of lansoprazole (*Prevacid*) on benzodiazepines needs further study, but it generally has less effect on hepatic drug metabolism than omeprazole.

MANAGEMENT OPTIONS:

➥ *Monitor.* Until data on the pharmacodynamics of this interaction are available, monitor for enhanced diazepam response if omeprazole is given concurrently.

REFERENCES:
1. Henry DA, et al. Omeprazole: effects on oxidative drug metabolism. *Br J Clin Pharmacol.* 1984;18:195.
2. Jensen JC, et al. Inhibition of human liver cytochrome P-450 by omeprazole. *Br J Clin Pharmacol.* 1986;21:328.
3. Gugler R, et al. Omeprazole inhibits oxidative drug metabolism: studies with diazepam and phenytoin in vivo and 7-ethoxycoumarin in vitro. *Gastroenterology.* 1985;89:1235.

Diazepam (eg, *Valium*)

Paroxetine (*Paxil*)

SUMMARY: Diazepam does not appear to affect the pharmacokinetics of paroxetine in healthy subjects, but the effect of paroxetine on diazepam has not been studied.

RISK FACTORS: No specific risk factors are known.

MECHANISM: No interaction.

CLINICAL EVALUATION: Twenty-four healthy subjects were given oral paroxetine 30 mg/day for 28 days, with oral diazepam 5 mg 3 times a day added from days 15 to 28 in 12 of the subjects.[1] Diazepam had no effect on the pharmacokinetics of paroxetine as measured by no change in the area under the paroxetine plasma concentration-time curve, half-life, elimination rate constant, or maximal plasma concentration. The effect of paroxetine on diazepam pharmacokinetics was not measured, nor was the possibility of a pharmacodynamic interaction between the 2 drugs.

RELATED DRUGS: No information is available.

MANAGEMENT OPTIONS: No interaction.

REFERENCES:
1. Bannister SJ, et al. Evaluation of the potential for interactions of paroxetine with diazepam, cimetidine, warfarin, and digoxin. *Acta Psychiatr Scand.* 1989;80(Suppl. 350):102.

 Diazepam (eg, *Valium*)

Propranolol (eg, *Inderal*)

SUMMARY: Propranolol may reduce slightly the metabolism of diazepam and may increase the pharmacodynamic effects of benzodiazepines.

RISK FACTORS: No specific risk factors are known.

MECHANISM: Propranolol appears to reduce the oxidative N-demethylation of diazepam. The glucuronidation of lorazepam and the hydroxylation of alprazolam are unaffected by propranolol.

CLINICAL EVALUATION: Propranolol administration 80 mg 3 times a day for 2 days reduced by 16% the mean clearance of a single 5 to 10 mg IV dose of diazepam.[1] Diazepam half-life was increased from 48.5 hr to 58.3 hr by propranolol administration and it appeared to slow the absorption rate of oral alprazolam (eg, *Xanax*). In subjects who were receiving oral diazepam 5 mg twice daily, the effects of propranolol 40 mg twice daily for 2 days followed by 80 mg twice daily for 3 days were similar to those after IV administration.[2] These changes may enhance the effects of diazepam in some patients.

RELATED DRUGS: Atenolol (eg, *Tenormin*) had no effect on diazepam pharmacokinetics or pharmacodynamics.[2] Propranolol had no effect on IV lorazepam (eg, *Ativan*) pharmacokinetics but increased the pharmacodynamic effects of oxazepam (eg, *Serax*) without affecting its pharmacokinetics.[3] Metoprolol (eg, *Lopressor*) produces a small reduction in the metabolism of diazepam.

MANAGEMENT OPTIONS: No specific action is required, but be alert for evidence of the interaction.

REFERENCES:

1. Ochs HR, et al. Propranolol interactions with diazepam, lorazepam, and alprazolam. *Clin Pharmacol Ther.* 1984;36:451.
2. Hawksorth G, et al. Diazepam/beta-adrenoceptor antagonist interactions. *Br J Clin Pharmacol.* 1984;17:69S.
3. Sonne J, et al. Single dose pharmacokinetics and pharmacodynamics of oral oxazepam during concomitant administration of propranolol and labetalol. *Br J Clin Pharmacol.* 1990;29:33.

Diazepam (eg, *Valium*)

Rifampin (eg, *Rifadin*)

SUMMARY: Rifampin appears to reduce the serum concentration of diazepam and perhaps other benzodiazepines.

RISK FACTORS: No specific risk factors are known.

MECHANISM: Rifampin probably enhances the hepatic metabolism (CYP3A4) of diazepam and nitrazepam[†].

CLINICAL EVALUATION: Rifampin 600 or 1,200 mg/day for a week increased the clearance of diazepam and nitrazepam by up to 80%.[1,2] The patients also appeared to eliminate desmethyldiazepam more rapidly.

RELATED DRUGS: Rifampin did not significantly increase the clearance of temazepam (eg, *Restoril*).[3] Rifampin increased nitrazepam clearance significantly. Rifampin also may reduce the effect of those benzodiazepines metabolized to desmethyldiazepam, such as halazepam (*Paxipam*), clorazepate (eg, *Tranxene*), and prazepam.

MANAGEMENT OPTIONS:

➡ *Monitor.* Monitor patients for evidence of reduced diazepam and nitrazepam effect when rifampin is given concurrently. The response to halazepam, clorazepate, and prazepam also may be reduced by rifampin.

REFERENCES:

1. Ochs HR, et al. Diazepam interaction with antituberculosis drugs. *Clin Pharmacol Ther.* 1981;29:671.
2. Ohnhaus EE, et al. The effect of antipyrine and rifampin on the metabolism of diazepam. *Clin Pharmacol Ther.* 1987;42:148.
3. Brockmeyer NH, et al. Comparative effects of rifampin or probenecid on the pharmacokinetics of temazepam and nitrazepam. *Int J Clin Pharmacol Ther Toxicol.* 1990;28:387.

† Not available in the United States.

Diazepam (eg, *Valium*)

Sertraline (*Zoloft*)

SUMMARY: Preliminary study in healthy subjects suggest that sertraline only slightly reduces diazepam elimination; the clinical importance of this effect is not established.

RISK FACTORS: No specific risk factors are known.

MECHANISM: Not established.

CLINICAL EVALUATION: Twenty healthy men were given single 10 mg IV doses of diazepam before and on day 21 of a 32-day regimen of sertraline, 50 mg/day titrated up to a dose of 200 mg/day (10 subjects), or placebo (10 subjects).[1] Sertraline was associated with a small reduction in clearance of diazepam and had only minimal effects on desmethyldiazepam, the active metabolite of diazepam. Although the results of this preliminary report suggest that sertraline is unlikely to affect the response to diazepam, additional study is needed to establish whether this interaction is clinically important.

RELATED DRUGS: Fluoxetine (*Prozac*) increases plasma diazepam concentrations somewhat, and fluvoxamine (*Luvox*) is known to inhibit CYP3A4, an isozyme important in the metabolism of diazepam.

MANAGEMENT OPTIONS: No specific action is required, but be alert for evidence of the interaction.

REFERENCES:
1. Gardner MJ, et al. The effects of sertraline on the pharmacokinetics of diazepam in healthy volunteers. *Biol Psychiatry*. 1991;29:354S.

 Diazepam (eg, *Valium*)

Succinylcholine (eg, *Anectine*)

SUMMARY: Diazepam reportedly reduces the duration of succinylcholine effect, but this has not been a consistent finding.

RISK FACTORS: No specific risk factors are known.

MECHANISM: Not established. Study in normal volunteers given diazepam indicates that the drug may directly inhibit the contractile mechanism of skeletal muscle.[4]

CLINICAL EVALUATION: In a preliminary clinical study, diazepam decreased the duration of succinylcholine activity and increased the duration of action of gallamine.[1] Subsequent studies[2,3] did not substantiate these findings, and diazepam itself probably does not significantly affect the response to neuromuscular blockers. When the injectable form of diazepam was given intra-arterially, neuromuscular blockade was inhibited presumably by the preservatives or solvents in this formulation. The effect of IV or IM doses of diazepam on the response to neuromuscular blockers under clinical conditions remains to be determined.

RELATED DRUGS: See Clinical Evaluation.

MANAGEMENT OPTIONS: No specific action is required, but be alert for evidence of the interaction.

REFERENCES:
1. Feldman SA, et al. Interaction of diazepam with the muscle-relaxant drugs. *BMJ*. 1970;2:336.
2. Dretchen K, et al. The interaction of diazepam with myoneural blocking agents. *Anesthesiology*. 1971;34:463.
3. Webb SN, et al. Diazepam and neuromuscular blocking drugs. *BMJ*. 1971;3:640.
4. Ludin HP, et al. Action of diazepam on muscular contraction in man. *Z Neurol*. 1971;199:30.

Diazepam (eg, *Valium*)

Tacrine (*Cognex*)

SUMMARY: Tacrine does not appear to affect the pharmacokinetics of diazepam.

RISK FACTORS: No specific risk factors are known.

MECHANISM: No interaction.

CLINICAL EVALUATION: Eleven or twelve (exact number not stated) older healthy subjects took a single oral 2 mg dose of diazepam with and without concurrent tacrine (20 mg every 6 hours).[1] Tacrine had no effect on diazepam pharmacokinetics, but the reverse interaction (effect of diazepam on tacrine) was not studied.

RELATED DRUGS: Little is known about possible interactions of tacrine with other benzodiazepines.

MANAGEMENT OPTIONS: No interaction.

REFERENCES:
1. de Vries TM, et al. Effect of multiple-dose tacrine administration on single-dose pharmacokinetics of digoxin, diazepam, and theophylline. *Pharm Res.* 1993;10:S333.

Diazepam (eg, *Valium*) 4

Valproic Acid (eg, *Depakene*)

SUMMARY: Valproic acid may increase serum diazepam concentrations, but the clinical importance of this effect is not established.

RISK FACTORS: No specific risk factors are known.

MECHANISM: Valproic acid appears to inhibit the hepatic metabolism of diazepam.

CLINICAL EVALUATION: Six healthy subjects received diazepam 10 mg intravenously with and without valproic acid 1.5 g orally.[1] Serum diazepam concentrations were higher in the presence of valproic acid, but the possibility of an enhanced diazepam effect was not studied.

RELATED DRUGS: The effect of valproic acid on the metabolism of other benzodiazepines is not known.

MANAGEMENT OPTIONS: No specific action is required, but be alert for evidence of the interaction.

REFERENCES:
1. Dhillon SA, et al. Valproic acid and diazepam interaction in vivo. *Br J Clin Pharmacol.* 1982;13(4):553-560.

Diazepam (eg, *Valium*)

Voriconazole (eg, *Vfend*)

SUMMARY: Voriconazole increases the plasma concentration of diazepam; increased adverse reactions, including sedation and ataxia, may occur.

RISK FACTORS:

➡ ***Pharmacogenetics.*** Patients who are poor metabolizers (PMs) of CYP2C19 will primarily metabolize diazepam via CYP3A4. Because voriconazole is also a substrate of CYP2C19, its plasma concentration will be elevated in PMs and may have a greater inhibitory effect on the CYP3A4 pathway of diazepam.

MECHANISM: Voriconazole inhibits both of the primary pathways of diazepam metabolism, CYP2C19 and CYP3A4.

CLINICAL EVALUATION: Twelve healthy subjects received a single oral dose of diazepam 5 mg alone and following voriconazole 400 mg twice daily on the first day and 200 mg twice daily on day 2.[1] The mean area under the concentration-time curve of diazepam was increased 2.1-fold during voriconazole dosing. Diazepam half-life increased from 31 to 61 hours during voriconazole coadministration. Because this study used only 2 days of voriconazole dosing, the magnitude of this interaction may differ with long-term voriconazole dosing. All of the subjects were either homozygous (n = 8) or heterozygous extensive metabolizers for CYP2C19, so no conclusions could be drawn on the possible role of CYP2C19 polymorphism in the magnitude of the interaction.

RELATED DRUGS: The metabolism of other benzodiazepines metabolized by CYP3A4 (eg, alprazolam [eg, *Xanax*], midazolam, and triazolam [eg, *Halcion*]) is also likely to be inhibited by voriconazole.

MANAGEMENT OPTIONS:

➡ ***Consider Alternative.*** Benzodiazepines (eg, lorazepam [eg, *Ativan*], oxazepam) that are not metabolized by CYP3A4 are unlikely to be affected by voriconazole. Consider using an antifungal that does not affect CYP3A4 or CYP2C9, such as terbinafine (eg, *Lamisil*).

➡ ***Monitor.*** Monitor patients receiving diazepam and voriconazole for evidence of increased diazepam effects.

REFERENCES:

    1. Saari TI, et al. Voriconazole and fluconazole increase the exposure to oral diazepam. *Eur J Clin Pharmacol.* 2007;63(10):941-949.

 Diazepam (eg, *Valium*)

Warfarin (eg, *Coumadin*)

SUMMARY: Diazepam appears to have little or no effect on the hypoprothrombinemic response to oral anticoagulants.

RISK FACTORS: No specific risk factors are known.

MECHANISM: No interaction.

CLINICAL EVALUATION: Although an early case report indicated that diazepam might interact with dicumarol,[1] subsequent studies have shown that diazepam probably has no significant effect on the action of warfarin.[2-4]

RELATED DRUGS: Diazepam may interact with dicumarol. Other benzodiazepines probably have little or no effect on oral anticoagulants.

MANAGEMENT OPTIONS: No interaction.

REFERENCES:

1. Taylor PJ. Hemorrhage while on anticoagulant therapy precipitated by drug interaction. *Ariz Med.* 1967;24(8):697-699.
2. Whitfield JB, et al. Changes in plasma gamma-glutamyl transpeptidase activity associated with alterations in drug metabolism in man. *Br Med J.* 1973;1(5849):316-318.
3. Solomon HM, et al. Mechanisms of drug interactions. *JAMA.* 1971;216(12):1997-1999.
4. DeCarolis PP, et al. Effect of tranquilizers on prothrombin time response to coumarin. *J Clin Pharmacol.* 1975;15:557.

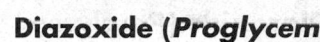

Diazoxide (*Proglycem*)

Hydralazine

SUMMARY: Severe hypotensive reactions have occurred with combined use of diazoxide and parenteral hydralazine.

RISK FACTORS: No specific risk factors are known.

MECHANISM: Diazoxide and hydralazine may exhibit additive hypotensive effects.

CLINICAL EVALUATION: Severe hypotensive reactions have occurred in several patients receiving diazoxide and hydralazine, usually within 1 to 2 hours of each other.[1,2,3]

RELATED DRUGS: No information is available.

MANAGEMENT OPTIONS:

➥ *Monitor.* Coadminister diazoxide and hydralazine with caution and with adequate monitoring for excessive hypotension.

REFERENCES:

1. Henrich WL, et al. Hypotensive sequelae of diazoxide and hydralazine therapy. *JAMA.* 1977;237(3):264-265.
2. Mizroch S, et al. Hypotension and bradycardia following diazoxide and hydralazine therapy. *JAMA.* 1977;237(23):2471-2471.
3. Romberg GP, et al. Hypotensive sequelae of diazoxide and hydralazine therapy. *JAMA.* 1977;238(10):1025.

Diazoxide (*Proglycem*)

Phenytoin (eg, *Dilantin*)

SUMMARY: Diazoxide has been associated with markedly decreased serum phenytoin concentrations in several children.

RISK FACTORS: No specific risk factors are known.

MECHANISM: Limited evidence suggests that diazoxide enhances phenytoin metabolism.

CLINICAL EVALUATION: Three children receiving phenytoin and diazoxide concomitantly developed very low serum phenytoin levels (in 2 cases phenytoin was undetectable).[1,2] Urinary excretion of the major metabolite of phenytoin (HPPH) was measured in 1 patient and found to be considerably increased during diazoxide administration.[2] In another patient, phenytoin half-life was only 3.5 hours during long-term diazoxide therapy, which is considerably shorter than normal.[1] Based on these 3 cases, patients receiving concomitant phenytoin and diazoxide may develop subtherapeutic phenytoin levels.

RELATED DRUGS: No information is available.

MANAGEMENT OPTIONS:

➡ **Monitor.** Monitor patients receiving concomitant phenytoin and diazoxide for increased seizure activity and decreased phenytoin levels.

REFERENCES:

1. Petro DJ, et al. Diazoxide-diphenylhydantoin interaction. *J Pediatr.* 1976;89(2):331-332.

2. Roe TF, et al. Drug interaction: diazoxide and diphenylhydantoin. *J Pediatr.* 1975;87(3):480-484.

Diazoxide (*Proglycem*)

Thiazides

SUMMARY: Combined use of thiazides and diazoxide may result in hyperglycemia.

RISK FACTORS: No specific risk factors are known.

MECHANISM: Both thiazides and diazoxide have hyperglycemic effects, and their combined use may be additive.[1] Diazoxide also may compete with thiazides for plasma protein binding sites,[2] but the clinical importance of this effect is unclear.

CLINICAL EVALUATION: The concomitant use of diazoxide and thiazides has resulted in enhanced hyperglycemic activity in a number of patients.[3] Keep this effect in mind when thiazides are used to treat diazoxide-induced sodium retention.

RELATED DRUGS: No information is available.

MANAGEMENT OPTIONS:

➡ **Monitor.** Monitor blood glucose during combined therapy with thiazides and diazoxide.

REFERENCES:

1. Wolff F. Diazoxide misunderstood. *N Engl J Med.* 1972;286(11):612.

2. Sellers EM, et al. Protein binding and vascular activity of diazoxide. *N Engl J Med.* 1969;281(21):1141-1145.

3. Seltzer HS, et al. Hyperglycemia and inhibition of insulin secretion during administration of diazoxide and trichlormethiazide in man. *Diabetes.* 1969;18(1):19-28.

Diazoxide (*Proglycem*)

Warfarin (eg, *Coumadin*)

SUMMARY: In vitro studies indicate that diazoxide may displace warfarin from plasma protein binding sites, but the clinical significance of this effect is not established.

RISK FACTORS: No specific risk factors are known.

MECHANISM: Diazoxide may displace warfarin from plasma protein binding.[1,2]

CLINICAL EVALUATION: Clinical examples of an interaction between diazoxide and warfarin have not appeared in the literature; however, theoretical considerations and in vitro studies suggest an interaction is possible. However, if displacement of warfarin from plasma protein binding sites does occur in vivo, the increase in hypoprothrombinemia is likely to be transient if no other mechanism is involved.

RELATED DRUGS: Oral anticoagulants other than warfarin also are extensively bound to plasma proteins, but it is not known if they interact with diazoxide.

MANAGEMENT OPTIONS: No specific action is required, but be alert for evidence of the interaction.

REFERENCES:

1. Sellers EM, Koch-Weser J. Displacement of warfarin from human albumin by diazoxide and ethacrynic, mefenamic, and nalidixic acids. *Clin Pharmacol Ther*. 1970;11(4):524-529.
2. Sellers EM, Koch-Weser J. Protein binding and vascular activity of diazoxide. *N Engl J Med*. 1969;281(21):1141-1145.

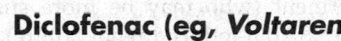

Diclofenac (eg, *Voltaren*)

Lithium (eg, *Eskalith*)

SUMMARY: A study in healthy subjects suggests that diclofenac, like most nonsteroidal anti-inflammatory drugs (NSAIDs), increases plasma lithium concentrations; one would expect this to increase the risks of lithium toxicity.

RISK FACTORS: No specific risk factors are known.

MECHANISM: Diclofenac inhibits the renal clearance of lithium. It has been proposed that renal tubular prostaglandins are involved in the excretion of lithium, and that the antiprostaglandin effects of NSAIDs thus interfere with renal lithium elimination; more study is needed.

CLINICAL EVALUATION: In 5 healthy women with steady-state plasma lithium concentrations, the addition of diclofenac 150 mg/day for 7 to 10 days increased lithium plasma concentrations by 26% and decreased lithium renal clearance by 23%.[1] However, it is possible that patients receiving this combination would manifest a greater increase in plasma lithium concentrations (ibuprofen [eg, *Motrin*] has been shown to produce a greater increase in plasma lithium levels in elderly patients than in young, healthy subjects).[2] Since several other NSAIDs have produced clinical evidence of lithium toxicity, it is reasonable to assume that diclofenac is also capable of doing so in at least some patients.

RELATED DRUGS: Most NSAIDs increase lithium serum concentrations, but sulindac (eg, *Clinoril*) and aspirin appear to have minimal effects.

MANAGEMENT OPTIONS:

➡ *Consider Alternative.* If appropriate for the patient, consider using an anti-inflammatory agent that is less likely to affect lithium, such as sulindac or aspirin.

➡ *Monitor.* If diclofenac therapy is initiated in a patient taking lithium, monitor serum lithium concentrations for evidence of lithium toxicity (eg, nausea, vomiting, diarrhea, anorexia, coarse tremor, slurred speech, vertigo, confusion, lethargy; in severe cases, seizures, stupor, coma, and cardiovascular collapse). In a patient stabilized on lithium and an NSAID, discontinuation of the NSAID may result in inadequate serum lithium concentrations.

REFERENCES:
1. Reimann IW, et al. Effects of diclofenac on lithium kinetics. *Clin Pharmacol Ther.* 1981;30:348.
2. Ragheb M, et al. Ibuprofen can increase serum lithium level in lithium-treated patients. *J Clin Psychiatry.* 1987;48:161.

 Diclofenac (eg, *Voltaren*)

Methotrexate (eg, *Rheumatrex*)

SUMMARY: One patient on high dose methotrexate developed severe methotrexate toxicity following the use of diclofenac.

RISK FACTORS:

➥ *Concurrent Diseases.* Particular caution is suggested in patients with pre-existing renal impairment (who may be more susceptible to nonsteroidal anti-inflammatory drug [NSAID]-induced renal failure).

➥ *Dosage Regimen.* The risk of adverse effects from this interaction is primarily in patients receiving antineoplastic doses of methotrexate, rather than the lower doses used to treat rheumatoid arthritis, psoriasis, and related diseases.

MECHANISM: It is widely held that NSAIDs interfere with renal secretion of methotrexate, either by inhibiting tubular secretion of methotrexate or by reducing renal blood flow by inhibiting prostaglandin synthesis. Alterations in plasma protein binding also have been proposed, but this is unlikely to be clinically significant because methotrexate is normally only 50% to 70% bound to plasma proteins. Pharmacokinetic studies involving several different NSAIDs have failed to consistently identify an alteration in methotrexate pharmacokinetics by NSAIDs;[1-8] however, even in studies where methotrexate pharmacokinetics remained unchanged overall, occasional patients appeared to exhibit reduced clearance of methotrexate after NSAID administration.[1,3]

CLINICAL EVALUATION: A patient developed severe methotrexate toxicity when diclofenac (150 mg/day IM) was started 1 day before the high-dose methotrexate cycle.[10] Although a causal relationship was not established, the severity of the reaction and the reports of similar reactions following other NSAIDs suggest that this potential interaction should not be ignored. Patients receiving low-dose methotrexate for rheumatoid arthritis frequently receive concurrent NSAIDs, and severe methotrexate toxicity in such patients is unusual.[11-13] Although these patients would appear to be at low risk, caution is warranted since NSAID use in patients on low-dose methotrexate occasionally is associated with severe methotrexate toxicity.[9,14]

RELATED DRUGS: Other NSAIDS appear to interact similarly with methotrexate, but the relative risk of one NSAID versus another is not established.

MANAGEMENT OPTIONS:

➥ *Avoid Unless Benefit Outweighs Risk.* Until more information is available on this interaction, it would be prudent to avoid diclofenac (as well as other NSAIDs) in patients receiving antineoplastic doses of methotrexate. Particular caution is suggested in patients with pre-existing renal impairment, who may be more susceptible to NSAID-induced renal failure.

➥ **Monitor.** If the combination is used, monitor for methotrexate toxicity. Findings in methotrexate toxicity can include stomatitis, severe gastrointestinal symptoms (eg, nausea, diarrhea, vomiting), bone marrow suppression, fever, bleeding, skin rashes, nephrotoxicity, and hepatotoxicity. Although decreasing the methotrexate dosage would be expected to reduce the likelihood of toxicity, the magnitude of the required reduction in methotrexate dosage has not been established.

REFERENCES:

1. Aherne A, et al. Methotrexate kinetics in rheumatoid arthritis: is there an interaction with nonsteroidal antiinflammatory drugs? *J Rheumatol.* 1988;15:1356.
2. Furst DE, et al. Effect of aspirin and sulindac on methotrexate clearance. *J Pharm Sci.* 1990;79:782.
3. Dupuis LL, et al. Methotrexate-nonsteroidal anti-inflammatory drug interaction in children with arthritis. *J Rheumatol.* 1990;17:1469.
4. Liegler DG, et al. The effect of organic acids on renal clearance of methotrexate in man. *Clin Pharmacol Ther.* 1969;10:849.
5. Skeith KJ, et al. Lack of significant interaction between low dose methotrexate and ibuprofen or flurbiprofen in patients with arthritis. *J Rheumatol.* 1990;17:1008.
6. Stewart CF, et al. Effect of aspirin (ASA) on the disposition of methotrexate (MTX) in patients with rheumatoid arthritis (RA). *Clin Pharmacol Ther.* 1990;47:139. Abstract PP-56.
7. Taylor JR, et al. Effect of sodium salicylate and indomethacin on methotrexate-serum albumin binding. *Arch Dermatol.* 1977;113:588.
8. Tracy FS, et al. The effect of NSAIDS on methotrexate disposition in patients with rheumatoid arthritis. *Clin Pharmacol Ther.* 1990;47:138. Abstract PP-54.
9. Daly HM, et al. Methotrexate toxicity precipitated by azapropazone. *Br J Dermatol.* 1986;114:733.
10. Thyss A, et al. Clinical and pharmacokinetic evidence of a life-threatening interaction between methotrexate and ketoprofen. *Lancet.* 1986;1:256.
11. Boh LE, et al. Low-dose weekly oral methotrexate therapy for inflammatory arthritis. *Clin Pharm.* 1986;5:503.
12. Anderson PA, et al. Weekly pulse methotrexate in rheumatoid arthritis: clinical and immunologic effects in a randomized, double-blind study. *Ann Intern Med.* 1985;103:489.
13. Tugwell P, et al. Methotrexate in rheumatoid arthritis: indications, contraindications, efficacy, and safety. *Ann Intern Med.* 1987;107:358.
14. Adams JD, et al. Drug interactions in psoriasis. *Aust J Dermatol.* 1976;17:39.

Diclofenac (eg, *Voltaren*)

Verapamil (eg, *Calan*)

SUMMARY: Diclofenac reduces the plasma concentration of verapamil; the clinical significance is unknown.

RISK FACTORS: No specific risk factors are known.

MECHANISM: Not established. Diclofenac may increase verapamil metabolism or reduce its absorption.

CLINICAL EVALUATION: Twenty-five patients with hypertension were administered sustained-release verapamil 240 mg/day for 2 weeks.[1] The patients were then randomized to receive either diclofenac 75 mg twice daily or naproxen (eg, *Naprosyn*) 375 mg twice daily for 4 weeks. Verapamil plasma concentrations were measured before and after weeks 1 and 4 of nonsteroidal anti-inflammatory drug (NSAID) coadministration. Diclofenac significantly reduced the mean area under the concentration-time curve of verapamil after 1 (26%) and 4 weeks (29%) of coadministration. Naproxen had no effect on verapamil concentrations.[2] While no pharmacodynamic data were presented, a reduction in verapamil concentration of this magnitude could reduce its efficacy in some situations (eg, the treatment of angina or arrhythmias).

RELATED DRUGS: Naproxen coadministration appears to have no effect on verapamil concentrations. The effects of other NSAIDs on verapamil are unknown. Diclofenac 50 mg administered once increased isradipine (*DynaCirc*) peak concentration by 20% but did not change its area under the concentration-time curve.[3] The clinical effects of this change would be minimal.

MANAGEMENT OPTIONS:

➡ *Consider Alternative.* Consider naproxen for patients taking verapamil.

➡ *Monitor.* Until more information is available, monitor patients stabilized on verapamil for reduced efficacy during concomitant therapy with diclofenac.

REFERENCES:

1. Peterson MS, et al. Differential effects of naproxen and diclofenac on verapamil pharmacokinetics. *Clin Pharmacol Ther.* 1991;49:129.

2. Houston MC, et al. The effects of nonsteroidal anti-inflammatory drugs on blood pressures of patients with hypertension controlled by verapamil. *Arch Intern Med.* 1995;155:1049.

3. Sommers DK, et al. Effects of diclofenac on isradipine pharmacokinetics and platelet aggregation in volunteers. *Eur J Clin Pharmacol.* 1993;44:391.

 Diclofenac (eg, *Voltaren*)

Warfarin (eg, *Coumadin*)

SUMMARY: A preliminary study indicates that diclofenac does not affect the hypoprothrombinemic response to oral anticoagulants; nonetheless, cotherapy requires caution because of possible detrimental effects of diclofenac on the gastric mucosa and platelet function.

RISK FACTORS:

➡ *Concurrent Diseases.* Patients with peptic ulcer disease or a history of gastrointestinal (GI) bleeding are probably at greater risk.

MECHANISM: Diclofenac-induced gastric erosions and inhibition of platelet function theoretically would increase the risk of bleeding in a patient receiving oral anticoagulants.

CLINICAL EVALUATION: In a crossover study of 32 patients receiving oral anticoagulants, diclofenac did not affect the hypoprothrombinemic response significantly.[1] Nevertheless, use any nonsteroidal anti-inflammatory drug (NSAID) cautiously in anticoagulated patients because NSAID-induced gastric erosions and possible platelet inhibition may lead to bleeding. In a retrospective cohort study, hospitalizations for hemorrhagic peptic ulcer disease were about 13 times higher in patients receiving warfarin plus an NSAID than in patients receiving neither drug.[2]

RELATED DRUGS: All NSAIDs inhibit platelet function, cause gastric erosions, and appear to have an additive effect with oral anticoagulants in increasing the risk of GI bleeding.

MANAGEMENT OPTIONS:

➡ *Avoid Unless Benefit Outweighs Risk.* Since all NSAIDs probably increase the risk of GI bleeding in patients on oral anticoagulants, use the combination only after careful consideration of the benefit versus risk. If the diclofenac is being used as an analgesic or antipyretic, acetaminophen is probably safer to use with oral anticoagulants. Nonacetylated salicylates (eg, choline salicylate, magnesium salicylate, salsalate, sodium salicylate) also are probably safer with oral anticoagulants than diclofenac since they have minimal effects on platelet function and the gastric mucosa.

➡ **Monitor.** If any NSAID is used with an oral anticoagulant, carefully monitor the prothrombin time and watch for evidence of bleeding, especially from the GI tract.

REFERENCES:
1. Michot F, et al. A double-blind clinical trial to determine if an interaction exists between diclofenac sodium and the oral anticoagulant acenocoumarol (*Nicoamalone*). *J Int Med Res*. 1975;3:153.
2. Shorr RI, et al. Concurrent use of nonsteroidal anti-inflammatory drugs and oral anticoagulants places elderly persons at high risk for hemorrhagic peptic ulcer disease. *Arch Intern Med*. 1993;153:1665.

Dicloxacillin (eg, *Dynapen*)

Warfarin (eg, *Coumadin*)

SUMMARY: Decreased anticoagulant response to warfarin has been reported in patients receiving dicloxacillin, but a study in other patients suggests that dicloxacillin has only a slight effect on warfarin response.

RISK FACTORS: No specific risk factors are known.

MECHANISM: Not established.

CLINICAL EVALUATION: One patient developed a reduction in the hypoprothrombinemic response to warfarin during therapy with dicloxacillin. When oral dicloxacillin was given to patients stabilized on warfarin, prothrombin times decreased only slightly by 2 to 3 seconds.[1,2] Warfarin concentrations were reduced 20% to 25% by dicloxacillin.[2] Further study is needed to define the significance of this interaction.

RELATED DRUGS: Nafcillin (eg, *Unipen*) also may inhibit the hypoprothrombinemic response to warfarin, but data are limited. The effect of other penicillinase-resistant penicillins such as cloxacillin (eg, *Cloxapen*), methicillin, and oxacillin (eg, *Bactocill*) on warfarin response is not established.

MANAGEMENT OPTIONS: No specific action is required, but be alert for evidence of the interaction.

REFERENCES:
1. Krstenansky PM, et al. Effect of dicloxacillin sodium on the hypoprothrombinemic response to warfarin sodium. *Clin Pharm*. 1987;6:804.
2. Mailloux AT, et al. Evaluation of the potential stereoselective interaction between warfarin and dicloxacillin. *Pharmacotherapy*. 1993;13:288.

Dicumarol

Ethchlorvynol (*Placidyl*)

SUMMARY: Ethchlorvynol appears to inhibit the hypoprothrombinemic response to dicumarol and possibly warfarin.

RISK FACTORS: No specific risk factors are known.

MECHANISM: Not established. Animal studies do not indicate that ethchlorvynol is an enzyme-inducing agent, but these data do not necessarily apply to humans.

CLINICAL EVALUATION: In a study of 6 patients on dicumarol, ethchlorvynol 1 g/day for 18 days inhibited the hypoprothrombinemic response.[2]

RELATED DRUGS: In 1 patient receiving warfarin (eg, *Coumadin*), a marked decrease in hypoprothrombinemic response followed ethchlorvynol administration.[1] Little is known about the effect of ethchlorvynol on the response to oral anticoagulants other than dicumarol or warfarin, but assume that they interact until it is proven otherwise. Benzodiazepines, such as diazepam (eg, *Valium*) or temazepam (eg, *Restoril*), are unlikely to affect oral anticoagulants.

MANAGEMENT OPTIONS:

➡ **Consider Alternative.** Consider using a benzodiazepine instead of ethchlorvynol as benzodiazepines are unlikely to affect oral anticoagulants.

➡ **Monitor.** Monitor for altered oral anticoagulant effect if ethchlorvynol is initiated, discontinued, or changed in dosage; adjustments of oral anticoagulant dosage may be needed.

REFERENCES:

1. Cullen SI, et al. Griseofulvin-warfarin antagonism. *JAMA*. 1967;199:582.
2. Johansson S. Apparent resistance to oral anticoagulant therapy and influence of hypnotics on some coagulation factors. *Acta Med Scand*. 1968;184:297.

Dicumarol[†]

Tolbutamide

SUMMARY: Dicumarol (but probably not warfarin) enhances the hypoglycemic response to tolbutamide. Most available evidence indicates that tolbutamide does not affect the hypoprothrombinemic response to oral anticoagulants.

RISK FACTORS: No specific risk factors are known.

MECHANISM: Dicumarol appears to inhibit the hepatic metabolism of tolbutamide.[1,2]

CLINICAL EVALUATION: Dicumarol produces an appreciable increase in the half-life of tolbutamide in both patients[2,3] and healthy subjects[1]; steady-state concentrations of tolbutamide also may be increased by dicumarol.[4] Several cases of hypoglycemic reactions have been reported with the concomitant use of these 2 drugs.[2,5]

Several cases of possible tolbutamide-induced enhancement of dicumarol response have been reported in the literature or to the manufacturer,[6,7] but no effect of tolbutamide on dicumarol response was found in 3 patients,[6] 4 healthy subjects,[4] or a retrospective study of patients.[7] In the retrospective study, however, the patients were maintained on tolbutamide and subsequently given an anticoagulant and therefore an interaction was not expected.

RELATED DRUGS: Tolbutamide metabolism[3] does not appear to be affected by warfarin (eg, *Coumadin*), phenindione,[†] or phenprocoumon.[†] Neither the half-life nor the plasma levels of phenprocoumon appear to be affected by tolbutamide, insulin, glyburide (eg, *DiaBeta*), or glibornuride[†] in diabetic patients, nondiabetic elderly patients, or healthy young volunteers.[8] Little is known regarding the effect of tolbutamide on warfarin response. It does not seem likely that oral anticoagulants would interact with insulin.

MANAGEMENT OPTIONS:

➥ *Consider Alternative.* Warfarin and phenprocoumon appear to be less likely than dicumarol to interact with tolbutamide.

➥ *Monitor.* If tolbutamide and dicumarol are used concurrently, monitor for altered hypoglycemic response when dicumarol is initiated, discontinued, or changed in dosage.

REFERENCES:

1. Solomon HM, Schrogie JJ. Effect of phenyramidol and bishydroxycoumarin on the metabolism of tolbutamide in human subjects. *Metabolism*. 1967;16(11):1029-1033.

2. Kristensen M, Hansen JM. Potentiation of the tolbutamide effect of dicoumarol. *Diabetes*. 1967;16(4):211-214.

3. Skovsted L, et al. The effect of different oral anticoagulants on diphenylhydantoin (DPH) and tolbutamide metabolism. *Acta Med Scand*. 1976;199(6):513-515.

4. Jähnschen E, et al. Pharmacokinetic analysis of the interaction between dicoumarol and tolbutamide in man. *Eur J Clin Pharmacol*. 1976;10(5):349-356.

5. Spurney OM, et al. Protracted tolbutamide-induced hypoglycemia. *Arch Intern Med*. 1965;115:53-56.

6. Chaplin H Jr, Casseu M. Studies on the possible relationship of tolbutamide to dicumarol in anticoagulant therapy. *Am J Med Sci*. 1958;235(6):706–716.

7. Poucher RL, Vecchio TJ. Absence of tolbutamide effect on anticoagulant therapy. *JAMA*. 1966;197(13):1069–1070.

8. Heine P, et al. The influence of hypoglycaemic sulphonylureas on elimination and efficacy of phenprocoumon following a single oral dose in diabetic patients. *Eur J Clin Pharmacol*. 1976;10:31.

† Not available in the United States.

Dicyclomine (eg, *Bentyl*) ▼ 3

Donepezil (eg, *Aricept*)

SUMMARY: Dicyclomine is an anticholinergic drug and may inhibit the therapeutic effect of donepezil in Alzheimer disease.

RISK FACTORS: No specific risk factors are known.

MECHANISM: Donepezil is a cholinesterase inhibitor and thus increases cholinergic activity; its efficacy is likely to be inhibited by anticholinergic drugs such as dicyclomine.[1]

CLINICAL EVALUATION: In a preliminary study of 69 patients with Alzheimer disease receiving donepezil 10 mg/day and followed for 2 years, 16 patients received concurrent therapy with anticholinergic drugs and 53 patients did not.[2] Mental functioning, as measured by the Mini-Mental State Exam (MMSE), was significantly lower in the patients receiving concomitant anticholinergic drugs. Also, the French Pharmacovigilance Database received 118 spontaneous reports of adverse reactions in patients receiving anticholinergic drugs with cholinesterase inhibitors (eg, donepezil, galantamine, rivastigmine). After evaluation by clinical pharmacologists, 24 were thought to be adverse drug interactions.[3] Although additional study is needed to establish the clinical importance of these interactions, the evidence is consistent with the known pharmacological effects of the drugs.

RELATED DRUGS: All cholinesterase inhibitors used to treat Alzheimer disease (donepezil, galantamine [eg, *Razadyne*], rivastigmine [eg, *Exelon*]) are expected to interact similarly with dicyclomine and other antispasmodic anticholinergics, such as atropine (eg, *Donnatal*), belladonna,† clidinium,† darifenacin (*Enablex*), festerodine (*Toviaz*), flavoxate, glycopyrrolate (eg, *Robinul*), hyosciamine (eg, *Anaspaz*), methscopolamine (eg, *Pamine*), oxybutynin (eg, *Ditropan*), propantheline, solifenacin (*Vesicare*), tolterodine (*Detrol*), and trospium (eg, *Sanctura*).

MANAGEMENT OPTIONS:

➥ **Consider Alternative.** If possible, use an alternative to the dicyclomine or other anticholinergic antispasmodics (see Related Drugs).

➥ **Monitor.** If dicyclomine or other anticholinergic antispasmodics are used with donepezil or other cholinesterase inhibitors, be alert for evidence of reduced mental functioning.

REFERENCES:

1. *Aricept* [package insert]. New York, NY: Pfizer; 2011.
2. Lu CJ, Tune LE. Chronic exposure to anticholinergic medications adversely affects the course of Alzheimer disease. *Am J Geriatr Psychiatry.* 2003;11(4):458-461.
3. Tavassoli N, et al. Drug interactions with cholinesterase inhibitors: an analysis of the French Pharmacovigilance Database and a comparison of two national drug formularies (Vidal, British National Formulary). *Drug Saf.* 2007;30(11):1063-1071.

† Not available in the United States.

5 | Didanosine (eg, *Videx*)

Fluconazole (eg, *Diflucan*)

SUMMARY: Fluconazole did not affect didanosine concentrations in HIV-infected patients.

RISK FACTORS: No specific risk factors are known.

MECHANISM: No interaction.

CLINICAL EVALUATION: Thirteen patients with HIV were receiving long-term didanosine therapy.[1] They were administered fluconazole 200 mg twice daily for 1 day followed by 200 mg daily for 6 days. Didanosine concentrations were not altered by coadministration with fluconazole. The effects of didanosine on fluconazole were not reported.

RELATED DRUGS: Didanosine administration is known to reduce ketoconazole (eg, *Nizoral*) absorption.

MANAGEMENT OPTIONS: No interaction.

REFERENCES:

1. Bruzzese VL, et al. Effect of fluconazole on pharmacokinetics of 2',3'-dideoxyinosine in persons seropositive for human immunodeficiency virus. *Antimicrob Agents Chemother.* 1995;39(5):1050-1053.

3 | Didanosine (eg, *Videx*)

Food

SUMMARY: Didanosine plasma concentrations are reduced by administration with food; the clinical significance of this is unknown, but the magnitude of the interaction indicates that loss of efficacy may result.

RISK FACTORS: No specific risk factors are known.

MECHANISM: Because didanosine is known to be acid labile, food may prolong didanosine contact with stomach acid, resulting in reduced bioavailability.

CLINICAL EVALUATION: Eight subjects received a single didanosine 375 mg chewable tablet while fasting and 5 minutes after a standard breakfast.[1] The area under the plasma concentration-time curve of didanosine was reduced 47% when the dose was taken with food. Peak plasma concentrations were nearly 54% less than those obtained during fasting. A similar reduction in didanosine bioavailability was noted when it was administered up to 2 hours after a meal.[2] The bioavailability of a sachet containing didanosine 375 mg, citrate-phosphate buffer 5 mg, and sucrose 14 mg was reduced from 31% to 17% when taken with a meal.[3] While neither study cited above evaluated clinical outcomes, it is likely that the efficacy of didanosine would be reduced by concomitant intake with food.

RELATED DRUGS: No information is available.

MANAGEMENT OPTIONS:

➡ *Circumvent/Minimize.* Administer didanosine in the fasting state (approximately 0.5 hour before or more than 2 hours after eating) to maximize its bioavailability.

➡ *Monitor.* If didanosine is coadministered with food, monitor patients for loss of antiviral efficacy.

REFERENCES:

1. Shyu WC, et al. Food-induced reduction in bioavailability of didanosine. *Clin Pharmacol Ther.* 1991;50(5, pt 1):503-507.

2. Knupp CA, et al. Effect of time of food administration on the bioavailability of didanosine from a chewable tablet formulation. *J Clin Pharmacol.* 1993;33(6):568-573.

3. Hartman NR, et al. Pharmacokinetics of 2′,3′-dideoxyinosine in patients with severe human immunodeficiency infection. II. The effects of different oral formulations and the presence of other medications. *Clin Pharmacol Ther.* 1991;50(3):278-285.

Didanosine (eg, *Videx*) 5

Foscarnet

SUMMARY: Based on a subchronic dosing study, didanosine and foscarnet do not appear to affect the pharmacokinetics of either drug.

RISK FACTORS: No specific risk factors are known.

MECHANISM: No interaction.

CLINICAL EVALUATION: Twelve HIV patients received 4 doses of foscarnet 90 mg/kg intravenously, 4 doses of didanosine 200 mg orally, or 4 doses of both agents.[1] No changes in the pharmacokinetics of didanosine or foscarnet were observed during combination therapy compared with single-drug administration.

RELATED DRUGS: No information is available.

MANAGEMENT OPTIONS: No interaction.

REFERENCES:

1. Aweeka FT, et al. Pharmacokinetics (PK) of concomitant foscarnet and didanosine in patients with HIV disease. *Clin Pharmacol Ther.* 1995;57:143.

Didanosine (eg, *Videx*)

Ganciclovir (*Cytovene*)

SUMMARY: Didanosine concentrations are increased during coadministration with ganciclovir; didanosine toxicity could occur in some patients.

RISK FACTORS: No specific risk factors are known.

MECHANISM: Not established. However, since both ganciclovir and didanosine are eliminated partially by renal secretion, this interaction could result from competitive inhibition of renal secretion.

CLINICAL EVALUATION: Eleven patients with human immunodeficiency virus were administered didanosine 200 mg twice daily alone and with oral ganciclovir 1 g 3 times a day, either simultaneously or separated by 2 hours.[1] Ganciclovir significantly affected the pharmacokinetics of didanosine in both instances. The area under the concentration-time curve of didanosine was increased over 70% while its peak plasma concentration increased nearly 60%. These changes in didanosine concentrations could lead to the development of toxicity (eg, pancreatitis, peripheral neuropathy).

RELATED DRUGS: No information is available.

MANAGEMENT OPTIONS:

➡ ***Monitor.*** Until further information regarding this interaction is available, monitor patients receiving didanosine carefully for toxicity, including peripheral neuropathy and pancreatitis, if ganciclovir is added.

REFERENCES:
1. Trapnell MD, et al. Altered didanosine pharmacokinetics with concomitant oral ganciclovir. *Clin Pharmacol Ther*. 1994;55:193.

Didanosine (eg, *Videx*)

Indinavir (*Crixivan*)

SUMMARY: Indinavir absorption can be reduced by coadministration of buffered didanosine; reduced antiviral efficacy is likely.

RISK FACTORS: No specific risk factors are known.

MECHANISM: Alkalinization of the stomach by didanosine buffers (magnesium hydroxide and dihydroaluminum sodium carbonate) reduces the absorption of indinavir.

CLINICAL EVALUATION: Although no data are provided, the manufacturer of didanosine reports an 84% decrease in indinavir plasma concentrations when the 2 drugs are coadministered.[1] This magnitude of an interaction is likely to inhibit the antiviral activity of indinavir. Taking a single didanosine (400 mg) dose 1 hour prior to a dose of indinavir (800 mg) eliminates the interaction even though the median gastric pH was measured to be somewhat elevated at 2.9.[2] The degree of gastric alkalinization needed to decrease the absorption of indinavir is unknown.

RELATED DRUGS: Other drugs that alkalinize the stomach will likely affect indinavir in a similar manner.

MANAGEMENT OPTIONS:

➡ *Circumvent/Minimize.* Administration of didanosine at least 1 hour before indinavir will minimize this interaction. Alternatively, the indinavir could be administered 2 hours prior to the didanosine. An enteric coated formulation of didanosine without buffers (*Videx EC*) does not affect indinavir absorption.[3]

➡ *Monitor.* If indinavir and buffered didanosine are coadministered, watch the patient for reduced indinavir plasma concentrations or antiviral activity.

REFERENCES:

1. Product information. Didanosine (*Videx*). Bristol-Myers Squibb Company. 2000.

2. Shelton MJ, et al. If taken 1 hour before indinavir (IDV), didanosine does not affect IDV exposure, despite persistent buffering effects. *Antimicrob Agents Chemother.* 2001;45:298-300.

3. Damle BD, et al. Lack of effect of simultaneously administered didanosine encapsulated enteric bead formulation (*Videx EC*) on oral absorption of indinavir, ketoconazole, or ciprofloxacin. *Antimicrob Agents Chemother.* 2002;46:385-391.

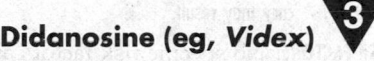

Didanosine (eg, *Videx*)

Itraconazole (*Sporanox*)

SUMMARY: Didanosine administration can significantly reduce the absorption of itraconazole; loss of antifungal efficacy may result.

RISK FACTORS: No specific risk factors are known.

MECHANISM: Alkalinization of the stomach by didanosine buffers (magnesium hydroxide and dihydroaluminum sodium carbonate) reduces the solubility and absorption of itraconazole.

CLINICAL EVALUATION: Six healthy subjects received a single 200 mg oral dose of itraconazole alone or with 300 mg of didanosine (ddI).[1] Four of the 6 subjects had detectable itraconazole in their serum following its administration without concomitant didanosine. Itraconazole was not detectable in any of the subjects following its administration with didanosine. A 25-year-old man taking itraconazole 200 mg twice daily for cryptococcal meningitis maintenance therapy developed a relapse of his meningitis after didanosine 200 mg twice daily was added to his regimen.[2] These reports suggest that the concomitant administration of didanosine and itraconazole might lead to a clinically important reduction in itraconazole plasma concentrations.

RELATED DRUGS: A similar effect of buffered didanosine on ketoconazole (eg, *Nizoral*) would be expected. Other drugs that alkalinize the stomach will affect itraconazole in a similar manner. Fluconazole (*Diflucan*) and voriconazole (*Vfend*) absorption does not appear to be affected by alkalinization of the stomach.

MANAGEMENT OPTIONS:

➡ *Circumvent/Minimize.* Administration of itraconazole at least 2 hours before didanosine will minimize this interaction. An enteric coated formulation of didanosine without buffers (*Videx EC*) would be unlikely to affect itraconazole absorption.[3] Consider using an alternative antifungal such as fluconazole or voriconazole.

➥ *Monitor.* If itraconazole- and didanosine-containing buffers are coadministered, watch the patient for loss of antifungal activity.

REFERENCES:

1. May DB, et al. Effect of simultaneous didanosine administration on itraconazole absorption in healthy volunteers. *Pharmacotherapy.* 1994;14:509-518.

2. Moreno F, et al. Itraconazole-didanosine excipient interaction. *JAMA.* 1993;269:1508.

3. Damle BD, et al. Lack of effect of simultaneously administered didanosine encapsulated enteric bead formulation (*Videx EC*) on oral absorption of indinavir, ketoconazole, or ciprofloxacin. *Antimicrob Agents Chemother.* 2002;46:385-391.

Didanosine (*Videx*)

Ketoconazole (eg, *Nizoral*)

SUMMARY: Didanosine administration can significantly reduce the absorption of ketoconazole; loss of antifungal efficacy may result.

RISK FACTORS: No specific risk factors are known.

MECHANISM: Alkalinization of the stomach by didanosine buffers (magnesium hydroxide and dihydroaluminum sodium carbonate) reduces the solubility and absorption of ketoconazole.

CLINICAL EVALUATION: Twelve patients with HIV were administered didanosine 375 mg twice daily alone, ketoconazole 200 mg alone, and the combination of both drugs with the ketoconazole administered 2 hours before the didanosine.[1] Each dosage regimen lasted 4 days. Ketoconazole caused a small (8%) reduction in the didanosine area under the concentration-time curve. Didanosine caused no changes in ketoconazole pharmacokinetics when administered 2 hours after ketoconazole. While not studied, the simultaneous administration of buffered didanosine and ketoconazole could result in a significant reduction in ketoconazole absorption.

RELATED DRUGS: Buffered didanosine has been reported to reduce the absorption of itraconazole (*Sporanox*). Other drugs that alkalinize the stomach will affect ketoconazole in a similar manner. Fluconazole (eg, *Diflucan*) and voriconazole (*Vfend*) absorption does not appear to be affected by alkalinization of the stomach.

MANAGEMENT OPTIONS:

➥ *Circumvent/Minimize.* Administration of ketoconazole at least 2 hours before didanosine will minimize this interaction. An enteric-coated formulation of didanosine without buffers (*Videx EC*) would be unlikely to affect ketoconazole absorption.[2] Consider using an alternative antifungal such as fluconazole or voriconazole.

➥ *Monitor.* If ketoconazole and buffered didanosine are coadministered, watch the patient for loss of antifungal activity.

REFERENCES:

1. Knupp CA, et al. Pharmacokinetics of didanosine and ketoconazole after coadministration to patients seropositive for the human immunodeficiency virus. *J Clin Pharmacol.* 1993;33:912-917.

2. Damle BD, et al. Lack of effect of simultaneously administered didanosine encapsulated enteric bead formulation (*Videx EC*) on oral absorption of indinavir, ketoconazole, or ciprofloxacin. *Antimicrob Agents Chemother.* 2002;46:385-391.

Didanosine (*Videx*)

Ranitidine (eg, *Zantac*)

SUMMARY: Ranitidine increased the serum concentration of didanosine slightly; and didanosine reduced ranitidine concentration slightly.

RISK FACTORS: No specific risk factors are known.

MECHANISM: Didanosine is acid labile and is formulated with citrate and phosphate buffers that enhance its bioavailability.[1] Coadministration with ranitidine may further enhance didanosine's bioavailability. The buffers present in the didanosine formulation may reduce the bioavailability of ranitidine.

CLINICAL EVALUATION: Didanosine 375 mg was administered alone to 12 patients infected with human immunodeficiency virus or 2 hours after a single 150 mg dose of ranitidine.[1] The area under the concentration-time curve (AUC) of didanosine was increased by ranitidine an average of 14%. This increase is unlikely to be clinically significant. The AUC of ranitidine fell 16% when didanosine was administered 2 hours after ranitidine compared with ranitidine alone. Again, this difference is unlikely to be clinically significant. The effect of chronic administration of these 2 agents is unknown.

RELATED DRUGS: The effects of other H$_2$-receptor antagonists (eg, cimetidine [eg, *Tagamet*], famotidine [eg, *Pepcid*], nizatidine [eg, *Axid*]) or proton pump inhibitors (eg, omeprazole [eg, *Prilosec*], lansoprazole [*Prevacid*]) on didanosine pharmacokinetics are unknown, but these drugs would be expected to interact in a similar manner if increased gastrointestinal pH is the mechanism for the interaction.

MANAGEMENT OPTIONS: No specific action is required, but be alert for evidence of the interaction.

REFERENCES:
1. Knupp CA, et al. Pharmacokinetic-interaction study of didanosine and ranitidine in patients seropositive for human immunodeficiency virus. *Antimicrob Agents Chemother*. 1992;36:2075-2079.

Didanosine (*Videx*)

Rifabutin (*Mycobutin*)

SUMMARY: Rifabutin does not alter didanosine concentrations significantly.

RISK FACTORS: No specific risk factors are known.

MECHANISM: Not established.

CLINICAL EVALUATION: Twelve patients taking didanosine 167 or 250 mg twice daily received rifabutin (300 mg/day in 8 patients and 600 mg/day in 4 patients) concomitantly for 12 days.[1] Didanosine plasma concentrations were measured the day before, and on the last day of, rifabutin administration. The area under the concentration-time curve of didanosine increased 13%, and peak didanosine concentrations increased 17% following rifabutin administration. These changes were not statistically significant and would not be expected to alter patient response to didanosine.

RELATED DRUGS: No information is available.

MANAGEMENT OPTIONS: No specific action is required, but be alert for evidence of the interaction.

REFERENCES:
1. Sahai J, et al. Rifabutin and didanosine interaction in AIDS patients. *Clin Pharmacol Ther.* 1993;53:197.

 Didanosine (*Videx*)

Ritonavir (*Norvir*)

SUMMARY: The coadministration of ritonavir and didanosine results in a small reduction in didanosine serum concentration that is unlikely to be of clinical significance.

RISK FACTORS: No specific risk factors are known.

MECHANISM: Ritonavir appears to reduce the bioavailability of didanosine.

CLINICAL EVALUATION: Twelve human immunodeficiency virus-positive men received ritonavir 600 mg every 12 hours, didanosine 200 mg every 12 hours, or the combination.[1] Each drug regimen was administered for 4 days. Didanosine administration did not change the serum concentrations of ritonavir compared with ritonavir administered alone. The peak concentration and area under the concentration-time curve of didanosine were reduced 16% and 13%, respectively, during ritonavir coadministration. The minor changes in didanosine serum concentrations observed in this study would not be expected to reduce the efficacy of didanosine.

RELATED DRUGS: The effects of other protease inhibitors on didanosine have not been reported. The labeling for indinavir (*Crixivan*) advises against taking it with didanosine because indinavir requires normal gastric pH for optimal absorption.[2]

MANAGEMENT OPTIONS: No specific action is required, but be alert for evidence of the interaction.

REFERENCES:
1. Cato A, et al. Evaluation of the pharmacokinetic interaction between ritonavir and didanosine. *Clin Pharmacol Ther.* 1996;59:144.
2. *Crixivan* [package insert]. White House Station, NJ: Merck and Co., Inc.; 1996.

5 **Didanosine (*Videx*)**

Stavudine (*Zerit*)

SUMMARY: Didanosine and stavudine coadministration does not affect the pharmacokinetics of either agent.

RISK FACTORS: No specific risk factors are known.

MECHANISM: No interaction.

CLINICAL EVALUATION: Ten patients with human immunodeficiency virus were administered single doses of didanosine 100 mg and stavudine 40 mg.[1] Each patient then received didanosine 100 mg twice daily and stavudine 40 mg twice daily for 9 doses. No differences in didanosine or stavudine pharmacokinetics were noted during coadministration compared with individual dosing.

RELATED DRUGS: No information is available.

MANAGEMENT OPTIONS: No interaction.

REFERENCES:

1. Seifert RD, et al. Pharmacokinetics of co-administered didanosine and stavudine in HIV-seropositive men. *Br J Clin Pharmacol.* 1994;38:405-410.

Didanosine (*Videx*) ▼ ③

Tenofovir (*Viread*)

SUMMARY: Tenofovir administration increases didanosine plasma concentrations; increased didanosine toxicity may occur.

RISK FACTORS:

➡ **Concurrent Diseases.** Patients with renal dysfunction may be particularly susceptible to the adverse effects of this interaction.

MECHANISM: Unknown. It appears that tenofovir increases the absorption of didanosine; no effect of tenofovir was noted on didanosine renal elimination.

CLINICAL EVALUATION: The coadministration of didanosine 250 or 400 mg 1 hour before tenofovir 300 mg daily for 7 days resulted in a mean increase in didanosine area under the plasma concentration time curve (AUC) of 44%. In a second study, 28 healthy subjects received didanosine 400 mg enteric-coated capsules followed 2 hours later by tenofovir 300 mg.[1] Didanosine mean peak concentrations and AUC both increased approximately 50% to 65% with tenofovir administration. Administering the drugs simultaneously with a meal did not reduce the effect of tenofovir on didanosine. Several cases of didanosine toxicity including acute renal failure, pancreatitis, and lactic acidosis have been reported in patients receiving tenofovir and didanosine.[2-5]

RELATED DRUGS: Ganciclovir (eg, *Cytovene*) and valganciclovir (*Valcyte*) have been reported to have a similar effect on didanosine.

MANAGEMENT OPTIONS:

➡ **Consider Alternative.** Based on the increased risk of didanosine toxicity, select alternative agents whenever possible.

➡ **Monitor.** If didanosine and tenofovir are coadministered, reduce the dose of didanosine. Because didanosine and tenofovir are eliminated by the kidneys, avoid the combination in patients with renal dysfunction. Be alert for evidence of didanosine toxicity, including pancreatitis and hepatitis.

REFERENCES:

1. Pecora Fulco P, et al. Effect of tenofovir on didanosine absorption in patients with HIV. *Ann Pharmacother.* 2003;37:1325-1328.
2. Murphy MD, et al. Fatal lactic acidosis and acute renal failure after addition of tenofovir to an antiretroviral regimen containing didanosine. *Clin Infect Dis.* 2003;36:1082-1085.
3. Callens S, et al. Pancreatitis in an HIV-infected person on a tenofovir, didanosine and stavudine containing highly active antiretroviral treatment. *J Infect.* 2003;47:188-189.
4. Martinez E, et al. Pancreatic toxic effects associated with co-administration of didanosine and tenofovir in HIV-infected adults. *Lancet.* 2004;364:65-67.
5. Blanchard JN, et al. Pancreatitis with didanosine and tenofovir disoproxil fumarate. *Clin Infect Dis.* 2003;37:e57-62.

4   Didanosine (*Videx*)

Zidovudine (*Retrovir*)

SUMMARY: Zidovudine modestly reduced the serum concentration of didanosine; the clinical significance of this change is probably limited.

RISK FACTORS: No specific risk factors are known.

MECHANISM: Not established.

CLINICAL EVALUATION: Eight children with human immunodeficiency virus received single doses of zidovudine 200 mg/m^2, didanosine 100 mg/m^2, and the combination on separate occasions.[1] Didanosine had no effect on the pharmacokinetics of zidovudine; however, the administration of zidovudine resulted in a 19% reduction in the area under the concentration-time curve of didanosine. This degree of reduction is not likely to alter the response to didanosine. The effects of chronic drug administration are unknown.

RELATED DRUGS: No information is available.

MANAGEMENT OPTIONS: No specific action is required, but be alert for evidence of the interaction.

REFERENCES:
1. Gibb D, et al. Pharmacokinetics of zidovudine and dideoxyinosine alone and in combination in children with HIV infection. *Br J Clin Pharmacol*. 1995;39:527-530.

5   Diethylpropion (eg, *Tenuate*)

Guanethidine (*Ismelin*)

SUMMARY: Preliminary data from a few patients indicate that diethylpropion does not affect the antihypertensive response to guanethidine.

RISK FACTORS: No specific risk factors are known.

MECHANISM: Not established.

CLINICAL EVALUATION: In 32 obese hypertensive patients receiving various antihypertensives (including guanethidine in some patients), diethylpropion reportedly did not interfere with the antihypertensive response.[1] Earlier animal studies had indicated that diethylpropion may inhibit the antihypertensive response to guanethidine.[2] More study is needed.

RELATED DRUGS: Guanadrel (*Hylorel*) is pharmacodynamically similar to guanethidine and probably has similar interactions.

MANAGEMENT OPTIONS: No interaction.

REFERENCES:
1. Seedat YK, et al. Letter: Diethylpropion hydrochloride (*Tenuate Dospan*) in the treatment of obese hypertensive patients. *S Afr Med J*. 1974;48:569.
2. Day MD, et al. Antagonism of guanethidine and bretylium by various agents. *Lancet*. 1962;2:1282-1283.

Diethylpropion (eg, *Tenuate*) 5

Methyldopa

SUMMARY: Diethylpropion does not appear to affect the response to methyldopa.

RISK FACTORS: No specific risk factors are known.

MECHANISM: No interaction.

CLINICAL EVALUATION: In 32 obese hypertensive patients (some of whom were receiving methyldopa), diethylpropion reportedly did not interfere with the antihypertensive response.[1] More study is needed to confirm these preliminary findings.

RELATED DRUGS: No information is available.

MANAGEMENT OPTIONS: No interaction.

REFERENCES:
1. Seedat YK, et al. Letter: Diethylpropion by hydrochloride (*Tenuate Dospan*) in the treatment of obese hypertensive patients. *S Afr Med J.* 1974;48:569.

Diflunisal (eg, *Dolobid*)   2

Warfarin (eg, *Coumadin*)

SUMMARY: Limited data indicate the diflunisal may enhance the hypoprothrombinemic response to oral anticoagulants in some patients; caution during cotherapy with these drugs also is required because of the detrimental effects of diflunisal on the gastric mucosa and platelet function.

RISK FACTORS:

➡ **Concurrent Diseases.** Patients with peptic ulcer disease or a history of gastrointestinal (GI) bleeding are probably at greater risk.

MECHANISM: Not established. Displacement from plasma protein binding may be involved. Diflunisal also can inhibit platelet function and cause gastric erosions.

CLINICAL EVALUATION: Five healthy subjects received a subtherapeutic dose of warfarin for 6 weeks; diflunisal 500 mg twice daily was added during the third and fourth weeks.[1] The hypoprothrombinemic response to warfarin was not affected during diflunisal administration; however, following discontinuation of the diflunisal, the hypoprothrombinemic response to warfarin was reduced substantially over several days and lasted for at least 2 weeks. Because this study used healthy subjects receiving subtherapeutic warfarin doses, the results do not apply necessarily to the clinical situation. In another study, the prothrombin time increased in 3 out of 6 patients stabilized on acenocoumarol when diflunisal 375 mg twice daily was added,[2] but details were not presented. Although diflunisal's effect appears to be less than that of aspirin on platelet function and the GI mucosa,[3-7] large doses of diflunisal can impair platelet function,[5] and the drug has been reported to cause GI hemorrhage occasionally.[3,8] In a retrospective cohort study, hospitalizations for hemorrhagic peptic ulcer disease were about 13 times higher in patients receiving warfarin plus a nonsteroidal anti-inflammatory drug (NSAID) than in patients receiving neither drug.[9]

RELATED DRUGS: All NSAIDs inhibit platelet function, cause gastric erosions, and probably increase the risk of GI bleeding. Some NSAIDs, however, such as ibuprofen (eg, *Advil*), naproxen (eg, *Naprosyn*), or may be less likely to increase oral anticoagulant-induced hypoprothrombinemia than other NSAIDs. Acenocoumarol appears to interact with diflunisal similarly.

MANAGEMENT OPTIONS:

➡ *Avoid Unless Benefit Outweighs Risk.* Since all NSAIDs probably increase the risk of GI bleeding in patients on oral anticoagulants, use the combination only after careful consideration of the benefit versus risk. If an NSAID must be used with an oral anticoagulant, it would be prudent to use NSAIDs that are unlikely to affect the hypoprothrombinemic response to oral anticoagulants (see Related Drugs). If the NSAID is being used as an analgesic or antipyretic, acetaminophen is probably safer to use with oral anticoagulants. Nonacetylated salicylates (eg, choline salicylate, magnesium salicylate, salsalate, sodium salicylate) are probably also safer with oral anti coagulants than NSAIDs, since such salicylates have minimal effects on platelet function and the gastric mucosa.

➡ *Monitor.* If any NSAID is used with an oral anticoagulant, carefully monitor the prothrombin time and watch for evidence of bleeding, especially from the GI tract.

REFERENCES:

1. Serlin MJ, et al. Interaction between diflunisal and warfarin. *Clin Pharmacol Ther.* 1980;28:493.

2. Tempero KF, et al. Diflunisal. A review of pharmacokinetic and pharmacodynamic properties, drug interactions and special tolerability studies in humans. *Br J Clin Pharmacol.* 1977;4:31S.

3. Davies RO. Review of the animal and clinical pharmacology of diflunisal. *Pharmacotherapy.* 1983;2(Suppl. 1):9S.

4. Rider JA. Comparison of fecal blood loss after use of aspirin and diflunisal. *Pharmacotherapy.* 1983;3(Suppl. 1):61S.

5. Green D, et al. Effects of diflunisal on platelet function and fetal blood loss. *Clin Pharmacol Ther.* 1981;30:378.

6. Petrillo M. Diflunisal, aspirin, and gastric mucosa. *Lancet.* 1979;2:638.

7. Ghosh ML, et al. Platelet aggregation in patients treated with diflunisal. *Curr Med Res Opin.* 1980;6:510.

8. Admani AK, et al. Gastrointestinal haemorrhage associated with diflunisal. *Lancet.* 1979;1:1247.

9. Shorr RI, et al. Concurrent use of nonsteroidal anti-inflammatory drugs and oral anticoagulants places elderly persons at high risk for hemorrhagic peptic ulcer disease. *Arch Intern Med.* 1993;153:1665.

Digitoxin†

Phenobarbital (eg, *Solfoton*)

SUMMARY: Phenobarbital administration may reduce digitoxin serum concentrations, but it is unknown how often this decreases the therapeutic response to digitoxin.

RISK FACTORS: No specific risk factors are known.

MECHANISM: Phenobarbital appears to enhance the metabolism of digitoxin, presumably caused by induction of hepatic microsomal enzymes.

CLINICAL EVALUATION: Decreased plasma digitoxin concentrations and a shortened digitoxin half-life have been demonstrated when phenobarbital is given to patients receiving digitoxin.[1] The increased conversion of digitoxin to digoxin and other metabolites could decrease the therapeutic effect, since digoxin has a much shorter half-life than digitoxin. Phenobarbital 60 mg 3 times a day has been reported to reduce steady-state serum digitoxin concentrations by 50%.[2] In a third study,[3] 10 subjects each received 0.4, 0.8, or 1 mg single doses of digitoxin. Plasma concentrations were measured repeatedly for 90 minutes following the digitoxin dose alone and after a week of pretreatment with phenobarbital 100 mg 3 times a day. Phenobarbital had no effect on digitoxin plasma concentrations during the 90 minutes following the dose. This sampling interval is too short to assess the effects of phenobarbital on the elimination of digitoxin but probably indicates no effect of phenobarbital on digitoxin absorption.

RELATED DRUGS: Digoxin (eg, *Lanoxin*) elimination is not likely to be affected by barbiturates to the same degree as digitoxin since it primarily is excreted renally.

MANAGEMENT OPTIONS:

➡ *Consider Alternative.* Digoxin would seem less likely to be affected by enzyme induction and may be preferable to digitoxin in patients taking chronic phenobarbital or other barbiturates.

➡ *Monitor.* Until further information is available, evaluate patients receiving digitoxin and a barbiturate for underdigitalization, and increase the digitoxin dose if necessary.

REFERENCES:

1. Jelliffe RW, et al. Effect of phenobarbital on digitoxin metabolism. *Clin Res*. 1966;14:160.
2. Solomon HM, et al. Interactions between digitoxin and other drugs in man. *Am Heart J*. 1972;83:277.
3. Kaldor A, et al. Interaction of heart glycosides and phenobarbital. *Int J Clin Pharmacol*. 1975;12:403.

† Not available in the United States.

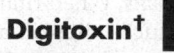

Digitoxin† 4

Phenylbutazone

SUMMARY: A single case report suggests that phenylbutazone may reduce the serum concentration of digitoxin.

RISK FACTORS: No specific risk factors are known.

MECHANISM: Not established. Phenylbutazone might interfere with the absorption of digitoxin. It seems unlikely that phenylbutazone increases digitoxin metabolism, since it is known to reduce the metabolism of other drugs.

CLINICAL EVALUATION: A decrease in plasma digitoxin concentrations was observed in 1 patient when phenylbutazone was administered.[1] Also, the ability of phenylbutazone or other nonsteroidal anti-inflammatory drugs (NSAIDs) to induce sodium retention should be considered carefully when this drug is contemplated for a patient receiving digitalis glycosides for congestive heart failure.

RELATED DRUGS: Other NSAIDs have been reported to increase serum digoxin concentrations. The effect of phenylbutazone on other digitalis glycosides is unknown.

MANAGEMENT OPTIONS: No specific action is required, but be alert for evidence of the interaction.

REFERENCES:

1. Solomon HM, et al. Interactions between digitoxin and other drugs in vitro and in vivo. *Ann NY Acad Sci*. 1971;179:362.

† Not available in the United States.

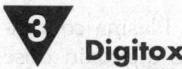

Digitoxin†

Rifampin (eg, *Rifadin*)

SUMMARY: Rifampin reduces the serum concentration of digoxin and digitoxin.

RISK FACTORS: No specific risk factors are known.

MECHANISM: Rifampin appears to enhance the hepatic metabolism of digitalis glycosides, presumably by inducing hepatic microsomal enzymes. Rifampin also possibly could increase the biliary secretion of digitalis.

CLINICAL EVALUATION: In a study of 6 healthy volunteers, the half-life of digitoxin 1 mg IV was reduced considerably (288 hours to 76 hours) by pretreatment with rifampin 1.2 g oral for 8 days.[1] Case reports of rifampin-induced reductions in serum digitoxin have appeared.[2,3] While rifampin also has been reported to reduce serum digoxin concentrations to subtherapeutic levels following oral or IV digoxin administration, expect digitoxin to be affected more than digoxin.[4,5]

RELATED DRUGS: Digoxin (eg, *Lanoxin*) is affected similarly by rifampin.

MANAGEMENT OPTIONS:

➡ *Circumvent/Minimize.* Dosage adjustments of digitalis glycosides (especially digitoxin) likely will be necessary when rifampin is added to or removed from a dosage regimen.

➡ *Monitor.* When rifampin and digitalis glycosides are used concomitantly, be alert for reduced digoxin and digitoxin efficacy.

REFERENCES:

1. Zilly W, et al. Pharmacokinetic interactions with rifampicin. *Clin Pharmacokinet*. 1977;2:61-70.
2. Boman G, et al. Acute cardiac failure during treatment with digitoxin—an interaction with rifampicin. *Br J Clin Pharmacol*. 1980;10:89-90.
3. Poor DM, et al. Interaction of rifampin and digitoxin. *Arch Intern Med*. 1983;143:599.
4. Gault H, et al. Digoxin-rifampin interaction. *Clin Pharmacol Ther*. 1984;35:750-754.
5. Novi C, et al. Rifampin and digoxin: possible drug interaction in a dialysis patient. *JAMA*. 1980;244:2521-2522.

† Not available in the United States.

Digoxin (eg, *Lanoxin*)

Diltiazem (eg, *Cardizem*)

SUMMARY: Diltiazem increases digoxin serum concentrations; digoxin toxicity may result.

RISK FACTORS: No specific risk factors are known.

MECHANISM: Diltiazem appears to inhibit the elimination of digoxin and may potentiate its negative dromotropic effects.

CLINICAL EVALUATION: Diltiazem may increase digoxin concentrations up to 50% in some, but not all, patients.[1-5] An increased risk of digoxin toxicity is likely to occur, particularly if high doses of diltiazem are administered.[2]

RELATED DRUGS: Verapamil (eg, *Calan*) and nitrendipine (investigational, *Baypress*) appear to reduce digoxin elimination. Digitoxin† is likely to be affected similarly.

Nifedipine (eg, *Procardia*),[1,2,6-8] isradipine (*DynaCirc*),[9] nicardipine (eg, *Cardene*),[10] felodipine (*Plendil*),[11] and amlodipine (eg, *Norvasc*)[12] do not appear to increase digoxin concentration.

MANAGEMENT OPTIONS:

➡ **Consider Alternative.** Nifedipine, isradipine, nicardipine, felodipine, and amlodipine do not appear to increase digoxin concentration and may be possible alternatives.

➡ **Circumvent/Minimize.** Digoxin dosages may need to be reduced when diltiazem is added to patients stabilized on digoxin.

➡ **Monitor.** Monitor patients for evidence of increased serum digitalis effects (eg, bradycardia, gastrointestinal upset, heart block, mental changes) in the presence of calcium channel blocker therapy.

REFERENCES:

1. Rameis H, et al. The diltiazem-digoxin interaction. *Clin Pharmacol Ther*. 1984;36:183-189.
2. Clarke WR, et al. Potentially serious drug interactions secondary to high-dose diltiazem used in the treatment of pulmonary hypertension. *Pharmacotherapy*. 1993;13:402-405.
3. Kuhlmann J. Effects of nifedipine and diltiazem on plasma levels and renal excretion of beta-acetyldigoxin. *Clin Pharmacol Ther*. 1985;37:150-156.
4. Boden WE, et al. No increase in serum digoxin concentration with high-dose diltiazem. *Am J Med*. 1986;81:425-428.
5. Andrejak M, et al. Diltiazem increases steady state digoxin serum levels in patients with cardiac disease. *J Clin Pharmacol*. 1987;27:967-970.
6. Belz GG, et al. Digoxin plasma concentrations and nifedipine. *Lancet*. 1981;1:844.
7. Schwartz JB, et al. Effect of nifedipine on serum digoxin concentration and renal digoxin clearance. *Clin Pharmacol Ther*. 1984;36:19-24.
8. Hutt HJ, et al. Dose-dependence of the nifedipine/digoxin interaction? *Arch Toxicol Suppl*. 1986;9:209-212.
9. Rodin SM, et al. Comparative effects of verapamil and isradipine on steady-state digoxin kinetics. *Clin Pharmacol Ther*. 1988;43:668-672.
10. Debruyne D, et al. Nicardipine does not significantly affect serum digoxin concentrations at the steady state of patients with congestive heart failure. *Int J Clin Pharmacol Res*. 1989;9:15-19.
11. Kirch W, et al. The felodipine/digoxin interaction. A placebo-controlled study in patients with heart failure. *Br J Clin Pharmacol*. 1988;26:644P.
12. Schwartz JB. Effects of amlodipine on steady-state digoxin concentrations and renal digoxin clearance. *J Cardiovasc Pharmacol*. 1988;12:1-5.

† Not available in the United States.

Digoxin (eg, *Lanoxin*) 4

Dipyridamole (*Persantine*)

SUMMARY: Dipyridamole administration results in a modest increase in digoxin concentrations; digoxin toxicity appears to be unlikely.

RISK FACTORS: No specific risk factors are known.

MECHANISM: Dipyridamole appears to inhibit the activity of p-glycoprotein, thus increasing the absorption of digoxin.

CLINICAL EVALUATION: Twelve subjects received dipyridamole 300 mg daily or placebo in divided doses, for 2 days.[1] On the third day, dipyridamole 150 mg or placebo was administered with the a single oral dose of digoxin 0.5 mg. The mean area under the plasma concentration-time curve (AUC) of digoxin over 24 hours was increased 13%. Most of the effect of dipyridamole on digoxin AUC was noted during the first 4 hours after administration. A limited increase in the renal clearance of digoxin was observed following dipyridamole administration. While the effect of chronic dipyridamole administration on digoxin plasma concentration is unknown, the results of this study suggest that the interaction will be of limited effect in most patients.

RELATED DRUGS: Digitoxin may be affected in a similar manner by dipyridamole.

MANAGEMENT OPTIONS:

➡ *Monitor.* Be alert for altered digoxin effects in patients who initiate or discontinue dipyridamole.

REFERENCES:

1. Verstuyft C, et al. Dipyridamole enhances digoxin bioavailability via P-glycoprotein inhibition.*Clin Pharmacol Ther.* 2003;73:51-60.

Digoxin (eg, *Lanoxin*)

Disopyramide (eg, *Norpace*)

SUMMARY: Disopyramide appears to have a minimal effect on digoxin pharmacokinetics but may somewhat inhibit digitalis-induced increases in cardiac contractility.

RISK FACTORS: No specific risk factors are known.

MECHANISM: Disopyramide may reduce positive inotropic effects of digoxin caused by its intrinsic negative inotropic activity.

CLINICAL EVALUATION: In 3 studies involving a total of 24 patients, disopyramide did not alter the disposition of digoxin.[1-3] In a subsequent study, however, the volume of distribution and half-life of digoxin were reduced in 5 healthy men given disopyramide 600 mg/day.[4] No change in the steady-state serum digoxin concentration was noted in this latter study since clearance did not change.

RELATED DRUGS: Disopyramide may cause a similar reaction with digitoxin[†].

MANAGEMENT OPTIONS: No specific action is required, but be alert for evidence of the interaction.

REFERENCES:

1. Leahey EB, et al. The effect of quinidine and other antiarrhythmic drugs on serum digoxin. A prospective study. *Ann Intern Med.* 1980;92:605-608.

2. Doering W. Quinidine-digoxin interaction. Pharmacokinetics, underlying mechanism and clinical implications. *N Engl J Med.* 1979;301:400-404.

3. Wellens HJ, et al. Effect of oral disopyramide on serum digoxin and disopyramide. A prospective study. *Am Heart J.* 1980;100:934-935.

4. Risler T, et al. On the interaction between digoxin and disopyramide. *Clin Pharmacol Ther.* 1983;34:176-180.

† Not available in the United States.

Digoxin (eg, *Lanoxin*)

Dronedarone (*Multaq*)

SUMMARY: Dronedarone increases the plasma concentration of digoxin; increased digoxin response is likely to occur.

RISK FACTORS: No specific risk factors are known.

MECHANISM: Dronedarone appears to inhibit the P-glycoprotein–mediated renal and non-renal elimination of digoxin. Dronedarone may also potentiate the negative dromotropic (conduction) effects of digoxin.

CLINICAL EVALUATION: While specific data are limited, the manufacturer of dronedarone notes that the coadministration of dronedarone with digoxin increased the mean area under the plasma concentration-time curve of digoxin approximately 2.5-fold.[1] Pending further data, observe patients receiving dronedarone and digoxin for increased digoxin effects, including arrhythmias, anorexia, nausea, and mental changes.

RELATED DRUGS: Amiodarone (eg, *Cordarone*) is also known to inhibit the elimination of digoxin.

MANAGEMENT OPTIONS:

➡ *Monitor.* Monitor patients taking dronedarone and digoxin for signs of digoxin toxicity and check digoxin plasma concentrations if dronedarone is added to or removed from their drug regimen.

REFERENCES:
1. *Multaq* [package insert]. Bridgewater, NJ: Sanofi-Aventis; 2009.

Digoxin (eg, *Lanoxin*)

Edrophonium (eg, *Enlon*)

SUMMARY: One case of asystole following edrophonium administration to a digitalized patient has been reported.

RISK FACTORS: No specific risk factors are known.

MECHANISM: It is proposed that the additive vagomimetic effects of digitalis glycosides and edrophonium may cause excessive slowing of heart rate.

CLINICAL EVALUATION: An 81-year-old woman taking large doses of digoxin developed increasing atrioventricular block, bradycardia, and, finally, asystole when edrophonium 10 mg intravenous was given.[1] It has been proposed that the adverse cardiac response represented the combined effects of digoxin and edrophonium.

RELATED DRUGS: No information is available.

MANAGEMENT OPTIONS: No specific action is required, but be alert for evidence of the interaction.

REFERENCES:
1. Gould L, et al. Cardiac arrest during edrophonium administration. *Am Heart J.* 1971;81(3):437-438.

Digoxin (eg, *Lanoxin*)

Erythromycin (eg, *Ery-Tab*)

SUMMARY: Erythromycin administration increases the plasma concentration of digoxin. Digoxin toxicity, including nausea, malaise, visual changes, and arrhythmias, may occur.

RISK FACTORS: No specific risk factors are known.

MECHANISM: Erythromycin may enhance the absorption of digoxin and/or reduce its renal and biliary elimination by inhibiting P-glycoprotein in the intestine, kidney, and liver.

CLINICAL EVALUATION: In a number of case studies, erythromycin has been reported to increase the plasma concentration of digoxin.[1-5] Digoxin concentrations may increase 100% in some cases. A larger effect has been noted with oral digoxin administration compared with intravenous digoxin.[6] This may be caused by erythromycin increasing the oral bioavailability of digoxin by inhibition of intestinal P-glycoprotein.

RELATED DRUGS: Digitoxin[†] is likely affected in a similar manner by erythromycin. Clarithromycin (eg, *Biaxin*) also increases digoxin plasma concentrations. There are few data on the effect of other macrolides on digoxin.

MANAGEMENT OPTIONS:

➥ *Consider Alternative.* Select an antibiotic known to have no effect on digoxin concentrations in patients receiving long-term digoxin therapy. If azithromycin (eg, *Zithromax*) or dirithromycin[†] is used, monitor for changes in digoxin concentrations.

➥ *Monitor.* In patients receiving digoxin, monitor for changes in digoxin concentrations when erythromycin is added to or removed from their drug regimen.

REFERENCES:

1. Doherty JE. A digoxin-antibiotic drug interaction. *N Engl J Med.* 1981;305(14):827-828.
2. Morton MR, et al. Erythromycin-induced digoxin toxicity. *DICP.* 1989;23(9):668-670.
3. Marik PE, et al. A case series of hospitalized patients with elevated digoxin levels. *Am J Med.* 1998;105(2):110-115.
4. Sutton A, et al. Digoxin toxicity and erythromycin. *BMJ.* 1989;298(6680):1101.
5. Maxwell DL, et al. Digoxin toxicity due to interaction of digoxin with erythromycin. *BMJ.* 1989;298(6673):572.
6. Rengelshausen J, et al. Contribution of increased oral bioavailability and reduced nonglomerular renal clearance of digoxin to the digoxin-clarithromycin interaction. *Br J Clin Pharmacol.* 2003;56(1):32-38.

† Not available in the United States.

Digoxin (eg, *Lanoxin*)

Exenatide (*Byetta*)

SUMMARY: Exenatide administration causes a small reduction in digoxin peak plasma concentrations; no change in digoxin clinical effect is anticipated.

RISK FACTORS: No specific risk factors are known.

MECHANISM: Exenatide is known to slow gastric motility, possibly resulting in an increase in digoxin degradation.

CLINICAL EVALUATION: The coadministration of exenatide 10 mcg twice daily decreased the peak plasma concentration of digoxin 17% and delayed its time to maximum concentration by 2.5 hours. No change in the steady-state area under the plasma concentration-time curve of digoxin was noted. These changes are not expected to produce a change in the clinical response to digoxin when exenatide is coadministered.[1]

RELATED DRUGS: None known.

MANAGEMENT OPTIONS:

➡ *Monitor.* Standard monitoring of digoxin response or plasma concentrations is adequate in patients receiving exenatide.

REFERENCES:

1. *Byetta* [package insert]. San Diego, CA: Amylin Pharmaceuticals, Inc; 2007.

Digoxin (eg, *Lanoxin*)

Famciclovir (eg, *Famvir*)

SUMMARY: Famciclovir administration produces a small increase in digoxin's peak plasma concentration; however, this change is not likely to enhance the patient response to digoxin.

RISK FACTORS: No specific risk factors are known.

MECHANISM: Not established.

CLINICAL EVALUATION: Twelve healthy men each received oral digoxin 0.5 mg alone or with famciclovir 500 mg.[1] The peak digoxin concentration increased 18% during famciclovir administration. While this was a single-dose study, it is not likely that the effect would be exacerbated significantly by long-term famciclovir dosing. No other digoxin pharmacokinetic parameters (area under the plasma concentration-time curve, trough concentration, time to peak concentration) were altered during famciclovir administration. The increase in digoxin peak concentration is not likely to result in any change in patient response.

RELATED DRUGS: No information is available.

MANAGEMENT OPTIONS: No specific action is required, but be alert for evidence of the interaction.

REFERENCES:

1. Pue MA, et al. An investigation of the potential interaction between digoxin and famciclovir in healthy male volunteers. *Br J Clin Pharmacol.* 1993;36:177P.

Digoxin (eg, *Lanoxin*)

Flecainide (eg, *Tambocor*)

SUMMARY: Flecainide may increase the serum digoxin concentration slightly; however, a change in clinical response is unlikely.

RISK FACTORS: No specific risk factors are known.

MECHANISM: Not established.

CLINICAL EVALUATION: When flecainide 200 mg twice daily was administered to 15 healthy subjects stabilized on digoxin 0.25 mg/day, trough digoxin concentrations increased 24%. PR intervals were increased slightly in some subjects when the 2 drugs were coadministered.[1] These results are similar to those reported in 8 healthy subjects who received flecainide 200 mg twice daily with and without single doses of digoxin.[2] In a study of 10 patients with heart failure who were receiving chronic digoxin and flecainide 100 or 200 mg twice daily for 1 to 4 weeks, no changes in digoxin concentrations were observed.[3]

RELATED DRUGS: It is likely that digitoxin[†] would interact in a similar manner.

MANAGEMENT OPTIONS: No specific action is required, but be alert for evidence of the interaction.

REFERENCES:

1. Weeks CE, et al. The effect of flecainide acetate, a new antiarrhythmic, on plasma digoxin levels. *J Clin Pharmacol*. 1986;26(1):27-31.
2. Tjandramaga TB, et al. Oral digoxin pharmacokinetics during multiple-dose flecainide treatment. *Arch Int Pharmacodyn Ther*. 1982;260(2):302-303.
3. McQuinn RL, et al. Digoxin levels in patients with congestive heart failure are not altered by flecainide. *Clin Pharmacol Ther*. 1988;43:150.

† Not available in the United States.

Digoxin (eg, *Lanoxin*)

Furosemide (eg, *Lasix*)

SUMMARY: Diuretic-induced hypokalemia may increase the risk of digitalis toxicity.

RISK FACTORS: No specific risk factors are known.

MECHANISM: Diuretics can produce potassium deficiency, which can predispose patients to digitalis toxicity and reduce digoxin renal clearance.[1] The drug-induced magnesium deficiency that can occur following diuretic therapy also may contribute to digitalis toxicity. The renal clearance of digoxin may be reduced by furosemide.[2]

CLINICAL EVALUATION: Within a given range of serum digoxin concentrations, the incidence of digitalis toxicity increases as serum potassium (and probably serum magnesium) levels decrease.[1,3-6] However, many patients on potassium-losing diuretics (eg, ethacrynic acid [*Edecrin*], bumetanide [eg, *Bumex*], chlorthalidone [eg, *Hygroton*], metolazone [eg, *Zaroxolyn*] , thiazides) do not develop clinically important potassium depletion for a variety of reasons such as low doses of diuretics and adequate potassium intake. Furosemide has been noted to increase digoxin concentrations.[7,8]

RELATED DRUGS: Ethacrynic acid, bumetanide, chlorthalidone, metolazone, and thiazides interact similarly. Torsemide (eg, *Demadex*) may produce a similar increased risk of digoxin toxicity. Patients taking digitoxin[†] also are at risk.

MANAGEMENT OPTIONS:

➡ *Consider Alternative.* Potassium-sparing diuretics can be considered as alternatives to potassium-wasting agents; however, note the interactions with amiloride (*Midamor*) and spironolactone (eg, *Aldactone*).

➥ *Monitor.* Monitor the potassium and magnesium status of patients on concomitant diuretic-digitalis therapy. Undertake replacement potassium or magnesium therapy if needed. Be alert for increased digoxin effects.

REFERENCES:

1. Steiness E. Suppression of renal excretion of digoxin in hypokalemic patients. *Clin Pharmacol Ther.* 1978;23(5):511-514.
2. Tsutsumi E, et al. Effect of furosemide on serum clearance and renal excretion of digoxin. *J Clin Pharmacol.* 1979;19(4):200-204.
3. Beller GA, et al. Correlation of serum magnesium levels and cardiac digitalis intoxication. *Am J Cardiol.* 1974;33(2):225-229.
4. Young IS, et al. Magnesium status and digoxin toxicity. *Br J Clin Pharmacol.* 1991;32(6):717-721.
5. Seller RH, et al. Digitalis toxicity and hypomagnesemia. *Am Heart J.* 1970;79(1):57-68.
6. Steiness E, et al. Cardiac arrhythmias induced by hypokalaemia and potassium loss during maintenance digoxin therapy. *Br Heart J.* 1976;38(2):167-172.
7. McAllister RG Jr, et al. Effect of intravenous furosemide on the renal excretion of digoxin. *J Clin Pharmacol.* 1976;16(2-3):110-117.
8. Malcolm AD, et al. Digoxin kinetics during furosemide administration. *Clin Pharmacol Ther.* 1977;21(5):567-574.

† Not available in the United States.

Digoxin (eg, *Lanoxin*) | 4

Grapefruit Juice

SUMMARY: Grapefruit juice produces a small increase in plasma digoxin concentrations.

RISK FACTORS: No specific risk factors are known.

MECHANISM: The mechanism responsible for the small changes in digoxin pharmacokinetics observed in this study are not known. The results do not seem to indicate that grapefruit juice is a potent inhibitor of intestinal P-glycoprotein, especially when digoxin's bioavailability is only minimally dependent on P-glycoprotein.

CLINICAL EVALUATION: Twelve healthy subjects received a single oral 0.5 mg dose of digoxin with 220 mL of water or grapefruit juice 30 minutes before and 7.5 and 11.5 hours after the digoxin dose.[1] Compared with administration with water, digoxin administration with grapefruit juice did not significantly increase the peak plasma concentration of digoxin. The mean area under the concentration-time curve of digoxin was increased 9% following grapefruit juice. Although specific data were not reported, the half-life of digoxin did not appear to be changed by grapefruit juice. These minor changes in digoxin concentrations would be unlikely to alter patient response. However, peak digoxin concentrations were increased about 50% by grapefruit juice in 2 subjects who concurrently demonstrated transient electrocardiographic changes (PR interval prolongation). The results of this study indicate that the coadministration of grapefruit juice and digoxin will be unlikely to alter a patient's response to digoxin, even if larger doses of grapefruit juice are ingested.

RELATED DRUGS: While no data are available, grapefruit juice would be expected to alter the plasma concentration of digitoxin in a similar manner.

MANAGEMENT OPTIONS:

➡ *Monitor.* Patients taking digoxin who consume grapefruit juice in moderate amounts should be at minimal risk for increased digoxin response.

REFERENCES:

1. Becquemont L, et al. Effect of grapefruit juice on digoxin pharmacokinetics in humans. *Clin Pharmacol Ther.* 2001;70:311-316.

 Digoxin (eg, *Lanoxin*)

Hydroxychloroquine (eg, *Plaquenil*)

SUMMARY: Hydroxychloroquine may increase serum digoxin concentrations, but the degree to which this increases the risk of digoxin toxicity is unknown.

RISK FACTORS: No specific risk factors are known.

MECHANISM: Not established.

CLINICAL EVALUATION: Two patients, 65 and 68 years of age, on chronic digoxin (0.25 mg/day) therapy developed increased serum digoxin concentrations (2.4 and 2.3 ng/mL, respectively) after hydroxychloroquine was given for rheumatoid arthritis.[1] Serum digoxin concentrations decreased to 0.7 and 0.6 ng/mL after discontinuation of hydroxychloroquine, supporting the contention that the increased serum digoxin concentrations were caused by hydroxychloroquine. These patients did not develop symptoms of digitalis toxicity; however, this magnitude of change in digoxin concentrations could result in toxicity in some patients.

RELATED DRUGS: No information is available.

MANAGEMENT OPTIONS:

➡ *Monitor.* Monitor digoxin concentration and patients observed for toxicity (eg, nausea, arrhythmia) when hydroxychloroquine is started in a patient receiving digoxin. Digoxin dosage may need to be altered.

REFERENCES:

1. Leden I. Digoxin-hydroxychloroquine interaction? *Acta Med Scand.* 1982;211:411-412.

 Digoxin (eg, *Lanoxin*)

Itraconazole (*Sporanox*)

SUMMARY: Itraconazole administration can result in elevated digoxin concentrations and symptoms of digoxin toxicity, including nausea, malaise, visual changes, and arrhythmias.

RISK FACTORS: No specific risk factors are known.

MECHANISM: Itraconazole may enhance the absorption of digoxin and/or reduce its renal and biliary elimination by inhibiting p-glycoprotein in the intestine, kidney, and liver.

CLINICAL EVALUATION: Ten healthy subjects received oral digoxin 0.25 mg daily for 20 days with itraconazole 200 mg or placebo coadministered twice daily for 10 days.[1] Mean digoxin concentrations were increased from 1.1 nmol/L to 1.8 nmol/L during itraconazole coadministration. Following a single dose of oral digoxin, itraconazole increased the plasma area under the concentration-time curve about 50% and reduce the renal clearance of digoxin 20%.[2] A number of cases of elevated digoxin plasma concentrations and toxicity have been reported in patients receiving itraconazole and digoxin.[3-5]

RELATED DRUGS: Ketoconazole (eg, *Nizoral*) is known to be an inhibitor of p-glycoprotein and would be expected to affect digoxin in a similar manner. It is likely that digitoxin[†] concentrations would also be increased by itraconazole administration. Voriconazole (*Vfend*) does not appear to alter digoxin plasma concentrations.

MANAGEMENT OPTIONS:

➡ *Consider Alternative.* Voriconazole does not affect digoxin concentrations and can be considered as an alternative.

➡ *Monitor.* Monitor patients stabilized on digoxin for changing digoxin concentrations and evidence of digoxin response if itraconazole is initiated, changed in dose, or discontinued from the regime.

REFERENCES:

1. Partanen J, et al. Itraconazole increases serum digoxin concentrations. *Pharmacol Toxicol.* 1996;79:274-276.
2. Jalava KM, et al. Itraconazole decreases renal clearance of digoxin. *Ther Drug Monit.* 1997;19:609-613.
3. Sachs MK, et al. Interaction of itraconazole and digoxin. *Clin Infect Dis.* 1993;16:400-403.
4. Alderman CP, et al. Digoxin-itraconazole interaction: possible mechanisms. *Ann Pharmacother.* 1997;31:438-440.
5. Lopez F, et al. Nausea and malaise during treatment of coccidioimycosis. *Hosp Pract.* 1997;32:21-22.

† Not available in the United States.

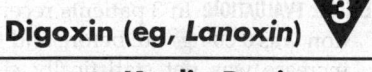

Digoxin (eg, *Lanoxin*)
Kaolin-Pectin

SUMMARY: Kaolin-pectin appears to reduce the bioavailability of digoxin tablets, but digoxin capsules do not appear to be affected.

RISK FACTORS:

➡ *Dosage Form.* Digoxin tablets (but not capsules) appear to be affected by kaolin-pectin.

MECHANISM: Kaolin-pectin appears to inhibit the GI absorption of digoxin.

CLINICAL EVALUATION: In 2 studies, the administration of kaolin-pectin resulted in a 40% to 60% reduction in digoxin absorption.[1,2] Serum digoxin concentrations were reduced in the presence of kaolin-pectin, as were the areas under the digoxin concentration-time curves and cumulative urinary digoxin excretion. In a subsequent study of 7 healthy subjects on chronic digoxin, kaolin-pectin reduced digoxin bioavailability 15% when the 2 drugs were given concurrently but not when the digoxin was given 2 hours before the kaolin-pectin.[3] In another study of 12 healthy subjects, kaolin-pectin reduced the bioavailability of digoxin tablets but not of digoxin capsules.[4]

RELATED DRUGS: Kaolin-pectin may be expected to affect digitoxin[†] in a similar manner.

MANAGEMENT OPTIONS:

➡ *Circumvent/Minimize.* Administer digoxin 2 hours before the kaolin-pectin to minimize the interaction. The use of digoxin capsules may help minimize the interaction.

➡ *Monitor.* Monitor patients receiving digoxin and kaolin-pectin for reduced digoxin concentrations and effect.

REFERENCES:

1. Brown DD, et al. Decreased bioavailability of digoxin due to antacids and kaolin-pectin. *N Engl J Med.* 1976;295:1034-1037.

2. Albert KS, et al. Influence of kaolin-pectin suspension on digoxin bioavailability. *J Pharm Sci.* 1978;67:1582-1586.

3. Albert KS, et al. Influence of kaolin-pectin suspension on steady-state plasma digoxin levels. *J Clin Pharmacol.* 1981;21:449-455.

4. Allen MD, et al. Effect of magnesium-aluminum hydroxide and kaolin-pectin on absorption of digoxin from tablets and capsules. *J Clin Pharmacol.* 1981;21:26-30.

† Not available in the United States.

 Digoxin (eg, *Lanoxin*)

Lidocaine (eg, *Xylocaine*)

SUMMARY: In a limited number of patients, lidocaine did not increase serum digoxin concentrations significantly.

RISK FACTORS: No specific risk factors are known.

MECHANISM: Not established.

CLINICAL EVALUATION: In 3 patients receiving digoxin, the mean serum digoxin concentration was 0.60 ng/mL before and 0.83 ng/mL during lidocaine administration.[1] The increase was not statistically significant, but too few patients were studied to determine whether an interaction occurs.

RELATED DRUGS: No information is available.

MANAGEMENT OPTIONS: No interaction.

REFERENCES:

1. Doering W. Quinidine-digoxin interaction: pharmacokinetics, underlying mechanism and clinical implications. *N Engl J Med.* 1979;301:400-404.

 Digoxin (eg, *Lanoxin*)

Metoclopramide (eg, *Reglan*)

SUMMARY: Metoclopramide reduces the serum digoxin concentration when it is coadministered with slowly dissolving digoxin tablets.

RISK FACTORS:

➡ *Dosage Form.* Patients taking slow dissolving digoxin preparations will be at increased risk of this interaction.

MECHANISM: The GI absorption of slowly dissolving brands of digoxin may be decreased by metoclopramide, which increases GI motility.[1]

CLINICAL EVALUATION: A rapidly dissolving digoxin preparation (eg, *Lanoxin*) does not appear to be affected by metoclopramide.[2] However, the addition of metoclopramide (30 mg/day for 10 days) resulted in a decreased serum digoxin concentration in 11 patients on maintenance therapy with a slowly dissolving digoxin preparation.[1] In a more recent study, metoclopramide reduced the area under the digoxin concentration-time curve by approximately 20%, but the brand of digoxin used was not specified.[3] Metoclopramide appears to have no effect on the absorption of digoxin capsules.[4]

RELATED DRUGS: Other drugs that increase GI motility (eg, cisapride†) also may affect digoxin absorption from slowly dissolving formulations.

MANAGEMENT OPTIONS:

➥ *Monitor.* In patients receiving chronic digoxin therapy, the addition of metoclopramide (or other drugs increasing GI motility) may result in decreased digoxin effect. The interaction probably can be minimized by using rapidly dissolving digoxin preparations (eg, *Lanoxin* tablets) or digoxin capsules (eg, *Lanoxicaps*).

REFERENCES:

1. Manninen V, et al. Altered absorption of digoxin in patients given propantheline and metoclopramide. *Lancet*. 1973;1(7800):398-400.

2. Johnson BF, et al. The influence of digoxin particle size on absorption of digoxin and the effect of propantheline and metoclopramide. *Br J Clin Pharmacol*. 1978;5(5):465-467.

3. Kirch W, et al. Effect of cisapride and metoclopramide on digoxin bioavailability. *Eur J Drug Metab Pharmacokinet*. 1986;11(4):249-250.

4. Johnson BF, et al. Effect of metoclopramide on digoxin absorption from tablets and capsules. *Clin Pharmacol Ther*. 1984;36(6):724-730.

† Not available in the United States.

Digoxin (eg, *Lanoxin*)

Mibefradil†

SUMMARY: Mibefradil produces a dose-dependent increase in digoxin concentrations; increased digoxin adverse reactions may occur at high mibefradil doses.

RISK FACTORS:

➥ *Dosage Regimen.* Mibefradil doses higher than 100 mg/day may increase the risk of interaction.

MECHANISM: Not established. Mibefradil appears to inhibit the elimination of digoxin.

CLINICAL EVALUATION: Forty-two healthy subjects were given a digoxin loading dose of 0.375 mg 3 times over 24 hours.[1] For the next week, each subject received digoxin 0.375 mg/day. During the next 7 days, the 42 subjects were divided into 3 groups. Group I received concomitant mibefradil 50 mg/day, group II 100 mg/day, and group III 150 mg/day. Digoxin pharmacokinetics and pharmacodynamics were determined on the first and seventh treatment day of each week. The coadministration of mibefradil 50, 100, and 150 mg/day increased the mean area under the concentration-time curve of digoxin by 8.2%, 7%, and 30.7%, respectively. The same doses of mibefradil increased mean peak digoxin concentrations by 21.7%, 25%, and 40.9%, respectively. The effect of mibefradil on digoxin half-life was not measured. The only significant pharmacodynamic effects noted were increased PQ intervals with the addition of mibefradil. This effect is likely due, at least in part, to mibefradil-induced prolongation of myocardial conduction. No changes in heart rate, blood pressure, or cardiac output were noted. The increase in digoxin concentrations, particularly with higher mibefradil doses, could lead to some increase in digoxin toxicity such as heart block, nausea, or palpitations in some patients. The administration of mibefradil 50 or 100 mg/day would be unlikely to produce clinically significant increases in digoxin concentrations in most patients.

RELATED DRUGS: Other calcium channel blockers, including verapamil (eg, *Calan*) and diltiazem (eg, *Cardizem*), are known to increase digoxin concentrations and may produce similar effects on cardiac conduction.

MANAGEMENT OPTIONS:

➥ *Monitor.* Observe patients taking digoxin and mibefradil, particularly if mibefradil doses exceed 100 mg/day, for evidence of increased digoxin concentrations or heart block.

REFERENCES:

1. Siepmann M, et al. The interaction of the calcium antagonist RO 40–5967 with digoxin. *Br J Clin Pharmacol.* 1995;39(5):491-496.

† Not available in the United States.

---

 4 **Digoxin (eg, *Lanoxin*)**

Moricizine (*Ethmozine*)

SUMMARY: While moricizine does not alter the serum concentration of digoxin, atrioventricular (AV) conduction defects or heart block may occur.

RISK FACTORS: No specific risk factors are known.

MECHANISM: No pharmacokinetic interaction has been noted; the potential for additive depression of AV conduction during combination therapy is possible because both drugs reduce AV conduction.

CLINICAL EVALUATION: Nine healthy subjects received digoxin 1 mg intravenously before and following 7 days of a 12-day course of moricizine 12 mg/kg/day.[1] No difference in digoxin pharmacokinetics was noted following pretreatment with moricizine. No electrophysiologic monitoring was attempted. In another study, 11 patients taking digoxin for heart failure or arrhythmias received moricizine 600 to 900 mg/day for 3 weeks or placebo.[2] Mean digoxin concentrations were not affected by moricizine administration. During concomitant digoxin and moricizine therapy, 4 patients developed arrhythmias, including AV-junctional rhythm and complete heart block. These arrhythmias resolved with the discontinuation of moricizine; it is unknown whether moricizine alone would have produced the arrhythmias in these patients. An additional report confirms the lack of pharmacokinetic interaction.[3]

RELATED DRUGS: Similar effects are expected with digitoxin† and moricizine.

MANAGEMENT OPTIONS: No specific action is required, but be alert for evidence of the interaction.

REFERENCES:

1. MacFarland RT, et al. Assessment of the potential pharmacokinetic interactions between digoxin and ethmozine. *J Clin Pharmacol.* 1985;25(2):138-143.

2. Antman EM, et al. Drug interactions with cardiac glycosides: evaluation of a possible digoxin-ethmozine pharmacokinetic interaction. *J Cardiovasc Pharmacol.* 1987;9(5):622-627.

3. Kennedy HL, et al. Serum digoxin concentrations during ethmozine antiarrhythmic therapy. *Am Heart J.* 1986;111(4):667-672.

† Not available in the United States.

Digoxin (eg, *Lanoxin*)

Nebivolol (*Bystolic*)

SUMMARY: Digoxin and nebivolol both reduce myocardial conduction; cardiac arrhythmias may occur. Nebivolol may also reduce the positive inotropic effects of digoxin.

RISK FACTORS: No specific risk factors are known.

MECHANISM: Both digoxin and nebivolol slow cardiac conduction.

CLINICAL EVALUATION: While specific data are not provided, the manufacturer of nebivolol notes to use caution in the coadministration of digoxin.[1] Pending further data, observe patients receiving nebivolol and digoxin for slowed cardiac conduction and reduced myocardial inotropic activity.

RELATED DRUGS: Other beta-blockers interact in a similar manner with digoxin.

MANAGEMENT OPTIONS:

➡ *Monitor.* Monitor patients receiving both nebivolol and digoxin for evidence of cardiac conduction disturbances and reduced cardiac output.

REFERENCES:

1. *Bystolic* [package insert]. St. Louis, MO: Forest Pharmaceuticals; 2007.

Digoxin (eg, *Lanoxin*)

Nefazodone

SUMMARY: Nefazodone produces a modest increase in digoxin serum concentrations; some patients may experience an increase in digoxin adverse reactions.

RISK FACTORS: No specific risk factors are known.

MECHANISM: Unknown.

CLINICAL EVALUATION: Eighteen healthy men received digoxin (as *Lanoxicaps*) 0.2 mg once daily, nefazodone 200 mg twice daily, or the combination of nefazodone and digoxin for 8 days.[1] During coadministration of nefazodone, mean trough digoxin concentrations increased approximately 30% and the area under the plasma concentration-time curve of digoxin increased approximately 15% compared with digoxin alone. No change in the renal clearance of digoxin was noted during nefazodone administration. No changes in heart rate, myocardial conduction, or adverse reactions were observed. Given the modest increases in digoxin concentrations observed in this study, some patients (eg, those with pre-nefazodone digoxin concentrations near the toxic level) may experience symptoms of digoxin toxicity (eg, nausea, arrhythmia, anorexia).

RELATED DRUGS: It is unknown if other antidepressants that inhibit serotonin uptake affect digoxin serum concentrations.

MANAGEMENT OPTIONS:

➥ *Monitor.* Monitor patients stabilized on digoxin for increased digoxin adverse reactions or serum concentrations following the addition of nefazodone. Because of digoxin's long half-life, 5 to 10 days may be required to reach a new steady-state digoxin concentration following the addition of nefazodone.

REFERENCES:

1. Dockens RC, et al. Assessment of pharmacokinetic and pharmacodynamic drug interactions between nefazodone and digoxin in healthy male volunteers. *J Clin Pharmacol*. 1996;36(2):160-167.

Digoxin (eg, *Lanoxin*)

Neomycin (eg, *Neo-Tabs*)

SUMMARY: Neomycin reduces digoxin serum concentrations.

RISK FACTORS: No specific risk factors are known.

MECHANISM: Neomycin (oral) appears to inhibit the gastrointestinal (GI) absorption of digoxin. However, oral aminoglycosides also might reduce the inactivation of digoxin by bacteria in the GI tract, thus counteracting the reduction in digoxin absorption. This latter mechanism occurs in only 10% of patients, whereas the inhibition of absorption is likely to occur more regularly.

CLINICAL EVALUATION: The administration of oral neomycin 1 to 3 g reduced digoxin absorption (both rate and amount).[1] Impaired digoxin absorption was noted when neomycin was given 3 to 6 hours before the digoxin. The magnitude of the decrease in serum digoxin is large enough that adverse clinical consequences might occur.

RELATED DRUGS: The potential for other orally administered aminoglycosides to inhibit digoxin absorption is unknown.

MANAGEMENT OPTIONS:

➥ *Circumvent/Minimize.* Administration of digoxin IV will avoid the interaction.

➥ *Monitor.* Since separating the doses of digoxin and antibiotic will not avoid the interaction, monitor patients receiving both drugs for reduced digoxin effect and serum concentrations.

REFERENCES:

1. Lindenbaum J, et al. Inhibition of digoxin absorption by neomycin. *Gastroenterology*. 1976;71:399.

Digoxin (eg, *Lanoxin*)

Nitrendipine (*Baypress*)

SUMMARY: Nitrendipine may cause a moderate increase in digoxin concentrations; digoxin toxicity is likely to be limited.

RISK FACTORS: No specific risk factors are known.

MECHANISM: Nitrendipine appears to inhibit the elimination of digoxin.

CLINICAL EVALUATION: Nitrendipine[1,3] and nisoldipine (*Sular*)[2] have been reported to increase digoxin concentrations by as much as 20%. This increase could produce digoxin toxicity in some patients but less commonly than with verapamil (eg, *Calan*) or diltiazem (eg, *Cardizem*).

RELATED DRUGS: Verapamil, bepridil (*Vascor*), and diltiazem appear to reduce digoxin elimination. Digitoxin (*Crystodigin*) is likely to be affected similarly.

MANAGEMENT OPTIONS: No specific action is required, but be alert for evidence of the interaction.

REFERENCES:

1. Kirch W, et al. Nitrendipine increases digoxin plasma levels dose dependently. *J Clin Pharmacol.* 1986;26:541.

2. Kirch W, et al. Influence of nisoldipine on haemodynamic effects and plasma levels of digoxin. *Br J Clin Pharmacol.* 1986;22:155.

3. Kirch W, et al. Effect of two different doses of nitrendipine on steadystate plasma digoxin level and systolic time intervals. *Eur J Clin Pharmacol.* 1986;31:391.

Digoxin (eg, *Lanoxin*) 3

Omeprazole (*Prilosec*)

SUMMARY: Omeprazole increases the serum concentration of digoxin. Digoxin effects may be increased, but the clinical importance is not established.

RISK FACTORS: No specific risk factors are known.

MECHANISM: Digoxin is hydrolyzed by gastric acid to metabolites with limited cardioactivity. Drugs that inhibit acid secretion (eg, omeprazole) increase the bioavailability of digoxin while increased acidity tends to decrease digoxin bioavailability.

CLINICAL EVALUATION: Six healthy subjects received 1 mg digoxin with placebo on the fourth of 5 days of omeprazole 40 mg/day or following pentagastrin (*Peptavlon*), 6 mcg/kg/hr IV for 1.5 hours.[1] Omeprazole administration increased digoxin urinary excretion by 32% while pentagastrin decreased urinary excretion by 37%. Electrocardiogram changes (suppression of Twave amplitude) were significantly greater following omeprazole and digoxin than after placebo and digoxin.[2] Ten healthy subjects taking digoxin 0.25 mg/day had slightly (10%) higher digoxin concentration (measured by radioimmunoassay) following omeprazole 20 mg/day for 8 days.[3] Patients taking chronic digoxin may have increased response to digoxin following the addition of omeprazole and a decreased digoxin response following increased gastric acidity produced by pentagastrin. The clinical significance of this interaction awaits further study.

RELATED DRUGS: Pentagastrin may reduce digoxin response. Lansoprazole (*Prevacid*) may produce similar effects on digoxin.

MANAGEMENT OPTIONS:

➡ *Monitor.* Until further information is available, monitor patients receiving digoxin for elevated digoxin concentrations and symptoms of toxicity if omeprazole is added and diminished effect if omeprazole is deleted from their regimen.

REFERENCES:

1. Cohen AF, et al. Influence of gastric acidity on the bioavailability of digoxin. *Ann Intern Med.* 1991;115:540.

2. Cohen AF, et al. Effects of gastric acidity on the bioavailability of digoxin. Evidence for a new mechanism for interactions with omeprazole. *Br J Clin Pharmacol.* 1991;31:565P.

3. Oosterhuis B, et al. Minor effect of multiple dose omeprazole on the pharmacokinetics of digoxin after a single oral dose. *Br J Clin Pharmacol.* 1991;32:569.

 Digoxin (eg, *Lanoxin*)

Penicillamine (eg, *Cuprimine*)

SUMMARY: Penicillamine has been reported to reduce digoxin serum concentrations, but the clinical importance of the effect is not established.

RISK FACTORS: No specific risk factors are known.

MECHANISM: Not established.

CLINICAL EVALUATION: Ten patients with heart failure who were stabilized on digoxin were given 1 g of oral penicillamine 2 hours after their normal daily dose of digoxin.[1] On 1 occasion the digoxin was administered orally; on a separate occasion it was administered IV. Digoxin serum concentrations 6 hours after administration were reduced about 40% and 65% following oral and IV digoxin dosing, respectively.

RELATED DRUGS: No information is available.

MANAGEMENT OPTIONS:

➡ **Monitor.** Monitor patients for evidence of reduced digoxin concentration and effect when penicillamine is initiated. Adjust the digoxin dosage as necessary.

REFERENCES:

1. Moezzi B, et al. The effect of penicillamine on serum digoxin levels. *Jpn Heart J.* 1978;19:366.

 Digoxin (eg, *Lanoxin*)

Pirmenol

SUMMARY: Pirmenol increases serum digoxin concentrations; the clinical significance is unknown but is likely to be limited in most patients.

RISK FACTORS: No specific risk factors are known.

MECHANISM: Digoxin renal clearance is reduced by pirmenol, resulting in a reduction in total body clearance.

CLINICAL EVALUATION: Thirteen healthy subjects took digoxin 0.25 mg/day for 20 days.[1] During days 11 to 20, pirmenol 150 mg twice daily was administered. Peak serum concentrations of digoxin increased 52% and the clearance after oral administration of digoxin was reduced 20% by pirmenol. The renal clearance of digoxin declined 20% during pirmenol coadministration. The clinical significance of these changes generally will be small, but some patients (eg, those with high-normal digoxin concentrations) could develop digoxin toxicity.

RELATED DRUGS: No information is available.

MANAGEMENT OPTIONS: No specific action is required, but be alert for evidence of the interaction.

REFERENCES:
1. Lebsack ME, et al. Pharmacokinetic interaction between pirmenol and digoxin. *Pharm Res.* 1988;5:S-175.

Digoxin (eg, *Lanoxin*)

Pravastatin (*Pravachol*)

SUMMARY: Neither pravastatin nor fluvastatin (*Lescol*) alter digoxin concentrations or pharmacodynamic effects. Digoxin produces an insignificant increase in pravastatin plasma concentrations.

RISK FACTORS: No specific risk factors are known.

MECHANISM: Not established.

CLINICAL EVALUATION: Eighteen healthy subjects each received 20 mg of pravastatin, 0.2 mg of digoxin, or both agents daily for 9 days.[1] Pravastatin administration had no effect on digoxin area under the plasma concentration-time curve (AUC), peak concentration, or urinary recovery. Digoxin administration resulted in a 22% (not statistically significant) increase in pravastatin AUC and a significant (25%) reduction in the AUC of pravastatin metabolite. It is not likely that these changes in pravastatin pharmacokinetics would result in any clinically important changes in drug effects.

RELATED DRUGS: A single dose of fluvastatin 40 mg or placebo was administered to 18 patients taking chronic digoxin.[2] Following fluvastatin dosing, digoxin peak concentrations and urinary excretion were increased by about 12%. These changes in digoxin plasma concentrations would not be expected to result in clinically significant changes in response. The effects of multiple doses of fluvastatin on digoxin are not known but are not likely to be significant. The effects of other hepatic hydroxymethylglutaryl coenzyme A reductase inhibitors on digoxin likely would be similar.

MANAGEMENT OPTIONS: No specific action is required, but be alert for evidence of the interaction.

REFERENCES:
1. Triscari J, et al. Steady state concentrations of pravastatin and digoxin when given in combination. *Br J Clin Pharmacol.* 1993;36:263.
2. Garnett WR, et al. Pharmacokinetic effects of fluvastatin in patients chronically receiving digoxin. *Am J Med.* 1994;96(Suppl. 6A):84S.

Digoxin (eg, *Lanoxin*)

Propafenone (*Rythmol*)

SUMMARY: Propafenone increases digoxin serum concentrations and potentially can cause toxicity.

RISK FACTORS: No specific risk factors are known.

MECHANISM: Propafenone appears to reduce the metabolic and renal clearance of digoxin.

CLINICAL EVALUATION: Propafenone doses of 450 to 900 mg/day produced increased serum digoxin concentrations by 14% to more than 80%.[1,3-5] Propafenone 300 mg every 8 hours significantly increased the digoxin area under the concentration-time curve by 29% and decreased the systemic clearance by 22%.[2] Ten patients receiving digoxin for at least 10 days were treated with propafenone 600 mg/day for 7 days.[6] Three of the subjects also received propafenone 750 mg/day and 900 mg/day for 7 day periods. Baseline mean digoxin concentrations averaged 0.97 ng/mL, increased to 1.54 ng/mL with propafenone 600 mg/day. The higher doses of propafenone did not increase the digoxin serum concentrations to a greater extent. However, increasing propafenone concentrations were correlated to the degree of increase in digoxin concentration in 9 patients treated with increasing doses (300 to 900 mg/day) of propafenone.[7] Similar effects of propafenone on digoxin have been noted in children.[8]

RELATED DRUGS: A similar effect may be seen with digitoxin (*Crystodigin*) but data are lacking.

MANAGEMENT OPTIONS:

➡ *Circumvent/Minimize.* The digoxin dosage may need to be reduced during propafenone coadministration.

➡ *Monitor.* Since propafenone may increase digoxin serum concentrations by 30% to 60%, some patients maintained on digoxin could develop toxicity following its addition. Monitor digoxin concentrations and response when propafenone is initiated or discontinued in a patient taking digoxin.

REFERENCES:

1. Salerno DM, et al. Controlled trial of propafenone for treatment of frequent and repetitive ventricular premature complexes. *Am J Cardiol.* 1984;53:77.
2. Nolan PE, et al. Effects of co-administration of propafenone on the pharmacokinetics of digoxin in healthy volunteer subjects. *J Clin Pharmacol.* 1989;29:46.
3. Cardaioli P, et al. Influence of propafenone on the pharmacokinetics of digoxin administered by the oral route:study on healthy volunteers. *G Ital Cardiol.* 1986;16:247.
4. Belz GG, et al. Interaction between digoxin and calcium antagonists and antiarrhythmic drugs. *Clin Pharmacol Ther.* 1983;33:410.
5. Hodges M, et al. Double-blind placebo-controlled evaluation of propafenone in suppressing ventricular ectopic activity. *Am J Cardiol.* 1984;54:45.
6. Calvo MV, et al. Interaction between digoxin and propafenone. *Ther Drug Monit.* 1989;11:10.
7. Bigot MC, et al. Serum digoxin levels related to plasma propafenone levels during concomitant treatment. *J Clin Pharmacol.* 1991;31:521.
8. Zalzstein E, et al. Interaction between digoxin and propafenone in children. *J Pediatr.* 1990;116:310.

5   Digoxin (eg, *Lanoxin*)

Propantheline (eg, *Pro-Banthine*)

SUMMARY: Propantheline administration may increase digoxin concentration, particularly when slowly dissolving dosage forms are used. Digoxin capsules do not appear to be affected.

RISK FACTORS: No specific risk factors are known.

MECHANISM: The gastrointestinal (GI) absorption of slowly dissolving brands of digoxin may be increased by propantheline, which decreases GI motility.[3] Other anticholinergic agents would be expected to produce a similar effect. *Lanoxin* brand of digoxin is not affected.

CLINICAL EVALUATION: In 13 patients on maintenance therapy with a slowly dissolving digoxin preparation, the addition of propantheline (15 mg/day for 10 days) resulted in an increased serum concentration (mean increase 30%) of digoxin in 9 of the patients.[3] In another study, digoxin administered as a solution did not appear to be affected by propantheline;[4] subsequent studies revealed that a more rapidly dissolving preparation (*Lanoxin*) was similarly unaffected by propantheline.[1,2]

RELATED DRUGS: No information is available.

MANAGEMENT OPTIONS: No interaction with *Lanoxin* brand of digoxin.

REFERENCES:

1. Manninen V, et al. Effect of propantheline and metoclopramide on absorption of digoxin. *Lancet.* 1973;1:1118.

2. Johnson BF, et al. The influence of digoxin particle size on absorption of digoxin and the effect of propantheline and metoclopramide. *Br J Clin Pharmacol.* 1978;5:465.

3. Manninen V, et al. Altered absorption of digoxin in patients given propantheline and metoclopramide. *Lancet.* 1973;1:398.

4. Brown DD, et al. A steady-state evaluation of the effects of propantheline bromide and cholestyramine on the bioavailability of digoxin when administered as tablets or capsules. *J Clin Pharmacol.* 1985;25:360.

Digoxin (eg, *Lanoxin*)

Propranolol (eg, *Inderal*)

SUMMARY: Bradycardia may be potentiated by the combination of digoxin and propranolol.

RISK FACTORS:

➡ **Concurrent Diseases.** Patients with concomitant myocardial conduction delays or those with renal dysfunction may be at greater risk.

MECHANISM: Myocardial conduction may be depressed in an additive manner by digoxin and beta-blockers. Propranolol also may reduce the positive inotropic effects of digoxin on myocardial contractility.

CLINICAL EVALUATION: The combination of propranolol or other beta-blockers with digoxin could lead to additive slowing of conduction through the atrioventricular node, potentially producing bradycardia or arrhythmias.[1] However, in some cases including atrial fibrillation or heart failure, the combination of digoxin and propranolol or other beta-blockers has proven useful.[2-4]

RELATED DRUGS: Most beta-blockers would be expected to have the potential for bradycardia when used with digoxin. Although specific data are lacking, beta-blockers with partial agonist activity may be less likely to produce bradycardia at rest. A similar interaction would be expected with digitoxin.

MANAGEMENT OPTIONS:

➡ **Monitor.** Monitor patients receiving beta-blockers and digoxin for reduced heart rate and the occurrence of arrhythmias.

REFERENCES:

1. LeWinter MM, Crawford MH, O'Rourke RA, Karliner JS. The effects of oral propranolol, digoxin and combination therapy on the resting and exercise electrocardiogram. *Am Heart J.* 1977;93:202-209.

2. Kochiadakis GE, Kanoupakis EM, Kalebubas MD, et al. Sotalol vs metoprolol for ventricular rate control in patients with chronic atrial fibrillation who have undergone digitalization: a single-blinded crossover study. *Europace.* 2001;3:73-79.

3. Klein L, O'Connor CM, Gattis WA, et al. Pharmacologic therapy for patients with chronic heart failure and reduced systolic function: review of trials and practical considerations. *Am J Cardiol.* 2003;91:18F-40F.

4. Foody JM, Farrell MH, Krumholz HM. Beta-blocker therapy in heart failure: scientific review. *JAMA.* 2002;287:883-889.

Digoxin (eg, *Lanoxin*)

Quinidine

SUMMARY: Quinidine increases the serum concentration of digoxin and digitoxin sufficiently to lead to digitalis toxicity in some patients.

RISK FACTORS:

➡ **Dosage Regimen.** Quinidine doses above 500 mg/day may increase digoxin serum concentration.

MECHANISM: Quinidine reduces the renal and nonrenal clearance (including biliary secretion) of digoxin by inhibition of P-glycoprotein and may possibly displace digoxin from tissue binding sites. Quinidine also can increase the rate (and possibly extent) of GI digoxin absorption, but the clinical importance of this mechanism is not clear. Quinidine primarily reduces the nonrenal clearance of digitoxin.

CLINICAL EVALUATION: Almost all (at least 90%) patients who receive digoxin and quinidine develop a 25% to 100% increase in serum digoxin concentrations.[1-10] A new steady-state serum digoxin concentration is achieved in 5 to 7 days, but this is likely to take longer in patients with chronic renal failure because their digoxin elimination half-life may be increased to a week or more. Quinidine doses of 400 to 500 mg/day can produce an increase that is generally one half or less of that seen with larger quinidine doses (eg, 1,000 to 1,200 mg/day). Although some clinicians contend that quinidine protects the patient against the adverse effects of the increased serum digoxin concentrations, clinical evidence shows that GI, central nervous system, and cardiac toxicity has been induced by quinidine administration.

RELATED DRUGS: The effect of quinidine on digitoxin disposition has been disputed, but the bulk of the evidence indicates that quinidine does increase serum digitoxin concentrations to a clinically significant degree.[11-13] Quinidine appears to reduce digitoxin nonrenal clearance but causes less change in its renal clearance and no change in the volume of distribution of digitoxin.

MANAGEMENT OPTIONS:

➡ **Circumvent/Minimize.** A reduction in digoxin dose when quinidine is started will reduce the likelihood of digoxin toxicity. However, because the magnitude of the interaction varies considerably from patient to patient, further adjustments in digoxin dose are likely to be necessary.

➡ **Monitor.** During the first 7 to 10 days of combined therapy, monitor the patient carefully for symptoms and electrocardiogram evidence of digoxin toxicity. In general, these precautions also would apply to the concurrent use of quinidine and digitoxin, although it may take longer to achieve a new steady-state serum digitoxin level after starting quinidine therapy.

REFERENCES:

1. Angelin B, Arvidsson A, Dahlqvist R, Hedman A, Schenck-Gustafsson K. Quinidine reduces biliary clearance of digoxin in man. *Eur J Clin Invest*. 1987;17:262-265.

2. Fenster PE, Hager WD, Perrier D, Powell JR, Graves PE, Michael VF. Digoxin-quinidine interaction in patients with chronic renal failure. *Circulation*. 1982;66:1277-1280.

3. Mungall DR, Robichaux RP, Perry W, et al. Effects of quinidine on serum digoxin concentration. *Ann Intern Med*. 1980;93:689.

4. Leahey EB, Bigger JT, Butler VP, et al. Quinidine-digoxin interaction: time course and pharmacokinetics. *Am J Cardiol*. 1981;48:1141-1146.

5. Ochs HR, Bodem G, Greenblatt DJ, et al. Impairment of digoxin clearance by co-administration of quinidine. *J Clin Pharmacol*. 1981;21:396-400.

6. Belz GG, Doering W, Aust PE, Heinz M, Matthews J, Schneider B. Quinidine-digoxin interaction: cardiac efficacy of elevated serum digoxin concentration. *Clin Pharmacol Ther*. 1982;31:548-554.

7. Schenck-Gustafsson K, Jogestrand T, Nordlander R, Dahlqvist R. Effect of quinidine on digoxin concentration in skeletal muscle and serum in patients with atrial fibrillation. *N Engl J Med*. 1981;305:209-211.

8. Williams JF, Mathew B. Effect of quinidine on positive inotropic action of digoxin. *Am J Cardiol*. 1981;47:1052-1055.

9. Pedersen KE, Christiansen BD, Klitgaard NA, Nielsen-Kudsk F. Effect of quinidine on digoxin bioavailability. *Eur J Clin Pharmacol*. 1983;24.41-47.

10. Schenck-Gustafsson K, Dahlqvist R. Pharmacokinetics of digoxin in patients subjected to the quinidine-digoxin interaction. *Br J Clin Pharmacol*. 1981;11:181-186.

11. Ochs HR, Pabst J, Greenblatt DJ, Dengler HJ. Noninteraction of digitoxin and quinidine. *N Engl J Med*. 1980;303:672-674.

12. Kuhlmann J, Dohrmann M, Marcin S. Effects of quinidine on pharmacokinetics and pharmacodynamics of digitoxin achieving steady-state conditions. *Clin Pharmacol Ther*. 1986;39:288-294.

13. Kuhlmann J. Effects of quinidine, verapamil and nifedipine on the pharmacokinetics and pharmacodynamics of digitoxin during steady state conditions. *Arzneimittelforschung*. 1987;37:545-548.

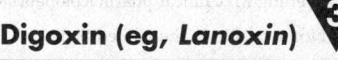

Digoxin (eg, *Lanoxin*)

Quinine

SUMMARY: Quinine potentially could increase digoxin concentrations, particularly when it is administered in high doses.

RISK FACTORS:

➡ ***Dosage Regimen.*** Quinine dosages of 600 mg/day or more could increase digoxin concentrations.

MECHANISM: Quinine reduces the clearance of digoxin.

CLINICAL EVALUATION: Serum digoxin concentration and digoxin half-life increased after quinine 200 mg every 8 hours was administered for 4 days.[1] The relatively large doses of quinine used in this study may produce digoxin intoxication; it is unknown whether the smaller doses of quinine used for leg cramps would influence digoxin serum concentrations, but it does not seem likely.

RELATED DRUGS: Digitoxin[+] also may be affected by large doses of quinine.

MANAGEMENT OPTIONS:

➡ ***Monitor.*** No digoxin dosage adjustment is likely to be required when quinine is administered in low doses. If large quinine doses are administered, monitor the patient for increased digoxin concentrations and signs of digoxin toxicity (eg, anorexia, arrhythmia, nausea).

REFERENCES:

1. Wandell M, et al. Effect of quinine on digoxin kinetics. *Clin Pharmacol Ther.* 1980;28(4):425-430.

† Not available in the United States.

Digoxin (eg, *Lanoxin*)

Ranolazine (*Ranexa*)

SUMMARY: Ranolazine administration may lead to elevated digoxin concentrations; select patients may experience some digoxin toxicity.

RISK FACTORS: No specific risk factors are known.

MECHANISM: Ranolazine is a P-glycoprotein inhibitor that may reduce the elimination of digoxin and enhance its absorption.

CLINICAL EVALUATION: Sixteen subjects received digoxin 0.125 mg daily for 14 days.[1] On days 7 through 14, they also received either placebo or ranolazine 1,000 mg twice daily. The mean area under the concentration-time curve of digoxin increased by 1.6-fold during the coadministration of ranolazine. This magnitude of increase in digoxin plasma concentrations could produce adverse reactions in some patients.

RELATED DRUGS: Digitoxin[†] is likely to be affected in a similar manner by ranolazine.

MANAGEMENT OPTIONS:

➡ *Monitor.* Observe patients taking digoxin for changes in response or digoxin plasma concentrations if ranolazine is initiated or discontinued.

REFERENCES:

1. Jerling M. Clinical pharmacokinetics of ranolazine. *Clin Pharmacokinet.* 2006;45(5):469-491.

† Not available in the United States.

Digoxin (eg, *Lanoxin*)

Rifampin (eg, *Rifadin*)

SUMMARY: Rifampin reduces digoxin plasma concentrations, particularly following oral digoxin dosing. A reduction in digoxin efficacy may result.

RISK FACTORS: No specific risk factors are known.

MECHANISM: Rifampin induces P-glycoprotein in the small intestine, resulting in a reduction in the absorption of digoxin.

CLINICAL EVALUATION: Eight healthy subjects received oral or intravenous digoxin 1 mg alone and on day 10 of 15 days of concurrent rifampin 600 mg/day.[1] The administration of rifampin reduced the bioavailability and the area under the plasma concentration-time curve (AUC) of digoxin about 30%. Most of the effect of rifampin was noted during the first 3 hours following digoxin administration. When digoxin was administered intravenously, rifampin treatment produced a 14% reduction in digoxin's AUC. The renal clearance of digoxin was not affected by rifampin, but the nonrenal clearance increased 217%. Digoxin half-life did not change during rifampin treatment. Some reduction in digoxin effect may result when rifampin is coadministered.

RELATED DRUGS: Digitoxin[†] is likely to be affected in a similar manner by rifampin. Rifabutin (*Mycobutin*) can be expected to reduce digoxin plasma concentrations.

MANAGEMENT OPTIONS:

➡ *Monitor.* Monitor patients stabilized on digoxin who require rifampin therapy for reduced digoxin plasma concentrations and diminished effect.

REFERENCES:

1. Greiner B, et al. The role of intestinal P-glycoprotein in the interaction of digoxin and rifampin. *J Clin Invest*. 1999;104(2):147-153.

† Not available in the United States.

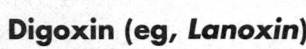

Digoxin (eg, *Lanoxin*)

Ritonavir (*Norvir*)

SUMMARY: Ritonavir appears to increase serum digoxin concentrations; digoxin toxicity may occur.

RISK FACTORS: No specific risk factors are known.

MECHANISM: Ritonavir may inhibit P-glycoprotein–mediated elimination of digoxin via the kidney and/or liver.

CLINICAL EVALUATION: A 61-year-old woman with HIV was stabilized on indinavir (*Crixivan*) 800 mg 3 times/day, lamivudine (*Epivir*) 150 mg twice daily, stavudine (*Zerit*) 40 mg twice daily, digoxin 0.25 mg/day, and warfarin (*Coumadin*) 5 mg alternating with 10 mg/day.[1] Ritonavir 200 mg twice daily was added to this regimen, and 3 days later the patient complained of nausea and vomiting. Digoxin concentration was 7.2 nmol/L (normal range, 1 to 2.6 nmol/L) five hours after the last dose. Digoxin and antiviral drugs were withheld. Twenty-two hours later, the digoxin concentration was 2.7 nmol/L. The next day her GI symptoms resolved. The patient had a pacemaker, and no cardiac symptoms of digoxin toxicity were noted. While no pre-ritonavir digoxin concentrations were reported, the long period of stabilized digoxin dosing (8 years) and time course of the GI symptoms associated with ritonavir administration support the occurrence of an interaction.

RELATED DRUGS: Digitoxin[†] is likely to be affected in a similar manner by ritonavir. The effect of other protease inhibitors on digoxin is unknown. However, indinavir did not appear to affect digoxin elimination in this patient.

MANAGEMENT OPTIONS:

➡ *Monitor.* Pending further data regarding this interaction, monitor patients stabilized on digoxin for altered serum concentrations if ritonavir is added to or removed from the drug regimen.

REFERENCES:

1 Phillips EJ, et al. Digoxin toxicity and ritonavir: a drug interaction mediated through p-glycoprotein? *AIDS*. 2003;17(10):1577-1578.

† Not available in the United States.

5   Digoxin (eg, *Lanoxin*)

Ropinirole (eg, *Requip*)

SUMMARY: The administration of ropinirole does not affect the plasma concentrations of digoxin.

RISK FACTORS: No specific risk factors are known.

MECHANISM: No interaction.

CLINICAL EVALUATION: Ten patients with Parkinson disease were administered digoxin 0.125 or 0.25 mg/day alone or concurrently with ropinirole up to 2 mg 3 times/day for 6 weeks.[1] The mean digoxin area under the concentration-time curve fell about 10% during ropinirole coadministration. No changes in patient response to digoxin were noted during ropinirole administration.

RELATED DRUGS: Ropinirole is not expected to produce a significant change in digitoxin[†] plasma concentrations.

MANAGEMENT OPTIONS: No interaction.

REFERENCES:

1. Taylor A, et al. The effect of steady-state ropinirole on plasma concentrations of digoxin in patients with Parkinson's disease. *Br J Clin Pharmacol.* 1999;47(2):219-222.

† Not available in the United States.

4   Digoxin (eg, *Lanoxin*)

Siberian Ginseng

SUMMARY: Coadministration of ginseng appeared to result in elevated concentrations of digoxin, although no signs of digoxin toxicity were noted.

RISK FACTORS: No specific risk factors are known.

MECHANISM: Unknown.

CLINICAL EVALUATION: A 74-year-old man had been taking digoxin for atrial fibrillation for several years.[1] His serum digoxin concentration was in the range of 0.9 to 2.2 nmol/L. Other medications included acetaminophen (eg, *Tylenol*), cimetidine (eg, *Tagamet*), and aspirin. A routine serum digoxin concentration was found to be elevated at 5.2 nmol/L (normal range, 0.6 to 2.6 nmol/L). He had been taking Siberian ginseng for several months (dose not stated). No signs or symptoms of digitalis intoxication were noted, and his electrocardiogram was normal. The digoxin dose was reduced and then stopped 10 days later, although the digoxin concentrations remained elevated. Ginseng was discontinued 16 days after the digoxin. Digoxin concentrations were within the normal range 17 days after ginseng discontinuation. He was restarted on digoxin with normal digoxin concentrations. Ginseng was restarted, and after 9 weeks, his digoxin concentration was again elevated to 3.2 nmol/L. Ginseng was again discontinued, while digoxin was maintained at the same dose. Within 2 weeks, the digoxin concentration had returned to the normal range. It is unclear why the digoxin concentrations fell more rapidly following the second exposure to ginseng. While there was a temporal relationship between ginseng administration and elevated digoxin concentrations, causation cannot be clearly established. No attempt was made to determine whether ginseng produced a false elevation of digoxin serum concentrations by assay interference, nor was it determined whether the purported ginseng actually contained Siberian ginseng. Analysis of the ginseng did not demonstrate the presence of any digoxin-like compounds.

RELATED DRUGS: None are known.

MANAGEMENT OPTIONS: Pending further study of this potential interaction, monitor patients for elevated digoxin concentrations if they are taking both ginseng and digoxin.

REFERENCES:

1. McRae S. Elevated serum digoxin levels in a patient taking digoxin and Siberian ginseng. *CMAJ.* 1996;155(3):293-295.

Digoxin (eg, *Lanoxin*)

Silodosin (*Rapaflo*)

SUMMARY: No interaction.

RISK FACTORS: No specific risk factors are known.

MECHANISM: None (no interaction).

CLINICAL EVALUATION: Sixteen men received digoxin 0.5 mg twice daily for 1 day followed by 0.25 mg daily for 14 days with silodosin 4 mg twice daily during the last 7 days of digoxin administration.[1] No change in digoxin pharmacokinetics was observed.

RELATED DRUGS: Silodosin is unlikely to affect digitoxin[†] pharmacokinetics. Tamsulosin (*Flomax*) does not appear to affect digoxin pharmacokinetics.

MANAGEMENT OPTIONS: No interaction.

REFERENCES:

1. *Rapaflo* [package insert]. Corona, CA: Watson Pharmaceuticals, Inc; 2008.

† Not available in the United States.

Digoxin (eg, *Lanoxin*)

Spironolactone (eg, *Aldactone*)

SUMMARY: Substantial evidence indicates that spironolactone may interfere with certain serum digoxin assays. More limited evidence suggests that spironolactone may produce a true increase in serum digoxin concentrations.

RISK FACTORS: No specific risk factors are known.

MECHANISM: Spironolactone may reduce the renal excretion of digoxin, falsely increase the plasma concentration of digoxin determined by some assay methods, and possibly inhibit the positive inotropic effect of digitalis glycosides.[1,2] Spironolactone also appears to enhance the metabolism of digitoxin.

CLINICAL EVALUATION: Several studies have demonstrated variable increases in serum digoxin concentrations following spironolactone administration.[3-5] The magnitude of the increase was variable from patient to patient; in 1 patient, the digoxin concentration increased from 1 to 3.5 ng/mL. Spironolactone did not appear to affect the assays used in these studies. However, several other studies have shown spironolactone produced false increases in some serum digoxin assays.[3,6-9] The presence of hepatic or renal dysfunction may exacerbate the effects of spironolactone or digoxin assays.[6,10] Digoxin assays using sheep antibody may be less likely to be affected by spironolactone than digoxin assays using rabbit antibody. However, spironolactone interference with digoxin assays cannot be ruled out unless the laboratory has performed serum digoxin assays on patients receiving chronic spironolactone in the absence of digoxin therapy.

RELATED DRUGS: No information is available.

MANAGEMENT OPTIONS:

➥ *Monitor.* In patients receiving digoxin and spironolactone, monitor the digoxin response by means other than serum digoxin concentrations, unless the digoxin assay used has been proven not to be affected by spironolactone therapy. Because there is some evidence that spironolactone may produce a small increase in serum digoxin concentration, watch for evidence of enhanced digoxin effect, such as nausea or arrhythmia.

REFERENCES:

1. Thomas RW, et al. The interaction of spironolactone and digoxin: a review and evaluation. *Ther Drug Monit.* 1981;3:117.

2. Hedman A, et al. Digoxin-interactions in man: spironolactone reduced renal but not biliary digoxin clearance. *Eur J Clin Pharmacol.* 1992;42:481.

3. Morris RG, et al. Spironolactone as a source of interference in commercial digoxin immunoassays. *Ther Drug Monit.* 1987;9:208.

4. Steiness E. Renal tubular secretion of digoxin. *Circulation.* 1974;50:103.

5. Waldorff S, et al. Spironolactone-induced changes in digoxin kinetics. *Clin Pharmacol Ther.* 1978;24:162.

6. DiPiro JT, et al. Spironolactone interference with digoxin radioimmunoassay in cirrhotic patients. *Am J Hosp Pharm.* 1980;37:1518.

7. Silber B, et al. Spironolactone-associated digoxin radioimmunoassay interference. *Clin Chem.* 1979;25:48.

8. Muller H, et al. Cross reactivity of digitoxin and spironolactone in two radioimmunoassays for serum digoxin. *Clin Chem.* 1978;24:706.

9. Paladino JA, et al. Influence of spironolactone on serum digoxin concentration. *JAMA.* 1984;251:470.

10. Morris RG, et al. The effect of renal and hepatic impairment and of spironolactone on digoxin immunoassays. *Eur J Clin Pharmacol.* 1988;34:233.

Digoxin (eg, *Lanoxin*)

St. John's Wort

SUMMARY: *Hypericum* extract, the main component of St. John's wort, reduces the plasma concentration of digoxin in a dose-dependent manner; some loss of digoxin efficacy may occur.

RISK FACTORS: No specific risk factors are known.

MECHANISM: Hyperforin from St. John's wort stimulates the expression of intestinal p-glycoprotein, resulting in a reduction of digoxin absorption.

CLINICAL EVALUATION: Several studies have demonstrated the effects of St. John's wort extract on digoxin concentrations.[1-3] The effect of the extract was increased with increased doses of *Hypericum*. Following 14 days of *Hypericum*, the mean area under the plasma concentration-time curve of digoxin increased from 18% to nearly 30%. Digoxin half-life was not altered by *Hypericum* administration. Some patients may experience a reduction in digoxin efficacy during St. John's wort administration.

RELATED DRUGS: St. John's wort may produce a similar reduction in digitoxin concentrations.

MANAGEMENT OPTIONS:

➠ *Monitor.* Patients stabilized on digoxin should be monitored for changing digoxin plasma concentrations if St. John's wort is added to or removed from the daily drug regimen.

REFERENCES:

1. Johne A, et al. Pharmacokinetic interaction of digoxin with an herbal extract from St. John's wort (*Hypericum perforatum*). *Clin Pharmacol Ther.* 1999;66:338-345.

2. Durr D, et al. St John's wort induces intestinal P-glycoprotein/MDR1 and intestinal and hepatic CYP3A4. *Clin Pharmacol Ther.* 2000;68:598-604.

3. Mueller SC, et al. Effect of St. John's wort dose and preparations on the pharmacokinetics of digoxin. *Clin Pharmacol Ther.* 2004;75:546-557.

Digoxin (eg, *Lanoxin*)

Succinylcholine (eg, *Anectine*)

SUMMARY: The administration of succinylcholine to digitalized patients may increase the risk of arrhythmias.

RISK FACTORS: No specific risk factors are known.

MECHANISM: Not established. Succinylcholine appears to potentiate the cardiac conduction effects of digitalis glycosides and may increase ventricular irritability. It has been proposed, but not proven, that this is caused by the effect on cholinergic receptors that release catecholamines. Also, depolarizing muscle relaxants may produce a sudden shift of potassium from inside to outside the muscle cell.[1] If this occurs in the digitalized myocardium, arrhythmias can result.

CLINICAL EVALUATION: Cardiac arrhythmias have occurred following administration of succinylcholine to fully digitalized patients.[2] However, more study is needed to assess the clinical significance of the interaction between succinylcholine and digitalis glycosides.

RELATED DRUGS: No information is available.

MANAGEMENT OPTIONS:

➠ *Monitor.* Cautiously use succinylcholine in digitalized patients. One succinylcholine manufacturer states that it should not be used in digitalized patients unless absolutely necessary.

REFERENCES:

1. Birch AA Jr, et al. Changes in serum potassium response to succinylcholine following trauma. *JAMA.* 1969;210:490-493.

2. Perez HR. Cardiac arrhythmia after succinylcholine. *Anesth Analg.* 1970;49:33-38.

4 Digoxin (eg, *Lanoxin*)

Sucralfate (eg, *Carafate*)

SUMMARY: A study in healthy subjects indicates that sucralfate slightly reduces the gastrointestinal absorption of digoxin.

RISK FACTORS: No specific risk factors are known.

MECHANISM: The mechanism for the reduced digoxin bioavailability is not established.

CLINICAL EVALUATION: Twelve healthy subjects were given a single dose of digoxin 0.75 mg under 3 conditions: alone, with sucralfate 1 g 4 times a day for 2 days (1 sucralfate dose was given with the digoxin), and with sucralfate 1 g 4 times a day for 2 days (the sucralfate dose that coincided with digoxin was given 2 hours after the digoxin).[1] Simultaneous administration of sucralfate reduced digoxin bioavailability 19%, but no interaction occurred when the digoxin was given 2 hours before the sucralfate. Pending multiple-dose studies, assume that coadministration of sucralfate will produce a small reduction in digoxin absorption.

RELATED DRUGS: Little is known regarding the effect of sucralfate on other digitalis glycosides, but consider the possibility of reduced bioavailability.

MANAGEMENT OPTIONS: No specific action is required, but be alert for evidence of the interaction.

REFERENCES:
   1. Giesing DH, et al. Lack of effect of sucralfate on digoxin pharmacokinetics. *Gastroenterology.* 1983;84:1165.

3 Digoxin (eg, *Lanoxin*)

Sulfasalazine (eg, *Azulfidine*)

SUMMARY: Sulfasalazine can reduce digoxin serum concentrations.

RISK FACTORS:

➥ **Dosage Regimen.** Sulfasalazine doses higher than 2 g/day can reduce digoxin serum concentrations.

MECHANISM: Sulfasalazine appears to reduce the bioavailability of coadministered digoxin.

CLINICAL EVALUATION: Ten healthy subjects were given digoxin elixir 0.5 mg with and without pretreatment with sulfasalazine.[1] Sulfasalazine pretreatment was associated with reduced serum digoxin concentrations and lower cumulative urinary digoxin excretion. These reductions were moderate but of sufficient magnitude to have a potential effect on the therapeutic response to digoxin. Subjects who received larger doses of sulfasalazine appeared to manifest larger decreases in digoxin bioavailability, while those who received only 2 g/day of sulfasalazine were not affected.

RELATED DRUGS: Digitoxin[+] may be less likely to interact with sulfasalazine.

MANAGEMENT OPTIONS:

➥ **Consider Alternative.** Digitoxin[+] may be preferable in sulfasalazine-treated patients.

➡ *Monitor.* It is not necessary to avoid the concomitant use of digoxin and sulfasalazine, but monitor patients for a decreased or inadequate therapeutic response to digoxin. Based on the response of 1 patient, separation of the doses of digoxin and sulfasalazine did not circumvent the interaction.

REFERENCES:

1. Juhl RP, et al. Effect of sulfasalazine on digoxin bioavailability. *Clin Pharmacol Ther.* 1976;20:387-394.

† Not available in the United States.

Digoxin (eg, *Lanoxin*)

Tacrine (*Cognex*)

SUMMARY: Tacrine does not appear to affect the pharmacokinetics of digoxin; both digoxin and tacrine can slow the heart rate, but the clinical importance of any additive effect is not established.

RISK FACTORS: No specific risk factors are known.

MECHANISM: Not established.

CLINICAL EVALUATION: Eleven or twelve (exact number is not stated) older healthy subjects took a single oral dose of digoxin 0.5 mg with and without concurrent tacrine 20 mg every 6 hours.[1] Tacrine had no effect on digoxin pharmacokinetics, but the reverse interaction (effect of digoxin on tacrine) was not studied. The cardiovascular effects of anticholinesterase agents, such as tacrine, are complex, but bradycardia can occur.[2,3] However, the degree to which tacrine and digitalis glycosides produce additive slowing of the heart and the clinical importance of any such effect are not known.

RELATED DRUGS: No information is available.

MANAGEMENT OPTIONS: No specific action is required, but be alert for evidence of the interaction.

REFERENCES:

1. de Vries TM, et al. Effect of multiple-dose tacrine administration on single-dose pharmacokinetics of digoxin, diazepam, and theophylline. *Pharm Res.* 1993;10(suppl 10):S333.

2. Taylor P. Agents acting at the neuromuscular junction and autonomic ganglia. In: Gilman AG, Rall TW, Nies AS, eds. *Goodman and Gilman's The Pharmacological Basis of Therapeutics.* 8th ed. New York, NY: Pergamon Press; 1990:166-186.

3. Hartvig P, et al. Pharmacokinetics and effects of 9-amino-1,2,3,4-tetrahydroacridine in the immediate postoperative period in neurosurgical patients. *J Clin Anesth.* 1991;3(2):137-142.

Digoxin (eg, *Lanoxin*)

Tamsulosin (eg, *Flomax*)

SUMMARY: Tamsulosin does not appear to affect the pharmacokinetics of digoxin.

RISK FACTORS: No specific risk factors are known.

MECHANISM: None (no interaction).

CLINICAL EVALUATION: Ten healthy subjects received digoxin 0.5 mg intravenous with or without pretreatment with tamsulosin 0.8 mg/day.[1] There was no effect on the pharmacokinetics of digoxin.

RELATED DRUGS: No information is available.

MANAGEMENT OPTIONS: No interaction.

REFERENCES:

1. Miyazawa Y, et al. Effects of the concomitant administration of tamsulosin (0.8 mg) on the pharmacokinetic and safety profile of intravenous digoxin (*Lanoxin*) in normal healthy subjects: a placebo-controlled evaluation. *J Clin Pharm Ther*. 2002;27(1):13-19.

Digoxin (eg, *Lanoxin*)

Telaprevir (*Incivek*)

SUMMARY: The coadministration of telaprevir increases the plasma concentration of digoxin; adverse reactions including bradycardia, GI upset, and arrhythmia may be more likely to occur.

RISK FACTORS: No specific risk factors are known.

MECHANISM: Telaprevir inhibits the P-glycoprotein–mediated elimination of digoxin.

CLINICAL EVALUATION: While specific data are limited, the manufacturer of telaprevir states that the coadministration of telaprevir 750 mg every 8 hours for 11 days increased the mean area under the plasma concentration-time curve of digoxin nearly 85%.[1] Pending further data, observe patients receiving telaprevir and digoxin for increased digoxin response.

RELATED DRUGS: Boceprevir (*Victrelis*) is potentially an inhibitor of P-glycoprotein; however, no data are available regarding its potential effect on digoxin pharmacokinetics. Indinavir (*Crixivan*), nelfinavir (*Viracept*), ritonavir (*Norvir*), and saquinavir (*Fortovase*) also inhibit P-glycoprotein and are expected to increase the plasma concentration of digoxin.

MANAGEMENT OPTIONS:

➡ *Monitor.* Monitor patients stabilized on digoxin for adverse reactions if telaprevir is coadministered.

REFERENCES:

1. *Incivek* [package insert]. Cambridge, MA: Vertex Pharmaceuticals Inc; 2011.

Digoxin (eg, *Lanoxin*)

Telithromycin (*Ketek*)

SUMMARY: Telithromycin causes a modest increase in digoxin concentrations.

RISK FACTORS: No specific risk factors are known.

MECHANISM: Unknown.

CLINICAL EVALUATION: While published data are limited, telithromycin increased digoxin's peak and trough concentrations 73% and 21%, respectively.[1] Digoxin's clinical effect is primarily related to its trough concentrations. It is possible that this magnitude of increase in digoxin concentration could lead to digoxin toxicity in some patients; however, it is likely to be limited. Because of digoxin's long half-life, prolonged administration of telithromycin may produce a larger change in digoxin plasma concentrations.

RELATED DRUGS: No information is available.

MANAGEMENT OPTIONS:

➡ *Monitor.* Monitor patients taking digoxin for increased digoxin effect (eg, arrhythmia, GI symptoms) during the administration of telithromycin.

REFERENCES:

1. *Ketek* [package insert]. Bridgewater, NJ: Aventis Pharmaceuticals Inc; 2004.

Digoxin (eg, *Lanoxin*)

Telmisartan (*Micardis*)

SUMMARY: Digoxin concentrations were increased modestly during telmisartan administration.

RISK FACTORS: No specific risk factors are known.

MECHANISM: Unknown.

CLINICAL EVALUATION: Although no data have been published, there is some information about this interaction. The coadministration of telmisartan and digoxin resulted in a mean increase in peak digoxin concentration of 49% and mean trough concentration of 20%.[1] Information was not provided on the doses or the duration of drug administration used in the study. The degree of increase in digoxin concentration is unlikely to cause digoxin toxicity in most patients. However, those patients with digoxin concentrations already near the toxic level could experience an increase in symptoms of toxicity (eg, arrhythmias, nausea, anorexia, visual changes) following the addition of telmisartan.

RELATED DRUGS: The effects of telmisartan on digitoxin[†] are unknown.

MANAGEMENT OPTIONS:

➡ *Monitor.* Monitor digoxin plasma concentrations, and be alert for signs of digoxin toxicity when telmisartan is administered to patients taking digoxin.

REFERENCES:

1. *Micardis* [package insert]. Ridgefield, CT: Boehringer Ingelheim Pharmaceuticals Inc; 1998.

† Not available in the United States.

Digoxin (eg, *Lanoxin*)

Tenidap†

SUMMARY: Tenidap did not cause any clinically significant change in digoxin pharmacokinetics.

RISK FACTORS: No specific risk factors are known.

MECHANISM: Not established.

CLINICAL EVALUATION: Tenidap 120 mg/day for 4 days had no effect on digoxin area under the concentration-time curve, renal clearance, or peak digoxin concentrations.[1] The time to peak digoxin concentration was increased from 0.7 to 1.2 hours following coadministration with tenidap. No change in patient response to digoxin is expected from this interaction.

RELATED DRUGS: No information is available.

MANAGEMENT OPTIONS: No interaction.

REFERENCES:

1. Dewland PM, et al. Effect of tenidap sodium on digoxin pharmacokinetics in healthy young men. *Br J Clin Pharmacol.* 1995;39(suppl 1):43S-46S.

† Not available in the United States.

5 Digoxin (eg, *Lanoxin*)

Terbinafine (eg, *Lamisil*)

SUMMARY: Terbinafine administration does not affect digoxin concentrations.

RISK FACTORS: No specific risk factors are known.

MECHANISM: No interaction.

CLINICAL EVALUATION: A single oral dose of digoxin 0.75 mg was administered to 16 healthy subjects on the eighth day of 12 days of placebo or terbinafine 250 mg/day.[1] The administration of digoxin following terbinafine produced no changes in digoxin area under the concentration-time curve or peak concentrations compared with placebo.

RELATED DRUGS: Itraconazole (eg, *Sporanox*), and perhaps other azole antifungal agents, may increase digoxin concentrations.

MANAGEMENT OPTIONS: No interaction.

REFERENCES:

1. Tarral A, et al. Effects of terbinafine on the pharmacokinetics of digoxin in healthy volunteers. *Pharmacotherapy.* 1997;17(4):791-795.

Digoxin (eg, *Lanoxin*)

Tetracycline

SUMMARY: Tetracycline can reduce bacterial gastrointestinal (GI) flora and increase digoxin concentrations in a minority of patients.

RISK FACTORS: No specific risk factors are known.

MECHANISM: Approximately 10% of patients treated with digoxin excrete substantial amounts of cardioinactive digoxin metabolites in their urine (at least 40% of the total urinary excretion of digoxin and its metabolites). The bacterial flora (especially *Eubacterium lentum*) of the intestine are involved in this process. Thus, tetracycline can decrease the bacterial metabolism of digoxin, which, in turn, results in higher digoxin serum concentrations.

CLINICAL EVALUATION: One subject who excreted substantial amounts of cardioinactive digoxin reduction products in his urine was given digoxin (two 0.25 mg tablets/day) for approximately 3 weeks.[1] Tetracycline 500 mg every 6 hours coadministered for 5 days reduced the excretion of cardioactive metabolites from 39% to 4% within 48 hours of antibiotic administration. Steady-state serum digoxin concentrations increased approximately 30%. The clinical significance of this interaction remains to be determined. Inactivation of digoxin by intestinal flora occurs only in a minority of patients, and the increase in serum digoxin resulting from concurrent antibiotics is greatest with digoxin products of poor bioavailability. Nevertheless, this interaction could result in digoxin toxicity in some patients.[1,2] The effect of antibiotics on the bacterial flora that inactivate digoxin appears to persist for several months.[1]

RELATED DRUGS: No information is available.

MANAGEMENT OPTIONS:

➡ *Monitor.* In the 1 patient in 10 who metabolizes substantial amounts of digoxin in the GI tract, concomitant tetracycline therapy can increase serum digoxin concentrations. Monitor for digoxin toxicity (eg, nausea, anorexia, arrhythmia) and reduce the dosage as needed.

REFERENCES:

1. Lindenbaum J, et al. Inactivation of digoxin by the gut flora: reversal by antibiotic therapy. *N Engl J Med.* 1981;305(14):789-794.

2. Norregaard-Hansen K, et al. The significance of the enterohepatic circulation on the metabolism of digoxin in patients with the ability of intestinal conversion of the drug. *Acta Med Scand.* 1986;220(1):89-92.

Digoxin (eg, *Lanoxin*)

Ticagrelor (*Brilinta*)

SUMMARY: Ticagrelor modestly increases the plasma concentration of digoxin; an increased risk of digoxin adverse events is possible in some patients.

RISK FACTORS: No specific risk factors are known.

MECHANISM: Ticagrelor appears to inhibit P-glycoprotein, the primary efflux transporter responsible for the elimination of digoxin.

CLINICAL EVALUATION: While specific data are limited, the manufacturer of ticagrelor notes that the coadministration of ticagrelor 400 mg once daily increased the mean area under the plasma concentration-time curve of digoxin by approximately 25%.[1] Pending further data, observe patients receiving ticagrelor and digoxin for increased digoxin plasma concentrations.

RELATED DRUGS: Prasugrel (*Effient*) has been noted to cause a slight reduction in digoxin plasma concentrations.[2]

MANAGEMENT OPTIONS:

➡ *Monitor.* Monitor patients stabilized on digoxin for changing plasma digoxin concentrations when ticagrelor is initiated or discontinued.

REFERENCES:

1. *Brilinta* [package insert]. Wilmington, DE: AstraZeneca LP; 2011.

2. Small DS, et al. Effect of intrinsic and extrinsic factors on the clinical pharmacokinetics and pharmacodynamics of prasugrel. *Clin Pharmacokinet.* 2010;49(12):777-798.

Digoxin (eg, *Lanoxin*)

Ticlopidine (eg, *Ticlid*)

SUMMARY: Ticlopidine appears to cause a small decrease in digoxin serum concentrations.

RISK FACTORS: No specific risk factors are known.

MECHANISM: Not established.

CLINICAL EVALUATION: Fifteen subjects were administered digoxin 0.125 to 0.5 mg/day for 15 days followed by coadministration of ticlopidine 250 mg twice daily for an additional 10 days.[1] Ticlopidine administration resulted in a 9% reduction in the digoxin area under the concentration-time curve. This magnitude of change is unlikely to be clinically significant.

RELATED DRUGS: No information is available.

MANAGEMENT OPTIONS: No specific action is required, but be alert for evidence of the interaction.

REFERENCES:
1. Vargas R, et al. Study of the effect of ticlopidine on digoxin blood levels. *Clin Pharmacol Ther.* 1988;43:176.

Digoxin (eg, *Lanoxin*)

Tolvaptan (*Samsca*)

SUMMARY: Tolvaptan administration has been noted to modestly increase the plasma concentration of digoxin.

RISK FACTORS: No specific risk factors are known.

MECHANISM: Tolvaptan inhibits P-glycoprotein, the primary active elimination pathway for digoxin.

CLINICAL EVALUATION: While specific data are limited, the manufacturer of tolvaptan notes that the coadministration of digoxin and tolvaptan (dose not stated) increased the mean area under the plasma concentration-time curve of digoxin approximately 1.3-fold.[1] While this change is likely to go unnoticed in many patients receiving tolvaptan and digoxin, a few may notice some increase in digoxin adverse reactions, such as cardiac conduction changes or GI upset.

RELATED DRUGS: No information is available.

MANAGEMENT OPTIONS:

➡ *Monitor.* If tolvaptan is administered with digoxin, monitor patients for evidence of digoxin adverse reactions or change in digoxin plasma concentration.

REFERENCES:
1. *Samsca* [package insert]. Rockville, MD: Otsuka America Pharmaceutical Inc; 2009.

Digoxin (eg, *Lanoxin*)

Trimethoprim (eg, *Proloprim*)

SUMMARY: Trimethoprim may increase serum digoxin concentrations modestly, particularly in elderly patients.

RISK FACTORS: No specific risk factors are known.

MECHANISM: Trimethoprim appears to reduce the tubular secretion of digoxin.

CLINICAL EVALUATION: Serum digoxin concentrations increased an average of 22% after trimethoprim was started in 9 elderly patients.[1] Serum creatinine also was increased during trimethoprim administration. In a study in healthy subjects (age range, 24 to 31 years), trimethoprim reduced the renal clearance of digoxin 17%

without affecting the glomerular filtration rate. Nonrenal digoxin clearance increased in these younger subjects.

RELATED DRUGS: Other trimethoprim-containing drugs such as trimethoprim-sulfamethoxazole (eg, *Bactrim*) are expected to produce a similar reaction.

MANAGEMENT OPTIONS: No specific action is required, but be alert for evidence of the interaction.

REFERENCES:

1. Petersen P, et al. Digoxin-trimethoprim interaction. *Acta Med Scand.* 1985;217(4):423-427.

Digoxin (eg, *Lanoxin*)

Verapamil (eg, *Calan*)

SUMMARY: Verapamil increases digoxin serum concentrations; digoxin toxicity may result.

RISK FACTORS:

➡ *Dosage Regimen.* Verapamil dosages greater than 160 mg/day produce larger increases in digoxin concentrations.[1]

MECHANISM: Verapamil appears to inhibit the renal and biliary secretion of digoxin.[2,3]

CLINICAL EVALUATION: Verapamil increases serum digoxin concentration an average of approximately 70%.[1,4-8] The increase in digoxin concentration may result in digoxin toxicity. Verapamil may add to the negative dromotropic and chronotropic effects of digoxin, possibly producing bradycardia or heart block.

RELATED DRUGS: Diltiazem (eg, *Cardizem*) and nitrendipine (*Baypress*) appear to reduce digoxin elimination. Digitoxin (*Crystodigin*[+]) is likely to be affected similarly. Nifedipine (eg, *Procardia*),[9-12] isradipine (eg, *DynaCirc*),[7] nicardipine (eg, *Cardene*),[13] felodipine,[14] and amlodipine (eg, *Norvasc*)[15] do not appear to increase digoxin concentrations.

MANAGEMENT OPTIONS:

➡ *Consider Alternative.* Nifedipine, isradipine, nicardipine, felodipine, and amlodipine do not appear to increase digoxin concentrations and may be suitable alternatives.

➡ *Circumvent/Minimize.* Digoxin dosages may need to be reduced when verapamil is added for a patient stabilized on digoxin.

➡ *Monitor.* Monitor patients for evidence of increased serum digitalis effects (eg, bradycardia, heart block, GI upset, mental changes) in the presence of verapamil therapy.

REFERENCES:

1. Klein HO, et al. The influence of verapamil on serum digoxin concentration. *Circulation.* 1982;65(5):998-1003.
2. Johnson BF, et al. The comparative effects of verapamil and a new dihydropyridine calcium channel blocker on digoxin pharmacokinetics. *Clin Pharmacol Ther.* 1987;42(1):66-71.
3. Hedman A. Inhibition by basic drugs of digoxin secretion into human bile. *Eur J Clin Pharmacol.* 1992;42(4):457-459.
4. Pedersen KE, et al. Digoxin-verapamil interaction. *Clin Pharmacol Ther.* 1981;30(3):311-316.
5. Klein HO, et al. Verapamil and digoxin: their respective effects on atrial fibrillation and their interaction. *Am J Cardiol.* 1982;50(4):894-902.

6. Belz GG, et al. Interaction between digoxin and calcium antagonists and antiarrhythmic drugs. *Clin Pharmacol Ther*. 1983;33(4):410-417.

7. Rodin SM, et al. Comparative effects of verapamil and isradipine on steady-state digoxin kinetics. *Clin Pharmacol Ther*. 1988;43(6):668-672.

8. Hedman A, et al. Digoxin-verapamil interaction: reduction of biliary but not renal digoxin clearance in humans. *Clin Pharmacol Ther*. 1991;49(3):256-262.

9. Belz GG, et al. Digoxin plasma concentrations and nifedipine. *Lancet*. 1981;1(8224):844-845.

10. Kuhlmann J. Effects of nifedipine and diltiazem on plasma levels and renal excretion of beta-acetyldigoxin. *Clin Pharmacol Ther*. 1985;37(2):150-156.

11. Schwartz JB, et al. Effect of nifedipine on serum digoxin concentration and renal digoxin clearance. *Clin Pharmacol Ther*. 1984;36(1):19-24.

12. Hutt HJ, et al. Dose-dependence of the nifedipine/digoxin interaction? *Arch Toxicol Suppl*. 1986;9:209-212.

13. Debruyne D, et al. Nicardipine does not significantly affect serum digoxin concentrations at the steady state of patients with congestive heart failure. *Int J Clin Pharmacol Res*. 1989;9(1):15-19.

14. Kirch W, et al. The felodipine/digoxin interaction. A placebo-controlled study in patients with heart failure. *Br J Clin Pharmacol*. 1988;26:644P.

15. Schwartz JB. Effects of amlodipine on steady-state digoxin concentrations and renal digoxin clearance. *J Cardiovasc Pharmacol*. 1988;12(1):1-5.

† = Not available in the United States.

5 Digoxin (eg, *Lanoxin*)

Voriconazole (*Vfend*)

SUMMARY: Voriconazole does not affect digoxin plasma concentrations.

RISK FACTORS: No specific risk factors are known.

MECHANISM: No interaction.

CLINICAL EVALUATION: Twenty-four healthy subjects were administered digoxin as a 1.5 mg oral loading dose over 2 days followed by 0.25 mg daily for 22 days.[1] On days 11 through 22 of digoxin dosing, placebo (13 subjects) or voriconazole 200 mg twice daily (12 subjects) was coadministered. Mean digoxin plasma concentrations on days 10 and 22 of digoxin administration were similar in the subjects taking placebo and those taking voriconazole. No significant change in digoxin concentration was noted in the voriconazole group between days 10 and 22 of digoxin dosing. This study indicates that voriconazole does not inhibit P-glycoprotein, the primary pathway of digoxin elimination.

RELATED DRUGS: Voriconazole is not expected to alter the pharmacokinetics of digitoxin (not available in the United States). Other azole antifungal drugs, including keto-conazole (eg, *Nizoral*) and itraconazole (eg, *Sporanox*), are known to increase digoxin plasma concentrations.

MANAGEMENT OPTIONS: No interaction.

REFERENCES:
1. Purkins L, et al. Voriconazole does not affect the steady-state pharmacokinetics of digoxin. *Br J Clin Pharmacol*. 2003;56:45-50.

Dihydrocodeine 4

Sildenafil (eg, *Viagra*)

SUMMARY: Isolated cases of prolonged erections have been reported following use of sildenafil in patients receiving dihydrocodeine, but a causal relationship was not established.

RISK FACTORS: No specific risk factors are known.

MECHANISM: Not established.

CLINICAL EVALUATION: Two patients receiving dihydrocodeine for the pain of soft tissue injuries developed prolonged (several hours) erections when they took sildenafil.[1] With previous use of sildenafil, erections had subsided immediately after orgasm for both patients. More evidence is needed to establish a causal relationship.

RELATED DRUGS: No information is available.

MANAGEMENT OPTIONS: No specific action is required, but be alert for evidence of the interaction.

REFERENCES:
1. Goldmeier D, Lamba H. Prolonged erections produced by dihydrocodeine and sildenafil. *BMJ.* 2002;324:1555.

Dihydroergotamine (eg, *Migranal*) 2

Sibutramine (*Meridia*)

SUMMARY: The risk of serotonin syndrome would theoretically increase when sibutramine is combined with other serotonergic drugs such as dihydroergotamine.

RISK FACTORS: No specific risk factors are known.

MECHANISM: Sibutramine inhibits serotonin reuptake; additive serotonergic effects may occur with dihydroergotamine.

CLINICAL EVALUATION: While no published data are available for evaluation, the manufacturer of sibutramine has made available some data on this interaction.[1] Because sibutramine has serotonergic effects, its concurrent use with other serotonergic drugs (eg, dihydroergotamine) may increase the risk of serotonin syndrome.[2] Although the actual risk of combining sibutramine with serotonergic drugs is unknown, the fact that serotonin syndrome can result in serious or fatal reactions must be considered.

RELATED DRUGS: No information is available.

MANAGEMENT OPTIONS:

➡ *Avoid Unless Benefit Outweighs Risk.* The manufacturer states that sibutramine should not be used with dihydroergotamine. This is a prudent recommendation until more information is available.

➡ *Monitor.* Serotonin syndrome can result in neurotoxicity (eg, myoclonus, tremors, rigidity, incoordination, restlessness, hyperreflexia, seizures, coma), psychiatric symptoms (eg, agitation, confusion, hypomania), and temperature regulation abnormalities (eg, fever, sweating). Note that mild forms of serotonin syndrome have also been reported, so consider any combination of the above symptoms possibly related to excessive serotonin activity.

REFERENCES:
1. *Meridia* [package insert]. Abbott Park, IL: Abbott; 1997.
2. Mills KC. Serotonin syndrome. A clinical update. *Crit Care Clin*. 1997;13:763-783.

 Dihydroergotamine (eg, *Migranal*)

AVOID **Sumatriptan (eg, *Imitrex*)**

SUMMARY: Do not administer sumatriptan or other triptans within 24 hours of dihydroergotamine.

RISK FACTORS: No specific risk factors are known.

MECHANISM: Additive pharmacodynamic effects.

CLINICAL EVALUATION: The product information for *Imitrex* (sumatriptan) states that it should not be used within 24 hours of dihydroergotamine because excessive (additive) vasoconstriction may occur.[1] Although this is based primarily on theoretical considerations, the adverse effect could be severe, and concurrent use may present medicolegal risks as well.

RELATED DRUGS: All other triptans, such as almotriptan (*Axert*), eletriptan (*Relpax*), frovatriptan (*Frova*), naratriptan (eg, *Amerge*), rizatriptan (*Maxalt*), and zolmitriptan (*Zomig*), are also contraindicated within 24 hours of dihydroergotamine or other ergot alkaloids.

MANAGEMENT OPTIONS:

➡ ***AVOID COMBINATION.*** Do not administer sumatriptan and other triptans within 24 hours of dihydroergotamine or other ergot alkaloids.

REFERENCES:
1. *Imitrex* [package insert]. Research Triangle Park, NC: GlaxoSmithKline; 2006.

 Diltiazem (eg, *Cardizem*)

Encainide†

SUMMARY: Diltiazem substantially increases serum encainide concentrations, but the clinical importance of this interaction is not established.

RISK FACTORS:

➡ ***Pharmacogenetics.*** Rapid encainide metabolizers are at risk.

MECHANISM: Diltiazem seems to decrease encainide's first-pass or systemic metabolism.

CLINICAL EVALUATION: Encainide 25 mg every 8 hours was administered for 7 days along with diltiazem 90 mg every 8 hours for 10 days to 8 extensive metabolizers of encainide.[1] The encainide area under the concentration-time curve following diltiazem administration increased 59% compared with that for encainide alone. No significant change was observed in the serum concentrations of encainide's active metabolites or in its pharmacodynamic effects.

RELATED DRUGS: The effect of other calcium channel blockers on encainide metabolism has not been studied; however, verapamil (eg, *Calan*) might produce similar effects because of its effects on drug metabolism.

MANAGEMENT OPTIONS:

➡ ***Monitor.*** Monitor patients maintained on encainide for possible toxicity (eg, arrhythmia, dizziness) or increased encainide concentrations when diltiazem is coadministered.

REFERENCES:

1. Kazierad DJ, et al. The effect of diltiazem on the disposition of encainide and its active metabolites. *Clin Pharmacol Ther*. 1989;46(6):668-673.

† Not available in the United States.

Diltiazem (eg, *Cardizem*)
Fentanyl (eg, *Duragesic*)

SUMMARY: The administration of diltiazem may enhance the effects of fentanyl.

RISK FACTORS: No specific risk factors are known.

MECHANISM: Diltiazem is known to inhibit CYP3A4, the enzyme primarily responsible for the metabolism of fentanyl, which could potentially cause increased serum concentrations of fentanyl.

CLINICAL EVALUATION: A patient receiving an intravenous drip of fentanyl at 25 mcg/h developed a supraventricular arrhythmia.[1] Diltiazem (dose not stated) was initiated to treat the arrhythmia. Three days later, the patient became delirious and somnolent and had pinpoint pupils, but no respiratory suppression was noted. The fentanyl drip was discontinued and the patient became more alert over the next few hours.

RELATED DRUGS: Verapamil (eg, *Calan*) may affect fentanyl in a similar manner. Alfentanil (eg, *Alfenta*) is also known to have its elimination reduced during diltiazem coadministration.

MANAGEMENT OPTIONS:

➡ ***Consider Alternative.*** Other drugs used to treat supraventricular arrhythmias, such as beta-blockers, are not expected to interact with fentanyl. Narcotics that are not substrates for CYP3A4 (eg, morphine [eg, *Roxanol*], hydromorphone [eg, *Dilaudid*], codeine) could be considered for use in patients requiring drugs known to inhibit CYP3A4.

➡ ***Monitor.*** Carefully monitor patients stabilized on fentanyl if diltiazem is added to or removed from their drug regimen.

REFERENCES:

1. Levin TT, et al. Case report: delirium due to a diltiazem-fentanyl CYP3A4 drug interaction. *Gen Hosp Psychiatry*. 2010;32(6):648.e9-648.e10.

4   Diltiazem (eg, *Cardizem*)

Grapefruit Juice

SUMMARY: The administration of a single glass of grapefruit juice with an immediate-release formulation of diltiazem produced a modest increase in diltiazem plasma concentrations.

RISK FACTORS: No specific risk factors are known.

MECHANISM: Grapefruit juice inhibits the activity of CYP3A4 in the intestinal wall, somewhat reducing the presystemic metabolism of diltiazem.

CLINICAL EVALUATION: Ten healthy subjects were administered a single immediate-release formulation of diltiazem 120 mg with water or with 250 mL of grapefruit juice.[1] The mean area under the plasma concentration-time curve (AUC) of diltiazem was increased 20%. The range of effect on the AUC was −5% to 81%. Diltiazem half-life was unaffected by grapefruit juice administration. While this study used a single dose of juice, another study using 200 mL of grapefruit juice for 5 doses after diltiazem reported less than a 10% increase in the mean AUC of diltiazem.[2] Some patients may experience an increased effect of diltiazem if it is administered with grapefruit juice, although the risk of adverse reactions appears to be limited.

RELATED DRUGS: Grapefruit juice is known to increase the plasma concentrations of other calcium channel blockers, including felodipine, nicardipine (eg, *Cardene*), verapamil (eg, *Calan*), and nifedipine (eg, *Procardia*).

MANAGEMENT OPTIONS:

➡ *Monitor.* Advise patients taking diltiazem to be alert for increased effect (hypotension or bradycardia) if grapefruit juice is consumed.

REFERENCES:

1. Christensen H, et al. Coadministration of grapefruit juice increases systemic exposure of diltiazem in healthy volunteers. *Eur J Clin Pharmacol*. 2002;58(8):515-520.
2. Sigusch H, et al. Lack of effect of grapefruit juice on diltiazem bioavailability in normal subjects. *Pharmazie*. 1994;49(9):675-679.

Diltiazem (eg, *Cardizem*)

Lovastatin (eg, *Mevacor*)

SUMMARY: Diltiazem administration produces a marked increase in lovastatin concentrations; increased toxicity may result.

RISK FACTORS: No specific risk factors are known.

MECHANISM: Diltiazem appears to inhibit the CYP3A4-mediated metabolism (particularly the first-pass metabolism) of lovastatin.

CLINICAL EVALUATION: Ten healthy subjects received a single dose of lovastatin before and after 2 weeks of administration of sustained-release diltiazem 120 mg twice daily.[1] Diltiazem pretreatment increased the area under the concentration-time curve of lovastatin 257% and the peak lovastatin concentration from 6 to 26 ng/mL. No change was observed in the half-life of lovastatin following diltiazem pretreatment. The pharmacokinetics of the active metabolite of lovastatin were not reported; however, it is likely that the metabolite concentrations also would be increased during diltiazem administration.

RELATED DRUGS: Simvastatin (eg, *Zocor*) is likely to be affected by diltiazem in a similar manner. Verapamil (eg, *Calan*) and mibefradil are likely to produce similar changes in lovastatin concentrations. Dihydropyridine calcium channel antagonists are less likely to alter lovastatin pharmacokinetics, although isradipine (eg, *DynaCirc*) was reported to decrease lovastatin concentrations.[2] Pravastatin (eg, *Pravachol*) metabolism is not altered by diltiazem. The effect of diltiazem on other HMG-CoA reductase inhibitors is unknown.

MANAGEMENT OPTIONS:

➡ *Consider Alternative.* Pravastatin is a good alternative for patients taking calcium channel blockers that inhibit CYP3A4 activity (eg, diltiazem, verapamil, mibefradil).

➡ *Monitor.* Carefully monitor patients taking lovastatin or simvastatin who receive diltiazem, verapamil, or mibefradil for evidence of myositis.

REFERENCES:

1. Agbim NE, et al. Interaction of diltiazem with lovastatin and pravastatin. *Clin Pharmacol Ther.* 1997;61:201.

2. Zhou LX, et al. Pharmacokinetic interaction between isradipine and lovastatin in normal, female and male volunteers. *J Pharmacol Exp Ther.* 1995;273(1):121-127.

Diltiazem (eg, *Cardizem*)

Methylprednisolone (eg, *Medrol*)

SUMMARY: Diltiazem administration increases the plasma concentration of methylprednisolone; increased glucocorticoid effects are likely to occur.

RISK FACTORS: No specific risk factors are known.

MECHANISM: Diltiazem inhibits CYP3A4, an enzyme known to metabolize methylprednisolone. Diltiazem is also an inhibitor of p-glycoprotein, a transmembrane efflux pump that acts to limit the absorption of methylprednisolone and may increase its excretion as well.

CLINICAL EVALUATION: Nine subjects received placebo or diltiazem 60 mg 3 times daily for 3 days.[1] On the third day of placebo or diltiazem administration, a single 16 mg dose of methylprednisolone was administered orally. The mean peak concentration of methylprednisolone increased 63%, while its mean area under the concentration-time curve increased approximately 2.6-fold. The half-life of methylprednisolone increased from a mean of 1.6 to 3.1 hours following diltiazem administration. The dose of methylprednisolone had a greater effect on suppressing plasma cortisol following diltiazem pretreatment. The administration of diltiazem with methylprednisolone may cause increased glucocorticoid effects (hyperglycemia, edema, weakness, or hypokalemia) including enhanced adrenal suppression.

RELATED DRUGS: Verapamil (eg, *Calan*) may also inhibit methylprednisolone metabolism. Dihydropyridine calcium channel antagonists (eg, amlodipine [*Norvasc*], felodipine [*Plendil*]) would not be expected to alter methylprednisolone metabolism. It is likely that other glucocorticoids would be affected in a similar manner by diltiazem administration.

MANAGEMENT OPTIONS:

➡ *Consider Alternative.* Consider using a dihydropyridine calcium channel antagonist instead of diltiazem.

➡ *Monitor.* Monitor patients receiving diltiazem and methylprednisolone for signs and symptoms of excess glucocorticoid effects.

REFERENCES:

1. Varis T, et al. Diltiazem and mibefradil increase the plasma concentrations and greatly enhance the adrenal-suppressant effect of oral methylprednisolone. *Clin Pharmacol Ther.* 2000;67(3):215-21.

Diltiazem (eg, *Cardizem*)

Midazolam (*Versed*)

SUMMARY: Diltiazem increases midazolam plasma concentrations and may prolong sedation and respiratory depression.

RISK FACTORS: No specific risk factors are known.

MECHANISM: Diltiazem appears to inhibit the metabolism (CYP3A4) of midazolam.

CLINICAL EVALUATION: Thirty patients undergoing coronary artery bypass surgery were given midazolam 0.1 mg/kg induction followed by 1 mcg/kg/min and alfentanil (*Alfenta*) 50 mcg/kg induction and 1 mcg/kg/min maintenance for anesthesia.[1] Fifteen of the patients were selected to receive placebo and 15 received diltiazem 60 mg orally 2 hours before induction and an infusion of 0.1 mg/kg/hr started at induction and continued for 23 hours. Mean total IV diltiazem dose was 169 mg. The 2 groups of patients were similar in other aspects of their surgeries. Coadministration of diltiazem prolonged the half-life of midazolam from a mean of 493 minutes to 704 minutes. The area under the concentration-time curve (AUC) of midazolam was increased by 15% in the diltiazem group. The awakening time was not statistically increased in the diltiazem group (125 min versus 17 min) but time to extubation was prolonged by an average of 2.5 hours. In a study of 9 subjects, diltiazem 60 mg 3 times a day for 2 days increased the AUC of midazolam (15 mg orally) by 275% and its half-life increased from 4.9 hr to 7.3 hr.[2]

RELATED DRUGS: Diltiazem has been noted to increase the concentrations of triazolam (eg, *Halcion*).[3,4] Verapamil (eg, *Isoptin*) may affect midazolam in a similar manner.[2] Mibefradil also would be expected to inhibit midazolam metabolism.

MANAGEMENT OPTIONS:

➡ *Consider Alternative.* The use of a dihydropyridine calcium channel blocker would probably avoid the interaction. Selection of a benzodiazepine such as lorazepam (*Ativan*) or temazepam (*Restoril*) that is not metabolized by CYP3A4 would prevent an interaction with diltiazem.

➡ *Monitor.* Monitor patients receiving diltiazem and midazolam for prolonged sedation and respiratory depression.

REFERENCES:

1. Ahonen J, et al. Effect of diltiazem on midazolam and alfentanil disposition in patients undergoing coronary artery bypass grafting. *Anesthesiology.* 1996;85:1246.

2. Backman JT, et al. Dose of midazolam should be reduced during diltiazem and verapamil treatments. *Br J Clin Pharmacol.* 1994;55:481.

3. Kosuge K, et al. Enhanced effect of triazolam with diltiazem. *Br J Clin Pharmacol.* 1997;43:367.

4. Varhe A, et al. Diltiazem enhances the effects of triazolam by inhibiting its metabolism. *Clin Pharmacol Ther*. 1996;59:369.

Diltiazem (eg, *Cardizem*)

Nifedipine (eg, *Procardia*)

SUMMARY: Diltiazem increases the serum concentration of nifedipine; nifedipine increases the serum concentration of diltiazem. Increased pharmacodynamic effects could occur.

RISK FACTORS:

➥ *Dosage Regimen.* Patients with daily diltiazem doses of greater than 270 mg are at particular risk.

MECHANISM: Diltiazem appears to inhibit the metabolism of nifedipine and increase its bioavailability; calcium channel blockers may exhibit additive pharmacodynamic effects. Nifedipine also appears to inhibit the metabolism of diltiazem, perhaps caused by competition for the same enzyme (CYP3A4) in the liver.

CLINICAL EVALUATION: Eleven patients with angina received diltiazem 30 mg 4 times a day, nifedipine 10 mg 4 times a day, and a combination of the 2 agents for 1 week.[1] Nifedipine serum concentrations increased from 34.8 ng/mL during monotherapy to 106.4 ng/mL when diltiazem was coadministered. Nifedipine did not alter diltiazem concentrations; however, in another study antianginal effects were greatest during administration of both drugs. In another study, 6 healthy subjects received diltiazem 30 mg and 90 mg 3 times a day for 4 days, and on the fourth day nifedipine 20 mg was administered.[2] The nifedipine mean area under the concentration-time curve (AUC) increased by 122% in the subjects who received 30 mg 3 times a day of diltiazem and by more than 200% in those who received 90 mg 3 times a day. Nifedipine half-life was prolonged from 2.5 hours to 3.5 hours. Diltiazem 60 mg 3 times a day reduced the clearance after oral administration of nifedipine by about 60% in healthy subjects.[3,5] Nifedipine 10 mg 3 times a day increased the peak diltiazem concentration and AUC by approximately 50% in healthy subjects.[6]

RELATED DRUGS: The combination of nitrendipine (*Baypress*) and diltiazem produced greater hypotensive effects than each drug alone; no pharmacokinetic data were evaluated.[7] The combination of amlodipine (*Norvasc*) and verapamil (eg, *Calan*) produced a greater increase in forearm blood flow than amlodipine alone.[4] Since the drugs were infused into the brachial artery for 3 minutes, this effect is likely caused by combined vasodilation.

MANAGEMENT OPTIONS:

➥ *Monitor.* Monitor patients receiving nifedipine and diltiazem for increased nifedipine effects such as hypotension or headache and increased diltiazem effects including bradycardia.

REFERENCES:

1. Toyosaki N, et al. Combination therapy with diltiazem and nifedipine in patients with effort angina pectoris. *Circulation*. 1988;77:1370.
2. Tateishi T, et al. Dose dependent effect of diltiazem on the pharmacokinetics of nifedipine. *J Clin Pharmacol*. 1989;29:994.
3. Ohashi K, et al. Effects of diltiazem on the pharmacokinetics of nifedipine. *J Caradiovasc Pharmacol*. 1990;15:96.

4. Kiowski W, et al. Arterial vasodilator effects of the dihydropyridine calcium antagonist amlodipine alone and in combination with verapamil in systemic hypertension. *Am J Cardiol*. 1990;66:1469.

5. Ohashi K, et al. The influence of pretreatment periods with diltiazem on nifedipine kinetics. *J Clin Pharmacol*. 1993;33:222.

6. Tateishi T, et al. The effect of nifedipine on the pharmacokinetics and dynamics of diltiazem: the preliminary study in normal volunteers. *J Clin Pharmacol*. 1993;33:738.

7. Andreyev N, et al. Comparison of diltiazem, nitrendipine, and their combination for systemic hypertension and stable angina pectoris. *J Cardiovasc Pharmacol*. 1991;18(Suppl. 9):S73.

Diltiazem (eg, *Cardizem*)

Nitroprusside (*Nipride*)

SUMMARY: Diltiazem administration reduces the dose of nitroprusside required to produce hypotension and may enhance nitroprusside-induced hypotension.

RISK FACTORS: No specific risk factors are known.

MECHANISM: Diltiazem may enhance the hypotensive effects of nitroprusside, and it appears to alter the metabolism of nitroprusside.

CLINICAL EVALUATION: Twenty surgical patients were administered nitroprusside at a rate that produced a mean arterial blood pressure of 55 to 60 mm Hg.[1] Ten of these patients were randomly selected also to receive diltiazem IV coadministered as an 80 mcg/kg bolus followed by 4.5 mcg/kg/min for 30 minutes and then 1.3 mcg/kg/min. This dosage regimen maintained diltiazem concentrations in the range of 70 to 90 ng/mL. The cumulative dose of nitroprusside was reduced by nearly 50% in the patients receiving diltiazem. Increased thiocyanate concentrations, tachycardia, and tachyphylaxis to nitroprusside response were absent in patients receiving diltiazem and nitroprusside.

RELATED DRUGS: Other calcium channel blockers may produce similar interactions with nitroprusside.

MANAGEMENT OPTIONS:

➡ *Monitor.* Patients stabilized on diltiazem may require reduced doses of nitroprusside to produce a controlled hypotension. This interaction could be advantageous in that the reduced thiocyanate formation could decrease the risk of cyanide toxicity in patients who require long-term infusions. Additional data are needed to assess this interaction over longer administration times.

REFERENCES:

1. Bernard JM, et al. Diltiazem reduces the nitroprusside doses for deliberate hypotension. *Anesthesiology*. 1992;77:A427.

Diltiazem (eg, *Cardizem*)

Phenytoin (*Dilantin*)

SUMMARY: Some clinical evidence suggests that diltiazem can increase phenytoin serum concentrations, but a causal relationship was not established.

RISK FACTORS: No specific risk factors are known.

MECHANISM: Not established, but diltiazem may reduce the metabolism of phenytoin. Theoretically, phenytoin may enhance the hepatic metabolism of diltiazem.

CLINICAL EVALUATION: In a retrospective analysis, 3 of 14 patients receiving diltiazem and phenytoin exhibited signs of phenytoin toxicity.[1] More study is needed to establish whether diltiazem affects phenytoin metabolism.

RELATED DRUGS: Nifedipine (eg, *Procardia*) also has been reported to cause phenytoin toxicity, but a causal relationship was not established. Little is known regarding other calcium channel blockers.

MANAGEMENT OPTIONS: No specific action is required, but be alert for evidence of the interaction.

REFERENCES:
1. Bahls F, et al. Interactions between calcium channel blockers and the anticonvulsants carbamazepine and phenytoin. *Neurology.* 1991;41:740.

Diltiazem (eg, *Cardizem*)

Pravastatin (*Pravachol*)

SUMMARY: Diltiazem administration does not affect pravastatin concentrations.

RISK FACTORS: No specific risk factors are known.

MECHANISM: No interaction.

CLINICAL EVALUATION: Ten normal subjects received a single dose of pravastatin before and after 2 weeks of administration of diltiazem SR 120 mg twice daily.[1] Diltiazem pretreatment produced no change in the half-life, area under the concentration-time curve, or peak concentration of pravastatin.

RELATED DRUGS: The metabolism of lovastatin (*Mevacor*) and simvastatin (*Zocor*) are likely to be reduced by diltiazem. Other calcium channel blockers would be unlikely to affect the metabolism of pravastatin.

MANAGEMENT OPTIONS: No interaction.

REFERENCES:
1. Agbim NE, et al. Interaction of diltiazem with lovastatin and pravastatin. *Clin Pharmacol Ther.* 1997;61:201.

Diltiazem (eg, *Cardizem*)

Propranolol (eg, *Inderal*)

SUMMARY: Diltiazem increases the plasma concentrations of propranolol and metoprolol (eg, *Lopressor*). Although the interaction may be used to advantage, some predisposed patients may experience adverse effects.

RISK FACTORS: No specific risk factors are known.

MECHANISM: Diltiazem has been shown to inhibit the hepatic metabolism of several beta blockers. Diltiazem has additive effects with beta blockers on cardiac conduction (slowing atrioventricular [AV] conduction) and may enhance the hypotensive effects of beta blockade.

CLINICAL EVALUATION: Diltiazem 30 mg 3 times a day administered for 3 to 4 days significantly increased the AUC of propranolol (48%)[2,4] and metoprolol (33%).[2] A report in 14 healthy subjects found that diltiazem 60 mg 3 times a day for 5 days reduced the clearance of oral propranolol by 40%.[1] Diltiazem reduces the clearance of both propranolol enantiomers by approximately 25%.[3]

RELATED DRUGS: Diltiazem had no effect on atenolol (eg, *Tenormin*) serum concentrations. Verapamil (eg, *Calan*) reduces the metabolism of several beta blockers, including metoprolol.

MANAGEMENT OPTIONS:

➤ *Circumvent/Minimize.* The use of beta blockers that are not metabolized (eg, atenolol) should minimize pharmacokinetic (but not pharmacodynamic) interactions with diltiazem.

➤ *Monitor.* Monitor patients receiving therapy with beta blockers and diltiazem for enhanced effects, particularly AV-conduction slowing, resulting from pharmacokinetic or pharmacodynamic interactions.

REFERENCES:

1. Dimmett DC, et al. Pharmacokinetics of cardizem and propranolol when administered alone and in combination. *Biopharm Drug Dispos.* 1991;12:515.
2. Tateishi T, et al. Effect of diltiazem on the pharmacokinetics of propranolol, metoprolol and atenolol. *Eur J Clin Pharmacol.* 1989;36:67.
3. Hunt BA, et al. Effects of calcium channel blockers on the pharmacokinetics of propranolol stereoisomers. *Clin Pharmacol Ther.* 1990;47:584.
4. Tateishi T, et al. The influence of diltiazem versus cimetidine on propranolol metabolism. *J Clin Pharmacol.* 1992;32:1099.

Diltiazem (eg, *Cardizem*)

Quinidine (eg, *Quinora*)

SUMMARY: Diltiazem increases the plasma concentration of quinidine at doses greater than 120 mg/day. Increased quinidine effect on myocardial conduction may occur.

RISK FACTORS: No specific risk factors are known.

MECHANISM: Diltiazem appears to inhibit the metabolism (CYP3A4) of quinidine.

CLINICAL EVALUATION: Ten healthy subjects received quinidine 600 mg twice daily for 7 days, diltiazem 120 mg/day for 7 days, and the combination of quinidine plus diltiazem for 7 days.[1] Details of the study are limited, but diltiazem did not alter the peak concentration or half-life of quinidine compared with quinidine administration alone. Quinidine did not alter the pharmacokinetics of diltiazem. In a second study, 12 healthy subjects received a single dose of diltiazem 60 mg or quinidine 200 mg alone. The doses were repeated after 2 days of pretreatment with diltiazem 90 mg twice daily (prior to quinidine) or quinidine 100 mg twice daily (prior to diltiazem).[2] Pretreatment with diltiazem increased the area under the concentration-time curve of quinidine 51% and increased its half-life 36%. The increased quinidine concentration was accompanied by increased pharmacodynamic effect (increased QTc). Quinidine pretreatment did not affect the pharmacokinetics of diltiazem. The increased effect observed in the second study may be caused by the larger dose of diltiazem employed.

RELATED DRUGS: Verapamil (eg, *Calan*) has been reported to inhibit the metabolism of quinidine. Dihydropyridine calcium channel antagonists (eg, amlodipine [*Norvasc*], felodipine [*Plendil*]) would not be expected to alter quinidine metabolism.

MANAGEMENT OPTIONS:

➡ *Circumvent/Minimize.* Patients taking quinidine could be treated with other calcium channel blockers such as amlodipine or felodipine that do not inhibit drug metabolism.

➡ *Monitor.* If quinidine and diltiazem are coadministered, monitor for increased quinidine effect such as prolonged QTc.

REFERENCES:

1. Matera MG, et al. Quinidine-Diltiazem: pharmacokinetic interaction in humans. *Curr Ther Res.* 1986;40:653-56.
2. Laganiere S, et al. Pharmacokinetic and pharmacodynamic interactions between diltiazem and quinidine. *Clin Pharmacol Ther.* 1996;60(3):255-64.

Diltiazem (eg, *Cardizem*)

Ranolazine (*Ranexa*)

SUMMARY: Diltiazem increases ranolazine plasma concentrations; some patients may experience adverse effects.

RISK FACTORS: No specific risk factors are known.

MECHANISM: Diltiazem inhibits CYP3A4, the primary pathway of ranolazine metabolism, reducing first-pass and systemic clearance of ranolazine.

CLINICAL EVALUATION: Diltiazem 60 mg 3 times daily or placebo was administered to 12 healthy subjects on 2 separate occasions: once for 7 days and again for 8 days.[1] Ranolazine 240 mg immediate release (IR) was coadministered 3 times daily from days 4 to 7. In the second study, ranolazine 500 mg sustained release (SR) was coadministered with diltiazem on days 4 to 8. The administration of diltiazem increased the mean area under the plasma concentration-time curve of IR and SR ranolazine about 85%. Increasing diltiazem doses from 180 to 360 mg daily increased the magnitude of its effect on ranolazine plasma concentrations. Ranolazine IR had no effect on diltiazem plasma concentrations. The manufacturer of ranolazine contraindicates its use with CYP3A4 inhibitors.[2]

RELATED DRUGS: Verapamil (eg, *Calan*) also is known to inhibit CYP3A4 and has been reported to increase ranolazine plasma concentrations.

MANAGEMENT OPTIONS:

➡ *Consider Alternative.* A calcium channel blocker that does not inhibit CYP3A4 (eg, amlodipine [*Norvasc*], felodipine [*Plendil*]) could be considered for patients receiving ranolazine.

➡ *Monitor.* Monitor patients taking ranolazine who also are prescribed diltiazem for evidence of ranolazine accumulation (eg, constipation, dizziness, headache, nausea).

REFERENCES:

1. Jerling M, et al. Studies to investigate the pharmacokinetic interactions between ranolazine and ketoconazole, diltiazem, or simvastatin during combined administration in healthy subjects. *J Clin Pharmacol.* 2005;45:422-433.
2. *Ranexa* [package insert]. Palo Alto, CA: CV Therapeutics; 2006.

Diltiazem (eg, *Cardizem*)

Rifampin (eg, *Rifadin*)

SUMMARY: Rifampin decreases diltiazem plasma concentrations; loss of therapeutic effect may result.

RISK FACTORS:

➡ *Route of Administration.* Oral administration of diltiazem will lead to a greater effect.

MECHANISM: Rifampin induces the metabolism (CYP3A), reduces the bioavailability, and increases the clearance after oral administration of diltiazem.

CLINICAL EVALUATION: Twelve subjects received a single dose of diltiazem 120 mg alone and another similar dose after receiving rifampin 600 mg/day for 8 days.[1] The mean diltiazem peak concentration of 186 ng/mL decreased to less than 8 ng/mL after rifampin. This magnitude of interaction is likely to reduce the efficacy of oral diltiazem.

RELATED DRUGS: Rifampin probably affects other calcium channel blockers in a similar manner.

MANAGEMENT OPTIONS:

➡ *Consider Alternative.* Because this interaction is likely to reduce the efficacy of diltiazem, consider an alternative to diltiazem. Other calcium channel blockers also may be affected. A therapeutic substitution of a different class of agent (noncalcium blocker) may be required.

➡ *Circumvent/Minimize.* Larger doses of calcium channel blocker (particularly those administered orally) may be required when rifampin is coadministered.

➡ *Monitor.* Monitor patients taking calcium channel blockers for a reduction in efficacy when rifampin is given.

REFERENCES:

1. Drda KD, et al. Effects of debrisoquine hydroxylation phenotype and enzyme induction with rifampin on diltiazem pharmacokinetics and pharmacodynamics. *Pharmacotherapy.* 1991;11:278.

Diltiazem (eg, *Cardizem*)

Saxagliptin (*Onglyza*)

SUMMARY: Saxagliptin hypoglycemic response may be enhanced during the coadministration of diltiazem; it is possible some patients may require a dose adjustment.

RISK FACTORS: No specific risk factors are known.

MECHANISM: Diltiazem may increase saxagliptin plasma concentrations by inhibition of CYP3A4, P-glycoprotein, or both.

CLINICAL EVALUATION: A single dose of saxagliptin 10 mg was administered alone and following long-acting diltiazem 360 mg daily for 9 days.[1] The pretreatment with diltiazem produced a 2-fold increase in the mean area under the concentration-time curve (AUC) of saxagliptin and reduced the AUC of its active metabolite 34%. It is not clear if this magnitude of change in saxagliptin pharmacokinetics will alter its hypoglycemic response.

RELATED DRUGS: Verapamil (eg, *Isoptin SR*) is expected to produce a similar change in the pharmacokinetics of saxagliptin. While sitagliptin (*Januvia*) is also a P-glycoprotein substrate, the potential for diltiazem to increase its plasma concentration is unknown.

MANAGEMENT OPTIONS:

➥ *Monitor.* Monitor patients stabilized on saxagliptin for changes in their blood glucose levels if diltiazem is initiated or discontinued from their drug regimen.

REFERENCES:

1. *Onglyza* [package insert]. Wilmington, DE: AstraZeneca Pharmaceuticals LP; 2011.

Diltiazem (eg, *Cardizem*)

Sildenafil (eg, *Viagra*)

SUMMARY: Diltiazem may increase the plasma concentrations of sildenafil; this could result in increased adverse reactions, particularly if another vasodilator is administered.

RISK FACTORS: No specific risk factors are known.

MECHANISM: Diltiazem is known to inhibit the activity of CYP3A4, one of the enzymes responsible for the metabolism of sildenafil.

CLINICAL EVALUATION: A 72-year-old man with stable angina had an elective coronary angiography.[1] His medications included metoprolol (eg, *Lopressor*) 50 mg twice daily, diltiazem 30 mg 3 times daily, and sublingual nitroglycerin as needed for angina. During the angiography, the patient reported chest pain and was administered half a sublingual nitroglycerin tablet. This was followed within 2 minutes by hypotension that gradually responded to fluids over the next 6 hours. The patient reported that he had taken a dose of sildenafil 50 mg 2 days prior to the angiography. While it is uncertain if the response to the nitroglycerin was exacerbated by the prior sildenafil exposure, it is possible that the diltiazem could reduce the first-pass or systemic metabolism of sildenafil. The presence of a beta-blocker may have also contributed by preventing a reflex tachycardia that may have helped to support the patient's blood pressure.

RELATED DRUGS: Verapamil (eg, *Isoptin SR*) is another calcium channel blocker known to inhibit CYP3A4. It may inhibit sildenafil metabolism.

MANAGEMENT OPTIONS:

➥ *Circumvent/Minimize.* Avoid using calcium channel blockers that inhibit CYP3A4 in patients taking sildenafil. Minimal interference of the metabolism of sildenafil is expected with dihydropyridine calcium channel blockers (eg, amlodipine [eg, *Norvasc*], felodipine). All calcium channel blockers may produce increased hypotensive effects when combined with sildenafil.

➥ *Monitor.* Be alert for hypotensive reactions if diltiazem is coadministered with sildenafil.

REFERENCES:

1. Khoury V, Kritharides L. Diltiazem-mediated inhibition of sildenafil metabolism may promote nitrate-induced hypotension. *Aust N Z J Med.* 2000;30(5):641-642.

Diltiazem (eg, *Cardizem*)

Sirolimus (*Rapamune*)

SUMMARY: Diltiazem administration increases sirolimus plasma concentrations; adverse reactions are likely to occur in some patients.

RISK FACTORS: No specific risk factors are known.

MECHANISM: Diltiazem is recognized as a CYP3A4 and P-glycoprotein inhibitor. One or both of these mechanisms may be responsible for the increase in sirolimus concentrations observed following diltiazem administration.

CLINICAL EVALUATION: A single dose of sirolimus 10 mg was administered orally to 18 subjects alone and 1 hour following diltiazem 120 mg immediate-release formulation.[1] The mean values for peak sirolimus concentration and area under the concentration-time curve increased 43% and 60%, respectively, following diltiazem dosing. Sirolimus half-life declined from 79 to 67 hours with diltiazem administration. The oral clearance of sirolimus was reduced 38% with diltiazem pretreatment. The apparent volume of distribution of sirolimus was also reduced 45% by diltiazem. Based on the effect of a single diltiazem dose, multiple-dose diltiazem administration is likely to result in altered sirolimus efficacy. Sirolimus did not affect diltiazem concentrations or pharmacologic effects.

RELATED DRUGS: Verapamil (eg, *Isoptin SR*) may affect sirolimus in a similar manner. Diltiazem is known to increase the concentrations of other immunosuppressants, including cyclosporine (eg, *Neoral*) and tacrolimus (eg, *Prograf*).

MANAGEMENT OPTIONS:

➡ **Monitor.** Pending studies of the effect of long-term diltiazem dosing on sirolimus plasma concentrations, carefully monitor patients receiving the drug combination.

REFERENCES:
1. Böttiger Y, et al. Pharmacokinetic interaction between single oral doses of diltiazem and sirolimus in healthy volunteers. *Clin Pharmacol Ther.* 2001;69(1):32-40.

Diltiazem (eg, *Cardizem*)

Tacrolimus (eg, *Prograf*)

SUMMARY: Tacrolimus concentrations increased during diltiazem administration, resulting in tacrolimus toxicity.

RISK FACTORS: No specific risk factors are known.

MECHANISM: Diltiazem is known to inhibit CYP3A4, the enzyme that primarily metabolizes tacrolimus. In addition, diltiazem may inhibit P-glycoprotein transport of tacrolimus, resulting in increased plasma concentration.

CLINICAL EVALUATION: A 68-year-old man, 4 months after orthotopic liver transplantation, developed atrial fibrillation.[1] In addition to tacrolimus 8 mg twice daily, he was treated with azathioprine (eg, *Imuran*), prednisone, sulfamethoxazole/trimethoprim (eg, *Bactrim*), ganciclovir (eg, *Cytovene*), digoxin (eg, *Lanoxin*), and multivitamins. His blood tacrolimus concentration was 12.9 ng/mL. Diltiazem was administered intravenously (5 to 10 mg/h) for 1 day and then switched to 30 mg orally every 8 hours. Three days after diltiazem was initiated, the patient developed delirium, confusion, and agitation. His tacrolimus concentration was 55 ng/mL. Tacrolimus and diltiazem were discontinued. The tacrolimus concentration was 6.7 ng/mL 3 days later and was accompanied by resolution of his mental symptoms. Tacrolimus was titrated to 5 mg twice daily, resulting in concentrations of 9 to 10 ng/mL.

RELATED DRUGS: Verapamil (eg, *Calan*) also may increase tacrolimus concentrations because it has been reported to inhibit CYP3A4.

MANAGEMENT OPTIONS:

➥ *Consider Alternative.* In patients taking tacrolimus who require cardioversion for atrial fibrillation, consider using digoxin, quinidine, or procainamide. Dihydropyridine calcium blockers (eg, amlodipine [*Norvasc*], nifedipine [eg, *Procardia*]) could be used to treat hypertension in patients taking tacrolimus.

➥ *Monitor.* In patients taking tacrolimus who are treated with diltiazem, carefully monitor their tacrolimus concentrations. Adjust doses to keep the tacrolimus concentration within the therapeutic range (approximately 5 to 15 ng/mL).

REFERENCES:

1. Hebert MF, Lam AY. Diltiazem increases tacrolimus concentrations. *Ann Pharmacother*. 1999;33(6):680-682.

Diltiazem (eg, *Cardizem*)

Ticagrelor (*Brilinta*)

SUMMARY: Diltiazem increases the plasma concentration of ticagrelor and reduces the concentration of its active metabolite; the net effect is likely to be increased antiplatelet activity.

RISK FACTORS: No specific risk factors are known.

MECHANISM: Diltiazem inhibits CYP3A4, the primary enzyme responsible for the metabolism of ticagrelor.

CLINICAL EVALUATION: While specific data are limited, the manufacturer of ticagrelor notes that the coadministration of diltiazem 240 mg once daily increased the mean area under the plasma concentration-time curve (AUC) of ticagrelor by 2- to 3-fold.[1] The AUC of ticagrelor's active metabolite (approximately equipotent to ticagrelor, but present at approximately 35% of the concentration of ticagrelor) was reduced during diltiazem coadministration. Pending further data, observe patients receiving ticagrelor and diltiazem for increased ticagrelor effects, including bleeding.

RELATED DRUGS: Diltiazem may reduce the metabolism of clopidogrel (*Plavix*) to its active metabolite. Verapamil (eg, *Calan*) may affect ticagrelor in a similar manner.

MANAGEMENT OPTIONS:

➥ *Consider Alternative.* Calcium channel blockers that do not inhibit CYP3A4 (eg, amlodipine [eg, *Norvasc*], nifedipine [eg, *Procardia*], felodipine) could be considered for patients taking ticagrelor. Prasugrel (*Effient*) antiplatelet activity may be less susceptible to alteration by diltiazem than ticagrelor.

➥ *Monitor.* Monitor patients stabilized on ticagrelor for altered antiplatelet effects if diltiazem is initiated or discontinued.

REFERENCES:

1. *Brilinta* [package insert]. Wilmington, DE: AstraZeneca LP; 2011.

4   Diltiazem (eg, *Cardizem*)

Tolbutamide

SUMMARY: Diltiazem produced a small increase in tolbutamide plasma concentrations; no change in hypoglycemic effect is expected. Tolbutamide did not affect the plasma concentrations of diltiazem.

RISK FACTORS: No specific risk factors are known.

MECHANISM: Unknown. Diltiazem is not thought to inhibit the metabolism of tolbutamide; however, it may alter tolbutamide's elimination by other pathways.

CLINICAL EVALUATION: Eight healthy subjects received diltiazem 60 mg daily, tolbutamide 500 mg daily, or the combination for 7 days.[1] The mean area under the tolbutamide plasma concentration-time curve increased 10% during diltiazem administration. Diltiazem pharmacokinetic parameters were not affected by tolbutamide coadministration. While the dose of diltiazem was low in this study, it is not expected that higher doses will cause a sufficient change in tolbutamide concentrations to alter blood glucose response.

RELATED DRUGS: No information is available.

MANAGEMENT OPTIONS:

➥ *Monitor.* No specific monitoring appears to be required beyond the usual blood glucose monitoring.

REFERENCES:

1. Dixit AA, et al. Pharmacokinetic interaction between diltiazem and tolbutamide. *Drug Metabol Drug Interact*. 1999;15(4):269-277.

Diltiazem (eg, *Cardizem*)

Triazolam (eg, *Halcion*)

SUMMARY: Diltiazem increases triazolam serum concentrations; expect increased triazolam effects (eg, sedation, ataxia).

RISK FACTORS: No specific risk factors are known.

MECHANISM: Diltiazem inhibits the CYP3A4-mediated metabolism of triazolam, resulting in increased bioavailability and reduced systemic clearance.

CLINICAL EVALUATION: The administration of diltiazem 180 mg/day resulted in a 2- to 3-fold increase in the serum concentrations of triazolam 0.25 mg orally.[1,2] The half-life of triazolam was increased 2-fold by diltiazem pretreatment. Pharmacodynamic assessment of benzodiazepine effects showed significant enhancement of triazolam effects in the presence of diltiazem. A study using a small (40 mg) dose of diltiazem did not find any effect on the hypnotic effects of triazolam or temazepam.[3]

RELATED DRUGS: Verapamil (eg, *Calan*) is expected to interact with triazolam in a similar manner. Other benzodiazepines that are metabolized by CYP3A4, such as alprazolam (eg, *Xanax*), midazolam, or halazepam, would likely interact with diltiazem.

MANAGEMENT OPTIONS:

➡ *Consider Alternative.* Other calcium channel blockers, except verapamil, are unlikely to interact with triazolam. Benzodiazepines that are not metabolized by CYP3A4 (eg, oxazepam, temazepam [eg, *Restoril*]) are not be likely to be affected by diltiazem.

➡ *Monitor.* Monitor patients when diltiazem is coadministered for evidence of increased triazolam effect.

REFERENCES:

1. Varhe A, et al. Diltiazem enhances the effects of triazolam by inhibiting its metabolism. *Clin Pharmacol Ther.* 1996;59(4):369-375.
2. Kosuge K, et al. Enhanced effect of triazolam with diltiazem. *Br J Clin Pharmacol.* 1997;43(4):367-372.
3. Scharf MB, et al. The effects of a calcium channel blocker on the effects of temazepam and triazolam. *Curr Ther Res Clin Exp.* 1990;48:516.

Diltiazem (eg, *Cardizem*)

Warfarin (eg, *Coumadin*)

SUMMARY: Diltiazem has minor effects on warfarin pharmacokinetics, but it does not appear to affect its hypoprothrombinemic response.

RISK FACTORS: No specific risk factors are known.

MECHANISM: Not established. Diltiazem may inhibit the hepatic metabolism of R-warfarin.

CLINICAL EVALUATION: Diltiazem inhibited the clearance of R-warfarin in healthy subjects, but had no effect on the more potent S-warfarin or hypoprothrombinemic response.[1]

RELATED DRUGS: The effect of diltiazem on oral anticoagulants other than warfarin is not established.

MANAGEMENT OPTIONS: No specific action is required, but be alert for evidence of the interaction.

REFERENCES:

1. Abernethy DR, et al. Selective inhibition of warfarin metabolism by diltiazem in humans. *J Pharmacol Exp Ther.* 1991;257(1):411-415.

Diphenhydramine (eg, *Benadryl*)

Donepezil (eg, *Aricept*)

SUMMARY: Diphenhydramine has anticholinergic properties and may inhibit the therapeutic effect of donepezil in Alzheimer disease.

RISK FACTORS: No specific risk factors are known.

MECHANISM: Donepezil is a cholinesterase inhibitor and its efficacy is likely to be inhibited by anticholinergic agents such as diphenhydramine.[1]

CLINICAL EVALUATION: In a preliminary study of 69 patients with Alzheimer disease receiving donepezil 10 mg/day and followed for 2 years, 16 patients received concurrent therapy with anticholinergic drugs and 53 patients did not.[2] Mental functioning, as measured by the Mini-Mental State Exam (MMSE), was significantly lower in the patients receiving concomitant anticholinergic drugs. Also, the French Pharmacovigilance Database received 118 spontaneous reports of adverse reactions in patients receiving anticholinergic drugs with cholinesterase inhibitors (eg, donepezil, galantamine, rivastigmine). After evaluation by clinical pharmacologists, 24 were thought to be adverse drug interactions.[3] Although additional study is needed to establish the clinical importance of these interactions, the evidence is consistent with the known pharmacological effects of the drugs. Short-term use of an anticholinergic antihistamine may not cause significant interaction.

RELATED DRUGS: All cholinesterase inhibitors used to treat Alzheimer disease (donepezil, galantamine [eg, *Razadyne*], rivastigmine [eg, *Exelon*]) are expected to interact similarly with diphenhydramine, as well as other antihistamines with anticholinergic effects, such as azatadine, azelastine (eg, *Astelin*), brompheniramine (eg, *Dimetapp*), chlorpheniramine (eg, *Chlor-Trimeton*), clemastine (eg, *Tavist*), cyproheptadine, dexchlorpheniramine, hydroxyzine (eg, *Vistaril*), phenindamine,[†]promethazine (eg, *Phenergan*), or triprolidine.[†]

MANAGEMENT OPTIONS:

➡ *Consider Alternative.* Use an alternative to diphenhydramine when possible. Antihistamines with little or no anticholinergic activity include cetirizine (eg, *Zyrtec*), desloratadine (*Clarinex*), ebastine,[†] fexofenadine (eg, *Allegra*), and loratadine (eg, *Claritin*).

➡ *Monitor.* If diphenhydramine or another anticholinergic antihistamine is used with donepezil or another cholinesterase inhibitor, be alert for evidence of reduced mental functioning.

REFERENCES:

1. *Aricept* [package insert]. New York, NY: Pfizer; 2011.
2. Lu CJ, Tune LE. Chronic exposure to anticholinergic medications adversely affects the course of Alzheimer disease. *Am J Geriatr Psychiatry.* 2003;11(4):458-461.
3. Tavassoli N, et al. Drug interactions with cholinesterase inhibitors: an analysis of the French Pharmacovigilance Database and a comparison of two national drug formularies (Vidal, British National Formulary). *Drug Saf.* 2007;30(11):1063-1071.

† Not available in the United States.

Diphenhydramine (eg, *Benadryl*)

Metoprolol (eg, *Lopressor*)

SUMMARY: Diphenhydramine increased the plasma concentration of metoprolol in patients who have high intrinsic CYP2D6 activity. Because of metoprolol's wide therapeutic range, toxicity is not likely to occur in most patients.

RISK FACTORS:

➡ *Pharmacogenetics.* Patients who have high CYP2D6 activity experience a greater reduction in their metoprolol metabolism than those with low CYP2D6 activity.

MECHANISM: Diphenhydramine appears to inhibit the CYP2D6-mediated metabolism of metoprolol.

CLINICAL EVALUATION: Nine subjects who had extensive CYP2D6 activity received placebo or diphenhydramine 50 mg 3 times daily for 3 days.[1] On day 3 of pretreatment, a single oral dose of metoprolol 100 mg was given. Compared with placebo, diphenhydramine administration reduced metoprolol oral clearance 40%. The partial clearance of metoprolol to alpha-hydroxymetoprolol was reduced 57% following diphenhydramine administration. Diphenhydramine had no significant effect (18% reduction) in metoprolol oral clearance when administered to 5 subjects with low CYP2D6 metabolic activity. Metoprolol's wide therapeutic range will mitigate the development of toxicity in most patients. Observe patients taking metoprolol for reduced heart rate or blood pressure if diphenhydramine is administered. While no data are available, diphenhydramine administered on an as-needed basis is expected to have less effect on metoprolol plasma concentrations.

RELATED DRUGS: Other beta-blockers that undergo CYP2D6 metabolism (eg, carvedilol [eg, *Coreg*], propranolol [eg, *Inderal*], timolol [eg, *Blocadren*]) will probably be affected by diphenhydramine in a similar manner. In vitro studies found that other classic antihistamines (eg, chlorpheniramine [eg, *Chlor-Trimeton*], promethazine [eg, *Phenergan*], tripelennamine) reduced the CYP2D6 metabolism of metoprolol.[2]

MANAGEMENT OPTIONS:

➡ *Consider Alternative.* Newer antihistamines (eg, fexofenadine [eg, *Allegra*], cetirizine [eg, *Zyrtec*], loratadine [eg, *Claritin*]) have not demonstrated any inhibitory action on CYP2D6. Beta-blockers not metabolized by CYP2D6 could be used in place of metoprolol in patients taking long-term diphenhydramine therapy. Atenolol (eg, *Tenormin*) is a beta-2 selective blocker that is not metabolized and is not expected to interact with diphenhydramine.

➡ *Monitor.* Monitor patients receiving metoprolol for bradycardia and hypotension when they are given diphenhydramine.

REFERENCES:

1. Hamelin BA, et al. Metoprolol/diphenhydramine interaction in men with high and low CYP2D6 activity. *Clin Pharmacol Ther.* 1999;65:157.

2. Hamelin BA, et al. Classic antihistamines inhibit metoprolol hydroxylation in vitro. *Clin Pharmacol Ther.* 1999;65:157.

Diphenhydramine (eg, *Benadryl*)

Tamoxifen

SUMMARY: Theoretically, diphenhydramine may reduce the efficacy of tamoxifen in the treatment of breast cancer.

RISK FACTORS: No specific risk factors are known.

MECHANISM: Tamoxifen is metabolized to 2 active metabolites by CYP2D6, the most important of which is endoxifen. By reducing endoxifen formation, CYP2D6 inhibitors, such as diphenhydramine, may reduce tamoxifen efficacy.[1-3]

CLINICAL EVALUATION: A study in patients with breast cancer found substantial reductions in endoxifen plasma concentrations in patients taking potent CYP2D6 inhibitors, such as fluoxetine and paroxetine.[4] Another tamoxifen study found a nearly 2-fold increase in the risk of breast cancer relapse in women with low CYP2D6 activity, either due to CYP2D6-inhibiting drugs or genetic deficiency.[5] Taken together, these and other results strongly suggest that CYP2D6 inhibitors reduce the efficacy of tamoxifen in the treatment of breast cancer. Diphenhydramine is a CYP2D6 inhibitor and may inhibit the anticancer effects of tamoxifen.

RELATED DRUGS: Other antihistamines that may inhibit CYP2D6 include chlorpheniramine (eg, *Chlor-Trimeton*), clemastine (eg, *Tavist*), tripelennamine, and promethazine (eg, *Phenergan*).

MANAGEMENT OPTIONS:

➡ *Consider Alternative.* If possible, use an antihistamine that is not known to inhibit CYP2D6 (see Related Drugs).

➡ *Monitor.* If a CYP2D6 inhibitor, such as diphenhydramine, is used with tamoxifen, cancer recurrence may be an indication that tamoxifen efficacy has been reduced. If this happens, consider discontinuing the CYP2D6 inhibitor.

REFERENCES:

1. Dezentjé VO, et al. Clinical implications of CYP2D6 genotyping in tamoxifen treatment for breast cancer. *Clin Cancer Res.* 2009;15(1):15-21.
2. Tan SH, et al. Pharmacogenetics in breast cancer therapy. *Clin Cancer Res.* 2008;14(24):8027-8041.
3. Newman WG, et al. Impaired tamoxifen metabolism reduces survival in familial breast cancer patients. *Clin Cancer Res.* 2008;14(18):5913-5918.
4. Borges S, et al. Quantitative effect of CYP2D6 genotype and inhibitors on tamoxifen metabolism: implication for optimization of breast cancer treatment. *Clin Pharmacol Ther.* 2006;80(1):61-74.
5. Goetz MP, et al. The impact of cytochrome P450 2D6 metabolism in women receiving adjuvant tamoxifen. *Breast Cancer Res Treat.* 2007;101(1):113-121.

 Diphenhydramine (eg, *Benadryl*)

Thioridazine

SUMMARY: Diphenhydramine may increase thioridazine serum concentrations, and thus may increase the risk of ventricular arrhythmias; avoid concurrent use.

RISK FACTORS:

➡ *Pharmacogenetics.* Only patients with the extensive metabolizer CYP2D6 phenotype would be expected to experience this interaction. Poor metabolizers do not have the gene for production of CYP2D6 and would likely already have high serum concentrations of thioridazine. Approximately 8% of the white population are deficient in CYP2D6, but the deficiency is rare in the Asian population, usually 1% or less.

➡ *Hypokalemia.* The corrected QT interval (QTc) may be prolonged in patients with hypokalemia, thus increasing the risk of this interaction. Any other factor that may prolong the QTc interval would also increase the risk of this interaction.

MECHANISM: Diphenhydramine probably inhibits the hepatic metabolism of thioridazine by CYP2D6.

CLINICAL EVALUATION: In a double-blind, randomized, crossover study of the pharmacodynamic effects of thioridazine alone, 9 healthy subjects received single oral doses of thioridazine (10 and 50 mg) compared with placebo.[1] The thioridazine 50 mg dose increased the QTc on the electrocardiogram (ECG) by 23 msec, and the 10 mg dose increased QTc by 9 msec. These results suggest that thioridazine produces a dose-related slowing of cardiac repolarization. Thus, drugs such as diphenhydramine that inhibit CYP2D6 would be expected to reduce the metabolism of thioridazine and increase the risk of excessive prolongation of the QTc and ventricular arrhythmias. Although this interaction is based primarily on theoretical consider-ations, the potential severity of the interaction suggests the combination should be avoided. Moreover, the combined use of thioridazine and CYP2D6 inhibitors is contraindicated[2]; thus, consider medicolegal issues also.

RELATED DRUGS: Other antihistamines are not known to inhibit CYP2D6. Although a number of antipsychotic drugs prolong the QT interval, clinical evidence suggests that thioridazine may produce the greatest risk.

MANAGEMENT OPTIONS:

➨ *Use Alternative.* Although the risk of this combination is not well established, use alternatives for one of the drugs (see Related Drugs).

➨ *Monitor.* If the combination must be used, monitor the ECG for evidence of QT prolongation and for clinical evidence of arrhythmias (eg, syncope).

REFERENCES:

1. Hartigan-Go K, et al. Concentration-related pharmacodynamic effects of thioridazine and its metabo-lites in humans. *Clin Pharmacol Ther.* 1996;60(5):543-553.
2. "Dear Doctor or Pharmacist" [letter]. East Hanover, NJ: Novartis Pharmaceuticals; July 7, 2000.

Diphenhydramine (eg, *Benadryl*)

Venlafaxine (*Effexor*)

SUMMARY: Preliminary results from a study in healthy subjects suggest that diphenhydramine increases venlafaxine serum concentrations, but the clinical importance of this effect is not established.

RISK FACTORS:

➨ *Pharmacogenetics.* This interaction is likely to occur only in patients who are exten-sive metabolizers (EMs) of CYP2D6. More than 90% of white Americans are EMs, while more than 98% of Chinese, Japanese, and Native Americans appear to be EMs.

MECHANISM: Diphenhydramine appears to inhibit the CYP2D6 metabolism of venlafax-ine in EMs of CYP2D6 but not in poor metabolizers (PMs) of CYP2D6.

CLINICAL EVALUATION: A preliminary report described 15 healthy subjects (9 EMs and 6 PMs of CYP2D6) who received 3 days of venlafaxine 18.75 mg twice daily alone and with concurrent diphenhydramine 50 mg twice daily.[1] Diphenhydramine decreased venlafaxine oral clearance by 59% in the EMs but had no effect in the PMs.

RELATED DRUGS: The effect of antihistamines other than diphenhydramine on CYP2D6 is not established.

MANAGEMENT OPTIONS: No specific action is required, but be alert for evidence of the interaction.

REFERENCES:

1. Lessard E. Venlafaxine-diphenhydramine interaction in subjects with extensive or poor CYP2D6 activ-ity. *Clin Pharmacol Ther.* 1999;65(2):171.

Diphenhydramine (eg, *Benadryl*)

Warfarin (eg, *Coumadin*)

SUMMARY: Animal studies indicate that diphenhydramine does not affect warfarin disposition.

RISK FACTORS: No specific risk factors are known.

MECHANISM: No interaction.

CLINICAL EVALUATION: Diphenhydramine had no effect on warfarin metabolism in dogs.[1] Anecdotal evidence indicates that diphenhydramine does not affect anticoagulant response in humans, but controlled human studies are needed to confirm this.

RELATED DRUGS: Although little is known regarding the effect of diphenhydramine on oral anticoagulants other than warfarin, there is no reason to suspect that they would interact.

MANAGEMENT OPTIONS: No interaction.

REFERENCES:
1. Hunninghake DB, et al. Drug interactions with warfarin. *Arch Intern Med*. 1968;121:349.

4 **Diphenoxylate (*Lomotil*)**

Quinidine

SUMMARY: Diphenoxylate lowers the peak quinidine serum concentration and delays the time required to reach a peak concentration, but it does not appear to reduce the total amount of quinidine absorbed.

RISK FACTORS: No specific risk factors are known.

MECHANISM: Diphenoxylate slows the absorption of quinidine.

CLINICAL EVALUATION: In 8 healthy subjects, 300 mg of quinidine sulfate was given alone or following 2-tablet doses of diphenoxylate with atropine 8 hours and 1 hour before the quinidine.[1] The time to reach peak quinidine concentration was significantly reduced 21% by diphenoxylate administration. No change in the total quinidine bioavailability (area under the concentration-time curve) was noted. These changes are not likely to be of clinical significance during chronic quinidine therapy.

RELATED DRUGS: No information is available.

MANAGEMENT OPTIONS: No specific action is required, but be alert for evidence of the interaction.

REFERENCES:
1. Ponzillo JJ, et al. Effect of diphenoxylate with atropine sulfate on the bioavailability of quinidine sulfate in healthy subjects. *Clin Pharm*. 1988;7:139.

5 **Dirithromycin (*Dynabac*)**

Terfenadine

SUMMARY: Dirithromycin does not alter terfenadine concentrations; no interaction occurs.

RISK FACTORS: No specific risk factors are known.

MECHANISM: No interaction.

CLINICAL EVALUATION: No changes in the pharmacokinetics of terfenadine (60 mg twice daily for 8 days) nor its acid metabolite were observed during dirithromycin (500 mg/day for 10 days) administration.[1] No changes in QT intervals were noted during the study. It appears that dirithromycin has no significant effect on terfenadine metabolism and can be administered safely with the antihistamine.

RELATED DRUGS: Other macrolides, such as erythromycin (eg, *E-Mycin*), inhibit terfenadine metabolism.

MANAGEMENT OPTIONS: No interaction.

REFERENCES:
1. Goldberg MJ, et al. Effect of dirithromycin on terfenadine pharmacokinetics and QTc in healthy men. *Clin Pharmacol Ther*. 1995;57:176.

Dirithromycin (*Dynabac*)

Theophylline (eg, *Theolair*)

SUMMARY: Dirithromycin caused a small reduction in theophylline plasma concentrations; clinical effects are likely to be limited.

RISK FACTORS: No specific risk factors are known.

MECHANISM: Dirithromycin does not appear to change the metabolism of theophylline. Unlike erythromycin, dirithromycin does not appear to bind to cytochrome P450 and inhibit metabolic activity.

CLINICAL EVALUATION: During dirithromycin administration, the mean peak and average theophylline concentrations were reduced 26% and 18%, respectively; no statistically significant change was observed in theophylline clearance after oral administration (15% increase).[1] Dirithromycin 500 mg/day had no significant effect on theophylline concentrations in patients with chronic pulmonary disease.[2] The minor change in theophylline concentrations noted in these studies is not likely to be clinically significant in patients with obstructive pulmonary disease.

RELATED DRUGS: Some macrolides, such as erythromycin, reduce theophylline metabolism. A related macrolide antibiotic, ponsinomycin, has no effect on theophylline metabolism.[3]

MANAGEMENT OPTIONS: No specific action is required, but be alert for evidence of the interaction.

REFERENCES:
1. Bachmann K, et al. Changes in the steady-state pharmacokinetics of theophylline during treatment with dirithromycin. *J Clin Pharmacol*. 1990;30:1001.

2. Bachmann K, et al. Steady-state pharmacokinetics of theophylline in COPD patients treated with dirithromycin. *J Clin Pharmacol*. 1993;33:861.

3. Couet W, et al. Lack of effect of ponsinomycin on the plasma pharmacokinetics of theophylline. *Eur J Clin Pharmacol*. 1989;37:101.

Disopyramide (eg, *Norpace*)

Clarithromycin (eg, *Biaxin*)

SUMMARY: Clarithromycin administration increases disopyramide concentrations; toxicity including hypoglycemia or delayed cardiac repolarization may result.

RISK FACTORS: No specific risk factors are known.

MECHANISM: Clarithromycin inhibits CYP3A4, the enzyme responsible for disopyramide metabolism. Elevated disopyramide plasma concentrations can block potassium channels leading to prolonged repolarization in the myocardium (long QTc interval) and enhanced insulin secretion with hypoglycemia. Clarithromycin also can prolong myocardial repolarization, particularly at elevated plasma concentrations.

CLINICAL EVALUATION: A patient with renal failure on hemodialysis was receiving disopyramide 50 mg/day for paroxysmal atrial fibrillation.[1] Clarithromycin 600 mg/day for chronic bronchitis was added to his regimen. On the 14th day of clarithromycin therapy, the patient became comatose and was noted to be severely hypoglycemic. Glucose administration corrected the coma, but he continued to have hypoglycemic episodes and again became comatose while receiving clarithromycin and disopyramide. At this time his serum disopyramide concentration was 8 mcg/mL. This concentration was an increase from 1.5 mcg/mL measured prior to clarithromycin dosing. His QTc interval was noted to be prolonged (490 ms) but a baseline value was not provided. His blood sugar and QTc interval returned to normal following discontinuation of clarithromycin and disopyramide. No further episodes of hypoglycemia were noted.

RELATED DRUGS: Erythromycin (eg, *Ery-Tab*) is known to inhibit the metabolism of disopyramide, and troleandomycin† is expected to inhibit disopyramide clearance as well. Erythromycin is also known to prolong the QTc interval, especially when administered intravenously.

MANAGEMENT OPTIONS:

➡ **Consider Alternative.** Azithromycin (eg, *Zithromax*) and dirithromycin† are unlikely to affect disopyramide metabolism. Consider alternative antiarrhythmic agents for patients who cannot avoid clarithromycin or erythromycin.

➡ **Monitor.** Carefully monitor patients taking disopyramide for prolonged QTc intervals and hypoglycemia if clarithromycin is coadministered.

REFERENCES:

1. Iida H, et al. Hypoglycemia induced by interaction between clarithromycin and disopyramide. *Jpn Heart J.* 1999;40(1):91-96.

† Not available in the United States.

Disopyramide (eg, *Norpace*)
Donepezil (eg, *Aricept*)

SUMMARY: Disopyramide has potent anticholinergic properties and may inhibit the therapeutic effect of donepezil in Alzheimer disease.

RISK FACTORS: No specific risk factors are known.

MECHANISM: Donepezil is a cholinesterase inhibitor and thus increases cholinergic activity; its efficacy is likely to be inhibited by anticholinergic drugs such as disopyramide.[1]

CLINICAL EVALUATION: In a preliminary study of 69 patients with Alzheimer disease receiving donepezil 10 mg/day and followed for 2 years, 16 patients received concurrent therapy with anticholinergic drugs and 53 patients did not.[2] Mental functioning, as measured by the Mini-Mental State Exam (MMSE), was significantly lower in the patients receiving concomitant anticholinergic drugs. Also, the French Pharmacovigilance Database received 118 spontaneous reports of adverse reactions in patients receiving anticholinergic drugs with cholinesterase inhibitors (eg, donepezil, galantamine, rivastigmine). After evaluation by clinical pharmacologists, 24 were thought to be adverse drug interactions.[3] Although additional study is needed to establish the clinical importance of these interactions, the evidence is consistent with the known pharmacological effects of the drugs.

RELATED DRUGS: All cholinesterase inhibitors used to treat Alzheimer disease (donepezil, galantamine [eg, *Razadyne*], rivastigmine [eg, *Exelon*]) are expected to interact similarly with disopyramide.

MANAGEMENT OPTIONS:

➥ **Consider Alternative.** If appropriate, use an alternative antiarrhythmic in place of the disopyramide.

➥ **Monitor.** If disopyramide is used with donepezil or another cholinesterase inhibitor, be alert for evidence of reduced mental functioning.

REFERENCES:

1. *Aricept* [package insert]. New York, NY: Pfizer; 2011.
2. Lu CJ, Tune LE. Chronic exposure to anticholinergic medications adversely affects the course of Alzheimer disease. *Am J Geriatr Psychiatry*. 2003;11(4):458-461.
3. Tavassoli N, et al. Drug interactions with cholinesterase inhibitors: an analysis of the French Pharmacovigilance Database and a comparison of two national drug formularies (Vidal, British National Formulary). *Drug Saf*. 2007;30(11):1063-1071.

Disopyramide (eg, *Norpace*)
Erythromycin (eg, *Ery-Tab*)

SUMMARY: In isolated case reports, erythromycin administration appeared to increase the serum disopyramide concentration, resulting in cardiac arrhythmias.

RISK FACTORS: No specific risk factors are known.

MECHANISM: Not established. Erythromycin may inhibit disopyramide clearance[1]; both drugs can prolong myocardial conduction.

CLINICAL EVALUATION: Two patients taking disopyramide for ventricular arrhythmias were treated with erythromycin.[2] The first patient was taking disopyramide 300 mg alternating with 150 mg every 6 hours when she was given erythromycin lactobionate 1 g every 6 hours intravenously. Less than 2 days later, the patient developed new arrhythmias. During continued erythromycin administration, discontinuation of disopyramide resulted in termination of the arrhythmia; reinstitution of disopyramide caused the arrhythmia to return. The second patient was taking disopyramide 200 mg 4 times/day when erythromycin base 500 mg 4 times/day orally was administered. Six days later, his electrocardiogram demonstrated a new arrhythmia. Disopyramide and erythromycin were discontinued with resolution of the arrhythmias. Resumption of disopyramide in the absence of erythromycin produced no further problems.

RELATED DRUGS: Other macrolides (eg, troleandomycin,[†] clarithromycin [eg, *Biaxin*]) may affect disopyramide similarly. Azithromycin (eg, *Zithromax*) and dirithromycin[†] are unlikely to inhibit disopyramide elimination.

MANAGEMENT OPTIONS:

➥ *Consider Alternative.* Azithromycin and dirithromycin[†] are unlikely to affect disopyramide metabolism. Consider alternative antiarrhythmic agents for patients who cannot avoid clarithromycin or erythromycin.

➥ *Monitor.* Monitor patients taking disopyramide for the development of arrhythmias if erythromycin is added to their regimen.

REFERENCES:

1. Echizen H, et al. A potent inhibitory effect of erythromycin and other macrolide antibiotics on the mono-N-dealkylation metabolism of disopyramide with human liver microsomes. *J Pharmacol Exp Ther.* 1993;264(3):1425-1431.

2. Ragosta M, et al. Potentially fatal interaction between erythromycin and disopyramide. *Am J Med.* 1989;86(4):465-466.

† Not available in the United States.

4   Disopyramide (eg, *Norpace*)

Insulin

SUMMARY: Disopyramide can cause hypoglycemia in some patients.

RISK FACTORS:

➥ *Concurrent Diseases.* Renal disease may predispose disopyramide-induced hypoglycemia.

MECHANISM: Not established.

CLINICAL EVALUATION: Isolated cases of hypoglycemia associated with disopyramide therapy, even without concurrent hypoglycemic therapy, have been reported.[1,2,3] Predisposing factors for disopyramide-induced hypoglycemia may include renal dysfunction associated with advanced age.[3]

RELATED DRUGS: No information is available.

MANAGEMENT OPTIONS: No specific action is required, but be alert for evidence of the interaction.

REFERENCES:

1. Nappi JM, et al. Severe hypoglycemia association with disopyramide. *West J Med.* 1983;138(1):95-97.

2. Goldberg IJ, et al. Disopyramide (*Norpace*)-induced hypoglycemia. *Am J Med*. 1980;69(3):463-466.

3. Strathman I, et al. Hypoglycemia in patients receiving disopyramide phosphate. *Drug Intell Clin Pharm*. 1983;17(9):635- 638.

Disopyramide (eg, *Norpace*)

Lidocaine (eg, *Xylocaine*)

SUMMARY: Combined use of lidocaine and disopyramide can induce arrhythmias or heart failure in predisposed patients.

RISK FACTORS: No specific risk factors are known.

MECHANISM: Both lidocaine and disopyramide alter myocardial conduction and may produce additive cardiodepressant effects.

CLINICAL EVALUATION: Isolated cases of impaired intraventricular conduction and ventricular asystole in patients receiving combined therapy with disopyramide and lidocaine have been reported.[1]

RELATED DRUGS: No information is available.

MANAGEMENT OPTIONS:

➡ **Monitor.** Closely monitor patients receiving combined therapy with disopyramide and lidocaine for arrhythmias and heart failure.

REFERENCES:

1. Ellrodt G, et al. Adverse effects of disopyramide (*Norpace*): toxic interactions with other antiarrhythmic agents. *Heart Lung*. 1980;9(3):469-474.

Disopyramide (eg, *Norpace*)

Mexiletine

SUMMARY: Mexiletine and disopyramide appear to be an effective antiarrhythmic combination; disopyramide plasma concentrations may be increased by mexiletine.

RISK FACTORS: No specific risk factors are known.

MECHANISM: Not established. Mexiletine may inhibit disopyramide elimination.

CLINICAL EVALUATION: Twenty-nine patients with ventricular premature beats received 1 week of therapy with disopyramide 100 mg every 8 hours, mexiletine 150 mg every 8 hours, or disopyramide 50 mg every 8 hours plus mexiletine 100 mg every 8 hours.[1] Both the single-drug and combination therapy significantly reduced the number of ventricular premature beats. The 33% reduction in the mexiletine dose when combined with disopyramide was accompanied by a mean 36% reduction in the average mexiletine plasma concentration. The 50% reduction in disopyramide dose produced a 30% decrease in plasma disopyramide concentration with combined therapy. Combinations of mexiletine and disopyramide could lead to increased disopyramide concentrations if doses are not adjusted.

RELATED DRUGS: No information is available.

MANAGEMENT OPTIONS: No specific action is required, but be alert for evidence of the interaction.

REFERENCES:

1. Tanabe T, et al. Evaluation of disopyramide and mexiletine used alone and in combination for ventricular arrhythmias in patients with and without overt heart disease. *Int J Cardiol.* 1991;32(3):303-312.

Disopyramide (eg, *Norpace*)

Phenobarbital (eg, *Solfoton*)

SUMMARY: Phenobarbital appears to reduce the serum concentrations of disopyramide, perhaps to subtherapeutic levels.

RISK FACTORS: No specific risk factors are known.

MECHANISM: Phenobarbital, a known stimulator of hepatic enzymes, appears to increase the metabolic clearance of disopyramide.

CLINICAL EVALUATION: Fourteen healthy subjects were given disopyramide 200 mg alone and after 21 days of phenobarbital therapy, 100 mg/day.[1] The disopyramide half-life was reduced by approximately 35% and the area under the concentration-time curve was increased by a similar amount after phenobarbital administration. Apparent clearance of disopyramide was increased by approximately 60%.

RELATED DRUGS: Other barbiturates probably have a similar effect on disopyramide, but little clinical evidence is available.

MANAGEMENT OPTIONS:

➥ *Monitor.* The changes in disopyramide clearance and half-life observed after phenobarbital administration could result in loss of arrhythmia control in some patients. Monitor disopyramide serum concentrations when phenobarbital is added to or removed from the drug regimen. Watch for dry mouth and urinary retention caused by increased metabolite serum concentrations.

REFERENCES:

1. Kapil RP, et al. Disopyramide pharmacokinetics and metabolism: effect of inducers. *Br J Clin Pharmacol.* 1987;24:781.

Disopyramide (eg, *Norpace*)

Phenytoin (*Dilantin*)

SUMMARY: Phenytoin increases the metabolism of disopyramide, potentially reducing its efficacy and increasing its toxicity to some extent.

RISK FACTORS: No specific risk factors are known.

MECHANISM: The hepatic metabolism of disopyramide is increased by phenytoin, resulting in decreased serum concentrations of disopyramide and increased concentrations of its metabolite.

CLINICAL EVALUATION: In several case reports, disopyramide clearance increased and antiarrhythmic efficacy was diminished with the coadministration of phenytoin.[1-5] A mean decrease (52%) in the area under the concentration-time curve (AUC) and a 51% reduction in the half-life of disopyramide were noted in 10 subjects who received phenytoin 300 mg/day.[6] The disopyramide AUC was reduced in all 10 subjects by more than 40%. Subjects also reported an increase in anticholinergic side effects following the coadministration of disopyramide and phenytoin, consistent with accumulation of a disopyramide metabolite. Thus, the increased metabolism of disopyramide may reduce its antiarrhythmic efficacy, while the accumulation of metabolite increases its anticholinergic side effects.

RELATED DRUGS: No information is available.

MANAGEMENT OPTIONS:

➥ *Monitor.* Closely monitor disopyramide serum concentrations and patient response (eg, control of arrhythmia) when phenytoin therapy is added to or removed from disopyramide therapy. Be alert for reduced antiarrhythmic efficacy and increased anticholinergic side effects such as dry mouth or urinary retention.

REFERENCES:

1. Ellrodt G, et al. Adverse effects of disopyramide (*Norpace*): toxic interactions with other antiarrhythmic agents. *Heart Lung.* 1980;9:469.
2. Aitio ML, et al. Enhanced metabolism and diminished efficacy of disopyramide by enzyme induction? *Br J Clin Pharmacol.* 1980;9:149.
3. Aitio ML, et al. The effect of enzyme induction on the metabolism of disopyramide in man. *Br J Clin Pharmacol.* 1981;11:279.
4. Kessler JM, et al. Disopyramide and phenytoin interaction. *Clin Pharm.* 1982;1:263.
5. Matos JA, et al. Disopyramide-phenytoin interaction. *Clin Res.* 1981;29:655A.
6. Nightingale J, et al. Effect of phenytoin on serum disopyramide concentrations. *Clin Pharm.* 1987;6:46.

Disopyramide (eg, *Norpace*)

Potassium

SUMMARY: Increased serum concentrations of potassium can enhance disopyramide effects on myocardial conduction.

RISK FACTORS:

➥ *Concurrent Diseases.* Renal dysfunction increases the risk of the interaction.

MECHANISM: Both hyperkalemia and disopyramide can slow myocardial conduction and produce cardiovascular depression.

CLINICAL EVALUATION: In 1 patient, the development of conduction disturbances and hypotension was attributed to the combined effects of disopyramide and potassium supplementation.[1] The serum disopyramide concentration was 10.8 mcg/mL (therapeutic range: 2 to 5 mcg/mL), and the serum potassium was 6.9 mEq/L. The potential for high serum potassium concentrations to predispose patients with therapeutic concentrations of disopyramide to disopyramide toxicity is not established. The likelihood of elevated serum levels of both disopyramide and potassium is greatest in patients with serious renal impairment.

RELATED DRUGS: The administration of potassium-sparing diuretics might cause a similar reaction with disopyramide.

MANAGEMENT OPTIONS:

➥ *Monitor.* Be alert for electrocardiographic evidence of disopyramide toxicity (eg, QRS widening) when potassium supplementation is given concurrently, especially if large doses of disopyramide and potassium are used or if renal function is impaired.

REFERENCES:

1. Maddux BD, et al. Toxic synergism of disopyramide and hyperkalemia. *Chest.* 1980;78:654.

 Disopyramide (eg, *Norpace*)

Practolol

SUMMARY: Disopyramide and beta blockers may produce additive negative inotropic effects on the heart.

RISK FACTORS:

➡ **Route of Administration.** IV administration of both drugs may produce the interaction.

MECHANISM: Combined pharmacologic effects may be involved with additive reduction in cardiac output resulting from the coadministration of beta blockers and disopyramide.

CLINICAL EVALUATION: Two patients with supraventricular tachycardia developed severe bradycardia after receiving practolol IV and then disopyramide IV.[1] One of the patients developed asystole and died. In studies of healthy subjects, no pharmacodynamic interactions on left ventricular function were noted with the combined use of propranolol (eg, *Inderal*) and disopyramide as compared with either drug alone.[2,4] Atenolol (eg, *Tenormin*) and disopyramide, when administered IV, produced additive effects on cardiac output.[5] Coadministration of disopyramide and propranolol does not appear to affect the pharmacokinetics of either drug;[3] however, atenolol coadministration reduced the clearance of disopyramide by 20%.[6]

RELATED DRUGS: Atenolol appears to interact with disopyramide similarly. Propranolol does not appear to interact.

MANAGEMENT OPTIONS:

➡ **Monitor.** Until more clinical information is available, administer disopyramide (especially if given IV) only with caution to patients receiving beta blockers. Monitor for bradycardia and reduced cardiac output.

REFERENCES:

1. Cumming AD, et al. Interaction between disopyramide and practolol. *BMJ.* 1979;2:1204.
2. Cathcart-Rake WF, et al. The pharmacodynamics of concurrent disopyramide and propranolol. *Clin Pharmacol Ther.* 1979;25:217.
3. Karim A, et al. Clinical pharmacokinetics of disopyramide. *J Pharmacokinet Biopharm.* 1982;10:465.
4. Cathcart-Rake WF, et al. The effect of concurrent oral administration of propranolol and disopyramide on cardiac function in healthy men. *Circulation.* 1980;61:938.
5. Bonde J, et al. Haemodynamic effects and kinetics of concomitant intravenous disopyramide and atenolol in patients with ischaemic heart disease. *Eur J Clin Pharmacol.* 1986;30:161.
6. Bonde J, et al. Atenolol inhibits the elimination of disopyramide. *Eur J Clin Pharmacol.* 1985;28:41.

Disopyramide (eg, *Norpace*) 4

Quinidine

SUMMARY: The serum concentrations of disopyramide are increased and quinidine are decreased to a minor extent when these 2 drugs are coadministered.

RISK FACTORS: No specific risk factors are known.

MECHANISM: The mechanism for small changes in serum concentrations of disopyramide and quinidine is not established. Cardiodepressant effects may be enhanced.

CLINICAL EVALUATION: In healthy subjects, quinidine administration produced small increases (less than 20%) in serum disopyramide concentrations, while disopyramide produced small decreases in serum quinidine concentrations.[1,2] Also, anticholinergic effects such as dry mouth, blurred vision, and urinary retention were more common with concurrent therapy than with either drug alone.[2] Significant additive electrocardiographic effects from disopyramide and quinidine were not noted in healthy subjects,[2] but this does not rule out such effects in patients with cardiac disease.

RELATED DRUGS: No information is available.

MANAGEMENT OPTIONS: No specific action is required, but be alert for evidence of the interaction.

REFERENCES:
1. Karim A, et al. Clinical pharmacokinetics of disopyramide. *J Pharmacokinet Biopharm*. 1982;10:465.
2. Baker B, et al. Concurrent use of quinidine and disopyramide: evaluation of serum concentrations and electrocardiographic effects. *Am Heart J*. 1983;105:12.

Disopyramide (eg, *Norpace*)

Rifampin (eg, *Rifadin*)

SUMMARY: Rifampin can lower serum disopyramide concentrations to subtherapeutic levels; loss of efficacy may result.

RISK FACTORS: No specific risk factors are known.

MECHANISM: Rifampin stimulates the hepatic metabolism of disopyramide.

CLINICAL EVALUATION: Twelve patients with tuberculosis were given disopyramide 200 to 300 mg as a single dose before and 2 weeks after starting rifampin therapy.[1] Plasma disopyramide concentrations were reduced to approximately 50% in the presence of rifampin, and the amount of disopyramide excreted unchanged in the urine fell to about one-fourth of that seen without rifampin. The study was complicated by the administration of isoniazid (known to inhibit the metabolism of several drugs) in addition to rifampin in some patients. A case report noted that a patient taking rifampin required a disopyramide dose of 250 to 300 mg every 8 hours to suppress an arrhythmia.[2] Rifampin-induced increases in disopyramide metabolism may lead to an increase in disopyramide metabolite concentration. Enhanced anticholinergic side effects (urinary retention, dry mouth) could result.

RELATED DRUGS: No information is available.

MANAGEMENT OPTIONS:

➥ *Monitor.* Monitor patients for re-emergence of arrhythmias when rifampin is added to disopyramide and disopyramide toxicity if rifampin is discontinued. Serum disopyramide concentrations would be useful to monitor this interaction.

REFERENCES:

1. Aitio ML, et al. The effect of enzyme induction on the metabolism of disopyramide in man. *Br J Clin Pharmacol.* 1981;11:279.

2. Staum JM, et al. Enzyme induction: rifampin-disopyramide interaction. *DICP.* 1990;24:701.

 Disopyramide (eg, *Norpace*)

Thioridazine (eg, *Mellaril*)

SUMMARY: Disopyramide may produce additive prolongation of the QT interval with thioridazine, and thus may increase the risk of ventricular arrhythmias; avoid concurrent use.

RISK FACTORS:

➥ *Hypokalemia.* The corrected QT interval (QTc) may be prolonged in patients with hypokalemia, thus increasing the risk of this interaction. Any other factor that may prolong the QTc interval would also increase the risk of this interaction.

MECHANISM: Both thioridazine and disopyramide can prolong the QT interval; additive effects may be seen.

CLINICAL EVALUATION: In a double-blind, randomized, crossover study of the pharmaco-dynamic effects of thioridazine alone, 9 healthy subjects received single oral doses of thioridazine (10 and 50 mg) compared with placebo.[1] The 50 mg dose of thioridazine increased the QTc on the ECG by 23 msec, and the 10 mg dose increased QTc by 9 msec. These results suggest that thioridazine produces a dose-related slowing of cardiac repolarization. Thus, drugs such as disopyramide that can independently prolong the QT interval may increase the risk of ventricular arrhythmias in patients taking thioridazine. Although this interaction is based primarily on theoretical considerations, the potential severity of the interaction suggests to avoid the combination. Moreover, the manufacturer's product information for *Mellaril* states that combined use of thioridazine with other drugs that are known to prolong the QT interval is contraindicated;[2] thus, consider medicolegal issues also.

RELATED DRUGS: Other antiarrhythmics such as amiodarone (eg, *Cordarone*), procain-amide (eg, *Procan SR*), and quinidine (*Quinora*) can also increase the QT interval, and may increase the risk of arrhythmias. Also, amiodarone, propafenone (*Rythmol*), and quinidine are know inhibitors of CYP2D6, and may increase thioridazine serum concentrations. Although a number of antipsychotic drugs, like thioridazine, have been shown to prolong the QT interval clinical evidence suggests that thioridazine may produce the greatest risk.

MANAGEMENT OPTIONS:

➥ *Use Alternative.* Although the risk of this combination is not well established, it would be prudent to use alternatives for 1 of the drugs (see Related Drugs).

➡ **Monitor.** If the combination must be used, monitor the ECG for evidence of QT prolongation and for clinical evidence of arrhythmias (eg, syncope).

REFERENCES:
1. Hartigan-Go K, et al. Concentration-related pharmacodynamic effects of thioridazine and its metabolites in humans. *Clin Pharmacol Ther*. 1996;60:543-53.
2. 'Dear Doctor of Pharmacist' Letter, Novartis Pharmaceuticals, July 7, 2000.

Disopyramide (eg, *Norpace*)

Warfarin (eg, *Coumadin*)

SUMMARY: There is little evidence to support an effect of disopyramide on warfarin response, but be aware of the possibility.

RISK FACTORS: No specific risk factors are known.

MECHANISM: Not established.

CLINICAL EVALUATION: A patient stabilized on warfarin 3 mg/day and disopyramide developed a two-fold increase in warfarin requirements when the disopyramide was discontinued.[1] Other causes for the increased warfarin requirements could not be found. However, disopyramide had little effect on the hypoprothrombinemic response to warfarin in 3 other patients.[2] It has been proposed that disopyramide-induced hemodynamic changes could increase hepatic clotting factor synthesis, thus reducing the prothrombin time.[2,3]

RELATED DRUGS: No information is available.

MANAGEMENT OPTIONS: No specific action is required, but be alert for evidence of the interaction.

REFERENCES:
1. Haworth E, et al. Disopyramide and warfarin interaction. *BMJ*. 1977;4:866.
2. Sylven C, et al. Evidence that disopyramide does not interact with warfarin. *BMJ*. 1983;286:1181.
3. Ryll C, et al. Warfarin-disopyramide interactions. *Drug Intell Clin Pharm*. 1979;13:260.

Disulfiram (eg, *Antabuse*)

Ethanol (*Ethyl Alcohol*) AVOID

SUMMARY: Disulfiram results in severe ethanol intolerance; patients must be warned to avoid all forms of ethanol.

RISK FACTORS: No specific risk factors are known.

MECHANISM: The disulfiram-ethanol reaction appears to result from accumulation of acetaldehyde as a result of disulfiram-induced inhibition of aldehyde dehydrogenase.[5]

CLINICAL EVALUATION: Among the signs and symptoms of the disulfiram-ethanol reaction are flushing, hypotension, nausea, tachycardia, vertigo, dyspnea, esophageal rupture, and blurred vision.[1-3] Myoclonus also has been reported in one case.[4] As little as 15 mL of ethanol has been reported to produce a mild reaction in some patients receiving disulfiram. Large amounts of ethanol may produce severe or even fatal reactions. Many oral liquid pharmaceutical preparations contain ethanol. Topically applied ethanol may also result in reactions, but the amount of ethanol required and the magnitude of the reaction require further study.

RELATED DRUGS: No information is available.

MANAGEMENT OPTIONS:

➡ *AVOID COMBINATION.* Warn patients about ethanol in foods and pharmaceuticals, as well as beverages. Advise patients receiving disulfiram to avoid oral liquid pharmaceuticals unless they are known to be ethanol-free.

REFERENCES:

1. Fernandez D. Another esophageal rupture after alcohol and disulfiram. *N Engl J Med.* 1972;286:610.
2. Elenbaas RM. Drug therapy reviews: management of the disulfiram/alcohol reaction. *Am J Hosp Pharm.* 1977;34:827.
3. Kitson TM. The disulfiram-ethanol reaction: a review. *J Stud Alcohol.* 1977;38:96.
4. Syed J, et al. An unusual presentation of a disulfiram-alcohol reaction. *Del Med J.* 1995;67:183.
5. Johansson B, et al. Dose-effect relationship of disulfiram in human volunteers. II. A study of the relation between the disulfiram-alcohol reaction and plasma concentrations of acetaldehyde, diethyldithiocarbamic acid methyl ester, and erythrocyte aldehyde dehydrogenase activity. *Pharmacol Toxicol.* 1991;68:166.

Disulfiram (eg, *Antabuse*)

Isoniazid (INH; eg, *Laniazid*)

SUMMARY: The combined use of disulfiram and INH may result in adverse CNS effects.

RISK FACTORS: No specific risk factors are known.

MECHANISM: Whittington, et al. have proposed that disulfiram and INH inhibit 2 of the 3 known metabolic pathways for dopamine.[2] Disulfiram inhibits betahydroxylase, and INH may inhibit monoamine oxidase. These authors hypothesize that this inhibition results in increased metabolism of dopamine by catechol-O-methyltransferase, and the resultant methylated metabolites of dopamine are responsible for the adverse mental changes and coordination problems.[2] Another possible factor is that both monoamine oxidase (possibly inhibited by INH) and aldehyde dehydrogenase (inhibited by disulfiram) are involved in the conversion of norepinephrine to 3,4-dihydroxymandelic acid. Thus, speculate that inhibition of both of these enzymes could increase levels of norepinephrine.

CLINICAL EVALUATION: Several possible examples of an interaction between disulfiram and INH have been presented.[2] Patients on concomitant INH and disulfiram therapy developed changes in effect and behavior as well as coordination difficulties. Although drug interaction seems likely to be involved in the adverse reactions, no definite conclusions can be drawn from the data presented because some of the patients received relatively large doses of INH, and other drugs also were being given. One case has been reported in which a patient receiving INH, disulfiram, and rifampin (eg, *Rifadin*) did not manifest signs of interaction.[1]

RELATED DRUGS: No information is available.

MANAGEMENT OPTIONS:

➡ *Avoid Unless Benefit Outweighs Risk.* Although evidence is somewhat limited, enough has been presented to warrant caution in the concomitant use of INH and disulfiram. It would be wise in most cases to avoid the use of disulfiram in patients receiving INH until more information is known about the interaction.

➡ *Monitor.* If combined use is necessary, monitor patients for adverse central nervous system effects (eg, altered mood, behavioral changes, ataxia).

REFERENCES:

1. Rothstein E. Rifampin with disulfiram. *JAMA.* 1972;219:1216.
2. Whittington HG, et al. Possible interaction between disulfiram and isoniazid. *Am J Psychiatry.* 1969;125:1725.

Disulfiram (eg, *Antabuse*)

Metronidazole (eg, *Flagyl*)

SUMMARY: The combined use of disulfiram and metronidazole may produce central nervous system toxicity.

RISK FACTORS: No specific risk factors are known.

MECHANISM: Not established. A combined inhibition of aldehyde dehydrogenase or other enzymes may be involved in the interaction between disulfiram and metronidazole.

CLINICAL EVALUATION: Psychotic episodes and confusional states in patients have been attributed to combined metronidazole-disulfiram therapy.[1-3] Although these reports involved only a few patients, the interaction may produce clinically significant adverse effects.

RELATED DRUGS: No information is available.

MANAGEMENT OPTIONS:

➡ *Consider Alternative.* Until the potential interaction between metronidazole and disulfiram is better described, it would be wise to avoid concomitant use of these drugs.

➡ *Monitor.* If the drugs are coadministered, watch for behavioral toxicity and confusion.

REFERENCES:

1. Rothstein E, et al. Toxicity of disulfiram combined with metronidazole. *N Engl J Med.* 1969;280:1006.
2. Goodhue WW Jr. Disulfiram-metronidazole (well identified) toxicity. *N Engl J Med.* 1969;280:1482.
3. Scher JM. Psychotic reaction to disulfiram. *JAMA.* 1967;201:1051.

Disulfiram (eg, *Antabuse*) 4

Omeprazole (*Prilosec*)

SUMMARY: A patient became confused and disoriented on two occasions when omeprazole was added to disulfiram therapy; more study is needed.

RISK FACTORS: No specific risk factors are known.

MECHANISM: Not established. Both disulfiram and omeprazole are known to inhibit the hepatic metabolism of drugs; perhaps the metabolism of one or both of these agents is inhibited by the other.

CLINICAL EVALUATION: A 40-year-old man on chronic omeprazole therapy was started on disulfiram, 500 mg/day.[1] Fifteen days later he was hospitalized because of confusion and disorientation that had gradually developed over the past nine days. Both omeprazole and disulfiram were discontinued on admission; the patient developed muscle rigidity, stared into space, and was unresponsive to verbal commands. He improved gradually over 7 days. Because a drug interaction between disulfiram and omeprazole was suspected, the patient was restarted on disulfiram 250 mg/day, and omeprazole 40 mg/day was started 2 weeks later. After 72 hours on combined therapy, the patient became confused and disoriented and reported nightmares. The drugs were stopped and the adverse effects abated over 72 hours. The fact that the patient was able to tolerate each drug alone but not together suggests that an interaction may have occurred. Nonetheless, one cannot rule out the possibility that a placebo effect contributed to the positive challenge because the patient presumably knew when the omeprazole was added. Additional study is needed to determine whether this potential interaction is clinically important.

RELATED DRUGS: The effect of lansoprazole (*Prevacid*) on disulfiram is not established.

MANAGEMENT OPTIONS: No specific action is required, but be alert for evidence of the interaction.

REFERENCES:
1. Hajela R, et al. Catatonic reaction to omeprazole and disulfiram in a patient with alcohol dependence. *Can Med Assoc J.* 1990;143:1207.

Disulfiram (eg, *Antabuse*)

Phenobarbital (eg, *Solfoton*)

SUMMARY: Disulfiram does not appear to affect serum phenobarbital concentrations.

RISK FACTORS: No specific risk factors are known.

MECHANISM: No interaction.

CLINICAL EVALUATION: Although disulfiram is known to increase phenytoin plasma levels, in at least 1 patient's serum phenobarbital was not altered by disulfiram administration.[1] More data are needed to establish the observation that phenobarbital is unaffected by disulfiram. The effect of phenobarbital on disulfiram was not assessed.

RELATED DRUGS: The effect of disulfiram on other barbiturates is not established.

MANAGEMENT OPTIONS: No interaction.

REFERENCES:
1. Olesen OV. The influence of disulfiram and calcium carbamide on the serum diphenylhydantoin. *Arch Neurol.* 1967;16:642.

Disulfiram (*Antabuse*)

Phenytoin (eg, *Dilantin*)

SUMMARY: Disulfiram consistently increases serum phenytoin concentrations; symptoms of phenytoin toxicity have occurred in some patients.

RISK FACTORS: No specific risk factors are known.

MECHANISM: Disulfiram inhibits the hepatic metabolism of phenytoin.[1-4] Serum concentrations of phenytoin are increased and urinary excretion of its major metabolite (HPPH) is decreased when disulfiram is given concurrently.

CLINICAL EVALUATION: Disulfiram 400 mg/day has increased serum phenytoin concentrations considerably in several patients. The effect was rapid, with increases in serum phenytoin beginning within 4 hours of the administration of the first dose of disulfiram.[2] The effect also was prolonged, requiring about 3 weeks after disulfiram withdrawal for the phenytoin concentration to return to normal. Similar results were obtained in normal volunteers given phenytoin before and after 4 days of disulfiram.[4] One patient developed phenytoin toxicity (ataxia, nystagmus) and a serum phenytoin concentration of 39.5 mg/mL following initiation of disulfiram therapy.[5]

RELATED DRUGS: No information is available.

MANAGEMENT OPTIONS:

➡ *Consider Alternative.* Consider using alternative treatment for alcohol abuse.

➡ *Circumvent/Minimize.* Reduction of the phenytoin dose may be necessary.

➡ *Monitor.* Monitor patients receiving phenytoin and disulfiram for evidence of phenytoin toxicity (eg, ataxia, nystagmus, mental impairment). Serum phenytoin determinations are useful to detect an interaction between these drugs. Monitor patients for a reduced phenytoin response when disulfiram therapy is discontinued.

REFERENCES:

1. Olesen OV. The influence of disulfiram and calcium carbamide on the serum diphenylhydantoin. *Arch Neurol.* 1967;16:642-644.
2. Olesen OV. Disulfiram (*Antabuse*) as inhibitor of phenytoin metabolism. *Acta Pharmacol Toxicol.* 1966;24:317.
3. Kiorboe E. Phenytoin intoxication during treatment with *Antabuse* (disulfiram). *Epilepsia.* 1966;7:246-249.
4. Svendsen TL, et al. The influence of disulfiram on the half life and metabolic clearance rate of diphenylhydantoin and tolbutamide in man. *Eur J Clin Pharmacol.* 1976;9:439-441.
5. Taylor JW, et al. Mathematical analysis of a phenytoin–disulfiram interaction. *Am J Hosp Pharm.* 1981;38:93-95.

Disulfiram (*Antabuse*)

Theophylline (eg, *Theolair*)

SUMMARY: Disulfiram increases serum theophylline concentrations; the magnitude of the effect appears sufficient to produce theophylline toxicity in at least some patients.

RISK FACTORS: No specific risk factors are known.

MECHANISM: Disulfiram inhibits the hepatic microsomal metabolism of several drugs; theophylline may be affected similarly. Both the hydroxylation and demethylation of theophylline appear to be inhibited, although the effect of hydroxylation is greater.

CLINICAL EVALUATION: Twenty recovering alcoholics received theophylline 5 mg/kg IV with and without pretreatment with disulfiram (10 patients received 250 mg/day and 10 received 500 mg/day).[1] The smaller dose of disulfiram reduced theophylline clearance 21%, and the 500 mg/day dose reduced it 31%. Given the results of this study and the known interactive properties of disulfiram and theophylline, it appears likely that the interaction is real. Nevertheless, because the study did not include a crossover design, it was not possible to rule out the contribution of a gradually dissipating stimulatory effect of alcohol on theophylline metabolism in these recovering alcoholics.

RELATED DRUGS: No information is available.

MANAGEMENT OPTIONS:

➡ **Monitor.** Monitor for altered theophylline effect if disulfiram therapy is initiated, discontinued, or if the disulfiram dosage is changed. Patients receiving disulfiram therapy may require lower theophylline dosages.

REFERENCES:

1. Loi CM, et al. Dose-dependent inhibition of theophylline metabolism by disulfiram in recovering alcoholics. *Clin Pharmacol Ther.* 1989;45:476-486.

5 Disulfiram (*Antabuse*)

Tolbutamide (eg, *Orinase*)

SUMMARY: No interaction occurs.

RISK FACTORS: No specific risk factors are known.

MECHANISM: No interaction.

CLINICAL EVALUATION: A study in 10 normal subjects demonstrated no effect of disulfiram on tolbutamide metabolic clearance.[1] The effect of disulfiram on other sulfonylureas or insulin was not studied.

RELATED DRUGS: The effect of disulfiram on other sulfonylureas is unknown.

MANAGEMENT OPTIONS: No interaction.

REFERENCES:

1. Svendsen TL, et al. The influence of disulfiram on the half life and metabolic clearance rate of diphe-nylhydantoin and tolbutamide in man. *Eur J Clin Pharmacol.* 1976;9:439-441.

3 Disulfiram (*Antabuse*)

Tranylcypromine (*Parnate*)

SUMMARY: A patient on disulfiram developed delirium following the addition of tranylcypromine, but a causal relationship was not established.

RISK FACTORS: No specific risk factors are known.

MECHANISM: Not established.

CLINICAL EVALUATION: A 48-year-old man on lithium (eg, *Eskalith*) and disulfiram was started on tranylcypromine 10 mg twice daily.[1] Two days later he was agitated, disoriented, incoherent, and had visual hallucinations; his symptoms cleared within 24 hours. The temporal relationship between starting the tranylcypromine and the onset of delirium suggests an interaction with disulfiram, but one cannot rule out an effect of tranylcypromine alone or a contribution of lithium to the reaction.

RELATED DRUGS: The effect of combining other nonselective monoamine oxidase (MAO) inhibitors with disulfiram is not established; assume that they may interact until proven otherwise.

MANAGEMENT OPTIONS:

➡ **Monitor.** Although data are limited, monitor for evidence of delirium if tranylcypromine or other nonselective MAO inhibitors are used with disulfiram.

REFERENCES:

1. Blansjaar BA, et al. Delirium in a patient treated with disulfiram and tranylcypromine. *Am J Psychiatry*. 1995;152:296.

Disulfiram (*Antabuse*)

Venlafaxine (*Effexor*)

SUMMARY: A patient on disulfiram developed acute hypertension after starting venlafaxine, but a causal relationship was not established.

RISK FACTORS: No specific risk factors are known.

MECHANISM: It was proposed that disulfiram inhibits venlafaxine metabolism, but no supporting evidence was given.

CLINICAL EVALUATION: A 37-year-old woman taking disulfiram was admitted with hypertensive crisis (220/140 mm Hg) 12 days after starting venlafaxine.[1] It was not possible to establish a causal relationship between the drug combination and the hypertensive crisis.

RELATED DRUGS: No information is available.

MANAGEMENT OPTIONS: No specific action is required, but be alert for evidence of the interaction.

REFERENCES:

1. Khurana RN, et al. Hypertensive crisis associated with venlafaxine. *Am J Med*. 2003;115:676-677.

Disulfiram (*Antabuse*)

Warfarin (eg, *Coumadin*)

SUMMARY: Disulfiram increases the hypoprothrombinemic response to warfarin in most patients receiving both drugs concurrently.

RISK FACTORS: No specific risk factors are known.

MECHANISM: Disulfiram inhibits the hepatic metabolism of warfarin.[1]

CLINICAL EVALUATION: Case reports, as well as study in healthy subjects, indicate that disulfiram increases the hypoprothrombinemic effect and plasma concentration of warfarin.[2-5] Research in healthy subjects indicates that most people receiving the combination show an increased response to warfarin.

RELATED DRUGS: Although little is known regarding the effect of disulfiram on oral anticoagulants other than warfarin, assume that they interact until evidence to the contrary is available.

MANAGEMENT OPTIONS:

➡ **Avoid Unless Benefit Outweighs Risk.** Avoid concomitant use of disulfiram and oral anticoagulants if possible. If oral anticoagulant therapy has begun in the patient receiving disulfiram, use conservative doses until the maintenance dose is established.

➡ **Monitor.** Monitor patients receiving oral anticoagulants for altered anticoagulant effect when disulfiram is started or stopped.

REFERENCES:

1. O'Reilly RA. Dynamic interaction between disulfiram and separated enantiomorphs of racemic warfarin. *Clin Pharmacol Ther.* 1981;29:332-336.
2. O'Reilly RA. Interaction of sodium warfarin and disulfiram (*Antabuse*) in man. *Ann Intern Med.* 1973;78:73-76.
3. Rothstein E. Warfarin effect enhanced by disulfiram. *JAMA.* 1968;206:1574-1575.
4. Rothstein E. Warfarin effect enhanced by disulfiram (*Antabuse*). *JAMA.* 1972;221:1052-1053.
5. O'Reilly RA. Potentiation of anticoagulant effect by disulfiram. *Clin Res.* 1971;19:180.

4   Diuretic, Herbal

Lithium (eg, *Eskalith*)

SUMMARY: A patient on lithium developed severe lithium toxicity following the use of an herbal diuretic, but a causal relationship was not established.

RISK FACTORS: No specific risk factors are known.

MECHANISM: Not established.

CLINICAL EVALUATION: A 26-year-old woman stabilized on lithium developed severe lithium intoxication 2 to 3 weeks after starting an herbal diuretic preparation containing a variety of substances, including equisetum, parsley, uva ursi, ovate buchu, corn silk, and juniper.[1] Her lithium level had increased from 1.1 to 4.5 mmol/L, and she had dizziness, grogginess, nausea, diarrhea, tremor, and unsteady gait. While it is not possible to establish a causal relationship between the herbal diuretic and the lithium toxicity, no other cause for the lithium toxicity could be found.

RELATED DRUGS: Thiazide diuretics are known to increase lithium concentrations and have caused lithium toxicity.

MANAGEMENT OPTIONS: No specific action is required, but be alert for evidence of the interaction. Lithium toxicity can produce nausea, vomiting, diarrhea, anorexia, coarse tremor, slurred speech, vertigo, confusion, lethargy; in severe cases, seizures, stupor, coma, and cardiovascular collapse can occur.

REFERENCES:

1. Pyevich D, et al. Herbal diuretics and lithium toxicity. *Am J Psychiatry.* 2001;158:1329.

5   Dofetilide (*Tikosyn*)

Digoxin (eg, *Lanoxin*)

SUMMARY: Dofetilide does not alter digoxin plasma concentrations.

RISK FACTORS: No specific risk factors are known.

MECHANISM: No interaction.

CLINICAL EVALUATION: Fourteen healthy subjects received digoxin (1 mg loading dose, then 0.25 mg/day) alone for 12 days.[1] On day 8, each subject was randomized to receive placebo or dofetilide 0.25 mg twice daily for 4 days. Digoxin plasma concentrations were measured on days 7 and 12 of digoxin administration. Subjects in the groups receiving placebo or dofetilide had similar digoxin concentrations. Digoxin concentrations were not affected by the administration of dofetilide.

RELATED DRUGS: It is expected that dofetilide would not alter the plasma concentrations of digitoxin.

MANAGEMENT OPTIONS: No interaction.

REFERENCES:

1. Kleinermans D, et al. Effect of dofetilide on the pharmacokinetics of digoxin. *Am J Cardiol.* 2001;87:248-250, A9-A10.

Dofetilide (*Tikosyn*)

Warfarin (eg, *Coumadin*)

SUMMARY: Dofetilide does not alter warfarin anticoagulation.

RISK FACTORS: No specific risk factors are known.

MECHANISM: No interaction.

CLINICAL EVALUATION: Fourteen healthy subjects received a single 40 mg dose of warfarin on day 5 of an 8-day treatment regimen of placebo or dofetilide 0.750 mg twice daily.[1] Prothrombin times were measured for 96 hours after warfarin administration. Subjects had similar prothrombin times following a single dose of warfarin whether receiving concurrent placebo or dofetilide.

RELATED DRUGS: No information is available.

MANAGEMENT OPTIONS: No interaction.

REFERENCES:

1. Nichols DJ, et al. Effect of dofetilide on the pharmacodynamics of warfarin and pharmacokinetics of digoxin. *J Clin Pharmacol.* 1999;39:972.

Dofetilide (*Tikosyn*)

Ziprasidone (*Geodon*)

SUMMARY: Ziprasidone and dofetilide can prolong the corrected QT (QTc) interval on the electrocardiogram. Theoretically, this could increase the risk of ventricular arrhythmias such as torsades de pointes.

RISK FACTORS:

➡ **Hypokalemia.** The QTc on the ECG may be prolonged in patients with hypokalemia, thus increasing the risk of this interaction.[1]

➡ **Miscellaneous.** Other factors that may prolong the QTc interval (eg, hypomagnesemia, bradycardia, impaired liver function, hypothyroidism) also may increase the risk of ventricular arrhythmias.[1]

MECHANISM: Possible additive prolongation of the QTc interval.

CLINICAL EVALUATION: In initial controlled trials, ziprasidone increased the QTc interval approximately 10 msec at the highest recommended dose of 160 mg/day. But because of concern that the QTc measurements were done when ziprasidone serum concentrations were low, the FDA recommended additional study.[2,3] In a subsequent study in patients with psychotic disorders, the QTc interval was measured following administration of several antipsychotic drugs (eg, ziprasidone, thioridazine, quetiapine, risperidone, haloperidol, olanzapine) when the antipsychotic drug concentrations were calculated to be at their peak. Ziprasidone increased the QTc by a mean of approximately 21 msec, which was less than thioridazine (36 msec) but about twice that of the other antipsychotics. Theoretically, the ability of dofetilide to prolong the QTc would be additive with ziprasidone, but the extent to which this would increase the risk of ventricular arrhythmias such as torsades de pointes is not known.

RELATED DRUGS: Available data suggest that ziprasidone produces less QTc prolongation than thioridazine (*Mellaril*), but about twice that of quetiapine (*Seroquel*), risperidone (*Risperdal*), haloperidol (*Haldol*), and olanzapine (*Zyprexa*).

MANAGEMENT OPTIONS:

➡ *Use Alternative.* Given the theoretical risk and the fact that dofetilide is listed in the ziprasidone product information as "contraindicated," it would be prudent to use an alternative to 1 of the drugs (see Related Drugs).

➡ *Monitor.* If dofetilide and ziprasidone are used concurrently, monitor for evidence of arrhythmias (eg, syncope) and for prolonged QT intervals.

REFERENCES:

1. De Ponti F, et al. QT-interval prolongation by non-cardiac drugs: lessons to be learned from recent experience. *Eur J Clin Pharmacol.* 2000;56:1-18.

2. Product information. Ziprasidone (*Geodon*). Pfizer Pharmaceuticals. 2001.

3. Briefing Information, Psychopharmacological Drugs Advisory Committee, U.S. Food and Drug Administration, July 19, 2000.

 Donepezil (eg, *Aricept*)

Digoxin (eg, *Lanoxin*)

SUMMARY: The combination of digoxin and donepezil may produce bradycardia in susceptible patients; digoxin may interact similarly with other cholinesterase inhibitors.

RISK FACTORS: No specific risk factors are known.

MECHANISM: Donepezil and other cholinesterase inhibitors increase vagal tone, predisposing to bradycardia. Digoxin may produce additive effects.

CLINICAL EVALUATION: The French Pharmacovigilance Database received 49 spontaneous reports of adverse reactions in patients receiving digoxin and cholinesterase inhibitors (eg, donepezil, galantamine, rivastigmine).[1] After evaluation by clinical pharmacologists, 19 were felt to be adverse drug interactions. Of the 73 patients who received cholinesterase inhibitors along with digoxin or other bradycardic drugs, there were 5 deaths due to syncope, bradycardia, arrhythmias, or cardiac arrest. Although additional study is needed to establish the clinical importance of these interactions, the potential severity of the reactions dictates caution. Study in healthy subjects found no effect of digoxin on donepezil pharmacokinetics or vice versa.[2]

RELATED DRUGS: Digoxin is expected to interact with all cholinesterase inhibitors, including galantamine (eg, *Razadyne*) and rivastigmine (eg, *Exelon*).

MANAGEMENT OPTIONS:

➡ *Consider Alternative.* If appropriate, use an alternative to either the cholinesterase inhibitor or digoxin.

➡ *Monitor.* If the combination is used, monitor for bradycardia, hypotension, and syncope.

REFERENCES:

1. Tavassoli N, et al. Drug interactions with cholinesterase inhibitors: an analysis of the French Pharmacovigilance Database and a comparison of two national drug formularies (Vidal, British National Formulary). *Drug Saf.* 2007;30(11):1063-1071.

2. Tiseo PJ, et al. Concurrent administration of donepezil HCl and digoxin: assessment of pharmacokinetic changes. *Br J Clin Pharmacol.* 1998;46(suppl 1):40-44.

Donepezil (eg, *Aricept*)

Ketoconazole (eg, *Nizoral*)

SUMMARY: Ketoconazole produces a modest increase in donepezil plasma concentrations; changes in patient response to donepezil would be limited.

RISK FACTORS:

➡ *Pharmacogenetics.* Poor metabolizers of CYP2D6. Donepezil is metabolized by CYP3A4 and CYP2D6. Patients who are poor metabolizers of CYP2D6 would be more dependent on CYP3A4 for donepezil elimination. Inhibitors of CYP3A4 may produce a larger effect in these patients.

MECHANISM: Donepezil is partially metabolized by CYP3A4. This pathway is inhibited by ketoconazole and may account for the increase in donepezil concentrations observed in this study.

CLINICAL EVALUATION: Eighteen healthy subjects received donepezil 5 mg/day, ketoconazole 200 mg/day, or the combination of donepezil and ketoconazole.[1] Each treatment was continued for 7 days. The mean plasma area under the concentration-time curve and peak concentration of doncepezil was increased approximately 27% following coadministration with ketoconazole. The half-life of donepezil was not altered by ketoconazole treatment. No significant differences in ketoconazole pharmacokinetics were noted when administered with donepezil.

RELATED DRUGS: Other antifungal drugs (eg, itraconazole [eg, *Sporanox*], fluconazole [eg, *Diflucan*]) that can be potent CYP3A4 inhibitors are expected to have a similar effect on donepezil pharmacokinetics.

MANAGEMENT OPTIONS:

➡ *Monitor.* Observe patients taking donepezil who are administered ketoconazole for adverse reactions, including nausea, vomiting, and abdominal pain.

REFERENCES:

1. Tiseo PJ, et al. Concurrent administration of donepezil HCl and ketoconazole: assessment of pharmacokinetic changes following single and multiple doses. *Br J Clin Pharmacol.* 1998;46(suppl 1):30-34.

Dopamine (eg, *Intropin*)

Ergonovine

SUMMARY: A case of gangrene with concurrent use of ergonovine and dopamine has been reported.

RISK FACTORS: No specific risk factors are known.

MECHANISM: The combined use of dopamine and ergot alkaloids may result in excessive peripheral vasoconstriction.

CLINICAL EVALUATION: One case report described a patient who developed gangrene of both hands and feet following administration of ergonovine (ergometrine) and dopamine infusions.[1] The gangrene was presumed to result from the combined effect of the drugs, although either drug alone in sufficient dosage can cause gangrene.

RELATED DRUGS: The effect of other combinations of ergot alkaloids and vasoconstricting sympathomimetics is unknown, but excessive vasoconstriction might occur.

MANAGEMENT OPTIONS:

➡ *Monitor.* Undertake the concurrent use of dopamine and ergot alkaloids such as ergonovine with caution; monitor for evidence of excessive vasoconstriction in the extremities (eg, cold, pale skin, pain).

REFERENCES:
1. Buchanan N, et al. Symmetrical gangrene of the extremities associated with the use of dopamine subsequent to ergometrine administration. *Intensive Care Med.* 1977;3:55.

 4

Dopamine (eg, *Intropin*)

Metoprolol (eg, *Lopressor*)

SUMMARY: Metoprolol administration may blunt dopamine-induced tachycardia and increase systolic blood pressure, but it does not appear to alter dopamine's renal effects.

RISK FACTORS: No specific risk factors are known.

MECHANISM: Metoprolol inhibits some of the beta-adrenergic effects of dopamine infusions.

CLINICAL EVALUATION: The effects of a single 100 mg dose of metoprolol on the hemodynamic and renal effects of a two-hour dopamine infusion (3 mcg/kg/min) was studied in 8 healthy subjects.[1] Metoprolol blunted the increases in heart rate and systolic blood pressure noted after dopamine, but dopamine-induced increases in cardiac output were not affected. Metoprolol had a minimal effect on the renal effects of dopamine. The significance of these effects awaits trials in patients; however, it seems likely that metoprolol would have little adverse effect on dopamine-induced hemodynamic changes.

RELATED DRUGS: Other beta blockers would be likely to produce similar changes in dopamine's response.

MANAGEMENT OPTIONS: No specific action is required, but be alert for evidence of the interaction.

REFERENCES:

1. Olsen NV, et al. Effects of acute beta-adrenoceptor blockade with metoprolol on the renal response to dopamine in normal humans. *Br J Clin Pharmacol.* 1994;37:347.

Dopamine (eg, *Intropin*)

Phenytoin (*Dilantin*)

SUMMARY: Case reports and animal studies indicate that patients receiving dopamine may be more susceptible to hypotension following IV phenytoin.

RISK FACTORS: No specific risk factors are known.

MECHANISM: Not established.

CLINICAL EVALUATION: Several patients requiring dopamine infusions to maintain blood pressure developed severe hypotension following IV phenytoin.[1] This response was reproduced in dogs. However, certain predisposing factors appear to be required because not all patients receiving IV phenytoin and dopamine develop such reactions. The effect of oral phenytoin in patients receiving dopamine is not established, but one would expect the risk of hypotension to be less.

RELATED DRUGS: No information is available.

MANAGEMENT OPTIONS:

➡ *Monitor.* In patients receiving IV dopamine, administer IV phenytoin only with careful monitoring of the cardiovascular status.

REFERENCES:

1. Bivins BA, et al. Dopamine-phenytoin interaction. *Arch Surg.* 1978;113:245.

Doxapram (eg, *Dopram*)

Phenelzine (*Nardil*)

SUMMARY: Phenelzine, a nonselective monoamine oxidase inhibitor (MAOI), reportedly enhances the cardiovascular effects of doxapram.

RISK FACTORS:

➡ *Concurrent Diseases.* Patients with pre-existing arrhythmias may be at increased risk.

MECHANISM: Not established.

CLINICAL EVALUATION: The adverse cardiovascular effects of doxapram (eg, hypertension, arrhythmias) are reportedly potentiated by nonselective MAOIs but no data are given.[1]

RELATED DRUGS: No information is available.

MANAGEMENT OPTIONS: No specific action is required, but be alert for evidence of the interaction.

REFERENCES:

1. Product information. (*Dopram*). 1996.

Doxazosin (*Cardura*)

Nifedipine (eg, *Procardia*)

SUMMARY: The combination of nifedipine with doxazosin can result in enhanced hypotensive effects.

RISK FACTORS: No specific risk factors are known.

MECHANISM: Additive pharmacodynamic effects without a change in pharmacokinetics probably account for the increased hypotensive effect of the combination.

CLINICAL EVALUATION: Twelve healthy subjects received nifedipine 20 mg and doxazosin 2 mg alone and in combination for 10 days.[1] No changes in the pharmacokinetics of either drug were noted during combination therapy. However, the combination did produce a mildly greater reduction in blood pressure than either drug alone. No adverse effects (orthostatic hypotension, reflex tachycardia) were noted. Further study in hypertensive patients is needed.

RELATED DRUGS: Other calcium channel blockers may have additive hypotensive effects when administered with doxazosin or other alpha blockers.

MANAGEMENT OPTIONS:

➡ *Monitor.* The combination of nifedipine and doxazosin appears to produce an increased antihypertensive effect. Monitor patients stabilized on 1 of these drugs for hypotension during the institution of the second drug.

REFERENCES:

1. Donnelly R, et al. The pharmacodynamics and pharmacokinetics of the combination of nifedipine and doxazosin. *Eur J Clin Pharmacol.* 1993;44:279.

Doxepin (eg, *Sinequan*)

Erythromycin (eg, *Erythrocin*)

SUMMARY: Erythromycin does not alter the concentration of doxepine.

RISK FACTORS: No specific risk factors are known.

MECHANISM: No interaction. Erythromycin inhibits a different cytochrome P450 than the one responsible for the majority of cyclic antidepressant metabolism.

CLINICAL EVALUATION: Eight patients taking cyclic antidepressants including desipramine (eg, *Norpramin*), imipramine (eg, *Tofranil*), doxepin, and nortriptyline (eg, *Pamelor*) were administered erythromycin stearate 250 mg 4 times a day for 6 days.[1] No change in antidepressant or active metabolite concentrations was noted following the addition of erythromycin.

RELATED DRUGS: Desipramine, imipramine, and nortriptyline do not appear to interact with erythromycin.

MANAGEMENT OPTIONS: No interaction.

REFERENCES:

1. Amsterdam JD, et al. Effect of erythromycin on tricyclic antidepressant metabolism. *J Clin Psychopharmacol.* 1991;11:203.

Doxepin (eg, *Sinequan*)

Propoxyphene (eg, *Darvocet-N*)

SUMMARY: Preliminary evidence suggests that propoxyphene increases serum concentrations of doxepin.

RISK FACTORS: No specific risk factors are known.

MECHANISM: Propoxyphene appears to inhibit the doxepin metabolism.

CLINICAL EVALUATION: An 89-year-old man on chronic doxepin therapy 150 mg/day developed a doubling of his plasma doxepin concentration following propoxyphene therapy 65 mg every 6 hours.[1] The increased plasma doxepin was associated with lethargy which reversed after propoxyphene therapy was discontinued. Ten healthy subjects were then given antipyrine 1.2 g IV with and without propoxyphene 65 mg every 4 hours for 8 doses, starting 8 hours before the antipyrine. Propoxyphene prolonged the antipyrine half-life from 12.2 hours to 15.2 hours and reduced the antipyrine clearance from 0.63 mL/min/kg body weight to 0.53 mL/min/kg body weight. These results are consistent with previous studies indicating that propoxyphene can impair the hepatic metabolism of carbamazepine (eg, *Tegretol*) and possibly other drugs. Note that the studies showing inhibition of drug metabolism caused by propoxyphene have involved propoxyphene doses of 65 mg 3 to 6 times daily. The effect of lower or sporadic doses of propoxyphene on drug metabolism is unclear, but such doses probably would be less likely to have an effect.

RELATED DRUGS: It is not known whether tricyclic antidepressants other than doxepin would be affected by propoxyphene, but it certainly seems possible. Propoxyphene impairs the hepatic metabolism of carbamazepine.

MANAGEMENT OPTIONS:

➡ *Monitor.* Monitor for altered doxepin effect if propoxyphene is initiated, discontinued, or changed in dosage; adjust doxepin dose as needed.

REFERENCES:

1. Abernethy DR, et al. Impairment of hepatic drug oxidation by propoxyphene. *Ann Intern Med.* 1982;97:223.

Doxepin (eg, *Sinequan*)

Tolazamide (eg, *Tolinase*)

SUMMARY: Doxepin may enhance the hypoglycemic effects of tolazamide or insulin.

RISK FACTORS: No specific risk factors are known.

MECHANISM: Doxepin and other cyclic antidepressants can alter a patient's response to hypoglycemia or increase the sensitivity to insulin; however, the actual mechanism has not been established.

CLINICAL EVALUATION: A 71-year-old diabetic patient who had been maintained on tolazamide 1 g/day for several years without a history of hypoglycemic episodes was found to be hypoglycemic 11 days after starting doxepin.[1] The doxepin dose was initiated at 25 mg/day and increased to 50 mg/day 4 days before admission.

When the tolazamide dose was reduced to 100 mg/day and the doxepin dose maintained, no further hypoglycemic episodes were experienced.

RELATED DRUGS: A patient who had been maintained on chlorpropamide (eg, *Diabinese*) 250 mg/day was found to have a blood glucose of 50 mg/dL 4 days after the initiation of nortriptyline (eg, *Pamelor*). Chlorpropamide was discontinued, and the patient remained normoglycemic. Nortriptyline has been reported to increase insulin sensitivity and lower blood glucose.[2] In other case reports, patients with diabetes developed hypoglycemia following the addition of amitriptyline (eg, *Elavil*),[3] imipramine (eg, *Tofranil*),[4] and maprotiline (eg, *Ludiomil*).[5]

MANAGEMENT OPTIONS:

➡ *Monitor.* Pending prospective evaluation of this interaction, diabetic patients should monitor their blood glucose daily when cyclic antidepressants are initiated or discontinued.

REFERENCES:

1. True BL, et al. Profound hypoglycemia with the addition of tricyclic antidepressant to maintenance sulfonylurea therapy. *Am J Psychiatry.* 1987;144:1220.
2. Grof E, et al. Effects of lithium, nortriptyline and dexamethasone on insulin sensitivity. *Prog Neuropsychopharmacol Biol Psychiatry.* 1984;8:687.
3. Sherman KE, et al. Amitriptyline and asymptomatic hypoglycemia. *Ann Intern Med.* 1988;109:683.
4. Shrivastava RK, et al. Hypoglycemia associated with imipramine. *Biol Psychiatry.* 1983;18:1509.
5. Zogno MG, et al. Hypoglycemia caused by maprotiline in a patient taking oral antidiabetics. *Ann Pharmacother.* 1994;28:406.

 Doxorubicin (eg, *Adriamycin*)

Phenobarbital (eg, *Solfoton*)

SUMMARY: Barbiturates may enhance the elimination of doxorubicin, but the clinical importance of this effect is not known.

RISK FACTORS: No specific risk factors are known.

MECHANISM: Not established. Barbiturates may enhance the hepatic metabolism of doxorubicin.

CLINICAL EVALUATION: Preliminary clinical evidence indicates that barbiturates increase the plasma clearance of doxorubicin,[1] but more data are needed to assess the incidence and magnitude of this purported interaction.

RELATED DRUGS: Theoretically, barbiturates other than phenobarbital also may increase doxorubicin elimination.

MANAGEMENT OPTIONS: No specific action is required, but be alert for evidence of the interaction.

REFERENCES:

1. Riggs CE, et al. Doxorubicin pharmacokinetics: prochlorperazine and barbiturate effects. *Clin Pharmacol Ther.* 1982;31:263.

Doxorubicin (eg, *Adriamycin*)

Verapamil (eg, *Calan*)

SUMMARY: Verapamil appears to increase doxorubicin serum concentrations.

RISK FACTORS: No specific risk factors are known.

MECHANISM: The hepatic metabolism of doxorubicin appears to be inhibited by verapamil.

CLINICAL EVALUATION: The effect of verapamil on the pharmacokinetics of doxorubicin was studied in 5 patients with lung cancer undergoing chemotherapy with multiple cytotoxic agents, including doxorubicin 40 mg/m^2.[1] Verapamil 80 mg 3 times a day for 3 days followed by 120 mg 4 times a day for 4 days was administered before 1 of the first 2 courses of chemotherapy. Doxorubicin clearance was reduced by an average of 33% (range: 8% to 79%), and its half-life increased from 23.6 hours to 32.5 hours. No increase in doxorubicin toxicity was noted in the patients.

RELATED DRUGS: The effect of calcium channel blockers other than verapamil on doxorubicin is not established.

MANAGEMENT OPTIONS:

➡ **Monitor.** Monitor for altered doxorubicin effect if verapamil is initiated, discontinued, or changed in dosage; adjust doxorubicin dose as needed.

REFERENCES:

1. Kerr DJ, et al. The effect of verapamil on the pharmacokinetics of Adriamycin. *Cancer Chemother Pharmacol.* 1986;18:239.

Doxycycline (eg, *Vibramycin*)

Ethanol (Ethyl Alcohol)

SUMMARY: Chronic alcohol ingestion may reduce the serum concentration of doxycycline.

RISK FACTORS: No specific risk factors are known.

MECHANISM: Chronic ingestion of large amounts of ethanol can induce hepatic microsomal enzymes. Because doxycycline is metabolized by the liver, its metabolism may be enhanced in alcoholic patients.

CLINICAL EVALUATION: Tetracycline (eg, *Sumycin*) and doxycycline were administered to 6 alcoholics and 6 healthy subjects to determine pharmacokinetic differences in the disposition of these 2 antibiotics in alcoholics compared with healthy subjects.[1] Doxycycline half-life was shorter in the alcoholics (10.5 hr) than in the healthy subjects (14.7 hr), whereas the half-life of tetracycline was the same in both groups.

RELATED DRUGS: Tetracycline does not appear to interact with ethanol.

MANAGEMENT OPTIONS:

➡ **Consider Alternative.** When a tetracycline is needed in an alcoholic patient, it may be preferable to use an agent other than doxycycline.

➡ *Monitor.* If doxycycline is used, be alert for diminished doxycycline effect.

REFERENCES:

1. Neuvonen PJ, et al. Effect of long-term alcohol consumption on the half-life of tetracycline and doxycycline in man. *Int J Clin Pharmacol.* 1976;14:303.

Doxycycline (eg, *Vibramycin*)

Methotrexate (eg, *Rheumatrex*)

SUMMARY: Doxycycline administration appears to increase methotrexate concentrations; methotrexate toxicity is likely.

RISK FACTORS: No specific risk factors are known.

MECHANISM: Unknown. Doxycycline may reduce the renal clearance of methotrexate.

CLINICAL EVALUATION: A patient with osteosarcoma was receiving postoperative methotrexate when she developed an abscess in her eye.[1] Oral doxycycline 100 mg every 12 hours was started. Several days later, she was given methotrexate 18 g by intravenous infusion over 12 hours with water loading and urinary alkalinization. This was the patient's eleventh cycle of methotrexate. The mean methotrexate clearance and half-life for the previous 10 cycles were 3.67 L/h and 2.96 hours, respectively. The clearance of methotrexate was reduced to 1.29 L/h and its half-life extended to 6.26 hours following administration after doxycycline. Doxycycline was discontinued 2 days after the methotrexate was administered, and leucovorin was administered 72 hours after the methotrexate infusion. The elevated methotrexate concentrations were accompanied by hematologic and GI toxicity. The effect of doxycycline on patients taking low doses of methotrexate is unknown.

RELATED DRUGS: Tetracycline (eg, *Sumycin*) may also increase methotrexate concentrations.

MANAGEMENT OPTIONS:

➡ *Consider Alternative.* Patients receiving high-dose methotrexate should avoid treatment with doxycycline. Select an alternative nontetracycline antibiotic. Note that some penicillins (eg, carbenicillin†) have been reported to increase the plasma concentration of methotrexate.

➡ *Monitor.* If patients being treated with high-dose methotrexate are administered doxycycline, carefully monitor methotrexate concentrations. Methotrexate dosage reduction may be necessary.

REFERENCES:

1. Tortajada-Ituren JJ, et al. High-dose methotrexate-doxycycline interaction. *Ann Pharmacother.* 1999;33(7-8):804–808.

† Not available in the United States.

Doxycycline (eg, *Vibramycin*)

Phenobarbital (eg, *Luminal*)

SUMMARY: Doxycycline serum concentrations may be reduced by the administration of phenobarbital.

RISK FACTORS: No specific risk factors are known.

MECHANISM: Phenobarbital presumably enhances the hepatic metabolism of doxycycline.

CLINICAL EVALUATION: Doxycycline half-life was decreased 27% following administration of phenobarbital 150 mg/day for 10 days in 5 patients.[1] Doxycycline half-life was reduced from 15.3 hours before to 11.1 hours after phenobarbital. Five additional patients on long-term barbiturate therapy had even shorter doxycycline half-lives (7.7 hours). The antibacterial efficacy of doxycycline could be decreased by coadministration of an enzyme inducer such as phenobarbital.

RELATED DRUGS: Other barbiturates may affect doxycycline in a similar manner. Theoretically, other tetracyclines are not affected by barbiturates such as phenobarbital.

MANAGEMENT OPTIONS:

➥ **Consider Alternative.** Theoretically, tetracyclines other than doxycycline are not affected by barbiturates because hepatic metabolism is not an important route of elimination.

➥ **Monitor.** If barbiturates cannot be avoided in patients receiving doxycycline, closely monitor the clinical response to doxycycline.

REFERENCES:

1. Neuvonen PJ, et al. Interaction between doxycycline and barbiturates. *Br Med J.* 1974;1(5907):535-536.

Doxycycline (eg, *Vibramycin*)

Phenytoin (eg, *Dilantin*)

SUMMARY: Phenytoin reduces doxycycline serum concentrations, but other tetracyclines do not appear to be affected.

RISK FACTORS: No specific risk factors are known.

MECHANISM: Phenytoin probably stimulates doxycycline metabolism.[1]

CLINICAL EVALUATION: The half-life of doxycycline was shorter in 7 patients on long-term phenytoin therapy (mean, 7. 2 hours) than in 9 control patients (mean, 15.1 hours).[2] A subsequent study by the same group produced similar results.[3] The effect of this shortened half-life on the clinical antibacterial effect of doxycycline was not assessed, but the magnitude of the differences in half-life suggests that the therapeutic effect of doxycycline may be reduced by phenytoin.

RELATED DRUGS: Chlortetracycline[+], demeclocycline (eg, *Declomycin*), and methacycline[+] do not appear to be affected by phenytoin administration. Theoretically, tetracycline (eg, *Sumycin*) is also unaffected by phenytoin.

MANAGEMENT OPTIONS:

➥ **Consider Alternative.** If possible, use a tetracycline other than doxycycline in patients receiving phenytoin (see Related Drugs).

➥ **Monitor.** If doxycycline is used with phenytoin, watch for reduced doxycycline efficacy and consider using larger doses of doxycycline.

REFERENCES:

1. Penttila O, et al. Interaction between doxycycline and some antiepileptic drugs. *Br Med J.* 1974;2(5917):470-472.

2. Neuvonen PJ, et al. Interaction between doxycycline and barbiturates. *Br Med J.* 1974;1(5907):535-536.

3. Neuvonen PJ, et al. Effect of antiepileptic drugs on the elimination of various tetracycline derivatives. *Eur J Clin Pharmacol.* 1975;9(2-3):147-154.

† Not available in the United States.

Doxycycline (eg, *Vibramycin*)

Warfarin (eg, *Coumadin*)

SUMMARY: Although doxycycline theoretically may increase the hypoprothrombinemic response to oral anticoagulants such as warfarin, clinical evidence is limited.

RISK FACTORS:

➡ **Concurrent Diseases.** The hypoprothrombinemic response to doxycycline may be larger in patients with deficient vitamin K intake.

MECHANISM: The following are proposed as mechanisms for this interaction: 1) intravenous tetracycline therapy may reduce plasma prothrombin activity, possibly by impairing prothrombin utilization;[1] 2) tetracyclines purportedly decrease vitamin K production by GI bacteria, but this effect is of questionable significance; 3) fever has been shown to enhance the catabolism of clotting factors; thus, the infection for which the tetracycline is used theoretically could enhance oral anticoagulant hypoprothrombinemia, an effect that should dissipate as the tetracycline lowers the fever.

CLINICAL EVALUATION: Oral doxycycline was associated with an increase in warfarin response and bleeding in 1 patient.[2,3] The effect of tetracyclines on vitamin K production by GI bacteria has not been shown to be a significant problem.[4]

RELATED DRUGS: Other tetracyclines may produce similar effects on oral anticoagulants.

MANAGEMENT OPTIONS:

➡ **Monitor.** Although the clinical evidence for an interaction between doxycycline and oral anticoagulants is limited, monitor patients for an enhanced anticoagulant effect when these drugs are used concurrently.

REFERENCES:

1. Searcy RL, et al. Blood clotting anomalies associated with intensive tetracycline therapy. *Clin Res.* 1964;12:230.

2. Westfall LK, et al. Potentiation of warfarin by tetracycline. *Am J Hosp Pharm.* 1980;37(12):1620, 1625.

3. Caraco Y, et al. Enhanced anticoagulant effect of coumarin derivatives induced by doxycycline coadministration. *Ann Pharmacother.* 1992;26(9):1084-1086.

4. Messinger WJ, et al. The effect of a bowel sterilizing antibiotic on blood coagulation mechanisms. The anti-cholesterol effect of paromomycin. *Angiology.* 1965;16:29-36.

Dronedarone (*Multaq*)

Grapefruit Juice

SUMMARY: Grapefruit juice increases the plasma concentration of dronedarone; increased dronedarone response may occur in some patients.

RISK FACTORS: No specific risk factors are known.

MECHANISM: Grapefruit juice appears to inhibit the metabolism (CYP3A4) of dronedarone.

CLINICAL EVALUATION: While specific data are limited, the manufacturer of dronedarone states that the coadministration of grapefruit juice (dose not stated) with dronedarone increased the mean area under the plasma concentration-time curve of dronedarone approximately 3-fold.[1] Pending further data, patients receiving dronedarone should avoid large amounts of grapefruit juice when possible.

RELATED DRUGS: Plasma concentrations of amiodarone (eg, *Cordarone*) are also known to be increased by the coadministration of grapefruit juice.

MANAGEMENT OPTIONS:

➡ *Monitor.* Monitor patients taking dronedarone and grapefruit juice for heart failure and arrhythmias.

REFERENCES:

1. *Multaq* [package insert]. Bridgewater, NJ: Sanofi-Aventis; 2009.

Dronedarone (*Multaq*)

Ketoconazole (eg, *Nizoral*)

SUMMARY: Ketoconazole markedly increases the plasma concentration of dronedarone; increased dronedarone response is likely to occur.

RISK FACTORS: No specific risk factors are known.

MECHANISM: Ketoconazole appears to inhibit the CYP3A4-mediated metabolism (probably first-pass and systemic) of dronedarone.

CLINICAL EVALUATION: While specific data are limited, the manufacturer of dronedarone states that the coadministration of ketoconazole with dronedarone increased the mean area under the plasma concentration-time curve of dronedarone approximately 17-fold.[1] Pending further data, avoid coadministration of ketoconazole in patients receiving dronedarone.

RELATED DRUGS: Other antifungal agents that inhibit CYP3A4 (eg, itraconazole [eg, *Sporanox*], voriconazole [*Vfend*], posaconazole [*Noxafil*], fluconazole [eg, *Diflucan*]) are expected to affect dronedarone in a similar manner.

MANAGEMENT OPTIONS:

➡ *Use Alternative.* Terbinafine (eg, *Lamisil*) can be considered as an alternative antifungal agent as it does not affect CYP3A4 activity. Amphotericin, caspofungin (*Cancidas*), and anidulafungin (*Eraxis*) do not appear to inhibit CYP3A4. The effect of potent CYP3A4 inhibitors on amiodarone (eg, *Cordarone*) is not well described so carefully monitor patients using amiodarone and ketoconazole.

➡ *Monitor.* Carefully monitor patients taking dronedarone and ketoconazole for signs of dronedarone toxicity, including heart failure and arrhythmias.

REFERENCES:

1. *Multaq* [package insert]. Bridgewater, NJ: Sanofi-Aventis; 2009.

Dronedarone (*Multaq*)

Metoprolol (eg, *Lopressor*)

SUMMARY: Dronedarone increases the plasma concentration and pharmacodynamic effects of metoprolol; increased metoprolol response is likely.

RISK FACTORS:

➡ *Pharmacogenetics.* Patients who are rapid metabolizers for CYP2D6 will have a larger reduction in metoprolol clearance during dronedarone coadministration than poor metabolizers.

MECHANISM: Dronedarone appears to inhibit the metabolism (CYP2D6) of metoprolol.

CLINICAL EVALUATION: Thirty-nine subjects (5 poor CYP2D6 metabolizers) received metoprolol 200 mg daily for 13 days.[1] On days 6 to 13, subjects also received either placebo or dronedarone 800, 1,200, or 1,600 mg daily. The mean metoprolol concentration increased from day 5 to 13 by 20%, 49%, 100%, and 115% in the subjects receiving concurrent placebo, dronedarone 800, 1,200, and 1,600 mg, respectively. Metoprolol concentrations in subjects who were poor metabolizers of CYP2D6 were not altered by dronedarone coadministration. The negative inotropic effects of metoprolol were increased during dronedarone administration.

RELATED DRUGS: Other beta-blockers metabolized by CYP2D6 (eg, carvedilol [eg, *Coreg*], propranolol (eg, *Inderal*), timolol) are expected to interact in a similar manner with dronedarone. Amiodarone (eg, *Cordarone*) is also known to be an inhibitor of CYP2D6 and can increase the plasma concentration of metoprolol.

MANAGEMENT OPTIONS:

➡ *Consider Alternative.* Beta-blockers that are not substrates for CYP2D6, such as atenolol (eg, *Tenormin*), may have less risk of adverse reactions when administered with dronedarone, but carefully monitor patients nevertheless.

➡ *Monitor.* Monitor patients taking dronedarone and metoprolol for decreased heart rate and cardiac output.

REFERENCES:

1. Damy T, et al. Pharmacokinetic and pharmacodynamic interactions between metoprolol and dronedarone in extensive and poor CYP2D6 metabolizers healthy subjects. *Fundam Clin Pharmacol.* 2004;18(1):113-123.

Dronedarone (*Multaq*)

Propranolol (eg, *Inderal*)

SUMMARY: Dronedarone increases the plasma concentration of propranolol; increased propranolol response is likely to occur in some patients.

RISK FACTORS:

➡ *Pharmacogenetics.* Patients who are rapid metabolizers for CYP2D6 are likely to have a larger reduction in propranolol clearance during dronedarone coadministration than poor metabolizers.

MECHANISM: Dronedarone appears to inhibit the metabolism (CYP2D6) of propranolol.

CLINICAL EVALUATION: While specific data are limited, the manufacturer of dronedarone states that the coadministration of dronedarone with propranolol increased the mean area under the plasma concentration-time curve of propranolol approximately 1.3-fold.[1] Pending further data, observe patients receiving dronedarone and propranolol for increased propranolol effect.

RELATED DRUGS: Other beta-blockers metabolized by CYP2D6 (eg, carvedilol [eg, *Coreg*], metoprolol, timolol) are expected to interact in a similar manner with dronedarone. Amiodarone (eg, *Cordarone*) is also known to be an inhibitor of CYP2D6 and may increase the concentration of propranolol.

MANAGEMENT OPTIONS:

➡ *Consider Alternative.* Beta-blockers that are not substrates for CYP2D6, such as atenolol (eg, *Tenormin*), may have less risk of adverse reactions when administered with dronedarone, but carefully monitor patients nevertheless.

➡ *Monitor.* Monitor patients taking dronedarone and propranolol for decreased heart rate and cardiac output.

REFERENCES:

1. *Multaq* [package insert]. Bridgewater, NJ: Sanofi-Aventis; 2009.

Dronedarone (*Multaq*)

Rifampin (eg, *Rifadin*)

SUMMARY: Rifampin markedly reduces the plasma concentration of dronedarone; reduction of dronedarone response is likely to occur in some patients.

RISK FACTORS: No specific risk factors are known.

MECHANISM: Rifampin appears to induce the metabolism (CYP3A4) of dronedarone.

CLINICAL EVALUATION: While specific data are limited, the manufacturer of dronedarone states that the coadministration of rifampin with dronedarone decreased the mean area under the plasma concentration-time curve of dronedarone approximately 80%.[1] This magnitude of reduction in dronedarone plasma concentration will reduce its efficacy; dose adjustments of dronedarone will be necessary to maintain desired response.

RELATED DRUGS: Rifabutin (*Mycobutin*) and rifapentine (*Priftin*) are known to induce CYP3A4 and are likely to affect dronedarone in a similar manner. Plasma concentrations of amiodarone (eg, *Cordarone*) are also known to be decreased by the coadministration of rifampin.

MANAGEMENT OPTIONS:

➡ *Monitor.* Carefully monitor patients taking dronedarone for a change in therapeutic response if rifampin is initiated or discontinued.

REFERENCES:

1. *Multaq* [package insert]. Bridgewater, NJ: Sanofi-Aventis; 2009.

Dronedarone (*Multaq*)

Simvastatin (eg, *Zocor*)

SUMMARY: Dronedarone increases the plasma concentration of simvastatin; increased simvastatin response is likely to occur.

RISK FACTORS: No specific risk factors are known.

MECHANISM: Dronedarone may inhibit the CYP3A4-mediated elimination of simvastatin.

CLINICAL EVALUATION: While specific data are limited, the manufacturer of dronedarone states that the coadministration of dronedarone with simvastatin increased the mean area under the plasma concentration-time curve of simvastatin approximately 4-fold.[1] Pending further data, observe patients receiving dronedarone and simvastatin for increased simvastatin effects, including muscle pain or weakness.

RELATED DRUGS: Lovastatin (eg, *Mevacor*) and atorvastatin (*Lipitor*) are also metabolized by CYP3A4, and are also likely to interact with dronedarone. Amiodarone (eg, *Cordarone*) is also known to inhibit the elimination of simvastatin.

MANAGEMENT OPTIONS:

➡ **Consider Alternative.** Pravastatin (eg, *Pravachol*), fluvastatin (*Lescol*), and rosuvastatin (*Crestor*) are unlikely to be affected by dronedarone.

➡ **Monitor.** Monitor patients taking dronedarone and simvastatin for signs of simvastatin toxicity.

REFERENCES:

1. *Multaq* [package insert]. Bridgewater, NJ: Sanofi-Aventis; 2009.

Dronedarone (*Multaq*)

Sirolimus (*Rapamune*)

SUMMARY: Dronedarone administration increases sirolimus plasma concentrations; some patients may experience increased sirolimus toxicity including renal dysfunction, pulmonary toxicity, or thrombocytopenia.

RISK FACTORS: No specific risk factors are known.

MECHANISM: Sirolimus is a substrate for CYP3A4 and P-glycoprotein, both of which are known to be inhibited by dronedarone.

CLINICAL EVALUATION: A kidney transplant patient stabilized on prednisone, mycophenolate mofetil, and sirolimus 5 mg daily developed atrial fibrillation during an episode of norovirus enteritis.[1] Dronedarone 400 mg twice daily was initiated. Following 3 days of dronedarone administration, the patient's sirolimus plasma concentration had increased to 38 ng/mL compared with a value of 13 ng/mL a week earlier. Dronedarone was continued, but the sirolimus dosage was eventually reduced to 1 mg daily with normalization of sirolimus concentrations.

RELATED DRUGS: Tacrolimus (eg, *Prograf*) and cyclosporine (eg, *Neoral*) are also substrates of CYP3A4 and P-glycoprotein and may interact in a similar manner with dronedarone. Amiodarone (eg, *Cordarone*) inhibits the elimination of cyclosporine and would probably exert a similar effect on sirolimus.

MANAGEMENT OPTIONS:

➡ *Consider Alternative.* Consider electrical cardioversion or acute diltiazem (eg, *Cardizem*) cardioversion for patients taking sirolimus who develop acute atrial fibrillation. Consider beta-blockers for long-term rate control because they are not expected to alter sirolimus concentrations.

➡ *Monitor.* Carefully monitor the sirolimus concentration and adjust the dose as needed if a CYP3A4 or P-glycoprotein inhibitor is added for a patient taking sirolimus.

REFERENCES:

    1. Tichy EM, et al. Significant sirolimus and dronedarone interaction in a kidney transplant patient. *Ann Pharmacother.* 2010;44(7-8):1338-1341.

Dronedarone (*Multaq*)
Verapamil (eg, *Isoptin*)

SUMMARY: Dronedarone increases the plasma concentration of verapamil, while verapamil increases the concentration of dronedarone.

RISK FACTORS: No specific risk factors are known.

MECHANISM: Dronedarone may inhibit the CYP3A4 and P-glycoprotein–mediated elimination of verapamil, and verapamil may inhibit the CYP3A4 and P-glycoprotein–mediated elimination of dronedarone.

CLINICAL EVALUATION: While specific data are limited, the manufacturer of dronedarone states that the coadministration of dronedarone with verapamil increased the mean area under the plasma concentration-time curve of verapamil approximately 1.5-fold.[1] In addition, verapamil appears to increase the concentration of dronedarone by a similar amount. Pending further data, observe patients receiving dronedarone and verapamil for increased effects of both drugs, particularly on cardiac conduction.

RELATED DRUGS: Diltiazem (eg, *Cardizem*) is reported to affect dronedarone in a similar manner. Dronedarone is also reported to increase the plasma concentration of diltiazem and nifedipine (eg, *Adalat*). Other calcium channel blockers that are CYP3A4 substrates (eg, amlodipine [eg, *Norvasc*], felodipine, isradipine [eg, *Dynacirc*]) are also likely to have reduced elimination during dronedarone administration. Amiodarone (eg, *Cordarone*) is likely to interact in a similar manner with calcium channel blockers.

MANAGEMENT OPTIONS:

➡ *Monitor.* Monitor patients taking dronedarone and verapamil for signs of toxicity, including hypotension and cardiac conduction disturbances.

REFERENCES:

    1. *Multaq* [package insert]. Bridgewater, NJ: Sanofi-Aventis; 2009.

4   Droperidol

Thioridazine

SUMMARY: A patient on thioridazine and droperidol died suddenly, but it was not possible to determine whether a drug interaction contributed.

RISK FACTORS: No specific risk factors are known.

MECHANISM: Not established. Both thioridazine and droperidol can prolong the QT interval, but an additive effect was not established in this case.

CLINICAL EVALUATION: A 68-year-old man with coronary artery disease was found dead after taking thioridazine.[1] The authors suggested that the death may have been caused by thioridazine-induced cardiac arrhythmia (torsades de pointes), with a possible contribution from carbamazepine (eg, *Tegretol*). But a subsequent letter suggested that a more likely contributing factor may have been the droperidol the patient received.[2] Given the lack of data on the cause of death, it is not possible to determine if a drug interaction, or an individual drug, was involved in the fatal reaction.

RELATED DRUGS: No information is available.

MANAGEMENT OPTIONS: No specific action is required, but be alert for evidence of the interaction.

REFERENCES:
1. Thomas SH, et al. Sudden death in a patient taking antipsychotic drugs. *Postgrad Med J.* 1998;74(873):445-446.

2. Hauben M. Sudden death in a patient taking antipsychotic drugs. *Postgrad Med J.* 1999;75(880):127.

Drospirenone (eg, *Angeliq*)

Enalapril (eg, *Vasotec*)

SUMMARY: Drospirenone tends to increase serum potassium somewhat, and may increase the risk of hyperkalemia when combined with enalapril or other angiotensin-converting enzyme (ACE) inhibitors.

RISK FACTORS:

➡ **Concurrent Diseases.** Patients with renal disease or diabetes may be at increased risk of hyperkalemia from this interaction. Drospirenone is contraindicated in patients with renal function impairment.

MECHANISM: Additive hyperkalemia.

CLINICAL EVALUATION: Drospirenone is an analog of spironolactone and has antialdosterone activity that may cause potassium retention. This may increase the risk of hyperkalemia in patients taking other drugs that can increase serum potassium, such as enalapril.[1]

RELATED DRUGS: Drospirenone may also increase the risk of hyperkalemia when combined with other ACE inhibitors, including benazepril (eg, *Lotensin*), captopril (eg, *Capoten*), fosinopril (eg, *Monopril*), lisinopril (eg, *Prinivil*), moexipril (eg, *Univasc*), quinapril (eg, *Accupril*), ramipril (*Altace*), and trandolapril (eg, *Mavik*).

MANAGEMENT OPTIONS:

➥ *Monitor.* Consider monitoring serum potassium concentrations, particularly during the first cycle of concurrent use.

REFERENCES:

1. *Angeliq* [package insert]. Wayne, NJ: Berlex, Inc; 2007.

Drospirenone (eg, *Angeliq*)

Heparin

SUMMARY: Drospirenone tends to increase serum potassium somewhat and may increase the risk of hyperkalemia when combined with heparin.

RISK FACTORS:

➥ *Concurrent Diseases.* Patients with renal disease or diabetes may be at increased risk of hyperkalemia from this interaction. Drospirenone is contraindicated in patients with renal function impairment.

MECHANISM: Additive hyperkalemia.

CLINICAL EVALUATION: Drospirenone is an analog of spironolactone and has antialdosterone activity that may cause potassium retention. This may increase the risk of hyperkalemia in patients taking other drugs that can increase serum potassium, such as heparin.[1]

RELATED DRUGS: No information available.

MANAGEMENT OPTIONS:

➥ *Monitor.* Consider monitoring serum potassium concentrations, particularly during the first cycle of concurrent use.

REFERENCES:

1. *Angeliq* [package insert]. Wayne, NJ: Berlex, Inc; 2007.

Drospirenone (eg, *Angeliq*)

Ibuprofen (eg, *Motrin*)

SUMMARY: Drospirenone tends to increase serum potassium somewhat and may increase the risk of hyperkalemia when combined with nonsteroidal anti-inflammatory drugs (NSAIDs) such as ibuprofen.

RISK FACTORS:

➥ *Concurrent Diseases.* Patients with renal disease or diabetes may be at increased risk of hyperkalemia from this interaction. Drospirenone is contraindicated in patients with renal function impairment.

MECHANISM: Additive hyperkalemia.

CLINICAL EVALUATION: Drospirenone is an analog of spironolactone and has antialdosterone activity that may cause potassium retention. This may increase the risk of hyperkalemia in patients taking other drugs that can increase serum potassium, such as ibuprofen.[1]

RELATED DRUGS: Drospirenone may also increase the risk of hyperkalemia when combined with other NSAIDs, including diclofenac (eg, *Voltaren*), diflunisal (*Dolobid*), etodolac, fenoprofen (eg, *Nalfon*), flurbiprofen (eg, *Ansaid*), indomethacin (eg, *Indocin*), ketoprofen, ketorolac, meclofenamate, meloxicam (eg, *Mobic*), nabumetone, naproxen (eg, *Aleve*), oxaprozin (eg, *Daypro*), piroxicam (eg, *Feldene*), sulindac (*Clinoril*), and tolmetin.

MANAGEMENT OPTIONS:

➡ **Monitor.** Consider monitoring serum potassium concentrations, particularly during the first cycle of concurrent use.

REFERENCES:
1. *Angeliq* [package insert]. Wayne, NJ: Berlex, Inc; 2007.

Drospirenone (eg, *Angeliq*)

Losartan (*Cozaar*)

SUMMARY: Drospirenone tends to increase serum potassium somewhat and may increase the risk of hyperkalemia when combined with losartan or other angiotensin II receptor blockers (ARBs).

RISK FACTORS:

➡ **Concurrent Diseases.** Patients with renal disease or diabetes may be at increased risk of hyperkalemia from this interaction. Drospirenone is contraindicated in patients with renal function impairment.

MECHANISM: Additive hyperkalemia.

CLINICAL EVALUATION: Drospirenone is an analog of spironolactone and has antialdosterone activity that may cause potassium retention. This may increase the risk of hyperkalemia in patients taking other drugs that can increase serum potassium, such as losartan.[1]

RELATED DRUGS: Drospirenone may also increase the risk of hyperkalemia when combined with other ARBs, including candesartan (*Atacand*), eprosartan (*Teveten*), irbesartan (*Avapro*), telmisartan (*Micardis*), and valsartan (*Diovan*).

MANAGEMENT OPTIONS:

➡ **Monitor.** Consider monitoring serum potassium concentrations, particularly during the first cycle of concurrent use.

REFERENCES:
1. *Angeliq* [package insert]. Wayne, NJ: Berlex, Inc; 2007.

Drospirenone (eg, *Angeliq*)

Potassium

SUMMARY: Drospirenone tends to increase serum potassium somewhat and may increase the risk of hyperkalemia when combined with potassium supplements.

RISK FACTORS:

➡ **Concurrent Diseases.** Patients with renal disease or diabetes may be at increased risk of hyperkalemia from this interaction. Drospirenone is contraindicated in patients with renal function impairment.

MECHANISM: Additive hyperkalemia.

CLINICAL EVALUATION: Drospirenone is an analog of spironolactone and has antialdosterone activity that may cause potassium retention. This may increase the risk of hyperkalemia in patients taking other drugs that can increase serum potassium, such as potassium supplements.[1]

RELATED DRUGS: No information available.

MANAGEMENT OPTIONS:

➡ **Monitor.** Consider monitoring serum potassium concentrations, particularly during the first cycle of concurrent use.

REFERENCES:

1. *Angeliq* [package insert]. Wayne, NJ: Berlex, Inc; 2007.

Drospirenone (eg, *Angeliq*)

Triamterene (*Dyrenium*)

SUMMARY: Drospirenone tends to increase serum potassium somewhat and may increase the risk of hyperkalemia when combined with triamterene or other potassium-sparing diuretics.

RISK FACTORS:

➡ **Concurrent Diseases.** Patients with renal disease or diabetes may be at increased risk of hyperkalemia from this interaction. Drospirenone is contraindicated in patients with renal function impairment.

MECHANISM: Additive hyperkalemia.

CLINICAL EVALUATION: Drospirenone is an analog of spironolactone and has antialdosterone activity that may cause potassium retention. This may increase the risk of hyperkalemia in patients taking other drugs that can increase serum potassium, such as triamterene.[1]

RELATED DRUGS: Drospirenone may also increase the risk of hyperkalemia when combined with other potassium-sparing diuretics, such as amiloride (*Midamor*), eplerenone (*Inspra*), and spironolactone (eg, *Aldactone*).

MANAGEMENT OPTIONS:

➡ *Monitor.* Consider monitoring serum potassium concentrations, particularly during the first cycle of concurrent use.

REFERENCES:

1. *Angeliq* [package insert]. Wayne, NJ: Berlex, Inc; 2007.

 Duloxetine (*Cymbalta*)

Ciprofloxacin (eg, *Cipro*)

SUMMARY: Ciprofloxacin theoretically may increase duloxetine serum concentrations, but clinical evidence is lacking.

RISK FACTORS: No specific risk factors are known.

MECHANISM: Ciprofloxacin is expected to inhibit the hepatic CYP1A2 metabolism of duloxetine.

CLINICAL EVALUATION: This interaction is based on theoretical considerations. The manufacturer of duloxetine reported a 5- to 6-fold increase in duloxetine serum concentrations when another CYP1A2 inhibitor (fluvoxamine) was coadministered in 14 subjects.[1] This suggests that other CYP1A2 inhibitors, such as ciprofloxacin, may also increase duloxetine serum concentrations. The product information for duloxetine recommends avoiding concurrent use with CYP1A2-inhibiting quinolone antibiotics, including ciprofloxacin and enoxacin.

RELATED DRUGS: Enoxacin[†] is a potent CYP1A2 inhibitor and is expected to increase duloxetine serum concentrations more than ciprofloxacin. Other quinolones, such as levofloxacin (*Levaquin*), lomefloxacin (*Maxaquin*), ofloxacin (eg, *Floxin*), and moxifloxacin (*Avelox*), have little effect on CYP1A2.

MANAGEMENT OPTIONS:

➡ *Consider Alternative.* The manufacturer recommends avoiding concurrent use of duloxetine with ciprofloxacin or enoxacin. Use a different quinolone antibiotic (see Related Drugs).

➡ *Monitor.* If duloxetine is used concurrently with either ciprofloxacin or enoxacin, monitor for evidence of duloxetine toxicity.

REFERENCES:

1. *Cymbalta* [package insert]. Indianapolis, IN: Eli Lilly and Company; 2007.

† Not available in the United States.

 Duloxetine (*Cymbalta*)

Desipramine (eg, *Norpramin*)

SUMMARY: Duloxetine may increase the serum concentrations of desipramine, but the clinical importance is not established.

RISK FACTORS:

➡ *Pharmacogenetics.* Patients who are deficient in CYP2D6 are not expected to manifest this interaction.

MECHANISM: Duloxetine probably inhibits the hepatic CYP2D6 metabolism of desipramine.

CLINICAL EVALUATION: The manufacturer of duloxetine has reported a 3-fold increase in desipramine serum concentrations following a single 50 mg dose given with duloxetine 60 mg twice daily.[1] Few details of the study were given, but duloxetine is known to be a moderate inhibitor of CYP2D6, and desipramine is metabolized by CYP2D6. Thus, the findings reported by the manufacturer are consistent with what is expected.

RELATED DRUGS: Other tricyclic antidepressants also are metabolized by CYP2D6, including amitriptyline, doxepin (eg, *Sinequan*), imipramine (eg, *Tofranil*), and nortriptyline (eg, *Pamelor*). They are expected to interact with duloxetine at least to some degree.

MANAGEMENT OPTIONS: No specific action is required, but be alert for evidence of the interaction.

REFERENCES:
1. *Cymbalta* [package insert]. Indianapolis, IN: Eli Lilly and Company; 2004

Duloxetine (*Cymbalta*)

Flecainide (eg, *Tambocor*)

SUMMARY: Theoretically, duloxetine may increase flecainide serum concentrations, but the clinical importance of this effect is not established.

RISK FACTORS:

➡ ***Pharmacogenetics.*** Patients who are deficient in CYP2D6 are not expected to manifest this interaction.

MECHANISM: Duloxetine may inhibit the hepatic CYP2D6 metabolism of flecainide.

CLINICAL EVALUATION: This potential interaction is based on theoretical considerations, and it is not known if the combination actually poses a risk. The manufacturer of duloxetine states that duloxetine and flecainide should be coadministered with caution.[1]

RELATED DRUGS: No information is available.

MANAGEMENT OPTIONS: No specific action is required, but be alert for evidence of the interaction.

REFERENCES:
1. *Cymbalta* [package insert]. Indianapolis, IN: Eli Lilly and Company; 2004.

Duloxetine (*Cymbalta*)

Fluvoxamine (eg, *Luvox*)

SUMMARY: Fluvoxamine markedly increases duloxetine plasma concentrations; avoid concurrent use or monitor closely.

RISK FACTORS: No specific risk factors are known.

MECHANISM: Fluvoxamine is likely to inhibit the CYP1A2 metabolism of duloxetine.

CLINICAL EVALUATION: In a study of 14 healthy subjects, fluvoxamine increased duloxetine area under the plasma concentration-time curve approximately 6-fold, and duloxetine half-life was increased approximately 3-fold.[1] An increase of this magnitude is expected to increase duloxetine toxicity. Consider increasing the dose of one of the selective serotonin reuptake inhibitors (SSRIs) instead of using them concurrently.

RELATED DRUGS: Duloxetine is metabolized by CYP1A2 and CYP2D6. Theoretically, SSRIs that do not significantly inhibit CYP1A2 and are not strong inhibitors of CYP2D6 are less likely to interact (eg, citalopram [eg, *Celexa*], escitalopram [*Lexapro*], sertraline [eg, *Zoloft*], venlafaxine [*Effexor*]). Paroxetine (eg, *Paxil*), a potent CYP2D6 inhibitor, has been shown to increase duloxetine serum concentrations. Fluoxetine (eg, *Prozac*), also a potent CYP2D6 inhibitor, may increase duloxetine plasma concentrations as well.

MANAGEMENT OPTIONS:

➡ *Avoid Unless Benefit Outweighs Risk.* Given the large magnitude of the interaction, avoid coadministration unless there is a compelling reason to do so. The manufacturer states that combined use of duloxetine and other SSRIs is not recommended.

➡ *Consider Alternative.* If it is necessary to use duloxetine with another SSRI, consider using an SSRI with minimal effects on CYP1A2 and CYP2D6 (see Related Drugs).

➡ *Circumvent/Minimize.* Consider increasing the dose of one of the SSRIs instead of using them concurrently.

➡ *Monitor.* If the combination is used, monitor for altered duloxetine effect if the dose of fluvoxamine is started, stopped, or changed.

REFERENCES:

    1. *Cymbalta* [package insert]. Indianapolis, IN: Eli Lilly; 2007.

Duloxetine (*Cymbalta*)

Lithium (eg, *Lithobid*)

SUMMARY: Theoretically, this combination may increase the risk of serotonin syndrome.

RISK FACTORS: No specific risk factors are known.

MECHANISM: Duloxetine and lithium may have additive serotonergic effects.

CLINICAL EVALUATION: The manufacturer warns that concurrent use of duloxetine with other serotonergic drugs, such as lithium, may increase the risk of serotonin syndrome.[1] This is based primarily on theoretical considerations, and it is not known how often serotonin syndrome would occur. Lithium is not a potent serotonergic drug.

RELATED DRUGS: Fluoxetine (eg, *Prozac*) has produced evidence of serotonin syndrome when combined with lithium. Theoretically, other selective serotonin reuptake inhibitors could have a similar effect.

MANAGEMENT OPTIONS:

➡ *Monitor.* Monitor for evidence of serotonin syndrome (eg, agitation, coma, confusion, fever, hypomania, incoordination, hyperreflexia, myoclonus, rigidity, seizures, shivering, sweating, tremor).

REFERENCES:

1. *Cymbalta* [package insert]. Indianapolis, IN: Eli Lilly; 2007.

Duloxetine (*Cymbalta*)

Paroxetine (eg, *Paxil*)

SUMMARY: Paroxetine moderately increases duloxetine plasma concentrations.

RISK FACTORS: No specific risk factors are known.

MECHANISM: Paroxetine probably inhibits the CYP2D6 metabolism of duloxetine.

CLINICAL EVALUATION: In a study of healthy subjects, paroxetine 20 mg/day increased duloxetine area under the plasma concentration-time curve about 60%.[1] Although the effect was modest, some patients may develop duloxetine toxicity, especially with doses of paroxetine larger than 20 mg/day. Consider increasing the dose of one of the selective serotonin reuptake inhibitors (SSRIs) instead of using them concurrently.

RELATED DRUGS: Fluvoxamine may produce marked increases in duloxetine serum concentrations. Fluoxetine (eg, *Prozac*), like paroxetine, is a potent inhibitor of CYP2D6 and may increase duloxetine plasma concentrations.

MANAGEMENT OPTIONS:

➡ *Avoid Unless Benefit Outweighs Risk.* Avoid coadministration unless there is a compelling reason to do so. The manufacturer states that combined use of duloxetine and other SSRIs is not recommended.

➡ *Circumvent/Minimize.* Consider increasing the dose of one of the SSRIs instead of using them concurrently.

➡ *Monitor.* If the combination is used, monitor for altered duloxetine effect if the dose of paroxetine is started, stopped, or changed.

REFERENCES:

1. *Cymbalta* [package insert]. Indianapolis, IN: Eli Lilly; 2007.

Duloxetine (*Cymbalta*)

Propafenone (eg, *Rythmol*)

SUMMARY: Theoretically, duloxetine may increase propafenone serum concentrations, but the clinical importance of this effect is not established.

RISK FACTORS:

➡ *Pharmacogenetics.* Patients who are deficient in CYP2D6 are not expected to manifest this interaction.

MECHANISM: Duloxetine may inhibit the hepatic CYP2D6 metabolism of propafenone.

CLINICAL EVALUATION: This potential interaction is based on theoretical considerations, and it is not known if the combination actually poses a risk. The manufacturer of duloxetine states that duloxetine and propafenone should be coadministered only with caution.[1]

RELATED DRUGS: No information is available.

MANAGEMENT OPTIONS: No specific action is required, but be alert for evidence of the interaction.

REFERENCES:
1. *Cymbalta* [package insert]. Indianapolis, IN: Eli Lilly and Company; 2004.

Duloxetine (*Cymbalta*)

Quinidine

SUMMARY: Quinidine is expected to increase duloxetine plasma concentrations.

RISK FACTORS: No specific risk factors are known.

MECHANISM: Duloxetine is metabolized partially by CYP2D6, and quinidine is a potent CYP2D6 inhibitor.

CLINICAL EVALUATION: The CYP2D6 inhibitor paroxetine moderately increased duloxetine plasma concentrations, and quinidine is expected to do the same.[1]

RELATED DRUGS: Other selective serotonin reuptake inhibitors are metabolized by CYP2D6 to varying extents, and quinidine is expected to interact with them as well.

MANAGEMENT OPTIONS:

➡ **Monitor.** If the combination is used, monitor for altered duloxetine effect if the dose of quinidine is started, stopped, or changed.

REFERENCES:
1. *Cymbalta* [package insert]. Indianapolis, IN: Eli Lilly; 2007.

Duloxetine (*Cymbalta*)

St. John's Wort

SUMMARY: Theoretically, the combination may increase the risk of serotonin syndrome.

RISK FACTORS: No specific risk factors are known.

MECHANISM: Duloxetine and St. John's wort may have additive serotonergic effects.

CLINICAL EVALUATION: The manufacturer warns that concurrent use of duloxetine with other serotonergic drugs, such as St. John's wort, may increase the risk of serotonin syndrome. This is based primarily on theoretical considerations, and there is debate about the extent to which St. John's wort actually exhibits serotonergic properties.[1]

RELATED DRUGS: St. John's wort used with other selective serotonin reuptake inhibitors (SSRIs) purportedly may increase the risk of serotonin syndrome, but the reactions have not been well documented.

MANAGEMENT OPTIONS:

➡ **Consider Alternative.** Consider using an alternative to St. John's wort in patients taking duloxetine or other SSRIs.

➡ **Monitor.** Monitor for evidence of serotonin syndrome (eg, myoclonus, rigidity, tremor, hyperreflexia, seizures, confusion, agitation, hypomania, incoordination, fever, sweating, shivering, coma).

REFERENCES:

1. *Cymbalta* [package insert]. Indianapolis, IN: Eli Lilly; 2007.

Duloxetine (*Cymbalta*)

Thioridazine AVOID

SUMMARY: Duloxetine may increase thioridazine serum concentrations, increasing the risk of ventricular arrhythmias. Avoid concurrent use.

RISK FACTORS:

➡ **Pharmacogenetics.** Patients who are deficient in CYP2D6 are not expected to manifest this interaction.

MECHANISM: Duloxetine may inhibit the hepatic CYP2D6 metabolism of thioridazine.

CLINICAL EVALUATION: Thioridazine may prolong the QT interval, which tends to be related to the thioridazine serum concentration. This interaction is based on theoretical considerations, but the potential danger (serious ventricular arrhythmias and sudden death) dictates that the combination be avoided. Also, the manufacturer of duloxetine states that duloxetine and thioridazine should not be coadministered, raising medicolegal considerations.[1]

RELATED DRUGS: No information is available.

MANAGEMENT OPTIONS:

➡ **AVOID COMBINATION.** Avoid the combined use of duloxetine and thioridazine.

REFERENCES:

1. *Cymbalta* [package insert]. Indianapolis, IN: Eli Lilly and Company; 2004.

Duloxetine (*Cymbalta*)

Tramadol (eg, *Ultram*)

SUMMARY: Theoretically, the combination may increase the risk of serotonin syndrome.

RISK FACTORS: No specific risk factors are known.

MECHANISM: Duloxetine and tramadol may have additive serotonergic effects, and duloxetine may inhibit the CYP2D6 metabolism of tramadol.

CLINICAL EVALUATION: The manufacturer warns that concurrent use of duloxetine with other serotonergic drugs, such as tramadol, may increase the risk of serotonin syndrome. This is based primarily on theoretical considerations, and it is not known how often serotonin syndrome would occur.[1]

RELATED DRUGS: Several selective serotonin reuptake inhibitors (SSRIs) have been reported to produce serotonin syndrome when combined with tramadol. Theoretically, SSRIs that are potent inhibitors of CYP2D6 (eg, fluoxetine [eg, *Prozac*], paroxetine [eg, *Paxil*]) are the highest risk, and moderate CYP2D6 inhibitors (eg, duloxetine) are more of a risk than the other SSRIs because CYP2D6 is an important enzyme in the metabolism of tramadol.

MANAGEMENT OPTIONS:

➡ *Consider Alternative.* Theoretically, using an SSRI with minimal effects on CYP2D6 (eg, citalopram [eg, *Celexa*], escitalopram [*Lexapro*], sertraline [eg, *Zoloft*], venlafaxine [*Effexor*]) would decrease the risk of serotonin syndrome.

➡ *Monitor.* Monitor for evidence of serotonin syndrome (eg, myoclonus, rigidity, tremor, hyperreflexia, seizures, confusion, agitation, hypomania, incoordination, fever, sweating, shivering, coma).

REFERENCES:

1. *Cymbalta* [package insert]. Indianapolis, IN: Eli Lilly; 2007.

 Duloxetine (*Cymbalta*)

AVOID **Tranylcypromine (eg, *Parnate*)**

SUMMARY: Severe or fatal reactions have been reported when nonselective monoamine oxidase inhibitors (MAOIs) such as tranylcypromine are coadministered with selective serotonin reuptake inhibitors (SSRIs) such as duloxetine. Avoid the combination.

RISK FACTORS: No specific risk factors are known.

MECHANISM: The exact mechanism is not established but probably involves additive serotonergic effect.

CLINICAL EVALUATION: Severe or fatal serotonin syndrome has been reported with combined use of MAOIs and SSRIs.[1] Although specific case reports with duloxetine combined with MAOIs have not been reported, it is highly likely that the combination is dangerous. All combinations of nonselective MAOIs and SSRIs are contraindicated.

RELATED DRUGS: Duloxetine is likely to interact with other MAOIs, including isocarboxazid (*Marplan*) and phenelzine (*Nardil*). Occasionally, the MAO-B inhibitor selegiline (eg, *Eldepryl*) may act as a nonselective MAOI, especially in larger doses.

MANAGEMENT OPTIONS:

➡ *AVOID COMBINATION.* Avoid the combined use of duloxetine and MAOIs. Wait at least 2 weeks after stopping an MAOI before starting duloxetine; wait at least 5 days after stopping duloxetine before starting an MAOI.

REFERENCES:

1. *Cymbalta* [package insert]. Indianapolis, IN: Eli Lilly and Company; 2004.

 Duloxetine (*Cymbalta*)

Tryptophan

SUMMARY: Theoretically, the combination may increase the risk of serotonin syndrome.

RISK FACTORS: No specific risk factors are known.

MECHANISM: Duloxetine and tryptophan may have additive serotonergic effects.

CLINICAL EVALUATION: The manufacturer warns that concurrent use of duloxetine with other serotonergic drugs, such as tryptophan, may increase the risk of serotonin syndrome. This is based primarily on theoretical considerations, and it is not known how often serotonin syndrome would occur.[1]

RELATED DRUGS: Fluoxetine (eg, *Prozac*) has been reported to produce evidence of serotonin syndrome when combined with tryptophan.

MANAGEMENT OPTIONS:

➥ *Monitor.* Monitor for evidence of serotonin syndrome (eg, myoclonus, rigidity, tremor, hyperreflexia, seizures, confusion, agitation, hypomania, incoordination, fever, sweating, shivering, coma).

REFERENCES:

1. *Cymbalta* [package insert]. Indianapolis, IN: Eli Lilly; 2007.

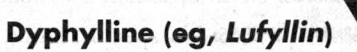

Dyphylline (eg, *Lufyllin*)

Probenecid

SUMMARY: Single-dose studies indicate that probenecid substantially increases serum dyphylline concentrations.

RISK FACTORS: No specific risk factors are known.

MECHANISM: Unlike theophylline, which is extensively metabolized by the liver, a substantial amount of dyphylline is eliminated by renal excretion. Probenecid appears to inhibit the renal excretion of dyphylline.

CLINICAL EVALUATION: In 12 healthy subjects, pretreatment with probenecid (1 g oral) approximately doubled the half-life of dyphylline and reduced dyphylline clearance about 50%.[1] If this interaction is sustained during multiple dosing, an excessive serum dyphylline concentration could result.

RELATED DRUGS: Unlike dyphylline, theophylline (eg, *Theochron*) does not appear to interact with probenecid.[2]

MANAGEMENT OPTIONS:

➥ *Consider Alternative.* Theophylline does not appear to interact with probenecid and may be a suitable alternative.

➥ *Monitor.* Monitor for evidence of altered dyphylline effect if probenecid therapy is initiated, discontinued, or changed in dosage.

REFERENCES:

1. May DC, et al. Effect of probenecid on dyphylline elimination. *Clin Pharmacol Ther.* 1983;33(6):822-825.
2. Chen TW, et al. Effect of probenecid on the pharmacokinetics of aminophylline. *Drug Intell Clin Pharm.* 1983;17(6):465-466.

4   Echinacea

Midazolam

SUMMARY: Echinacea may slightly reduce midazolam plasma concentrations, but the clinical importance of this effect is not established.

RISK FACTORS: No specific risk factors are known.

MECHANISM: Echinacea appears to increase CYP3A4 activity, resulting in reduced midazolam serum concentrations.

CLINICAL EVALUATION: Twelve healthy subjects received oral and intravenous midazolam with and without pretreatment with echinacea 400 mg 4 times daily for 8 days.[1] Echinacea modestly reduced midazolam area under the concentration-time curve, but it is not clear if this effect would produce any adverse reactions.

RELATED DRUGS: No information is available.

MANAGEMENT OPTIONS: No specific action is required, but be alert for evidence of the interaction.

REFERENCES:
1. Gorski JC, et al. The effect of echinacea (*Echinacea purpurea* root) on cytochrome P450 activity in vivo. *Clin Pharmacol Ther.* 2004;75(1):89-100.

Echothiophate Iodide (*Phosphate Iodide*)

Succinylcholine (eg, *Anectine*)

SUMMARY: Echothiophate prolongs the neuromuscular blocking effects of succinylcholine; if possible, avoid succinylcholine in patients taking echothiophate.

RISK FACTORS: No specific risk factors are known.

MECHANISM: Prolonged ophthalmic use of echothiophate reduced the activity of pseudocholinesterase, the enzyme responsible for the metabolism of succinylcholine. Pralidoxime (*Protopam Chloride*) may reverse the lowered pseudocholinesterase levels without affecting the control of glaucoma by echothiophate.

CLINICAL EVALUATION: Prolonged apnea is possible with the administration of succinylcholine to patients with echothiophate-induced depression of pseudocholinesterase.[1-7] This reduction is more likely to occur in patients on long-term echothiophate therapy and may be most significant with short procedures (eg, electroshock therapy).

RELATED DRUGS: No information is available.

MANAGEMENT OPTIONS:

➡ *Avoid Unless Benefit Outweighs Risk.* A neuromuscular blocker other than succinylcholine is preferred in most patients taking echothiophate.

➡ *Monitor.* If succinylcholine is used, carefully monitor for prolonged neuromuscular blockade. Serum pseudocholinesterase determinations would be useful to identify patients at highest risk.

REFERENCES:
1. Mone JG, et al. Qualitative defects of pseudocholinesterase activity. *Anaesthesia.* 1967;22:55-68.

2. Cavallaro RJ, et al. Effect of echothiophate therapy on the metabolism of succinylcholine in man. *Anesth Analg.* 1968;47(5):570-574.

3. Kinyon GE. Anticholinesterase eye drops—need for caution. *N Engl J Med.* 1969;280(1):53.

4. Lipson ML, et al. Oral administration of pralidoxime chloride in echothiophate iodide therapy. *Arch Ophthalmol.* 1969;82(6):830-835.

5. Cohen PJ, et al. A simple test for abnormal pseudocholinesterase. *Anesthesiology.* 1970;32(3):281-282.

6. Kothary SP, et al. Plasma cholinesterase activity in relation to the safe use of succinylcholine in myasthenic patients on chronic anticholinesterase treatment. *Clin Pharmacol Ther.* 1977;21:108.

7. Eilderton TE, et al. Reduction in plasma cholinesterase levels after prolonged administration of echothiophate iodide eyedrops. *Can Anaesth Soc J.* 1968;15(3):291-296.

Efavirenz (*Sustiva*)

Indinavir (*Crixivan*)

SUMMARY: Efavirenz administration reduces indinavir concentrations, even when ritonavir (*Norvir*) is coadministered with indinavir to inhibit the metabolism of indinavir.

RISK FACTORS: No specific risk factors are known.

MECHANISM: Efavirenz appears to increase the metabolism of indinavir, probably by increasing CYP3A4 activity.

CLINICAL EVALUATION: Eighteen healthy subjects took a combination of indinavir 800 mg and ritonavir 100 mg every day for 30 days.[1] On days 15 through 29, efavirenz 600 mg/day was coadministered. Indinavir area under the plasma concentration-time curve was reduced 25% and its trough and peak concentrations were reduced 50% and 17%, respectively, following efavirenz coadministration. The half-life of indinavir was not changed. The administration of efavirenz to patients receiving the combination of indinavir and ritonavir may result in plasma concentrations of indinavir below effective antiviral levels.

RELATED DRUGS: Efavirenz reduces the plasma concentration of ritonavir. Its effect on other protease inhibitors metabolized by CYP3A4 (eg, nelfinavir [*Viracept*], saquinavir [*Invirase*]) is likely to be similar.

MANAGEMENT OPTIONS:

➡ *Circumvent/Minimize.* It may be possible to circumvent the effects of efavirenz on indinavir by increasing the dose of ritonavir that is coadministered. The added inhibitory effect of ritonavir on CYP3A4 may lessen or reverse the induction effect of efavirenz.

➡ *Monitor.* Monitor patients taking indinavir and ritonavir who are prescribed efavirenz for reduced indinavir concentrations and possible loss of antiviral efficacy.

REFERENCES:

1. Aarnoutse RE, et al. The influence of efavirenz on the pharmacokinetics of a twice-daily combination of indinavir and low-dose ritonavir in healthy volunteers. *Clin Pharmacol Ther.* 2002;71(1):57-67.

Efavirenz (*Sustiva*)

Ketoconazole (eg, *Nizoral*)

SUMMARY: Efavirenz reduces ketoconazole plasma concentrations; a reduction in antifungal efficacy is likely to result.

RISK FACTORS: No specific risk factors are known.

MECHANISM: Efavirenz induces the metabolism of ketoconazole, probably via the CYP3A4 pathway.

CLINICAL EVALUATION: Twelve patients with HIV received a single dose of ketoconazole 400 mg alone and following 2 weeks of combination therapy with efavirenz 600 mg daily, lamivudine 150 mg twice daily, and stavudine 30 or 40 mg twice daily.[1] The mean ketoconazole area under the plasma concentration-time curve was reduced by 72% and its half-life shortened by nearly 60% following efavirenz administration. This degree of reduction in ketoconazole plasma concentrations is likely to reduce or eliminate its antifungal efficacy. Although not assessed in this study, it is possible that ketoconazole will decrease the metabolism of efavirenz, resulting in elevated plasma efavirenz concentrations. Efavirenz-induced reduction in ketoconazole plasma concentrations would tend to mitigate the effect of ketoconazole on efavirenz.

RELATED DRUGS: Itraconazole (eg, *Sporanox*) is also metabolized by CYP3A4 and is expected to interact in a similar manner as ketoconazole with efavirenz.

MANAGEMENT OPTIONS:

➡ **Consider Alternative.** Terbinafine (eg, *Lamisil*) could be considered as an alternative antifungal agent because it does not appear to be a substrate for CYP3A4. Amphotericin (eg, *Amphotec*), caspofungin (*Cansidas*), and anidulafungin (*Eraxis*) also do not appear to be substrates for CYP3A4.

➡ **Monitor.** Monitor patients receiving efavirenz and ketoconazole for reduced ketoconazole efficacy. A dose increase of ketoconazole may be necessary. Also, be alert for efavirenz adverse reactions caused by the potential for ketoconazole to increase efavirenz plasma concentrations.

REFERENCES:

1. Sriwiriyajan S, et al. Effect of efavirenz on pharmacokinetics of ketoconazole in HIV-infected patients. *Eur J Clin Pharmacol.* 2007;63(5):479-483.

Efavirenz (*Sustiva*)

Maraviroc (*Selzentry*)

SUMMARY: Efavirenz administration reduces maraviroc plasma concentrations; a reduction in the antiviral effect of maraviroc is likely to occur.

RISK FACTORS: No specific risk factors are known.

MECHANISM: Efavirenz is known to induce CYP3A4 activity, thus increasing the clearance of maraviroc.

CLINICAL EVALUATION: Twelve healthy subjects received maraviroc 100 mg twice a day for 21 days with either placebo or efavirenz 600 mg daily coadministered on days 8 to

21.[1] The maraviroc mean area under the concentration-time curve (AUC) was reduced approximately 50% during efavirenz dosing. Increasing the maraviroc dosage to 200 mg twice a day during concurrent efavirenz returned the maraviroc AUC to values observed with the 100 mg twice-daily dosage of maraviroc without efavirenz.

RELATED DRUGS: None known.

MANAGEMENT OPTIONS:

➡ *Monitor.* Monitor for reduced maraviroc efficacy if efavirenz is coadministered. A dose increase of maraviroc is likely to be required.

REFERENCES:

1. Abel S, et al. Effects of CYP3A4 inducers with and without CYP3A4 inhibitors on the pharmacokinetics of maraviroc in healthy volunteers. *Br J Clin Pharmacol.* 2008;65(suppl 1):38-46.

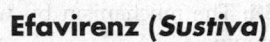

Efavirenz (*Sustiva*)

Methadone (eg, *Dolophine*)

SUMMARY: Efavirenz reduces methadone plasma concentrations; methadone withdrawal or loss of analgesic effect may occur.

RISK FACTORS: No specific risk factors are known.

MECHANISM: Efavirenz appears to increase the metabolism of methadone via induction of the CYP3A4 isozyme. An effect of efavirenz on P-glycoprotein cannot be ruled out.

CLINICAL EVALUATION: Methadone plasma concentrations were measured in 11 patients on long-term methadone maintenance therapy (35 to 100 mg/day) before and following 2 to 3 weeks of antiretroviral therapy, including efavirenz 600 mg/day plus stavudine (*Zerit*) and didanosine (eg, *Videx*), stavudine and lamivudine (*Epivir*), stavudine and abacavir (*Ziagen*), or zidovudine (eg, *Retrovir*) and lamivudine.[1] During concomitant efavirenz therapy, methadone area under the plasma concentration-time curve decreased 57%, and peak methadone concentrations fell 48%. Nine of the 11 patients complained of methadone withdrawal symptoms following 8 to 10 days of efavirenz administration. Methadone doses were increased an average of 22% to alleviate withdrawal symptoms.

RELATED DRUGS: Nevirapine (*Viramune*) has also been reported to reduce methadone plasma concentrations and precipitate methadone withdrawal symptoms. Other narcotic analgesics metabolized by CYP3A4 (eg, fentanyl [eg, *Actiq*]) may be similarly affected by efavirenz.

MANAGEMENT OPTIONS:

➡ *Consider Alternative.* Consider the use of an analgesic that is not a substrate for CYP3A4 (eg, codeine, morphine) in patients taking efavirenz.

➡ *Monitor.* Be alert for symptoms of methadone withdrawal if efavirenz is initiated in patients taking methadone maintenance regimens. Discontinuation of efavirenz may result in excessive methadone effects (respiratory depression, sedation).

Methadone dosage adjustments may be necessary whenever efavirenz is added to or removed from the regimen of patients maintained on methadone.

REFERENCES:
1. Clarke SM, et al. The pharmacokinetics of methadone in HIV-positive patients receiving the nonnucleoside reverse transcriptase inhibitor efavirenz. *Br J Clin Pharmacol.* 2001;51(3):213-217.

 Efavirenz (*Sustiva*)

Pravastatin (eg, *Pravachol*)

SUMMARY: Pravastatin plasma concentrations are reduced during efavirenz coadministration; some reduction in the lipid-lowering effect of pravastatin may occur.

RISK FACTORS: No specific risk factors are known.

MECHANISM: The mechanism by which efavirenz lowers pravastatin concentrations is unknown.

CLINICAL EVALUATION: Fourteen healthy subjects received pravastatin 40 mg daily for 4 days before and following 14 days of efavirenz 600 mg daily.[1] After efavirenz coadministration, the mean area under the plasma concentration-time curve of pravastatin was reduced 40%, compared with the concentration when pravastatin was administered alone. The low-density lipoprotein (LDL)–lowering effect of pravastatin tended to lessen following efavirenz pretreatment. Monitor for reduced hypolipemic efficacy in patients requiring efavirenz therapy who are taking pravastatin.

RELATED DRUGS: Lovastatin (eg, *Mevacor*), simvastatin (eg, *Zocor*), and atorvastatin (*Lipitor*) may be affected in a similar manner.

MANAGEMENT OPTIONS:

➡ **Consider Alternative.** Ezetimibe (*Zetia*) is not known to be affected by CYP3A4 inducers.

➡ **Monitor.** After the addition or discontinuation of efavirenz, monitor LDL concentrations of patients stabilized on pravastatin.

REFERENCES:
1. Gerber JG, et al. Effect of efavirenz on the pharmacokinetics of simvastatin, atorvastatin, and pravastatin: results of AIDS Clinical Trials Group 5108 Study. *J Acquir Immune Defic Syndr.* 2005;39(3):307-312.

 Efavirenz (*Sustiva*)

Proguanil (*Malarone*)

SUMMARY: Efavirenz increases the plasma concentration of proguanil by approximately 2-fold; some patients may experience signs of proguanil toxicity.

RISK FACTORS:

➡ **Pharmacogenetics.** Patients who are rapid metabolizers of CYP2C19 will have a larger reduction in proguanil clearance during efavirenz coadministration than poor metabolizers.

MECHANISM: Efavirenz is an inhibitor of CYP2C19, the enzyme primarily responsible for the metabolism of proguanil to its active metabolite.

CLINICAL EVALUATION: Fifteen subjects took a single dose of proguanil 300 mg alone and following efavirenz 400 mg daily for 11 days.[1] The mean area under the concentration-time curve of proguanil was increased approximately 2-fold, and its half-life increased from 16 to 23 hours after pretreatment with efavirenz. However, the concentration of proguanil's active metabolite was reduced 38% by efavirenz. Thus, the antimalarial efficacy of proguanil may be reduced in some patients.

RELATED DRUGS: Delavirdine (*Rescriptor*) is also known to inhibit CYP2C19 and may interact in a similar manner with proguanil.

MANAGEMENT OPTIONS:

➡ *Monitor.* Monitor patients receiving both proguanil and efavirenz for adequate antimalarial response to proguanil.

REFERENCES:
1. Soyinka JO, Onyeji CO. Alteration of pharmacokinetics of proguanil in healthy volunteers following concurrent administration of efavirenz. *Eur J Pharm Sci.* 2010;39(4):213-218.

Efavirenz (*Sustiva*)

Raltegravir (*Isentress*)

SUMMARY: Efavirenz administration decreases the plasma concentration of raltegravir; some loss of raltegravir's antiviral effect may occur.

RISK FACTORS: No specific risk factors are known.

MECHANISM: Unknown. Efavirenz is known to induce several metabolizing enzymes, and it may similarly affect raltegravir elimination.

CLINICAL EVALUATION: While specific data are limited, the manufacturer of raltegravir notes that the coadministration of efavirenz 600 mg daily prior to a single 400 mg dose of raltegravir reduced the mean area under the plasma concentration-time curve of raltegravir by approximately 35%.[1] Pending further data, patients receiving raltegravir and efavirenz should be observed for reduced raltegravir response.

RELATED DRUGS: None known.

MANAGEMENT OPTIONS:

➡ *Monitor.* Monitor patients taking raltegravir and efavirenz for signs of reduced raltegravir antiviral activity.

REFERENCES:
1. *Isentress* [package insert]. Whitehouse Station, NJ: Merck & Co; 2010.

Efavirenz (*Sustiva*)

Rifabutin (*Mycobutin*)

SUMMARY: Efavirenz may reduce the plasma concentration of rifabutin; rifabutin may reduce the concentration of efavirenz.

RISK FACTORS: No specific risk factors are known.

MECHANISM: Both efavirenz and rifabutin are substrates and inducers of CYP3A4. It is possible that each drug could induce the metabolism of the other, resulting in lower plasma concentrations of both.

CLINICAL EVALUATION: While data are limited, the manufacturer of efavirenz notes that efavirenz 600 mg daily for 7 days reduced the mean area under the concentration-time curve of rifabutin 38% and its peak concentration 32%.[1] However, rifabutin 300 mg daily for 14 days or 600 mg twice weekly for an average of 2 weeks did not affect the plasma concentration of efavirenz.[1,2] In a separate report, a patient taking rifabutin 450 mg with efavirenz 800 mg daily had low efavirenz plasma concentrations.[3] Concurrent rifabutin has been reported to result in lower efavirenz concentrations compared with efavirenz administered alone.[4] The clinical significance of this interaction is not well defined; loss of therapeutic efficacy may occur.

RELATED DRUGS: Rifampin (eg, *Rifadin*) is known to reduce the plasma concentration of efavirenz.

MANAGEMENT OPTIONS:

➡ **Monitor.** Carefully monitor patients taking efavirenz and rifabutin for loss of therapeutic efficacy.

REFERENCES:

1. *Sustiva* [package insert]. Princeton, NJ: Bristol-Myers Squibb Company; 2005.
2. Weiner M, et al. Evaluation of the drug interaction between rifabutin and efavirenz in patients with HIV infection and tuberculosis. *Clin Infect Dis.* 2005;41(9):1343-1349.
3. Hsu O, et al. Decreased plasma efavirenz concentrations in a patient receiving rifabutin. *Am J Health Syst Pharm.* 2010;67(19):1611-1614.
4. Lewthwaite P, et al. Efavirenz, rifampicin and rifabutin—a case for therapeutic drug monitoring. *Antivir Ther.* 2003;8(suppl 1):S424.

Efavirenz (*Sustiva*)

Rifampin (eg, *Rifadin*)

SUMMARY: Efavirenz plasma concentrations may be reduced during rifampin coadministration; monitor for reduced antiviral effect.

RISK FACTORS: No specific risk factors are known.

MECHANISM: Rifampin appears to increase the metabolism of efavirenz, possibly via induction of CYP2B6.

CLINICAL EVALUATION: While data are limited, the manufacturer notes that rifampin 600 mg daily for 7 days reduced the mean area under the plasma concentration-time curve (AUC) of efavirenz 600 mg daily for 7 days by 26%.[1] A second study noted that rifampin reduced the AUC of efavirenz by 22%.[2] One report noted that increasing the dose of efavirenz in patients receiving rifampin, isoniazid, pyrazinamide, and ethambutol (eg, *Myambutol*) resulted in elevated efavirenz plasma concentrations and efavirenz toxicity in 7 of 9 patients.[3] It is not known why these patients did not demonstrate the expected degree of induction in efavirenz metabolism.

RELATED DRUGS: Rifabutin (*Mycobutin*) may also reduce efavirenz plasma concentrations.

MANAGEMENT OPTIONS:

➡ *Monitor.* Pending more complete data, carefully monitor patients receiving efavirenz when rifampin is added to or removed from the drug regimen.

REFERENCES:

1. *Sustiva* [package insert]. Princeton, NJ: Bristol-Myers Squibb Company; 2005.

2. López-Cortés LF, et al. Pharmacokinetic interactions between efavirenz and rifampicin in HIV-infected patients with tuberculosis. *Clin Pharmacokinet.* 2002;41(9):681-690.

3. Brennan-Benson P, et al. Pharmacokinetic interactions between efavirenz and rifampicin in the treatment of HIV and tuberculosis: one size does not fit all. *AIDS.* 2005;19(14):1541-1543.

Efavirenz (*Sustiva*)

Ritonavir (*Norvir*)

SUMMARY: Efavirenz reduces the plasma concentration of ritonavir; reduction of antiviral effect may occur.

RISK FACTORS: No specific risk factors are known.

MECHANISM: Efavirenz appears to increase the metabolism of ritonavir, probably by increasing CYP3A4 activity.

CLINICAL EVALUATION: Eighteen healthy subjects took a daily combination of indinavir (*Crixivan*) 800 mg and ritonavir 100 mg for 30 days.[1] On days 15 through 29, efavirenz 600 mg/day was coadministered. Ritonavir area under the plasma concentration-time curve was reduced 34%, and its trough and peak concentrations were reduced 39% and 34%, respectively, following efavirenz coadministration. The half-life of ritonavir was not changed. The administration of efavirenz to patients receiving the combination of indinavir and ritonavir may reduce the plasma concentrations of ritonavir below levels necessary to inhibit the metabolism of indinavir. The effect of efavirenz on larger doses of ritonavir is not known.

RELATED DRUGS: Efavirenz reduces the plasma concentration of indinavir. Its effect on other protease inhibitors metabolized by CYP3A4 (eg, nelfinavir [*Viracept*], saquinavir [*Invirase*]) may be similar.

MANAGEMENT OPTIONS:

➡ *Monitor.* Monitor patients taking ritonavir for reduced ritonavir concentrations and possible loss of efficacy during efavirenz coadministration.

REFERENCES:

1. Aarnoutse RE, et al. The influence of efavirenz on the pharmacokinetics of a twice-daily combination of indinavir and low-dose ritonavir in healthy volunteers. *Clin Pharmacol Ther.* 2002;71(1):57-67.

Efavirenz (*Sustiva*)

Saquinavir (*Invirase*)

SUMMARY: Efavirenz reduces the plasma concentration of saquinavir; reduction of antiviral effect may occur.

RISK FACTORS: No specific risk factors are known.

MECHANISM: Efavirenz induces the metabolism of saquinavir via the CYP3A4 pathway.

CLINICAL EVALUATION: While data are limited, the manufacturer notes that administration of saquinavir 1,200 mg every 8 hours plus efavirenz 600 mg daily for 10 days reduced the saquinavir area under the plasma concentration-time curve (AUC) 62% compared with saquinavir alone.[1] Saquinavir coadministration also reduced the efavirenz AUC 12%. A reduction in the antiviral effect of saquinavir may occur. While no direct comparison was made, the addition of ritonavir (*Norvir*) 100 mg daily may lessen or reverse the effect of efavirenz on saquinavir.[2]

RELATED DRUGS: Efavirenz reduces the plasma concentrations of ritonavir and indinavir (*Crixivan*). Other protease inhibitors metabolized by CYP3A4 may be affected in a similar manner by efavirenz.

MANAGEMENT OPTIONS:

➡ *Monitor.* Monitor patients taking saquinavir for reduced plasma concentrations and possible reduced antiviral efficacy during efavirenz coadministration.

REFERENCES:

1. *Sustiva* [package insert]. Princeton, NJ: Bristol-Myers Squibb Company; 2005.

2. López-Cortés LF, et al. Once-daily saquinavir-sgc plus low-dose ritonavir (1200/100 mg) in combination with efavirenz: pharmacokinetics and efficacy in HIV-infected patients with prior antiretroviral therapy. *J Acquir Immune Defic Syndr*. 2003;32(2):240-242.

 Efavirenz (*Sustiva*)

Simvastatin (eg, *Zocor*)

SUMMARY: Simvastatin plasma concentrations are reduced during efavirenz coadministration; some reduction in the lipid-lowering effect of simvastatin may occur.

RISK FACTORS: No specific risk factors are known.

MECHANISM: Efavirenz is an inducer of CYP3A4, the primary pathway of simvastatin metabolism.

CLINICAL EVALUATION: Fourteen healthy subjects received simvastatin 40 mg daily for 4 days before and following 14 days of efavirenz 600 mg daily.[1] The mean area under the plasma concentration-time curve of simvastatin after efavirenz was about 60% lower than when the simvastatin was administered alone. The low-density lipoprotein (LDL)–lowering effect of simvastatin was lessened following efavirenz pretreatment. Monitor for reduced hypolipemic efficacy in patients requiring efavirenz therapy and taking simvastatin.

RELATED DRUGS: Nevirapine (*Viramune*) is also known to induce CYP3A4 and is likely to reduce simvastatin plasma concentrations. Lovastatin (eg, *Mevacor*), atorvastatin (*Lipitor*), and pravastatin (eg, *Pravachol*) may be affected in a similar manner.

MANAGEMENT OPTIONS:

➡ *Consider Alternative.* Ezetimibe (*Zetia*) is not known to be affected by CYP3A4 inducers.

➡ *Monitor.* Following the addition or discontinuation of efavirenz, monitor LDL concentrations in patients stabilized on simvastatin.

REFERENCES:

1. Gerber JG, et al. Effect of efavirenz on the pharmacokinetics of simvastatin, atorvastatin, and pravastatin: results of AIDS Clinical Trials Group 5108 Study. *J Acquir Immune Defic Syndr*. 2005;39(3):307-312.

Efavirenz (*Sustiva*)

Tipranavir (*Aptivus*)

SUMMARY: The administration of efavirenz with ritonavir (*Norvir*)—boosted tipranavir resulted in a reduction in tipranavir plasma concentrations; some loss of antiviral effect may occur.

RISK FACTORS: No specific risk factors are known.

MECHANISM: Unknown. Efavirenz may induce the metabolism of tipranavir.

CLINICAL EVALUATION: While specific data are limited, the manufacturer of tipranavir notes that coadministration of multiple doses of efavirenz 600 mg daily with tipranavir/ritonavir 500/100 mg twice daily reduced the mean area under the plasma concentration-time curve of tipranavir about 30% and its trough concentration 40%.[1] Pending further data, observe patients receiving tipranavir and efavirenz for reduced tipranavir effects.

RELATED DRUGS: Efavirenz is known to reduce the plasma concentrations of indinavir (*Crixivan*) and ritonavir. Its effect on other protease inhibitors that are metabolized by CYP3A4 (eg, nelfinavir [*Viracept*], saquinavir [*Invirase*]) may be similar.

MANAGEMENT OPTIONS:

➡ ***Monitor.*** Carefully observe patients receiving efavirenz and tipranavir for reduced antiviral effect.

REFERENCES:
1. *Aptivus* [package insert]. Ridgefield, CT: Boehringer Ingelheim Pharmaceuticals, Inc; 2005.

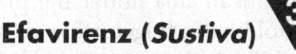

Efavirenz (*Sustiva*)

Voriconazole (*Vfend*)

SUMMARY: Efavirenz administration reduces voriconazole plasma concentrations while voriconazole increases efavirenz concentrations.

RISK FACTORS: No specific risk factors are known.

MECHANISM: Efavirenz induces the metabolism of voriconazole, perhaps via CYP2C19, CYP2C9, and/or CYP3A4. Voriconazole inhibits the CYP3A4-mediated metabolism of efavirenz.

CLINICAL EVALUATION: The coadministration of efavirenz and voriconazole results in a 2-way drug interaction that affects both drugs.[1,2] The administration of efavirenz reduces the area under the plasma concentration-time curve (AUC) of voriconazole by 55% to 80%. This is likely to lead to a loss of voriconazole antifungal efficacy. Voriconazole administration with efavirenz results in an increase in efavirenz AUC from about 20% to 43%. Some patients may experience increased efavirenz adverse reactions such as dizziness, insomnia, and somnolence.

RELATED DRUGS: Ketoconazole (*Nizoral*), fluconazole (eg, *Diflucan*), itraconazole (eg, *Sporanox*), and posaconazole (*Noxafil*) also inhibit the activity of CYP3A4 and are expected to increase the plasma concentrations of efavirenz.

MANAGEMENT OPTIONS:

➡ **Consider Alternative.** Consider terbinafine (*Lamisil*) as an alternative antifungal agent because it does not affect CYP3A4 activity. Amphotericin (eg, *Amphotec*), caspofungin (*Cansidas*), and anidulafungin (*Eraxis*) do not appear to inhibit CYP3A4.

➡ **Monitor.** Carefully monitor patients requiring the coadministration of voriconazole and efavirenz for reduced voriconazole efficacy and increased efavirenz adverse reactions.

REFERENCES:

1. Liu P, et al. Pharmacokinetic interaction between voriconazole and efavirenz at steady state in healthy male subjects. *J Clin Pharmacol.* 2008;48(1):73-84.

2. Damle B, et al. Pharmacokinetic interactions of efavirenz and voriconazole in healthy volunteers. *Br J Clin Pharmacol.* 2008;65(4):523-530.

 Eletriptan (*Relpax*)

Erythromycin (eg, *Ery-Tab*)

SUMMARY: Erythromycin administration increases eletriptan plasma concentrations; be alert for signs of excess eletriptan, such as vasospasm or ischemia.

RISK FACTORS: No specific risk factors are known.

MECHANISM: Erythromycin inhibits CYP3A4, the enzyme primarily responsible for the metabolism of eletriptan.

CLINICAL EVALUATION: While specific data are limited, the manufacturer of eletriptan notes that coadministration of erythromycin prior to a single dose of eletriptan increased the mean area under the plasma concentration-time curve of eletriptan by about 4-fold.[1] Pending further data, patients receiving eletriptan should avoid erythromycin coadministration. If the drugs are coadministered, watch for signs of excess eletriptan response.

RELATED DRUGS: Clarithromycin (eg, *Biaxin*) and troleandomycin[†] are likely to inhibit the metabolism of eletriptan in a similar manner.

MANAGEMENT OPTIONS:

➡ **Use Alternative.** Consider azithromycin (eg, *Zithromax*) as an alternative to erythromycin in patients receiving eletriptan because it does not inhibit CYP3A4. Consider a triptan that is primarily metabolized by monoamine oxidase (eg, rizatriptan [*Maxalt*], sumatriptan [*Imitrex*]) as a substitute for eletriptan in patients requiring erythromycin.

➡ **Monitor.** If patients taking erythromycin (or another drug known to inhibit CYP3A4) are administered eletriptan, monitor carefully for dizziness, nausea, and excessive vasoconstriction.

REFERENCES:

1. *Relpax* [package insert]. New York, NY: Pfizer Inc; 2006.

† Not available in the United States.

Eletriptan (*Relpax*)

Fluconazole (eg, *Diflucan*)

SUMMARY: Fluconazole administration increases eletriptan plasma concentrations; be alert for increased signs of excess eletriptan such as vasospasm or ischemia.

RISK FACTORS: No specific risk factors are known.

MECHANISM: Fluconazole inhibits CYP3A4, the enzyme primarily responsible for the metabolism of eletriptan.

CLINICAL EVALUATION: While specific data are limited, the manufacturer of eletriptan notes that coadministration of fluconazole prior to a single dose of eletriptan increased the mean area under the plasma concentration-time curve of eletriptan about 2-fold.[1] Pending further data, patients receiving eletriptan should avoid fluconazole coadministration. If the drugs are coadministered, watch for signs of excess eletriptan response.

RELATED DRUGS: Ketoconazole (eg, *Nizoral*) is known to markedly increase eletriptan plasma concentrations. Other antifungal agents that inhibit CYP3A4 (eg, itraconazole [*Sporanox*], voriconazole [*Vfend*], posaconazole [*Noxafil*]) are expected to affect eletriptan in a similar manner and should be avoided.

MANAGEMENT OPTIONS:

➡ *Consider Alternative.* Consider amphotericin, anidulafungin (*Eraxis*), caspofungin (*Cancidas*), or terbinafine (*Lamisil*) as alternative antifungal agents because they do not affect CYP3A4 activity. Consider a triptan that is primarily metabolized by monoamine oxidase (eg, rizatriptan [*Maxalt*], sumatriptan [*Imitrex*]) as a substitute for eletriptan in patients requiring fluconazole.

➡ *Monitor.* If patients taking fluconazole or another drug known to inhibit CYP3A4 are administered eletriptan, carefully monitor for dizziness, nausea, and excessive vasoconstriction.

REFERENCES:

1. *Relpax* [package insert]. New York, NY: Pfizer Inc.; 2006.

Eletriptan (*Relpax*)

Ketoconazole (eg, *Nizoral*)

SUMMARY: Ketoconazole administration produces a marked increase in eletriptan plasma concentrations; be alert for signs of excess eletriptan such as vasospasm or ischemia.

RISK FACTORS: No specific risk factors are known.

MECHANISM: Ketoconazole inhibits CYP3A4, the enzyme primarily responsible for the metabolism of eletriptan.

CLINICAL EVALUATION: While specific data are limited, the manufacturer of eletriptan notes that the coadministration of ketoconazole prior to a single dose of eletriptan increased the mean area under the plasma concentration-time curve of eletriptan about 6-fold.[1] Pending further data, do not administer ketoconazole to patients receiving eletriptan.

RELATED DRUGS: Fluconazole (eg, *Diflucan*) is known to increase eletriptan plasma concentrations. Other antifungal agents that inhibit CYP3A4 (eg, itraconazole [eg, *Sporanox*], voriconazole [*Vfend*], posaconazole [*Noxafil*]) are expected to affect eletriptan in a similar manner and should be avoided.

MANAGEMENT OPTIONS:

➡ *Use Alternative.* Use amphotericin, anidulafungin (*Eraxis*), caspofungin (*Cancidas*), or terbinafine (*Lamisil*) as alternative antifungal agents because they do not affect CYP3A4 activity. Use a triptan that is primarily metabolized by monoamine oxidase (eg, rizatriptan [*Maxalt*], sumatriptan [*Imitrex*]) as a substitute for eletriptan in patients requiring ketoconazole.

➡ *Monitor.* If patients taking ketoconazole or another drug known to inhibit CYP3A4 are administered eletriptan, carefully monitor for dizziness, nausea, and excessive vasoconstriction.

REFERENCES:

   1. *Relpax* [package insert]. New York, NY: Pfizer Inc.; 2006.

Eletriptan (*Relpax*)

Verapamil (eg, *Calan*)

SUMMARY: Verapamil administration increases eletriptan plasma concentrations; be alert for signs of excess eletriptan such as vasospasm or ischemia.

RISK FACTORS: No specific risk factors are known.

MECHANISM: Verapamil inhibits CYP3A4, the enzyme primarily responsible for the metabolism of eletriptan.

CLINICAL EVALUATION: While specific data are limited, the manufacturer of eletriptan notes that coadministration of verapamil prior to a single dose of eletriptan increased the mean area under the plasma concentration-time curve of eletriptan by about 3-fold.[1] Pending further data, patients receiving eletriptan should avoid verapamil coadministration. If the drugs are coadministered, watch for signs of excess eletriptan response.

RELATED DRUGS: Diltiazem (eg, *Cardizem*) may affect eletriptan in a similar manner.

MANAGEMENT OPTIONS:

➡ *Consider Alternative.* Consider calcium channel blockers that do not inhibit CYP3A4 (eg, amlodipine [eg, *Norvasc*], felodipine [*Plendil*], nifedipine [eg, *Procardia*]) for patients taking eletriptan. Consider a triptan that is primarily metabolized by monoamine oxidase (eg, rizatriptan [*Maxalt*], sumatriptan [*Imitrex*]) as a substitute for eletriptan in patients taking verapamil.

➡ *Monitor.* If patients taking verapamil or another drug known to inhibit CYP3A4 are administered eletriptan, carefully monitor for dizziness, nausea, and excessive vasoconstriction.

REFERENCES:

   1. *Relpax* [package insert]. New York, NY: Pfizer Inc.; 2006.

Enalapril (eg, *Vasotec*)

Furosemide (eg, *Lasix*)

SUMMARY: Initiation of angiotensin-converting enzyme (ACE) inhibitor therapy in the presence of intensive diuretic therapy results in a precipitous fall in blood pressure (BP) in some patients. ACE inhibitors may induce renal insufficiency in the presence of diuretic-induced sodium depletion.

RISK FACTORS:

➡ ***Concurrent Diseases.*** Preexisting high BP, secondary hypertension, high circulating levels of renin and angiotensin II, and congestive heart failure (CHF) may increase the risk of acute hypotensive episodes.[1-3]

➡ ***Dosage Regimen.*** Hypovolemia caused by diuretic therapy may predispose hypotensive reactions or acute renal failure.[2,4,5]

MECHANISM: Patients with diuretic-induced sodium depletion and hypovolemia appear to be most susceptible to an acute hypotensive episode following initiation of ACE inhibitor therapy.[6] Pentopril may impair the renal excretion of furosemide[7]; captopril (eg, *Capoten*)[8] and enalapril[9] do not appear to do so.

CLINICAL EVALUATION: Acute hypotensive episodes have occurred within 2 to 3 hours of initial doses of ACE inhibitors in patients with hypertension or CHF. Although acute hypotensive episodes can occur when ACE inhibitors are initiated in the presence of diuretic-induced hypovolemia, chronic therapy with ACE inhibitors plus loop or thiazide diuretics appears safe and effective.[10-12] Renal function may be affected by ACE inhibitors in the presence of diuretic-induced sodium depletion. In a randomized, double-blind, placebo-controlled study of 73 patients with hypertensive nephrosclerosis, 8 patients receiving enalapril developed reversible renal insufficiency; none of the patients receiving placebo developed this effect.[13] The 8 patients who developed renal insufficiency were receiving diuretics (usually furosemide). Volume depletion was a factor in 3 of the 8 patients affected. Heat may have contributed to the volume depletion in 6 of the 8 patients. Another patient with moderate renal insufficiency and CHF developed renal failure when enalapril was given during furosemide-induced severe sodium depletion.[14] In postmarketing surveillance, hypotension associated with captopril was more frequent in patients taking concurrent diuretics.

RELATED DRUGS: Other loop diuretics (eg, bumetanide [eg, *Bumex*], torsemide [*Demadex*], ethacrynic acid [*Edecrin*]) probably interact with ACE inhibitors in the same way as furosemide. All ACE inhibitors most likely interact in a similar way with diuretics.

MANAGEMENT OPTIONS:

➡ ***Circumvent/Minimize.*** Some recommend that CHF patients on furosemide should be kept supine for 3 hours after the first dose of ACE inhibitors; this especially refers to elderly patients.[15]

➡ ***Monitor.*** Initiate ACE inhibitor therapy cautiously in patients receiving diuretics, especially if there is evidence of hypovolemia. Monitor BP carefully for at least

3 hours after the ACE inhibitor is given. In some patients, it may be desirable to withdraw the diuretic temporarily before starting the ACE inhibitor.

REFERENCES:

1. Hodsman GP, et al. Factors related to first dose hypotensive effect of captopril: prediction and treatment. *Br Med J.* 1983;286:832-834.

2. Mandal AK, et al. Diuretics potentiate angiotensin converting enzyme inhibitor-induced acute renal failure. *Clin Nephrol.* 1994;42:170-174.

3. MacFayden RJ. The response to the first dose of an ACE inhibitor in essential hypertension: a placebo-controlled study utilizing ambulatory blood pressure recording. *Br J Clin Pharmacol.* 1991;31:568P.

4. Atkinson AB, et al. Captopril in a hyponatremic hypertensive: need for caution in initiating therapy. *Lancet.* 1979;1:557-558.

5. Vlasses PH, et al. Captopril: clinical pharmacology and benefit-to-risk ratio in hypertension and congestive heart failure. *Pharmacotherapy.* 1982;2:1-17.

6. Chalmers D, et al. Postmarketing surveillance of captopril for hypertension. *Br J Clin Pharmacol.* 1992;34:215-223.

7. Rakhit A, et al. Pharmacokinetics and pharmacodynamics of pentopril, a new angiotensin-converting-enzyme inhibitor in humans. *J Clin Pharmacol.* 1986;26:156-164.

8. Fujimura A, et al. Influence of captopril on urinary excretion of furosemide in hypertensive subjects. *J Clin Pharmacol.* 1990;30:538-542.

9. Van Hecken AM, et al. Absence of a pharmacokinetic interaction between enalapril and furosemide. *Br J Clin Pharmacol.* 1987;23:84-87.

10. Gluck Z, et al. Long-term effects of captopril on renal function in hypertensive patients. *Eur J Clin Pharmacol.* 1984;26:315-323.

11. Clementy J, et al. Comparative study of the efficacy and tolerance of capozide and moduretic administered in a single daily dose for the treatment of chronic moderate arterial hypertension. *Postgrad Med J.* 1986;62(suppl 1):132-134.

12. Pandhi P, et al. Low-dose captopril alone and in combination with hydrochlorothiazide in treatment of mild to moderate essential hypertension. *Int J Clin Pharmacol Ther Toxicol.* 1986;24:294-297.

13. Toto RD, et al. Reversible renal insufficiency due to angiotensin converting enzyme inhibitors in hypertensive nephrosclerosis. *Ann Intern Med.* 1991;115:513-519.

14. Funck-Brentano C, et al. Reversible renal failure after combined treatment with enalapril and furosemide in a patient with congestive heart failure. *Br Heart J.* 1986;55:596-598.

15. Mets T, et al. First-dose hypotension, ACE inhibitors, and heart failure in the elderly. *Lancet.* 1992;339:1487.

Enalapril (eg, *Vasotec*)

Indomethacin (eg, *Indocin*)

SUMMARY: Indomethacin, and probably other nonsteroidal anti-inflammatory drugs (NSAIDs), inhibits the antihypertensive effects of enalapril and likely other angiotensin-converting enzyme (ACE) inhibitors.

RISK FACTORS: No specific risk factors are known.

MECHANISM: Not established. Enalapril-induced inhibition of renal prostaglandins may be involved.

CLINICAL EVALUATION: In a double-blind, crossover study of patients on amlodipine (n = 24) and enalapril (n = 25), indomethacin 50 mg twice daily or placebo was given for 3 weeks. Indomethacin increased blood pressure by 10.1/4.9 mm Hg and reduced the pulse rate by 5.6 bpm. The antihypertensive effect of amlodipine was not affected.[1]

RELATED DRUGS: Theoretically, any combination of an ACE inhibitor and an NSAID would result in inhibition of the antihypertensive effect of the ACE inhibitor.

MANAGEMENT OPTIONS:

➥ *Consider Alternative.* Antihypertensive agents other than ACE inhibitors (eg, amlodipine [eg, *Norvasc*]) may be less affected by NSAIDs.

➥ *Monitor.* If indomethacin or other NSAIDs are used with enalapril or other ACE inhibitors, monitor blood pressure carefully.

REFERENCES:

1. Morgan TO, et al. Effect of indomethacin on blood pressure in elderly people with essential hypertension well controlled on amlodipine or enalapril. *Am J Hypertens.* 2000;13:1161-1167.

Enalapril (eg, *Vasotec*)

Iron

SUMMARY: Three patients on enalapril developed systemic reactions (GI symptoms, hypotension) following intravenous (IV) iron; more study is needed to establish a causal relationship.

RISK FACTORS:

➥ *Route of Administration.* The IV administration of iron appears more likely to interact with enalapril than oral iron.

MECHANISM: Not established. It is possible that angiotensin-converting enzyme (ACE) inhibitors potentiate anaphylaxis by decreasing the breakdown of kinins.[1]

CLINICAL EVALUATION: Three of 18 patients developed systemic reactions (ie, erythema, nausea, vomiting, diarrhea, fever, hypotension) during or soon after IV ferrigluconate. All 3 patients were receiving enalapril, while none of the other 15 patients was receiving an ACE inhibitor.[1] One of the patients tolerated both drugs alone with no systemic reaction. This suggests, but does not prove, that enalapril increases the risk of systemic reactions to IV iron.

RELATED DRUGS: Oral iron has not been associated with these reactions in patients receiving other ACE inhibitors.

MANAGEMENT OPTIONS:

➥ *Consider Alternative.* This potential interaction is not well established, but given the severity of the reactions, consider alternatives to IV iron or the ACE inhibitor.

➥ *Monitor.* If IV iron is given to a patient on an ACE inhibitor, monitor for systemic reactions and be prepared to treat anaphylaxis.

REFERENCES:

1. Rolla G, et al. Systemic reactions to intravenous iron therapy in patients receiving angiotensin converting enzyme inhibitor. *J Allergy Clin Immunol.* 1994;93(6):1074-1075.

Enalapril (eg, *Vasotec*)

Rofecoxib†

SUMMARY: A patient on enalapril developed hyperkalemia after starting rofecoxib, but it is not known how often this problem occurs.

RISK FACTORS: No specific risk factors are known, but it seems likely that renal impairment or diabetes would increase the risk of hyperkalemia.

MECHANISM: Probably additive. Both enalapril and rofecoxib can reduce renal potassium elimination.

CLINICAL EVALUATION: A 77-year-old woman on long-term enalapril developed fatal hyperkalemia 5 days after starting rofecoxib 25 mg/day.[1] She had also been taking additional potassium in her diet. It seems likely that the drug combination contributed to her hyperkalemia.

RELATED DRUGS: It is likely that rofecoxib could also increase the risk of hyperkalemia in patients receiving other angiotensin-converting enzyme (ACE) inhibitors, such as benazepril (eg, *Lotensin*), captopril (eg, *Capoten*), fosinopril (eg, *Monopril*), lisinopril (eg, *Prinivil*), moexipril (eg, *Univasc*), quinapril (eg, *Accupril*), ramipril (eg, *Altace*), and trandolapril (eg, *Mavik*).

MANAGEMENT OPTIONS:

➡ *Monitor.* In patients receiving rofecoxib and an ACE inhibitor, monitor serum potassium and renal function, particularly if the patient has 1 or more risk factors, such as diabetes or renal impairment.

REFERENCES:

1. Hay E, et al. Fatal hyperkalemia related to combined therapy with a COX-2 inhibitor, ACE inhibitor and potassium rich diet. *J Emerg Med.* 2002;22(4):349-352.

† Not available in the United States.

---

4   Enalapril (eg, *Vasotec*)

Tamsulosin (eg, *Flomax*)

SUMMARY: Tamsulosin does not appear to affect the antihypertensive response to enalapril.

RISK FACTORS: No specific risk factors are known.

MECHANISM: Theoretically, additive hypotension could occur but does not appear to be a problem clinically.

CLINICAL EVALUATION: Eight hypertensive subjects stabilized on enalapril for at least 3 months were given tamsulosin 0.4 mg/day for 7 days followed by 0.8 mg/day for 7 days.[1] According to documentation, tamsulosin did not produce any clinically significant effects on blood pressure or pulse rate compared with placebo.

RELATED DRUGS: Tamsulosin did not affect the hypotensive response to nifedipine (eg, *Procardia*) or atenolol (eg, *Tenormin*).

MANAGEMENT OPTIONS: No specific action is required, but be alert for evidence of the interaction.

REFERENCES:

1. *Flomax* [package insert]. Ridgefield, CT: Boehringer Ingelheim; 2009.

Enalapril (eg, *Vasotec*)

Trimethoprim/Sulfamethoxazole (eg, *Bactrim*)

SUMMARY: The risk of developing hyperkalemia is markedly increased in patients receiving trimethoprim and angiotensin-converting enzyme (ACE) inhibitors.

RISK FACTORS:

➡ **Concurrent Diseases.** Diseases associated with reduced kidney function, including acute or chronic renal failure, diabetes mellitus, and heart failure, other drugs that reduce potassium excretion, and advancing age are likely to increase the risk.

MECHANISM: Both enalapril and trimethoprim inhibit renal potassium excretion.

CLINICAL EVALUATION: Trimethoprim administered with enalapril or other ACE inhibitors has been reported to produce hyperkalemia in both case reports and case-controlled studies.[1-3] In a case-control study of patients receiving therapy with ACE inhibitors or angiotensin receptor blockers, the risk of hospitalization for hyperkalemia within 14 days of antibiotic therapy was increased nearly 7-fold by trimethoprim/sulfamethoxazole compared with amoxicillin or any other antibiotic.[3] Severe hyperkalemia has been reported in patients receiving high-dose trimethoprim for the treatment of *Pneumocystis carinii*.[1]

RELATED DRUGS: All other ACE inhibitors, such as benazepril (eg, *Lotensin*), fosinopril (eg, *Monopril*), and lisinopril (eg, *Prinivil*), as well as all angiotensin receptor blockers, including candesartan (*Atacand*), losartan (eg, *Cozaar*), and valsartan (*Diovan*), are expected to interact in a similar manner as enalapril.

MANAGEMENT OPTIONS:

➡ **Monitor.** Carefully monitor patients receiving ACE inhibitors or angiotensin receptor blockers with trimethoprim, particularly if any of the risk factors listed in Risk Factors are present, for serum potassium concentrations.

REFERENCES:

1. Bugge JF. Severe hyperkalemia induced by trimethoprim in combination with an angiotensin-converting enzyme inhibitor in a patient with transplanted lungs. *J Intern Med.* 1996;240(4):249-251.
2. Marinella MA. Trimethoprim-induced hyperkalemia: an analysis of reported cases. *Gerontology.* 1999;44:209-212.
3. Antoniou T, et al. Tmp-sulfamethoxazole-induced hyperkalemia in patients receiving inhibitors of the renin-angiotensin system. *Arch Intern Med.* 2010;170:1-5.

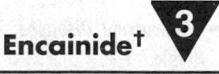

Encainide†

Quinidine

SUMMARY: Quinidine can substantially increase encainide serum concentrations in patients who are extensive (rapid) encainide metabolizers. However, because of the opposing effects of quinidine on the serum concentrations of encainide and its active metabolites, the clinical outcome is likely to be limited.

RISK FACTORS:

➡ **Pharmacogenetics.** Rapid encainide metabolizers are at greater risk.

MECHANISM: Quinidine reduces the hepatic clearance of encainide in extensive metabolizers (EMs) but not in poor metabolizers of encainide.

CLINICAL EVALUATION: Eleven healthy subjects received encainide 60 mg orally with a 4.5 mg intravenous (IV) dose of radiolabeled encainide alone.[1] These subjects also received the IV dose of encainide following 5 days of quinidine 50 mg every 6 hours. In EMs of encainide, quinidine reduced the mean clearance of encainide from 935 to 190 mL/min, increased the encainide plasma concentration more than 3-fold, and significantly reduced the serum concentration of the 2 active metabolites of encainide. Quinidine also reversed the pharmacodynamic effects of encainide as measured by electrocardiographic wave (QRS) and PR interval prolongation. In 10 patients with ventricular arrhythmias, quinidine 60 mg every 8 hours significantly decreased encainide clearance and increased mean encainide concentrations from 21 to 240 ng/mL.[2] Both enantiomers of encainide appear to be equally inhibited by quinidine.[3] No effects of quinidine on encainide pharmacokinetics or pharmacodynamics were observed in slow encainide metabolizers. Because most patients are encainide EMs, increases in encainide serum concentrations and decreases in the serum concentration of encainide's active metabolites are expected when quinidine is administered.

RELATED DRUGS: No information is available.

MANAGEMENT OPTIONS:

➡ **Monitor.** Monitor patients maintained on encainide for changes in antiarrhythmic efficacy when quinidine is added or deleted.

REFERENCES:

1. Funck-Brentano C, et al. Effect of low dose quinidine on encainide pharmacokinetics and pharmacodynamics. Influence of genetic polymorphism. *J Pharmacol Exp Ther*. 1989;249(1):134-142.

2. Turgeon J, et al. Genetically determined steady-state interaction between encainide and quinidine in patients with arrhythmias. *J Pharmacol Exp Ther*. 1990;255(2):642-649.

3. Turgeon J, et al. Genetically determined stereoselective excretion of encainide in humans and electrophysiologic effects of its enantiomers in canine cardiac Purkinje fibers. *Clin Pharmacol Ther*. 1991;49(5):488-496.

† Not available in the United States.

Enoxacin†

Fenbufen†

SUMMARY: The combination of enoxacin and fenbufen has been reported to produce seizures.

RISK FACTORS:

➡ **Concurrent Diseases.** Patients with epilepsy or a history of convulsions are at greater risk.

MECHANISM: Gamma-aminobutyric acid (GABA) is an endogenous CNS depressant. It is inhibited by both quinolones and some nonsteroidal anti-inflammatory drugs (NSAIDs). It has been suggested that the combination of enoxacin and the NSAID fenbufen or its metabolite particularly inhibits GABA activity, resulting in cerebral stimulation and seizures.[1,2]

CLINICAL EVALUATION: A few case reports of convulsions during the administration of enoxacin and fenbufen have been noted. Preliminary evidence suggests that fenbufen is the most likely NSAID to cause this interaction, but other factors may contribute.[3-5] Pefloxacin† has been reported to cause seizures in the absence of

NSAID administration. More study is needed to determine causation and the risk, if any, from other NSAIDs.

RELATED DRUGS: Ciprofloxacin (eg, *Cipro*) and diclofenac (eg, *Cataflam*) do not appear to interact,[6,7] nor do ketoprofen, pefloxacin, or ofloxacin (eg, *Floxin*).

MANAGEMENT OPTIONS:

➡ *Consider Alternative.* Consider using a quinolone, which is less likely to interact (eg, ciprofloxacin, ketoprofen, pefloxacin, ofloxacin, diclofenac).

➡ *Monitor.* Until more data are available, carefully observe patients with a history of convulsions when they are prescribed quinolones and NSAIDs. Special precautions are not necessary for most patients.

REFERENCES:

1. Akahane K, et al. Possible intermolecular interaction between quinolones and biphenylacetic acid inhibits gamma-aminobutyric acid receptor sites. *Antimicrob Agents Chemother.* 1994;38:2323-2329.

2. Halliwell RF, et al. Antagonism of GABA$_A$ receptors by 4-quinolones. *J Antimicrob Chemother.* 1993;31:457-462.

3. Christ W, et al. Interactions of quinolones with opioids and fenbufen, a NSAID: involvement of dopaminergic neurotransmission. *Rev Infect Dis.* 1989;11(suppl 5):S1393.

4. Davies BI, et al. Drug interactions with quinolones. *Rev Infect Dis.* 1989;11(suppl 5):S1083-S1090.

5. Hori, et al. A study on enhanced epileptogenicity of new quinolones in the presence of anti-inflammatory drugs [abstract]. In: Abstracts of the 26th Interscience Conference on Antimicrobial Agents and Chemotherapy; September 28-October 1, 1986; New Orleans, LA.

6. Segev S, et al. Quinolones, theophylline, and diclofenac interactions with the gamma-aminobutyric acid receptor. *Antimicrob Agents Chemother.* 1988;32:1624-1626.

7. Fillastre JP, et al. Lack of effect of ketoprofen on the pharmacokinetics of pefloxacin and ofloxacin. *J Antimicrob Chemother.* 1993;31:805-806.

† Not available in the United States.

Enoxacin† 4

Probenecid

SUMMARY: Probenecid may increase the serum concentration of some quinolones; the clinical significance of this appears to be limited.

RISK FACTORS: No specific risk factors are known.

MECHANISM: Probenecid inhibits the renal tubular secretion of quinolones.

CLINICAL EVALUATION: The half-life of enoxacin following a 600 mg dose plus probenecid 2.5 g was increased from 3 to 7 hours; enoxacin renal clearance fell from 374 to 171 mL/min.[1]

RELATED DRUGS: The clinical significance of this interaction is likely to be greater in quinolones where renal elimination comprises most of the body clearance (eg, ofloxacin [eg, *Floxin*]). Other quinolones that are renally eliminated may be affected by probenecid.

MANAGEMENT OPTIONS: No specific action is required, but be alert for evidence of the interaction.

REFERENCES:

1. Wijnands WJ, et al. Pharmacokinetics of enoxacin and its penetration into bronchial secretions and lung tissue. *J Antimicrob Chemother.* 1988;21(suppl B):67-77.

† Not available in the United States.

Enoxacin[†]

Ramelteon (*Rozerem*)

SUMMARY: Ramelteon is very sensitive to inhibition of CYP1A2; theoretically enoxacin would produce substantial increases in ramelteon plasma concentrations.

RISK FACTORS: No specific risk factors are known.

MECHANISM: Ramelteon is metabolized primarily by CYP1A2, and enoxacin is a potent CYP1A2 inhibitor.

CLINICAL EVALUATION: In healthy subjects, fluvoxamine 100 mg twice daily for 3 days produced a 190-fold increase in ramelteon plasma concentrations and a 70-fold increase in the ramelteon maximal plasma concentrations.[1] Enoxacin is also a potent CYP1A2 inhibitor, and substantial increases in ramelteon plasma concentrations are expected. Administer ramelteon with caution with CYP1A2 inhibitors.[1]

RELATED DRUGS: Ciprofloxacin is a moderate inhibitor of CYP1A2 and should generally be avoided with ramelteon. Other fluoroquinolones have little effect on CYP1A2 and theoretically would not be expected to interact significantly with ramelteon, such as levofloxacin (*Levaquin*), lomefloxacin (*Maxaquin*), ofloxacin (eg, *Floxin*), gatifloxacin (*Zymar*), and moxifloxacin (*Avelox*).

MANAGEMENT OPTIONS:

➡ ***Use Alternative.*** If a fluoroquinolone is needed, avoid enoxacin or ciprofloxacin, and use an alternative that has little effect on CYP1A2 (see Related Drugs).

REFERENCES:

1. *Rozerem* [package insert]. Lincolnshire, IL: Takeda Pharmaceuticals; 2006.

† Not available in the United States.

Enoxacin (*Penetrex*)

Ranitidine (eg, *Zantac*)

SUMMARY: Ranitidine administration reduces the plasma concentrations of enoxacin; failure of antibiotic efficacy could result.

RISK FACTORS: No specific risk factors are known.

MECHANISM: Reduction of gastric acidity by ranitidine appears to reduce the absorption of orally administered enoxacin resulting in lower plasma concentrations.

CLINICAL EVALUATION: Enoxacin peak concentration and area under the plasma concentration-time curve were reduced 38% and 26%, respectively, following ranitidine administration.[1] No change in the renal clearance of enoxacin was noted following ranitidine. Adding pentagastrin to ranitidine abolished ranitidine's effect on gastric pH and enoxacin pharmacokinetics. In another study enoxacin bioavailability was reduced 40% following 50 mg IV ranitidine.[2]

RELATED DRUGS: The effects of other H_2-receptor antagonists (eg, cimetidine [eg, *Tagamet*], famotidine [eg, *Pepcid*], nizatidine [*Axid*]) or proton pump inhibitors (eg, lansoprazole [*Prevacid*], omeprazole [*Prilosec*]) on orally administered enoxacin are unknown but would be expected to be similar to those of ranitidine.

MANAGEMENT OPTIONS:

➡ *Consider Alternative.* Separation of the doses of ranitidine and oral enoxacin will probably have little effect on this interaction since the pH tends to stay somewhat elevated during therapy with H_2-receptor antagonists or omeprazole. The administration of IV enoxacin or an alternative antibiotic may be necessary in patients requiring gastric acid suppression.

➡ *Monitor.* Observe patients receiving enoxacin and drugs that alkalinize the gut for loss of antibiotic efficacy.

REFERENCES:

1. Lebsack ME, et al. Effect of gastric acidity on enoxacin absorption. *Clin Pharmacol Ther.* 1992;52:252.
2. Grasela TH, et al. Inhibition of enoxacin absorption by antacids or ranitidine. *Antimicrob Agents Chemother.* 1989;33:615.

Enoxacin (*Penetrex*)
Tacrine (*Cognex*)

SUMMARY: In vitro studies suggest that enoxacin is a potent inhibitor of tacrine metabolism. Given the major effect that enoxacin has on theophylline metabolism (which is metabolized by the same enzyme [CYP1A2] as tacrine), it seems likely that enoxacin has a similar effect on tacrine.

RISK FACTORS: No specific risk factors are known.

MECHANISM: Enoxacin is a potent inhibitor of cytochrome CYP1A2, the isozyme primarily responsible for the metabolism of tacrine. Other quinolones appear to have varying effects on CYP1A2 activity.

CLINICAL EVALUATION: In an in vitro study of microsomes pooled from 6 human livers, enoxacin inhibited all routes of tacrine metabolism. Nonetheless, additional study is needed to establish what effect, if any, quinolones have on tacrine metabolism clinically. Moreover, the clinical outcome of the inhibition of tacrine metabolism is not established.

RELATED DRUGS: Expect the various quinolones to affect tacrine metabolism in a manner similar to their effects on theophylline. If that proves to be true, enoxacin would have a marked effect on tacrine metabolism, ciprofloxacin (*Cipro*) a moderate effect, and norfloxacin (*Noroxin*) a small effect. Theoretically, quinolones such as lomefloxacin (*Maxaquin*) and ofloxacin (*Floxin*) would be less likely to interact with tacrine.

MANAGEMENT OPTIONS:

➡ *Consider Alternative.* Consider using a quinolone, which is less likely to interact (eg, lomefloxacin, ofloxacin).

➡ *Monitor.* If quinolones and tacrine are used together, monitor for tacrine toxicity (eg, nausea, vomiting, anorexia, diarrhea, abdominal pain). However, some evidence suggests that tacrine hepatotoxicity results from reactive tacrine metabolites.[1] Thus, if quinolones are found to inhibit tacrine metabolism clinically, possibly expect the effect to reduce the risk of hepatotoxicity.

REFERENCES:

1. Madden S, et al. An investigation into the formation of stable, proteinreactive, and cytotoxic metabolites from tacrine in vitro. Studies with human and rat liver microsomes. *Biochem Pharmacol.* 1993;46:13.

 Enoxacin (*Penetrex*)

Theophylline (eg, *Theolair*)

SUMMARY: Enoxacin markedly increases the serum concentrations of theophylline and may result in the development of theophylline toxicity.

RISK FACTORS:

➡ ***Dosage Regimen.*** Higher doses of enoxacin produce a greater risk.

MECHANISM: Enoxacin presumably inhibits the N-demethylation of theophylline by CYP1A2.

CLINICAL EVALUATION: Chronic oral enoxacin 600 to 1,200 mg/day increased theophylline plasma concentrations 40% to 243% and decreased the theophylline clearance 40% to 74%.[1-7] The theophylline plasma concentration appears to increase over approximately 3 days after the antibiotic is started. Theophylline concentrations could increase 2- to 4-fold during enoxacin therapy resulting in toxicity. Human liver microsome studies indicate that enoxacin is a more potent inhibitor of theophylline than its 4-oxo metabolite.[8] Theophylline does not alter enoxacin serum concentrations.[9]

RELATED DRUGS: Quinolones reported to inhibit the metabolism of drugs include ciprofloxacin (*Cipro*), enoxacin, norfloxacin (*Noroxin*), pipemidic acid, and pefloxacin.[†] Quinolones reported to produce no or minor changes in theophylline pharmacokinetics include fleroxacin,[†] lomefloxacin (*Maxaquin*), ofloxacin (*Floxin*), rufloxacin,[†] and sparfloxacin (eg, *Zagam*).

MANAGEMENT OPTIONS:

➡ ***Use Alternative.*** Enoxacin should not be administered with theophylline. Use a quinolone known to have no or minor effect on theophylline pharmacokinetics (eg, fleroxacin, lomefloxacin, ofloxacin, rufloxacin, sparfloxacin).

REFERENCES:

1. Wijnands WJA, et al. Enoxacin raises plasma theophylline concentrations. *Lancet.* 1984;2:108.

2. Wijnands WJA, et al. The effect of the 4-quinolone enoxacin on plasma theophylline concentrations. *Pharm Weekly [Sci].* 1986;8:42.

3. Wijnands WJA, et al. The influence of quinolone derivatives on theophylline clearance. *Br J Clin Pharmacol.* 1986;22:677.

4. Koup JR, et al. Theophylline dosage adjustment during enoxacin coadministration. *Anitmicrob Agents Chemother.* 1990;34:803.

5. Beckmann EW, et al. Enoxacin—a potent inhibitor of theophylline metabolism. *Eur J Clin Pharmacol.* 1987;33:227.

6. Rogge MC, et al. The theophylline-enoxacin interaction: I. Effect of enoxacin dose size on theophylline disposition. *Clin Pharmacol Ther.* 1988;44:579.

7. Sano M, et al. Effects of enoxacin, ofloxacin, and norfloxacin on theophylline disposition in humans. *Eur J Clin Pharmacol.* 1988;35:161.

8. Sarkar M, et al. In vitro effect of fluoroquinolones of theophylline metabolism in human liver microsomes. *Antimicrob Agents Chemother.* 1990;34:594.

9. Wijnands WJA, et al. Steady-state kinetics of the quinolone derivatives ofloxacin, enoxacin, ciprofloxacin, and pefloxacin during maintenance treatment with theophylline. *Drugs.* 1987;34(Suppl. 1):159.

† Not available in the United States.

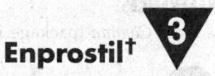

Enprostil†

Ethanol (Ethyl Alcohol)

SUMMARY: Enprostil appears to increase instead of decrease the gastric mucosal damage produced by ethanol.

RISK FACTORS: No specific risk factors are known.

MECHANISM: Not established.

CLINICAL EVALUATION: In 8 healthy subjects, 100 mL of 80% ethanol was sprayed on the gastric mucosa with and without pretreatment with enprostil 10 mL sprayed on gastric mucosa.[1] Gastroscopy showed a marked increase in ethanol-induced mucosal injury with enprostil compared with control (the vehicle). The significance of these findings to patients taking oral enprostil who drink alcohol is not established.

RELATED DRUGS: The effect of ethanol combined with prostaglandins other than enprostil is not established.

MANAGEMENT OPTIONS:

➡ *Circumvent/Minimize.* Until more information is available, it would be prudent for patients taking enprostil (and possibly other prostaglandins) to minimize their alcohol intake.

➡ *Monitor.* Monitor for evidence of GI intolerance if the combination is used.

REFERENCES:

1. Cohen MM, et al. Human antral damage induced by alcohol is potentiated by enprostil. *Gastroenterology.* 1990;99:45.

† Not available in the United States.

Entacapone (*Comtan*)

Bitolterol (*Tornalate*)

SUMMARY: Theoretically, entacapone may inhibit bitolterol metabolism and increase the risk of bitolterol toxicity.

RISK FACTORS: No specific risk factors are known.

MECHANISM: Bitolterol is metabolized by catechol-O-methyltransferase (COMT), and entacapone is a COMT inhibitor.

CLINICAL EVALUATION: A single dose of entacapone 400 mg increased the effect of intravenous isoproterenol (eg, *Isuprel*) on heart rate by 50% compared with isoproterenol alone.[1] Because bitolterol is also metabolized by COMT, it may interact similarly. The manufacturer states that the interaction also may occur with inhalation bitolterol.

RELATED DRUGS: Isoetharine is also metabolized by COMT and may interact similarly with entacapone.

MANAGEMENT OPTIONS:

➡ *Avoid Unless Benefit Outweighs Risk.* The manufacturer recommends caution if the drugs are used concurrently.

➡ *Monitor.* If the combination is used, monitor cardiovascular status carefully.

REFERENCES:

1. *Comtan* [package insert]. Parsippany NJ: Novartis Pharmaceuticals; 2008.

 Entacapone (*Comtan*)

Dobutamine

SUMMARY: Theoretically, entacapone may inhibit dobutamine metabolism and increase the risk of dobutamine toxicity.

RISK FACTORS: No specific risk factors are known.

MECHANISM: Dobutamine is metabolized by catechol-O-methyltransferase (COMT), and entacapone is a COMT inhibitor.

CLINICAL EVALUATION: Entacapone increased the heart rate effect of epinephrine (eg, *EpiPen*) and isoproterenol (eg, *Isuprel*) (both are COMT substrates).[1] Because dobutamine is also metabolized by COMT, it may interact as well.

RELATED DRUGS: Epinephrine, norepinephrine (eg, *Levopred*), and isoproterenol are all metabolized by COMT and may interact with entacapone.

MANAGEMENT OPTIONS:

➡ *Avoid Unless Benefit Outweighs Risk.* The manufacturer recommends caution if the drugs are used concurrently.

➡ *Monitor.* If the combination is used, monitor cardiovascular status carefully.

REFERENCES:

1. *Comtan* [package insert]. Parsippany NJ: Novartis Pharmaceuticals; 2008.

 Entacapone (*Comtan*)

Ephedrine

SUMMARY: A patient on entacapone developed acute hypertensive episodes after receiving ephedrine.

RISK FACTORS: No specific risk factors are known.

MECHANISM: Ephedrine acts directly and indirectly by causing release of catecholamines; entacapone may inhibit the metabolism of the released catecholamines by catechol-O-methyltranferase (COMT).

CLINICAL EVALUATION: A 76-year-old woman with Parkinson disease on entacapone 200 mg/day developed repeated hypertensive episodes (up to 240/130 mm Hg) after ephedrine 3 mg intravenous (IV) was given during surgery. Several doses of hydralazine (eg, *Apresoline*) were needed to correct the hypertension.[1] In a study done by the manufacturer, a single dose of entacapone 400 mg increased the effect of IV epinephrine on heart rate by 80% compared with epinephrine alone.[2] Therefore, it is possible that the entacapone potentiated norepinephrine and epinephrine released by the ephedrine in this patient.

RELATED DRUGS: Many adrenergic agents are metabolized by COMT and may interact with entacapone, such as epinephrine (eg, *EpiPen*), norepinephrine (eg, *Levobid*), isoproterenol (eg, Isuprel), dobutamine, bitolterol (*Tornalate*), and isoetharine.

MANAGEMENT OPTIONS:

➡ ***Avoid Unless Benefit Outweighs Risk.*** Although this interaction is not well documented, it is consistent with the interactive properties of the 2 drugs, and the adverse outcome may be severe.

➡ ***Consider Alternative.*** Research suggests that diluted phenylephine may be preferable if a vasopressor is needed intraoperatively in a patient on entacapone.[1]

REFERENCES:

1. Renfrew, C et al. Severe hypertension following ephedrine administration in a patient receiving entacapone. *Anesthesiology*. 2000;93(6):1562.

2. *Comtan* [package insert]. Parsippany NJ: Novartis Pharmaceuticals; 2008.

Entacapone (*Comtan*)

Epinephrine (eg, *EpiPen*)

SUMMARY: Entacapone may substantially increase the effect of epinephrine on the heart rate.

RISK FACTORS: No specific risk factors are known.

MECHANISM: Epinephrine is metabolized by catechol-O-methyltransferase (COMT), and entacapone is a COMT inhibitor.

CLINICAL EVALUATION: A single dose of entacapone 400 mg increased the effect of intravenous epinephrine on heart rate by 80% compared with epinephrine alone.[1] One 32-year-old healthy subject developed ventricular tachycardia following the combination. Theoretically, small amounts of epinephrine used with local anesthetics are unlikely to interact.

RELATED DRUGS: Isoproterenol's (eg, *Isuprel*) effect on heart rate was also increased by entacapone. Norepinephrine (eg, *Levophed*) is also metabolized by COMT and may interact similarly.

MANAGEMENT OPTIONS:

➡ ***Avoid Unless Benefit Outweighs Risk.*** The manufacturer recommends caution if the drugs are used concurrently.

➡ ***Monitor.*** If the combination is used, monitor cardiovascular status carefully.

REFERENCES:

1. *Comtan* [package insert]. Parsippany NJ: Novartis Pharmaceuticals; 2008.

Entacapone (*Comtan*)

Isoproterenol (eg, *Isuprel*)

SUMMARY: Entacapone may substantially increase the effect of isoproterenol on the heart rate.

RISK FACTORS: No specific risk factors are known.

MECHANISM: Isoproterenol is metabolized by catechol-O-methyltransferase (COMT), and entacapone is a COMT inhibitor.

CLINICAL EVALUATION: A single dose of entacapone 400 mg increased the effect of intravenous isoproterenol on heart rate by 50%, compared with isoproterenol alone.[1]

RELATED DRUGS: Epinephrine's (eg, *EpiPen*) effect on heart rate was also increased by entacapone. Norepinephrine (eg, *Levophed*) is also metabolized by COMT and may interact similarly.

MANAGEMENT OPTIONS:

➡ *Avoid Unless Benefit Outweighs Risk.* The manufacturer recommends caution if the drugs are used concurrently.

➡ *Monitor.* If the combination is used, monitor cardiovascular status carefully.

REFERENCES:

   1. *Comtan* [package insert]. Parsippany NJ: Novartis Pharmaceuticals; 2008.

Entacapone (*Comtan*)

Methyldopa

SUMMARY: Theoretically, entacapone may inhibit methyldopa metabolism and increase the risk of methyldopa toxicity.

RISK FACTORS: No specific risk factors are known.

MECHANISM: Methyldopa is metabolized by catechol-O-methyltransferase (COMT), and entacapone is a COMT inhibitor.

CLINICAL EVALUATION: Entacapone increased the pharmacologic effects of epinephrine (eg, *EpiPen*) and isoproterenol (eg, *Isuprel*) (both are COMT substrates).[1] Methyldopa is also metabolized by COMT and may interact similarly.

RELATED DRUGS: No information available.

MANAGEMENT OPTIONS:

➡ *Avoid Unless Benefit Outweighs Risk.* The manufacturer recommends caution if the drugs are used concurrently.

➡ *Monitor.* If the combination is used, monitor cardiovascular status carefully.

REFERENCES:

   1. *Comtan* [package insert]. Parsippany NJ: Novartis Pharmaceuticals; 2008.

Entacapone (*Comtan*)

Phenelzine (*Nardil*)

SUMMARY: The combined use of these drugs could inhibit both major pathways for catcholamine metabolism, thus increasing catecholamine response.

RISK FACTORS: No specific risk factors are known.

MECHANISM: Entacapone is a catechol-O-methyltransferase (COMT) inhibitor, and phenelzine is a monoamine oxidase (MAO) inhibitor; because COMT and MAO are the 2 primary pathways of catecholamine metabolism, excessive catecholamine effect could occur.

CLINICAL EVALUATION: This theoretical interaction is based on the potential danger of inhibiting both major pathways for catecholamine metabolism in the body.[1] Although not based on clinical evidence, it is reasonable to assume that the combination may cause adverse reactions.

RELATED DRUGS: Tranylcypromine (eg, *Parnate*), like phenelzine, is a nonselective MAO inhibitor, and may interact similarly with entacapone.

MANAGEMENT OPTIONS:

➡ *Avoid Unless Benefit Outweighs Risk.* This combination is not recommended.

➡ *Monitor.* If the combination is used, monitor cardiovascular status carefully.

REFERENCES:

1. *Comtan* [package insert]. Parsippany NJ: Novartis Pharmaceuticals; 2008.

Ephedrine ▼3

Guanethidine (*Ismelin*)

SUMMARY: Preliminary evidence indicates that ephedrine inhibits the antihypertensive response to guanethidine.

RISK FACTORS: No specific risk factors are known.

MECHANISM: Ephedrine probably antagonizes the adrenergic neuron blockade produced by guanethidine.

CLINICAL EVALUATION: An interaction between ephedrine and guanethidine has been described in several hypertensive patients and is likely to be clinically significant.[1,2,3] Although the effect is not as large as that with amphetamines, it is likely to be sufficient to interfere with control of hypertension.

RELATED DRUGS: Theoretically, one would expect guanadrel (eg, *Hylorel*), a drug pharmacologically similar to guanethidine, to be similarly affected by ephedrine.

MANAGEMENT OPTIONS:

➡ *Monitor.* If ephedrine must be used in a patient receiving guanethidine, closely watch the patient for rising blood pressure. If the guanethidine dosage is increased to compensate for this effect, watch for hypotension when ephedrine is discontinued.

REFERENCES:

1. Starr KJ, et al. Drug interactions in patients on long-term oral anticoagulant and antihypertensive adrenergic neuron-blocking drugs. *BMJ.* 1972;4:133-135.
2. Day MD, et al. Antagonism of guanethidine and bretylium by various agents. *Lancet.* 1962;2:1282.
3. Gulati OD, et al. Antagonism of adrenergic neuron blockade in hypertensive subjects. *Clin Pharmacol Ther.* 1966;7:510-514.

Ephedrine 4

Methyldopa (eg, *Aldomet*)

SUMMARY: Limited clinical information indicates that methyldopa may inhibit the ocular response to ephedrine; whether this applies to other ephedrine effects is unknown.

RISK FACTORS: No specific risk factors are known.

MECHANISM: Methyldopa appears to reduce the amount of norepinephrine available for neuronal release because alpha-methylnorepinephrine acts as a "false" neurotransmitter. Most of ephedrine's sympathomimetic activity is mediated indirectly through the release of norepinephrine. Thus, ephedrine would be expected to be less active in methyldopa-treated patients.

CLINICAL EVALUATION: Clinically, the only descriptions of this interaction have been concerned with the eye, where methyldopa treatment decreased the mydriasis induced by topical ephedrine.[1] Presumably, methyldopa could inhibit the effect of systemically administered ephedrine as well.

RELATED DRUGS: No information is available.

MANAGEMENT OPTIONS: No specific action is required, but be alert for evidence of the interaction.

REFERENCES:
1. Sneddon JM, et al. Ephedrine mydriasis in hypertension and the response to treatment. *Clin Pharmacol Ther.* 1969;10:64-71.

 Ephedrine

Moclobemide†

SUMMARY: Moclobemide substantially enhances the pressor response to ephedrine, and increases the risk of palpitations, headache, and lightheadedness.

RISK FACTORS: No specific risk factors are known.

MECHANISM: Moclobemide inhibits monoamine oxidase-A, an enzyme involved in the metabolism of norepinephrine. Thus, like older nonselective monoamine oxidase inhibitors such as phenelzine (*Nardil*), moclobemide would be expected to increase norepinephrine stores in sympathetic neurons. This increases the response to sympathomimetics with "indirect" activity (such as ephedrine), which causes release of norepinephrine from storage sites resulting in pharmacologic action upon receptors.

CLINICAL EVALUATION: In a randomized, placebo-controlled, crossover study, 12 healthy subjects received 100 mg oral ephedrine (two 50 mg doses 4 hours apart) alone and after pretreatment with moclobemide (300 mg twice daily for 7 to 8 days).[1] Ephedrine in the absence of moclobemide moderately increased both systolic and diastolic blood pressures by up to 30 and 20 mm Hg, respectively. After moclobemide pretreatment, the pressor effect of ephedrine was increased about threefold. In 1 representative subject, the blood pressure increased to 170/100 mm Hg. Palpitations, lightheadedness, and headache were more common with combined therapy than with either drug alone. Although the dose of ephedrine used in this study was relatively large, it was within the recommended therapeutic range.

RELATED DRUGS: Theoretically, the pressor response to other sympathomimetics with significant indirect activity (eg, pseudoephedrine [eg, *Sudafed*]) also would be increased in patients receiving moclobemide.

MANAGEMENT OPTIONS:

➧ *Use Alternative.* Based upon available data, avoid ephedrine in patients receiving moclobemide. Until safety data are available, avoid other indirect acting sympathomimetics (eg, pseudoephedrine) with agents that inhibit MAO-A.

REFERENCES:

1. Dingemanse J. An update of recent moclobemide interaction data. *Int Clin Psychopharmacol.* 1993;7:167-180.

† Not available in the United States.

Ephedrine

Reserpine (eg, *Serpalan*)

SUMMARY: Limited clinical evidence indicates that reserpine may inhibit the pharmacologic effects of ephedrine; more study is needed.

RISK FACTORS: No specific risk factors are known.

MECHANISM: Reserpine depletes norepinephrine from the adrenergic neuron. Much of ephedrine's sympathomimetic activity is mediated indirectly through the release of norepinephrine. Thus, ephedrine would be expected to be less active in reserpine-treated patients.

CLINICAL EVALUATION: Clinically, reserpine treatment has been shown to decrease the mydriasis of topical ephedrine, and it was thought that reserpine also could inhibit, somewhat, the effect of systemically administered ephedrine.[1] However, more clinical information is needed.

RELATED DRUGS: No information is available.

MANAGEMENT OPTIONS: No specific action is required, but be alert for evidence of the interaction.

REFERENCES:

1. Sneddon JM, et al. Ephedrine mydriasis in hypertension and the response to treatment. *Clin Pharmacol Ther.* 1969;10:64-71.

Ephedrine

Theophylline (eg, *Theolair*)

SUMMARY: In 1 study, ephedrine increased theophylline toxicity, but this has not been a consistent finding.

RISK FACTORS: No specific risk factors are known.

MECHANISM: Not established.

CLINICAL EVALUATION: In a study of asthmatic children, the addition of ephedrine to theophylline therapy considerably increased the incidence of adverse reactions such as insomnia, nervousness, and GI complaints.[1] Although ephedrine appeared to increase theophylline side effects, it did not increase the efficacy of treatment. In a subsequent study in 16 asthmatic children, ephedrine enhanced the bronchodilating effects of theophylline but did not enhance its toxicity.[2] The latter study used lower doses of ephedrine than the former, which may account for the conflicting results. More study is needed to assess the clinical importance of the interactions between theophylline and ephedrine. In any case, avoiding fixed-dose combinations of ephedrine and theophylline would facilitate achieving the optimal dose of each drug.

RELATED DRUGS: No information is available.

MANAGEMENT OPTIONS: No specific action is required, but be alert for evidence of the interaction.

REFERENCES:
1. Weinberger M, et al. Interaction of ephedrine and theophylline. *Clin Pharmacol Ther.* 1975;17:586.
2. Tinkelman DG, et al. Ephedrine therapy in asthmatic children. *JAMA.* 1977;237:553.

 Epinephrine (eg, *Adrenalin*)

Imipramine (eg, *Tofranil*)

SUMMARY: The pressor response to IV epinephrine may be markedly enhanced in patients receiving tricyclic antidepressants (TCAs) like imipramine.

RISK FACTORS: No specific risk factors are known.

MECHANISM: Not established.

CLINICAL EVALUATION: IV epinephrine infusions to healthy subjects receiving imipramine resulted in 2- to 4-fold increases in the pressor response to epinephrine.[1,3] In addition, several instances of cardiac dysrhythmias were observed. In another study of 6 healthy subjects, pretreatment with protriptyline (eg, *Vivactil*) 60 mg/day for 4 days enhanced the pressor response to epinephrine infusions considerably.[2] The effect TCA pretreatment would have on the response to epinephrine administered by other routes or in smaller doses is unknown. Little is known about the response to epinephrine when used to treat or prevent anaphylaxis in patients receiving TCAs. Theoretically, the benefit of using epinephrine in such patients would outweigh the risk of a hypertensive reaction; however, clinical evidence is lacking.

RELATED DRUGS: Little is known about the use of epinephrine with other TCAs; assume they interact until proved otherwise.

MANAGEMENT OPTIONS:

➡ ***Avoid Unless Benefit Outweighs Risk.*** Give patients receiving TCAs IV epinephrine only with close monitoring of blood pressure. Some caution should also be exercised if the epinephrine is administered by other routes. However, when epinephrine is used to prevent or treat anaphylaxis, consider the real possibility that the benefit of giving epinephrine will outweigh the risks in such patients.

➡ ***Monitor.*** If IV epinephrine is given to patients receiving TCAs, monitor blood pressure carefully and adjust epinephrine dose as needed.

REFERENCES:
1. Boakes AJ, et al. Interactions between sympathomimetic amines and antidepressant agents in man. *BMJ.* 1973;1:311.
2. Svedmyr N. The influence of a tricyclic antidepressant agent (protriptyline) on some of the circulatory effects of noradrenaline and adrenaline in man. *Life Sci.* 1968;7:77.
3. Boakes AJ. Sympathomimetic amines and antidepressant agents. *BMJ.* 1973;2:114.

Epinephrine (eg, *Adrenalin*)

Phenelzine (*Nardil*)

SUMMARY: Epinephrine does not appear to be potentiated significantly by nonselective monoamine oxidase inhibitors (MAOIs).

RISK FACTORS: No specific factors are known.

MECHANISM: The termination of the pharmacologic response to epinephrine is not primarily dependent upon MAO. Thus, exogenous epinephrine should not be appreciably affected by administration of an MAOI. The small enhancement of epinephrine that sometimes occurs when an MAOI is coadministered may be caused by "denervation supersensitivity" induced by the MAOI.[2-4]

CLINICAL EVALUATION: In 1 study involving 4 healthy subjects, 2 receiving phenelzine and 2 receiving tranylcypromine (*Parnate*), the administration of epinephrine did not affect heart rate or blood pressure significantly.[1]

RELATED DRUGS: Tranylcypromine does not appear to interact.

MANAGEMENT OPTIONS: No specific action is required, but be alert for evidence of the interaction.

REFERENCES:

1. Boakes AJ, et al. Interactions between sympathomimetic amines and antidepressant agents in man. *BMJ.* 1973;1:311.
2. Boakes AJ. Sympathomimetic amines and antidepressant agents. *BMJ.* 1973;2:114.
3. Goldberg LI. Monoamine oxidase inhibitors. Adverse reactions and possible mechanisms. *JAMA.* 1964;190:456.
4. Sjoqvist F. Psychotropic drugs (2). Interaction between monoamine oxidase (MAO) inhibitors and other substances. *Proc R Soc Med.* 1965;58:967.

Epinephrine (eg, *Adrenalin*)

Propranolol (eg, *Inderal*)

SUMMARY: Noncardioselective beta-blockers enhance the pressor response to epinephrine, resulting in hypertension and bradycardia.

RISK FACTORS: No specific risk factors are known.

MECHANISM: Epinephrine alone exerts both alpha-effects (vasoconstriction) and beta-effects (eg, vasodilation, cardiac stimulation). These effects usually result in a mild increase in heart rate and minimal changes in mean arterial pressure. However, when the beta-effects of epinephrine are blocked by propranolol, the alpha-effects predominate. Hypertension and a reflex increase in vagal tone leading to bradycardia are the clinical outcomes.

CLINICAL EVALUATION: There is convincing evidence from studies in hypertensive patients, patients with angina, and healthy subjects that propranolol enhances the pressor response to epinephrine, usually with accompanying bradycardia.[1-6] Severe hypertensive reactions also have been noted following infiltration of lidocaine with epinephrine in plastic surgery patients on chronic propranolol therapy.[7] Propranolol inhibits the pressor and bronchodilator response of epinephrine in patients with anaphylaxis.[8-10] Thus, patients receiving propranolol who develop anaphylaxis may respond poorly to epinephrine injections. Large amounts of IV fluids were required for stabilization in several patients.[10]

RELATED DRUGS: Other nonspecific beta-blockers (eg, alprenolol,[†] nadolol [eg, *Corgard*], pindolol [eg, *Visken*], timolol [eg, *Blocadren*]) would produce a similar effect. Labetalol (eg, *Trandate*, which is a nonspecific beta-blocker as well as an alpha$_1$-blocker) increases the diastolic pressure and slows the heart rate during epinephrine infusions,[11] but acute hypertensive reactions appear unlikely.[12] Metoprolol (eg, *Lopressor*), and perhaps other cardioselective beta-blockers, have minimal effects on the pressor response to epinephrine even at doses of 200 to 300 mg/day.[2-4]

MANAGEMENT OPTIONS:

➡ **Consider Alternative.** Selective beta$_1$-blockers (eg, metoprolol) may be less likely than propranolol to result in hypertension and bradycardia when epinephrine is administered or when endogenous epinephrine is released.

➡ **Monitor.** Administer epinephrine with caution in patients receiving propranolol or other nonselective beta-blockers, and monitor blood pressure carefully. If the epinephrine is used to treat anaphylaxis, the response to epinephrine may be poor and vigorous supportive care (eg, volume replacement) may be needed.

REFERENCES:

1. Gandy W. Severe epinephrine-propranolol interaction. *Ann Emerg Med*. 1989;18:98-99.

2. Houben H, et al. Effect of low-dose epinephrine infusion on hemodynamics after selective and nonselective beta-blockade in hypertension. *Clin Pharmacol Ther*. 1982;31:685-690.

3. Houben H, et al. Influence of selective and non-selective beta-adrenoreceptor blockade on the haemodynamic effect of adrenaline during combined antihypertensive drug therapy. *Clin Sci*. 1979;57(suppl 5):397s-399s.

4. van Herwaarden CL, et al. Haemodynamic effects of adrenaline during treatment of hypertensive patients with propranolol and metoprolol. *Eur J Clin Pharmacol*. 1977;12:397-402.

5. Hansbrough JF. Propranolol-epinephrine antagonism with hypertension and stroke. *Ann Intern Med*. 1980;92:717.

6. Lampman RM, et al. Cardiac arrhythmias during epinephrine-propranolol infusions for measurement of in vivo insulin resistance. *Diabetes*. 1981;30:618-620.

7. Foster CA, et al. Propranolol-epinephrine interaction: a potential disaster. *Plast Reconstr Surg*. 1983;72:74-78.

8. Newman BR, et al. Epinephrine-resistant anaphylaxis in a patient taking propranolol hydrochloride. *Ann Allergy*. 1981;47:35-37.

9. Jacobs RL, et al. Potentiated anaphylaxis in patients with drug-induced beta-adrenergic blockade. *J Allergy Clin Immunol*. 1981;68:125-127.

10. Hannaway PJ, et al. Severe anaphylaxis and drug-induced beta-blockade. *N Engl J Med*. 1983;308:1536.

11. Richards DA, et al. Circulatory effects of noradrenaline and adrenaline before and after labetalol. *Br J Clin Pharmacol*. 1979;7:371-378.

12. Doshi BS, et al. Effects of labetalol and propranolol on responses to adrenaline infusion in healthy volunteers. *Int J Clin Pharmacol Res*. 1984;4:29-33.

† Not available in the United States.

Eplerenone (*Inspra*)

Candesartan (*Atacand*)

SUMMARY: Combining eplerenone with candesartan or other angiotensin II receptor blockers (ARBs) may increase the risk of hyperkalemia, especially in patients with 1 or more risk factors.

RISK FACTORS:

➡ **Other Drugs.** CYP3A4 inhibitors such as itraconazole, ketoconazole, erythromycin, clarithromycin, diltiazem, verapamil, and protease inhibitors may increase eplerenone serum concentrations and may increase the risk of hyperkalemia. Also, the addition of other hyperkalemic drugs may increase the risk of hyperkalemia in patients on eplerenone and ARBs. Hyperkalemic drugs include ACE inhibitors, potassium supplements, cyclosporine, tacrolimus, NSAIDs, COX-2 inhibitors, non-selective beta-adrenergic blockers, trimethoprim, and pentamidine.

➡ **Concurrent Diseases.** Diseases that increase the risk of hyperkalemia for this interaction include diabetes and significant renal impairment.

➡ **Diet/Food.** A diet high in potassium may increase the risk of hyperkalemia from this interaction. Salt substitutes may contain potassium.

MECHANISM: Both eplerenone and ARBs tend to increase serum potassium, and their effects are additive.

CLINICAL EVALUATION: Forty-four cases of life-threatening hyperkalemia in patients receiving either ARBs or ACE inhibitors in combination with spironolactone have been described.[1] It is likely that eplerenone would also increase the risk of hyperkalemia when combined with ARBs or ACE inhibitors, especially in patients with 1 or more risk factors.

RELATED DRUGS: Eplerenone can be expected to increase the risk of hyperkalemia when combined with other ARBs, including eprosartan (*Teveten*), irbesartan (*Avapro*), losartan (*Cozaar*), telmisartan (*Micardis*), and valsartan (*Diovan*).

MANAGEMENT OPTIONS:

➡ **Monitor.** In patients receiving eplerenone and an ARB, monitor serum potassium and renal function, particularly if the patient has 1 or more of the risk factors listed above.

REFERENCES:
1. Wrenger E, et al. Interaction of spironolactone with ACE inhibitors or antiogensin receptor blockers: analysis of 44 cases. *BMJ*. 2003;327:147-149.

Eplerenone (*Inspra*)

Enalapril (eg, *Vasotec*)

SUMMARY: Combining eplerenone with enalapril or other ACE inhibitors may increase the risk of hyperkalemia, especially in patients with 1 or more risk factors.

RISK FACTORS:

➡ ***Other Drugs.*** In patients on eplerenone and ACE inhibitors, the addition of other hyperkalemic drugs can increase the risk. Such drugs include potassium supplements, nonselective beta-adrenergic blockers, cyclosporine, tacrolimus, NSAIDs, COX-2 inhibitors, trimethoprim, and pentamidine.

➡ ***Concurrent Diseases.*** Diseases that increase the risk of hyperkalemia for this interaction include diabetes and significant renal impairment.

➡ ***Diet/Food.*** A diet high in potassium may increase the risk of hyperkalemia from this interaction. Some salt substitutes contain potassium.

MECHANISM: Both eplerenone and ACE inhibitors tend to increase serum potassium, and their effects are additive.

CLINICAL EVALUATION: Most of the cases of hyperkalemia in patients receiving concurrent therapy with potassium-sparing diuretics and ACE inhibitors have involved spironolactone. The RALES study, which involved the use of spironolactone and ACE inhibitors, found only a 2% risk of hyperkalemia.[1] But reports of severe and fatal hyperkalemia have started to appear, especially in patients with risk factors.[2-6] The difference is likely caused by the fact that patients in the RALES study were much more carefully monitored and received lower doses of spironolactone. There is not as much information on concurrent use of eplerenone and ACE inhibitors, but it is likely that such combinations also increase the risk of hyperkalemia in predisposed patients.

RELATED DRUGS: Eplerenone would also be expected to interact with other ACE inhibitors, including benazepril (*Lotensin*), captopril (eg, *Capoten*), fosinopril (*Monopril*), lisinopril (eg, *Prinivil*), moexipril (eg, *Univasc*), quinapril (*Accupril*), ramipril (*Altace*), and trandolapril (*Mavik*).

MANAGEMENT OPTIONS:

➡ ***Monitor.*** In patients receiving eplerenone and an ACE inhibitor, monitor serum potassium and renal function, particularly if the patient has 1 or more of the risk factors listed above.

REFERENCES:

1. Pitt B, Zannad F, Remme WJ, et al. The effect of spironolactone on morbidity and mortality in patients with severe heart failure. Randomized Aldactone Evaluation Study Investigators. *New Engl J Med.* 1999;341:709-717.

2. Schepkens H, et al. Life-threatening hyperkalemia during combined therapy with angiotensin-converting enzyme inhibitors and spironolactone. *Am J Med.* 2001;110:438-441.

3. Berry C, McMurray J. Life-threatening hyperkalemia during combined therapy with angiotensin-converting enzyme inhibitors and spironolactone. *Am J Med.* 2001;111:587.

4. Blaustein DA, et al. Estimation of glomerular filtration rate to prevent life-threatening hyperkalemia due to combined therapy with spironolactone and antiotensin-converting enzyme inhibition or antiotensin receptor blockade. *Am J Cardiol.* 2002;90:662-663.

5. Wrenger E, et al. Interaction of spironolactone with ACE inhibitors or antiogensin receptor blockers: analysis of 44 cases. *BMJ.* 2003;327:147-149.

6. Weber EW, et al. Incidence of hyperkalemia in chronic heart failure patients taking spironolactone in a VA medical center. *Pharmacotherapy*. 2003;23:391.

Eprosartan (*Teveten*) 5

Fluconazole (*Diflucan*)

SUMMARY: The coadministration of fluconazole and eprosartan does not alter the pharmacokinetics of eprosartan. No change in pharmacodynamic response is likely.

RISK FACTORS: No specific risk factors are known.

MECHANISM: No interaction.

CLINICAL EVALUATION: Sixteen healthy subjects received eprosartan 300 mg/day for 20 days.[1] On days 11 through 20, they also received fluconazole 200 mg/day. Eprosartan pharmacokinetics were estimated on days 10 and 20. The pharmacokinetics of eprosartan on day 20, following 10 days of concomitant fluconazole, were unchanged compared with those on day 10. No change in the response to eprosartan would be expected.

RELATED DRUGS: Fluconazole has been reported to increase the plasma concentrations of losartan (*Cozaar*), a related angiotensin II inhibitor. The effects of other antifungal agents on eprosartan are unknown, but they would not be expected to affect eprosartan pharmacokinetics or clinical efficacy. Eprosartan does not appear to be metabolized by the cytochrome P450 enzyme system.

MANAGEMENT OPTIONS: No interaction.

REFERENCES:

1. Kazierad DJ, et al. Effect of fluconazole on the pharmacokinetics of eprosartan and losartan in healthy male volunteers. *Clin Pharmacol Ther*. 1997;62:417-425.

Ergotamine (*Ergomar*)

Indinavir (*Crixivan*)

SUMMARY: Indinavir is likely to increase the plasma concentrations of ergotamine, possibly leading to toxicity including vasospasm and cyanosis.

RISK FACTORS: No specific risk factors are known.

MECHANISM: Indinavir inhibits the activity of CYP3A4, the enzyme known to metabolize ergotamine.

CLINICAL EVALUATION: A patient with HIV was treated with lamivudine (*Epivir*), stavudine (*Zerit*), indinavir, and co-trimoxazole (eg, *Bactrim*).[1] He was prescribed 2 tablets containing ergotamine 1 mg and caffeine 100 mg/day for migraine. He took the ergotamine for 3 days. Five days following the last dose of ergotamine, he presented with cyanosis and numbness in the toes on one foot. This was followed by cramps and intermittent claudication of the same limb. Translumbar aortography demonstrated vasospasm consistent with ergotism. Three days after discontinuing the antiretroviral therapy, his symptoms were relieved.

RELATED DRUGS: Other protease inhibitors such as ritonavir (*Norvir*), amprenavir (*Agenerase*), nelfinavir (*Viracept*), and saquinavir (eg, *Fortovase*) would be expected to affect ergotamine in a similar manner.

MANAGEMENT OPTIONS:

➡ *Use Alternative.* If possible, avoid ergot derivatives in patients taking protease inhibitors.

➡ *Monitor.* If ergotamine is administered to a patient taking a protease inhibitor, start the patient on low doses of ergotamine and monitor carefully for any signs of ergotism.

REFERENCES:

1. Rosenthal E, et al. Ergotism related to concurrent administration of ergotamine tartrate and indinavir. *JAMA.* 1999;281:987.

  Ergotamine (*Ergomar*)

Nitroglycerin (*eg, Nitrostat*)

SUMMARY: Ergotamine may oppose the coronary vasodilation of nitrates.

RISK FACTORS: No specific risk factors are known.

MECHANISM: Ergotamine can precipitate angina, and nitroglycerin can reduce the first-pass hepatic metabolism of dihydroergotamine (eg, *Migranol*).

CLINICAL EVALUATION: Ergotamine is known to precipitate angina pectoris and is used as a provocative agent in angina studies. Also, nitroglycerin markedly enhanced the bioavailability of dihydroergotamine in a study of 6 patients with orthostatic hypotension.[1]

RELATED DRUGS: No information is available.

MANAGEMENT OPTIONS:

➡ *Avoid Unless Benefit Outweighs Risk.* Patients receiving nitroglycerin for angina pectoris should avoid ergotamine if at all possible.

➡ *Monitor.* If the combination is used, monitor patients for enhanced ergotamine effect and lower the ergot dosage as needed.

REFERENCES:

1. Bobik A, et al. Low oral bioavailability of dihydroergotamine and first-pass extraction in patients with orthostatic hypotension. *Clin Pharmacol Ther.* 1981;30:673-679.

  Ergotamine (*Ergomar*)

Propranolol (eg, *Inderal*)

SUMMARY: In some patients, propranolol may enhance the vasoconstrictive action of ergotamine.

RISK FACTORS: No specific risk factors are known.

MECHANISM: Some have proposed that propranolol blocks the natural pathway for vasodilation in patients receiving vasoconstrictors such as ergotamine.[1] The potential adverse result of this combination would be excessive vasoconstriction.

CLINICAL EVALUATION: A patient with migraine headaches who was taking ergotamine-caffeine (eg, *Cafergot*) suppositories, developed purple and painful feet after being placed on propranolol 30 mg/day.[1] This case may represent ergotism from excessive ergotamine use rather than a drug interaction. Additional cases describing patients taking ergotamine and propranolol who developed peripheral ischemia,[2] exacerbation of migraine attacks[3] (refractory to *Cafergot*), and hypertension with chest pain[4] have been reported. A number of patients have received ergotamine plus propranolol with no obvious ill effects.[1,5] If an interaction between propranolol and ergotamine does exist, it occurs rarely.

RELATED DRUGS: A similar interaction may occur with other beta-blockers.

MANAGEMENT OPTIONS: No specific action is required, but be alert for evidence of an interaction.

REFERENCES:

1. Baumrucker JF. Drug-interaction—propranolol and cafergot. *N Engl J Med.* 1973;288:916-917.
2. Venter CP, et al. Severe peripheral ischaemia during concomitant use of beta blockers and ergot alkaloids. *Br Med J.* 1984;289:288-289.
3. Blank NK, Rieder MJ. Letter: Paradoxical response to propranolol in migraine. *Lancet.* 1973;2:1336.
4. Gandy W. Dihydroergotamine interaction with propranolol. *Ann Emerg Med.* 1990;19:221.
5. Diamond S. Propranolol and ergotamine tartrate. *N Engl J Med.* 1973;289:159.

Ergotamine (*Ergomar*)

Ritonavir (*Norvir*)

SUMMARY: Ritonavir is likely to increase the plasma concentrations of ergotamine, possibly leading to toxicity including vasospasm and cyanosis.

RISK FACTORS: No specific risk factors are known.

MECHANISM: Ritonavir inhibits the activity of CYP3A4, the enzyme known to metabolize ergotamine.

CLINICAL EVALUATION: A patient with HIV and migraine headaches was taking ergotamine 1 to 2 mg/day for several years. His HIV therapy was changed to include zidovudine (eg, *Retrovir*), didanosine (eg, *Videx*), and ritonavir 600 mg twice daily.[1] Approximately 1 week after the change in HIV therapy, he developed pain, paresthesias, and cyanosis of both arms and hands with absence of blood flow in both the radial and ulnar arteries. Following discontinuation of ritonavir, ergotamine, and vasodilator therapy, the symptoms resolved.

RELATED DRUGS: Other protease inhibitors such as indinavir (*Crixivan*), amprenavir (*Agenerase*), nelfinavir (*Viracept*), and saquinavir (*Invirase*) are likely to affect ergotamine in a similar manner.

MANAGEMENT OPTIONS:

➡ *Use Alternative.* If possible, avoid ergot derivatives in patients taking protease inhibitors.

➡ *Monitor.* If ergotamine is administered to a patient taking a protease inhibitor, start the patient on low doses of ergotamine and monitor carefully for any signs of ergotism.

REFERENCES:

1. Caballero-Granado FJ, et al. Ergotism related to concurrent administration of ergotamine tartrate and ritonavir in an AIDS patient. *Antimicrob Agents Chemother.* 1997;41:1207.

Ergotamine (*Ergomar*)

AVOID **Sumatriptan (*Imitrex*)**

SUMMARY: Do not administer sumatriptan or other triptans within 24 hours of ergotamine.

RISK FACTORS: No specific risk factors are known.

MECHANISM: Additive pharmacodynamic effects.

CLINICAL EVALUATION: The product information for *Imitrex* (sumatriptan) states that it should not be used within 24 hours of ergotamine because excessive (additive) vasoconstriction may occur.[1] Although this is based primarily on theoretical considerations, the adverse effect could be severe, and concurrent use may present medicolegal risks as well.

RELATED DRUGS: All other triptans such as almotriptan (*Axert*), eletriptan (*Relpax*), frovatriptan (*Frova*), naratriptan (*Amerge*), rizatriptan (*Maxalt*), and zolmitriptan (*Zomig*) are also contraindicated within 24 hours of ergotamine or other ergot alkaloids.

MANAGEMENT OPTIONS:

➡ ***AVOID COMBINATION.*** Do not administer sumatriptan and other triptans within 24 hours of ergotamine or other ergot alkaloids.

REFERENCES:
1. *Imitrex* [package insert]. Research Triangle Park, NC: GlaxoSmithKline; 2006.

 Ergotamine (*Ergomar*)

Tacrolimus (*Prograf*)

SUMMARY: Drug interaction studies using human liver microsomes in vitro suggest that ergotamine inhibits the metabolism of tacrolimus; watch for excessive tacrolimus if the drugs are used concurrently.

RISK FACTORS: No specific risk factors are known.

MECHANISM: Tacrolimus is metabolized by CYP3A4, and ergotamine appears to inhibit this process.

CLINICAL EVALUATION: Thirty-four drugs were tested for interactions with tacrolimus using in vitro human liver microsomal preparations.[1] Ergotamine was found to inhibit tacrolimus metabolism. Although the clinical importance of this finding is not established, in vitro human microsomal studies have been remarkably accurate in predicting which drugs will interact in the clinical setting.

RELATED DRUGS: The effect of ergotamine on cyclosporine (eg, *Sandimmune*) is not established, but cyclosporine and tacrolimus tend to have similar drug interactions.

MANAGEMENT OPTIONS: No specific action is required, but be alert for evidence of the interaction.

REFERENCES:
1. Christians U, et al. Identification of drugs inhibiting the in vitro metabolism of tacrolimus by human liver microsomes. *Br J Clin Pharmacol.* 1996;41(3):187-190.

Ergotamine (*Ergomar*)

Voriconazole (*Vfend*)

SUMMARY: Elevated ergotamine concentrations and toxicity may occur if voriconazole and ergotamine are coadministered.

RISK FACTORS: No specific risk factors are known.

MECHANISM: Voriconazole is known to inhibit CYP3A4, the enzyme responsible for ergotamine metabolism.

CLINICAL EVALUATION: While specific data are lacking, the manufacturer of voriconazole contraindicates the coadministration of ergotamine and voriconazole.[1] Coadministration may lead to hypertension or cyanosis.

RELATED DRUGS: Other ergot drugs, including dihydroergotamine (eg, *Migranal*) and methylergonovine (*Methergine*), may be affected in a similar manner by voriconazole. Itraconazole (eg, *Sporanox*), ketoconazole (eg, *Nizoral*), and fluconazole (eg, *Diflucan*) may produce increased ergotamine plasma concentrations, thus increasing the risk of toxicity.

MANAGEMENT OPTIONS:

➡ *Use Alternative.* Do not administer voriconazole or any antifungal agent known to inhibit CYP3A4 to patients receiving ergotamine. Consider terbinafine (eg, *Lamisil*) as an alternative because it does not affect CYP3A4 activity.

➡ *Monitor.* If voriconazole is coadministered with ergotamine, monitor the patient for evidence of excess vasoconstriction.

REFERENCES:

1. *Vfend* [package insert]. New York, NY: Pfizer, Inc; 2003.

Erlotinib (*Tarceva*)

Atazanavir (*Reyataz*)

SUMMARY: The coadministration of erlotinib and atazanavir may result in increased erlotinib plasma concentrations; be alert for erlotinib toxicity.

RISK FACTORS: No specific risk factors are known.

MECHANISM: Atazanavir inhibits CYP3A4, the enzyme primarily responsible for erlotinib metabolism.

CLINICAL EVALUATION: Ketoconazole (eg, *Nizoral*) was shown to substantially increase the erlotinib area under the plasma concentration-time curve.[1] Other CYP3A4 inhibitors, such as atazanavir, are expected to have a similar effect.

RELATED DRUGS: Other HIV drugs that inhibit CYP3A4 and may interact with erlotinib include darunavir (*Prezista*), delavirdine (*Rescriptor*), fosamprenavir (*Lexiva*), indinavir (*Crixivan*), nelfinavir (*Viracept*), ritonavir (*Norvir*), and saquinavir (*Invirase*).

MANAGEMENT OPTIONS:

➡ *Consider Alternative.* If possible, avoid atazanavir or other CYP3A4 inhibitors in patients taking erlotinib.

➡️ **Monitor.** If the combination is used, monitor patients for increased erlotinib toxicity (eg, diarrhea, rash, stomatitis). Erlotinib dosage may need to be adjusted.

REFERENCES:

1. *Tarceva* [package insert]. South San Francisco, CA: Genentech, Inc; 2008.

Erlotinib (*Tarceva*)

Carbamazepine (eg, *Tegretol*)

SUMMARY: The coadministration of erlotinib and carbamazepine may result in decreased erlotinib plasma concentrations; be alert for reduced erlotinib efficacy.

RISK FACTORS: No specific risk factors are known.

MECHANISM: Carbamazepine induces CYP3A4, the enzyme primarily responsible for the metabolism of erlotinib.

CLINICAL EVALUATION: Rifampin (eg, *Rifadin*) reduced the erlotinib area under the plasma concentration-time curve by 66%.[1] It is likely that other enzyme inducers, such as carbamazepine, would have a similar effect (although probably lesser in magnitude).

RELATED DRUGS: Other enzyme-inducing anticonvulsants that theoretically may also reduce erlotinib efficacy include barbiturates, oxcarbazepine (eg, *Trileptal*), primidone (eg, *Mysoline*), and phenytoin (eg, *Dilantin*).

MANAGEMENT OPTIONS:

➡️ **Consider Alternative.** If possible, avoid enzyme inducers in patients receiving erlotinib. Consider the use of valproic acid or other agents that do not induce CYP3A4.

➡️ **Monitor.** If the combination is used, monitor patients for reduced erlotinib efficacy.

REFERENCES:

1. *Tarceva* [package insert]. South San Francisco, CA: Genentech, Inc; 2008.

Erlotinib (*Tarceva*)

Clarithromycin (eg, *Biaxin*)

SUMMARY: The coadministration of erlotinib and clarithromycin may result in increased erlotinib plasma concentrations; be alert for erlotinib toxicity.

RISK FACTORS: No specific risk factors are known.

MECHANISM: Clarithromycin inhibits CYP3A4, the enzyme primarily responsible for the metabolism of erlotinib.

CLINICAL EVALUATION: Ketoconazole (eg, *Nizoral*) was shown to substantially increase the erlotinib area under the plasma concentration-time curve.[1] Other CYP3A4 inhibitors, such as clarithromycin, are expected to have a similar effect, although the magnitude may be less in some cases.

RELATED DRUGS: Erythromycin (eg, *EryTab*), telithromycin (*Ketek*), and troleandomycin[+] are moderate to potent inhibitors of CYP3A4 and may interact with erlotinib. However, azithromycin (eg, *Zithromax*) has little effect on CYP3A4.

MANAGEMENT OPTIONS:

➡ *Consider Alternative.* Avoid clarithromycin or other CYP3A4 inhibitors in patients taking erlotinib. Theoretically, azithromycin would be less likely to interact.

➡ *Monitor.* If the combination is used, monitor patients for increased erlotinib toxicity (eg, diarrhea, rash, stomatitis). Erlotinib dosage may need to be adjusted.

REFERENCES:

1. *Tarceva* [package insert]. South San Francisco, CA: Genentech, Inc; 2008.

† Not available in the United States.

Erlotinib (*Tarceva*)

Grapefruit Juice

SUMMARY: The coadministration of erlotinib and grapefruit juice or grapefruit may result in increased erlotinib plasma concentrations; be alert for erlotinib toxicity.

RISK FACTORS: No specific risk factors are known.

MECHANISM: Grapefruit juice inhibits CYP3A4, the enzyme primarily responsible for erlotinib metabolism.

CLINICAL EVALUATION: Ketoconazole (eg, *Nizoral*) was shown to substantially increase erlotinib area under the plasma concentration-time curve.[1] Other CYP3A4 inhibitors, such as grapefruit juice, are expected to have a similar effect.

RELATED DRUGS: Theoretically, orange juice would not be expected to interact with erlotinib.

MANAGEMENT OPTIONS:

➡ *Consider Alternative.* Avoid grapefruit juice in patients taking erlotinib.

➡ *Monitor.* Monitor patients receiving erlotinib for increased toxicity (eg, diarrhea, rash, stomatitis) if grapefruit juice is taken concomitantly.

REFERENCES:

1. *Tarceva* [package insert]. South San Francisco, CA: Genentech, Inc; 2008.

Erlotinib (*Tarceva*)

Ketoconazole (eg, *Nizoral*)

SUMMARY: The coadministration of erlotinib and ketoconazole results in an increase in erlotinib plasma concentrations; be alert for erlotinib-associated adverse reactions.

RISK FACTORS: No specific risk factors are known.

MECHANISM: Ketoconazole inhibits CYP3A4, the enzyme primarily responsible for erlotinib metabolism.

CLINICAL EVALUATION: While specific data are limited, the manufacturer of erlotinib notes that the coadministration of ketoconazole increased the area under the plasma concentration-time curve of erlotinib 66%.[1] Monitor patients taking erlotinib for adverse reactions (eg, diarrhea, rash, stomatitis) while they are receiving ketoconazole or other potent inhibitors of CYP3A4.

RELATED DRUGS: Other antifungal agents that inhibit CYP3A4 (eg, itraconazole [eg, *Sporanox*], voriconazole [*Vfend*], fluconazole [eg, *Diflucan*]) are likely to affect erlotinib in a similar manner.

MANAGEMENT OPTIONS:

➡ *Consider Alternative.* Terbinafine (eg, *Lamisil*) does not affect CYP3A4 activity and could be an alternative antifungal agent.

➡ *Monitor.* Monitor patients receiving erlotinib who require antifungal therapy with ketoconazole for possible increased adverse reactions.

REFERENCES:

1. *Tarceva* [package insert]. Melville, NY: OSI Pharmaceuticals; 2004.

Erlotinib (*Tarceva*)

Nefazodone

SUMMARY: The coadministration of erlotinib and nefazodone may result in increased erlotinib plasma concentrations; be alert for erlotinib toxicity.

RISK FACTORS: No specific risk factors are known.

MECHANISM: Nefazodone inhibits CYP3A4, the enzyme primarily responsible for the metabolism of erlotinib.

CLINICAL EVALUATION: Ketoconazole substantially increases erlotinib area under the plasma concentration-time curve.[1] Other CYP3A4 inhibitors, such as nefazodone, are expected to have a similar effect.

RELATED DRUGS: Most antidepressants other than nefazodone, such as selective serotonin reuptake inhibitors or tricyclic antidepressants, have little or no effect on CYP3A4, but mild to moderate inhibition of CYP3A4 can occur with fluoxetine (eg, *Prozac*) or fluvoxamine (eg, *Luvox CR*).

MANAGEMENT OPTIONS:

➡ *Consider Alternative.* Avoid nefazodone in patients taking erlotinib. Most other antidepressants are less likely to interact (see Related Drugs).

➡ *Monitor.* If the combination is used, monitor patients for increased erlotinib toxicity (eg, diarrhea, rash, stomatitis). Erlotinib dosage may need to be adjusted.

REFERENCES:

1. *Tarceva* [package insert]. South San Francisco, CA: Genentech, Inc; 2008.

Erlotinib (*Tarceva*)

Omeprazole (eg, *Prilosec*)

SUMMARY: Omeprazole administration decreased the plasma concentration of erlotinib; patients may experience a decrease in the efficacy of erlotinib.

RISK FACTORS: No specific risk factors are known.

MECHANISM: Omeprazole appears to reduce the absorption of erlotinib, probably by increasing gastric pH.

CLINICAL EVALUATION: While specific data are limited, the coadministration of erlotinib and omeprazole (dose not stated) decreased the mean area under the plasma concentration-time curve of erlotinib 46%.[1] Peak erlotinib concentrations were reduced 61%. Pending further data, monitor patients receiving erlotinib and omeprazole for reduced erlotinib efficacy.

RELATED DRUGS: Esomeprazole (*Nexium*), pantoprazole (eg, *Protonix*), rabeprazole (*Aciphex*), and lansoprazole (*Prevacid*) are expected to interact with erlotinib in a similar manner. H_2-receptor antagonists and antacids may also reduce the absorption of erlotinib.

MANAGEMENT OPTIONS:

➡ *Monitor.* Be alert for reduced erlotinib efficacy in patients taking proton pump inhibitors or H_2-receptor antagonists. If antacids are used, separate the dose of the antacid and erlotinib by several hours to minimize the potential interaction.

REFERENCES:

1. *Tarceva* [package insert]. South San Francisco, CA: Genentech USA Inc; 2008.

Erlotinib (*Tarceva*)

Rifampin (eg, *Rifadin*)

SUMMARY: The coadministration of erlotinib and rifampin results in a decrease in erlotinib plasma concentrations; be alert for reduced erlotinib efficacy.

RISK FACTORS: No specific risk factors are known.

MECHANISM: Rifampin induces CYP3A4, the enzyme primarily responsible for erlotinib metabolism.

CLINICAL EVALUATION: While specific data are limited, the coadministration of erlotinib and rifampin reduced the area under the plasma concentration-time curve of erlotinib 66% and increased the clearance of erlotinib 3-fold.[1] Monitor patients receiving rifampin or other CYP3A4 inducers while taking erlotinib for reduced therapeutic effect. An increased dose of erlotinib may be required during rifampin coadministration.

RELATED DRUGS: Rifabutin (*Mycobutin*) may affect erlotinib in a similar manner.

MANAGEMENT OPTIONS:

➡ *Monitor.* Monitor patients receiving erlotinib with rifampin for reduced efficacy.

REFERENCES:

1. *Tarceva* [package insert]. Melville, NY: OSI Pharmaceuticals; 2004.

Erlotinib (*Tarceva*)

St. John's Wort

SUMMARY: The coadministration of erlotinib and St. John's wort may result in decreased erlotinib plasma concentrations; be alert for reduced erlotinib efficacy.

RISK FACTORS: No specific risk factors are known.

MECHANISM: St. John's wort induces CYP3A4, the enzyme primarily responsible for the metabolism of erlotinib.

CLINICAL EVALUATION: Rifampin reduced the erlotinib area under the plasma concentration-time curve 66%,[1] and it is likely that other enzyme inducers, such as St. John's wort, would have a similar effect (although probably lesser in magnitude).

RELATED DRUGS: No information is available.

MANAGEMENT OPTIONS:

➥ *Consider Alternative.* Given questions about the efficacy of St. John's wort, it may be advisable to use an alternative in patients taking erlotinib.

➥ *Monitor.* Monitor patients receiving erlotinib for reduced efficacy if St. John's wort is taken concomitantly. Note that herbal medications are often not standardized, and different herbal brands may interact differently because of varying content of the active ingredient or additional ingredients not mentioned on the label. Moreover, different lots of the same brand may vary substantially in content.

REFERENCES:
1. *Tarceva* [package insert]. South San Francisco, CA: Genentech Inc; 2008.

Ertapenem (*Invanz*)

Valproic Acid (eg, *Depakene*)

SUMMARY: The administration of ertapenem reduces the serum concentration of valproic acid; loss of seizure control is possible.

RISK FACTORS: No specific risk factors are known.

MECHANISM: The mechanism of this interaction is unclear, but it appears that ertapenem inhibits valproic acid–glucuronidase, an enzyme that converts valproic acid–glucuronide back into valproic acid.

CLINICAL EVALUATION: A patient stabilized on divalproex 2,000 mg daily had a serum valproic acid concentration of 120 to 130 mcg/mL.[1] Six days after initiation of ertapenem 1 g daily, the patient experienced a recurrence of seizures and his valproic acid concentration was noted to be 70 mcg/mL. Despite increased divalproex dosage, his valproic acid levels continued to fall, reaching a nadir of 10.7 mcg/mL. Ertapenem was discontinued and his valproic acid concentrations increased back to therapeutic levels over the following 5 days.

RELATED DRUGS: Other drugs in the carbapenem class, such as meropenem (*Merrem*), imipenem (eg, *Primaxin*), and panipenem, have also been implicated in reducing valproic acid concentration.[2-4]

MANAGEMENT OPTIONS:

➥ *Consider Alternative.* If possible, consider an alternative antibiotic to a carbapenem if the patient is also taking valproic acid.

➥ ***Monitor.*** If ertapenem is administered with valproic acid, monitor valproic acid concentrations and adjust doses as necessary.

REFERENCES:

1. Lunde JL, et al. Acute seizures in a patient receiving divalproex sodium after starting ertapenem therapy. *Pharmacotherapy*. 2007;27(8):1202-1205.
2. Mori H, et al. Interaction between valproic acid and carbapenem antibiotics. *Drug Metab Rev*. 2007;39(4):647-657.
3. Haroutiunian S, et al. Valproic acid plasma concentration decreases in a dose-independent manner following administration of meropenem: a retrospective study. *J Clin Pharmacol*. 2009;49(11):1363-1369.
4. Nakamura Y, et al. Decreased valproate level caused by VPA-glucuronidase inhibition by carbapenem antibiotics. *Drug Metab Lett*. 2008;2(4):280-285.

Erythromycin 3

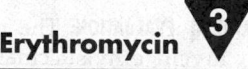

Clopidogrel (*Plavix*)

SUMMARY: Erythromycin appears to inhibit the antiplatelet effects of clopidogrel, but the extent to which the therapeutic effects of clopidogrel are reduced is not known.

RISK FACTORS: No specific risk factors are known.

MECHANISM: Clopidogrel is a prodrug, and CYP3A4 appears to be the primary isozyme involved in formation of the active metabolite.[1] Erythromycin is a CYP3A4 inhibitor, and probably inhibits the conversion of clopidogrel to its active metabolite.

CLINICAL EVALUATION: Nineteen healthy subjects were given clopidogrel (75 mg/day for 6 days) alone and with erythromycin (250 mg 4 times daily).[2] Erythromycin was associated with a reduction in the ability of clopidogrel to inhibit platelet aggregation. With clopidogrel alone, platelet aggregation was 42%, but with concurrent erythromycin, platelet aggregation increased to 55% of control. It is not known if this modest inhibition of clopidogrel effect would reduce the therapeutic effects of clopidogrel.

RELATED DRUGS: Troleandomycin (*TAO*) also appears to inhibit the antiplatelet effects of clopidogrel. Clarithromycin (Biaxin) is also an inhibitor of CYP3A4 and would theoretically interact with clopidogrel in a similar manner.

MANAGEMENT OPTIONS:

➥ ***Consider Alternative.*** Theoretically, azithromycin (*Zithromax*) and dirithromycin (*Dynabac*) would be unlikely to interact with clopidogrel since they do not inhibit CYP3A4.

➥ ***Monitor.*** Consider monitoring platelet function if erythromycin is initiated or discontinued. Adjustments in clopidogrel dose may be needed.

REFERENCES:

1. Clarke TA, et al. The metabolism of clopidogrel is catalyzed by human cytochrome P450 3A and is inhibited by atorvastatin. *Drug Metab Dispos*. 2003;31:53-59.
2. Lau WC, et al. Atorvastatin reduces the ability of clopidogrel to inhibit platelet aggregation: a new drug-drug interaction. *Circulation*. 2003;107:32-37.

Erythromycin (eg, *EryPed*)

Ethanol (*Ethyl Alcohol*)

SUMMARY: Erythromycin ethylsuccinate plasma concentrations are reduced by ethanol coadministration; clinically significant changes are unlikely.

RISK FACTORS: No specific risk factors are known.

MECHANISM: Ethanol appears to reduce the rate and extent of erythromycin ethylsuccinate absorption, perhaps by decreasing GI motility. Erythromycin may increase ethanol absorption when low doses of ethanol are administered.

CLINICAL EVALUATION: The mean peak erythromycin concentration following erythromycin ethylsuccinate 500 mg was decreased 15% and the area under the concentration-time curve (AUC) was decreased 27% following ethanol administration of 250 mg/kg.[1] One subject experienced decreased erythromycin absorption following water administration and an increased AUC (almost 2-fold) after ethanol administration. Other studies have found either no effect of erythromycin on alcohol (0.8 g/kg orally) or an increased alcohol (0.5 g/kg orally) concentration after erythromycin.[2,3] Differences between studies also may be accounted for by the dose of erythromycin used and route of administration. The clinical significance of these effects requires further study.

RELATED DRUGS: No information is available.

MANAGEMENT OPTIONS:

➡ *Circumvent/Minimize.* Counsel patients taking erythromycin ethylsuccinate to avoid ingesting alcoholic beverages with the antibiotic. An increase in ethanol effects may be noted in some patients.

➡ *Monitor.* Alert patients for enhanced ethanol effects during coadministration of erythromycin.

REFERENCES:

1. Morasso MI, et al. Influence of alcohol consumption on erythromycin ethylsuccinate kinetics. *Int J Clin Pharmacol Ther Toxicol.* 1990;28:426-429.
2. Min DI, et al. Effect of erythromycin on ethanol's pharmacokinetics and perception of intoxication. *Pharmacotherapy.* 1995;15:164-169.
3. Edelbroek MA, et al. Effects of erythromycin on gastric emptying, alcohol absorption and small intestinal transit in normal subjects. *J Nucl Med.* 1993;34:582-188.

Erythromycin (eg, *E-Mycin*)

Felbamate (*Felbatol*)

SUMMARY: Erythromycin did not alter felbamate plasma concentrations.

RISK FACTORS: No specific risk factors are known.

MECHANISM: No interaction.

CLINICAL EVALUATION: Twelve patients with epilepsy taking felbamate 3 or 3.6 g/day were administered erythromycin 333 mg 3 times/day for 9 days.[1] Plasma concentrations of felbamate were measured before and after erythromycin coadministration. No changes in felbamate pharmacokinetic parameters were noted following the concurrent erythromycin therapy. No change in felbamate dosing is necessary when erythromycin is administered.

RELATED DRUGS: Other macrolide antibiotics including clarithromycin (eg, *Biaxin*) and azithromycin (*Zithromax*) would not be expected to affect felbamate pharmacokinetics.

MANAGEMENT OPTIONS: No interaction.

REFERENCES:

1. Sachdeo RC, et al. Evaluation of the potential interaction between felbamate and erythromycin in patients with epilepsy. *J Clin Pharmacol.* 1998;38:184-190.

Erythromycin (eg, *E-Mycin*)

Felodipine (*Plendil*)

SUMMARY: Erythromycin administration resulted in elevated felodipine concentrations accompanied by flushing, edema, and tachycardia. More information is needed to establish a causal relationship.

RISK FACTORS: No specific risk factors are known.

MECHANISM: Not established. Erythromycin may inhibit the metabolism or increase the bioavailability of felodipine.

CLINICAL EVALUATION: A patient with hypertension receiving felodipine 10 mg/day developed flushing, ankle and leg edema, and tachycardia after starting erythromycin 250 mg.[1] Felodipine concentrations declined and symptoms abated after discontinuation of the erythromycin.

RELATED DRUGS: Troleandomycin (*TAO*) also may inhibit the metabolism of calcium channel blockers. Because other calcium channel blockers are metabolized similarly to felodipine, erythromycin also may affect their metabolism.

MANAGEMENT OPTIONS:

➥ *Monitor.* Until further information is available, observe patients taking felodipine, and perhaps other calcium channel blockers, for adverse effects (eg, hypotension, headache, arrythmias) during the coadministration of erythromycin.

REFERENCES:

1. Liedholm H, et al. Erythromycin-felodipine interaction. *DICP.* 1991;25:1007-1008.

Erythromycin (eg, *Ery-Tab*)

Fentanyl (eg, *Duragesic*)

SUMMARY: Fentanyl concentrations are likely to increase during erythromycin administration; increased narcotic effects may occur.

RISK FACTORS: No specific risk factors are known.

MECHANISM: Erythromycin is known to inhibit the enzyme (CYP3A4) responsible for the metabolism of fentanyl.

CLINICAL EVALUATION: While specific data are limited, the manufacturer of fentanyl notes that the coadministration of fentanyl and erythromycin should be undertaken with caution.[1] Pending further data, observe patients receiving fentanyl and erythromycin for evidence of increased fentanyl effect, including prolonged sedation and possible respiratory depression.

RELATED DRUGS: The metabolism of alfentanil (eg, *Alfenta*) and sufentanil (eg, *Sufenta*) is reduced by erythromycin. Clarithromycin (eg, *Biaxin*) and troleandomycin[+] are likely to inhibit the metabolism of fentanyl in a manner similar to erythromycin.

MANAGEMENT OPTIONS:

➥ *Consider Alternative.* Azithromycin (eg, *Zithromax*) does not inhibit CYP3A4 and may be considered as an alternative to erythromycin in patients receiving fentanyl. Narcotics not metabolized by CYP3A4, such as morphine or oxycodone, may also be considered as alternatives.

➥ *Monitor.* Monitor patients for excess sedation and respiratory depression if fentanyl is coadministered with a CYP3A4 inhibitor.

REFERENCES:

1. *Duragesic* [package insert]. Titusville, NJ: Janssen LP; 2008.

† Not available in the United States.

Erythromycin (eg, *Ery-Tab*)

Food

SUMMARY: Food has variable effects on erythromycin bioavailability; some formulations increase, decrease, or have no change in bioavailability when administered with food.

RISK FACTORS: No specific risk factors are known.

MECHANISM: Not established.

CLINICAL EVALUATION: Food has variable effects on different erythromycin salts and formulations of the same salt. For example, food reduced the area under the concentration-time curve (AUC) 35% and peak serum concentration 43% of one tablet formation of erythromycin ethylsuccinate.[1] However, the bioavailability of erythromycin ethylsuccinate granules or pediatric suspension was not affected in other studies.[2,3] Food has been reported to increase the AUC (64%) and peak serum concentrations (82%) of erythromycin estolate,[3] while the bioavailability of erythromycin base appears to be unaltered.[3-5] Erythromycin stearate has been reported to have increased bioavailability when given immediately before food[4] and decreased bioavailability when given immediately after food.[5] The clinical significance of these findings is undetermined and may be formulation specific.[6,7]

RELATED DRUGS: See Clinical Evaluation.

MANAGEMENT OPTIONS:

➥ *Circumvent/Minimize.* Because the results of studies on the effects of food on erythromycin bioavailability are variable, follow the manufacturer's recommendations concerning the timing of specific erythromycin products in relationship to meals.

➥ *Monitor.* Counsel patients to follow label directions carefully when taking erythromycin.

REFERENCES:

1. Thompson PJ, et al. Influence of food on absorption of erythromycin ethyl succinate. *Antimicrob Agents Chemother*. 1980;18(5):829-831.

2. Coyne TC, et al. Bioavailability of erythromycin ethylsuccinate in pediatric patients. *J Clin Pharmacol*. 1987;18(4):194-202.

3. Bechtol LD, et al. The influence of food on the absorption of erythromycin esters and enteric-coated erythromycin in single-dose studies. *Curr Ther Res*. 1979;25:618-625.

4. Malmborg AS. Effect of food on absorption of erythromycin: a study of two derivatives, the stearate and the base. *J Antimicrob Chemother*. 1979;5(5):591-599.

5. Clayton D, et al. The bioavailability of erythromycin stearate vs enteric-coated erythromycin base when taken immediately before and after food. *J Int Med Res*. 1981;9(6):470-477.

6. Hovi T, et al. Effect of concomitant food intake on absorption kinetics of erythromycin in healthy volunteers. *Eur J Clin Pharmacol*. 1985;28(2):231-233.

7. Randinitis EJ, et al. Effect of a high-fat meal on the bioavailability of a polymer-coated erythromycin particle tablet formulation. *J Clin Pharmacol*. 1989;29(1):79-84.

Erythromycin (eg, *Ery-Tab*)

Loratadine (eg, *Claritin*)

SUMMARY: Erythromycin increases loratadine plasma concentrations, but these changes do not appear to result in increased toxicity.

RISK FACTORS: No specific risk factors are known.

MECHANISM: Loratadine is partially metabolized by CYP3A4 enzymes. Erythromycin is known to inhibit CYP3A4 metabolism and probably increases loratadine concentrations by this mechanism.

CLINICAL EVALUATION: In a study of healthy men, the area under the concentration-time curve of loratadine and its descarboethoxyloratadine metabolite was increased approximately 140% following erythromycin 500 mg every 8 hours.[1] No change in corrected QT or other toxicity was observed. While loratadine appears to be susceptible to metabolic inhibition, it does not seem to cause conduction changes in the myocardium as has been observed with other nonsedating antihistamines. Loratadine has not been reported to produce electrocardiogram changes, even when administered in high doses.[2]

RELATED DRUGS: Other CYP3A4 inhibitors (eg, ketoconazole [eg, *Nizoral*], troleandomycin[†], clarithromycin [eg, *Biaxin*]) are also expected to inhibit loratadine's metabolism. Do not use terfenadine[†] and astemizole[†] in place of loratadine. Azithromycin (eg, *Zithromax*) and dirithromycin[†] are not likely to alter loratadine metabolism.

MANAGEMENT OPTIONS: No specific action is required, but be alert for evidence of the interaction.

REFERENCES:

1. Brannan MD, et al. Effects of various cytochrome P450 inhibitors on the metabolism of loratadine. *Clin Pharmacol Ther*. 1995;57:193.

2. Affrime MB, et al. Three month evaluation of electrocardiographic effects of loratadine in humans. *J Allergy Clin Immunol*. 1993;91:259.

† Not available in the United States.

5   Erythromycin (eg, *Ery-Tab*)

Losartan (*Cozaar*)

SUMMARY: Erythromycin administration does not affect the pharmacokinetics of losartan; no change in response to losartan is likely to occur.

RISK FACTORS: No specific risk factors are known.

MECHANISM: No interaction.

CLINICAL EVALUATION: Ten healthy subjects received losartan 50 mg/day for 1 week alone or with erythromycin 500 mg 3 or 4 times daily.[1] The administration of erythromycin had no effect on the area under the concentration-time curve or half-life of losartan or its active metabolite. Expect no change in hypotensive response to losartan when erythromycin is coadministered.

RELATED DRUGS: Other macrolide antibiotics are not expected to affect losartan plasma concentrations or clinical response. Eprosartan (*Teveten*), a related angiotensin II receptor inhibitor, is not metabolized by the CYP-450 system and is not expected to interact with erythromycin.

MANAGEMENT OPTIONS: No interaction.

REFERENCES:
1. Williamson KM, et al. Effects of erythromycin or rifampin on losartan pharmacokinetics in healthy volunteers. *Clin Pharmacol Ther.* 1998;63(3):316-323.

2   Erythromycin (eg, *Ery-Tab*)

Lovastatin (eg, *Mevacor*)

SUMMARY: Erythromycin increases the plasma concentration of lovastatin; myopathy or rhabdomyolysis may occur.

RISK FACTORS: No specific risk factors are known.

MECHANISM: Erythromycin inhibits the metabolism of lovastatin via CYP3A4 and the elimination of lovastatin via the efflux transporter P-glycoprotein.

CLINICAL EVALUATION: While clinical data are limited, lovastatin is known to be dependent on CYP3A4 for its metabolism and has a very low bioavailability (less than 5%). The coadministration of inhibitors of CYP3A4 may result in marked elevations of lovastatin and the possible development of myopathy or rhabdomyolysis.[1,2]

RELATED DRUGS: Simvastatin (eg, *Zocor*) and atorvastatin (*Lipitor*) are also metabolized by CYP3A4 and are known to interact with erythromycin. Azithromycin (eg, *Zithromax*) does not inhibit CYP3A4 and may be considered as an alternative to erythromycin in patients receiving lovastatin.

MANAGEMENT OPTIONS:

➡ **Use Alternative.** Pravastatin (eg, *Pravachol*), fluvastatin (*Lescol*), and rosuvastatin (*Crestor*) are unlikely to be affected by erythromycin.

➡ *Monitor.* Counsel patients taking lovastatin to report any muscle pain or weakness, particularly if receiving a CYP3A4 inhibitor.

REFERENCES:

1. East C, et al. Rhabdomyolysis in patients receiving lovastatin after cardiac transplantation. *N Engl J Med.* 1988;318(1):47-48.
2. Williams D, et al. Pharmacokinetic-pharmacodynamic drug interactions with HMG-CoA reductase inhibitors. *Clin Pharmacokinet.* 2002;41(5):343-370.

Erythromycin (eg, *Ery-Tab*)

Midazolam

SUMMARY: Erythromycin administration appears to increase the plasma concentrations and effect of midazolam.

RISK FACTORS:

➡ *Route of Administration.* Oral midazolam is much more affected than parenteral midazolam.

MECHANISM: Administration of erythromycin may inhibit the cytochrome P450 (CYP-450) isozyme (IIIA) responsible for the metabolism of midazolam. Midazolam's first-pass clearance may also be decreased, resulting in increased bioavailability.[1]

CLINICAL EVALUATION: After erythromycin administration, peak midazolam concentrations increased 170%, area under the concentration-time curve increased 3.5-fold, and half-life increased from 144 to 342 minutes.[2] Increased drowsiness during erythromycin-midazolam dosing has been reported in another study and clinical experience.[3,4]

RELATED DRUGS: Three days of erythromycin administration reduced the clearance of triazolam (eg, *Halcion*) 52%. Triazolam is metabolized by the same CYP-450 isozyme as midazolam.[5] Troleandomycin[†] and clarithromycin (eg, *Biaxin*) also may inhibit the metabolism of midazolam and triazolam. Other benzodiazepines also may be affected by erythromycin, clarithromycin, or troleandomycin. Azithromycin (eg, *Zithromax*) and dirithromycin[†] are less likely to affect midazolam metabolism.

MANAGEMENT OPTIONS:

➡ *Monitor.* Until further information is available, monitor patients taking erythromycin for increased response (eg, drowsiness, sedation) to midazolam and triazolam.

REFERENCES:

1. Kronbach T, et al. Oxidation of midazolam and triazolam by human liver cytochrome P450IIIA4. *Mol Pharmacol.* 1989;36(1):89-96.
2. Olkkola KT, et al. A potentially hazardous interaction between erythromycin and midazolam. *Clin Pharmacol Ther.* 1993;53(3):298-305.
3. Hiller A, et al. Unconsciousness associated with midazolam and erythromycin. *Br J Anaesth.* 1990;65(6):826-828.
4. Mattila MJ, et al. Oral single doses of erythromycin and roxithromycin may increase the effects of midazolam on human performance. *Pharmacol Toxicol.* 1993;73(3):180-185.
5. Phillips JP, et al. A pharmacokinetic drug interaction between erythromycin and triazolam. *J Clin Psychopharmacol.* 1986;6(5):297-299.

† Not available in the United States.

4 **Erythromycin (eg, *Ery-Tab*)**

Nadolol (eg, *Corgard*)

SUMMARY: Antibiotics that reduce bowel flora may increase peak nadolol concentrations and reduce its half-life, but the clinical importance of these effects is not established.

RISK FACTORS: No specific risk factors are known.

MECHANISM: Reduction of GI flora may increase the bioavailability of nadolol while reducing its enterohepatic reabsorption.

CLINICAL EVALUATION: Two days of oral therapy with erythromycin 0.5 g 4 times daily and neomycin 0.5 g 4 times daily more than doubled the mean peak plasma nadolol concentration following a single 80 mg oral dose and reduced its half-life from 17.3 hours to 11.6 hours.[1] The clinical importance of these findings is not established.

RELATED DRUGS: No information is available.

MANAGEMENT OPTIONS: No specific action is required, but be alert for evidence of the interaction.

REFERENCES:
1. du Souich P, et al. Enhancement of nadolol elimination by activated charcoal and antibiotics. *Clin Pharmacol Ther*. 1983;33(5):585-590.

3 **Erythromycin (eg, *Ery-Tab*)**

Penicillin G

SUMMARY: Erythromycin may inhibit the antibacterial activity of penicillins.

RISK FACTORS:

➡ ***Dosage Regimen.*** Low doses of both agents may interfere with antibacterial activity.

MECHANISM: Theoretically, a bacteriostatic antibiotic (eg, erythromycin) may interfere with the action of a bactericidal agent (eg, penicillin) Because penicillin acts by inhibiting cell wall synthesis, agents that inhibit protein synthesis (eg, erythromycin) could potentially mask the bactericidal effect of penicillin.

CLINICAL EVALUATION: Some researchers have noted that because antibiotic antagonism occurs only under specific conditions of dose, order of therapy, or indication, it probably plays a minor role in clinical medicine.[1-3] Although clinical evidence exists for erythromycin-penicillin antagonism in patients with group A hemolytic streptococcal pharyngitis, erythromycin is bactericidal against *streptococci* when high doses are used. Thus, it may act synergistically with penicillins under these conditions.[4] Erythromycin plus ampicillin in the treatment of pulmonary nocardiosis has been used with apparently favorable bacteriologic and clinical results.[5] Thus, the possibility of antagonism between erythromycin and penicillins exists, but it has not been sufficiently documented in clinical studies.

RELATED DRUGS: Other macrolides (eg, azithromycin [eg, *Zithromax*], clarithromycin [eg, *Biaxin*]) may interact in a similar manner.

MANAGEMENT OPTIONS:

➡ *Monitor.* Use combination therapy with antibiotics only when necessary. Indications for the concomitant use of penicillin and erythromycin should be rare. If a penicillin is used with erythromycin, observe the following points: 1) be sure that appropriate doses of each agent are given (antagonism is most likely when small doses of each are given); 2) begin administration of the penicillin at least a few hours before the erythromycin.

REFERENCES:

1. Jawetz E. The use of combinations of antimicrobial drugs. *Ann Rev Pharmacol.* 1968;8:151-170.
2. Mills J, et al. Clinical use of antimicrobials. In: Katzung BG. *Basic and Clinical Pharmacology.* Los Altos, CA: Lange Medical Publications;1982:538–552.
3. Jawetz E. Synergism and antagonism among antimicrobial drugs, a personal perspective. *West J Med.* 1975;123(2):87-91.
4. Kabins SA. Interactions among antibiotics and other drugs. *JAMA.* 1972;219(2):206-212.
5. Bach MC, et al. Pulmonary nocardiosis. Therapy with minocycline and with erythromycin plus ampicillin. *JAMA.* 1973;224(10):1378-1381.

Erythromycin (eg, *Ery-Tab*)

Pitavastatin (eg, *Livalo*)

SUMMARY: Erythromycin has been reported to increase the concentrations of pitavastatin; increased adverse reactions may occur in some patients.

RISK FACTORS: No specific risk factors are known.

MECHANISM: Unknown. Pitavastatin is a substrate for the organic anion-transporting polypeptide (OATP) and erythromycin is known to inhibit this transporter. Inhibition of OATP would reduce the uptake of pitavastatin into hepatocytes where it is metabolized.

CLINICAL EVALUATION: While specific data are limited, coadministration of erythromycin 500 mg 4 times a day for 6 days prior to a single 4 mg dose of pitavastatin increased the mean area under the plasma concentration-time curve of pitavastatin by about 2.8-fold.[1] Pending further data, patients receiving pitavastatin and erythromycin should be observed for increased pitavastatin effect. Pitavastatin labeling recommends limiting the dosage of pitavastatin to 1 mg daily during erythromycin coadministration.

RELATED DRUGS: Clarithromycin (eg, *Biaxin*) may also increase pitavastatin plasma concentrations.

MANAGEMENT OPTIONS:

➡ *Monitor.* Monitor patients receiving pitavastatin who require erythromycin for signs of pitavastatin toxicity, including muscle weakness and myalgia.

REFERENCES:

1. *Livalo* [package insert]. Montgomery, AL: Kowa Pharmaceuticals America, Inc; 2009.

5   Erythromycin (eg, *Ery-Tab*)

Pravastatin (eg, *Pravachol*)

SUMMARY: Erythromycin does not affect pravastatin concentrations.

RISK FACTORS: No specific risk factors are known.

MECHANISM: No interaction.

CLINICAL EVALUATION: Twelve subjects received pravastatin 40 mg alone or concomitantly with erythromycin 500 mg 3 times daily for 7 days.[1] Erythromycin administration did not change the serum concentration or pharmacokinetics of pravastatin. It appears that no significant interaction occurs.

RELATED DRUGS: Erythromycin is known to increase lovastatin (*Mevacor*) and atorvastatin (*Lipitor*) concentrations and may increase the risk of rhabdomyolysis. The effect of erythromycin on other HMG-CoA reductase inhibitors is unknown. Other macrolide antibiotics are not expected to alter pravastatin's pharmacokinetics.

MANAGEMENT OPTIONS: No interaction.

REFERENCES:

1. Bottorff MB, et al. Differences in metabolism of lovastatin and pravastatin as assessed by CYP3A4 inhibition with erythromycin. *Pharmacotherapy.* 1997;17:41.

Erythromycin (eg, *Ery-Tab*)

Quetiapine (*Seroquel*)

SUMMARY: Erythromycin increases quetiapine plasma concentrations; increased adverse reactions can be expected in some patients.

RISK FACTORS: No specific risk factors are known.

MECHANISM: Erythromycin inhibits the metabolism (CPY3A4) of quetiapine, causing elevated quetiapine plasma concentrations.

CLINICAL EVALUATION: Nineteen patients received quetiapine titrated to 200 mg twice daily over 4 days and continued at that dosage for 3 more days.[1] Starting on the eighth day of quetiapine, erythromycin 500 mg 3 times daily was coadministered for 5 days. Mean quetiapine area under the concentration-time curve during erythromycin coadministration was 129% greater (range, approximately 15% to 300% increase) than that measured when quetiapine was administered alone. Quetiapine half-life was increased from 7 to 16.1 hours by erythromycin administration. This degree of increase in quetiapine plasma concentrations is likely to increase the incidence of adverse reactions, including dizziness, dry mouth, hypotension, and somnolence.

RELATED DRUGS: Clarithromycin (eg, *Biaxin*) is likely to affect quetiapine in a similar manner.

MANAGEMENT OPTIONS:

➡ *Consider Alternative.* Consider macrolide antibiotics that do not inhibit CYP3A4 (eg, azithromycin [eg, *Zithromax*], dirithromycin[†]) for patients taking quetiapine.

➥ *Monitor.* Monitor patients taking quetiapine who require erythromycin for increased somnolence, dizziness, and hypotension.

REFERENCES:

1. Li KY, et al. Effect of erythromycin on metabolism of quetiapine in Chinese suffering from schizophrenia. *Eur J Clin Pharmacol.* 2005;60(11):791-795.

† Not available in the United States.

Erythromycin (eg, *E-Mycin*)

Quinidine (eg, *Quinora*)

SUMMARY: Erythromycin increased quinidine concentrations; cardiac arrhythmias could result.

RISK FACTORS:

➥ *Concurrent Diseases.* Patients with preexisting cardiac disease are at greater risk.

MECHANISM: Erythromycin may inhibit the metabolism of quinidine by CYP3A4 isozymes.

CLINICAL EVALUATION: A 74-year-old man was taking quinidine 200 mg every 6 hours and had a quinidine concentration of 2.8 mg/L.[1] Erythromycin lactobionate 500 mg every 6 hours IV and ceftriaxone (*Rocephin*) were administered. Quinidine concentrations increased to 4.2 mg/L. The dose of erythromycin was increased to 1 g every 6 hours and metronidazole (*MetroGel–Vaginal*) 500 mg IV every 8 hours was added. Five days later the quinidine concentration was 5.8 mg/L. Following discontinuation of the erythromycin and metronidazole, the quinidine concentration returned to baseline. The patient developed arrhythmias, and although a causal relationship to the elevated quinidine was not established, the arrhythmia was noted to be consistent with elevated quinidine concentrations. Both quinidine and erythromycin can prolong QT intervals. The role of metronidazole, if any, in this case is unknown.

RELATED DRUGS: Other macrolides that inhibit CYP3A4 (eg, troleandomycin [*TAO*], clarithromycin [*Biaxin*]) also may inhibit quinidine metabolism. Azithromycin (*Zithromax*) and dirithromycin (*Dynabac*) are unlikely to affect quinidine concentrations.

MANAGEMENT OPTIONS:

➥ *Consider Alternative.* The use of azithromycin or a nonmacrolide antibiotic would likely avoid the interaction with quinidine.

➥ *Monitor.* If quinidine and erythromycin are coadministered, monitor for signs of quinidine cardiac toxicity (prolonged QRS and QT intervals).

REFERENCES:

1. Spinler SA, et al. Possible inhibition of hepatic metabolism of quinidine by erythromycin. *Clin Pharmacol Ther.* 1995;57:89.

Erythromycin (eg, *E-Mycin*)

Ritonavir (*Norvir*)

SUMMARY: Ritonavir may inhibit erythromycin metabolism; erythromycin may inhibit ritonavir metabolism. The clinical significance of this potential interaction is unknown.

RISK FACTORS: No specific risk factors are known.

MECHANISM: Ritonavir probably inhibits erythromycin metabolism; erythromycin may inhibit ritonavir metabolism. Both ritonavir and erythromycin are metabolized by CYP3A4 and both drugs are known to inhibit CYP3A4 activity.

CLINICAL EVALUATION: While no data have been published on this interaction, the manufacturer has included it in their labeling.[1] It would be expected that the coadministration of ritonavir and erythromycin could lead to elevated concentrations of both drugs. In patients receiving ritonavir who are prescribed erythromycin, ritonavir would be expected to reduce the metabolism of erythromycin and thus limit the formation of its CYP3A4 enzyme-inhibiting metabolite. Elevated erythromycin concentrations could result in GI upset or possibly QT prolongation. Patients on ritonavir who are administered erythromycin may develop elevated ritonavir concentrations and experience toxic symptoms including nausea, vomiting, diarrhea, or paresthesias.

RELATED DRUGS: Clarithromycin (*Biaxin*) serum concentrations are increased by ritonavir and clarithromycin produces a small increase in ritonavir concentrations.[1] Other protease inhibitors such as indinavir (*Crixivan*), saquinavir (eg, *Invirase*), and nelfinavir (*Viracept*) may affect erythromycin in a similar manner. Since azithromycin (*Zithromax*) is not metabolized and is not a CYP3A4 inhibitor, ritonavir would not be expected to interact with azithromycin. Ritonavir concentrations are increased by clarithromycin, and troleandomycin (*TAO*) would be expected to have a similar effect. Dirithromycin (*Dynabac*) would not be expected to have much effect on ritonavir although it could reduce ritonavir concentrations. The effect of ritonavir on dirithromycin concentrations is unknown.

MANAGEMENT OPTIONS:

➡ ***Consider Alternative.*** Azithromycin would probably be a noninteracting alternative to erythromycin for patients receiving ritonavir.

➡ ***Monitor.*** Monitor for evidence of erythromycin or ritonavir toxicity when the 2 drugs are coadministered.

REFERENCES:
1. Product information. Ritonavir (*Norvir*). Abbott Laboratories. 1996.

Erythromycin (eg, *E-Mycin*)

Sertindole (*Serlect*)

SUMMARY: Three days of erythromycin dosing has a limited effect on sertindole pharmacokinetics; the effect of longer periods of erythromycin administration is unknown.

RISK FACTORS: No specific risk factors are known.

MECHANISM: Erythromycin increases the rate of sertindole absorption; its potential effects on sertindole metabolism await further study with a longer erythromycin pretreatment period.

CLINICAL EVALUATION: Ten healthy subjects received sertindole 4 mg alone and after 3 days of erythromycin 250 mg every 6 hours.[1] Erythromycin was continued for 10 days at the same dose. Following erythromycin pretreatment, no change was observed in sertindole oral clearance or half-life. Peak sertindole concentrations increased 15%, while the time to peak was reduced from 12 to 8 hours. The somewhat short duration of erythromycin treatment prior to the dose of sertindole (3 days) may not have been long enough to assess erythromycin's full potential to inhibit the sertindole metabolism. Erythromycin is metabolized to a potent inhibitor of CYP3A4, and the metabolite requires several days to accumulate. Assess the effects of erythromycin on sertindole pharmacokinetics following 7 to 10 days of therapy before making a final evaluation of this interaction.

RELATED DRUGS: The effect of other macrolides on sertindole is unknown.

MANAGEMENT OPTIONS:

➡ *Monitor.* Pending studies with longer exposure to erythromycin, monitor patients receiving sertindole and erythromycin for increased sertindole effects.

REFERENCES:

1. Wong SL, et al. The effect of erythromycin on the CYP3A component of sertindole clearance in healthy volunteers. *J Clin Pharmacol.* 1997;37:1056–61.

Erythromycin (eg, *E-Mycin*)
Sertraline (*Zoloft*)

SUMMARY: A patient developed an apparent serotonin syndrome following the addition of erythromycin to a chronic dose of sertraline.

RISK FACTORS: No specific risk factors are known.

MECHANISM: Erythromycin is known to inhibit CYP3A4, the isozyme responsible for the metabolism of sertraline. A reduction in sertraline first-pass metabolism or reduced systemic clearance may have resulted in an increase in sertraline plasma concentrations.

CLINICAL EVALUATION: A 12-year-old boy with obsessive-compulsive disorder was receiving sertraline 37.5 mg/day.[1] Four days after starting a course of erythromycin 200 mg twice daily, the boy began to feel nervous. His symptoms worsened over the next 10 days and included agitation, confusion, tremors, and paresthesia. Both drugs were stopped, and the symptoms resolved over the following 3 days. Plasma concentrations of sertraline were not measured. The mechanism and clinical relevance of this purported interaction requires additional study.

RELATED DRUGS: Clarithromycin (*Biaxin*) and troleandomycin (*TAO*) are other macrolide antibiotics known to inhibit CYP3A4 metabolism and could affect sertraline similarly. Azithromycin (*Zithromax*) and dirithromycin (*Dynabac*) would not be expected to interact with sertraline. It is likely that other SSRIs that are metabolized by CYP3A4 (eg, citalopram [*Celexa*], nefazodone [*Serzone*]) would be affected in a similar manner by erythromycin, clarithromycin, and troleandomycin. Paroxetine (*Paxil*) is primarily metabolized by CYP2D6 and would be unlikely to be affected by erythromycin.

MANAGEMENT OPTIONS:

➥ *Consider Alternative.* The use of a non-CYP3A4-inhibiting macrolide such as azithromycin or dirithromycin would probably avoid any potential to induce the serotonin syndrome in patients taking SSRIs.

➥ *Monitor.* Monitor patients taking any SSRI metabolized by CYP3A4 for signs of excess serotonin effect if CYP3A4 inhibitors are coadministered.

REFERENCES:

1. Lee DO, et al. Serotonin syndrome in a child associated with erythromycin and sertraline. *Pharmacotherapy.* 1999;19:894–96.

Erythromycin (eg, *E-Mycin*)

Sildenafil (*Viagra*)

SUMMARY: Erythromycin administration produces a large increase in sildenafil plasma concentrations; increased side effects are possible.

RISK FACTORS: No specific risk factors are known.

MECHANISM: Erythromycin inhibits the first-pass and systemic metabolism (CYP3A4) of sildenafil, resulting in elevated plasma concentrations and a prolonged half-life.

CLINICAL EVALUATION: While no published data are available for evaluation, the manufacturer of sildenafil has made available some data on this interaction.[1] Twenty-four healthy men received a single dose of sildenafil 100 mg on study day 1. On days 2 through 6, twelve subjects received erythromycin 500 mg orally twice daily and 12 subjects received placebo. On day 6, all subjects were again administered a single 100 mg dose of sildenafil. Placebo had no effect on the pharmacokinetics of sildenafil. Following erythromycin administration, the area under the concentration-time curve of sildenafil increased 158% and its peak plasma concentration increased 108%. The half-life of sildenafil was prolonged from 3.5 hours to 4.1 hours following erythromycin administration. These increases in sildenafil concentrations could result in an increased incidence of side effects such as headache, abnormal vision, or flushing.

RELATED DRUGS: Other macrolides that inhibit CYP3A4 [eg, clarithromycin (*Biaxin*), troleandomycin (*TAO*) would be likely to affect sildenafil in a similar manner. Noninhibiting macrolides such as azithromycin (*Zithromax*) or dirithromycin (*Dynabac*) would be unlikely to alter the plasma concentration of sildenafil.

MANAGEMENT OPTIONS:

➥ *Circumvent/Minimize.* Use small doses of sildenafil (eg, 25 mg) when patients are taking macrolides that inhibit CYP3A4 metabolism. Noninhibiting macrolides (eg, azithromycin, dirithromycin) would be unlikely to alter sildenafil concentrations.

➥ *Monitor.* Counsel patients to use a low dose of sildenafil during the administration of erythromycin or other macrolides that inhibit CYP3A4 metabolism. Be alert for increased side effects including headache, abnormal vision, or flushing.

REFERENCES:

1. Product information. Sildenafil (*Viagra*). Pfizer Pharmaceuticals. 1998.

Erythromycin (eg, *E-Mycin*)

Simvastatin (*Zocor*)

SUMMARY: Erythromycin administration may markedly increase simvastatin concentrations; avoid using the drugs together to avoid the risk of increased side effects.

RISK FACTORS: No specific risk factors are known.

MECHANISM: Erythromycin reduces the intrinsic and first-pass metabolism of simvastatin by inhibition of CYP3A4, the enzyme responsible for simvastatin's metabolism in the intestinal wall and liver.

CLINICAL EVALUATION: A single dose of simvastatin 40 mg was administered to 12 healthy subjects after 2 days of placebo or erythromycin 500 mg 3 times daily.[1] The area under the concentration-time curve of simvastatin and its active metabolite simvastatin acid were increased 6.2-fold and 3.9-fold, respectively, by erythromycin pretreatment. The half-life of simvastatin increased from 1.2 hours during placebo to 2.1 hours following erythromycin. The increase was not statistically significant, although only 4 subjects in the control phase had half-life determinations. A longer duration of therapy with erythromycin may result in an increased magnitude of the effect on simvastatin pharmacokinetics. These erythromycin-induced increases in simvastatin concentrations could increase the potential for side effects including myalgias and rhabdomyolysis.

RELATED DRUGS: Erythromycin will likely affect lovastatin (*Mevacor*) plasma concentrations in a similar manner. Atorvastatin (*Lipitor*) plasma concentrations are increased to a lesser degree by erythromycin administration. While no data are available, erythromycin may also increase the plasma concentrations of cerivastatin (*Baycol*). Clarithromycin (*Biaxin*) and troleandomycin (*TAO*) would probably reduce the metabolism of simvastatin. Azithromycin (*Zithromax*) and dirithromycin (*Dynabac*) would not likely inhibit the metabolism of simvastatin. The metabolism of pravastatin (*Pravachol*) and fluvastatin (*Lescol*) would not be expected to be affected by erythromycin.

MANAGEMENT OPTIONS:

➡ ***Use Alternative.*** Consider the use of a HMG-CoA reductase inhibitor other than simvastatin or lovastatin for patients receiving erythromycin. Atorvastatin and cerivastatin plasma concentrations are likely to be increased by a smaller amount during erythromycin coadministration. Pravastatin and fluvastatin metabolism should not be altered by erythromycin. Azithromycin or dirithromycin are macrolides that will not affect simvastatin metabolism.

REFERENCES:

1. Kantola T, et al. Erythromycin and verapamil considerably increase serum simvastatin and simvastatin acid concentrations. *Clin Pharmacol Ther.* 1988;64:177.

Erythromycin (eg, *E-Mycin*)

Sufentanil (eg, *Sufenta*)

SUMMARY: Erythromycin administration for 7 days had no effect on sufentanil serum concentrations.

RISK FACTORS: No specific risk factors are known.

MECHANISM: No interaction.

CLINICAL EVALUATION: Six healthy men were administered IV sufentanil 3 mc/kg on 3 separate days: following no concomitant drug, 1 oral dose of erythromycin base 500 mg, and after 7 days of erythromycin 500 mg twice daily.[1] Unlike alfentanil[2] the administration of erythromycin had no effect on the apparent clearance or half-life of sufentanil.

RELATED DRUGS: Alfentanil (eg, *Alfenta*) affects erythromycin pharmacokinetics.

MANAGEMENT OPTIONS: No interaction.

REFERENCES:

1. Barkowski RR, et al. Sufentanil disposition. Is it affected by erythromycin? *Anesthesiology*. 1993;78:260.
2. Barkowski RR, et al. Inhibition of alfentanil metabolism by erythromycin. *Clin Pharmacol Ther*. 1989;46:99.

Erythromycin (eg, *E-Mycin*)

Tacrolimus (*Prograf*)

SUMMARY: Patients receiving tacrolimus developed increased concentrations and nephrotoxicity following coadministration with erythromycin.

RISK FACTORS: No specific risk factors are known.

MECHANISM: Not established. Erythromycin inhibits the metabolism of some drugs and could also inhibit the metabolism of tacrolimus.

CLINICAL EVALUATION: A liver transplant patient treated with tacrolimus 6 mg twice daily was administered erythromycin 250 mg every 6 hours.[1] The patient's tacrolimus concentration increased over 4 days of erythromycin therapy. His serum creatinine concentration also increased over these 4 days. The erythromycin and tacrolimus were discontinued and the patient's serum creatinine and tacrolimus concentrations decreased over the following week. Tacrolimus was reinstituted without apparent evidence of renal toxicity. Other case reports noted erythromycin-induced increases in tacrolimus concentrations up to 8-fold.[2,3]

RELATED DRUGS: Erythromycin also is known to inhibit cyclosporine (eg, *Sandimmune*) metabolism. The effects of other macrolides on tacrolimus concentration are unknown, but troleandomycin (*TAO*) and clarithromycin (*Biaxin*) might produce similar changes in tacrolimus. While no data is available, azithromycin (*Zithromax*) would appear to be less likely to interact with tacrolimus.

MANAGEMENT OPTIONS:

➡ **Monitor.** Pending further investigation of this interaction, patients should have their tacrolimus and creatinine serum concentrations monitored if they are coadministered erythromycin.

REFERENCES:

1. Shaeffer MS, et al. Interaction between FK506 and erythromycin. *Ann Pharmacother*. 1994;28:280.
2. Jensen C, et al. Interaction between tacrolimus and erythromycin. *Lancet*. 1994;344:825.
3. Furlan V, et al. Interactions between FK506 and rifampicin or erythromycin in pediatric liver recipients. *Transplantation*. 1995;59:1217.

Erythromycin (eg, *Ery-Tab*)

Tamsulosin (*Flomax*)

SUMMARY: Theoretically, the tamsulosin effect may be increased by erythromycin and other CYP3A4 inhibitors, but the clinical importance of this effect is not established.

RISK FACTORS: No specific risk factors are known.

MECHANISM: Tamsulosin is metabolized by CYP3A4 and erythromycin is a CYP3A4 inhibitor; theoretically, erythromycin would inhibit tamsulosin metabolism.

CLINICAL EVALUATION: Although the interaction is based on theoretical considerations, use caution when tamsulosin is coadministered with drugs that may affect tamsulosin metabolism.[1]

RELATED DRUGS: Clarithromycin (eg, *Biaxin*), telithromycin (*Ketek*), and troleandomycin[†] are moderate to potent inhibitors of CYP3A4 and may interact with tamsulosin, but azithromycin (eg, *Zithromax*) has little effect on CYP3A4.

MANAGEMENT OPTIONS: No specific action is required, but be alert for evidence of the interaction.

REFERENCES:

1. *Flomax* [package insert]. Ridgefield, CT: Boehringer Ingelheim; 2009.

† Not available in the United States.

Erythromycin (eg, *E-Mycin*)

Temazepam (eg, *Restoril*)

SUMMARY: Erythromycin does not alter the metabolism of temazepam.

RISK FACTORS: No specific risk factors are known.

MECHANISM: No interaction.

CLINICAL EVALUATION: Ten healthy subjects were administered temazepam 20 mg orally alone and after 6 days of erythromycin base 500 mg 3 times daily.[1] Erythromycin administration had no effect on temazepam pharmacokinetics. Temazepam primarily is metabolized by conjugation to a glucuronide and would not be expected to be affected by erythromycin, a potent inhibitor of CYP3A4 oxidation reactions.

RELATED DRUGS: Other macrolides would be unlikely to affect temazepam metabolism. Lorazepam (eg, *Ativan*), triazolam (eg, *Halcion*), and oxazepam (eg, *Serax*) are metabolized in a manner similar to temazepam and would not be likely to interact with erythromycin. The metabolism of benzodiazepines that are metabolized by CYP3A4 (eg, diazepam [eg, *Valium*] or midazolam [*Versed*]) is inhibited by erythromycin. (Also, see Erythromycin/Midazolam monograph.)

MANAGEMENT OPTIONS: No interaction.

REFERENCES:

1. Luurila H, et al. Lack of interaction of erythromycin with temazepam. *Ther Drug Monit.* 1994;16:548.

Erythromycin (eg, *E-Mycin*)

AVOID **Terfenadine (*Seldane*)**

SUMMARY: Erythromycin administration may cause cardiac arrythmias in patients taking terfenadine.

RISK FACTORS: No specific risk factors are known.

MECHANISM: Erythromycin inhibits the metabolism of terfenadine to its carboxylic acid metabolite and may also inhibit the further metabolism of the metabolite. Erythromycin administration alone has been noted to prolong QT intervals.

CLINICAL EVALUATION: Erythromycin administration causes an accumulation of terfenadine and its active metabolite.[1,4,5] Electrocardiographic changes (prolonged QT interval, ventricular arrhythmia) may be noted.[1,3,5] In another study, erythromycin 333 mg 3 times daily for 5 days did not alter the concentration of terfenadine or its metabolite following a single 120 mg dose.[2]

RELATED DRUGS: The manufacturer of terfenadine has received case reports of an interaction between troleandomycin (*TAO*) and terfenadine that resulted in cardiac arrhythmias.

MANAGEMENT OPTIONS:

➡ *AVOID COMBINATION.* Patients taking terfenadine should avoid concomitant use of erythromycin or troleandomycin. Until further data are available, careful observation is warranted during the administration of terfenadine and other macrolides. Loratadine (*Claritin*) or cetirizine (*Zyrtec*) may be acceptable alternatives for terfenadine.

REFERENCES:
1. Honig PK, et al. Erythromycin changes terfenadine pharmacokinetics and electrocardiographic pharmacodynamics. *Clin Pharmacol Ther.* 1992;51:156.
2. Mathews DR, et al. Torsades de pointes occurring in association with terfenadine use. *JAMA.* 1991;266:2375.
3. Biglin KE, et al. Drug-induced torsades de pointes: a possible interaction of terfenadine and erythromycin. *Ann Pharmacother.* 1994;28:282.
4. Eller M, et al. Effect of erythromycin on terfenadine metabolite pharmacokinetics. *Clin Pharmacol Ther.* 1993;53:161.
5. Honig PK, et al. Comparison of the effect of the macrolide antibiotics erythromycin, clarithromycin and azithromycin on terfenadine steady-state pharmacokinetics and electrocardiographic parameters. *Drug Invest.* 1994;7:148.

 Erythromycin (eg, *E-Mycin*)

Theophylline (eg, *Theolair*)

SUMMARY: Erythromycin can increase theophylline serum concentrations and may produce toxicity; theophylline can reduce the concentration of erythromycin.

RISK FACTORS: No specific risk factors are known.

MECHANISM: Erythromycin inhibits the metabolism of theophylline. Theophylline increases the renal clearance of erythromycin.

CLINICAL EVALUATION: In several clinical studies and case reports, erythromycin reduced theophylline clearance and increased serum theophylline concentrations.[1-6,8,9] This interaction usually occurred only after several days of erythromycin therapy. Other studies failed to note an interaction,[10,11] but in some cases this may have been caused by the short duration of erythromycin therapy, low erythromycin doses, or a possible inhibitory effect of smoking on the interaction. Serum erythromycin concentrations may be lowered by the administration of theophylline, possibly to subtherapeutic levels.[1,6,7]

RELATED DRUGS: Troleandomycin (*TAO*) and clarithromycin (*Biaxin*) also may inhibit the metabolism of theophylline.

MANAGEMENT OPTIONS:

➡ *Consider Alternative.* Azithromycin (*Zithromax*) does not appear to alter theophylline concentrations.

➡ *Monitor.* Closely monitor patients when erythromycin therapy is initiated. Although some clinicians suggest lowering the dose of theophylline 25% when erythromycin is initiated, this precaution may excessively complicate the management of low-risk patients (ie, those likely to have a low serum theophylline concentration). Be aware that a reduction in erythromycin serum concentration by theophylline may also be observed.

REFERENCES:

1. Pasic J, et al. The interaction between chronic oral slow-release theophylline and single-dose intravenous erythromycin. *Xenobiotica.* 1987;17:493.
2. Branigan TA, et al. The effect of erythromycin on the absorption and disposition kinetics of theophylline. *Eur J Clin Pharmacol.* 1981;21:115.
3. Zarowitz BJM, et al. Effect of erythromycin base on the theophylline kinetics. *Clin Pharmacol Ther.* 1981;29:601.
4. Renton KW, et al. Depression of theophylline elimination by erythromycin. *Clin Pharmacol Ther.* 1981;30:422.
5. LaForce CF, et al. Effect of erythromycin on theophylline clearance in asthmatic children. *J Pediatr.* 1981;99:153.
6. Iliopoulou A, et al. Pharmacokinetic interaction between theophylline and erythromycin. *Br J Clin Pharmacol.* 1982;14:495.
7. Paulsen O, et al. The interaction of erythromycin with theophylline. *Eur J Clin Pharmacol.* 1987;32:493.
8. Reisz G, et al. The effect of erythromycin on theophylline pharmacokinetics in chronic bronchitis. *Am Rev Resp Dis.* 1982;127:581.
9. Paulsen O, et al. The interaction of erythromycin with theophylline. *Eur J Clin Pharmacol.* 1987;32:493.
10. Melethil S, et al. Steady state urinary excretion of theophylline and its metabolites in the presence of erythromycin. *Res Commun Chem Pathol Pharmacol.* 1982;35:341.
11. Hildebrandt R, et al. Lack of clinically important interaction between erythromycin and theophylline. *Eur J Clin Pharmacol.* 1984;26:485.

Erythromycin (eg, *E-Mycin*)

Triazolam (eg, *Halcion*)

SUMMARY: Erythromycin causes considerable increases in triazolam plasma concentrations.

RISK FACTORS: No specific risk factors are known.

MECHANISM: Erythromycin appears to inhibit the enzymes responsible for the metabolism of triazolam, thereby reducing its systemic clearance. Triazolam's first-pass clearance may also be reduced, resulting in increased bioavailability. These changes are probably responsible for the marked increases in triazolam concentrations that have been reported.

CLINICAL EVALUATION: In normal volunteers, the area under the triazolam plasma concentration-time curve increased 106%, the apparent clearance of triazolam was reduced 52%, and its half-life increased from 3.5 hours to 5.9 hours following erythromycin administration.[1] Peak plasma concentrations were increased approximately 50% by the pretreatment with erythromycin. Psychomotor impairment, memory dysfunction, and drowsiness were increased during erythromycin coadministration.

RELATED DRUGS: Troleandomycin (*TAO*) and clarithromycin (*Biaxin*) also may inhibit the metabolism of triazolam; theoretically, azithromycin (*Zithromax*) would be unlikely to interact. Other benzodiazepines that undergo oxidative metabolism are likely to be affected similarly.

MANAGEMENT OPTIONS:

➡ *Monitor.* Carefully observe patients receiving triazolam who are prescribed erythromycin for enhanced triazolam effects. Several days may be required for the maximum effect of erythromycin to become evident, and triazolam dosages may require adjustment after addition of the antibiotic and again when it is discontinued.

REFERENCES:

1. Philips JP, et al. A pharmacokinetic drug interaction between erythromycin and triazolam. *J Clin Psychopharmacol.* 1986;6:297.

Erythromycin (eg, *Ery-Tab*)

Valproic Acid (eg, *Depakene*)

SUMMARY: In 1 patient, valproic acid plasma concentrations increased after the addition of erythromycin, resulting in symptoms of valproic acid toxicity.

RISK FACTORS: No specific risk factors are known.

MECHANISM: Not established. Erythromycin probably inhibits the hepatic metabolism of valproic acid.

CLINICAL EVALUATION: In a patient on long-term valproic acid and lithium therapy, valproic acid concentrations increased from 89 mg/L 2 months before admission to 260 mg/L after erythromycin 250 mg 4 times daily was added for an upper respiratory tract infection.[1] The patient developed symptoms of valproic acid toxicity (eg, ataxia, nausea, sedation).

RELATED DRUGS: Troleandomycin[†] and clarithromycin (eg, *Biaxin*) also may inhibit the metabolism of valproic acid.

MANAGEMENT OPTIONS:

➡ *Monitor.* Monitor patients for altered responses to valproic acid when erythromycin dosage is initiated, discontinued, or changed.

REFERENCES:

1. Redington K, et al. Erythromycin and valproate interaction. *Ann Intern Med.* 1992;116(10):877-878.

† Not available in the United States.

Erythromycin (eg, *Ery-Tab*)

Vardenafil (*Levitra*)

SUMMARY: Erythromycin increases the plasma concentration of vardenafil; increased vardenafil adverse reactions may occur.

RISK FACTORS: No specific risk factors are known.

MECHANISM: Erythromycin inhibits the metabolism of vardenafil via CYP3A4; increased vardenafil bioavailability and reduced clearance would be expected.

CLINICAL EVALUATION: While specific data are limited, the coadministration of erythromycin 500 mg 3 times daily prior to a single dose of vardenafil 5 mg increased the mean area under the plasma concentration-time curve of vardenafil approximately 4-fold.[1]

RELATED DRUGS: Clarithromycin (eg, *Biaxin*) and troleandomycin[†] are likely to inhibit the metabolism of vardenafil in a similar manner. Sildenafil (eg, *Viagra*) and tadalafil (eg, *Cialis*) are likely to be affected in a similar manner by erythromycin.

MANAGEMENT OPTIONS:

➡ **Consider Alternative.** Azithromycin (eg, *Zithromax*) does not inhibit CYP3A4 and may be considered as an alternative to erythromycin in patients receiving vardenafil.

➡ **Circumvent/Minimize.** Pending further data, observe patients receiving vardenafil and erythromycin for increased vardenafil effect, and limit the dosage of vardenafil to 5 mg every 24 hours.

➡ **Monitor.** Be alert for signs of excessive vardenafil effects (eg, hypotension) if erythromycin is coadministered.

REFERENCES:

1. *Levitra* [package insert]. West Haven, CT: Bayer Pharmaceuticals Corporation; 2008.

† Not available in the United States.

Erythromycin (eg, *Ery-Tab*)

Verapamil (eg, *Calan*)

SUMMARY: Erythromycin can increase verapamil plasma concentrations; some patients may experience verapamil-induced adverse reactions, including hypotension and bradycardia.

RISK FACTORS: No specific risk factors are known.

MECHANISM: Erythromycin inhibits the metabolism of verapamil via the CYP3A4 enzyme and can potentially enhance its absorption by inhibiting P-glycoprotein.

CLINICAL EVALUATION: A patient with a history of diabetes mellitus, hypertension, left ventricular hypertrophy, and obstructive lung disease was being treated with verapamil sustained-release 240 mg daily.[1] Because of the development of an upper respiratory tract infection, she was placed on erythromycin 2,000 mg daily. One week later, she complained of dizziness and lethargy. She was found to be hypotensive and bradycardic with complete heart block. Erythromycin and verapamil were stopped, and the cardiac symptoms resolved over the next week. Similar cases have been noted with the concurrent use of verapamil with clarithromycin (eg, *Biaxin*) or telithromycin (*Ketek*).[2,3]

RELATED DRUGS: Diltiazem (eg, *Cardizem*) is likely to be affected in a similar manner by macrolide antibiotics that inhibit CYP3A4 and P-glycoprotein.

MANAGEMENT OPTIONS:

➥ *Consider Alternative.* Azithromycin (eg, *Zithromax*) does not inhibit CYP3A4 and could be considered as an alternative to erythromycin in patients receiving verapamil.

➥ *Monitor.* Carefully monitor patients taking verapamil if erythromycin is initiated or discontinued from their drug regimen.

REFERENCES:

1. Goldschmidt N, et al. Compound cardiac toxicity of oral erythromycin and verapamil. *Ann Pharmacother.* 2001;35(11):1396-1399.

2. Kaeser YA, et al. Severe hypotension and bradycardia associated with verapamil and clarithromycin. *Am J Health-Syst Pharm.* 1998;55(22):2417-2418.

3. Reed M, et al. Verapamil toxicity resulting from a probable interaction with telithromycin. *Ann Pharmacother.* 2005;39(2):357-360.

Erythromycin (eg, *Ery-Tab*)

Warfarin (eg, *Coumadin*)

SUMMARY: Erythromycin markedly increases the hypoprothrombinemic response to warfarin in some patients, but the incidence of the interaction in patients receiving both drugs is unknown.

RISK FACTORS:

➥ *Concurrent Diseases.* Fever may enhance the catabolism of clotting factors.

➥ *Diet/Food.* A diet low in vitamin K may contribute to the risk of this interaction.

MECHANISM: Inhibition of warfarin metabolism by erythromycin is probably the primary factor in its enhancement of the hypoprothrombinemic response. However, fever also may enhance the catabolism of clotting factors[1]; thus, the infection for which erythromycin is used could theoretically enhance the effect of the oral anticoagulant. This effect should dissipate as erythromycin lowers the fever.

CLINICAL EVALUATION: Several case reports describe patients who developed marked increases in the hypoprothrombinemic response to warfarin and bleeding following administration of a variety of erythromycin salts in dosages of 1 to 2 mg/day (except 2 patients who received 3 to 4 mg/day).[2-7] However, some patients did not manifest a clinically important increase in the prothrombin time following erythromycin administration.[8,9] In a randomized study, erythromycin produced a modest (14%) reduction in the clearance of warfarin.[10] These small increases appear to be inconsistent with the dramatic increases noted in the case reports.

RELATED DRUGS: Little is known regarding the effect of erythromycin on oral anticoagulants other than warfarin. A study in 6 healthy subjects found no effect of ponsinomycin[+] on the pharmacokinetics of a single dose of acenocoumarol[+]. Troleandomycin[+] or clarithromycin (eg, *Biaxin*) may alter warfarin elimination, but specific information is not available.

MANAGEMENT OPTIONS:

➡ *Consider Alternative.* Early evidence suggests that azithromycin (eg, *Zithromax*) is not likely to be an enzyme inhibitor and the manufacturer states that it did not affect the hypoprothrombinemic response to a single dose of warfarin.[11]

➡ *Monitor.* Be alert for evidence of an increased response to oral anticoagulants when erythromycin therapy is initiated and the converse when erythromycin is discontinued. The anticoagulant dose may need to be adjusted.

REFERENCES:

1. Loeliger EA, et al. The biological disappearance rate of prothrombin and factors VII, IX and X from plasma in hypothyroidism, hyperthyroidism, and during fever. *Thromb Diath Haemorrh.* 1964;10:267-277.
2. Schwartz J, et al. Interaction between warfarin and erythromycin. *South Med J.* 1983;76(1):91-93.
3. Bartle WR. Possible warfarin-erythromycin interaction. *Arch Intern Med.* 1980;140(7):985-987.
4. Husserl FE. Erythromycin-warfarin interaction. *Arch Intern Med.* 1983;143(9):1831, 1836.
5. Sato RI, et al. Warfarin interaction with erythromycin. *Arch Intern Med.* 1984;144(12):2413-2414.
6. Grau E, et al. Erythromycin-oral anticoagulants interaction. *Arch Intern Med.* 1986;146(8):1639.
7. Bussey HI, et al. Warfarin-erythromycin interaction. *Arch Intern Med.* 1985;145(9):1736-1737.
8. Bachmann K, et al. The effect of erythromycin on the disposition kinetics of warfarin. *Pharmacology.* 1984;28(3):171-176.
9. Couet W, et al. Lack of effect of ponsinomycin on the pharmacokinetics of nicoumalone enantiomers. *Br J Clin Pharmacol.* 1990;30(4):616-620.
10. Weibert RT, et al. Effect of erythromycin in patients receiving long-term warfarin therapy. *Clin Pharm.* 1989;8(3):210-214.
11. *Zithromax* [package insert]. New York, NY: Pfizer Labs; 2007.

† Not available in the United States.

Erythromycin (eg, *Ery-Tab*) ▼ 3
Zafirlukast (*Accolate*)

SUMMARY: Erythromycin coadministration reduces the plasma concentrations of zafirlukast; reduced efficacy may result.

RISK FACTORS: No specific risk factors are known.

MECHANISM: Not established. Erythromycin may reduce the bioavailability of zafirlukast.

CLINICAL EVALUATION: While no published data are available for evaluation, the manufacturer of zafirlukast has made available some data on this interaction.[1] In a study of 11 asthmatic patients, the administration of a single dose of zafirlukast 40 mg with erythromycin 500 mg 3 times daily for 5 days resulted in a 40% reduction in zafirlukast plasma concentrations. This degree of reduction in zafirlukast concentrations could result in a reduction in efficacy.

RELATED DRUGS: The effect of other macrolides on zafirlukast is unknown.

MANAGEMENT OPTIONS:

➡ *Monitor.* Be alert for reduced zafirlukast efficacy when it is administered with erythromycin.

REFERENCES:

1. *Accolate* [package insert]. Wilmington, DE: Astrazeneca LP; 1997.

Erythromycin (eg, *Ery-Tab*)

Zopiclone†

SUMMARY: The administration of erythromycin with zopiclone resulted in increased plasma concentrations and pharmacodynamic effects.

RISK FACTORS: No specific risk factors are known.

MECHANISM: Not established. The increases in zopiclone plasma concentrations following erythromycin administration may be the result of enhanced zopiclone absorption caused by an erythromycin-induced increase in gastric emptying or reduced zopiclone metabolism.

CLINICAL EVALUATION: In 10 healthy subjects, the peak concentration of zopiclone increased 40%, the area under the concentration-time curve increased 80%, and the time to peak concentration was reduced from 2 hours to 1 hour following erythromycin.[1] The pharmacodynamic effects of the hypnotic zopiclone were enhanced for 2 hours following coadministration. These changes in zopiclone pharmacokinetics and pharmacodynamics are likely to lead to enhanced hypnotic response.

RELATED DRUGS: Other macrolides (eg, clarithromycin [eg, *Biaxin*], troleandomycin†) may affect zopiclone in a similar manner.

MANAGEMENT OPTIONS:

➡ **Monitor.** Patients receiving zopiclone may experience increased sedation following the addition of erythromycin therapy. Zopiclone dosage adjustment may be required to avoid morning sedation.

REFERENCES:
   1. Aranko K, et al. The effect of erythromycin on the pharmacokinetics and pharmacodynamics of zopiclone. *Br J Clin Pharmacol.* 1994;38(4):363-367.

   † Not available in the United States.

Escitalopram (*Lexapro*)

Metoprolol (*Lopressor*)

SUMMARY: Escitalopram increases the plasma concentrations of metoprolol; however, little change in patient response is likely to be seen in most patients taking metoprolol.

RISK FACTORS:

➡ **Pharmacogenetics.** Only patients who are rapid CYP2D6 genotypes are susceptible to the interaction.

MECHANISM: Escitalopram inhibits CYP2D6, the enzyme responsible for the metabolism of metoprolol.

CLINICAL EVALUATION: The administration of escitalopram 20 mg/day for 21 days resulted in a 82% increase in the area under the concentration-time curve and a 50% increase in the peak concentration of metoprolol (single 100 mg dose).[1] No further detail is available regarding this interaction. Because of the relatively wide therapeutic window for metoprolol, few patients should experience a significant change in their response to the beta blocker.

RELATED DRUGS: Propranolol (*Inderal*), timolol (*Betimol*), and carvedilol (*Coreg*) are at least partially metabolized by CYP2D6 and would probably demonstrate increased plasma concentrations if coadministered with escitalopram. Citalopram (*Celexa*) is known to inhibit the metabolism of metoprolol. Other antidepressants that inhibit CYP2D6 (eg, paroxetine [*Paxil*], fluoxetine [*Prozac*]), would also be expected to increase metoprolol plasma concentrations.

MANAGEMENT OPTIONS:

➡ *Monitor.* Patients stabilized on metoprolol who are administered escitalopram should be watched for any evidence of increased beta blockade such as bradycardia, hypotension, or heart failure.

REFERENCES:

1. Product information. *Lexapro* (Escitalopram). Forest Laboratories, Inc. 2002.

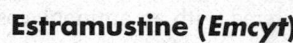

Estramustine (*Emcyt*)

Food

SUMMARY: Food and milk cause significant reductions in estramustine serum concentrations; loss of efficacy could result.

RISK FACTORS: No specific risk factors are known.

MECHANISM: Not established, but estramustine may form a poorly soluble complex with calcium or other divalent cations found in food and milk.

CLINICAL EVALUATION: Six patients with prostatic carcinoma were given three 420 mg doses of estramustine.[1] The estramustine doses were taken with 200 mL of water, milk (240 mg calcium), or a standardized breakfast. The bioavailability and peak serum concentration of estramustine were reduced by approximately 60% and approximately 70%, respectively, following concomitant milk ingestion. Administration with food produced similar effects (40% reduction in bioavailability). While no outcome studies are available, this magnitude of a reduction in bioavailability could lead to a reduction in efficacy.

RELATED DRUGS: No information is available.

MANAGEMENT OPTIONS:

➡ *Circumvent/Minimize.* Administer estramustine in a fasting state.

➡ *Monitor.* Monitor for reduced estramustine effect if the patient takes it with food or milk.

REFERENCES:

1. Gunnarsson PO, et al. Impairment of estramustine phosphate absorption by concurrent intake of milk and food. *Eur J Clin Pharmacol.* 1990;38:189.

Ethacrynic Acid (*Edecrin*)

Gentamicin (eg, *Garamycin*)

SUMMARY: The risk of ototoxicity increases when ethacrynic acid and aminoglycosides are coadministered.

RISK FACTORS:

➡ *Concurrent Diseases.* Impaired renal function increases the risk of interaction.

MECHANISM: Ethacrynic acid can produce ototoxicity that may add to or potentiate the ototoxicity of aminoglycoside antibiotics.[2,3]

CLINICAL EVALUATION: In several reported cases, ethacrynic acid appeared to enhance the ototoxicity of agents such as kanamycin (eg, *Kantrex*), neomycin (eg, *Neo-Tabs*), gentamicin, and streptomycin.[1] The presence of impaired renal function markedly enhances the danger of ototoxicity from any of these agents.

RELATED DRUGS: Furosemide (*Lasix*), torsemide (*Demadex*), or bumetanide (eg, *Bumex*) are less likely to produce an increase in nephrotoxicity when used with an aminoglycoside. Other aminoglycosides, such as kanamycin, neomycin, and streptomycin, are likely to produce ototoxicity with ethacrynic acid.

MANAGEMENT OPTIONS:

➥ *Use Alternative.* Select an alternative diuretic such as furosemide, torsemide, or bumetanide, which are less likely to produce increased nephrotoxicity when coadministered with an aminoglycoside.

REFERENCES:

1. Mathog RH, et al. Ototoxicity of ethacrynic acid and aminoglycoside antibiotics in uremia. *N Engl J Med*. 1969;280:1223.
2. Pillay VKG, et al. Transient and permanent deafness following treatment with ethacrynic acid in renal failure. *Lancet*. 1969;1:77.
3. Meriwether WD, et al. Deafness following standard intravenous dose of ethacrynic acid. *JAMA*. 1971;216:795.

---

4   **Ethacrynic Acid (*Edecrin*)**

Lithium (eg, *Eskalith*)

SUMMARY: Ethacrynic acid appears to have little effect on lithium concentrations in most patients.

RISK FACTORS: No specific risk factors are known.

MECHANISM: Sustained ethacrynic acid therapy can cause sodium depletion, which in turn, can decrease lithium excretion.

CLINICAL EVALUATION: Acute experiments failed to demonstrate an effect of ethacrynic acid on lithium excretion.[2] However, 1 case report described lithium intoxication apparently caused by furosemide plus dietary sodium restriction.[1] It seems reasonable that ethacrynic acid could have a similar effect, particularly if administered with a sodium-restricted diet.

RELATED DRUGS: Thiazides consistently increase serum lithium concentrations, but furosemide (*Lasix*) appears less likely to do so.

MANAGEMENT OPTIONS: No specific action is required, but be alert for evidence of the interaction.

REFERENCES:

1. Hurtig HI, et al. Lithium toxicity enhanced by diuresis. *N Engl J Med*. 1974;290:748.
2. Thomsen K, et al. Renal lithium excretion in man. *Am J Physiol*. 1968;215:823.

Ethacrynic Acid (*Edecrin*) 4

Warfarin (eg, *Coumadin*)

SUMMARY: Isolated case reports and in vitro protein-binding studies indicate that ethacrynic acid may increase the hypoprothrombinemic response to warfarin; more study is needed.

RISK FACTORS:

➡ **Concurrent Diseases.** In at least 1 of the cases, hypoalbuminemia was present, which may have predisposed the patient to the enhanced hypoprothrombinemia.[2] Renal insufficiency also might be expected to increase the likelihood of this interaction.

➡ **Dosage Regimen.** Large doses of ethacrynic acid might be expected to increase the risk of interaction.

MECHANISM: Ethacrynic acid has been shown, in vitro, to displace warfarin from human albumin binding sites, but the clinical significance of this finding is unclear.[5] If protein displacement does occur in vivo, any increase in oral anticoagulant-induced hypoprothrombinemia is likely to be transient, since increasing free anticoagulant serum concentrations would tend to result in a compensatory increase in its elimination.

CLINICAL EVALUATION: The clinical evidence to support this interaction between ethacrynic acid and oral anticoagulants consists primarily of occasional case reports.[1,2] If this interaction is real, other anticoagulants would be expected to interact with ethacrynic acid as well. Ethacrynic acid also may increase the risk of GI bleeding in patients receiving oral anticoagulants.[3]

RELATED DRUGS: Furosemide (eg, *Lasix*) appears to have little effect on warfarin.[4]

MANAGEMENT OPTIONS: No specific action is required, but be alert for evidence of the interaction.

REFERENCES:

1. Koch-Weser J. Hemorrhagic reactions and drug interactions in 500 warfarin-treated patients. *Clin Pharmacol Ther.* 1973;14:139.
2. Petrick RJ, et al. Interaction between warfarin and ethacrynic acid. *JAMA.* 1975;231:843.
3. Slone D, et al. Intravenously given ethacrynic acid and gastrointestinal bleeding: a finding resulting from comprehensive drug surveillance. *JAMA.* 1969;209:1668.
4. Nilsson CM, et al. The effect of furosemide and bumetanide on warfarin metabolism and anticoagulant response. *J Clin Pharmacol.* 1978;18:91.
5. Sellers EM, et al. Displacement of warfarin from human albumin by diazoxide and ethacrynic, mefenamic and nalidixic acids. *Clin Pharmacol Ther.* 1970;11:524.

Ethanol (*Ethyl Alcohol*) 4

Contraceptives, Oral (eg, *Ortho-Novum*)

SUMMARY: Oral contraceptives may slightly reduce the elimination rate of ethanol, but the clinical importance is not established.

RISK FACTORS: No specific risk factors are known.

MECHANISM: Not established. Oral contraceptives may inhibit the hepatic metabolism of ethanol.

CLINICAL EVALUATION: A moderate dose of ethanol (0.52 g/kg) was given to 20 women taking oral contraceptives (various levels of estrogen content) and 20 controls who were not taking oral contraceptives.[1] The ethanol elimination rate was 13% lower in the women taking oral contraceptives than in those who were not, but peak blood alcohol concentrations tended to be slightly lower in women on oral contraceptives. An interaction of this magnitude would not be expected to substantially increase the pharmacodynamic effect of ethanol. Nonetheless, it is important to remember that the 13% reduction in ethanol elimination is an average value and some women will manifest a larger effect.

RELATED DRUGS: No information is available.

MANAGEMENT OPTIONS: No specific action is required, but be alert for evidence of the interaction.

REFERENCES:
1. Jones M, et al. Ethanol metabolism in women taking oral contraceptives. *Alcoholism*. 1984;8:24.

 Ethanol (*Ethyl Alcohol*)

Famotidine (eg, *Pepcid*)

SUMMARY: Available evidence suggests that famotidine does not affect blood alcohol concentrations, but patients receiving famotidine for peptic ulcers or gastroesophageal reflux should minimize their alcohol intake to avoid worsening their disease.

RISK FACTORS: No specific risk factors are known.

MECHANISM: No interaction.

CLINICAL EVALUATION: Several studies in both fed and fasting healthy subjects have found that famotidine in doses of 40 mg/day does not affect blood alcohol concentrations.[1-7] However, the total number of subjects studied is not as large as the number studied for alcohol plus cimetidine or alcohol plus ranitidine.

RELATED DRUGS: Other H_2-receptor antagonists, such as cimetidine (eg, *Tagamet*), ranitidine (eg, *Zantac*), and nizatidine (*Axid*), appear to have minimal effects on the response to ethanol.

MANAGEMENT OPTIONS: No interaction.

REFERENCES:
1. Tanaka, et al. Effects of H_2-receptor antagonists on ethanol metabolism in Japanese volunteers. *Br J Clin Pharmacol*. 1988;26:96.
2. Hernandez-Munoz R, et al. Human gastric alcohol dehydrogenase; its inhibition by H_2-receptor antagonists, and its effect on the bioavailability of ethanol. *Alcohol Clin Exp Res*. 1990;14:946.
3. Guram M, et al. Further evidence for an interaction between alcohol and certain H_2-receptor antagonists. *Alcohol Clin Exp Res*. 1991;15:1084.
4. Fraser AG, et al. The effect of ranitidine, cimetidine, or famotidine on low-dose post-prandial alcohol absorption. *Aliment Pharmacol Ther*. 1991;5:263.
5. DiPadova C, et al. Effects of ranitidine on blood alcohol levels after ethanol ingestion: comparison with other H_2-receptor antagonists. *JAMA*. 1992;267:3.
6. Gugler R. H_2-antagonists and alcohol: do they interact? *Drug Safety*. 1994;10:271.
7. Levitt MD. Review article: lack of clinical significance of the interaction between H_2-receptor antagonists and ethanol. *Aliment Pharmacol Ther*. 1993;7:131.

Ethanol (Ethyl Alcohol)

Fluoxetine (*Prozac*)

SUMMARY: Studies in healthy subjects suggest that fluoxetine does not enhance the impairment of psychomotor or cognitive function that follows moderate doses of ethanol, but depressed patients probably should limit their ethanol intake.

RISK FACTORS: No specific risk factors are known.

MECHANISM: No interaction.

CLINICAL EVALUATION: Six healthy men were given single or multiple doses of fluoxetine (30 or 60 mg) with and without concurrent ingestion of ethanol in a dose of 45 mL absolute ethanol per 70 kg body weight (equivalent to approximately 2 double shots of whiskey). Fluoxetine alone did not affect psychomotor tests, and it did not affect the psychomotor impairment produced by the alcohol.[1] Fluoxetine also had no effect on blood alcohol concentrations. In another study, 12 healthy subjects were given a moderate dose of ethanol (mean blood ethanol: 77 mg/dL) with and without pretreatment with fluoxetine for 1 week.[2] Fluoxetine had only minimal effects on the adverse psychomotor effects of ethanol. Another study of 8 healthy subjects found no effect of fluoxetine (40 mg/day) on the adverse psychomotor effects or pharmacokinetics of ethanol (blood alcohol: 80 to 100 mg/dL).[3] Thus, it does not appear that patients taking fluoxetine would manifest additive detrimental effects on psychomotor function if they consumed moderate amounts of ethanol. Nonetheless, acute ethanol intoxication impairs the hepatic metabolism of many drugs, and it is possible that fluoxetine would be affected similarly. Since excessive alcohol intake can worsen depression, such patients would do well to limit their alcohol intake regardless of what antidepressant they are receiving. Fluoxetine also has been used to reduce alcohol craving in patients who abuse alcohol, but its role in treating alcohol abuse is still under study.

RELATED DRUGS: Other selective serotonin reuptake inhibitors [eg, fluvoxamine (*Floxyfral*), paroxetine (*Paxil*), sertraline (*Zoloft*)] also appear to have little effect on alcohol response.

MANAGEMENT OPTIONS: No interaction.

REFERENCES:

1. Lemberger L, et al. Effect of fluoxetine on psychomotor performance, physiologic response, and kinetics of ethanol. *Clin Pharmacol Ther.* 1985;37:658.
2. Allen D, et al. Interactions of alcohol with amitriptyline, fluoxetine and placebo in normal subjects. *Int Clin Psychopharmacol.* 1989;4:7.
3. Hamilton CA, et al. Interaction of fluoxetine (F) and amitriptyline (A) with ethanol. *Clin Pharmacol Ther.* 1987;41:231.

Ethanol (Ethyl Alcohol) 5

Fluvoxamine (*Floxyfral*)

SUMMARY: Studies in healthy subjects suggest that fluvoxamine does not enhance the impairment of psychomotor or cognitive function that follows moderate doses of ethanol, but In any case depressed patients probably should limit their ethanol intake.

RISK FACTORS: No specific risk factors are known.

MECHANISM: No interaction.

CLINICAL EVALUATION: In 12 healthy subjects fluvoxamine 50 mg orally (both single and multiple doses) did not affect either the pharmacokinetics or the cognitive impairment produced by a 40 g dose of ethanol given orally or IV.[1] In fact, some of the adverse effects of ethanol on cognitive function appeared to be slightly antagonized by fluvoxamine. In another study of 10 healthy subjects, fluvoxamine in single doses of 50 or 100 mg was given alone and concurrently with ethanol (0.8 g/kg).[2] Fluvoxamine did not affect blood ethanol concentrations, nor did it affect the psychomotor or cognitive impairment produced by ethanol. Thus, it does not appear that patients taking fluvoxamine would manifest additive detrimental effects on psychomotor function if they consumed moderate amounts of ethanol. Nonetheless, acute ethanol intoxication impairs the hepatic metabolism of many drugs, and it is possible that fluvoxamine would be affected similarly. Some selective serotonin reuptake inhibitors (SSRIs) have been used to reduce alcohol craving in patients who abuse alcohol, but their role in treating alcohol abuse is still under study.

RELATED DRUGS: Other SSRIs [eg, fluoxetine (*Prozac*), paroxetine (*Paxil*), sertraline (*Zoloft*)] also do not appear to enhance ethanol-induced impairment of psychomotor function.

MANAGEMENT OPTIONS: No interaction.

REFERENCES:
1. van Harten J, et al. Fluvoxamine does not interact with alcohol or potentiate alcohol-related impairment of cognitive function. *Clin Pharmacol Ther.* 1992;52:427.
2. Linnoila M, et al. Effects of fluvoxamine, alone and in combination with ethanol, on psychomotor and cognitive performance and on autonomic nervous system reactivity in healthy volunteers. *J Clin Psychopharmacol.* 1993;13:175.

Ethanol (Ethyl Alcohol)

Furazolidone (*Furoxone*)

SUMMARY: A disulfiram-like reaction may occur when patients taking furazolidone ingest alcohol.

RISK FACTORS: No specific risk factors are known.

MECHANISM: It is possible that furazolidone inhibits aldehyde dehydrogenase, resulting in accumulation of acetaldehyde following ethanol ingestion.

CLINICAL EVALUATION: A disulfiram-like reaction reportedly may occur following ethanol ingestion by patients receiving furazolidone.[1-3] Symptoms (eg, flushing, dyspnea, lacrimation, lightheadedness) occur within 1 hour of ethanol ingestion and last less than 1 hour. The incidence of this reaction is unknown.

RELATED DRUGS: No information is available.

MANAGEMENT OPTIONS:

➡ *Monitor.* Warn patients on furazolidone that a disulfiram-like reaction (eg, flushing, nausea, sweating) may occur following ethanol ingestion.

REFERENCES:
1. Todd RG, ed. Extra Pharmacopoeia-Martindale. 25th ed. London: The Pharmaceutical Press; 1967:844-45.
2. Kolodny AL. Side-effects produced by alcohol in a patient receiving furazolidone. *Maryland State Med J.* 1962;11:248.
3. Calesnick B. Antihypertensive action of the antimicrobial agent furazolidone. *Am J Med Sci.* 1958;236:736.

Ethanol (Ethyl Alcohol)

Glutethimide

SUMMARY: The combined use of ethanol and glutethimide may cause excessive central nervous system (CNS) depression and impaired psychomotor performance.

RISK FACTORS: No specific risk factors are known.

MECHANISM: Additive CNS depression is likely to occur.

CLINICAL EVALUATION: The combined use of ethanol and glutethimide has been shown to increase the blood ethanol concentration and decrease the plasma glutethimide concentration.[1] Although these effects may prove to have clinical significance, it probably is more important to remember that both drugs are CNS depressants.

RELATED DRUGS: Alcohol would be expected to increase the CNS depression of all sedative-hypnotic drugs.

MANAGEMENT OPTIONS:

➡ *Circumvent/Minimize.* Patients on glutethimide should limit their intake of ethanol to avoid excessive CNS depression.

➡ *Monitor.* Monitor for excessive CNS depression if the combination is used.

REFERENCES:

1. Mould GP, et al. Interaction of glutethimide and phenobarbitone with ethanol in man. *J Pharm Pharmacol.* 1972;24:894.

Ethanol (Ethyl Alcohol)

Isoniazid (INH)

SUMMARY: Alcoholics have a higher incidence of INH-induced hepatitis.

RISK FACTORS:

➡ *Dosage Regimen.* Daily alcohol consumption can increase the risk of interaction.

MECHANISM: Not established.

CLINICAL EVALUATION: Patients taking isoniazid have an increased risk of hepatotoxicity if they chronically consume alcohol on a daily basis.[1]

RELATED DRUGS: No information is available.

MANAGEMENT OPTIONS:

➡ *Circumvent/Minimize.* Avoiding the combination of alcohol and isoniazid would be prudent, but because alcoholism and tuberculosis often coexist, it may not be possible in some cases.

➡ *Monitor.* Monitor alcoholic patients carefully for INH hepatitis if they are administered isoniazid.

REFERENCES:

1. Isoniazid [package insert]. Princeton, NJ: Apothecon, Inc.; 1996.

Ethanol (Ethyl Alcohol)

Ketoconazole (eg, *Nizoral*)

SUMMARY: Ethanol consumption during ketoconazole therapy may result in a disulfiram-like reaction.

RISK FACTORS: No specific risk factors are known.

MECHANISM: Not established.

CLINICAL EVALUATION: A patient taking ketoconazole 200 mg/day experienced disulfiram-like reactions on 3 occasions after ingesting ethanol.[1] After completing the course of ketoconazole therapy, ethanol consumption was not associated with a disulfiram-like reaction.

RELATED DRUGS: No information is available.

MANAGEMENT OPTIONS:

➡ *Circumvent/Minimize.* Advise patients taking ketoconazole to minimize their alcohol intake.

➡ *Monitor.* Counsel patients taking ketoconazole that ethanol consumption might cause flushing, nausea, and headache and should avoid ethanol while taking ketoconazole.

REFERENCES:
  1. Magnasco AJ, et al. Interaction of ketoconazole and ethanol. *Clin Pharm.* 1986;5:522.

 Ethanol (Ethyl Alcohol)

Meperidine (eg, *Demerol*)

SUMMARY: Ethanol and narcotic analgesics are likely to exhibit additive central nervous system (CNS) depressant effects. Ethanol also may affect the distribution of meperidine, but the clinical importance of this effect is not established.

RISK FACTORS: No specific risk factors are known.

MECHANISM: Both ethanol and narcotic analgesics are CNS depressants; additive effects may occur.[1]

CLINICAL EVALUATION: The combined CNS depressant effects of ethanol and narcotic analgesics may result in excessive sedation and impaired psychomotor performance. A study involving the IV injection of meperidine in surgical patients and volunteers indicated that the volume of distribution (Vd) of meperidine increased with increasing ethanol consumption.[2] It was proposed that this increase in Vd might produce a *decrease* in the pharmacologic response to meperidine, but this remains speculative.

RELATED DRUGS: Ethanol also would be expected to add to the CNS depressant effects of narcotic analgesics other than meperidine.

MANAGEMENT OPTIONS:

➡ *Circumvent/Minimize.* Patients taking narcotic analgesics should limit their use of alcohol, especially if performing tasks requiring alertness.

➡ *Monitor.* Monitor for excessive CNS depression in patients receiving the combination.

REFERENCES:
1. Linnoila M, et al. Effects of diazepam and codeine, alone and in combination with alcohol, on simulated driving. *Clin Pharmacol Ther.* 1974;15:368.
2. Mather LE, et al. Meperidine kinetics in man. Intravenous injection in surgical patients and volunteers. *Clin Pharmacol Ther.* 1975;17:21.

Ethanol (Ethyl Alcohol)

Meprobamate (eg, *Equanil*)

SUMMARY: Concurrent use of ethanol and meprobamate results in enhanced CNS depression.

RISK FACTORS: No specific risk factors are known.

MECHANISM: Both meprobamate and ethanol are CNS depressants, and additive effects would be expected.[2,4] Moreover, acute intoxication with ethanol appears to inhibit meprobamate metabolism,[3] while chronic ethanol ingestion appears to induce hepatic microsomal enzymes, resulting in enhanced meprobamate metabolism.[1]

CLINICAL EVALUATION: The simultaneous use of ethanol and meprobamate may result in synergistic CNS depression. If the doses of 1 or both agents are large, the degree of CNS depression may be dangerous. The enhanced drug metabolism observed with chronic ethanol intake[1] may partially explain the tolerance to CNS depressants in chronic alcoholics.

RELATED DRUGS: Alcohol would be expected to increase the CNS depression of all sedative-hypnotics.

MANAGEMENT OPTIONS:

➡ *Circumvent/Minimize.* Make patients aware that the combined use of ethanol and meprobamate can cause excessive CNS depression. Patients on meprobamate should avoid ingesting moderate to large amounts of ethanol.

➡ *Monitor.* Monitor for excessive CNS depression in patients receiving the combination.

REFERENCES:
1. Misra PS, et al. Increase of ethanol, meprobamate and pentobarbital metabolism after chronic ethanol administration in man and in rats. *Am J Med.* 1971;41:346.
2. Valsrub S. Alcohol-induced sensitivity and tolerance. *JAMA.* 1972;219:508. Editorial.
3. Rubin E, et al. Inhibition of drug metabolism by acute ethanol intoxication: a hepatic microsomal mechanism. *Am J Med.* 1970;49:801.
4. Ashford JR, et al. Drug interactions. The effects of alcohol and meprobamate applied singly and jointly in human subjects. III. *J Stud Alcohol.* 1975;7(Suppl.):140.
5. Cobby JM, et al. Drug interactions. The effect of alcohol and meprobamate applied singly and jointly in human subjects. IV. *J Stud Alcohol.* 1975;7(Suppl.):162.
6. Ashford JR, et al. Drug interactions. The effects of alcohol and meprobamate applied singly and jointly in human subjects. V. *J Stud Alcohol.* 1975;7(Suppl.):177.

Ethanol (Ethyl Alcohol)

AVOID **Methotrexate (eg, _Rheumatrex_)**

SUMMARY: Some evidence indicates that ethanol may increase the likelihood of methotrexate-induced liver injury, but a causal relationship has not been established.

RISK FACTORS: No specific risk factors are known.

MECHANISM: Not established; additive hepatotoxicity may be involved.

CLINICAL EVALUATION: In 1 study of 5 cases of methotrexate-induced cirrhosis,[1] 1 patient ingested 28 to 85 g/week of ethanol and 2 ingested more than 85 g/week. This finding is consistent with the contention of others that ethanol may enhance the liver toxicity of methotrexate[2,3] but certainly does not establish such an association. Also, a single case has been reported in which a patient on methotrexate developed respiratory failure and coma following a cocktail.[4] However, a causal relationship was not established.

RELATED DRUGS: No information is available.

MANAGEMENT OPTIONS:

➥ **AVOID COMBINATION.** Avoid ethanol in patients receiving methotrexate.[2] The manufacturer of methotrexate also recommends the avoidance of ethanol.[4] Even though the evidence for additive hepatotoxic effects is not conclusive, alcohol restriction probably is appropriate for most patients receiving methotrexate.

REFERENCES:

1. Tobias H, et al. Hepatotoxicity of long-term methotrexate therapy for psoriasis. _Arch Intern Med_. 1973;132:391.
2. Pai SH, et al. Severe liver damage caused by treatment of psoriasis with methotrexate. _NY State J Med_. 1973;73:2585.
3. Methotrexate. Product Information. Wayne, NJ: Lederle Laboratories; 1988.
4. Glassner J. Methotrexate and psoriasis. _JAMA_. 1970;210:1925.

 Ethanol (Ethyl Alcohol)

Metoclopramide (eg, _Reglan_)

SUMMARY: Metoclopramide may enhance the sedative effects of ethanol, but the clinical importance of this effect is not established.

RISK FACTORS: No specific risk factors are known.

MECHANISM: Ethanol and metoclopramide may produce additive sedative effects. Metoclopramide also may increase the absorption rate of oral ethanol, probably by speeding gastric emptying.

CLINICAL EVALUATION: A study of 7 healthy subjects indicated that metoclopramide 10 mg IV may enhance the sedative effect of ethanol 70 mg/kg body weight.[1] In 5 healthy subjects, oral ethanol 0.35 g/kg body weight was absorbed much more rapidly following pretreatment with 20 mg of oral or IV metoclopramide.[2] The effect of this change on the pharmacodynamic effects of ethanol was not assessed.

RELATED DRUGS: No information is available.

MANAGEMENT OPTIONS:

➤ *Circumvent/Minimize.* Until more is known about this purported interaction, advise patients taking metoclopramide that alcohol may have a greater than expected effect.

➤ *Monitor.* Monitor for excessive central nervous system depression in patients receiving the combination.

REFERENCES:

1. Bateman DN, et al. Pharmacokinetic and concentration-effect studies with intravenous metoclopramide. *Br J Clin Pharmacol.* 1978;6:401.

2. Gibbons DO, et al. Effects of intravenous and oral propantheline and metoclopramide on ethanol absorption. *Clin Pharmacol Ther.* 1975;17:578.

Ethanol (Ethyl Alcohol)

Metronidazole (eg, *Flagyl*)

SUMMARY: Alcohol ingestion during metronidazole therapy may lead to a disulfiram-like reaction in some patients.

RISK FACTORS: No specific risk factors are known.

MECHANISM: Metronidazole presumably acts in a manner similar to that of disulfiram by inhibiting the activity of aldehyde dehydrogenase.

CLINICAL EVALUATION: A disulfiram-like reaction was reported after the combined administration of IV trimethoprim-sulfamethoxazole (eg, *Bactrim*) and metronidazole.[1] IV TMP-SMX uses 10% ethanol as a solubilizing agent. No reaction occurred with orally administered TMP-SMX in patients receiving metronidazole.

RELATED DRUGS: The coadministration of metronidazole and other IV drugs containing ethanol (eg, phenytoin [eg, *Dilantin*], trimethoprim-sulfamethoxazole, phenobarbital [eg, *Solfoton*], diazepam [eg, *Valium*], and nitroglycerin [eg, *Tridil*]) may result in flushing and vomiting.

MANAGEMENT OPTIONS:

➤ *Circumvent/Minimize.* Warn patients receiving metronidazole about the possibility of reactions following ethanol ingestion and avoid ethanol or ethanol-containing drugs.

➤ *Monitor.* If ethanol is taken by a patient receiving metronidazole, watch for flushing, nausea, and vomiting.

REFERENCES:

1. Edwards DL, et al. Disulfiram-like reaction associated with intravenous trimethoprim-sulfamethoxazole and metronidazole. *Clin Pharm.* 1986;5:999.

Ethanol (*Ethyl Alcohol*)

Nicotinic Acid (eg, *Niacin*)

SUMMARY: A man receiving niacin for hyperlipidemia developed delirium and lactic acidosis after drinking a bottle of wine, but a causal relationship between the reaction and an interaction between alcohol and niacin was not established.

RISK FACTORS: No specific risk factors are known.

MECHANISM: Not established. It was proposed that the reaction was caused by use of alcohol in the presence of niacin-induced hepatic dysfunction.

CLINICAL EVALUATION: A 44-year-old man on chronic therapy with niacin 3 g/day developed delirium and lactic acidosis the morning after ingesting approximately 1 L of red wine.[1] He was aggressive, paranoid, and combative; his lactic acid concentration was 9.5 mmol/L (normal: 7.35 to 7.45) and hepatic enzymes were elevated. He was admitted to the hospital and given thiamine, magnesium, and hydration. His mental status and lactic acid returned to normal within 10 hours. Although it is possible that the reaction was caused by a combined effect of niacin and alcohol, it is difficult to assess without a rechallenge of alcohol with and without niacin pretreatment. Note that patients with some types of hyperlipidemias need to minimize or eliminate ethanol regardless of whether they are on niacin because ethanol worsens their hyperlipidemia (particularly hypertriglyceridemia).

RELATED DRUGS: No information is available.

MANAGEMENT OPTIONS: No specific action is required, but be alert for evidence of the interaction.

REFERENCES:
1. Schwab RA, et al. Delirium and lactic acidosis caused by ethanol and niacin coingestion. *Am J Emer Med.* 1991;9:363-65.

Ethanol (Ethyl Alcohol)

Nitroglycerin

SUMMARY: Additive vasodilation could cause hypotension when ethanol is consumed by patients taking nitroglycerin.

RISK FACTORS: No specific risk factors are known.

MECHANISM: Hypotension can occur following the combined use of ethanol and nitroglycerin,[1] presumably caused by additive vasodilatory effects.[2]

CLINICAL EVALUATION: Although clinical reports are lacking, hypotensive reactions may result from the combination of alcohol and nitroglycerin.[1] Unless the clinician is aware of this interaction, the hypotensive episode may be attributed to coronary insufficiency or occlusion.

RELATED DRUGS: No information is available.

MANAGEMENT OPTIONS:

➡ *Circumvent/Minimize.* Until further information is available, advise patients receiving nitroglycerin to limit their alcohol intake.

➡ *Monitor.* Be alert for evidence of hypotension (eg, lightheadedness, fainting) in patients receiving the combination.

REFERENCES:
1. Shafer N. Hypotension due to nitroglycerin combined with alcohol. *N Engl J Med.* 1965;273:1169.

2. Allison RD, et al. Effects of alcohol and nitroglycerin on vascular responses in man. *Angiology.* 1971;22:211.

Ethanol (Ethyl Alcohol) 4

Nizatidine (*Axid*)

SUMMARY: Limited clinical information indicates that nizatidine may increase blood alcohol concentrations under certain conditions, but this has not been shown to be clinically important. Patients receiving nizatidine for peptic ulcers or gastroesophageal reflux should minimize their alcohol intake to avoid worsening their disease.

RISK FACTORS:

➡ **Dosage Regimen.** H_2-receptor antagonists have a greater effect on blood alcohol if a small amount of alcohol is taken. An interaction is unlikely with 2 to 3 drinks or more.

➡ **Diet/Food.** Increased alcohol levels are more likely after a meal.

➡ **Gender.** Increased alcohol levels are more likely in men.

➡ **Time of Day.** Some evidence suggests that the interaction is more likely to occur in the morning than in the evening.

MECHANISM: It has been proposed that nizatidine inhibits gastric alcohol dehydrogenase,[4] which theoretically could inhibit the first-pass metabolism of alcohol.

CLINICAL EVALUATION: Relatively little information is available on potential interactions between nizatidine and alcohol. In a crossover study, 6 fed subjects were given 0.75 g/kg alcohol with and without nizatidine (300 mg/day for 7 days). Nizatidine increased the area under the blood alcohol concentrationtime curve (AUC) approximately 20%, and the maximum blood alcohol concentration (C_{max}) approximately 19%.[1] However, in a subsequent crossover study of 23 fed subjects, nizatidine (300 mg/day for 7 days) had no effect on either AUC or C_{max} of alcohol (0.3 g/kg).[2] Moreover, the combination of nizatidine and alcohol did not appear to adversely affect psychomotor function in 10 subjects.[3] Nonetheless, additional study is needed to assess the effect of nizatidine on blood alcohol.[5,6] Most patients receiving nizatidine should minimize their alcohol intake because alcohol can worsen both peptic ulcer disease and gastroesophageal reflux disease. Although nizatidine-induced increases in blood alcohol concentrations are unlikely to be clinically important in most patients, this is another reason (albeit a minor one) for restricting alcohol intake in such patients.

RELATED DRUGS: Other H_2-receptor antagonists (eg, cimetidine [eg, *Tagamet*], famotidine [eg, *Pepcid*], ranitidine [eg, *Zantac*]) appear to have minimal effects on the response to ethanol.

MANAGEMENT OPTIONS: No specific action is required, but be alert for evidence of the interaction.

REFERENCES:

1. Guram M, et al. Further evidence for an interaction between alcohol and certain H_2-receptor antagonists. *Alcoholism Clin Exp Res.* 1991;15:1084.
2. Raufman JP, et al. Histamine-H_2-receptor antagonists do not alter serum ethanol levels in fed, nonalcoholic men. *Am J Gastroenterol.* 1992;87:1344.
3. Hindmarch I, et al. The lack of CNS effects of nizatidine with and without alcohol on psychomotor ability and cognitive function. *Hum Psychopharmacol.* 1990;5:25.
4. Caballeria J, et al. Effect of H_2-receptor antagonists on gastric alcohol dehydrogenase activity. *Dig Dis Sci.* 1991;36:1673.

5. Gugler R. H$_2$-antagonists and alcohol: do they interact? *Drug Safety.* 1994;10:271.

6. Levitt MD. Review article: lack of clinical significance of the interaction between H$_2$-receptor antagonists and ethanol. *Aliment Pharmacol Ther.* 1993;7:131.

5 Ethanol (Ethyl Alcohol)

Omeprazole (*Prilosec*)

SUMMARY: Omeprazole does not appear to affect ethanol metabolism.

RISK FACTORS: No specific risk factors are known.

MECHANISM: No interaction.

CLINICAL EVALUATION: Several studies have shown that omeprazole (20 to 40 mg/day) does not affect the metabolism of alcohol in fasting or fed subjects.[1-4]

RELATED DRUGS: The effect of lansoprazole (*Prevacid*) on ethanol is not established.

MANAGEMENT OPTIONS: No interaction.

REFERENCES:

1. Roine R, et al. Effect of omeprazole on first-pass metabolism of ethanol. *Dig Dis Sci.* 1992;37:891.

2. Jonsson K, et al. Lack of an effect of omeprazole, cimetidine, and ranitidine on the pharmacokinetics of ethanol in fasting male volunteers. *Eur J Clin Pharmacol.* 1992;42:209.

3. Guram M, et al. Further evidence for an interaction between alcohol and certain H$_2$-receptor antagonists. *Alcohol Clin Exp Res.* 1991;15:1084.

4. Terpin MM, et al. Antisecretive drugs and interactions of ethanol metabolism. *Ital J Gastroenterol.* 1990;22:266.

5 Ethanol (Ethyl Alcohol)

Orlistat (*Xenical*)

SUMMARY: Concurrent use of orlistat and alcohol did not affect the pharmacokinetics of either drug.

RISK FACTORS: No specific risk factors are known.

MECHANISM: No interaction.

CLINICAL EVALUATION: In a randomized, double-blind, parallel study, 3 groups of 10 healthy subjects received orlistat 120 mg 3 times daily and multiple doses of alcohol alone and together.[1] Alcohol had no effect on orlistat-induced increase in fecal fat excretion or orlistat plasma concentrations, and orlistat had no effect on alcohol pharmacokinetics.

RELATED DRUGS: No related drugs.

MANAGEMENT OPTIONS: No interaction.

REFERENCES:

1. Melia AT, et al. The interaction of the lipase inhibitor orlistat with ethanol in healthy volunteers. *Eur J Clin Pharmacol.* 1998;54:773–77.

Ethanol (Ethyl Alcohol) 4

Paroxetine (*Paxil*)

SUMMARY: Studies in healthy subjects suggest that paroxetine has only minimal effects on ethanol-induced impairment of psychomotor function, but in any case depressed patients probably should limit their ethanol intake.

RISK FACTORS: No specific risk factors are known.

MECHANISM: Not established.

CLINICAL EVALUATION: Six healthy subjects received a single 30 mg dose of paroxetine or placebo with and without 50 g of ethanol using a randomized, double-blind, Latin square design.[1] Numerous psychomotor tests were performed after each treatment. Paroxetine alone had no effect on the psychomotor tests and increased the effect of ethanol on only 1 of the psychomotor tests (attentiveness). In another study, 10 healthy subjects received a single 30 mg dose of paroxetine with and without ethanol (0.5 g/kg body weight) in a randomized crossover study.[2] Paroxetine alone did not affect any of the psychomotor tests and increased the effect of ethanol on only 1 of the psychomotor tests (reaction time). Thus, it appears that patients taking paroxetine would manifest only small increases in ethanol-induced impairment of psychomotor function when only small to moderate amounts of ethanol are ingested. Nonetheless, acute ethanol intoxication impairs the hepatic metabolism of many drugs, and it is possible that paroxetine would be affected similarly. Some selective serotonin reuptake inhibitors (SSRIs) have been used to reduce alcohol craving in patients who abuse alcohol, but their role in treating alcohol abuse is still under study.

RELATED DRUGS: Other SSRIs also do not appear to enhance ethanol-induced impairment of psychomotor function.

MANAGEMENT OPTIONS: No specific action is required, but be alert for evidence of the interaction.

REFERENCES:

1. Cooper SM, et al. The psychomotor effects of paroxetine alone and in combination with haloperidol, amylobarbitone, oxazepam, or alcohol. *Acta Psychiatr Scand.* 1989;80(Suppl. 350):53.
2. Hindamarch L, et al. The effects of paroxetine and other antidepressants in combination with alcohol on psychomotor activity related to car driving. *Acta Psychiatr Scand.* 1989;80(Suppl. 350):45.

Ethanol (Ethyl Alcohol) 1

Phenelzine (*Nardil*)

SUMMARY: Alcoholic beverages containing tyramine may induce a severe hypertensive response in patients taking nonselective monoamine oxidase inhibitors (MAOIs).

RISK FACTORS: No specific risk factors are known.

MECHANISM: There is no known mechanism for any interaction between ethanol itself and MAOIs. However, some alcoholic beverages (eg, Chianti wine and some beer) may contain considerable amounts of tyramine. In the presence of an MAOI, the normally rapid metabolism of tyramine in the intestine and liver is impaired, resulting in a markedly enhanced pressor response to tyramine.

CLINICAL EVALUATION: Although the effect of ethanol itself may be enhanced somewhat in the presence of MAOIs, too little information is available to assess the clinical significance of this interaction.[1,2] Although most alcoholic beverages that have been tested do not contain significant amounts of tyramine, the danger of tyramine-containing alcoholic beverages is definite; fatal hypertensive crises may result when persons taking an MAOI ingest such beverages.[3]

RELATED DRUGS: All nonselective MAOIs including isocarboxazid (*Marplan*) and tranylcypromine (*Parnate*) interact with tyramine-containing alcoholic beverages.

MANAGEMENT OPTIONS:

➡ *AVOID COMBINATION.* Because it is difficult to assess the tyramine content of a given drink (especially drinks with many ingredients), advise patients receiving MAOIs to avoid all alcoholic beverages. If alcohol is ingested, the patient should use products that are unlikely to contain significant amounts of tyramine (eg, vodka, white wine) and ingest small amounts initially.[4] Assume that the effects of nonselective monoamine oxidase inhibitors to persist for 2 weeks after they are discontinued.

REFERENCES:

1. Sjoqvist F. Psychotropic drugs (2). Interaction between monoamine oxidase (MAO) inhibitors and other substances. *Proc R Soc Med.* 1965;58:967.
2. Ellis J, et al. Modification by monoamine oxidase inhibitors of the effect of some sympathomimetics on blood pressure. *BMJ.* 1967;2:75.
3. MacLeod I. Fatal reaction to phenelzine. *BMJ.* 1965;1:1554.
4. Shulman KI, et al. Dietary restriction, tyramine, and the use of monoamine oxidase inhibitors. *J Clin Psychopharmacol.* 1989;9:397.

Ethanol (Ethyl Alcohol)

Phenobarbital (eg, *Solfoton*)

SUMMARY: Ethanol and barbiturates like phenobarbital have additive depressant effects on the CNS; combined use is dangerous in patients performing tasks requiring alertness and may be fatal in overdose.

RISK FACTORS: No specific risk factors are known.

MECHANISM: The mechanisms of this interaction are: 1) *Effect on Ethanol.* Phenobarbital appears to enhance the disappearance of ethanol from the blood, resulting in somewhat decreased blood ethanol concentrations.[1,6] The mechanism for this effect is unknown. It may involve factors other than a direct increase in the hepatic metabolism of ethanol. 2) *Effect on Barbiturates.* Acute intoxication with ethanol appears to inhibit pentobarbital metabolism,[5] while chronic ethanol ingestion appears to enhance the hepatic metabolism of pentobarbital.[3] It also has been proposed that ethanol may promote the penetration of barbiturates into tissues.[10] 3) Combined CNS depression.[2,4,7,9]

CLINICAL EVALUATION: It is clear from the mechanisms described above that the interrelationships between ethanol and barbiturates are quite complex. Clinically, the most important considerations are that they are both CNS depressants and that acute ethanol intoxication may impair barbiturate metabolism. Also, the enhanced drug metabolism with chronic ethanol intake[3] may partially explain the tolerance to barbiturates seen in chronic alcoholics.

RELATED DRUGS: All barbiturates are likely to result in additive CNS depressant effects with ethanol. Acute ethanol intoxication appears to inhibit pentobarbital (eg, nembutal) metabolism.

MANAGEMENT OPTIONS:

➥ *Circumvent/Minimize.* Warn patients receiving barbiturates that the combined use of ethanol can lead to excessive CNS depression.

➥ *Monitor.* Monitor for excessive CNS depression in patients receiving the combination.

REFERENCES:

1. Mould GP, et al. Interaction of glutethimide and phenobarbitone with ethanol in man. *J Pharm Pharmacol.* 1972;24:894.
2. Lieber CS. Hepatic and metabolic effects of alcohol (1966 to 1973). *Gastroenterology.* 1973;65:821.
3. Misra PS, et al. Increase of ethanol, meprobamate and pentobarbital metabolism after chronic ethanol administration in man and in rats. *Am J Med.* 1971;43:346.
4. Valsrub S. Alcohol-induced sensitivity and tolerance. *JAMA.* 1972;219:508. Editorial.
5. Rubin E, et al. Inhibition of drug metabolism by acute ethanol intoxication: a hepatic microsomal mechanism. *Am J Med.* 1970;49:801.
6. Mezey E, et al. Effects of phenobarbital administration on rates of ethanol clearance and on ethanol-oxidizing enzymes in man. *Gastroenterology.* 1974;66:248.
7. Johnstone RF, et al. Respiratory interaction of alcohol. *JAMA.* 1975;233:770.
8. Mezey E. Effect of phenobarbital administration on ethanol oxidizing enzymes and on rates of ethanol degradation. *Biochem Pharmacol.* 1971;20:508.
9. Milner G. Interaction between barbiturates, alcohol and some psychotropic drugs. *Med J Aust.* 1970;1:1204.
10. Stead AH, et al. Quantification of the interaction between barbiturates and alcohol and interpretation of fatal blood concentrations. *Hum Toxicol.* 1983;2:5.

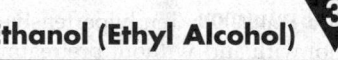

Ethanol (Ethyl Alcohol)

Phenytoin (eg, *Dilantin*)

SUMMARY: Chronic ethanol abuse may reduce serum phenytoin concentrations, but the clinical importance of this effect is not established.

RISK FACTORS: No specific risk factors are known.

MECHANISM: Ethanol induces the production of hepatic microsomal enzymes, resulting in enhanced phenytoin metabolism.

CLINICAL EVALUATION: Alcoholics (while sober) metabolize phenytoin more rapidly than control subjects.[1] Theoretically, prolonged excessive ethanol ingestion could result in seizures in an epileptic patient controlled on phenytoin. Whether smaller amounts of ethanol would affect phenytoin metabolism is unknown, but it is unlikely to be substantial. Note that alcohol withdrawal in a chronic alcoholic may result in seizures in nonepileptic patients, and phenytoin has been recommended to treat such seizures.[2]

RELATED DRUGS: No information is available.

MANAGEMENT OPTIONS:

➡ *Monitor.* Monitor epileptic patients receiving phenytoin who also drink heavily for a decreased anticonvulsant effect.

REFERENCES:

1. Kater RMH, et al. Increased rate of clearance of drugs from the circulation of alcoholics. *Am J Med Sci.* 1969;258:35.
2. Finer MJ. Diphenylhydantoin in alcohol withdrawal. *JAMA.* 1971;217:211.

 Ethanol

Prazosin (*Minipress*)

SUMMARY: Prazosin enhanced alcohol-induced hypotension in Asian hypertensive patients; limit alcohol intake in such patients.

RISK FACTORS:

➡ *Pharmacogenetics.* Japanese and other Asians may be more susceptible to this interaction because Asians are more likely than Whites to be deficient in aldehyde dehydrogenase. When such patients ingest alcohol, the vasodilatory alcohol metabolite, acetaldehyde, accumulates and reduces the blood pressure. Thus, patients who develop flushing with alcohol ingestion may be more susceptible to the interaction with prazosin.

MECHANISM: Not established. Normally, the tendency for alcohol to produce a hypotensive effect is attenuated by an increase in sympathetic activity and stimulation of α_1-adrenergic receptors. In the presence of an α_1-adrenergic blocker such as prazosin, alcohol may produce a greater hypotensive effect.

CLINICAL EVALUATION: Ten hypertensive Japanese men received a single oral dose of alcohol with and without pretreatment with a relatively small dose of prazosin (1 mg 3 times daily for 5 to 7 days).[1] Alcohol-induced hypotension was greater in the presence of prazosin. The extent to which the enhanced hypotensive response would lead to adverse consequences is not clear. One would expect that the interaction would be larger in patients on larger doses of prazosin, but data are not available.

RELATED DRUGS: Theoretically, one would expect a similar interaction with alcohol with other α_1-adrenergic blockers, such as doxazosin (eg, *Cardura*) and terazosin (eg, *Hytrin*).

MANAGEMENT OPTIONS:

➡ *Circumvent/Minimize.* Patients (especially those who flush after alcohol ingestion) should limit their alcohol intake while on prazosin or other alpha$_1$-adrenergic blockers.

REFERENCES:

1. Kawano Y, et al. Interaction of alcohol and an α_1-blocker on ambulatory blood pressure in patients with essential hypertension. *Am J Hypertens.* 2000;13:307.

Ethanol (Ethyl Alcohol)

Procainamide (eg, *Procan SR*)

SUMMARY: Acute ethanol administration reduces procainamide concentrations and increases N-acetylprocainamide concentrations.

RISK FACTORS: No specific risk factors are known.

MECHANISM: Not established. Ethanol appears to enhance the acetylation of procainamide in the liver.

CLINICAL EVALUATION: Procainamide 10 mg/kg orally was given to 11 healthy subjects with and without ethanol (0.73 g/kg body weight at 1.5 hours after procainamide and then 0.11 g/kg body weight hourly for 6 doses).[1] In 8 other subjects, ethanol administration was started 2 hours before procainamide. In both experiments, ethanol administration was associated with an increase in procainamide clearance and an increase in the concentration of the active procainamide metabolite, N-acetylprocainamide. The clinical consequences of these changes are unknown.

RELATED DRUGS: No information is available.

MANAGEMENT OPTIONS: No specific action is required, but be alert for evidence of the interaction.

REFERENCES:
1. Olsen H, et al. Ethanol-induced increase in procainamide acetylation in man. *Br J Clin Pharmacol.* 1982;13:203.

Ethanol (Ethyl Alcohol)

Procarbazine (*Matulane*) AVOID

SUMMARY: Ingestion of ethanol by patients receiving procarbazine may result in a disulfiram-like reaction: flushing, headache, nausea, and hypotension.

RISK FACTORS: No specific risk factors are known.

MECHANISM: Studies in animals have shown that procarbazine inhibits aldehyde dehydrogenase, similar to disulfiram.[1]

CLINICAL EVALUATION: In several trials with procarbazine, patients who consumed alcohol developed a "flushing syndrome" after the consumption of alcohol.[2-4] Their faces became hot and red for a short period of time. Other patients have reported a potentiation of the effect of alcohol.[4]

RELATED DRUGS: No information is available.

MANAGEMENT OPTIONS:

➡ **AVOID COMBINATION.** Advise patients receiving procarbazine to avoid alcohol.

REFERENCES:
1. Vasiliou V, et al. The mechanism of alcohol intolerance produced by various therapeutic agents. *Acta Pharmacol et Toxicol.* 1986;58:305.
2. Brul G, et al. N-isopropyl-a-(2-methylhydrazino)-p-toluamide, hydrochloride (NSC-77213) in treatment of solid tumors. *Cancer Chemother Rep.* 1965;44:31.
3. Math G, et al. Methyl-hydrazine in treatment of Hodgkin's disease and various forms of haematosarcoma and leukaemia. *Lancet.* 1963;2:1077.
4. Todd IDH. Natulan in management of late Hodgkin's disease, other lymphoreticular neoplasms, and malignant melanoma. *BMJ.* 1965;628.

Ethanol (Ethyl Alcohol)

Propofol (*Diprivan*)

SUMMARY: Alcoholic patients may require a larger dose of propofol.

RISK FACTORS: No specific risk factors are known.

MECHANISM: Not established.

CLINICAL EVALUATION: Twenty-six patients with chronic alcoholism and 20 patients with small alcohol intake were studied. Induction of general anesthesia with propofol required approximately a 30% larger dose in the alcoholic patients.[1]

RELATED DRUGS: No information is available.

MANAGEMENT OPTIONS:

➥ *Monitor.* Be alert for the need to use larger doses of propofol in alcoholic patients.

REFERENCES:

1. Fassoulaki A, et al. Chronic alcoholism increases the induction dose of propofol in humans. *Anesth Analg.* 1993;77:553.

 Ethanol (Ethyl Alcohol)

Propoxyphene (eg, *Darvocet-N*)

SUMMARY: Overdoses of propoxyphene combined with ethanol have been associated with fatal reactions, but there is little evidence of danger when alcohol is combined with therapeutic doses of propoxyphene.

RISK FACTORS:

➥ *Dosage Regimen.* The danger of this interaction occurs primarily when large amounts of alcohol are ingested.

MECHANISM: Alcohol appears to increase propoxyphene bioavailability, possibly by reducing its first-pass metabolism. The mechanism for the apparent ethanol-induced increase in the risk of propoxyphene overdoses is unclear.

CLINICAL EVALUATION: Twelve healthy subjects were given propoxyphene 130 mg orally and ethanol 0.5 g/kg body weight alone and together in a double-blind 3-way crossover design.[1] Ethanol enhanced the bioavailability of propoxyphene 25%, but the bioavailability of ethanol was not affected by propoxyphene. The combination did not affect performance measures any more than ethanol alone. In another study, 6 healthy subjects received propoxyphene 65 mg orally with and without concurrent alcohol (enough to maintain breath alcohol concentrations between 800 to 1000 mg/L).[2] Ethanol was associated with a statistically insignificant 10% increase in propoxyphene bioavailability. Thus, when propoxyphene is taken in therapeutic doses, available evidence does not suggest that small amounts of alcohol will cause difficulties. Nonetheless, studies with multiple therapeutic doses of propoxyphene or larger doses of alcohol would be needed to assess this interaction more fully. Propoxyphene overdoses are a different matter; a number of fatalities have occurred in patients taking overdoses of propoxyphene along with alcohol.[3]

RELATED DRUGS: No information is available.

MANAGEMENT OPTIONS:

➡ *Circumvent/Minimize.* It does not appear that patients taking propoxyphene need to abstain from alcohol, but warn them to avoid acute alcohol intoxication.

➡ *Monitor.* Monitor for excessive central nervous system depression in patients receiving the combination.

REFERENCES:

1. Girre C, et al. Enhancement of propoxyphene bioavailability by ethanol: relation to psychomotor and cognitive function in healthy volunteers. *Eur J Clin Pharmacol.* 1991;41:147.

2. Sellers EM, et al. Pharmacokinetic interaction of propoxyphene with ethanol. *Br J Clin Pharmacol.* 1985;19:398.

3. Finkle BS, et al. A national assessment of propoxyphene in postmortem medicolegal investigation 1972–1975. *J Forensic Sci.* 1976;21:706.

Ethanol (Ethyl Alcohol) 4

Propranolol (eg, *Inderal*)

SUMMARY: Ethanol appears to have little clinical effect on propranolol.

RISK FACTORS: No specific risk factors are known.

MECHANISM: Not established. Ethanol-induced increases in hepatic blood flow or metabolism might be involved.

CLINICAL EVALUATION: Short-term studies in normal subjects indicate that ethanol increases both the elimination rate and bioavailability of propranolol; it also slightly reduces the elimination rate of sotalol (*Betapace*).[1,2,3] However, the changes in beta blocker pharmacokinetics were not large, and the studies did not typify the clinical situation. More study is needed to assess the clinical significance of these effects.

RELATED DRUGS: Ethanol slightly reduces sotalol's elimination rate. The effects of ethanol on other beta blockers are unknown.

MANAGEMENT OPTIONS: No specific action is required, but be alert for evidence of the interaction.

REFERENCES:

1. Sotaniemi EA, et al. Propranolol and sotalol metabolism after a drinking party. *Clin Pharmacol Ther.* 1981;29:705.

2. Grabowski BS, et al. Effects of acute alcohol administration on propranolol absorption. *Int J Clin Pharmacol Ther Toxicol.* 1980;18:317.

3. Dorian P, et al. Propranolol-ethanol pharmacokinetic interaction. *Clin Pharmacol Ther.* 1982;31:219.

Ethanol (Ethyl Alcohol)

Quetiapine (*Seroquel*)

SUMMARY: Patients on quetiapine who ingest alcohol may develop excessive impairment of cognitive and motor function; the manufacturer advises patients on quetiapine to avoid the consumption of alcohol.

RISK FACTORS: No specific risk factors are known.

MECHANISM: Probably additive CNS depression.

CLINICAL EVALUATION: While no published data are available for evaluation, the manufacturer of quetiapine has made available some data on this interaction. Quetiapine is reported to enhance the cognitive and motor effects of alcohol.[1] Because the details of the study were not presented, it is not possible to assess its validity. Nonetheless, quetiapine alone can cause many of the same effects as alcohol (eg, somnolence, impaired cognitive, motor function), and it is likely that at least additive effects would be seen.

RELATED DRUGS: No information is available.

MANAGEMENT OPTIONS:

➡ *Circumvent/Minimize.* Advise patients receiving quetiapine to avoid alcohol. If alcohol is ingested, it should be in small amounts and operation of automobiles or machinery should be avoided.

REFERENCES:
1. *Seroquel* [package insert]. Wilmington, DE: Zeneca Pharmaceuticals; 1997.

 Ethanol (Ethyl Alcohol)

Ramelteon (*Rozerem*)

SUMMARY: Ramelteon and alcohol may have some additive pharmacodynamic effects.

RISK FACTORS: No specific risk factors are known.

MECHANISM: Not established.

CLINICAL EVALUATION: When single doses of ramelteon (32 mg) and alcohol (0.6 g/kg) were given alone and in combination, additive effects on certain psychomotor performance tests were observed.[1] The ramelteon product information warns against concurrent use of ramelteon and alcohol.

RELATED DRUGS: No information available.

MANAGEMENT OPTIONS:

➡ *Avoid Unless Benefit Outweighs Risk.* Generally, avoid concurrent use of ramelteon and alcohol.

REFERENCES:
1. *Rozerem* [package insert]. Lincolnshire, IL: Takeda Pharmaceuticals; 2006.

 Ethanol (Ethyl Alcohol)

Sertraline (*Zoloft*)

SUMMARY: Studies in healthy subjects suggest that sertraline does not affect ethanol-induced impairment of psychomotor function, but depressed patients should limit their ethanol intake.

RISK FACTORS: No specific risk factors are known.

MECHANISM: No interaction.

CLINICAL EVALUATION: Ten healthy women were given sertraline in increasing doses (up to 200 mg/day) for 9 days with ethanol 0.5 g/kg given 6 hours after the last dose.[1] Sertraline alone did not affect cognitive or psychomotor performance and did not produce additive CNS effects when combined with a moderate dose of ethanol.

Some selective serotonin reuptake inhibitors (SSRIs) have been used to reduce alcohol craving in patients who abuse alcohol, but their role in treating alcohol abuse is still under study.

RELATED DRUGS: Other SSRIs also do not appear to enhance ethanol-induced impairment of psychomotor function.

MANAGEMENT OPTIONS: No interaction.

REFERENCES:
1. Hindmarch I, et al. The effects of sertraline on psychomotor performance in elderly volunteers. *J Clin Psychiatry.* 1990;51(suppl B):34-36.

Ethanol (Ethyl Alcohol)

Tacrolimus (*Prograf*)

SUMMARY: Tacrolimus ointment may increase the risk of alcohol-induced facial flushing; warn patients of this adverse reaction.

RISK FACTORS: No specific risk factors are known.

MECHANISM: Not established.

CLINICAL EVALUATION: Six non-Asian patients who had reported alcohol-induced facial flushing during treatment with tacrolimus ointment were given 100 mL of white wine after 4 days of applying tacrolimus 0.1% ointment twice a day for 4 days.[1] All 6 patients developed facial flushing 5 to 15 minutes after alcohol ingestion. Previous large studies of tacrolimus ointment had reported alcohol-induced facial flushing in 6% to 7% of patients.

RELATED DRUGS: No information is available.

MANAGEMENT OPTIONS:

➠ *Circumvent/Minimize.* Advise patients using tacrolimus ointment to inform their health care provider if they experience alcohol-induced facial flushing.

REFERENCES:
1. Milingou M, et al. Alcohol intolerance and facial flushing in patients treated with topical tacrolimus. *Arch Dermatol.* 2004;140:1542-1544.

Ethanol (Ethyl Alcohol)

Tinidazole (*Tindamax*)

SUMMARY: Alcohol ingestion during tinidazole therapy may lead to a disulfiram-like reaction in some patients.

RISK FACTORS: No specific risk factors are known.

MECHANISM: Tinidazole appears to act in a manner similar to that of disulfiram by inhibiting the activity of aldehyde dehydrogenase.

CLINICAL EVALUATION: Although data are limited, the manufacturer of tinidazole recommends avoiding alcohol or preparations with propylene glycol during therapy with tinidazole and for 3 days following its discontinuation.[1]

RELATED DRUGS: Metronidazole (eg, *Flagyl*) is known to cause a similar disulfiram-like reaction with alcohol.

MANAGEMENT OPTIONS:

➡ *Circumvent/Minimize.* Warn patients receiving tinidazole about the possibility of reactions following ethanol ingestion and to avoid ethanol and ethanol-containing drugs.

➡ *Monitor.* Monitor patients who take tinidazole and consume alcohol for flushing, nausea, and vomiting.

REFERENCES:

    1. *Tindamax* [package insert]. Arlington Heights, IL: Presutti Laboratories, Inc.; 2004.

 Ethanol (Ethyl Alcohol)

Tizanidine (eg, *Zanaflex*)

SUMMARY: Alcohol increases the sedative effects of tizanidine; patients should be warned accordingly.

RISK FACTORS: No specific risk factors are known.

MECHANISM: Tizanidine and alcohol are CNS depressants, and alcohol appears to somewhat increase tizanidine plasma concentrations.

CLINICAL EVALUATION: The manufacturer of tizanidine states that alcohol modestly increases tizanidine plasma concentrations, and also increases the sedative effects of tizanidine.[1]

RELATED DRUGS: No information is available.

MANAGEMENT OPTIONS:

➡ *Circumvent/Minimize.* Warn patients taking tizanidine to minimize alcohol intake and avoid alcohol completely when alertness is required.

REFERENCES:

    1. *Zanaflex* [package insert]. Hawthorne, NY: Acorda Therapeutics; March 2005.

 Ethanol (Ethyl Alcohol)

AVOID **Tolbutamide (eg, *Orinase*)**

SUMMARY: Excessive ethanol intake may lead to altered glycemic control, most commonly hypoglycemia. An *Antabuse*-like reaction may occur in patients taking sulfonylureas.

RISK FACTORS: No specific risk factors are known.

MECHANISM: The mechanisms for this interaction are as follows: 1) Ethanol may exhibit intrinsic hypoglycemic activity, although hyperglycemia also has been noted; 2) chlorpropamide and, to a lesser extent, other sulfonylureas may provoke an *Antabuse*-like reaction (eg, flushing, headache) to ethanol[1,2]; and 3) prolonged heavy intake of ethanol markedly decreases the half-life of tolbutamide, probably by induction of hepatic enzymes.[3-5]

CLINICAL EVALUATION: Acute ingestion of ethanol by patients on any antidiabetic carries the risk of severe hypoglycemia, especially in fasting patients.[6-8] The increased tolbutamide metabolism in alcoholic patients probably decreases its hypoglycemic effect, although the intrinsic hypoglycemic activity of ethanol may somewhat counteract the effects.

RELATED DRUGS: Excessive ethanol produced hypoglycemia in patients taking insulin or other oral hypoglycemic agents. Two patients receiving chlorpropamide (eg, *Diabinese*) for diabetes insipidus developed polyuria and polydipsia following ethanol intake, presumably caused by ethanol inhibition of chlorpropamide-induced antidiuresis.[9] Ethanol ingestion may contribute to lactic acidosis in patients receiving phenformin.[10,11]

MANAGEMENT OPTIONS:

➡ *AVOID COMBINATION.* Because an *Antabuse* reaction may occur following ethanol ingestion in patients receiving sulfonylureas, inform patients of this possibility when therapy is initiated. Advise patients on antidiabetics to avoid ingestion of moderate to large amounts of ethanol because of the possible adverse effects of alcohol on diabetic control.

REFERENCES:

1. Asaad MM, et al. Studies on the biochemical aspects of the "disulfiram-like" reaction induced by oral hypoglycemics. *Eur J Pharmacol.* 1976;35:301-307.
2. Wardle EN, et al. Alcohol and glibenclamide. *BMJ.* 1971;3:309.
3. Kater RM, et al. Increased rate of tolbutamide metabolism in alcoholic patients. *JAMA.* 1969;207:363-365.
4. Carulli N, et al. Alcohol-drugs interaction in man: alcohol and tolbutamide. *Eur J Clin Invest.* 1971;1:421-424.
5. Sotaniemi EA, et al. Half life of intravenous tolbutamide in the serum of patients in medical wards. *Ann Clin Res.* 1974;6:146-154.
6. Arky RA, et al. Irreversible hypoglycemia. A complication of alcohol and insulin. *JAMA.* 1968;206:575-578.
7. Hartling SG, et al. Interaction of ethanol and glipizide in humans. *Diabetes Care.* 1987;10:683-686.
8. Baruh S, et al. Fasting hypoglycemia. *Med Clin North Am.* 1973;57:1441-1462.
9. Yamamoto LT. Letter: Diabetes insipidus and drinking alcohol. *N Engl J Med.* 1976;294:55-56.
10. Johnson HK, et al. Relationship of alcohol and hyperlactatemia in diabetic subjects treated with phenformin. *Am J Med.* 1968;45:98-104.
11. Kreisberg RA, et al. Hyperlacticacidemia in man: ethanol-phenformin synergism. *J Clin Endocrinol Metab.* 1972;34:29-35.

Ethanol (Ethyl Alcohol)

Verapamil (eg, *Calan*)

SUMMARY: Consumption of ethanol following the chronic administration of verapamil results in increased ethanol concentrations with the possibility of prolonged and increased levels of intoxication.

RISK FACTORS: No specific risk factors are known.

MECHANISM: Not established. Verapamil appears to inhibit the metabolism of ethanol; it also may decrease the first-pass metabolism of ethanol.

CLINICAL EVALUATION: Ten healthy subjects received verapamil 80 mg every 8 hours or placebo for 6 days in a crossover study.[1] On the morning of the 6th day, ethanol 0.8 mg/kg was administered. Compared to placebo administration, verapamil increased the peak ethanol serum concentrations 16.7% and the ethanol area under the concentration-time curve approximately 30%. A study of a single 80 or 160 mg dose of verapamil reported no effect of verapamil on ethanol concentrations or intoxication.[4]

RELATED DRUGS: Ethanol was reported to increase the hypotensive response of a 5 mg dose of felodipine (*Plendil*) in 10 hypertensive patients.[2] The ethanol was administered in doublestrength grapefruit juice which has been demonstrated to increase felodipine concentrations.[3] Therefore, it is uncertain whether ethanol affects felodipine or if the changes were caused by an interaction between grapefruit juice and felodipine. Ethanol administration resulted in a 53% increase in nifedipine (eg, *Procardia*) area under the concentration-time curve in healthy subjects; nifedipine-induced blood pressure changes were not affected by ethanol.[5]

MANAGEMENT OPTIONS:

➠ *Avoid Unless Benefit Outweighs Risk.* Avoid or reduce ethanol intake while taking verapamil. Verapamil may enhance the psychomotor effects of ethanol.

➠ *Monitor.* Caution patients taking verapamil regarding the consumption of ethanol. Serum ethanol concentrations may be higher than normally experienced when the patient is not taking verapamil.

REFERENCES:

1. Bauer LA, et al. Verapamil inhibits ethanol elimination and prolongs the perception of intoxication. *Clin Pharmacol Ther.* 1992;52:6.
2. Bailey DG, et al. Ethanol enhances the hemodynamic effect of felodipine. *Clin Invest Med.* 1989;12:357.
3. Bailey DG, et al. Interaction of citrus juices with felodipine and nifedipine. *Lancet.* 1991;337:268.
4. Perez-Reyes M, et al. Interaction between ethanol and calcium channel blockers in humans. *Alcohol Clin Exp Res.* 1992;16:769.
5. Qureshi S, et al. Effect of an acute dose of alcohol on the pharmacokinetics of oral nifedipine in humans. *Pharm Res.* 1992;9:683.

 Ethanol (Ethyl Alcohol)

Vitamin C

SUMMARY: Vitamin C may slightly increase the elimination of ethanol.

RISK FACTORS: No specific risk factors are known.

MECHANISM: The activity of alcohol dehydrogenase may be enhanced by increasing ascorbic acid saturation.

CLINICAL EVALUATION: In healthy volunteers, the clearance of ethanol was slightly enhanced by ascorbic acid administration (1 g/day for 2 weeks).[1] These results were confirmed in another study of 13 healthy men who were given 0.5 and 0.8 g/kg of alcohol with and without short- and long-term use of ascorbic acid therapy. Both short- and long-term use of ascorbic acid enhanced the plasma clearance of alcohol.

RELATED DRUGS: No information is available.

MANAGEMENT OPTIONS: No specific action is required, but be alert for evidence of the interaction.

REFERENCES:

1. Krasner N, et al. Ascorbic-acid saturation and ethanol metabolism. *Lancet.* 1974;2:693.
2. Chen MF, et al. Effect of ascorbic acid on plasma alcohol clearance. *J Am Coll Nutr.* 1990;9:185.

Ethanol (Ethyl Alcohol)

Warfarin (eg *Coumadin*)

SUMMARY: Enhanced hypoprothrombinemic response to oral anticoagulants has been reported following acute ethanol intoxication.

RISK FACTORS:

➡ ***Dosage Regimen.*** Enhanced anticoagulant effect appears to occur primarily with acute alcohol intoxication; small amounts of ethanol (eg, 2 or fewer drinks per day) seem to have little effect on most patients.

MECHANISM: Not established. The ability of acute ethanol intoxication to enhance the hypoprothrombinemic response to oral anticoagulants may be caused by inhibition of anticoagulant metabolism. The apparent increase in warfarin metabolism in heavy drinkers (when they are sober) is probably caused by ethanol-induced stimulation of hepatic microsomal enzymes.[1,6] The late stages of ethanol-induced hepatic damage may be accompanied by reduced hepatic production of vitamin K-dependent clotting factors.

CLINICAL EVALUATION: Ethanol-induced increases in the hypoprothrombinemic response to oral anticoagulants have been noted clinically for many years, but few cases have been reported. It is clear, however, that most patients on oral anticoagulants are not affected by moderate ethanol intake. In 1 study of 10 patients on chronic warfarin therapy, only 1 developed enhanced hypoprothrombinemia following 8 oz/day of vodka for 2 weeks.[2] Furthermore, daily ingestion of 592 mL of table wine or 296 mL of fortified wine (20% ethanol) did not affect the hypoprothrombinemic response to warfarin in healthy subjects.[4,5] Enhanced metabolism of warfarin may occur in alcoholics,[1] but this would be expected to occur only when the patient is not intoxicated.

RELATED DRUGS: Until we have evidence to the contrary, expect all oral anticoagulants to be affected by alcohol intoxication. In another study, 80 g of ethanol did not affect the hypoprothrombinemic response in healthy subjects maintained on phenprocoumon.[3†] Additional study in patients with coronary disease indicated a slight increase in hypoprothrombinemic response to phenprocoumon in some patients following administration of moderate amounts of ethanol.

MANAGEMENT OPTIONS:

➡ ***Circumvent/Minimize.*** Patients on oral anticoagulants should avoid large amounts of ethanol, but 2 or 3 drinks/day or less are unlikely to affect warfarin response.

➡ ***Monitor.*** Monitor for altered hypoprothrombinemic response if a patient takes greater than 3 drinks per day or if alcohol intake changes considerably.

REFERENCES:

1. Kater RHM, et al. Increased rate of clearance of drugs from the circulation of alcoholics. *Am J Med Sci.* 1969;258:35.

2. Udall JA. Drug interference with warfarin therapy. *Clin Med.* 1970;77:20.

3. Waris E. Effect of ethyl alcohol on some coagulation factors in man during anticoagulant therapy. *Ann Med Exp Biol Fenn.* 1963;41:45.

4. O'Reilly RA. Lack of effect of mealtime wine on the hypoprothrombinemia of oral anticoagulants. *Am J Med Sci.* 1979;277:189.

5. O'Reilly RA. Lack of effect of fortified wine ingested during fasting and anticoagulant therapy. *Arch Intern Med*. 1981;141:458.

6. Breckenridge A. Pathophysiological factors influencing drug kinetics. *Acta Pharmacol Toxicol*. 1971;29(Suppl. 3):225.

† Not available in the United States.

Ethinyl Estradiol (eg, *Ortho-Novum*)

Grapefruit Juice

SUMMARY: Grapefruit juice appears to increase ethinyl estradiol serum concentrations somewhat, but the clinical importance of this effect is not established.

RISK FACTORS:

➡ *Route of Administration.* This interaction most likely occurs only with oral administration of ethinyl estradiol.

MECHANISM: Not established. Grapefruit juice probably inhibits the presystemic metabolism of ethinyl estradiol by intestinal CYP3A4.[1]

CLINICAL EVALUATION: In a randomized, crossover study in healthy women, grapefruit juice increased the ethinyl estradiol area under the plasma concentration-time curve 28%.[2] The effect was highly variable between subjects, ranging from a 19% decrease to an 80% increase. Although it is not known how often this interaction will result in a clinically important alteration in ethinyl estradiol effect, it does appear that grapefruit juice can contribute to variations in ethinyl estradiol plasma concentrations. It is reasonable to expect that concurrent ingestion of ethinyl estradiol and grapefruit juice (especially if the grapefruit juice ingestion is sporadic) may complicate the titration of ethinyl estradiol in some patients. Theoretically, orange juice is not expected to interact with ethinyl estradiol.

RELATED DRUGS: The effect of grapefruit juice on other estrogens is not established, but because many hormonal steroids undergo metabolism by CYP3A4, it is possible that other estrogens (given orally) would be similarly affected. Theoretically, non-oral administration of estrogens (eg, transdermal patches) would not interact with grapefruit juice.

MANAGEMENT OPTIONS:

➡ *Consider Alternative.* Orange juice does not appear to inhibit CYP3A4 and is not expected to interact with ethinyl estradiol.

➡ *Circumvent/Minimize.* Although it is not known how often this interaction will cause adverse reactions, patients taking ethinyl estradiol (and perhaps other estrogens) should avoid taking the estrogen with or within several hours after grapefruit products. If grapefruit juice is used, attempt to keep the dosing interval between the ethinyl estradiol and the grapefruit juice the same each day.

REFERENCES:

1. Schubert W, et al. Flavonoids in grapefruit juice inhibit the in vitro hepatic metabolism of 17 beta-estradiol. *Eur J Drug Metab Pharmacokinet*. 1995;20(3):219-224.

2. Weber A, et al. Can grapefruit juice influence ethinylestradiol bioavailability? *Contraception*. 1996;53(1):41-47.

Ethinyl Estradiol (eg, *Ortho-Novum 1/35*)

Indinavir (*Crixivan*)

SUMMARY: Indinavir administration resulted in a small increase in ethinyl estradiol and norethindrone concentrations; no change in clinical response is likely.

RISK FACTORS: No specific risk factors are known.

MECHANISM: Not established. Indinavir may inhibit the metabolism of estrogens via the CYP3A4 pathway.

CLINICAL EVALUATION: While no published data are available for evaluation, the manufacturer of indinavir has made available some data on this interaction. Indinavir 800 mg every 8 hours was administered with a combination of ethinyl estradiol/norethindrone 1/35 for 7 days. There was a 24% increase in ethinyl estradiol area under the plasma concentration-time curve (AUC) and a 26% increase in norethindrone AUC.[1]

RELATED DRUGS: Ritonavir (*Norvir*) reduces the concentration of ethinyl estradiol. While no data are available, saquinavir (*Invirase*) and nelfinavir (*Viracept*) may be less likely to affect oral contraceptive concentrations.

MANAGEMENT OPTIONS: No specific action is required, but be alert for evidence of the interaction.

REFERENCES:
1. *Crixivan* [package insert]. Whitehouse Station, NJ: Merck & Company, Inc; 1996.

Ethinyl Estradiol (eg, *Ortho-Novum 1/35*) ▼3

Tipranavir (*Aptivus*)

SUMMARY: Ethinyl estradiol plasma concentrations are reduced during administration of the combination tipranavir/ritonavir; loss of contraceptive efficacy or hormone replacement response may occur.

RISK FACTORS: No specific risk factors are known.

MECHANISM: Unknown. Ethinyl estradiol is metabolized by CYP3A4 and glucuronidation and is a substrate of P-glycoprotein. It appears that the induction of glucuronidation and/or P-glycoprotein by tipranavir is responsible for the reduction in ethinyl estradiol plasma concentrations.

CLINICAL EVALUATION: While specific data are limited, the manufacturer of tipranavir notes that the coadministration of tipranavir 500 to 750 mg with ritonavir 100 to 200 mg twice daily and ethinyl estradiol 0.035 mg daily decreased the mean area under the plasma concentration-time curve of ethinyl estradiol 48% compared with ethinyl estradiol administered alone.[1]

RELATED DRUGS: Tipranavir does not appear to alter the plasma concentration of norethindrone. Indinavir (*Crixivan*) administration produced a small increase (22%) in ethinyl estradiol concentrations.[2]

MANAGEMENT OPTIONS:

➡ ***Consider Alternative.*** Pending additional study, consider an alternative contraceptive method or hormone replacement therapy for patients taking ethinyl estradiol while being treated with the combination of tipranavir/ritonavir.

➡ ***Monitor.*** Watch for reduced contraceptive efficacy, breakthrough bleeding, or other signs of hormone therapy failure when tipranavir/ritonavir is coadministered with ethinyl estradiol.

REFERENCES:

1. *Aptivus* [package insert]. Ridgefield, CT: Boehringer Ingelheim Pharmaceuticals, Inc; 2007.
2. *Crixivan* [package insert]. Whitehouse Station, NJ: Merck & Company, Inc; 1996.

 Ethyl Biscoumacetate

Methylphenidate (eg, *Ritalin*)

SUMMARY: Methylphenidate does not appear to affect hypoprothrombinemic response to ethyl biscoumacetate.

RISK FACTORS: No specific risk factors are known.

MECHANISM: No interaction.

CLINICAL EVALUATION: The results of a preliminary study in 4 volunteers showing that methylphenidate prolonged the half-life of ethyl biscoumacetate[1] were not confirmed in a double-blind study of 12 healthy volunteers.[2] Thus, the available evidence does not support the existence of a clinically significant interaction between these drugs.

RELATED DRUGS: The effect of methylphenidate on warfarin (eg, *Coumadin*) or other oral anticoagulants is not established, but there is no reason to suspect an interaction.

MANAGEMENT OPTIONS: No interaction.

REFERENCES:

1. Garrettson LK, et al. Methylphenidate interaction with both anticonvulsants and ethyl biscoumacetate. *JAMA.* 1969;207(11):2053-2056.
2. Hague DE, et al. The effect of methylphenidate and prolintane on the metabolism of ethyl biscoumacetate. *Clin Pharmacol Ther.* 1971;12(2):259-262.

 Etintidine†

Propranolol (eg, *Inderal*)

SUMMARY: Serum concentrations of propranolol and other beta-blockers that undergo significant hepatic metabolism may be increased by etintidine administration.

RISK FACTORS: No specific risk factors are known.

MECHANISM: Etintidine is a chemical analog of cimetidine and probably shares cimetidine's ability to inhibit oxidative metabolism in the liver.

CLINICAL EVALUATION: Twelve healthy subjects received a single oral dose of propranolol 40 mg following 4 days of etintidine 400 mg twice daily or a matching placebo.[1] Following etintidine pretreatment, the area under the propranolol concentration-time curve increased nearly 300%, the clearance for oral propranolol fell from 440 to 103 L/hr, and the maximum serum concentration and half-life doubled. A change in clearance of this magnitude is likely to produce a clinically significant alteration in a patient's response to propranolol.

RELATED DRUGS: Cimetidine (eg, *Tagamet*) is known to inhibit the metabolism of propranolol and other beta-blockers (eg, labetalol [eg, *Normodyne*], metoprolol [eg, *Lopressor*]) that undergo hepatic metabolism. Etintidine might affect them similarly. Other H_2-receptor antagonists (famotidine [eg, *Pepcid*], nizatidine [eg, *Axid*], ranitidine [eg, *Zantac*]) have little effect on propranolol.

MANAGEMENT OPTIONS:

➭ *Consider Alternative.* If possible, administer atenolol (eg, *Tenormin*) or nadolol (eg, *Corgard*) instead of hepatically metabolized beta-blockers. Ranitidine, famotidine, nizatidine, antacids, or sucralfate (eg, *Carafate*) also may be suitable alternatives to etintidine, but separate beta-blocker doses from antacids or sucralfate to minimize the possibility of impaired absorption of the beta-blocker.

➭ *Monitor.* Etintidine administration may result in large increases in propranolol serum concentrations. Monitor patients stabilized on propranolol for altered response to beta-blockade if etintidine is started or stopped.

REFERENCES:

1. Huang SM, et al. Etintidine-propranolol interaction study in humans. *J Pharmacokinet Biopharm.* 1987;15(6):557-568.

† Not available in the United States.

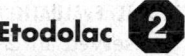

Etodolac ❷

Warfarin (eg, *Coumadin*)

SUMMARY: Preliminary data suggest that etodolac does not affect the hypoprothrombinemic response to warfarin, but cotherapy requires caution because of possible detrimental effects of etodolac on the gastric mucosa and platelet function.

RISK FACTORS:

➭ *Concurrent Diseases.* Patients with peptic ulcer disease (PUD) or a history of GI bleeding probably are at greater risk.

MECHANISM: Pharmacokinetic studies suggest a minor displacement of warfarin from plasma protein binding by etodolac but minimal effects on warfarin response.

CLINICAL EVALUATION: Etodolac did not affect warfarin hypoprothrombinemic response or unbound clearance in a randomized, crossover study of healthy subjects.[1] Nevertheless, use nonsteroidal anti-inflammatory drugs (NSAIDs) cautiously in anticoagulated patients because NSAID-induced gastric erosions and possible platelet inhibition may lead to bleeding. In a retrospective cohort study, hospitalizations for hemorrhagic PUD were approximately 13 times higher in patients receiving warfarin plus an NSAID than in patients receiving either drug alone.[2]

RELATED DRUGS: All NSAIDs inhibit platelet function, cause gastric erosions, and probably increase the risk of GI bleeding.

MANAGEMENT OPTIONS:

➭ *Avoid Unless Benefit Outweighs Risk.* Because all NSAIDs probably increase the risk of GI bleeding in patients on oral anticoagulants, use the combination only after careful consideration of benefit versus risk. If NSAIDs are used as analgesics or antipyretics, acetaminophen (eg, *Tylenol*) is probably safer to use with oral anticoagulants. Nonacetylated salicylates (eg, choline salicylate, magnesium salicylate, salsalate, sodium salicylate) are probably also safer with oral anticoagulants than NSAIDs because they have minimal effects on platelet function and gastric mucosa.

➡ **Monitor.** If NSAIDs are used with oral anticoagulants, carefully monitor prothrombin time and watch for evidence of bleeding, especially from the GI tract.

REFERENCES:

1. Ermer JC, et al. Concomitant etodolac affects neither the unbound clearance nor the pharmacologic effect of warfarin. *Clin Pharmacol Ther*. 1994;55(3):305-316.

2. Shorr RI, et al. Concurrent use of nonsteroidal anti-inflammatory drugs and oral anticoagulants places elderly persons at high risk for hemorrhagic peptic ulcer disease. *Arch Intern Med*. 1993;153(14):1665-1670.

4 Etomidate (eg, *Amidate*)

Verapamil (eg, *Calan*)

SUMMARY: Two cases of prolonged anesthesia occurred in patients who received verapamil before etomidate.

RISK FACTORS: No specific risk factors are known.

MECHANISM: Not established.

CLINICAL EVALUATION: Prolonged anesthesia with Cheyne-Stokes respirations was observed in 2 patients after they received etomidate 300 to 400 mcg/kg.[1] One patient was taking chronic verapamil, and the other received an intravenous dose of verapamil 10 mg before the anesthetic. Anesthesia appeared to be extended by 3 to 25 minutes. Whether the interaction is responsible for the clinical observations requires further study.

RELATED DRUGS: No information is available.

MANAGEMENT OPTIONS: No specific action is required, but be alert for evidence of the interaction.

REFERENCES:

1. Moore CA, et al. Potentiation of etomidate anesthesia by verapamil: a report of two cases. *Hosp Pharm*. 1989;24(1):24-25.

3 Etravirine (*Intelence*)

Omeprazole (eg, *Prilosec*)

SUMMARY: Omeprazole administration increased etravirine plasma concentrations; some patients may experience increased etravirine adverse reactions, such as rash or nausea.

RISK FACTORS:

➡ **Pharmacogenetics.** Patients who are poor metabolizers of CYP2C19 are unlikely to be affected by this interaction.

MECHANISM: Etravirine is partially metabolized by CYP2C19. The activity of this enzyme is inhibited by omeprazole, which reduces the metabolism of etravirine.

CLINICAL EVALUATION: While specific data are limited, the coadministration of omeprazole 40 mg once daily with etravirine resulted in an increase in the mean area under the plasma concentration-time curve of etravirine of approximately 40%.[1] Pending further data, observe patients receiving omeprazole and etravirine for increased etravirine effects.

RELATED DRUGS: Esomeprazole (*Nexium*) is expected to affect etravirine in a similar manner.

MANAGEMENT OPTIONS:

➥ *Consider Alternative.* Pantoprazole (eg, *Protonix*), rabeprazole (*Aciphex*), and lansoprazole (*Prevacid*) are not expected to interact with etravirine because they do not inhibit CYP2C19.

➥ *Monitor.* Monitor for etravirine adverse reactions when omeprazole is coadministered.

REFERENCES:

1. *Intelence* [package insert]. Raritan, NJ: Tibotec Therapeutics; 2008.

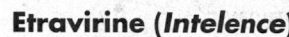

Etravirine (*Intelence*)

Sildenafil (eg, *Viagra*)

SUMMARY: The coadministration of sildenafil and etravirine reduced the plasma concentration of sildenafil; some patients may experience a reduction in sildenafil effectiveness.

RISK FACTORS: No specific risk factors are known.

MECHANISM: Etravirine appears to increase the metabolism of sildenafil via CYP3A4.

CLINICAL EVALUATION: While specific data are limited, the coadministration of etravirine 800 mg twice daily and a single dose of sildenafil 50 mg resulted in a decrease in the mean area under the plasma concentration-time curve of sildenafil by nearly 60%.[1] Pending further data, patients receiving etravirine and sildenafil should be counseled regarding the potential for reduced sildenafil response.

RELATED DRUGS: Tadalafil (*Cialis*) and vardenafil (*Levitra*) probably interact in a similar manner with etravirine.

MANAGEMENT OPTIONS:

➥ *Monitor.* Monitor patients taking etravirine and sildenafil for reduced sildenafil response. Sildenafil doses may need to be increased.

REFERENCES:

1. *Intelence* [package insert]. Raritan, NJ: Tibotec Therapeutics; 2008.

Etravirine (*Intelence*)

Tipranavir (*Aptivus*)

SUMMARY: The coadministration of tipranavir and etravirine reduced the plasma concentration of etravirine; some patients may experience a reduction in etravirine antiviral efficacy.

RISK FACTORS: No specific risk factors are known.

MECHANISM: Tipranavir appears to increase the elimination of etravirine via CYP3A4.

CLINICAL EVALUATION: While specific data are limited, the coadministration of tipranavir 500 mg plus ritonavir 200 mg twice daily decreased the mean area under the plasma concentration-time curve (AUC) of etravirine approximately 75%.[1] Etravirine administration had no affect on tipranavir plasma concentrations. In a separate study, tipranavir 200 mg twice daily reduced the AUC of etravirine 19%.[2] Pending further data, patients receiving etravirine and tipranavir should be monitored for reduced etravirine response.

RELATED DRUGS: Efavirenz (*Sustiva*) has been noted to reduce the plasma concentration of tipranavir.

MANAGEMENT OPTIONS:

➡ **Monitor.** Monitor patients taking etravirine and tipranavir for reduced etravirine response.

REFERENCES:

1. *Intelence* [package insert]. Raritan, NJ: Tibotec Therapeutics; 2008.
2. Fulco PP, et al. Etravirine and rilpivirine: nonnucleoside reverse transcriptase inhibitors with activity against human immunodeficiency virus type 1 strains resistant to previous nonnucleoside agents. *Pharmacotherapy*. 2009;29(3):281-294.

Everolimus†

Erythromycin (eg, *Ery-Tab*)

SUMMARY: Erythromycin increases everolimus plasma concentrations; increased toxicity may occur.

RISK FACTORS: No specific risk factors are known.

MECHANISM: Erythromycin appears to inhibit the metabolism (CYP3A4) and/or the P-glycoprotein transport of everolimus.

CLINICAL EVALUATION: Sixteen healthy subjects received a single oral dose of everolimus 2 mg alone and on day 5 of a 9-day course of erythromycin 500 mg 3 times daily.[1] During erythromycin administration, the mean area under the plasma concentration-time curve of everolimus was increased 4.4-fold (range, 2- to 12.6-fold), and the half-life of everolimus was increased from 32 to 44 hours. A population pharmacokinetic evaluation found a modest effect of erythromycin on everolimus metabolism.[2] Increased everolimus adverse reactions are possible in some patients exposed to both drugs. The single dose of everolimus appeared to have no effect on erythromycin concentrations.

RELATED DRUGS: Clarithromycin (eg, *Biaxin*) and troleandomycin† may affect everolimus in a similar manner. Erythromycin is known to increase the concentrations of cyclosporine (eg, *Neoral*) and tacrolimus (*Prograf*).

MANAGEMENT OPTIONS:

➤ **Consider Alternative.** Macrolide antibiotics that do not inhibit CYP3A4 (eg, azithromycin [eg, *Zithromax*], dirithromycin†) could be considered for patients taking everolimus.

➤ **Monitor.** During erythromycin cotherapy, observe patients for everolimus-associated toxicity and monitor everolimus plasma concentrations, if possible. Everolimus doses may require reduction during coadministration with erythromycin.

REFERENCES:

1. Kovarik JM, et al. Effect of multiple-dose erythromycin on everolimus pharmacokinetics. *Eur J Clin Pharmacol.* 2005;61(1):35-38.

2. Kovarik JM, et al. Population pharmacokinetics of everolimus in de novo renal transplant patients: impact of ethnicity and comedications. *Clin Pharmacol Ther.* 2001;70(3):247-254.

† Not available in the United States.

Everolimus† 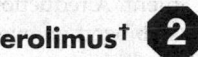 2

Ketoconazole (eg, *Nizoral*)

SUMMARY: Ketoconazole administration causes marked increases in everolimus plasma concentrations; everolimus toxicity is likely to occur.

RISK FACTORS: No specific risk factors are known.

MECHANISM: Ketoconazole is a known inhibitor of CYP3A4, the enzyme responsible for everolimus metabolism. In addition, everolimus is a substrate for the efflux transporter P-glycoprotein, which also is inhibited by ketoconazole.

CLINICAL EVALUATION: A single dose of everolimus 2 mg was administered to 12 healthy subjects alone and on day 4 of an 8-day regimen of ketoconazole 200 mg twice daily.[1] The mean area under the plasma concentration-time curve of everolimus was increased nearly 15-fold, while its peak concentration was increased 4-fold. Everolimus half-life increased from 30 to 56 hours. Everolimus did not alter ketoconazole concentrations.

RELATED DRUGS: Ketoconazole also inhibits tacrolimus (*Prograf*), sirolimus (*Rapamune*), and cyclosporine (eg, *Neoral*) metabolism. Itraconazole (eg, *Sporanox*), voriconazole (*Vfend*), and fluconazole (eg, *Diflucan*) are likely to increase everolimus plasma concentrations and increase the risk of toxicity.

MANAGEMENT OPTIONS:

➤ **Consider Alternative.** Consider terbinafine (eg, *Lamisil*) as an alternative because it does not affect CYP3A4 activity.

➤ **Monitor.** If ketoconazole is coadministered with everolimus, monitor for evidence of everolimus toxicity.

REFERENCES:

1. Kovarik JM, et al. Blood concentrations of everolimus are markedly increased by ketoconazole. *J Clin Pharmacol.* 2005;45(5):514-518.

† Not available in the United States.

Everolimus†

Rifampin (eg, *Rifadin*)

SUMMARY: Rifampin reduces the plasma concentration of everolimus; a reduction in everolimus efficacy may occur.

RISK FACTORS: No specific risk factors are known.

MECHANISM: Rifampin appears to induce the CYP3A4 metabolism of everolimus, resulting in an increased first-pass and systemic clearance of everolimus.

CLINICAL EVALUATION: Twelve healthy subjects received a single oral dose of everolimus 4 mg alone and after pretreatment with rifampin 600 mg daily for 8 days.[1] The mean area under the plasma concentration-time curve of everolimus was reduced 67%. The oral clearance of everolimus increased an average of 172% (range, 0% to 451%). Everolimus half-life was reduced from 32 to 24 hours by rifampin treatment. A reduction of efficacy is likely when rifampin is coadministered to patients stabilized on everolimus; dose increases may be necessary.

RELATED DRUGS: Rifabutin (*Mycobutin*) also is likely to increase the clearance of everolimus. Rifampin is known to increase the clearance of other immunosuppressants, including cyclosporine (eg, *Neoral*), tacrolimus (*Prograf*), and caspofungin (*Cancidas*).

MANAGEMENT OPTIONS:

➧ **Monitor.** Monitor patients stabilized on everolimus for changing plasma concentrations and clinical effect if rifampin is added to or removed from their drug regimen.

REFERENCES:
1. Kovarik JM, et al. Effect of rifampin on apparent clearance of everolimus. *Ann Pharmacother.* 2002;36(6):981-985.

† Not available in the United States.

Everolimus†

Verapamil (eg, *Calan*)

SUMMARY: Verapamil increases everolimus plasma concentrations; increased toxicity may occur.

RISK FACTORS: No specific risk factors are known.

MECHANISM: Verapamil appears to inhibit the first-pass metabolism (CYP3A4) or P-glycoprotein transport of everolimus. Everolimus may inhibit the metabolism of verapamil.

CLINICAL EVALUATION: Sixteen healthy subjects received a single dose of everolimus 2 mg alone and on day 2 of a 6-day course of verapamil 80 mg 3 times daily.[1] During verapamil administration, the mean area under the plasma concentration-time curve of everolimus was increased 3.5-fold (range, 2.2- to 6.3-fold), but the half-life of everolimus was nearly unchanged. Increased everolimus adverse reactions are possible in some patients exposed to both drugs. The single dose of everolimus resulted in a mean 2.3-fold increase in the trough plasma concentrations of verapamil. More data are necessary to evaluate the potential effect of everolimus on verapamil.

RELATED DRUGS: Diltiazem (eg, *Cardizem*) may affect everolimus in a similar manner. If everolimus inhibits the metabolism of verapamil, other calcium channel blockers would be affected in a similar manner. Verapamil is known to increase cyclosporine (eg, *Neoral*) blood concentrations.

MANAGEMENT OPTIONS:

➥ *Consider Alternative.* Consider calcium channel blockers that do not inhibit CYP3A4 (eg, amlodipine [eg, *Norvasc*], nifedipine [eg, *Procardia*], felodipine [eg, *Plendil*]) for patients taking everolimus. However, as noted, everolimus may inhibit their metabolism.

➥ *Monitor.* Observe patients for everolimus- associated toxicity. Everolimus doses may require reduction during coadministration with verapamil.

REFERENCES:

1. Kovarik JM, et al. Pharmacokinetic interaction between verapamil and everolimus in healthy subjects. *Br J Clin Pharmacol.* 2005;60(4):434-437.

† Not available in the United States.

Exemestane (*Aromasin*)

Carbamazepine (eg, *Tegretol*)

SUMMARY: Theoretically, carbamazepine may produce substantial reductions in exemestane plasma concentrations; an increase in the exemestane dose is recommended.

RISK FACTORS: No specific risk factors are known.

MECHANISM: Exemestane is extensively metabolized by CYP3A4, and carbamazepine is an inducer of CYP3A4.

CLINICAL EVALUATION: Rifampin (eg, *Rifadin*) was shown to substantially reduce exemestane plasma concentrations, and it is likely that other CYP3A4 inducers, such as carbamazepine, also reduce exemestane concentrations.[1]

RELATED DRUGS: Oxcarbazepine (eg, *Trileptal*) is also an enzyme inducer, and is expected to reduce exemestane plasma concentrations.

MANAGEMENT OPTIONS:

➥ *Circumvent/Minimize.* If patients taking exemestane require enzyme inducers such as carbamazepine, the manufacturer recommends that the exemestane dose be increased to 50 mg daily after a meal.

REFERENCES:

1. *Aromasin* [package insert]. New York, NY: Pharmacia & Upjohn; 2007.

Exemestane (*Aromasin*)

Nevirapine (*Viramune*)

SUMMARY: Theoretically, nevirapine may produce substantial reductions in exemestane plasma concentrations; an increase in the exemestane dose is recommended.

RISK FACTORS: No specific risk factors are known.

MECHANISM: Exemestane is extensively metabolized by CYP3A4, and nevirapine is an inducer of CYP3A4.

CLINICAL EVALUATION: Rifampin (eg, *Rifadin*) was shown to substantially reduce exemestane plasma concentrations, and it is likely that other CYP3A4 inducers, such as nevirapine, also reduce exemestane concentrations.[1]

RELATED DRUGS: Efavirenz (*Sustiva*) is also an enzyme inducer, and is expected to reduce exemestane plasma concentrations.

MANAGEMENT OPTIONS:

➡ *Circumvent/Minimize.* If patients taking exemestane require enzyme inducers such as nevirapine, the manufacturer recommends that the exemestane dose be increased to 50 mg daily after a meal.

REFERENCES:

1. *Aromasin* [package insert]. New York, NY: Pharmacia & Upjohn; 2007.

Exemestane (*Aromasin*)

Phenobarbital (eg, *Solfoton*)

SUMMARY: Theoretically, phenobarbital may produce substantial reductions in exemestane plasma concentrations; an increase in the exemestane dose is recommended.

RISK FACTORS: No specific risk factors are known.

MECHANISM: Exemestane is extensively metabolized by CYP3A4, and phenobarbital is an inducer of CYP3A4.

CLINICAL EVALUATION: Rifampin (eg, *Rifadin*) was shown to substantially reduce exemestane plasma concentrations, and it is likely that other CYP3A4 inducers, such as phenobarbital, also reduce exemestane concentrations.[1]

RELATED DRUGS: Other barbiturates and other enzyme inducers are also expected to reduce exemestane plasma concentrations.

MANAGEMENT OPTIONS:

➡ *Circumvent/Minimize.* If patients taking exemestane require enzyme inducers such as phenobarbital, the manufacturer recommends that the exemestane dose be increased to 50 mg daily after a meal.

REFERENCES:

1. *Aromasin* [package insert]. New York, NY: Pharmacia & Upjohn; 2007.

Exemestane (*Aromasin*)

Phenytoin (eg, *Dilantin*)

SUMMARY: Theoretically, phenytoin may produce substantial reductions in exemestane plasma concentrations; an increase in the exemestane dose is recommended.

RISK FACTORS: No specific risk factors are known.

MECHANISM: Exemestane is extensively metabolized by CYP3A4, and phenytoin is an inducer of CYP3A4.

CLINICAL EVALUATION: Rifampin (eg, *Rifadin*) was shown to substantially reduce exemestane plasma concentrations, and it is likely that other CYP3A4 inducers, such as phenytoin, also reduce exemestane concentrations.[1]

RELATED DRUGS: Other enzyme inducers are also expected to reduce exemestane plasma concentrations.

MANAGEMENT OPTIONS:

➡ *Circumvent/Minimize.* If patients taking exemestane require phenytoin, the manufacturer recommends that the exemestane dose be increased to 50 mg daily after a meal.

REFERENCES:

1. *Aromasin* [package insert]. New York, NY: Pharmacia & Upjohn; 2007.

Exemestane (*Aromasin*)

Primidone (eg, *Mysoline*)

SUMMARY: Theoretically, primidone may produce substantial reductions in exemestane plasma concentrations; an increase in the exemestane dose is recommended.

RISK FACTORS: No specific risk factors are known.

MECHANISM: Exemestane is extensively metabolized by CYP3A4, and primidone is an inducer of CYP3A4.

CLINICAL EVALUATION: Rifampin (eg, *Rifadin*) was shown to substantially reduce exemestane plasma concentrations, and it is likely that other CYP3A4 inducers, such as primidone, also reduce exemestane concentrations.[1]

RELATED DRUGS: Other enzyme inducers are also expected to reduce exemestane plasma concentrations.

MANAGEMENT OPTIONS:

➡ *Circumvent/Minimize.* If patients taking exemestane require enzyme inducers such as primidone, the manufacturer recommends that the exemestane dose be increased to 50 mg daily after a meal.

REFERENCES:

1. *Aromasin* [package insert]. New York, NY: Pharmacia & Upjohn; 2007.

Exemestane (*Aromasin*)

Rifampin (eg, *Rifadin*)

SUMMARY: Rifampin may produce substantial reductions in exemestane plasma concentrations; an increase in the exemestane dose is recommended.

RISK FACTORS: No specific risk factors are known.

MECHANISM: Exemestane is extensively metabolized by CYP3A4, and rifampin is a potent inducer of CYP3A4.

CLINICAL EVALUATION: In 10 healthy postmenopausal women, pretreatment with rifampin (600 mg/day for 14 days) reduced exemestane area under the plasma concentration-time curve 54%.[1] The magnitude of this reduction is expected to reduce the efficacy of exemestane.

RELATED DRUGS: Rifabutin (*Mycobutin*) is a less potent enzyme inducer than rifampin, but is also expected to reduce exemestane plasma concentrations, as are other enzyme inducers.

MANAGEMENT OPTIONS:

➡ *Circumvent/Minimize.* If patients taking exemestane require rifampin, the manufacturer recommends that the exemestane dose be increased to 50 mg daily after a meal.

REFERENCES:

1. *Aromasin* [package insert]. New York, NY: Pharmacia & Upjohn; 2007.

Exemestane (*Aromasin*)

St. John's Wort

SUMMARY: Theoretically, St. John's wort may produce substantial reductions in exemestane plasma concentrations; an increase in the exemestane dose is recommended.

RISK FACTORS: No specific risk factors are known.

MECHANISM: Exemestane is extensively metabolized by CYP3A4, and St. John's wort is an inducer of CYP3A4.

CLINICAL EVALUATION: Rifampin (eg, *Rifadin*) was shown to substantially reduce exemestane plasma concentrations, and it is likely that other CYP3A4 inducers, such as St. John's wort, also reduce exemestane concentrations.[1]

RELATED DRUGS: Other enzyme inducers are also expected to reduce exemestane plasma concentrations.

MANAGEMENT OPTIONS:

➡ *Consider Alternative.* Because the efficacy of St. John's wort is not well established, use of an alternative treatment in patients receiving exemestane is recommended.

➡️ *Circumvent/Minimize.* If patients taking exemestane also take enzyme inducers such as St. John's wort, the manufacturer recommends that the exemestane dose be increased to 50 mg daily after a meal.

REFERENCES:

1. *Aromasin* [package insert]. New York, NY: Pharmacia & Upjohn; 2007.

Exenatide (*Byetta*)

Lovastatin (eg, *Mevacor*)

SUMMARY: Coadministration of exenatide reduced the plasma concentrations of lovastatin; reduced lipid-lowering effect could occur in some patients.

RISK FACTORS: No specific risk factors are known.

MECHANISM: Exenatide reduces gastric motility; reduction of lovastatin bioavailability may occur.

CLINICAL EVALUATION: While specific data are limited, the manufacturer of exenatide notes that administration of lovastatin prior to a single dose of exenatide reduced the mean area under the plasma concentration-time curve of lovastatin about 40% and reduced its mean peak concentration 28%.[1] Pending further data, observe patients receiving exenatide and lovastatin concurrently for reduced lovastatin effect.

RELATED DRUGS: While no data are available, it is possible that other statins will demonstrate a reduced bioavailability if administered with exenatide.

MANAGEMENT OPTIONS:

➡️ *Monitor.* Instruct patients taking exenatide to take other orally administered drugs 1 hour prior to exenatide dosing to avoid delayed absorption of the oral medication. It is not known how long the observed delay in gastric emptying will last following a dose of exenatide.

REFERENCES:

1. *Byetta* [package insert]. San Diego, CA: Amylin Pharmaceuticals; 2006.

Ezetimibe (*Zetia*)

Atorvastatin (*Lipitor*)

SUMMARY: A patient taking atorvastatin developed myopathy after starting ezetimibe, but a causal relationship was not established.

RISK FACTORS: No specific risk factors are known.

MECHANISM: Unknown.

CLINICAL EVALUATION: A 43-year-old man on chronic therapy with atorvastatin 80 mg/day developed severe muscle pain and elevated creatine kinase (CK) activity 3 weeks after ezetimibe 10 mg/day was added.[1] Both drugs were withdrawn and the symptoms resolved. Later, atorvastatin 80 mg/day was restarted with no evidence of myopathy. The clinical importance of this purported interaction is not clear. Many patients have received concurrent therapy with ezetimibe and statins without any evidence of myopathy. More data are needed to establish whether a causal relationship exists.

RELATED DRUGS: A case of elevated CK levels has been reported with ezetimibe and fluvastatin (*Lescol*), but a causal relationship was not established.

MANAGEMENT OPTIONS: No specific action is required, but be alert for evidence of the interaction.

REFERENCES:

1. Fux R, et al. Ezetimibe and statin-associated myopathy. *Ann Intern Med.* 2004;140(8):671-672.

 4 **Ezetimibe (*Zetia*)**

Fluvastatin (*Lescol*)

SUMMARY: A patient taking fluvastatin developed myopathy after starting ezetimibe, but a causal relationship was not established.

RISK FACTORS: No specific risk factors are known.

MECHANISM: Unknown.

CLINICAL EVALUATION: A 52-year-old man on chronic therapy with fluvastatin 80 mg/day developed elevated creatine kinase (CK) activity 8 weeks after ezetimibe 10 mg/day was added.[1] The fluvastatin therapy was continued, but the ezetimibe was withdrawn. The CK returned to normal within 4 weeks. The clinical importance of this purported interaction is not clear. Many patients have received concurrent therapy with ezetimibe and statins without any evidence of myopathy. More data are needed to establish whether a causal relationship exists.

RELATED DRUGS: A case of myopathy has been reported with ezetimibe and atorvastatin (*Lipitor*), but a causal relationship was not established.

MANAGEMENT OPTIONS: No specific action is required, but be alert for evidence of the interaction.

REFERENCES:

1. Fux R, et al. Ezetimibe and statin-associated myopathy. *Ann Intern Med.* 2004;140(8):671-672.

Famotidine (eg, *Pepcid*) 4

Probenecid

SUMMARY: Probenecid substantially increases serum famotidine concentrations, but the interaction is unlikely to result in adverse reactions.

RISK FACTORS: No specific risk factors are known.

MECHANISM: Probenecid inhibits the renal clearance of famotidine, apparently through inhibition of famotidine renal tubular secretion.

CLINICAL EVALUATION: Eight healthy subjects received single doses of oral famotidine 20 mg with and without coadministration of probenecid 1,500 mg.[1] Probenecid increased the famotidine area under the serum concentration-time curve 81% and reduced famotidine renal clearance 64%. These changes are expected to increase famotidine-induced inhibition of gastric acid secretion, but this has not been studied. Because famotidine has little dose-related toxicity, it seems unlikely that the interaction would result in adverse reactions.

RELATED DRUGS: Other H_2-receptor antagonists, such as cimetidine (eg, *Tagamet HB*), ranitidine (eg, *Zantac*), and nizatidine (eg, *Axid*), also undergo extensive renal excretion and are expected to be affected similarly by probenecid.

MANAGEMENT OPTIONS: No specific action is required, but be alert for evidence of the interaction.

REFERENCES:
1. Inotsume N, et al. The inhibitory effect of probenecid on renal excretion of famotidine in young, healthy volunteers. *J Clin Pharmacol*. 1990;30(1):50-56.

Febuxostat (*Uloric*) 5

Colchicine

SUMMARY: Febuxostat and colchicine do not appear to interact in a clinically significant way.

RISK FACTORS: No specific risk factors are known.

MECHANISM: None (no interaction).

CLINICAL EVALUATION: When febuxostat and colchicine were coadministered, only small and clinically insignificant changes were observed in the plasma concentrations of both drugs.[1]

RELATED DRUGS: No information is available.

MANAGEMENT OPTIONS: No interaction.

REFERENCES:
1. *Uloric* [package insert]. Deerfield, IL: Takeda Pharmaceuticals America Inc; 2009.

Febuxostat (*Uloric*)

Indomethacin (eg, *Indocin*)

SUMMARY: Febuxostat does not appear to interact with indomethacin.

RISK FACTORS: No specific risk factors are known.

MECHANISM: None (no interaction).

CLINICAL EVALUATION: In a multiple-dose, crossover study in healthy subjects, indomethacin had no effect on febuxostat pharmacokinetics, and febuxostat had no effect on indomethacin pharmacokinetics.[1]

RELATED DRUGS: No information is available.

MANAGEMENT OPTIONS: No interaction.

REFERENCES:
1. Khosravan R, et al. Pharmacokinetic interactions of concomitant administration of febuxostat and NSAIDs. *J Clin Pharmacol*. 2006;46(8):855-866.

 Febuxostat (*Uloric*)

AVOID **Mercaptopurine (eg, *Purinethol*)**

SUMMARY: Febuxostat theoretically increases the risk of serious mercaptopurine toxicity; avoid the combination.

RISK FACTORS: No specific risk factors are known.

MECHANISM: Mercaptopurine is metabolized by xanthine oxidase and febuxostat is a xanthine oxidase inhibitor; plasma concentrations of mercaptopurine are likely to increase.

CLINICAL EVALUATION: Although this interaction is based on theoretical considerations, an interaction is likely to occur and mercaptopurine toxicity is potentially fatal. The combination is considered contraindicated.[1] Another xanthine oxidase inhibitor (allopurinol [eg, *Zyloprim*]) has been used intentionally with mercaptopurine (or azathioprine [eg, *Imuran*]) to improve efficacy and reduce hepatotoxicity in patients with inflammatory bowel disease, but this is only done with mercaptopurine dose reductions and careful monitoring for bone marrow suppression.[2,3]

RELATED DRUGS: Any other xanthine oxidase inhibitor (eg, allopurinol) is likely to increase the effect of both mercaptopurine and azathioprine.

MANAGEMENT OPTIONS:

➡ ***AVOID COMBINATION.*** Avoid concurrent use of mercaptopurine and febuxostat.

REFERENCES:
1. *Uloric* [package insert]. Deerfield, IL: Takeda Pharmaceuticals America Inc; 2009.
2. Sparrow MP, et al. Effect of allopurinol on clinical outcomes in inflammatory bowel disease nonresponders to azathioprine or 6-mercaptopurine. *Clin Gastroenterol Hepatol*. 2007;5(2):209-214.
3. Ansari A, et al. Long-term outcome of using allopurinol co-therapy as a strategy for overcoming thiopurine hepatotoxicity in treating inflammatory bowel disease. *Aliment Pharmacol Ther*. 2008;28(6):734-741.

Febuxostat (*Uloric*) 4

Naproxen (eg, *Aleve*)

SUMMARY: Naproxen produces small increases in febuxostat plasma concentrations, but the clinical significance is probably minimal.

RISK FACTORS: No specific risk factors are known.

MECHANISM: Not established.

CLINICAL EVALUATION: In a multiple-dose, crossover study in healthy subjects, naproxen produced a 40% increase in the febuxostat area under the plasma concentration-time curve.[1] Febuxostat had no effect on plasma concentrations of naproxen. The increased febuxostat concentrations are unlikely to produce adverse consequences, but more data are needed to establish the safety of the combination.

RELATED DRUGS: No information is available.

MANAGEMENT OPTIONS: No special precautions are necessary.

REFERENCES:

1. Khosravan R, et al. Pharmacokinetic interactions of concomitant administration of febuxostat and NSAIDs. *J Clin Pharmacol.* 2006;46(8):855-866.

Febuxostat (*Uloric*)

Theophylline (eg, *Theochron*)

SUMMARY: Febuxostat theoretically increases the risk of theophylline toxicity; avoid the combination.

RISK FACTORS: No specific risk factors are known.

MECHANISM: Theophylline is partially metabolized by xanthine oxidase and febuxostat is a xanthine oxidase inhibitor; plasma concentrations of theophylline are likely to increase.

CLINICAL EVALUATION: Although this interaction is based on theoretical considerations, the combination may increase the risk of theophylline toxicity. The actual risk of theophylline toxicity is not known, but the combination is considered contraindicated.[1]

RELATED DRUGS: Allopurinol (eg, *Zyloprim*) is also a xanthine oxidase inhibitor and increases theophylline plasma concentrations.

MANAGEMENT OPTIONS:

➥ *Avoid Unless Benefit Outweighs Risk.* Given the contraindication in the product information, avoid concurrent use of theophylline and febuxostat.

➥ *Monitor.* If the combination is used, monitor closely for evidence of theophylline toxicity.

REFERENCES:

1. *Uloric* [package insert]. Deerfield, IL: Takeda Pharmaceuticals America, Inc; 2009.

Febuxostat (*Uloric*)

Warfarin (eg, *Coumadin*)

SUMMARY: Febuxostat does not appear to interact with warfarin.

RISK FACTORS: No specific risk factors are known.

MECHANISM: None (no interaction).

CLINICAL EVALUATION: When febuxostat and warfarin were coadministered, there was no effect on warfarin pharmacokinetics or hypoprothrombinemic response.[1]

RELATED DRUGS: No information is available.

MANAGEMENT OPTIONS: No interaction.

REFERENCES:
1. *Uloric* [package insert]. Deerfield, IL: Takeda Pharmaceuticals America, Inc; 2009.

Felbamate (*Felbatol*)

Phenobarbital (eg, *Solfoton*)

SUMMARY: Felbamate increases phenobarbital concentrations and may result in toxicity.

RISK FACTORS: No specific risk factors are known.

MECHANISM: Felbamate increased phenobarbital concentrations by inhibiting the formation of its hydroxylated metabolite, parahydroxphenobarbital. Phenobarbital may decrease felbamate concentrations by stimulating the metabolism of felbamate.

CLINICAL EVALUATION: A case report describes a patient with an elevated phenobarbital plasma concentration following the addition of felbamate.[1] A double-blind, placebo-controlled study in 24 healthy volunteers demonstrated that felbamate increased phenobarbital plasma concentrations 20% to 25% after 9 days of felbamate. This was caused by decreased phenobarbital metabolism. This study underestimated the magnitude of the potential interaction because steady-state concentrations of phenobarbital could not have been reached for at least 1 month. Therefore, the extent of the interaction has not been established. Phenobarbital may have reduced felbamate concentrations in this study.[2]

RELATED DRUGS: No information is available.

MANAGEMENT OPTIONS:

➡ *Consider Alternative.* Given the serious toxicity that has been reported with felbamate, it is reserved for carefully selected patients. Thus, use alternatives to felbamate if possible, whether or not the patient is on interacting drugs.

➡ *Circumvent/Minimize.* Because patients may have an increase in serum phenobarbital concentrations when felbamate therapy is added, consider reducing the phenobarbital dose 20% to 25% when felbamate is added. Conversely, an increase in phenobarbital dosage may be required if felbamate is discontinued. It is not clear whether an alteration in felbamate dosage is needed when phenobarbital therapy is initiated or discontinued.

➡ *Monitor.* Monitor symptoms of phenobarbital toxicity for at least 1 month after felbamate is added.

REFERENCES:

1. Gidal BE, et al. Potential pharmacokinetic interaction between felbamate and phenobarbital. *Ann Pharmacother*. 1994;28(4):455-458.

2. Reidenberg P, et al. Effects of felbamate on the pharmacokinetics of phenobarbital. *Clin Pharmacol Ther*. 1995;58(3):279-287.

Felbamate (*Felbatol*)

Phenytoin (eg, *Dilantin*)

SUMMARY: Felbamate consistently increases serum phenytoin concentrations; phenytoin toxicity may occur in some patients. Phenytoin appears to decrease serum felbamate concentrations, but the clinical importance of this effect is not established.

RISK FACTORS: No specific risk factors are known.

MECHANISM: The mechanism of the effect of felbamate on phenytoin is not established, but felbamate may inhibit the metabolism of phenytoin. Phenytoin probably stimulates the hepatic metabolism of felbamate.

CLINICAL EVALUATION: In a double-blind, placebo-controlled crossover study involving 32 patients, addition of felbamate was associated with a 10% to 32% reduction in phenytoin dosage to maintain stable phenytoin concentrations.[1] In 2 case reports, the addition of felbamate resulted in evidence of phenytoin toxicity and a need to reduce the phenytoin dose.[2,3] The evidence suggests that felbamate consistently increases serum phenytoin concentrations in patients receiving both drugs, but the magnitude of the effect varies from patient to patient. In 8 patients, receiving either carbamazepine (eg, *Tegretol*) or phenytoin, the half-life of felbamate was 14 hours, which is shorter than what is seen in healthy subjects (20 hours).[3] Tapering of phenytoin and then carbamazepine in 4 patients receiving all 3 drugs (felbamate, carbamazepine, and phenytoin) resulted in a decreased felbamate clearance and necessitated a reduction in the felbamate dose.[4]

RELATED DRUGS: No information is available.

MANAGEMENT OPTIONS:

➡ *Consider Alternative.* Given the serious toxicity that has been reported with felbamate, it is reserved for carefully selected patients. Thus, use alternatives to felbamate if possible, whether or not the patient is on interacting drugs.

➡ *Circumvent/Minimize.* Because almost all patients appear to manifest an increase in serum phenytoin concentrations when felbamate therapy is added, consider reducing the phenytoin dose by 25% when felbamate is added. Conversely, an increase in phenytoin dosage may be required if felbamate is discontinued. It is not clear whether an alteration in felbamate dosage is needed when phenytoin therapy is initiated or discontinued.

➡ *Monitor.* When the 2 agents are used together, monitor for symptoms of phenytoin toxicity.

REFERENCES:

1. Graves NM, et al. Effects of felbamate on phenytoin and carbamazepine serum concentrations. *Epilepsia*. 1989;30(2):225–229.

2. Fuerst RH, et al. Felbamate increases phenytoin but decreases carbamazepine concentrations. *Epilepsia*. 1988;29(4):488–491.

3. Wilensky AJ, et al. Pharmacokinetics of W-554 (ADD 03055) in epileptic patients. *Epilepsia*. 1985;26(6):602–606.

4. Wagner ML, et al. Discontinuation of phenytoin and carbamazepine in patients receiving felbamate. *Epilepsia*. 1991;32(3):398–406.

Felbamate (*Felbatol*)

Valproic Acid (eg, *Depakene*)

SUMMARY: Preliminary evidence suggests that felbamate consistently increases serum valproic acid concentrations, but the magnitude of the effect varies from patient to patient.

RISK FACTORS: No specific risk factors are known.

MECHANISM: Not established. Felbamate may inhibit the hepatic metabolism of valproic acid.

CLINICAL EVALUATION: Ten patients with epilepsy stabilized on valproic acid 10 to 26 mg/kg/day received felbamate 1,200 and 2,400 mg/day in a randomized, crossover design.[1] The patients had initially received felbamate 2,400 to 3,600 mg/day, but the doses of felbamate had to be reduced because of GI and cognitive adverse effects. Felbamate 1,200 and 2,400 mg/day substantially increased steady-state serum concentrations of valproic acid 28% and 54%, respectively.

RELATED DRUGS: No information is available.

MANAGEMENT OPTIONS:

➡ *Consider Alternative.* Given the serious toxicity that has been reported with felbamate, it is reserved for carefully selected patients. Thus, use alternatives to felbamate if possible, whether or not the patient is on interacting drugs.

➡ *Circumvent/Minimize.* In patients stabilized on valproic acid, titrating felbamate slowly may reduce the risk of adverse reactions. If felbamate is rapidly added to valproic acid, it may be necessary to reduce valproic acid doses. Also be aware that discontinuing felbamate may affect valproic acid requirements.

➡ *Monitor.* Monitor for symptoms of valproic toxicity, such as tremor, confusion, irritability, and restlessness.

REFERENCES:
1. Wagner ML, et al. The effect of felbamate on valproic acid disposition. *Clin Pharmacol Ther*. 1994;56(5):494–502.

Felbamate (*Felbatol*)

Warfarin (eg, *Coumadin*)

SUMMARY: A patient developed a marked increase in the hypoprothrombinemic response to warfarin after starting felbamate, but a causal relationship was not established.

RISK FACTORS: No specific risk factors are known.

MECHANISM: Not established.

CLINICAL EVALUATION: A 62-year-old man who was on a weekly dosage of warfarin 35 mg ($\pm$ 5 mg) to maintain an international normalized ratio (INR) of 2.5 to 3.5 was also receiving carbamazepine (eg, *Tegretol*) 1,200 mg/day, phenobarbital (eg, *Solfoton*) 30 mg/day, and valproic acid (eg, *Depakene*) 400 mg/day.[1] Because of inadequate seizure control, the 3 anticonvulsants were replaced with felbamate 2,400 mg/day (increased to 3,200 mg/day after 2 weeks). After 2 weeks of felbamate, the INR had increased to 7.8, and later increased to 18.2. Determination of the cause of the excessive hypoprothrombinemic response in this patient is difficult because 2 enzyme-inducing anticonvulsants (carbamazepine and phenobarbital) were discontinued at the same time the felbamate was started. Both carbamazepine and phenobarbital enhance the metabolism of warfarin, and it is expected that discontinuation would increase warfarin response in most patients. Although the patient's warfarin requirements reportedly were not altered when the carbamazepine and phenobarbital were initially started, details were not provided. It is possible that the marked increase in INR was related to discontinuation of carbamazepine and phenobarbital, and the initiation of felbamate therapy.

RELATED DRUGS: The effect of felbamate on other oral anticoagulants is not established.

MANAGEMENT OPTIONS: No specific action is required, but be alert for evidence of the interaction.

REFERENCES:
1. Tisdel KA, et al. Warfarin-felbamate interaction: first report. *Ann Pharmacother.* 1994;28(6):805.

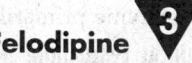

Felodipine

Itraconazole (eg, *Sporanox*)

SUMMARY: Itraconazole increases felodipine concentrations and enhances its vasodilatory effects; excessive hypotensive response could result.

RISK FACTORS: No specific risk factors are known.

MECHANISM: Itraconazole is known to inhibit the activity of CYP3A4, the enzyme that is responsible for the first-pass and hepatic metabolism of felodipine. Itraconazole administration is likely to increase the bioavailability of felodipine and reduce its intrinsic clearance.

CLINICAL EVALUATION: Nine healthy subjects received placebo or itraconazole 200 mg/day for 4 days.[1] On the fourth day, each took a single oral dose of felodipine 5 mg. Itraconazole administration increased the mean peak concentration of felodipine from 1.2 to 9.3 ng/mL. The mean area under the concentration-time curve of felodipine increased over 6-fold following itraconazole administration. The effects of felodipine on blood pressure and heart rate were significantly increased following itraconazole pretreatment.

RELATED DRUGS: The bioavailability and metabolism of other calcium channel blockers that undergo CYP3A4 metabolism are likely to be affected by itraconazole. Other azole antifungal agents, such as ketoconazole (eg, *Nizoral*), miconazole (eg, *Monistat*), and fluconazole (eg, *Diflucan*), would also be expected to reduce the metabolism of felodipine. Terbinafine (eg, *Lamisil*) may be less likely to affect felodipine clearance.

MANAGEMENT OPTIONS:

➥ *Consider Alternative.* Although there are no specific data, terbinafine may be less likely to affect felodipine clearance. Because most calcium channel blockers will likely be affected to some extent, the use of a noncalcium blocker may be appropriate during treatment with an azole antifungal agent.

➥ *Circumvent/Minimize.* A reduction in the dose of felodipine may be necessary to avoid excessive pharmacologic effects.

➥ *Monitor.* Monitor patients receiving the combination of itraconazole and felodipine carefully for excessive hypotension.

REFERENCES:

1. Jalava KM, et al. Itraconazole greatly increases plasma concentrations and effects of felodipine. *Clin Pharmacol Ther.* 1997;61(4):410–415.

Felodipine

Menthol

SUMMARY: Menthol appears to produce only small increases in felodipine plasma concentrations, and adverse reactions from the interaction are probably minimal.

RISK FACTORS: No specific risk factors are known.

MECHANISM: Not established. Menthol might produce a mild inhibition of CYP3A4, the enzyme primarily responsible for the metabolism of felodipine.

CLINICAL EVALUATION: In a randomized crossover study of 11 healthy subjects, menthol 200 mg over 7 hours had no effect on the pharmacokinetics of a single oral dose of felodipine 10 mg.[1] In another study of 12 healthy subjects, menthol (in the form of peppermint oil) modestly increased the felodipine area under the plasma concentration-time curve.[2] The second study involved larger amounts of menthol, which might explain the differing results. In any case, it does not appear that menthol is likely to result in an increase in felodipine toxicity.

RELATED DRUGS: No information is available.

MANAGEMENT OPTIONS: No specific action is required, but be alert for evidence of the interaction.

REFERENCES:

1. Gelal A, et al. Effect of menthol on the pharmacokinetics and pharmacodynamics of felodipine in healthy subjects. *Eur J Clin Pharmacol.* 2005;60(11):785-790.

2. Dresser GK, et al. Evaluation of peppermint oil and ascorbyl palmitate as inhibitors of cytochrome P4503A4 activity in vitro and in vivo. *Clin Pharmacol Ther.* 2002;72(3):247-255.

Felodipine

Nelfinavir (*Viracept*)

SUMMARY: Nelfinavir may increase the hypotensive effects of felodipine.

RISK FACTORS: No specific risk factors are known.

MECHANISM: Nelfinavir appears to inhibit CYP3A4, the enzyme that metabolizes felodipine.

CLINICAL EVALUATION: A patient with hypertension was taking metoprolol 50 mg and felodipine 5 mg daily for several years. Three days after starting therapy with zidovudine, lamivudine, and nelfinavir 2,000 mg daily, the patient experienced an orthostatic episode and leg edema. Following discontinuation of the metoprolol and felodipine, the leg edema and orthostatic hypotension abated. The effect of long-term nelfinavir on felodipine is unknown.[1]

RELATED DRUGS: Nelfinavir could affect other calcium channel blockers in a similar manner.

MANAGEMENT OPTIONS:

➡ *Consider Alternative.* If necessary, select an alternative antihypertensive agent that is not metabolized in the same manner as felodipine (eg, angiotensin-converting enzyme inhibitor, diuretic).

➡ *Monitor.* If nelfinavir is initiated or discontinued in a patient taking felodipine, watch for altered hypotensive response.

REFERENCES:

1. Izzedine H, et al. Nelfinavir and felodipine: a cytochrome P450 3A4-mediated drug interaction. *Clin Pharmacol Ther.* 2004;75(4):362-363.

Felodipine

Warfarin (eg, *Coumadin*)

SUMMARY: Felodipine does not appear to affect warfarin response.

RISK FACTORS: No specific risk factors are known.

MECHANISM: No interaction.

CLINICAL EVALUATION: Extended-release felodipine did not affect the pharmacokinetics or pharmacodynamics of warfarin in 12 healthy subjects.[1]

RELATED DRUGS: The effect of felodipine on oral anticoagulants other than warfarin is not established.

MANAGEMENT OPTIONS: No interaction.

REFERENCES:

1. Grind M, et al. Method for studying drug-warfarin interactions. *Clin Pharmacol Ther.* 1993;54(4):381–387.

Fenfluramine (*Pondimin*)

Fluoxetine (eg, *Prozac*)

SUMMARY: Cotherapy with fenfluramine and selective serotonin reuptake inhibitors (SSRIs) such as fluoxetine theoretically could result in serotonin syndrome.

RISK FACTORS: No specific risk factors are known.

MECHANISM: Fenfluramine releases serotonin and inhibits its uptake. Because SSRIs are also serotonergic, combined use theoretically increases the risk of serotonin syndrome. Also, fluoxetine and paroxetine are potent inhibitors of CYP2D6, an isozyme important in the metabolism of fenfluramine. Sertraline and fluvoxamine are much weaker inhibitors of CYP2D6.

CLINICAL EVALUATION: Although this interaction is based primarily on theoretical considerations, the potential outcome is serious. Serotonin syndrome has occurred when
SSRIs such as fluoxetine have been combined with other serotonergic agents such
as nonselective monoamine oxidase inhibitors. Serotonin syndrome can result in
severe toxicity; fatalities have occurred. Given the potential severity of the reaction, the product information for the related drug, dexfenfluramine (*Redux*), states
that dexfenfluramine should not be used with SSRIs or any other serotonergic
agent.[1] Dexfenfluramine is the S-enantiomer of the racemate fenfluramine, so the
2 drugs probably interact in a similar way with SSRIs. Anecdotal evidence suggests that many patients have received fenfluramine plus SSRIs without manifesting serious adverse consequences, but such evidence does not rule out an
occasional serious reaction. Fenfluramine serum concentrations are likely to be
higher in: a) patients who are genetically deficient in CYP2D6 (deficiency occurs
in about 5% to 10% of white patients and black patients, no more than 1% of Asian
patients)[2]; b) patients who are taking potent inhibitors of CYP2D6 such as fluoxetine or paroxetine; or c) patients whose urinary pH is more alkaline. However, it
is not known whether patients with higher levels of fenfluramine are more likely
to manifest an adverse drug interaction with SSRIs.

RELATED DRUGS: Avoid dexfenfluramine (*Redux*) in combination with other SSRIs such as
paroxetine (eg, *Paxil*), sertraline (*Zoloft*), and fluvoxamine (eg, *Luvox*).

MANAGEMENT OPTIONS:

➡ *Avoid Unless Benefit Outweighs Risk.* Avoid using SSRIs with fenfluramine or dexfenfluramine unless the combinations are found to be safe in well-controlled clinical trials. There also is a medicolegal risk in using the combinations; the manufacturer's
information states that cotherapy should be avoided.

➡ *Monitor.* If the combination is used, be alert for evidence of serotonin syndrome,
which can result in neurotoxicity (eg, myoclonus, tremors, rigidity, incoordination,
restlessness, hyperreflexia, seizures, coma), psychiatric symptoms (eg, agitation,
confusion, hypomania), and temperature regulation abnormalities (eg, fever,
sweating).

REFERENCES:

1. *Redux* [package insert]. Philadelphia, PA; Wyeth-Ayerst Laboratories; 1996.
2. Gross AS, et al. The influence of the sparteine/debrisoquine genetic polymorphism on the disposition
   of dexfenfluramine. *Br J Clin Pharmacol.* 1996;41:311-317.

4   Fenfluramine[†]

Insulin

SUMMARY: Fenfluramine may enhance the hypoglycemic activity of antidiabetic treatments; the clinical significance
probably is limited.

RISK FACTORS: No specific risk factors are known.

MECHANISM: Fenfluramine appears to increase the uptake of glucose by skeletal muscle
without affecting insulin secretion.

CLINICAL EVALUATION: Initial experiments indicate that fenfluramine has intrinsic hypoglycemic activity when given immediately before a meal[1] or in the fasting state.[2] It
appears to lower postprandial blood glucose levels in diabetic patients maintained
on insulin, tolbutamide (eg, *Orinase*), or diet alone.[2,3]

RELATED DRUGS: Tolbutamide appears to be affected similarly. The effect of fenfluramine on other hypoglycemic agents is unknown, but a similar effect may occur.

MANAGEMENT OPTIONS: No specific action is required, but be alert for evidence of the interaction.

REFERENCES:
1. Turtle JR, Burgess JA. Hypoglycemic action of fenfluramine in diabetes mellitus. *Diabetes*. 1973;22:858-867.
2. Pestell RG, Crock PA, Ward GM, Alford FP, Best JD. Fenfluramine increases insulin action in patients with NIDDM. *Diabetes Care*. 1989;12:252.
3. Kesson CM, Ireland JT. Phenformin compared with fenfluramine in the treatment of obese diabetic patients. *Practitioner*. 1976;216:577-580.
† Not available in the United States.

Fenfluramine†

Phenelzine (eg, *Nardil*) AVOID

SUMMARY: Cotherapy with fenfluramine and nonselective monamine oxidase (MAO) inhibitors such as phenelzine theoretically could result in serotonin syndrome.

RISK FACTORS: No specific risk factors are known.

MECHANISM: Fenfluramine releases serotonin and inhibits its uptake. Because nonselective MAO inhibitors are also serotonergic, combined use theoretically increases the risk of serotonin syndrome.

CLINICAL EVALUATION: Although this interaction is based primarily on theoretical considerations, the potential outcome is serious. Serotonin syndrome has occurred when nonselective MAO inhibitors such as phenelzine and tranylcypromine have been combined with other serotonergic agents. Serotonin syndrome can result in neurotoxicity (myoclonus, tremors, rigidity, incoordination, restlessness, hyperreflexia, seizures, coma); psychiatric symptoms (agitation, confusion, hypomania); and temperature regulation abnormalities (fever, sweating). Fatalities have occurred. Given the potential severity of the reaction, the product information states that combined use of fenfluramine and MAO inhibitors is contraindicated.[1] Fenfluramine serum concentrations are likely to be higher in patients who are genetically deficient in CYP2D6 (about 5% to 10% of white and black patients, 1% or fewer of Asian patients),[2] and also in patients whose urinary pH is more alkaline. However, it is not known whether patients with higher levels of fenfluramine are more likely to manifest an adverse drug interaction with nonselective MAO inhibitors.

RELATED DRUGS: Fenfluramine also is contraindicated with other nonselective MAO inhibitors such as tranylcypromine (eg, *Parnate*) and isocarboxazid (*Marplan*). Given that selegiline (eg, *Eldepryl*) also can act as a nonselective MAO inhibitors (especially if given in large doses), it also might interact adversely with fenfluramine. Dexfenfluramine is the S-enantiomer of the racemate fenfluramine, so the 2 drugs probably interact in a similar way with nonselective MAO inhibitors.

MANAGEMENT OPTIONS:

➡ *AVOID COMBINATION.* Patients should avoid any combination of a nonselective MAO inhibitors with fenfluramine or dexfenfluramine.

REFERENCES:
1. Product information. Fenfluramine (*Pondimin*). A. H. Robins Company, 1996.
2. Gross AS, et al. The influence of the sparteine/debrisoquine genetic polymorphism on the disposition of dexfenfluramine. *Br J Clin Pharmacol*. 1996;41:311-317.
† Not available in the United States.

Fenofibrate (eg, *Tricor*)

Rosuvastatin (*Crestor*)

SUMMARY: Fenofibrate and rosuvastatin appear to have minimal effects on the pharmacokinetics of each other.

RISK FACTORS: None (no interaction).

MECHANISM: None (no interaction).

CLINICAL EVALUATION: In a randomized 3-way crossover study in healthy subjects, fenofibrate (67 mg 3 times/day) and rosuvastatin (10 mg/day) were given alone and together in a multiple-dose study.[1] The pharmacokinetics of rosuvastatin and fenofibrate were similar when the drugs were given alone or in combination. The slight changes observed are of minimal clinical importance.

RELATED DRUGS: Pravastatin (*Pravachol*) also appears to be unaffected by fenofibrate, and available evidence suggests that, in general, fenofibrate is less likely to interact with HMG-CoA reductase inhibitors than gemfibrozil (eg, *Lopid*). Gemfibrozil may increase the risk of myopathy when combined with lovastatin (eg, *Mevacor*), simvastatin (*Zocor*), and probably atorvastatin (*Lipitor*), but pravastatin and fluvastatin (*Lescol*) appear less likely to interact with gemfibrozil to produce myopathy.

MANAGEMENT OPTIONS: No interaction.

REFERENCES:
1. Martin PD, Dane AL, Schneck DW, Warwick MJ. An open-label, randomized, three-way crossover trial of the effects of coadministration of rosuvastatin and fenofibrate on the pharmacokinetic properties of rosuvastatin and fenofibric acid in healthy male volunteers. *Clin Ther*. 2003;25:459-471.

 Fenofibrate (eg, *Tricor*)

Warfarin (eg, *Coumadin*)

SUMMARY: Based on case reports, it appears that fenofibrate increases the anticoagulant effect of warfarin.

RISK FACTORS: No specific risk factors are known.

MECHANISM: Not established.

CLINICAL EVALUATION: Two men, 47 and 56 years of age, developed increased hypoprothrombinemic response to warfarin during coadministration of fenofibrate.[1] The 47-year-old man agreed to rechallenge with fenofibrate in the presence of warfarin therapy; it was positive on 2 occasions. Thus, it seems likely that the fenofibrate was responsible for the increased anticoagulant effect.

RELATED DRUGS: Clofibrate (*Atromid-S*) and gemfibrozil (eg, *Lopid*) have also been reported to increase the hypoprothrombinemic response of warfarin.

MANAGEMENT OPTIONS:

➡ *Monitor.* Closely monitor the hypoprothrombinemic response to warfarin if fenofibrate is initiated, discontinued, or changed in dosage.

REFERENCES:
1. Ascah KJ, Rock GA, Wells PS. Interaction between fenofibrate and warfarin. *Ann Pharmacother*. 1998;32:765-768.

Fenoprofen (eg, *Nalfon*)

Warfarin (eg, *Coumadin*)

SUMMARY: Although little is known regarding the effect of fenoprofen on the hypoprothrombinemic response to oral anticoagulants, cotherapy requires caution because of possible detrimental effects of fenoprofen on gastric mucosa and platelet function.

RISK FACTORS:

➡ ***Concurrent Diseases.*** Patients with peptic ulcer disease (PUD) or a history of GI bleeding may be at greater risk.

MECHANISM: Fenoprofen-induced gastric erosions and inhibition of platelet function theoretically could increase the risk of bleeding in a patient receiving oral anticoagulants. Fenoprofen is strongly bound to plasma albumin and may displace warfarin from protein-binding sites in high concentrations.[1]

CLINICAL EVALUATION: Although fenoprofen may displace warfarin from protein-binding sites, little is known about the effect of fenoprofen on the hypoprothrombinemic response to oral anticoagulants. Moreover, any competition for plasma protein-binding sites is likely to result in only a transient increase in the hypoprothrombinemic response to the oral anticoagulant. However, the ability of fenoprofen to cause GI bleeding and inhibit platelet function theoretically could increase the risk of serious bleeding in patients receiving oral anticoagulants. In a retrospective cohort study, hospitalizations for hemorrhagic PUD were about 13 times higher in patients receiving warfarin plus a nonsteroidal anti-inflammatory drug (NSAID) than in patients receiving either drug.[2]

RELATED DRUGS: All NSAIDs inhibit platelet function, cause gastric erosions, and probably increase the risk of GI bleeding. However, some NSAIDs such as ibuprofen (eg, *Advil*), naproxen (eg, *Anaprox*), or diclofenac (eg, *Voltaren*) may be less likely to increase oral anticoagulant-induced hypoprothrombinemia than other NSAIDs.

MANAGEMENT OPTIONS:

➡ ***Avoid Unless Benefit Outweighs Risk.*** Because all NSAIDs may increase the risk of GI bleeding in patients on oral anticoagulants, use the combination only after careful consideration of the benefit versus risk. If an NSAID must be used with an oral anticoagulant, use NSAIDs that are unlikely to affect the hypoprothrombinemic response to oral anticoagulants. If the NSAID is being used as an analgesic or antipyretic, acetaminophen may be safer to use with oral anticoagulants. Non-acetylated salicylates (eg, choline salicylate, magnesium salicylate, salsalate, sodium salicylate) may also be safer with oral anticoagulants than NSAIDs, because these salicylates have minimal effects on platelet function and the gastric mucosa.

➡ ***Monitor.*** If any NSAID is used with an oral anticoagulant, carefully monitor the prothrombin time and watch for evidence of bleeding, especially from the GI tract.

REFERENCES:

1. Rubin A, et al. Physiological disposition of fenoprofen in man. 3. Metabolism and protein binding of fenoprofen. *J Pharmacol Exp Ther.* 1972;183:449-457.

2. Shorr RI, et al. Concurrent use of nonsteroidal anti-inflammatory drugs and oral anticoagulants places elderly persons at high risk for hemorrhagic peptic ulcer disease. *Arch Intern Med.* 1993;153:1665-1670.

Fentanyl (eg, *Duragesic*)

Fluconazole (eg, *Diflucan*)

SUMMARY: The administration of fluconazole to patients receiving transdermal fentanyl may result in respiratory depression.

RISK FACTORS: No specific risk factors are known.

MECHANISM: Fluconazole is known to inhibit the enzyme that metabolizes fentanyl, CYP3A4.

CLINICAL EVALUATION: A patient was receiving fentanyl transdermal patch 150 mcg/hr for 3 weeks.[1] Fluconazole 50 mg daily was initiated for oral fungal infection. Three days later, the patient died in his sleep. Postmortem examination found elevated fentanyl concentrations. Cause of death was thought to be respiratory depression and circulatory failure. While data in this case are limited, fluconazole is expected to inhibit the metabolism of fentanyl.

RELATED DRUGS: Other antifungal agents that inhibit CYP3A4 (eg, itraconazole [eg, *Sporanox*], voriconazole [*Vfend*], ketoconazole [eg, *Nizoral*]) are expected to inhibit fentanyl metabolism in a similar manner. The metabolism of alfentanil (eg, *Alfenta*) is inhibited by fluconazole.

MANAGEMENT OPTIONS:

➥ ***Consider Alternative.*** Consider terbinafine (*Lamisil*) as an alternative antifungal agent because it does not affect CYP3A4 activity.

➥ ***Monitor.*** Closely monitor patients receiving transdermal fentanyl for signs of respiratory depression or excess sedation if fluconazole is coadministered.

REFERENCES:

1. Hallberg P, et al. Possible fluconazole-fentanyl interaction-a case report. *Eur J Clin Pharmacol.* 2006;62:491-492.

 Fentanyl (eg, *Sublimaze*)

Lidocaine (eg, *Xylocaine*)

SUMMARY: A patient who received morphine (eg, *Duramorph*) and fentanyl during anesthetic induction developed respiratory depression and lost consciousness after receiving intravenous (IV) lidocaine; carefully monitor patients receiving opioids and lidocaine for excessive opioid effects.

RISK FACTORS:

➥ ***Route of Administration.*** The observed reaction occurred following IV use of lidocaine. Theoretically, an interaction with opioids would be unlikely to occur with lidocaine administration routes that do not result in lidocaine reaching the CNS.

MECHANISM: Not established. The authors propose that lidocaine may enhance opioid effects by reducing calcium concentrations in selected CNS sites.

CLINICAL EVALUATION: A 74-year-old man underwent coronary artery bypass surgery with fentanyl and morphine employed for anesthetic induction.[1] He was transferred to the surgical intensive care unit, breathing spontaneously. He was then administered lidocaine 200 mg IV bolus and 2 mg/min infusion for treatment of ventricular tachycardia. During the next 5 minutes, he developed progressive slowing of the respiratory rate, lost consciousness, and required reintubation. Spontaneous ventilation and consciousness returned within 1 to 2 minutes of administering naloxone (eg, *Narcan*) 0.2 mg. The rapid reversal with naloxone is consistent with the authors' contention that lidocaine enhances opioid effects, but more study is needed to establish the clinical importance of this interaction.

RELATED DRUGS: Theoretically, lidocaine would enhance the effect of any opioid.

MANAGEMENT OPTIONS:

➡ *Monitor.* If lidocaine is used concurrently with opioids, monitor for excessive opioid effects (eg, CNS depression, respiratory depression). Based on a case report, administration of an opioid antagonist such as naloxone may be effective in reversing the reaction.

REFERENCES:

1. Jensen E, et al. Potentiation of narcosis after intravenous lidocaine in a patient given spinal opioids. *Anesth Analg*. 1999;89:758-759.

Fentanyl (eg, *Sublimaze*)

Quinidine

SUMMARY: Quinidine increases fentanyl plasma concentrations and pharmacologic effects.

RISK FACTORS:

➡ *Route of Administration.* The magnitude of this interaction will be greater with oral administration of fentanyl compared with intravenous (IV) or transdermal administration.

MECHANISM: Quinidine appears to increase fentanyl plasma concentrations by inhibiting P-glycoprotein. This may increase fentanyl absorption (oral) and/or reduce its elimination.

CLINICAL EVALUATION: Twenty-four healthy subjects received a single dose of immediate-release quinidine 600 mg.[1] In 2 separate studies, 12 of the subjects were administered IV fentanyl 2.5 mcg/kg and 12 subjects received 2.5 mcg/kg orally. In both studies, the fentanyl was administered 1 hour after the dose of quinidine. Quinidine pretreatment increased the mean area under the plasma concentration-time curve of fentanyl by 56% following IV administration and 160% when oral fentanyl was administered. Increased pharmacodynamics (maximal pupil miosis, self-assessed sedation, nausea) reflected the pharmacokinetic changes following quinidine coadministration. The effects of multiple doses or extended-release formulations of quinidine on fentanyl are not known.

RELATED DRUGS: Propafenone (eg, *Rythmol*) also is an inhibitor of P-glycoprotein. It may affect fentanyl absorption or elimination. The effect of quinidine on other analgesic opioids is unknown.

MANAGEMENT OPTIONS:

➥ *Monitor.* Pending further data, monitor patients receiving fentanyl for increased opioid effect if quinidine is coadministered.

REFERENCES:

1. Kharasch E, et al. Quinidine as a probe for the role of P-glycoprotein in the intestinal absorption and clinical effects of fentanyl. *J Clin Pharmacol.* 2004;44:224-233.

Fentanyl (eg, *Sublimaze*)

Rifampin (eg, *Rifadin*)

SUMMARY: Rifampin reduces fentanyl plasma concentrations; reduced analgesic effect is likely to occur during coadministration.

RISK FACTORS: No specific risk factors known.

MECHANISM: Rifampin's induction of CYP3A4, the enzyme that metabolizes fentanyl, will result in lower fentanyl plasma concentrations.

CLINICAL EVALUATION: A patient being treated with transdermal fentanyl experienced a loss of analgesia following coadministration of rifampin 300 mg daily.[1] Fentanyl doses were increased nearly 4-fold to regain pain control. Fentanyl plasma concentrations were reduced by the coadministration of rifampin and returned to therapeutic levels only after the fentanyl dose was increased.

RELATED DRUGS: Rifampin is known to induce the metabolism of alfentanil (eg, *Alfenta*). Rifabutin may have a similar effect on fentanyl concentrations.

MANAGEMENT OPTIONS:

➥ *Consider Alternative.* Consider using an analgesic that is not a CYP3A4 substrate (eg, morphine [eg, *MS Contin*]) for patients taking rifampin.

➥ *Monitor.* Monitor patients receiving fentanyl for diminished analgesic efficacy if rifampin is administered concurrently.

REFERENCES:

1. Takane H, et al. Rifampin reduces the analgesic effect of transdermal fentanyl. *Ann Pharmacother.* 2005;39:2139-2140.

Fentanyl (eg, *Sublimaze*)

Ritonavir (*Norvir*)

SUMMARY: Ritonavir administration results in large increases in fentanyl concentrations; increased analgesic effects and side effects may occur during concurrent therapy.

RISK FACTORS: No specific risk factors are known.

MECHANISM: Ritonavir appears to inhibit the CYP3A4-mediated metabolism of fentanyl.

CLINICAL EVALUATION: Twelve healthy subjects were given placebo or ritonavir for 3 days.[1] On day 1, the dose was 200 mg 3 times daily, on day 2, the dose was 300 mg 3 times daily, and a final dose was given on the morning of day 3. On day 2, approximately 2 hours after the second daily dose of ritonavir, intravenous fentanyl 5 mcg/kg was given over 2 minutes. Naloxone (eg, *Narcan*) was administered to prevent respiratory depression. The clearance of fentanyl was reduced 66% following pretreatment with ritonavir. This produced an approximately 3-fold increase in the area under the concentration-time curve of fentanyl and just over a 2-fold increase in its half-life. Higher doses of ritonavir over a longer period may have different effects on fentanyl plasma concentrations. Patients taking ritonavir may be at risk of increased sedation or respiratory depression if usual doses of fentanyl are administered.

RELATED DRUGS: Other protease inhibitors such as indinavir (*Crixivan*), saquinavir (*Invirase*), and nelfinavir (*Viracept*) may affect fentanyl in a similar manner. Alfentanil (eg, *Alfenta*) may be affected in a similar manner by ritonavir. Ritonavir has been reported to reduce methadone effects following 1 week of concurrent therapy.

MANAGEMENT OPTIONS:

➡ **Monitor.** Monitor patients taking ritonavir for increased narcotic effects (eg, respiratory depression, sedation) following the administration of fentanyl.

REFERENCES:

1. Olkkola KT, et al. Ritonavir's role in reducing fentanyl clearance and prolonging its half-life. *Anesthesiology.* 1999;91:681-685.

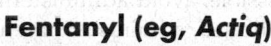

Fentanyl (eg, Actiq)

Troleandomycin†

SUMMARY: Troleandomycin administration increases fentanyl plasma concentrations; increased sedation and respiratory depression may occur.

RISK FACTORS: No specific risk factors are known.

MECHANISM: Troleandomycin inhibits the metabolism of fentanyl by inhibiting the CYP3A4 enzyme. Most of the effect appears to occur during first-pass metabolism of fentanyl.

CLINICAL EVALUATION: Twelve healthy subjects were administered a single dose of transmucosal fentanyl 10 mcg/kg alone and following troleandomycin 500 mg 3 hours before and again 9 hours later.[1] The mean area under the concentration-time curve of fentanyl increased nearly 80% following troleandomycin coadministration. Fentanyl half-life was not changed. This increase in fentanyl concentration is likely to result in increased respiratory depression and sedation in some patients.

RELATED DRUGS: Clarithromycin (eg, *Biaxin*) and erythromycin (eg, *Ery-Tab*) would likely inhibit the metabolism of fentanyl in a similar manner. Alfentanil's (eg, *Alfenta*) metabolism is reduced by troleandomycin.

MANAGEMENT OPTIONS:

➡ **Consider Alternative.** Azithromycin (eg, *Zithromax*) and dirithromycin† do not inhibit CYP3A4 and may be considered as alternatives to troleandomycin in patients receiving fentanyl.

➡ **Monitor.** If a macrolide that inhibits CYP3A4 is administered with fentanyl, be alert for increased sedation and respiratory depression.

REFERENCES:

1. Kharasch ED, et al. Influence of hepatic and intestinal cytochrome P4503A activity on the acute disposition and effects of oral transmucosal fentanyl citrate. *Anesthesiology.* 2004;101(3):729-737.

† Not available in the United States.

Ferrous Sulfate (eg, *Feosol*)

Trovafloxacin†

SUMMARY: Ferrous sulfate reduces the bioavailability of trovafloxacin; a loss of therapeutic efficacy may occur.

RISK FACTORS: No specific risk factors are known.

MECHANISM: Ferrous sulfate reduces the bioavailability of trovafloxacin.

CLINICAL EVALUATION: While no published data are available for evaluation, there are some data on this interaction from the manufacturer.[1] Like other quinolone antibiotics, the absorption of trovafloxacin is reduced when administered with ferrous sulfate. The area under the concentration-time curve of trovafloxacin was reduced 40% when administered with ferrous sulfate (elemental iron 120 mg).

RELATED DRUGS: Ferrous sulfate affects other quinolones similarly (eg, ciprofloxacin [eg, *Cipro*], ofloxacin [eg, *Floxin*]).

MANAGEMENT OPTIONS:

➡ **Circumvent/Minimize.** Administer the antibiotic at least 2 hours before ferrous sulfate. If possible, avoid administering iron products to patients receiving trovafloxacin. If indicated, administer parenteral iron.

➡ **Monitor.** Observe patients who take iron products for a potential reduction in antibiotic effect when trovafloxacin is taken.

REFERENCES:

1. *Trovan* [package insert]. New York, NY: Pfizer Inc; 1998.

† Not available in the United States.

Fesoterodine (*Toviaz*)

Ketoconazole (eg, *Nizoral*)

SUMMARY: Ketoconazole administration increases the plasma concentration of the active metabolite of fesoterodine; increased adverse reactions may occur in some patients.

RISK FACTORS: No specific risk factors are known.

MECHANISM: Ketoconazole inhibits one of the enzymes (CYP3A4) known to metabolize the active metabolite of fesoterodine. The renal clearance of fesoterodine was also reduced by ketoconazole; the mechanism of this observation is unknown.

CLINICAL EVALUATION: Seventeen healthy subjects received a single dose of fesoterodine 8 mg alone or on day 4 of a 5-day regimen of ketoconazole 200 mg twice daily.[1] Because fesoterodine is metabolized by CYP3A4 and CYP2D6, each subject's CYP2D6 phenotype was determined. When administered with ketoconazole, the mean area under the concentration-time curve of the active metabolite of fesoterodine (5-HMT) was increased 2.3- and 2.5-fold in subjects who were extensive metabolizers (EMs) (n = 11) and poor metabolizers (PMs) for CYP2D6, respectively. While the ketoconazole-induced increase in 5-HMT was similar for CYP2D6 EMs and PMs, the plasma concentration of the active metabolite was over twice as high in the PMs regardless of the presence of ketoconazole. The manufacturer reports that a similar study using ketoconazole 200 mg once daily increased the levels of fesoterodine by about 2-fold.[2] An increase in fesoterodine adverse reactions (eg, dry mouth, headache) may occur in patients receiving ketoconazole. The manufacturer recommends fesoterodine doses of 4 mg or less in patients taking ketoconazole.[2]

RELATED DRUGS: Fluconazole (eg, *Diflucan*), itraconazole (eg, *Sporanox*), posaconazole (*Noxafil*), and voriconazole (*Vfend*) also inhibit the activity of CYP3A4 and would be expected to increase the plasma concentrations of fesoterodine.

MANAGEMENT OPTIONS:

➥ *Consider Alternative.* Terbinafine (eg, *Lamisil*) may be considered as an alternative antifungal agent because it does not affect CYP3A4 activity. However, terbinafine does inhibit CYP2D6 and may increase fesoterodine concentrations. Amphotericin, caspofungin (*Cancidas*), and anidulafungin (*Eraxis*) do not appear to inhibit CYP3A4.

➥ *Monitor.* Monitor for increased adverse reactions in patients receiving fesoterodine who are coprescribed ketoconazole.

REFERENCES:

1. Malhotra B, et al. Evaluation of drug-drug interactions with fesoterodine. *Eur J Clin Pharmacol.* 2009;65(6):551-560.

2. *Toviaz* [package insert]. New York, NY: Pfizer Labs; 2008.

Fesoterodine (*Toviaz*)

Rifampin (eg, *Rifadin*)

SUMMARY: Rifampin administration reduces the plasma concentration of the active metabolite of fesoterodine; reduced effectiveness of fesoterodine may occur in some patients.

RISK FACTORS: No specific risk factors are known.

MECHANISM: Rifampin increases the activity of one of the enzymes (CYP3A4) know to metabolize the active metabolite of fesoterodine.

CLINICAL EVALUATION: Twelve healthy subjects received a single dose of fesoterodine 8 mg alone or on day 9 of a 10-day regimen of rifampin 600 mg daily.[1] Because fesoterodine is metabolized by CYP3A4 and CYP2D6, each subject's CYP2D6 phenotype was determined. When administered with rifampin, the mean area under the concentration-time curve of the active metabolite of fesoterodine (5-HMT) was reduced about 75% in extensive metabolizers (n = 8) and poor metabolizers for CYP2D6. A decrease in fesoterodine efficacy may occur in patients receiving concurrent rifampin.

RELATED DRUGS: Rifabutin (*Mycobutin*) and rifapentine (*Priftin*) are known to induce CYP3A4 and would likely affect fesoterodine in a similar manner.

MANAGEMENT OPTIONS:

➥ *Monitor.* Monitor for reduced fesoterodine efficacy in patients receiving fesoterodine who are coprescribed rifampin.

REFERENCES:

1. Malhotra B, et al. Evaluation of drug-drug interactions with fesoterodine. *Eur J Clin Pharmacol.* 2009;65(6):551-560.

Fexofenadine (eg, *Allegra*)

Itraconazole (eg, *Sporanox*)

SUMMARY: Itraconazole administration markedly increases fexofenadine plasma concentrations; be alert for increased antihistamine effects.

RISK FACTORS: No specific risk factors are known.

MECHANISM: Itraconazole appears to inhibit P-glycoprotein–mediated elimination of fexofenadine, enhance its oral absorption, or both.

CLINICAL EVALUATION: Ten subjects were administered a single dose of fexofenadine 180 mg 1 hour after placebo or a single dose of itraconazole 200 mg.[1] The mean area under the plasma concentration-time curve and peak plasma concentration of fexofenadine increased 2.1- and 2.7-fold, respectively, following the coadministration of itraconazole. Because the adverse reactions associated with nonsedating antihistamines are mild, the clinical significance of this interaction is probably limited.

RELATED DRUGS: Ketoconazole is also an inhibitor of P-glycoprotein and would likely increase fexofenadine plasma concentrations. Other nonsedating antihistamines, including cetirizine (eg, *Zyrtec*), loratadine (eg, *Claritin*), and desloratadine (*Clarinex*), are substrates for P-glycoprotein. Their plasma concentrations would likely increase during ketoconazole coadministration.

MANAGEMENT OPTIONS:

➡ **Monitor.** Monitor patients taking fexofenadine for increased antihistamine effects, including sedation, if itraconazole is coadministered.

REFERENCES:
1. Shon J, et al. Effect of itraconazole on the pharmacokinetics and pharmacodynamics of fexofenadine in subjects with known genotype of MDR1 3435C>T allele. *Clin Pharmacol Ther.* 2003;73(2):P58.

Fexofenadine (eg, *Allegra*)

Rifampin (eg, *Rifadin*)

SUMMARY: Rifampin reduces the bioavailability of fexofenadine, resulting in lower plasma concentrations; some loss of therapeutic effect may occur.

RISK FACTORS: No specific risk factors are known.

MECHANISM: Rifampin appears to induce P-glycoprotein expression in the small intestine. P-glycoprotein, and possibly other transporters, limit the absorption of fexofenadine. Increasing P-glycoprotein expression would have the effect of reducing the bioavailability and plasma concentration of fexofenadine.

CLINICAL EVALUATION: Twenty-four subjects received oral fexofenadine 60 mg alone and after treatment with rifampin 600 mg/day for 6 days.[1] Subjects included younger and elderly volunteers. No differences were noted between the groups in the effects of rifampin on fexofenadine pharmacokinetics. Rifampin administration increased fexofenadine oral clearance 2- to 3-fold. Fexofenadine half-life was not altered by rifampin administration, although the volume of distribution of fexofenadine was increased. Some patients may experience a reduction in the antihistaminic activity of fexofenadine.

RELATED DRUGS: No information is available.

MANAGEMENT OPTIONS:

➡ *Monitor.* Watch for a reduction of antihistaminic effect in patients taking fexofenadine during coadministration of rifampin.

REFERENCES:

1. Hamman MA, et al. The effect of rifampin administration on the disposition of fexofenadine. *Clin Pharmacol Ther.* 2001;69(3):114-121.

Fexofenadine (eg, *Allegra*)

Verapamil (eg, *Calan*)

SUMMARY: Verapamil substantially increases fexofenadine plasma concentrations, but the risk of adverse outcomes appears small.

RISK FACTORS: No specific risk factors are known.

MECHANISM: Fexofenadine is a P-glycoprotein substrate, and verapamil is a known P-glycoprotein inhibitor; other mechanisms may also be involved.

CLINICAL EVALUATION: In a randomized crossover study, 13 healthy subjects received a single dose of fexofenadine 120 mg with and without pretreatment with verapamil 240 mg/day for 6 days.[1] Verapamil almost tripled the plasma concentrations of S(-)-fenofexadine, and more than doubled the concentrations of R(+)-fexofenadine. None of the subjects reported any adverse outcomes during the study, and, given the relative lack of dose-dependent adverse reactions of fexofenadine, it does not seem likely that this interaction would often produce adverse outcomes.

RELATED DRUGS: Theoretically, other calcium-channel blockers that inhibit P-glycoprotein, such as diltiazem (eg, *Cardizem*), may interact with fexofenadine.

MANAGEMENT OPTIONS: No specific action is required, but be alert for evidence of the interaction.

REFERENCES:

1. Sakugawa T, et al. Enantioselective disposition of fexofenadine with the P-glycoprotein inhibitor verapamil. *Br J Clin Pharmacol.* 2009;67(5):535-540.

Fingolimod (*Gilenya*)

Ketoconazole (eg, *Nizoral*)

SUMMARY: Ketoconazole administration increases fingolimod plasma concentrations; an increased incidence of adverse reactions, including arrhythmias, neutropenia, or pulmonary toxicity, may result.

RISK FACTORS: No specific risk factors are known.

MECHANISM: Ketoconazole appears to reduce the metabolism of fingolimod by inhibiting the enzyme CYP4F2.[1]

CLINICAL EVALUATION: Twenty-two healthy subjects received a single oral dose of fingolimod 5 mg alone and on day 4 of a 9-day regimen of ketoconazole 200 mg twice daily.[2] The area under the concentration-time curve of fingolimod was increased approximately 70% during concomitant ketoconazole dosing. The half-life (6 to 9 days) of fingolimod was not altered in this study. While data are limited, this degree of increase in fingolimod plasma concentration could result in an increase in adverse reactions.

RELATED DRUGS: None known.

MANAGEMENT OPTIONS:

➡ *Monitor.* Monitor patients receiving fingolimod for adverse reactions if ketoconazole is coadministered.

REFERENCES:

1. Jin Y, et al. CYP4F enzymes are responsible for the elimination of fingolimod (FTY720), a novel treatment of relapsing multiple sclerosis. *Drug Metab Dispos.* 2011;39(2):191-198.
2. Kovarik JM, et al. Ketoconazole increases fingolimod blood levels in a drug interaction via CYP4F2 inhibition. *J Clin Pharmacol.* 2009;49(2):212-218.

Fish Oil

Warfarin (eg, *Coumadin*)

SUMMARY: A patient developed increased warfarin response after increasing her dose of fish oil, but a causal relationship was not established.

RISK FACTORS: No specific risk factors are known.

MECHANISM: Not established.

CLINICAL EVALUATION: A 67-year-old woman stabilized on long-term warfarin therapy developed a doubling of her international normalized ratio (INR) after doubling her daily dose of fish oil.[1] The INR declined after fish oil use was reduced. More data are needed to establish the effect of fish oil on warfarin response. Moreover, different brands of fish oil may have different effects on warfarin.

RELATED DRUGS: No information is available.

MANAGEMENT OPTIONS: No specific action is required, but be alert for evidence of the interaction.

REFERENCES:

1. Buckley MS, et al. Fish oil interaction with warfarin. *Ann Pharmacother.* 2004;38(1):50-52.

Flecainide (eg, *Tambocor*)

Paroxetine (eg, *Paxil*)

SUMMARY: Paroxetine administration can increase the plasma concentration of flecainide; increased effects on cardiac conduction may occur.

RISK FACTORS:

➡ *Pharmacogenetics.* Patients who are rapid metabolizers of CYP2D6 are likely to be at greatest risk.

MECHANISM: Paroxetine inhibits the CYP2D6-mediated metabolism of flecainide.

CLINICAL EVALUATION: A patient stabilized on paroxetine 40 mg daily was started on flecainide 100 mg twice daily for atrial fibrillation.[1] The patient developed confusion, paranoia, and delirium. Flecainide plasma concentration was elevated. Within 3 days of reducing the flecainide dosage to 50 mg daily and stopping the paroxetine, the patient's mental status improved with complete resolution of her symptoms. In a study of 21 healthy subjects, the pharmacokinetics of a single dose of flecainide 200 mg were evaluated before and after the administration of paroxetine 20 mg daily for 7 days.[2] In the rapid metabolizers of CYP2D6, paroxetine increased the mean area under the concentration-time curve of flecainide by 28% and its half-life by 20%.[3] No effect of paroxetine was noted in CYP2D6 poor metabolizers. The increased flecainide plasma concentrations associated with paroxetine administration were accompanied by an increase in the QTc interval of about 7 msec compared with flecainide administered alone.

RELATED DRUGS: Fluoxetine (eg, *Prozac*) and duloxetine (*Cymbalta*) are also known to inhibit CYP2D6 and are expected to increase flecainide plasma concentrations.

MANAGEMENT OPTIONS:

➡ *Consider Alternative.* Consider using selective serotonin reuptake inhibitors (SSRIs) that do not affect CYP2D6, such as escitalopram (*Lexapro*), in patients receiving flecainide.

➡ *Monitor.* If flecainide is coadministered with a CYP2D6 inhibitor, monitor flecainide plasma concentrations, as well as the electrocardiogram , for evidence of excessive inhibition of cardiac conduction.

REFERENCES:

1. Tsao YY, et al. Delirium in a patient with toxic flecainide plasma concentrations: the role of a pharmacokinetic drug interaction with paroxetine. *Ann Pharmacother.* 2009;43(7):1366-1369.
2. Lim KS, et al. Pharmacokinetic interaction of flecainide and paroxetine in relation to the CYP2D6*10 allele in healthy Korean subjects. *Br J Clin Pharmacol.* 2008;66(5):660-666.
3. Lim KS, et al. Changes in the QTc interval after administration of flecainide acetate, with and without coadministered paroxetine, in relation to cytochrome P450 2D6 genotype: data from an open-label, two-period, single-sequence crossover study in healthy Korean male subjects. *Clin Ther.* 2010;32(4):659-666.

Flecainide (eg, *Tambocor*)

Propranolol (eg, *Inderal*)

SUMMARY: Flecainide increases the serum concentration of propranolol; propranolol increases the concentration of flecainide. Coadministration of these drugs produces additive negative inotropic effects.

RISK FACTORS: No specific risk factors are known.

MECHANISM: Not established; however, it appears that each of the 2 agents inhibits the metabolism of the other, and both have negative inotropic effects that may be additive.

CLINICAL EVALUATION: Propranolol 80 mg 3 times daily and flecainide 200 mg twice daily were administered alone and together to healthy subjects.[1] Propranolol increased flecainide's area under the concentration-time curve (AUC) 20% and flecainide increased propranolol's AUC 31%. Both drugs significantly decreased the left ventricular ejection fraction, and this effect was additive when the 2 drugs were combined; however, it is not known how often these effects result in adverse reactions in patients receiving concomitant flecainide and propranolol.

RELATED DRUGS: It is probable that other beta-blockers will exert additive negative inotropic effects with flecainide, but little is known regarding a pharmacokinetic interaction between flecainide and other beta-blockers.

MANAGEMENT OPTIONS:

➥ **Monitor.** Monitor patients taking propranolol and flecainide for increased effects of both drugs and additive negative inotropic effects on the heart.

REFERENCES:

1. Holtzman JL, et al. The pharmacodynamic and pharmacokinetic interaction of flecainide acetate with propranolol: effects on cardiac function and drug clearance. *Eur J Clin Pharmacol.* 1987;33(1):97-99.

 Flecainide (eg, *Tambocor*)

Quinidine Sulfate

SUMMARY: Quinidine increases the serum concentration of flecainide; the clinical importance of this effect is not established.

RISK FACTORS:

➥ **Pharmacogenetics.** Rapid metabolizers of flecainide are at particular risk.

MECHANISM: Quinidine, a potent CYP2D6 inhibitor, reduces the metabolism of flecainide.

CLINICAL EVALUATION: Six subjects received flecainide 150 mg intravenously before and after a single dose of quinidine 50 mg.[1] The mean flecainide clearance was reduced 23%, and flecainide metabolite formation was inhibited by quinidine. There were no significant changes in flecainide volume of distribution or renal clearance. It is not known how often this interaction would result in flecainide toxicity. Quinidine 50 mg every 6 hours for 5 days reduced flecainide metabolic clearance 28% and increased renal clearance 21%; total clearance after oral administration decreased approximately 14%.[2] Only the R(-)-flecainide enantiomer (both enantiomers have equivalent activity) was affected by quinidine. Minimal changes were noted in electrocardiographic wave intervals during combined therapy.

RELATED DRUGS: No information is available.

MANAGEMENT OPTIONS: No specific action is required, but be alert for evidence of the interaction.

REFERENCES:

1. Munafo A, et al. Disposition of flecainide in subjects taking quinidine. *Clin Pharmacol Ther.* 1990;47:156.

2. Birgersdotter UM, et al. Stereoselective genetically-determined interaction between chronic flecainide and quinidine in patients with arrhythmias. *Br J Clin Pharmacol.* 1992;33(3):275-280.

Flecainide (*Tambocor*) 4

Quinine

SUMMARY: Quinine increases flecainide serum concentrations; the clinical significance is unknown.

RISK FACTORS:

➠ *Pharmacogenetics.* Rapid metabolizers of flecainide are at particular risk.

MECHANISM: Quinine inhibits the hepatic metabolism of flecainide.

CLINICAL EVALUATION: The clinical significance of the interaction is unknown. Ten healthy subjects received 150 mg flecainide IV alone, and after the first of 3 doses of quinine 500 mg every 12 hours.[1] Flecainide clearance was reduced 16%, and its area under the concentration-time curve increased 21% following quinine coadministration. Electrocardiograms tended to show increased PR and QRS prolongation during coadministration of quinine and flecainide, but it is not clear if these changes were caused by quinine itself or resulted from the elevated flecainide concentrations.

RELATED DRUGS: No information is available.

MANAGEMENT OPTIONS: No specific action is required, but be alert for evidence of the interaction.

REFERENCES:

1. Munafo A, et al. Altered flecainide disposition in healthy volunteers taking quinine. *Eur J Clin Pharmacol.* 1990;38:269:

Flecainide (*Tambocor*) 3

Sodium Bicarbonate

SUMMARY: Increases in urine pH will increase the serum concentrations of flecainide; the clinical significance of this interaction is unclear.

RISK FACTORS: No specific risk factors are known.

MECHANISM: The urinary clearance of flecainide is increased at acidic pH and reduced at alkaline pH. An increase in urine pH tends to unionize flecainide molecules resulting in increased reabsorption and higher plasma concentration.

CLINICAL EVALUATION: The mean half-life of flecainide ranged from 10 to 18 hours during coadministration of ammonium chloride or sodium bicarbonate to adjust the urinary pH between 5.1 and 8.1.[1,2] Significant increases in flecainide area under the concentration-time curve (50%) and decreases in urinary clearance (70%) accompany urinary alkalinization.[1-3] While no studies are available in patients receiving flecainide, the magnitude of the changes observed in these studies suggests that clinically significant changes in flecainide serum concentrations could occur with changes in urine pH.

RELATED DRUGS: Drugs that alter urinary pH such as sodium bicarbonate, acetazolamide (eg, *Diamox*), ammonium chloride, or large doses of antacids will be likely to affect flecainide clearance.

MANAGEMENT OPTIONS:

➡ *Monitor.* Monitor flecainide concentrations in patients receiving drugs likely to alter their urinary pH such as sodium bicarbonate, acetazolamide (*Diamox*), ammonium chloride, or large doses of antacids.

REFERENCES:

1. Johnston A, et al. Flecainide pharmacokinetics in healthy volunteers: the influence of urinary pH. *Br J Clin Pharmacol.* 1985;20:333.

2. Hertrampf R, et al. Elimination of flecainide as a function of urinary flow rate and pH. *Eur J Clin Pharmacol.* 1991;41:61.

3. Muhiddin KA, et al. The influence of urinary pH on flecainide excretion and its serum pharmacokinetics. *Br J Clin Pharmacol.* 1984;17:447.

Flecainide (*Tambocor*)

Sotalol (*Betapace*)

SUMMARY: A case report notes sinus bradycardia, atrioventricular (AV) block, and cardiac arrest following a switch from flecainide to sotalol therapy for ventricular arrhythmia, but a causal relationship was not established.

RISK FACTORS: No specific risk factors are known.

MECHANISM: Not established. Both sotalol and flecainide can depress myocardial conduction, and their combined use may have led to cardiac arrest.

CLINICAL EVALUATION: A 72-year-old man with nonsustained ventricular tachycardia was treated with flecainide 100 mg twice daily.[1] Three days later, the return of the arrhythmia prompted a change in therapy to sotalol 40 mg. The first sotalol dose was administered 4 hours after the last flecainide dose, and a second sotalol dose followed 2 hours later. The patient suffered sinus bradycardia, AV block, and a cardiac arrest 3 hours after the second sotalol dose. Since sotalol can produce sinus bradycardia and has a negative inotropic effect, causation was not established.

RELATED DRUGS: Propranolol (eg, *Inderal*) and other beta blockers may cause similar reactions with flecainide.

MANAGEMENT OPTIONS:

➡ *Circumvent/Minimize.* It may be prudent to avoid the administration of sotalol for several days to patients previously receiving drugs that depress myocardial conduction.

➡ *Monitor.* Until further information is available, carefully monitor patients receiving sotalol and flecainide for reduced myocardial conduction (eg, bradycardia).

REFERENCES:

1. Warren R, et al. Serious interactions of sotalol with amiodarone and flecainide. *Med J Aust.* 1990;152:227.

Flecainide (*Tambocor*)

Verapamil (eg, *Calan*)

SUMMARY: Data indicate that the combination of verapamil and flecainide prolongs both QRS intervals in patients with arrhythmias and atrioventricular (AV) conduction in normal subjects; the clinical significance is unknown.

RISK FACTORS: No specific risk factors are known.

MECHANISM: Not established.

CLINICAL EVALUATION: A preliminary report described 14 patients with arrhythmias who received a combination of flecainide and verapamil (no doses stated).[1] Flecainide concentration was not altered by verapamil. The combination of drugs prolonged the QRS interval but had no other significant effect on myocardial conduction. Eight healthy subjects received single oral doses of flecainide 200 mg or verapamil 120 mg, or a combination of flecainide and verapamil in crossover trials.[2] Flecainide had no effect on verapamil pharmacokinetics; verapamil caused a small (4%) reduction in flecainide clearance after oral administration. The combination produced a small negative inotropic effect that primarily was caused by flecainide and an additive decrease in AV conduction velocity.

RELATED DRUGS: Diltiazem (eg, *Cardizem*) may produce similar reactions when administered with flecainide. Dihydropyridine calcium blockers (eg, amlodipine [*Norvasc*], felodipine [*Plendil*], nifedipine [eg, *Procardia*]) would be unlikely to interact with flecainide.

MANAGEMENT OPTIONS: No specific action is required, but be alert for evidence of the interaction.

REFERENCES:

1. Landau S, et al. The combined administration of verapamil and flecainide. *J Clin Pharmacol.* 1988;28:909.
2. Holtzman JL, et al. The pharmacodynamic and pharmacokinetic interaction between single doses of flecainide acetate and verapamil: effects on cardiac function and drug clearance. *Clin Pharmacol Ther.* 1989;46:26.

Fluconazole (eg, *Diflucan*) **5**

Contraceptives, Oral (eg, *Ortho-Novum*)

SUMMARY: Low doses (50 mg/day) of fluconazole do not significantly alter the endocrinological response to oral contraceptives.

RISK FACTORS: No specific risk factors are known.

MECHANISM: No interaction.

CLINICAL EVALUATION: Eighteen healthy women taking a variety of oral contraceptives were studied before and after taking fluconazole 50 mg/day for 3 to 4 weeks.[1] Fluconazole administration had no effect on serum estradiol concentrations or other endocrinological measures. A similar study found no change in ethinyl estradiol or norgestrel concentrations following fluconazole 50 mg/day for 10 days.[2] Low doses of fluconazole appear to be safe in women taking oral contraceptives. The effect of higher doses of fluconazole is unknown.

RELATED DRUGS: The effect of other imidazole antifungals on oral contraceptives is not known.

MANAGEMENT OPTIONS: No interaction.

REFERENCES:

1. Devenport MH, et al. Metabolic effects of low-dose fluconazole in healthy female users and non-users of oral contraceptives. *Br J Clin Pharmacol.* 1989;27:851-859.
2. Lazar JD, et al. Drug interactions with fluconazole. *Rev Infect Dis.* 1990;12(suppl 3):S327-S333.

Fluconazole (eg, *Diflucan*)

Flurbiprofen (eg, *Ansaid*)

SUMMARY: Fluconazole administration increases the plasma concentration of flurbiprofen; the clinical significance of this interaction is unclear.

RISK FACTORS: No specific risk factors known.

MECHANISM: Fluconazole inhibits the enzyme CYP2C9 that is responsible for the metabolism of flurbiprofen.

CLINICAL EVALUATION: In a study of 14 healthy subjects, a single dose of flurbiprofen 100 mg was administered following 2 doses, 8 to 10 hours apart, of placebo or fluconazole 200 mg.[1] The mean area under the plasma concentration-time curve of flurbiprofen was increased 81% following the 2 doses of fluconazole, and the half-life of flurbiprofen increased from 3.3 to 5.3 hours. Chronic administration of fluconazole may result in a larger change in flurbiprofen plasma concentrations. The clinical implications of fluconazoles effect on flurbiprofen are unknown.

RELATED DRUGS: Other nonsteroidal anti-inflammatory drugs are also metabolized by CYP2C9 and would be expected to interact in a similar manner with fluconazole.

MANAGEMENT OPTIONS: No specific action is required, but be alert for evidence of the interaction.

REFERENCES:
1. Greenblatt DJ, et al. Interaction of flurbiprofen with cranberry juice, grape juice, tea, and fluconazole: in vitro and clinical studies. *Clin Pharmacol Ther.* 2006;79:125-133.

 Fluconazole (eg, *Diflucan*)

Fluvastatin (*Lescol*)

SUMMARY: Fluconazole administration increases the plasma concentration of fluvastatin. An increased risk of toxicity may occur.

RISK FACTORS: No specific risk factors are known.

MECHANISM: Fluvastatin is metabolized by CYP2C9, an enzyme that is inhibited by fluconazole. Fluconazole appears to reduce the systemic clearance of fluvastatin and may also decrease its first-pass metabolism.

CLINICAL EVALUATION: Twelve healthy subjects were administered a single dose of fluvastatin 40 mg following 4 days of placebo or fluconazole 400 mg on day 1 and 200 mg on days 2 through 4.[1] The mean area under the concentration-time curve (AUC) of fluvastatin increased 84% (range, 10% to 190%), and its peak concentration increased 44% following fluconazole pretreatment. The mean half-life of fluvastatin was prolonged from 1.5 to 2.7 hours. Some patients taking this combination may be at increased risk of fluvastatin toxicity such as myopathy.

RELATED DRUGS: The effect of fluconazole on other HMG-CoA reductase inhibitors is unknown. However, because of the ability of fluconazole to inhibit CYP3A4, other HMG-CoA reductase inhibitors (eg, simvastatin [*Zocor*], lovastatin [eg, *Mevacor*], atorvastatin [*Lipitor*]) may be affected to some extent. Fluconazole administration produced a nonsignificant (36%) increase in pravastatin (*Pravachol*) AUC. No other antifungal agents are known to inhibit CYP2C9 and would not be expected to interact with fluvastatin.

MANAGEMENT OPTIONS:

➡ *Circumvent/Minimize.* Temporarily discontinue fluvastatin during fluconazole administration. Because fluconazole has a long half-life, hold fluvastatin for several days after fluconazole is discontinued.

➡ *Monitor.* Monitor patients who are prescribed fluconazole and taking fluvastatin for fluvastatin side effects, including muscle pain.

REFERENCES:

1. Kantola T, et al. Effect of fluconazole on plasma fluvastatin and pravastatin concentrations. *Eur J Clin Pharmacol.* 2000;56:225-229.

Fluconazole (eg, *Diflucan*)

Food

SUMMARY: Food has no effect on fluconazole serum concentrations.

RISK FACTORS: No specific risk factors are known.

MECHANISM: No interaction.

CLINICAL EVALUATION: The administration of a meal with fluconazole had no effect on fluconazole concentrations compared with fasting administration.[1] Fluconazole can be taken without regard of food.

RELATED DRUGS: No information is available.

MANAGEMENT OPTIONS: No interaction.

REFERENCES:

1. Zimmermann T, et al. Influence of concomitant food intake on the oral absorption of two triazole antifungal agents, itraconazole and fluconazole. *Eur J Clin Pharmacol.* 1994;46(2):147-150.

Fluconazole (eg, *Diflucan*)

Glimepiride (eg, *Amaryl*)

SUMMARY: Fluconazole increases plasma concentrations of glimepiride.

RISK FACTORS: No specific risk factors are known.

MECHANISM: Fluconazole-induced inhibition of glimepiride's metabolism by CYP2C9 may be responsible for the reduction in the elimination of glimepiride.

CLINICAL EVALUATION: Fluconazole 400 mg was administered to 12 healthy subjects on day 1.[1] This was followed by 3 more days of fluconazole 200 mg/day. On day 4, a single 0.5 mg dose of glimepiride was given. Compared with placebo administration, fluconazole pretreatment resulted in a 138% increase in the mean area under the concentration-time curve of glimepiride. Mean peak glimepiride concentration increased 50%. The half-life of glimepiride increased from 2 to 2.3 hours following fluconazole pretreatment. No change in glimepiride's effect on blood glucose was noted following fluconazole. The effect of this interaction in patients with diabetes is unknown, but the magnitude of the interaction suggests an increased hypoglycemic effect when fluconazole and glimepiride are coadministered. The administration of a single dose of fluconazole is expected to reduce the magnitude of its effect on glimepiride.

RELATED DRUGS: Fluconazole has been noted to reduce the metabolism of tolbutamide, resulting in increased tolbutamide plasma concentrations. Other hypoglycemic drugs that are substrates for CYP2C9, such as glipizide (eg, *Glucotrol*) and glyburide (eg, *DiaBeta*), may be similarly affected by fluconazole, but with limited effect on plasma glucose concentrations.[2]

MANAGEMENT OPTIONS:

➡ **Monitor.** Until more information is available, monitor patients stabilized on glimepiride when fluconazole is initiated or discontinued.

REFERENCES:

1. Niemi M, et al. Effects of fluconazole and fluvoxamine on the pharmacokinetics and pharmacodynamics of glimepiride. *Clin Pharmacol Ther*. 2001;69(4):194-200.
2. Rowe BR, et al. Safety of fluconazole in women taking oral hypoglycaemic agents. *Lancet*. 1992;339(8787):255-256.

Fluconazole (eg, *Diflucan*)

Glipizide (eg, *Glucotrol*)

SUMMARY: Fluconazole administration can increase the risk of hypoglycemia in patients taking glipizide.

RISK FACTORS: No specific risk factors are known.

MECHANISM: Fluconazole inhibits the enzyme CYP2C9, which is known to be the primary pathway of glipizide metabolism.

CLINICAL EVALUATION: The risk of developing hypoglycemia while taking glipizide was compared between patients prescribed fluconazole or cephalexin (eg, *Keflex*) within 10 days of the hypoglycemic episode.[1] Compared with cephalexin, patients prescribed fluconazole demonstrated a 2- to 3-fold increased risk of hypoglycemia. Cephalexin was used as a comparator to eliminate the effect of an infection on the risk of hypoglycemia.

RELATED DRUGS: Voriconazole (eg, *Vfend*) also inhibits CYP2C9 and is expected to interact with glipizide. Other hypoglycemic drugs that are metabolized by CYP2C9 (glyburide [eg, *DiaBeta*], chlorpropamide, tolbutamide) may be similarly affected by fluconazole.

MANAGEMENT OPTIONS:

➡ **Consider Alternative.** Terbinafine (eg, *Lamisil*) may be an alternative antifungal agent because it does not affect CYP2C9 activity. Consider hypoglycemic agents that are not substrates for CYP2C9 (metformin [eg, *Glucophage*], insulin) for patients who require long-term treatment with a CYP2C9 inhibitor.

➡ **Monitor.** During the coadministration of fluconazole and glipizide, watch blood glucose values closely for unusual changes.

REFERENCES:

1. Schelleman H, et al. Anti-infectives and the risk of severe hypoglycemia in users of glipizide or glyburide. *Clin Pharmacol Ther*. 2010;88(2):214-222.

Fluconazole (eg, *Diflucan*)

Glyburide (eg, *DiaBeta*)

SUMMARY: Fluconazole administration can increase the risk of hypoglycemia in patients taking glyburide.

RISK FACTORS: No specific risk factors are known.

MECHANISM: Fluconazole inhibits the enzyme CYP2C9, which is known to be the primary pathway of glyburide metabolism.

CLINICAL EVALUATION: The risk of developing hypoglycemia while taking glyburide was compared between patients being prescribed fluconazole or cephalexin (eg, *Keflex*) within 10 days of the hypoglycemic episode.[1] Compared with cephalexin, patients prescribed fluconazole demonstrated a 2-fold increased risk of hypoglycemia. Cephalexin was used as a comparator to eliminate the effect of an infection on the risk of hypoglycemia.

RELATED DRUGS: Voriconazole (eg, *Vfend*) also inhibits CYP2C9 and is expected to interact with glyburide. Other hypoglycemic drugs that are metabolized by CYP2C9 (glipizide [eg, *Glucotrol*], chlorpropamide, tolbutamide) may be similarly affected by fluconazole.

MANAGEMENT OPTIONS:

➡ **Consider Alternative.** Terbinafine (eg, *Lamisil*) may be an alternative antifungal agent because it does not affect CYP2C9 activity. Consider hypoglycemic agents that are not substrates for CYP2C9 (metformin [eg, *Glucophage*], insulin) for patients who require long-term treatment with a CYP2C9 inhibitor.

➡ **Monitor.** During the coadministration of fluconazole and glyburide, watch blood glucose values closely for unusual changes.

REFERENCES:

1. Schelleman H, et al. Anti-infectives and the risk of severe hypoglycemia in users of glipizide or glyburide. *Clin Pharmacol Ther.* 2010;88(2):214-222.

Fluconazole (eg, *Diflucan*)

Halofantrine†

SUMMARY: A low dose of fluconazole had minimal effect on halofantrine; however, be alert for increased halofantrine toxicity.

RISK FACTORS: No specific risk factors are known.

MECHANISM: Halofantrine is metabolized by CYP3A4. Fluconazole, particularly in dosages above 100 mg daily, can inhibit this enzyme.

CLINICAL EVALUATION: Fifteen healthy subjects received a single oral dose of halofantrine 500 mg alone and with a single dose of fluconazole 50 mg.[1] The coadministration of fluconazole only affected the half-life of halofantrine, increasing it by 25%. The concentration of the major metabolite of halofantrine was reduced approximately 40% by fluconazole administration. Because of the low doses of fluconazole and halofantrine used in this study, the results may underestimate the true potential for fluconazole to increase halofantrine plasma concentrations. Until studies with higher fluconazole doses are reported, it would be prudent to assume this interaction could produce elevated halofantrine concentrations and increase its risk for adverse events, including arrhythmias.

RELATED DRUGS: Ketoconazole (eg, *Nizoral*), itraconazole (eg, *Sporanox*), posaconazole (*Noxafil*), and voriconazole (eg, *Vfend*) also inhibit the activity of CYP3A4 and are expected to increase the plasma concentrations of halofantrine.

MANAGEMENT OPTIONS:

➠ *Monitor.* Carefully monitor patients taking halofantrine for cardiac toxicity (prolonged QT intervals) if therapeutic doses of fluconazole are coadministered.

REFERENCES:

1. Babalola CP, et al. Effect of fluconazole on the pharmacokinetics of halofantrine in healthy volunteers. *J Clin Pharm Ther*. 2009;34(6):677-682.

† Not available in the United States.

 Fluconazole (eg, *Diflucan*)

Indinavir (*Crixivan*)

SUMMARY: Fluconazole coadministration produced a small reduction in indinavir serum concentrations. The clinical significance of this reduction appears to be limited.

RISK FACTORS: No specific risk factors are known.

MECHANISM: Not established.

CLINICAL EVALUATION: While no published data are available for evaluation, the manufacturer of indinavir has made available some data on this interaction. The administration of indinavir 1,000 mg every 4 hours with fluconazole 400 mg/day for 7 days resulted in a 19% reduction in the indinavir area under the concentration-time curve.[1] Indinavir produced no change in fluconazole concentrations. The clinical significance of this change in indinavir concentration is likely to be limited.

RELATED DRUGS: Fluconazole has been reported to increase ritonavir (*Norvir*) concentrations. The effect of fluconazole on other protease inhibitors is unknown. Ketoconazole (eg, *Nizoral*) increases indinavir serum concentrations.

MANAGEMENT OPTIONS: No specific action is required, but be alert for evidence of the interaction.

REFERENCES:

1. *Crixivan* [package insert]. Whitehouse Station, NJ: Merck & Company Inc; 1996.

 Fluconazole (*Diflucan*)

Losartan (*Cozaar*)

SUMMARY: Fluconazole reduces the concentration of losartan's active metabolite; reduction of losartan's antihypertensive efficacy may result.

RISK FACTORS: No specific risk factors are known.

MECHANISM: Losartan is converted by the hepatic enzyme CYP2C9 to an active metabolite. Fluconazole inhibits CYP2C9 resulting in an accumulation of losartan and a reduction in the concentration of its active metabolite.

CLINICAL EVALUATION: Sixteen healthy subjects received losartan 100 mg/day for 20 days.[1] Fluconazole 200 mg/day was added to the losartan on days 11 through 20. Losartan plasma concentrations were assessed on days 10 and 20. The area under the concentration-time curve (AUC) of losartan was increased nearly 70% following fluconazole coadministration. The AUC of losartan's active metabolite was reduced 41% by fluconazole. No pharmacodynamic data were presented but the reduction in active metabolite concentration could lead to a reduction in efficacy.

RELATED DRUGS: Antifungal agents that do not inhibit CYP2C9 (eg, terbinafine [*Lamisil*]) are unlikely to interact. The effect of other antifungal agents on losartan is unknown but is likely to be less than the effect seen with fluconazole. The effects of fluconazole on other angiotensin receptor antagonists are unknown.

MANAGEMENT OPTIONS:

➥ **Consider Alternative.** An antifungal agent that does not inhibit CYP2C9 could be selected for patients stabilized on losartan. Patients taking fluconazole could be treated with an angiotensin-converting enzyme inhibitor.

➥ **Monitor.** Monitor patients stabilized on losartan for a reduction in blood pressure control if fluconazole is administered.

REFERENCES:

1. Kazierad DJ, et al. Fluconazole significantly alters the pharmacokinetics of losartan but not eprosartan. *Clin Pharmacol Ther.* 1997;61:203.

Fluconazole (*Diflucan*)

Methadone (eg, *Dolophine*)

SUMMARY: Fluconazole administration increases the plasma concentration of methadone; some patients may experience increased narcotic effects.

RISK FACTORS: No specific risk factors are known.

MECHANISM: Methadone has been reported to be metabolized by CYP3A4. Fluconazole is known to inhibit both CYP3A4 and CYP2C9 isozymes.

CLINICAL EVALUATION: Twenty-five patients receiving chronic methadone (20 mg/day to 90 mg/day) were studied. Twelve patients were randomized to receive placebo, and 13 received fluconazole 200 mg/day for 2 weeks.[1] In the group receiving fluconazole, mean methadone area under the concentration-time curve increased 35% and the peak methadone concentration increased 27%. No patients experienced adverse effects caused by the increase in methadone concentrations. Higher doses of fluconazole may produce a greater reduction in the clearance of methadone and could result in toxicity in some patients.

RELATED DRUGS: Other azole antifungal agents including ketoconazole (eg, *Nizoral*) and itraconazole (*Sporanox*) may affect methadone in a similar manner. Since terbinafine (*Lamisil*) does not inhibit CYP3A4 metabolism, it would not be expected to affect the metabolism of methadone. Narcotic analgesics that are not metabolized by CYP3A4 such as morphine (eg, *MSIR*) or codeine derivatives are not likely to interact with fluconazole.

MANAGEMENT OPTIONS:

➡ *Consider Alternative.* Consider an antifungal agent that does not inhibit CYP3A4 (eg, terbinafine) for patients receiving methadone. Consider alternative analgesics such as codeine or morphine in patients receiving fluconazole.

➡ *Monitor.* Monitor patients receiving methadone and fluconazole for enhanced narcotic effects including sedation.

REFERENCES:

1. Cobb MN, Desai J, Brown LS, Zannikos PN, Rainey PM. The effect of fluconazole on the clinical pharmacokinetics of methadone. *Clin Pharmacol Ther.* 1998;63:655-662.

Fluconazole (*Diflucan*)

Midazolam (eg, *Versed*)

SUMMARY: Fluconazole administration appears to increase the concentrations and effects of midazolam.

RISK FACTORS: No specific risk factors are known.

MECHANISM: Fluconazole appears to inhibit the metabolism of midazolam.

CLINICAL EVALUATION: The pharmacodynamic effects of single 10 mg or 15 mg doses of midazolam were increased by the coadministration of a single dose of fluconazole 150 mg.[1] In a second study in 5 subjects, administration of a single dose of fluconazole 150 mg resulted in about a 30% increase in the concentration of midazolam. The effects of chronic fluconazole dosing or larger doses await further study. The increased midazolam concentrations are likely to produce enhanced effects including prolonged sedation in patients taking fluconazole.

RELATED DRUGS: Ketoconazole (eg, *Nizoral*) and itraconazole (*Sporanox*) also may inhibit midazolam metabolism. Other benzodiazepines including diazepam (eg, *Valium*) and triazolam (eg, *Halcion*) are likely to be affected in a similar manner by fluconazole.

MANAGEMENT OPTIONS:

➡ *Monitor.* Monitor patients requiring midazolam and fluconazole for increased sedation.

REFERENCES:

1. Mattila MJ, et al. Fluconazole moderately increases midazolam effects on performance. *Br J Clin Pharmacol.* 1995;39:567P.

Fluconazole (eg, *Diflucan*)

Nateglinide (*Starlix*)

SUMMARY: Fluconazole increases the serum concentration of nateglinide; some diabetic patients may be at increased risk for hypoglycemic episodes.

RISK FACTORS: No specific risk factors are known.

MECHANISM: Nateglinide is metabolized primarily by CYP2C9 and to a lesser extent by CYP3A4. Fluconazole is known to inhibit both CYP2C9 and CYP3A4.

CLINICAL EVALUATION: Ten healthy subjects received a single nateglinide 30 mg dose following 4 days of placebo or fluconazole 200 mg/day (400 mg was administered on day 1).[1] The mean area under the concentration-time curve of nateglinide increased 48% following fluconazole pretreatment. The half-life of nateglinide was prolonged from 1.6 to 1.9 hours. While no significant change in blood glucose was noted in the healthy subjects, patients with diabetes may be at increased risk for hypoglycemia.

RELATED DRUGS: Voriconazole (*Vfend*) also inhibits CYP2C9 and CYP3A4 and may produce a similar interaction with nateglinide. Itraconazole (eg, *Sporanox*) and ketoconazole (eg, *Nizoral*) are CYP3A4 inhibitors and may produce some inhibition of nateglinide. Other oral hypoglycemics that are metabolized by CYP2C9 or CYP3A4 (eg, tolbutamide [eg, *Orinase*], glipizide [eg, *Glucotrol*], glyburide [eg, *DiaBeta*]) may interact similarly with fluconazole.

MANAGEMENT OPTIONS:

➡ *Monitor.* Carefully observe patients taking nateglinide for altered blood glucose control when fluconazole is added to or removed from the drug regimen.

REFERENCES:

1. Niemi M, et al. Effect of fluconazole on the pharmacokinetics and pharmacodynamics of nateglinide. *Clin Pharmacol Ther*. 2003;74(1):25-31.

Fluconazole (eg, *Diflucan*)

Nevirapine (*Viramune*)

SUMMARY: Fluconazole administration increases the plasma concentration of nevirapine; some patients may experience increased adverse reactions.

RISK FACTORS: No specific risk factors are known.

MECHANISM: Fluconazole is known to inhibit CYP3A4, an enzyme partially responsible for nevirapine metabolism.

CLINICAL EVALUATION: The potential effect of fluconazole administration on nevirapine has been reported in 2 studies of HIV patients receiving nevirapine. In the first, patients either received nevirapine 200 mg twice daily alone or with the coadministration of fluconazole 200 or 400 mg daily.[1] Compared with patients taking only nevirapine, patients concurrently receiving fluconazole had trough plasma nevirapine concentrations that were 60% and 100% higher during fluconazole 200 and 400 mg daily, respectively. In a second study of HIV-infected patients, the coadministration of fluconazole 200 mg 3 times weekly resulted in nevirapine plasma concentrations that were approximately 30% higher than in patients taking nevirapine alone.[2] Higher doses of fluconazole are expected to produce a greater increase in nevirapine plasma concentrations.

RELATED DRUGS: Ketoconazole (eg, *Nizoral*), itraconazole (eg, *Sporanox*), posaconazole (*Noxafil*), and voriconazole (*Vfend*) also inhibit the activity of CYP3A4 and are expected to increase the plasma concentrations of nevirapine. The metabolism of other related antiviral agents (eg, delavirdine [*Rescriptor*], etravirine [*Intelence*]) is likely to be inhibited by fluconazole.

MANAGEMENT OPTIONS:

➡ *Monitor.* Monitor patients taking nevirapine for potential toxicity (eg, hepatic dysfunction) if fluconazole is coadministered.

REFERENCES:

1. Manosuthi W, et al. Plasma nevirapine levels, adverse events and efficacy of antiretroviral therapy among HIV-infected patients concurrently receiving nevirapine-based antiretroviral therapy and fluconazole. *BMC Infectious Diseases.* 2007;7:14.

2. Wakeham K, et al. Co-administration of fluconazole increases nevirapine concentrations in HIV-infected Ugandans. *J Antimicrob Chemother.* 2010;65(2):316-319.

Fluconazole (eg, *Diflucan*)

Phenytoin (eg, *Dilantin*)

SUMMARY: Fluconazole may substantially increase plasma phenytoin concentrations, resulting in phenytoin toxicity in some patients.

RISK FACTORS: No specific risk factors are known.

MECHANISM: Not established. Fluconazole probably inhibits the hepatic metabolism of phenytoin.[1]

CLINICAL EVALUATION: Several case reports have documented increased phenytoin concentrations resulting in signs of phenytoin toxicity after fluconazole therapy was initiated.[2-4] For example, a 23-year-old woman taking phenytoin 500 mg/day was treated with fluconazole 100 mg/day for 3 days followed by 200 mg/day.[2] On the seventh day of fluconazole therapy, the patient developed nausea, double vision, sweating, light-headedness, bilateral nystagmus, and dizziness. The phenytoin blood level had increased dramatically to 37 mcg/L (desired range, 10 to 20 mcg/L). The phenytoin was discontinued and the fluconazole continued. This resulted in a blood phenytoin concentration that remained in the toxic range for several more days. In a randomized, placebo-controlled pharmacokinetic study of this interaction in 19 healthy subjects, fluconazole 200 mg/day for 16 days resulted in a 75% increase in the phenytoin serum area under the concentration-time curve (AUC).[5,6] Phenytoin did not appear to affect trough serum fluconazole concentrations.[6] A similar pharmacokinetic study in 9 healthy subjects found a 33% increase in the phenytoin AUC. Thus, the clinical evidence suggests that fluconazole markedly increases serum phenytoin concentrations and can produce phenytoin toxicity.

RELATED DRUGS: Available evidence suggests that ketoconazole (eg, *Nizoral*) does not affect phenytoin pharmacokinetics.

MANAGEMENT OPTIONS:

➡ *Monitor.* Monitor patients carefully for phenytoin toxicity (eg, nystagmus, ataxia, confusion, dizziness, slurred speech, involuntary muscular movements) when fluconazole is started in the presence of phenytoin therapy. Serum phenytoin determinations would also be useful. When fluconazole therapy is stopped in the presence of phenytoin therapy, monitor the patient for a reduced phenytoin effect.

REFERENCES:

1. Lazar JD, et al. Drug interactions with fluconazole. *Rev Infect Dis.* 1990;12(suppl 3):S327-S333.

2. Howitt KM, et al. Phenytoin toxicity induced by fluconazole. *Med J Aust.* 1989;151(10):603-604.

3. Mitchell AS, et al. Fluconazole and phenytoin: a predictable interaction. *BMJ.* 1989;298(6683):1315.

4. Cadle RM, et al. Fluconazole-induced symptomatic phenytoin toxicity. *Ann Pharmacother*. 1994;28(2):191-195.

5. Blum RA, et al. Effect of fluconazole on the disposition of phenytoin. *Clin Pharmacol Ther*. 1991;49(4):420-425.

6. Touchette M, et al. Contrasting effects of fluconazole and ketoconazole on phenytoin and testosterone disposition in man. *Br J Clin Pharmacol*. 1992;34(1):75–78.

Fluconazole (eg, *Diflucan*)

Pravastatin (*Pravachol*)

SUMMARY: Fluconazole administration had no significant effect on pravastatin plasma concentrations.

RISK FACTORS: No specific risk factors are known.

MECHANISM: No interaction.

CLINICAL EVALUATION: Twelve healthy subjects were administered a single dose of pravastatin 40 mg following 4 days of placebo or fluconazole 400 mg on day 1 and 200 mg on days 2 through 4.[1] The mean area under the concentration-time curve (AUC) of pravastatin increased 36%, and its peak concentration increased 34% following fluconazole pretreatment. Neither of these changes was statistically significant. The mean half-life of pravastatin was unchanged. The small changes noted in pravastatin plasma concentrations are not likely to be clinically important.

RELATED DRUGS: Fluconazole administration produced an 83% increase in the mean AUC of fluvastatin (*Lescol*). The effect of fluconazole on other 3-hydroxy-3-methylglutaryl coenzyme A reductase inhibitors is unknown. However, because of the ability of fluconazole to inhibit CYP3A4, other statins (eg, simvastatin [*Zocor*], lovastatin [eg, *Mevacor*], atorvastatin [*Lipitor*]) may be affected to some extent. Other antifungal agents such as itraconazole (eg, *Sporanox*) have shown little affect on pravastatin plasma concentrations.

MANAGEMENT OPTIONS: No interaction.

REFERENCES:
1. Kantola T, et al. Effect of fluconazole on plasma fluvastatin and pravastatin concentrations. *Eur J Clin Pharmacol*. 2000;56:225-229.

Fluconazole (eg, *Diflucan*)

Ramelteon (*Rozerem*)

SUMMARY: Fluconazole increases ramelteon plasma concentrations; increased sedation may occur in some patients.

RISK FACTORS: No specific risk factors are known.

MECHANISM: Fluconazole is known to inhibit CYP3A4 and CYP2C9, enzymes partially responsible for the metabolism of ramelteon.

CLINICAL EVALUATION: While specific data are limited, the manufacturer of ramelteon notes that the coadministration of fluconazole prior to a single dose of ramelteon increased the mean area under the plasma concentration-time curve of ramelteon about 150%.[1] Pending further data, patients receiving ramelteon and fluconazole should be observed for increased ramelteon effect.

RELATED DRUGS: Ketoconazole (eg, *Nizoral*) also inhibits the metabolism of ramelteon. Itraconazole (eg, *Sporanox*) and voriconazole (*Vfend*) also would be expected to increase the plasma concentrations of ramelteon.

MANAGEMENT OPTIONS:

➡ **Consider Alternative.** Consider using an antifungal that does not affect CYP1A2, CYP3A4, or CYP2C9, such as terbinafine (*Lamisil*), or a sedative that is not metabolized by CYP3A4 or CYP2C9, such as oxazepam (eg, *Serax*) or lorazepam (eg, *Ativan*).

➡ **Monitor.** If fluconazole and ramelteon are coadministered, monitor patients for increased ramelteon effects, including excess sedation.

REFERENCES:

1. *Rozerem* [package insert]. Lincolnshire, IL: Takeda Pharmaceutical Company Limited; 2005.

Fluconazole (*Diflucan*)

Rifabutin (*Mycobutin*)

SUMMARY: Fluconazole administration increases rifabutin plasma concentrations; increased side effects including uveitis, rash, and liver or bone marrow toxicity may occur.

RISK FACTORS: No specific risk factors are known.

MECHANISM: Fluconazole inhibits the metabolism of rifabutin via the CYP3A4 pathway.

CLINICAL EVALUATION: Fluconazole 200 mg daily was administered for 2 weeks to 12 HIV-infected patients alone and in combination with rifabutin 300 mg daily.[1] The mean area under the concentration-time curve (AUC) of rifabutin increased 82% and the mean AUC of the active rifabutin metabolite increased more than 200%. In a study of 10 HIV-infected patients, 1 week of coadministration of rifabutin 300 mg daily and fluconazole 200 mg daily resulted in increases in the mean AUC of rifabutin 76%.[2] The effect of a single fluconazole dose on rifabutin pharmacokinetics has not been reported, but the effect would probably be modest. The administration of rifabutin 300 mg daily did not affect the pharmacokinetics of fluconazole.[3]

RELATED DRUGS: Other antifungal agents including itraconazole (*Sporanox*), ketoconazole (eg, *Nizoral*), and voriconazole (*Vfend*) also inhibit CYP3A4 and is expected to affect rifabutin in a similar manner. Terbinafine (*Lamisil*) does not inhibit CYP3A4 and is not expected to affect rifabutin metabolism.

MANAGEMENT OPTIONS:

➡ **Consider Alternative.** Consider terbinafine as an alternative antifungal in patients taking rifabutin.

➡ **Monitor.** Carefully monitor patients taking rifabutin for signs of rifabutin toxicity (uveitis, rash, and liver or bone marrow toxicity) if fluconazole is coadministered.

REFERENCES:

1. Trapnell CB, et al. Increased plasma rifabutin levels with concomitant fluconazole therapy in HIV-infected patients. *Ann Intern Med*. 1996;124:573-576.

2. Jordan MK, et al. Effects of fluconazole and clarithromycin on rifabutin and 25-O-desacetylrifabutin pharmacokinetics. *Antimicrob Agents Chemother*. 2000;44:2170-2172.

3. Trapnell CB, et al. Rifabutin does not alter fluconazole pharmacokinetics. *Clin Pharmacol Ther*. 1993;53:196.

Fluconazole (*Diflucan*)
Rifampin (eg, *Rifadin*)

SUMMARY: Chronic rifampin administration reduces fluconazole plasma concentrations; the clinical significance of this interaction is unknown.

RISK FACTORS: No specific risk factors are known.

MECHANISM: It appears that rifampin increases fluconazole elimination.

CLINICAL EVALUATION: The fluconazole area under the concentration-time curve was reduced significantly (23%) in subjects receiving fluconazole plus rifampin 600 mg/day for 7 days.[1] Fluconazole's half-life was reduced from 33 to 26 hours. Three patients treated with fluconazole for cryptococcal meningitis had recurrence of symptoms following the administration of antitubercular therapy that included rifampin.[2] Causation was not established. The clinical significance of these changes has not been defined clearly.

RELATED DRUGS: Rifampin reduces the concentration of fluconazole, itraconazole (*Sporanox*), and ketoconazole (eg, *Nizoral*). Rifabutin (*Mycobutin*) does not affect fluconazole.

MANAGEMENT OPTIONS:

➥ *Circumvent/Minimize.* A limited increase in fluconazole dose may be warranted in patients requiring high fluconazole concentrations.

➥ *Monitor.* Until further information is available, be aware of potentially reduced fluconazole plasma concentrations when rifampin is coadministered.

REFERENCES:

1. Apseloff G, et al. Induction of fluconazole metabolism by rifampin: *in vivo* study in humans. *J Clin Pharmacol.* 1991;31:358-361.
2. Coker RJ, et al. Interaction between fluconazole and rifampicin. *BMJ.* 1990;301:818.

Fluconazole (*Diflucan*)
Ritonavir (*Norvir*)

SUMMARY: Fluconazole administration produced a small increase in ritonavir plasma concentrations.

RISK FACTORS: No specific risk factors are known.

MECHANISM: Fluconazole is known to inhibit CYP3A4, an enzyme responsible for ritonavir's metabolism. It would appear that fluconazole has only limited effect on ritonavir, perhaps because of ritonavir's very high affinity for the CYP3A4 enzyme.

CLINICAL EVALUATION: While no published data are available for evaluation, the manufacturer of ritonavir has made available some data on this interaction. Thirteen healthy subjects received ritonavir 200 mg 4 times daily alone or in combination with fluconazole, 400 mg on day 1 and 200 mg on days 2 to 5.[1] During coadministration, the area under the concentration-time curve and peak plasma concentration of ritonavir increased 12% and 15%, respectively. This small increase in ritonavir concentration is unlikely to be of clinical significance.

RELATED DRUGS: The effects of ketoconazole (eg, *Nizoral*) or itraconazole (*Sporanox*) on ritonavir are unknown. Other protease inhibitors such as indinavir (*Crixivan*), saquinavir (eg, *Invirase*), and nelfinavir (*Viracept*) may be affected by fluconazole in a similar manner.

MANAGEMENT OPTIONS: No specific action is required, but be alert for evidence of the interaction.

REFERENCES:
1. *Norvir* [package insert]. Abbott Park, IL: Abbott Laboratories. 1996.

 ## Fluconazole (*Diflucan*)

Saquinavir (eg, *Fortovase*)

SUMMARY: Fluconazole administration increases the plasma concentration of saquinavir; some patients could experience an increase in side effects when fluconazole and saquinavir are coadministered.

RISK FACTORS: No specific risk factors are known.

MECHANISM: Fluconazole is known to inhibit CYP3A4, the enzyme responsible for saquinavir metabolism. It would appear that fluconazole predominately affects the first-pass metabolism of saquinavir.

CLINICAL EVALUATION: Five patients with HIV infection taking saquinavir were studied before and after 7 days of fluconazole coadministration.[1] Fluconazole 400 mg was administered on the first day followed by 200 mg for 6 more days. The mean area under the concentration-time curve of saquinavir was increased 50% following fluconazole dosing. The mean peak plasma concentration of saquinavir increased 56%, but its half-life did not change after the fluconazole administration. The administration of a single dose of fluconazole would be expected to reduce the magnitude of its effect on saquinavir.

RELATED DRUGS: Other antifungal drugs (ketoconazole [eg, *Nizoral*], itraconazole [*Sporanox*]) that inhibit CYP3A4 would increase saquinavir plasma concentrations. Other protease inhibitors such as indinavir (*Crixivan*) and nelfinavir (*Viracept*) may also be affected by fluconazole. Fluconazole has been reported to have minimal effect on the kinetics of ritonavir (*Norvir*).[2,3]

MANAGEMENT OPTIONS:

➡ *Monitor.* No specific action is required, but be alert for evidence of the interaction. In patients taking ritonavir (*Norvir*) with saquinavir, the inhibition of saquinavir metabolism produced by ritonavir will be much greater than that of fluconazole; little added effect would be expected to occur.

REFERENCES:
1. Koks CH, et al. The effect of fluconazole on ritonavir and saquinavir pharmacokinetics in HIV-1-infected individuals. *Br J Clin Pharmacol.* 2001;51:631-635.
2. *Norvir* [package insert]. Abbott Park, IL: Abbott Laboratories. 1996.
3. Cato A, et al. Evaluation of the effect of fluconazole on the pharmacokinetics of ritonavir. *Drug Metab Dispos.* 1997;25:1104-1106.

Fluconazole (eg, *Diflucan*)

Simvastatin (eg, *Zocor*)

SUMMARY: The coadministration of fluconazole and simvastatin has been associated with rhabdomyolysis.

RISK FACTORS: No specific risk factors are known.

MECHANISM: Fluconazole inhibits CYP3A4, the enzyme known to metabolize simvastatin.

CLINICAL EVALUATION: An 83-year-old man stabilized on simvastatin 40 mg daily for 2 years was placed on fluconazole 400 mg daily as prophylactic therapy for neutropenia.[1] Seven days later, he was admitted to the hospital with severe muscle weakness and elevated creatine kinase. Simvastatin and fluconazole were discontinued, and his symptoms gradually reversed over the next 2 weeks. An earlier case reported rhabdomyolysis following simvastatin and fluconazole.[2] Single or lower doses of fluconazole are not expected to produce as much inhibition to simvastatin metabolism, but no data are available.

RELATED DRUGS: Other antifungal agents that inhibit CYP3A4 (eg, itraconazole [eg, *Sporanox*], voriconazole [*Vfend*], ketoconazole [eg, *Nizoral*]) are known to affect simvastatin in a similar manner. The metabolism of lovastatin (eg, *Mevacor*) and, to a lesser extent, atorvastatin (*Lipitor*) also may be inhibited by fluconazole. Fluvastatin (*Lescol*) and rosuvastatin (*Crestor*) are metabolized by CYP2C9, an enzyme that is inhibited by fluconazole.

MANAGEMENT OPTIONS:

➡ **Consider Alternative.** Pravastatin (eg, *Pravachol*) metabolism is unlikely to be affected by fluconazole.

➡ **Monitor.** Monitor patients taking statins that are CYP3A4 or CYP2C9 substrates for muscle pain and weakness if fluconazole is coadministered.

REFERENCES:

1. Shaukat A, et al. Simvastatin-fluconazole causing rhabdomyolysis. *Ann Pharmacother.* 2003;37(7-8):1032-1035.

2. Moro H, et al. Rhabdomyolysis after simvastatin in an HIV-infected patient with chronic renal failure. *AIDS Patient Care STDS.* 2004;18(12):687-690.

Fluconazole (eg, *Diflucan*)

Sirolimus (*Rapamune*)

SUMMARY: The coadministration of fluconazole with sirolimus may result in elevated plasma concentrations of sirolimus and possible adverse effects.

RISK FACTORS: No specific risk factors are known.

MECHANISM: Fluconazole is known to be an inhibitor of CYP3A4, the enzyme that is responsible for sirolimus metabolism.

CLINICAL EVALUATION: A kidney transplant patient who was taking sirolimus 4 mg daily was started on fluconazole 200 mg daily.[1] The sirolimus dose was reduced from 4 to 3 mg daily when the fluconazole was started. Even with subsequent reductions in the sirolimus dose to 2 mg daily, the plasma concentrations of sirolimus increased from 10 mcg/L to more than 35 mcg/L during fluconazole coadministration.

RELATED DRUGS: Ketoconazole (eg, *Nizoral*), itraconazole (eg, *Sporanox*), posaconazole (*Noxafil*), and voriconazole (*Vfend*) also inhibit the activity of CYP3A4 and would be expected to increase the plasma concentrations of sirolimus. The elimination of tacrolimus (*Prograf*) and cyclosporine (eg, *Neoral*) would be reduced by fluconazole.

MANAGEMENT OPTIONS:

➡ *Consider Alternative.* Terbinafine (*Lamisil*) could be considered as an alternative antifungal agent since it does not affect CYP3A4 activity. Amphotericin, caspofungin (*Cansidas*), and anidulafungin (*Eraxis*) do not appear to inhibit CYP3A4.

➡ *Monitor.* Monitor sirolimus plasma concentrations in patients being treated with sirolimus and fluconazole.

REFERENCES:
1. Cervelli MJ. Fluconazole-sirolimus drug interaction. *Transplantation*. 2002;74(10):1477-1478.

 Fluconazole (eg, *Diflucan*)

Sulfamethoxazole (SMZ)

SUMMARY: Fluconazole inhibits the formation of a metabolite of sulfamethoxazole that is thought to be associated with sulfamethoxazole toxicity; no dosage adjustment is necessary.

RISK FACTORS: No specific risk factors are known.

MECHANISM: Fluconazole is known to inhibit the activity of the isozyme CYP2C9. Sulfamethoxazole is partially metabolized by this enzyme.

CLINICAL EVALUATION: Sulfamethoxazole is partially metabolized to a reactive intermediate, N4-hydroxy sulfamethoxazole (SMZ-NOH). This metabolite, or a subsequent nitroso metabolite, is considered to be associated with some of the adverse reactions observed with sulfamethoxazole administration, including fever, rashes, hepatic toxicity, and bone marrow toxicity. A single dose of cotrimoxazole (sulfamethoxazole 800 mg and trimethoprim 160 mg) was administered to 10 subjects alone or 1 hour after a single dose of fluconazole 150 mg.[1] Three of the subjects followed a similar protocol but ingested fluconazole 400 mg. Following sulfamethoxazole dosing, SMZ-NOH elimination accounted for 1.6% of the dose. After pretreatment with fluconazole, this metabolite accounted for only 0.8% of the dose. The administration of the higher dose of fluconazole did not produce a greater effect in the 3 subjects. Fluconazole did not affect the formation of acetyl-sulfamethoxazole or sulfamethoxazole glucuronide, the major metabolites of sulfamethoxazole, so dose adjustments are unnecessary. The significance of the decrease in the production of SMZ-NOH is unknown. It may potentially reduce the toxicity of sulfamethoxazole.

RELATED DRUGS: Ketoconazole (eg, *Nizoral*) did not affect the metabolism of sulfamethoxazole. The effect of other antifungal agents on sulfamethoxazole is unknown, but would likely be minimal.

MANAGEMENT OPTIONS: No specific action is required, but be alert for evidence of the interaction.

REFERENCES:
1. Gill HJ, et al. The effect of fluconazole and ketoconazole on the metabolism of sulphamethoxazole. *Br J Clin Pharmacol.* 1996;42(3):347-353.

Fluconazole (*Diflucan*)

Tacrolimus (*Prograf*)

SUMMARY: Fluconazole administration significantly increases tacrolimus concentrations and can increase the risk of nephrotoxicity.

RISK FACTORS:

➡ **Dosage Regimen.** Fluconazole doses greater than 100 mg/day will increase the risk of an interaction.

MECHANISM: Fluconazole appears to inhibit the metabolism (CYP3A4) of tacrolimus. This could result in elevated plasma concentrations caused by increased bioavailability, reduced systemic clearance, or both.

CLINICAL EVALUATION: Twenty transplant patients were receiving tacrolimus (FK506) doses that were adjusted to maintain tacrolimus plasma concentrations between 0.5 and 2.0 ng/mL.[1] Fluconazole doses of either 100 mg/day (12 patients) or 200 mg/day (8 patients) were administered for an average of 14 days. After just 1 day of fluconazole, tacrolimus concentrations increased by 1.4-fold and 3.1-fold in patients receiving 100 mg/day and 200 mg/day of fluconazole, respectively. In 1 of the patients, the administration of fluconazole resulted in a 58% increase in the area under the plasma concentration-time curve (AUC) of tacrolimus. In another report, a liver transplant patient receiving tacrolimus and fluconazole developed an increased serum creatinine.[2] Tacrolimus was discontinued and the serum creatinine concentration returned to baseline over the following week. This patient was later rechallenged with 7 days of fluconazole 400 mg/day while receiving 1 mg/day of tacrolimus. The AUC of tacrolimus increased by 152% and 506% after 3 and 7 days, respectively, of concomitant fluconazole. This large increase in the AUC of tacrolimus may have been the result of the larger dose of fluconazole that was used in this single-patient trial.

RELATED DRUGS: Fluconazole also inhibits cyclosporine (eg, *Sandimmune*) metabolism. Other oral antifungal agents (eg, ketoconazole [eg, *Nizoral*], itraconazole [*Sporanox*]) also may inhibit tacrolimus metabolism.

MANAGEMENT OPTIONS:

➡ **Monitor.** Patients receiving tacrolimus should have their plasma concentrations monitored during the coadministration of fluconazole. A reduction in the dose of tacrolimus is likely to be necessary to avoid nephrotoxicity.

REFERENCES:
1. Manez R, et al. Fluconazole therapy in transplant recipients receiving FK506. *Transplantation.* 1994;57:1521.
2. Assan R, et al. FK 506/ fluconazole interaction enhances FK 506 nephrotoxicity. *Diabetes Metab.* 1994;20:49.

Fluconazole (*Diflucan*)

Terfenadine (*Seldane*)

SUMMARY: The plasma concentration of terfenadine is increased by large doses of fluconazole; the concentration of the active, carboxylic acid metabolite of terfenadine is increased, but this is without apparent significance.

RISK FACTORS:

➠ **Dosage Regimen.** Fluconazole doses above 200 mg/day may lead to terfenadine accumulation.

MECHANISM: Fluconazole appears to inhibit terfenadine's metabolism (CYP3A4) or the elimination of the carboxylic acid metabolite of terfenadine.

CLINICAL EVALUATION: Six healthy subjects received terfenadine 60 mg twice daily for 6 days alone and concomitantly with fluconazole 200 mg/day.[1] The area under the plasma concentration-time curve (AUC) of the active acid metabolite of terfenadine increased by 34%. None of the subjects demonstrated an accumulation of terfenadine nor change in their electrocardiogram (QTc) during fluconazole administration. Another study found a similar lack of effect following 200 mg/day of fluconazole, but administration of 800 mg/day of fluconazole increased the AUC of terfenadine by 52%[2] Thus, high fluconazole doses used to treat systemic fungal infections may lead to terfenadine accumulation and possible cardiac (prolonged QT interval) toxicity.

RELATED DRUGS: Ketoconazole (eg, *Nizoral*) and itraconazole (*Sporanox*) also inhibit the metabolism of terfenadine. Loratadine (*Claritin*), fexofenadine (eg, *Allegra*), and cetirizine (*Zyrtec*) would be less likely to interact with fluconazole and cause toxicity.

MANAGEMENT OPTIONS:

➠ **Circumvent/Minimize.** Until additional studies of the interaction between fluconazole and terfenadine are available, it would be prudent to avoid giving the 2 drugs together. The use of sedating antihistamines or perhaps loratadine or cetirizine instead of terfenadine would seem to be preferred in patients taking fluconazole or other oral antifungal agents.

➠ **Monitor.** Watch for cardiotoxicity in patients receiving terfenadine and fluconazole.

REFERENCES:

1. Honig PK, et al. The effect of fluconazole on the steady-state pharmacokinetics and electrocardiographic pharmacodynamics of terfenadine in humans. *Clin Pharmacol Ther.* 1993;53:630.

2. Cantilena LR, et al. Fluconazole alters terfenadine pharmacokinetics and electrocardiographic pharmacodynamics. *Clin Pharmacol Ther.* 1995;57:185.

Fluconazole (*Diflucan*) | 4

Testosterone

SUMMARY: Fluconazole administration may result in an increase in serum testosterone concentrations; the clinical significance of these changes is unknown.

RISK FACTORS:

➥ *Dosage Regimen.* Fluconazole doses above 200 mg daily may increase testosterone concentrations.

MECHANISM: Not established. Fluconazole may increase the biosynthesis of testosterone or inhibit its metabolism.

CLINICAL EVALUATION: The administration of fluconazole 400 mg daily for 6 days resulted in a 33% increase in serum testosterone concentrations in 9 subjects.[1] Others have noted an increase in testosterone concentrations during administration of fluconazole 200 to 400 mg daily.[2] Fluconazole doses of 25 to 50 mg were reported to have no effect on testosterone.[3] The clinical significance of these changes is unknown.

RELATED DRUGS: No information is available.

MANAGEMENT OPTIONS: No specific action is required, but be alert for evidence of the interaction.

REFERENCES:

1. Touchette MA, et al. Contrasting effects of fluconazole and ketoconazole on phenytoin and testosterone disposition in man. *Br J Clin Pharmacol.* 1992;34:75.
2. Lazar JD, et al. Drug interactions with fluconazole. *Rev Infect Dis.* 1990;12:S327.
3. Hanger DP, et al. Fluconazole and testosterone: *in vivo* and in vitro studies. *Antimicrob Agents Chemother.* 1988;32:646.

Fluconazole (eg, *Diflucan*) | 5

Theophylline (eg, *Theochron*)

SUMMARY: Fluconazole 200 mg/day did not produce a significant change in theophylline plasma concentrations or elimination.

RISK FACTORS: No specific risk factors are known.

MECHANISM: No interaction.

CLINICAL EVALUATION: Five healthy subjects received a single oral dose of theophylline 300 mg alone and following 3 days of fluconazole 100 mg twice daily.[1] The mean oral clearance of theophylline was reduced 16%. This degree of decrease in theophylline clearance was not statistically significant because of the small sample size used in the study. Nevertheless, the potential for fluconazole at a dose of 200 mg/day to produce a clinically significant change appears to be minimal. Because theophylline metabolism is primarily via the CYP1A2 pathway with CYP3A4 also contributing, it appears that fluconazole does not affect the CYP1A2 enzyme. The effect of larger doses of fluconazole on theophylline metabolism is unknown, but a somewhat larger effect is likely because of greater inhibition of CYP3A4-mediated theophylline metabolism.

RELATED DRUGS: Ketoconazole (eg, *Nizoral*), an antifungal agent with potent CYP3A4 inhibition, does not appear to affect theophylline clearance.

MANAGEMENT OPTIONS: No interaction.

REFERENCES:
1. Konishi H, et al. Effect of fluconazole on theophylline disposition in humans. *Eur J Clin Pharmacol.* 1994;46(4):309-312.

Fluconazole (eg, *Diflucan*)

Tipranavir (*Aptivus*)

SUMMARY: Limited data suggest that fluconazole can increase tipranavir plasma concentrations; some increase in toxicity may occur.

RISK FACTORS: No specific risk factors are known.

MECHANISM: Fluconazole is known to inhibit CYP3A4, the enzyme responsible for the metabolism of tipranavir.

CLINICAL EVALUATION: While specific data are limited, the manufacturer of tipranavir notes that a loading dose of fluconazole 200 mg followed by 100 mg daily for 13 days increased the mean area under the plasma concentration-time curve of tipranavir 56%, compared with historical controls.[1] Some patients may experience an increased risk of tipranavir toxicity. Two of the 20 subjects in the combination study experienced elevated hepatic enzymes.

RELATED DRUGS: Ketoconazole (eg, *Nizoral*), itraconazole (eg, *Sporanox*), posaconazole (*Noxafil*), and voriconazole (*Vfend*) also inhibit the activity of CYP3A4 and are likely to increase the plasma concentration of tipranavir.

MANAGEMENT OPTIONS:

➡ **Consider Alternative.** Consider using an antifungal agent that does not affect CYP3A4, such as amphotericin (eg, *Amphocin*), anidulafungin (*Eraxis*), caspofungin (*Cancidas*), or terbinafine (eg, *Lamisil*).

➡ **Monitor.** If agents that inhibit CYP3A4 are coadministered with tipranavir, monitor for signs of tipranavir toxicity (eg, hepatic function impairment, bleeding).

REFERENCES:
1. *Aptivus* [package insert]. Ridgefield, CT: Boehringer Ingelheim Pharmaceuticals, Inc; 2007.

Fluconazole (*Diflucan*)

Tolbutamide (eg, *Orinase*)

SUMMARY: Fluconazole increases the plasma concentration of tolbutamide; the clinical significance of this interaction in diabetic patients is unknown.

RISK FACTORS: No specific risk factors are known.

MECHANISM: Fluconazole appears to inhibit the metabolism of tolbutamide.

CLINICAL EVALUATION: Thirteen healthy subjects received tolbutamide 500 mg alone and following fluconazole 100 mg/day for 7 days.[1] Tolbutamide area under the concentration-time curve was increased 108% following fluconazole administration. The half-life of tolbutamide was increased from about 8 hours to 15 hours.

RELATED DRUGS: Fluconazole 50 mg/day for 14 days did not affect the glycosylated hemoglobin or fructosamine concentrations in 14 diabetic women taking glipizide (eg, *Glurotrol*) or glyburide (eg, *DiaBeta*).[2] Although glycosylated hemoglobin concentrations may not reflect short-term changes in blood glucose, no patient had symptoms of hypoglycemia. No pharmacokinetic data were presented; higher fluconazole doses may alter glipizide or glyburide pharmacokinetics. Other azole antifungal agents (eg, ketoconazole [eg, *Nizoral*], miconazole [eg, *Monistat*], itraconazole [*Sporanox*]) may inhibit the metabolism of tolbutamide.

MANAGEMENT OPTIONS:

➡ *Monitor.* Until further information is available, observe patients maintained on tolbutamide for reduced glucose concentrations when fluconazole is started or increased glucose when fluconazole is discontinued.

REFERENCES:

1. Lazar J, et al. Drug interactions with fluconazole. *Rev Infect Dis.* 1990;12(Suppl. 3):S327.
2. Rowe BR, et al. Safety of fluconazole in women taking oral hypoglycemic agents. *Lancet.* 1992;339:255.

Fluconazole (*Diflucan*)

Triazolam (eg, *Halcion*)

SUMMARY: Fluconazole increases the serum concentration of triazolam and may increase its pharmacodynamic effects such as sedation.

RISK FACTORS:

➡ *Dosage Regimen.* While the authors did not do a dose response study, fluconazole is known to produce a greater magnitude of metabolic inhibition when administered in doses above 100 mg/day.

MECHANISM: Fluconazole inhibits the metabolism of triazolam by the CYP3A4 enzyme.

CLINICAL EVALUATION: Twelve healthy subjects received fluconazole 100 mg/day or placebo for 4 days.[1] On the fourth day, each subject was administered a single oral dose of triazolam 0.25 mg. The peak concentration of triazolam increased 25% and its area under the concentration-time curve increased over 200% following pretreatment with fluconazole. Triazolam half-life increased from 3.7 hours to 6.8 hours. Pharmacodynamic effects including drowsiness and body sway also were increased during the coadministration of diazepam and fluconazole.

RELATED DRUGS: Fluconazole inhibits the metabolism of midazolam (*Versed*) (also see Fluconazole/Midazolam monograph) and could affect diazepam (eg, *Valium*) in a similar manner. A benzodiazepine such as lorazepam (eg, *Ativan*), which is not metabolized by CYP3A4 may be less likely to interact. Other antifungal agents such as ketoconazole (eg, *Nizoral*) or itraconazole (*Sporanox*) similarly inhibit the metabolism of triazolam; however, terbinafine does not appear to inhibit triazolam metabolism.

MANAGEMENT OPTIONS:

➡ *Use Alternative.* Avoid the combination of fluconazole and triazolam. A benzodiazepine such as lorazepam that is not metabolized by CYP3A4 would be a potential alternative anxiolytic agent. The antifungal agent terbinafine does not appear to inhibit the metabolism of triazolam.

REFERENCES:

1. Varhe A, et al. Fluconazole, but not terbinafine, enhances the effects of triazolam by inhibiting its metabolism. *Br J Clin Pharmacol.* 1996;41:319.

Fluconazole (*Diflucan*)

Warfarin (eg, *Coumadin*)

SUMMARY: Case reports and clinical studies show that fluconazole enhances the hypoprothrombinemic response to warfarin; adjustments in warfarin dose may be needed.

RISK FACTORS:

➡ **Dosage Regimen.** Although the ability of fluconazole to inhibit drug metabolism by CYP3A4 has been shown to require large doses of fluconazole, doses of 100 mg/day can inhibit warfarin metabolism (metabolized by CYP2C9).

MECHANISM: Fluconazole exerts its antifungal effect by inhibiting fungal cytochrome P450; human cytochrome P450 appears to be affected as well. Fluconazole appears to inhibit the hepatic metabolism of warfarin.[3] The magnitude of the effect suggests inhibition of CYP2C9 (the primary isozyme that metabolizes S-warfarin).

CLINICAL EVALUATION: A 68-year-old woman stabilized on warfarin developed an increase in her prothrombin time from 19 seconds to 65 seconds 8 days after she started fluconazole 200 mg/day.[2] Several other cases of increased warfarin response following fluconazole have been reported.[4-7] In 7 men stabilized on warfarin, the addition of fluconazole (100 mg/day for 7 days) resulted in a 38% increase in prothrombin time.[8] Six healthy subjects were given a single oral dose of warfarin (0.75 mg/kg) with and without oral fluconazole 400 mg/day for 7 days.[3] Fluconazole was associated with a 44% increase in the area under the prothrombin-time curve; the clearances of (R)- and (S)-warfarin were reduced 54% and 68%, respectively. Smaller increases in warfarin response were noted in a single-dose warfarin study in healthy subjects given 200 mg/day of fluconazole.[1]

RELATED DRUGS: The effect of fluconazole on oral anticoagulants other than warfarin is unknown, but consider the possibility. However, phenprocoumon[†] is metabolized primarily by glucuronidation and, theoretically, would be less likely to interact with cytochrome P450 inhibitors such as fluconazole. Ketoconazole (eg, *Nizoral*) and itraconazole (*Sporanox*) also may increase the effect of oral anticoagulants.

MANAGEMENT OPTIONS:

➡ **Monitor.** Monitor for altered oral anticoagulant effect if fluconazole is initiated, discontinued, or changed in dosage. Adjust the anticoagulant dose as needed.

REFERENCES:

1. Lazar JD, et al. Drug interactions with fluconazole. *Rev Infect Dis.* 1990;12(Suppl. 3):S327.
2. Seaton TL, et al. Possible potentiation of warfarin by fluconazole. *DICP.* 1990;24:1177.
3. Black DJ, et al. An evaluation of the effect of fluconazole (F) on the stereoselective metabolism of warfarin (W). *Clin Pharmacol Ther.* 1992;51:184.
4. Gericke KR. Possible interaction between warfarin and fluconazole. *Pharmacotherapy.* 1993;13:508.
5. Baciewicz AM, et al. Fluconazole-warfarin interaction. *Ann Pharmacother.* 1994.28:1111.
6. Kerr HD. Case report: potentiation of warfarin by fluconazole. *Am J Med Sci.* 1993;305:164.

7. Tett S, et al. Drug interactions with fluconazole. *Med J Aust.* 1992;156:365.

8. Crussel-Porter LL, et al. Low-dose fluconazole therapy potentiates the hypoprothrombinemic response of warfarin sodium. *Arch Intern Med.* 1993;153:102.

† Not available in the United States.

Fluconazole (*Diflucan*)

Zidovudine (*Retrovir*)

SUMMARY: Fluconazole administration increases zidovudine serum concentrations; the clinical significance is not established.

RISK FACTORS: No specific risk factors are known.

MECHANISM: Not established. Fluconazole appears to inhibit the metabolism of zidovudine, possibly via zidovudine's glucuronidation pathway.

CLINICAL EVALUATION: Twelve patients with HIV received oral zidovudine 200 mg every 8 hours for 7 days alone and in combination with oral fluconazole 400 mg/day.[1] During fluconazole administration, the clearance of zidovudine after oral administration was reduced 43%, while its area under the concentration-time curve increased 74%. The half-life of zidovudine increased from 1.5 to 3.4 hours during fluconazole administration. It is unknown whether smaller doses of fluconazole produces similar effects, but it is likely that the magnitude of the interaction would be reduced. The clinical significance of this interaction is not established; however, monitor patients for zidovudine toxicity (eg, anemia).

RELATED DRUGS: No information is available.

MANAGEMENT OPTIONS: No specific action is required, but be alert for evidence of the interaction.

REFERENCES:

1. Sahai J, et al. Effect of fluconazole on zidovudine pharmacokinetics in patients infected with human immunodeficiency virus. *J Infect Dis.* 1994;169:1103-1107.

Fluconazole (*Diflucan*)

Zolpidem (*Ambien*)

SUMMARY: Fluconazole produces a minor increase in zolpidem concentrations; increased sedation is unlikely to occur.

RISK FACTORS: No specific risk factors are known.

MECHANISM: Fluconazole minimally reduces the clearance of zolpidem, probably by inhibiting the CYP3A4 metabolism of zolpidem.

CLINICAL EVALUATION: Twelve healthy subjects received a single oral dose of zolpidem 5 mg alone and 1 hour after the third of 4 doses of fluconazole 100 mg twice daily.[1] The fluconazole treatment increased the area under the plasma concentration-time curve for zolpidem 31% and reduced its apparent oral clearance 20%. Neither of these changes was statistically significant. Zolpidem's half-life increased from 1.86 hours when administered alone to 1.98 hours (not significant) when coadministered with fluconazole. Most patients taking zolpidem are at a limited risk of suffering increased sedation if fluconazole is prescribed. However, higher doses of fluconazole can produce a more profound inhibition of zolpidem.

RELATED DRUGS: Ketoconazole (eg, *Nizoral*) has been reported to significantly reduce the clearance of zolpidem. Itraconazole (*Sporanox*) has been noted to produce a minimal increase in zolpidem plasma concentrations.

MANAGEMENT OPTIONS:

➡ *Monitor.* Observe patients taking fluconazole and zolpidem for a slight risk of enhanced sedation.

REFERENCES:

1. Greenblatt DJ, et al. Kinetic and dynamic interaction study of zolpidem with ketoconazole, itraconazole, and fluconazole. *Clin Pharmacol Ther.* 1998;64:661-671.

Fluorouracil (5-FU)

Metronidazole (eg, *Flagyl*)

SUMMARY: Metronidazole enhances the toxicity of fluorouracil without increasing its efficacy.

RISK FACTORS: No specific risk factors are known.

MECHANISM: Metronidazole appears to reduce the clearance of fluorouracil, resulting in increased plasma concentrations.

CLINICAL EVALUATION: Twenty-seven patients with metastatic colorectal cancer were treated with a combination of fluorouracil (600 mg/m^2/day) and metronidazole (750 mg/m^2).[1] Toxicity appeared frequently and included granulocytopenia (74%), oral ulceration (34%), anemia (41%), and nausea and vomiting (22%). Fluorouracil clearance decreased an average of 27% when taken with metronidazole. Metronidazole administration did not modify the cytotoxicity of fluorouracil against colon cancer cells, despite the apparently increased toxicity. Based on these limited data, metronidazole administration to patients taking fluorouracil is unlikely to enhance fluorouracil antitumor activity, but appears to increase its plasma concentration and toxicity.

RELATED DRUGS: No information is available.

MANAGEMENT OPTIONS:

➡ *Avoid Unless Benefit Outweighs Risk.* Patients taking fluorouracil should generally avoid metronidazole administration.

➡ *Monitor.* Monitor patients for enhanced toxicity when metronidazole is coadministered.

REFERENCES:

1. Bardakji Z, et al. 5-fluorouracil-metronidazole combination therapy in metastatic colorectal cancer. *Cancer Chemother Pharmacol.* 1986;18:140-144.

Fluorouracil (5-FU)

Phenytoin (eg, *Dilantin*)

SUMMARY: Limited clinical evidence suggests that fluorouracil can increase phenytoin serum concentrations.

RISK FACTORS: No specific risk factors are known.

MECHANISM: Fluorouracil probably inhibits the metabolism of phenytoin via CYP2C9.

CLINICAL EVALUATION: Several cases have been reported of phenytoin toxicity after initiation of fluorouracil therapy.[1-3] Given these cases and the strong theoretical basis for the interaction, expect increases in phenytoin plasma concentrations if fluorouracil therapy is initiated.

RELATED DRUGS: Capecitabine (*Xeloda*) is an oral prodrug for fluorouracil, and phenytoin toxicity also has been reported after capecitabine.[2]

MANAGEMENT OPTIONS:

➥ *Monitor.* In patients given phenytoin and fluorouracil, monitor phenytoin serum concentrations and be alert for evidence of phenytoin toxicity. Adjustments in phenytoin dose may be needed if fluorouracil is initiated, discontinued, or changed in dosage.

REFERENCES:

1. Gilbar PJ, et al. Phenytoin and fluorouracil interaction. *Ann Pharmacother.* 2001;35:1367-1370.
2. Brickell K, et al. Phenytoin toxicity due to fluoropyrimidines (5-FU/capecitabine): three case reports. *Br J Cancer.* 2003;89:615-616.
3. Rosemergy I, Findlay M. Phenytoin toxicity as a result of 5-fluorouracil administration. *N Z Med J.* 2002;115:U124.

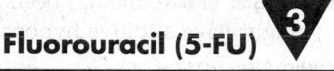

Fluorouracil (5-FU)

Warfarin (eg, *Coumadin*)

SUMMARY: Case reports suggest that fluorouracil may increase the hypoprothrombinemic response to warfarin; monitor for altered warfarin response.

RISK FACTORS: No specific risk factors are known.

MECHANISM: Not established.

CLINICAL EVALUATION: A 73-year-old man stabilized on warfarin was started on 5-fluorouracil and levamisole for colon cancer.[1] The international normalized ratio (INR) was 3 prior to chemotherapy, and 4 weeks later it had increased to almost 40. A positive dechallenge and rechallenge supports a causal relationship between the chemotherapy and the increased warfarin effect. Because fluorouracil and levamisole were used together, it is not possible to determine whether the increased warfarin effect was caused by 1 of the drugs acting alone or by a combination of the 2 drugs. A 75-year-old man on warfarin therapy developed an excessive prothrombin time after starting fluorouracil, an effect not seen when either drug was used alone.[2] Based on these cases, it appears that the increased hypoprothrombinemic response can begin after a few days of fluorouracil, but it may continue to increase gradually over several weeks. In both cases, the prothrombin time continued to increase for several days after fluorouracil was discontinued. Five patients on warfarin required a mean 44% reduction in warfarin dose after starting fluorouracil therapy.[3]

RELATED DRUGS: Capecitabine (*Xeloda*) is an oral prodrug for fluorouracil, and increased warfarin response has been reported after capecitabine.

MANAGEMENT OPTIONS:

➥ *Monitor.* Monitor for altered warfarin effect if fluorouracil is initiated, discontinued, or changed in dosage; adjustments of warfarin dosage may be needed. If warfarin is initiated in the presence of fluorouracil therapy, it would be prudent to begin with conservative doses of warfarin.

REFERENCES:

1. Scarfe MA, et al. Possible drug interaction between warfarin and combination of levamisole and fluorouracil. *Ann Pharmacother.* 1994;28:464-467.

2. Wajima T, et al. Possible interactions between warfarin and 5-fluorouracil. *Am J Hematol.* 1992;40:238.

3. Kolesar JM, et al. Warfarin-5-FU interaction—a consecutive case series. *Pharmacotherapy.* 1999;19:1445-1449.

Fluoxetine (*Prozac*)

Furosemide (eg, *Lasix*)

SUMMARY: Two patients receiving fluoxetine and furosemide died unexpectedly, and it was proposed that the combination of these 2 drugs may have contributed to their deaths. However, a causal relationship was not established.

RISK FACTORS: No specific risk factors are known.

MECHANISM: Fluoxetine has been associated with occasional cases of hyponatremia and might have additive hyponatremic effects with loop diuretics such as furosemide.

CLINICAL EVALUATION: Three seriously ill elderly women died from unexplained causes within 10 days of starting fluoxetine.[1] Two of the 3 were receiving furosemide, and it was proposed that the combined effects of fluoxetine and furosemide might have contributed to the reactions. All 3 patients developed hyponatremia. Fluoxetine has been associated with hyponatremia in several patients, presumably because of a syndrome of inappropriate secretion of antidiuretic hormone (SIADH).[2,3] However, 2 of the patients also were receiving angiotensin-converting enzyme inhibitors, agents that can cause severe hypotension in the presence of hyponatremia. One of the patients received metolazone (eg, *Zaroxolyn*) along with high-dose furosemide therapy, a particularly potent diuretic combination. Thus, it is possible that several of their drugs contributed to the fatal reactions, but the lack of definitive information on the cause of death makes it difficult to establish a causal relationship.

RELATED DRUGS: If the furosemide-fluoxetine combination did, in fact, contribute to the fatal reactions, expect other loop diuretics such as bumetanide (eg, *Bumex*) and torsemide (*Demadex*) to produce the same effect. Little is known regarding the ability of other selective serotonin reuptake inhibitors (SSRIs) to produce SIADH. Sertraline (*Zoloft*) has been reported to produce hyponatremia caused by SIADH in one 73-year-old man,[4] and cases of paroxetine (*Paxil*)-induced hyponatremia have been reported to the manufacturer.[5] It is possible that other SSRIs have a similar effect.

MANAGEMENT OPTIONS:

➥ **Monitor.** Monitor for evidence of hyponatremia if fluoxetine is used in patients undergoing vigorous diuresis or others at risk of hyponatremia. The relative likelihood of SIADH in patients receiving fluoxetine vs other SSRIs or tricyclic antidepressants is not established. Thus, it is not known if any of them would be preferable to fluoxetine in a patient prone to hyponatremia.

REFERENCES:
1. Spier SA, et al. Unexpected deaths in depressed medical inpatients treated with fluoxetine. *J Clin Psychiatry.* 1991;52:377.
2. Hwang AS, et al. Syndrome of inappropriate secretion of antidiuretic hormone due to fluoxetine. *Am J Psychiatry.* 1989;146:399.
3. Cohen BJ, et al. More cases of SIADH with fluoxetine. *Am J Psychiatry.* 1990;147:948.
4. Crews JR, et al. Hyponatremia in a patient treated with sertraline. *Am J Psychiatry.* 1993;150:1564.
5. Product Information. Paroxetine (*Paxil*). SmithKline Beecham. 1993.

Fluoxetine (*Prozac*)

Grapefruit Juice

SUMMARY: A patient on fluoxetine developed possible serotonin syndrome after eating large amounts of grapefruit, but a causal relationship was not established.

RISK FACTORS: No specific risk factors are known.

MECHANISM: Fluoxetine and its active metabolite norfluoxetine are metabolized primarily by CYP2D6, but grapefruit juice is a CYP3A4 inhibitor. In a patient lacking CYP2D6; however, other cytochrome P450 isozymes (eg, CYP3A4, CYP2C9, CYP2C19) may become important in the metabolism of fluoxetine.

CLINICAL EVALUATION: A 57-year-old HIV-infected man on indinavir, stavudine, and lamivudine also was receiving fluoxetine, trazodone, benazepril, and co-trimoxazole.[1] He developed dizziness, confusion, visual changes, and syncope. Further investigation revealed that the patient had visited Florida, and brought back 5 crates of grapefruit, which he was consuming at a high rate. His symptoms resolved after he stopped eating grapefruit. While this may have resulted from inhibition of fluoxetine metabolism in a CYP2D6 deficient patient, the CYP2D6 status of this patient was not assessed. Moreover, trazodone is metabolized by CYP3A4, and trazodone serum concentrations may have been elevated. More study is needed to establish whether grapefruit juice can result in fluoxetine toxicity.

RELATED DRUGS: No information is available.

MANAGEMENT OPTIONS: No specific action is required, but be alert for evidence of the interaction.

REFERENCES:
1. DeSilva KE, et al. Serotonin syndrome in HIV-infected individuals receiving antiretroviral therapy and fluoxetine. *AIDS.* 2001;15:1281.

Fluoxetine (eg, *Prozac*)

Haloperidol (eg, *Haldol*)

SUMMARY: A woman on haloperidol developed severe extrapyramidal symptoms after starting fluoxetine, but a causal relationship was not established.

RISK FACTORS: No specific risk factors are known.

MECHANISM: Not established. Haloperidol is metabolized by CYP2D6, and both fluoxetine and norfluoxetine are potent inhibitors of CYP2D6.

CLINICAL EVALUATION: A 39-year-old woman with bipolar disorder who had been taking haloperidol 2 to 5 mg/day for 2 years, developed only occasional, mild extrapyramidal symptoms.[1] Five days after fluoxetine was started (fluoxetine dose was increased to 40 mg twice daily over several days), the patient developed mild oral-buccal movement abnormalities. The haloperidol was stopped, and the fluoxetine was continued at the same dose. Nine days later she took 5 mg haloperidol on 2 consecutive mornings and soon developed severe tongue stiffness, parkinsonism, and akathisia. The haloperidol and fluoxetine were discontinued, and she was hospitalized; she recovered gradually over approximately 1 week. She later received up to 30 mg/day of haloperidol (combined with benztropine); this was associated with a slight parkinsonian gait but no other extrapyramidal symptoms. The fact that the patient received haloperidol both before and after the fluoxetine without manifesting a severe reaction suggests that the fluoxetine may have predisposed her to haloperidol-induced severe extrapyramidal symptoms. Nevertheless, more study will be required to establish a causal relationship. Because of the long half-life of fluoxetine (2 to 3 days) and its active metabolite norfluoxetine (7 to 9 days), fluoxetine interactions theoretically could occur weeks after fluoxetine is discontinued.

RELATED DRUGS: The effect of fluoxetine on other neuroleptics is not established. Paroxetine (*Paxil*) also is a potent inhibitor of CYP2D6 and also might inhibit haloperidol metabolism. Sertraline (*Zoloft*) appears to be a less potent CYP2D6 inhibitor, but it may have some effect.

MANAGEMENT OPTIONS:

➡ *Monitor.* Until more information is available, monitor patients for extrapyramidal symptoms if fluoxetine is used concomitantly with haloperidol (and possibly other neuroleptics).

REFERENCES:

1. Tate JL. Extrapyramidal symptoms in a patient taking haloperidol and fluoxetine. *Am J Psychiatry.* 1989;146:399-400.

Fluoxetine (eg, *Prozac*)

Ibuprofen (eg, *Motrin*)

SUMMARY: The combined use of fluoxetine (or other selective serotonin reuptake inhibitors [SSRIs]) with ibuprofen (or other nonsteroidal anti-inflammatory drugs [NSAIDs]) appears to increase the risk of upper gastrointestinal bleeding.

RISK FACTORS: No specific risk factors are known.

MECHANISM: NSAIDs impair the defenses of the gastric mucosa, which can lead to gastric erosions and bleeding. Also, both NSAIDs and SSRIs can impair platelet function. Serotonin appears to play a role in platelet function, but platelets do not synthesize serotonin. SSRIs such as fluoxetine inhibit the uptake of serotonin by platelets, and may add to the antiplatelet effects of NSAIDs.

CLINICAL EVALUATION: In a 5-year, case-control study of 1651 cases of serious GI bleeding compared to 10,000 matched controls, there was a 3-fold increase in GI bleeding in users of SSRIs (without NSAIDs) compared with nonusers.[1] NSAIDs without SSRIs increase the risk about 4-fold, but patients receiving both an SSRI and a NSAID had an almost 16-fold increase of GI bleeding. A subsequent population-based cohort study of 26,005 antidepressant users found similar results. SSRIs alone increased the risk of serious GI bleeding by 3.6-fold, but patients on both an SSRI and NSAID had over a 12-fold increase in risk.[2] Given the plausible biological mechanism (see Mechanism), and the consistent findings from 2 studies, one should assume that the combination of SSRIs and NSAIDs substantially increases the relative risk of upper GI bleeding. Nonetheless, note that the absolute risk of GI bleeding was not high; GI bleeding occurred in only 17 of 4107 patients receiving SSRIs and NSAIDs.[2] Given the low absolute risk, there could be situations in which the benefit of the combination would outweigh the risk.

The increase in GI bleeding risk appeared to correlate with the potency of the antidepressant as a serotonin reuptake inhibitor.[2] Antidepressants with less serotonergic effect than SSRIs such as imipramine (*Tofranil*), amitriptyline (*Elavil*), and doxepin (*Adapin*) appeared somewhat less likely to be associated with GI bleeding than SSRIs, although the risk was increased. Antidepressants with minimal serotonergic effects such as desipramine (*Norpramin*), trimipramine (*Surmontil*), nortriptyline (*Aventyl*), maprotiline (*Ludiomil*), and mianserin did not appear to increase the risk of GI bleeding.

RELATED DRUGS: Assume that all other drugs that inhibit serotonin reuptake (citalopram [*Effexor*], clomipramine [*Anafranil*], fluvoxamine [*Luvox*], nefazodone [*Serzone*], paroxetine [*Paxil*], sertraline [*Zoloft*], and venlafaxine [*Effexor*]) would interact with all NSAIDs: diclofenac (*Voltaren*), diflunisal (*Dolobid*), etodolac (*Lodine*), fenoprofen (*Nalfon*), flurbiprofen (*Ansaid*), ibuprofen (*Motrin*), indomethacin (*Indocin*), ketoprofen (*Orudis*), ketorolac (*Toradol*), meclofenamate (*Meclomen*), mefenamic acid (*Ponstel*), meloxicam (*Mobic*), nabumetone (*Relafen*), naproxen (*Aleve*), oxaprozin (*Daypro*), piroxicam (*Feldene*), sulindac (*Clinoril*), tolmetin (*Tolectin*).

MANAGEMENT OPTIONS:

➥ ***Consider Alternative.*** Consider using a non-NSAID analgesic such as acetaminophen. If an NSAID is needed, consider a non-acetylated salicylate such as choline magnesium trisalicylate (*Trilisate*), salsalate (*Disalcid*), or magnesium salicylate (*Doan's*) since these products have minimal effects on platelets and the gastric mucosa. It is not known whether COX-2 inhibitors such as celecoxib (*Celebrex*), rofecoxib (*Vioxx*), or valdecoxib (*Bextra*) would be less likely to cause GI bleeding with SSRIs. Antidepressants with less effect on serotonin (see Clinical Evaluation) may reduce the risk of GI bleeding when combined with NSAIDs.

➥ ***Monitor.*** Patients receiving both a SSRI and NSAID should be alert for evidence of GI bleeding.

REFERENCES:

1. de Abajo FJ, et al. Association between selective serotonin reuptake inhibitors and upper gastrointestinal bleeding: population based case-control study. *BMJ*. 1999;319:1106-1109.

2. Dalton SO, et al. Use of selective serotonin reuptake inhibitors and risk of upper gastrointestinal tract bleeding: a population-based cohort study. *Arch Intern Med*. 2003;163:59-64.

Fluoxetine (eg, *Prozac*)

Linezolid (*Zyvox*)

SUMMARY: Isolated cases of possible serotonin syndrome have been reported with concurrent linezolid and fluoxetine. Although the incidence of this reaction is not established, the linezolid prescribing information recommends careful monitoring if linezolid is used with drugs that inhibit serotonin uptake.

RISK FACTORS: No specific risk factors are known.

MECHANISM: Linezolid is a weak nonselective monoamine oxidase inhibitor (MAOI), but in some patients it may increase the risk of serotonin syndrome when combined with serotonergic drugs, such as fluoxetine.

CLINICAL EVALUATION: A 4-year-old girl developed evidence of serotonin syndrome after linezolid was added to her fluoxetine therapy.[1] The fentanyl she also received may have contributed to the serotonin syndrome. A 39-year-old woman who had stopped taking fluoxetine 18 days earlier developed serotonin syndrome after linezolid was started.[2] Although it appears that most patients who receive linezolid and selective serotonin reuptake inhibitors (SSRIs) do not develop serotonin syndrome,[3] the manufacturer of linezolid states that serotonin reuptake inhibitors are contraindicated with linezolid unless the patient can be carefully observed for evidence of serotonin syndrome.[4]

RELATED DRUGS: Other SSRIs may interact similarly, including citalopram (eg, *Celexa*), escitalopram (*Lexapro*), fluvoxamine (eg, *Luvox*), paroxetine (eg, *Paxil*), and sertraline (eg, *Zoloft*). Selective serotonin/norepinephrine reuptake inhibitors may also interact, including clomipramine (eg, *Anafranil*), desvenlafaxine (*Pristiq*), duloxetine (*Cymbalta*), imipramine (eg, *Tofranil*), and venlafaxine (eg, *Effexor*).

MANAGEMENT OPTIONS:

➡ *Monitor.* Monitor for evidence of serotonin syndrome (eg, agitation, coma, confusion, fever, hyperreflexia, hypomania, incoordination, myoclonus, rigidity, seizures, shivering, sweating, tachycardia, tremor). Because fluoxetine and particularly its active metabolite, norfluoxetine, have very long half-lives, monitor patients if linezolid is started within 5 weeks of stopping fluoxetine.

REFERENCES:

1. Thomas CR, et al. Serotonin syndrome and linezolid. *J Am Acad Child Adolesc Psychiatry.* 2004;43(7):790.
2. Morales N, et al. Serotonin syndrome associated with linezolid treatment after discontinuation of fluoxetine. *Psychosomatics.* 2005;46(3):274-275.
3. Taylor JJ, et al. Linezolid and serotonergic drug interactions: a retrospective survey. *Clin Infect Dis.* 2006;43(2):180-187.
4. *Zyvox* [package insert]. New York, NY: Pfizer, Inc; 2008.

Fluoxetine (eg, *Prozac*)

Lithium (eg, *Lithobid*)

SUMMARY: Some patients receiving lithium and fluoxetine have developed neurotoxicity, but the incidence of this reaction is unknown.

RISK FACTORS: No specific risk factors are known.

MECHANISM: Not established.

CLINICAL EVALUATION: Several cases of neurotoxicity have been reported in patients receiving fluoxetine and lithium.[1-4] The toxicity generally occurred within a few days of starting concurrent therapy and consisted of absence seizures, ataxia, confusion, dizziness, dysarthria, stiffness of arms and legs, and tremor. The order of drug administration did not appear to be a factor in these cases. In one case, the neurotoxicity was associated with an increase in the serum lithium concentration from approximately 1 to 1.7 mEq/L,[4] but in another case the lithium did not reach toxic levels.[3] The latter patient subsequently achieved good results with lithium plus nortriptyline (eg, *Aventyl*).[3] However, some patients appear to tolerate lithium plus fluoxetine without difficulty. No adverse reactions were noted in a study of 5 patients with refractory depression given the combination.[5]

RELATED DRUGS: Theoretically, other selective serotonin reuptake inhibitors would interact with lithium in a similar manner.

MANAGEMENT OPTIONS:

➡ **Monitor.** Until additional information is available, monitor for evidence of neurotoxicity in patients receiving lithium and fluoxetine. Symptoms have included absence seizures, ataxia, confusion, dizziness, dysarthria, and tremor. If symptoms occur, consider using a tricyclic antidepressant (eg, imipramine [eg, *Tofranil*], nortriptyline) with lithium.

REFERENCES:

1. Sacristan JA, et al. Absence seizures induced by lithium: possible interaction with fluoxetine. *Am J Psychiatry.* 1991;148(1):146-147.
2. Austin LS, et al. Toxicity resulting from lithium augmentation of antidepressant treatment in elderly patients. *J Clin Psychiatry.* 1990;51(8):344-345.
3. Noveske FG, et al. Possible toxicity of combined fluoxetine and lithium. *Am J Psychiatry.* 1989;146(11):1515.
4. Salama AA, Shafey M. A case of severe lithium toxicity induced by combined fluoxetine and lithium carbonate. *Am J Psychiatry.* 1989;146(2):278.
5. Pope HG Jr, et al. Possible synergism between fluoxetine and lithium in refractory depression. *Am J Psychiatry.* 1988;145(10):1292-1294.

Fluoxetine (eg, *Prozac*)

Meperidine (eg, *Demerol*)

SUMMARY: A patient developed some symptoms of serotonin toxicity after receiving fluoxetine and meperidine.

RISK FACTORS: No specific risk factors are known.

MECHANISM: Probably additive serotonergic effects.

CLINICAL EVALUATION: A 43-year-old man who had been on fluoxetine developed symptoms of serotonin toxicity after being given meperidine during endoscopy.[1] Although the symptoms were not classic serotonin toxicity (no myoclonus, tremor, or rigidity),[2,3] both drugs are serotonergic, and it is possible that the reaction resulted from additive serotonergic effects.

RELATED DRUGS: Theoretically, other antidepressants that inhibit serotonin reuptake (citalopram [eg, *Celexa*], clomipramine [eg, *Anafranil*], duloxetine [*Cymbalta*], escitalopram [*Lexapro*], fluvoxamine [eg, *Luvox*], imipramine [eg, *Tofranil*], paroxetine [eg,

Paxil], sertraline [eg, *Zoloft*], venlafaxine [eg, *Effexor*]) may also increase the risk of serotonin toxicity when combined with meperidine.

MANAGEMENT OPTIONS:

➡ *Monitor.* If the combination is used, monitor for symptoms of serotonin toxicity, including agitation, coma, confusion, fever, hyperreflexia, hypomania, incoordination, myoclonus, rigidity, seizures, shivering, sweating, and tremor.

REFERENCES:

1. Tissot TA. Probable meperidine-induced serotonin syndrome in a patient with a history of fluoxetine use. *Anesthesiology.* 2003;98(6):1511-1512.

2. Isbister GK, et al. Serotonin toxicity: a practical approach to diagnosis and treatment. *Med J Aust.* 2007;187(6):361-365.

3. Boyer EW, Shannon M. The serotonin syndrome. *N Engl J Med.* 2005;352(11):1112-1120.

 Fluoxetine (eg, *Prozac*)

AVOID **Methylene Blue (eg, *Urolene Blue*)**

SUMMARY: Giving methylene blue to patients receiving fluoxetine or other serotonergic drugs may result in serotonin syndrome; avoid the combination.

RISK FACTORS: No specific risk factors are known.

MECHANISM: Methylene blue appears to be a strong inhibitor of monoamine oxidase type A (MAO-A, and a weak inhibitor of MAO-B.[1,2] Selective serotonin reuptake inhibitors (SSRIs), such as fluoxetine, and selective serotonin-norepinephrine reuptake inhibitors (SNRIs) may cause severe serotonin syndrome when combined with MAO inhibitors.

CLINICAL EVALUATION: A 60-year-old woman on long-term fluoxetine therapy was given methylene blue prior to parathyroid surgery. In the recovery room she developed symptoms of serotonin syndrome, including agitation, hyperreflexia, muscle jerking, profuse sweating, and rigidity.[3] Virtually all cases of serotonin syndrome following administration of methylene blue have occurred in patients receiving SSRIs or SNRIs, which is consistent with the view that a drug interaction is involved. (SSRIs and SNRIs given alone rarely produce serious serotonin toxicity, even when taken in overdose.)

RELATED DRUGS: Methylene blue has been associated with serotonin syndrome in patients receiving other SSRIs, such as citalopram (eg, *Celexa*) and paroxetine (eg, *Paxil*), and also in patients receiving SNRIs, such as clomipramine (eg, *Anafranil*) and venlafaxine (eg, *Effexor*). Methylene blue is likely to also interact with other SSRIs, such as escitalopram (*Lexapro*), fluvoxamine (eg, *Luvox*), and sertraline (eg, *Zoloft*), and other SNRIs, such as desvenlafaxine (*Pristiq*), duloxetine (*Cymbalta*), and imipramine (eg, *Tofranil*).

MANAGEMENT OPTIONS:

➡ *AVOID COMBINATION.* Given that serotonin syndrome can be life-threatening, avoid the combination.[4] Because the effects of fluoxetine have a long duration (because of its active metabolite), stop fluoxetine 5 weeks before using methylene blue. Stopping other SSRIs or SNRIs for 2 weeks before using methylene blue would minimize the risk. Available evidence suggests that the interaction cannot be avoided by decreasing the dose of methylene blue.[1,5]

REFERENCES:

1. Stanford SC, et al. Risk of severe serotonin toxicity following co-administration of methylene blue and serotonin reuptake inhibitors: an update on a case report of post-operative delirium [published online ahead of print May 7, 2009]. *J Psychopharmacol.* doi:10.1177/0269881109105450.

2. Ramsay RR, et al. Methylene blue and serotonin toxicity: inhibition of monoamine oxidase A (MAO A) confirms a theoretical prediction. *Br J Pharmacol.* 2007;152(6):946-951.

3. Martindale SJ, Stedeford JC. Neurological sequelae following methylene blue injection for parathyroidectomy. *Anaesthesia.* 2003;58(10):1041-1042.

4. Pollack G, et al. Parathyroid surgery and methylene blue: a review with guidelines for safe intraoperative use [published online ahead of print May 13, 2009]. *Laryngoscope.* doi:10.1002/lary.20581.

5. Schwiebert C, et al. Small doses of methylene blue, previously considered safe, can precipitate serotonin toxicity. *Anaesthesia.* 2009;64(8):924.

Fluoxetine (eg, *Prozac*)

Midazolam

SUMMARY: Fluoxetine and its metabolite, norfluoxetine, may inhibit the metabolism of midazolam, but the clinical importance of this effect is not established.

RISK FACTORS:

➡ *Route of Administration.* This interaction is likely to be more important when the midazolam is given orally, because midazolam undergoes extensive presystemic metabolism.

MECHANISM: Fluoxetine and its active metabolite, norfluoxetine, inhibit the hydroxylation of midazolam by CYP3A4 in vitro.[1] Clinical studies of fluoxetine given with other CYP3A4 substrates (eg, alprazolam [eg, *Xanax*], carbamazepine [eg, *Tegretol*]) suggest that it inhibits CYP3A4 in vivo.[2]

CLINICAL EVALUATION: Although in vitro study in human liver microsomes suggests that fluoxetine inhibits midazolam metabolism, a study in healthy subjects given oral midazolam after 12 days of fluoxetine failed to find an interaction.[3] Because norfluoxetine appears to be much more potent than the parent drug as an inhibitor of midazolam metabolism, it would theoretically take several weeks before the maximal effect on midazolam metabolism would be seen. This is because norfluoxetine has a half-life of about 1 week and can accumulate for 1 month or more.

RELATED DRUGS: Fluvoxamine is known to inhibit CYP3A4, and a study in healthy subjects found a trend toward increased midazolam plasma concentrations with fluvoxamine treatment.[3] Citalopram (eg, *Celexa*), escitalopram (*Lexapro*), paroxetine (eg, *Paxil*), sertraline (eg, *Zoloft*), and venlafaxine (eg, *Effexor*) appear to have little effect on CYP3A4.

MANAGEMENT OPTIONS: No specific action is required, but be alert for evidence of the interaction.

REFERENCES:

1. von Moltke LL, et al. Midazolam hydroxylation by human liver microsomes in vitro: inhibition by fluoxetine, norfluoxetine, and by azole antifungal agents. *J Clin Pharmacol.* 1996;36(9):783-791.

2. Greenblatt DJ, et al. Inhibition of human cytochrome P450-3A isoforms by fluoxetine and norfluoxetine: in vitro and in vivo studies. *J Clin Pharmacol.* 1996;36(9):792-798.

3. Lam YW, et al. Pharmacokinetic and pharmacodynamic interactions of oral midazolam with ketoconazole, fluoxetine, fluvoxamine, and nefazodone. *J Clin Pharmacol.* 2003;43(11):1274-1282.

4   Fluoxetine (eg, *Prozac*)

Moclobemide[†]

SUMMARY: Preliminary data suggest that fluoxetine reduces the clearance of moclobemide after oral administration, but adverse effects do not appear to be increased. Theoretically, combined overdose of both drugs could be dangerous.

RISK FACTORS: No specific risk factors are known.

MECHANISM: Not established. It is possible that fluoxetine inhibits the hepatic metabolism of moclobemide, but more data are needed. Fluoxetine is a selective serotonin reuptake inhibitor (SSRI) and moclobemide is a selective inhibitor of monoamine oxidase (MAO)-A, the form of MAO that metabolizes serotonin. Theoretically, the combination could result in excessive serotonin effects, but available evidence suggests that serotonin syndrome does not occur, at least at therapeutic doses.

CLINICAL EVALUATION: In a preliminary report of a randomized crossover study, 18 healthy subjects received fluoxetine (40 mg/day for 7 days, followed by 20 mg/day for 16 days) with increasing doses of moclobemide (100 to 600 mg/day) or placebo added on day 14.[1] Fluoxetine reduced moclobemide apparent clearance to approximately one third of the value seen before fluoxetine administration. The reduction in clearance reportedly was not associated with excessive accumulation of moclobemide, but no data were presented. There was no evidence of serotonin syndrome or other adverse reactions not seen with either drug alone. This data suggest that it is not necessary to have a washout period when switching from fluoxetine to moclobemide or vice versa, but more information is needed to establish the safety of immediately replacing one with the other. Moreover, these data do not preclude the possibility that excessive doses or overdoses of the combination could result in serotonin syndrome.

RELATED DRUGS: Three people died following a combined overdose of citalopram (*Celexa*) and moclobemide.[2] Combining fluoxetine with nonselective MAO inhibitors such as tranylcypromine (*Parnate*) or phenelzine (*Nardil*) has resulted in fatalities, even at therapeutic doses.[3,4] Little is known regarding the combined use of moclobemide with other SSRIs.

MANAGEMENT OPTIONS: No specific action is required, but be alert for evidence of the interaction.

REFERENCES:

1. Dingemanse J, et al. Pharmacodynamic and pharmacokinetic interactions between fluoxetine and moclobemide. *Clin Pharmacol Ther*. 1993;53:178.

2. Neuvonen PJ, Pohjola-Sintonen S, Tacke U, Vuori E. Five fatal cases of serotonin syndrome after moclobemide-citalopram or moclobemide-clomipramine overdoses. *Lancet*. 1993;342:1419.

3. Sternbach H. Danger of MAOI therapy after fluoxetine withdrawal. *Lancet*. 1988;2:850-851.

4. Feighner JP, Boyer WF, Tyler DL, Neborsky RJ. Adverse consequences of fluoxetine-MAOI combination therapy. *J Clin Psychiatry*. 1990;51:222-225.

† Not available in the United States.

Fluoxetine (eg, *Prozac*)

Nefazodone (*Serzone*)

SUMMARY: A patient on fluoxetine developed serotonin syndrome after nefazodone was added without discontinuation of the fluoxetine.

RISK FACTORS: No specific risk factors are known.

MECHANISM: The serotonin syndrome probably resulted from the additive serotonergic effects of fluoxetine and nefazodone.

CLINICAL EVALUATION: A 50-year-old man on fluoxetine 60 mg/day added nefazodone 100 mg twice daily 2 days after the fluoxetine dose was reduced to 40 mg/day.[1] He failed to discontinue the fluoxetine after 4 days as instructed, and about 6 days later he developed lethargy, ataxia, disorientation, vomiting, myoclonus, hyperreflexia, and visual hallucinations. These symptoms suggest that the patient had serotonin syndrome. His failure to discontinue the fluoxetine probably contributed to the reaction, but he might have had excessive serotonergic effects even if he had followed the directions. Fluoxetine and its active metabolite have a very long half-life, and their effects can last for weeks after discontinuation of fluoxetine.

RELATED DRUGS: Serotonin syndrome also has been reported in a patient receiving paroxetine (*Paxil*) plus nefazodone. All selective serotonin reuptake inhibitors (SSRIs) can be expected to have additive serotonergic effects with nefazodone.

MANAGEMENT OPTIONS:

➥ *Circumvent/Minimize.* When switching from fluoxetine to another serotonergic drug, be aware that the serotonergic effects of fluoxetine and its active metabolite can last for several weeks.

➥ *Monitor.* Be alert for evidence of serotonin syndrome when nefazodone is used concurrently or sequentially with SSRIs. Serotonin syndrome can result in neurotoxicity (myoclonus, tremors, rigidity, incoordination, hyperreflexia, seizures, coma), psychiatric symptoms (agitation, confusion, hypomania, restlessness), and autonomic dysfunction (fever, sweating, tachycardia, hypertension).

REFERENCES:

1. Smith DL, Wenegrat BG. A case report of serotonin syndrome associated with combined nefazodone and fluoxetine. *J Clin Psychiatry.* 2000;61:146.

Fluoxetine (eg, *Prozac*)

Nifedipine (eg, *Procardia XL*)

SUMMARY: Some patients may experience increased calcium blocker effects when fluoxetine is coadministered.

RISK FACTORS: No specific risk factors are known.

MECHANISM: Fluoxetine has been reported to be a mild inhibitor of CYP3A4, the enzyme that metabolizes nifedipine.

CLINICAL EVALUATION: Several case reports have noted that patients stabilized on nifedipine developed symptoms of nifedipine toxicity including palpitations, weakness, hypotension, and tachycardia following the addition of fluoxetine.[1,2] Symptoms occurred from 7 to 18 days after fluoxetine was added. The combined use of verapamil (eg, *Calan*) and fluoxetine has also been reported to produce headaches and edema.[1] Because these case reports are limited and difficult to evaluate, additional prospective studies would be helpful to define the nature and magnitude of this interaction.

RELATED DRUGS: While no data are available, nefazodone (*Serzone*) is a more potent inhibitor of CYP3A4 than fluoxetine and might be expected to inhibit the metabolism of nifedipine, verapamil, or other calcium blockers.

MANAGEMENT OPTIONS: No specific action is required, but monitor patients stabilized on calcium channel blockers for increased effect if fluoxetine is coadministered.

REFERENCES:
1. Sternbach H. Fluoxetine-associated potentiation of calcium-channel blockers. *J Clin Psychopharmacol.* 1991;11:390-391.
2. Azaz-Livshits TL, Danenberg HD. Tachycardia, orthostatic hypotension and profound weakness due to concomitant use of fluoxetine and nifedipine. *Pharmacopsychiatry.* 1997;30:274-275.

 Fluoxetine (eg, *Prozac*)

Pentazocine (*Talwin*)

SUMMARY: A patient taking fluoxetine developed an excitatory neurologic reaction soon after taking a single dose of pentazocine, but a causal relationship was not established.

RISK FACTORS: No specific risk factors are known.

MECHANISM: Not established.

CLINICAL EVALUATION: A 39-year-old man taking fluoxetine 40 mg/day developed light-headedness, anxiety, nausea, flushing, tremor, diaphoresis, paresthesias, and hypertension within 30 minutes of receiving oral pentazocine 100 mg.[1] Although the reaction may have been caused by an interaction between fluoxetine and pentazocine, one cannot rule out the possibility that the reaction resulted from pentazocine alone.

RELATED DRUGS: The effect of combining other selective serotonin reuptake inhibitors with pentazocine is not established.

MANAGEMENT OPTIONS: No specific action is required, but be alert for evidence of the interaction.

REFERENCES:
1. Hansen TE, Dieter K, Keepers GA. Interaction of fluoxetine and pentazocine. *Am J Psychiatry.* 1990;147:949-950.

 Fluoxetine (eg, *Prozac*)

Phenytoin (eg, *Dilantin*)

SUMMARY: Several case reports have been published describing phenytoin toxicity with concurrent use of fluoxetine.

RISK FACTORS: No specific risk factors are known.

MECHANISM: Fluoxetine appears to inhibit the metabolism of phenytoin.

CLINICAL EVALUATION: A patient with epilepsy treated with phenytoin at a concentration of 18 mcg/L was started on fluoxetine 20 mg/day. After 2 weeks of fluoxetine, the patient presented with tremor, headache, impaired cognition, abnormal thinking, and increased partial seizure activity with a phenytoin concentration of 30 mcg/L. Her phenytoin level returned to normal range 2 weeks after discontinuing the fluoxetine.[1] Two other case reports described similar increases in phenytoin concentrations with the addition of fluoxetine therapy.[2]

RELATED DRUGS: The effect of selective serotonin reuptake inhibitors other than fluoxetine on phenytoin is not established.

MANAGEMENT OPTIONS:

➡ *Monitor.* Carefully monitor patients for phenytoin toxicity (eg, nystagmus, ataxia, confusion, dizziness, slurred speech, involuntary muscular movements) when fluoxetine is started. Serum phenytoin determinations would be useful. Monitor the patient for a reduced phenytoin effect when fluoxetine therapy is stopped during phenytoin therapy.

REFERENCES:

1. Woods DJ, et al. Interaction of phenytoin and fluoxetine. *N Z Med J.* 1994;107:19.
2. Jalil P. Toxic reaction following the combined administration of fluoxetine and phenytoin: two case reports. *J Neurol Neurosurg Psychiatry.* 1992;55:412.

Fluoxetine (eg, *Prozac*)

Propafenone (eg, *Rythmol*)

SUMMARY: Fluoxetine increases the plasma concentration of propafenone; increased effect on myocardial conduction may occur including the induction of arrhythmias.

RISK FACTORS:

➡ *Pharmacogenetics.* Patients who are rapid metabolizers (CYP2D6) of propafenone are more susceptible to this interaction than poor CYP2D6 metabolizers.

MECHANISM: Propafenone metabolism is mediated via CYP2D6. Fluoxetine and its metabolite norfluoxetine inhibit the CYP2D6 metabolism of propafenone resulting in increased plasma concentrations.

CLINICAL EVALUATION: Nine healthy subjects, with the extensive metabolizer phenotype for CYP2D6, received a single oral dose of propafenone 400 mg before and after pretreatment with fluoxetine 20 mg/day for 10 days.[1] Pretreatment with fluoxetine reduced the oral clearance of propafenone approximately 35%. Fluoxetine displayed some stereoselective effects on propafenone pharmacokinetics; the peak concentration of R-propafenone increased 71% while the peak concentration of S-propafenone increased only 39%. The increase in propafenone concentrations resulting from fluoxetine coadministration could result in increased effect and possibly toxicity (eg, cardiac arrhythmias). Because of the long half-life of fluoxetine and its active metabolite, norfluoxetine, the maximum effect of fluoxetine on propafenone would require several weeks to occur. Thus, this study design may have underestimated the typical magnitude of this interaction. Observe caution if propafenone is administered to patients in whom fluoxetine was discontinued in the past 3 to 4 weeks.

RELATED DRUGS: Paroxetine (*Paxil*) is another antidepressant with significant CYP2D6 inhibitory activity; it would be expected to interact in a similar manner as fluoxetine. Sertraline (*Zoloft*) is a weaker inhibitor of CYP2D6 but may affect the metabolism of propafenone at daily doses greater than 150 mg.

MANAGEMENT OPTIONS:

➥ *Consider Alternative.* Selecting antidepressants that do not inhibit CYP2D6 (eg, citalopram [*Celexa*], nefazodone [*Serzone*], venlafaxine [*Effexor*]) would avoid the interaction.

➥ *Monitor.* If fluoxetine is coadministered, carefully monitor patients taking propafenone for increased effect on myocardial conduction.

REFERENCES:

1. Cai WM, et al. Fluoxetine impairs the CYP2D6-mediated metabolism of propafenone enantiomers in healthy Chinese volunteers. *Clin Pharmacol Ther*. 1999;66:516.

Fluoxetine (eg, *Prozac*)

Propranolol (eg, *Inderal*)

SUMMARY: Fluoxetine increases the beta-adrenergic blocking effects of some beta blockers; cardiac toxicity may result.

RISK FACTORS: No specific risk factors are known.

MECHANISM: Not established. However, fluoxetine or norfluoxetine probably inhibits the activity of the hepatic isozyme CYP2D6 which is partially responsible for the metabolism of propranolol and metoprolol.[1] Thus, the administration of fluoxetine probably could inhibit the metabolism and increase the bioavailability of both beta blockers, leading to elevated plasma concentrations and toxicity.

CLINICAL EVALUATION: A 53-year-old patient taking propranolol 40 mg twice daily developed complete heart block that was associated with a pulse of 30 beats/minute and a syncopal episode 2 weeks after starting fluoxetine 20 mg/day.[2] Two days after the fluoxetine and propranolol were discontinued, he converted to sinus rhythm with a complete left bundle branch block thought to be a chronic conduction defect. A second case report noted a patient with angina taking metoprolol (eg, *Lopressor*) 100 mg/day for 1 month who developed bradycardia 2 days after starting fluoxetine 20 mg/day.[3] The substitution of sotalol (eg, *Betapace*) for metoprolol with continuation of fluoxetine did not result in bradycardia. Fluoxetine can increase the plasma concentrations and pharmacodynamic effects of metoprolol and perhaps other beta blockers.

RELATED DRUGS: Metoprolol interacts similarly with fluoxetine, while sotalol appears unaffected. While the effects of other selective serotonin reuptake inhibitors on beta blocker clearance is not known, fluvoxamine (eg, *Luvox*) and sertraline (*Zoloft*) appear to be less potent inhibitors of CYP2D6 than fluoxetine.

MANAGEMENT OPTIONS:

➥ *Consider Alternative.* Although specific data are lacking, beta blockers that are renally eliminated (eg, atenolol [eg, *Tenormin*]) may be a safer choice.

➥ *Monitor.* Monitor patients stabilized on propranolol or metoprolol for toxicity (eg, bradycardia, conduction defects, hypotension, heart failure, CNS disturbances) if fluoxetine is coadministered. The long half-life of fluoxetine (24 hours) and its metabolite norfluoxetine (half-life 7 days and also known to be a metabolic inhibitor) explains why this interaction may take several weeks to reach its maximum effect. Exercise caution when administering a beta blocker to a patient who has stopped taking fluoxetine within the past 2 weeks.

REFERENCES:

1. Otton SV, et al. Inhibition by fluoxetine of cytochrome P450 2D6 activity. *Clin Pharmacol Ther.* 1993;53:401.
2. Drake WM, et al. Heart block in a patient on propranolol and fluoxetine. *Lancet.* 1994;343:425.
3. Walley T, et al. Interaction of metoprolol and fluoxetine. *Lancet.* 1993;341:967.

Fluoxetine (eg, *Prozac*)

Rasagiline (*Azilect*)

SUMMARY: Theoretically, the concomitant use of rasagiline and selective serotonin reuptake inhibitors (SSRIs) such as fluoxetine could increase the risk of serotonin syndrome.

RISK FACTORS: No specific risk factors known.

MECHANISM: The combination may have additive serotonergic effects.

CLINICAL EVALUATION: Severe serotonin syndrome-like reactions (including fatalities) have occurred when SSRIs were used in patients on nonselective monoamine oxidase inhibitors or selegiline. Thus, combining rasagiline with SSRIs could increase the risk of serotonin syndrome.[1,2] Nonetheless, over 100 patients in rasagiline clinical trials received concomitant SSRIs apparently without evidence of serotonin syndrome. Thus, it appears likely that most patients receiving rasagiline and SSRIs concurrently would not develop a severe adverse drug interaction.

RELATED DRUGS: All SSRIs and selective serotonin/norepinephrine reuptake inhibitors (SNRIs) are expected to interact similarly with rasagiline. Other SSRIs include citalopram (eg, *Celexa*), escitalopram (*Lexapro*), fluvoxamine, paroxetine (eg, *Paxil*), and sertraline (*Zoloft*). SNRIs include duloxetine (*Cymbalta*) and venlafaxine (*Effexor*). Fluvoxamine is contraindicated with rasagiline because, in addition to being an SSRI, it is a potent inhibitor of CYP1A2, the isozyme primarily responsible for the metabolism of rasagiline.

MANAGEMENT OPTIONS:

➡ *Avoid Unless Benefit Outweighs Risk.* Although it is difficult to assess the risk of this interaction, consider the severity of the interaction if it occurs. Rasagiline product information recommends avoiding SSRIs or SNRIs concurrently or within 2 weeks of stopping rasagiline. Because fluoxetine and its active metabolite have such long half-lives, wait at least 5 weeks after stopping fluoxetine before starting rasagiline.

➡ *Monitor.* If SSRIs or SNRIs are used with rasagiline, monitor for symptoms of serotonin syndrome such as agitation, coma, confusion, fever, hyperreflexia, hypomania, incoordination, myoclonus, rigidity, seizures, shivering, sweating, and tremor.

REFERENCES:

1. Chen JJ, et al. Rasagiline: A second-generation monoamine oxidase type-B inhibitor for the treatment of Parkinson's disease. *Am J Health Syst Pharm.* 2006;63:915-928.
2. *Azilect* [package insert]. Kansas City, MO: Teva Neuroscience, Inc.; 2006.

Fluoxetine (*Prozac*)

Risperidone (*Risperdal*)

SUMMARY: A patient on fluoxetine and risperidone developed tardive dyskinesia, but a causal relationship was not established.

RISK FACTORS: No specific risk factors are known.

MECHANISM: Not established. Fluoxetine is known to inhibit the activity of some cytochrome P450 isozymes (eg, CYP2D6 and possibly CYP3A4). It is possible that fluoxetine affects risperidone metabolism.

CLINICAL EVALUATION: An 18-year-old man on fluoxetine and risperidone developed extrapyramidal symptoms followed by persistent tardive dyskinesia (dyskinetic tongue movements).[1] It was proposed that the dyskinesia was related to the combination of fluoxetine and risperidone, but more study is needed to establish a causal relationship.

RELATED DRUGS: The effect of selective serotonin reuptake inhibitors other than fluoxetine on risperidone is not established.

MANAGEMENT OPTIONS: No specific action is required, but be alert for evidence of the interaction.

REFERENCES:
1. Daniel DG, et al. Probably neuroleptic induced tardive dyskinesia in association with combined SSRI and risperidone treatment. *Schizophrenia Res.* 1996;18:149.

4 **Fluoxetine (*Prozac*)**

Ritonavir (*Norvir*)

SUMMARY: Fluoxetine increases ritonavir plasma concentrations in some patients.

RISK FACTORS:

➥ **Pharmacogenetics.** Patients who are extensive CYP2D6 metabolizers would be at greater risk.

MECHANISM: Fluoxetine is an inhibitor of CYP2D6, an enzyme partially responsible for ritonavir metabolism.

CLINICAL EVALUATION: While no published data are available for evaluation, the manufacturer of ritonavir has made available some data on this interaction. Sixteen subjects received single 600 mg doses of ritonavir alone and after fluoxetine 30 mg twice daily for 8 days.[1] The mean area under the concentration time curve of ritonavir increased by 19% when administered following fluoxetine pretreatment. The clinical significance of this increase is unknown, but may produce increased toxicity (eg, nausea, vomiting, diarrhea, paresthesias) in some patients, particularly those who are extensive metabolizers of CYP2D6 substrates.

RELATED DRUGS: The effect of fluoxetine on other protease inhibitors is unknown. Other serotonin reuptake inhibitors may affect ritonavir in a similar manner.

MANAGEMENT OPTIONS: No specific action is required, but be alert for evidence of the interaction.

REFERENCES:

1. Abbott Laboratories. Ritonavir (*Norvir*) package insert. 1996.

Fluoxetine (*Prozac*)

Selegiline (eg, *Eldepryl*)

SUMMARY: Isolated cases suggest that combined therapy with selegiline and fluoxetine may result in mania or hypertension, but a causal relationship has not been established.

RISK FACTORS: No specific risk factors are known.

MECHANISM: Not established. Selegiline is a selective inhibitor of MAO-B, but serotonin is metabolized by MAO-A. Thus, one would not expect that selegiline would produce additive serotonergic effects with selective serotonin reuptake inhibitors (SSRIs). However, the selectivity of selegiline is not absolute, and doses over 10 mg/day may become somewhat nonselective.

CLINICAL EVALUATION: In 2 patients taking selegiline and fluoxetine 20 mg/day, one developed mania and the other hypertension and vasoconstriction.[1]

RELATED DRUGS: The manufacturer of selegiline recommends that it not be used with SSRIs, including fluoxetine, paroxetine (*Paxil*), sertraline (*Zoloft*), and fluvoxamine (*Luvox*).[2]

MANAGEMENT OPTIONS:

➡ **Avoid Unless Benefit Outweighs Risk.** Although the risk of combined use is not established, the potential adverse effects are severe.

➡ **Monitor.** Monitor for evidence of hypertension or mania if the combination is used.

REFERENCES:

1. Suchowersky O, et al. Interaction of fluoxetine and selegiline. *Can J Psychiatry.* 1990;35:571.
2. Product information. Selegiline (*Eldepryl*). Solvay Pharmaceuticals. 1996.

Fluoxetine (*Prozac*)

Sibutramine (*Meridia*)

SUMMARY: The risk of serotonin syndrome would theoretically increase when sibutramine is combined with other serotonergic drugs such as fluoxetine.

RISK FACTORS: No specific risk factors are known.

MECHANISM: Sibutramine inhibits serotonin reuptake; additive serotonergic effects may occur with fluoxetine.

CLINICAL EVALUATION: While no published data are available for evaluation, the manufacturer of sibutramine has made available some data on this interaction.[1] Since sibutramine has serotonergic effects, its concurrent use with other serotonergic drugs (eg, fluoxetine) may increase the risk of serotonin syndrome.[1] Although the actual risk of combining sibutramine with serotonergic drugs is unknown, the fact that serotonin syndrome can result in serious or fatal reactions must be considered.

RELATED DRUGS: Other selective serotonin reuptake inhibitors such as paroxetine (*Paxil*), sertraline (*Zoloft*), and fluvoxamine (*Luvox*) would be expected to interact with sibutramine as well.

MANAGEMENT OPTIONS:

➡ *Avoid Unless Benefit Outweighs Risk.* The manufacturer states that sibutramine should not be used with fluoxetine. This is a prudent recommendation until more information is available.

➡ *Monitor.* Serotonin syndrome can result in neurotoxicity (eg, myoclonus, tremors, rigidity, incoordination, restlessness, hyperreflexia, seizures, coma), psychiatric symptoms (eg, agitation, confusion, hypomania), and temperature regulation abnormalities (eg, fever, sweating). Note that mild forms of serotonin syndrome have also been reported, so consider any combination of the above symptoms possibly related to excessive serotonin activity.

REFERENCES:

1. Product information. Sibutramine (*Meridia*). Knoll Pharmaceuticals. 1997.
2. Mills KC. Serotonin syndrome: a clinical update. *Crit Care Clin.* 1997;13:763.

Fluoxetine (eg, *Prozac*)

Sumatriptan (eg, *Imitrex*)

SUMMARY: The risk of serotonin syndrome may be increased when fluoxetine is used with sumatriptan or other triptans.

RISK FACTORS: No specific risk factors are known.

MECHANISM: Not established. It has been proposed that triptans may have additive serotonergic effects with selective serotonin reuptake inhibitors (SSRIs) or serotonin-norepinephrine reuptake inhibitors (SNRIs).

CLINICAL EVALUATION: Cases of possible serotonin syndrome have occasionally been reported with combined use of triptans and SSRIs, such as fluoxetine and paroxetine (eg, *Paxil*).[1,2] These cases notwithstanding, clinical studies of the combined use of triptans with SSRIs have generally found little evidence of an increased risk of serotonin syndrome. In a prospective study of 12,339 patients who received sumatriptan for migraine, evidence of serotonin syndrome was not seen in the 1,023 patients receiving fluoxetine concurrently.[3] In a randomized, double-blind, crossover study of 20 healthy subjects, fluoxetine did not affect the pharmacokinetics, pharmacodynamics, or adverse reactions of zolmitriptan (*Zomig*).[4] In another randomized, double-blind, crossover study of 12 healthy subjects, paroxetine did not affect the pharmacokinetics, pharmacodynamics, or adverse reactions of rizatriptan (*Maxalt*).[5] Taken together, this information suggests that the combined use of triptans and SSRIs usually does not result in adverse drug interactions, but that it is possible for that serotonin syndrome to occur in certain susceptible individuals.

However, in July 2006, the Food and Drug Administration issued a public health advisory stating that combined use of triptans with SSRIs or SNRIs can result in serotonin syndrome.[6] Few details were presented on the nature of the information that led to this advisory.

RELATED DRUGS: Theoretically, the risk of serotonin syndrome may be increased by any combination of a triptan (almotriptan [*Axert*], eletriptan [*Relpax*], frovatriptan [*Frova*], naratriptan [*Amerge*], rizatriptan, sumatriptan, zolmitriptan) with an SSRI (citalopram [eg, *Celexa*], escitalopram [*Lexapro*], fluoxetine [eg, *Prozac*], fluvoxamine [eg, *Luvox*], paroxetine [eg, *Paxil*], sertraline [eg, *Zoloft*]) or an SNRI (clomipramine [eg, *Anafranil*], duloxetine [*Cymbalta*], imipramine [eg, *Tofranil*], venlafaxine [*Effexor*]).

MANAGEMENT OPTIONS:

➡ *Monitor.* Patients receiving fluoxetine (or other SSRIs or SNRIs) should watch for evidence of serotonin syndrome if they take sumatriptan (or other triptans). Symptoms of serotonin syndrome include agitation, coma, confusion, fever, hyperreflexia, hypomania, incoordination, myoclonus, rigidity, seizures, shivering, sweating, and tremor. Advise patients to contact their health care provider if any of these symptoms occur.

REFERENCES:

1. Hendrix Y, et al. Serotonin syndrome as a result of concomitant use of paroxetine and sumatriptan [in Dutch]. *Ned Tijdschr Geneeskd*. 2005;149(16):888-890.
2. Mathew NT, et al. Serotonin syndrome complicating migraine pharmacotherapy. *Cephalalgia*. 1996;16(5):323-327.
3. Putnam GP, et al. Migraine polypharmacy and the tolerability of sumatriptan: a large-scale, prospective study. *Cephalalgia*. 1999;19(7):668-675.
4. Smith DA, et al. Zolmitriptan (311C90) does not interact with fluoxetine in healthy volunteers. *Int J Clin Pharmacol Ther*. 1998;36(6):301-305.
5. Goldberg MR, et al. Lack of pharmacokinetic and pharmacodynamic interaction between rizatriptan and paroxetine. *J Clin Pharmacol*. 1999;39(2):192-199.
6. FDA Public Health Advisory. Combined Use of 5-Hydroxytryptamine Receptor Agonists (Triptans), Selective Serotonin Reuptake Inhibitors (SSRIs) or Selective Serotonin/Norepinephrine Reuptake Inhibitors (SNRIs) May Result in Life-threatening Serotonin Syndrome. Center for Drug Evaluation and Research (CDER), U.S. Food and Drug Administration. http://www.fda.gov/CDER/DRUG/advisory/SSRI_SS200607.htm. Published July 19, 2006. Updated November 24, 2006. Accessed September 7, 2006.

Fluoxetine (eg, *Prozac*)

Tamoxifen (eg, *Soltamox*)

SUMMARY: CYP2D6 inhibitors, such as fluoxetine, appear to reduce the efficacy of tamoxifen in the treatment of breast cancer.

RISK FACTORS: No specific risk factors are known.

MECHANISM: Tamoxifen is metabolized to 2 active metabolites by CYP2D6, the most important of which is endoxifen. By reducing endoxifen formation, CYP2D6 inhibitors, such as fluoxetine, may reduce tamoxifen efficacy.[1-5]

CLINICAL EVALUATION: A study in patients with breast cancer found substantial reductions in endoxifen plasma concentrations in patients taking potent CYP2D6 inhibitors, such as fluoxetine and paroxetine (eg, *Paxil*), while weak inhibitors, such as sertraline and citalopram (eg, *Celexa*), produced only small reductions.[6] In a preliminary study of 12 women on tamoxifen, the addition of paroxetine 10 mg/day for 4 weeks resulted in a 56% decrease in endoxifen plasma concentrations.[7] A subsequent study in 80 patients starting tamoxifen therapy found that those on CYP2D6 inhibitor antidepressants had substantially lower endoxifen concentrations.[8] The reduction in endoxifen was greatest with paroxetine, intermediate with sertraline, and minimal with venlafaxine (*Effexor*). Venlafaxine had no effect on endoxifen concentrations. Another tamoxifen study found a nearly 2-fold increase in the risk of breast cancer relapse in women with low CYP2D6 activity, either due to CYP2D6-inhibiting drugs or genetic deficiency.[9] Taken together, these results strongly suggest that CYP2D6 inhibitors reduce the efficacy of tamoxifen in the treatment of breast cancer.

RELATED DRUGS: Paroxetine, like fluoxetine, is a potent CYP2D6 inhibitor; duloxetine (*Cymbalta*) and bupropion (eg, *Wellbutrin*) also inhibit CYP2D6. Weaker inhibitors of CYP2D6 include citalopram, escitalopram (*Lexapro*), desvenlafaxine (*Pristiq*), and sertraline. Venlafaxine and mirtazapine (eg, *Remeron*) appear to have little or no effect on CYP2D6 and are unlikely to interact.

MANAGEMENT OPTIONS:

➡️ *Use Alternative.* Patients taking tamoxifen should avoid fluoxetine, paroxetine, duloxetine, and bupropion. Although other SSRIs, such as citalopram and sertraline, are weaker inhibitors of CYP2D6, they can somewhat reduce endoxifen concentrations and may reduce tamoxifen efficacy in some patients. Available evidence suggests that venlafaxine does not affect endoxifen concentrations, so it may be preferable. Mirtazapine has been used effectively for hot flashes in breast cancer survivors, and theoretically it would be unlikely to interact with tamoxifen.[10]

➡️ *Monitor.* If a CYP2D6 inhibitor, such as fluoxetine, is used with tamoxifen, cancer recurrence may be an indication that tamoxifen efficacy has been reduced. If this happens, consider whether the CYP2D6 inhibitor should be stopped.

REFERENCES:

1. Dezentje VO, et al. Clinical implications of CYP2D6 genotyping in tamoxifen treatment for breast cancer. *Clin Cancer Res.* 2009;15(1):15-21.
2. Tan SH, et al. Pharmacogenetics in breast cancer therapy. *Clin Cancer Res.* 2008;14(24):8027-8041.
3. Newman WG, et al. Impaired tamoxifen metabolism reduces survival in familial breast cancer patients. *Clin Cancer Res.* 2008;14(18):5913-5918.
4. Henry NL, et al. Drug interactions and pharmacogenomics in the treatment of breast cancer and depression. *Am J Psychiatry.* 2008;165(10):1251-1255.
5. Algeciras-Schimnich A, et al. Pharmacogenomics of tamoxifen and irinotecan therapies. *Clin Lab Med.* 2008;28(4):553-567.
6. Borges S, et al. Quantitative effect of CYP2D6 genotype and inhibitors on tamoxifen metabolism: implication for optimization of breast cancer treatment. *Clin Pharmacol Ther.* 2006;80(1):61-74.
7. Stearns V, et al. Active tamoxifen metabolite plasma concentrations after coadministration of tamoxifen and the selective serotonin reuptake inhibitor paroxetine. *J Natl Cancer Inst.* 2003;95(23):1758-1764.
8. Jin Y, et al. CYP2D6 genotype, antidepressant use, and tamoxifen metabolism during adjuvant breast cancer treatment. *J Natl Cancer Inst.* 2005;97(1):30-39.
9. Goetz MP, et al. The impact of cytochrome P450 2D6 metabolism in women receiving adjuvant tamoxifen. *Breast Cancer Res Treat.* 2007;101(1):113-121.
10. Biglia N, et al. Mirtazapine for the treatment of hot flushes in breast cancer survivors: a prospective pilot trial. *Breast J.* 2007;13(5):490-495.

Fluoxetine (eg, *Prozac*)

Tamsulosin (*Flomax*)

SUMMARY: Theoretically, the tamsulosin effect may be increased by fluoxetine and other CYP2D6 inhibitors, but the clinical importance of this effect is not established.

RISK FACTORS: No specific risk factors are known.

MECHANISM: Tamsulosin is partially metabolized by CYP2D6 and fluoxetine is a CYP2D6 inhibitor; theoretically, fluoxetine would inhibit tamsulosin metabolism.

CLINICAL EVALUATION: Although the interaction is based on theoretical considerations, tamsulosin should be used with caution with moderate to strong inhibitors of CYP2D6 (eg, fluoxetine).[1]

RELATED DRUGS: Theoretically, other selective serotonin reuptake inhibitors (SSRIs) that are potent or moderate inhibitors of CYP2D6 (eg, duloxetine, paroxetine) would produce a similar effect. SSRIs with minimal effects on CYP2D6 would theoretically decrease the risk of interaction (eg, citalopram [eg, *Celexa*], escitalopram [*Lexapro*], sertraline [eg, *Zoloft*], venlafaxine [*Effexor*]).

MANAGEMENT OPTIONS: No specific action is required, but be alert for evidence of the interaction.

REFERENCES:

1. *Flomax* [package insert]. Ridgefield, CT: Boehringer Ingelheim; 2009.

Fluoxetine (eg, *Prozac*) 2

Terfenadine†

SUMMARY: A patient receiving fluoxetine and terfenadine developed possible cardiac rhythm disturbances, but a causal relationship was not established.

RISK FACTORS: No specific risk factors are known.

MECHANISM: Not established. Limited evidence suggests that fluoxetine (perhaps because of its active metabolite, norfluoxetine) can inhibit CYP3A4, the enzyme responsible for detoxifying terfenadine.

CLINICAL EVALUATION: A 41-year-old man was awakened with shortness of breath and sensation of irregular heartbeat approximately 1 month after fluoxetine 20 mg/day was added to his terfenadine therapy (60 mg twice daily).[1] He also was taking ibuprofen (eg, *Advil*), misoprostol (eg, *Cytotec*), ranitidine (eg, *Zantac*), and a combination of acetaminophen, dichloralphenazone, and isometheptene (eg, *Midrin*). An electrocardiogram upon admission revealed normal sinus rhythm, but there was no mention of a prolonged QT interval (which is expected if excessive terfenadine serum concentrations were present). A Holter monitor placed 12 days later revealed intermittent frequent sinus tachycardia, isolated atrial premature contractions, and 3 couplets. However, the terfenadine had been discontinued "a few days" earlier, so it is likely that little terfenadine remained in the blood at this point. The patient was taking a sympathomimetic (isometheptene) on an as-required basis, which also complicated the assessment of the cardiac findings in this case. Thus, consider a causal relationship tentative.

RELATED DRUGS: Astemizole,[†] like terfenadine, is metabolized by CYP3A4 and can cause ventricular arrhythmias; its interactions appear similar to terfenadine. Loratadine (eg, *Claritin*), fexofenadine (eg, *Allegra*), and cetirizine (eg, *Zyrtec*) do not appear to produce cardiotoxicity and may be safer in patients on fluoxetine. Fluvoxamine (eg, *Luvox*) is known to inhibit CYP3A4 and is contraindicated with terfenadine or astemizole.

MANAGEMENT OPTIONS:

➡ *Avoid Unless Benefit Outweighs Risk.* Although evidence for an interaction between terfenadine and fluoxetine is unconfirmed, avoid concurrent use when possible until more information is available.

➡ *Monitor.* If the combination is used, monitor for evidence of cardiac arrhythmias (eg, fainting, palpitations, shortness of breath).

REFERENCES:

   1. Swims MP. Potential terfenadine-fluoxetine interaction. *Ann Pharmacother.* 1993;27(11):1404-1405.

   † Not available in the United States.

 Fluoxetine (eg, *Prozac*)

Thioridazine

SUMMARY: Fluoxetine may increase thioridazine serum concentrations, and thus may increase the risk of ventricular arrhythmias; avoid concurrent use.

RISK FACTORS:

➡ *Pharmacogenetics.* Extensive metabolizers (EMs) of the CYP2D6 phenotype are expected to experience this interaction to a greater extent than poor metabolizers (PMs) who do not have the gene for production of CYP2D6. PMs would likely already have high serum concentrations of thioridazine, but, theoretically, inhibition of CYP2C19 by fluoxetine might increase levels further. Approximately 8% of whites are deficient in CYP2D6, but the deficiency is rare in Asians, usually 1% or fewer.

➡ *Hypokalemia.* The corrected QT interval (QTc) on the electrocardiogram (ECG) may be prolonged in patients with hypokalemia, thus increasing the risk of this interaction. Any other factor that may prolong the QTc interval would also increase the risk of this interaction.

MECHANISM: Fluoxetine may inhibit the hepatic metabolism of thioridazine by CYP2D6 and possibly also by CYP2C19.

CLINICAL EVALUATION: In a double-blind, randomized, crossover study of the pharmacodynamic effects of thioridazine alone, 9 healthy subjects received single oral doses of thioridazine (10 and 50 mg) compared with placebo.[1] Thioridazine 50 mg increased the QTc by 23 msec, and the 10 mg dose increased QTc by 9 msec. These results suggest that thioridazine produces a dose-related slowing of cardiac repolarization. Thus, drugs such as fluoxetine that inhibit CYP2D6 would be expected to reduce the metabolism of thioridazine and increase the risk of excessive prolongation of the QTc interval and ventricular arrhythmias. Although this interaction is based primarily on theoretical considerations, the potential severity of the interaction suggests to avoid the combination. Moreover, the manufacturer's product information for *Mellaril* states that combined use of thioridazine and fluoxetine is contraindicated;[2] therefore, consider medicolegal issues.

RELATED DRUGS: Paroxetine (eg, *Paxil*), like fluoxetine, is a potent inhibitor of CYP2D6, and is expected to increase the risk of arrhythmias. Fluvoxamine, although not a significant CYP2D6 inhibitor, also increases thioridazine serum concentrations, possibly by inhibiting CYP2C19 and CYP1A2. Other selective serotonin reuptake inhibitors, such as citalopram (eg, *Celexa*) and sertraline (*Zoloft*), are less likely to significantly inhibit CYP2D6, CYP2C19, or CYP1A2. Theoretically, they would be less likely to interact with thioridazine, but little clinical information is available. Although a number of antipsychotic drugs such as thioridazine have been shown to prolong the QT interval, clinical evidence suggests that thioridazine may produce the greatest risk.

MANAGEMENT OPTIONS:

➡ *Use Alternative.* Although the risk of this combination is not well established, use alternatives for 1 of the drugs when possible (see Related Drugs).

➡ *Monitor.* If the combination must be used, monitor the ECG for evidence of QT prolongation and for clinical evidence of arrhythmias (eg, syncope).

REFERENCES:

1. Hartigan-Go K, et al. Concentration-related pharmacodynamic effects of thioridazine and its metabolites in humans. *Clin Pharmacol Ther.* 1996;60:543-553.
2. 'Dear Doctor or Pharmacist' [letter]. East Hanover, NJ: Novartis Pharmaceuticals; July 7, 2000.

Fluoxetine (eg, *Prozac*)

Tolterodine (*Detrol*)

SUMMARY: Fluoxetine increases tolterodine plasma concentrations, but the effect is not thought to be clinically important.

RISK FACTORS:

➡ *Pharmacogenetics.* The interaction is greater in patients with 2 functional CYP2D6 genes than in patients with 1 or no functional CYP2D6 genes.

MECHANISM: Tolterodine is metabolized by CYP2D6 to an active metabolite, 5-hydroxymethyl tolterodine. Because fluoxetine is a potent inhibitor of CYP2D6, it is likely to inhibit this pathway. Tolterodine also is metabolized by CYP3A4 (normally a minor pathway), but under conditions of CYP2D6 deficiency (genetic or pharmacological) CYP3A4 probably serves a greater role in tolterodine elimination.

CLINICAL EVALUATION: Nine women with depression or anxiety and urinary incontinence received tolterodine 2 mg twice daily for 2.5 days, then fluoxetine 20 mg/day for 21 days, then both drugs for an additional 2.5 days.[1] In the 3 patients with 2 functional CYP2D6 genes (EM2), the area under the plasma concentration-time curves of the active moiety (tolterodine plus its active metabolite, 5-HM) increased 2.1-fold, but fluoxetine had no effect on the active moiety in the 4 patients with 1 functional CYP2D6 gene. It was concluded that the effects on tolterodine serum concentrations were within normal variation, and thus unlikely to be clinically important.[1,2]

RELATED DRUGS: Paroxetine (eg, *Paxil*) is also a CYP2D6 inhibitor and would probably produce a similar effect on tolterodine metabolism. Other selective serotonin reuptake inhibitors such as sertraline (eg, *Zoloft*) and citalopram (eg, *Celexa*) are weak CYP2D6 inhibitors, while fluvoxamine appears to have little or no effect on CYP2D6.

MANAGEMENT OPTIONS: No specific action is required, but be alert for evidence of the interaction.

REFERENCES:

1. Brynne N, et al. Fluoxetine inhibits the metabolism of tolterodine-pharmacokinetic implications and proposed clinical relevance. *Br J Clin Pharmacol*. 1999;48(4):553-563.

2. Short DD. Tolterodine, a new antimuscarinic drug for treatment of bladder overactivity–a comment. *Pharmacotherapy*. 1999;19(10):1188.

Fluoxetine (eg, *Prozac*)

Tramadol (eg, *Ultram*)

SUMMARY: Isolated cases of possible serotonin syndrome have occurred in patients taking fluoxetine and tramadol.

RISK FACTORS: No specific risk factors are known.

MECHANISM: Both tramadol and fluoxetine have serotonergic effects, and they may be additive.

CLINICAL EVALUATION: Two cases of possible serotonin syndrome have been reported in women (31 and 72 years of age) who started tramadol in the presence of chronic fluoxetine therapy.[1,2] The 72-year-old patient also had evidence of mania. Based on the standard diagnostic methods, the patient probably had serotonin toxicity.[3,4]

RELATED DRUGS: Isolated cases of serotonin syndrome have been reported when tramadol was combined with other selective serotonin reuptake inhibitors (SSRIs) such as paroxetine (eg, *Paxil*) and sertraline (eg, *Zoloft*). Combining fluoxetine with meperidine or fentanyl theoretically may increase the risk of serotonin toxicity.

MANAGEMENT OPTIONS:

➡ *Consider Alternative.* In patients taking fluoxetine or other SSRIs, consider using an analgesic other than tramadol, meperidine, or fentanyl.

➡ *Monitor.* If the combination is used, monitor for symptoms of serotonin toxicity, including myoclonus, tremor, hyperreflexia, muscle rigidity, fever, sweating, agitation, confusion, hypomania, incoordination, seizures, and coma.

REFERENCES:

1. Gonzalez-Pinto A, et al. Mania and tramadol-fluoxetine combination. *Am J Psychiatry*. 2001;158(6):964-965.

2. Kesavan S, et al. Serotonin syndrome with fluoxetine plus tramadol. *J R Soc Med*. 1999;92(9):474-475.

3. Isbister GK, et al. Serotonin toxicity: a practical approach to diagnosis and treatment. *Med J Aust*. 2007;187(6):361-365.

4. Boyer EW, et al. The serotonin syndrome. *N Engl J Med*. 2005;352(11):1112-1120.

Fluoxetine (eg, *Prozac*)

Tranylcypromine (eg, *Parnate*) AVOID

SUMMARY: Severe or fatal reactions have been reported when nonselective monoamine oxidase inhibitors (MAOIs) are coadministered with selective serotonin reuptake inhibitors (SSRIs) such as fluoxetine; avoid the combination.

RISK FACTORS: No specific risk factors are known.

MECHANISM: Not established. It probably involves increased CNS serotonergic effect.

CLINICAL EVALUATION: The use of fluoxetine and MAOIs together or in close sequence can produce signs and symptoms of serotonin syndrome, including hypomania, confusion, hypertension, and tremor.[1] Several cases of serious or fatal reactions to tranylcypromine have occurred when tranylcypromine was initiated after fluoxetine had been discontinued.[2,3] A 31-year-old woman with depression, anxiety, and obsessional thinking was given a trial of fluoxetine 20 mg/day, but it was discontinued after 2 weeks because of nausea and restlessness.[3] Two days later she was started on tranylcypromine 10 mg/day. On the fourth day of tranylcypromine therapy, she decided to take tranylcypromine 20 mg; within 2 to 3 hours she developed severe shivering, nausea, double vision, anxiety, and confusion. Her blood pressure and temperature were normal. Tranylcypromine was discontinued, and the symptoms resolved within 24 hours. Because of the long half-life of fluoxetine (2 to 3 days) and its active metabolite norfluoxetine (7 to 9 days), fluoxetine interactions theoretically could occur weeks after fluoxetine is discontinued.

RELATED DRUGS: All combinations of nonselective MAOIs (eg, phenelzine [*Nardil*], isocarboxazid [*Marplan*]) and SSRIs (eg, fluvoxamine, paroxetine [eg, *Paxil*], sertraline [eg, *Zoloft*]) are contraindicated.

MANAGEMENT OPTIONS:

➡ ***AVOID COMBINATION.*** Avoid the combined use of fluoxetine and MAOIs. Wait at least 2 weeks after stopping an MAOI before starting fluoxetine or any other SSRI; wait 5 weeks after stopping fluoxetine before starting an MAOI.

REFERENCES:

1. Feighner JP, et al. Adverse consequences of fluoxetine-MAOI combination therapy. *J Clin Psychiatry.* 1990;51(6):222-225.
2. Kline SS, et al. Serotonin syndrome versus neuroleptic malignant syndrome as a cause of death. *Clin Pharm.* 1989;8(7):510-514.
3. Sternbach H. Danger of MAOI therapy after fluoxetine withdrawal. *Lancet.* 1988;2(8615):850-851.

Fluoxetine (eg, *Prozac*)

Trazodone (eg, *Desyrel*)

SUMMARY: A patient developed anxiety and tremor after therapy with trazodone and fluoxetine, but a causal relationship was not established.

RISK FACTORS: No specific risk factors are known.

MECHANISM: Not established. Additive serotonergic effects are possible, as is fluoxetine-induced inhibition of trazodone metabolism by CYP2D6 and to a lesser extent, CYP3A4.

CLINICAL EVALUATION: A 39-year-old man on chronic therapy with trazodone 50 mg/day developed anxiety and worsening hand tremor after fluoxetine 20 mg/day was added to his therapy and his trazodone dose was increased to 100 mg/day.[1] The tremor resolved after both drugs were stopped. The reaction may have resulted from the combined serotonergic effects of trazodone and fluoxetine, but one cannot rule out that it was caused by the increased trazodone dose alone.

RELATED DRUGS: No information is available.

MANAGEMENT OPTIONS: No specific action is required, but be alert for evidence of the interaction.

REFERENCES:

1. Darko W, et al. Myoclonus secondary to the concurrent use of trazodone and fluoxetine. *Vet Hum Toxicol.* 2001;43:214.

 Fluoxetine (eg, *Prozac*)

Triazolam (eg, *Halcion*)

SUMMARY: Fluoxetine does not appear to affect the pharmacokinetics of triazolam in healthy subjects, but more study is needed.

RISK FACTORS: No specific risk factors are known.

MECHANISM: No interaction.

CLINICAL EVALUATION: In 19 healthy subjects, a single oral 0.25 mg dose of triazolam was given with and without pretreatment with fluoxetine 60 mg/day for 8 days.[1] Fluoxetine had no effect on the pharmacokinetics of triazolam as measured by area under the triazolam plasma concentration-time curve, clearance, or half-life. However, 8 days of fluoxetine does not rule out the possibility of an interaction with triazolam. Psychomotor performance tests were not performed, so one cannot exclude the possibility of a pharmacodynamic interaction between the 2 drugs.

RELATED DRUGS: The effect of selective serotonin reuptake inhibitors other than fluoxetine on triazolam is not established, but fluvoxamine (eg, *Luvox*) is known to inhibit CYP3A4, an important isozyme in the metabolism of triazolam.

MANAGEMENT OPTIONS: No interaction.

REFERENCES:

1. Wright CE, et al. A pharmacokinetic evaluation of the combined administration of triazolam and fluoxetine. *Pharmacotherapy.* 1992;12:103.

 Fluoxetine (eg, *Prozac*)

Tryptophan†

SUMMARY: Several patients on fluoxetine developed symptoms of agitation, restlessness, poor concentration, and nausea when tryptophan was added to their therapy; the symptoms resolved when the tryptophan was discontinued.

RISK FACTORS: No specific risk factors are known.

MECHANISM: Not established. Fluoxetine inhibits the reuptake of serotonin into neurons, and tryptophan is a precursor for serotonin. An excessive serotonin effect may be involved.

CLINICAL EVALUATION: Five patients receiving fluoxetine for obsessive-compulsive disorder were started on tryptophan 2 g/day. The dose was increased by 2 g every 5 days in an attempt to enhance the response to fluoxetine.[1] All 5 patients developed agitation after starting tryptophan; other symptoms included restlessness, poor concentration, nausea, diarrhea, and worsening of their obsessive-compulsive disorders. The symptoms usually occurred a few days after starting the tryptophan. All adverse symptoms resolved when tryptophan was discontinued, but improvement occurred over a few weeks. Some patients had taken tryptophan previously without adverse effects. The temporal relationship between the onset and offset of symptoms, the initiation and discontinuation of tryptophan, and the fact that neither drug alone produced the symptoms suggest that the combination was responsible for the reactions in these patients. Nonetheless, more study is needed to determine the incidence and magnitude of this interaction in the general population of patients likely to receive these drugs. Because of the long half-life of fluoxetine (2 to 3 days) and its active metabolite norfluoxetine (7 to 9 days), interactions could require 2 to 4 weeks to dissipate.

RELATED DRUGS: Pending additional study, assume that all selective serotonin reuptake inhibitors (SSRIs) interact with tryptophan.

MANAGEMENT OPTIONS:

➡ *Avoid Unless Benefit Outweighs Risk.* Until more information on safety and efficacy is available, avoid concurrent use of fluoxetine or other SSRIs with tryptophan.

➡ *Monitor.* If the combination is used, monitor patients for the symptoms previously described and for a reduced therapeutic response to fluoxetine. It may be necessary to discontinue tryptophan if the reaction occurs.

REFERENCES:

1. Steiner W, et al. Toxic reaction following the combined administration of fluoxetine and L-tryptophan: five case reports. *Biol Psychiatry.* 1986;21:1067-1071.

2. FDA. *Drug Bull.* 1990;20:2.

† The FDA requested a nationwide recall of all nonprescription supplements that contain L-tryptophan as the sole major component because of a possible link with eosinophilia myalgia.[2] However, it may still be available in some supplements or natural products.

Fluoxetine (eg, *Prozac*)

Warfarin (eg, *Coumadin*)

SUMMARY: Limited clinical evidence suggests fluoxetine does not affect the hypoprothrombinemic response to warfarin, but more study is needed. Isolated reports suggest that fluoxetine alone can increase the risk of bleeding in some patients.

RISK FACTORS: No specific risk factors are known.

MECHANISM: Not established. Some evidence suggests fluoxetine may have an intrinsic inhibitory effect on hemostasis, perhaps by inhibiting platelet aggregation.[1] Fluoxetine has been reported to increase serum concentrations of phenytoin, a drug metabolized by the same isozyme (CYP2C9) as warfarin.

CLINICAL EVALUATION: Three healthy subjects received a single oral dose of warfarin 20 mg on the following 3 occasions: alone, 3 hours after a single fluoxetine 30 mg dose, and after 1 week of fluoxetine 30 mg/day.[2] Fluoxetine had no effect on the hypoprothrombinemic response or the half-life of warfarin. However, because of the small number of subjects and the fact that warfarin enantiomers were not measured, additional study is needed to determine whether fluoxetine affects the pharmacokinetics or pharmacodynamics of warfarin. Another report briefly mentions a patient in whom severe bruising occurred after receiving fluoxetine and warfarin concomitantly. However, the authors did not conclude that a causal relationship was established between the bleeding and combined effect of the 2 drugs.[3] Moreover, they found no evidence of an increase in warfarin response in a retrospective analysis of 6 other patients who had received fluoxetine and warfarin concomitantly. Although the limited clinical evidence available suggests that fluoxetine does not increase the hypoprothrombinemic response to warfarin, it is possible that it could increase the risk of bleeding through some other mechanism. Bleeding has been reported in a number of patients receiving fluoxetine in the absence of warfarin.[4,5] A 40-year-old woman developed ecchymoses and menorrhagia after starting fluoxetine; the bleeding improved after fluoxetine was discontinued but reappeared when the patient restarted the fluoxetine about a month later.[4] At least 8 other patients also have developed bleeding while taking fluoxetine, most of whom were taking fluoxetine 80 mg/day.[5] No further episodes of bleeding were reported by any of the 8 patients after the fluoxetine was discontinued. An epidemiologic study did not find an increase in hospitalization for upper GI bleeding when selective serotonin reuptake inhibitors were added to patients receiving chronic warfarin therapy.[6]

RELATED DRUGS: Although little is known regarding the use of fluoxetine with oral anticoagulants other than warfarin, the same precautions would apply until data are available. Based on limited data, other selective serotonin reuptake inhibitors also may increase the risk of bleeding in patients receiving oral anticoagulants.

MANAGEMENT OPTIONS:

➡ *Monitor.* Although evidence for a fluoxetine-induced increase in the hypoprothrombinemic response to warfarin is limited, monitor for altered warfarin effect if fluoxetine is initiated, discontinued, or changed in dosage. Adjust warfarin dosage as needed. Note that the risk of bleeding might be increased even if the hypoprothrombinemic response is in the desired range.

REFERENCES:

1. Alderman CP, et al. Abnormal platelet aggregation associated with fluoxetine therapy. *Ann Pharmacother.* 1992;26:1517-1519.
2. Rowe H, et al. The effects of fluoxetine on warfarin metabolism in the rat and man. *Life Sci.* 1978;23:807-811.
3. Claire RJ, et al. Potential interaction between warfarin sodium and fluoxetine. *Am J Psychiatry.* 1991;148:1604.
4. Aranth J, et al. Bleeding, a side effect of fluoxetine. *Am J Psychiatry.* 1992;149:412.
5. Yaryura-Tobias JA, et al. Fluoxetine and bleeding in obsessive-compulsive disorder. *Am J Psychiatry.* 1991;148:949.
6. Kurdyak PA, et al. Antidepressants, warfarin, and the risk of hemorrhage. *J Clin Psychopharmacol.* 2005;25:561-564.

Fluphenazine Decanoate (eg, *Prolixin*)

Imipramine (eg, *Tofranil*)

SUMMARY: Phenothiazines may increase serum concentrations of some tricyclic antidepressants (TCAs), and TCAs may increase neuroleptic serum concentrations. These changes would be expected to increase both the therapeutic and toxic effects of each drug, but the degree to which these interactions alter the therapeutic and toxic responses to each drug is not well established.

RISK FACTORS: No specific risk factors are known.

MECHANISM: It is proposed that neuroleptics may inhibit the metabolism of TCAs.[1,2] Evidence also has been presented indicating that TCAs may inhibit neuroleptic metabolism.[3,4] Finally, neuroleptics and TCAs may exhibit additive anticholinergic effects.

CLINICAL EVALUATION: Phenothiazines and TCAs have been used together for many years, often with apparently positive results. Nevertheless, there is considerable evidence that the drugs affect each other's pharmacokinetics. Studies indicate that in schizophrenic patients, TCA plasma concentrations are increased and urinary excretion is decreased when neuroleptics are given concomitantly.[1] In 1 study of 4 patients, extremely high TCA concentrations were found during concurrent therapy with imipramine and fluphenazine decanoate,[5] although there was a curious absence of adverse effects from these elevated levels. In 82 depressed patients, the 35 who were receiving concurrent neuroleptic therapy had 40% higher plasma desipramine concentrations than the 47 who were not receiving neuroleptics.[6] In another report, extremely high desipramine (eg, *Norpramin*) plasma concentrations associated with deterioration of therapeutic response were seen in 2 patients on concurrent therapy with trifluoperazine and chlorpromazine (eg, *Thorazine*).[7] There is also evidence to suggest that overdoses of TCAs plus neuroleptics produce more severe adverse cardiac effects than overdoses of TCAs alone.[8] Tricyclic antidepressants also have been reported to increase plasma concentrations of neuroleptics. In a study of 8 patients, butaperazine plasma concentrations were higher when desipramine was given concomitantly.[3] The effect was seen in the 6 patients who received at least 150 mg/day of desipramine but not in the 2 patients who received less than 150 mg/day. In 7 schizophrenic patients receiving chlorpromazine 300 mg/day, the addition of nortriptyline (eg, *Pamelor*) 150 mg/day increased plasma chlorpromazine concentrations, reduced blood pressure, and markedly reduced the therapeutic response to chlorpromazine as measured by the Inpatient Multidimensional Psychiatric Scale.[4] In 4 patients, perphenazine prolonged the half-life and reduced the clearance of nortriptyline.[9]

Nevertheless, combination products containing both a neuroleptic and a TCA (eg, *Etrafon, Triavil*) have been used for many years. More study is needed to ascertain whether the purported benefit of combined use outweighs the risk.

RELATED DRUGS: No information is available.

MANAGEMENT OPTIONS:

➡ *Monitor.* In patients receiving combined therapy with neuroleptics and TCAs, be alert for evidence of increased toxicity and altered therapeutic response.

REFERENCES:

1. Gram LF, et al. Drug interaction: inhibitory effect of neuroleptics on metabolism of tricyclic antidepressants in man. *Br Med J.* 1972;1:463-465.
2. Gram LF, et al. Influence of neuroleptics and benzodiazepines on metabolism of tricyclic antidepressants in man. *Am J Psychiatry.* 1974;131:863-866.
3. el-Yousef MK, et al. Letter: Tricyclic antidepressants and phenothiazines. *JAMA.* 1974;229:1419.
4. Loga S, et al. Interaction of chlorpromazine and nortriptyline in patients with schizophrenia. *Clin Pharmacokinet.* 1981;6:454-462.
5. Siris SG, et al. Plasma imipramine concentrations in patients receiving concomitant fluphenazine decanoate. *Am J Psychiatry.* 1982;139:104-106.
6. Bock JL, et al. Desipramine hydroxylation: variability and effect of antipsychotic drugs. *Clin Pharmacol Ther.* 1983;33:322-328.
7. Conrad CD, et al. Symptom exacerbation in psychotically depressed adolescents due to high desipramine plasma concentrations. *J Clin Psychopharmacol.* 1986;6:161-164.
8. Wilens TE, et al. Adverse cardiac effects of combined neuroleptic ingestion and tricyclic antidepressant overdose. *J Clin Psychopharmacol.* 1990;10:51-54.
9. Overo KF, et al. Interaction of perphenazine with the kinetics of nortriptyline. *Acta Pharmacol Toxicol.* 1977;40:97-105.

4 Fluphenazine (eg, *Prolixin*)

Olanzapine (*Zyprexa*)

SUMMARY: A man developed neuroleptic malignant syndrome after olanzapine was added to his regimen, but a causal relationship was not established.

RISK FACTORS: No specific risk factors are known.

MECHANISM: Not established.

CLINICAL EVALUATION: A 57-year-old man on fluphenazine developed neuroleptic malignant syndrome 1 month after olanzapine was added to his regimen.[1] It is not clear, however, that the reaction resulted from the combined effects of the 2 drugs. Rifampin, a potent enzyme inducer, was discontinued 2 weeks before the neuroleptic malignant syndrome occurred. This could result in increasing plasma concentrations for several of his medications, and could have contributed to the neuroleptic malignant syndrome.

RELATED DRUGS: No information is available.

MANAGEMENT OPTIONS: No specific action is required, but be alert for evidence of the interaction.

REFERENCES:

1. Tofler IT, Ahmed B. Atypical (olanzapine) plus conventional (fluphenazine) neuroleptic treatment associated with the neuroleptic malignant syndrome. *J Clin Psychopharmacol.* 2003;23:672-674.

Flurazepam (eg, *Dalmane*) 5

Warfarin (eg, *Coumadin*)

SUMMARY: Flurazepam does not appear to affect the hypoprothrombinemic response to warfarin.

RISK FACTORS: No specific risk factors are known.

MECHANISM: No interaction.

CLINICAL EVALUATION: In a study of 8 normal subjects, flurazepam did not affect plasma warfarin levels.[1] A slight decrease in the hypoprothrombinemic effect of warfarin seen in these subjects was not substantiated by subsequent observations of 12 patients maintained on chronic warfarin therapy. The lack of interaction found in this published study is consistent with numerous informal observations of patients receiving this combination.

RELATED DRUGS: The effect of flurazepam on oral anticoagulants other than warfarin is not established, but there is no reason to expect that they interact.

MANAGEMENT OPTIONS: No interaction.

REFERENCES:

1. Robinson DS, et al. Interaction of benzodiazepines with warfarin in man. Paper presented at: Annual Symposium on Benzodiazepines; November 1971; Milan, Italy.

Flurbiprofen (eg, *Ansaid*)

Methotrexate (eg, *Rheumatrex*)

SUMMARY: A case report suggested flurbiprofen increased methotrexate toxicity; prospective study failed to demonstrate an interaction.

RISK FACTORS: No specific risk factors are known.

MECHANISM: Some nonsteroidal anti-inflammatory drugs appear to reduce the renal clearance or renal tubular secretion of methotrexate, but the effect of flurbiprofen on methotrexate is not established.

CLINICAL EVALUATION: A patient with rheumatoid arthritis taking methotrexate 2.5 mg 3 times weekly developed neutropenia, thrombocytopenia, and GI bleeding within 2 weeks of adding flurbiprofen 100 mg/day to her regimen, but a causal relationship was not established.[1] In a study of 5 patients with rheumatoid arthritis, flurbiprofen 300 mg/day for 7 days had no effect on methotrexate administered IM (15 mg) or PO (20 mg).[2]

RELATED DRUGS: Several nonsteroidal anti-inflammatory drugs and aspirin have been shown to increase methotrexate plasma concentrations. Acetaminophen (eg, *Tylenol*) has not been shown to affect methotrexate response.

MANAGEMENT OPTIONS:

➡ *Consider Alternative.* Until more information is available on this interaction, it is preferable to avoid flurbiprofen (as well as other NSAIDs) in patients receiving antineoplastic doses of methotrexate. If possible, use a non-NSAID analgesic instead.

➡ **Monitor.** If the combination is used, observe the patient for signs of methotrexate toxicity including mucosal ulceration, renal dysfunction, and blood dyscrasias. Decreasing the methotrexate dosage may be required.

REFERENCES:

1. Frenia ML, et al. Methotrexate and nonsteroidal antiinflammatory drug interactions. *Ann Pharmacother*. 1992;26:234-237.

2. Skeith KJ, et al. Lack of significant interaction between low dose methotrexate and ibuprofen or flurbiprofen in patients with arthritis. *J Rheumatol*. 1990;17:1008-1110.

 Flurbiprofen

Phenprocoumon†

SUMMARY: Some patients receiving oral anticoagulants developed excessive hypoprothrombinemia and bleeding after flurbiprofen was initiated.

RISK FACTORS:

➡ **Concurrent Diseases.** Patients with peptic ulcer disease or a history of GI bleeding are probably at greater risk.

MECHANISM: Not established. In 1 study, flurbiprofen did not affect the serum concentrations of phenprocoumon[1]; little is known regarding effects on warfarin (eg, *Coumadin*). Flurbiprofen-induced inhibition of platelet function might contribute to an increased bleeding tendency.

CLINICAL EVALUATION: Three of 19 patients stabilized on phenprocoumon developed excessive hypoprothrombinemia when flurbiprofen 150 mg/day was started, and 2 patients had bleeding episodes.[1] In another report, 2 patients stabilized on acenocoumarol† developed bleeding and excessive hypoprothrombinemia within 2 to 3 days of starting flurbiprofen 150 to 300 mg/day.[2] Thus, some patients receiving this combination are likely to develop an enhanced hypoprothrombinemic response, although the available data are insufficient to determine the incidence of the interaction.

RELATED DRUGS: All nonsteroidal anti-inflammatory drugs (NSAIDs) inhibit platelet function, cause gastric erosions, and probably increase the risk of GI bleeding. However, some NSAIDs, such as ibuprofen (eg, *Advil*), naproxen (eg, *Naprosyn*), or diclofenac (eg, *Cataflam*), may be less likely to increase oral anticoagulant–induced hypoprothrombinemia than other NSAIDs. The degree to which warfarin interacts with flurbiprofen has not been established, but assume that an interaction will occur until evidence to the contrary is available. In a retrospective cohort study, hospitalizations for hemorrhagic peptic ulcer disease were approximately 13 times higher in patients receiving warfarin plus an NSAID than in patients receiving neither drug.[3] Acenocoumarol interacts similarly.

MANAGEMENT OPTIONS:

➡ **Avoid Unless Benefit Outweighs Risk.** Because all NSAIDs probably increase the risk of GI bleeding in patients taking oral anticoagulants, use the combination only after careful consideration of the benefit versus risk. If an NSAID must be used with an oral anticoagulant, use NSAIDs that are unlikely to affect the hypoprothrombinemic response to oral anticoagulants (see Related Drugs). If the NSAID is being used as an analgesic or antipyretic, acetaminophen is probably safer to use with oral anticoagulants. Nonacetylated salicylates (eg, choline salicylate, magnesium salicylate, salsalate, sodium salicylate) also are probably safer with oral anticoagulants than NSAIDs because they have minimal effects on platelet function and the gastric mucosa.

➡ *Monitor.* If any NSAID is used with an oral anticoagulant, carefully monitor the prothrombin time and watch for evidence of bleeding, especially from the GI tract.

REFERENCES:
1. Marbet GA, et al. Interaction study between phenoprocoumon and flurbiprofen. *Curr Med Res Opin.* 1977;5(1):26-31.
2. Stricker BH, et al. Interaction between flurbiprofen and coumarins. *Br Med J.* 1982;285(6344):812-813.
3. Shorr RI, et al. Concurrent use of nonsteroidal anti-inflammatory drugs and oral anticoagulants places elderly persons at high risk for hemorrhagic peptic ulcer disease. *Arch Intern Med.* 1993;153(14):1665-1670.

† Not available in the United States.

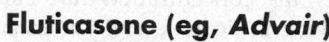

Fluticasone (eg, *Advair*)

Itraconazole (eg, *Sporanox*)

SUMMARY: Itraconazole may increase the fluticasone effect, leading to Cushing syndrome and other evidence of corticosteroid toxicity.

RISK FACTORS: No specific risk factors are known.

MECHANISM: Itraconazole appears to inhibit the CYP3A4 metabolism of fluticasone.

CLINICAL EVALUATION: After observing Cushing syndrome in 4 lung transplant patients given itraconazole with inhaled fluticasone, a study of the interaction was done in 17 lung transplant patients on fluticasone. In 10 patients given concurrent itraconazole for 14 days, plasma fluticasone concentrations were more than 2.5 times higher than in the 7 patients who were not given itraconazole.[1] Another report describes a 55-year-old man with asthma who, after having itraconazole added to his inhaled fluticasone, developed Cushing syndrome (moon face, acne, easy bruising, buffalo hump, myopathy, and impaired glucose tolerance).[2] It took many months for the symptoms to resolve and for the adrenal suppression to abate.

RELATED DRUGS: Fluconazole (eg, *Diflucan*), ketoconazole (eg, *Nizoral*), posaconazole (*Noxafil*), and voriconazole (*Vfend*) also inhibit the activity of CYP3A4 and are expected to increase the plasma concentrations of budesonide. Other corticosteroids that are metabolized by CYP3A4 and also may interact with CYP3A4 inhibitors include budesonide (eg, *Pulmicort*), dexamethasone (eg, *Baycadron*), and methylprednisolone (eg, *Medrol*).

MANAGEMENT OPTIONS:

➡ *Consider Alternative.* Consider using an alternative to one of the drugs (see Related Drugs).

➡ *Monitor.* If fluticasone and itraconazole are used concurrently, monitor for Cushing syndrome. Other evidence of corticosteroid toxicity includes increased blood glucose, hypertension, bone fractures, muscle weakness, cataracts, glaucoma, mood swings, and poor wound healing.

REFERENCES:
1. Naef R, et al. Itraconazole comedication increases systemic levels of inhaled fluticasone in lung transplant patients. *Respiration.* 2007;74(4):418-422.
2. Woods DR, et al. Cushings syndrome without excess cortisol. *BMJ.* 2006;332(7539):469-470.

Fluticasone (eg, *Advair*)

Ketoconazole (eg, *Nizoral*)

SUMMARY: Ketoconazole administration increases fluticasone concentrations; some patients may experience toxicity.

RISK FACTORS: No specific risk factors are known.

MECHANISM: Fluticasone metabolism via CYP3A4 is inhibited by ketoconazole.

CLINICAL EVALUATION: While specific data are limited, the manufacturer of fluticasone notes that in 8 healthy volunteers, the coadministration of a single dose of orally inhaled fluticasone propionate 1,000 mcg with multiple doses of ketoconazole 200 mg to steady state resulted in increased plasma fluticasone propionate exposure (amount of increase not noted), but had no effect on plasma cortisol area under the concentration-time curve.[1] Pending further data, observe patients receiving fluticasone and ketoconazole for the potential of increased fluticasone effects.

RELATED DRUGS: Fluconazole (eg, *Diflucan*), itraconazole (eg, *Sporanox*), posaconazole (*Noxafil*), and voriconazole (*Vfend*) also inhibit the activity of CYP3A4 and are expected to increase the plasma concentrations of fluticasone.

MANAGEMENT OPTIONS:

➡ ***Monitor.*** Monitor patients taking fluticasone for evidence of toxicity if ketoconazole or other potent CYP3A4 inhibitors are coadministered.

REFERENCES:
1. *Advair Diskus* [package insert]. Research Triangle Park, NC: GlaxoSmithKline; 2008.

 Fluticasone (eg, *Advair*)

Ritonavir (*Norvir*)

SUMMARY: Ritonavir administration increases fluticasone concentrations; some patients may experience toxicity.

RISK FACTORS: No specific risk factors are known.

MECHANISM: Fluticasone metabolism via CYP3A4 is inhibited by ritonavir.

CLINICAL EVALUATION: The manufacturer of fluticasone nasal spray reported marked increases in fluticasone plasma concentrations with concurrent ritonavir (100 mg twice daily for 7 days).[1] This was accompanied by an 86% decrease in the serum cortisol area under the curve. Also numerous cases of Cushing syndrome have been reported following combined use of ritonavir with fluticasone (inhaled or nasal).[2-10] The interaction appears to be both large and predictable; therefore, generally avoid the combination.

RELATED DRUGS: Other protease inhibitors including amprenavir†, atazanavir (*Reyataz*), darunavir (*Prezista*), fosamprenavir (*Lexiva*), indinavir (*Crixivan*), nelfinavir (*Viracept*), and saquinavir (eg, *Invirase*) also inhibit the activity of CYP3A and are expected to increase the plasma concentration of fluticasone. Other corticosteroids that are metabolized by CYP3A4 and also may interact with CYP3A4 inhibitors include budesonide (*Pulmicort*), dexamethasone (eg, *Baycadron*), and methylprednisolone (eg, *Medrol*).

MANAGEMENT OPTIONS:

➠ *Consider Alternative.* Consider using an alternative to one of the drugs (see Related Drugs).

➠ *Monitor.* If fluticasone and ritonavir are used concurrently, monitor for Cushing syndrome (eg, moon face, acne, easy bruising, increased facial hair, buffalo hump). Other evidence of corticosteroid toxicity includes increased blood glucose, hypertension, bone fractures, muscle weakness, cataracts, glaucoma, mood swings, and poor wound healing.

REFERENCES:

1. *Advair Diskus* [package insert]. Research Triangle Park, NC: GlaxoSmithKline; 2008.
2. Hillebrand-Haverkort ME, et al. Ritonavir-induced Cushing's syndrome in a patient treated with nasal fluticasone. *AIDS.* 1999;13(13):1803.
3. Chen F, et al. Cushing's syndrome and severe adrenal suppression in patients treated with ritonavir and inhaled nasal fluticasone. *Sex Transm Infect.* 1999;75(4):274.
4. Gupta SK, et al. Exogenous cushing syndrome mimicking human immunodeficiency virus lipodystrophy. *Clin Infect Dis.* 2002;35(6):E69-E71.
5. Clevenbergh P, et al. Iatrogenic Cushing's syndrome in an HIV-infected patient treated with inhaled corticosteroids (fluticasone propionate) and low dose ritonavir enhanced PI containing regimen. *J Infect.* 2002;44(3):194-195.
6. Rouanet I, et al. Cushing's syndrome in a patient treated by ritonavir/lopinavir and inhaled fluticasone. *HIV Med.* 2003;4(2):149-150.
7. Samaras K, et al. Iatrogenic Cushing's syndrome with osteoporosis and secondary adrenal failure in human immunodeficiency virus-infected patients receiving inhaled corticosteroids and ritonavir-boosted protease inhibitors: six cases. *J Clin Endocrinol Metab.* 2005;90(7):4394-4398.
8. Foisy MM, et al. Adrenal suppression and Cushing's syndrome secondary to an interaction between ritonavir and fluticasone: a review of the literature. *HIV Med.* 2008;9(6):389-396.
9. Dupont C, et al. Cushing's syndrome induced by combined treatment with inhaled fluticasone and oral ritonavir. *Rev Mal Respir.* 2009;26(7):779-782.
10. Valin N, et al. Iatrogenic Cushing's syndrome in HIV-infected patients receiving ritonavir and inhaled fluticasone: description of 4 new cases and review of the literature. *J Int Assoc Physicians AIDS Care.* 2009;8(2):113-121.

† Not available in the United States.

Fluvastatin (*Lescol*) 4

Glyburide (eg, *DiaBeta*)

SUMMARY: Fluvastatin administration produces a minor change in glyburide concentrations; a minimal change in patient hypoglycemic response is expected.

RISK FACTORS: No specific risk factors are known.

MECHANISM: Unknown.

CLINICAL EVALUATION: Sixteen healthy subjects received fluvastatin 40 mg/day for 15 days.[1] A single dose of glyburide 3.5 mg was administered on days 1 and 15 of fluvastatin dosing. The area under the concentration-time curve and peak concentration of glyburide were increased about 20% by fluvastatin administration. Oral glucose tolerance tests administered 1.5 hours after glyburide administration were not changed by fluvastatin coadministration. Glyburide administration did not alter fluvastatin concentrations. The changes in glyburide concentrations are not likely to affect glucose control.

RELATED DRUGS: Simvastatin (eg, *Zocor*) produces a similar change in glyburide concentrations. The effect of other HMG-CoA inhibitors on glyburide is unknown. Fluvastatin produced a similar effect on tolbutamide (eg, *Orinase*) concentrations.

MANAGEMENT OPTIONS: No specific action is required, but be alert for evidence of the interaction.

REFERENCES:
1. Appel S, et al. Lack of interaction between fluvastatin and oral hypoglycemic agents in healthy subjects and patients with non-insulin-dependent diabetes mellitus. *Am J Cardiol.* 1995;76(2):29A-32A.

5   Fluvastatin (*Lescol*)

Itraconazole (eg, *Sporanox*)

SUMMARY: No interaction.

RISK FACTORS: No specific risk factors are known.

MECHANISM: No interaction.

CLINICAL EVALUATION: Ten healthy subjects received placebo or itraconazole 100 mg/day for 4 days. A single dose of fluvastatin 40 mg was administered on day 4. No change in fluvastatin area under the concentration-time curve or peak concentration was noted following itraconazole administration.[1]

RELATED DRUGS: Ketoconazole (eg, *Nizoral*) is not expected to interact with fluvastatin. Fluconazole (eg, *Diflucan*) has been reported to inhibit the enzyme responsible for the metabolism of fluvastatin (CYP2C9) and may increase fluvastatin concentrations.

MANAGEMENT OPTIONS: No interaction.

REFERENCES:
1. Kivisto KT, et al. Different effects of itraconazole on the pharmacokinetics of fluvastatin and lovastatin. *Br J Clin Pharmacol.* 1998;46(1):49-53.

Fluvastatin (*Lescol*)

Rifampin (eg, *Rifadin*)

SUMMARY: Rifampin administration reduces fluvastatin plasma concentrations; reduction of fluvastatin's cholesterol-lowering effect is likely.

RISK FACTORS: No specific risk factors are known.

MECHANISM: Rifampin may increase the metabolism of fluvastatin via the CYP2C9 pathway. A reduction in fluvastatin bioavailability and systemic clearance may result.

CLINICAL EVALUATION: While few details of the interaction have been published for evaluation, the magnitude of the interaction merits careful patient observation.[1,2] Rifampin pretreatment (dose and duration not stated) reduced the mean area under the concentration-time curve and peak plasma concentration of fluvastatin 50% and 59%, respectively. Oral clearance was increased 95%. While no data are provided on the effect of the interaction on fluvastatin's cholesterol-lowering activity, a decrease of this extent in fluvastatin plasma concentration would be expected to reduce its efficacy. Combined therapy with rifampin that was limited to a few weeks would not be expected to produce long-term adverse effects caused by the temporary reduction in fluvastatin concentrations.

RELATED DRUGS: Rifampin is known to reduce the plasma concentrations of other cholesterol lowering drugs, especially those that are CYP3A4 substrates (eg, simvastatin, [*Zocor*], lovastatin [*Mevacor*]). Other statins that are metabolized by CYP3A4 (cerivastatin [*Baycol*], atorvastatin [*Lipitor*]) probably would be affected by rifampin but perhaps to a lesser extent. Because pravastatin (*Pravachol*) is not a CYP3A4 substrate, rifampin may have limited effect on its pharmacokinetics.

MANAGEMENT OPTIONS:

➡ *Consider Alternative.* For patients taking rifampin, select cholesterol-lowering drugs that are not dependent on CYP3A4 or CYP2C9 for their metabolism.

➡ *Monitor.* Monitor serum cholesterol in patients taking fluvastatin when rifampin is administered for more than a few weeks.

REFERENCES:

1. Jokubaitis, LA. Updated clinical safety experience with fluvastatin. *Am J Cardiol.* 1994;73:18D. Review.
2. Product information. Fluvastatin (*Lescol*). Novartis Pharmaceuticals. 1999.

Fluvastatin (*Lescol*)

Tolbutamide (eg, *Orinase*)

SUMMARY: Fluvastatin administration produces a minor increase in tolbutamide plasma concentrations; a minimal change in patient hypoglycemic response would be expected.

RISK FACTORS: No specific risk factors are known.

MECHANISM: Unknown.

CLINICAL EVALUATION: Sixteen healthy subjects received fluvastatin 40 mg/day for 15 days.[1] A single oral dose of tolbutamide 1 g was administered on days 1 and 15 of fluvastatin dosing. The area under the concentration-time curve and peak concentration of tolbutamide were increased about 10% to 20%, respectively, by fluvastatin administration. Oral glucose tolerance tests administered 1.5 hours after tolbutamide administration were not changed by fluvastatin coadministration. Tolbutamide administration did not alter fluvastatin concentrations. The changes in tolbutamide concentrations are not likely to affect glucose control.

RELATED DRUGS: Simvastatin (*Zocor*) produces a similar, limited change in tolbutamide concentrations. The effect of other HMG-CoA inhibitors on tolbutamide is unknown. Fluvastatin produced a similar effect on glyburide (eg, *DiaBeta*) concentrations.

MANAGEMENT OPTIONS: No specific action is required, but be alert for evidence of the interaction.

REFERENCES:

1. Appel S, et al. Lack of interaction between fluvastatin and oral hypoglycemic agents in healthy subjects and patients with non-insulin-dependent diabetes mellitus. *Am J Cardiol.* 1995;76:29A-32A.

Fluvoxamine

Lansoprazole (*Prevacid*)

SUMMARY: Fluvoxamine increases the plasma concentrations of lansoprazole, but the clinical importance of this effect is not established.

RISK FACTORS:

→ **Pharmacogenetics.** Only extensive metabolizers (EMs) of CYP2C19 (homozygous or heterozygous) are susceptible to fluvoxamine inhibition; poor metabolizers (PMs) of CYP2C19 are not affected by this interaction.

MECHANISM: Fluvoxamine inhibits CYP2C19, the enzyme responsible for the majority of lansoprazole's metabolism.

CLINICAL EVALUATION: In 18 healthy subjects with various CYP2C19 genotypes (6 homozygous EMs, 6 heterozygous EMs, and 6 PMs), single doses of lansoprazole were given with and without pretreatment with fluvoxamine 50 mg/day for 6 days.[1] Fluvoxamine substantially increased the lansoprazole area under the plasma concentration-time curve in homozygous EMs and heterozygous EMs but had no effect on lansoprazole in PMs. The extent to which this would increase adverse reactions to lansoprazole is not known, but the risk is probably small.

RELATED DRUGS: Omeprazole (eg, *Prilosec*) is similarly affected by fluvoxamine; theoretically, esomeprazole (*Nexium*) and pantoprazole (*Protonix*) are likely to be affected in a similar manner. Because CYP2C19 is a minor pathway for rabeprazole (*Aciphex*), fluvoxamine coadministration would be expected to have little effect on rabeprazole concentrations.

MANAGEMENT OPTIONS: No specific action is required, but be alert for evidence of the interaction.

REFERENCES:

1. Yasui-Furukori N, et al. Effects of fluvoxamine on lansoprazole pharmacokinetics in relation to CYP2C19 genotypes. *J Clin Pharmacol.* 2004;44:1223-1229.

 Fluvoxamine

Lithium (eg, *Eskalith*)

SUMMARY: Isolated cases of adverse neurological effects have been reported in patients receiving fluvoxamine and lithium, but a causal relationship is not established.

RISK FACTORS: No specific risk factors are known.

MECHANISM: It has been proposed that the side effects are related to excessive serotonin effects, because lithium increases serotonin synthesis and fluvoxamine increases synaptic serotonin concentrations.[1]

CLINICAL EVALUATION: A 39-year-old woman developed severe somnolence within 24 hours after starting lithium 400 mg at night.[1] She became difficult to awake and fell asleep almost immediately after she was aroused. Previous reports to the Committee on Safety of Medicines (UK) cited tremor, seizures, nausea, and hyperarousal associated with the combined use of fluvoxamine and lithium. Nonetheless, it is not possible to determine whether an interaction between fluvoxamine and lithium produced the adverse effects noted in these patients on the basis of the data presented.

RELATED DRUGS: Other selective serotonin reuptake inhibitors may interact with lithium in a similar manner.

MANAGEMENT OPTIONS:

➡ *Monitor.* Until more information is available, monitor patients for adverse neurologic effects if fluvoxamine and lithium are used concurrently.

REFERENCES:

1. Evans M, et al. Fluvoxamine and lithium: an unusual interaction. *Br J Psychiatry.* 1990;156:286.

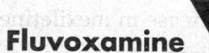

Fluvoxamine

Methadone (eg, *Dolophine*)

SUMMARY: Fluvoxamine may increase methadone serum concentrations, increasing the risk of methadone toxicity.

RISK FACTORS: No specific risk factors are known.

MECHANISM: Not established. Fluvoxamine can inhibit CYP1A2, CYP2C19, and CYP3A4; methadone may be metabolized by at least 1 of these isozymes.

CLINICAL EVALUATION: A pharmacokinetic study in 5 patients demonstrated substantial increases in methadone serum concentrations following fluvoxamine 50 to 250 mg/day.[1] A 28-year-old woman on chronic methadone treatment (70 mg/day) was started on fluvoxamine 100 mg/day.[2] Three weeks later, she was admitted to the hospital with respiratory depression, resulting in hypoxemia and hypercapnia. Fluvoxamine-induced elevations in methadone serum concentrations may have been responsible for the reaction. The patient was also taking diazepam (eg, *Valium*) 2 mg twice daily. It is possible that fluvoxamine inhibited the metabolism of diazepam, thus enhancing respiratory depression. Fluvoxamine inhibits 2 of the isozymes involved in the metabolism of diazepam (CYP2C19 and CYP3A4).

RELATED DRUGS: Fluvoxamine is the only selective serotonin reuptake inhibitor (SSRI) that inhibits CYP1A2 and CYP3A4, although fluoxetine (eg, *Prozac*) inhibits CYP2C19 and is a weak CYP3A4 inhibitor. Other SSRIs, such as paroxetine (eg, *Paxil*), sertraline (*Zoloft*), and citalopram (eg, *Celexa*), do not appear to have much effect on CYP1A2 or CYP3A4, although paroxetine is a potent CYP2D6 inhibitor. Because the isozyme(s) involved in this interaction are not known, sertraline and citalopram would probably be the least likely to interact with methadone.

MANAGEMENT OPTIONS:

➡ *Consider Alternative.* Sertraline and citalopram may be less likely to interact with methadone.

➡ *Monitor.* If fluvoxamine and methadone are used concurrently, monitor the patient for evidence of excessive methadone effect (eg, respiratory depression).

REFERENCES:

1. Bertschy G, et al. Probable metabolic interaction between methadone and fluvoxamine in addict patients. *Ther Drug Monit.* 1994;16:42-45.
2. Alderman CP, et al. Fluvoxamine-methadone interaction. *Aust N Z J Psychiatry.* 1999;33:99-101.

Fluvoxamine (*Luvox*)

Mexiletine (*Mexitil*)

SUMMARY: Fluvoxamine administration increases the plasma concentrations of mexiletine; increased side effects could occur.

RISK FACTORS:

➡ **Pharmacogenetics.** Slow metabolizers of CYP2D6. Since mexiletine is mainly metabolized by CYP2D6, patients who are deficient in this enzyme are dependent on CYP1A2 for mexiletine metabolism. If CYP1A2 activity is inhibited, a large increase in mexiletine concentration is likely to occur.

MECHANISM: Fluvoxamine is an inhibitor of CYP1A2. Mexiletine metabolism is dependent on CYP2D6 and CYP1A2. Inhibition of CYP1A2 by fluvoxamine will result in an increase in mexiletine plasma concentrations.

CLINICAL EVALUATION: Six subjects received a single oral dose of mexiletine 200 mg alone and following 7 days of fluvoxamine 50 mg twice daily.[1] The mean oral clearance of mexiletine was reduced approximately 40% (range, 25% to 52%) by fluvoxamine pretreatment. The mean mexiletine area under the concentration-time curve increased more than 50% after fluvoxamine dosing. While no pharmacodynamic monitoring was reported in this study, this degree of change in mexiletine clearance could produce unwanted changes in cardiac conduction.

RELATED DRUGS: While no data are currently available, fluoxetine (eg, *Prozac*) and paroxetine (*Paxil*) are CYP2D6 inhibitors and would be expected to increase mexiletine plasma concentrations.

MANAGEMENT OPTIONS:

➡ **Monitor.** Monitor patients stabilized on mexiletine for altered plasma concentrations if fluvoxamine is initiated or discontinued.

REFERENCES:

1. Kusumoto M, et al. Effect of fluvoxamine on the pharmacokinetics of mexiletine in healthy Japanese men. *Clin Pharmacol Ther.* 2001;69:104-107.

Fluvoxamine (eg, *Luvox*)

Moclobemide†

SUMMARY: A short-term study in healthy subjects suggests that the combined use of fluvoxamine and moclobemide is not dangerous but might increase the risk of adverse reactions, such as headache and fatigue. More study is needed.

RISK FACTORS: No specific risk factors are known.

MECHANISM: Monoamine oxidase type A (MAO-A) is primarily responsible for the oxidative deamination of serotonin in the brain. There has been concern that combined use of an MAO-A inhibitor (eg, moclobemide) and a selective serotonin reuptake inhibitor (eg, fluvoxamine) might result in excessive serotonergic effect (serotonin syndrome).

CLINICAL EVALUATION: In a randomized, placebo-controlled parallel study, 25 healthy subjects received fluvoxamine 100 mg/day on days 1 through 9, with a placebo or moclobemide (50 mg/day increasing to 400 mg/day) given on days 7 through 10.[1] The addition of moclobemide did not result in clinically relevant changes in safety parameters, such as vital signs, electrocardiogram, neurological examination, and clinical laboratory tests. Nonetheless, there was a tendency for patients on the combination to have more adverse reactions than those receiving fluvoxamine alone: headache (77% vs 22%), fatigue (62% vs 22%), dizziness (23% vs 0%). Because none of the subjects received moclobemide alone, it cannot be ruled out that the possibility of increase in adverse reactions was primarily caused by moclobemide rather than an interaction between moclobemide and fluvoxamine. There was no evidence of a serotonin syndrome in these patients, but additional data are needed to establish the safety of this combination. In this study, the dose of fluvoxamine was at the low end of the therapeutic range, and the drugs were combined for only a few days. The results of this study suggest that a washout period is not necessary when switching therapy from fluvoxamine to moclobemide. However, the value of combined therapy with fluvoxamine and moclobemide is not established.

RELATED DRUGS: Fluoxetine (eg, *Prozac*) may reduce moclobemide clearance, but the clinical importance is not established.

MANAGEMENT OPTIONS: No specific action is required, but be alert for evidence of the interaction.

REFERENCES:

1. Dingemanse J. An update of recent moclobemide interaction data. *Int Clin Psychopharmacol.* 1993;7(3-4):167-180.

† Not available in the United States.

Fluvoxamine (eg, *Luvox*)

Olanzapine (*Zyprexa*)

SUMMARY: Fluvoxamine may substantially increase olanzapine serum concentrations.

RISK FACTORS: No specific risk factors are known.

MECHANISM: Fluvoxamine probably inhibits the hepatic metabolism of olanzapine by CYP1A2.

CLINICAL EVALUATION: Patients taking olanzapine plus fluvoxamine (n = 10) had a 2.3-fold higher concentration/daily dose ratio than patients receiving olanzapine without fluvoxamine (n = 134).[1] One patient manifested a greater than 4-fold increase in olanzapine serum concentration following addition of fluvoxamine. With an interaction this large, at least some patients are expected to manifest olanzapine toxicity in the presence of fluvoxamine therapy. Cases of extrapyramidal symptoms and excessive salivation have been attributed to this interaction.[2,3]

RELATED DRUGS: Fluvoxamine is the only selective serotonin reuptake inhibitor (SSRI) that is a potent inhibitor of CYP1A2, so other SSRIs, such as fluoxetine (eg, *Prozac*), paroxetine (eg, *Paxil*), sertraline (eg, *Zoloft*), and citalopram (eg, *Celexa*), are not expected to interact to the same degree. Indeed, sertraline (n = 21) was not associated with increased olanzapine serum concentrations in the current study.[1]

MANAGEMENT OPTIONS:

➥ *Consider Alternative.* SSRIs other than fluvoxamine are probably less likely to interact with olanzapine.

➥ *Monitor.* If fluvoxamine is used with olanzapine, monitor for evidence of excessive olanzapine serum concentrations.

REFERENCES:

1. Weigmann H, et al. Fluvoxamine but not sertraline inhibits the metabolism of olanzapine: evidence from a therapeutic drug monitoring service. *Ther Drug Monit.* 2001;23(4):410-413.

2. de Jong, et al. Interaction of olanzapine with fluvoxamine. *Psychopharmacology.* 2001;155(2):219-220.

3. Hori T, et al. Hypersalivation induced by olanzapine with fluvoxamine. *Prog Neuropsychopharmacol Biol Psychiatry.* 2006;30(4):758-760.

 Fluvoxamine (eg, *Luvox*)

Omeprazole (eg, *Prilosec*)

SUMMARY: Fluvoxamine increases the plasma concentration of omeprazole in extensive metabolizers.

RISK FACTORS: Only extensive metabolizers of CYP2C19 are susceptible to fluvoxamine inhibition; poor CYP2C19 metabolizers will not be affected by the interaction.

MECHANISM: Fluvoxamine inhibits CYP2C19, the enzyme responsible for the majority of omeprazole's metabolism.

CLINICAL EVALUATION: Eighteen subjects received fluvoxamine 50 mg or placebo daily for 6 days.[1] On day 6, a single dose of omeprazole 40 mg was administered. The subjects included 6 homozygous extensive metabolizers, 6 heterozygous extensive metabolizers, and 6 poor metabolizers of CYP2C19, the primary enzyme that metabolizes omeprazole. Following fluvoxamine, the mean area under the plasma concentration-time curve (AUC) of omeprazole was increased 6-fold and 2.4-fold in the homozygous and heterozygous rapid metabolizers, respectively. The change in the omeprazole AUC seen in the poor CYP2C19 metabolizers following fluvoxamine was not significant. Doses of fluvoxamine as low as 10 mg daily for a week have been shown to significantly increase omeprazole concentrations.[2]

RELATED DRUGS: Esomeprazole (*Nexium*), pantoprazole (*Protonix*), and lansoprazole (eg, *Prevacid*) are likely to be affected in a similar manner by fluvoxamine. CYP2C19 is a minor pathway for rabeprazole (*AciPhex*) metabolism, so fluvoxamine coadministration is expected to have little effect on rabeprazole concentrations.

MANAGEMENT OPTIONS:

➥ *Monitor.* Monitor patients taking omeprazole for increased adverse reactions (eg, headache, GI pain) during fluvoxamine coadministration.

REFERENCES:

1. Yasui-Furukori N, et al. Different inhibitory effect of fluvoxamine on omeprazole metabolism between CYP2C19 genotypes. *Br J Clin Pharmacol.* 2004;57(4):487-494.

2. Christensen M, et al. Low daily 10-mg and 20-mg doses of fluvoxamine inhibit the metabolism of both caffeine (cytochrome P4501A2) and omeprazole (cytochrome P4502C19). *Clin Pharmacol Ther.* 2002;71(3):141-152.

Fluvoxamine ▼ ③

Oxycodone (eg, *OxyContin*)

SUMMARY: Isolated case reports suggest that concurrent therapy with oxycodone and fluvoxamine (or other selective serotonin reuptake inhibitors [SSRIs]) may increase the risk of serotonin syndrome; more information is needed to establish a causal relationship.

RISK FACTORS: No specific risk factors are known.

MECHANISM: Not established. Initial therapy or increasing doses of oxycodone might initiate a release of serotonin, resulting in additive effects with SSRIs.

CLINICAL EVALUATION: A 70-year-old woman receiving fluvoxamine 200 mg/day and doxepin 50 mg/day developed evidence of serotonin syndrome after starting oxycodone.[1] Her symptoms (confusion, fever, hyperreflexia, hypertonia, myoclonus, nausea, shivering, tachycardia) clearly established a diagnosis of serotonin syndrome. Because serotonin syndrome is essentially a drug-induced phenomenon, the most likely explanation is an interaction between oxycodone and the serotonergic effects of fluvoxamine. Another case of possible serotonin syndrome was described in a patient on sertraline who dramatically increased his dose of oxycodone.[2] The combination of escitalopram and oxycodone has also caused serotonin syndrome.[3] Because SSRIs and oxycodone are widely used, it is likely that many people have received the combination. Thus, the lack of reports may indicate that adverse drug interactions in patients receiving these combinations are not common.

RELATED DRUGS: If a causal interaction exists, oxycodone is expected to interact with other SSRIs such as citalopram (eg, *Celexa*), escitalopram (*Lexapro*), fluoxetine (eg, *Prozac*), paroxetine (eg, *Paxil*), and sertraline (*Zoloft*), as well as serotonin-norepinephrine reuptake inhibitors (SNRIs) such as clomipramine (eg, *Anafranil*), duloxetine (*Cymbalta*), imipramine (eg, *Tofranil*), and venlafaxine (*Effexor*).

MANAGEMENT OPTIONS:

➡ *Monitor.* Patients receiving fluvoxamine (or other SSRIs or SNRIs) should be alert for evidence of serotonin syndrome if oxycodone is coadministered. Symptoms of serotonin syndrome include agitation, coma, confusion, fever, hyperreflexia, hypomania, incoordination, myoclonus, rigidity, seizures, shivering, sweating, and tremor.

REFERENCES:

1. Karunatilake H, et al. Serotonin syndrome induced by fluvoxamine and oxycodone. *Ann Pharmacother.* 2006;40:155-157.

2. Rosebraugh CJ, et al. Visual hallucination and tremor induced by sertraline and oxycodone in a bone marrow transplant patient. *J Clin Pharmacol.* 2001;41:224-227.

3. Gnanadesigan N, et al. Interaction of serotonergic antidepressants and opioid analgesics: Is serotonin syndrome going undetected? *J Am Med Dir Assoc.* 2005;6:265-269.

Fluvoxamine

Phenytoin (eg, *Dilantin*)

SUMMARY: A patient developed phenytoin toxicity after starting fluvoxamine therapy.

RISK FACTORS: No specific risk factors are known.

MECHANISM: Fluvoxamine may inhibit the metabolism of phenytoin by CYP2C9 and CYP2C19.

CLINICAL EVALUATION: A 45-year-old woman with epilepsy was on chronic therapy with phenytoin 300 mg/day.[1] About 1 month after fluvoxamine 50 mg/day was added, the patient developed ataxia and her phenytoin serum concentration increased from 16.6 mcg/mL (before fluvoxamine) to 49.1 mcg/mL. Genotyping of the patient showed that she did not have mutations for CYP2C9 or CYP2C19. A causal relationship is supported by the temporal relationship between the initiation of fluvoxamine and phenytoin toxicity, as well as the known inhibitory effect of fluvoxamine on CYP2C9 and CYP2C19. However, additional clinical information is needed to confirm this interaction.

RELATED DRUGS: In vitro studies suggest that fluvoxamine is the most potent inhibitor of phenytoin hydroxylation among selective serotonin reuptake inhibitors (SSRIs). Nonetheless, fluoxetine (eg, *Prozac*) appears to increase phenytoin serum concentrations in some patients; numerous cases of phenytoin toxicity have been reported. Isolated cases of sertraline (*Zoloft*)-induced phenytoin toxicity have been reported, but a causal relationship was not established.

MANAGEMENT OPTIONS:

➨ *Consider Alternative.* Consider using an SSRI other than fluvoxamine or fluoxetine (see Related Drugs).

➨ *Monitor.* If fluvoxamine is added to phenytoin therapy, monitor phenytoin serum concentrations and for clinical evidence of phenytoin toxicity.

REFERENCES:

1. Mamiya K, et al. Phenytoin intoxication induced by fluvoxamine. *Ther Drug Monit.* 2001;23:75-77.

Fluvoxamine

Quinidine

SUMMARY: Fluvoxamine administration produces a modest increase in quinidine concentrations; increased quinidine effect or toxicity could result.

RISK FACTORS: No specific risk factors are known.

MECHANISM: Fluvoxamine may inhibit the CYP3A4 metabolism of quinidine.

CLINICAL EVALUATION: Six healthy subjects took a single dose of quinidine sulfate 200 mg alone and following 5 days of pretreatment with fluvoxamine 100 mg/day.[1] Median quinidine oral clearance was reduced approximately 30% by pretreatment with fluvoxamine. Quinidine's half-life increased from 8.1 to 9 hours following fluvoxamine, but its renal clearance was not altered. While no electrocardiographic data were presented, some patients may experience increased quinidine effects, particularly if quinidine concentrations are near the upper limit of normal prior to fluvoxamine administration or if higher fluvoxamine doses are administered.

RELATED DRUGS: Nefazodone inhibits CYP3A4 and is expected to interact with quinidine, perhaps to an even greater extent than fluvoxamine.

MANAGEMENT OPTIONS:

➡ *Consider Alternative.* Consider alternative antidepressants that do not affect CYP3A4 metabolism, such as paroxetine (eg, *Paxil*) or venlafaxine (*Effexor*), for patients taking quinidine. Other antiarrhythmics not metabolized by CYP3A4, such as procainamide (eg, *Procanbid*), could be considered, depending on the arrhythmia.

➡ *Monitor.* If fluvoxamine is coadministered with quinidine, monitor the electrocardiogram for evidence of increased quinidine concentrations (eg, prolonged QRS) and monitor quinidine serum concentrations.

REFERENCES:

1. Damkier P, et al. Effect of fluvoxamine on the pharmacokinetics of quinidine. *Eur J Clin Pharmacol.* 1999;55:451-456.

Fluvoxamine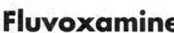

Ramelteon (*Rozerem*)

SUMMARY: Fluvoxamine produces enormous increases in ramelteon plasma concentrations; avoid the combination.

RISK FACTORS: No specific risk factors are known.

MECHANISM: Ramelteon is metabolized primarily by CYP1A2, and fluvoxamine is a potent CYP1A2 inhibitor.

CLINICAL EVALUATION: In healthy subjects, fluvoxamine 100 mg twice daily for 3 days produced a 190-fold increase in ramelteon plasma concentrations and a 70-fold increase in the ramelteon maximal plasma concentrations.[1] An interaction of this magnitude indicates that concurrent use of these drugs is unwise because of potential ramelteon toxicity.

RELATED DRUGS: Fluvoxamine is the only selective serotonin reuptake inhibitor (SSRI) available that is a potent inhibitor of CYP1A2; therefore, use other SSRIs, such as citalopram (eg, *Celexa*), escitalopram (*Lexapro*), fluoxetine (eg, *Prozac*), paroxetine (eg, *Paxil*), or sertraline (*Zoloft*), when coadministering ramelteon.

MANAGEMENT OPTIONS:

➡ *AVOID COMBINATION.* Do not use fluvoxamine concomitantly with ramelteon.

REFERENCES:

1. *Rozerem* [package insert]. Lincolnshire, IL: Takeda Pharmaceuticals; 2006.

Fluvoxamine

Rasagiline (*Azilect*) AVOID

SUMMARY: Fluvoxamine is likely to markedly increase rasagiline plasma concentrations; avoid the combination.

RISK FACTORS: No specific risk factors known.

MECHANISM: Rasagiline is metabolized primarily by CYP1A2, and fluvoxamine is a potent inhibitor of this isozyme. The combination also may have additive serotonergic effects.

CLINICAL EVALUATION: Severe serotonin syndrome–like reactions (including fatalities) have occurred when selective serotonin reuptake inhibitors (SSRIs) were used in patients on nonselective monoamine oxidase inhibitors or selegiline. Thus, combining rasagiline with SSRIs theoretically may increase the risk of serotonin syndrome.[1,2] But given the ability of fluvoxamine to dramatically inhibit CYP1A2 activity, it is also likely to substantially increase rasagiline plasma concentrations.

RELATED DRUGS: Fluvoxamine is the only currently available SSRI that is a potent inhibitor of CYP1A2.

MANAGEMENT OPTIONS:

➥ *AVOID COMBINATION.* Do not use rasagiline and fluvoxamine concurrently. If an SSRI is used with rasagiline, use an SSRI other than fluvoxamine.

REFERENCES:
1. Chen JJ, et al. Rasagiline: A second-generation monoamine oxidase type-B inhibitor for the treatment of Parkinson's disease. *Am J Health Syst Pharm.* 2006;63:915-928.

2. *Azilect* [package insert]. Kansas City, MO: Teva Neuroscience, Inc.; 2006.

 Fluvoxamine

Sildenafil (eg, *Viagra*)

SUMMARY: Fluvoxamine may increase plasma sildenafil concentrations; use conservative initial doses of sildenafil.

RISK FACTORS: No specific risk factors are known.

MECHANISM: Fluvoxamine may inhibit the CYP3A4 metabolism of sildenafil.

CLINICAL EVALUATION: In a double-blind, crossover study of healthy subjects, pretreatment with fluvoxamine increased the plasma concentrations of a single dose of sildenafil 50 mg by 40%.[1] The combination was well tolerated in these healthy subjects, and sildenafil was used successfully in at least 1 patient for fluvoxamine-induced erectile dysfunction.[2] Nonetheless, the magnitude of the interaction appears sufficient to produce adverse reactions in some patients.

RELATED DRUGS: The effect of fluvoxamine on tadalafil (*Cialis*) and vardenafil (*Levitra*) is not established, but theoretically these drugs may interact with fluvoxamine in a similar manner.

MANAGEMENT OPTIONS:

➥ *Consider Alternative.* Other selective serotonin reuptake inhibitors, such as citalopram (eg, *Celexa*), escitalopram (*Lexapro*), paroxetine (eg, *Paxil*), sertraline (*Zoloft*), and venlafaxine (*Effexor*), appear to have little effect on CYP3A4 and may be less likely to interact with sildenafil.

➥ *Circumvent/Minimize.* In patients taking fluvoxamine, start with sildenafil 25 mg and increase the dose only if 25 mg is insufficient.

REFERENCES:
1. Hesse C, et al. Fluvoxamine affects sildenafil kinetics and dynamics. *J Clin Psychopharmacol.* 2005;25:589-592.

2. Balon R. Fluvoxamine-induced erectile dysfunction responding to sildenafil. *J Sex Marital Ther.* 1998;24:313-317.

Fluvoxamine (eg, *Luvox*) 2

Tacrine (*Cognex*)

SUMMARY: Fluvoxamine markedly increases tacrine serum concentrations and may increase tacrine adverse effects; avoid the combination if possible.

RISK FACTORS: No specific risk factors are known.

MECHANISM: Fluvoxamine probably inhibits the hepatic metabolism of tacrine by CYP1A2.

CLINICAL EVALUATION: In a randomized, crossover study of healthy subjects given a single oral dose of tacrine with and without pretreatment with fluvoxamine 100 mg/day for 6 days, tacrine area under the plasma concentration-time curve increased more than 700%.[1] The combination also appeared to increase the risk of GI side effects from tacrine (eg, nausea, vomiting, diarrhea). Although tacrine-induced hepatotoxicity is known to be dose related, the relative role played by tacrine vs its metabolites in these reactions is not yet established. Nonetheless, it is possible that the marked increases in tacrine plasma concentrations observed in this study could increase the risk of tacrine hepatotoxicity.

RELATED DRUGS: The effect of other selective serotonin reuptake inhibitors such as fluoxetine (eg, *Prozac*), paroxetine (eg, *Paxil*), and sertraline (*Zoloft*) on tacrine is not established, but none of these drugs is known to inhibit CYP1A2. The effect of fluvoxamine on donepezil (*Aricept*) is not established.

MANAGEMENT OPTIONS:

➡ *Use Alternative.* Until more data are available, it is preferable to use an alternative selective serotonin reuptake inhibitor such as fluoxetine, paroxetine, or sertraline in patients taking tacrine. If the combination is used, monitor for adverse tacrine GI effects and for tacrine-induced hepatotoxicity.

REFERENCES:

1. Becquemont L, et al. Influence of the CYP1A2 inhibitor fluvoxamine on tacrine pharmacokinetics in humans. *Clin Pharmacol Ther.* 1997;61:619.

Fluvoxamine (eg, *Luvox*) 1

Terfenadine† AVOID

SUMMARY: Fluvoxamine appears to inhibit the enzyme that metabolizes terfenadine, which theoretically could result in increased unchanged serum terfenadine concentrations and cardiac arrhythmias; avoid the combination.

RISK FACTORS: No specific risk factors are known.

MECHANISM: Theoretically, fluvoxamine may inhibit the first-pass hepatic metabolism of terfenadine by cytochrome P4503A4.

CLINICAL EVALUATION: Fluvoxamine has been shown to substantially inhibit the metabolism of alprazolam, a drug that is metabolized by CYP3A4.[1] Thus fluvoxamine also may inhibit the metabolism of other drugs metabolized by CYP3A4, such as terfenadine. Terfenadine undergoes extensive first-pass hepatic metabolism by

CYP3A4, and most people therefore have minimal concentrations of unmetabolized terfenadine in the plasma. Inhibitors of CYP3A4, such as ketoconazole (eg, *Nizoral*), have been shown to increase parent terfenadine serum concentrations, leading to electrocardiographic changes (QT prolongation) and, in some cases, life-threatening ventricular arrhythmias (torsades de pointes). Although it is not known whether fluvoxamine would inhibit the metabolism of terfenadine enough to increase the risk of arrhythmias, it is theoretically possible.

RELATED DRUGS: Astemizole[†] also is metabolized by CYP3A4 and can cause the same types of cardiac arrhythmias when combined with CYP3A4 inhibitors; thus, it also may interact adversely with fluvoxamine. Loratadine (eg, *Claritin*) also may be metabolized by CYP3A4, but it does not appear to produce cardiotoxicity when given with drugs that inhibit its metabolism.

MANAGEMENT OPTIONS:

➡ *AVOID COMBINATION.* Although this interaction is based largely upon theoretical considerations, generally avoid the combination of terfenadine and fluvoxamine.[2] The potential adverse effects of the interaction can be life-threatening, and terfenadine is generally used for symptomatic relief of allergic disorders. Theoretically, loratadine is a safer nonsedating antihistamine in the presence of fluvoxamine.

REFERENCES:

1. Fleishaker JC, et al. A pharmacokinetic and pharmacodynamic evaluation of the combined administration of alprazolam and fluvoxamine. *Eur J Clin Pharmacol.* 1994;46:35-39.

2. *Luvox* [package insert]. Marietta, GA: Solvay Pharmaceuticals; 1996.

† Not available in the United States.

 Fluvoxamine (eg, *Luvox*)

Theophylline (eg, *Theolair*)

SUMMARY: Several cases of theophylline toxicity caused by fluvoxamine have been reported. Although more study is needed to establish a causal relationship, the interaction is consistent with the interactive properties of the 2 drugs.

RISK FACTORS: No specific risk factors are known.

MECHANISM: Cytochrome P4501A2 (CYP1A2) is an important enzyme in the metabolism of theophylline, and drugs that inhibit CYP1A2 (eg, quinolone antibiotics) are known to inhibit the metabolism of theophylline. An in vitro study using human hepatic microsomal enzymes suggests that fluvoxamine is a potent inhibitor of CYP1A2.[1]

CLINICAL EVALUATION: An 11-year-old boy on chronic theophylline therapy (*Theo-Dur* 300 mg twice daily) was started on fluvoxamine 25 mg twice daily.[2] Within a week of starting fluvoxamine, he developed severe headaches, tiredness, and vomiting. Thinking the reaction was caused by the fluvoxamine alone, they reduced the dose of fluvoxamine to 25 mg/day. He continued to vomit. A serum theophylline concentration measured in an emergency room was 27.4 mg/L (the level before fluvoxamine was 14.2 mg/L). When the theophylline later was restarted in the absence of fluvoxamine, the level was 10.5 mg/L. In another report, a 70-year-old man on theophylline 1,200 mg/day developed dizziness, blurred vision, and ventricular tachycardia after his fluvoxamine dose was increased from 50 mg/day to 100 mg/day.[3] There were several positive dechallenges and rechallenges in this patient, supporting the authors' contention that fluvoxamine was responsible for the theophylline toxicity. A third case of elevated theophylline concentrations caused by fluvoxamine has been reported in the French literature.[4] The time course of this interaction is not well established, but most drugs that inhibit theophylline metabolism result in a new steady-state serum theophylline concentration within the first 2 days of therapy.

RELATED DRUGS: Based on in vitro studies in human hepatic microsomes, other selective serotonin reuptake inhibitors (SSRIs) such as citalopram (*Celexa*), fluoxetine (eg, *Prozac*), paroxetine (eg, *Paxil*), and sertraline (*Zoloft*) are less likely to interact with theophylline.[1]

MANAGEMENT OPTIONS:

➡ *Use Alternative.* Given the magnitude of the interaction and the potential toxicity of theophylline, use an alternative to fluvoxamine (eg, citalopram, fluoxetine, paroxetine, sertraline). Until clinical evidence is available, however, be alert for evidence of theophylline toxicity when therapy with any SSRI is started. If the combination is used, monitor for altered serum theophylline concentrations and clinical evidence of theophylline toxicity if fluvoxamine is initiated, discontinued, or changed in dosage. Evidence of theophylline toxicity includes nausea, vomiting, diarrhea, restlessness, irritability, and insomnia. Higher serum concentrations can result in cardiac arrhythmias or seizures. Permanent brain damage and death have been reported in severe cases. Note that nausea is also a common side effect of fluvoxamine,[5] so measuring the theophylline serum concentration may be needed to determine whether nausea is caused by fluvoxamine or theophylline toxicity.

REFERENCES:

1. Brosen K, et al. Fluvoxamine is a potent inhibitor of cytochrome P4501A2. *Biochem Pharmacol.* 1993;45:1211.
2. Sperber AD. Toxic interaction between fluvoxamine and sustained release theophylline in an 11-year-old boy. *Drug Safety.* 1991;6:460.
3. Thomson AH, et al. Interaction between fluvoxamine and theophylline. *Pharmaceutical J.* 1992;249:137.
4. Diot P, et al. Possible interaction between theophylline and fluvoxamine. *Therapie.* 1991;46:470.
5. Benfield P, et al. Fluvoxamine: a review of its pharmacodynamic and pharmacokinetic properties, and therapeutic efficacy in depressive illness. *Drugs.* 1986;32:313.

Fluvoxamine

Thioridazine

SUMMARY: Fluvoxamine increases thioridazine serum concentrations, and thus may increase the risk of ventricular arrhythmias; avoid concurrent use.

RISK FACTORS:

➡ *Hypokalemia.* The corrected QT interval (QTc) may be prolonged in patients with hypokalemia, thus increasing the risk of this interaction. Any other factor that may prolong the QTc interval also increases the risk of this interaction.

MECHANISM: Fluvoxamine probably inhibits the hepatic metabolism of thioridazine by CYP2C19 and possibly also by CYP1A2.

CLINICAL EVALUATION: Ten schizophrenic men on thioridazine were given fluvoxamine 50 mg/day for 7 days.[1] Fluvoxamine was associated with a 3-fold increase in serum concentrations of thioridazine and its 2 active metabolites. In a double-

blind, randomized, crossover study of the pharmacodynamic effects of thioridazine, 9 healthy subjects received single oral doses (10 and 50 mg) compared with
placebo.[2] The 50 mg dose of thioridazine increased the QTc on the electrocardiogram (ECG) by 23 msec, and the 10 mg dose increased the QTc by 9 msec. These
2 studies suggest that thioridazine produces a dose-related slowing of cardiac
repolarization and that fluvoxamine substantially increases thioridazine serum
concentrations. Fluvoxamine is expected to increase the risk of excessive prolongation of the QTc interval with the attendant increase in the risk of ventricular
arrhythmias. Although case reports of arrhythmias appear to be lacking, the
potential severity of the interaction suggests avoiding the combination. The manufacturer's product information for *Mellaril* (not available in the United States)
stated that combined use of thioridazine and fluvoxamine was contraindicated[3];
thus, also consider medicolegal issues.

RELATED DRUGS: Fluoxetine (eg, *Prozac*) and paroxetine (eg, *Paxil*) are potent inhibitors of
CYP2D6, and are expected to increase the risk of arrhythmias. Other selective
serotonin reuptake inhibitors such as citalopram (eg, *Celexa*) and sertraline (*Zoloft*)
are less likely to significantly inhibit CYP2D6, CYP2C19, or CYP1A2. Theoretically,
they are less likely to interact with thioridazine, but little clinical information is
available. Although a number of antipsychotic drugs have been shown to prolong
the QT interval, clinical evidence suggests that thioridazine may produce the
greatest risk.

MANAGEMENT OPTIONS:

➡ ***Use Alternative.*** Although the risk of this combination is not well established, use an
alternative for 1 of the drugs (see Related Drugs).

➡ ***Monitor.*** If the combination must be used, monitor the ECG for evidence of QT
prolongation and for clinical evidence of arrhythmias (eg, syncope).

REFERENCES:

1. Carrillo JA, et al. Pharmacokinetic interaction of fluvoxamine and thioridazine in schizophrenic
   patients. *J Clin Psychopharmacol*. 1999;19:494-499.

2. Hartigan-Go K, et al. Concentration-related pharmacodynamic effects of thioridazine and its metabolites in humans. *Clin Pharmacol Ther*. 1996;60:543-553.

3. "Dear Doctor or Pharmacist" Letter, Novartis Pharmaceuticals, July 7, 2000. FDA Web site. MedWatch.
   Available at: www.fda.gov/medwatch/safety/2000/mellar.htm. Accessed June 9, 2005.

 Fluvoxamine

Tizanidine (eg, *Zanaflex*)

SUMMARY: Fluvoxamine dramatically increased tizanidine plasma concentrations in healthy subjects; other selective
serotonin reuptake inhibitors (SSRIs) are probably less likely to interact.

RISK FACTORS: No specific risk factors are known.

MECHANISM: Not established. Fluvoxamine probably inhibits the metabolism of tizanidine via CYP1A2. In vitro study suggests that tizanidine is metabolized primarily
by CYP1A2, and fluvoxamine is a known inhibitor of this enzyme. The changes in
tizanidine pharmacokinetics following fluvoxamine correlated with changes in the
caffeine/paraxanthine concentration ratio, a finding that further supports the role
of CYP1A2 in this interaction.[1]

CLINICAL EVALUATION: Ten healthy subjects received a single oral dose of tizanidine 4 mg with and without pretreatment with fluvoxamine 100 mg daily for 4 days.[1] Fluvoxamine increased the tizanidine area under the plasma concentration-time curve (AUC) 33-fold; 1 subject had a 103-fold increase in tizanidine AUC. The elevated tizanidine plasma concentrations during fluvoxamine therapy were associated with hypotension, somnolence, and dizziness. In patients, the combined use of fluvoxamine and tizanidine has been associated with bradycardia, dizziness, hypothermia, and hypotension.[2]

RELATED DRUGS: Fluvoxamine is one of the most potent inhibitors of CYP1A2 known. Other SSRIs are not known to inhibit CYP1A2 and are theoretically less likely to interact with tizanidine.

MANAGEMENT OPTIONS:

➡ **Avoid Unless Benefit Outweighs Risk.** Given the large magnitude of the interaction, avoid concurrent use of fluvoxamine and tizanidine.

➡ **Use Alternative.** Other SSRIs and related drugs that are theoretically less likely to interact with tizanidine include citalopram (*Celexa*), escitalopram (*Lexapro*), fluoxetine (eg, *Prozac*), paroxetine (eg, *Paxil*), sertraline (*Zoloft*), mirtazapine (eg, *Remeron*), trazodone (eg, *Desyrel*), and venlafaxine (eg, *Effexor*).

➡ **Monitor.** If the combination is used, monitor for hypotension and excessive CNS depression.

REFERENCES:

1. Granfors MT, et al. Fluvoxamine drastically increases concentrations and effects of tizanidine: a potentially hazardous interaction. *Clin Pharmacol Ther*. 2004;75:331-341.
2. Momo K, et al. Drug interaction of tizanidine and fluvoxamine. *Clin Pharmacol Ther*. 2004;76:509-510.

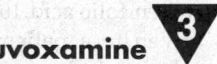

Fluvoxamine

Warfarin (eg, *Coumadin*)

SUMMARY: Preliminary data suggest that fluvoxamine increases the hypoprothrombinemic response to warfarin; more study is needed.

RISK FACTORS: No specific risk factors are known.

MECHANISM: Not established.

CLINICAL EVALUATION: In healthy subjects taking warfarin, the addition of fluvoxamine for 2 weeks purportedly resulted in a 65% increase in warfarin plasma concentrations and an increase in the hypoprothrombinemic response.[1] This information is based on unpublished data on file with the manufacturer, so it is not possible to assess the scientific validity of the study. Moreover, the lack of information on the relative effect of fluvoxamine on the R- and S-enantiomers of warfarin makes it difficult to interpret the clinical importance of the 65% increase in warfarin plasma concentrations.

RELATED DRUGS: The effect of fluvoxamine on the response to other oral anticoagulants is not established. Some evidence suggests that other selective serotonin reuptake inhibitors (SSRIs) also may increase the bleeding risk of warfarin, in some cases without affecting the hypoprothrombinemic response.

MANAGEMENT OPTIONS:

➡ **Monitor.** Although data are lacking, be alert for evidence of altered hypoprothrombinemic response to warfarin (or other anticoagulants) if fluvoxamine is initiated, discontinued, or changed in dosage. Although not reported for fluvoxamine, some SSRIs may impair hemostasis; be alert for evidence of bleeding even if the hypoprothrombinemic response is in the desired range.

REFERENCES:

1. Benfield P, et al. Fluvoxamine. A review of its pharmacodynamic and pharmacokinetic properties, and therapeutic efficacy in depressive illness. *Drugs*. 1986;32:313-334.

Folic Acid (eg, *Folvite*)

Phenytoin (eg, *Dilantin*)

SUMMARY: Folic acid may decrease serum phenytoin concentrations to a clinically significant degree in an occasional patient. Whether folic acid is capable of directly antagonizing the anticonvulsant effects of phenytoin is not established.

RISK FACTORS:

➡ **Dosage Regimen.** Small amounts of folic acid found in multiple vitamins are not likely to have much effect.

MECHANISM: Replacement of folic acid in folate-deficient patients taking phenytoin may increase the metabolism of phenytoin with a resultant decrease in serum phenytoin concentrations.[1-15]

CLINICAL EVALUATION: Decreases in serum phenytoin were noted in 3 of 4 normal subjects when folic acid 10 mg/day was added to phenytoin 300 mg/day.[11] Also, folic acid given to a patient on phenytoin therapy was followed by a decrease in serum phenytoin concentrations to subtherapeutic levels and an increase in seizure frequency.[8] However, most patients manifest relatively small decreases in serum phenytoin with folic acid therapy.[3,8,16] Available evidence suggests that the fall in serum phenytoin is greatest in those patients with higher initial serum phenytoin concentrations.[16] In a study evaluating the effect of folic acid on recurrence of phenytoin-induced gingival overgrowth, 8 patients were randomly assigned to receive either folic acid 5 mg/day or placebo. Free phenytoin plasma concentrations were monitored at baseline, 2 weeks, 3 months, and 6 months. There were no significant differences in free phenytoin plasma concentrations between groups or within each group.[17] The ability of folic acid to antagonize the anticonvulsant effect of phenytoin directly is not well established, but occasional patients stabilized on chronic phenytoin manifest decreased seizure control when folic acid is given. In 1 study, very small doses of folic acid (5 mg/week) corrected phenytoin-induced folate deficiency without affecting seizure control.[18]

RELATED DRUGS: No information is available.

MANAGEMENT OPTIONS:

➡ **Monitor.** When folic acid is given to patients receiving phenytoin, watch for decreased seizure control (although most patients are probably not significantly affected).

REFERENCES:

1. Reynolds EH. Anticonvulsants, folic acid, and epilepsy. *Lancet*. 1973;1:1376.

2. Smith DB, et al. Folate metabolism and the anticonvulsant efficacy of phenobarbital. *Arch Neurol.* 1973;28:18-22.

3. Jensen ON, et al. Subnormal serum folate due to anticonvulsive therapy. A double-blind study of the effect of folic acid treatment in patients with drug-induced subnormal serum folates. *Arch Neurol.* 1970;22:181-182.

4. Norris JW, et al. A controlled study of folic acid in epilepsy. *Neurology.* 1971;21:659-664.

5. Spaans F. No effect of folic acid supplement on CSF folate and serum vitamin B12 in patients on anticonvulsants. *Epilepsia.* 1970;11:403-411.

6. Ralston AJ, et al. Effects of folic acid on fit-frequency and behaviour of epileptics on anticonvulsants. *Lancet.* 1970;1:867-868.

7. Scott RB, et al. Reduced absorption of vitamin B12 in two patients with folic acid deficiency. *Ann Intern Med.* 1968;69:111-114.

8. Baylis EM, et al. Influence of folic acid on blood-phenytoin levels. *Lancet.* 1971;1:62-64.

9. Houben PF, et al. Anticonvulsant drugs and folic acid in young mentally retarded epileptic patients. *Epilepsia.* 1971;12:235-247.

10. Kariks J, et al. Serum folic acid and phenytoin levels in permanently hospitalized epileptic patients receiving anticonvulsant drug therapy. *Med J Aust.* 1971;2:368-371.

11. Glazko AJ. Antiepileptic drugs: biotransformation, metabolism, and serum half-life. *Epilepsia.* 1975;16:367-391.

12. Reynolds EH. Folate metabolism and anticonvulsant therapy. *Proc R Soc Med.* 1974;67:68.

13. Ch'ien LT, et al. Harmful effect of megadoses of vitamins: electroencephalogram abnormalities and seizures induced by intravenous folate in drug-treated epileptics. *Am J Clin Nutr.* 1975;28:51-58.

14. Strauss RG, et al. Folic acid and dilantin antagonism in pregnancy. *Obstet Gynecol.* 1974;44:345-348.

15. MacCosbe PE, et al. Interaction of phenytoin and folic acid. *Clin Pharm.* 1983;2:362.

16. Furlanut M, et al. Effects of folic acid on phenytoin kinetics in healthy subjects. *Clin Pharmacol Ther.* 1978;24:294-297.

17. Poppell TD, et al. Effect of folic acid on recurrence of phenytoin-induced gingival overgrowth following gingivectomy. *J Clin Periodontol.* 1991;18:134-139.

18. Inoue F. Clinical implications of anticonvulsant induced folate deficiency. *Clin Pharm.* 1982;1:372-373.

Folic Acid (eg, *Folvite*)

Pyrimethamine (*Daraprim*)

SUMMARY: Folic acid potentially can interfere with the efficacy of pyrimethamine.

RISK FACTORS: No specific risk factors are known.

MECHANISM: Because pyrimethamine interferes with folic acid metabolism in certain parasitic and other diseases, folic acid theoretically could inhibit its efficacy.

CLINICAL EVALUATION: Folic acid reportedly interferes with the action of pyrimethamine against toxoplasmosis. However, because malarial parasites are unable to use preformed folic acid, the antimalarial effect of pyrimethamine should not be affected by folic acid. In patients with leukemia who received pyrimethamine for *Pneumocystis carinii* infections, folic acid administration worsened the leukemic condition.[1]

RELATED DRUGS: No information is available.

MANAGEMENT OPTIONS:

➥ *Avoid Unless Benefit Outweighs Risk.* Until more information is available, do not administer folic acid to patients receiving pyrimethamine for treatment of toxoplasmosis or in patients with leukemia.

➡ *Monitor.* If folic acid is used, monitor for loss of pyrimethamine efficacy.

REFERENCES:
1. Tong MJ, et al. Supplemental folates in the therapy of *Plasmodium falciparum* malaria. *JAMA.* 1970;214:2330-2333.

 Food

Gatifloxacin (eg, *Tequin*)

SUMMARY: Food appears to minimally affect the absorption of gatifloxacin.

RISK FACTORS: No specific risk factors are known.

MECHANISM: Unknown.

CLINICAL EVALUATION: Several studies have determined the effect of various foods on the absorption of gatifloxacin. Administration with a high-fat meal delayed the absorption (time to peak concentration) of gatifloxacin from 0.75 to 2 hours and reduced the mean area under the plasma concentration-time curve (AUC) and peak concentration less than 10%.[1] The administration of gatifloxacin 400 mg with *Ensure* 120 mL every 30 minutes for 5 doses resulted in a 26% reduction in gatifloxacin AUC and a 44% reduction in its peak concentration compared with administration with water.[2] Twelve ounces of calcium-fortified orange juice, orange juice, or water were administered with a single dose of gatifloxacin 400 mg to 16 subjects.[3] The calcium-fortified orange juice reduced the AUC of gatifloxacin 12%. Neither interrupted nor continuous tube feedings altered the bioavailability of gatifloxacin in 16 patients.[4] A case report noted apparent therapeutic failure of gatifloxacin when administered with a product containing calcium carbonate, iron, magnesium, and zinc.[5] Overall, the effects of food on gatifloxacin bioavailability appear small and unlikely to be of clinical significance.

RELATED DRUGS: Most quinolone antibiotics appear to be unaffected by food.

MANAGEMENT OPTIONS:

➡ *Monitor.* No special monitoring is required when gatifloxacin is administered with food. Pending more information, administer gatifloxacin doses 2 to 3 hours before *Ensure* or products containing calcium and minerals.

REFERENCES:
1. Fish DN et al. Gatifloxacin, an advanced 8-methoxy fluoroquinolone. *Pharmacotherapy.* 2001;21:35-59.
2. Kays M, et al. Effect of ensure on the oral bioavailability of gatifloxacin. *Pharmacotherapy.* 2003;23:1344.
3. Wallace AW, et al. Lack of bioequivalence of gatifloxacin when coadministrated with calcium-fortified orange juice in healthy volunteers. *J Clin Pharmacol.* 2003;43:92-96.
4. Kanji S, et al. Bioavailability of gatifloxacin by gastric tube administration with and without concomitant enteral feeding in critically ill patients. *Crit Care Med.* 2003;31:1347-1352.
5. Mallet L, et al. Coadministration of gatifloxacin and multivitamin preparation containing minerals: potential treatment failure in an elderly patient. *Ann Pharmacother.* 2005;39:150-152.

Food **4**

Griseofulvin (eg, *Gris-PEG*)

SUMMARY: Food increases the serum concentration of griseofulvin; the clinical significance of this effect is probably limited.

RISK FACTORS: No specific risk factors are known.

MECHANISM: Dissolution of griseofulvin is probably enhanced in the presence of a fatty meal, thus enhancing GI absorption.

CLINICAL EVALUATION: A high-fat meal can increase the absorption of griseofulvin.[1] Griseofulvin serum concentrations following a high-fat meal were approximately double the concentrations in the fasting state.[1] Subsequent study using microsize griseofulvin yielded similar results.[2] These findings might be used to advantage in patients whose clinical resistance is caused by inadequate GI absorption.[1]

RELATED DRUGS: Food also increases the serum concentration of itraconazole (*Sporanox*).

MANAGEMENT OPTIONS: No specific action is required, but be alert for evidence of the interaction.

REFERENCES:

1. Crounse RG. Human pharmacology of griseofulvin: the effect of fat intake on gastrointestinal absorption. *J Invest Dermatol*. 1961;37:529-533.
2. Crounse RG. Effective use of griseofulvin. *Arch Dermatol*. 1963;87:176-178.

Food **3**

Indinavir (*Crixivan*)

SUMMARY: The administration of indinavir with food reduces the serum concentration; loss of efficacy may result.

RISK FACTORS: No specific risk factors are known.

MECHANISM: Not established.

CLINICAL EVALUATION: The administration of indinavir with a high-fat, high-protein meal reduced the area under the concentration-time curve of indinavir 77%.[1] This degree of reduction in serum concentrations is likely to result in a reduction in the efficacy of indinavir. Small meals appear to have little effect on indinavir serum concentrations.

RELATED DRUGS: Food produces a small increase (15%) in ritonavir (*Norvir*) serum concentrations[2] and a large increase (2- to 5-fold) in saquinavir (eg, *Invirase*) concentrations.[3]

MANAGEMENT OPTIONS:

➡ *Circumvent/Minimize.* Administer indinavir on an empty stomach or after a small snack.

➡ *Monitor.* Monitor for reduced indinavir effect in patients taking the drug with meals.

REFERENCES:

1. *Crixivan* [package insert]. White House Station, NJ: Merck and Company, Inc.; 1996.
2. *Norvir* [package insert]. Abbott Park, IL: Abbott Laboratories; 1996.
3. *Invirase* [package insert]. Nutley, NJ: Roche Laboratories; 1995.

 **Food**

Isoniazid (INH)

SUMMARY: Food may reduce INH concentrations, and some cheeses may cause a reaction in patients taking INH.

RISK FACTORS: No specific risk factors are known.

MECHANISM: The mechanism for inhibition of INH absorption by food is not established. The reaction to cheese in patients taking INH may be caused by inhibition of monoamine oxidase by INH.

CLINICAL EVALUATION: A study in 9 healthy men demonstrated that the peak serum concentrations and the total amount of INH absorbed were lower when the drug was taken with food than when it was taken in the fasting state.[1] The decreases were considerable in many cases, indicating that the therapeutic response to INH could be impaired. Also, patients have reported reactions including flushing, chills, headache, tachycardia, and hypertension after eating cheese.[2,3]

RELATED DRUGS: No information is available.

MANAGEMENT OPTIONS:

➡ *Circumvent/Minimize.* For optimal absorption, give INH on an empty stomach.

➡ *Monitor.* Watch for "cheese reactions" (eg, flushing, chills, headache, tachycardia, hypertension) in patients on INH.

REFERENCES:
1. Melander A, et al. Reduction of isoniazid bioavailability in normal men by concomitant intake of food. *Acta Med Scand.* 1976;200:93.
2. Smith CK, et al. Isoniazid and reaction to cheese. *Ann Intern Med.* 1978;88:520.
3. Lejonc JL, et al. Isoniazid and reaction to cheese. *Ann Intern Med.* 1979;91:793.

 Food

Itraconazole (*Sporanox*)

SUMMARY: The administration of itraconazole following a meal greatly enhances its bioavailability.

RISK FACTORS: No specific risk factors are known.

MECHANISM: Not established.

CLINICAL EVALUATION: Six healthy subjects took itraconazole 100 mg fasting and following a standard breakfast.[1] The area under the concentration-time curve for itraconazole increased 160%, and peak concentrations more than tripled following administration with food. Relative bioavailability compared to itraconazole solution increased from 40% to 100% when the capsules were taken with food. Similar results were observed in a study of 27 healthy subjects receiving single and multiple doses of itraconazole.[3] A low stomach pH and slow stomach emptying also enhance itraconazole absorption.[2] This interaction may be utilized to increase itraconazole serum concentrations.

RELATED DRUGS: Food also increases the serum concentration of griseofulvin (eg, *Grisactin*).

MANAGEMENT OPTIONS:

➡ *Monitor.* Administer itraconazole capsules following a meal to obtain maximum serum concentration.

REFERENCES:

1. Van Peer A, et al. The effects of food and dose on the oral systemic availability of itraconazole in healthy subjects. *Eur J Clin Pharmacol.* 1989;36:423.

2. Zimmerman T, et al. Influence of concomitant food intake on the oral absorption of two triazole anti-fungal agents, itraconazole and fluconazole. *Eur J Clin Pharmacol.* 1994;46:147.

3. Barone JA, et al. Food interaction and steady-state pharmacokinetics of itraconazole capsules in healthy male volunteers. *Antimicrob Agents Chemother.* 1993;37:778.

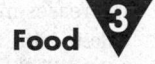

Food

Levodopa (eg, *Larodopa*)

SUMMARY: Some evidence suggests that high-protein diets inhibit the efficacy of levodopa in parkinsonism.

RISK FACTORS: No specific risk factors are known.

MECHANISM: Although it has been proposed that large, neutral amino acids may compete with levodopa for intestinal absorption, there is evidence to suggest that the competition is more likely for transport across the blood brain barrier.[1-3]

CLINICAL EVALUATION: In 8 patients with parkinsonism, high protein intakes (2 g/kg body weight/day) tended to cancel the therapeutic effects of levodopa, whereas low protein intakes (0.5 g/kg body weight/day) tended to potentiate and stabilize the therapeutic effects of the drug.[3] These data suggest that there may be loss of clinical improvement in patients receiving levodopa who ingest large amounts of protein daily. Peak plasma concentrations of levodopa were lower in a patient following a small protein meal (milk and crackers) than in other patients taking the drug in the fasting state.[2] However, in 8 healthy subjects neither a high-nor a low-protein meal affected levodopa absorption when compared to the fasting state.[4]

RELATED DRUGS: No information is available.

MANAGEMENT OPTIONS:

➡ *Circumvent/Minimize.* Although it is usually recommended that levodopa be taken with meals to slow absorption and thus reduce the central emetic effect, patients on levodopa should probably avoid high-protein diets as well as diets with widely fluctuating protein content.

➡ *Monitor.* Monitor for reduced levodopa effect if high-protein foods are taken.

REFERENCES:

1. Mena I, et al. Protein treatment of Parkinson's disease with levodopa. *N Engl J Med.* 1975;292:181.

2. Morgan JP, et al. Metabolism of levodopa in patients with Parkinson's disease. *Arch Neurol.* 1971;25:39.

3. Gillespie NG, et al. Diets affecting treatment of parkinsonism with levodopa. *J Am Diet Assoc.* 1973;62:525.

4. Robertson DRC, et al. The influence of protein on the absorption of levodopa. *Br J Clin Pharmacol.* 1990;29:608P.

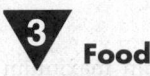

Food

Lincomycin (eg, *Lincocin*)

SUMMARY: Food significantly reduced lincomycin serum concentrations.

RISK FACTORS: No specific risk factors are known.

MECHANISM: Food reduces lincomycin absorption.

CLINICAL EVALUATION: In single-dose studies of healthy subjects, the GI absorption of lincomycin taken after food has been poor and erratic, with significant delays and decreases in absorption.[2-4] Average serum concentrations of lincomycin when it is taken with food appear to be about one-half the serum concentrations when it is taken in the fasting state.

RELATED DRUGS: Diet foods or drinks with sodium cyclamate decrease the serum concentrations of clindamycin (eg, *Cleocin*) by up to 80%.[1]

MANAGEMENT OPTIONS:

➡ **Circumvent/Minimize.** For optimal absorption, nothing should be given by mouth except water for 1 to 2 hours before and after oral lincomycin.

➡ **Monitor.** Monitor patients receiving lincomycin with food for loss of antibiotic effect.

REFERENCES:

1. DeHaan RM, et al. Clindamycin serum concentrations after administration of clindamycin palmitate with food. *J Clin Pharmacol*. 1972;12:205.
2. McCall CE, et al. Lincomycin: activity *in vitro* and absorption and excretion in normal young men. *Am J Med Sci*. 1967;254:144.
3. Kaplan K, et al. Microbiological, pharmacological and clinical studies of lincomycin. *Am J Med Sci*. 1965;250:137.
4. McGehee RF, et al. Comparative studies of antibacterial activity *in vitro* and absorption and excretion of lincomycin and clindamycin. *Am J Med Sci*. 1968;256:279.

Food

Melphalan (*Alkeran*)

SUMMARY: Food markedly reduces the bioavailability and plasma concentrations of melphalan.

RISK FACTORS: No specific risk factors are known.

MECHANISM: The mechanism of this interaction is not established, but food may compete with melphalan for active transport across the lumen of the small intestine.

CLINICAL EVALUATION: In 5 patients with multiple myeloma, peak concentrations of melphalan and area under the concentration-time curve (AUC) were compared when the drug was given intravenously (IV), orally after fasting, and orally after breakfast.[1] The doses were given in random order on consecutive days. Mean peak melphalan concentrations after oral administration were 195 ng/mL after fasting and 65 ng/mL when the melphalan was taken with breakfast. Based on the AUCs, melphalan bioavailability was 93% following administration in the fasting state and 49% after breakfast. In a second report, 10 patients with neoplastic diseases received melphalan in the fasting state and after a standard breakfast.[2] Eight of these patients also received IV melphalan. Bioavailability averaged 85% in the fasting state, but only averaged 58% when melphalan was coadministered with food. Melphalan absorption also may be more variable following administration with food.

RELATED DRUGS: No information is available.

MANAGEMENT OPTIONS:

➡ *Circumvent/Minimize.* Do not administer melphalan with food. The marked reduction in its bioavailability could result in loss of efficacy.

➡ *Monitor.* Monitor patients receiving multiple courses of melphalan who are switched from postprandial to fasting administration for increased toxicity.

REFERENCES:

1. Bosanquet AG, et al. Comparison of the fed and fasting states on the absorption of melphalan in multiple myeloma. *Cancer Chemother Pharmacol.* 1984;12(3):183-186.
2. Reece PA, et al. The effect of food on oral melphalan absorption. *Cancer Chemother Pharmacol.* 1986;16(2):194-197.

Food

Nifedipine (eg, *Procardia*)

SUMMARY: Food reduces the peak plasma concentration of immediate-release nifedipine; concentrations of sustained-release nifedipine may be increased by food.

RISK FACTORS: No specific risk factors are known.

MECHANISM: Not established.

CLINICAL EVALUATION: The area under the concentration-time curve (AUC) of nifedipine after a single 10 mg dose was not altered by food; however, the peak nifedipine concentration was reduced 25% and 47% following high-fat and low-fat meals, respectively.[1] The time to peak nifedipine concentration was prolonged from 1 hour to 1.9 hours following the low-fat meal. Following a breakfast meal, significant increases were noted in mean sustained-release nifedipine peak concentration (103%) and the AUC (31%).[2] Blood pressures were significantly lower than under fasting conditions. A smaller (28%) increase in the peak nifedipine concentration without a change in AUC has been reported with a controlled-release formulation of nifedipine following administration with food compared with fasting conditions.[3]

RELATED DRUGS: No information is available.

MANAGEMENT OPTIONS:

➡ *Circumvent/Minimize.* The absorption of sustained-release nifedipine appears to be increased by food. Thus, administer sustained-release dosage forms in the fasting state to avoid altering the release characteristics of the formulation. However, controlled-release nifedipine appears to minimally be affected by food and can be taken without regard for meals.

➡ **Monitor.** Patients taking immediate-release nifedipine capsules will have reduced peak concentrations when taking doses with food. This may help minimize adverse reactions associated with elevated peak serum concentrations of nifedipine.

REFERENCES:
1. Reitberg DP, et al. Effect of food on nifedipine pharmacokinetics. *Clin Pharmacol Ther*. 1987;42(1):72-75.
2. Ueno K, et al. Effect of food on nifedipine sustained-release preparation. *DICP*. 1989;23(9):662-665.
3. Chung M, et al. Clinical pharmacokinetics of nifedipine gastrointestinal therapeutic system. A controlled-release formulation of nifedipine.*Am J Med*. 1987;83(6B):10-14.

 Food

Nilotinib (*Tasigna*)

SUMMARY: High-fat meals can increase nilotinib plasma concentration; increased risk of toxicity may occur.

RISK FACTORS: No specific risk factors are known.

MECHANISM: Unknown.

CLINICAL EVALUATION: While specific data are limited, the manufacturer of nilotinib notes that the administration of nilotinib 30 minutes after a high-fat meal increased the mean area under the plasma concentration-time curve of nilotinib by about 82%.[1] Pending further data, patients receiving nilotinib should be counseled to avoid food for at least 2 hours before and 1 hour after taking a dose. Because nilotinib is metabolized by CYP3A4, it would be particularly prudent to avoid grapefruit juice.

RELATED DRUGS: The absorption of dasatinib (*Sprycel*) is minimally affected by food.

MANAGEMENT OPTIONS:

➡ **Monitor.** Advise patients taking nilotinib to avoid administration near meal times. Be alert for signs of adverse reactions, including nausea, pruritus, rash, hematological toxicity, and arrhythmias.

REFERENCES:
1. *Tasigna* [package insert]. East Hanover, NJ: Novartis Pharmaceuticals Corporation; 2007.

 Food

Ofloxacin (eg, *Floxin*)

SUMMARY: The administration of ofloxacin with milk or yogurt has little effect on ofloxacin absorption.

RISK FACTORS: No specific risk factors are known.

MECHANISM: The calcium ions in dairy products chelate to the quinolone molecule and reduce its absorption.

CLINICAL EVALUATION: Seven healthy subjects received ofloxacin with 300 mL of water, milk (calcium 360 mg), or yogurt (calcium 450 mg). Milk and yogurt had no effect on ofloxacin absorption.[1] Eight ounces of milk or a standard breakfast were found to have no significant effect on the area under the plasma concentration-time curve of ofloxacin; food reduced the peak concentration of ofloxacin by 20%.[2]

RELATED DRUGS: Calcium ions may produce similar interactions with other quinolones.

MANAGEMENT OPTIONS: No specific action is required, but be alert for evidence of the interaction.

REFERENCES:

1. Neuvonen PJ, et al. Milk and yoghurt do not impair the absorption of ofloxacin. *Br J Clin Pharmacol.* 1992;33(3):346-348.

2. Dudley MN, et al. The effect of food or milk on the absorption kinetics of ofloxacin. *Eur J Clin Pharmacol.* 1991;41(6):569-571.

Food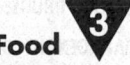

Propafenone (eg, *Rythmol*)

SUMMARY: Meals can substantially increase the peak serum concentrations of propafenone.

RISK FACTORS:

➥ ***Pharmacogenetics.*** Rapid propafenone metabolizers tend to have a greater increase in propafenone bioavailability if it is taken with food.

MECHANISM: Meals may reduce the first-pass metabolism of propafenone, resulting in increased bioavailability.

CLINICAL EVALUATION: The pharmacokinetics of a single oral dose of propafenone 300 mg administered in the fasting state and following a standard breakfast were compared in 23 healthy subjects.[1] Overall, the mean maximum propafenone concentration was increased by 50%; however, the increase in mean total area under the concentration-time curve (AUC) was insignificant (7%). When data for 4 subjects who were slow metabolizers of propafenone were excluded from analysis, peak concentrations increased by 91%, and the mean AUC increased by 55%. Propafenone half-life was not changed by food. Although the intersubject variation was large, subjects with the highest clearance after oral propafenone administration had the greatest percent increase in AUC following the meal.

RELATED DRUGS: No information is available.

MANAGEMENT OPTIONS:

➥ ***Monitor.*** Until data are available describing the effect of food on multiple-dose propafenone administration, advise patients to maintain a consistent relationship between propafenone administration and meals.

REFERENCES:

1. Axelson JE, et al. Food increases the bioavailability of propafenone. *Br J Clin Pharmacol.* 1987;23(6):735-741.

Food

Stavudine (eg, *Zerit*)

SUMMARY: Peak concentrations of stavudine were reduced during administration with a high-fat meal; the clinical significance is likely to be limited.

RISK FACTORS: No specific risk factors are known.

MECHANISM: Not established.

CLINICAL EVALUATION: Fifteen patients with HIV were administered a single dose of stavudine 70 mg while fasting, 1 hour before or immediately after a high-fat meal.[1] While the area under the concentration-time curve (AUC) of stavudine was unchanged by administration with food, the peak stavudine concentration was reduced by nearly 50%, and the time to peak concentration increased from 0.65 to 1.73 hours. The effect of a reduced peak concentration without a change in the AUC of stavudine on patient response is not known.

RELATED DRUGS: No information is available.

MANAGEMENT OPTIONS: No specific action is required, but be alert for evidence of the interaction.

REFERENCES:
1. MacLeod CM, et al. Effect of food on oral absorption of stavudine. *J Clin Pharmacol*. 1994;34(10):1025.

Food

Tetracycline (eg, *Sumycin*)

SUMMARY: Food and dairy products containing high concentrations of cations may reduce the serum concentration of tetracycline; reduced clinical efficacy may result.

RISK FACTORS: No specific risk factors are known.

MECHANISM: Cations, such as calcium and magnesium, in food can chelate with tetracyclines, thus impairing absorption of these drugs. Other factors are probably involved as well.

CLINICAL EVALUATION: It is well established that milk and dairy products can reduce the absorption of some tetracyclines. For example, ingestion of 240 to 300 mL of milk with various tetracyclines (eg, tetracycline, oxytetracycline,[+] methacycline,[+] demeclocycline [eg, *Declomycin*]) has been shown to reduce drug serum concentrations by approximately 50% or more.[1-5] Calcium in the diet (145 to 235 mg) reduced tetracycline bioavailability up to 50%.[6]

RELATED DRUGS: Food and dairy products seem to minimally affect doxycycline (eg, *Vibramycin*)[3-5] and minocycline (eg, *Minocin*) absorption.[7] Food reduces tetracycline, oxytetracycline, methacycline, and demeclocycline serum concentrations.

MANAGEMENT OPTIONS:

➡ **Consider Alternative.** Doxycycline and minocycline appear to be minimally affected and may be possible alternatives.

➡ **Circumvent/Minimize.** For optimal absorption, administer tetracycline as far apart as possible from milk and other dairy products high in cation content.

➡ **Monitor.** If tetracycline and food or dairy products containing large amounts of cations are coadministered, be alert for reduced antibiotic effects.

REFERENCES:
1. Scheiner J, et al. Experimental study of factors inhibiting absorption and effective therapeutic levels of declomycin. *Surg Gynecol Obstet*. 1962;114:9-14.
2. Neuvonen PJ. Interactions with the absorption of tetracyclines. *Drugs*. 1976;11(1):45-54.
3. *Minocin* [package insert]. Madison, NJ: Lederle Pharmaceuticals; 1993.
4. Rosenblatt JE, et al. Comparison of *in vitro* activity and clinical pharmacology of doxycycline with other tetracyclines. *Antimicrob Agents Chemother (Bethesda)*. 1966;6:134-141.

5. Welling PG, et al. Bioavailability of tetracycline and doxycycline in fasted and nonfasted subjects. *Antimicrob Agents Chemother*. 1977;11(3):462-469.

6. Cook HJ, et al. Influence of the diet on bioavailability of tetracycline. *Biopharm Drug Dispos*. 1993;14(6):549-553.

7. Mattila MJ, et al. Interference of iron preparations and milk with the absorption of tetracyclines. In: International Congress Series No. 254: Toxological Problems of Drug Combinations. Amsterdam: Exerpta Medica; 1972:129-133.

† Not available in the United States.

Food

Zidovudine (eg, *Retrovir*)

SUMMARY: Administration of zidovudine with meals lowers its plasma concentrations and could result in loss of efficacy.

RISK FACTORS:

➡ **Diet/Food.** High-fat meals may increase the bioavailability of a sustained-release formulation of zidovudine.

MECHANISM: It appears that the rate and extent of immediate-release zidovudine absorption are reduced by administration with meals. High-fat meals may increase the bioavailability of a sustained-release formulation of zidovudine.

CLINICAL EVALUATION: Eight patients with AIDS were given zidovudine in a fasting state or immediately following a high-fat meal.[1] Zidovudine concentrations following administration of a fatty meal were 57% lower than those observed when administered during the fasting state. The time to peak concentration was also significantly extended from 0.68 to 1.93 hours. The administration of zidovudine with breakfast resulted in a 25% to 35% reduction in the mean area under the concentration-time curve and greater interindividual variability, compared with administration in the fasting state.[2,3] However, some studies found little change in zidovudine absorption following high-fat[4] or high-protein[5] meals. These changes in zidovudine availability may lead to reduced efficacy. A high-fat meal was noted to increase (mean, 28%) the bioavailability of a sustained-release formulation of zidovudine.[6]

RELATED DRUGS: No information is available.

MANAGEMENT OPTIONS:

➡ **Circumvent/Minimize.** Administer zidovudine 1 to 2 hours before a meal; it should be taken in a consistent manner in relationship to meals.

➡ **Monitor.** If immediate-release zidovudine is administered with meals, monitor for loss of efficacy.

REFERENCES:

1. Unadkat JD, et al. Pharmacokinetics of oral zidovudine (ZDV) when administered with and without a high-fat meal. *Clin Pharmacol Ther*. 1989;45(2):165.

2. Lotterer E, et al. Decreased and variable systemic availability of zidovudine in patients with AIDS if administered with a meal. *Eur J Clin Pharmacol*. 1991;40(3):305-308.

3. Ruhnke M, et al. Effects of standard breakfast on pharmacokinetics of oral zidovudine in patients with AIDS. *Antimicrob Agents Chemother*. 1993;37(10):2153-2158.

4. Shelton MJ, et al. Prolonged, but not diminished, zidovudine absorption induced by a high-fat breakfast. *Pharmacotherapy*. 1994;14(6):671-677.

5. Sahai J, et al. The effect of a protein meal on zidovudine pharmacokinetics in HIV-infected patients. *Br J Clin Pharmacol.* 1992;33(6):657-660.

6. Hollister AS, et al. The effects of a high fat meal on the serum pharmacokinetics of sustained-release zidovudine. *Clin Pharmacol Ther.* 1994;55(2):193.

 4   **Fosamprenavir (*Lexiva*)**

Ranitidine (eg, *Zantac*)

SUMMARY: The administration of ranitidine reduced the plasma concentration of amprenavir following fosamprenavir dosing; the clinical significance is likely to be limited.

RISK FACTORS: No specific risk factors are known.

MECHANISM: Unknown; increased gastric pH may reduce the absorption of fosamprenavir.

CLINICAL EVALUATION: Twenty-four healthy subjects were administered a single dose of fosamprenavir 1,400 mg alone or 1 hour after a single dose of ranitidine 300 mg.[1] The administration of ranitidine reduced the mean area under the concentration-time curve of amprenavir by 26%. The effect of esomeprazole (*Nexium*) on the absorption of fosamprenavir was studied during chronic dosing of both drugs.[2] No change in plasma amprenavir was noted during 14 days of concurrent fosamprenavir and esomeprazole dosing. A single case report also noted no effect of esomeprazole on amprenavir plasma concentrations resulting from the administration of fosamprenavir/ritonavir.[3] Similarly, omeprazole (eg, *Prilosec*) 20 mg daily had no effect on amprenavir plasma concentrations following fosamprenavir plus ritonavir.[4] Based on these studies, it does not appear that the administration of gastric acid suppressants results in a significant alteration in amprenavir concentrations following fosamprenavir dosing.

RELATED DRUGS: Other H_2-receptor antagonists and proton pump inhibitors are not expected to alter the absorption of fosamprenavir. Some protease inhibitors (eg, atazanavir [*Reyataz*]) demonstrate reduced absorption if taken with gastric acid suppressors.

MANAGEMENT OPTIONS:

➡ ***Monitor.*** No special monitoring appears to be necessary when patients taking fosamprenavir are also administered H_2-receptor antagonists.

REFERENCES:

1. Ford SL, et al. Effect of antacids and ranitidine on the single-dose pharmacokinetics of fosamprenavir. *Antimicrob Agents Chemother.* 2005;49(1):467-469.

2. Shelton MJ, et al. Coadministration of esomeprazole with fosamprenavir has no impact on steady-state plasma amprenavir pharmacokinetics. *J Acquir Immune Defic Syndr.* 2006;42(1):61-67.

3. Kiser JJ, et al. Effects of esomeprazole on the pharmacokinetics of atazanavir and fosamprenavir in a patient with human immunodeficiency virus infection. *Pharmacotherapy.* 2006;26(4):511-514.

4. Luber AD, et al. Steady-state pharmacokinetics of once-daily fosamprenavir/ritonavir and atazanavir/ritonavir alone and in combination with 20 mg omeprazole in healthy volunteers. *HIV Med.* 2007;8(7):457-464.

Foscarnet

Ganciclovir (eg, *Cytovene*)

SUMMARY: The combined administration of foscarnet and ganciclovir does not appear to alter the plasma concentrations of either drug.

RISK FACTORS: No specific risk factors are known.

MECHANISM: No interaction.

CLINICAL EVALUATION: Thirteen patients with cytomegalovirus retinitis were treated with 2 weeks of ganciclovir 3.75 mg/kg and foscarnet 60 mg/kg daily or ganciclovir 6 mg/kg and foscarnet 120 mg/kg on alternating days.[1] The pharmacokinetics of foscarnet and ganciclovir were unchanged by either dosage regimen compared with the single administration of each drug.

RELATED DRUGS: Foscarnet does not appear to affect zidovudine (eg, *Retrovir*) concentrations.

MANAGEMENT OPTIONS: No interaction.

REFERENCES:
1. Aweeka FT, et al. Foscarnet and ganciclovir pharmacokinetics during concomitant or alternating maintenance therapy for AIDS-related cytomegalovirus retinitis. *Clin Pharmacol Ther.* 1995;57(4):403-412.

Foscarnet (*Foscavir*)

Zalcitabine (*Hivid*)

SUMMARY: The coadministration of foscarnet and zalcitabine does not affect the serum concentration of either drug.

RISK FACTORS: No specific risk factors are known.

MECHANISM: No interaction.

CLINICAL EVALUATION: Twelve patients each received multiple doses (duration not specified) of foscarnet 90 mg/kg IV, zalcitabine 0.75 mg, and the combination of both drugs.[1] No significant change in zalcitabine kinetics were observed during the coadministration of foscarnet vs zalcitabine alone. Similarly, coadministration of zalcitabine did not alter the kinetics of foscarnet following its administration alone.

RELATED DRUGS: No information is available.

MANAGEMENT OPTIONS: No interaction.

REFERENCES:
1. Botwin KJ, et al. Pharmacokinetics of concomitantly administered foscarnet and dideoxycytidine. *Clin Pharmacol Ther.* 1996;59:200.

Foscarnet (*Foscavir*) **5**

Zidovudine (*Retrovir*)

SUMMARY: The coadministration of foscarnet and zidovudine has no effect on the pharmacokinetics of either drug.

RISK FACTORS: No specific risk factors are known.

MECHANISM: No interaction.

CLINICAL EVALUATION: Five men with HIV taking zidovudine 200 mg every 4 hours orally for at least 2 weeks were administered foscarnet 30 mg/kg every 8 hours IV for 14 days.[1] Zidovudine plasma concentrations were measured before and after the 14 days of foscarnet. Prior to the coadministration of both drugs, zidovudine was discontinued for 2 days so that foscarnet concentrations could be obtained in the absence of zidovudine. The pharmacokinetic parameters of foscarnet were not affected by zidovudine administration. Similarly, foscarnet administration had no effect on the pharmacokinetics of zidovudine.

RELATED DRUGS: Foscarnet does not appear to affect the pharmacokinetics of ganciclovir (*Cytovene*) or didanosine (*Videx*).

MANAGEMENT OPTIONS: No interaction.

REFERENCES:
1. Aweeka FT, et al. Pharmacokinetics of concomitantly administered foscarnet and zidovudine for treatment of human immunodeficiency virus infection (AIDS clinical trials group protocol 053). *Antimicrob Agents Chemother*. 1992;36:1773.

  Furosemide (eg, *Lasix*)

Gentamicin (eg, *Garamycin*)

SUMMARY: Studies have produced little persuasive evidence that furosemide increases the toxicity of aminoglycosides.

RISK FACTORS: No specific risk factors are known.

MECHANISM: Furosemide has been reported to have variable effects on the clearance of aminoglycosides.

CLINICAL EVALUATION: A retrospective study found no greater incidence of nephrotoxicity or ototoxicity in patients receiving aminoglycosides plus furosemide compared to those taking aminoglycosides alone.[1] Furosemide has been reported to both increase and decrease the clearance of aminoglycosides.[2,3] In addition, furosemide may reduce the volume of distribution of an aminoglycoside in edematous patients.[4] More studies are needed to determine the incidence and magnitude of this interaction.

RELATED DRUGS: See Clinical Evaluation.

MANAGEMENT OPTIONS: No specific action is required, but be alert for evidence of the interaction.

REFERENCES:
1. Smith CR, et al. Effect of furosemide on aminoglycoside-induced nephrotoxicity and auditory toxicity in humans. *Antimicrob Agents Chemother*. 1983;23:133.
2. Tilstone WJ, et al. Effects of furosemide on glomerular filtration rate and clearance of practolol, digoxin, cephaloridine, and gentamicin. *Clin Pharmacol Ther*. 1977;22:389.
3. Whiting PH, et al. The effect of furosemide and piretanide on the renal clearance of gentamicin in man. *Br J Clin Pharmacol*. 1981;12:795.
4. Kaka JS, et al. Tobramycin-furosemide interaction. *Drug Intel Clin Pharm*. 1984;15:235.

Furosemide (eg, *Lasix*)

Ginseng

SUMMARY: Ginseng appeared to inhibit the diuretic response to furosemide in 1 patient, but the clinical importance of this effect is not established.

RISK FACTORS: No specific risk factors are known.

MECHANISM: Not established. The authors propose that germanium (a constituent of many ginseng preparations) may exert a toxic effect on the loop of Henle in the kidney.

CLINICAL EVALUATION: A 63-year-old man with membranous glomerulonephritis who was taking furosemide and cyclosporine (eg, *Neoral*) was hospitalized with edema and hypertension approximately 10 days after starting 10 to 12 tablets/day of a ginseng preparation (*Uncle Hsu's Korean Ginseng*).[1] He responded to high-dose IV furosemide and discontinuation of the ginseng preparation; he was sent home on furosemide 80 mg twice daily. He resumed his intake of ginseng, and over the next 14 days gained 27 pounds. He was readmitted, and 48 hours after stopping the ginseng, IV furosemide again became effective. The temporal relationship between the ingestion of ginseng and the resistance to furosemide suggests that ginseng may have inhibited the diuretic effects of furosemide, but additional clinical evidence is needed to assess the clinical importance of this purported interaction.

RELATED DRUGS: The effect of ginseng on other diuretics is not established, but consider the possibility.

MANAGEMENT OPTIONS: No specific action is required, but be alert for evidence of the interaction.

REFERENCES:

1. Becker BN, et al. Ginseng-induced diuretic resistance. *JAMA*. 1996;276:607.

Furosemide (eg, *Lasix*) ▼

Indomethacin (eg, *Indocin*)

SUMMARY: Indomethacin administration reduces the diuretic and antihypertensive efficacy of furosemide.

RISK FACTORS:

➡ *Concurrent Diseases.* Patients with hyponatremia may be at greatest risk for reduced glomerular filtration when nonsteroidal anti-inflammatory drugs (NSAIDs) are administered.

MECHANISM: Indomethacin reduces renal sodium excretion and inhibits the increase in prostaglandins that accompanies the administration of furosemide.[1]

CLINICAL EVALUATION: Indomethacin inhibits the antihypertensive and diuretic effects of furosemide in normal subjects and hypertensive patients.[6-8] In addition, patients with congestive heart failure maintained on furosemide have become worse after the addition of indomethacin therapy,[4,5] particularly if they had low sodium concentrations.[3] In a study of 8 patients with rheumatoid arthritis, furosemide 40 mg PO was associated with lower plasma indomethacin concentrations following a single dose of indomethacin 50 mg PO.[2] However, since indomethacin plasma concentrations were measured for only 3 hours, it cannot be concluded that the total effect of indomethacin would be decreased.

RELATED DRUGS: Some evidence indicates that other NSAIDs, including naproxen (eg, *Naprosyn*), ibuprofen (eg, *Advil*), piroxicam (eg, *Feldene*), flurbiprofen (eg, *Ansaid*), sulindac (eg, *Clinoril*), and large doses of salicylates have similar effects.[9,14-16] Some clinical evidence suggests that sulindac may be less likely than other NSAIDs to interfere with the response to furosemide,[10-12,16] but the difference may be only relative.[13,15]

MANAGEMENT OPTIONS:

➡ *Monitor.* Monitor patients for evidence of reduced response to furosemide when indomethacin or another NSAID is coadministered. If increasing the dose of furosemide does not achieve the desired response, consider a different NSAID such as sulindac or salicylates, which may not affect furosemide to the same degree.

REFERENCES:

1. Davis A, et al. Interactions between non-steroidal anti-inflammatory drugs and antihypertensive and diuretics. *Aust NZ J Med*. 1986;16:537.

2. Brooks PM, et al. The effect of furosemide on indomethacin plasma levels. *Br J Clin Pharmacol*. 1974;1:485.

3. Dzau VJ, et al. Prostaglandins in severe congestive heart failure in relation to activation of the renin-angiotensin system and hyponatremia. *N Engl J Med*. 1984;310:347.

4. Allan SG, et al. Interaction between diuretics and indomethacin. *Br Med J*. 1981;283:1611.

5. Poe TE, et al. Interaction of indomethacin with furosemide. *J Fam Pract*. 1983;16:610.

6. Brater DC. Analysis of the effect of indomethacin on the response to furosemide in man: effect of dose of furosemide. *J Pharmacol Exp Ther*. 1979;210:386.

7. Smith DE, et al. Attenuation of furosemide's diuretic effect by indomethacin: pharmacokinetic evaluation. *J Pharmacokinet Biopharm*. 1979;7:265.

8. Patak RV, et al. Antagonism of the effects of furosemide by indomethacin in normal and hypertensive man. *Prostaglandins*. 1975;10:649.

9. Rawles JM. Antagonism between non-steroidal anti-inflammatory drugs and diuretics. *Scott Med J*. 1982;27:37.

10. Ciabattoni G, et al. Renal effects of anti-inflammatory drugs. *Eur J Rheumatol Inflamm*. 1980;3:210.

11. Bunning RD, et al. Sulindac: a potentially renal-sparing nonsteroidal anti-inflammatory drug. *JAMA*. 1982;248:2864.

12. Wong DG, et al. Non-steroidal antiinflammatory drugs (NSAIDs) vs placebo in hypertension treated with diuretic and beta-blocker. *Clin Pharmacol Ther*. 1984;35:284.

13. Roberts DG, et al. Comparative effects of sulindac and indomethacin in humans. *Clin Pharmacol Ther*. 1984;35:269.

14. Wilkins MR, et al. The effects of selective and nonselective inhibition of cyclo-oxygenase on furosemide-stimulated natriuresis. *Int J Clin Pharmacol Ther Toxicol*. 1986;24:55.

15. Brater DC, et al. Sulindac does not spare the kidney. *Clin Pharmacol Ther*. 1984;35:258.

16. Eriksson L-O, et al. Renal function and tubular transport effects of sulindac and naproxen in chronic heart failure. *Clin Pharmacol Ther*. 1987;42:646.

Furosemide (eg, *Lasix*) 4

Lithium (eg, *Eskalith*)

SUMMARY: Isolated cases of lithium toxicity associated with furosemide have been reported, but furosemide appears to have little effect on lithium concentrations in most patients.

RISK FACTORS:

➡ ***Diet/Food.*** Patients on a sodium-restricted diet may be at higher risk.

MECHANISM: Sustained furosemide therapy can cause sodium depletion, which in turn can decrease lithium excretion.

CLINICAL EVALUATION: Although both acute[1] and chronic[2] experiments failed to demonstrate an effect of furosemide on lithium excretion, 1 case report described lithium intoxication that apparently resulted from furosemide plus dietary sodium restriction.[3] Another case of a purported furosemide-induced lithium intoxication has been reported,[4] but it is not clear that furosemide was responsible. In a study of 5 normal subjects stabilized on lithium, furosemide 40 mg/day for 2 weeks did not affect serum lithium concentrations, but a significant rise in serum lithium occurred during treatment with hydrochlorothiazide 50 mg/day for 2 weeks.[5] Larger doses of furosemide were not studied. Thus, relatively little evidence exists to indicate that furosemide affects serum lithium concentrations, but it is possible that the interaction occurs under certain circumstances.

RELATED DRUGS: Thiazides consistently increase serum lithium concentrations, but little is known about the effect of other loop diuretics on lithium.

MANAGEMENT OPTIONS: No specific action is required, but be alert for evidence of the interaction.

REFERENCES:

1. Thomsen K, et al. Renal lithium excretion in man. *Am J Physiol.* 1968;215:823.
2. Shalmi M, et al. Effect of chronic oral furosemide administration on the 24-hour cycle of lithium clearance and electrolyte excretion in humans. *Eur J Clin Pharmacol.* 1990;38:275.
3. Hurtig HI, et al. Lithium toxicity enhanced by diuresis. *N Engl J Med.* 1974;290:748.
4. Oh TE. Furosemide and lithium toxicity. *Anaesth Intensive Care.* 1977;5:60.
5. Jefferson JW, et al. Serum lithium levels and long-term diuretic use. *JAMA.* 1979;214:1134.

Furosemide (eg, *Lasix*) 4

Lomefloxacin (*Maxaquin*)

SUMMARY: Furosemide administration results in a small increase in lomefloxacin plasma concentrations; changes in patient response to lomefloxacin are likely to be minimal.

RISK FACTORS: No specific risk factors are known.

MECHANISM: Not established. Lomefloxacin is eliminated primarily via the kidney by both glomerular filtration and tubular secretion. It is possible that furosemide competes for renal tubular secretion with lomefloxacin resulting in a reduced renal clearance of lomefloxacin.

CLINICAL EVALUATION: Furosemide 40 mg increased the area under the plasma concentration-time curve of lomefloxacin by 12%.[1] The renal clearance of lomefloxacin was reduced 33% during the coadministration of furosemide. Lomefloxacin administration had no effect on the pharmacokinetics of furosemide. The clinical significance of the changes observed in lomefloxacin concentrations are likely to be minimal.

RELATED DRUGS: The effect of furosemide on the elimination of other quinolone antibiotics is unknown, but probably would be limited to those quinolones that are eliminated renally (eg, ofloxacin [*Floxin*]). The effect of other loop diuretics might be similar.

MANAGEMENT OPTIONS: No specific action is required, but be alert for evidence of the interaction.

REFERENCES:

1. Sudoh T, et al. Renal clearance of lomefloxacin is decreased by furosemide. *Eur J Clin Pharmacol.* 1994;46:267.

Furosemide (eg, *Lasix*)

Oxcarbazepine (*Trileptal*)

SUMMARY: A patient on oxcarbazepine developed hyponatremia with encephalopathy following addition of furosemide; monitor electrolytes and mental status.

RISK FACTORS: No specific risk factors are known.

MECHANISM: Not established. Oxcarbazepine can decrease serum sodium concentrations, and furosemide increases urinary sodium elimination. It is possible that the hyponatremia in this patient resulted from the combined hyponatremic effect of oxcarbazepine and furosemide.

CLINICAL EVALUATION: A 64-year-old woman on oxcarbazepine for complex partial seizures was started on furosemide 25 mg/day for mild hypertension.[1] About a month later she developed confusion, hallucinations, and delirium along with hyponatremia (sodium 115 mEq/L). Her sodium was measured at 138 mEq/L before the furosemide was added. Both drugs were stopped and valproic acid 1 g/day was added. Twenty days later, the sodium returned to normal and her symptoms had resolved.

RELATED DRUGS: Theoretically, other loop diuretics may also increase the risk of hyponatremia in patients on oxcarbazepine.

MANAGEMENT OPTIONS:

➥ *Monitor.* In patients receiving oxcarbazepine with furosemide or other loop diuretics, monitor serum sodium and for evidence of hyponatremic encephalopathy (eg, confusion, delirium, hallucinations).

REFERENCES:

1. Siniscalchi A, et al. Acute encephalopathy induced by oxcarbazepine and furosemide. *Ann Pharmacother.* 2004;38:509-510.

Furosemide (eg, *Lasix*)

Phenytoin (eg, *Dilantin*)

SUMMARY: Studies in patients and healthy subjects indicate that phenytoin may reduce the diuretic response to furosemide.

RISK FACTORS: No specific risk factors are known.

MECHANISM: Phenytoin appears to inhibit the GI absorption of furosemide.[2] An additional inhibitory effect of phenytoin on the diuretic response to furosemide is possible.[1]

CLINICAL EVALUATION: Following the clinical observation that patients on anticonvulsant therapy responded poorly to diuretics, the diuretic response to furosemide was studied in a group of epileptic patients and normal subjects. The diuretic response to furosemide was significantly smaller and delayed in the 17 patients receiving anticonvulsants (phenytoin and phenobarbital (eg, *Solfoton*), with some also receiving other anticonvulsants).[1] In a subsequent study in 5 normal subjects, phenytoin 300 mg/day for 10 days reduced oral furosemide absorption by about 50% without affecting its serum clearance.[2]

RELATED DRUGS: The effect of phenytoin on other loop diuretics is not established. Phenobarbital affects furosemide similarly.

MANAGEMENT OPTIONS:

➡ **Monitor.** In patients taking phenytoin, be alert for an impaired diuretic response to furosemide; larger furosemide doses may be required. It is not known if separating the doses of the drugs would minimize the interaction.

REFERENCES:

1. Ahmad S. Renal insensitivity to furosemide caused by chronic anticonvulsant therapy. *Br Med J.* 1974;3:657.
2. Fine A, et al. Malabsorption of furosemide caused by phenytoin. *Br Med J.* 1977;4:1061.

Furosemide (eg, *Lasix*)

Probenecid (*Benemid*)

SUMMARY: Probenecid may increase the serum concentration of furosemide but has less effect on furosemide-induced renal sodium excretion.

RISK FACTORS: No specific risk factors are known.

MECHANISM: Furosemide is excreted primarily by active renal tubular secretion, which may be inhibited by concomitant probenecid therapy.

CLINICAL EVALUATION: Several studies have demonstrated an ability of probenecid to reduce the renal clearance of furosemide considerably (25% to 35%).[1-3] However, the ability of furosemide to increase urinary sodium excretion was minimally affected.

RELATED DRUGS: Probenecid also appears to have minimal effects on the response to bumetanide (eg, *Bumex*).

MANAGEMENT OPTIONS: No specific action is required, but be alert for evidence of the interaction.

REFERENCES:

1. Honari J, et al. Effects of probenecid on furosemide kinetics and natriuresis in man. *Clin Pharmacol Ther.* 1977;22:395.
2. Homeida M, et al. Influence of probenecid and spironolactone on furosemide kinetics and dynamics in man. *Clin Pharmacol Ther.* 1977;22:402.
3. Sommers DK, et al. The influence of co-administered organic acids on the kinetics and dynamics of furosemide. *Br J Clin Pharmacol.* 1991;32:489.

4 Furosemide (eg, *Lasix*)

Propranolol (eg, *Inderal*)

SUMMARY: Furosemide may increase plasma propranolol concentrations, but the clinical importance of this effect is not established.

RISK FACTORS: No specific risk factors are known.

MECHANISM: Not established.

CLINICAL EVALUATION: Propranolol 40 mg was given with and without furosemide 25 mg to 10 subjects.[3] Concurrent furosemide was associated with a considerable increase in plasma propranolol concentrations and increased beta blockade.

RELATED DRUGS: Practolol (*Pravachol*) renal clearance is reduced by furosemide,[1] but atenolol (eg, *Tenormin*) does not appear to be affected by concurrent furosemide treatment.[2] The effect of furosemide on other beta blockers is not established. The common combination of beta blockers and furosemide suggests that adverse effects from this interaction are very uncommon.

MANAGEMENT OPTIONS: No specific action is required, but be alert for evidence of the interaction.

REFERENCES:

1. Tilstone WJ, et al. Effects of furosemide on glomerular filtration rate and clearance of practolol, digoxin, cephaloridine, and gentamicin. *Clin Pharmacol Ther.* 1977;22:389.
2. Kirch W, et al. Interaction of atenolol with furosemide and calcium and aluminum salts. *Clin Pharmacol Ther.* 1981;30:429.
3. Chiariello M, et al. Effect of furosemide on plasma concentration and beta blockade by propranolol. *Clin Pharmacol Ther.* 1979;26:433.

Furosemide (eg, *Lasix*)

Terbutaline (eg, *Brethaire*)

SUMMARY: The administration of furosemide and terbutaline produces additive hypokalemia; the clinical significance of this interaction is not well defined.

RISK FACTORS:

➡ *Other Drugs.* Patients taking potassium-depleting corticosteroids may be more prone to hypokalemia from this interaction.

➡ *Concurrent Diseases.* Patients with low basal serum potassium may be at increased risk for arrhythmia when treated with combinations of furosemide and terbutaline.

MECHANISM: Both furosemide and the beta₂-agonist terbutaline can produce hypokalemia. When administered together, their effects on serum potassium concentrations appear to be additive.

CLINICAL EVALUATION: Fifteen healthy subjects received a placebo or furosemide 40 mg/day for at least 4 days in a cross-over design.[1] Following pretreatment with a placebo or diuretic, a 1,000 mcg dose of terbutaline was administered via a metered dose inhaler. Blood samples and electrocardiogram (ECG) were obtained 30 minutes later. Mean baseline serum potassium concentration was 3.88 mmol/L. Furosemide and terbutaline lowered the serum potassium concentration to 3.58 mmol/L and 3.35 mmol/L, respectively. The combination of terbutaline and furosemide reduced the serum potassium concentration 3.13 mmol/L. T wave amplitude fell during hypokalemia and terbutaline increased the heart rate. Triamterene (*Dyrenium*) 50 mg administered with furosemide or terbutaline only attenuated the hypokalemia associated with furosemide. The potential significance of this magnitude of change in serum potassium awaits patient trials.

RELATED DRUGS: It is likely that other combinations of potassium-wasting diuretics and beta₂-agonists also would tend to reduce serum potassium concentrations.

MANAGEMENT OPTIONS:

➡ *Circumvent/Minimize.* In patients who appear predisposed to hypokalemia, triamterene or potassium supplementation may be given to prevent excessive reduction in serum potassium concentrations.

➡ *Monitor.* Monitor patients treated with combinations of potassium-wasting diuretics and beta₂-agonists for signs of hypokalemia including ECG changes, fatigue, and muscle pains.

REFERENCES:

1. Newnham DM, et al. The effects of furosemide and terbutaline on the hypokalemic and electrocardiographic responses to inhaled terbutaline. *Br J Clin Pharmacol.* 1991;32:630.

4　**Furosemide (eg, *Lasix*)**

Theophylline (eg, *Theolair*)

SUMMARY: Single dose furosemide administration increased the serum theophylline concentration; clinically significant changes in theophylline concentrations appear to be unlikely.

RISK FACTORS: No specific risk factors are known.

MECHANISM: Not established. Furosemide administration may reduce the volume of distribution of theophylline and increase its serum concentrations.

CLINICAL EVALUATION: Ten patients with pulmonary diseases were treated with IV aminophylline for 48 hours before the serum theophylline concentration was measured.[1] After 48 hours, a 40 mg dose of furosemide IV was administered; 4 hours later, theophylline serum concentration was measured again. Theophylline concentrations measured following the furosemide dose were on average 2.9 mcg/mL higher than those measured before furosemide administration. None of the patients developed symptoms of theophylline toxicity.

RELATED DRUGS: The effect of loop diuretics other than furosemide on theophylline is not established.

MANAGEMENT OPTIONS: No specific action is required, but be alert for evidence of the interaction.

REFERENCES:

1. Conion PF, et al. Effect of intravenous furosemide on serum theophylline concentrations. *Am J Hosp Pharm.* 1981;38:1345.

　Furosemide (eg, *Lasix*)

Tubocurarine

SUMMARY: Furosemide appears to prolong the neuromuscular blockade following tubocurarine.

RISK FACTORS: No specific risk factors are known.

MECHANISM: Not established.

CLINICAL EVALUATION: Three patients given tubocurarine during surgery developed enhanced neuromuscular blockade following administration of furosemide.[1] Although mannitol was given concomitantly in most cases, it seems likely that the furosemide was primarily responsible. Animal studies indicate that low doses of furosemide enhance the neuromuscular blockade of tubocurarine, whereas high doses (1 to 4 mg/kg body weight) of furosemide antagonized the neuromuscular blockade.[2]

RELATED DRUGS: No information is available.

MANAGEMENT OPTIONS:

➡ ***Monitor.*** Monitor patients for altered dosage requirements for neuromuscular blocking agents when receiving furosemide.

REFERENCES:

1. Miller RD, et al. Enhancement of d-tubocurarine neuromuscular blockade by diuretics in man. *Anesthesiology.* 1976;45:442.
2. Scappaticci KA, et al. Effects of furosemide on the neuromuscular junction. *Anesthesiology.* 1982;57:381.

Furosemide (eg, *Lasix*) 5

Warfarin (eg, *Coumadin*)

SUMMARY: Furosemide probably has minimal effect on the hypoprothrombinemic response to oral anticoagulants.

RISK FACTORS: No specific risk factors are known.

MECHANISM: No interaction.

CLINICAL EVALUATION: In a study of 11 normal subjects, furosemide did not affect the warfarin half-life or hypoprothrombinemic response.[1]

RELATED DRUGS: Furosemide theoretically might have minor effects on the hypoprothrombinemic response to oral anticoagulants as do thiazides; however, any such effects are of questionable clinical significance. Warfarin also appears unaffected by bumetanide (eg, *Bumex*). Thiazides may slightly reduce warfarin effect.

MANAGEMENT OPTIONS: No interaction.

REFERENCES:

1. Nilsson CM, et al. The effect of furosemide and bumetanide on warfarin metabolism and anticoagulant response. *J Clin Pharmacol*. 1978;18:91.

Gamma Globulin

Phenytoin (eg, *Dilantin*)

SUMMARY: A patient on phenytoin therapy developed a hypersensitivity myocarditis (HM) and died after receiving gamma globulin, but a causal relationship was not established.

RISK FACTORS: No specific risk factors are known.

MECHANISM: Not established. Phenytoin has been associated with HM, and it was proposed that the gamma globulin may have promoted the development of phenytoin-induced HM.

CLINICAL EVALUATION: A 43-year-old man on chronic therapy with phenytoin, nizatidine, and acetaminophen developed Guillain-Barré syndrome, and was given IV gamma globulin 0.4 g/kg/day for 5 days.[1] Two days after completing the gamma globulin therapy, he developed abdominal pain and aching shoulders and back. He died during a hypotensive episode, and an autopsy revealed HM. It was proposed that the HM resulted from combined therapy with phenytoin and gamma globulin, and that the HM produced a fatal arrhythmia. However, a causal relationship was not established.

RELATED DRUGS: No information is available.

MANAGEMENT OPTIONS:

➠ *Consider Alternative.* Although a causal relationship between HM and combined phenytoin-gamma globulin therapy is not established, the severity of the reaction dictates that the benefit-risk of using this combination be considered carefully.

➠ *Monitor.* If gamma globulin is given in the presence of phenytoin therapy, be alert for evidence of hypersensitivity (eg, fever, skin rash, eosinophilia) and cardiac findings (eg, tachycardia, ECG changes, enzyme elevations).

REFERENCES:
1. Koehler PJ, et al. Lethal hypersensitivity myocarditis associated with the use of intravenous gamma globulin for Guillain-Barré syndrome, in combination with phenytoin. *J Neurol.* 1996;243:366-367.

 Ganciclovir (eg, *Cytovene*)

AVOID **Zidovudine (*Retrovir*)**

SUMMARY: Combination therapy with ganciclovir and zidovudine in the treatment of cytomegalovirus (CMV) disease increases hematological toxicity.

RISK FACTORS: No specific risk factors are known.

MECHANISM: Not established. The toxicity appears to be the result of combined pharmacodynamic effects, rather than the result of a pharmacokinetic interaction between ganciclovir and zidovudine.

CLINICAL EVALUATION: Patients with acquired immunodeficiency syndrome-related CMV disease were treated with zidovudine 1,200 mg/day (n = 10) or zidovudine 600 mg/day (n = 29) plus ganciclovir 5 mg/kg IV twice daily for 14 days followed by 5 mg/kg/day for 5 days/week.[1] All 10 patients treated with ganciclovir and high-dose zidovudine developed severe hematologic toxicity over several weeks. About 80% of the patients receiving the smaller dose of zidovudine required further dosage reduction because of anemia, neutropenia, or GI toxicity. In approximately 80% of the patients receiving combination therapy, the CMV infection worsened or new infections developed necessitating withdrawal of therapy. No significant differences were noted in the pharmacokinetics of either drug when used in combination compared to monotherapy.[1,2]

RELATED DRUGS: No information is available.

MANAGEMENT OPTIONS:

➥ *AVOID COMBINATION.* Until more information is available, avoid this combination of drugs. Foscarnet (*Foscavir*) may be a reasonable alternative to ganciclovir for the treatment of CMV retinitis in patients treated with zidovudine.[3]

REFERENCES:

1. Hochster H, et al. Toxicity of combined ganciclovir and zidovudine for cytomegalovirus disease associated with AIDS. *Ann Intern Med.* 1990;113:111-117.

2. Burger DM, et al. Pharmacokinetic variability of zidovudine in HIV-infected individuals: subgroup analysis and drug interactions. *AIDS.* 1994;8:1683-1689.

3. Jacobson MA, et al. Foscarnet therapy for ganciclovir-resistant cytomegalovirus retinitis in patients with AIDS. *J Infect Dis.* 1991;163:1348-1351.

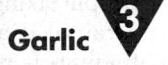

Garlic

Saquinavir (eg, *Fortovase*)

SUMMARY: Garlic administration reduces saquinavir plasma concentrations; reduction in antiviral effect may occur.

RISK FACTORS: No specific risk factors are known.

MECHANISM: Garlic appears to reduce the bioavailability of saquinavir. It is unknown if this effect is caused by induction of CYP450 enzymes, alteration of saquinavir active transporters, or both.

CLINICAL EVALUATION: Healthy subjects received saquinavir 1,200 mg 3 times daily with meals for 3 days and following 20 days of garlic (equivalent to about 8 g of fresh garlic cloves daily) given with breakfast and dinner.[1] Saquinavir and garlic were discontinued for 10 days and a final 3-day course of saquinavir was administered, again without garlic pretreatment. When administered following garlic, the area under the concentration-time curve (AUC) and peak plasma concentration of saquinavir decreased 51% and 54%, respectively. When saquinavir was re-administered 10 days after the discontinuation of garlic, the mean AUC was still about 35% below the pregarlic values. Shorter exposure to garlic or lower doses may be less likely to affect saquinavir. Reduced saquinavir concentrations may result in decreased antiviral effect in some patients.

RELATED DRUGS: Garlic administration for 4 days produced an insignificant reduction in ritonavir (*Norvir*) concentrations. The effect of garlic on other protease inhibitors is unknown.

MANAGEMENT OPTIONS:

➥ *Circumvent/Minimize.* Patients taking saquinavir should avoid chronic, high-dose garlic administration.

➡ *Monitor.* Observe patients taking saquinavir, and perhaps other protease inhibitors, for reduced antiviral plasma concentrations if garlic is ingested chronically.

REFERENCES:

1. Piscitelli SC, et al. The effect of garlic supplements on the pharmacokinetics of saquinavir. *Clin Infect Dis.* 2002;34:234-238.

 Garlic

Warfarin (eg, *Coumadin*)

SUMMARY: Isolated reports suggest that garlic may increase the risk of bleeding in patients on oral anticoagulants, but a causal relationship has not been established.

RISK FACTORS: No specific risk factors are known.

MECHANISM: Reports of garlic-induced inhibition of platelet function have appeared,[1-4] but it is not known if this represents a clinically important finding. One randomized, double-blind study failed to find any effect of garlic on platelet aggregation.[5]

CLINICAL EVALUATION: Several anecdotal cases of bleeding episodes have been reported in people taking garlic, with or without concurrent warfarin therapy.[6-8] Nonetheless, a causal relationship has not been established; the clinical importance of these findings is not established.[9,10] The available data are not sufficient to warrant a warning for patients on warfarin to avoid eating garlic in foods or taking garlic supplements. As with any herbal drug, there are likely to be substantial differences in the content, depending on the product used.

RELATED DRUGS: No information is available.

MANAGEMENT OPTIONS: No specific action is required, but be alert for evidence of the interaction.

REFERENCES:

1. Srivastava KC. Evidence for the mechanism by which garlic inhibits platelet aggregation. *Prostaglandins Leukot Med.* 1986;22(3):313-321.
2. Srivastava KC, et al. Effects of a garlic-derived principle (ajoene) on aggregation and arachidonic acid metabolism in human blood platelets. *Prostaglandins Leukot Essent Fatty Acids.* 1993;49(2):587-595.
3. Bordia A, et al. Effect of garlic on platelet aggregation in humans: a study in healthy subjects and patients with coronary artery disease. *Prostaglandins Leukot Essent Fatty Acids.* 1996;55(3):201-205.
4. Bordia A, et al. Effect of garlic (*Allium sativum*) on blood lipids, blood sugar, fibrinogen and fibrinolytic activity in patients with coronary artery disease. *Prostaglandins Leukot Essent Fatty Acids.* 1998;58(4):257-263.
5. Morris J, et al. Effects of garlic extract on platelet aggregation: a randomized placebo-controlled double-blind study. *Clin Exp Pharmacol Physiol.* 1995;22(6-7):414-417.
6. Sunter WH. Warfarin and garlic. *Pharm J.* 1991;246:722.
7. Rose KD, et al. Spontaneous spinal epidural hematoma with associated platelet dysfunction from excessive garlic ingestion: a case report. *Neurosurgery.* 1990;26(5):880-882.
8. Burnham BE. Garlic as a possible risk for postoperative bleeding. *Plast Reconstr Surg.* 1995;95(1):213.
9. Vaes LP, et al. Interactions of warfarin with garlic, ginger, ginkgo, or ginseng: nature of the evidence. *Ann Pharmacother.* 2000;34(12):1478-1482.
10. Miller LG. Herbal medicinals: selected clinical considerations focusing on known or potential drugherb interactions. *Arch Intern Med.* 1998;158(20):2200-2211.

Gatifloxacin (*Zymar*)

Glyburide (eg, *DiaBeta*)

SUMMARY: The administration of gatifloxacin to patients with diabetes may result in episodes of hypoglycemia.

RISK FACTORS: No specific risk factors are known.

MECHANISM: Unknown. It is thought that gatifloxacin may increase insulin secretion from the pancreas.[1]

CLINICAL EVALUATION: Several case reports have noted hypoglycemia occurring within the first 2 days of gatifloxacin coadministration in patients with diabetes. Most of these patients were being treated with oral hypoglycemic agents, including glyburide, metformin (eg, *Glucophage*), repaglinide (*Prandin*), and pioglitazone (*Actos*).[2-4] A 10-day study of the coadministration of gatifloxacin and glyburide did not demonstrate a change in fasting glucose concentrations in patients with type 2 diabetes.[5] Pending additional study, be alert for hypoglycemia in patients with diabetes who are started on gatifloxacin.

RELATED DRUGS: Ciprofloxacin (eg, *Cipro*) has been associated with hypoglycemia in patients taking oral hypoglycemic agents. If gatifloxacin stimulates insulin secretion, any hypoglycemic agent could produce additive hypoglycemia.

MANAGEMENT OPTIONS:

➡ *Monitor.* Pending further data, monitor blood glucose concentrations carefully during gatifloxacin administration to patients with diabetes.

REFERENCES:

1. Gajjar DA, et al. Effect of multiple-dose gatifloxacin or ciprofloxacin on glucose homeostasis and insulin production in patients with noninsulin-dependent diabetes mellitus maintained with diet and exercise. *Pharmacotherapy.* 2000;20(6 pt 2):76S-86S.
2. Hussein G, et al. Gatifloxacin-induced hypoglycemia: a case report and review of the literature. *Clin Res Regul Aff.* 2002;19(4):333-339.
3. Baker SE, et al. Possible gatifloxacin-induced hypoglycemia. *Ann Pharmacother.* 2002;36(11):1722-1726.
4. Menzies DJ, et al. Severe and persistent hypoglycemia due to gatifloxacin interaction with oral hypoglycemic agents. *Am J Med.* 2002;113(3):232-234.
5. *Tequin* [package insert]. Princeton, NJ: Bristol-Meyers Squibb Company; 2000.

Gefitinib (*Iressa*)

Itraconazole (eg, *Sporanox*)

SUMMARY: Itraconazole coadministration with gefitinib can cause an increase in gefitinib plasma concentrations; increased toxicity is likely to occur unless dosage adjustments are made.

RISK FACTORS: No specific risk factors are known.

MECHANISM: Itraconazole inhibits the activity of CYP3A4, the enzyme primarily responsible for the metabolism of gefitinib.

CLINICAL EVALUATION: Forty-seven healthy subjects received a single dose of gefitinib 250 or 500 mg alone and on day 4 of a 10-day course of itraconazole 200 mg daily.[1] The mean area under the plasma concentration-time curve of gefitinib was increased 80% and 57% following the 250 and 500 mg doses, respectively, during itraconazole coadministration. The half-life of gefitinib was prolonged from 31 to 35 hours to 38 to 43 hours following itraconazole administration. This degree of increase in gefitinib plasma concentration is likely to result in increased adverse reactions.

RELATED DRUGS: Other antifungal agents that inhibit CYP3A4 (eg, fluconazole [eg, *Diflucan*], ketoconazole [eg, *Nizoral*], posaconazole [*Noxafil*], voriconazole [*Vfend*]) are expected to affect gefitinib in a similar manner.

MANAGEMENT OPTIONS:

➡ ***Consider Alternative.*** Terbinafine (eg, *Lamisil*) could be considered as an alternative antifungal agent because it does not affect CYP3A4 activity. Amphotericin (eg, *Amphocin*), caspofungin (*Cancidas*), and anidulafungin (*Eraxis*) do not appear to inhibit CYP3A4.

➡ ***Monitor.*** Monitor patients who must receive itraconazole and gefitinib for adverse reactions (eg, diarrhea, nausea, skin rash, vomiting). A reduction in gefitinib dosage may be necessary.

REFERENCES:

1. Swaisland HC, et al. Pharmacokinetic drug interactions of gefitinib with rifampicin, itraconazole and metoprolol. *Clin Pharmacokinet*. 2005;44(10):1067-1081.

 Gefitinib (*Iressa*)

Metoprolol (eg, *Lopressor*)

SUMMARY: Gefitinib coadministration with metoprolol can cause a modest increase in metoprolol plasma concentrations; some increase in metoprolol-induced adverse reactions may occur.

RISK FACTORS: No specific risk factors are known.

MECHANISM: Gefitinib may reduce the activity of CYP2D6, the enzyme primarily responsible for the metabolism of metoprolol.

CLINICAL EVALUATION: Fifteen cancer patients received a single dose of metoprolol 50 mg alone and on day 15 of a 28-day course of gefitinib 500 mg daily.[1] The mean area under the plasma concentration-time curve of metoprolol was increased 50% during coadministration of gefitinib. The half-life of metoprolol was increased from a mean of 3.5 to 3.8 hours during gefitinib coadministration. This change in metoprolol plasma concentration is not likely to cause significant adverse reactions in most patients.

RELATED DRUGS: Other beta-blockers metabolized by CYP2D6 (eg, carvedilol [*Coreg*], propranolol [eg, *Inderal*], timolol [eg, *Blocadren*]) also may be affected by gefitinib coadministration.

MANAGEMENT OPTIONS:

➡ ***Monitor.*** Monitor patients receiving metoprolol and gefitinib for evidence of increased beta-blockade, including bradycardia and hypotension.

REFERENCES:

1. Swaisland HC, et al. Pharmacokinetic drug interactions of gefitinib with rifampicin, itraconazole and metoprolol. *Clin Pharmacokinet*. 2005;44(10):1067-1081.

Gefitinib (*Iressa*)

Ranitidine (eg, *Zantac*)

SUMMARY: Drugs that increase the gastric pH may reduce the plasma concentrations of gefitinib.

RISK FACTORS: No specific risk factors are known.

MECHANISM: Unknown. It appears that gefitinib may have a lower bioavailability when the gastric pH is elevated.

CLINICAL EVALUATION: While specific data are limited, the manufacturer of gefitinib notes that coadministration of agents that significantly elevate gastric pH may reduce the plasma concentrations of gefitinib.[1] Pending further data to clarify the clinical significance of this interaction, observe patients receiving gefitinib and gastric acid suppressants for decreased gefitinib therapeutic effect.

RELATED DRUGS: Other H$_2$-receptor antagonists (cimetidine [eg, *Tagamet*], famotidine [eg, *Pepcid*], nizatidine [*Axid*]) and antacids also may reduce gefitinib plasma concentrations. Omeprazole (eg, *Prilosec*), esomeprazole (*Nexium*), pantoprazole (*Protonix*), rabeprazole (*Aciphex*), and lansoprazole (*Prevacid*) are also expected to interact in a similar manner with gefitinib.

MANAGEMENT OPTIONS:

➡ **Monitor.** Carefully monitor patients who receive a gastric acid suppressant and gefitinib for adequate clinical response to gefitinib. An increase in gefitinib dosage may be necessary.

REFERENCES:

1. *Iressa* [package insert]. Wilmington, DE: AstraZeneca Pharmaceuticals LP; 2004.

Gefitinib (*Iressa*) ▼

Rifampin (eg, *Rifadin*)

SUMMARY: Rifampin coadministration with gefitinib can cause a large reduction in gefitinib plasma concentrations; loss of gefitinib efficacy is likely unless dosage adjustments are made.

RISK FACTORS: No specific risk factors are known.

MECHANISM: Rifampin induces the activity of CYP3A4, the enzyme primarily responsible for the metabolism of gefitinib.

CLINICAL EVALUATION: Eighteen healthy subjects received a single dose of gefitinib 500 mg alone and on day 10 of a 16-day course of rifampin 600 mg daily.[1] The mean area under the plasma concentration-time curve of gefitinib was reduced 83% during coadministration of rifampin. The half-life of gefitinib was reduced from a mean of 34 to 21 hours following rifampin administration. This degree of reduction in gefitinib plasma concentration is likely to significantly reduce its therapeutic effects.

RELATED DRUGS: Rifabutin (*Mycobutin*) is known to induce CYP3A4 and is expected to increase the elimination of gefitinib.

MANAGEMENT OPTIONS:

➡ *Monitor.* Carefully monitor patients who must receive rifampin and gefitinib for adequate clinical response to gefitinib. An increase in gefitinib dosage may be necessary.

REFERENCES:

1. Swaisland HC, et al. Pharmacokinetic drug interactions of gefitinib with rifampicin, itraconazole and metoprolol. *Clin Pharmacokinet.* 2005;44(10):1067-1081.

Gemcitabine (*Gemzar*)

Warfarin (eg, *Coumadin*)

SUMMARY: A patient on warfarin developed increased anticoagulant effect when gemcitabine was given concurrently. A causal effect appears likely in this patient, but the general incidence and magnitude of this interaction are not established.

RISK FACTORS: No specific risk factors are known.

MECHANISM: Not established. A pharmacokinetic interaction seems unlikely because gemcitabine is not metabolized by CYP-450 isoenzymes and is minimally bound to plasma proteins. It is possible that gemcitabine-induced impairment of hepatic function reduces the production of clotting factors, but this possibility has not been investigated.

CLINICAL EVALUATION: A 63-year-old man developed an increased hypoprothrombinemic response to warfarin on 2 occasions during gemcitabine therapy.[1] Each time the gemcitabine was stopped, the effect dissipated. This phenomenon indicated that there may be a causal relationship between the changes in international normalized ratio (INR) and the starting and stopping of gemcitabine.

RELATED DRUGS: The effect of gemcitabine on other oral anticoagulants is not known. Nonetheless, if the mechanism is pharmacodynamic, all oral anticoagulants are expected to interact in a similar manner.

MANAGEMENT OPTIONS:

➡ *Monitor.* Monitor the hypoprothrombinemic response more frequently in patients taking warfarin or other oral anticoagulants if gemcitabine is given concurrently. Weekly INR measurements should be sufficient.[1]

REFERENCES:

1. Kinikar SA, et al. Identification of a gemcitabine-warfarin interaction. *Pharmacotherapy.* 1999;19(11):1331-1333.

Gemfibrozil (eg, *Lopid*)

Glimepiride (eg, *Amaryl*)

SUMMARY: Gemfibrozil administration to healthy subjects resulted in a modest increase in glimepiride plasma concentrations; no change in blood sugar concentration was noted.

RISK FACTORS: No specific risk factors are known.

MECHANISM: Gemfibrozil appears to modestly reduce the metabolism of glimepiride, probably by inhibiting CYP2C9 activity.

CLINICAL EVALUATION: Gemfibrozil 600 mg/day or placebo was administered to 10 healthy subjects for 2 days.[1] On the third day, a single dose of glimepiride 0.5 mg was administered orally 1 hour after the dose of gemfibrozil. The pretreatment of gemfibrozil increased the mean area under the concentration-time curve of glimepiride 23% and prolonged its half-life from 2.1 to 2.3 hours. Serum insulin and glucose concentrations were not altered. While no data were presented, this interaction is not expected to significantly alter the blood glucose response in patients with diabetes.

RELATED DRUGS: Gemfibrozil may affect other oral hypoglycemic drugs that are primarily metabolized by CYP2C9 (eg, tolbutamide [eg, *Orinase*], glyburide [eg, *DiaBeta*], glipizide [eg, *Glucotrol*], nateglinide [*Starlix*]) in a similar manner.

MANAGEMENT OPTIONS:

➡ **Monitor.** Monitor patients with diabetes mellitus who are taking glimepiride for potential changes in glycemic control if gemfibrozil is coadministered.

REFERENCES:
1. Niemi M, et al. Effect of gemfibrozil on the pharmacokinetics and pharmacodynamics of glimepiride. *Clin Pharmacol Ther.* 2001;70(5):439-445.

Gemfibrozil (eg, *Lopid*)

Glyburide (eg, *DiaBeta*)

SUMMARY: Gemfibrozil appeared to cause hypoglycemia in a patient receiving glyburide; a causal relationship is likely in this patient, but more study is needed.

RISK FACTORS: No specific risk factors are known.

MECHANISM: Not established. Gemfibrozil is highly protein bound and could displace glyburide from its protein-binding sites. Alteration of glyburide metabolism by gemfibrozil cannot be ruled out.

CLINICAL EVALUATION: A patient with diabetes was taking glyburide 5 mg/day.[1] After 3 weeks of cotherapy with gemfibrozil 1,200 mg/day, the patient experienced symptoms of hypoglycemia. The glyburide dosage was reduced to 1.25 mg/day with no further hypoglycemic attacks. Following the discontinuation of gemfibrozil, hyperglycemia developed over the next 2 weeks, and the glyburide dose was increased to 5 mg/day. Several months later, gemfibrozil was started again and hypoglycemia returned after 3 days. Reduction of the glyburide dosage to 1.25 mg/day corrected the hypoglycemia.

RELATED DRUGS: It is possible that other sulfonylureas are affected similarly by gemfibrozil.

MANAGEMENT OPTIONS:

➡ **Circumvent/Minimize.** The glyburide dose may need to be reduced during concomitant gemfibrozil and glyburide therapy.

➡ **Monitor.** Monitor patients receiving gemfibrozil and glyburide for symptoms of hypoglycemia (eg, tachycardia, sweating, tremor).

REFERENCES:
1. Ahmad S. Gemfibrozil: interaction with glyburide. *South Med J.* 1991;84(1):102.

2   Gemfibrozil (eg, *Lopid*)

Lovastatin (eg, *Mevacor*)

SUMMARY: Case reports suggest that gemfibrozil increases the likelihood of lovastatin-induced myopathy, but the incidence of the reaction is not established.

RISK FACTORS: No specific risk factors are known.

MECHANISM: Not established. Both lovastatin and gemfibrozil alone have been associated with myopathy, and it is possible that they have additive effects. Pharmacokinetic interactions between lovastatin and gemfibrozil have not been ruled out.

CLINICAL EVALUATION: The US Food and Drug Administration received 12 spontaneous reports of severe myopathy or rhabdomyolysis associated with coadministration of lovastatin and gemfibrozil.[1] Five of the patients developed acute renal failure. Other apparent causes of myopathy were absent, and discontinuation of both drugs was followed by decreases in the creatine kinase (CK) and clinical improvement. In another report, 4 of 6 cardiac transplant patients on cyclosporine developed severe rhabdomyolysis following the use of lovastatin for 6 weeks to 16 months.[2] Two of the patients with rhabdomyolysis also were receiving gemfibrozil, but the role that gemfibrozil played in the reactions is unclear. Several cases of lovastatin-associated myopathy reported to the manufacturer involved concurrent use of gemfibrozil.[3] Another patient stabilized on lovastatin 20 mg twice daily developed rhabdomyolysis and renal failure 2 weeks after gemfibrozil 600 mg twice daily was added to his therapy.[4] The temporal relationship of the reaction with the gemfibrozil and the lack of myopathy with lovastatin alone support the contention that gemfibrozil precipitated lovastatin-induced muscle damage. Other cases of myopathy associated with the combined use of lovastatin and gemfibrozil have been reported.[5-7] Nevertheless, the reaction does not occur in all patients; in 1 study of 34 patients with hyperlipidemia, none of those receiving gemfibrozil and lovastatin combination therapy developed myopathy or elevated CK levels.[8] Similarly, in a retrospective study, 70 patients received lovastatin (51 on 20 mg/day, 17 on 40 mg/day, and 2 on 60 mg/day) plus gemfibrozil 1,200 mg/day[9]; 5 patients developed mild elevations in CK, but none developed muscle weakness or pain. Thus, myopathy appears to occur only in certain predisposed individuals.

RELATED DRUGS: Available evidence suggests that pravastatin (eg, *Pravachol*) is less likely to cause myopathy than lovastatin, either when given alone or when combined with other drugs such as gemfibrozil.[2] Nonetheless, comparative studies will be required to confirm these findings. Little is known regarding the likelihood of myopathy with simvastatin (eg, *Zocor*) plus gemfibrozil, but assume that it is similar to lovastatin plus gemfibrozil until information is available. Because the safety of combined use of lovastatin and clofibrate is also not known, apply the same precautions as with lovastatin plus gemfibrozil.

MANAGEMENT OPTIONS:

➥ *Avoid Unless Benefit Outweighs Risk.* Some experts recommend against using combined lovastatin and gemfibrozil therapy. The manufacturers suggest that the benefits of combined therapy are not likely to outweigh the risk of myopathy and rhabdomyolysis.[10]

➤ **Monitor.** If the combination is used, advise patients to report muscular symptoms such as pain, tenderness, or weakness; measure CK in patients with such symptoms. Early recognition of these symptoms is important because they may progress to acute renal failure in some patients if the drugs are not discontinued promptly. The same precautions may apply to combined use of lovastatin and clofibrate.

REFERENCES:

1. Pierce LR, et al. Myopathy and rhabdomyolysis associated with lovastatin-gemfibrozil combination therapy. *JAMA*. 1990;264(1):71-75.

2. East C, et al. Rhabdomyolysis in patients receiving lovastatin after cardiac transplantation. *N Engl J Med*. 1988;318(1):47-48.

3. Tobert JA. HMG-CoA reductase inhibitors, gemfibrozil, and myopathy. *Am J Cardiol*. 1995; 75(12):862.

4. Marais GE, et al. Rhabdomyolysis and acute renal failure induced by combination lovastatin and gemfibrozil therapy. *Ann Intern Med*. 1990;112(3):228-230.

5. Kogan AD, et al. Lovastatin-induced acute rhabdomyolysis. *Postgrad Med J*. 1990;66(774):294-296.

6. Manoukian AA, et al. Rhabdomyolysis secondary to lovastatin therapy. *Clin Chem*. 1990;36(12):2145-2147.

7. Goldman JA, et al. The role of cholesterol-lowering agents in drug-induced rhabdomyolysis and polymyositis. *Arthritis Rheum*. 1989;32(3):358-359.

8. East C, et al. Combination drug therapy for familial combined hyperlipidemia. *Ann Intern Med*. 1988;109(1):25-32.

9. Wirebaugh SR, et al. A retrospective review of the use of lipid-lowering agents in combination, specifically, gemfibrozil and lovastatin. *Pharmacotherapy*. 1992;12(6):445-450.

10. *Mevacor* [package insert]. Whitehouse Station, NJ: Merck; 1993.

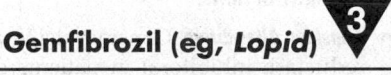

Gemfibrozil (eg, *Lopid*)

Montelukast (*Singlulair*)

SUMMARY: Gemfibrozil markedly increases montelukast plasma concentrations, but the clinical importance of this interaction requires further study.

RISK FACTORS: No specific risk factors are known.

MECHANISM: Gemfibrozil is a potent inhibitor of CYP2C8 and montelukast is a CYP2C8 substrate; therefore, gemfibrozil probably inhibits montelukast metabolism.

CLINICAL EVALUATION: In a randomized, crossover study, 10 healthy subjects received montelukast 10 mg with and without pretreatment with gemfibrozil 600 mg twice daily for 3 days.[1] Gemfibrozil was associated with a 4.5-fold increase in montelukast area under the plasma concentration-time curve and a 3-fold increase in montelukast half-life. The extent to which these increases would lead to adverse outcomes is not known.

RELATED DRUGS: No information is available.

MANAGEMENT OPTIONS:

➤ **Circumvent/Minimize.** Consider using conservative doses of montelukast in the presence of gemfibrozil therapy.

➥ **Monitor.** If the combination is used, be alert for evidence of adverse effects.

REFERENCES:

1. Karonen T, et al. Gemfibrozil markedly increases the plasma concentrations of montelukast: a previously unrecognized role for CYP2C8 in the metabolism of montelukast. *Clin Pharmacol Ther*. 2010;88(2):223-230.

Gemfibrozil (eg, *Lopid*)

Pioglitazone (*Actos*)

SUMMARY: Gemfibrozil increases pioglitazone plasma concentrations; enhanced hypoglycemic effect may occur.

RISK FACTORS: No specific risk factors are known.

MECHANISM: Gemfibrozil appears to inhibit the metabolism (CYP2C8) of pioglitazone.

CLINICAL EVALUATION: Gemfibrozil 600 mg or placebo was administered twice daily to 12 subjects for 4 days.[1] On day 3, each subject received a single dose of pioglitazone 15 mg. The coadministration of gemfibrozil resulted in a mean 3.2-fold increase in the area under the plasma concentration-time curve of pioglitazone. Pioglitazone's mean half-life increased from 8.3 to 22.7 hours following gemfibrozil. The magnitude of this interaction indicates that some patients stabilized on pioglitazone may develop hypoglycemia if gemfibrozil is added to their regimen.

RELATED DRUGS: Gemfibrozil also inhibits the metabolism of repaglinide (*Prandin*).

MANAGEMENT OPTIONS:

➥ **Consider Alternative.** Consider using alternative lipid-lowering drugs (eg, HMG-CoA reductase inhibitors) in patients stabilized on pioglitazone. The effect of fenofibrate (eg, *Tricor*) on pioglitazone is unknown, but, pending further study, it could be considered as an alternative to gemfibrozil. Alternative oral hypoglycemic agents not metabolized by CYP2C8 (eg, glipizide [eg, *Glucotrol*], tolbutamide) may be considered for patients requiring gemfibrozil.

➥ **Monitor.** Observe patients taking pioglitazone for altered glycemic control if gemfibrozil is added to or discontinued from the drug regimen.

REFERENCES:

1. Jaakkola T, et al. Effects of gemfibrozil, itraconazole, and their combination on the pharmacokinetics of pioglitazone. *Clin Pharmacol Ther*. 2005;77(5):404-414.

Gemfibrozil (eg, *Lopid*)

Pravastatin (*Pravachol*)

SUMMARY: Most patients appear to tolerate the combined use of pravastatin and gemfibrozil well, but it is possible that myopathy may occasionally develop (as has been reported with lovastatin and gemfibrozil).

RISK FACTORS: No specific risk factors are known.

MECHANISM: Not established.

CLINICAL EVALUATION: In a double-blind study, 290 patients with hypercholesterolemia were randomized to 1 of 4 treatments for 12 weeks: pravastatin 40 mg 4 times/day, gemfibrozil 600 mg twice daily, both pravastatin and gemfibrozil, or placebo.[1] When both drugs were used, additive hypolipidemic effects were observed; low density lipoprotein-cholesterol decreased 37%, high density lipoprotein-cholesterol increased, and very low density lipoprotein-cholesterol decreased 49%. Four patients on the combination developed creatine kinase levels over 4 times pretreatment values, compared with 2 on gemfibrozil alone and 1 each on pravastatin alone and placebo. The differences were not statistically different and none of the patients developed myopathy. Thus, combined therapy of pravastatin and gemfibrozil appears safe in most patients, but an occasional predisposed patient may develop myopathy.

RELATED DRUGS: Available evidence suggests that pravastatin is less likely to cause myopathy than lovastatin (eg, *Mevacor*), either when given alone or when combined with other drugs such as gemfibrozil.[2] Nonetheless, comparative studies will be required to confirm these findings. Little is known regarding the likelihood of myopathy with simvastatin (*Zocor*) plus gemfibrozil, but assume that it is similar to lovastatin plus gemfibrozil until information is available. One patient developed myopathy when clofibrate was added to well-tolerated pravastatin therapy; the myopathy resolved when the clofibrate was discontinued and the pravastatin therapy was continued.

MANAGEMENT OPTIONS:

➡ *Consider Alternative.* Although the combination of pravastatin and gemfibrozil is well tolerated in most patients, generally avoid the routine use of this combination until more evidence of safety is available.[1,3]

➡ *Monitor.* If the combination is used, alert patients for muscular symptoms such as pain, tenderness, or weakness; measure creatine kinase in patients with such symptoms.

REFERENCES:

1. Wiklund O, et al. Pravastatin and gemfibrozil alone and in combination for the treatment of hypercholesterolemia. *Am J Med.* 1993;94:13-20.

2. Jungnickel PW, et al. Pravastatin: a new drug for the treatment of hypercholesterolemia. *Clin Pharm.* 1992;11:677-689.

3. *Pravachol* [package insert]. Princeton, NJ: Bristol-Myers Squibb; 1993.

Gemfibrozil (eg, *Lopid*)

Repaglinide (*Prandin*)

SUMMARY: Gemfibrozil markedly increases serum concentrations of repaglinide; enhanced hypoglycemic effects are likely to result.

RISK FACTORS: No specific risk factors are known.

MECHANISM: Repaglinide is thought to be metabolized predominately by CYP2C8 and to a lesser extent by CYP3A4. Gemfibrozil appears to inhibit the CYP2C8-mediated metabolism of repaglinide.

CLINICAL EVALUATION: Twelve healthy subjects received a single dose of repaglinide 0.25 mg following placebo or gemfibrozil 600 mg twice daily for 3 days.[1] The mean area under the plasma concentration-time curve of repaglinide was increased 8-fold (range, 5- to 15-fold), and the half-life of repaglinide increased from 1.3 to 3.7 hours following pretreatment with gemfibrozil. Enhanced and prolonged effects on blood glucose, serum insulin, and C-peptide concentrations accompanied these increases in repaglinide concentrations. Patients with diabetes may experience hypoglycemia if gemfibrozil and repaglinide are coadministered.

RELATED DRUGS: No information is available; however, the elimination of other oral hypoglycemic agents (eg, pioglitazone [*Actos*], rosiglitazone [*Avandia*]) metabolized by CYP2C8 may be reduced by gemfibrozil coadministration.

MANAGEMENT OPTIONS:

➡ *Consider Alternative.* Consider using alternative lipid-lowering drugs (eg, HMG-CoA reductase inhibitors) in patients stabilized on repaglinide. Alternative oral hypoglycemic agents not metabolized by CYP2C8 (eg, glipizide [eg, *Glucotrol*], tolbutamide) could be considered for use in patients requiring gemfibrozil.

➡ *Monitor.* Monitor patients taking repaglinide for changes in blood glucose concentrations if gemfibrozil is added to or discontinued from the drug regimen.

REFERENCES:

1. Niemi M, et al. Effects of gemfibrozil, itraconazole, and their combination on the pharmacokinetics and pharmacodynamics of repaglinide: potentially hazardous interaction between gemfibrozil and repaglinide. *Diabetologia.* 2003;46(3):347-351.

 Gemfibrozil (eg, *Lopid*)

Warfarin (eg, *Coumadin*)

SUMMARY: Gemfibrozil appeared to increase the hypoprothrombinemic response to warfarin in 1 patient, but more study is needed to confirm this effect.

RISK FACTORS: No specific risk factors are known.

MECHANISM: Not established.

CLINICAL EVALUATION: A 38-year-old woman stabilized on warfarin 5 mg/day developed a marked increase in her hypoprothrombinemic response and began bleeding after starting gemfibrozil 1,200 mg/day.[1] A dechallenge of the gemfibrozil without reducing the warfarin dose was not possible. Gemfibrozil is chemically and pharmacologically similar to clofibrate, a drug that is known to enhance the hypoprothrombinemic response to warfarin. Moreover, the manufacturer of gemfibrozil presents a strong warning about the risk of increased hypoprothrombinemic response to oral anticoagulants.[2]

RELATED DRUGS: The effect of gemfibrozil on oral anticoagulants other than warfarin is not established, but consider the possibility of an interaction until clinical studies are performed. Clofibrate,[+] lovastatin (eg, *Mevacor*), and simvastatin (eg, *Zocor*) also may increase the effect of oral anticoagulants, while cholestyramine (eg, *Questran*) and colestipol (eg, *Colestid*) may reduce their effect.

MANAGEMENT OPTIONS:

➡ *Avoid Unless Benefit Outweighs Risk.* Avoid concomitant therapy with gemfibrozil and oral anticoagulants if possible. If oral anticoagulant therapy is started in a patient receiving gemfibrozil, conservatively administer anticoagulant doses until the maintenance dose is established.

➥ *Monitor.* Monitor patients for altered oral anticoagulant effect if gemfibrozil is initiated, discontinued, or changed in dosage.

REFERENCES:
1. Ahmad S. Gemfibrozil interaction with warfarin sodium (*Coumadin*). *Chest.* 1990;98(4):1041-1042.

2. *Lopid* [package insert]. New York, NY: Parke-Davis (a Pfizer company); 1993.

† Not available in the United States.

Gemifloxacin (*Factive*)
Probenecid

SUMMARY: Probenecid increases the plasma concentration of gemifloxacin; however, little added risk of adverse reactions is expected.

RISK FACTORS: No specific risk factors are known.

MECHANISM: Probenecid appears to inhibit 1 or more transporters, particularly in the kidney, that secrete gemifloxacin from the body.

CLINICAL EVALUATION: Seventeen healthy subjects took a single oral dose of gemifloxacin 320 mg alone and during the coadministration of probenecid.[1] Probenecid dosing was a total of 4.5 g started 10 hours before gemifloxacin dosing and ending 60 hours after gemifloxacin dosing. The administration of probenecid reduced the renal clearance of gemifloxacin by 51% and its nonrenal clearance by 19%; mean total body clearance of gemifloxacin was reduced 31%. Gemifloxacin half-life increased from 8 to 9.5 hours when probenecid was coadministered. The authors estimated that the mean area under the concentration-time curve of gemifloxacin would be increased approximately 20% when typical probenecid doses (500 mg twice daily) were administered. These changes in gemifloxacin concentration are not likely to be clinically significant.

RELATED DRUGS: Probenecid has been reported to increase the concentration of other quinolone antibiotics, such as ciprofloxacin (eg, *Cipro*), levofloxacin (eg, *Levaquin*), and enoxacin.†

MANAGEMENT OPTIONS:

➥ *Monitor.* No special monitoring is required for patients taking gemifloxacin plus probenecid.

REFERENCES:
1. Landersdorfer CB, et al. Competitive inhibition of renal tubular secretion of gemifloxacin by probenecid. *Antimicrob Agents Chemother.* 2009;53(9):3902-3907.

† Not available in the United States.

Gentamicin (eg, *Garamycin*)

Indomethacin (eg, *Indocin*)

SUMMARY: Indomethacin appears to reduce the renal clearance of gentamicin and amikacin in premature infants, resulting in increased gentamicin serum concentrations.

RISK FACTORS:

➡ **Effects of Age.** The glomerular filtration rate for preterm newborns is only 0.7 to 0.8 mL/min compared to 2 to 4 mL/min or 10 to 20 mL/min/1.73 m² for full-term newborns.

MECHANISM: Aminoglycosides are eliminated primarily by glomerular filtration. A transient reduction in glomerular filtration by indomethacin can reduce aminoglycoside clearance and increase aminoglycoside serum concentrations. Aspirin-induced inhibition of renal prostaglandins can increase the nephrotoxicity of gentamicin in animals.[1]

CLINICAL EVALUATION: Twenty preterm infants were treated with either gentamicin or amikacin (eg, *Amikin*).[2] Each infant also received indomethacin to treat patent ductus arteriosus. Indomethacin was started after at least 3 days of aminoglycoside therapy. The concentrations of both amikacin and gentamicin were significantly increased on the day after the administration of indomethacin compared to the values obtained the day before indomethacin administration. Mean peak concentrations increased 17% and 33%, and troughs climbed 29% and 48% for amikacin and gentamicin, respectively. In addition, the serum creatinine concentration increased 17%, urine output decreased, and serum sodium concentration was reduced.

RELATED DRUGS: Amikacin interacts similarly. Other aminoglycosides may be affected by indomethacin. Other nonsteroidal anti-inflammatory drugs also may reduce the renal clearance of aminoglycosides.

MANAGEMENT OPTIONS:

➡ **Monitor.** If aminoglycosides and indomethacin are administered to infants, monitor plasma antibiotic concentrations and renal function. The potential for this interaction in adults is unknown.

REFERENCES:
1. Gagliardi L. Possible indomethacin-aminoglycoside interaction in preterm infants. *J Pediatr.* 1985;106:991.
2. Zarfin Y, et al. Possible indomethacin-aminoglycoside interaction in preterm infants. *J Pediatr.* 1985;106:511.

Gentamicin (eg, *Garamycin*)

Methoxyflurane (*Penthrane*)

SUMMARY: Methoxyflurane appears to enhance the renal toxicity of aminoglycoside antibiotics.

RISK FACTORS: No specific risk factors known.

MECHANISM: Aminoglycoside antibiotics and methoxyflurane may have additive or synergistic nephrotoxic effects.

CLINICAL EVALUATION: Several cases of nephrotoxicity occurred after the administration of kanamycin (eg, *Kantrex*) or gentamicin to patients who recently had received methoxyflurane.[1] In these cases, nephrotoxicity appeared to occur at doses lower than those ordinarily associated with renal impairment. More study is needed to determine causation.

RELATED DRUGS: The nephrotoxicity of other aminoglycosides including kanamycin also may be enhanced by methoxyflurane.

MANAGEMENT OPTIONS:

➥ *Consider Alternative.* Avoid nephrotoxic antibiotics such as aminoglycosides in patients who have recently received methoxyflurane.

➥ *Monitor.* If aminoglycosides are administered with methoxyflurane, monitor for renal dysfunction.

REFERENCES:
1. Churchill D. Persisting renal insufficiency after methoxyflurane anesthesia. Report of two cases and review of literature. *Am J Med.* 1974;56:575.

Gentamicin (eg, *Garamycin*)

Vancomycin (eg, *Vancocin*)

SUMMARY: The combination of vancomycin and aminoglycosides may lead to increased nephrotoxicity in some patients.

RISK FACTORS:

➥ *Concurrent Diseases.* Individuals with pre-existing renal failure are at risk.

➥ *Dosage Regimen.* Individuals with increased antibiotic concentrations, undergoing prolonged therapy, or receiving other nephrotoxic drugs are at increased risk.

MECHANISM: Not established, although tobramycin does not appear to alter the renal elimination of vancomycin during shortterm coadministration.[7] Alanine amino-peptidase (AAP) renal excretion, an indicator of renal cell injury, was measured after therapy with vancomycin and gentamicin administered alone and concurrently.[2] The combination of vancomycin and gentamicin for 5 days significantly increased AAP compared to vancomycin administration alone.

CLINICAL EVALUATION: Nephrotoxicity has been noted more frequently in patients taking aminoglycosides and vancomycin than in those taking only vancomycin or an aminoglycoside.[1,4,5] The incidence of nephrotoxicity in 224 patients receiving vancomycin alone, an aminoglycoside alone, or the combination was 5%, 11%, and 22%, respectively.[6] The association is less consistent in studies of short duration or when vancomycin concentrations are not markedly elevated.[3]

RELATED DRUGS: Other aminoglycosides administered with vancomycin may increase the risk of nephrotoxicity.

MANAGEMENT OPTIONS:

➥ *Monitor.* If aminoglycosides and vancomycin are coadministered, monitor renal function and maintain antibiotic concentrations in the normal range.

REFERENCES:
1. Farber BF, et al. Retrospective study of the toxicity of preparations of vancomycin from 1974 to 1981. *Antimicrob Agents Chemother.* 1983;23:138.

2. Rybak MJ, et al. Alanine aminopeptidase and beta$_2$ microglobulin excretion in patients receiving vancomycin and gentamicin. *Antimicrob Agents Chemother.* 1987;31:1461.

3. Cimino MA, et al. Relationship of serum antibiotic concentrations to nephrotoxicity in cancer patients receiving concurrent aminoglycoside and vancomycin therapy. *Am J Med.* 1987;83:1091.

4. Downs NJ, et al. Mild nephrotoxicity associated with vancomycin use. *Arch Intern Med.* 1989;149:1777.

5. Pauly DJ, et al. Risk of nephrotoxicity with combination vancomycinaminoglycoside therapy. *Pharmacotherapy.* 1990;10:378.

6. Rybak MJ, et al. Nephrotoxicity of vancomycin, alone and with an aminoglycoside. *J Antimicrob Chemother.* 1990;25:679.

7. Munar MY, et al. The effect of tobramycin on the renal handling of vancomycin. *J Clin Pharmacol.* 1991;31:618.

4 Ginger

Warfarin (eg, *Coumadin*)

SUMMARY: Some reports suggest that ginger may inhibit platelet function, but the clinical importance of this effect is not established.

RISK FACTORS: No specific risk factors are known.

MECHANISM: Ginger purportedly inhibits platelet aggregation, thus increasing the risk of bleeding in patients on oral anticoagulants such as warfarin.[1,2]

CLINICAL EVALUATION: Reports of ginger-induced inhibition of platelet function in healthy subjects have appeared,[3-5] but others have failed to confirm this effect.[6,7] It is not known whether ginger increases the risk of bleeding in patients on oral anticoagulants, but it seems unlikely based on current evidence. As with any herbal drug, there are likely to be substantial differences in the content, depending on the product used.

RELATED DRUGS: A case of increased phenprocoumon effect purportedly caused by ginger has also been reported.[8]

MANAGEMENT OPTIONS: No specific action is required, but be alert for evidence of the interaction.

REFERENCES:

1. Vaes LP, et al. Interactions of warfarin with garlic, ginger, ginkgo, or ginseng: nature of the evidence. *Ann Pharmacother.* 2000;34:1478-1482.

2. Miller LG. Herbal medicinals: selected clinical considerations focusing on known or potential drug-herb interactions. *Arch Intern Med.* 1998;158:2200-2211.

3. Srivastava KC. Effect of onion and ginger consumption on platelet tromooxane production in humans. *Prostaglandins Leukot Essent Fatty Acids.* 1989;35:183-185.

4. Verma SK, et al. Effect of ginger on platelet aggregation in man. *Indian J Med Res.* 1993;98:240-242.

5. Bordia A, et al. Effect of ginger (*Zingiber officinale* Rosc.) and fenugreek (*Trigonella foenumgraecum* L.) on blood lipids, blood sugar and platelet aggregation in patients with coronary artery disease. *Prostaglandins Leukot Essent Fatty Acids.* 1997;56:379-384.

6. Janssen PL, et al. Consumption of ginger (*Zingiber officinale* roscoe) does not affect ex vivo platelet thromboxane production in humans. *Eur J Clin Nutr.* 1996;50:772-774.

7. Lumb AB. Effect of dried ginger on human platelet function. *Thromb Haemost.* 1994;71:110-111.

8. Kruth P, et al. Ginger-associated overanticoagulation by phenprocoumon. *Ann Pharmacother.* 2004;38:257-260.

Ginkgo Biloba

Nifedipine (eg, *Procardia*)

SUMMARY: Ginkgo biloba increases the plasma concentration of nifedipine; some increase in pharmacologic activity may result.

RISK FACTORS: No specific risk factors are known.

MECHANISM: Ginkgo biloba appears to inhibit the metabolism of nifedipine, perhaps by inhibiting the enzyme CYP3A4.

CLINICAL EVALUATION: Twenty-two subjects received nifedipine 10 mg alone and after 18 days of ginkgo biloba 120 mg daily.[1] Nifedipine plasma concentration was sampled 0.5 hours after its administration. Ginkgo biloba administration increased the nifedipine concentration 53%. While no data on nifedipine area under the concentration-time curve or clinical effect were provided, an increase of nifedipine concentration of this magnitude may produce some change in pharmacologic response in some patients.

RELATED DRUGS: Ginkgo biloba would likely inhibit the metabolism of other calcium channel blockers because all are metabolized by CYP3A4.

MANAGEMENT OPTIONS:

➡ *Monitor.* Pending more complete data on this interaction, monitor patients for increase in nifedipine effect if ginkgo biloba is coadministered.

REFERENCES:
1. Smith M, et al. An open trial of nifedipine-herb interactions: nifedipine with St. John's wort, ginseng or ginkgo biloba. *Clin Pharmacol Ther.* 2001;69:P86.

Ginkgo Biloba **2**

Warfarin (eg, *Coumadin*)

SUMMARY: Isolated cases of bleeding have been reported following use of ginkgo biloba with and without concurrent warfarin therapy, but the contribution of ginkgo to the bleeding was not established.

RISK FACTORS: No specific risk factors are known.

MECHANISM: In vitro evidence suggests that ginkgo inhibits platelet aggregation, but the clinical relevance of this effect is not established.

CLINICAL EVALUATION: A 78-year-old woman taking warfarin developed worsening cognitive deficits and an inability to feed herself.[1] A brain computed tomography scan showed left parietal hemorrhage, but the prothrombin time was not excessive (16.9 seconds). Her daughter had been giving her ginkgo for the previous 2 months, but it was not possible to determine if it contributed to the bleeding. Other cases of bleeding (eg, ocular, subdural hematoma) have been reported in patients receiving ginkgo in the absence of warfarin, but again, a cause-and-effect relationship was not established in these cases.[2]

RELATED DRUGS: If ginkgo proves to increase the risk of bleeding in patients receiving warfarin because of inhibition of platelet function, it will probably have the same effect with all other oral anticoagulants.

MANAGEMENT OPTIONS:

➥ *Use Alternative.* Although the risk of serious bleeding associated with the addition of ginkgo to warfarin therapy is not established, generally avoid the combination because a) the benefit of ginkgo as a "memory aid" is questionable and b) the potential adverse outcome of the interaction is life-threatening.

REFERENCES:

1. Matthews MK Jr. Association of ginkgo biloba with intracerebral hemorrhage. *Neurology*. 1998;50:1933-1934.

2. Rosenblatt M, et al. Spontaneous hyphema associated with ingestion of ginkgo biloba extract. *N Engl J Med*. 1997;336:1108.

Ginseng

Nifedipine (eg, *Procardia*)

SUMMARY: Ginseng increases the plasma concentration of nifedipine; some increase of activity may result.

RISK FACTORS: No specific risk factors are known.

MECHANISM: Ginseng appears to inhibit the metabolism of nifedipine, perhaps by inhibiting the enzyme CYP3A4.

CLINICAL EVALUATION: Twenty-two subjects received nifedipine 10 mg alone and after 18 days of ginseng 200 mg/day.[1] Nifedipine plasma concentration was sampled 0.5 hours after its administration. Ginseng administration increased nifedipine concentration 29%. While no data on nifedipine area under the concentration-time curve or clinical effect were provided, an increase of nifedipine concentration of this magnitude would be expected to produce only small changes in response in some patients.

RELATED DRUGS: Ginseng would likely inhibit the metabolism of other calcium channel blockers because all are metabolized by CYP3A4.

MANAGEMENT OPTIONS:

➥ *Monitor.* Pending more complete data on this interaction, monitor patients for increase in nifedipine effect if ginseng is coadministered.

REFERENCES:

1. Smith M, et al. An open trial of nifedipine-herb interactions: nifedipine with St. John's wort, ginseng or *ginkgo biloba*. *Clin Pharmacol Ther*. 2001;69:P86.

Ginseng

Warfarin (eg, *Coumadin*)

SUMMARY: Case reports and controlled studies suggest that ginseng can reduce the anticoagulant response of warfarin, but the effect is likely to be highly variable, depending on the patient and the ginseng product used.

RISK FACTORS: No specific risk factors are known.

MECHANISM: A mechanism for reduced warfarin response caused by ginseng is not known. Evidence indicates that ginseng does not induce CYP1A2 or CYP3A4, although induction of CYP2C9 (the most important warfarin-metabolizing isozyme) cannot be ruled out.[1,2] Animal data suggest that ginseng may inhibit platelet function (which could increase the risk of bleeding without affecting the international normalized ratio [INR] or prothrombin time), but the clinical importance of this purported effect is not established.[3]

CLINICAL EVALUATION: A 47-year-old man stabilized on warfarin (INR = 3.1) started taking ginseng capsules (*Ginsana*) 3 times daily.[4] Two weeks later, his INR had declined to 1.5, and the ginseng was discontinued. Two weeks after stopping the ginseng, the INR increased to 3.3. The positive dechallenge suggests that the ginseng affected the warfarin in this patient. Another patient on warfarin developed thrombosis in a prosthetic aortic valve after starting ginseng.[5] These cases are consistent with the results of a randomized, double-blind study in 20 healthy subjects given warfarin for 3 days with and without 2 weeks of ginseng administration.[6] Ginseng was associated with a modest reduction in INR and warfarin plasma concentrations. Another study found no effect of ginseng on warfarin serum concentrations or effect,[7] but this study involved fewer subjects, was less well controlled, and only involved 7 days of ginseng use (which may have been insufficient to demonstrate the interaction). This study also used a different ginseng product, which also could account for the differing results. Therefore, the bulk of evidence suggests that at least some ginseng products may reduce warfarin effect, although the magnitude of the effect probably varies widely from no effect to a substantial and clinically important reduction.

RELATED DRUGS: No information is available.

MANAGEMENT OPTIONS:

➡ ***Consider Alternative.*** Considering the benefit vs risk, it would be prudent for patients on warfarin to avoid taking any ginseng products, even though most patients could probably take the combination without harm. Even taking a consistent dose of the same ginseng product would not eliminate the risk because there is no guarantee that the interaction would remain constant over time from lot to lot of the same product.

➡ ***Monitor.*** If ginseng is used with warfarin, monitor the anticoagulant response any time ginseng is started, stopped, changed in dosage, or the product is changed.

REFERENCES:

1. Anderson GD, et al. Drug interaction potential of soy extract and *Panax ginseng*. *J Clin Pharmacol*. 2003;43:643-648.

2. Gurley BJ, et al. Cytochrome P450 phenotypic ratios for predicting herb-drug interactions in humans. *Clin Pharmacol Ther*. 2002;72:276-287.

3. Teng CM, et al. Antiplatelet actions of panaxynol and ginsenosides isolated from ginseng. *Biochim Biophys Acta*. 1989;990:315-320.

4. Janetzky K, et al. Probable interaction between warfarin and ginseng. *Am J Health Syst Pharm*. 1997;54:692-693.

5. Rosado MF. Thrombosis of a prosthetic aortic valve disclosing a hazardous interaction between warfarin and a commercial ginseng product. *Cardiology*. 2003;99:111.

6. Yuan CS, et al. Brief communication: American ginseng reduces warfarin's effect in healthy patients. A randomized, controlled trial. *Ann Intern Med*. 2004;141:23-27.

7. Jiang X, et al. Effect of St. John's wort and ginseng on the pharmacokinetics and pharmacodynamics of warfarin in healthy subjects. *Br J Clin Pharmacol*. 2004;57:592-599.

4   **Glimepiride (Amaryl)**

Propranolol (eg, Inderal)

SUMMARY: Propranolol increases the plasma concentrations of glimepiride; an increase in its hypoglycemic effect may occur.

RISK FACTORS: No specific risk factors are known.

MECHANISM: Unknown.

CLINICAL EVALUATION: Based on limited data provided by the manufacturer, propranolol 40 mg 3 times daily increased the area under the concentration-time curve of glimepiride by an average of 22%.[1] Glimepiride plasma clearance was reduced 18%. While blood glucose concentrations were not reported, the limited effect of propranolol on glimepiride pharmacokinetics would be expected to have minimal effect on glucose levels.

RELATED DRUGS: No data are available on the potential effects of other beta-blockers on glimepiride pharmacokinetics.

MANAGEMENT OPTIONS:

➡ **Monitor.** Be alert for altered glucose concentrations if propranolol therapy is initiated, discontinued, or changed in dosage in patients taking glimepiride. Beta-blockers also are known to suppress the tachycardia associated with hypoglycemia.

REFERENCES:

1. *Amaryl* [package insert]. Bridgewater, NJ: Aventis Pharmaceuticals; 2001.

4   **Glimepiride (Amaryl)**

Rifampin (eg, Rimactane)

SUMMARY: Rifampin reduces the plasma concentrations of glimepiride; a reduction in its hypoglycemic effect may occur.

RISK FACTORS: No specific risk factors are known.

MECHANISM: Rifampin appears to increase the metabolism of glimepiride, probably by induction of CYP2C9, the enzyme known to metabolize glimepiride.

CLINICAL EVALUATION: A single 1 mg dose of glimepiride was administered to 10 healthy subjects following 5 days of placebo or rifampin 600 mg/day.[1] The mean area under the concentration-time curve of glimepiride was reduced 34% (range, 14% to 41%) after rifampin. Glimepiride half-life was reduced from 2.6 to 2 hours with rifampin pretreatment. While blood glucose concentrations were not significantly different during rifampin and placebo pretreatment, the effect of this magnitude of reduction in glimepiride concentration in diabetic patients is unknown.

RELATED DRUGS: Rifampin is known to increase the metabolism of other oral hypoglycemic drugs that are also metabolized by CYP2C9 including tolbutamide (*Orinase*), glipizide (eg, *Glucotrol*), and glyburide (eg, *DiaBeta*). Rifabutin (*Mycobutin*) also may induce the metabolism of glimepiride; however, no data are available.

MANAGEMENT OPTIONS:

➤ *Monitor.* Be alert for altered glucose concentrations if rifampin therapy is initiated, discontinued, or changed in dosage in patients taking glimepiride.

REFERENCES:

1. Niemi M, et al. Effect of rifampicin on the pharmacokinetics and pharmacodynamics of glimepiride. *Br J Clin Pharmacol.* 2000;50:591-595.

Glipizide (eg, *Glucotrol*) ▼ 3

Ranitidine (eg, *Zantac*)

SUMMARY: Ranitidine may increase the serum concentration of glipizide and enhance its hypoglycemic effects. Ranitidine may have independent effects on serum glucose.

RISK FACTORS: No specific risk factors are known.

MECHANISM: Not established. Ranitidine may increase the bioavailability of glipizide by increasing gastric pH.

CLINICAL EVALUATION: Ranitidine increases glipizide concentrations and enhances its hypoglycemic effect.[1,2] Ranitidine administered alone to healthy subjects significantly increased plasma glucose following an oral glucose load. The hyperglycemia persisted even when 5 mg glyburide (eg, *Micronase*) was administered with the H_2-receptor antagonist. The significance of these changes in diabetic patients is unknown.

RELATED DRUGS: Ranitidine does not alter tolbutamide (eg, *Orinase*)[3,4] or glyburide (eg, *DiaBeta*)[5] pharmacokinetics. Cimetidine (eg, *Tagamet*) increases the concentrations of tolbutamide, glipizide, and glyburide.[6] The effect of famotidine (eg, *Pepcid*) and nizatidine (*Axid*) on sulfonylurea pharmacokinetics is unknown, but they may interact if increased gastric pH is involved in the observed changes with cimetidine and ranitidine. Proton pump inhibitors (eg, omeprazole [*Prilosec*], lansoprazole [*Prevacid*]) may affect glipizide in a similar manner.

MANAGEMENT OPTIONS:

➤ *Consider Alternative.* Sucralfate (eg, *Carafate*) may be a good alternative therapy for the treatment of ulcer disease in diabetic patients because it appears unlikely to alter glycemic control to a clinically significant degree.[7]

➤ *Monitor.* Observe diabetic patients stabilized on any hypoglycemic therapy (and especially glipizide) in whom H_2-receptor antagonist therapy is initiated or discontinued for altered glycemic responses.

REFERENCES:

1. Feely J, et al. Potentiation of the hypoglycaemic response to glipizide in diabetic patients by histamine H_2-receptor antagonists. *Br J Clin Pharmacol.* 1993;35:321.
2. MacWalter RS, et al. Potentiation by ranitidine of the hypoglycaemic response to glipizide in diabetic patients. *Br J Clin Pharmacol.* 1985;19:121P.
3. Cate EW, et al. Inhibition of tolbutamide elimination by cimetidine but not ranitidine. *J Clin Pharmacol.* 1986;26:372.
4. Toon S, et al. Effects of cimetidine, ranitidine and omeprazole on tolbutamide pharmacokinetics. *J Pharm Pharmacol.* 1995;47:85.
5. Kubacka RT, et al. The paradoxical effect of cimetidine and ranitidine on glibenclamide pharmacokinetics and pharmacodynamics. *Br J Clin Pharmacol.* 1987;23:743.

6. Adebayo GI, et al. Lack of efficacy of cimetidine and ranitidine as inhibitors of tolbutamide metabolism. *Eur J Clin Pharmacol*. 1988;34:653.

7. Letendre PW, et al. Effect of sucralfate on the absorption and pharmacokinetics of chlorpropamide. *J Clin Pharmacol*. 1986;26:622.

 ## Glipizide (eg, *Glucotrol*)

Rifampin (eg, *Rifadin*)

SUMMARY: Rifampin reduces glipizide concentrations; reduction in hypoglycemic response may occur.

RISK FACTORS: No specific risk factors are known.

MECHANISM: Rifampin appears to increase the elimination of glipizide by induction of CYP2C9, the enzyme responsible for glipizide metabolism in the liver. The mechanism responsible for the apparent increase in glipizide peak concentration is unclear.

CLINICAL EVALUATION: Ten healthy subjects received rifampin 600 mg or placebo daily for 5 days.[1] On day 6, a single oral dose of 2.5 mg glipizide was administered. Following rifampin pretreatment, the mean area under the concentration-time curve of glipizide was reduced 22% and its half-life reduced from 3 to 1.9 hours. The peak concentration of glipizide was increased (mean, 18%) by rifampin administration. The hypoglycemic effect produced by glipizide when administered with placebo was unaffected following rifampin.

RELATED DRUGS: The hypoglycemic efficacy of tolbutamide (*Orinase*) and glyburide (*DiaBeta*) may be reduced by rifampin. Rifabutin (*Mycobutin*) might increase the metabolism of glipizide in a similar manner.

MANAGEMENT OPTIONS:

➡ **Monitor.** When rifampin is coadministered with glipizide and possibly other sulfonylureas, watch for reduced hypoglycemic efficacy. Discontinuation of rifampin in a patient stabilized on glipizide and rifampin therapy could result in hypoglycemia.

REFERENCES:

1. Niemi M, et al. Effects of rifampin on the pharmacokinetics and pharmacodynamics of glyburide and glipizide. *Clin Pharmacol Ther*. 2001;69:400-406.

Glipizide (eg, *Glucotrol*)

Trimethoprim-Sulfamethoxazole (eg, *Bactrim*)

SUMMARY: Trimethoprim-sulfamethoxazole appears to have minimal effect on glipizide pharmacokinetics and pharmacodynamics.

RISK FACTORS: No specific risk factors are known.

MECHANISM: Unknown.

CLINICAL EVALUATION: Eight healthy subjects received 1 tablet of glipizide 10 mg with no pretreatment or following 1 co-trimoxazole (trimethoprim 160 mg and sulfamethoxazole 800 mg) tablet every 12 hours for 7 days.[1] The area under the concentration-time curve of glipizide was increased 11% following co-trimoxazole. While this change was statistically significant, little clinical effect would be expected. No other pharmacokinetic parameters of glipizide were affected by pretreatment with co-trimoxazole. Serum glucose concentrations were similar following glipizide alone or after pretreatment with co-trimoxazole. A prior case report without pharmacokinetic evaluation noted an apparent change in glucose response to glipizide during coadministration of co-trimoxazole.[2] It is possible that some patients may experience an increase in glipizide concentrations that could result in change in glucose control.

RELATED DRUGS: Co-trimoxazole increases tolbutamide (eg, *Orinase*) concentrations. Glyburide (eg, *DiaBeta*) does not appear to be affected by coadministration with trimethoprim-sulfamethoxazole.

MANAGEMENT OPTIONS: No specific action is required, but be alert for evidence of the interaction.

REFERENCES:

1. Kradjan WA, et al. Lack of interaction between glipizide and co-trimoxazole. *J Clin Pharmacol.* 1994;34:997-1002.

2. Johnson JF, et al. Symptomatic hypoglycemia secondary to a glipizide-trimethoprim/sulfamethoxazole drug interaction. *DICP.* 1990;24:250-251.

Glucagon

Propranolol (eg, *Inderal*)

SUMMARY: Propranolol may blunt the hyperglycemic action of glucagon.

RISK FACTORS: No specific risk factors are known.

MECHANISM: Propranolol partially inhibits the hyperglycemic effect of glucagon. The mechanism for this effect is not established, but those proposed include: 1) propranolol inhibition of the hyperglycemic response to catecholamines released by the glucagon and 2) propranolol-induced decrease in hepatic gluconeogenesis.[1]

CLINICAL EVALUATION: Five healthy subjects were given glucagon with and without propranolol; the hyperglycemic response to glucagon was partially inhibited by the propranolol.[2] Propranolol did not reduce the large increases in plasma cyclic adenosine monophosphate seen following glucagon administration, leading to the conclusion that glucagon and beta-agonists such as isoproterenol (eg, *Isuprel*) act on independent receptor sites. This proposal is consistent with previously reported data indicating that glucagon may be effective in reversing the myocardial depressant effects of propranolol.[3]

RELATED DRUGS: Little is known regarding the interactions of other beta blockers and glucagon, but other beta blockers would be expected to interact in a similar manner.

MANAGEMENT OPTIONS: No specific action is required, but be alert for evidence of the interaction.

REFERENCES:

1. Mills GA, et al. Beta-blockers and glucose control. *Drug Intell Clin Pharm.* 1985;19:246-251.

2. Messerli FH, et al. Effects of beta-adrenergic blockade on plasma cyclic AMP and blood sugar responses to glucagon and isoproterenol in man. *Int J Clin Pharmacol Biopharm.* 1976;14:189-194.

3. Kosinski EJ, et al. Glucagon and isoproterenol in reversing propranolol toxicity. *Arch Intern Med.* 1973;132:840-843.

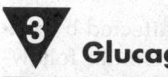 **Glucagon**

Warfarin (eg, *Coumadin*)

SUMMARY: Glucagon appears to enhance the hypoprothrombinemic response to warfarin, and possibly other oral anti-coagulants, causing bleeding in some patients. Adjustment of the oral anticoagulant dose may be needed in patients receiving both drugs.

RISK FACTORS: No specific risk factors are known.

MECHANISM: Not established.

CLINICAL EVALUATION: In 8 patients who received glucagon for 2 or longer days in a total dose of more than 50 mg, marked enhancement of the hypoprothrombinemic response to warfarin was noted.[1] Three of these 8 patients had bleeding episodes, presumably as a result of the interaction. The risk of 1 or 2 doses of glucagon to treat hypoglycemia in a patient receiving warfarin is not known, but it is probably not large.

RELATED DRUGS: Little is known regarding the effect of glucagon on oral anticoagulants other than warfarin. Assume that an interaction occurs until information to the contrary appears. A potentiating effect of acenocoumarol† by glucagon has been demonstrated in animals.[2]

MANAGEMENT OPTIONS:

➡ *Monitor.* Monitor for altered oral anticoagulant effect if glucagon is given concurrently. Adjust the anticoagulant dose as needed.

REFERENCES:

1. Koch-Weser J. Potentiation by glucagon of the hypoprothrombinemic action of warfarin. *Ann Intern Med.* 1970;72:331-335.
2. Weiner M, et al. The effect of glucagon and insulin on the prothrombin response to coumarin anticoagulants. *Proc Soc Exp Biol Med.* 1968;127:761-763.

† Not available in the United States.

 Glutethimide

Warfarin (eg, *Coumadin*)

SUMMARY: Glutethimide inhibits the hypoprothrombinemic response to warfarin, and probably other oral anticoagulants; the dose of the oral anticoagulant may have to be increased during coadministration of these drugs.

RISK FACTORS:

➡ *Dosage Regimen.* Since the onset and offset of enzyme induction is gradual, this interaction would be expected to take place over a week or more and to continue for a week or more after glutethimide is stopped.

MECHANISM: Glutethimide appears to increase the metabolism of oral anticoagulants by inducing hepatic microsomal enzymes.

CLINICAL EVALUATION: Glutethimide decreases plasma warfarin levels and the hypoprothrombinemic response in patients and healthy subjects.[1-3] These effects of glutethimide appear to be similar in magnitude to those of barbiturates. Also, glutethimide is like barbiturates in that some patients do not appear to manifest the interaction with oral anticoagulants.

RELATED DRUGS: Although little is known regarding the effect of glutethimide on oral anticoagulants other than warfarin, assume that an interaction exists until information to the contrary appears.

MANAGEMENT OPTIONS:

➡ *Use Alternative.* Benzodiazepines such as flurazepam (eg, *Dalmane*), temazepam (eg, *Restoril*), and triazolam (eg, *Halcion*) are preferable to glutethimide in patients on oral anticoagulants. If glutethimide is used, monitor for altered oral anticoagulant effect if glutethimide is initiated, discontinued, or changed in dosage. Adjust the anticoagulant dose as needed. Note that it may take up to 2 weeks or more for the maximal effect of glutethimide on warfarin to develop, and a similar time for the effect to fully dissipate.

REFERENCES:

1. Corn M. Effect of phenobarbital and glutethimide on biological halflife of warfarin. *Thromb Diath Haemorrh*. 1966;16:606-612.

2. MacDonald MG, et al. The effects of phenobarbital, chloral betaine, and glutethimide administration on warfarin plasma levels and hypoprothrombinemic responses in man. *Clin Pharmacol Ther*. 1969;10:80-84.

3. Udall JA. Clinical implications of warfarin interactions with five sedatives. *Am J Cardiol*. 1975;35:67-71.

Glyburide (eg, *DiaBeta*)

Orlistat (*Xenical*)

SUMMARY: Orlistat did not alter the pharmacokinetics or pharmacodynamics of glyburide.

RISK FACTORS: No specific risk factors are known.

MECHANISM: No interaction.

CLINICAL EVALUATION: The administration of orlistat 80 mg 3 times daily for 4 days to healthy subjects had no effect on the pharmacokinetics or pharmacodynamics of a single 5 mg dose of glyburide.[1] Studies in patients with diabetes are needed to assure the safety of this combination.

RELATED DRUGS: No information is available.

MANAGEMENT OPTIONS: No interaction.

REFERENCES:

1. Zhi J, et al. The influence of orlistat on the pharmacokinetics and pharmacodynamics of glyburide in healthy volunteers. *J Clin Pharmacol*. 1995;35:521-525.

Glyburide (eg, *DiaBeta*)

Rifampin (eg, *Rifadin*)

SUMMARY: Rifampin reduces glyburide concentrations; reduction in hypoglycemic response is likely to occur.

RISK FACTORS: No specific risk factors are known.

MECHANISM: Rifampin appears to increase the elimination of glyburide by induction of CYP2C9 or p-glycoprotein, or both.

CLINICAL EVALUATION: Ten healthy subjects received rifampin 600 mg or placebo daily for 5 days.[1] On day 6, a single oral dose of 1.75 mg glyburide was administered. Following rifampin pretreatment, the mean area under the concentration-time curve of glyburide was reduced 39% and its half-life reduced from 2 to 1.7 hours. The hypoglycemic effect produced by glyburide when administered with placebo was reduced more than 40% following rifampin. Previous reports have noted a reduction in glyburide plasma concentrations and patient response during rifampin coadministration.[2,3]

RELATED DRUGS: The hypoglycemic efficacy of tolbutamide (*Orinase*) and glipizide (*Glucotrol*) may be reduced by rifampin. Rifabutin (*Mycobutin*) might affect glyburide in a similar manner.

MANAGEMENT OPTIONS:

➠ *Monitor.* When rifampin is coadministered with glyburide and possibly other sulfonylureas, watch for reduced hypoglycemic efficacy. Discontinuation of rifampin could result in hypoglycemia in a patient stabilized on glyburide and rifampin therapy.

REFERENCES:

1. Niemi M, et al. Effects of rifampin on the pharmacokinetics and pharmacodynamics of glyburide and glipizide. *Clin Pharmacol Ther*. 2001;69:400-406.
2. Self TH, et al. Interaction of rifampin and glyburide. *Chest*. 1989;96:1443-1444.
3. Surekha V, et al. Drug interaction: rifampicin and glibenclamide. *Natl Med J India*. 1997;10:11-12.

---

4   Glyburide (eg, *DiaBeta*)

Simvastatin (eg, *Zocor*)

SUMMARY: Simvastatin administration produces a minor change in glyburide concentrations; a minimal change in patient hypoglycemic response is expected.

RISK FACTORS: No specific risk factors are known.

MECHANISM: Unknown.

CLINICAL EVALUATION: Sixteen healthy subjects received simvastatin 20 mg/day for 15 days.[1] A single dose of glyburide 3.5 mg was administered on days 1 and 15 of simvastatin dosing. The area under the concentration-time curve and peak concentration of glyburide were increased 20% to 28% by simvastatin administration. Oral glucose tolerance tests administered 1.5 hours after glyburide administration were not changed by simvastatin coadministration. Glyburide administration did not alter simvastatin concentrations. The changes in glyburide concentrations are not likely to affect glucose control.

RELATED DRUGS: Fluvastatin (*Lescol*) produces a similar change in glyburide concentrations. The effect of other HMG-CoA inhibitors on glyburide is unknown. Simvastatin produced a minimal effect on tolbutamide concentrations.

MANAGEMENT OPTIONS: No specific action is required, but be alert for evidence of the interaction.

REFERENCES:

1. Appel S, et al. Lack of interaction between fluvastatin and oral hypoglycemic agents in healthy subjects and patients with non-insulin-dependent diabetes mellitus. *Am J Cardiol*. 1995;76(2):29A-32A.

Glyburide (eg, *DiaBeta*)

Trimethoprim/Sulfamethoxazole (eg, *Bactrim*)

SUMMARY: Trimethoprim/sulfamethoxazole administration can increase the risk of hypoglycemia in patients taking glyburide.

RISK FACTORS: No specific risk factors are known.

MECHANISM: Trimethoprim/sulfamethoxazole inhibits the enzyme CYP2C9, which is known to be the primary pathway of glyburide metabolism.

CLINICAL EVALUATION: The risk of hypoglycemia while taking glyburide was evaluated in patients prescribed trimethoprim/sulfamethoxazole or cephalexin within 10 days of the hypoglycemic episode.[1] Compared with cephalexin, patients prescribed trimethoprim/sulfamethoxazole demonstrated a 2.7-fold increased risk of hypoglycemia. Cephalexin was used as a comparator to control for the effect of an infection on the risk of hypoglycemia.

RELATED DRUGS: Other hypoglycemic drugs that are metabolized by CYP2C9 (glipizide [eg, *Glucotrol*], chlorpropamide [*Diabinese*], and tolbutamide) may be similarly affected by trimethoprim/sulfamethoxazole administration.

MANAGEMENT OPTIONS:

➥ *Consider Alternative.* Consider antibiotics that do not inhibit CYP2C9 (eg, ampicillin, cephalexin) in patients stabilized on glyburide. Hypoglycemic agents that are not substrates for CYP2C9 (insulin, sitagliptin [*Januvia*], nateglinide [eg, *Starlix*]) are unlikely to interact with trimethoprim/sulfamethoxazole.

➥ *Monitor.* Watch patients stabilized on glyburide for changes in blood glucose levels if trimethoprim/sulfamethoxazole is initiated or discontinued.

REFERENCES:
1. Schelleman H, et al. Anti-infectives and the risk of severe hypoglycemia in users of glipizide or glyburide. *Clin Pharmacol Ther.* 2010;88(2):214-222.

Glyburide (eg, *DiaBeta*)

Warfarin (eg, *Coumadin*)

SUMMARY: A patient taking warfarin developed a marked increase in warfarin response and bleeding after starting glyburide, but a causal relationship was not established.

RISK FACTORS: No specific risk factors are known.

MECHANISM: Not established. If glyburide were to inhibit warfarin metabolism, the increase in international normalized ratio (INR) would not be expected to be so dramatic or so rapid (48 hours after starting glyburide).

CLINICAL EVALUATION: One 77-year-old woman well stabilized on warfarin developed bleeding and an increase in her hypoprothrombinemic response (INR increased from 2.3 to 6.6) 48 hours after starting glyburide.[1] More study is needed to determine whether glyburide affects warfarin response. In another study, phenprocoumon⁺ half-life and plasma levels were not affected by tolbutamide, insulin, glyburide, or glibornuride[†] in diabetic patients, nondiabetic elderly patients, or healthy young volunteers.[2]

RELATED DRUGS: An interaction between oral anticoagulants and insulin is unlikely.

MANAGEMENT OPTIONS:

➡ *Monitor.* Although this interaction is poorly documented, the potential severity of the adverse outcome suggests that warfarin response should be monitored if glyburide is initiated, discontinued, or changed in dosage.

REFERENCES:

1. Warfarin potentiated by proguanil. *BMJ.* 1991;303(6805):789.
2. Heine P, et al. The influence of hypoglycaemic sulphonylureas on elimination and efficacy of phenprocoumon following a single oral dose in diabetic patients. *Eur J Clin Pharmacol.* 1976;10:31.

† Not available in the United States.

 ## Glycopyrrolate (eg, *Robinul*)

Potassium

SUMMARY: Anticholinergics may facilitate gastric mucosal damage after ingestion of wax matrix potassium chloride tablets, but the clinical importance of this effect is not established.

RISK FACTORS: No specific risk factors are known.

MECHANISM: Anticholinergic-induced slowing of GI motility may increase the contact time of solid potassium chloride dosage forms within the GI mucosa.

CLINICAL EVALUATION: Forty-eight healthy subjects received potassium chloride (2.4 g 3 times daily for 7 days) as a wax matrix or microencapsulated (*Micro-K*) product with and without concurrent treatment with 2 mg 3 times daily of glycopyrrolate.[1] The anticholinergic agent (glycopyrrolate) was associated with a considerable increase in upper GI lesions detected by endoscopy following use of the wax matrix preparation. The microencapsulated product was associated with less mucosal injury overall and did not appear to be affected by concurrent glycopyrrolate therapy. It has been proposed that glycopyrrolate itself may produce gastric mucosal damage.[2] More study is needed on this interaction.

RELATED DRUGS: Based on the mechanism, all anticholinergics are expected to interact similarly with potassium chloride.

MANAGEMENT OPTIONS: No specific action is required, but be alert for evidence of the interaction.

REFERENCES:

1. McMahon FG, et al. Upper gastrointestinal lesions after potassium chloride supplements: a controlled clinical trial. *Lancet.* 1982;2(8307):1059-1061.
2. Alsop WR, et al. The effects of five potassium chloride preparations on the upper gastrointestinal mucosa in healthy subjects receiving glycopyrrolate. *J Clin Pharmacol.* 1984;24(5-6):235-239.

Glycyrrhizin 4

Prednisolone (eg, *Prelone*)

SUMMARY: Three traditional Chinese herbal medicines containing the licorice glycoside, glycyrrhizin, were given with prednisolone to healthy subjects. Serum concentrations of prednisolone were slightly decreased by Sho-saiko-To, slightly increased by Saiboku-To, and unchanged by Sairei-To.

RISK FACTORS: No specific risk factors are known.

MECHANISM: Glycyrrhizin is known to inhibit 11-beta-hydroxysteroid dehydrogenase, the enzyme that converts the active prednisolone to inactive prednisone. Thus, agents that affect the activity of this enzyme could affect prednisolone response.

CLINICAL EVALUATION: The effects of 3 important traditional Chinese medicines (Sho-saiko-To, Saiboku-To, and Sairei-To) on prednisolone pharmacokinetics were studied in healthy subjects.[1] All 3 of these Chinese medicines contain *Glycerhiza glabra*, which in turn contains the glycoside, glycyrrhizin. In 6 subjects, Sho-saiko-To 7.5 g/day for 3 days was associated with a slight decrease in the prednisolone area under the serum concentration-time curve (AUC) following a single oral dose of prednisolone 10 mg. In 9 subjects, Saiboku-To 7.5 g/day for 3 days was associated with a slight increase in the prednisolone AUC, and, in 7 subjects, Sairei-To 9 g/day had no effect on prednisolone AUC. Because all 3 herbal medicines had roughly equivalent amounts of glycyrrhizin in the doses used, other components of the herbal medicines may have affected the results. Although the changes in prednisolone pharmacokinetics were small, it is possible that alterations in prednisolone effect would occur in an occasional patient.

RELATED DRUGS: The effect of glycyrrhizin on corticosteroids other than prednisolone is not established.

MANAGEMENT OPTIONS: No specific action is required, but be alert for evidence of the interaction.

REFERENCES:
1. Homma M, et al. Different effects of traditional Chinese medicines containing similar herbal constituents on prednisolone pharmacokinetics. *J Pharm Pharmacol.* 1995;47:687-692.

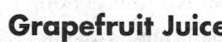**Grapefruit Juice** 3

Felodipine (*Plendil*)

SUMMARY: Grapefruit juice increases felodipine plasma concentrations; increased hypotensive effects or headaches may occur.

RISK FACTORS: No specific risk factors are known.

MECHANISM: Grapefruit juice inhibits intestinal CYP3A4 metabolism of felodipine, leading to increased bioavailability and plasma concentrations.

CLINICAL EVALUATION: A number of studies have demonstrated the ability of grapefruit juice to increase the plasma concentrations of felodipine.[1-5] Increases in plasma felodipine area under the concentration-time curve typically have ranged from 150% to 350%. Felodipine half-life usually is not altered by grapefruit juice administration. The increased felodipine plasma concentrations have resulted in an increased hypotensive effect. A single glass of grapefruit juice exerts an effect on felodipine that continues for about 12 hours. Multiple doses of grapefruit juice tend to produce greater and longer-lasting effects on felodipine pharmacokinetics. Some patients maintained on felodipine may experience increased hypotensive response or side effects such as headache when grapefruit juice is consumed.

RELATED DRUGS: Grapefruit juice has been demonstrated to inhibit the intestinal metabolism of most calcium channel blockers.

MANAGEMENT OPTIONS:

➡ *Circumvent/Minimize.* The use of calcium channel blockers with less first-pass metabolism (eg, amlodipine [eg, *Norvasc*]) would be less affected by grapefruit juice. Other fruit juices may be substituted for grapefruit juice to avoid the interaction with calcium channel blockers.

➡ *Monitor.* Monitor patients stabilized on felodipine for orthostatic hypotension and tachycardia if grapefruit juice is administered, particularly if the juice is consumed daily.

REFERENCES:

1. Lundahl J, et al. Effects of grapefruit juice ingestion—pharmacokinetics and haemodynamics of intravenously and orally administered felodipine in healthy men. *Eur J Clin Pharmacol.* 1997;52:139-145.
2. Bailey DG, et al. Erythromycin-felodipine interaction: magnitude, mechanism, and comparison with grapefruit juice. *Clin Pharmacol Ther.* 1996;60:25-33.
3. Lown KS, et al. Grapefruit juice increases felodipine oral availability in humans by decreasing intestinal CYP3A4 protein expression. *J Clin Invest.* 1997;99:2545-2553.
4. Bailey DG, et al. Grapefruit juice-felodipine interaction: reproducibility and characterization with the extended release drug formulation. *Br J Clin Pharmacol.* 1995;40:135-140.
5. Dresser GK, et al. Grapefruit juice—felodipine interaction in the elderly. *Clin Pharmacol Ther.* 2000;68:28-34.

5 Grapefruit Juice

Fentanyl (*Actiq*)

SUMMARY: Grapefruit juice did not affect the amount of oral transmucosal fentanyl absorbed.

RISK FACTORS: No specific risk factors are known.

MECHANISM: No interaction.

CLINICAL EVALUATION: Twelve healthy subjects received a single dose of oral transmucosal fentanyl 10 mcg/kg alone and following 250 mL of regular-strength grapefruit juice the night before the study and 100 mL of double-strength grapefruit juice 1 hour before the study.[1] The drug was administered as a lozenge, and the subjects were instructed to rub the lozenge across the buccal mucosa and to minimize swallowing. This would allow maximum transmucosal absorption. Grapefruit juice did not affect plasma fentanyl concentrations. The lack of effect may have been caused by the doses of grapefruit juice administered or the attempt to minimize the amount of fentanyl swallowed and absorbed from the intestinal tract.

RELATED DRUGS: None known.

MANAGEMENT OPTIONS: No Interaction.

REFERENCES:

1. Kharasch ED, et al. Influence of hepatic and intestinal cytochrome P4503A activity on the acute disposition and effects of oral transmucosal fentanyl citrate. *Anesthesiology.* 2004;101:729-737.

Grapefruit Juice ▼ 3

Fexofenadine (*Allegra*)

SUMMARY: Ingestion of large amounts of grapefruit juice reduces the absorption of fexofenadine, and may reduce fexofenadine efficacy.

RISK FACTORS: No specific risk factors are known.

MECHANISM: In vitro studies suggest that grapefruit juice inhibits organic anion transporting polypeptide, a transporter involved in the intestinal absorption of fexofenadine.

CLINICAL EVALUATION: In a randomized, crossover study of 10 healthy subjects, a single oral dose of fexofenadine 120 mg was given with water and with grapefruit juice (1.2 L over 3 hours).[1] Grapefruit juice was associated with a 69% reduction in fexofenadine plasma concentrations. The magnitude of this effect appears sufficient to reduce the efficacy of fexofenadine in at least some patients. The amount of grapefruit juice used in this study was larger than most people consume; smaller amounts of grapefruit juice would probably have less effect.

RELATED DRUGS: Apple juice and orange juice also appear to reduce fexofenadine bioavailability.

MANAGEMENT OPTIONS:

➡ *Circumvent/Minimize.* Until more data are available, take fexofenadine with water rather than with grapefruit juice or other fruit juices.

REFERENCES:

1. Dresser GK, et al. Fruit juices inhibit organic anion transporting polypeptide-mediated drug uptake to decrease the oral availability of fexofenadine. *Clin Pharmacol Ther*. 2002;71:11-20.

Grapefruit Juice 2

Halofantrine†

SUMMARY: Grapefruit juice increases the plasma concentration of halofantrine and the potential for halofantrine-induced prolongation of cardiac repolarization.

RISK FACTORS: No specific risk factors are known.

MECHANISM: Grapefruit juice inhibits the first-pass metabolism (via CYP3A4) of halofantrine, resulting in increased halofantrine plasma concentrations.

CLINICAL EVALUATION: Twelve healthy subjects received a single dose of halofantrine 500 mg with water, orange juice, and with 250 mL of grapefruit juice. Grapefruit juice was administered daily for 3 days and again 12 hours prior to the dose of halofantrine.[1] Compared with water, grapefruit juice increased the mean area under the concentration-time curve of halofantrine by 2.8-fold and its peak concentration by more than 3-fold. The half-life of halofantrine was not altered by grapefruit juice pretreatment. The maximal QTc prolongation compared with baseline was 17 msec during halofantrine plus water and 31 msec during halofantrine plus grapefruit juice. Orange juice did not alter the pharmacokinetics or pharmacodynamics of halofantrine. While the halofantrine dose was modest in this study, grapefruit juice can significantly increase the plasma concentration of halofantrine and increase its potential to produce arrhythmias. The effect of a single dose of grapefruit juice on halofantrine pharmacokinetics is unknown; a smaller effect is expected.

RELATED DRUGS: None known.

MANAGEMENT OPTIONS:

➡ *Use Alternative.* Patients taking halofantrine should avoid grapefruit juice. Orange juice appears to be a safe alternative.

➡ *Monitor.* Carefully monitor patients taking halofantrine for changes in cardiac conduction (QT interval) if grapefruit juice is consumed.

REFERENCES:

1. Charbit B, et al. Pharmacokinetic and pharmacodynamic interaction between grapefruit juice and halofantrine. *Clin Pharmacol Ther.* 2002;72(5):514-523.

† Not available in the United States.

4 Grapefruit Juice

Indinavir (*Crixivan*)

SUMMARY: Grapefruit juice appears to reduce the absorption of indinavir; the clinical significance of this is unknown.

RISK FACTORS: No specific risk factors are known.

MECHANISM: Not established.

CLINICAL EVALUATION: While no published data are available for evaluation, the manufacturer of indinavir has made some data on this interaction available. The administration of a single dose of indinavir 400 mg with 240 mL of grapefruit juice decreased the area under the concentration-time curve (AUC) of indinavir an average of 26%.[1] This outcome is unusual in view of the known CYP3A4 metabolism of indinavir and the ability of grapefruit juice to inhibit intestinal wall CYP3A4 activity. However, if the prehepatic metabolism of indinavir is small, the effect of grapefruit juice on the AUC of indinavir would be limited. Indinavir's bioavailability is known to be decreased by food. Grapefruit juice also may affect indinavir's bioavailability in a similar manner.

RELATED DRUGS: The effect of grapefruit juice on the bioavailability of other protease inhibitors is unknown. Because saquinavir (*Invirase*) has a very low bioavailability (4%), grapefruit juice could increase its bioavailability; however, no information is available.

MANAGEMENT OPTIONS: No specific action is required, but be alert for evidence of the interaction.

REFERENCES:

1. *Crixivan* [package insert]. Whitehouse Station, NJ: Merck & Co Inc; 1996.

Grapefruit Juice

Itraconazole (eg, *Sporanox*)

SUMMARY: Grapefruit juice administered with itraconazole reduces itraconazole plasma concentrations; antifungal efficacy may be reduced.

RISK FACTORS: No specific risk factors are known.

MECHANISM: Unknown. Grapefruit juice appears to reduce the absorption of itraconazole.

CLINICAL EVALUATION: Eleven healthy subjects took a single dose of itraconazole 200 mg after breakfast with 240 mL of water or double-strength grapefruit juice.[1] Two hours later, an additional dose of water or grapefruit juice was administered. The administration of grapefruit juice resulted in a 43% average reduction in itraconazole area under the plasma concentration-time curve (AUC) compared with administration with water. The AUC of itraconazole's metabolite, hydroxyitraconazole, was similarly reduced. Mean peak itraconazole concentration was reduced 35% when grapefruit juice was administered. In a second study, itraconazole concentrations were not significantly different in subjects who took itraconazole with water compared with another group of subjects who took itraconazole with single-strength grapefruit juice.[2] The potential for reduced itraconazole therapeutic effect may occur with coadministration of grapefruit juice.

RELATED DRUGS: Although no data exist, grapefruit juice also may affect ketoconazole (eg, *Nizoral*) in a similar manner. Orange juice reduced itraconazole bioavailability in 1 study.[2]

MANAGEMENT OPTIONS:

➡ *Consider Alternative.* Counsel patients taking itraconazole to avoid drinking grapefruit juice.

➡ *Monitor.* Monitor patients who take itraconazole and grapefruit juice for subtherapeutic itraconazole concentrations and possible loss of efficacy.

REFERENCES:

1. Penzak SR, et al. Grapefruit juice decreases the systemic availability of itraconazole capsules in healthy volunteers. *Ther Drug Monit.* 1999;21:304-309.
2. Kawakami M, et al. Effect of grapefruit juice on pharmacokinetics of itraconazole in healthy subjects. *Int J Clin Pharmacol Ther.* 1998;36:306-308.

Grapefruit Juice **4**

Levothyroxine (eg, *Synthroid*)

SUMMARY: Grapefruit juice slightly reduced levothyroxine serum concentrations, but the effect is unlikely to be clinically important.

RISK FACTORS: No specific risk factors are known.

MECHANISM: Not established.

CLINICAL EVALUATION: In a randomized crossover study, 10 healthy subjects were given a single dose of levothyroxine 600 mcg with and without multiple doses of grapefruit juice.[1] Grapefruit juice slightly reduced levothyroxine serum concentrations but did not affect the levothyroxine-induced reduction in serum thyroid-stimulating hormone. The magnitude of the effect does not appear likely to result in clinically important changes in levothyroxine response.

RELATED DRUGS: No information is available.

MANAGEMENT OPTIONS: No specific action is required, but be alert for evidence of the interaction.

REFERENCES:

1. Lilja JJ, et al. Effects of grapefruit juice on the absorption of levothyroxine. *Br J Clin Pharmacol.* 2005;60:337-341.

Grapefruit Juice

Lovastatin (eg, *Mevacor*)

SUMMARY: Repeated doses of grapefruit juice markedly increased lovastatin serum concentrations in healthy subjects.

RISK FACTORS: No specific risk factors are known.

MECHANISM: Lovastatin undergoes extensive first-pass metabolism by CYP3A4 in the small intestine and liver, resulting in about 5% bioavailability. Grapefruit juice inhibits intestinal CYP3A4, thus increasing the bioavailability of lovastatin.

CLINICAL EVALUATION: Ten healthy subjects received a single oral dose of lovastatin 80 mg with and without repeated doses of grapefruit juice (200 mL, double strength).[1] Grapefruit juice increased the mean area under the serum concentration-time curve (AUC) for lovastatin and lovastatin acid (the active metabolite) by 15- and 5-fold, respectively. The effect was highly variable from patient to patient; the range of increase in lovastatin AUC following grapefruit juice was 5- to 20-fold. Therefore, it appears that some patients would be expected to have an increased risk of lovastatin-induced myopathy. However, the subjects ingested a large amount of grapefruit juice; the effect of a more normal amount of grapefruit juice on lovastatin probably would be less than that observed in this study. Thus, the risk associated with a single glass of normal-strength grapefruit juice in a patient receiving lovastatin is probably not high.

RELATED DRUGS: Simvastatin (*Zocor*), like lovastatin, undergoes extensive first-pass metabolism in the gut wall and liver; it is similarly affected by grapefruit juice.[2] Atorvastatin (*Lipitor*) is also metabolized by CYP3A4, and would be expected to interact with grapefruit juice (but to a lesser extent than lovastatin and simvastatin). Pravastatin (*Pravachol*) and fluvastatin (*Lescol*) are not metabolized by CYP3A4 and are not likely to be affected by grapefruit juice.

MANAGEMENT OPTIONS:

➡ **Consider Alternative.** Orange juice does not inhibit CYP3A4 and would not be expected to interact with lovastatin.

➡ **Circumvent/Minimize.** Patients taking lovastatin should only ingest grapefruit juice occasionally.

REFERENCES:

1. Kantola T, et al. Grapefruit juice greatly increases serum concentrations of lovastatin and lovastatin acid. *Clin Pharmacol Ther.* 1998;63:397-402.

2. Lilja JJ, et al. Grapefruit juice-simvastatin interaction: effect on serum concentrations of simvastatin, simvastatin acid, and HMG-CoA reductase inhibitors. *Clin Pharmacol Ther.* 1998;64:477-483.

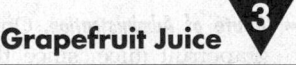

Grapefruit Juice

Methadone (eg, *Methadose*)

SUMMARY: Grapefruit juice may produce a modest increase in methadone serum concentrations; although the effect is not likely to produce adverse effects in most patients, advise patients to avoid grapefruit juice if on methadone maintenance.

RISK FACTORS: No specific risk factors are known.

MECHANISM: Not established. Grapefruit juice may inhibit first-pass metabolism of methadone by CYP3A4.

CLINICAL EVALUATION: Eight patients on methadone maintenance therapy were given methadone for one 5-day period with grapefruit juice and for another 5-day period without grapefruit juice.[1] Grapefruit juice was associated with a small increase in methadone bioavailability, but the magnitude of the increase (17%) is not likely to result in methadone toxicity in most patients. Nonetheless, in some patients, the effect may be large enough to increase methadone effects in a clinically important way.

RELATED DRUGS: No information is available.

MANAGEMENT OPTIONS:

➡ ***Circumvent/Minimize.*** Although the effect is modest, advise patients on methadone maintenance to avoid grapefruit juice.

➡ ***Monitor.*** Monitor patients on methadone maintenance for altered methadone effect if they start or stop drinking grapefruit juice.

REFERENCES:

1. Benmebarek M, et al. Effects of grapefruit juice on the pharmacokinetics of the enantiomers of methadone. *Clin Pharmacol Ther*. 2004;76:55-63.

Grapefruit Juice

Methylprednisolone (eg, *Medrol*)

SUMMARY: Grapefruit juice increases methylprednisolone plasma concentrations; the extent to which this increases the risk of methylprednisolone toxicity is not established.

RISK FACTORS: No specific risk factors are known.

MECHANISM: Grapefruit juice probably inhibits the presystemic CYP3A4 metabolism of methylprednisolone in the small intestine; with high grapefruit doses, the systemic metabolism of methylprednisolone is probably also inhibited.

CLINICAL EVALUATION: In a randomized, crossover study, 10 healthy subjects took a single oral dose of methylprednisolone with and without pretreatment with grapefruit juice (200 mL double strength 3 times daily for 2 days, and 3 more 200 mL doses around the time of methylprednisolone administration).[1] Grapefruit juice increased the methylprednisolone area under the plasma concentration-time curve 75%, but the plasma cortisol concentrations were not affected. The lack of effect on plasma cortisol suggests that most patients on this combination would not experience methylprednisolone toxicity, but it seems likely that toxicity would occur in the sensitive patient.

RELATED DRUGS: Theoretically, dexamethasone (eg, *Decadron*) would interact with grapefruit juice in a manner similar to methylprednisolone, but prednisone does not appear to be affected.[2]

MANAGEMENT OPTIONS:

➡ *Circumvent/Minimize.* Because grapefruit juice is a mechanism-based (suicide) inhibitor, this interaction cannot be completely avoided by separating the doses of methylprednisolone from grapefruit juice. But, it seems unlikely that a fresh grapefruit half would have enough juice to interact with methylprednisolone in a clinically important way.

➡ *Monitor.* If a patient on methylprednisolone drinks grapefruit juice, monitor for methylprednisolone toxicity.

REFERENCES:

1. Varis T, et al. Grapefruit juice can increase the plasma concentrations of oral methylprednisolone. *Eur J Clin Pharmacol.* 2000;56:489-493.

2. Hollander AA, et al. The effect of grapefruit juice on cyclosporine and prednisone metabolism in transplant patients. *Clin Pharmacol Ther.* 1995;57:318-324.

Grapefruit Juice

Midazolam (*Versed*)

SUMMARY: Grapefruit juice increases oral midazolam serum concentrations and pharmacodynamic effects, but does not appear to affect intravenous midazolam. Although the clinical importance of this effect is not established, it seems likely that some patients would be adversely affected when oral midazolam is taken with grapefruit juice.

RISK FACTORS:

➡ *Route of Administration.* Only oral midazolam would be expected to interact with grapefruit juice, since the effect of grapefruit juice is primarily on intestinal CYP3A4.

MECHANISM: Grapefruit juice inhibits the presystemic metabolism of midazolam by intestinal CYP3A4. Flavonoids found in grapefruit juice (ie, kaempferol, naringenin, quercetin) have been shown to inhibit midazolam metabolism in vitro,[1] but more study is needed to establish which component(s) in grapefruit juice inhibit midazolam metabolism.

CLINICAL EVALUATION: A study in healthy subjects found an approximately 50% increase in oral midazolam area under the plasma concentration-time curve and enhanced impairment of psychomotor impairment when it was given with grapefruit juice.[2] Grapefruit juice did not interact with IV midazolam. Another study in healthy subjects found grapefruit juice increased midazolam serum concentrations and pharmacodynamic effects of oral midazolam.[3] Although the effects were not large, these results in healthy subjects receiving single doses cannot necessarily be applied to predisposed patients receiving multiple doses of oral midazolam (in those countries where it is used orally). Thus, it seems likely that at least some patients would be adversely affected by combining oral midazolam with grapefruit juice (and probably other forms of grapefruit).

RELATED DRUGS: Alprazolam (*Xanax*) and triazolam (*Halcion*) are also metabolized by CYP3A4. When given orally, they would also be expected to interact with grapefruit juice. Diazepam (*Valium*) is partially metabolized by CYP3A4, but would not be expected to interact to the same degree. Most other benzodiazepines are metabolized primarily by enzymes other than CYP3A4 and would not be expected to interact.

MANAGEMENT OPTIONS:

➠ *Consider Alternative.* Orange juice does not appear to inhibit CYP3A4 and would not be expected to interact with midazolam. Also, one could use a benzodiazepine other than midazolam, alprazolam, or triazolam such as diazepam.

➠ *Circumvent/Minimize.* Warn patients taking oral midazolam to avoid taking it with or within several hours after grapefruit products.

➠ *Monitor.* If the combination is used, be alert for evidence of excessive midazolam effect (eg, drowsiness).

REFERENCES:

1. Ha HR, et al. In vitro inhibition of midazolam and quinidine metabolism by flavonoids. *Eur J Clin Pharmacol.* 1995;48:367-371.
2. Kupferschmidt HH, et al. Interaction between grapefruit juice and midazolam in humans. *Clin Pharmacol Ther.* 1995;58:20-28.
3. Vanakoski J, et al. Grapefruit juice does not enhance the effects of midazolam and triazolam in man. *Eur J Clin Pharmacol.* 1996;50:501-508.

Grapefruit Juice **4**

Nicardipine (*Cardene*)

SUMMARY: Grapefruit juice increases nicardipine plasma concentrations; some patients may experience increased response.

RISK FACTORS: No specific risk factors are known.

MECHANISM: Grapefruit juice appears to inhibit the metabolism of nicardipine by CYP3A4 in the small intestine without affecting its hepatic metabolism.

CLINICAL EVALUATION: Six healthy subjects received 40 mg nicardipine orally with water or 300 mL of concentrated grapefruit juice 30 minutes before the nicardipine. Each subject also received 2 mg nicardipine IV with water or grapefruit juice as described above.[1] Following oral nicardipine administration, grapefruit juice caused a 1.4- and 1.8-fold increase in the area under the concentration-time curve of (+)- and (-)-nicardipine, respectively. Following grapefruit juice, the oral clearance was reduced and the bioavailability was increased for both nicardipine enantiomers. Grapefruit juice affected the presystemic metabolism of (-)-nicardipine to a greater degree than (+)-nicardipine. This is expected, as the presystemic metabolism of (-)-nicardipine is greater than (+)-nicardipine under control conditions. No changes in nicardipine half-life or nicardipine enantiomer pharmacokinetics following its IV administration were noted with grapefruit juice treatment. The increased nicardipine concentrations were well tolerated by the subjects in this study. Patients consuming larger amounts of grapefruit juice may experience increased calcium channel blocker response including decreased blood pressure and tachycardia.

RELATED DRUGS: Several other calcium channel blockers are substrates for CYP3A4 and grapefruit juice has been shown to reduce their first-pass metabolism.

MANAGEMENT OPTIONS:

➡ *Monitor.* Patients taking nicardipine may experience some increase in response (eg, decreased blood pressure) if grapefruit juice is consumed. Be particularly alert for changes in response in patients consuming large quantities of grapefruit juice.

REFERENCES:

1. Uno T, et al. Effects of grapefruit juice on the stereoselective disposition of nicardipine in humans: evidence for dominant presystemic elimination at the gut site. *Eur J Clin Pharmacol.* 2000;56:643-649.

Grapefruit Juice

Nifedipine (eg, *Procardia*)

SUMMARY: Grapefruit juice increases the serum concentrations of several dihydropyridine calcium channel blockers; increased toxicity could occur in some patients.

RISK FACTORS:

➡ *Dosage Regimen.* Double-strength grapefruit juice (diluted with half the usual amount of water) increased the risk of toxicity.

MECHANISM: Grapefruit juice appears to inhibit the gut wall metabolism (CYP3A4) of calcium channel blockers and increase their bioavailability. This effect appears to be caused by the presence of metabolic inhibitors (eg, flavonoid, sesquiterpenoid compounds) in the grapefruit juice.[1-3]

CLINICAL EVALUATION: The area under the concentration-time curve (AUC) of orally administered nifedipine was increased from 46% to 57% following ingestion of nifedipine 10 mg with double-strength grapefruit juice (diluted with 50% the usual amount of water).[3,4] Grapefruit juice increased the AUC of felodipine (*Plendil*) nearly 200%[1,5-8] and nifedipine 34%[1] compared with administration with water. Hypotensive effects of felodipine were increased following its administration with grapefruit juice.

RELATED DRUGS: Grapefruit juice increases felodipine's AUC. Orange juice had no effect on felodipine.[1] A single dose of grapefruit juice caused a 40% increase in the AUC of nitrendipine,[+,9] while multiple doses produced a 106% increase in the AUC.[10] The combination of nisoldipine (eg, *Sular*) and grapefruit juice produced a 2-fold increase in nisoldipine AUC and an approximate 4-fold increase in its peak concentration.[11] Other dihydropyridine calcium channel blockers may be affected similarly by grapefruit juice.

MANAGEMENT OPTIONS:

➡ *Consider Alternative.* Patients should avoid taking calcium channel blockers with grapefruit juice. Orange juice does not affect calcium channel blocker metabolism.

➡ *Monitor.* Monitor patients who drink grapefruit juice while taking calcium channel blockers for increased response to the calcium channel blocker.

REFERENCES:

1. Bailey DG, et al. Interaction of citrus juices with felodipine and nifedipine. *Lancet.* 1991;337(8736):268-269.

2. Chayen R, et al. Interaction of citrus juices with felodipine and nifedipine. *Lancet.* 1991;337(8745):854.

3. Rashid TJ, et al. Factors affecting the absolute bioavailability of nifedipine. *Br J Clin Pharmacol.* 1995;40(1):51-58.

4. Rashid J, et al. Quercetin, an *in vitro* inhibitor of CYP3A4, does not contribute to the interaction between nifedipine and grapefruit juice. *Br J Clin Pharmacol.* 1993;36(5):460-463.

5. Edgar B, et al. Formulation dependent interaction between felodipine and grapefruit juice. *Clin Pharmacol Ther.* 1990;47:181.

6. Bailey DG, et al. Grapefruit juice—felodipine interaction: mechanism, predictability, and effect of naringin. *Clin Pharmacol Ther.* 1993;53(6):637-642.

7. Edgar B, et al. Acute effects of drinking grapefruit juice on the pharmacokinetics and dynamics of felodipine—and its potential clinical relevance. *Eur J Clin Pharmacol.* 1992;42(3):313-317.

8. Lundahl J, et al. Relationship between time of intake of grapefruit juice and its effect on pharmacokinetics and pharmacodynamics of felodipine in healthy subjects. *Eur J Clin Pharmacol.* 1995;49(1-2):61-67.

9. Bailey DG, et al. Grapefruit juice and naringin interaction with nitrendipine. *Clin Pharmacol Ther.* 1992;51:156.

10. Soons PA, et al. Grapefruit juice and cimetidine inhibit stereoselective metabolism of nitrendipine in humans. *Clin Pharmacol Ther.* 1991;50(4):394-403.

11. Bailey DG, et al. Effect of grapefruit juice and naringin on nisoldipine pharmacokinetics. *Clin Pharmacol Ther.* 1993;54(6):589-594.

† Not available in the United States.

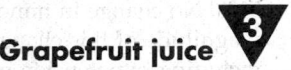

Grapefruit juice

Nilotinib (*Tasigna*)

SUMMARY: Grapefruit juice may increase nilotinib serum concentrations; increased nilotinib toxicity might occur in some patients.

RISK FACTORS: No specific risk factors are known.

MECHANISM: Grapefruit juice probably increases the bioavailability of nilotinib by inhibiting CYP3A4 in the intestine, and possibly also by inhibiting intestinal P-glycoprotein.

CLINICAL EVALUATION: In a crossover study of 21 healthy subjects, a single oral dose of nilotinib 400 mg was given with and without 240 mL of double-strength grapefruit juice.[1] Grapefruit juice was associated with a modest 29% increase in nilotinib area under the serum concentration-time curve (AUC) with no change in nilotinib half-life. Although the mean increase in AUC was not large, there was considerable variability from one subject to another; 1 subject developed a 188% increase in nilotinib AUC. Thus, some patients may manifest adverse outcomes from this interaction.

RELATED DRUGS: Many other tyrosine kinase inhibitors are also CYP3A4 substrates, including dasatinib (*Sprycel*), erlotinib (*Tarceva*), gefitinib (*Iressa*), imatinib (*Gleevec*), lapatinib (*Tykerb*), pazopanib (*Votrient*), sorafenib (*Nexavar*), and sunitinib (*Sutent*). These drugs may also interact with grapefruit juice.

MANAGEMENT OPTIONS:

➡ **Consider Alternative.** Advise patients to avoid grapefruit juice when taking nilotinib or other tyrosine kinase inhibitors. Orange juice does not appear to affect CYP3A4 or P-glycoprotein.

➤ *Monitor.* If the combination is used, monitor for increased nilotinib effect.

REFERENCES:

1. Yin OQ, et al. Effect of grapefruit juice on the pharmacokinetics of nilotinib in healthy participants. *J Clin Pharmacol.* 2010;50(2):188-194.

Grapefruit Juice

Nimodipine (eg, *Nimotop*)

SUMMARY: Grapefruit juice increases the plasma concentration of nimodipine; increased pharmacodynamic effects may occur.

RISK FACTORS: No specific risk factors are known.

MECHANISM: Grapefruit juice inhibits the CYP3A4-mediated intestinal metabolism of nimodipine, increasing its bioavailability.

CLINICAL EVALUATION: Eight healthy subjects received a single dose of nimodipine 30 mg with water or 250 mL of grapefruit juice.[1] Compared with water, the administration of nimodipine with grapefruit juice resulted in an increased bioavailability of 51%. No change in nimodipine half-life was noted following grapefruit juice. The magnitude of this change could result in an increase in the effects of nimodipine, including hypotension or headache.

RELATED DRUGS: Other calcium channel blockers, including felodipine and nifedipine (eg, *Procardia*), are similarly affected by grapefruit juice. Orange juice does not affect CYP3A4 activity in the intestinal wall. Grapefruit juice has little effect on amlodipine (eg, *Norvasc*).

MANAGEMENT OPTIONS:

➤ *Consider Alternative.* Advise patients receiving nimodipine to avoid drinking grapefruit juice. Substitute with orange juice or another fruit juice.

➤ *Monitor.* Monitor patients who take nimodipine and ingest grapefruit juice for increased hypotensive effects and possible adverse reactions such as headache.

REFERENCES:

1. Fuhr U, et al. Grapefruit juice increases oral nimodipine bioavailability. *Int J Clin Pharmacol Ther.* 1998;36(3):126-132.

Grapefruit Juice

Nisoldipine (*Sular*)

SUMMARY: Grapefruit juice administered just before or with nisoldipine increases the plasma concentration and pharmacodynamic effect of nisoldipine.

RISK FACTORS: No specific risk factors are known.

MECHANISM: Grapefruit juice inhibits the CYP3A4 metabolism of nisoldipine in the wall of the small intestine. Prolonged administration of grapefruit juice also may affect hepatic CYP3A4 activity.

CLINICAL EVALUATION: Eight healthy subjects received nisoldipine 10 mg with water alone, concurrently with 250 mL of grapefruit juice, 1 hour before 250 mL of grapefruit juice, and 1 hour after 250 mL of grapefruit juice.[1] It appears that a single dose of regular-strength grapefruit juice was used. Administration of nisoldipine concurrently or 1 hour after the grapefruit juice produced significant increases (approximately 3.7-fold) in the nisoldipine area under the concentration-time curve (AUC). Taking nisoldipine 1 hour prior to grapefruit juice resulted in a nonsignificant trend toward an increase in nisoldipine AUC. Grapefruit juice administered with or 1 hour prior to the calcium channel blocker also increased the peak concentration and half-life of nisoldipine. The hypotensive effect of nisoldipine was increased by grapefruit juice administration. The effect of multiple doses of grapefruit juice on nisoldipine is expected to be somewhat greater than the results reported in this study.

RELATED DRUGS: Other calcium channel blockers are likely to be affected by grapefruit juice in a similar manner.

MANAGEMENT OPTIONS:

➡ *Consider Alternative.* Orange juice could be substituted for grapefruit juice to avoid the interaction. Calcium channel blockers with low first-pass metabolism such as amlodipine (eg, *Norvasc*) will be less affected by grapefruit juice.

➡ *Monitor.* Watch for increased hypotensive effects or side effects (eg, headache, hypotension) when patients taking calcium channel blockers consume grapefruit juice.

REFERENCES:

1. Azuma J, et al. Effects of grapefruit juice on the pharmacokinetics of the calcium channel blockers nifedipine and nisoldipine. *Curr Ther Res*. 1998;59:619-634.

Grapefruit Juice

Primaquine

SUMMARY: Grapefruit juice may increase the plasma concentrations of primaquine; however, most patients will not be at increased risk of side effects.

RISK FACTORS: No specific risk factors are known.

MECHANISM: Grapefruit juice appears to reduce the CYP3A4-mediated metabolism of primaquine during intestinal first-pass metabolism.

CLINICAL EVALUATION: Twenty healthy subjects received a single dose of primaquine 30 mg with water and with a single dose of 50% grapefruit juice 300 mL.[1] Compared with administration with water, grapefruit juice increased the mean area under the concentration-time curve of primaquine 19% (range, −29% to 218%). It is unclear if this degree of increase in primaquine's plasma concentration will increase the risk of side effects in patients taking primaquine.

RELATED DRUGS: None known.

MANAGEMENT OPTIONS:

➡ *Monitor.* Advise patients taking primaquine to avoid drinking grapefruit juice.

REFERENCES:

1. Cuong BT, et al. Does gender, food or grapefruit juice alter the pharmacokinetics of primaquine in healthy subjects? *Br J Clin Pharmacol*. 2006;61:682-689.

Grapefruit Juice

Quinidine

SUMMARY: Grapefruit juice appears to produce a slight change in the metabolism of quinidine; the clinical significance of these changes is limited.

RISK FACTORS: No specific risk factors are known.

MECHANISM: Grapefruit juice may reduce the gut wall metabolism (CYP3A4) of quinidine without altering its hepatic metabolism.

CLINICAL EVALUATION: Twelve healthy subjects were administered a single oral dose of quinidine sulfate 400 mg with 240 mL of water or grapefruit juice.[1] Grapefruit juice did not alter the area under the concentration-time curve (AUC), peak concentration, or half-life of quinidine. The time to peak quinidine concentration was extended from 1.6 to 3.3 hours when administered with grapefruit juice. The AUC of the quinidine metabolite 3-hydroxyquinidine was reduced 33% following grapefruit juice administration compared with water. The effect of quinidine administration on the electrocardiogram QT interval was unchanged by grapefruit juice, except that the maximum QT effect was delayed.

RELATED DRUGS: No information is available.

MANAGEMENT OPTIONS: No specific action is required, but be alert for evidence of the interaction.

REFERENCES:
1. Min DI, et al. Effect of grapefruit juice on the pharmacokinetics and pharmacodynamics of quinidine in healthy volunteers. *J Clin Pharmacol*. 1996;36:469-476.

4 **Grapefruit Juice**

Repaglinide (*Prandin*)

SUMMARY: Grapefruit juice causes a small increase in the plasma concentration of repaglinide; no alteration in glycemic control is anticipated.

RISK FACTORS: No specific risk factors are known.

MECHANISM: Grapefruit juice appears to inhibit the CYP3A4-mediated intestinal wall metabolism of repaglinide. Because repaglinide also is metabolized by CYP2C8, inhibition of intestinal CYP3A4 does not produce a large change in repaglinide's total clearance.

CLINICAL EVALUATION: The administration of 300 mL of grapefruit juice 2 hours before a single dose of repaglinide 2 mg produced a mean increase in repaglinide's area under the plasma concentration-time curve of 18% compared with administration with water.[1] No change was observed in repaglinide half-life. Blood glucose concentrations were not affected.

RELATED DRUGS: Pioglitazone (*Actos*) and nateglinide (*Starlix*) are partially metabolized by CYP3A4; however, it is unlikely that grapefruit juice would cause a large enough change in their total clearance to result in altered glycemic control.

MANAGEMENT OPTIONS: No specific action is required, but be alert for evidence of the interaction.

REFERENCES:

1. Bidstrup TB, et al. The impact of CYP2C8 polymorphism and grapefruit juice on the pharmacokinetics of repaglinide. *Br J Clin Pharmacol.* 2005;61:49-57.

Grapefruit Juice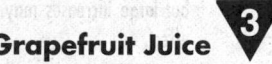

Saquinavir (eg, *Fortovase*)

SUMMARY: Grapefruit juice increases saquinavir plasma concentrations; increased saquinavir efficacy and toxicity may occur.

RISK FACTORS: No specific risk factors are known.

MECHANISM: Grapefruit juice inhibits the CYP3A4-mediated, first-pass metabolism of saquinavir, resulting in increased bioavailability. Grapefruit juice may also inhibit P-glycoprotein-mediated efflux of saquinavir in the small intestine.[1,2]

CLINICAL EVALUATION: Eight subjects received a single dose of saquinavir 600 mg orally or 12 mg IV alone and following 400 mL of grapefruit juice administered during the 45 minutes prior to the saquinavir dose.[3] Grapefruit juice had no effect on the pharmacokinetics of saquinavir administered IV. The mean area under the plasma concentration-time curve of saquinavir administered orally was increased 50% following grapefruit juice, the result of saquinavir's bioavailability increasing from 0.7% to 1.4%. The magnitude of the effect of grapefruit juice on saquinavir would likely vary with the amount of grapefruit juice consumed. The effect of grapefruit juice on the absorption of saquinavir in patients receiving other CYP3A4 inhibitors such as ritonavir is unknown.

RELATED DRUGS: Grapefruit juice also increases the plasma concentration of indinavir. Other protease inhibitors that are CYP3A4 substrates are also likely to be effected by grapefruit juice.

MANAGEMENT OPTIONS:

➥ *Monitor.* Observe patients receiving saquinavir for increased plasma concentrations if they consume grapefruit juice more than just occasionally.

REFERENCES:

1. Eagling VA, et al. Inhibition of the CYP3A4-mediated metabolism and P-glycoprotein-mediated transport of the HIV-I protease inhibitor saquinavir by grapefruit juice components. *Br J Clin Pharmacol.* 1999;48:543-552.

2. Tian R, et al. Effects of grapefruit juice and orange juice on the intestinal efflux of P-glycoprotein substrates. *Pharm Res.* 2002;19:802-809.

3. Kupferschmidt HH, et al. Grapefruit juice enhances the bioavailability of the HIV protease inhibitor saquinavir in man. *Br J Clin Pharmacol.* 1998;54:355-359.

Grapefruit Juice

Sildenafil (*Viagra*)

SUMMARY: Study in healthy subjects suggests that grapefruit juice modestly increases sildenafil plasma concentrations, but large increases may be seen in some patients. Grapefruit juice also may slow the onset of sildenafil effect.

RISK FACTORS: No specific risk factors are known.

MECHANISM: Grapefruit juice probably inhibits the CYP3A4 metabolism of sildenafil in the intestine, thus increasing sildenafil bioavailability.

CLINICAL EVALUATION: In a randomized, crossover study, 24 healthy subjects received a single oral dose of sildenafil 50 mg with and without concurrent grapefruit juice (250 mL 1 hour before and 250 mL with the sildenafil).[1] Grapefruit juice produced a 23% increase in sildenafil area under the plasma concentration-time curve (AUC) and delayed by 15 minutes the time to reach peak sildenafil plasma concentrations. Although the mean increase in sildenafil AUC was modest, there was considerable variability among subjects; 1 subject had a 2.6-fold increase in sildenafil concentrations with grapefruit juice. Although most patients would probably not develop sildenafil toxicity caused by grapefruit juice, an occasional patient may be at risk. Moreover, the delay in peak sildenafil plasma concentrations may be a disadvantage in that it could delay onset of sildenafil effect. Because grapefruit juice is a mechanism-based inhibitor of CYP3A4, theoretically, it could affect sildenafil even if the administration is separated by many hours. Given the variability in response, it would not be prudent to use grapefruit juice as a sildenafil-sparing agent.

RELATED DRUGS: No information is available.

MANAGEMENT OPTIONS:

➡ *Circumvent/Minimize.* Patients who take sildenafil should probably avoid grapefruit juice completely.

REFERENCES:

1. Jetter A, et al. Effects of grapefruit juice on the pharmacokinetics of sildenafil. *Clin Pharmacol Ther.* 2002;71:21-29.

Grapefruit Juice

Simvastatin (*Zocor*)

SUMMARY: Repeated doses of grapefruit juice markedly increased simvastatin serum concentrations in healthy subjects.

RISK FACTORS: No specific risk factors are known.

MECHANISM: Simvastatin undergoes extensive first-pass metabolism by CYP3A4 in the small intestine and liver, resulting in approximately 5% bioavailability. Grapefruit juice inhibits intestinal CYP3A4, thus increasing the bioavailability of simvastatin.

CLINICAL EVALUATION: Ten healthy subjects received a single oral dose of simvastatin 60 mg with and without repeated doses of grapefruit juice (200 mL, double strength).[1] Grapefruit juice increased the mean area under the serum concentration-time curve (AUC) for simvastatin and simvastatin acid (the active metabolite) by 16- and 7-fold, respectively. The effect was highly variable from patient to patient; 1 patient had a 38-fold increase in simvastatin AUC following grapefruit juice. Therefore, it appears that at least some patients would be expected to have an increased risk of simvastatin-induced myopathy. However, note that the subjects ingested a large amount of grapefruit juice; the effect of a more normal amount of grapefruit juice on simvastatin would probably be less than that observed in this study. Thus, the risk associated with a single glass of normal-strength grapefruit juice in a patient receiving simvastatin is probably not high.

RELATED DRUGS: Lovastatin (eg, *Mevacor*), like simvastatin, undergoes extensive first-pass metabolism in the gut wall and liver; it is similarly affected by grapefruit juice.[2] Atorvastatin (*Lipitor*) is also metabolized by CYP3A4 and would be expected to interact with grapefruit juice (but to a lesser extent than lovastatin and simvastatin). Pravastatin (*Pravachol*) and fluvastatin (*Lescol*) are not metabolized by CYP3A4 and are not likely to be affected by grapefruit juice.

MANAGEMENT OPTIONS:

➡ *Consider Alternative.* Orange juice does not inhibit CYP3A4 and would not be expected to interact with simvastatin.

➡ *Circumvent/Minimize.* Patients taking simvastatin should ingest grapefruit juice only occasionally.

REFERENCES:

1. Lilja JJ, et al. Grapefruit juice-simvastatin interaction: effect on serum concentrations of simvastatin, simvastatin acid, and HMG-CoA reductase inhibitors. *Clin Pharmacol Ther.* 1998;64:477-483.

2. Kantola T, et al. Grapefruit juice greatly increases serum concentrations of lovastatin and lovastatin acid. *Clin Pharmacol Ther.* 1998;63:397-402.

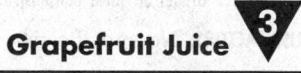

Grapefruit Juice

Terfenadine†

SUMMARY: Grapefruit juice increases the amount of oral terfenadine reaching the systemic circulation intact. Although the clinical importance of this effect is not established, it is possible that the risk of cardiac arrhythmias may increase in predisposed individuals.

RISK FACTORS: No specific risk factors are known.

MECHANISM: Grapefruit juice appears to increase the bioavailability of terfenadine by inhibiting gut wall CYP3A4.

CLINICAL EVALUATION: Twelve healthy subjects were given terfenadine 60 mg twice daily for 14 days with grapefruit juice added for the last 7 days.[1] Six subjects took the grapefruit juice simultaneously with each dose of terfenadine, and 6 took the grapefruit juice delayed by 2 hours after each dose of terfenadine. Quantifiable plasma terfenadine was not found in the 12 subjects during baseline, but was found in all 6 subjects during simultaneous grapefruit juice and in 2 of 6 subjects during delayed grapefruit juice. Terfenadine with simultaneous grapefruit juice (but not delayed grapefruit juice) increased the QT interval in the electrocardiogram compared with terfenadine alone. Similar results were found in another study of terfenadine and simultaneous grapefruit juice involving 6 poor metabolizers of terfenadine.[2] It is not likely that this interaction would result in adverse reactions because terfenadine-induced ventricular arrhythmias appear rare even when terfenadine is given with CYP3A4 inhibitors that are more potent than grapefruit juice. Nonetheless, the possibility cannot be ruled out that an occasional patient would be adversely affected.

RELATED DRUGS: Astemizole[†] is likely to interact with grapefruit juice in a similar manner, but adverse reactions are not expected when grapefruit juice is given with the nonsedating antihistamines loratadine (eg, *Claritin*) and fexofenadine (eg, *Allegra*), or the low-sedating agent cetirizine (eg, *Zyrtec*).

MANAGEMENT OPTIONS:

➡ *Circumvent/Minimize.* Although the clinical significance of this interaction is not established, given the potentially serious nature of the adverse reaction, warn patients to avoid grapefruit products while taking terfenadine or astemizole.

➡ *Monitor.* If terfenadine or astemizole is taken with grapefruit, monitor for evidence of ventricular arrhythmias (eg, palpitations, syncope).

REFERENCES:

1. Benton RE, et al. Grapefruit juice alters terfenadine pharmacokinetics, resulting in prolongation of repolarization on the electrocardiogram. *Clin Pharmacol Ther*. 1996;59(4):383-388.

2. Honig PK, et al. Grapefruit juice alters the systemic bioavailability and cardiac repolarization of terfenadine in poor metabolizers of terfenadine. *J Clin Pharmacol*. 1996;36(4):345-351.

† Not available in the United States.

4 · Grapefruit Juice

Tolvaptan (*Samsca*)

SUMMARY: Grapefruit juice administration has been noted to increase the plasma concentration of tolvaptan.

RISK FACTORS: No specific risk factors are known.

MECHANISM: Grapefruit inhibits enterocyte CYP3A4, the primary enzyme that metabolizes tolvaptan as it passes through the intestinal wall during absorption.

CLINICAL EVALUATION: While specific data are limited, the coadministration of grapefruit juice (dose not stated) and tolvaptan increased the mean area under the plasma concentration-time curve of tolvaptan by approximately 1.8-fold.[1] Pending further data, patients receiving tolvaptan and grapefruit juice should be observed for increased tolvaptan adverse reactions, including constipation, dry mouth, and hyperglycemia. However, as with most grapefruit juice interactions, it is likely that high-dose, long-term coadministration of grapefruit juice and tolvaptan would be required to produce adverse reactions.

RELATED DRUGS: No information is available.

MANAGEMENT OPTIONS:

➡ *Monitor.* If grapefruit juice is administered with tolvaptan, monitor patients for evidence of tolvaptan adverse reactions.

REFERENCES:

1. *Samsca* [package insert]. Rockville, MD: Otsuka America Pharmaceutical Inc; 2009.

Grapefruit Juice ▼3

Triazolam (eg, *Halcion*)

SUMMARY: Grapefruit juice increases triazolam serum concentrations. Although the clinical importance of this effect is not established, it seems likely that some patients would be adversely affected.

RISK FACTORS:

→ *Effects of Age.* Elderly patients are known to be more sensitive to triazolam and are likely to be at greater risk of this interaction.

MECHANISM: Grapefruit juice inhibits the presystemic metabolism of triazolam by intestinal CYP3A4.

CLINICAL EVALUATION: Studies in healthy subjects have found grapefruit juice to produce approximately 50% increase in triazolam serum concentrations, but only a small increase in triazolam-induced psychomotor impairment.[1,2] Thus, under the conditions of these studies involving young healthy subjects, the interaction appears to be of minimal clinical importance. However, triazolam can produce significant dose-dependent toxicity (especially in elderly patients), and it cannot be assumed that the results of these studies apply to patients taking triazolam therapeutically. A 50% increase in triazolam serum concentrations caused by grapefruit juice (and probably other forms of grapefruit) is likely to produce adverse outcomes in at least some predisposed individuals.

RELATED DRUGS: Alprazolam (eg, *Xanax*) and midazolam are metabolized by CYP3A4. When given orally, they are expected to interact with grapefruit juice. Diazepam (eg, *Valium*) is partially metabolized by CYP3A4 but is not expected to interact to the same degree. Most other benzodiazepines are metabolized primarily by enzymes other than CYP3A4 and are not expected to interact.

MANAGEMENT OPTIONS:

→ *Consider Alternative.* Orange juice does not appear to inhibit CYP3A4 and is not expected to interact with triazolam. Also, a benzodiazepine other than triazolam, alprazolam, or midazolam could be used, such as diazepam.

→ *Circumvent/Minimize.* Warn patients taking triazolam to avoid taking it with or within several hours after grapefruit. Ingesting grapefruit in the morning and taking the triazolam in the evening would theoretically minimize the interaction, but there may still be a small effect.

→ *Monitor.* If the combination is used, be alert for excessive triazolam effect (eg, drowsiness).

REFERENCES:

1. Hukkinen SK, et al. Plasma concentrations of triazolam are increased by concomitant ingestion of grapefruit juice. *Clin Pharmacol Ther.* 1995;58(2):127-131.

2. Vanakoski J, et al. Grapefruit juice does not enhance the effects of midazolam and triazolam in man. *Eur J Clin Pharmacol.* 1996;50(6):501-508.

4   Grapefruit Juice

Verapamil (eg, *Isoptin SR*)

SUMMARY: Repeated doses of grapefruit juice can produce modest increases in verapamil plasma concentrations; changes in clinical response are likely to be limited.

RISK FACTORS: No specific risk factors are known.

MECHANISM: Grapefruit juice appears to moderately inhibit the metabolism of verapamil by CYP3A4 in the small intestine without affecting its hepatic metabolism.

CLINICAL EVALUATION: Ten patients with hypertension taking chronic verapamil received 200 mL water or normal strength grapefruit juice 1 hour before and with their morning dose of immediate-release verapamil on 2 separate days.[1] All subjects received the grapefruit juice treatment on the second study day. The mean area under the concentration-time curve (AUC) of verapamil was increased 17% following grapefruit juice; however, this increase was not statistically significant. No other pharmacokinetic parameters of verapamil were significantly altered by grapefruit juice administration compared with water. In a second randomized, crossover study, 9 healthy subjects received 200 mL of grapefruit juice or orange juice as a control twice daily for 5 days prior to the pharmacokinetics study.[2] They received sustained-release verapamil 120 mg twice daily for 3 days before the pharmacokinetic study day. On the pharmacokinetic study day, a single 120 mg dose of verapamil was administered, as was the twice-daily juice. Grapefruit juice increased the mean AUC of S- and R-verapamil 36% and 28%, respectively. The peak concentration of S-verapamil was increased an average of 57% following grapefruit juice. Verapamil half-life and renal clearance were not altered by grapefruit juice administration. The use of a sustained-release formulation of verapamil may lessen the effect of grapefruit juice since some drug may not be released from the dosage form until it has passed the small intestine, which is the purported site of grapefruit juice inhibition of verapamil first-pass metabolism.

RELATED DRUGS: Several other calcium channel blockers are substrates for CYP3A4 and grapefruit juice has been shown to reduce their first-pass metabolism.

MANAGEMENT OPTIONS:

➡ *Monitor.* Patients taking verapamil may experience some increase in effect if grapefruit juice is chronically consumed. The consumption of 1 serving/day or less would not be expected to produce significant changes in the response to verapamil in most patients.

REFERENCES:

1. Zaidenstein, R et al. The effect of grapefruit juice on the pharmacokinetics of orally administered verapamil. *Eur J Clin Pharmacol.* 1998;54:337-340.
2. Ho PC, et al. Effect of grapefruit juice on pharmacokinetics and pharmacodynamics of verapamil enantiomers in healthy volunteers. *Eur J Clin Pharmacol.* 2000;56:693-698.

Grapefruit Juice

Warfarin (eg, *Coumadin*)

SUMMARY: Grapefruit juice does not appear to affect the hypoprothrombinemic response to warfarin.

RISK FACTORS: No specific risk factors are known.

MECHANISM: No interaction.

CLINICAL EVALUATION: Ten patients stabilized on warfarin therapy took grapefruit juice 240 mL 3 times a week for 1 week.[1] Grapefruit juice did not affect the prothrombin time or INR.

RELATED DRUGS: None.

MANAGEMENT OPTIONS: No interaction.

REFERENCES:

1. Sullivan DM, et al. Grapefruit juice and the response to warfarin. *Am J Health Syst Pharm.* 1998;55:1581–1583.

Griseofulvin

Contraceptives, Oral (eg, *Ortho-Novum*)

SUMMARY: Griseofulvin may induce menstrual irregularities or increase the risk of pregnancy in women taking oral contraceptives.

RISK FACTORS: No specific risk factors are known.

MECHANISM: Griseofulvin is believed to enhance the hepatic metabolism of contraceptive steroids, but this hypothesis has not been studied.

CLINICAL EVALUATION: Menstrual irregularities (breakthrough bleeding or amenorrhea) were noted in 20 women receiving oral contraceptives and griseofulvin.[1] In 4 of the women, a rechallenge with griseofulvin resulted in a recurrence of the menstrual disorder. Two women became pregnant after concurrent therapy with griseofulvin and oral contraceptives; however, they also were receiving sulfonamides, which theoretically could have reduced contraceptive efficacy. An additional patient, who developed irregular menses and oligomenorrhea while on oral contraceptives and griseofulvin, responded to an increase in the estrogen component of the contraceptive with resolution of the menstrual problems.[2]

RELATED DRUGS: Other antifungal agents may affect oral contraceptives similarly.

MANAGEMENT OPTIONS:

➡ *Circumvent/Minimize.* Patients on low-estrogen oral contraceptives may need a contraceptive with a higher estrogen dose when taking griseofulvin.

➡ *Monitor.* Women taking oral contraceptives should consider using additional contraceptives during and for 1 cycle after griseofulvin therapy. The development of menstrual irregularities (eg, spotting, breakthrough bleeding) may indicate that the interaction is occurring and warrants particular caution.

REFERENCES:

1. van Dijke CP, et al. Interaction between oral contraceptives and griseofulvin. *Br Med J.* 1984;288.1125-1126.
2. McDaniel PA, et al. Oral contraceptives and griseofulvin interaction. *Drug Intell Clin Pharm.* 1986;20:384.

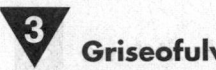

Griseofulvin

Phenobarbital (eg, *Solfoton*)

SUMMARY: Phenobarbital may reduce the serum concentration of griseofulvin, but the clinical significance of this effect is not established.

RISK FACTORS: No specific risk factors are known.

MECHANISM: Phenobarbital appears to impair the absorption of griseofulvin without increasing its metabolism.

CLINICAL EVALUATION: Although decreased plasma concentrations of griseofulvin following administration of phenobarbital are well documented, the effect of these decreases on the therapeutic response to griseofulvin has not been established.[1] Treatment failures caused by phenobarbital are reported uncommonly; more study is needed to assess the clinical significance of this interaction.[2,3]

RELATED DRUGS: Other barbiturates may produce a similar reaction with griseofulvin or other antifungal agents.

MANAGEMENT OPTIONS:

➡ *Circumvent/Minimize.* It has been suggested that divided griseofulvin doses (eg, 3 times/day) may be absorbed better than larger doses taken less often.[2]

➡ *Monitor.* Until further information is available, monitor patients for lack of griseofulvin efficacy. Whether an increase in the daily dosage of griseofulvin is warranted when phenobarbital is coadministered requires further study.

REFERENCES:

1. Busfield D, et al. An effect of phenobarbitone on blood-levels of griseofulvin in man. *Lancet.* 1963;13:1042-1043.
2. Riegelman S, et al. Griseofulvin-phenobarbital interaction in man. *JAMA.* 1970;213:426-431.
3. Lorenc E. A new factor in griseofulvin treatment failures. *MO Med.* 1967;64:32-33.

Griseofulvin

Warfarin (eg, *Coumadin*)

SUMMARY: Griseofulvin appears to inhibit the hypoprothrombinemic response to warfarin and possibly other oral anticoagulants. An adjustment in the oral anticoagulant dose may be required in patients receiving both drugs.

RISK FACTORS:

➡ *Dosage Regimen.* Some evidence suggests that the effect of griseofulvin on warfarin is very gradual, so it may take several weeks or longer for the maximal effect to be seen.

MECHANISM: Not established. Some evidence suggests that griseofulvin induces hepatic microsomal enzymes.

CLINICAL EVALUATION: One report describes 3 patients in whom griseofulvin appeared to inhibit the effect of warfarin, but no effect was seen in a healthy volunteer given the combination.[1] In another case study, a 61-year-old man on chronic warfarin therapy gradually developed a 41% increase in warfarin requirement over a 3-month period after starting griseofulvin.[2] Udall found that only 4 of 10 patients on chronic warfarin therapy developed decreased prothrombin times (mean, 4.2 seconds) when placed on griseofulvin 1 g/day for 2 weeks.[3] However, if the interaction occurs gradually, as reported for the 61-year-old patient, a greater effect might have been seen with longer administration of griseofulvin (which is required for treatment of some infections). Although the evidence indicates that an interaction between warfarin and griseofulvin does occur, how often it would be clinically important in patients receiving the combination is unclear.

RELATED DRUGS: Little is known regarding the effect of griseofulvin on oral anticoagulants other than warfarin; however, assume that an interaction exists until information to the contrary appears.

MANAGEMENT OPTIONS:

➡ *Monitor.* Monitor for altered oral anticoagulant effect if griseofulvin is initiated, discontinued, or changed in dosage. Because the effect of griseofulvin may be very gradual, monitor the hypoprothrombinemic response until it is stable, adjusting the anticoagulant dose as needed.

REFERENCES:

1. Cullen SI, et al. Griseofulvin-warfarin antagonism. *JAMA*. 1967;199:582-583.
2. Okino K, et al. Warfarin-griseofulvin interaction. *Drug Intell Clin Pharm*. 1986;20:291-293.
3. Udall JA. Drug interference with warfarin therapy. *Clin Med*. 1970;77:20.

Guanethidine (*Ismelin*)

Haloperidol (eg, *Haldol*)

SUMMARY: Haloperidol has been associated with inhibition of the antihypertensive effect of guanethidine in a few patients.

RISK FACTORS: No specific risk factors are known.

MECHANISM: Not established. Haloperidol might inhibit the uptake of guanethidine by adrenergic neurons in a manner similar to that of the tricyclic antidepressants.

CLINICAL EVALUATION: In 3 hypertensive patients stabilized on guanethidine, haloperidol 6 to 9 mg/day was associated with a mean blood pressure increase of about 15 to 20 mm Hg.[1]

RELATED DRUGS: Guanadrel (*Hylorel*) is pharmacologically similar to guanethidine and also may be inhibited by haloperidol.

MANAGEMENT OPTIONS:

➡ *Consider Alternative.* Consider using an antihypertensive other than guanethidine (or drugs related to guanethidine such as guanadrel).

➡ *Monitor.* If the combination is used, monitor blood pressure for inhibition of antihypertensive effect. Increasing the guanethidine dose may overcome the interaction.[1]

REFERENCES:

1. Janowsky DS, et al. Antagonism of guanethidine by chlorpromazine. *Am J Psychiatry*. 1973;130:808-812.

Guanethidine (*Ismelin*)

Levodopa (eg, *Larodopa*)

SUMMARY: Isolated cases of an enhanced hypotensive effect of guanethidine associated with levodopa have been reported, but a causal relationship has not been established.

RISK FACTORS: No specific risk factors are known.

MECHANISM: Not established.

CLINICAL EVALUATION: The hypotensive effect of guanethidine appeared to be enhanced by levodopa in 2 patients,[1] but more study is needed to confirm these observations.

RELATED DRUGS: Although little is known regarding the effect of the guanethidine-like drug, guanadrel (*Hylorel*), consider the possibility that it interacts similarly with levodopa until clinical information is available.

MANAGEMENT OPTIONS: No specific action is required, but be alert for evidence of the interaction.

REFERENCES:
1. Hunter KR, et al. Use of levodopa with other drugs. *Lancet*. 1970;2:1283.

Guanethidine (*Ismelin*)

Methylphenidate (eg, *Ritalin*)

SUMMARY: Methylphenidate appears to inhibit the antihypertensive effect of guanethidine.

RISK FACTORS: No specific risk factors are known.

MECHANISM: Methylphenidate probably antagonizes the adrenergic blockade produced by guanethidine. Amphetamines inhibit the antihypertensive effect of guanethidine (and probably also guanadrel).

CLINICAL EVALUATION: The inhibition of guanethidine's hypotensive effect by methylphenidate is not as great as that caused by amphetamines, but it may be sufficient to interfere with hypertension control.[1-3] A patient receiving both methylphenidate and guanethidine developed ventricular tachycardia, apparently as a result of this drug interaction.[3]

RELATED DRUGS: Guanadrel (*Hylorel*) is pharmacologically similar to guanethidine and also may be inhibited by methylphenidate.

MANAGEMENT OPTIONS:

➡ *Consider Alternative.* Consider using antihypertensive agents other than guanethidine or guanadrel in patients who require methylphenidate therapy.

➡ *Monitor.* If the combination is used, monitor blood pressure and heart rate.

REFERENCES:
1. Day MD, et al. Antagonism of guanethidine and bretylium by various agents. *Lancet*. 1962;2:1282.
2. Gulati OD, et al. Antagonism of adrenergic neuron blockade in hypertensive subjects. *Clin Pharmacol Ther*. 1966;7:510.
3. Deshmankar BS, et al. Ventricular tachycardia associated with the administration of methylphenidate during guanethidine therapy. *Can Med Assoc J*. 1967;97:1166.

Guanethidine (eg, *Ismelin*)

Norepinephrine (*Levophed*)

SUMMARY: Patients on guanethidine have an exaggerated pressor response to norepinephrine.

RISK FACTORS: No specific risk factors are known.

MECHANISM: Possible mechanisms include increased sensitivity of the adrenergic receptor to norepinephrine and inhibition of norepinephrine uptake and subsequent inactivation by the adrenergic neuron.

CLINICAL EVALUATION: The increased pressor effect of norepinephrine in patients receiving guanethidine is well documented and of sufficient magnitude to be clinically significant.[1,2] In addition, there appears to be an increased tendency for cardiac arrhythmias to occur in guanethidine-treated patients who are given norepinephrine.

RELATED DRUGS: Guanadrel (*Hylorel*) is pharmacologically similar to guanethidine and also may enhance the pressor response to norepinephrine.

MANAGEMENT OPTIONS:

➡️ *Monitor.* In patients receiving guanethidine or guanadrel, use conservative doses of norepinephrine (and other sympathomimetics); monitor blood pressure carefully.

REFERENCES:

1. Muelheims GH, et al. Increased sensitivity of the heart to catecholamine-induced arrhythmias following guanethidine. *Clin Pharmacol Ther*. 1965;6:757.
2. Dollery CT. Physiological and pharmacological interactions of antihypertensive drugs. *Proc R Soc Med*. 1965;58:983.

Guanethidine (*Ismelin*)

Phenelzine (*Nardil*)

SUMMARY: Monoamine oxidase inhibitors (MAOIs) may inhibit the antihypertensive response to guanethidine.

RISK FACTORS: No specific risk factors known.

MECHANISM: MAOIs reportedly antagonize the antihypertensive effect of guanethidine,[1,2,4] possibly by counteracting guanethidine-induced neuronal catecholamine depletion. In a patient receiving an MAOI, the initial release of norepinephrine following guanethidine therapy may produce a greater response because of MAOI-induced increased norepinephrine stores.[3]

CLINICAL EVALUATION: Limited clinical evidence suggests that nonselective MAOIs inhibit the hypotensive effect of guanethidine. More study is needed to determine the magnitude and significance of this interaction.

RELATED DRUGS: All nonselective MAOIs including isocarboxazid (*Marplan*) and tranylcypromine (*Parnate*) would be expected to inhibit guanethidine effect. Guanadrel (*Hylorel*) is pharmacologically similar to guanethidine and also may be inhibited by MAOIs.

MANAGEMENT OPTIONS:

➡ **Monitor.** Until more information is available, watch patients receiving guanethidine for hypertension if an MAOI is administered. Watch patients receiving MAOI therapy for a pressor response upon initiation of guanethidine therapy. Assume the effects of nonselective MAOIs to persist for 2 weeks after they are discontinued.

REFERENCES:

1. Day MD, et al. Antagonism of guanethidine and bretylium by various agents. *Lancet.* 1962;2:1282.
2. Gulati OD, et al. Antagonism of adrenergic neuron blockade in hypertensive subjects. *Clin Pharmacol Ther.* 1966;7:510.
3. Goldberg LI. Monoamine oxidase inhibitors: adverse reactions and possible mechanisms. *JAMA.* 1964;190:456.
4. Esbenshade JH Jr, et al. A long-term evaluation of pargyline hydrochloride in hypertension. *Am J Med Sci.* 1966;251:119.

Guanethidine (*Ismelin*)

Phenylephrine (eg, *Neo-Synephrine*)

SUMMARY: Guanethidine enhances the pupillary response to phenylephrine; other phenylephrine effects also might be enhanced.

RISK FACTORS: No specific risk factors are known.

MECHANISM: Phenylephrine, like norepinephrine, is a direct-acting sympathomimetic and is probably more active in patients receiving guanethidine because of the increased sensitivity of the receptor.

CLINICAL EVALUATION: A marked increase in the pupillary response to phenylephrine eyedrops has been noted following guanethidine eyedrops[1,2] and long-term oral guanethidine therapy.[3] It appears likely that the cardiovascular response to systemic phenylephrine would be similarly enhanced by guanethidine, but clinical studies are not available to support this possibility.

RELATED DRUGS: Guanadrel[†] is pharmacologically similar to guanethidine and also may interact with phenylephrine.

MANAGEMENT OPTIONS:

➡ **Monitor.** Monitor for excessive phenylephrine response in patients receiving guanethidine; adjust phenylephrine dose as needed.

REFERENCES:

1. Jablonski J. Guanethidine (*Ismelin*) as an adjuvant in pharmacological mydriasis. *Ophthalmologica.* 1974;168(1):27-38.
2. Sneddon JM, et al. The interactions of local guanethidine and sympathomimetic amines in the human eye. *Arch Ophthalmol.* 1969;81(5):622-627.
3. Cooper B. Neo-Synephrine (10%) eye drops. *Med J Aust.* 1968;55(2):240.

† Not available in the United States.

Guanethidine[†]

Thiothixene (eg, *Navane*)

SUMMARY: Thiothixene appeared to substantially inhibit the antihypertensive response to guanethidine in 1 patient; other neuroleptics may have a similar effect.

RISK FACTORS: No specific risk factors are known.

MECHANISM: Not established. Thiothixene might inhibit the uptake of guanethidine into sites of action in a manner similar to that of phenothiazines and tricyclic antidepressants.

CLINICAL EVALUATION: In a hypertensive patient stabilized on guanethidine, thiothixene 60 mg/day was associated with a mean blood pressure increase of 30 mm Hg.[1] Study in additional patients is needed to assess the clinical significance of this interaction.

RELATED DRUGS: The effect of another thioxanthine, chlorprothixene,[†] on guanethidine is not established, but it may interact in a similar way. Guanadrel[†] is pharmacologically similar to guanethidine and also may be inhibited by thiothixene.

MANAGEMENT OPTIONS:

➡ **Monitor.** Although evidence for an interaction is insufficient at present, closely monitor patients taking guanethidine therapy for a decreased antihypertensive response if thioxanthines also are prescribed.

REFERENCES:

1. Janowsky DS, et al. Antagonism of guanethidine by chlorpromazine. *Am J Psychiatry*. 1973;130(7):808-812.

† Not available in the United States.

Guanfacine (eg, *Intuniv*)

Ketoconazole (eg, *Nizoral*)

SUMMARY: Ketoconazole administration increases the plasma concentration of guanfacine; increased adverse reactions, including hypotension, bradycardia, and sedation, are likely in some patients.

RISK FACTORS: No specific risk factors are known.

MECHANISM: Ketoconazole inhibits the metabolism of guanfacine via the enzyme CYP3A4.

CLINICAL EVALUATION: While specific data are limited, the manufacturer of guanfacine notes that the coadministration of ketoconazole increased the mean area under the plasma concentration-time curve of guanfacine by approximately 3-fold.[1] Pending further data, observe patients receiving guanfacine and ketoconazole for increased guanfacine adverse reactions.

RELATED DRUGS: Fluconazole (eg, *Diflucan*), itraconazole (eg, *Sporanox*), posaconazole (*Noxafil*), and voriconazole (*Vfend*) also inhibit the activity of CYP3A4 and are expected to increase the plasma concentrations of guanfacine.

MANAGEMENT OPTIONS:

➥ *Monitor.* Carefully monitor patients taking guanfacine for changes in response if ketoconazole is initiated or discontinued.

REFERENCES:

1. *Intuniv* [package insert]. Wayne, PA: Shire US Inc; 2009.

Halofenate 4

Propranolol (eg, *Inderal*)

SUMMARY: Limited data suggest that halofenate may reduce propranolol concentrations.

RISK FACTORS: No specific risk factors are known.

MECHANISM: Not established.

CLINICAL EVALUATION: In a crossover study of 4 heathy subjects, halofenate 1 g/day for 21 days markedly decreased steady-state plasma propranolol concentrations as compared with placebo.[1] In addition to the reduced propranolol plasma concentrations, there was a corresponding decrease in beta-blocking activity as measured by the heart rate response to isoproterenol (*Isuprel*).

RELATED DRUGS: No information is available.

MANAGEMENT OPTIONS: No specific action is required, but be alert for evidence of the interaction.

REFERENCES:
1. Huffman DH, et al. The interaction between halofenate and propranolol. *Clin Pharmacol Ther*. 1976;19:807.

Halofenate

Tolbutamide (eg, *Orinase*)

SUMMARY: Halofenate appears to increase the serum concentrations of tolbutamide and reduce blood glucose concentrations.

RISK FACTORS: No specific risk factors are known.

MECHANISM: Unknown. Some have proposed that halofenate displaces sulfonylureas from plasma protein binding; however, this would not account for chronic increases in the serum concentrations or hypoglycemic activity of sulfonylureas.

CLINICAL EVALUATION: Six of 9 diabetic patients receiving tolbutamide required a reduction in antidiabetic drug dosage when halofenate was added.[1] Halofenate increased tolbutamide serum concentrations and decreased serum glucose in 12 healthy subjects.[1] Others have noted a similar enhancement of chlorpropamide (eg, *Diabinese*) response with halofenate.[2] The enhanced hypoglycemic response appears to take several weeks to fully develop.[1]

RELATED DRUGS: Chlorpropamide interacts similarly.

MANAGEMENT OPTIONS:

➥ *Monitor.* Concomitant use of halofenate and oral hypoglycemics need not be avoided; however, alert patients to the need for blood glucose monitoring and the possible necessity of altering dosages of hypoglycemic agents when halofenate is taken concurrently.

REFERENCES:
1. Jain AK, et al. Potentiation of hypoglycemic effect of sulfonylureas by halofenate. *N Engl J Med*. 1975;293:1283.
2. Kudzma DJ, et al. Potentiation of hypoglycemic effect of chlorpropamide and phenformin by halofenate. *Diabetes*. 1977;26:291.

Haloperidol (eg, *Haldol*)

Imipramine (eg, *Tofranil*)

SUMMARY: Haloperidol may inhibit the metabolism of some tricyclic antidepressants (TCAs), but reports of adverse effects are lacking.

RISK FACTORS: No specific risk factors are known.

MECHANISM: Unknown. Haloperidol may inhibit the metabolism of some TCAs.

CLINICAL EVALUATION: In 2 schizophrenic patients, haloperidol 12 to 20 mg/day resulted in a decrease in total urinary radioactivity after oral administration of ^{14}C-imipramine.[1] In another study,[2] the metabolism of nortriptyline (*Pamelor*) appeared to be inhibited in a patient receiving haloperidol 16 mg/day. However, the clinical importance of these effects is not established.

RELATED DRUGS: Several combinations of phenothiazines and TCAs, including haloperidol and nortriptyline, have been shown to inhibit each other's hepatic metabolism.

MANAGEMENT OPTIONS: No specific action is required, but be alert for evidence of the interaction.

REFERENCES:

1. Gram LF, et al. Drug interaction: inhibitory effect of neuroleptics on metabolism of tricyclic antidepressants in man. *BMJ.* 1972;1:463.
2. Gram LF, et al. Influence of neuroleptics and benzodiazepines on metabolism of tricyclic antidepressants in man. *Am J Psychiatry.* 1974;131:863.

Haloperidol (eg, *Haldol*)

Indomethacin (eg, *Indocin*)

SUMMARY: A preliminary study suggested that the combination of indomethacin and haloperidol resulted in a high incidence of adverse effects such as drowsiness, tiredness, and confusion compared with indomethacin alone, but the role of drug interaction in the reactions was not established.

RISK FACTORS: No specific risk factors are known.

MECHANISM: Not established.

CLINICAL EVALUATION: In 40 patients with osteoarthritis, a study was planned to give indomethacin 25 mg 3 times/day for 42 days with haloperidol 5 mg/day or placebo. The latter were to be given for the last 28 days in a randomized, crossover manner.[1] The study was terminated; however, when 13 of the first 20 patients failed to complete the trial, primarily because patients receiving the indomethacin-haloperidol combination experienced adverse effects such as drowsiness, tiredness, and confusion. The absence of similar adverse reactions in the indomethacin-placebo group suggests that the adverse effects resulted from the combined use of indomethacin and haloperidol. Nevertheless, one cannot rule out the possibility that the effects were caused only by haloperidol.

RELATED DRUGS: It is unknown whether other combinations of nonsteroidal anti-inflammatory drugs (NSAIDs) and neuroleptics would result in a higher incidence of adverse effects over either agent alone. Since indomethacin alone has a relatively high incidence of adverse CNS effects compared with most other NSAIDs, it may be that NSAIDs other than indomethacin would be less likely to produce such effects when combined with haloperidol.

MANAGEMENT OPTIONS:

➥ *Monitor.* Monistor patients receiving indomethacin and haloperidol for adverse effects such as drowsiness and confusion. If such effects are observed, consider the use of an NSAID other than indomethacin or a neuroleptic other than haloperidol.

REFERENCES:

1. Bird HA, et al. Drowsiness due to haloperidol/indomethacin in combination. *Lancet.* 1983;1:830.

Haloperidol (eg, *Haldol*)

Lithium (eg, *Eskalith*)

SUMMARY: A number of patients have developed severe neurotoxic extrapyramidal symptoms while receiving lithium and haloperidol, but many other patients have received the combination without such adverse effects.

RISK FACTORS:

➥ *Other Drugs.* Concurrent use of anticholinergic antiparkinsonian drugs can increase the risk.

➥ *Concurrent Diseases.* Presence of acute mania; pre-existing brain damage; the presence of other physiologic disturbances such as infection, fever, or dehydration; or a history of extrapyramidal symptoms with neuroleptic therapy alone can increase the risk of an interaction occurring.

➥ *Dosage Regimen.* Large doses of one or both drugs and failure to discontinue drugs when adverse effects occur can increase the risk of an interaction.

MECHANISM: Unknown. It has been proposed that haloperidol and lithium could have a combined inhibitory effect on striatal adenylate cyclase.[1]

CLINICAL EVALUATION: Four patients with mania developed encephalopathy (eg, lethargy, fever, confusion, extrapyramidal symptoms) following the combined use of lithium carbonate and high doses of haloperidol.[2] Two of the patients developed permanent brain damage and the other two developed persistent dyskinesias. A similar case of severe rigidity, fever, mutism, and an irreversible dyskinesia was associated with the combined use of lithium and haloperidol.[3] Extrapyramidal symptoms also were noted in 10 other patients who received combined therapy with haloperidol (maximum dose: 30 mg/day) and lithium (serum lithium is always less than 1.2 mmol/L).[4] Another report described 7 patients who developed an unexpected degree of extrapyramidal symptoms while receiving lithium and haloperidol.[5] Several other reports have described examples of the lithium-haloperidol interaction.[6-10] Most of these reported cases were relatively isolated events that occurred within a much larger group of lithium-haloperidoltreated patients who did not manifest such effects. Further, several epidemiological studies have failed to detect evidence supporting an adverse lithium-haloperidol interaction.[11-14] However, negative epidemiological evidence does not disprove the occurrence of this interaction in specific, predisposed persons.

RELATED DRUGS: No information available.

MANAGEMENT OPTIONS:

➡ **Circumvent/Minimize.** It has been recommended that neuroleptics such as haloperidol be used alone for initial control of acute mania symptoms and that lithium be added as the neuroleptic dosage is reduced.[4,15] Avoid excessive doses of either agent.

➡ **Monitor.** If haloperidol and lithium are used concomitantly, monitor carefully for signs of neurotoxicity, particularly in the presence of one or more of the risk factors described above.

REFERENCES:

1. Geisler A, et al. Combined effect of lithium and flupenthixol on striatal adenylate cyclase. *Lancet.* 1977;1:430.

2. Cohen WF, et al. Lithium carbonate, haloperidol and irreversible brain damage. *JAMA.* 1974;230:1283.

3. Spring G, Frankel M. New data on lithium and haloperidol incompatibility. *Am J Psychiatry.* 1981;138:818.

4. Kamlana SH, et al. Lithium: some drug interactions. *Practitioner.* 1980;224:1291.

5. Louden JB, et al. Toxic reactions to lithium and haloperidol. *Lancet.* 1976;2:1088.

6. Strayhorn JM, et al. Severe neurotoxicity despite "therapeutic" serum lithium levels. *Dis Nerv Syst.* 1977;38:107.

7. Fetzer J, et al. Lithium encephalopathy: a clinical, psychiatric, and EEG evaluation. *Am J Psychiatry.* 1981;138:1622.

8. Thomas CJ. Brain damage with lithium/haloperidol. *Br J Psychiatry.* 1979;134:552.

9. Thornton WE, et al. Lithium intoxication: a report of two cases. *Can Psychiatr Assoc J.* 1975;20:281.

10. Thomas C, et al. Lithium/haloperidol combinations and brain damage. *Lancet.* 1982;1:626.

11. Baastrup P, et al. Adverse reactions in treatment with lithium carbonate and haloperidol. *JAMA.* 1976;236:2645.

12. Juhl RP, et al. Concomitant administration of haloperidol and lithium carbonate in acute mania. *Dis Nerv Syst.* 1977;38:675.

13. Carman JS, et al. Lithium combined with neuroleptics in chronic schizophrenic and schizoaffective patients. *J Clin Psychiatry.* 1981;42:124.

14. Biederman J, et al. Combination of lithium carbonate and haloperidol in schizo-affective disorder. *Arch Gen Psychiatry.* 1979;36:327.

15. Tupin JP, et al. Lithium and haloperidol incompatibility reviewed. *Psychiat J Univ Ottawa.* 1978;3:245.

4 **Haloperidol (eg, *Haldol*)**

Methyldopa (eg, *Aldomet*)

SUMMARY: Isolated case reports indicate that the combination of haloperidol and methyldopa may result in dementia; in an uncontrolled study, the combination had a favorable effect on schizophrenia.

RISK FACTORS: No specific risk factors are known.

MECHANISM: Not established. A combined inhibitory effect on dopamine in the central nervous system has been proposed.[2]

CLINICAL EVALUATION: Two patients on chronic methyldopa therapy developed dementia (eg, slowed mentation, disorientation) within 1 week of starting haloperidol therapy.[2] Symptoms cleared within 72 hours when haloperidol was discontinued. A similar case was subsequently reported.[3] The symptoms appear to be due to a drug interaction in these 3 patients, but more information is needed to assess the incidence and severity of this reaction. A favorable therapeutic response to methyldopa plus haloperidol was reported in 10 schizophrenic patients, but the study was uncontrolled.[1]

RELATED DRUGS: No information is available.

MANAGEMENT OPTIONS: No specific action is required, but be alert for evidence of the interaction.

REFERENCES:

1. Chouinard G, et al. Potentiation of haloperidol by alpha-methyldopa in the treatment of schizophrenic patients. *Curr Ther Res*. 1973;15:473.
2. Thornton WE. Dementia induced by methyldopa with haloperidol. *N Engl J Med*. 1976;294:1222.
3. Nadel I, et al. Drug interaction between haloperidol and methyldopa. *Br J Psychiatry*. 1979;135:484.

Haloperidol (eg, *Haldol*)

Olanzapine (*Zyprexa*)

SUMMARY: A patient on combined therapy with haloperidol and olanzapine developed severe parkinsonism, but the clinical importence of this effect is not established.

RISK FACTORS: No specific risk factors are known.

MECHANISM: Not established. It is possible that the small amount of dopamine blockade produced by olanzapine may be additive with that of haloperidol. It is also possible that olanzapine and haloperidol might compete for metabolism via CYP2D6, although there is little clinical evidnece to support such competition.

CLINICAL EVALUATION: A 67–year-old man with bipolar disorder developed increased parkinsonism several days after olanzapine therapy was initiated in the presence of haloperidol 10 mg/day.[1] His symptoms resolved within 3 days after stopping haloperidol in the presence of continued olanzapine therapy. However, the extent to which the reaction resulted from the combined effects of olanzapine and haloperidol is not clear.

RELATED DRUGS: No information is available.

MANAGEMENT OPTIONS: No specific action is required, but be alert for evidence of the interaction.

REFERENCES:

1. Gomberg RF. Interaction between olanzapine and haloperidol. *J Clin Psychopharmacol*. 1999;19;272–73.

Haloperidol (eg, *Haldol*)

Phenindione†

SUMMARY: Haloperidol appeared to inhibit the hypoprothrombinemic response to phenindione in one patient, but a causal relationship was not established.

RISK FACTORS: No specific risk factors are known.

MECHANISM: Not established.

CLINICAL EVALUATION: A single case has been reported in which haloperidol administration was associated with a marked increase in the dosage requirement for phenindione.[1] When the haloperidol was stopped, the anticoagulant requirements returned to the pre-haloperidol levels. More study is needed to assess the clinical significance of this interaction and to determine whether anticoagulants other than phenindione interact with haloperidol.

RELATED DRUGS: No information is available.

MANAGEMENT OPTIONS: No specific action is required, but be alert for evidence of the interaction.

REFERENCES:

1. Oakley DP, et al. Haloperidol and anticoagulant treatment. *Lancet.* 1963;2:1231.

† Not available in the U nited States.

Haloperidol (eg, *Haldol*)

Quinidine (eg, *Quinora*)

SUMMARY: Quinidine administration increases haloperidol concentrations, potentially increasing the risk of haloperidol toxicity.

RISK FACTORS: No specific risk factors are known.

MECHANISM: Unknown. Quinidine may alter the volume of distribution of haloperidol and its reduced metabolite. Further, quinidine may decrease the elimination of reduced haloperidol, indirectly increasing the concentration of haloperidol.

CLINICAL EVALUATION: Single 5 mg doses of haloperidol and its reduced metabolite were administered to 12 healthy subjects alone and 1 hour after 250 mg quinidine bisulfate.[1] Following quinidine administration, the area under the plasma concentration-time curve (AUC) and peak plasma concentration of haloperidol increased approximately twofold. The AUC of the metabolite also was increased following quinidine dosing. The half-life of haloperidol was not altered by quinidine. This interaction is complicated by the metabolic interconversion of haloperidol and its reduced metabolite. The clinical significance of this interaction is unknown, but increased haloperidol concentrations could lead to toxicity including extrapyramidal side effects.

RELATED DRUGS: No information is available.

MANAGEMENT OPTIONS:

➡ *Monitor.* Until further studies are available, patients taking haloperidol should be monitored for extrapyramidal symptoms, sedation, and hypotension if quinidine is co-administered.

REFERENCES:

1. Young D, et al. Effect of quinidine on the interconversion kinetics between haloperidol and reduced haloperidol in humans: implications for the involvement of cytochrome P450IID6. *Eur J Clin Pharmacol.* 1993;44:433.

Haloperidol (eg, *Haldol*)

Rifampin (eg, *Rifadin*)

SUMMARY: Rifampin may reduce haloperidol concentrations.

RISK FACTORS: No specific risk factors are known.

MECHANISM: Rifampin may increase haloperidol metabolism or reduce its bioavailability.

CLINICAL EVALUATION: Haloperidol serum concentrations were compared in patients maintained on haloperidol alone or in combination with isoniazid, rifampin, or ethambutol.[1] Those on haloperidol and rifampin had lower haloperidol serum concentrations and a shorter haloperidol half-life. The significance of these data are limited by the lack of a crossover-study design and the small number of subjects.

RELATED DRUGS: No information is available.

MANAGEMENT OPTIONS: No specific action is required, but be alert for evidence of the interaction.

REFERENCES:

1. Tekeda M, et al. Serum haloperidol levels of schizophrenics receiving treatment for tuberculosis. *Clin Neuropharmacol.* 1986;9:386.

Haloperidol (eg, *Haldol*) 4

Sertraline (*Zoloft*)

SUMMARY: Sertraline may produce a modest increase in haloperidol plasma concentrations, but the clinical importance of this effect is not established.

RISK FACTORS:

➡ **Pharmacogenetics.** If this interaction is due to sertraline-induced inhibition of CYP2D6, patients with a genetic deficiency of CYP2D6 would not be expected to manifest a change in haloperidol plasma concentrations.

MECHANISM: Not established. Sertraline is a weak inhibitor of CYP2D6 and may inhibit the metabolism of haloperidol (a CYP2D6 substrate).

CLINICAL EVALUATION: Sixteen schizophrenic patients with inadequate response to antipsychotics had sertraline 50 mg/day for 2 weeks added to their stable dosage of haloperidol (2 to 3.5 mg/day).[1] Sertraline was associated with a 28% increase in haloperidol plasma concentrations, but changes in clinical symptoms were not measured. Given the modest increases in haloperidol concentrations, one would not expect many patients to be clinically affected by this interaction. Nonetheless, some patients with insufficient haloperidol concentrations might manifest improvement in schizophrenic symptoms, while those with high preexisting haloperidol concentrations might manifest adverse effects.

RELATED DRUGS: Fluoxetine (*Prozac*) and paroxetine (*Paxil*) are both potent inhibitors of CYP2D6 and can substantially increase CYP2D6 substrates such as haloperidol. Citalopram (*Celexa*), like sertraline, is a weak CYP2D6 inhibitor and would be expected to produce small increases in haloperidol plasma concentrations, while fluvoxamine (*Luvox*) has very little effect on CYP2D6 and would not be expected to affect haloperidol concentrations.

MANAGEMENT OPTIONS: No specific action is required, but be alert for evidence of the interaction.

REFERENCES:

1. Lee MS, et al. Co-administration of sertraline and haloperidol. *Psychiatry Clin Neurosci.* 1998;52(Suppl)S193–98.

4 **Haloperidol (eg, *Haldol*)**

Tacrine (*Cognex*)

SUMMARY: A patient taking haloperidol developed parkinsonian symptoms after starting tacrine, but a causal relationship between the reaction and a drug interaction was not established.

RISK FACTORS: No specific risk factors are known.

MECHANISM: Tacrine is a cholinergic agent, and haloperidol is a dopamine inhibitor. Both effects tend to increase the risk of parkinsonian symptoms, and additive effects theoretically may occur.

CLINICAL EVALUATION: An 87-year-old man receiving haloperidol 5 mg/day for dementia was started on tacrine 10 mg 4 times a day. Within 72 hours he developed severe parkinsonian symptoms (eg, akinesia/bradykinesia, masked facies, shuffling gait, rigidity).[1] His symptoms resolved about 8 hours after both medications were stopped. Because both haloperidol and tacrine can produce parkinsonism, it is proposed that this patient's symptoms resulted from an additive effect of the 2 drugs. Nonetheless, tacrine alone can exacerbate parkinsonism, and the possibility that tacrine alone may have produced parkinsonian symptoms should not be ruled out.

RELATED DRUGS: No information is available.

MANAGEMENT OPTIONS: No specific action is required, but be alert for evidence of the interaction.

REFERENCES:
1. McSwain ML, et al. Severe parkinsonian symptom development on combination treatment with tacrine and haloperidol. *J Clin Psychopharmacol*. 1995;15(4):284.

  Haloperidol (eg, *Haldol*)

Tamoxifen (eg, *Soltamox*)

SUMMARY: Theoretically, haloperidol may reduce the efficacy of tamoxifen in the treatment of breast cancer.

RISK FACTORS: No specific risk factors are known.

MECHANISM: Tamoxifen is metabolized to 2 active metabolites by CYP2D6, the most important of which is endoxifen. By reducing endoxifen formation, CYP2D6 inhibitors such as haloperidol may reduce tamoxifen efficacy.[1-3]

CLINICAL EVALUATION: A study in patients with breast cancer found substantial reductions in endoxifen plasma concentrations in patients taking potent CYP2D6 inhibitors, such as fluoxetine and paroxetine.[4] Another tamoxifen study found a nearly 2-fold increase in risk of breast cancer relapse in women with low CYP2D6 activity, either due to CYP2D6-inhibiting drugs or genetic deficiency.[5] Taken together, these and other results strongly suggest that CYP2D6 inhibitors reduce the efficacy of tamoxifen in treatment of breast cancer. Haloperidol is a CYP2D6 inhibitor and may inhibit the anticancer effects of tamoxifen.

RELATED DRUGS: Thioridazine, chlorpromazine, and perphenazine are also CYP2D6 inhibitors, and may reduce the efficacy of tamoxifen.

MANAGEMENT OPTIONS:

➡ *Consider Alternative.* If possible, use an alternative to chlorpromazine, haloperidol, perphenazine, or thioridazine.

➡ *Monitor.* If a CYP2D6 inhibitor such as haloperidol is used with tamoxifen, cancer recurrence may be an indication that tamoxifen efficacy has been reduced. If this happens, consider discontinuing the CYP2D6 inhibitor.

REFERENCES:

1. Dezentjé VO, et al. Clinical implications of CYP2D6 genotyping in tamoxifen treatment for breast cancer. *Clin Cancer Res.* 2009;15(1):15-21.
2. Tan SH, et al. Pharmacogenetics in breast cancer therapy. *Clin Cancer Res.* 2008;14(24):8027-8041.
3. Newman WG, et al. Impaired tamoxifen metabolism reduces survival in familial breast cancer patients. *Clin Cancer Res.* 2008;14(18):5913-5918.
4. Borges S, et al. Quantitative effect of CYP2D6 genotype and inhibitors on tamoxifen metabolism: implication for optimization of breast cancer treatment. *Clin Pharmacol Ther.* 2006;80(1):61-74.
5. Goetz MP, et al. The impact of cytochrome P450 2D6 metabolism in women receiving adjuvant tamoxifen. *Breast Cancer Res Treat.* 2007;101(1):113-121.

Halothane 4

Phenytoin (eg, *Dilantin*)

SUMMARY: Halothane was associated with phenytoin toxicity in 1 patient.

RISK FACTORS: No specific risk factors are known.

MECHANISM: Halothane may produce hepatotoxicity, thus impairing the hepatic metabolism of phenytoin.

CLINICAL EVALUATION: One patient developed symptoms of phenytoin toxicity following exposure to halothane.[1] The patient had been stabilized on phenytoin, and it appeared that the halothane-induced hepatic dysfunction was responsible for the elevated phenytoin plasma concentrations.

RELATED DRUGS: No information is available.

MANAGEMENT OPTIONS: No specific action is required, but be alert for evidence of the interaction.

REFERENCES:

1. Karlin JM, et al. Acute diphenylhydantoin intoxication following halothane anesthesia. *J Pediatr.* 1970;76(6):941-944.

Halothane 4

Rifampin (eg, *Rifadin*)

SUMMARY: The combined use of rifampin and halothane may increase the risk of hepatotoxicity.

RISK FACTORS: No specific risk factors are known.

MECHANISM: Not established.

CLINICAL EVALUATION: A single case report describes a patient who was started on rifampin and isoniazid therapy immediately following halothane anesthesia and subsequently developed nearly fatal hepatotoxicity.[1] The authors assumed that this reaction was due to the combined hepatotoxic effects of halothane and rifampin, but more study is needed to establish causation. This case could be the result of the hepatotoxicity of either drug alone.

RELATED DRUGS: No information is available.

MANAGEMENT OPTIONS: No specific action is required, but be alert for evidence of the interaction.

REFERENCES:
1. Most JA, et al. A nearly fatal hepatotoxic reaction to rifampin after halothane anesthesia. *Am J Surg.* 1974;127(5):593-595.

Heparin

Streptokinase[†]

SUMMARY: Post–myocardial infarction patients treated with streptokinase appear to require larger heparin doses than patients not treated with streptokinase.

RISK FACTORS: No specific risk factors are known.

MECHANISM: Streptokinase may inhibit heparin activity by increasing thrombin activity.

CLINICAL EVALUATION: Patients diagnosed with acute myocardial infarctions who were treated with heparin were reviewed retrospectively.[1] Patients were placed into 2 groups: those who received streptokinase (0.75 or 1.5 million units) and those who did not. The amount of heparin required to produce an activated partial thromboplastin time (aPTT) of more than 65 seconds was significantly higher (20.5%) in the group receiving streptokinase. Five days of heparin therapy were required to reach the goal aPTT in the streptokinase group compared with 3 days in the group not receiving streptokinase. The aPTTs also tended to be lower (17%) in the streptokinase group despite the higher doses of streptokinase administered. This suggests that streptokinase-induced thrombolysis increases heparin requirements.

RELATED DRUGS: The effect of other thrombolytic agents on heparin activity is not established.

MANAGEMENT OPTIONS: No specific action is required, but be alert for evidence of the interaction.

REFERENCES:
1. Zahger D, et al. Partial resistance to anticoagulation after streptokinase treatment for acute myocardial infarction. *Am J Cardiol.* 1990;66(1):28-30.

† Not available in the United States.

Heparin

Warfarin (eg, *Coumadin*)

SUMMARY: Warfarin may prolong the activated partial thromboplastin time (aPTT) in patients receiving heparin, and heparin may prolong the prothrombin time (PT) in patients receiving warfarin. Consider these when assessing the anticoagulant effect of each agent.

RISK FACTORS: No specific risk factors are known.

MECHANISM: Additive anticoagulant effects produce this interaction.

CLINICAL EVALUATION: In 18 patients with deep vein thrombosis given heparin (5,000 units bolus, followed by a constant infusion), the addition of warfarin substantially lowered the dose of heparin required to maintain the same aPTT response.[1] It is not known, however, whether prolongation of the aPTT with heparin plus warfarin is therapeutically equivalent to that achieved by using heparin alone. Warfarin alone also has been shown to prolong the aPTT.[2] Bolus intravenous (IV) administration of heparin prolongs the PT considerably, whereas subcutaneous administration of the same dose (eg, 10,000 units) results in only a small prolongation (1 or 2 seconds).[3] Consider this effect when drawing blood samples to assess the hypoprothrombinemic response to oral anticoagulants.

RELATED DRUGS: All oral anticoagulants probably interact with heparin in a similar way.

MANAGEMENT OPTIONS:

➡ **Monitor.** In patients receiving both heparin and an oral anticoagulant, monitor for oral anticoagulant–induced increases in aPTT. To minimize the interference of heparin with PT determinations, do not draw blood samples for PTs within about 5 or 6 hours of administration of a bolus of IV heparin.

REFERENCES:

1. Mungall D, et al. Bayesian forecasting of APTT response to continuously infused heparin with and without warfarin administration. *J Clin Pharmacol.* 1989;29(11):1043-1047.
2. Hauser VM, et al. Effect of warfarin on the activated partial thromboplastin time. *Drug Intell Clin Pharm.* 1986;20(12):964-967.
3. Moser KM, et al. Effect of heparin on the one-stage prothrombin time. Source of artifactual "resistance" to prothrombinopenic therapy. *Ann Intern Med.* 1967;66(6):1207-1213.

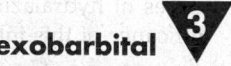

Hexobarbital

Rifampin (eg, *Rifadin*)

SUMMARY: Hexobarbital serum concentrations are reduced by the administration of rifampin.

RISK FACTORS: No specific risk factors are known.

MECHANISM: Rifampin stimulates the hepatic metabolism of hexobarbital enantiomers.

CLINICAL EVALUATION: The half-life of hexobarbital is considerably shortened by rifampin in both healthy subjects[1-3] and patients with hepatic disease.[2] Rifampin markedly increases the oral clearance of hexobarbital.[4]

RELATED DRUGS: The effect of rifampin administration on the disposition of other barbiturates has not been established, but it is possible that they are similarly affected by rifampin.

MANAGEMENT OPTIONS:

➡ **Monitor.** Watch for reduced barbiturate effect. It does not seem necessary to avoid concomitant use of rifampin and barbiturates. However, when patients fail to respond to barbiturates, consider rifampin a potential cause if it is being taken concurrently.

REFERENCES:

1. Zilly W, et al. Induction of drug metabolism in man after rifampicin treatment measured by increased hexobarbital and tolbutamide clearance. *Eur J Clin Pharmacol.* 1975;9:219-227.
2. Miguet JP, et al. Induction of hepatic microsomal enzymes after brief administration of rifampicin in man. *Gastroenterology.* 1977;72(5 pt 1):924-926.

3. Breimer DD, et al. Influence of rifampicin on drug metabolism: differences between hexobarbital and antipyrine. *Clin Pharmacol Ther*. 1977;21:470-481.

4. Zilly W, et al. Stimulation of drug metabolism by rifampicin in patients with cirrhosis or cholestasis measured by increased hexobarbital and tolbutamide clearance. *Eur J Clin Pharmacol*. 1977;11:287-293.

5. Smith DA, et al. Age-dependent stereoselective increase in the oral clearance of hexobarbitone isomers caused by rifampicin. *Br J Clin Pharmacol*. 1991;32:735-739.

Hydralazine (eg, *Apresoline*)

Indomethacin (eg, *Indocin*)

SUMMARY: Indomethacin has been shown to inhibit the antihypertensive response to hydralazine in healthy subjects.

RISK FACTORS: No specific risk factors are known.

MECHANISM: Not established. Indomethacin-induced inhibition of prostaglandins may be involved.

CLINICAL EVALUATION: Nine healthy subjects were given 2 IV doses of hydralazine 0.15 mg/kg, with and without oral indomethacin (eg, *Indocin*) pretreatment 200 mg.[1] Pretreatment with indomethacin abolished the decrease in mean arterial pressure seen after the first dose of hydralazine plus placebo and more than halved the blood pressure decrease after the second hydralazine dose. Although a previous study failed to find an effect of indomethacin on the antihypertensive response to hydralazine, this may have been because smaller doses of both drugs were used in the earlier study.[2] Studies of hypertensive patients on multiple oral doses of hydralazine and indomethacin will be needed to assess the clinical significance of this interaction.

RELATED DRUGS: Nonsteroidal anti-inflammatory drugs (NSAIDs) other than indomethacin would be expected to produce a similar effect.

MANAGEMENT OPTIONS:

➡ *Monitor.* Monitor for a reduced antihypertensive response when indomethacin or other NSAIDs are given with hydralazine.

REFERENCES:

1. Cinquegrani MP, et al. Indomethacin attenuates the hypotensive action of hydralazine. *Clin Pharmacol Ther*. 1986;39:564-570.

2. Jackson SH, et al. Indomethacin does not attenuate the effects of hydralazine in normal subjects. *Eur J Clin Pharmacol*. 1983;25:303-305.

Hydralazine (eg, *Apresoline*)

Propranolol (eg, *Inderal*)

SUMMARY: Hydralazine can substantially increase propranolol bioavailability under fasting conditions, but the clinical importance of this effect is not established.

RISK FACTORS:

➡ *Dosage Regimen.* Coadministration in the fasting state can increase the risk.

MECHANISM: Hydralazine reduces the first-pass metabolism of propranolol by reducing hepatic metabolism or increasing hepatic blood flow.

CLINICAL EVALUATION: The bioavailability of propranolol and metoprolol (eg, *Lopressor*) are increased up to 75% when administered to fasting subjects with 100 mg oral hydralazine.[1] Propranolol bioavailability was increased by approximately 75%. Hydralazine may not affect propranolol bioavailability under nonfasting conditions, possibly because the food already has increased propranolol bioavailability.[2] Sustained-release propranolol formulations are not likely to be affected by hydralazine.[3,4]

RELATED DRUGS: Metoprolol interacts similarly. Hydralazine did not affect the bioavailability of nadolol (eg, *Corgard*) or acebutolol (eg, *Sectral*).[5]

MANAGEMENT OPTIONS: No specific action is required, but be alert for evidence of the interaction.

REFERENCES:

1. Jack DB, et al. The effect of hydralazine on the pharmacokinetics of three different beta adrenoceptor antagonists: metoprolol, nadolol, and acebutolol. *Biopharm Drug Dispos.* 1982;3:47-54.

2. Schafer-Korting M, et al. Pharmacokinetics of bendroflumethiazide alone and in combination with propranolol and hydralazine. *Eur J Clin Pharmacol.* 1982;21:315-323.

3. Byrne AJ, et al. Stable oral availability of sustained release propranolol when coadministered with hydralazine or food: evidence implicating substrate delivery rate as a determinant of presystemic drug interactions. *Br J Clin Pharmacol.* 1984;17:45S-50S.

4. McLean AJ, et al. The effect of hydralazine on the metabolism of oral propranolol during first-pass hepatic clearance. *Clin Pharmacol Ther.* 1986;43:209.

5. McLean AJ, et al. Interaction between oral propranolol and hydralazine. *Clin Pharmacol Ther.* 1980;27:726-732.

Hydrocortisone (eg, *Cortef*) | 4

Theophylline (eg, *Theolair*)

SUMMARY: Although hydrocortisone and other systemic corticosteroids have been associated with increased theophylline serum concentrations, the bulk of the evidence suggests that corticosteroids have minimal effects on theophylline in most patients.

RISK FACTORS: No specific risk factors are known.

MECHANISM: Not established.

CLINICAL EVALUATION: In 3 patients with status asthmaticus receiving theophylline, IV hydrocortisone (500 mg, followed in 6 hours by three 200 mg doses, 2 hours apart) was associated with approximately a doubling of the serum theophylline concentrations.[1] A fourth patient with status asthmaticus who was given saline instead of the hydrocortisone had no change in serum theophylline concentration. Opposite results were obtained in a study of 7 healthy subjects receiving sustained-release theophylline who were randomly given the following IV treatments (twice, 4 hours apart): methylprednisolone (eg, *Medrol*) 1.6 mg/kg; hydrocortisone (eg, *Cortef*) 8 mg/kg; saline.[2] The mean theophylline clearance was more than 21% in the presence of the corticosteroids compared with saline. In 9 outpatients with chronic airflow obstruction, theophylline pharmacokinetics (after a single IV dose of aminophylline 5.6 mg/kg) were not affected by oral prednisolone (eg, *Prelone*) 20 mg/day for 3 weeks.[3] In another study, only 1 of 3 healthy subjects developed an increase in theophylline clearance (after a single IV dose of aminophylline 6 mg/kg) with methylprednisolone pretreatment (1 mg/kg oral, 1 and 8 hours before aminophylline).[4] Considering all of the data, it appears that corticosteroids have minimal effects on theophylline pharmacokinetics in most patients. Nonetheless, it is possible that corticosteroids affect theophylline elimination under certain circumstances, such as in patients with severe airway obstruction or other acute disorders.

The pattern of theophylline metabolites in the plasma was studied in 9 premature infants, 4 of whom had been exposed to betamethasone (*Celestone*) prenatally.[5] Those infants exposed to betamethasone demonstrated demethylation and oxidation of theophylline in the first week of life, suggesting that the betamethasone activated hepatic microsomal enzymes. The clinical importance of this effect is not clear.

RELATED DRUGS: Prednisolone (eg, *Prelone*), methylprednisolone (eg, *Medrol*), and betamethasone (*Celestone*) interact similarly with theophylline.

MANAGEMENT OPTIONS: No specific action is required, but be alert for evidence of the interaction.

REFERENCES:

1. Buchanan N, et al. Asthma–a possible interaction between hydrocortisone and theophylline. *S Afr Med J.* 1979;56:1147-1148.
2. Leavengood DC, et al. The effect of corticosteroids on theophylline metabolism. *Ann Allergy.* 1983;50:249-251.
3. Fergusson RJ, et al. Effect of prednisolone on theophylline pharmacokinetics in patients with chronic airflow obstruction. *Thorax.* 1987;42:195-198.
4. Squire EN, et al. Corticosteroids and theophylline clearance. *N Engl Reg Allergy Proc.* 1987;8:113-115.
5. Jager-Roman E, et al. Increased theophylline metabolism in premature infants after prenatal betamethasone administration. *Dev Pharmacol Ther.* 1982;5:127-135.

Hydroxychloroquine (eg, *Plaquenil*)

Methotrexate (eg, *Trexall*)

SUMMARY: Coadministration of hydroxychloroquine increases the plasma concentration of methotrexate; both an increase in methotrexate efficacy and toxicity may occur.

RISK FACTORS: No specific risk factors are known.

MECHANISM: Unknown. Because methotrexate primarily is eliminated via the kidneys, hydroxychloroquine may reduce the renal elimination of methotrexate.

CLINICAL EVALUATION: Ten healthy subjects received a single oral dose of methotrexate 15 mg alone and together with an oral dose of hydroxychloroquine 200 mg.[1] The mean area under the plasma concentration-time curve (AUC) of methotrexate was increased 52% during concurrent hydroxychloroquine administration, while the mean peak methotrexate concentration was reduced 17%. The effects of multiple doses of both drugs have not been studied. The increase in methotrexate concentration following coadministration of hydroxychloroquine partially may explain the effectiveness of this combination over methotrexate alone in the treatment of rheumatoid arthritis. However, carefully monitor patients receiving this combination for evidence of methotrexate toxicity, such as reduced renal function.

RELATED DRUGS: Chloroquine (eg, *Aralen*) has been demonstrated to reduce the peak concentration and total AUC of methotrexate. It is unclear why chloroquine and hydroxychloroquine produce different effects on the AUC of methotrexate.

MANAGEMENT OPTIONS:

➡ *Monitor.* Monitor patients being treated with methotrexate and hydroxychloroquine for evidence of methotrexate toxicity, including reduced renal function.

REFERENCES:

1. Carmichael SJ, et al. Combination therapy with methotrexate and hydroxychloroquine for rheumatoid arthritis increases exposure to methotrexate. *J Rheumatol.* 2002;29:2077-2083.

Hydroxychloroquine (eg, *Plaquenil*)

Metoprolol (eg, *Lopressor*)

SUMMARY: Hydroxychloroquine administration increases metoprolol plasma concentrations; some increase in beta blockade may occur.

RISK FACTORS:

➡ *Pharmacogenetics.* Extensive metabolizers of CYP2D6.

MECHANISM: Hydroxychloroquine appears to increase the bioavailability of metoprolol by inhibiting the CYP2D6 metabolism of metoprolol.

CLINICAL EVALUATION: Seven healthy subjects (6 homozygous and 1 heterozygous extensive CYP2D6 metabolizers) were administered hydroxychloroquine 400 mg or placebo twice daily for 8 days.[1] On day 9, subjects ingested a single dose of metoprolol 100 mg. The mean area under the concentration-time curve of metoprolol was increased 65% following hydroxychloroquine pretreatment. Metoprolol half-life did not change following hydroxychloroquine dosing. It is possible that some patients may experience an increase in beta blockade during metoprolol and hydroxychloroquine coadministration. It is of interest that dextromethorphan (commonly considered a marker drug for CYP2D6) metabolism was not altered by hydroxychloroquine administration in this study. Further study is needed to elucidate the reason for this apparent lack of effect.

RELATED DRUGS: Propranolol (eg, *Inderal*) and timolol (eg, *Blocadren*) are metabolized by CYP2D6 and are expected to interact in a similar manner with hydroxychloroquine. Beta-blockers eliminated by the kidney, such as atenolol (eg, *Tenormin*), nadolol (eg, *Corgard*), and sotalol (eg, *Betapace*), are unlikely to be affected by hydroxychloroquine.

MANAGEMENT OPTIONS:

➡ *Monitor.* Observe patients taking metoprolol for increased beta blockade (eg, bradycardia, hypotension) when hydroxychloroquine is coadministered.

REFERENCES:

1. Somer M, et al. Influence of hydroxychloroquine on the bioavailability of oral metoprolol. *Br J Clin Pharmacol.* 2000;49:549-554.

Ibuprofen (eg, *Motrin*)

Fluconazole (eg, *Diflucan*)

SUMMARY: Fluconazole administration increases the plasma concentration of ibuprofen; ibuprofen adverse reactions may increase.

RISK FACTORS: No specific risk factors are known.

MECHANISM: Fluconazole inhibits CYP2C9, the enzyme primarily responsible for the metabolism of the more active enantiomer of ibuprofen (S-ibuprofen).

CLINICAL EVALUATION: Twelve healthy subjects received a single dose of ibuprofen 400 mg alone and 1 hour after the last of 2 days of fluconazole dosing.[1] The fluconazole was dosed as 400 mg on day 1 and 200 mg on day 2. The mean area under the plasma concentration-time curve of ibuprofen was increased 83% following the 2 days of fluconazole pretreatment. The half-life of ibuprofen was prolonged 34% after fluconazole. Some increase in ibuprofen adverse reactions might occur if fluconazole is coadministered.

RELATED DRUGS: Most other NSAIDs are substrates for CYP2C9, including ketoprofen, naproxen (eg, *Aleve*), and diclofenac (eg, *Voltaren*), and are expected to be affected by fluconazole in a similar manner. Voriconazole (*Vfend*) also inhibits the activity of CYP2C9 and is known to inhibit the metabolism of ibuprofen and probably other NSAIDs.

MANAGEMENT OPTIONS:

➡ ***Consider Alternative.*** Ketoconazole (eg, *Nizoral*), itraconazole (eg, *Sporanox*), and terbinafine (*Lamisil*) could be considered as alternative antifungal agents because they do not affect CYP2C9 activity.

➡ ***Monitor.*** Observe patients taking NSAIDs, particularly chronic, high-dose regimens, for evidence of NSAID toxicity during coadministration of fluconazole.

REFERENCES:
    1. Hynninen VV, et al. Effects of the antifungals voriconazole and fluconazole on the pharmacokinetics of S-(+)- and R-(-)-Ibuprofen. *Antimicrob Agents Chemother*. 2006;50:1967-1972.

Ibuprofen (eg, *Motrin*)

Lithium (eg, *Eskalith*)

SUMMARY: Ibuprofen increases lithium serum concentrations and may increase the risk of lithium toxicity; the magnitude of the effect appears to vary considerably from patient to patient.

RISK FACTORS:

➡ ***Effects of Age.*** It has been proposed that older patients may be more susceptible to the interaction,[1] which may explain the difference in the magnitude of the interaction noted in the studies.

MECHANISM: Ibuprofen, like other nonsteroidal anti-inflammatory drugs (NSAIDs), inhibits the renal clearance of lithium.[2] It has been proposed that renal tubular prostaglandins are involved in the excretion of lithium and that the antiprosta-glandin effects of NSAIDs interfere with renal lithium elimination. More study is needed.

CLINICAL EVALUATION: Nine men (mean age, 65 years) with bipolar affective disorder or schizoaffective disorder and steady-state lithium serum concentrations were given ibuprofen 1,800 mg/day for 6 days.[1] The ibuprofen was associated with an aver-age increase in serum lithium concentration of 34%, but there was considerable variation from patient to patient (12% to 67%). Three patients developed increased tremors and 1 became drowsy with the addition of ibuprofen; the symptoms abated after the ibuprofen was stopped. In another study of 11 healthy subjects with steady-state lithium plasma concentrations, ibuprofen 1,600 mg/day for 9 days increased mean minimum lithium concentrations only 15%.[3] Although the frequency of adverse reactions (eg, decreased ability to concentrate, fatigue, light-headedness) was greater during ibuprofen therapy, the symptoms could have been caused by the ibuprofen alone rather than by an interaction with lithium. In another study of 3 patients with steady-state lithium concentrations, ibuprofen 1,200 to 2,400 mg/day for 7 days did not consistently increase serum lithium con-centrations. Some patients are likely to develop sufficient increases in lithium plasma concentrations resulting in clinical evidence of toxicity.

RELATED DRUGS: Most NSAIDs increase lithium serum concentrations, but sulindac (eg, *Clinoril*) and aspirin appear to have minimal effects.

MANAGEMENT OPTIONS:

➡ *Consider Alternative.* If appropriate, consider using an anti-inflammatory agent that is less likely to affect lithium, such as sulindac or aspirin.

➡ *Circumvent/Minimize.* Advise patients receiving lithium to avoid ibuprofen-containing products unless approved by the prescriber.

➡ *Monitor.* If ibuprofen therapy is initiated, monitor for lithium toxicity (eg, anorexia, coarse tremor, confusion, diarrhea, lethargy, nausea, slurred speech, vertigo, vom-iting; in severe cases, cardiovascular collapse, coma, seizures, stupor) and elevated serum lithium concentrations. In patients stabilized on lithium and an NSAID, discontinuation of the NSAID may result in inadequate serum lithium concentra-tions.

REFERENCES:

1. Ragheb M. Ibuprofen can increase serum lithium level in lithium-treated patients. *J Clin Psychiatry.* 1987;48:161-163.

2. Ragheb M, et al. Interaction of indomethacin and ibuprofen with lithium in manic patients under a steady-state lithium level. *J Clin Psychiatry.* 1980;41:397-398.

3. Kristoff CA, et al. Effect of ibuprofen on lithium plasma and red blood cell concentrations. *Clin Pharm.* 1986;5:51-55.

Ibuprofen (eg, *Motrin*)

Methotrexate (eg, *Rheumatrex*)

SUMMARY: Ibuprofen has been reported to increase the serum concentrations of methotrexate, but this has not been a consistent finding. It is not known how often this would result in adverse reactions.

RISK FACTORS: No specific risk factors are known.

MECHANISM: Some nonsteroidal anti-inflammatory drugs (NSAIDs) appear to reduce the renal clearance or renal tubular secretion of methotrexate, but the effect of ibuprofen on methotrexate is not established.

CLINICAL EVALUATION: Seven patients with rheumatoid arthritis were given methotrexate and ibuprofen 40 mg/kg/day.[1] The renal clearance of methotrexate was reduced approximately 50% and the area under the methotrexate concentration-time curve doubled compared with methotrexate administered with acetaminophen. Conversely, in a study of 5 patients with rheumatoid arthritis, ibuprofen 800 mg 3 times/day for 7 days had no effect on methotrexate administered intramuscularly (15 mg) or orally (20 mg).[2]

RELATED DRUGS: Several NSAIDs and aspirin have been shown to increase methotrexate plasma concentrations. Acetaminophen (eg, *Tylenol*) has not been shown to affect methotrexate response.

MANAGEMENT OPTIONS:

➡ *Consider Alternative.* Until more information is available, avoid ibuprofen (as well as other NSAIDs) in patients receiving antineoplastic doses of methotrexate.

➡ *Monitor.* If methotrexate and ibuprofen are used concurrently, monitor for signs of methotrexate toxicity, including mucosal ulceration, renal dysfunction, and blood dyscrasias. A reduced methotrexate dosage may be required.

REFERENCES:

1. Tracy TS, et al. The effect of NSAIDs on methotrexate disposition in patients with rheumatoid arthritis. *Clin Pharmacol Ther.* 1990;47:138.
2. Skeith KJ, et al. Lack of significant interaction between low dose methotrexate and ibuprofen or flurbiprofen in patients with arthritis. *J Rheumatol.* 1990;17(8):1008-1010.

Ibuprofen (eg, *Motrin*)

Milnacipran (*Savella*)

SUMMARY: The combined use of nonsteroidal anti-inflammatory drugs (NSAIDs), such as ibuprofen, with serotonin-norepinephrine reuptake inhibitors (SNRIs), such as milnacipran, has been associated with an increased risk of GI bleeding.

RISK FACTORS: No specific risk factors are known.

MECHANISM: SNRIs and selective serotonin reuptake inhibitors (SSRIs) appear to inhibit platelet function by inhibiting the uptake of serotonin by platelets. When this effect is combined with the platelet inhibition and GI toxicity of NSAIDs, an increased risk of GI bleeding may occur.

CLINICAL EVALUATION: This interaction is based largely on epidemiological studies with SNRIs and SSRIs other than milnacipran, and it is not known how often adverse outcomes would be observed. Nonetheless, given the potential severity of the GI bleeding, consider this risk when deciding whether to use this combination.[1]

RELATED DRUGS: Theoretically, milnacipran would also interact with NSAIDs other than ibuprofen, including diclofenac (eg, *Voltaren*), diflunisal, etodolac, fenoprofen (eg, *Nalfon*), flurbiprofen (eg, *Ansaid*), indomethacin (eg, *Indocin*), ketoprofen, ketorolac, meclofenamate, mefenamic acid (*Ponstel*), meloxicam (eg, *Mobic*), nabumetone, oxaprozin (eg, *Daypro*), piroxicam (eg, *Feldene*), sulindac (eg, *Clinoril*), and tolmetin.

MANAGEMENT OPTIONS:

➡ *Consider Alternative.* If possible, use an alternative to one of the drugs.

➡ *Monitor.* If the combination is used, monitor for evidence of GI bleeding.

REFERENCES:

1. *Savella* [package insert]. St. Louis, MO: Forest Pharmaceuticals; 2010.

Ibuprofen (eg, *Motrin*)

Sucralfate (eg, *Carafate*)

SUMMARY: A study in healthy subjects indicates that sucralfate does not affect the GI absorption of ibuprofen.

RISK FACTORS: No specific risk factors are known.

MECHANISM: No interaction.

CLINICAL EVALUATION: In a randomized, crossover study, 9 healthy subjects were given a single oral dose of ibuprofen 600 mg with and without sucralfate 1 g 4 times/day for 5 doses; the last sucralfate dose was given 60 minutes before the ibuprofen.[1] Sucralfate did not affect the bioavailability of ibuprofen. Although the results of a single-dose study in healthy subjects cannot automatically be applied to patients on long-term ibuprofen therapy, it appears unlikely that the drugs interact in a clinically important way.

RELATED DRUGS: The effect of sucralfate on other nonsteroidal anti-inflammatory drugs (NSAIDs) is not established; nevertheless, the lack of sucralfate effect on the absorption of ibuprofen and aspirin lowers the index of suspicion that other NSAIDs would be affected.

MANAGEMENT OPTIONS: No interaction.

REFERENCES:

1. Pugh MC, et al. Effect of sucralfate on ibuprofen absorption in normal volunteers. *Clin Pharm.* 1984;3 (6):630-633.

Ibuprofen (eg, *Motrin*)

Tacrine (*Cognex*)

SUMMARY: A patient taking tacrine developed delirium when ibuprofen was added, but a causal relationship was not established.

RISK FACTORS: No specific risk factors are known.

MECHANISM: Not established.

CLINICAL EVALUATION: A 71-year-old woman developed delirium while taking tacrine 40 mg 4 times daily, which gradually resolved when the dosage was reduced to 20 mg 4 times daily.[1] Symptoms included delusions, dizziness, fluctuating awareness, and hallucinations. The delirium returned 8 months later when ibuprofen 600 mg daily was added to tacrine. Both drugs were stopped, and the delirium resolved. Given the lack of dechallenge or rechallenge, it was not possible to establish whether the delirium was caused by a drug interaction, the ibuprofen alone, or some other factor.

RELATED DRUGS: The effect of tacrine combined with other nonsteroidal anti-inflammatory drugs (NSAIDs) is not established, but it may not be unusual for tacrine-treated patients to receive NSAIDs because both tend to be used in older patients.

MANAGEMENT OPTIONS: No specific action is required, but be alert for evidence of the interaction.

REFERENCES:

1. Hooten WM, et al. Delirium caused by tacrine and ibuprofen interaction. *Am J Psychiatry.* 1996;153(6):842.

Ibuprofen (eg, *Motrin*)

Voriconazole (*Vfend*)

SUMMARY: Voriconazole administration increases the plasma concentration of ibuprofen; ibuprofen adverse reactions may increase.

RISK FACTORS: No specific risk factors are known.

MECHANISM: Voriconazole inhibits CYP2C9, the enzyme primarily responsible for the metabolism of the more active enantiomer of ibuprofen (S-ibuprofen).

CLINICAL EVALUATION: Twelve healthy subjects received a single dose of ibuprofen 400 mg alone and 1 hour after the last of 2 daily voriconazole doses.[1] The voriconazole was dosed as 400 mg twice daily on day 1 and 200 mg twice daily on day 2. The mean area under the plasma concentration-time curve of ibuprofen was increased more than 100% following the 2 days of voriconazole pretreatment. The half-life of ibuprofen was prolonged 43% after voriconazole. Some increase in ibuprofen adverse reactions might occur if voriconazole is coadministered.

RELATED DRUGS: Most other nonsteroidal anti-inflammatory drugs (NSAIDs) are substrates for CYP2C9, including ketoprofen, naproxen (eg, *Aleve*), and diclofenac (eg, *Voltaren*), and are expected to be affected by voriconazole in a similar manner. Fluconazole (eg, *Diflucan*) also inhibits the activity of CYP2C9 and is known to inhibit the metabolism of ibuprofen and probably other NSAIDs.

MANAGEMENT OPTIONS:

➡ ***Consider Alternative.*** Ketoconazole (eg, *Nizoral*), itraconazole (eg, *Sporanox*), and terbinafine (eg, *Lamisil*) could be considered as alternative antifungal agents because they do not affect CYP2C9 activity.

➡ ***Monitor.*** Observe patients taking NSAIDs, particularly long-term, high-dose regimens, for evidence of NSAID toxicity during coadministration of voriconazole.

REFERENCES:

1. Hynninen VV, et al. Effects of the antifungals voriconazole and fluconazole on the pharmacokinetics of S-(+)- and R-(-)-Ibuprofen. *Antimicrob Agents Chemother.* 2006;50(6):1967-1972.

Ibuprofen (eg, *Motrin*)

Warfarin (eg, *Coumadin*)

SUMMARY: Ibuprofen does not appear to affect the hypoprothrombinemic response to warfarin or phenprocoumon,[†] but cotherapy requires caution because of possible detrimental effects of ibuprofen on gastric mucosa and platelet function.

RISK FACTORS:

➡ **Concurrent Diseases.** Patients with peptic ulcer disease (PUD) or a history of GI bleeding are probably at higher risk for this interaction.

MECHANISM: Although ibuprofen does not appear to enhance the hypoprothrombinemic response to oral anticoagulants, ibuprofen-induced gastric erosions and inhibition of platelet function theoretically could increase the risk of bleeding in anticoagulated patients.

CLINICAL EVALUATION: Ibuprofen in doses up to 2,400 mg/day in anticoagulated patients and healthy subjects did not affect the hypoprothrombinemic response to phenprocoumon[1,2] or warfarin.[3] One case of an apparent drug interaction between warfarin and ibuprofen has been reported, but the only detail provided concerned a coagulation defect.[4] Thus, most available evidence indicates that the hypoprothrombinemic response to oral anticoagulants is not affected by ibuprofen. However, as with any nonsteroidal anti-inflammatory drug (NSAID), the possible detrimental effects of ibuprofen on GI mucosa and platelet function must be considered. In a retrospective cohort study, hospitalizations for hemorrhagic PUD were about 13 times higher in patients receiving warfarin plus an NSAID than in patients receiving neither drug.[5]

RELATED DRUGS: Phenprocoumon interacts similarly. All NSAIDs inhibit platelet function, cause gastric erosions, and probably increase the risk of GI bleeding.

MANAGEMENT OPTIONS:

➡ **Avoid Unless Benefit Outweighs Risk.** Because NSAIDs may increase the risk of GI bleeding in patients taking oral anticoagulants, use the combination only after careful consideration of benefit versus risk. As an analgesic or antipyretic, acetaminophen is the best choice for safer use with oral anticoagulants. Nonacetylated salicylates (eg, choline salicylate, magnesium salicylate, salsalate, sodium salicylate) also are probably safer with oral anticoagulants than NSAIDs because they have minimal effects on platelet function and gastric mucosa.

➡ **Monitor.** If any NSAID is used with an oral anticoagulant, carefully monitor the prothrombin time and watch for evidence of bleeding, especially from the GI tract.

REFERENCES:

1. Boekhout-Mussert MJ, et al. Influence of ibuprofen on oral anticoagulation with phenprocoumon. *J Int Med Res.* 1974;2:279.
2. Thilo D, et al. A study of the effects of the anti-rheumatic drug ibuprofen (*Rufen*) on patients being treated with the oral anticoagulant phenprocoumon (*Marcoumar*). *J Int Med Res.* 1974;2:276.
3. Penner JA, et al. Lack of interaction between ibuprofen and warfarin. *Curr Ther Res Clin Exp.* 1975;18:862-871.
4. McQueen EG. New Zealand Committee on Adverse Drug Reactions: Tenth Annual Report 1975. *N Z Med J.* 1975;82:308-309.
5. Shorr RI, et al. Concurrent use of nonsteroidal anti-inflammatory drugs and oral anticoagulants places elderly persons at high risk for hemorrhagic peptic ulcer disease. *Arch Intern Med.* 1993;153:1665-1670.

† Not available in the United States.

Imatinib (*Gleevec*)

Lansoprazole (*Prevacid*)

SUMMARY: A patient developed cutaneous reactions during concurrent use of imatinib and lansoprazole, but a causal relationship was not established.

RISK FACTORS: No specific risk factors are known.

MECHANISM: Not established.

CLINICAL EVALUATION: A 60-year-old woman taking imatinib for 2 months developed various cutaneous reactions (eg, edema, generalized rash, hyperemic conjunctivae, Stevens-Johnson syndrome) on 3 occasions when receiving imatinib and lansoprazole concurrently.[1] Nonetheless, it is possible that the reactions were caused by lansoprazole alone rather than by an interaction between lansoprazole and imatinib.

RELATED DRUGS: No information is available.

MANAGEMENT OPTIONS: No specific action is required, but be alert for evidence of the interaction.

REFERENCES:

1. Severino G, et al. Adverse reactions during imatinib and lansoprazole treatment in gastrointestinal stromal tumors. *Ann Pharmacother*. 2005;39:162-164.

 Imatinib (*Gleevec*)

Levothyroxine

SUMMARY: Imatinib may reduce the response to levothyroxine and increase levothyroxine dosage requirements.

RISK FACTORS:

➥ **Concurrent Diseases.** Based on current evidence, this interaction appears to occur only in patients who have had thyroidectomy.

MECHANISM: Not established.

CLINICAL EVALUATION: Thyroid function was monitored in 11 patients on imatinib (9 patients had undergone thyroidectomy and were taking levothyroxine, while 3 had not had thyroidectomy).[1] All 9 thyroidectomy patients had symptoms of hypothyroidism and markedly increased thyrotropin levels following use of imatinib, but the other 3 patients remained euthyroid. Although more study is needed, it appears that imatinib consistently reduces levothyroxine effect.

RELATED DRUGS: No information is available.

MANAGEMENT OPTIONS:

➥ **Monitor.** If levothyroxine and imatinib are used concurrently, monitor thyroid function. Levothyroxine dosage may need to be adjusted if imatinib is started, stopped, or changed.

REFERENCES:

1. de Groot JW, et al. Imatinib induces hypothyroidism in patients receiving levothyroxine. *Clin Pharmacol Ther*. 2005;78:433-438.

Imatinib (*Gleevec*)

Rifampin (eg, *Rifadin*)

SUMMARY: Rifampin reduced the plasma concentrations of imatinib; some loss of efficacy is likely to occur.

RISK FACTORS: No specific risk factors are known.

MECHANISM: Rifampin induces the metabolism (CYP3A4) of imatinib; it also may increase the effect of P-glycoprotein on imatinib, further lowering plasma concentrations.

CLINICAL EVALUATION: Fourteen healthy subjects received a single oral dose of imatinib 400 mg alone and on day 8 of an 11-day course of rifampin 600 mg once daily.[1] During rifampin coadministration, the mean area under the plasma concentration-time curve of imatinib was reduced 74%, and its half-life declined from 16.7 to 8.8 hours. A reduction in the efficacy of imatinib is likely to occur during rifampin coadministration.

RELATED DRUGS: Rifabutin (*Mycobutin*), and any other CYP3A4 inducer, is likely to affect imatinib in a similar manner.

MANAGEMENT OPTIONS:

➡ *Monitor.* Carefully monitor patient response to imatinib if rifampin is added or removed from the drug regimen. Increased doses of imatinib may be necessary during rifampin administration.

REFERENCES:

1. Bolton AE, et al. Effect of rifampicin on the pharmacokinetics of imatinib mesylate (*Gleevec*, STI571) in healthy subjects. *Cancer Chemother Pharmacol*. 2004;53(2):102-106.

Imatinib (*Gleevec*)

St. John's Wort

SUMMARY: A study in healthy subjects found reduced imatinib plasma concentrations following use of St. John's wort.

RISK FACTORS: No specific risk factors are known.

MECHANISM: St. John's wort probably increases the metabolism of imatinib via CYP3A4.

CLINICAL EVALUATION: In 12 healthy subjects given imatinib with and without pretreatment with St. John's wort for 11 days, St. John's wort reduced imatinib area under the plasma concentration-time curve (AUC) 30%.[1] A similar study in 10 healthy subjects found a 32% decrease in imatinib AUC with concurrent use of St. John's wort.[2] Because the magnitude of this interaction may be sufficient to reduce imatinib efficacy in some patients, and because imatinib is used for life-threatening diseases, avoid concurrent use.

RELATED DRUGS: No information is available.

MANAGEMENT OPTIONS:

➡ *Avoid Unless Benefit Outweighs Risk.* In most patients receiving imatinib, the risk of using St. John's wort is likely to outweigh the benefit.

➡ *Circumvent/Minimize.* Advise patients taking imatinib to avoid taking St. John's wort.

➡ *Monitor.* If the combination is used, monitor for reduced imatinib response.

REFERENCES:

1. Frye RF, et al. Effect of St. John's wort on imatinib mesylate pharmacokinetics. *Clin Pharmacol Ther.* 2004;76(4):323-329.

2. Smith P, et al. The influence of St. John's wort on the pharmacokinetics and protein binding of imatinib mesylate. *Pharmacotherapy.* 2004;24(11):1508-1514.

Imatinib (*Gleevec*)

Tamoxifen (eg, *Soltamox*)

SUMMARY: Theoretically, imatinib may reduce the efficacy of tamoxifen in the treatment of breast cancer.

RISK FACTORS: No specific risk factors are known.

MECHANISM: Tamoxifen is metabolized to 2 active metabolites by CYP2D6, the most important of which is endoxifen. By reducing endoxifen formation, CYP2D6 inhibitors such as imatinib may reduce tamoxifen efficacy.[1-3]

CLINICAL EVALUATION: A study in patients with breast cancer found substantial reductions in endoxifen plasma concentrations in patients taking potent CYP2D6 inhibitors such as fluoxetine and paroxetine.[4] Another tamoxifen study found a nearly 2-fold increase in risk of breast cancer relapse in women with low CYP2D6 activity, either due to CYP2D6-inhibiting drugs or genetic deficiency.[5] Taken together, these and other results strongly suggest that CYP2D6 inhibitors reduce the efficacy of tamoxifen in treatment of breast cancer. Imatinib is a CYP2D6 inhibitor, and may inhibit the anticancer effects of tamoxifen.

RELATED DRUGS: No information available.

MANAGEMENT OPTIONS:

➡ *Consider Alternative.* If possible, use an alternative for one of the drugs.

➡ *Monitor.* If a CYP2D6 inhibitor such as imatinib is used with tamoxifen, cancer recurrence may be an indication that tamoxifen efficacy has been reduced. If this happens, consider discontinuing the CYP2D6 inhibitor.

REFERENCES:

1. Dezentjé VO, et al. Clinical implications of CYP2D6 genotyping in tamoxifen treatment for breast cancer. *Clin Cancer Res.* 2009;15(1):15-21.

2. Tan SH, et al. Pharmacogenetics in breast cancer therapy. *Clin Cancer Res.* 2008;14(24):8027-8041.

3. Newman WG, et al. Impaired tamoxifen metabolism reduces survival in familial breast cancer patients. *Clin Cancer Res.* 2008;14(18):5913-5918.

4. Borges S, et al. Quantitative effect of CYP2D6 genotype and inhibitors on tamoxifen metabolism: implication for optimization of breast cancer treatment. *Clin Pharmacol Ther.* 2006;80(1):61-74.

5. Goetz MP, et al. The impact of cytochrome P450 2D6 metabolism in women receiving adjuvant tamoxifen. *Breast Cancer Res Treat.* 2007;101(1):113-121.

Imipenem (*Primaxin*)

Theophylline (eg, *Theo-24*)

SUMMARY: Several patients receiving theophylline developed generalized seizures following the addition of imipenem, but more study is needed to establish a causal relationship.

RISK FACTORS: No specific risk factors are known.

MECHANISM: Unknown. Additive CNS stimulation by theophylline and imipenem may have induced seizures.

CLINICAL EVALUATION: Four patients taking theophylline (concentrations 11.5 to 21.8 mcg/mL) experienced generalized seizures 2 to 6 days after the administration of imipenem 1,500 to 2,000 mg/day.[1] Theophylline concentrations did not appear to increase following imipenem. While these cases do not prove causation, it is possible that the concurrent use of imipenem and theophylline may increase the risk of seizures.

RELATED DRUGS: No information is available.

MANAGEMENT OPTIONS:

➥ *Circumvent/Minimize.* Make appropriate dosage adjustments in patients with reduced renal function to avoid potentially toxic concentrations.

➥ *Monitor.* Until more information is known about this interaction, monitor patients for appropriate theophylline and imipenem dosage. Be alert for signs of CNS stimulation or seizures.

REFERENCES:
1. Semel JD, et al. Seizures in patients simultaneously receiving theophylline and imipenem or ciprofloxacin or metronidazole. *South Med J*. 1991;84(4):465-468.

Imipramine (eg, *Tofranil*)

Contraceptives, Oral (eg, *Ortho-Novum*)

SUMMARY: Limited evidence indicates that oral contraceptives or estrogens may alter the response to tricyclic antidepressants (TCAs), such as imipramine, but the clinical importance of this effect is not established.

RISK FACTORS: No specific risk factors are known.

MECHANISM: It has been proposed that estrogens may affect the metabolism of TCAs,[1] but direct evidence for such a mechanism is lacking.

CLINICAL EVALUATION: Women taking low-dose oral contraceptives had an imipramine bioavailability of 44% compared with 27% in women who were not taking oral contraceptives.[2] Ethinyl estradiol 50 mcg/day may impair the response to imipramine 150 mg/day and increase adverse reactions, while lower doses of estrogen 25 mcg/day may have a favorable effect.[3] A case was described[4] that reportedly represented an example of this interaction; however, an adverse interaction between oral contraceptives and clomipramine (eg, *Anafranil*) was not found, possibly because the oral contraceptive estrogen doses were lower than those in previous studies.[5] More evidence is needed to evaluate the clinical significance of this interaction.

RELATED DRUGS: Clomipramine interacts similarly. The effect of oral contraceptives on other TCAs is not established.

MANAGEMENT OPTIONS: No specific action is required, but be alert for evidence of the interaction.

REFERENCES:
1. Somani SM, et al. Mechanism of estrogen-imipramine interaction. *JAMA*. 1973;223(5):560.
2. Abernethy DR, et al. Imipramine disposition in users of oral contraceptive steroids. *Clin Pharmacol Ther*. 1984;35(6):792-797.
3. Prange AJ Jr. Estrogen may well affect response to antidepressant. *JAMA*. 1972;219:143-144.
4. Khurana RC. Estrogen-imipramine interaction. *JAMA*. 1972;222(6):702-703.
5. Beaumont G. Drug interactions with clomipramine (*Anafranil*). *J Int Med Res*. 1973;1:480-484.

Imipramine (eg, *Tofranil*)

Ketoconazole (eg, *Nizoral*)

SUMMARY: Ketoconazole causes a small increase in imipramine concentrations; imipramine toxicity is not likely to occur.

RISK FACTORS: No specific risk factors are known.

MECHANISM: Ketoconazole inhibits the CYP3A4 metabolism of imipramine. However, several other enzymes that are not inhibited by ketoconazole (eg, CYP2D6) also metabolize imipramine, limiting the magnitude of this interaction.

CLINICAL EVALUATION: Six healthy subjects received a single dose of imipramine 100 mg alone and on day 10 of a 14–day regimen of ketoconazole 200 mg/day.[1] Pretreatment with ketoconazole resulted in a 20% increase in the area under the plasma concentration-time curve of imipramine. Imipramine half-life increased 15%. Clinically significant changes in a patient's response to imipramine are unlikely.

RELATED DRUGS: Itraconazole (*Sporanox*) and fluconazole (*Diflucan*) may inhibit imipramine in a similar manner. Ketoconazole does not affect the metabolism of desipramine (eg, *Norpramin*) or nortriptyline (eg, *Pamelor*), tricyclics that are not metabolized by CYP3A4.

MANAGEMENT OPTIONS: No specific action is required, but be alert for evidence of the interaction.

REFERENCES:
1. Spina E, et al. Effect of ketoconazole on the pharmacokinetics of imipramine and desipramine in healthy subjects. *Br J Clin Pharmacol*. 1997;43:315–18.

Imipramine (eg, *Tofranil*)

Labetalol (eg, *Normodyne*)

SUMMARY: Labetalol increases imipramine serum concentration, but the significance of this effect is not established.

RISK FACTORS: No specific risk factors are known.

MECHANISM: It appears that labetalol reduces the metabolism of imipramine.

CLINICAL EVALUATION: Imipramine 100 mg was administered to 13 healthy subjects alone or on the fourth of 7 days of labetalol treatment 200 mg every 12 hours.[1] Impramine clearance was reduced 38% and peak concentrations increased by 83%. The clinical significance of this effect is not established.

RELATED DRUGS: While no data are available, it is possible that labetalol affects other antidepressants. There are no data suggesting other beta blockers affect imipramine metabolism.

MANAGEMENT OPTIONS: No specific action is required, but be alert for evidence of the interaction.

REFERENCES:

1. Krol TF, et al. Comparison of verapamil, diltiazem and labetalol on the oral clearance and metabolism of imipramine. *Pharmacotherapy.* 1989;9:184.

Imipramine (eg, *Tofranil*)

Levodopa (eg, *Larodopa*)

SUMMARY: Preliminary evidence indicates that imipramine may lower serum levodopa concentrations, but the clinical importance of this effect is not established.

RISK FACTORS: No specific risk factors are known.

MECHANISM: Unknown. Imipramine may slow gastric emptying, thus enhancing the degradation of levodopa to inactive products within the stomach.

CLINICAL EVALUATION: The absorption of a single levodopa dose was studied before and after imipramine 100 mg/day for 3 days.[1] The results suggested that the bioavailability of intact levodopa was impaired in the presence of imipramine, although definite conclusions could not be reached. An inhibitory effect of imipramine on levodopa absorption would be consistent with the effect of other anticholinergics on levodopa absorption, but the clinical importance of this purported interaction is not established.

RELATED DRUGS: Other tricyclic antidepressants with anticholinergic effects (eg, amitriptyline [eg, *Elavil*], amoxapine [eg, *Asendin*], doxepin [eg, *Sinequan*], nortriptyline [eg, *Pamelor*], protriptyline [eg, *Vivactil*]) theoretically would affect levodopa similarly.

MANAGEMENT OPTIONS: No specific action is required, but be alert for evidence of the interaction.

REFERENCES:

1. Morgan JP, et al. Imipramine-mediated interference with levodopa absorption from the gastrointestinal tract in man. *Neurology.* 1975;25:1029.

Imipramine (eg, *Tofranil*)

Methylphenidate (eg, *Ritalin*)

SUMMARY: Methylphenidate may increase serum concentrations of imipramine and other tricyclic antidepressants (TCAs) appreciably, but reports of adverse effects from the interaction are lacking.

RISK FACTORS: No specific risk factors are known.

MECHANISM: Methylphenidate appears to inhibit the metabolism of TCAs.

CLINICAL EVALUATION: Clinical studies suggest that methylphenidate can increase serum concentrations of TCAs. In some reports, the methylphenidate-induced increases in cyclic antidepressant serum concentrations have resulted in an improved antidepressant response.[3] Some patients apparently do not manifest elevated TCA levels following methylphenidate administration.[1,2] Although this interaction theoretically could result in TCA toxicity, clinical examples are lacking.

RELATED DRUGS: Other TCAs may be affected similarly.

MANAGEMENT OPTIONS: No specific action is required, but be alert for evidence of the interaction.

REFERENCES:

1. Zeidenberg P, et al. Clinical and metabolic studies with imipramine in man. *Am J Psychiatry*. 1971;127:1321.
2. Drimmer EJ, et al. Desipramine and methylphenidate combination treatment for depression: case report. *Am J Psychiatry*. 1983;140:241.
3. Wharton RN, et al. A potential clinical use for the interaction of methylphenidate with tricyclic antidepressants. *Am J Psychiatry*. 1971;127:1619.

 Imipramine (eg, *Tofranil*)

Norepinephrine (eg, *Levophed*)

SUMMARY: Imipramine and other tricyclic antidepressants can markedly enhance the pressor response to norepinephrine.

RISK FACTORS: No specific risk factors are known.

MECHANISM: The increased pressor response is probably due to TCA-induced inhibition of the uptake of norepinephrine into the adrenergic neuron.[4,5]

CLINICAL EVALUATION: Intravenous (IV) infusions of norepinephrine to healthy subjects receiving imipramine resulted in four-to eightfold increases in the pressor response to norepinephrine.[1] Similarly, Mitchell et al.[2] found a several-fold increase in the pressor response to norepinephrine in patients receiving desipramine (eg, *Norpramin*), amitriptyline (eg, *Elavil*), or protriptyline (eg, *Vivactil*).[2] In another study of 6 healthy subjects, pretreatment with protriptyline 60 mg/day for 4 days markedly increased the pressor response to infusion of norepinephrine.[3] Thus, this interaction appears to be well documented with a variety of tricyclic antidepressants.

RELATED DRUGS: Desipramine, amitriptyline, and protriptyline interact similarly. Assume that all TCAs will interact with norepinephrine until proven otherwise.

MANAGEMENT OPTIONS:

➡ *Avoid Unless Benefit Outweighs Risk.* If IV norepinephrine is used, begin with conservative doses.

➡ *Monitor.* Monitor blood pressure carefully if the combination is used.

REFERENCES:

1. Boakes AJ, et al. Interactions between sympathomimetic amines and antidepressant agents in man. *Br Med J*. 1973;1:311.
2. Mitchell JR, et al. Guanethidine and related agents. III. Antagonism by drugs which inhibit the norepinephrine pump in man. *J Clin Invest*. 1970;49:1596.
3. Svedmyr N. The influence of a tricyclic antidepressant agent (protriptyline) on some of the circulatory effects of noradrenaline and adrenaline in man. *Life Sci*. 1968;7:77.

4. Boakes AJ. Sympathomimetic amines and antidepressant agents. *Br Med J.* 1973;2:114. Letter.
5. Ghose K. Sympathomimetic amines and tricyclic antidepressant drugs. *Neuropharmacology.* 1980;19:1251.

Imipramine (eg, *Tofranil*)

Phenelzine (*Nardil*)

SUMMARY: Severe reactions have occurred in patients receiving combined therapy with tricyclic antidepressants (TCAs) and phenelzine or other nonselective monoamine oxidase inhibitors (MAOIs), but some combinations can be used safely with appropriate precautions.

RISK FACTORS:

➡ *Dosage Regimen.* Large doses of one or both drugs appear to increase the risk.

➡ *Order of Drug Administration.* Most reactions occurred when the cyclic agent was added to established MAOI therapy.

MECHANISM: Not established. Excessive serotonergic effects appear involved in some cases.

CLINICAL EVALUATION: Severe reactions have been reported with the concomitant administration of these two drug classes; this usually occurs when the cyclic agent is added to established MAOI therapy. Findings include excitation, hyperpyrexia, mania, disseminated intravascular coagulation,[12] and convulsions; fatalities also have occurred. In most reported cases of severe reactions, excessive doses of one or both drugs were used, the TCA was given parenterally or other psychotropic drugs also were being given.[1-4] Still, there is convincing evidence[1,5-11] that an MAOI and some tricyclic antidepressants an be given together safely in most patients if the following precautions are observed: 1) avoid large doses; 2) give the drugs orally; 3) avoid clomipramine and imipramine; and 4) monitor the patient closely. Thus, although adverse reactions sometimes occur following the combined use of MAOIs and TCAs, the incidence and severity of such reactions appear lower than previously suspected.

RELATED DRUGS: Antidepressants that inhibit serotonin reuptake such as clomipramine (eg, *Anafranil*), amitriptyline (eg, *Elavil*), desipramine (eg, *Norpramin*), and trazodone (eg, *Desyrel*) may be more likely to result in serotonin syndrome than other tricyclic antidepressants.

MANAGEMENT OPTIONS:

➡ *Avoid Unless Benefit Outweighs Risk.* Some MAOIs and some tricyclics can be used together; however, when cotherapy is contemplated, any possible benefit of the combination should be weighed against the potential hazards. Moreover, it should be noted that the product information for both MAOIs and TCAs states that concurrent use is contraindicated, which may have medicolegal implications. Finally, be aware that a potentially lethal combination (in overdose) will be at the disposal of suicide-prone patients.

➡ *Monitor.* If the combination is used, monitor for evidence of excitation, fever, mania, seizures, or other unexpected adverse effects.

REFERENCES:
1. Kline NS. Experimental use of monoamine oxidase inhibitors with tricyclic antidepressants (Questions and Answers). *JAMA.* 1974;227:807.

2. De La Fuente RJ, et al. Mania induced by tricyclic-MAOI combination therapy in bipolar treatment-resistant disorder: case reports. *J Clin Psychiatry.* 1986;47:40.

3. Beaumont G. Drug interactions with clomipramine (Anafranil). *J Int Med Res.* 1973;1:480.

4. White K, et al. The combined use of MAOIs and tricyclics. *J Clin Psychiatry.* 1984;45:67.

5. Winston F. Combined antidepressant therapy. *Br J Psychiatry.* 1971;118:301.

6. Schuckit U et al. Tricyclic antidepressants and monoamine oxidase inhibitors. Combination therapy in the treatment of depression. *Arch Gen Psychiatry.* 1971;24:509.

7. Spiker DG, et al. Combining tricyclic and monoamine oxidase inhibitor antidepressants. *Arch Gen Psychiatry.* 1976;33:828.

8. Ananth J, et al. A review of combined tricyclic and MAOI therapy. *Compr Psychiatry.* 1977;18:221.

9. White K. Tricyclic overdose in a patient given combined tricyclic MAOI treatment. *Am J Psychiatry.* 1978;135:1411.

10. Young JPR, et al. Controlled trial of trimipramine, monoamine oxidase inhibitors, and combined treatment in depressed outpatients. *Br Med J.* 1979;2:1315.

11. White K. Combined tricyclic and monoamine-oxidase inhibitor antidepressant treatment. *West J Med.* 1983;138:406.

12. Tackley RM, et al. Fatal disseminated intravascular coagulation following a monoamine oxidase inhibitor/tricyclic interaction. *Anaesthesia.* 1987;42:760.

Imipramine (eg, *Tofranil*)

Phenylephrine (eg, *Neo-Synephrine*)

SUMMARY: Imipramine and possibly other tricyclic antidepressants (TCAs) may enhance the pressor response to IV phenylephrine; the effect on oral or nasal phenylephrine is not established.

RISK FACTORS: No specific risk factors are known.

MECHANISM: Not established.

CLINICAL EVALUATION: IV infusions of phenylephrine to healthy subjects receiving imipramine resulted in 2- to 3-fold increases in the pressor response to phenylephrine.[1,2] The effect of imipramine pretreatment on the response to oral or nasal phenylephrine is unknown, but one would expect the interaction to be less (particularly with nasal use in FDA-approved doses).

RELATED DRUGS: Until additional information is available, assume that other TCAs would produce a similar effect if combined with IV phenylephrine.

MANAGEMENT OPTIONS:

➥ *Monitor.* Patients receiving TCAs should be given parenteral phenylephrine only with caution and careful monitoring of the blood pressure. Until additional information is available, be alert for enhanced pressor responses to oral phenylephrine.

REFERENCES:

1. Boakes AJ, et al. Interactions between sympathomimetic amines and antidepressant agents in man. *BMJ.* 1973;1:311-315.

2. Boakes AJ. Sympathomimetic amines and antidepressant agents. *BMJ.* 1973;2:114.

Imipramine (eg, *Tofranil*)

Quinidine (eg, *Quinora*)

SUMMARY: Quinidine markedly increases imipramine and desipramine serum concentrations; toxicity may result.

RISK FACTORS:

➥ **Pharmacogenetics.** Extensive metabolizers of the antidepressants are at greater risk.[1]

MECHANISM: Quinidine inhibits cytochrome P4502D6 that is responsible for the hydroxylation of imipramine and desipramine.

CLINICAL EVALUATION: The effect of quinidine 200 mg/day for 12 days on single-dose pharmacokinetics of imipramine 100 mg and desipramine (eg, *Norpramin*) 100 mg was evaluated and compared with the antidepressants administered alone. Imipramine clearance was reduced 35%, and desipramine clearance was reduced 85%.[2] Quinidine primarily affects the 2-hydroxylation of the antidepressants. The metabolism of nortriptyline (eg, *Pamelor*) was inhibited by a single 50 mg dose of quinidine.[3] The magnitude of this interaction in extensive metabolizers is likely to be of clinical significance.

RELATED DRUGS: Desipramine and nortriptyline concentrations are increased by quinidine. Other cyclic antidepressants may be affected by this interaction but little clinical information is available.

MANAGEMENT OPTIONS:

➥ **Monitor.** Monitor patients maintained on cyclic antidepressants for increased side effects (eg, sedation, arrhythmia, confusion) if quinidine is added to their drug therapy.

REFERENCES:

1. Steiner E, et al. Inhibition of desipramine 2-hydroxylation by quinidine and quinine. *Clin Pharmacol Ther.* 1988;43:577.
2. Brosen K, et al. Quinidine inhibits the 2-hydroxylation of imipramine and desipramine but not the demethylation of imipramine. *Eur J Clin Pharmacol.* 1989;37:155.
3. Pfandl B, et al. Stereoselective inhibition of nortriptyline hydroxylation in man by quinidine. *Xenobiotica.* 1992;22:721.

Imipramine (*Tofranil*)

Venlafaxine (eg, *Effexor*)

SUMMARY: Study in healthy subjects suggests that venlafaxine increases imipramine serum concentrations, but the extent to which this increases the risk of imipramine toxicity is not established.

RISK FACTORS:

➥ **Pharmacogenetics.** Only patients who have CYP2D6 would be expected to experience this interaction.

MECHANISM: Venlafaxine probably reduces the CYP2D6 metabolism of imipramine and desipramine.

CLINICAL EVALUATION: Six subjects took a single oral dose of imipramine 100 mg with and without pretreatment with venlafaxine 50 mg 3 times daily for 3 days.[1] Venlafaxine increased imipramine area under the plasma concentration-time curve (AUC)

28%, but the AUC of desipramine (an active metabolite of imipramine) was increased 40%. Because the plasma concentrations of imipramine and desipramine are increased, it is possible that some patients may experience tricyclic antidepressant (TCA) toxicity. Nonetheless, the clinical importance of this interaction is not established.

RELATED DRUGS: Theoretically, other TCAs that are metabolized by CYP2D6, such as amitriptyline (*Elavil*), would be similarly affected.

MANAGEMENT OPTIONS:

➡ *Monitor.* Monitor for altered imipramine effect if venlafaxine is initiated, discontinued, or changed in dosage.

REFERENCES:
1. Albers LJ, et al. Effect of venlafaxine on imipramine metabolism. *Psychiatry Res.* 2000;96:235-243.

Imipramine (eg, *Tofranil*)

Verapamil (eg, *Calan*)

SUMMARY: Verapamil and diltiazem appear to increase imipramine serum concentrations; the clinical significance is unknown.

RISK FACTORS: No specific risk factors are known.

MECHANISM: Verapamil and diltiazem appear to decrease the metabolism of imipramine.

CLINICAL EVALUATION: Thirteen subjects received verapamil 120 mg every 8 hours, diltiazem (eg, *Cardizem*) 90 mg every 8 hours, or placebo for 7 days[1]; imipramine 100 mg was added to these regimens on the fourth day. Imipramine oral clearance was decreased 25% and 35% by verapamil and diltiazem, respectively. The peak imipramine concentration was significantly increased (35%) by diltiazem but not by verapamil. The clinical importance of this interaction is unknown.

RELATED DRUGS: Verapamil and diltiazem likely would affect other cyclic antidepressants in a similar manner. The effects of other calcium channel blockers on cyclic antidepressants are unknown.

MANAGEMENT OPTIONS:

➡ *Monitor.* Monitor patients maintained on imipramine for increased serum imipramine concentrations (eg, sedation, dry mouth, tachycardia) if verapamil or diltiazem is initiated concurrently.

REFERENCES:
1. Hermann DJ, et al. Comparison of verapamil, diltiazem, and labetalol on the bioavailability and metabolism of imipramine. *J Clin Pharmacol.* 1992;32:176-183.

Indinavir (*Crixivan*)

Colchicine

SUMMARY: Based on the interactive properties of the 2 drugs, it is likely that indinavir substantially increases colchicine plasma concentrations. Avoid the combination if possible.

RISK FACTORS: No specific risk factors are known.

MECHANISM: Colchicine is a P-glycoprotein and CYP3A4 substrate, and indinavir inhibits both P-glycoprotein and CYP3A4; colchicine plasma concentrations are likely to increase.[1]

CLINICAL EVALUATION: Although the interaction is based primarily on theoretical considerations, it is likely that indinavir would increase the risk of colchicine toxicity. Given that colchicine toxicity can be fatal, even a theoretical interaction warrants close attention.

RELATED DRUGS: Other protease inhibitors that inhibit both P-glycoprotein and CYP3A4 include nelfinavir (*Viracept*), ritonavir (*Norvir*), and saquinavir (*Invirase*); these drugs are also likely to interact similarly with colchicine. HIV drugs that inhibit CYP3A4 include atazanavir (*Reyataz*), darunavir (*Prezista*), delavirdine (*Rescriptor*); these drugs may also increase colchicine plasma concentrations.

MANAGEMENT OPTIONS:

➡ *Avoid Unless Benefit Outweighs Risk.* Given that colchicine toxicity can be life-threatening, use the combination only if it is likely to provide therapeutic benefits that cannot be achieved with noninteracting alternatives.

➡ *Use Alternative.* If possible, avoid colchicine in patients receiving indinavir or other HIV drugs that inhibit P-glycoprotein and/or CYP3A4.

➡ *Monitor.* If the combination must be used, monitor carefully for colchicine toxicity such as diarrhea, vomiting, fever, abdominal pain, and muscle pain. Advise the patient to immediately contact a health care provider if any of these symptoms occur. Colchicine-induced pancytopenia can result in infections, bleeding, and anemia, and is often the cause of death in fatal cases.

REFERENCES:

1. Rautio J, et al. In vitro p-glycoprotein inhibition assays for assessment of clinical drug interaction potential of new drug candidates: a recommendation for probe substrates. *Drug Metab Dispos.* 2006;34(5):786-792.

Indinavir (*Crixivan*)

Ketoconazole (eg, *Nizoral*)

SUMMARY: Ketoconazole increases the serum concentration of indinavir; increased toxicity may result.

RISK FACTORS: No specific risk factors are known.

MECHANISM: Indinavir is primarily metabolized by CYP3A4, an isoenzyme that is known to be inhibited by ketoconazole and other azole antifungal drugs.

CLINICAL EVALUATION: While no published data are available for evaluation, the manufacturer of indinavir has made available some data on this interaction. The administration of a dose of ketoconazole 400 mg with indinavir resulted in a 68% increase in the area under the concentration-time curve of indinavir.[1] The effects of chronic ketoconazole dosing are not known. This degree of increase in indinavir concentrations could result in an increase in adverse reactions.

RELATED DRUGS: Other protease inhibitors, including ritonavir (*Norvir*), saquinavir (*Invirase*), and nelfinavir (*Viracept*), may be affected by ketoconazole in a similar manner. Itraconazole (eg, *Sporanox*), miconazole (eg, *Monistat*), and fluconazole (eg, *Diflucan*) also are likely to inhibit the metabolism of indinavir. Terbinafine (eg,

Lamisil) does not appear to affect CYP3A4 activity and may be less likely to affect indinavir metabolism.

MANAGEMENT OPTIONS:

➥ *Circumvent/Minimize.* Pending further clinical studies, the dose or dosing interval of indinavir may need to be altered. The manufacturer has suggested a reduced dosage of indinavir to 600 mg every 8 hours during concomitant ketoconazole administration.

➥ *Monitor.* Watch for indinavir toxicity (eg, nephrolithiasis, hyperbilirubinemia, nausea).

REFERENCES:

1. *Crixivan* [package insert]. Whitehouse Station, NJ: Merck & Company Inc; 1996.

Indinavir (*Crixivan*)

Methadone (eg, *Methadose*)

SUMMARY: No interaction.

RISK FACTORS: No specific risk factors are known.

MECHANISM: No interaction.

CLINICAL EVALUATION: Twelve patients on methadone maintenance received either indinavir 800 mg every 8 hours or placebo for 8 days.[1] Indinavir administration did not alter any pharmacokinetic parameter of methadone or its pyrrolidine metabolite. No change in clinical response is likely to occur when indinavir and methadone are coadministered.

RELATED DRUGS: Ritonavir (*Norvir*) has been noted to reduce methadone plasma concentrations.

MANAGEMENT OPTIONS: No interaction.

REFERENCES:

1. Cantilena L, et al. Lack of a pharmacokinetic interaction between indinavir and methadone. *Clin Pharmacol Ther*. 1999:65:135.

Indinavir (*Crixivan*)

Nelfinavir (*Viracept*)

SUMMARY: Chronic administration of indinavir and nelfinavir produces a modest increase in indinavir concentrations; lower doses or less frequent administration may be a possible solution. Nelfinavir plasma concentrations during chronic dosing appear to be minimally affected by chronic indinavir administration.

RISK FACTORS: No specific risk factors are known.

MECHANISM: Both single- and multiple-dose studies suggest that nelfinavir reduces the metabolism (CYP3A4) of indinavir. Single-dose studies also demonstrate an inhibitory effect of indinavir on nelfinavir metabolism. However, with multiple dosing of both drugs, this effect appears to be diminished. Competition for CYP3A4 enzymes between indinavir and nelfinavir metabolites, nelfinavir autoinduction, or a shift of nelfinavir metabolism to the CYP2C19 pathway during chronic dosing may mitigate the effect of indinavir on the elimination of nelfinavir during chronic administration.

CLINICAL EVALUATION: Based on limited data in 6 subjects, nelfinavir 750 mg every 8 hours for 7 days increased the mean area under the concentration-time curve (AUC) following a single dose of indinavir 800 mg by about 51%.[1] Indinavir 800 mg every 8 hours for 7 days increased the AUC of nelfinavir by 83% following a single 750 mg dose.[1]

In a study of patients with HIV infection, the plasma concentrations resulting from the combination of indinavir (1,000 or 1,250 mg twice daily) and nelfinavir (750, 1,000, and 1,250 mg twice daily) were compared.[2] While the pharmacokinetics of indinavir and nelfinavir administered alone were not evaluated in this study, the combination of indinavir and nelfinavir given twice daily resulted in indinavir concentrations similar to those reported in patients taking indinavir 800 mg 3 times/day without nelfinavir. This may reflect a modest inhibition of indinavir during chronic administration of both indinavir and nelfinavir. The chronic administration of indinavir and nelfinavir had little effect, however, on nelfinavir concentrations.

RELATED DRUGS: Other antiretroviral drugs that are known to inhibit CYP32A4 (eg, ritonavir [*Norvir*]) may reduce indinavir and nelfinavir metabolism.

MANAGEMENT OPTIONS:

➡ **Monitor.** Monitor patients receiving combinations of antiretroviral drugs for adequate response and drug toxicity if the doses or combinations are changed.

REFERENCES:

1. *Viracept.* [package insert] New York, NY: Pfizer; 2001.
2. Riddler SA, et al. Coadministration of indinavir and nelfinavir in human immunodeficiency virus type 1-infected adults: safety, pharmacokinetics, and antiretroviral activity. *Antimicrob Agents Chemother.* 2002;46(12):3877-3882.

Indinavir (*Crixivan*)

Omeprazole (eg, *Prilosec*)

SUMMARY: Omeprazole reduces the absorption of indinavir; loss of antiviral efficacy may result.

RISK FACTORS: No specific risk factors are known.

MECHANISM: Indinavir solubility decreases as pH increases. The acid suppression of omeprazole may reduce the solubility of indinavir, resulting in reduced GI absorption.

CLINICAL EVALUATION: The indinavir plasma concentrations in 9 patients taking indinavir and omeprazole 20 to 40 mg/day were compared with those of 15 patients taking the same dose of indinavir (800 mg 3 times/day) without omeprazole coadministration.[1] Four of the 9 patients taking indinavir and omeprazole had indinavir concentrations below the 95% confidence interval of the 15 patients not taking omeprazole. In 1 patient, the indinavir concentration was reduced more than 50% following the addition of omeprazole. Other patients required an increase of their indinavir dose to 1,000 mg 3 times/day following the addition of omeprazole. A reduction of indinavir concentration may result in a reduction of antiviral effect or the development of resistance.

RELATED DRUGS: Other proton pump inhibitors (eg, lansoprazole [*Prevacid*], rabeprazole [*Aciphex*], pantoprazole [eg, *Protonix*]) are expected to produce similar effects on indinavir plasma concentrations. The effect of omeprazole on other protease inhibitors (eg, saquinavir [*Invirase*], ritonavir [*Norvir*], nelfinavir [*Viracept*]) is unknown.

MANAGEMENT OPTIONS:

➡ *Monitor.* Monitor patients treated with indinavir for reduced antiviral efficacy if omeprazole or other proton pump inhibitors are coadministered.

REFERENCES:
1. Burger DM, et al. Pharmacokinetic interaction between the proton pump inhibitor omeprazole and the HIV protease inhibitor indinavir. *AIDS*. 1998;12(15):2080-2082.

Indinavir (*Crixivan*)

Rifabutin (*Mycobutin*)

SUMMARY: Indinavir markedly increases rifabutin serum concentrations, while rifabutin lowers indinavir serum concentrations. Rifabutin toxicity and reduction of indinavir efficacy may result.

RISK FACTORS: No specific risk factors are known.

MECHANISM: Indinavir appears to inhibit the metabolism of rifabutin. Rifabutin appears to induce the metabolism (CYP3A4) of indinavir.

CLINICAL EVALUATION: Indinavir 800 mg every 8 hours and rifabutin 300 mg/day were administered alone and together for 10 days.[1] Indinavir increased the area under the concentration-time curve (AUC) of rifabutin more than 200%. This degree of increase may result in rifabutin toxicity. Rifabutin administration reduced the AUC of indinavir 32%, a change that may result in reduced indinavir efficacy. The indinavir-induced increase in rifabutin serum concentrations likely would increase the magnitude of rifabutin effect on indinavir. Although few details are available, the combined use of indinavir and rifabutin is likely to affect the response to both drugs.

RELATED DRUGS: Rifabutin decreases the AUC of saquinavir (*Invirase*) and is expected to affect ritonavir (*Norvir*) similarly. Ritonavir increases rifabutin concentrations. Rifampin (eg, *Rifadin*) may affect saquinavir in a similar manner.

MANAGEMENT OPTIONS:

➡ *Circumvent/Minimize.* The dose of rifabutin may require reduction to avoid toxicity; the dose of indinavir may require an increase to maintain efficacy.

➡ *Monitor.* Monitor for rifabutin toxicity (eg, GI upset, skin rash) and loss of indinavir efficacy.

REFERENCES:
1. *Crixivan* [package insert]. Whitehouse Station, NJ: Merck & Company; 1996.

Indinavir (*Crixivan*)

Rifapentine (*Priftin*)

SUMMARY: Rifapentine administration reduces the plasma concentration of indinavir; reduction of indinavir's antiviral effect may occur.

RISK FACTORS: No specific risk factors are known.

MECHANISM: Rifapentine is an inducer of CYP3A4, the enzyme primarily responsible for the metabolism of indinavir.

CLINICAL EVALUATION: While specific data are limited, the manufacturer of rifapentine notes that the coadministration of rifapentine 600 mg twice weekly for 28 days with the administration of indinavir 800 mg 3 times daily for days 14 through 28 resulted in a reduction of the peak plasma indinavir concentration by 55%. The area under the plasma concentration-time curve of indinavir was reduced 70% by coadministration of rifapentine.[1] Pending further data, patients receiving indinavir and rifapentine should be observed for reduced indinavir antiviral effect.

RELATED DRUGS: Rifampin (eg, *Rifadin*) is expected to affect indinavir in a similar manner. Other protease inhibitors that are metabolized by CYP3A4 such as atazanavir (*Reyataz*), darunavir (*Prezista*), nelfinavir (*Viracept*), and saquinavir (*Invirase*) are likely to be affected in a similar manner by rifapentine.

MANAGEMENT OPTIONS:

➡ *Monitor.* Carefully monitor patients taking indinavir and rifapentine for reduced antiviral effect.

REFERENCES:
1. *Priftin* [package insert]. Kansas City, MO: Aventis Pharmaceuticals; 2000.

Indinavir (*Crixivan*)

Ritonavir (*Norvir*)

SUMMARY: Indinavir plasma concentrations are increased during ritonavir coadministration; less frequent dosage administration may be possible.

RISK FACTORS: No specific risk factors are known.

MECHANISM: Ritonavir appears to reduce the first-pass and systemic clearance of indinavir by inhibiting CYP3A4.

CLINICAL EVALUATION: The effects of chronically dosed ritonavir on indinavir pharmacokinetics were studied in a total of 39 healthy subjects divided into 5 study groups.[1] The pharmacokinetics of indinavir were estimated in each subject following a single dose (400 to 800 mg) in the absence of ritonavir coadministration. Following the single-dose indinavir study, ritonavir 200 to 400 mg every 12 hours or placebo was administered for 2 weeks. At the end of the 2 weeks of ritonavir dosing, a single dose of indinavir was again administered, and pharmacokinetic parameters were estimated. The area under the plasma concentration-time curve of indinavir increased from 185% to 475% during concurrent ritonavir dosing. Mean indinavir half-life increased from 1.2 to 2.7 hours. Ritonavir did not affect indinavir renal clearance. The reduced indinavir clearance during concomitant ritonavir dosing may enable the administration of indinavir twice daily.

RELATED DRUGS: Ritonavir had been reported to increase saquinavir (*Invirase*) concentrations more than 50-fold. The effect of ritonavir on other protease inhibitors is not established.

MANAGEMENT OPTIONS:

➡ *Circumvent/Minimize.* Because it is likely that ritonavir and indinavir will be used together in some patients, a reduction in the dose or frequency of indinavir administration is advisable. Guide dosage by monitoring indinavir plasma concentrations, if possible.

➡ *Monitor.* Monitor patients for signs of possible indinavir toxicity (eg, neurological or hematological impairment) during combined indinavir/ritonavir therapy.

REFERENCES:
1. Hsu A, et al. Pharmacokinetic interaction between ritonavir and indinavir in healthy volunteers. *Antimicrob Agents Chemother.* 1998;42(11):2784-2791.

Indinavir (*Crixivan*)

Sildenafil (eg, *Viagra*)

SUMMARY: Indinavir increases sildenafil plasma concentrations; increased toxic effects may occur.

RISK FACTORS: No specific risk factors are known.

MECHANISM: Indinavir inhibits the metabolism of sildenafil by the isoenzyme CYP3A4, resulting in an increase in sildenafil bioavailability and reduced systemic clearance.

CLINICAL EVALUATION: Six HIV-positive men chronically taking indinavir 800 mg 3 times daily were studied.[1] Other drugs being taken by the patients included zidovudine (*Retrovir*), lamivudine (*Epivir*), stavudine (*Zerit*), and didanosine (*Videx*). Each patient was administered a single dose of sildenafil 25 mg. All 6 patients experienced adverse reactions (eg, headache, flushing, hypotension, dyspepsia, rhinitis) following sildenafil administration. Sildenafil plasma concentrations from the 6 patients were compared with plasma concentration data obtained in studies of the pharmacokinetics of sildenafil in healthy subjects. The area under the plasma concentration-time curve and peak sildenafil concentration in the HIV-positive patients who had taken a 25 mg dose with indinavir were similar to those produced following a dose of sildenafil 100 mg in healthy subjects. The large apparent increase in sildenafil concentrations that may be associated with indinavir administration could produce sildenafil toxicity.

RELATED DRUGS: Other protease inhibitors such as ritonavir (*Norvir*), saquinavir (*Invirase*), and nelfinavir (*Viracept*) are known to inhibit CYP3A4 activity and are expected to interact with sildenafil.

MANAGEMENT OPTIONS:

➡ *Circumvent/Minimize.* Because of the potential for serious adverse reactions, counsel patients taking protease inhibitors that are CYP3A4 inhibitors to avoid concurrent sildenafil administration.

➡ **Monitor.** Carefully monitor patients treated with indinavir for adverse reactions if sildenafil is prescribed.

REFERENCES:

1. Merry C, et al. Interaction of sildenafil and indinavir when co-administered to HIV-positive patients *AIDS*. 1999;13(15):F101-F107.

Indinavir (*Crixivan*)

St. John's Wort AVOID

SUMMARY: The main component of St. John's wort, hypericum extract, significantly reduced the plasma concentration of indinavir; reduction of antiviral efficacy may occur in some patients. Avoid this combination.

RISK FACTORS: No specific risk factors are known.

MECHANISM: Hypericum extract appears to be an inducer of CYP3A4 and may also induce P-glycoprotein. Both mechanisms lead to reduced plasma concentrations of indinavir.

CLINICAL EVALUATION: Eight subjects received 4 dosages of indinavir 800 mg every 8 hours alone and following hypericum extract (containing 0.3% hypericin) 300 mg 3 times a day for 14 days.[1] Pretreatment with hypericum extract reduced the area under the concentration-time curve of indinavir 57% and the 8-hour trough concentration 81%. The effect of hypericum extract on the half-life of indinavir was not stated. The hypericum extract–induced decline in indinavir plasma concentration is expected to reduce indinavir's antiviral efficacy and increase the risk for the development of resistance.

RELATED DRUGS: Other protease inhibitors (eg, ritonavir [*Norvir*], saquinavir [*Invirase*], nelfinavir [*Viracept*]) are likely to be affected in a similar manner by hypericum extract.

MANAGEMENT OPTIONS:

➡ **AVOID COMBINATION.** Advise patients taking indinavir or other antiviral agents that are metabolized by CYP3A4 to avoid taking St. John's wort.

REFERENCES:

1. Piscitelli SC, et al. Indinavir concentrations and St. John's wort. *Lancet*. 2000;355(9203):547-548.

Indinavir (*Crixivan*)

Vardenafil (*Levitra*)

SUMMARY: Indinavir increases the plasma concentration of vardenafil; increased vardenafil adverse reactions may occur.

RISK FACTORS: No specific risk factors are known.

MECHANISM: Indinavir inhibits the metabolism of vardenafil via CYP3A4; increased vardenafil bioavailability and reduced clearance are expected.

CLINICAL EVALUATION: While specific data are limited, the manufacturer of vardenafil notes that the coadministration of indinavir 800 mg 3 times daily prior to a single dose of vardenafil 10 mg increased the mean area under the plasma concentration-time curve of vardenafil by about 16-fold.[1]

RELATED DRUGS: Atazanavir (*Reyataz*), darunavir (*Prezista*), nelfinavir (*Viracept*), saquinavir (*Invirase*), and ritonavir (*Norvir*) also inhibit the activity of CYP3A4 and are expected to increase the plasma concentrations of vardenafil. Sildenafil (eg, *Viagra*) and tadalafil (*Cialis*) are likely to be affected in a similar manner by indinavir.

MANAGEMENT OPTIONS:

➡ *Circumvent/Minimize.* Pending further data, observe patients receiving vardenafil and indinavir for increased vardenafil effect, and limit the dosage of vardenafil to 2.5 mg every 24 hours.

➡ *Monitor.* Be alert for signs of excessive vardenafil effects such as hypotension if indinavir is coadministered.

REFERENCES:

1. *Levitra* [package insert]. West Haven, CT: Bayer Pharmaceuticals Corporation; 2008.

 Indinavir (*Crixivan*)

Zidovudine (eg, *Retrovir*)

SUMMARY: Zidovudine administration produced a limited increase in indinavir serum concentrations; indinavir may moderately increase zidovudine concentrations. No change in patient response to either drug is likely to be observed.

RISK FACTORS: No specific risk factors are known.

MECHANISM: Not established.

CLINICAL EVALUATION: While no published data are available for evaluation, the manufacturer of indinavir has made available some data on this interaction. The administration of indinavir 1,000 mg every 8 hours with zidovudine 200 mg every 8 hours for 7 days increased the indinavir area under the concentration-time curve (AUC) 13% and increased the zidovudine AUC 17%.[1] In a second study, indinavir 800 mg every 8 hours administered with both zidovudine 200 mg every 8 hours and lamivudine (*Epivir*) 150 mg twice daily for 7 days had no effect on the serum concentration of indinavir, but a 36% increase in zidovudine concentration was noted.[1] While no information regarding the clinical effects of the changes in serum zidovudine concentrations was provided, the changes are limited and increased adverse reactions are not likely to be observed.

RELATED DRUGS: Ritonavir (*Norvir*) has been reported to reduce zidovudine serum concentrations, while saquinavir (*Invirase*) does not appear to alter zidovudine concentrations. Stavudine (*Zerit*) administration did not affect indinavir; indinavir increased stavudine concentrations.

MANAGEMENT OPTIONS: No specific action is required, but be alert for evidence of the interaction.

REFERENCES:

1. *Crixivan* [package insert]. Whitehouse Station, NJ: Merck & Company; 1996.

Indomethacin (eg, *Indocin*)

Lithium (eg, *Eskalith*)

SUMMARY: Indomethacin may increase plasma lithium concentrations.

RISK FACTORS: No specific risk factors are known.

MECHANISM: Indomethacin reduces renal lithium excretion, probably due to indomethacin-induced prostaglandin inhibition. The resulting reduction in renal sodium excretion may lead to increased lithium reabsorption from the renal tubule.

CLINICAL EVALUATION: Indomethacin 150 mg/day reduces renal lithium clearance and increases plasma lithium concentrations.[1,2] The magnitude of the increases appears sufficient to cause lithium toxicity in some patients. If the mechanism of the interaction is prostaglandin inhibition, most other nonsteroidal anti-inflammatory drugs (NSAIDs) would be expected to increase plasma lithium concentrations as well.

RELATED DRUGS: Most NSAIDs increase lithium serum concentrations, but sulindac (eg, *Clinoril*) and aspirin appear to have minimal effects.

MANAGEMENT OPTIONS:

➡ *Consider Alternative.* If appropriate for the patient, consider using an anti-inflammatory agent that is less likely to affect lithium, such as sulindac or aspirin.

➡ *Monitor.* plasma lithium concentrations carefully if indomethacin (or another NSAID) is initiated or discontinued in patients on lithium therapy. Monitor also for lithium toxicity (eg, nausea, vomiting, diarrhea, anorexia, coarse tremor, slurred speech, vertigo, confusion, lethargy; in severe cases, seizures, stupor, coma, cardiovascular collapse).

REFERENCES:

1. Frolich JC, et al. Indomethacin increases plasma lithium. *Br Med J.* 1978;1:1115.
2. Ragheb M, et al. Interaction of indomethacin and ibuprofen with lithium in manic patients under a steady-state lithium level. *J Clin Psychiatry.* 1980;41:397.

Indomethacin (eg, *Indocin*)

Methotrexate (eg, *Rheumatrex*)

SUMMARY: Isolated cases indicate that indomethacin may increase the toxicity of antineoplastic doses of methotrexate.

RISK FACTORS:

➡ *Concurrent Diseases.* Particular caution is suggested in patients with pre-existing renal impairment (who may be more susceptible to nonsteroidal anti-inflammatory drug [NSAID]-induced renal failure).

➡ *Dosage Regimen.* The risk of adverse effects from this interaction is primarily in patients receiving antineoplastic doses of methotrexate rather than the lower doses used to treat rheumatoid arthritis, psoriasis, and related diseases.

MECHANISM: It is widely held that NSAIDs interfere with renal secretion of methotrexate, either by inhibiting tubular secretion of methotrexate or by reducing renal blood flow by inhibiting prostaglandin synthesis. Alterations in plasma protein binding also have been proposed, but this is unlikely to be clinically significant because methotrexate is normally only 50% to 70% bound to plasma proteins. Pharmacokinetic studies involving several different NSAIDs have failed to identify consistently an alteration in methotrexate pharmacokinetics by NSAIDs[1-8]; however, even in studies where methotrexate pharmacokinetics remained unchanged overall, occasional patients appeared to exhibit reduced clearance of methotrexate after NSAID administration.[1-3]

CLINICAL EVALUATION: Two patients receiving methotrexate and fluorouracil developed intractable nausea, vomiting, and renal failure about 2 weeks after starting indomethacin; both patients died.[14] Another patient receiving indomethacin (90 mg/day) developed higher than expected serum methotrexate concentrations, acute renal failure, severe nausea and vomiting, confusion, and weakness.[15] Although a causal relationship was not established, the severity of the reactions and the reports of similar reactions following other NSAIDs suggest that this potential interaction should not be ignored. Patients receiving low-dose methotrexate for rheumatoid arthritis frequently receive concurrent NSAIDs, and severe methotrexate toxicity in such patients is unusual.[10-12] Although these patients would appear to be at low risk, caution is warranted since NSAID use in patients on low-dose methotrexate is occasionally associated with severe methotrexate toxicity.[9,13]

RELATED DRUGS: See Clinical Evaluation.

MANAGEMENT OPTIONS:

➡ *Avoid Unless Benefit Outweighs Risk.* Until more information is available on this interaction, it would be prudent to avoid indomethacin (as well as other NSAIDs) in patients receiving antineoplastic doses of methotrexate. Particular caution is suggested in patients with pre-existing renal impairment who may be more susceptible to NSAID-induced renal failure.

➡ *Monitor.* If the combination is used, monitor for methotrexate toxicity. Findings in methotrexate toxicity can include stomatitis, severe gastrointestinal symptoms (eg, nausea, diarrhea, vomiting), bone marrow suppression, fever, bleeding, skin rashes, nephrotoxicity, and hepatotoxicity. Although decreasing the methotrexate dosage would be expected to reduce the likelihood of toxicity, the magnitude of the required reduction in methotrexate dosage has not been established.

REFERENCES:

1. Aherne A, et al. Methotrexate kinetics in rheumatoid arthritis: is there an interaction with nonsteroidal antiinflammatory drugs? *J Rheumatol*. 1988;15:1356.
2. Furst DE, et al. Effect of aspirin and sulindac on methotrexate clearance. *J Pharm Sci*. 1990;79:782.
3. Dupuis LL, et al. Methotrexate-nonsteroidal antiinflammatory drug interaction in children with arthritis. *J Rheumatol*. 1990;17:1469.
4. Leigler DG, et al. The effect of organic acids on renal clearance of methotrexate in man. *Clin Pharmacol Ther*. 1969;10:849.
5. Skeith KJ, et al. Lack of significant interaction between low dose methotrexate and ibuprofen or flurbiprofen in patients with arthritis. *J Rheumatol*. 1990;17:1008.
6. Stewart CF et al. Effect of aspirin (ASA) on disposition of methotrexate (MTX) in patients with rheumatoid arthritis (RA). *Clin Pharmacol Ther*. 1990;47:139. Abstract PP-56.
7. Taylor JR et al. Effect of sodium salicylate and indomethacin on methotrexate-serum albumin binding. *Arch Dermatol*. 1977;113:588.
8. Tracy FS et al. The effect of NSAIDs on methotrexate disposition in patients with rheumatoid arthritis. *Clin Pharmacol Ther*. 1990;47:138. Abstract PP-54.
9. Daly HM et al. Methotrexate toxicity precipitated by azapropazone. *Br J Dermatol*. 1986;114:733.

10. Boh LE et al. Low-dose weekly oral methotrexate therapy for inflammatory arthritis. *Clin Pharm.* 1986;5:503.

11. Anderson PA et al. Weekly pulse methotrexate in rheumatoid arthritis: clinical and immunologic effects in a randomized, double-blind study. *Ann Intern Med.* 1985;103:489.

12. Tugwell P et al. Methotrexate in rheumatoid arthritis: indications, contraindications, efficacy, and safety. *Ann Intern Med.* 1987;107:358.

13. Adams JD et al. Drug interactions in psoriasis. *Aust J Dermatol.* 1976;17:39.

14. Ellison NM et al. Acute renal failure and death following sequential intermediate-dose methotrexate and 5-FU: a possible adverse effect due to concomitant indomethacin administration. *Cancer Treat Rep.* 1985;69:342.

15. Maiche AG. Acute renal failure due to concomitant action of methotrexate and indomethacin. *Lancet.* 1986;1:1390.

Indomethacin (eg, *Indocin*)

Nifedipine (eg, *Procardia*)

SUMMARY: Short-term use of indomethacin does not appear to alter the hypotensive response to calcium channel blockers like nifedipine.

RISK FACTORS: No specific risk factors are known.

MECHANISM: No interaction.

CLINICAL EVALUATION: Twelve hypertensive patients chronically treated with nifedipine 20 mg twice daily received indomethacin 50 mg twice daily or a placebo for 1 week.[1] Indomethacin did not alter the hypotensive response to nifedipine.

RELATED DRUGS: Twelve healthy subjects took a single dose of felodipine (*Plendil*) 10 mg following pretreatment with placebo or indomethacin 25 mg 4 times/day for 3 days.[2] Felodipine pharmacokinetics, pharmacodynamics, and hypotensive effects were unchanged by indomethacin administration. No change in nimodipine (*Nimotop*) response was noted in subjects receiving concomitant indomethacin 25 mg twice daily for 5 days compared with nimodipine alone, although nimodipine area under the concentration-time curve was increased 8%.[3] Indomethacin 75 mg SR twice daily produced no changes in verapamil (eg, *Calan*) pharmacokinetics or hypotensive efficacy.[4] The short-term use of other nonsteroidal anti-inflammatory drugs would be unlikely to affect the hypotensive effect of nifedipine.

MANAGEMENT OPTIONS: No interaction.

REFERENCES:

1. Salvetti A, et al. Calcium antagonists: interactions in hypertension. *Am J Nephrol.* 1986;6(suppl 1):95-99.

2. Hardy BG, et al. Effect of indomethacin on the pharmacokinetics and pharmacodynamics of felodipine. *Br J Clin Pharmacol.* 1988;26:557-562.

3. Muck W, et al. Steady-state pharmacokinetics of nimodipine during chronic administration of indomethacin in elderly healthy volunteers. *Arzneimittelforschung.* 1995;45:460-462.

4. Perreault MM, et al. Effect of indomethacin on the pharmacodynamics and on the stereoselective pharmacokinetics of verapamil and nor-verapamil in hypertensive patients. *Pharmacotherapy.* 1995;15:109.

Indomethacin (eg, *Indocin*)

Prazosin (eg, *Minipress*)

SUMMARY: In some patients indomethacin may inhibit the antihypertensive response to prazosin; the effect of other nonsteroidal anti-inflammatory drugs (NSAIDs) is not known, but they may produce a similar effect.

RISK FACTORS: No specific risk factors are known.

MECHANISM: Inhibition of prostaglandin synthesis by NSAIDs is probably responsible for the inhibition of the antihypertensive effect of prazosin.

CLINICAL EVALUATION: Indomethacin pretreatment may have inhibited the hypotensive effect of a single 5 mg dose of prazosin in 4 of 9 healthy subjects.[1] The effect of chronic therapy with both drugs is not known.

RELATED DRUGS: The effect of other NSAIDs on prazosin has not been studied, but they probably produce a similar response. Ibuprofen (eg, *Motrin*) in a dose of 400 mg 3 times/day for 3 weeks has been shown to increase the mean blood pressure by approximately 5 to 7 mm Hg in a parallel trial of 45 hypertensive patients receiving a variety of antihypertensive drugs.[2] Doxazosin (eg, *Cardura*) and terazosin (eg, *Hytrin*) probably interact with NSAIDs in a similar manner.

MANAGEMENT OPTIONS:

➡ **Consider Alternative.** Sulindac (eg, *Clinoril*) appears less likely than other NSAIDs to inhibit the antihypertensive response to beta-blockers, captopril (eg, *Capoten*), and thiazides. It is possible that sulindac also would have less effect on prazosin.

➡ **Monitor.** Monitor for reduced hypotensive response to prazosin (or other antihypertensive agents) when NSAIDs are given concurrently. If blood pressure increases, alteration in antihypertensive drug dosage or the use of alternative antihypertensive agents may be required.

REFERENCES:

1. Rubin P, et al. Studies on the clinical pharmacology of prazosin. II: The influence of indomethacin and of propranolol on the action and disposition of prazosin. *Br J Clin Pharmacol*. 1980;10:33-39.
2. Radack KL, et al. Ibuprofen interferes with the efficacy of antihypertensive drugs: a randomized, double-blind, placebo-controlled trial of ibuprofen compared with acetaminophen. *Ann Intern Med*. 1987;107:628-635.

Indomethacin (eg, *Indocin*)

Prednisone (eg, *Deltasone*)

SUMMARY: The combined effects of prednisone and indomethacin may result in an increased incidence or severity of GI ulceration; other combinations of nonsteroidal anti-inflammatory drugs (NSAIDs) and corticosteroids probably produce a similar effect.

RISK FACTORS: No specific risk factors are known.

MECHANISM: NSAIDs and corticosteroids have been implicated in producing damage to the GI mucosa; the effects may be additive. Indomethacin apparently does not displace cortisol from protein binding[1] as was previously suggested.

CLINICAL EVALUATION: The use of prednisone in conjunction with indomethacin appeared to increase the tendency for gastric ulceration in 6 patients, but a cause-and-effect relationship was not established.[2]

RELATED DRUGS: If indomethacin does increase GI toxicity of corticosteroids, other NSAIDs would be expected to act similarly.

MANAGEMENT OPTIONS:

➡ *Circumvent/Minimize.* Consider the concurrent use of misoprostol (*Cytotec*).

➡ *Monitor.* Be particularly alert for evidence of GI ulceration and bleeding in patients receiving combinations of NSAIDs and corticosteroids.

REFERENCES:

1. Hvidberg E, et al. Influence of indomethacin on the distribution of cortisol in man. *Eur J Clin Pharmacol.* 1971;3:102.

2. Emmanuel JH, et al. Gastric ulcer and the anti-arthritic drugs. *Postgrad Med J.* 1971;47:227-232.

Indomethacin (eg, *Indocin*)

Probenecid

SUMMARY: Probenecid increases plasma indomethacin concentrations, but the interaction has not been shown to be detrimental; some patients may manifest an increased therapeutic response to indomethacin with concomitant probenecid.

RISK FACTORS: No specific risk factors are known.

MECHANISM: Indomethacin appears to undergo renal tubular secretion that may be blocked by probenecid.

CLINICAL EVALUATION: In one study of 6 subjects, indomethacin serum levels were increased considerably by concomitant probenecid administration.[1] The half-life of indomethacin alone was 10.1 hours, and it increased to 17.6 hours when probenecid also was given. Preliminary results from another study were similar.[2] The increased plasma indomethacin levels may be associated with an increased therapeutic response without a corresponding increase in side effects.[3] Thus, the interaction between probenecid and indomethacin may be favorable in at least some patients.

RELATED DRUGS: Probenecid also inhibits the elimination of some other nonsteroidal anti-inflammatory drugs (eg, ketoprofen [eg, *Orudis*], naproxen [eg, *Naprosyn*]).

MANAGEMENT OPTIONS: No specific action is required, but be alert for evidence of the interaction.

REFERENCES:

1. Skeith MD, et al. The renal excretion of indomethacin and its inhibition by probenecid. *Clin Pharmacol Ther.* 1968;9:89.

2. Emori W, et al. The pharmacokinetics of indomethacin in serum. *Clin Pharmacol Ther.* 1973;14:134.

3. Baber N, et al. The interaction between indomethacin and probenecid: a clinical and pharmacokinetic study. *Clin Pharmacol Ther.* 1978;24:298.

Indomethacin (eg, *Indocin*)

Propranolol (eg, *Inderal*)

SUMMARY: Indomethacin and many other nonsteroidal anti-inflammatory drugs (NSAIDs) can reduce the hypotensive effect of propranolol and other beta blockers.

RISK FACTORS:

➡ ***Dosage Regimen.*** Chronic administration of an NSAID may inhibit antihypertensive response.

MECHANISM: Not established. It is proposed that the antihypertensive action of beta blockers may involve prostaglandins and related substances which are in turn affected by prostaglandin inhibitors, such as indomethacin.

CLINICAL EVALUATION: In hypertensive patients given beta blockers (including propranolol, pindolol [eg, *Visken*], labetalol [eg, *Normodyne*], and atenolol [eg, *Tenormin*] the administration of indomethacin was associated with inhibition of the antihypertensive response.[1,2,6,7,12] In other studies the antihypertensive response to oxprenolol was reduced 50% by indomethacin 100 mg/day[8] and also reversed by sulfinpyrazone (eg, *Anturane*) 400 mg twice daily.[11] Piroxicam (eg, *Feldene*)[3,4] and perhaps naproxen (eg, *Naprosyn*)[4,5] also may reduce the antihypertensive effects of beta blockers. Sulindac (eg, *Clinoril*) appears least likely to interfere with the antihypertensive effects of beta blockers.[2-5,10,13] Indomethacin has been reported to increase coronary and systemic artery resistance.[9,14] It is not known whether this property of indomethacin would affect adversely patients receiving beta blockers for angina. The use of NSAIDs for less than 1 week probably will have little effect on beta blocker efficacy in most patients.

RELATED DRUGS: Other beta blockers may be affected similarly. Other NSAIDs probably produce a similar effect, but there may be differences in the magnitude of the interaction with different NSAIDs. (See Clinical Evaluation.)

MANAGEMENT OPTIONS:

➡ ***Circumvent/Minimize.*** Using the shortest duration of NSAID therapy will minimize the magnitude of the interaction. Using an antihypertensive other than a beta blocker may not circumvent the interaction because NSAIDs generally tend to inhibit the effect of antihypertensives.

➡ ***Monitor.*** Patients should be monitored for altered antihypertensive or antianginal response to beta blockers when indomethacin is initiated or discontinued. Short-term NSAID use requires no special precautions.

REFERENCES:

1. Ylitalo P, et al. Inhibition of prostaglandin synthesis by indomethacin interacts with the antihypertensive effect of atenolol. *Clin Pharmacol Ther*. 1985;38:443.
2. Salvetti A, et al. The influence of indomethacin and sulindac on some pharmacological actions of atenolol in hypertensive patients. *Br J Clin Pharmacol*. 1984;17:108S.
3. Ebel DL, et al. Effect of sulindac, piroxicam and placebo on the hypotensive effect of propranolol in patients with mild to moderate essential hypertension. *Scand J Rheumatol*. 1986;62:41.
4. Chalmers JP, et al. Effects of indomethacin, sulindac, naproxen, aspirin, and paracetamol in treated hypertensive patients. *Clin Exp Hypertens*. 1984;6:1077.
5. Wong DG, et al. Nonsteroidal antiinflammatory drugs (NSAIDs) vs. placebo in hypertension treated with diuretic and beta blocker. *Clin Pharmacol Ther*. 1984;35:284.

6. Sugimoto K, et al. Influence of indomethacin on a reduction in forearm blood flow induced by pro-pranolol in healthy subjects. *J Clin Pharmacol.* 1989;29:307.

7. Watkins J, et al. Attenuation of hypotensive effect of propranolol and thiazide diuretics by indometha-cin. *Br J Med.* 1980;218:702.

8. Salvetti A, et al. Interaction between oxprenolol and indomethacin on blood pressure in essential hypertensive patients. *Eur J Clin Pharmacol.* 1982;22:197.

9. Friedman PL, et al. Coronary vasoconstrictor effect of indomethacin in patients with coronary-artery disease. *N Engl J Med.* 1981;305:1171.

10. Wong DG, et al. Effect of non-steroidal anti-inflammatory drugs on control of hypertension by beta-blockers and diuretics. *Lancet.* 1986;1:997.

11. Ferrara LA, et al. Interference by sulphinpyrazone with the antihypertensive effects of oxprenolol. *Eur J Clin Pharmacol.* 1986;29:717.

12. Abate MA, et al. Interaction of indomethacin and sulindac with labetalol. *Br J Clin Pharmacol.* 1991;31:363.

13. Schuna AA, et al. Lack of interaction between sulindac or naproxen and propranolol in hypertensive patients. *J Clin Pharmacol.* 1989;29:524.

14. Forman MB, et al. Effects of indomethacin on systemic coronary hemodynamics in patients with coro-nary artery disease. *Am Heart J.* 1985;110:311.

Indomethacin (eg, *Indocin*)

Thiazides (eg, chlorothiazide)

SUMMARY: Indomethacin and other nonsteroidal anti-inflammatory drugs (NSAIDs) appear to cause a mild reduction in the antihypertensive action of thiazides.

RISK FACTORS: No specific risk factors are known.

MECHANISM: Because thiazides have limited vasodilatory effects and induce little prostaglandin production, the NSAIDs generally exert less influence on thiazide hypotensive effects than on those of furosemide. However, NSAID-induced sodium and water retention may reduce the effectiveness of thiazides.[4]

CLINICAL EVALUATION: Indomethacin and sulindac (eg, *Clinoril*) have been found to have little effect on the antihypertensive effect of thiazides.[1-3] Indomethacin was reported to reverse the reduction in plasma potassium and increase the renin con-centrations that follow thiazide administration.[3]

RELATED DRUGS: Until proved otherwise, assume that all combinations of a thiazide and an NSAID would interact similarly. Sulindac has been reported to reduce the renal clearance of hydrochlorothiazide[2] but appears to have no effect on thiazide anti-hypertensive effects.[6] Ibuprofen (eg, *Motrin*) 3200 mg/day[5] or 1200 mg/day[6] also has been shown to have little effect on the antihypertensive effect of thiazide diuretics.

MANAGEMENT OPTIONS: No specific action is required, but be alert for evidence of the interaction.

REFERENCES:

1. Koopmans PP, et al. Influence of non-steroidal anti-inflammatory drugs on diuretic treatment of mild to moderate essential hypertension. *Br Med J.* 1984;289:1492.

2. Koopmans PP, et al. Effects of indomethacin and sulindac on hydrochlorothiazide kinetics. *Clin Phar-macol Ther.* 1985;37:625.

3. Koopmans PP, et al. The effects of sulindac and indomethacin on the antihypertensive and diuretic action of hydrochlorothiazide in patients with mild to moderate essential hypertension. *Br J Clin Pharmacol.* 1986;21:417.

4. Dixey JJ, et al. The effects of naproxen and sulindac on renal function and their interaction with hydrochlorothiazide and piretanide in man. *Br J Clin Pharmacol.* 1987;23:55.

5. Wright JT, et al. The effect of high-dose short-term ibuprofen on antihypertensive control with hydrochlorothiazide. *Clin Pharmacol Ther.* 1989;46:440.

6. Koopmans PP, et al. The influence of ibuprofen, diclofenac and sulindac on the blood pressure lowering effect of hydrochlorothiazide. *Eur J Clin Pharmacol.* 1987;31:553.

Indomethacin (eg, *Indocin*)

Triamterene (*Dyrenium*)

SUMMARY: Some patients develop acute renal failure when indomethacin and triamterene are administered concurrently.

RISK FACTORS: No specific risk factors are known.

MECHANISM: Indomethacin may inhibit the normal secretion of prostaglandins which protect against triamterene-induced nephrotoxicity.

CLINICAL EVALUATION: In one study 4 healthy subjects were given triamterene 200 mg/day for 3 days with and without indomethacin 150 mg/day before and during triamterene therapy.[1] Two of the subjects developed substantial reductions (62% and 72%) in creatinine clearance with concurrent administration of the drugs but not with either drug alone. Triamterene was associated with 60% and 69% reductions in urinary indomethacin excretion in these 2 subjects. The magnitude of the reductions in renal function in the 2 affected subjects following concurrent use of triamterene and indomethacin is sufficient to question the advisability of using the combination in practice. Additional case reports of this interaction between triamterene and indomethacin have appeared.[2,3]

RELATED DRUGS: Nephrotoxicity was not seen when indomethacin was combined with furosemide (eg, *Lasix*), hydrochlorothiazide (eg, *Dyazide*), or spironolactone (eg, *Aldactone*)[1] Cases of reduced renal function have been reported with triamterene combined with other nonsteroidal anti-inflammatory drugs (NSAIDs), one involving diclofenac (eg, *Voltaren*) and triamterene[4] and one involving ibuprofen (eg, *Motrin*) and triamterene.[5] Other NSAIDs also may interact, but little information is available.

MANAGEMENT OPTIONS:

➡ ***Consider Alternative.*** It is possible that spironolactone and amiloride are less likely than triamterene to interact adversely with indomethacin, but this has not been established clinically.

➡ ***Monitor.*** Carefully monitor renal function in patients on combined therapy with triamterene and indomethacin (or other NSAIDs).

REFERENCES:

1. Favre L, et al. Reversible acute renal failure from combined triamterene and indomethacin: a study in healthy subjects. *Ann Intern Med.* 1982;96:317.

2. McCarthy JT, et al. Acute intrinsic renal failure induced by indomethacin. *Mayo Clin Proc.* 1982;57:289.

3. Weinberg MS, et al. Anuric renal failure precipitated by indomethacin and triamterene. *Nephron.* 1985;40:216.

4. Harkonen M, et al. Reversible deterioration of renal function after diclofenac in patient receiving triamterene. *Br Med J.* 1986;293:698.

5. Gehr TWB, et al. Interaction of triamterene-hydrochlorothiazide and ibuprofen. *Clin Pharmacol Ther.* 1990;47:200. Abstract.

Indomethacin (*Indocin*)

Vancomycin (*Vancocin*)

SUMMARY: Indomethacin administration may increase the concentration of vancomycin in neonates; vancomycin toxicity may result.

RISK FACTORS: No specific risk factors known.

MECHANISM: Not established; however, indomethacin may reduce the renal clearance of vancomycin.

CLINICAL EVALUATION: Vancomycin pharmacokinetics were studied in 6 neonates with patent ductus arteriosus (PDA) who had received indomethacin and 5 control neonates without PDA who did not receive indomethacin.[1] Vancomycin clearance was approximately 50% lower and its half-life 3 times greater (25 vs 7 hours) in the indomethacin-treated neonates compared to the control neonates.

RELATED DRUGS: Other nonsteroidal anti-inflammatory drugs may affect vancomycin in a similar manner.

MANAGEMENT OPTIONS:

➡ *Circumvent/Minimize.* Vancomycin dosage may need to be reduced during indomethacin coadministration.

➡ *Monitor.* Vancomycin concentrations should be monitored in neonates receiving indomethacin.

REFERENCES:

1. Spivey MJ, et al. Vancomycin pharmacokinetics in neonates. *Am J Dis Child.* 1986;149:859.

Indomethacin (eg, *Indocin*)

Warfarin (eg, *Coumadin*)

SUMMARY: Although isolated case reports of indomethacin-induced increases in the hypoprothrombinemic response to warfarin have appeared, most patients do not manifest an enhanced anticoagulant effect. Nonetheless, caution is indicated during cotherapy with these drugs because of possible detrimental effects of indomethacin on the gastric mucosa and platelet function.

RISK FACTORS:

➡ *Concurrent Diseases.* Patients with peptic ulcer disease (PUD) or a history of gastrointestinal (GI) bleeding are probably at greater risk.

MECHANISM: Indomethacin does not affect the hypoprothrombinemic response to oral anticoagulants in most patients, but indomethacin-induced gastric erosions and inhibition of platelet function[1] theoretically could increase the risk of bleeding in patients receiving oral anticoagulants. The significance of any displacement of oral anticoagulants from plasma protein binding by indomethacin is not clear.[2]

CLINICAL EVALUATION: In one study, when indomethacin 25 mg 3 times a day for 3 weeks was given to 16 patients stabilized on phenprocoumon, no mean change in the hypoprothrombinemic response to phenprocoumon was observed during indomethacin administration.[3] In another study indomethacin 100 mg/day for 5 days failed to affect the hypoprothrombinemic response to warfarin given chronically to 16 healthy subjects, and indomethacin 100 mg/day for 11 days also failed to affect either the hypoprothrombinemic response or plasma half-life of single doses of warfarin in 19 healthy subjects.[4] These studies indicate that indomethacin is not likely to affect the hypoprothrombinemic response to oral anticoagulants, at least in doses up to 100 mg/day. Nevertheless, since isolated cases of possible indomethacin-induced increases in warfarin hypoprothrombinemia have been reported,[5-8,10,11] one should recognize the possibility that such a reaction may occur in rare instances. In a retrospective cohort study, hospitalizations for hemorrhagic PUD were approximately 13 times higher in patients receiving warfarin plus a nonsteroidal anti-inflammatory drug (NSAID) than in patients receiving neither drug.[9]

RELATED DRUGS: All NSAIDs inhibit platelet function, cause gastric erosions, and probably increase the risk of GI bleeding. Some NSAIDs, however, such as ibuprofen (eg, *Motrin*), naproxen (eg, *Naprosyn*), or diclofenac (eg, *Voltaren*) may be less likely to increase oral anticoagulant-induced hypoprothrombinemia than other NSAIDs.

MANAGEMENT OPTIONS:

➡ *Avoid Unless Benefit Outweighs Risk.* Since all NSAIDs probably increase the risk of GI bleeding in patients on oral anticoagulants, use the combination only after careful consideration of the benefit versus risk. If an NSAID must be used with an oral anticoagulant, it would be prudent to use NSAIDs that are unlikely to affect the hypoprothrombinemic response to oral anticoagulants. If the NSAID is being used as an analgesic or antipyretic, acetaminophen is probably safer to use with oral anticoagulants. Non-acetylated salicylates (eg, choline salicylate, magnesium salicylate, salsalate, sodium salicylate) also are probably safer with oral anticoagulants than NSAIDs since such salicylates have minimal effects on platelet function and the gastric mucosa.

➡ *Monitor.* If any NSAID is used with an oral anticoagulant, one should carefully monitor the prothrombin time and watch for evidence of bleeding, especially from the GI tract.

REFERENCES:

1. Zucker MB, et al. Effect of acetylsalicylic acid, other nonsteroidal antiinflammatory agents, and dipyridamole on human blood platelets. *J Lab Clin Med.* 1970;76:66.

2. Hoffbrand BI, et al. Potentiation of anticoagulants. *Br Med J.* 1967;2:838. Letter.

3. Frost H, et al. Concomitant administration of indomethacin and anticoagulants. International Symposium on Inflammation, Freiburg Im Breisgau. Germany. 1966, May.

4. Vesell ES, et al. Failure of indomethacin and warfarin to interact in normal human volunteers. *J Clin Pharmacol.* 1975;15:486.

5. Koch-Weser J. Hemorrhagic reactions and drug interactions in 500 warfarin-treated patients. *Clin Pharmacol Ther.* 1973;14:139. Abstract.

6. Self TH, et al. Drug-enhancement of warfarin activity. *Lancet.* 1975;2:557. Letter.

7. McQueen EG. New Zealand committee on adverse drug reactions; tenth annual report, 1975. *N Z Med J.* 1975;82:308.

8. Self TH, et al. Possible interaction of indomethacin and warfarin. *DICP.* 1978;12:580.

9. Shorr RI, et al. Concurrent use of nonsteroidal anti-inflammatory drugs and oral anticoagulants places elderly persons at high risk hemorrhagic peptic ulcer disease. *Arch Intern Med.* 1993;153:1665.

10. Chan TYK, et al. Adverse interaction between warfarin and indomethacin. *Drug Safety.* 1994;10:267.

11. Day R, et al. Adverse interaction between warfarin and indomethacin. *Drug Safety.* 1994;1:213.

Influenza Vaccine ▼3

Phenytoin (eg, *Dilantin*)

SUMMARY: Some patients appear to develop an increase in total serum phenytoin concentrations following vaccination, but reductions in free serum phenytoin concentrations also have been reported. The clinical importance of these findings is not established.

RISK FACTORS: No specific risk factors are known.

MECHANISM: Not established; inhibition of phenytoin hepatic metabolism has been proposed.

CLINICAL EVALUATION: In 7 patients stabilized on phenytoin, influenza vaccination was associated with a slight decrease in plasma phenytoin concentrations.[1] When 15 elderly patients on chronic phenytoin were given inactivated whole-virion trivalent influenza vaccine, mean serum phenytoin concentrations did not change at day 7 or 14, but 4 patients had 46% to 170% increases in serum phenytoin.[2] The same vaccine did not appear to affect serum phenytoin in 31 men on chronic phenytoin.[3] In 8 mentally retarded patients on chronic phenytoin, influenza vaccine (types A and B, whole virus) was associated with a 60% increase in serum phenytoin 7 days after vaccination; phenytoin levels returned to baseline by day 14.[4] In 8 patients receiving phenytoin monotherapy for seizures, influenza vaccination (trivalent types A and B, subvirion) was followed by a slight and transient increase in total serum phenytoin followed by a somewhat larger decrease in free serum phenytoin 14 days after vaccination.[5] No change in seizure frequency was seen. The reason for the disparate results in the various studies is not clear, but it probably relates to differences in the vaccine used and the types of patients involved. In any case, clinical evidence of an alteration in phenytoin response due to influenza vaccination is minimal.

RELATED DRUGS: No information is available.

MANAGEMENT OPTIONS:

➡ *Monitor.* Although patients should be monitored for evidence of phenytoin toxicity following influenza vaccination, an adjustment in phenytoin dosage rarely is needed. If the phenytoin dose is changed, additional adjustments should be anticipated as the effect of the vaccine dissipates (this has taken as little as 2 weeks but may take much longer).

REFERENCES:

1. Sawchuk RJ, et al. Effect of influenza vaccination on plasma phenytoin concentration. *Ther Drug Monit.* 1979;1:285.

2. Levine M, et al. Increased serum phenytoin concentration following influenza vaccination. *Clin Pharm.* 1984;3:505.

3. Levine M, et al. Phenytoin therapy and immune response to influenza vaccine. *Clin Pharm.* 1985;4:191.

4. Jann MW, et al. Effect of influenza vaccine on serum anticonvulsant concentrations. *Clin Pharm.* 1986;5:817.

5. Smith CD, et al. Effect of influenza vaccine on serum concentrations of total and free phenytoin. *Clin Pharm.* 1988;7:828.

4 Influenza Vaccine

Theophylline (eg, *Theo-Dur*)

SUMMARY: Some influenza vaccines may increase serum theophylline concentrations, but the effect is usually not clinically significant.

RISK FACTORS: No specific risk factors are known.

MECHANISM: Some preparations of influenza vaccine may be capable of inhibiting the metabolism of theophylline, especially when the vaccine contains proteins from the virus or culture media that can act as interferon stimulators.

CLINICAL EVALUATION: Theophylline half-life was increased in subjects given single doses of theophylline before and after administration of influenza vaccine.[1] Patients with upper respiratory viral infections can have a reduced clearance of theophylline[2] and antipyrine.[3] In another study of patients taking chronic theophylline, however, no changes in theophylline concentrations were observed 24 hours following the administration of influenza vaccine.[4] Fischer et al, measured theophylline concentrations repeatedly over 2 weeks after an influenza vaccination in patients taking *Theo-Dur* and also reported no changes in serum concentrations.[5] The discrepant findings reported in these studies may be explained partially by the variety of patients and protocols used. More importantly, differences among vaccines may contribute to variations in the occurrence and extent of the interaction. Interferon induction by actual viral infections or by agents that stimulate interferon production can reduce hepatic metabolism.[6] Patients vaccinated with trivalent, subvirion vaccine (Wyeth Laboratories) had no increase in interferon levels and no alteration in their theophylline pharmacokinetics.[7] The use of newer, purified subvirion influenza vaccines in place of disrupted whole virion vaccines appears to reduce substantially the risk of an interaction between vaccine and theophylline.[8] It must be remembered, however, that viral illnesses also are associated with increased interferon production and can reduce theophylline metabolism; thus theophylline dosage may have to be decreased in patients with these illnesses.

RELATED DRUGS: The use of purified subvirion vaccines, which induce an antibody response but do not stimulate interferon production does not appear to alter theophylline metabolism.

MANAGEMENT OPTIONS: No specific action is required, but be alert for evidence of the interaction.

REFERENCES:

1. Renton KW, et al. Decreased elimination of theophylline after influenza vaccination. *Can Med Assoc J.* 1980;23:288.
2. Kraemer MJ, et al. Altered theophylline clearance during an influenza outbreak. *Pediatrics.* 1982;69:476.
3. Forsyth JS, et al. The effect of fever on antipyrine metabolism in children. *Br J Clin Pharmacol.* 1982;13:811.
4. Goldstein RS, et al. Decreased elimination of theophylline after influenza vaccination. *Can Med Assoc J.* 1982;126:470.
5. Fischer R, et al. Influence of trivalent influenza vaccine on serum theophylline levels. *Can Med Assoc J.* 1982;126:1312.
6. Renton K, et al. Depression of hepatic cytochrome P-450 dependent monooxygenase systems with administered interferon inducing agents. *Biochem Biophys Res Commun.* 1976;73:343.

7. Stults BM, et al. Influenza vaccination and theophylline pharmacokinetics in patients with chronic obstructive lung-disease. *West J Med*. 1983;139:651.

8. Winstanley PA, et al. Lack of effect of highly purified subunit influenza vaccination of theophylline metabolism. *Br J Clin Pharmacol*. 1985;20:47.

Influenza Vaccine 4

Warfarin (eg, *Coumadin*)

SUMMARY: Although isolated cases of an altered hypoprothrombinemic response to oral anticoagulants have occurred following influenza vaccination, most patients do not appear to be affected.

RISK FACTORS: No specific risk factors are known.

MECHANISM: Some have proposed that influenza vaccination may inhibit the hepatic metabolism of warfarin; yet serum warfarin concentrations do not appear to be increased by the vaccine.[1] Because fever increases the degradation of clotting factors,[2] patients who develop vaccination-induced pyrexia theoretically could manifest a transient increase in the hypoprothrombinemic response to oral anticoagulants.

CLINICAL EVALUATION: In a study of 8 patients on chronic warfarin, influenza vaccine (trivalent, types A and B) tended to increase the hypoprothrombinemic response but did not affect serum warfarin concentrations; warfarin half-life also was unaffected in 12 subjects for up to 3 weeks following the influenza vaccination.[1] In another study of 33 patients on chronic warfarin therapy, influenza vaccination (trivalent, types A and B) slightly decreased the hypoprothrombinemic response.[9] Several other studies in anticoagulated patients found that influenza vaccine had little or no effect on warfarin or acenocoumarol half-life or hypoprothrombinemic response.[3-7,10] Thus, in most patients, influenza vaccination probably will affect the hypoprothrombinemic response to warfarin only slightly or not at all. Nonetheless, the possibility that an occasional predisposed patient will manifest a clinically significant effect cannot be ruled out; isolated cases of severe bleeding have occurred in warfarin-treated patients following influenza vaccination.[1,8]

RELATED DRUGS: Acenocoumarol[+] may interact similarly. It also has been reported that intramuscular injection of influenza vaccine in patients receiving anticoagulants can result in large hematomas,[1] but this has not been a consistent finding.[11]

MANAGEMENT OPTIONS: No specific action is required, but be alert for evidence of the interaction.

REFERENCES:

1. Kramer P, et al. Effect of influenza vaccine on warfarin anticoagulation. *Clin Pharmacol Ther*. 1984;35:416.

2. Loeliger EA, et al. The biological disappearance rate of prothrombin and factors VII, IX and X from plasma in hypothyroidism, hyperthyroidism and during fever. *Thromb Diath Haemorrh*. 1964;10:267.

3. Lipsky BA, et al. Influenza vaccination and warfarin anticoagulation. *Ann Intern Med*. 1984;100:835.

4. Gomolin IH, et al. Lack of effect of influenza vaccine on theophylline levels and warfarin anticoagulation in the elderly. *J Am Geriatr Soc*. 1985;33:269.

5. Weibert RT, et al. Effect of influenza vaccine in patients receiving long-term warfarin therapy. *Clin Pharm*. 1986;5:499.

6. Bussey III, et al. Influence of influenza vaccine on warfarin therapy. *DICP*. 1986;20:460.

7. Gomolin IH. Lack of effect of influenza vaccine on warfarin anticoagulation in the elderly. *Can Med Assoc J*. 1986;135:39.

8. Sumner HW, et al. Drug induced liver disease.*Geriatrics.* 1981;36:83.

9. Bussey HI, et al. Effect of influenza vaccine on chronic warfarin therapy. *DICP.* 1988;22:198.

10. Souto JC, et al. Lack of effect of influenza vaccine on anticoagulation by acenocoumarol. *Ann Pharmacother.* 1993;27:365.

11. Delafuente JC, et al. A comparison of subcutaneous and intramuscular routes of administration of influenza vaccine in warfarin anticoagulated elderly patients. *Pharmacotherapy.* 1993;13:275. Abstract.

† Not available in the United States.

  Insulin

Contraceptives, Oral (eg, *Ortho-Novum*)

SUMMARY: Oral contraceptives have been noted to impair glucose tolerance, but this effect may be infrequent with preparations containing less than 50 mcg of estrogen.

RISK FACTORS:

➡ ***Dosage Regimen.*** Ethinyl estradiol content above 50 mcg may impair glucose tolerance.

MECHANISM: Not established.

CLINICAL EVALUATION: Several studies have found that oral contraceptives with estrogen content more than 50 mcg can produce a small impairment in glucose tolerance in patients with and without a predisposition to diabetes.[2-4] A patient receiving acetohexamide (*Dymelor*) developed a worsening of diabetic control after starting an oral contraceptive containing norethynodrel 2.5 mg with mestranol 0.1 mg. In 1 study, the glucose intolerance was greatest with 75 mcg of estrogen. less with 50 mcg estrogen, and lowest with 35 mcg of estrogen.[5] Similarly, a small study found minimal alteration in oral glucose tolerance tests after 6 months of treatment with an oral contraceptive containing 0.4 mg norethindrone and 35 mcg of ethinyl estradiol.[6] Small increases in fasting glucose have been noted in patients taking progestin-only contraceptives.[7]

RELATED DRUGS: Acetohexamide may be affected similarly by oral contraceptives. Diethylstilbestrol (DES) has been reported both to increase and decrease blood glucose.[1] Conjugated estrogens (*Premarin*) may effect the serum glucose concentration in a manner similar to oral contraceptives.

MANAGEMENT OPTIONS:

➡ ***Monitor.*** No specific action is required, but be alert for evidence of this interaction.

REFERENCES:

1. Sotaniemi EA, et al. Effect of diethylstilbestrol on blood glucose of prostatic cancer patients. *Invest Urol.* 1973;10:438.

2. Wynn V, et al. Some effects of oral contraceptives on carbohydrate metabolism. *Lancet.* 1969;2:761.

3. Wingerd J, et al. Oral contraceptive use and other factors in the standard glucose tolerance test. *Diabetes.* 1977;26:1024.

4. Posner NA, et al. Changes on carbohydrate tolerance during long-term oral contraception. *Am J Obstet Gynecol.* 1975;123:119.

5. Wynn V, et al. Comparison of effects of different combined oral-contraceptive formulations on carbohydrate and lipid metabolism. *Lancet.* 1979;1:1045.

6. Spellacy WN, et al. The effects of "low-estrogen" oral contraceptive on carbohydrate metabolism during six months of treatment: a preliminary report of blood glucose and plasma insulin values. *Fertil Steril.* 1977;28:885.

7. Goldman JA, et al. Blood glucose levels and glucose tolerance in prediabetic and subclinical diabetic women on a low dose progestogen contraceptive. *Isr J Med Sci.* 1970;6:703.

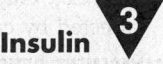

Insulin

Marijuana

SUMMARY: Marijuana use may increase serum glucose concentrations.

RISK FACTORS: No specific risk factors are known.

MECHANISM: Not established.

CLINICAL EVALUATION: Preliminary evidence indicates that marijuana use may impair glucose tolerance.[2] A patient with diabetes developed a threefold increase in insulin requirements following the use of amphetamines and marijuana.[1] Whether either drug was individually responsible for the effect on insulin requirements in this case was not determined. In another case, diabetic ketoacidosis followed the oral ingestion of large amounts of marijuana in a 21-year-old man.[3] In a study of 6 subjects, delta-9-tetrahydrocannabinol (6 mg IV) impaired glucose tolerance.[4]

RELATED DRUGS: Marijuana may affect glucose tolerance in patients taking oral hypoglycemic agents.

MANAGEMENT OPTIONS:

➡ *Monitor.* Diabetic patients should be aware that marijuana use might affect glucose tolerance.

REFERENCES:

1. Lockhart JG. Effects of "speed" and "pot" on the juvenile diabetic (Questions and Answers). *JAMA.* 1970;214:2065.

2. Pololsky S, et al. Effect of marijuana on the glucose-tolerance test. *Ann NY Acad Sci.* 1971;191:54.

3. Hughes JE, et al. Marijuana and the diabetic coma. *JAMA.* 1970;214:1113.

4. Hollister LE, et al. Delta-9-tetrahydrocannabinol and glucose tolerance. *Clin Pharmacol Ther.* 1974;16:297.

Insulin

Nifedipine (eg, *Procardia*)

SUMMARY: Calcium channel blockers like nifedipine have little effect on antidiabetic agents or on blood glucose concentrations in noninsulin-dependent diabetics.

RISK FACTORS: No specific risk factors are known.

MECHANISM: Not established. Some have suggested that calcium channel blockers inhibit insulin secretion or alter cell permeability to glucose.

CLINICAL EVALUATION: The effects of calcium channel blockers on glucose metabolism have been studied in patients taking multiple doses of nifedipine,[1-3] verapamil (eg, *Calan*),[4,5] nitrendipine (*Baypress*),[6] or nimodipine (*Nimotop*).[10] The results of these studies are diverse and somewhat contradictory. A loss of glycemic control during concurrent calcium channel blocker administration has been reported in anecdotal cases[7-9]; however, it is rare or noninsulin-dependent diabetics taking chronic calcium channel blockers to demonstrate a reduction in glucose tolerance.

RELATED DRUGS: Nimodipine, nitrendipine, and verapamil interact similarly with insulin. It is possible that patients taking other hypoglycemic agents (eg, tolbutamide [eg, *Orinase*], chlorpropamide [eg, *Diabinese*], glipizide [eg, *Glucotrol*]) also might be affected by calcium channel blockers; however, data are limited.

MANAGEMENT OPTIONS: No specific action is required, but be alert for evidence of the interaction.

REFERENCES:

1. Donnelly T, et al. Effect of nifedipine on glucose tolerance and insulin secretion in diabetic and non-diabetic patients. *Curr Med Res Opin.* 1980;6:690.
2. Guigliano D, et al. Impairment of insulin secretion in man by nifedipine. *Eur J Clin Pharmacol.* 1980;18:395.
3. Kanatsuna T, et al. Effects of nifedipine on insulin secretion and glucose metabolism in rats and in hypertensive type 2 (non-insulin dependent) diabetics. *Arzneimittelforschung.* 1985;35:514.
4. Rojdmark S, et al. Influence of verapamil on glucose tolerance. *Acta Med Scand.* 1984;681(Suppl.): 37.
5. Andersson DEH, et al. Improvement of glucose tolerance by verapamil in patients with non-insulin dependent diabetes mellitus. *Acta Med Scand.* 1981;210:27.
6. Trost BN, et al. Effects of nitrendipine and other calcium antagonists on glucose metabolism in man. *J Cardiovasc Pharmacol.* 1984;6:S986.
7. Heyman SN, et al. Diabetogenic effect of nifedipine. *DICP, Ann of Pharmacother.* 1989;23:236.
8. Shoen RE, et al. Hormonal metabolic effects of calcium channel antagonists in man. *Am J Med.* 1988;84:492.
9. Zezulka AV, et al. Diabetogenic effects of nifedipine. *Br J Med.* 1984;289:437.
10. Muck W, et al. The effect of multiple oral dosing of nimodipine on glibenclamide pharmacodynamics and pharmacokinetics in elderly patients with type-2 diabetes mellitus. *Int J Clin Pharmacol Ther.* 1995;33:89.

Insulin

Prednisone (eg, *Deltasone*)

SUMMARY: Corticosteroids like prednisone may increase blood glucose in patients with diabetes.

RISK FACTORS:

➡ **Dosage Regimen.** Chronic administration of corticosteroids can increase glucose concentrations.

MECHANISM: Corticosteroids may increase blood sugar by several possible mechanisms including increased hepatic glucose production secondary to stimulation of gluconeogenesis, mobilization of fatty acids from tissue stores, or decreased affinity of tissue receptors for insulin.

CLINICAL EVALUATION: The hyperglycemic effect of corticosteroids is well documented and may occur in up to 14% of patients taking steroids over several weeks. The incidence appears to be increased with prolonged use of both oral and topical steroids. Unlike idiopathic diabetes mellitus, steroid-induced diabetes rarely produces acidosis or ketonuria even when blood sugars are very high.[1-3]

RELATED DRUGS: All corticosteroids can increase glucose concentrations during chronic dosing.

MANAGEMENT OPTIONS:

➡ *Monitor.* Patients should be observed for evidence of altered diabetic control when corticosteroids are initiated, discontinued or changed in dosage.

REFERENCES:

1. Gomez EC, et al. Induction of glycosuria and hyperglycemia by topical corticosteroid therapy. *Arch Dermatol.* 1976;112:1559.

2. Hunder GG, et al. Daily and alternate-day corticosteroid regimens in treatment of giant cell arteritis. Comparison in a prospective study. *Ann Intern Med.* 1975;82:613.

3. McMahon M, et al. Effects of glucocorticoids on carbohydrate metabolism. *Diabetes Metab Rev.* 1988;4:17.

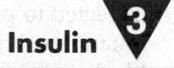

Insulin

Propranolol (eg, *Inderal*)

SUMMARY: Propranolol and other beta blockers may alter the response to hypoglycemia by prolonging the recovery of normoglycemia, causing hypertension and blocking tachycardia. They also may increase blood glucose concentrations and impair peripheral circulation.

RISK FACTORS: No specific risk factors are known.

MECHANISM: The mechanisms for this interaction are as follows: 1) Beta blockers delay recovery from insulin-induced hypoglycemia by inhibiting the hyperglycemic response to epinephrine released during hypoglycemia. 2) Hypertension during hypoglycemia results from blockade of the beta-2 (vasodilator) effects of epinephrine released in response to hypoglycemia; this leaves alpha (vasoconstrictor) effects of epinephrine unopposed, which increases the blood pressure. 3) Beta blockers inhibit the tachycardia during hypoglycemia by reducing the cardiac stimulatory effect of the epinephrine released in response to the hypoglycemia. 4) Beta blockers may inhibit insulin secretion and decrease tissue sensitivity to insulin, leading to a hyperglycemic effect under certain conditions.

CLINICAL EVALUATION: *Delayed Glucose Recovery During Hypoglycemia.* Propranolol inhibits recovery following insulin-induced hypoglycemia. The cardioselective beta blockers (eg, metoprolol [eg, *Lopressor*], atenolol [eg, *Tenormin*], penbutolol [*Levatol*], and acebutolol [eg, *Sectral*]) exhibit minimal or no effect on insulin-induced hypoglycemia.[4-7] Timolol (eg, *Blocadren*) eye drops purportedly contributed to hypoglycemic episodes in 1 patient; however, the significance of this is not clear.[16]

Hypertension During Hypoglycemia. A number of case reports and clinical studies have described increased blood pressure and bradycardia during hypoglycemia in the presence of propranolol treatment.[2] Other nonselective beta blockers, such as alprenolol,[8] nadolol (eg, *Corgard*), and timolol, would be expected to produce a similar effect. Cardioselective beta blockers (eg, metoprolol and atenolol) are less likely to produce hypertension during hypoglycemia[1,2,8]; however, in 1 patient, large doses of metoprolol (100 mg twice daily) caused hypertension in this setting.[9]

Inhibition of the Symptoms of Hypoglycemia. Propranolol and metoprolol inhibit the tachycardia that normally accompanies hypoglycemia.[2] Other beta blockers that have inhibited hypoglycemia-induced tachycardia include atenolol, acebutolol,[4,5] penbutolol,[7] and alprenolol,[8] and it is likely that all beta blockers have this property. Sweating as a sign of hypoglycemia is not inhibited by beta blockers and may actually be prolonged.[2,3]

Inhibition of Insulin Secretion. Beta blockers inhibit the insulin response to glucose or tolbutamide.[1,10,11] Long-term propranolol therapy (especially when combined with thiazides) has been associated with reduced glucose tolerance.[2,12-14] Metoprolol appears to be less likely than propranolol to impair glucose tolerance.[14,15] Because stimulation of beta-2-receptors in the pancreas tends to increase insulin secretion, cardioselective beta blockers should have less inhibitory effect on insulin secretion than nonselective beta blockers.

RELATED DRUGS: (Also see Clinical Evaluation.) Nonselective beta blockers would be expected to produce results similar to propranolol when administered to patients taking insulin. Oral hypoglycemic agents may interact with the nonselective beta blockers but, since they are less likely to produce hypoglycemia than insulin, the incidence and magnitude of reactions associated with hypoglycemic episodes will be reduced.

MANAGEMENT OPTIONS:

➡ *Consider Alternative.* Cardioselective beta blockers (eg, metoprolol, acebutolol, atenolol) are preferable in diabetic patients, especially if the patient is prone to hypoglycemic episodes. The increased safety of cardioselective agents is only relative, as they may exhibit nonselective beta blockade at higher doses.

➡ *Monitor.* Diabetic patients receiving beta blockers should be aware that hypoglycemic episodes may not result in the expected tachycardia, but hypoglycemic-induced sweating will occur or even may be increased.

REFERENCES:

1. Mills GA, et al. Beta-blockers and glucose control. *DICP.* 1985;19:246.
2. Hansten PD. Beta-blocking agents and antidiabetic drugs. *DICP.* 1980;14:46.
3. Molnar GW, et al. Propranolol enhancement of hypoglycemic sweating. *Clin Pharmacol Ther.* 1974;15:490.
4. Newman RJ. Comparison of propranolol, metoprolol, and acebutolol on insulin-induced hypoglycaemia. *Br Med J.* 1976;2:447.
5. Deacon SP, et al. Acebutolol, atenolol, and propranolol and metabolic responses to acute hypoglycaemia in diabetics. *Br Med J.* 1977;2:1255.
6. Deacon SP, et al. Comparison of atenolol and propranolol during insulin-induced hypoglycaemia. *Br Med J.* 1976;2:272.
7. Sharma SD, et al. Comparison of penbutolol and propranolol during insulin-induced hypoglycaemia. *Curr Ther Res.* 1979;26:252.
8. Ostman J, et al. Effect of metoprolol and alprenolol on the metabolic, hormonal, and haemodynamic response to insulin-induced hypoglycaemia in hypertensive, insulin-dependent diabetics. *Acta Med Scand.* 1982;211:381.
9. Shepherd AMM, et al. Hypoglycemia-induced hypertension in a diabetic patient on metoprolol. *Ann Intern Med.* 1981;94:357.
10. Meyers MG, et al. Effect of d-and dl-propranolol on glucose-stimulated insulin release. *Clin Pharmacol Ther.* 1979;25:303.
11. Pollare T, et al. Sensitivity to insulin during treatment with atenolol and metoprolol; a randomized, double blind study of effects of carbohydrate and lipoprotein metabolism in hypertensive patients. *Br Med J.* 1989;298:1152.
12. Mohler H, et al. Glucose intolerance during chronic beta-adrenergic blockade in man. *Clin Pharmacol Ther.* 1979;25:237.
13. Nardone DA, et al. Hyperglycemia and diabetic coma; possible relationship to diuretic-propranolol therapy. *South Med J.* 1979;72:1607.

14. Groop L, et al. Influence of beta-blocking drugs on glucose metabolism in patients with non-insulin dependent diabetes mellitus. *Acta Med Scand*. 1982;211:7.

15. Reeves RL, et al. The effect of metoprolol and propranolol on pancreatic insulin release. *Clin Pharmacol Ther*. 1982;31:262.

16. Angelo-Nelsen K, et al. Timolol topically and diabetes mellitus. *JAMA*. 1980;244:2263.

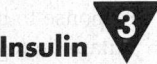

Insulin

Thiazides (eg, chlorothiazide)

SUMMARY: Thiazides tend to increase blood glucose and may increase the dosage requirements of antidiabetic drugs.

RISK FACTORS:

➡ **Dosage.** Thiazide dosage greater than 50 mg/day may increase blood glucose.

MECHANISM: The mechanisms for this interaction are: 1) The diabetogenic effect of thiazides may be due partially to potassium depletion, resulting in a reduced insulin response to elevated glucose. It also has been proposed that thiazide-induced hypokalemia may inhibit insulin secretion[1] or decrease tissue sensitivity to insulin.[2,3] 2) Thiazides and chlorpropamide can produce hyponatremia, probably by different mechanisms.[4]

CLINICAL EVALUATION: Thiazides tend to elevate blood glucose in diabetic and prediabetic patients and thus may antagonize the hypoglycemic effect of antidiabetic drugs.[5-7] However, in most patients this effect does not cause significant clinical problems.

RELATED DRUGS: Thiazides may inhibit the hypoglycemic effect of chlorpropamide (eg, *Diabinese*) and other oral hypoglycemic agents.

MANAGEMENT OPTIONS:

➡ **Monitor.** Watch for decreased diabetic control when thiazide therapy is started in a patient receiving any antidiabetic drug.

REFERENCES:

1. Levine R. Mechanisms of insulin secretion. *N Engl J Med*. 1970;283:522.

2. Grunfeld C, et al. Hypokalemia and diabetes mellitus. *Am J Med*. 1983;75:553.

3. Helderman JH, et al. Prevention of the glucose intolerance of thiazide diuretics by maintenance of body potassium. *Diabetes*. 1983;32:106.

4. Fichman MP, et al. Diuretic-induced hyponatremia. *Ann Intern Med*. 1971;75:853.

5. Amery A, et al. Glucose tolerance during diuretic therapy. Results of trial by the European Working Party on Hypertension in the Elderly. *Lancet*. 1978;1:681.

6. Murphy MB, et al. Glucose intolerance in hypertensive patients treated with diuretics: a fourteen-year follow-up. *Lancet*. 1982;2:1293.

7. Lowder NK, et al. Clinically significant diuretic-induced glucose intolerance. *DICP*. 1988;22:969.

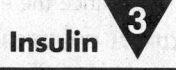

Insulin

Tranylcypromine (*Parnate*)

SUMMARY: Excessive hypoglycemia may occur when tranylcypromine, and other monoamine oxidase inhibitors (MAOIs), are administered to patients with diabetes.

RISK FACTORS: No specific risk factors are known.

MECHANISM: Some have proposed that MAOIs interfere with the compensatory adrenergic response to hypoglycemia,[1] but others have failed to confirm this mechanism.[2] Tranylcypromine stimulates insulin secretion in animals, probably through beta-adrenergic stimulation.[3]

CLINICAL EVALUATION: Clinically, type A MAOIs enhance or prolong the hypoglycemic response to both insulin and sulfonylurea (eg, chlorpropamide [eg, *Diabinese*], tolbutamide (eg, [*Orinase*]) hypoglycemics.[1-6] This effect may be of sufficient magnitude to produce unexpected hypoglycemic episodes if it is not anticipated. However, some patients may be expected to benefit from the enhanced hypoglycemic response.

RELATED DRUGS: Sulfonylureas such as chlorpropamide and tolbutamide interact with type A MAOIs like tranylcypromine similarly. While it is likely that all type A MAOIs will interact in a similar manner, the effect of type B MAOIs (eg, selegiline [eg, *Eldepryl*]) on glucose tolerance is not established.

MANAGEMENT OPTIONS:

➡ *Monitor.* Until further information on this interaction is available, diabetic patients should be warned about possible hypoglycemic reactions when MAOI therapy is started. Be alert for deterioration of glycemic control when MAOI therapy is discontinued.

REFERENCES:

1. Cooper AJ, et al. Modification of insulin and sulfonylurea hypoglycemia by monoamine-oxidase inhibitor drugs. *Diabetes.* 1967;16:272.
2. Adnitt PI. Hypoglycemic action of monoamine oxidase inhibitors (MAOI's). *Diabetes.* 1968;17:628.
3. Bressler R, et al. Tranylcypromine: a potent insulin secretagogue and hypoglycemic agent. *Diabetes.* 1968;17:617.
4. Cooper AJ, et al. Potentiation of insulin hypoglycaemia by MAOI antidepressant drugs. *Lancet.* 1966;1:407.
5. Barrett AM. Modification of the hypoglycaemic response to tolbutamide and insulin by mebanazine, an inhibitor of monoamine oxidase. *J Pharm Pharmacol.* 1965;17:19.
6. Whickstrom L, et al. Treatment of diabetics with monoamine-oxidase inhibitors. *Lancet.* 1964;2:995.

4   Interferon (eg, *Roferon-A*)

Melphalan (*Alkeran*)

SUMMARY: Interferon appears to reduce plasma concentrations of melphalan; the clinical significance of this is unknown.

RISK FACTORS: No specific risk factors are known.

MECHANISM: Not established. It is postulated that interferon-induced fever may enhance the elimination of melphalan.

CLINICAL EVALUATION: Ten patients with multiple myeloma were treated with oral melphalan 0.25 mg/kg alone and 5 hours after IM interferon alpha 7×10^6 units/m^2.[1] The area under the concentration-time curve (AUC) for melphalan was slightly reduced (13%) following interferon administration. The melphalan AUC displayed a significant negative correlation with body temperature: the higher the temperature, the lower the AUC. This could suggest that fever is partially responsible for the reduced plasma concentrations of melphalan following interferon.

RELATED DRUGS: No information is available.

MANAGEMENT OPTIONS: No specific action is required, but be alert for evidence of the interaction.

REFERENCES:

1. Ehrsson H, et al. Oral melphalan pharmacokinetics: influence of interferon-induced fever. *Clin Pharmacol Ther.* 1990;47:86.

Interferon (eg, *Roferon-A*)

Prednisone (eg, *Deltasone*)

SUMMARY: Corticosteroids like prednisone may inhibit some of the biologic effects of interferon, but the clinical importance of this inhibition is not established.

RISK FACTORS: No specific risk factors are known.

MECHANISM: Not established.

CLINICAL EVALUATION: Because patients receiving corticosteroids appear to be more susceptible to life-threatening viral infections, a study was designed to determine if prednisone inhibits the biologic response to interferon. Eight healthy subjects received a single dose of recombinant human interferon 18×10^6 units IM, with oral prednisone 40 mg/day 1 day before through 6 days after the interferon.[1] Responses to interferon plus prednisone were compared with a group of subjects receiving interferon alone. Prednisone reduced the biologic response to interferon as shown by a 56% attenuation in interferon induction of 2'-5'-oligoadenylate synthetase. However, prednisone did not affect another measure of the biologic response to interferon, resistance to vesicular stomatitis virus infection. Prednisone did not ameliorate interferon side effects such as chills, headache, myalgia, or fatigue.

RELATED DRUGS: Corticosteroids other than prednisone may have a similar effect when combined with interferon, but little information is available.

MANAGEMENT OPTIONS: No specific action is required, but be alert for evidence of the interaction.

REFERENCES:

1. Witter FR, et al. Effects of prednisone, aspirin, and acetaminophen on an in vivo biologic response to interferon in humans. *Clin Pharmacol Ther.* 1988;44:239.

Interferon (eg, *Roferon-A*)

Theophylline (eg, *Theo-Dur*)

SUMMARY: Interferon alpha may increase theophylline plasma concentrations, especially in patients with high pre-existing theophylline clearance (ie, those who smoke); the degree to which this increases the risk of theophylline toxicity is not known.

RISK FACTORS:

➡ **Habits.** Limited evidence suggests that the reduction in theophylline clearance by interferon is greater in patients who have high pre-existing theophylline clearance due to smoking.[1]

MECHANISM: Pharmacokinetic studies suggest that interferon alpha inhibits the hepatic metabolism of theophylline. Interferon alpha has been shown to reduce the activity of drug metabolizing enzymes in the liver.[2]

CLINICAL EVALUATION: Eleven healthy subjects received IV aminophylline 4 mg/kg with and without pretreatment with interferon-alfa-2a 3 MU/day for 3 days.[3] Interferon was associated with a small (18%) increase in the area under the theophylline plasma concentration-time curve and a 10% reduction in theophylline clearance. In another study of 4 healthy subjects and 5 patients with chronic active hepatitis B, a single dose of 9 MU of interferon-alfa-2a reduced the clearance of theophylline (5 mg/kg IV) 33% to 81% in 8 of the 9 subjects.[1] Repeat study in the healthy subjects 4 weeks after the interferon showed that the effect on theophylline clearance had dissipated. It is possible that the greater effect on theophylline seen in the latter study was because of the larger daily dose of interferon (single dose of 9 MU) compared to 3 MU/day for 3 days in the earlier study. Probably more important, however, was the inclusion of patients with high theophylline clearance in the latter study. The reduction in theophylline clearance by interferon was much greater in the 3 patients who had high preexisting theophylline clearance because of smoking, and it is possible that the risk of theophylline toxicity is increased in such patients. The other subjects and patients in the study experienced only modest reductions in theophylline clearance. Studies of the effect of interferon on theophylline in patients on chronic theophylline therapy are needed to determine the clinical importance of this interaction. Although interferon-alfa-2a (*Roferon-A*) was used in the studies cited, assume that interferon-alfa-2b (*Intron A*) interacts in a similar manner (as might other interferons such as beta and gamma).

RELATED DRUGS: See Clinical Evaluation.

MANAGEMENT OPTIONS:

➡ *Monitor.* Monitor for excessive theophylline response if interferon is given, especially in theophylline-treated patients who smoke or other patients in whom theophylline clearance may be high (eg, those on enzyme inducers such as barbiturates, carbamazepine [eg, *Tegretol*], phenytoin [eg, *Dilantin*], primidone [eg, *Mysoline*], and rifampin [eg, *Rifadin*]). The effect of interferon on theophylline elimination appears to occur rapidly; expect to see increased plasma theophylline concentrations within 1 to 2 days of interferon administration.

REFERENCES:
1. Williams SJ, et al. Inhibition of theophylline metabolism by interferon. *Lancet*. 1987;2:939-941.
2. Okuno H, et al. Depression of drug metabolizing activity in the human liver by interferon-alpha. *Eur J Clin Pharmacol*. 1990;39:365-367.
3. Jonkman JH, et al. Effects of alpha-interferon on theophylline pharmacokinetics and metabolism. *Br J Clin Pharmacol*. 1989;27:795-802.

Interferon (eg, *Betaseron*)

Zidovudine (eg, *Retrovir*)

SUMMARY: Beta interferon markedly increases the plasma concentrations of zidovudine.

RISK FACTORS: No specific risk factors are known.

MECHANISM: It appears that beta interferon inhibits the glucuronidation of zidovudine.

CLINICAL EVALUATION: Patients with AIDS were treated with oral zidovudine 200 mg every 4 hours for 8 weeks before the coadministrations of SC recombinant beta interferon 90×10^6 units/day.[1] After 3 days the zidovudine clearance was reduced 66%; after 15 days the clearance was reduced 93%. Zidovudine's half-life increased by 2 to 3 times the baseline values. One group studied the effects of interleukin-2 (IL-2) on zidovudine pharmacokinetics and found no significant changes following 4 weeks of continuous IV infusion (0.25×10^6 U/m^2/day).[2] IL-2 is believed to stimulate the production of gamma interferon, which has been reported to inhibit oxidative metabolism but not glucuronidation.

RELATED DRUGS: Interleukin-2 interacts similarly.

MANAGEMENT OPTIONS:

➡ **Circumvent/Minimize.** Patients taking zidovudine who are given beta interferon should be given reduced doses of zidovudine. If additional studies substantiate the large degree of metabolic inhibition, zidovudine doses could be reduced 75% or more.

➡ **Monitor.** Monitor for altered zidovudine effect if beta interferon is initiated, discontinued, or changed in dosage; adjust zidovudine dose as needed.

REFERENCES:

1. Nolta M, et al. Molecular interaction of recombinant beta interferon and zidovudine (AZT): alternations of AZT pharmacokinetics in HIV-infected patients. Fifth International Conference on AIDS. Quebec; 1989:278.

2. Skinner MH, et al. IL-2 does not alter zidovudine kinetics. *Clin Pharmacol Ther*. 1989;45:128.

Intrauterine Progesterone System (IUDs) (*Progestasert*)

Prednisone (eg, *Deltasone*)

SUMMARY: Corticosteroids like prednisone have been reported to decrease the efficacy of IUDs, but a causal relationship has not been established.

RISK FACTORS: No specific risk factors are known.

MECHANISM: Not established. The contraceptive efficacy of IUDs may be related to an inflammatory reaction that would be inhibited by corticosteroids.

CLINICAL EVALUATION: Isolated cases of unwanted pregnancy during IUD use have occurred in women taking anti-inflammatory drugs such as corticosteroids.[1,2] However, it has not been established that the anti-inflammatory drugs were responsible for the contraceptive failure.

RELATED DRUGS: If this interaction is real, it would be expected to occur with other corticosteroids as well.

MANAGEMENT OPTIONS:

➡ **Circumvent/Minimize.** Until more information is available, women using IUDs should consider using another form of contraception during short-term therapy with corticosteroids or other anti-inflammatory drugs. If the anti-inflammatory drug is used chronically, the possibility that the IUD failure rate may be increased somewhat should be considered when selecting a contraceptive method.

➥ *Monitor.* Because pregnancy is the potential outcome, monitoring guidelines are not applicable.

REFERENCES:

1. Inkeles DM, et al. Unexpected pregnancy in a woman using an intrauterine device and receiving steroid therapy. *Ann Ophthalmol.* 1982;14:975.

2. Zerner J, et al. Failure of an intrauterine device concurrent with administration of corticosteroids. *Fertil Steril.* 1976;27:1467-1468.

4 Irbesartan (*Avapro*)

Fluconazole (eg, *Diflucan*)

SUMMARY: Fluconazole increases irbesartan plasma concentrations; increased hypotensive effect may occur.

RISK FACTORS: No specific risk factors are known.

MECHANISM: Fluconazole inhibits CYP2C9, the enzyme primarily responsible for the metabolism of irbesartan.

CLINICAL EVALUATION: Fifteen subjects received irbesartan 150 mg daily for 20 days with concomitant fluconazole 200 mg daily administered on days 11 to 20.[1] The mean area under the plasma concentration-time curve was increased 63% during fluconazole coadministration. Because irbesartan is an active angiotensin II receptor antagonist, the degree of increase in plasma concentration may increase the hypotensive effect of irbesartan in some patients.

RELATED DRUGS: Fluconazole inhibits the metabolism of losartan (*Cozaar*) to its active metabolite; a reduction in hypotensive response is possible with this combination. Telmisartan (*Micardis*) does not appear to undergo CYP2C9 metabolism and would not likely be affected by fluconazole administration.

MANAGEMENT OPTIONS:

➥ *Monitor.* It is unlikely that a large increase in hypotensive effect would be observed during the coadministration of fluconazole (particularly with single-dose fluconazole regimens) with irbesartan. Nevertheless, monitor for changes in blood pressure control if fluconazole is added to or removed from a patient's regimen.

REFERENCES:

1. Kovasc SJ, et al. Steady state (SS) pharmacokinetics (PK) of irbesartan alone and in combination with fluconazole (F). *Clin Pharmacol Ther.* 1999;65(2):132.

 ## Irinotecan (*Camptosar*)

Phenytoin (eg, *Dilantin*)

SUMMARY: Irinotecan may exhibit reduced efficacy in patients receiving phenytoin or other enzyme-inducing anticonvulsants; increased irinotecan dosage may be required.

RISK FACTORS: No specific risk factors are known.

MECHANISM: Phenytoin is likely to enhance the metabolism of irinotecan to inactive metabolites, but an effect of phenytoin on ABC transporters may also be involved.

CLINICAL EVALUATION: In a 28-year-old patient with a malignant glioma given irinotecan with phenytoin 100 mg 3 times daily, plasma concentrations of the active metabolite of irinotecan (SN-38) were reduced 10-fold.[1] In another study of 102 patients given irinotecan, some patients were taking concurrent enzyme-inducing anticonvulsants, such as phenytoin, and other patients were not.[2] Those taking anticonvulsants had substantially lower plasma concentrations of irinotecan and SN-38. Given the magnitude of the reduction in irinotecan and SN-38 concentrations, a reduction in the efficacy of irinotecan in such patients is expected.

RELATED DRUGS: Enzyme-inducing anticonvulsants other than phenytoin, such as barbiturates, carbamazepine, and primidone, may also reduce irinotecan effect.

MANAGEMENT OPTIONS:

➡ *Circumvent/Minimize.* Patients receiving phenytoin or other enzyme-inducing anticonvulsants may require larger doses of irinotecan. Refer to the most recent dosing recommendations and latest prescribing information before starting irinotecan therapy in patients taking enzyme-inducing anticonvulsants.

➡ *Monitor.* Monitor for altered irinotecan response if enzyme-inducing anticonvulsants are given concurrently; when available, pharmacokinetic monitoring may be useful.

REFERENCES:

1. Mathijssen RH, et al. Altered irinotecan metabolism in a patient receiving phenytoin. *Anticancer Drugs.* 2002;13(2):139-140.

2. Kuhn JG. Influence of anticonvulsants on the metabolism and elimination of irinotecan. A North American Brain Tumor Consortium preliminary report. *Oncology* (Williston Park). 2002;16(8)(suppl 7):33-40.

Irinotecan (*Camptosar*)

St. John's Wort AVOID

SUMMARY: St. John's wort may reduce irinotecan effect; avoid the combination.

RISK FACTORS: No specific risk factors are known.

MECHANISM: St. John's wort is likely to increase the hepatic metabolism of irinotecan by CYP3A4.

CLINICAL EVALUATION: Five patients with cancer were given irinotecan with and without pretreatment with St. John's wort (3 times daily for 14 days).[1] St. John's wort was associated with a 42% reduction in the area under the plasma concentration-time curve for SN-38, the active metabolite of irinotecan. The myelosuppressive effects of irinotecan were markedly reduced in the presence of St. John's wort. These findings suggest that St. John's wort could substantially reduce the antineoplastic activity of irinotecan.

RELATED DRUGS: Theoretically, topotecan may interact similarly with St. John's wort.

MANAGEMENT OPTIONS:

➡ *AVOID COMBINATION.* Given the potential risk of reduced irinotecan activity and the questionable efficacy of St. John's wort, avoid the combination at this time.

REFERENCES:

1. Mathijssen RH, et al. Effects of St. John's wort on irinotecan metabolism. *J Natl Cancer Inst.* 2002;94(16):1247-1249.

Iron

Gemifloxacin (*Factive*)

SUMMARY: When the administration of iron salts is separated from gemifloxacin, only a slight reduction in gemifloxacin plasma concentrations occurs; diminution of antibiotic effect is unlikely.

RISK FACTORS: No specific risk factors are known.

MECHANISM: Iron appears to cause some reduction in the absorption of gemifloxacin, probably by forming poorly absorbed chelates.

CLINICAL EVALUATION: Twenty-seven healthy subjects received a single oral dose of gemifloxacin 320 mg alone, or 3 hours after or 2 hours before a single dose of ferrous sulfate 325 mg.[1] In both cases, when the administration of ferrous sulfate was separated from the dose of gemifloxacin, the area under the concentration-time curve of gemifloxacin was reduced by only 10%. This is unlikely to lead to loss of antibacterial efficacy. Although not studied, avoid coadministration of iron and gemifloxacin because a greater reduction in the bioavailability of gemifloxacin is likely.

RELATED DRUGS: Most quinolones have reduced bioavailability when administered with iron salts.

MANAGEMENT OPTIONS:

➡ ***Circumvent/Minimize.*** Administer gemifloxacin 2 hours before oral iron salts. Iron could be administered parenterally to avoid the interaction.

➡ ***Monitor.*** Monitor patients receiving gemifloxacin and iron for adequate anti-infective response.

REFERENCES:

1. Allen A, et al. The effect of ferrous sulphate and sucralfate on the bioavailability of oral gemifloxacin in healthy volunteers. *Int J Antimicrob Agents.* 2000;15(4):283-289.

Iron

Levodopa

SUMMARY: Oral iron reduced levodopa bioavailability 50% in a single-dose study of healthy subjects; the importance of this interaction in patients with Parkinson disease on long-term levodopa therapy is not established.

RISK FACTORS: No specific risk factors are known.

MECHANISM: Iron appears to bind levodopa in the GI tract, thus inhibiting the absorption of levodopa. In vitro studies indicate that ferric ions chelate with levodopa within the pH range commonly found in the small bowel.[1]

CLINICAL EVALUATION: Eight healthy subjects received a single tablet of levodopa 250 mg with and without coadministration of a single tablet of ferrous sulfate 325 mg.[1] The iron tablet reduced levodopa bioavailability 51% and reduced peak levodopa plasma concentrations 55%. If similar reductions in levodopa bioavailability occur with long-term use of levodopa and iron, a clinically important reduction in levodopa effect would be expected to occur.

RELATED DRUGS: Theoretically, other oral iron preparations would reduce levodopa absorption; however, the small amounts of iron found in most vitamin-mineral products are likely to be insufficient to produce much of aninteraction.

MANAGEMENT OPTIONS:

➥ *Circumvent/Minimize.* Until more information is available, separate the doses of iron and levodopa as much as possible; monitor for inadequate levodopa response.

➥ *Monitor.* Monitor for reduced levodopa response if the combination is used.

REFERENCES:

1. Campbell NR, et al. Ferrous sulfate reduces levodopa bioavailability: chelation as a possible mechanism. *Clin Pharmacol Ther*. 1989;45(3):220-225.

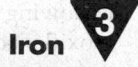

Iron

Methyldopa (eg, *Aldomet*)

SUMMARY: Pharmacokinetic studies in healthy subjects and blood pressure measurements in hypertensive patients both indicate that oral iron may inhibit the antihypertensive response to methyldopa.

RISK FACTORS: No specific risk factors are known.

MECHANISM: Oral iron appears to reduce the extent of methyldopa absorption.

CLINICAL EVALUATION: Twelve healthy subjects received a 500 mg tablet of methyldopa with and without coadministration of ferrous sulfate 325 mg in a randomized crossover trial.[1] The percentage of methyldopa absorbed was 29% with methyldopa alone and was reduced to 8% with ferrous sulfate coadministration. When the study was repeated using ferrous gluconate 600 mg in place of the ferrous sulfate, a similar reduction in methyldopa absorption was observed. When 5 hypertensive patients stabilized on chronic methyldopa therapy were given ferrous sulfate 325 mg 3 times a day for 2 weeks, systolic blood pressure increased in all patients (in 3 patients, the increases were more than 15 mm Hg). Blood pressure returned to preiron levels within 7 days of stopping the iron administration. It is unknown if separating doses of iron and methyldopa negates this interaction.

RELATED DRUGS: Although the effect of oral iron salts other than ferrous sulfate and ferrous gluconate on methyldopa is not known, assume that they interact until proven otherwise. The amount of iron in most multivitamins may not be sufficient to inhibit methyldopa absorption, but clinical studies are needed to confirm this. Parenteral iron would not be expected to interact, but this has not been studied. Little is known regarding the effect of iron on antihypertensives other than methyldopa.

MANAGEMENT OPTIONS:

➥ *Consider Alternative.* Methyldopa has disadvantages compared with many other antihypertensives; consider alternative therapy.

➥ *Circumvent/Minimize.* Give methyldopa 2 hours before or 6 hours after oral iron.

➥ *Monitor.* Monitor for reduced antihypertensive response when oral iron and methyldopa are used concurrently.

REFERENCES:

1. Campbell N, et al. Alteration of methyldopa absorption, metabolism, and blood pressure control caused by ferrous sulfate and ferrous gluconate. *Clin Pharmacol Ther*. 1988;43:381.

Iron

Moxifloxacin (*Avelox*)

SUMMARY: Iron administration reduces moxifloxacin plasma concentrations; a reduction in antibiotic activity may occur.

RISK FACTORS: No specific risk factors are known.

MECHANISM: Iron appears to inhibit the absorption of moxifloxacin from the GI tract.

CLINICAL EVALUATION: A single 400 mg oral dose of moxifloxacin was administered to 12 healthy subjects alone and concurrently with iron sulfate equivalent to 100 mg of elemental iron.[1] A second dose of iron was administered 24 hours after the first. Following iron coadministration, the area under the concentration-time curve of moxifloxacin was reduced 39% while its peak concentration fell 59%. This magnitude of a reduction in moxifloxacin concentration could result in a reduction of its antibiotic efficacy in some patients.

RELATED DRUGS: Other quinolone antibiotics such as ciprofloxacin (*Cipro*) and norfloxacin (*Noroxin*) are affected in a similar manner by iron.

MANAGEMENT OPTIONS:

➡ **Consider Alternative.** Patients taking moxifloxacin should not take oral iron salts concurrently because of the risk of subtherapeutic moxifloxacin concentrations.

➡ **Circumvent/Minimize.** IV iron could be considered to avoid the interaction. If moxifloxacin is administered to patients taking oral iron, give the antibiotic at least 2 hours before the iron.

➡ **Monitor.** Watch for reduced antibiotic efficacy if moxifloxacin and iron salts are coadministered.

REFERENCES:
1. Stass H, et al. Effects of iron supplements on the oral bioavailability of moxifloxacin, a novel 8-methoxyfluoroquinolone, in humans. *Clin Pharmacokinet.* 2001;40(suppl 1):57.

Iron

Mycophenolate Mofetil (*CellCept*)

SUMMARY: Oral iron appears to markedly reduce the bioavailability of mycophenolate mofetil; avoid concurrent use or carefully separate doses.

RISK FACTORS:

➡ **Route of Administration.** The interaction is likely to occur only with oral administration of iron.

MECHANISM: Iron appears to bind with mycophenolate mofetil in the GI tract, probably by chelation.

CLINICAL EVALUATION: Seven healthy subjects took a single dose of mycophenolate mofetil (1 g orally) with and without concurrent ferrous sulfate (two 525 mg tablets).[1] The iron reduced the mycophenolate mofetil area under the serum concentration-time curve to approximately 10% of that seen with mycophenolate mofetil given alone. When mycophenolate mofetil was given alone, the absorption was rapid, with maximal serum concentrations at approximately 1 hour after dosing. Thus, giving iron 2 hours or more after mycophenolate mofetil would theoretically minimize the interaction.

RELATED DRUGS: All oral iron preparations would be expected to interact with mycophenolate mofetil.

MANAGEMENT OPTIONS:

➡ *Circumvent/Minimize.* Until more information is available, it would be prudent to give oral iron 4 to 6 hours before or 2 hours after mycophenolate mofetil. Also, warn patients on mycophenolate to avoid taking *otc* iron preparations.

➡ *Monitor.* If oral iron must be used with mycophenolate mofetil, monitor for altered mycophenolate mofetil effect if oral iron is initiated, discontinued, changed in dosage, or if the interval between doses of the 2 drugs is changed.

REFERENCES:

1. Morii M, et al. Impairment of mycophenolate mofetil absorption by iron ion. *Clin Pharmacol Ther.* 2000;68:613.

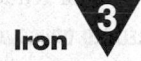

Iron

Norfloxacin (*Noroxin*)

SUMMARY: The administration of iron salts with norfloxacin lowers the antibiotic serum concentration and may lead to therapeutic failure.

RISK FACTORS: No specific risk factors are known.

MECHANISM: Iron salts inhibit norfloxacin absorption by binding to it in the GI tract.

CLINICAL EVALUATION: The administration of iron has been reported to reduce the absorption of norfloxacin from 65% to greater than 70%.[1-3] The efficacy of norfloxacin is likely to be reduced by coadministration with iron.

RELATED DRUGS: Other quinolones (eg, ciprofloxacin [*Cipro*]) have been reported to be affected similarly by iron.[2,4-6] Ofloxacin (*Floxin*) absorption may be less affected by iron.[2,5]

MANAGEMENT OPTIONS:

➡ *Consider Alternative.* Patients taking norfloxacin should not take oral iron concurrently because serum norfloxacin concentrations may be subtherapeutic.

➡ *Circumvent/Minimize.* The administration of norfloxacin at least 2 hours before oral iron would theoretically reduce the magnitude of the interaction. IV iron could be used to avoid the interaction.

➡ *Monitor.* If the drugs are used together, watch for lessened antibiotic effect.

REFERENCES:

1. Campbell NR, et al. Norfloxacin interaction with antacids and minerals. *Br J Clin Pharmacol.* 1992;33:115.

2. Lehto P, et al. The effect of ferrous sulphate on the absorption of norfloxacin, ciprofloxacin and ofloxacin. *Br J Clin Pharmacol.* 1994;37:82.

3. Okhamafe AO, et al. Pharmacokinetic interactions of norfloxacin with some metallic medicinal agents. *Int J Pharmacol.* 1991;68:11.

4. Polk RE, et al. Effect of ferrous sulfate and multivitamins with zinc on absorption of ciprofloxacin in normal volunteers. *Antimicrob Agents Chemother.* 1989;33:1841.

5. Akerele JO, et al. Influence of oral co-administered metallic drugs on ofloxacin pharmacokinetics. *J Antimicrob Chemother.* 1991;28:87.

6. Kara M, et al. Clinical and chemical interactions between iron preparations and ciprofloxacin. *Br J Clin Pharmacol.* 1991;31:257.

 Iron

Ofloxacin (*Floxin*)

SUMMARY: The administration of iron salts with ofloxacin produces minimal effect on antibiotic concentrations.

RISK FACTORS: No specific risk factors are known.

MECHANISM: Iron salts appear to inhibit ofloxacin absorption by binding to it in the GI tract.

CLINICAL EVALUATION: In one study, iron administration produced a 25% reduction in the ofloxacin area under the concentration-time curve.[1] Another study found only a small reduction in ofloxacin urinary excretion.[2]

RELATED DRUGS: Other quinolones (eg, norfloxacin [*Noroxin*], ciprofloxacin [*Cipro*]) have been reported to be affected by iron.[1]

MANAGEMENT OPTIONS: No specific action is required, but be alert for evidence of the interaction.

REFERENCES:

1. Lehto P, et al. The effect of ferrous sulphate on the absorption of norfloxacin, ciprofloxacin and ofloxacin. *Br J Clin Pharmacol.* 1994;37:82.

2. Akerele JO, et al. Influence of oral co-administered metallic drugs on ofloxacin pharmacokinetics. *J Antimicrob Chemother.* 1991;28:87.

 Iron

Pancreatic Extracts

SUMMARY: Pancreatic extracts may inhibit iron absorption, but the extent of this effect is unknown.

RISK FACTORS: No specific risk factors are known.

MECHANISM: Pancreatic extracts apparently contain a substance that inhibits iron absorption.

CLINICAL EVALUATION: Not established. One preliminary study indicates that the serum iron response to oral iron is decreased by coadministration of various pancreatic extracts and purified pancreatic enzymes.[1]

RELATED DRUGS: No information is available.

MANAGEMENT OPTIONS: No specific action is required, but be alert for evidence of the interaction.

REFERENCES:

1. Dietze F, et al. Inhibition of iron absorption by pancreatic extracts. *Lancet.* 1970;1:424.

Iron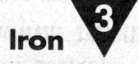

Penicillamine (eg, *Cuprimine*)

SUMMARY: Oral iron may reduce plasma penicillamine concentrations substantially; reduced therapeutic response to penicillamine may occur in some patients.

RISK FACTORS: No specific risk factors are known.

MECHANISM: Oral iron preparations appear to inhibit the absorption of penicillamine.

CLINICAL EVALUATION: In a study using increased urinary copper excretion as a measure of penicillamine effect, 5 healthy subjects were given iron alone, penicillamine alone, and iron plus penicillamine.[1] Iron reduced the pharmacologic effect of penicillamine on urinary copper excretion, presumably by reducing oral absorption of penicillamine. In another study in 6 healthy men, ferrous sulfate 300 mg orally reduced plasma penicillamine levels to 35% of control values.[2]

RELATED DRUGS: No information is available.

MANAGEMENT OPTIONS:

➡ *Circumvent/Minimize.* Patients receiving penicillamine (eg, for rheumatoid arthritis) should separate penicillamine ingestion from oral iron to minimize mixing in the GI tract. Theoretically, giving the penicillamine a few hours before the iron would minimize the interaction.

➡ *Monitor.* Be alert for evidence of reduced penicillamine response, and adjust the penicillamine dosage as needed.

REFERENCES:

1. Lyle WH. Penicillamine and iron. *Lancet*. 1976;2:420.
2. Osman MA, et al. Reduction in oral penicillamine absorption by food, antacid, and ferrous sulfate. *Clin Pharmacol Ther*. 1983;33:465.

Iron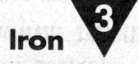

Tetracycline (eg, *Achromycin V*)

SUMMARY: Oral iron products may reduce the serum concentrations and, possibly, the antibacterial efficacy of tetracycline.

RISK FACTORS: No specific risk factors are known.

MECHANISM: Oral ferrous sulfate appears to impair the gastrointestinal (GI) absorption of various tetracyclines, possibly because of chelation or other type of binding in the GI tract.

CLINICAL EVALUATION: In one study, the absorption of tetracycline, oxytetracycline (eg, *Terramycin*), methacycline (*Rondomycin*), and doxycycline (eg, *Vibramycin*) was decreased considerably by the concomitant oral administration of 200 mg of ferrous sulfate.[3] The absorption of methacycline and doxycycline was decreased to a greater degree than that of tetracycline and oxytetracycline. Enteric-coated ferrous sulfate may be less likely to interfere with doxycycline absorption than sugar-coated ferrous sulfate.[1,2] Because doxycycline undergoes enterohepatic circulation, iron may bind this drug even when doxycycline is given parenterally.[4]

RELATED DRUGS: Oxytetracycline, methacycline, and doxycycline interact similarly with oral iron products.

MANAGEMENT OPTIONS:

➡ *Consider Alternative.* On the basis of current evidence, iron preparations should not be administered simultaneously with oral tetracyclines. When possible, a different antibiotic should be chosen if iron is administered.

➡ *Circumvent/Minimize.* If both need to be given to a patient, ferrous sulfate should be administered 3 hours before or 2 hours after tetracycline to minimize the interaction between them.[1] However, the separation of doses may not circumvent interactions between doxycycline and iron preparations.

➡ *Monitor.* If tetracycline and iron are coadministered, be alert for reduced antibiotic effects.

REFERENCES:

1. Mattila MJ, et al. Interference of iron preparations and milk with the absorption of tetracyclines. In: Exerpta Medica International Congress Series No. 254. Amsterdam: Exerpta Medica; 1972:128–33.

2. Bateman FJA. Effects of tetracyclines. *Br Med J.* 1970;4:802.

3. Neuvonen P, et al. Interference of iron with the absorption of tetracyclines in man. *Br Med J.* 1970;4:532.

4. Neuvonen PJ, et al. Effect of oral ferrous sulphate on the half-life of doxycycline in man. *Eur J Clin Pharmacol.* 1974;7:361.

Iron

Vitamin E

SUMMARY: Vitamin E may impair the hematologic response to iron therapy in children with iron-deficiency anemia.

RISK FACTORS: No specific risk factors are known.

MECHANISM: Not established.

CLINICAL EVALUATION: Of 26 children with iron-deficiency anemia receiving daily iron dextran injections, the 9 children who received concurrent vitamin E (200 units/day) had a diminished hematologic response to the iron.[1] More study is needed to confirm this finding.

RELATED DRUGS: No information is available.

MANAGEMENT OPTIONS:

➡ *Monitor.* Patients with iron-deficiency anemia who are receiving iron therapy should be observed for impaired hematologic response if vitamin E is given concomitantly.

REFERENCES:

1. Melhorn DK, et al. Relationships between iron-dextran and vitamin E in an iron deficiency anemia in children. *J Lab Clin Med.* 1969;74:789.

Isocarboxazid (*Marplan*)

Venlafaxine (*Effexor*) AVOID

SUMMARY: Severe serotonin syndrome can occur when venlafaxine is used with or within 2 weeks of discontinuation of isocarboxazid or other nonselective monoamine oxidase inhibitor (MAOI). The combination should be strictly avoided.

RISK FACTORS: No specific risk factors are known.

MECHANISM: Additive. Isocarboxazid, a nonselective MAOI, inhibits serotonin metabolism, and venlafaxine is a potent inhibitor of serotonin reuptake.

CLINICAL EVALUATION: A 43-year-old man on isocarboxazid 30 mg per day started add-on therapy with venlafaxine.[1] After the second dose of venlafaxine he developed agitation, diaphoresis, dilated pupils, hypomania, and shivering. The symptoms abated after the venlafaxine was stopped. Several months later he again added venlafaxine to his isocarboxazid therapy, and quickly developed agitation, myoclonus, diaphoresis, hyperreflexia, and increased muscle tone (ie, a classic case of serotonin syndrome). He responded to supportive therapy and the serotonin antagonist, cyproheptadine, in a dose of 4 mg every 6 hrs.

RELATED DRUGS: All nonselective MAOIs should be expected to result in serotonin syndrome if combined with venlafaxine. This would include phenelzine (*Nardil*) and tranylcypromine (*Parnate*); selegiline (eg, *Eldepryl*) can act as a nonselective MAOI in some patients, especially if large doses are used.

MANAGEMENT OPTIONS:

➥ *AVOID COMBINATION.* Combined use of venlafaxine with isocarboxazid (or any other nonselective MAOI) should be avoided. This would include the use of venlafaxine within 2 weeks of discontinuation of a monoamine oxidase inhibitor.

REFERENCES:

1. Klysner R, et al. Toxic interaction of venlafaxine and isocarboxazide. *Lancet.* 1995;346:1298.

Isoniazid (INH) (eg, *Laniazid*)

Phenytoin (eg, *Dilantin*)

SUMMARY: INH predictably increases serum phenytoin concentrations; phenytoin intoxication is possible in patients who receive the combination.

RISK FACTORS:

➥ *Pharmacogenetics.* Patients who are slow metabolizers of INH are at increased risk for the interaction.

MECHANISM: INH inhibits the hepatic metabolism of phenytoin so that serum concentrations of phenytoin are increased and urinary excretion of its major metabolite is decreased.

CLINICAL EVALUATION: Administration of INH alone as well as in combination with aminosalicylic acid has resulted in phenytoin intoxication.[1,2] Epidemiological data also indicate that toxic central nervous system effects are considerably more common in patients receiving INH and phenytoin than in those receiving phenytoin without INH.[3]

RELATED DRUGS: No information available.

MANAGEMENT OPTIONS:

➡ *Monitor.* Patients receiving both INH and phenytoin should be watched closely for signs of phenytoin toxicity (eg, ataxia, nystagmus, mental impairment, involuntary muscular movements, seizures); the phenytoin dose should be decreased if necessary. If INH is discontinued, monitor the patient for a decreased therapeutic response to phenytoin and increase the dose as needed.

REFERENCES:

1. Kutt H, et al. Diphenylhydantoin intoxication. A complication of isoniazid therapy. *Am Rev Respir Dis.* 1970;101:377.
2. Brennan RW, et al. Diphenylhydantoin intoxication attendant to slow inactivation of isoniazid. *Neurology.* 1970;20:687.
3. Miller RR, et al. Clinical importance of the interaction of phenytoin and isoniazid. *Chest.* 1979;75:356.

Isoniazid (INH) (eg, *Laniazid*)

Prednisolone (eg, *Prelone*)

SUMMARY: Prednisolone may reduce the plasma concentrations of INH.

RISK FACTORS:

➡ *Pharmacogenetics.* Patients who are rapid INH acetylators are at increased risk for the interaction.

MECHANISM: Not established. Enhanced hepatic INH metabolism and/or enhanced renal excretion of INH may be involved. Also, INH may reduce the hepatic metabolism of corticosteroids.

CLINICAL EVALUATION: In 26 patients, prednisolone therapy was associated with a 25% decrease in plasma INH concentrations in slow INH acetylators and a 40% decrease in rapid INH acetylators.[1] Plasma INH concentrations were not reduced by prednisolone in the presence of rifampin. In another study, there was evidence of INH-induced reduction in the hepatic microsomal oxidation of endogenous cortisol, raising the possibility that exogenous corticosteroids might be similarly affected.[2] The clinical significance of these interactions is not established.

RELATED DRUGS: Other corticosteroids might be similarly affected (see Clinical Evaluation).

MANAGEMENT OPTIONS:

➡ *Monitor.* In patients receiving concurrent INH and corticosteroids, watch for evidence of reduced INH effect and enhanced corticosteroid effect.

REFERENCES:

1. Sarma GR, et al. Effect of prednisone and rifampin on isoniazid metabolism in slow and rapid inactivators of isoniazid. *Antimicrob Agents Chemother.* 1980;18:661.
2. Brodie MJ, et al. Effect of isoniazid on vitamin D metabolism and hepatic monooxygenase activity. *Clin Pharmacol Ther.* 1981;30:363.

Isoniazid (INH) (eg, *Laniazid*) 4

Primidone (eg, *Mysoline*)

SUMMARY: INH appeared to increase serum primidone concentrations in 1 patient, but the clinical importance of this effect is not established.

RISK FACTORS: No specific risk factors are known.

MECHANISM: INH may inhibit the metabolism of primidone to its metabolites, phenobarbital and phenylethylmalonamide.

CLINICAL EVALUATION: In a patient taking primidone and INH, serum primidone concentrations were high and serum phenobarbital concentrations were lower than expected.[1] Subsequent study of this patient with and without INH indicated that INH inhibited primidone metabolism. More study is needed to determine the incidence of this interaction in patients receiving both drugs.

RELATED DRUGS: No information is available.

MANAGEMENT OPTIONS: No specific action is required, but be alert for evidence of the interaction.

REFERENCES:

1. Sutton G, et al. Isoniazid as an inhibitor of primidone metabolism. *Neurology*. 1975;25:1179.

Isoniazid (INH) (eg, *Laniazid*) 4

Procainamide (eg, *Pronestyl*)

SUMMARY: The half-life of INH is slightly prolonged by procainamide administration, but the clinical importance of this effect is not established.

RISK FACTORS: No specific risk factors are known.

MECHANISM: Not established.

CLINICAL EVALUATION: In a study of 4 normal subjects, INH half-life was slightly prolonged by concomitant ingestion of procainamide (6 mg/kg every 4 hours).[1] However, procainamide acetylation rate, as measured by its half-life, did not appear to be affected by INH. This interaction is not definitely established. The clinical effect of a prolonged INH half-life is not clear from the data provided but probably is not significant.

RELATED DRUGS: No information is available.

MANAGEMENT OPTIONS: No specific action is required, but be alert for evidence of the interaction.

REFERENCES:

1. Schneck D, et al. Effect of procainamide and isoniazid on each other's acetylation pathway in normal subjects. *Clin Pharmacol Ther*. 1977;21:116.

Isoniazid (INH) (eg, *Laniazid*)

Rifampin (eg, *Rifadin*)

SUMMARY: Although rifampin may increase the hepatic toxicity of INH in certain predisposed patients, the combination does not cause hepatotoxicity in the vast majority of patients.

RISK FACTORS:

➡ *Concurrent Diseases.* Patients with pre-existing liver disease and those having recently undergone general anesthesia are at increased risk of the interaction.

➡ *Pharmacogenetics.* Patients who are slow INH acetylators are at increased risk for the interaction.

MECHANISM: Rifampin enhances the conversion of INH to a hepatotoxic metabolite (hydrazine) and rarely may increase the risk of hepatitis in patients taking both drugs.[2,4]

CLINICAL EVALUATION: There is some clinical evidence to indicate that the combined use of INH and rifampin may result in more frequent hepatotoxicity than when either drug is given alone.[1,3-7]

RELATED DRUGS: No information is available.

MANAGEMENT OPTIONS:

➡ *Monitor.* Patients receiving INH and rifampin should be monitored for evidence of hepatotoxicity, especially if they are known to be slow acetylators of INH or have pre-existing liver disease.

REFERENCES:

1. Lal S, et al. Effect of rifampicin and isoniazid on liver function. *Br Med J.* 1972;1:148.
2. Beever IW, et al. Circulating hydrazine during treatment with isoniazid and rifampicin in man. *Br J Clin Pharmacol.* 1982;13:599.
3. Pessayre D, et al. Isoniazid-rifampin fulminant hepatitis. A possible consequence of the enhancement of isoniazid hepatotoxicity by enzyme induction. *Gastroenterology.* 1977;72:284.
4. Sarma GR, et al. Rifampin-induced release of hydrazine from isoniazid. *Am Rev Resp Dis.* 1986;133:1072.
5. Bistritzer T, et al. Isoniazid-rifampin-induced fulminant liver disease in an infant. *J Pediatr.* 1980;97:480.
6. Llorens J, et al. Pharmacodynamic interference between rifampicin and isoniazid. *Chemotherapy.* 1978;24:97.
7. Steele MA, et al. Toxic hepatitis with isoniazid and rifampin. A metaanalysis. *Chest.* 1991;99:465.

Isoniazid (INH) (eg, *Laniazid*)

Theophylline (eg, *Theo-Dur*)

SUMMARY: Theophylline plasma concentrations increased following several weeks of INH administration; some patients may develop theophylline toxicity.

RISK FACTORS: No specific risk factors are known.

MECHANISM: INH appears to gradually decrease the clearance of theophylline during chronic administration.

CLINICAL EVALUATION: Studies in healthy subjects have noted an 8% to 21% reduction in theophylline clearance (Isoniazid dose: 400 mg/day to 10 mg/kg/day).[2,5] Several case reports have noted increased theophylline concentrations and occasional symptoms of theophylline toxicity.[3,4] One small study found an increase in theophylline clearance following INH (300 mg/day).[1]

RELATED DRUGS: No information is available.

MANAGEMENT OPTIONS:

➡ *Monitor.* Patients stabilized on theophylline should be monitored for increased theophylline concentrations when INH is administered. The interaction may require several weeks to reach its full potential.

REFERENCES:

1. Thompson JR, et al. Isoniazid-induced alternations in theophylline pharmacokinetics. *Curr Ther Res.* 1982;32:921.
2. Hoglund P, et al. Interaction between isoniazid and theophylline. *Eur J Respir Dis.* 1987;70:110.
3. Torrent J, et al. Theophylline-isoniazid interaction. *DICP.* 1989;23:143.
4. Dal Nergo R, et al. Rifampicin-isoniazid and delayed elimination of theophylline: a case report. *Int J Clin Pharm Res.* 1988;8:275.
5. Samigun M, et al. Lowering of theophylline clearance by isoniazid in slow and rapid acetylators. *Br J Clin Pharmacol.* 1990;29:570.

Isoniazid (INH) (eg, *Laniazid*)

Triazolam (eg, *Halcion*)

SUMMARY: INH may increase triazolam serum concentrations; the clinical significance is unknown.

RISK FACTORS: No specific risk factors are known.

MECHANISM: INH probably inhibits the hepatic metabolism of some benzodiazepines.

CLINICAL EVALUATION: Preliminary evidence indicates that triazolam metabolism may be reduced by INH.[1] Since INH is known to inhibit the metabolism of diazepam, one would expect a similar interaction with triazolam. More study is needed to define the significance of this interaction.

RELATED DRUGS: INH inhibits the metabolism of diazepam (eg, *Valium*).

MANAGEMENT OPTIONS:

➡ *Monitor.* Watch for evidence of increased sedation when triazolam is administered with INH.

REFERENCES:

1. Ochs HR, et al. Interaction of triazolam with ethanol and isoniazid. *Clin Pharmacol Ther.* 1983;33:241.

Isoniazid (INH) (eg, *Laniazid*)

Valproic Acid (eg, *Depakene*)

SUMMARY: In 1 patient, valproic acid plasma concentrations increased after the addition of INH resulting in symptoms of valproic acid toxicity.

RISK FACTORS:

➡ ***Pharmacogenetics.*** Patients who are slow acetylators of INH are at increased risk for the interaction.

MECHANISM: Not established. INH probably inhibits the hepatic metabolism of valproic acid.

CLINICAL EVALUATION: In a patient on chronic valproic acid therapy, valproic acid concentrations increased after INH was administered. The patient was identified as a slow acetylator of INH. A 62% decrease in valproic acid dose was required to maintain valproic acid plasma concentrations after addition of the INH.[1]

RELATED DRUGS: No information is available.

MANAGEMENT OPTIONS:

➡ ***Monitor.*** Patients should be monitored for changes in response to valproic acid when INH is started (ie, nausea, sedation) or stopped (ie, reduced seizure control).

REFERENCES:

1. Jonville AP, et al. Interaction between isoniazid and valproate: a case of valproate overdosage. *Eur J Clin Pharmacol.* 1991;40:197.

 Isoniazid (INH) (eg, *Laniazid*)

Warfarin (eg, *Coumadin*)

SUMMARY: Isolated case reports and theoretical considerations indicate that INH may enhance the effect of oral anticoagulants such as warfarin, but the incidence and clinical significance of this interaction are unknown.

RISK FACTORS: No specific risk factors are known.

MECHANISM: Not established. INH is known to inhibit the metabolism of phenytoin which, like warfarin, is metabolized by CYPZC9.

CLINICAL EVALUATION: A patient stabilized on warfarin developed excessive hypoprothrombinemia and bleeding approximately 10 days after his INH dose was increased from 300 to 600 mg/day.[1] Slow INH acetylators who take large doses of the drug would appear to be at greatest risk. Furthermore, INH alone has resulted in severe bleeding in several patients; this phenomenon is related to the production of a substance that inhibits fibrin stabilization.[2] This effect probably is quite rare but should be considered in patients on INH who develop bleeding.

RELATED DRUGS: Other oral anticoagulants may be similarly affected.

MANAGEMENT OPTIONS:

➡ ***Monitor.*** Patients stabilized on oral anticoagulants should be monitored for increased hypoprothrombinemic response when INH therapy is initiated and decreased response when it is discontinued. Initiation of oral anticoagulant therapy in a patient already on chronic INH should not pose difficulties because the patient can be titrated to the proper dose of anticoagulant.

REFERENCES:
1. Rosenthal AR, et al. Interaction of isoniazid and warfarin. *JAMA*. 1977;238:2177.
2. Otis PT, et al. An acquired inhibitor of fibrin stabilization associated with isoniazid therapy: clinical and biochemical observations. *Blood*. 1974;44:771.

Isoproterenol (eg, *Isuprel*)

Propranolol (eg, *Inderal*)

SUMMARY: Propranolol and other beta blockers, particularly nonselective agents, may reduce the effectiveness of isoproterenol and other beta agonists in the treatment of asthma.

RISK FACTORS:

➡ *Concurrent Diseases.* Patients with asthma are at increased risk for the interaction.

MECHANISM: Beta-adrenergic blockers can antagonize the beta-adrenergic effects (including bronchodilation, hypotension, and tachycardia) of isoproterenol.

CLINICAL EVALUATION: Asthmatic patients pretreated with propranolol are resistant to the bronchodilating effects of isoproterenol as measured by the forced expiratory volume in 1 second (FEV_1).[2,4] The selective β_1-receptor blockers, such as metoprolol (eg, *Lopressor*) and practolol, appear to be less likely to inhibit isoproterenol-induced increases in FEV_1.[1,2,4] Nevertheless, metoprolol reduced FEV_1 and the response to isoproterenol in patients with asthma, while labetalol (eg, *Normodyne*) had no such effect.[1] Propranolol and other beta blockers also have inhibited (in normal subjects) isoproterenol-induced increases in pulse rate, decreases in diastolic blood pressure, and increases in plasma cyclic AMP.[3,5]

RELATED DRUGS: See Clinical Evaluation. Beta blockers, such as metoprolol and practolol, would be expected to inhibit the bronchodilating activity of all beta agonists. Labetalol appears to have a lesser effect on isoproterenol response.

MANAGEMENT OPTIONS:

➡ *Consider Alternative.* The mutually antagonistic effects of propranolol and isoproterenol indicate that their concomitant use would seldom be justified. If beta agonists such as isoproterenol are being used to treat asthma, propranolol and other nonselective beta blockers probably should be avoided. No beta blocker should be considered absolutely safe in patients with asthma.

➡ *Monitor.* If a beta blocker is used in a patient with asthma, carefully monitor for adverse pulmonary effects.

REFERENCES:
1. Falliers CJ, et al. Effect of single doses of labetalol, metoprolol, and placebo on ventilatory function in patients with bronchial asthma: interaction with isoproterenol. *J Asthma*. 1986;23:251.
2. Johnson G, et al. Effects of intravenous propranolol and metoprolol and their interaction with isoprenaline on pulmonary function, heart rate, and blood pressure in asthmatics. *Eur J Clin Pharmacol*. 1975;8:175.
3. Messerli FH, et al. Effects of beta-adrenergic blockade on plasma cyclic AMP and blood sugar responses to glucagon and isoproterenol in man. *Int J Clin Pharmacol*. 1976;14:189.
4. Thiringer G, et al. Interaction of orally administered metoprolol, practolol and propranolol in asthmatics. *Eur J Clin Pharmacol*. 1976;10:163.
5. Perruca E, et al. Effect of atenolol, metoprolol, and propranolol on isoproterenol-induced tremor and tachycardia in normal subjects. *Clin Pharmacol Ther*. 1981;29:425.

Isosorbide Mononitrate (ISMO)

AVOID **Sildenafil (*Viagra*)**

SUMMARY: Systolic and diastolic blood pressure may be markedly reduced by the coadministration of sildenafil and isosorbide mononitrate.

RISK FACTORS: No specific risk factors are known.

MECHANISM: Unknown. Additive hypotensive effects due to vasodilation appear to be at least partially responsible.

CLINICAL EVALUATION: Eighteen subjects with stable angina who were being treated with nitrates received isosorbide mononitrate 20 mg/day for 5 to 7 days.[1] A single dose of placebo or sildenafil 50 mg was administered with the isosorbide. The maximal reduction in systolic blood pressure with sildenafil exceeded placebo by 19 mm Hg and 27 mm Hg in the sitting and standing positions, respectively. Sitting and standing diastolic blood pressure fell by 13 mm Hg and 14 mm Hg, respectively. The exaggerated hypotensive effect persisted for several hours following sildenafil administration. These reductions could result in dizziness or syncope.

RELATED DRUGS: It is expected that a similar result would occur with other forms of nitrates including nitroglycerin (eg, *Nitro Dur*) and isosorbide dinitrate (eg, *Isordil*).

MANAGEMENT OPTIONS:

➡ ***AVOID COMBINATION.*** Sildenafil should not be used by patients taking nitrates due to the risk of hypotension.

REFERENCES:

1. Pfizer Pharmaceuticals. Sildenafil (*Viagra*) product information. 1998.

4   **Isotretinoin (eg, *Accutane*)**

Warfarin (eg, *Coumadin*)

SUMMARY: A patient developed reduced warfarin response after starting isotretinoin, but the clinical importance of this effect is not established.

RISK FACTORS: No specific risk factors are known.

MECHANISM: Not established.

CLINICAL EVALUATION: A 61-year-old man well stabilized on chronic warfarin therapy developed reduced warfarin effect after he was started on oral isotretinoin 30 mg/day.[1] His warfarin requirements increased from 2.5 to 3.75 mg/day after isotretinoin was added and returned to 2.5 mg/day after isotretinoin was stopped. The positive dechallenge supports the suspicion that isotretinoin was responsible, but more study is needed to establish a causal relationship.

RELATED DRUGS: Reduced warfarin effect also has been reported following etretinate[†], but a causal relationship was not established.

MANAGEMENT OPTIONS: No specific action is required, but be alert for evidence of the interaction.

REFERENCES:

1. Fiallo P. Reduced therapeutic activity of warfarin during treatment with oral isotretinoin. *Br J Dermatol.* 2004;150(1):164.

† Not available in the United States.

Isradipine (eg, *DynaCirc*)

Lovastatin (eg, *Mevacor*)

SUMMARY: Isradipine decreases lovastatin plasma concentrations; the clinical significance of this reduction is unknown, but reduction of efficacy is possible.

RISK FACTORS: No specific risk factors are known.

MECHANISM: Not established. Isradipine appears to increase the clearance after oral administration of lovastatin, perhaps by increasing hepatic blood flow. Based on available data, reduced lovastatin absorption cannot be ruled out.

CLINICAL EVALUATION: Five healthy subjects received isradipine 5 mg alone, lovastatin 20 mg alone, or the combination for 5 days.[1] Drug clearances were determined on days 1 and 5 of each regimen. Isradipine clearance was not significantly affected by lovastatin administration. During isradipine coadministration, lovastatin clearance after oral administration was increased 67% and 78% on days 1 and 5, respectively, compared with lovastatin monotherapy. In another study, isradipine 5 mg twice daily for 5 days reduced lovastatin concentrations and activity in more men than women.[2] The clinical efficacy of lovastatin could be diminished by the reduced plasma concentrations.

RELATED DRUGS: The effect of isradipine on other HMG-CoA inhibitors is unknown, but they may be similarly affected.

MANAGEMENT OPTIONS:

➡ *Monitor.* Until more information is available, monitor patients taking lovastatin for reduced effects during isradipine coadministration.

REFERENCES:

1. Holtzman JL, et al. Interaction between isradipine and lovastatin in normal male volunteers. *Clin Pharmacol Ther.* 1993;53:164.

2. Zhou LX, et al. Pharmacokinetic interaction between isradipine and lovastatin in normal, female and male volunteers. *J Pharmacol Exper Ther.* 1995;273(1):121-127.

Itraconazole (eg, *Sporanox*)

Colchicine

SUMMARY: Based on the interactive properties of the 2 drugs, it is likely that itraconazole substantially increases colchicine plasma concentrations. Avoid the combination if possible.

RISK FACTORS: No specific risk factors are known

MECHANISM: Colchicine is a P-glycoprotein substrate, and itraconazole is a P-glycoprotein inhibitor, so colchicine plasma concentrations are likely to increase.[1,2] Itraconazole is also a CYP3A4 inhibitor, and may inhibit the CYP3A4 metabolism of colchicine.

CLINICAL EVALUATION: Although the interaction is based primarily on theoretical considerations, it is likely that itraconazole would increase the risk of colchicine toxicity. Given that colchicine toxicity can be fatal, even a theoretical interaction warrants close attention.

RELATED DRUGS: Ketoconazole (eg, *Nizoral*) and posaconazole (*Noxafil*) may also inhibit P-glycoprotein and CYP3A4, and are expected to increase the risk of colchicine toxicity. Fluconazole (eg, *Diflucan*) and voriconazole (*Vfend*) inhibit CYP3A4 and may also increase colchicine plasma concentrations.

MANAGEMENT OPTIONS:

➡ ***Avoid Unless Benefit Outweighs Risk.*** Given that colchicine toxicity can be life-threatening, use itraconazole only if it is likely to provide therapeutic benefits that cannot be achieved with noninteracting alternatives.

➡ ***Use Alternative.*** If possible, use an alternative to itraconazole that does not inhibit P-glycoprotein, or use an alternative to colchicine.

➡ ***Monitor.*** If the combination must be used, monitor carefully for colchicine toxicity such as diarrhea, vomiting, fever, abdominal pain, and muscle pain. Advise the patient to immediately contact a health care provider if any of these symptoms occur. Colchicine-induced pancytopenia can result in infections, bleeding, and anemia, and is often the cause of death in fatal cases.

REFERENCES:

1. Rautio J, et al. In vitro p-glycoprotein inhibition assays for assessment of clinical drug interaction potential of new drug candidates: a recommendation for probe substrates. *Drug Metab Dispos*. 2006;34(5):786-792.

2. Shimizu M, et al. Effects of itraconazole and diltiazem on the pharmacokinetics of fexofenadine, a substrate of P-glycoprotein. *Br J Clin Pharmacol*. 2006;61(5):538-544.

Itraconazole (eg, *Sporanox*)

Fentanyl (eg, *Actiq*)

SUMMARY: Itraconazole administration may increase the plasma concentrations of fentanyl.

RISK FACTORS: No specific risk factors are known.

MECHANISM: Fentanyl is metabolized by CYP3A4, an enzyme that is inhibited by itraconazole.

CLINICAL EVALUATION: A case report noted opioid toxicity (agitated delirium and myoclonus of the muscles in the hand) 1 day after itraconazole 200 mg twice daily was administered to a patient who had been receiving transdermal fentanyl 50 mcg/h.[1] Symptoms resolved 2 days following the discontinuation of fentanyl. While this interaction is expected on a theoretical basis, this case report does not provide much data for evaluation. Further study is needed.

RELATED DRUGS: Other antifungal agents that inhibit CYP3A4 (eg, fluconazole [eg, *Diflucan*], ketoconazole [eg, *Nizoral*], voriconazole [*Vfend*]) are expected to affect fentanyl in a similar manner. Itraconazole is likely to decrease the elimination of methadone.

MANAGEMENT OPTIONS:

➡ *Consider Alternative.* Consider using analgesics not metabolized by CYP3A4 (eg, codeine, morphine, tramadol [eg, *Ultram*]) in patients requiring itraconazole.

➡ *Monitor.* Monitor patients receiving fentanyl and itraconazole for increased sedation, respiratory depression, and nausea.

REFERENCES:

1. Mercadante S, et al. Itraconazole-fentanyl interaction in a cancer patient. *J Pain Symptom Manage.* 2002;24(3):284-286.

Itraconazole (eg, *Sporanox*)

Haloperidol (eg, *Haldol*)

SUMMARY: Itraconazole may increase the plasma concentrations of haloperidol; monitor patients for signs of toxicity.

RISK FACTORS:

➡ *Pharmacogenetics.* Patients who have a deficiency in CYP2D6 enzyme activity may be more susceptible to the inhibitory effect of itraconazole on haloperidol metabolism.

MECHANISM: Haloperidol is metabolized by CYP2D6 as well as by CYP3A4 and perhaps CYP1A2. In patients lacking normal CYP2D6 activity, CYP3A4 may take on a greater role in the metabolism of haloperidol. Itraconazole is a potent inhibitor of CYP3A4 and may cause an increase in the plasma concentration of haloperidol.

CLINICAL EVALUATION: Thirteen patients with schizophrenia were being treated with haloperidol 12 or 24 mg daily.[1] Itraconazole 200 mg was added for 7 days. Mean haloperidol plasma concentrations were increased 30% following itraconazole coadministration. Neurologic side effects appeared to increase during itraconazole coadministration. Healthy subjects received single doses of haloperidol 5 mg following 7 days of itraconazole or placebo.[2] Mean haloperidol clearance was reduced 31% following itraconazole pretreatment. The effect of itraconazole was greater (mean 50% reduction) in patients who were identified as deficient in the CYP2D6 enzyme. This suggests that CYP3A4 may play a more important role in the metabolism of haloperidol in patients genetically deficient in the primary enzyme (CYP2D6) that metabolizes haloperidol. No side effects, such as QT prolongation, were observed in this single-dose study. However, patients with low CYP2D6 clearance of haloperidol may be at increased risk of haloperidol toxicity (eg, arrhythmia, sedation) during itraconazole coadministration.

RELATED DRUGS: Fluconazole (eg, *Diflucan*), ketoconazole (eg, *Nizoral*), and voriconazole (*Vfend*) also may produce a reduction in the clearance of haloperidol.

MANAGEMENT OPTIONS:

➡ *Consider Alternative.* Terbinafine (*Lamisil*) does not inhibit CYP3A4 but does inhibit CYP2D6, the major pathway for haloperidol metabolism in most patients. It may be a suitable alternative to itraconazole in patients known to be deficient in CYP2D6.

➡ **Monitor.** Patients taking potent CYP3A4 inhibitors may be at increased risk for toxicity from haloperidol, particularly if large doses of haloperidol are required or in slow metabolizers of CYP2D6 substrates.

REFERENCES:

1. Yasui N, et al. Effects of itraconazole on the steady-state plasma concentrations of haloperidol and its reduced metabolite in schizophrenic patients: in vivo evidence of the involvement of CYP3A4 for haloperidol metabolism. *J Clin Psychopharmacol.* 1999;19:149-154.

2. Park J, et al. The effects of CHYP2D6*10 and itraconazole on the disposition and adverse effects of haloperidol (HAL) in normal subjects. *Clin Pharmacol Ther.* 2002;71:P87.

 Itraconazole (*Sporanox*)

Lovastatin (eg, *Mevacor*)

SUMMARY: Itraconazole administration produces a large increase in lovastatin concentrations; toxicity, including rhabdomyolysis, may occur. Avoid concurrent use.

RISK FACTORS: No specific risk factors are known.

MECHANISM: Lovastatin is metabolized to an active metabolite, lovastatin acid, by hydrolysis that is not dependent on the enzyme CYP3A4. Lovastatin also is metabolized to inactive metabolites by CYP3A4. Itraconazole inhibits the metabolism of lovastatin to its inactive metabolites (notably during first pass in the intestinal wall and liver), resulting in higher lovastatin concentrations and an increase in lovastatin acid concentrations as the parent drug is converted by non-CYP3A4 dependent metabolism. This results in accumulation of lovastatin and its active metabolite during itraconazole administration.

CLINICAL EVALUATION: A case report noted a 63-year-old woman who for years had been receiving lovastatin 80 mg and niacin 3 g/day for the treatment of hypercholesterolemia.[1] She also was taking timolol and aspirin. Itraconazole 100 mg twice daily was added to her regimen. Two weeks later she developed weakness, painful muscles, and elevated serum enzymes (eg, aldolase, creatine kinase) indicative of rhabdomyolysis. Her symptoms cleared when the itraconazole, lovastatin, and niacin were discontinued. In a study of 12 subjects, single doses of lovastatin 40 mg were administered alone and following itraconazole 200 mg/day for 4 days.[2] The mean peak lovastatin concentration increased more than 20-fold during the itraconazole phase. The mean area under the concentration-time curve of lovastatin increased from less than 15 ng/mL/hr to 546 ng/mL/hr. The concentrations of the active metabolite of lovastatin, lovastatin acid, were increased to a similar degree. The plasma creatine kinase concentration increased in 1 subject during the itraconazole phase but not when lovastatin was administered alone. Patients taking lovastatin and itraconazole are at increased risk for rhabdomyolysis.

RELATED DRUGS: Simvastatin (*Zocor*) and atorvastatin (*Lipitor*) are metabolized in a similar manner to lovastatin and their metabolism probably would be inhibited by itraconazole. Pravastatin (*Pravachol*) may not be as dependent on CYP3A4 metabolism and, therefore, may not be inhibited to the same extent by itraconazole. The safety of fluvastatin (*Lescol*) has not been established. Ketoconazole (eg, *Nizoral*), miconazole (eg, *Monistat*), and fluconazole (eg, *Diflucan*) would be expected to inhibit the metabolism of some HMG-CoA reductase inhibitors. Terbinafine (*Lamisil*) may have minimal effect on the metabolism of HMG-CoA reductase inhibitors.

MANAGEMENT OPTIONS:

➡ *Use Alternative.* Pending further studies on other HMG-CoA reductase inhibitors, lovastatin and probably simvastatin should not be administered with itraconazole or other inhibitors of CYP3A4. The safety of pravastatin or fluvastatin when combined with itraconazole has not been established. Terbinafine may have minimal effect on the metabolism of the HMG-CoA reductase inhibitors because it does not appear to inhibit CYP3A4 activity. Carefully monitor patients receiving HMG-CoA reductase inhibitors, especially lovastatin or simvastatin, for muscle pain or weakness when any drug known to inhibit the activity of CYP3A4 is administered.

REFERENCES:

1. Lees RS, et al. Rhabdomyolysis from the coadministration of lovastatin and the antifungal agent itraconazole. *N Engl J Med.* 1995;333:664-665.

2. Neuvonen PJ, et al. Itraconazole drastically increases plasma concentrations of lovastatin and lovastatin acid. *Clin Pharmacol Ther.* 1996;60:54-61.

Itraconazole (*Sporanox*)

Methylprednisolone (eg, *Medrol*)

SUMMARY: Itraconazole increases the plasma concentrations of methylprednisolone; increased side effects associated with corticosteroid use may occur.

RISK FACTORS: No specific risk factors are known.

MECHANISM: Itraconazole inhibits the metabolism of methylprednisolone, a substrate for CYP3A4 metabolism.

CLINICAL EVALUATION: Ten healthy subjects received 200 mg itraconazole or placebo once daily for 4 days.[1] On day 4, they were administered 16 mg oral methylprednisolone. Compared with placebo, itraconazole increased the area under the concentration-time curve of methylprednisolone by approximately 4-fold, and its half-life increased from 1.9 to 4.4 hours. The concentration of endogenous cortisol was reduced approximately 87% during concurrent methylprednisolone and itraconazole compared with methylprednisolone and placebo. A case report noted the development of myopathy and diabetes in a transplant patient receiving methylprednisolone and itraconazole.[2]

RELATED DRUGS: The effect of other azole antifungals that inhibit CYP3A4 would likely be similar. Ketoconazole (eg, *Nizoral*) has been noted to increase the concentration of IV methylprednisolone 135%. Fluconazole (*Diflucan*) is a weak CYP3A4 inhibitor, except in high doses. Terbinafine (*Lamisil*) is not known to inhibit CYP3A4 activity. The effect of itraconazole on other corticosteroids has not been established, but the metabolism of prednisone (*Deltasone*) and prednisolone (*Delta-Cortef*) is likely to be reduced by CYP3A4 inhibition.

MANAGEMENT OPTIONS:

➡ *Circumvent/Minimize.* Patients receiving concurrent itraconazole may require reduced doses of methylprednisolone.

➡ **Monitor.** Monitor patients for steroid-induced side effects including myopathy, weakness, and glucose intolerance.

REFERENCES:

1. Varis T, et al. Plasma concentrations and effects of oral methylprednisolone are considerably increased by itraconazole. *Clin Pharmacol Ther.* 1998;64:363-368.
2. Linthoudt H, et al. The association of itraconazole and methylprednisolone may give rise to important steroid-related side effects. *J Heart Lung Transplant.* 1996;15:1165.

Itraconazole (*Sporanox*)

Midazolam (*Versed*)

SUMMARY: Itraconazole administration causes a large increase in oral midazolam plasma concentrations and pharmacodynamic effects; increased side effects are likely.

RISK FACTORS:

➡ **Route of Administration.** Plasma midazolam concentrations will increase to a greater extent following oral administration than after IV midazolam dosing.

MECHANISM: Itraconazole inhibits the CYP3A4 metabolism of midazolam. This results in an increase in midazolam's bioavailability following oral dosing and a reduction in its systemic clearance after oral and IV dosing.

CLINICAL EVALUATION: Twelve healthy subjects received placebo or itraconazole 100 mg/day for 4 days.[1] On the fourth day, a single dose of midazolam 7.5 mg was administered orally 2 hours after the placebo or itraconazole. Compared with placebo, itraconazole increased the peak concentration of midazolam 155% and its area under the concentration-time curve 475%. Midazolam's half-life increased from 3.8 to 7.3 hours. Other studies have demonstrated equally large changes during the coadministration of oral midazolam and itraconazole.[2,3] Itraconazole has been shown to reduce the clearance of IV midazolam 70%.[3] The psychomotor effects of midazolam were increased by coadministration with itraconazole.

RELATED DRUGS: Ketoconazole (eg, *Nizoral*) and fluconazole (*Diflucan*) also reduce the metabolism of midazolam. Terbinafine (*Lamisil*) does not affect midazolam pharmacokinetics. Other benzodiazepines metabolized by CYP3A4 also will be affected by itraconazole, including alprazolam (eg, *Xanax*) and triazolam (eg, *Halcion*). Benzodiazepines that are metabolized by glucuronidation (eg, oxazepam [eg, *Serax*], lorazepam [eg, *Ativan*], temazepam [eg, *Restoril*]) will likely be minimally affected by itraconazole.

MANAGEMENT OPTIONS:

➡ **Consider Alternative.** Prescribe an oral benzodiazepine that is not metabolized via the CYP3A4 enzyme for patients maintained on itraconazole (see Related Drugs). Patients stabilized on midazolam requiring antifungal therapy might be candidates for terbinafine.

➡ **Monitor.** Carefully monitor patients receiving oral midazolam and itraconazole for increased sedation and reduced psychomotor performance.

REFERENCES:

1. Ahonen J, et al. Effect of itraconazole and terbinafine on the pharmacokinetics and pharmacodynamics of midazolam in healthy volunteers. *Br J Clin Pharmacol.* 1995;40:270-272.

2. Olkkola KT, et al. Midazolam should be avoided in patients receiving the systemic antimycotics keto-conazole and itraconazole. *Clin Pharmacol Ther*. 1994;55:481-485.

3. Olkkola KT, et al. The effects of the systemic antimycotics, itraconazole and fluconazole, on the phar-macokinetics and pharmacodynamics of intravenous and oral midazolam. *Anesth Analg*. 1996;82:511-516.

Itraconazole (*Sporanox*)

Nifedipine (eg, *Procardia*)

SUMMARY: Itraconazole administration produced increased nifedipine concentrations and enhanced the hypotensive effects of the calcium channel blocker.

RISK FACTORS: No specific risk factors are known.

MECHANISM: Itraconazole is known to inhibit CYP3A4, the enzyme responsible for the metabolism of nifedipine.

CLINICAL EVALUATION: A patient with pedal onychomycosis was treated with itraconazole 200 mg twice daily 1 week/month for 3 months.[1] The patient's chronic medications included medroxyprogesterone (eg, *Provera*), conjugated estrogen (*Premarin*), nifedipine, and atenolol (eg, *Tenormin*) (doses not stated). During the first and second courses of itraconazole, the patient developed ankle edema starting 2 to 3 days after initiation of itraconazole and resolving 2 to 3 days after the itracona-zole pulse dose was completed. Trough serum nifedipine concentrations were measured during the third itraconazole pulse and increased from 12.7 ng/mL before itraconazole was administered to 56.1 ng/mL at the end of the treatment week. A drop in blood pressure accompanied this increase in nifedipine concentration.

RELATED DRUGS: It is likely that ketoconazole (eg, *Nizoral*) would inhibit the metabolism of nifedipine in a similar manner. Fluconazole (*Diflucan*) is a weak CYP3A4 inhibitor except in high doses. Terbinafine (*Lamisil*) is not known to inhibit CYP3A4 activity. Other calcium channel blockers would likely be affected by azole antifungals that inhibit CYP3A4.

MANAGEMENT OPTIONS:

➡ **Consider Alternative.** If excessive calcium channel blocker effect is observed with con-comitant itraconazole therapy, a non-calcium channel blocker antihypertensive agent could be substituted for nifedipine. Consider terbinafine in place of itra-conazole if appropriate.

➡ **Monitor.** Monitor patients receiving nifedipine or other calcium channel blockers for exaggerated effect (eg, hypotension, peripheral edema) during the coadministra-tion of itraconazole.

REFERENCES:

1. Tailor SA, et al. Peripheral edema due to nifedipine-itraconazole interaction: a case report. *Arch Dermatol*. 1996;132:350-352.

Itraconazole (eg, *Sporanox*)

Omeprazole (eg, *Prilosec*)

SUMMARY: Omeprazole administration markedly reduces the plasma concentration of itraconazole; loss of antifungal effect may occur.

RISK FACTORS:

➡ ***Pharmacogenetics.*** Patients who are slow CYP2C19 metabolizers of omeprazole likely will be affected to a higher degree.

MECHANISM: Itraconazole requires an acidic media in the stomach for complete dissolution of the drug. Increasing the gastric pH will decrease the amount of itraconazole absorbed.

CLINICAL EVALUATION: Eleven healthy subjects received a single oral dose of itraconazole 200 mg after breakfast and again following 2 weeks of omeprazole 40 mg/day.[1] The coadministration of omeprazole resulted in a reduction in the mean area under the concentration-time curve and peak plasma concentration of itraconazole 64% and 66%, respectively. Loss of antifungal efficacy could result. Although not examined in this study, it is likely that itraconazole would inhibit the metabolism of omeprazole (via CYP3A4) as has been noted when ketoconazole (eg, *Nizoral*) and omeprazole are administered together.

RELATED DRUGS: Ketoconazole is also dependent on an acidic gastric pH for complete absorption. All proton pump inhibitors (eg, esomeprazole [*Nexium*], lansoprazole [eg, *Prevacid*], pantoprazole [eg, *Protonix*], rabeprazole [*Aciphex*]) will reduce the absorption of itraconazole and ketoconazole. Fluconazole (eg, *Diflucan*) and voriconazole (*Vfend*) absorption does not appear to be affected by alkalinization of the stomach.

MANAGEMENT OPTIONS:

➡ ***Circumvent/Minimize.*** The administration of acidic drinks such as *Coca-Cola* or *Pepsi* (both have a pH of 2.5) increases the absorption of itraconazole and ketoconazole in patients with an elevated gastric pH.[2,3] Theoretically, an oral solution of itraconazole would not be affected by changes in gastric pH, although no data are available. Consider using an alternative antifungal, such as fluconazole or voriconazole.

➡ ***Monitor.*** Monitor patients taking itraconazole for possible loss of antifungal efficacy if drugs that can increase gastric pH are coadministered.

REFERENCES:

1. Jaruratanasirikul S, et al. Effect of omeprazole on the pharmacokinetics of itraconazole. *Eur J Clin Pharmacol*. 1998;54(2):159-161.
2. Lange D, et al. The effect of coadministration of a cola beverage on the bioavailability of itraconazole in patients with acquired immunodeficiency syndrome. *Curr Ther Res Clin Exp*. 1997;58:202-212.
3. Jaruratanasirikul S, et al. Influence of an acidic beverage (*Coca-Cola*) on the absorption of itraconazole. *Eur J Clin Pharmacol*. 1997;52(3):235-237.

Itraconazole (eg, *Sporanox*)

Oxybutynin (eg, *Ditropan*)

SUMMARY: Itraconazole may increase oxybutynin serum concentrations, but the clinical importance of this effect appears minimal.

RISK FACTORS: No specific risk factors are known.

MECHANISM: Itraconazole probably inhibits the CYP3A4 metabolism of oxybutynin.

CLINICAL EVALUATION: In a double-blind randomized study in healthy subjects, itraconazole 200 mg daily for 4 days produced about a doubling of oxybutynin serum concentrations.[1] However, there was little change in the serum concentrations of the active metabolite of oxybutynin, N-desethoxybutynin. Because most of the pharmacodynamic effect of oxybutynin is caused by the active metabolite, the interaction does not appear likely to result in adverse outcomes.

RELATED DRUGS: No information is available.

MANAGEMENT OPTIONS: No specific action is required, but be alert for evidence of the interaction.

REFERENCES:
1. Lukkari E, et al. Itraconazole moderately increases serum concentrations of oxybutynin but does not affect those of the active metabolite. *Eur J Clin Pharmacol.* 1997;52(5):403-406.

Itraconazole (eg, *Sporanox*)

Oxycodone (eg, *Oxycontin*)

SUMMARY: Itraconazole administration increases oxycodone plasma concentrations; enhanced narcotic effects are likely to occur in some patients.

RISK FACTORS:

➡ ***Pharmacogenetics.*** Patients who are poor metabolizers of CYP2D6 are likely to be at increased risk.

MECHANISM: Itraconazole inhibits the CYP3A4-mediated metabolism of oxycodone.

CLINICAL EVALUATION: Oral oxycodone 10 mg and intravenous (IV) oxycodone 0.1 mg/kg were administered alone and on day 4 of a 5-day course of itraconazole 200 mg daily.[1] Itraconazole increased the mean area under the concentration-time curve (AUC) of IV oxycodone 50% and prolonged its half-life from 3.8 to 5.5 hours. With oral administration of oxycodone, its mean AUC increased 244%, bioavailability increased 56%, and its half-life was prolonged approximately 48%. The concentration of oxymorphone, a metabolite of oxycodone, was increased 4.6-fold after oral oxycodone plus itraconazole. These increases in oxycodone exposure are likely to result in enhanced narcotic effects.

RELATED DRUGS: Ketoconazole (eg, *Nizoral*), fluconazole (eg, *Diflucan*), posaconazole (*Noxafil*), and voriconazole (*Vfend*) also inhibit the activity of CYP3A4 and are expected to increase the plasma concentrations of oxycodone. Other narcotic analgesics metabolized by CYP3A4 (eg, fentanyl) will also be affected in a similar manner by itraconazole.

MANAGEMENT OPTIONS:

➠ *Consider Alternative.* Consider analgesics that are not CYP3A4 substrates (codeine or morphine) for use in patients taking itraconazole.

➠ *Monitor.* Carefully monitor patients taking oxycodone and itraconazole for signs of increased narcotic activity, including sedation and respiratory depression.

REFERENCES:

1. Saari TI, et al. Effects of itraconazole on the pharmacokinetics and pharmacodynamics of intravenously and orally administered oxycodone. *Eur J Clin Pharmacol.* 2010;66(4):387-397.

 Itraconazole (eg, *Sporanox*)

Phenytoin (eg, *Dilantin*)

SUMMARY: Phenytoin dramatically reduces itraconazole serum concentrations and is likely to reduce its therapeutic response.

RISK FACTORS: No specific risk factors are known.

MECHANISM: Phenytoin likely enhances the first-pass metabolism and hepatic metabolism of itraconazole by CYP3A4.

CLINICAL EVALUATION: In healthy subjects, phenytoin 300 mg/day reduced itraconazole area under the serum concentration-time curve more than 90%.[1] The magnitude of this effect is likely to result in therapeutic failure with itraconazole unless its dose is increased dramatically. Itraconazole slightly increased phenytoin serum concentrations, but this effect is not likely to be clinically important in most patients.[1]

RELATED DRUGS: Enzyme inducers other than phenytoin also have been shown to reduce itraconazole serum concentrations.

MANAGEMENT OPTIONS:

➠ *Use Alternative.* Given the marked reduction in itraconazole serum concentrations, use an alternative antifungal agent in patients taking phenytoin. Ketoconazole (eg, *Nizoral*) metabolism also is increased by enzyme inducers and is not a suitable alternative. Phenytoin is not likely to substantially affect fluconazole (eg, *Diflucan*), which is eliminated primarily unchanged by the kidneys, but fluconazole can inhibit phenytoin metabolism (via inhibition of CYP2C9). Thus, monitor for increased phenytoin effect if fluconazole is used.

REFERENCES:

1. Ducharme MP, et al. Itraconazole and hydroxyitraconazole serum concentrations are reduced more than tenfold by phenytoin. *Clin Pharmacol Ther.* 1995;58(6):617-624.

 Itraconazole (eg, *Sporanox*)

Pioglitazone (*Actos*)

SUMMARY: No interaction.

RISK FACTORS: No specific risk factors are known.

MECHANISM: No interaction.

CLINICAL EVALUATION: After an initial dose of itraconazole 200 mg, itraconazole 100 mg or placebo were administered to 12 subjects twice daily for 4 days.[1] On day 3, each subject received a single dose of pioglitazone 15 mg. Itraconazole did not alter the pharmacokinetics of pioglitazone. Based on this study, it appears that CYP3A4 does not play a major role in the metabolism of pioglitazone.

RELATED DRUGS: Itraconazole inhibits the metabolism of repaglinide (*Prandin*).

MANAGEMENT OPTIONS: No interaction.

REFERENCES:

1. Jaakkola T, et al. Effects of gemfibrozil, itraconazole, and their combination on the pharmacokinetics of pioglitazone. *Clin Pharmacol Ther.* 2005;77(5):404-414.

Itraconazole (eg, *Sporanox*)

Pravastatin (*Pravachol*)

SUMMARY: Itraconazole does not affect the plasma concentration of pravastatin.

RISK FACTORS: No specific risk factors are known.

MECHANISM: No interaction.

CLINICAL EVALUATION: Ten healthy subjects received placebo or itraconazole 200 mg/day for 4 days followed by a single dose of pravastatin 40 mg.[1] No significant changes occurred in the plasma concentrations of pravastatin following itraconazole administration.

RELATED DRUGS: Lovastatin (eg, *Mevacor*) and simvastatin (*Zocor*) are known to be affected by itraconazole. Itraconazole is not expected to alter fluvastatin (*Lescol*) metabolism.

MANAGEMENT OPTIONS: No interaction.

REFERENCES:

1. Neuvonen PJ, et al. Simvastatin but not pravastatin is very susceptible to interaction with the CYP3A4 inhibitor itraconazole. *Clin Pharmacol Ther.* 1998;63:332-341.

Itraconazole (eg, *Sporanox*)

Quinidine

SUMMARY: Itraconazole administration increases quinidine plasma concentrations; cardiac toxicity could result.

RISK FACTORS: No specific risk factors are known.

MECHANISM: Itraconazole inhibits the intrinsic and renal clearance of quinidine. The intrinsic clearance is reduced because of the inhibition of CYP3A4 by itraconazole. Itraconazole-induced reduction in renal P-glycoprotein activity appears to be responsible for reduced quinidine renal clearance.

CLINICAL EVALUATION: Itraconazole 200 mg or placebo was administered to 9 healthy subjects for 4 days.[1] On day 4, each subject received a single dose of quinidine 100 mg 1 hour after itraconazole or placebo. The administration of itraconazole increased the area under the concentration-time curve and half-life of quinidine 242% and 158%, respectively. The renal clearance of quinidine was reduced 51% during itraconazole coadministration. Patients taking therapeutic doses of quinidine could experience toxicity, including arrhythmias, during itraconazole coadministration.

RELATED DRUGS: Ketoconazole (eg, *Nizoral*) is known to reduce quinidine clearance; fluconazole (eg, *Diflucan*) is also likely to increase quinidine concentrations. Terbinafine (*Lamisil*) does not affect CYP3A4 and would not be expected to alter quinidine concentrations.

MANAGEMENT OPTIONS:

➡ *Consider Alternative.* Consider the use of an antifungal agent that does not reduce CYP3A4 activity, such as terbinafine, for patients taking quinidine.

➡ *Monitor.* Observe patients taking quinidine for increased plasma concentrations and electrocardiographic changes, including increased QTc intervals.

REFERENCES:
1. Kaukonen KM, et al. Itraconazole increases plasma concentrations of quinidine. *Clin Pharmacol Ther.* 1997;62:510-517.

Itraconazole (eg, *Sporanox*)

Ranitidine (eg, *Zantac*)

SUMMARY: Ranitidine reduces the absorption of itraconazole; loss of antifungal activity may result.

RISK FACTORS: No specific risk factors are known.

MECHANISM: Itraconazole solubility is reduced when gastric pH is increased, resulting in a decrease in itraconazole bioavailability.

CLINICAL EVALUATION: Thirty subjects received a single dose of itraconazole 200 mg alone or following ranitidine 150 mg twice daily for 3 days.[1] Gastric pH was maintained at 6 or greater for 6 hours following the itraconazole-ranitidine dosing phase. The mean area under the plasma concentration-time curve of itraconazole was reduced 47% when administered after ranitidine. Ranitidine reduced the peak concentration of itraconazole over 50%. The administration of a cola drink (pH 2.3) with itraconazole in subjects pretreated with ranitidine returned the absorption to baseline levels. It is likely that patients taking itraconazole and ranitidine will have a reduction in antifungal efficacy.

RELATED DRUGS: Any drug that increases gastric pH, including H_2-receptor antagonists and proton pump inhibitors, will reduce the absorption of itraconazole. The absorption of ketoconazole (eg, *Nizoral*) is decreased by agents increasing gastric pH.

MANAGEMENT OPTIONS:

➡ *Consider Alternative.* Antifungal agents not affected by changes in gastric pH include fluconazole (eg, *Diflucan*), terbinafine (*Lamisil*), and voriconazole (*Vfend*). The absorption of the oral solution formulation of itraconazole does not appear to be affected by changes in the gastric pH.

➡ *Circumvent/Minimize.* The administration of an acid (eg, cola drinks) concurrently with itraconazole can increase its absorption.

➥ *Monitor.* Monitor patients taking itraconazole for reduced absorption if acid suppressing drugs are coadministered.

REFERENCES:

1. Lange D, et al. Effect of a cola beverage on the bioavailability of itraconazole in the presence of H_2 blockers. *J Clin Pharmacol.* 1997;37:535-540.

Itraconazole (eg, *Sporanox*)
Repaglinide (*Prandin*)

SUMMARY: Itraconazole increases the serum concentration of repaglinide; enhanced hypoglycemic effects may result.

RISK FACTORS: No specific risk factors are known.

MECHANISM: Repaglinide is thought to be metabolized predominately by CYP2C8 and, to a lesser extent, by CYP3A4. Itraconazole inhibits the CYP3A4-mediated metabolism of repaglinide.

CLINICAL EVALUATION: Twelve healthy subjects received a single dose of repaglinide 0.25 mg following placebo or itraconazole 200 mg for the first dose and then 100 mg twice daily for 3 days.[1] The mean area under the plasma concentration-time curve of repaglinide was increased 1.4-fold (range, 1- to 1.9-fold). The half-life of repaglinide did not change following itraconazole coadministration. Patients with diabetes may have an increased risk of hypoglycemia if itraconazole and repaglinide are coadministered. The magnitude of this interaction is somewhat limited by the alternative pathway of elimination (CYP2C8) available to metabolize repaglinide.

RELATED DRUGS: The elimination of other oral hypoglycemic agents (eg, pioglitazone [*Actos*]) metabolized by CYP3A4 may be reduced by itraconazole coadministration. Fluconazole (eg, *Diflucan*), ketoconazole (eg, *Nizoral*), and voriconazole (*Vfend*) also inhibit CYP3A4 activity and may increase repaglinide serum concentrations.

MANAGEMENT OPTIONS:

➥ *Consider Alternative.* Consider using alternative lipid-lowering drugs not metabolized by CYP3A4 (eg, fluvastatin [*Lescol*] or pravastatin [*Pravachol*]) in patients receiving itraconazole. Terbinafine (*Lamisil*) does not inhibit CYP3A4 and could be considered as an alternative antifungal agent.

➥ *Monitor.* Monitor patients taking repaglinide for changes in blood glucose concentrations if itraconazole is added to or discontinued from the drug regimen.

REFERENCES:

1. Niemi M, et al. Effects of gemfibrozil, itraconazole, and their combination on the pharmacokinetics and pharmacodynamics of repaglinide: potentially hazardous interaction between gemfibrozil and repaglinide. *Diabetologia.* 2003;46:347-351.

Itraconazole (eg, *Sporanox*)

Rifampin (eg, *Rifadin*)

SUMMARY: Rifampin appears to reduce itraconazole plasma concentrations; the interaction may reduce the efficacy of itraconazole.

RISK FACTORS: No specific risk factors are known.

MECHANISM: It appears that rifampin induces the metabolism or reduces the bioavailability of itraconazole.

CLINICAL EVALUATION: A patient taking rifampin 600 mg/day and isoniazid 300 mg/day was treated with itraconazole 200 mg/day.[1] Two weeks later, itraconazole plasma concentrations were low (less than 0.02 mg/L), and the dose was increased to 400 mg/day; plasma concentrations were still less than 0.1 mg/L. Following discontinuation of antituberculosis therapy, itraconazole 300 mg/day resulted in itraconazole plasma concentrations of 3.2 mg/L. Clinical improvement was noted. Several patients treated with itraconazole 400 mg/day had markedly reduced itraconazole concentrations during administration of rifampin 600 mg/day.[2,3] Clinically significant reductions in itraconazole concentrations appear to result from rifampin coadministration.

RELATED DRUGS: Rifampin also reduces the concentration of fluconazole (eg, *Diflucan*) and ketoconazole (eg, *Nizoral*).

MANAGEMENT OPTIONS:

➡ **Monitor.** Until further information is available, monitor patients for reduced itraconazole concentrations and response when rifampin is coadministered.

REFERENCES:
1. Blomley M, et al. Itraconazole and anti-tuberculosis drugs. *Lancet*. 1990;336:1255.
2. Tucker RM, et al. Interaction of azoles with rifampin, phenytoin, and carbamazepine: in vitro and clinical observations. *Clin Infect Dis*. 1992;14:165-174.
3. Drayton J, et al. Coadministration of rifampin and itraconazole leads to undetectable levels of serum itraconazole. *Clin Infect Dis*. 1994;18:266.

Itraconazole (eg, *Sporanox*)

Risperidone (*Risperdal*)

SUMMARY: Itraconazole increases risperidone plasma concentrations; an increased incidence of risperidone-induced adverse reactions is possible.

RISK FACTORS: No specific risk factors are known.

MECHANISM: Risperidone is metabolized by CYP2D6 and, to a lesser extent, CYP3A4. It may also be a substrate for P-glycoprotein. Itraconazole is known to inhibit the activity of CYP3A4 and P-glycoprotein.

CLINICAL EVALUATION: Nineteen patients with schizophrenia receiving doses of risperidone 2 to 8 mg daily for at least 2 months were coadministered itraconazole 200 mg daily for 7 days.[1] Following itraconazole administration, mean risperidone plasma concentrations increased over 80% and the concentration of its active metabolite increased 70%. A similar effect of itraconazole was observed in patients genotyped as rapid or slow CYP2D6 metabolizers. The development of risperidone adverse reactions may occur in some patients treated with itraconazole and risperidone. Longer exposure to itraconazole may produce greater changes in risperidone plasma concentrations.

RELATED DRUGS: Other antifungal agents that inhibit CYP3A4 (eg, fluconazole [eg, *Diflucan*], ketoconazole [eg, *Nizoral*], and voriconazole [*Vfend*]) may affect risperidone in a similar manner. Terbinafine (*Lamisil*) inhibits CYP2D6 activity and may also interact with risperidone.

MANAGEMENT OPTIONS:

➡ *Consider Alternative.* Antifungal drugs that do not inhibit CYP3A4 or CYP2D6 (eg, amphotericin, caspofungin [*Cancidas*], anidulafungin [*Eraxis*]) could be considered.

➡ *Monitor.* Monitor patients receiving risperidone and itraconazole for changes in mental status and extrapyramidal symptoms.

REFERENCES:

1. Jung SM, et al. Cytochrome P450 3A inhibitor itraconazole affects plasma concentrations of risperidone and 9-hydroxyrispiridone in schizophrenic patients. *Clin Pharmacol Ther.* 2005;78:520-528.

Itraconazole (eg, *Sporanox*)

Simvastatin (*Zocor*)

SUMMARY: Itraconazole increases the plasma concentrations of simvastatin and simvastatin acid; skeletal muscle toxicity could result.

RISK FACTORS: No specific risk factors are known.

MECHANISM: Itraconazole inhibits the first-pass metabolism (CYP3A4) of simvastatin during passage through the intestinal wall and liver. The intrinsic metabolism of simvastatin also appears to be reduced by itraconazole. In addition, itraconazole may increase bioavailability of simvastatin by inhibiting P-glycoprotein in the wall of the intestine.

CLINICAL EVALUATION: Ten healthy subjects received placebo or itraconazole 200 mg/day for 4 days followed by a single dose of simvastatin 40 mg.[1] The mean area under the concentration-time curve (AUC) of simvastatin was increased approximately 10-fold following itraconazole treatment. The AUC of the active form of simvastatin, simvastatin acid, was increased 19-fold, while half-life was prolonged 25% by itraconazole pretreatment. The large increases in simvastatin and simvastatin acid could lead to skeletal muscle toxicity.

RELATED DRUGS: Lovastatin (eg, *Mevacor*) undergoes metabolism similar to simvastatin and would likely be affected in a similar manner. Other antifungal agents (eg, fluconazole [eg, *Diflucan*], ketoconazole [eg, *Nizoral*]) are likely to increase simvastatin concentrations. Pravastatin (*Pravachol*) and fluvastatin (*Lescol*) are not metabolized by CYP3A4 and would not be expected to interact with itraconazole.

MANAGEMENT OPTIONS:

➡ *Use Alternative.* Give fluvastatin or pravastatin to patients taking itraconazole who require an HMG-CoA reductase inhibitor.

REFERENCES:

1. Neuvonen PJ, et al. Simvastatin but not pravastatin is very susceptible to interaction with the CYP3A4 inhibitor itraconazole. *Clin Pharmacol Ther.* 1998;63:332-341.

Itraconazole (eg, *Sporanox*)

Sirolimus (*Rapamune*)

SUMMARY: Itraconazole increases sirolimus plasma concentrations; increased sirolimus toxicity may result.

RISK FACTORS: No specific risk factors are known.

MECHANISM: Itraconazole is known to inhibit CYP3A4, the enzyme that metabolizes sirolimus.

CLINICAL EVALUATION: A renal transplant patient was receiving sirolimus, mycophenolate mofetil, and corticosteroids.[1] The diagnosis of a renal fungal infection prompted the administration of itraconazole 600 mg for 1 day followed by 400 mg daily. On the day itraconazole was initiated, the sirolimus dosage was increased from 5 to 10 mg daily. Sirolimus plasma concentrations increased from 6.8 to 82.5 ng/mL after 6 days of concurrent therapy. Several other case reports have been published describing patients who had elevated sirolimus concentrations following itraconazole administration.[2,3]

RELATED DRUGS: Other antifungal agents that inhibit CYP3A4 (eg, fluconazole [eg, *Diflucan*], ketoconazole [eg, *Nizoral*], voriconazole [*Vfend*]) would be expected to affect sirolimus in a similar manner. Itraconazole is known to inhibit the metabolism of cyclosporine (eg, *Neoral*) and tacrolimus (*Prograf*).

MANAGEMENT OPTIONS:

➡ **Consider Alternative.** Consider terbinafine (*Lamisil*) as an alternative antifungal agent because it does not affect CYP3A4 activity.

➡ **Monitor.** Carefully monitor sirolimus plasma concentrations during itraconazole coadministration. Because of itraconazole's long half-life, its inhibitory effect on sirolimus metabolism is likely to take a week or more to abate following discontinuation of itraconazole.

REFERENCES:

1. Kuypers DR, et al. Drug interaction between itraconazole and sirolimus in a primary renal allograft recipient. *Transplantation*. 2005;79:737.
2. Sadaba B, et al. Clinical relevance of sirolimus drug interactions in transplant patients. *Transplant Proc*. 2004;36:3226-3228.
3. Said A, et al. Sirolimus-itraconazole interaction in a hematopoietic stem cell transplant recipient. *Pharmacotherapy*. 2006;26:289-295.

Itraconazole (*Sporanox*)

Tacrolimus (*Prograf*)

SUMMARY: Itraconazole administration appears to increase tacrolimus concentrations; adjust tacrolimus dosage as required.

RISK FACTORS: No specific risk factors are known.

MECHANISM: Tacrolimus is a CYP3A4 substrate whose metabolism would be expected to be inhibited by itraconazole, resulting in a likely reduction in the first-pass and intrinsic clearance of tacrolimus.

CLINICAL EVALUATION: A hepato-pulmonary transplant patient was noted to require lower doses of tacrolimus (0.02 mg/kg twice daily) during the administration of itraconazole 600 mg twice daily. Following the discontinuation of itraconazole, the patient's tacrolimus dosage was increased to 0.08 mg/kg twice daily to maintain blood concentrations in the therapeutic range (5 to 15 ng/ml). The concentration-to-dose ratio for tacrolimus was 6 times greater during concomitant itraconazole administration in this patient and in 7 others. Elevated tacrolimus concentrations and potential toxicity should be anticipated when itraconazole is coadministered. The effect of lower doses of itraconazole on tacrolimus concentrations is unknown.

RELATED DRUGS: Other antifungal agents (eg, ketoconazole [eg, *Nizoral*], fluconazole [*Diflucan*]) are likely to increase tacrolimus concentrations. Cyclosporine (eg, *Neoral*) concentrations have been noted to increase when it is administered with itraconazole.

MANAGEMENT OPTIONS:

➠ *Consider Alternative.* Consider the use of an antifungal agent that does not inhibit CYP3A4 (eg, terbinafine [*Lamisil*]).

➠ *Monitor.* The concentration of tacrolimus should be monitored during coadministration of itraconazole. Be alert for evidence of tacrolimus toxicity including nephrotoxicity, hypertension, or hyperkalemia.

REFERENCES:

1. Billaud EM, et al. Evidence for a pharmacokinetic interaction between itraconazole and tacrolimus in organ transplant patients. *Br J Clin Pharmacol.*1998;46:271–74.

Itraconazole (*Sporanox*)

Temazepam (eg, *Restoril*)

SUMMARY: Itraconazole administration produced a small increase in temazepam serum concentrations. Minimal change in response to temazepam would be expected.

RISK FACTORS: No specific risk factors are known.

MECHANISM: Temazepam is primarily metabolized by conjugation to temazepam glucuronide. A minor metabolic pathway for temazepam is via demethylation to oxazepam, probably via the CYP3A4 enzyme.

CLINICAL EVALUATION: Ten healthy subjects received placebo or itraconazole 200 mg 4 times a day for 4 days.[1] A single oral 20 mg dose of temazepam was administered on the 4th day of placebo and itraconazole administration. The area under the concentration time curve of temazepam was increased approximately 14% following itraconazole pretreatment. The half-life of temazepam was not altered, nor were concentrations of its metabolite oxazepam. Itraconazole did not significantly affect any of temazepam's pharmacodynamic effects.

RELATED DRUGS: Itraconazole is known to inhibit triazolam (eg, *Halcion*) and diazepam (eg, *Valium*) metabolism. It also is likely to reduce the metabolism of chlordiazepoxide (eg, *Librium*) and midazolam (*Versed*). Other antifungal agents such as ketoconazole (eg, *Nizoral*) and fluconazole (*Diflucan*) would be likely to produce a similar, limited inhibition of the metabolism of temazepam.

MANAGEMENT OPTIONS: No specific action is required, but be alert for evidence of the interaction (eg, drowsiness, sedation).

REFERENCES:

1. Anonen J, et al. Lack of effect of antimycotic itraconazole on the pharmacokinetics or pharmacodynamics of temazepam. *Ther Drug Monit.* 1996;18:124.

 Itraconazole (Sporanox)

AVOID **Terfenadine†**

SUMMARY: Itraconazole administration produces elevated plasma concentrations of terfenadine that can lead to prolonged QTc intervals and ventricular arrhythmias. Terfenadine should not be taken by patients requiring itraconazole for antifungal therapy.

RISK FACTORS: No specific risk factors are known.

MECHANISM: Itraconazole appears to inhibit the metabolism (CYP3A4) of terfenadine leading to its accumulation and potential cardiotoxicity.

CLINICAL EVALUATION: Itraconazole 200 mg/day for 7 days administered to 6 healthy subjects resulted in increased concentrations of terfenadine and its metabolite and prolonged their QTc intervals.[1] Case reports of patients taking terfenadine and itraconazole have noted cardiac toxicity including syncopal episodes, prolonged QTc intervals, bradycardia, and torsades de pointes.[2,3] The symptoms resolved after discontinuation of terfenadine and itraconazole.

RELATED DRUGS: Other antifungal agents, including ketoconazole (*Nizoral*) and fluconazole (*Diflucan*), have been noted to increase terfenadine concentrations. Astemizole† concentrations have been noted to increase when it is administered with antifungal agents. Cetirizine (*Zyrtec*) and loratadine (*Claritin*) appear to be less likely to interact with itraconazole and produce cardiotoxicity.

MANAGEMENT OPTIONS:

➥ *AVOID COMBINATION.* Until more information on the interaction between itraconazole and terfenadine is available, it would be prudent to avoid giving the 2 drugs together. The use of sedating antihistamines or perhaps loratadine instead of terfenadine would seem to be preferred in patients taking itraconazole or other oral antifungal agents.

REFERENCES:

1. Honig PK, et al. Itraconazole affects single-dose terfenadine pharmacokinetics and cardiac repolarization pharmacodynamics. *J Clin Pharmacol.* 1993;33:1201.

2. Crane JK, et al. Syncope and cardiac arrhythmia due to an interaction between itraconazole and terfenadine. *Am J Med.* 1993;95:445.

3. Pohjola-Sintonen S et al. Itraconazole prevents terfenadine metabolism and increases risk of torsades de pointes ventricular tachycardia. *Eur J Clin Pharmacol.* 1993;45:191.

† Not available in the United States.

Itraconazole (*Sporanox*)

Triazolam (eg, *Halcion*)

SUMMARY: Itraconazole administration produces large increases in triazolam concentrations and pharmacologic effects.

RISK FACTORS:

➡ ***Route of Administration.*** Oral administration of triazolam increases the risk for the interaction.

MECHANISM: Itraconazole inhibits the first-pass metabolism and hepatic clearance (CYP3A4) of triazolam.

CLINICAL EVALUATION: Four days' administration of itraconazole 200 mg/day increased the area under the plasma concentration time curve of triazolam (0.25 mg) 27-fold.[1] Triazolam half-life increased from 3.3 to 22.3 hours after itraconazole administration. The increased triazolam concentrations were accompanied by increased sedation and a reduced ability to complete psychomotor tests. Patients receiving both drugs may experience prolonged amnesia and drowsiness.

RELATED DRUGS: Midazolam (*Versed*) and diazepam (eg, *Valium*) concentrations are likely to be increased by itraconazole. Ketoconazole (*Nizoral*) or fluconazole (*Diflucan*) administration may result in increased triazolam concentrations.

MANAGEMENT OPTIONS:

➡ ***Avoid Unless Benefit Outweighs Risk.*** The concomitant administration of triazolam and itraconazole should be avoided.

➡ ***Monitor.*** Patients receiving triazolam and itraconazole should be monitored for increased triazolam effects including drowsiness and prolonged amnesia. Reduced doses of triazolam should be considered in patients taking itraconazole.

REFERENCES:

1. Varhe A, et al. Oral triazolam is potentially hazardous to patients receiving systemic antimycotics ketoconazole or itraconazole. *Clin Pharmacol Ther.* 1994;56:601.

Itraconazole (eg, *Sporanox*)

Vincristine (eg, *Vincasar*)

SUMMARY: Patients with hematological malignancies being treated with vincristine have an increased risk of developing vincristine toxicity if itraconazole or other azole antifungals are coadministered.

RISK FACTORS: No specific risk factors are known.

MECHANISM: Itraconazole inhibits the CYP3A4 metabolism of vincristine as well as the P-glycoprotein mediated efflux of vincristine.

CLINICAL EVALUATION: Itraconazole has been implicated in causing vincristine toxicity in patients with lymphoblastic leukemia and malignant lymphoma.[1,2] Symptoms occurred as soon as the second dose of vincristine was administered with itraconazole and included myalgia, arthralgia, paresthesias, weakness, constipation, and paralytic ileus. Other azoles, including fluconazole (eg, *Diflucan*), voriconazole (*Vfend*), and posaconazole (*Noxafil*), have also been associated with vincristine neurotoxicity.[3] In this report, vincristine doses were reduced due to toxicity by an average of 46% in nearly 60% of the patients receiving azole antifungal therapy with vincristine. The symptoms of toxicity usually abate 10 to 15 days after discontinuation of itraconazole.

RELATED DRUGS: In addition to the azoles noted above, ketoconazole (eg, *Nizoral*) is also likely to interact with vincristine. Vinblastine and vinorelbine (eg, *Navelbine*) are also substrates of CYP3A and their metabolism may be inhibited by itraconazole or other azole antifungals.

MANAGEMENT OPTIONS:

➡ *Consider Alternative.* Terbinafine (eg, *Lamisil*) could be considered as an alternative antifungal agent because it does not affect CYP3A4 activity. Amphotericin (eg, *Abelcet*), caspofungin (*Cancidas*), and anidulafungin (*Eraxis*) do not appear to inhibit CYP3A4.

➡ *Monitor.* Carefully monitor patients taking vincristine and ritonavir for signs of neurotoxicity, including paralytic ileus.

REFERENCES:

1. Böhme A, et al. Aggravation of vincristine-induced neurotoxicity by itraconazole in the treatment of adult ALL. *Ann Hematol.* 1995;71(6):311-312.

2. Takahashi N, et al. Itraconazole oral solution enhanced vincristine neurotoxicity in five patients with malignant lymphoma. *Intern Med.* 2008;47(7):651-653.

3. Harnicar S, et al. Modification of vincristine dosing during concomitant azole therapy in adult acute lymphoblastic leukemia patients. *J Oncol Pharm Pract.* 2009;15(3):175-182.

 Itraconazole (eg, *Sporanox*)

Vinorelbine (eg, *Navelbine*)

SUMMARY: Itraconazole appears to reduce the metabolism of vinorelbine; significant toxicity may result.

RISK FACTORS: No specific risk factors are known.

MECHANISM: Itraconazole is an inhibitor of CYP3A4, the enzyme that appears to be responsible for the metabolism of vinorelbine.

CLINICAL EVALUATION: A patient with adenocarcinoma of the lung and fungal pneumonia was started on itraconazole (dose not stated).[1] Shortly following the start of itraconazole, vinorelbine was added to treat the adenocarcinoma. Within a week of the first dose of vinorelbine, the patient developed mucositis, vomiting, and granulocytopenia. The patient later died of complications related to his pneumonia and drug toxicity. While data are limited regarding this case, vinorelbine has been reported to be a CYP3A4 substrate and is likely susceptible to interactions with drugs that alter CYP3A4 activity.[2]

RELATED DRUGS: Ketoconazole (eg, *Nizoral*), fluconazole (eg, *Diflucan*), posaconazole (*Noxafil*), and voriconazole (*Vfend*) also inhibit the activity of CYP3A4 and are expected to increase the plasma concentrations of vinorelbine. Vincristine (eg, *Vincasar*) and vinblastine are likely to be affected in a similar manner by itraconazole.

MANAGEMENT OPTIONS:

➡ *Use Alternative.* Terbinafine (eg, *Lamisil*) may be considered as an alternative antifungal agent because it does not affect CYP3A4 activity. Amphotericin (eg, *Abelcet*), caspofungin (*Cancidas*), and anidulafungin (*Eraxis*) do not appear to inhibit CYP3A4.

➡ *Monitor.* Carefully monitor patients receiving vinorelbine for increased toxicity if any CYP3A4 inhibitor is prescribed

REFERENCES:

1. Bosque E. Possible drug interaction between itraconazole and vinorelbine tartrate leading to death after one dose of chemotherapy. *Ann Intern Med.* 2001;134(5):427.

2. Kajita J, et al. CYP3A4 is mainly responsible for the metabolism of a new vinca alkaloid, vinorelbine, in human liver microsomes. *Drug Metab Dispos.* 2000;28(9):1121-1127.

Itraconazole (*Sporanox*)

Warfarin (eg, *Coumadin*)

SUMMARY: A patient stabilized on warfarin developed excessive hypoprothrombinemia and severe bleeding after itraconazole was added to her regimen.

RISK FACTORS: No specific risk factors are known.

MECHANISM: Not established. Itraconazole is known to inhibit cytochrome P450 enzymes, and it is possible that it reduces the hepatic metabolism of warfarin.

CLINICAL EVALUATION: A 61-year-old woman on chronic warfarin therapy (5 mg/day) was also on stable chronic doses of omeprazole, quinine, ipratropium bromide, albuterol, and budesonide.[1] Four days after she was started on itraconazole (200 mg twice daily) for oral candidiasis, she developed bruising and recurrent nose bleeds; her INR had increased to 8. Even though warfarin and itraconazole were discontinued, the next day she developed intractable bleeding and generalized bruising. She was treated successfully with fresh frozen plasma and subsequently was stabilized on her previous warfarin dose of 5 mg/day. Although a rigorous attempt to rule out other possible causes of an increase in warfarin response was apparently not conducted (eg, changes in compliance, acute alcohol ingestion, nonprescription drugs, thyroid disease), the temporal relationship between the administration of itraconazole and the excessive warfarin response is consistent with a warfarin-itraconazole interaction. Nonetheless, more study is needed to establish the incidence and magnitude of this interaction.

RELATED DRUGS: Other azole antifungal agents such as fluconazole (*Diflucan*), ketoconazole (*Nizoral*), and miconazole (eg, *Monistat*) also have been reported to increase the hypoprothrombinemic response to warfarin. The effect of itraconazole on oral anticoagulants other than warfarin is unknown, but theoretically phenprocoumon would be less likely to interact.

MANAGEMENT OPTIONS:

➡ *Monitor.* Monitor for altered oral anticoagulant effect if itraconazole is initiated, discontinued, or changed in dosage. Adjust the anticoagulant dose as needed.

REFERENCES:

1. Yeh J, et al. Potentiation of action of warfarin by itraconazole. *Br Med J.* 1990;301:669.

Itraconazole (*Sporanox*)

Zidovudine (*Retrovir*)

SUMMARY: Itraconazole does not appear to alter zidovudine concentrations.

RISK FACTORS: No specific risk factors are known.

MECHANISM: No interaction.

CLINICAL EVALUATION: Seven patients treated with zidovudine 3 mg/kg/day for at least 48 weeks received itraconazole 200 mg/day for 2 weeks.[1] No changes in zidovudine pharmacokinetics were observed following itraconazole therapy.

RELATED DRUGS: No information is available.

MANAGEMENT OPTIONS: No interaction.

REFERENCES:
1. Henrivaux P, et al. Pharmacokinetics of AZT among HIV infected patients treated with itraconazole. Fifth International Conference on AIDS. Quebec; 1989:278. Abstract.

Itraconazole (*Sporanox*)

Zolpidem (*Ambien*)

SUMMARY: Itraconazole produces a minor increase in zolpidem concentration; increased sedation is unlikely to occur.

RISK FACTORS: No specific risk factors are known.

MECHANISM: Itraconazole minimally reduces the clearance of zolpidem. probably by inhibiting the CYP3A4 metabolism of zolpidem.

CLINICAL EVALUATION: Twelve healthy subjects received a single oral dose of zolpidem 5 mg alone and 1 hour after the third of 4 doses of itraconazole 100 mg twice daily.[1] The itraconazole treatment increased the area under the plasma concentration-time curve (AUC) for zolpidem 32% and reduced its apparent oral clearance 24%. Neither of these changes was statistically significant. Zolpidem's half-life increased from 1.86 hours when administered alone to 1.95 hours when coadministered with itraconazole. In a second study, itraconazole 200 mg/day for 4 days increased the AUC of a 10 mg single dose of zolpidem 34%.[2] A small change in zolpidem pharmacodynamic effects was observed following the coadministration of itraconazole. Most patients taking zolpidem are at little risk of suffering increased sedation if itraconazole is prescribed.

RELATED DRUGS: Ketoconazole (eg, *Nizoral*) has been reported to significantly reduce the clearance of zolpidem. Fluconazole (*Diflucan*) has been noted to produce a minimal increase in zolpidem plasma concentrations.

MANAGEMENT OPTIONS:

➡ **Monitor.** Observe patients taking itraconazole and zolpidem for a slight risk of enhanced sedation.

REFERENCES:
1. Greenblatt DJ, et al. Kinetic and dynamic interaction study of zolpidem with ketoconazole, itraconazole, and fluconazole. *Clin Pharmacol Ther.* 1998;64:661–71.
2. Luurila H, et al. Effect of itraconazole on the pharmacokinetics and pharmacodynamics of zolpidem. *Eur J Clin Pharmacol.* 1998;54:163–66.

Ixabepilone (*Ixempra*)

Ketoconazole (eg, *Nizoral*)

SUMMARY: Ketoconazole administration increased the plasma concentration and adverse effects of ixabepilone.

RISK FACTORS: No specific risk factors are known.

MECHANISM: Ketoconazole inhibits the CYP3A4 metabolism of ixabepilone.

CLINICAL EVALUATION: Twenty-two patients with metastatic cancer received a single dose (ranging from 10 to 30 mg/m^2) of ixabepilone on day 2 of a 6-day regimen of ketoconazole 400 mg daily.[1] Patients received a dose of ixabepilone 40 mg/m^2 alone during their second cycle of therapy. The coadministration of ketoconazole increased the dose-adjusted area under the concentration-time curve of ixabepilone by 79% compared with the ixabepilone administered alone. The peak concentration of ixabepilone was not increased by ketoconazole administration. Ixabepilone adverse reactions (eg, fatigue, nausea, mucositis, neutropenia) were more common in patients taking ixabepilone plus ketoconazole compared with ixabepilone alone, particularly when the ixabepilone dose exceeded 25 mg/m^2. Reduce ixabepilone doses if patients are taking CYP34 inhibitors.

RELATED DRUGS: Fluconazole (*Diflucan*), itraconazole (*Sporanox*), posaconazole (*Noxafil*), and voriconazole (*Vfend*) also inhibit the activity of CYP3A4 and would be expected to increase the plasma concentrations of ixabepilone.

MANAGEMENT OPTIONS:

➡ *Consider Alternative.* Terbinafine (*Lamisil*) may be considered as an alternative antifungal agent because it does not affect CYP3A4 activity. Amphotericin, caspofungin (*Cancidas*), and anidulafungin (*Eraxis*) do not appear to inhibit CYP3A4.

➡ *Monitor.* Carefully monitor patients receiving ixabepilone for adverse effects if ixabepilone is administered with ketoconazole or other potent CYP3A4 inhibitors.

REFERENCES:

1. Goel S, et al. The effect of ketoconazole on the pharmacokinetics and pharmacodynamics of ixabepilone: a first in class epothilone B analogue in late-phase clinical development. *Clin Cancer Res.* 2008;14(9):2701-2709.

Ixabepilone (*Ixempra*)

St. John's Wort

SUMMARY: St. John's wort is expected to reduce the plasma concentration and efficacy of ixabepilone.

RISK FACTORS: No specific risk factors are known.

MECHANISM: St. John's wort is known to induce CYP3A4, the primary enzyme that metabolizes ixabepilone.

CLINICAL EVALUATION: While specific data are limited, the manufacturer of ixabepilone notes that the coadministration of St. John's wort may decrease the plasma concentration of ixabepilone and should be avoided[1] Pending further data, advise patients receiving ixabepilone to avoid taking St. John's wort.

RELATED DRUGS: None known.

MANAGEMENT OPTIONS:

➥ **Use Alternative.** Avoid St. John's wort use in patients treated with ixabepilone. Use an alternative antidepressant.

➥ **Monitor.** Carefully monitor patients taking St. John's wort and ixabepilone concurrently for reduced ixabepilone response.

REFERENCES:

1. *Ixempra* [package insert]. Princeton, NJ: Bristol-Myers Squibb Company; 2009.

Kaolin-Pectin 2

Lincomycin (*Lincocin*)

SUMMARY: Kaolin-pectin mixtures may reduce the antibacterial efficacy of lincomycin.

RISK FACTORS: No specific risk factors are known.

MECHANISM: Kaolin-pectin mixtures inhibit the absorption of orally administered lincomycin.

CLINICAL EVALUATION: When kaolin-pectin and lincomycin are given concurrently, serum concentrations of lincomycin are about 10% of those produced when lincomycin is given alone.[1-3]

RELATED DRUGS: Clindamycin (eg, *Cleocin*) may be similarly affected by kaolin-pectin.

MANAGEMENT OPTIONS:

➡ *Avoid Unless Benefit Outweighs Risk.* Do not generally administer kaolin-pectin to patients taking lincomycin.

➡ *Monitor.* Monitor for reduced lincomycin efficacy if administered with kaolin-pectin.

REFERENCES:

1. Wagner JG. Pharmacokinetics. 1. Definitions, modeling and reasons for measuring blood levels and urinary excretion. *Drug Intell.* 1968;2:38.
2. McCall CE, et al. Lincomycin: activity in vitro and absorption and excretion in normal young men. *Am J Med Sci.* 1967;254:144-155.
3. McGehee RF Jr, et al. Comparative studies of antibacterial activity in vitro and absorption and excretion of lincomycin and clindamycin. *Am J Med Sci.* 1968;256:279-292.

Kaolin-Pectin 4

Pseudoephedrine (eg, *Sudafed*)

SUMMARY: Kaolin may slightly reduce the extent of pseudoephedrine absorption, but this reduction probably is not clinically significant.

RISK FACTORS: No specific risk factors are known.

MECHANISM: Kaolin probably has the ability to absorb pseudoephedrine, thus inhibiting its GI absorption.

CLINICAL EVALUATION: In a study of 6 healthy subjects, pseudoephedrine absorption (as measured by cumulative urinary excretion) was slightly decreased by coadministration of a kaolin suspension.[1] The magnitude of the effect is unlikely to diminish pseudoephedrine's therapeutic action.

RELATED DRUGS: No information is available.

MANAGEMENT OPTIONS: No specific action is required, but be alert for evidence of the interaction.

REFERENCES:

1. Lucarotti RL, et al. Enhanced pseudoephedrine absorption by concurrent administration of aluminum hydroxide gel in humans. *J Pharm Sci.* 1972;61:903-905.

Kaolin-Pectin

Quinidine

SUMMARY: Kaolin-pectin reduces quinidine plasma concentrations when the 2 drugs are coadministered.

RISK FACTORS: No specific risk factors are known.

MECHANISM: Kaolin-pectin appears to absorb quinidine in the GI tract and reduce its bioavailability.

CLINICAL EVALUATION: Four healthy subjects received quinidine 100 mg alone or with kaolin-pectin 30 mL. The maximum concentration of quinidine was reduced 53%, and the area under the quinidine concentration-time curve (bioavailability) was reduced 59%.[1]

RELATED DRUGS: No information is available.

MANAGEMENT OPTIONS:

➡ *Circumvent/Minimize.* Although no data are available on the effect of separating the doses of quinidine and kaolin-pectin, it would be prudent to administer kaolin-pectin suspension several hours after quinidine to minimize this interaction.

➡ *Monitor.* Monitor quinidine concentrations and diminished antiarrhythmic efficacy if kaolin-pectin is coadministered.

REFERENCES:
1. Moustafa MA, et al. Decreased bioavailability of quinidine sulphate due to interactions with adsorbent antacids and antidiarrheal mixtures. *Int J Pharm.* 1987;34:207.

 Kava

Levodopa (*Larodopa*)

SUMMARY: Kava appeared to reduce levodopa efficacy in a patient with Parkinson disease, but the clinical importance of this effect is not established.

RISK FACTORS: No specific risk factors are known.

MECHANISM: Not established.

CLINICAL EVALUATION: A patient with Parkinson disease developed reduced levodopa efficacy after using kava for 10 days, but a causal relationship was not established.[1] Herbal medications are generally not standardized, so herbal brands may interact differently because of varying amounts of active ingredient, additional ingredients not on the label, and, in some cases, no active ingredients at all. Moreover, different lots of the same brand may vary substantially as well.

RELATED DRUGS: The effect of kava on other anti-Parkinson drugs is not known, but be alert for the possibility.

MANAGEMENT OPTIONS: No specific action is required, but be alert for evidence of the interaction.

REFERENCES:
1. Schelosky L, et al. Kava and dopamine antagonism. *J Neurol Neurosurg Psychiat.* 1995;58:639-640.

Ketamine (eg, *Ketalar*) [4]

Thyroid

SUMMARY: Adverse cardiovascular effects occurred in 2 patients on thyroid replacement therapy who were given ketamine, but a causal relationship was not established.

RISK FACTORS: No specific risk factors are known.

MECHANISM: Not established.

CLINICAL EVALUATION: In 2 patients receiving thyroid replacement therapy, the administration of ketamine was followed by marked hypertension and tachycardia.[1] Although less severe increases in blood pressure and heart rate may occur following ketamine alone, the thyroid replacement therapy was suspected in these cases. Propranolol (eg, *Inderal*) may be useful in controlling hypertension and tachycardia.[1] More study is needed to assess the clinical significance of this possible interaction.

RELATED DRUGS: No information is available.

MANAGEMENT OPTIONS: No specific action is required, but be alert for evidence of the interaction.

REFERENCES:
1. Kaplan JA, et al. Alarming reactions to ketamine in patients taking thyroid medication—treatment with propranolol. *Anesthesiology*. 1971;35:229-230.

Ketoconazole (eg, *Nizoral*)

Lapatinib (*Tykerb*)

SUMMARY: Coadministration of ketoconazole markedly increases the plasma concentration of lapatinib; some increase in adverse reactions can be expected.

RISK FACTORS: No specific risk factors are known.

MECHANISM: Ketoconazole inhibits the enzyme (CYP3A4) primarily responsible for the metabolism of lapatinib.

CLINICAL EVALUATION: Twenty-one healthy subjects received a single dose of lapatinib 100 mg alone or on day 4 of a 7-day regimen of ketoconazole 200 mg twice daily.[1] Following ketoconazole administration, the mean area under the concentration-time curve of lapatinib was increased 3.57-fold, while its half-life increased from 9.6 to 16 hours. Because lapatinib is known to inhibit its own metabolism, long-term lapatinib dosing may alter the magnitude of this interaction.

RELATED DRUGS: Other antifungal agents that inhibit CYP3A4 (eg, itraconazole [eg, *Sporanox*], voriconazole [*Vfend*], posaconazole [*Noxafil*], fluconazole [eg, *Diflucan*]) are expected to affect lapatinib in a similar manner. Dasatinib (*Sprycel*), erlotinib (*Tarceva*), gefitinib (*Iressa*), imatinib (*Gleevec*), nilotinib (*Tasigna*), pazopanib (*Votrient*), sorafenib (*Nexavar*), and sunitinib (*Sutent*) may be affected in a similar manner by ketoconazole.

MANAGEMENT OPTIONS:

➦ *Consider Alternative.* Terbinafine (eg, *Lamisil*) could be considered as an alternative antifungal agent because it does not affect CYP3A4 activity. Amphotericin, caspofungin (*Cancidas*), and anidulafungin (*Eraxis*) do not appear to inhibit CYP3A4.

➦ *Monitor.* Carefully observe patients taking lapatinib who require ketoconazole for evidence of lapatinib toxicity, including diarrhea, hepatotoxicity, nausea, rash, or vomiting.

REFERENCES:

    1. Smith DA, et al. Effects of ketoconazole and carbamazepine on lapatinib pharmacokinetics in healthy subjects. *Br J Clin Pharmacol.* 2009;67(4):421-426.

Ketoconazole (eg, *Nizoral*)

Loratadine (eg, *Claritin*)

SUMMARY: Ketoconazole administration increases loratadine plasma concentrations; the clinical significance of this effect is unknown.

RISK FACTORS: No specific risk factors are known.

MECHANISM: Ketoconazole appears to inhibit the metabolism (CYP3A4) of loratadine and its active metabolite.

CLINICAL EVALUATION: The administration of ketoconazole produced a 4-fold increase in the steady-state loratadine area under the concentration-time curve.[1] Concentrations of loratadine's active metabolite also were increased during ketoconazole administration. Details of the study were not provided. The clinical significance of this interaction is unknown.

RELATED DRUGS: Other antifungal agents (eg, miconazole [eg, *Monistat*], itraconazole [eg, *Sporanox*], fluconazole [eg, *Diflucan*]) are likely to increase loratadine concentrations.

MANAGEMENT OPTIONS:

➦ *Monitor.* Monitor patients receiving ketoconazole and loratadine for increased loratadine effects.

REFERENCES:

    1. Brannan MD, et al. Effects of various cytochrome P450 inhibitors on the metabolism of loratadine. *Clin Pharmacol Ther.* 1995;57:193.

Ketoconazole (eg, *Nizoral*)

Losartan (eg, *Cozaar*)

SUMMARY: No interaction.

RISK FACTORS: No specific risk factors are known.

MECHANISM: No interaction.

CLINICAL EVALUATION: Eleven healthy subjects received a single dose of losartan 30 mg intravenous on day 5 of a 6-day treatment with placebo or ketoconazole 400 mg/day.[1] There was no change in the clearance of losartan or its active metabolite following ketoconazole pretreatment compared with placebo. The conversion of losartan to its active metabolite is mediated via CYP2C9, an enzyme that is not affected by ketoconazole. Thus, ketoconazole is not expected to alter the efficacy of losartan.

RELATED DRUGS: Expect itraconazole (eg, *Sporanox*) to affect the metabolism of losartan. Fluconazole (eg, *Diflucan*) has been reported to reduce the conversion of losartan to its active metabolite (via inhibition of CYP2C9) and may reduce losartan's therapeutic efficacy.

MANAGEMENT OPTIONS: No interaction.

REFERENCES:

1. McCrea JB, et al. Ketoconazole does not affect the systemic conversion of losartan to E-3174. *Clin Pharmacol Ther.* 1996;59:169.

Ketoconazole (eg, *Nizoral*)

Lovastatin (eg, *Mevacor*)

SUMMARY: Like itraconazole, ketoconazole administration may produce very large increases in lovastatin concentrations; toxicity, including rhabdomyolysis, may occur. Avoid concurrent use.

RISK FACTORS: No specific risk factors are known.

MECHANISM: Lovastatin is metabolized to an active metabolite, lovastatin acid, by hydrolysis that is not dependent on the enzyme CYP3A4. Lovastatin is also metabolized to inactive metabolites by CYP3A4. Ketoconazole probably inhibits the metabolism of lovastatin to its inactive metabolites (notably during first-pass in the intestinal wall and liver), resulting in higher lovastatin concentrations and an increase in lovastatin acid concentrations as the parent drug is converted by non-CYP3A4 metabolism.

CLINICAL EVALUATION: While there are no case reports of an interaction between ketoconazole and lovastatin, based on the major effect noted with itraconazole on lovastatin metabolism (see Itraconazole-Lovastatin), a similar interaction is likely with ketoconazole.[1] Excessive lovastatin concentrations and toxicity (rhabdomyolysis) are expected to occur in patients receiving lovastatin and ketoconazole.

RELATED DRUGS: Simvastatin (eg, *Zocor*) and atorvastatin (*Lipitor*) are also metabolized by CYP3A4 and interact with CYP3A4 inhibitors. Pravastatin (eg, *Pravachol*), rosuvastatin (*Crestor*), and fluvastatin (*Lescol*) are not CYP3A4 substrates and are minimally affected by CYP3A4 inhibitors. Itraconazole (eg, *Sporanox*), miconazole (eg, *Monistat*), and fluconazole (eg, *Diflucan*) are expected to inhibit the metabolism of some HMG-CoA reductase inhibitors. Terbinafine (eg, *Lamisil*) may have a minimal effect on the metabolism of HMG-CoA reductase inhibitors.

MANAGEMENT OPTIONS:

➡ *Use Alternative.* Pending studies on other HMG-CoA reductase inhibitors, lovastatin and probably simvastatin should not be administered with ketoconazole or other inhibitors of CYP3A4. The safety of pravastatin or fluvastatin when combined with ketoconazole has not been established. Terbinafine may have minimal effect on the metabolism of the HMG-CoA reductase inhibitors because it does not appear to inhibit CYP3A4 activity. Carefully monitor patients receiving HMG-CoA reductase inhibitors, especially lovastatin or simvastatin, for muscle pain or weakness when any drug known to inhibit the activity of CYP3A4 is administered.

REFERENCES:
   1. Neuvonen PJ, Jalava KM. Itraconazole drastically increases plasma concentrations of lovastatin and lovastatin acid. *Clin Pharmacol Ther.* 1996;60(1):54-61.

 Ketoconazole (eg, *Nizoral*)

Lurasidone (*Latuda*)

SUMMARY: Ketoconazole administration produces very large increases in lurasidone plasma concentrations; avoid coadministration of the drugs.

RISK FACTORS: No specific risk factors are known.

MECHANISM: Ketoconazole is an inhibitor of CYP3A4, the primary pathway of elimination for lurasidone.

CLINICAL EVALUATION: While specific data are limited, the manufacturer of lurasidone notes that the coadministration of ketoconazole 400 mg daily for 5 days prior to a single dose of lurasidone 10 mg increased the mean area under the plasma concentration-time curve of lurasidone by approximately 900%.[1] Pending further data, patients receiving lurasidone should avoid taking ketoconazole.

RELATED DRUGS: Fluconazole (eg, *Diflucan*), itraconazole (eg, *Sporanox*), posaconazole (*Noxafil*), and voriconazole (eg, *Vfend*) also inhibit the activity of CYP3A4, and are expected to increase the plasma concentrations of lurasidone.

MANAGEMENT OPTIONS:

➡ ***Use Alternative.*** Terbinafine (eg, *Lamisil*) may be an alternative antifungal agent because it does not affect CYP3A4 activity. Amphotericin,† caspofungin (*Cancidas*), and anidulafungin (*Eraxis*) do not appear to inhibit CYP3A4.

➡ ***Monitor.*** If a CYP3A4 inhibitor is administered with lurasidone, carefully monitor for signs of elevated lurasidone plasma concentrations, including somnolence, akathisia, nausea, and agitation.

REFERENCES:
   1. *Latuda* [package insert]. Marlborough, MA: Sunovion Pharmaceuticals Inc; 2010.

   † Not available in the United States.

 Ketoconazole (eg, *Nizoral*)

Maraviroc (*Selzentry*)

SUMMARY: Ketoconazole inhibits the metabolism of maraviroc, causing a marked increase in maraviroc plasma concentrations and potential toxicity.

RISK FACTORS: No specific risk factors are known.

MECHANISM: Ketoconazole appears to inhibit the CYP3A4 metabolism of maraviroc, the P-glycoprotein transport of maraviroc, or both.

CLINICAL EVALUATION: Twelve healthy men received maraviroc 100 mg twice daily for 7 days with placebo or ketoconazole 400 mg daily for 9 days.[1] The coadministration of ketoconazole resulted in a mean increase in the area under the concentration-time curve and maximum plasma concentration of maraviroc by 501% and 338%, respectively. The half-life of maraviroc was not significantly altered by ketoconazole administration. The increase in maraviroc concentration is likely to produce an increase in adverse reactions (eg, dizziness, pyrexia, rash) in some patients. Maraviroc doses may require reduction.

RELATED DRUGS: Other antifungal agents that inhibit CYP3A4 (eg, itraconazole [eg, *Sporanox*], voriconazole [eg, *Vfend*], posaconazole [*Noxafil*], fluconazole [eg, *Diflucan*]) are expected to affect maraviroc in a similar manner.

MANAGEMENT OPTIONS:

➡ *Consider Alternative.* Terbinafine (eg, *Lamisil*) may be considered as an alternative antifungal agent because it does not affect CYP3A4 activity. Amphotericin,† caspofungin (*Cancidas*), and anidulafungin (*Eraxis*) do not appear to inhibit CYP3A4.

➡ *Monitor.* Monitor patients taking maraviroc for changing maraviroc response if ketoconazole is initiated or discontinued.

REFERENCES:

1. Abel S, et al. Effects of CYP3A4 inhibitors on the pharmacokinetics of maraviroc in healthy volunteers. *Br J Clin Pharmacol.* 2008;65(suppl 1):27-37.

† Not available in the United States.

Ketoconazole (eg, *Nizoral*)

Mefloquine (eg, *Lariam*)

SUMMARY: Ketoconazole administration increases plasma concentrations of mefloquine; be alert for increased mefloquine toxicity.

RISK FACTORS: No specific risk factors are known.

MECHANISM: Ketoconazole is known to be an inhibitor of CYP3A4, the enzyme responsible for mefloquine's metabolism.

CLINICAL EVALUATION: A single dose of mefloquine 500 mg was administered alone or following ketoconazole 400 mg daily for 10 days.[1] The mean area under the plasma concentration-time curve of mefloquine was increased nearly 80% and its half-life 40% by pretreatment with ketoconazole.

RELATED DRUGS: Other antifungal agents that inhibit CYP3A4 (eg, fluconazole [eg, *Diflucan*], itraconazole [eg, *Sporanox*], voriconazole [*Vfend*]) are expected to affect mefloquine in a similar manner.

MANAGEMENT OPTIONS:

➡ *Consider Alternative.* Terbinafine (eg, *Lamisil*) may be considered as an alternative antifungal agent because it does not affect CYP3A4 activity.

➡ *Monitor.* Monitor patients for increased dizziness, GI adverse reactions, and headache if ketoconazole is coadministered with mefloquine.

REFERENCES:

1. Ridtitid W, et al. Ketoconazole increases plasma concentrations of antimalarial mefloquine in healthy human volunteers. *J Clin Pharm Ther.* 2005;30(3):285-290.

Ketoconazole (eg, *Nizoral*)

Methylprednisolone (eg, *Medrol*)

SUMMARY: Ketoconazole increases methylprednisolone concentrations and enhances methylprednisolone-induced suppression of cortisol secretion.

RISK FACTORS: No specific risk factors are known.

MECHANISM: Ketoconazole may inhibit hepatic enzymes responsible for the metabolism of methylprednisolone.

CLINICAL EVALUATION: Ketoconazole 200 mg/day for 6 or 7 days reduced the clearance of methylprednisolone 50% to 60% in healthy subjects.[1,2] Endogenous cortisol secretion was inhibited by methylprednisolone, and the inhibition was enhanced by the addition of ketoconazole despite reduction in the methylprednisolone dose.

RELATED DRUGS: Ketoconazole has been reported to inhibit the metabolism of prednisolone.

MANAGEMENT OPTIONS:

➥ ***Monitor.*** Patients receiving methylprednisolone may require dosage adjustments when ketoconazole is added to or removed from their drug regimens.

REFERENCES:

1. Glynn AM, et al. Effects of ketoconazole on methylprednisolone pharmacokinetics and cortisol secretion. *Clin Pharmacol Ther.* 1986;39(6):654-659.
2. Kandrotas RJ, et al. Ketoconazole effects on methylprednisolone disposition and their joint suppression of endogenous cortisol. *Clin Pharmacol Ther.* 1987;42(4):465-470.

Ketoconazole (eg, *Nizoral*)

Midazolam

SUMMARY: Oral midazolam concentrations were markedly increased following ketoconazole administration; expect increased sedation and psychomotor impairment.

RISK FACTORS:

➥ ***Route of Administration.*** Plasma midazolam concentrations will increase to a greater extent following oral administration than after intravenous dosing.

MECHANISM: Ketoconazole inhibits the metabolism (CYP3A4) of midazolam in the intestine and liver following oral administration.

CLINICAL EVALUATION: Nine healthy subjects took a single oral dose of midazolam 7.5 mg alone and following ketoconazole 400 mg/day for 4 days.[1] The area under the concentration-time curve of midazolam was increased approximately 16-fold, and its peak plasma concentration increased 4-fold. Midazolam half-life was prolonged from 2.8 to 8.7 hours following ketoconazole pretreatment. These increased midazolam plasma concentrations were associated with enhanced sedation and increased impairment of psychomotor performance.

RELATED DRUGS: Itraconazole (eg, *Sporanox*), fluconazole (eg, *Diflucan*), and miconazole (eg, *Monistat*) are likely to reduce midazolam's metabolism. Ketoconazole is likely to inhibit other benzodiazepines metabolized by CYP3A4, such as alprazolam (eg,

Xanax) and triazolam (eg, *Halcion*). Benzodiazepines not metabolized via the CYP3A4 enzyme (eg, lorazepam [eg, *Ativan*], oxazepam, temazepam [eg, *Restoril*]) are less likely to be affected.

MANAGEMENT OPTIONS:

➡ *Consider Alternative.* Prescribe a benzodiazepine not metabolized via the CYP3A4 enzyme to patients maintained on ketoconazole (see Related Drugs). Consider prescribing terbinafine to patients stabilized on midazolam who require antifungal therapy.

➡ *Monitor.* Carefully monitor patients coadministered midazolam and ketoconazole for increased sedation and reduced psychomotor performance.

REFERENCES:

1. Olkkola KT, et al. Midazolam should be avoided in patients receiving the systemic antimycotics ketoconazole or itraconazole. *Clin Pharmacol Ther.* 1994;55(5):481-485.

Ketoconazole (eg, *Nizoral*)

Nelfinavir (*Viracept*)

SUMMARY: Ketoconazole administration increases the serum concentration of nelfinavir; the clinical significance of the increase is likely to be limited.

RISK FACTORS: No specific risk factors are known.

MECHANISM: Nelfinavir is partially metabolized by CYP3A4, an enzyme that ketoconazole is known to inhibit.

CLINICAL EVALUATION: Nelfinavir 500 mg every 8 hours was administered for 5 days alone and concomitantly with ketoconazole 400 mg/day for 7 days to 12 healthy subjects.[1] During ketoconazole coadministration, the oral clearance of nelfinavir was reduced approximately 30%. This degree of change in nelfinavir clearance is not expected to result in adverse reactions.

RELATED DRUGS: Ketoconazole is known to inhibit the metabolism of indinavir (*Crixivan*) and saquinavir (*Invirase*) and is likely to inhibit ritonavir (*Norvir*) metabolism as well. Other azole antifungal agents, including itraconazole (eg, *Sporanox*), miconazole (eg, *Monistat*), and fluconazole (eg, *Diflucan*), are likely to affect nelfinavir in a similar manner.

MANAGEMENT OPTIONS: No specific action is required, but be alert for evidence of the interaction.

REFERENCES:

1. Kerr BM, et al. The pharmacokinetics (PK) of nelfinavir administered alone and with ketoconazole (K) in healthy volunteers [abstract]. *Program and Abstracts of the Ninety-Eighth Annual Meeting of the American Society Congress for Clinical Pharmacology and Therapeutics*; March 5-8, 1997; San Diego, CA.

Ketoconazole (eg, *Nizoral*)

Nilotinib (*Tasigna*)

SUMMARY: Ketoconazole administration will increase the plasma concentration of nilotinib; increased adverse reactions are likely to occur in some patients.

RISK FACTORS: No specific risk factors are known.

MECHANISM: Ketoconazole inhibits the CYP3A4 metabolism of nilotinib.

CLINICAL EVALUATION: While specific data are limited, the coadministration of ketoconazole 400 mg daily for 6 days increased the mean area under the plasma concentration-time curve of nilotinib by approximately 3-fold.[1] Pending further data, observe patients receiving nilotinib and ketoconazole for increased nilotinib adverse reactions, including hematological toxicity, nausea, pruritus, and rash.

RELATED DRUGS: Fluconazole (eg, *Diflucan*), itraconazole (eg, *Sporanox*), posaconazole (*Noxafil*), and voriconazole (*Vfend*) also inhibit the activity of CYP3A4 and are expected to increase the plasma concentrations of nilotinib. The metabolism of dasatinib (*Sprycel*) is also inhibited by ketoconazole.

MANAGEMENT OPTIONS:

➡ **Consider Alternative.** Consider terbinafine (*Lamisil*) as an alternative antifungal agent because it does not affect CYP3A4 activity. Amphotericin (eg, *AmBisome*), caspofungin (*Cancidas*), and anidulafungin (*Eraxis*) do not appear to inhibit CYP3A4.

➡ **Monitor.** If nilotinib is coadministered with ketoconazole, monitor for signs of adverse reactions, including arrhythmias, hematological toxicity, nausea, pruritus, and rash.

REFERENCES:

1. *Tasigna* [package insert]. East Hanover, NJ: Novartis Pharmaceuticals Corporation; 2007.

Ketoconazole (eg, *Nizoral*)

Nisoldipine (eg, *Sular*)

SUMMARY: Ketoconazole markedly increases nisoldipine concentrations; increased hypotensive effects may occur.

RISK FACTORS: No specific risk factors are known.

MECHANISM: Nisoldipine has a very low bioavailability (5% to 10%) because of presystemic CYP3A4 metabolism. Ketoconazole inhibits CYP3A4 activity, resulting in a marked increase in nisoldipine bioavailability and plasma concentrations. It is possible that the systemic clearance of nisoldipine is also reduced by ketoconazole administration.

CLINICAL EVALUATION: Seven healthy subjects received a single oral dose of immediate-release nisoldipine 5 mg alone or following 5 daily doses of ketoconazole 200 mg.[1] The mean area under the concentration-time curve of nisoldipine increased 24-fold, while its peak plasma concentration increased 11-fold following ketoconazole. Compared with the administration of nisoldipine alone, pretreatment with ketoconazole resulted in an increase in heart rate and decrease in blood pressure.

Patients stabilized on nisoldipine for hypertension or angina may experience orthostatic hypotension if ketoconazole is added to their therapy.

RELATED DRUGS: Expect other antifungal drugs (eg, itraconazole [eg, *Sporanox*], fluconazole [eg, *Diflucan*]) that can inhibit CYP3A4 to have a similar effect on nisoldipine pharmacokinetics. Several other calcium channel blockers are substrates for CYP3A4, and ketoconazole reduces their first-pass metabolism and increases their plasma concentrations.

MANAGEMENT OPTIONS:

➡ *Circumvent/Minimize.* Calcium channel blockers with less first-pass metabolism (eg, amlodipine [eg, *Norvasc*]) are less affected by ketoconazole; however, be alert for increased hypotensive effects. Terbinafine (eg, *Lamisil*) does not appear to inhibit CYP3A4 activity and may be considered as an alternative antifungal agent in patients taking nisoldipine.

➡ *Monitor.* Monitor patients stabilized on nisoldipine for orthostatic hypotension and tachycardia if ketoconazole is administered.

REFERENCES:
1. Heinig R, et al. The effect of ketoconazole on the pharmacokinetics, pharmacodynamics and safety of nisoldipine. *Eur J Clin Pharmacol.* 1999;55(1):57-60.

Ketoconazole (eg, *Nizoral*)

Omeprazole (eg, *Prilosec*)

SUMMARY: Omeprazole markedly reduces the bioavailability of ketoconazole; loss of antifungal effect may occur. Ketoconazole increases omeprazole concentrations; some patients may experience increased adverse reactions.

RISK FACTORS:

➡ *Pharmacogenetics.* Patients who are slow CYP2C19 metabolizers of omeprazole will likely be affected to a greater degree, both for the effect of omeprazole on ketoconazole absorption and the effect of ketoconazole on omeprazole metabolism.

MECHANISM: Ketoconazole requires an acidic media in the stomach for complete dissolution of the drug to occur. Increasing gastric pH will decrease the amount of ketoconazole absorbed. Ketoconazole inhibits one of the enzymes (CYP3A4) that metabolizes omeprazole.

CLINICAL EVALUATION: Nine healthy subjects took a single dose of ketoconazole 200 mg alone and 6 to 8 hours following a single dose of omeprazole 60 mg.[1] The mean area under the concentration-time curve (AUC) for ketoconazole administered following omeprazole was reduced over 80% compared with ketoconazole alone. A similar reduction in the mean peak ketoconazole concentration also was observed. This marked reduction in ketoconazole concentration will reduce its antifungal efficacy. Therapeutic failure is likely to occur in some patients. The administration of ketoconazole with *Coca-Cola* following pretreatment with omeprazole resulted in a decrease in the mean ketoconazole AUC of about 45% compared with ketoconazole alone.[1]

The effect of varying dosages of ketoconazole (50, 100, and 200 mg/day for 4 days) on the metabolism of a single dose of omeprazole 20 mg was studied in 10 healthy subjects.[2] Both rapid and slow metabolizers (CYP2C19) of omeprazole were included. Patients who have limited CYP2C19 activity metabolize omeprazole primarily via CYP3A4. The administration of ketoconazole 200 mg/day increased the mean AUC of omeprazole 36% and 99% in the rapid and slow metabolizers (CYP2C19), respectively. Smaller increases were observed following the 50 and 100 mg doses. None of the subjects developed adverse reactions, although chronic administration of omeprazole and ketoconazole may cause adverse reactions in some patients.

RELATED DRUGS: Itraconazole (eg, *Sporanox*) also is dependent on an acidic gastric pH for absorption. All proton pump inhibitors (PPIs) will reduce the absorption of ketoconazole and itraconazole. Esomeprazole (*Nexium*), lansoprazole (*Prevacid*), and pantoprazole (*Protonix*) are metabolized partially by CYP2C19 and CYP3A4, and they are expected to interact with ketoconazole and other azole antifungal agents that inhibit CYP3A4 (eg, fluconazole [eg, *Diflucan*], itraconazole, voriconazole [*Vfend*]). Rabeprazole (*Aciphex*) has minimal CYP3A4 metabolism and is not likely to be affected to a significant degree by azole antifungal agents.

MANAGEMENT OPTIONS:

➥ *Circumvent/Minimize.* The administration of acidic drinks such as *Coca-Cola* or *Pepsi* (both have a pH of 2.5) will increase the absorption of ketoconazole and itraconazole in patients who have elevated gastric pH.[3] Theoretically, a solution formulation of the azole antifungal agent (eg, itraconazole oral solution) will not be affected by changes in gastric pH, although no data are available.

➥ *Monitor.* Monitor patients taking ketoconazole for possible loss of antifungal efficacy if drugs that can increase gastric pH are coadministered. While the PPIs are generally well tolerated, be alert for increased side effects (eg, diarrhea, headache) if ketoconazole is administered to patients taking PPIs metabolized by CYP3A4.

REFERENCES:
1. Chin TW, et al. Effects of an acidic beverage (*Coca-Cola*) on absorption of ketoconazole. *Antimicrob Agents Chemother*. 1995;39:1671-1675.
2. Bottiger Y, et al. Inhibition of the sulfoxidation of omeprazole by ketoconazole in poor and extensive metabolizers of S-mephenytoin. *Clin Pharmacol Ther*. 1997;62:384-391.
3. Lange D, et al. The effect of coadministration of a cola beverage on the bioavailability of itraconazole in patients with acquired immunodeficiency syndrome. *Curr Ther Res*. 1997;8:202-212.

Ketoconazole (eg, *Nizoral*)

Paricalcitol (*Zemplar*)

SUMMARY: The administration of ketoconazole may result in elevated concentrations of paricalcitol and potentially may produce adverse effects.

RISK FACTORS: No specific risk factors are known.

MECHANISM: Ketoconazole is known to inhibit the activity of CYP3A4, an enzyme partially responsible for the metabolism of paricalcitol.

CLINICAL EVALUATION: Data regarding this interaction are limited; however, the manufacturer notes that paricalcitol plasma concentrations were doubled during coadministration with ketoconazole 200 mg twice daily.[1] The mean half-life of paricalcitol increased from 9.8 to 17 hours during ketoconazole administration. It is possible that excessive paricalcitol effect may occur during ketoconazole administration.

RELATED DRUGS: Other antifungal agents that inhibit CYP3A4 (eg, fluconazole [eg, *Diflucan*], itraconazole [eg, *Sporanox*], voriconazole [*Vfend*]) are expected to affect paricalcitol in a similar manner.

MANAGEMENT OPTIONS:

➡ *Consider Alternative.* Consider terbinafine (*Lamisil*) as an alternative antifungal agent because it does not affect CYP3A4 activity.

➡ *Monitor.* Be alert for signs of excess vitamin D activity, including hypercalcemia, hypercalciuria, hyperphosphatemia, and excess suppression of parathyroid hormone.

REFERENCES:

1. *Zemplar* [package insert]. North Chicago, IL: Abbott Laboratories; 2005.

Ketoconazole (eg, *Nizoral*)

Phenytoin (eg, *Dilantin*)

SUMMARY: Ketoconazole does not appear to alter the pharmacokinetics of orally administered phenytoin.

RISK FACTORS: No specific risk factors are known.

MECHANISM: No interaction.

CLINICAL EVALUATION: Nine healthy men received a single dose of oral phenytoin with and without ketoconazole 200 mg twice daily. There was no significant difference in the areas under the plasma concentration-time curve between control and ketoconazole treatment.[1]

RELATED DRUGS: No information is available.

MANAGEMENT OPTIONS: No interaction.

REFERENCES:

1. Touchette MA, et al. Contrasting effects of fluconazole and ketoconazole on phenytoin and testosterone disposition in man. *Br J Clin Pharmacol.* 1992;34:75-78.

Ketoconazole (eg, *Nizoral*)

Pimozide (*Orap*)

SUMMARY: Elevated pimozide concentrations and cardiac arrhythmias may occur if pimozide and ketoconazole are coadministered.

RISK FACTORS: No specific risk factors are known.

MECHANISM: Ketoconazole is a known inhibitor of CYP3A4, the enzyme responsible for the metabolism of pimozide. The coadministration of pimozide and ketoconazole may lead to ventricular arrhythmias, including torsades de pointes.

CLINICAL EVALUATION: While specific data are lacking, the manufacturer of pimozide contraindicates the coadministration of pimozide and ketoconazole.[1] Patients with bradycardia, hypokalemia, or hypomagnesemia may be at increased risk of developing torsades de pointes.

RELATED DRUGS: Itraconazole (eg, *Sporanox*) is also likely to produce increased pimozide plasma concentrations. Fluconazole (eg, *Diflucan*) and voriconazole (*Vfend*) are less potent CYP3A4 inhibitors but may result in increased pimozide plasma concentrations, increasing the risk of QTc prolongation.

MANAGEMENT OPTIONS:

➡ **Use Alternative.** Do not administer ketoconazole or any antifungal agent that is known to inhibit CYP3A4 to patients receiving pimozide. Consider terbinafine (eg, *Lamisil*) as an alternative because it does not affect CYP3A4 activity.

➡ **Monitor.** If ketoconazole is coadministered with pimozide, monitor the electrocardiogram for evidence of QTc prolongation.

REFERENCES:
1. *Orap* [package insert]. North Wales, PA: Gate Pharmaceuticals; 1999.

 Ketoconazole (eg, *Nizoral*)

Pioglitazone (*Actos*)

SUMMARY: Ketoconazole administration modestly increases pioglitazone plasma concentrations; the effect on blood glucose concentrations is unknown.

RISK FACTORS: No specific risk factors are known.

MECHANISM: Pioglitazone is partially metabolized by CYP3A4, an enzyme that is inhibited by ketoconazole.

CLINICAL EVALUATION: While specific data are limited, the manufacturer of pioglitazone notes that coadministration of ketoconazole 200 mg twice daily for 7 days prior to a single dose of pioglitazone increased the mean area under the plasma concentration-time curve of pioglitazone approximately 34%.[1] Pending further data, observe patients receiving pioglitazone and ketoconazole for increased pioglitazone effect.

RELATED DRUGS: Other antifungal agents that inhibit CYP3A4 (eg, itraconazole [eg, *Sporanox*], voriconazole [*Vfend*], posaconazole [*Noxafil*], fluconazole [eg, *Diflucan*]) are expected to affect pioglitazone in a similar manner.

MANAGEMENT OPTIONS:

➡ **Monitor.** In patients stabilized on pioglitazone, monitor blood glucose if ketoconazole is added or removed from the drug regimen.

REFERENCES:
1. *Actos* [package insert]. Indianapolis, IN: Eli Lilly and Company; 2004.

 Ketoconazole (eg, *Nizoral*)

Prednisolone (eg, *Prelone*)

SUMMARY: Ketoconazole increases prednisolone concentrations; the clinical significance is unknown.

RISK FACTORS: No specific risk factors are known.

MECHANISM: Ketoconazole may inhibit hepatic enzymes responsible for the metabolism of prednisolone.

CLINICAL EVALUATION: Ketoconazole 200 mg/day for 6 days had no significant effect (8% reduction) on prednisolone clearance after oral administration in healthy subjects following prednisolone 20 mg.[1,2] A study of 10 healthy subjects found a 27% reduction in prednisolone clearance following ketoconazole 200 mg/day for 7 days.[3] The urinary excretion of 6-betahydroxyprednisolone, a metabolite of prednisolone, was significantly reduced. The clinical significance of these changes is unknown but is likely to be minor.

RELATED DRUGS: Ketoconazole has been reported to inhibit the metabolism of methylprednisolone (eg, *Medrol*).

MANAGEMENT OPTIONS: No specific action is required, but be alert for evidence of the interaction.

REFERENCES:

1. Ludwig EA, et al. Steroid-specific effects of ketoconazole on corticosteroid disposition: unaltered prednisolone elimination. *DICP*. 1989;23(11):858-861.
2. Yamashita SK, et al. Lack of pharmacokinetic and pharmacodynamic interactions between ketoconazole and prednisolone. *Clin Pharmacol Ther*. 1991;49(5):558-570.
3. Zurcher RM, et al. Impact of ketoconazole on the metabolism of prednisolone. *Clin Pharmacol Ther*. 1989;45(4):366-372.

Ketoconazole (eg, *Nizoral*)

Quetiapine (*Seroquel*)

SUMMARY: Ketoconazole increases quetiapine plasma concentrations; expect increased adverse reactions in some patients.

RISK FACTORS: No specific risk factors are known.

MECHANISM: Ketoconazole inhibits the metabolism (CYP3A4) of quetiapine, causing elevated quetiapine plasma concentrations.

CLINICAL EVALUATION: Twenty-seven patients with schizophrenia were administered quetiapine 375 mg twice daily alone and with ketoconazole 200 mg/day for 5 days.[1] Ketoconazole coadministration reduced the oral clearance of quetiapine 84% and increased the mean quetiapine plasma concentration 335%. This degree of increase in quetiapine plasma concentrations is likely to increase the incidence of adverse reactions, including dizziness, dry mouth, hypotension, and somnolence.

RELATED DRUGS: Itraconazole (eg, *Sporanox*), fluconazole (eg, *Diflucan*), and voriconazole (*Vfend*) also may increase quetiapine plasma concentrations. Some other atypical antipsychotics (eg, ziprasidone [*Geodon*], clozapine [eg, *Clozaril*]) that are at least partially metabolized by CYP3A4 may be affected similarly by ketoconazole.

MANAGEMENT OPTIONS:

➡ *Consider Alternative.* Terbinafine (eg, *Lamisil*) does not inhibit CYP3A4 and is not expected to interact with quetiapine. An antipsychotic agent that is not metabolized by CYP3A4 (eg, olanzapine [*Zyprexa*]) might be considered for patients requiring an antifungal that inhibits this enzyme.

➡️ *Monitor.* Monitor for increased dizziness, hypotension, and somnolence in patients who take quetiapine and require ketoconazole.

REFERENCES:
1. *Seroquel* [package insert]. Wilmington, DE: AstraZeneca; 2004.

Ketoconazole (eg, *Nizoral*)

Quinidine

SUMMARY: In a patient stabilized on quinidine, ketoconazole was associated with a marked increase in quinidine plasma concentrations.

RISK FACTORS: No specific risk factors are known.

MECHANISM: Ketoconazole inhibits CYP3A4 metabolism, the enzyme responsible for quinidine metabolism.

CLINICAL EVALUATION: A patient taking quinidine 300 mg 4 times/day was started on keto-conazole 200 mg/day.[1] Before the addition of ketoconazole, the patient's quinidine plasma concentration ranged from 1.4 to 2.7 mg/L. After 7 days of ketoconazole therapy, the quinidine concentration increased to 6.9 mg/L, and its apparent half-life was 25 hours. The quinidine dosage was reduced to 200 mg twice daily, but it had to be increased to 300 mg every 6 hours over the following 4 weeks during continued ketoconazole administration. No signs of quinidine toxicity were noted. Ketoconazole did not interfere with the assay for quinidine. The transient effect on quinidine is unusual and not readily explainable based on the data presented.

RELATED DRUGS: Other azole CYP3A4-inhibiting antifungals (eg, fluconazole [eg, *Diflucan*], miconazole [eg, *Monistat*], itraconazole [eg, *Sporanox*]) are expected to have similar effects on quinidine metabolism.

MANAGEMENT OPTIONS:

➡️ *Monitor.* Until more definitive studies are available, observe patients stabilized on quinidine for increased plasma concentrations and electrocardiographic changes (prolonged QRS) when ketoconazole is added to the regimen.

REFERENCES:
1. McNulty RM, et al. Transient increase in plasma quinidine concentrations during ketoconazole-quinidine therapy. *Clin Pharm.* 1989;8(3):222-225.

Ketoconazole (eg, *Nizoral*)

Quinine

SUMMARY: Ketoconazole administration increases the plasma concentrations of quinine.

RISK FACTORS: No specific risk factors are known.

MECHANISM: Ketoconazole inhibits the metabolism of quinine, probably by inhibiting the activity of CYP3A4.

CLINICAL EVALUATION: Nine subjects were administered a single dose of quinine 500 mg alone and following the first 2 doses of ketoconazole 100 mg administered twice daily for 3 days.[1] Ketoconazole reduced the mean oral clearance of quinine 31% and prolonged the half-life from 13.8 to 16.1 hours. The formation of the quinine metabolite 3-hydroxyquinine was reduced by ketoconazole administration. While no data are available, higher doses of ketoconazole may produce a greater effect on quinine pharmacokinetics. Some patients may experience quinine toxicity if ketoconazole is coadministered.

RELATED DRUGS: Other antifungal agents that inhibit CYP3A4 (eg, itraconazole [eg, *Sporanox*], voriconazole [*Vfend*], fluconazole [eg, *Diflucan*]) are expected to affect quinine in a similar manner.

MANAGEMENT OPTIONS:

➡ *Monitor.* Monitor patients receiving quinine and ketoconazole for signs of quinine toxicity (eg, nausea, thrombocytopenia, tinnitus).

REFERENCES:

1. Mirghani RA, et al. The roles of cytochrome P450 3A4 and 1A2 in the 3-hydroxylation of quinine in vivo. *Clin Pharmacol Ther*. 1999;66(5):454-460.

Ketoconazole (eg, *Nizoral*)

Ramelteon (*Rozerem*)

SUMMARY: Ketoconazole increases ramelteon plasma concentrations; increased sedation may occur in some patients.

RISK FACTORS: No specific risk factors are known.

MECHANISM: Ketoconazole is known to inhibit CYP3A4, an enzyme partially responsible for the metabolism of ramelteon.

CLINICAL EVALUATION: While specific data are limited, the manufacturer of ramelteon notes that administration of ketoconazole 200 mg twice daily for 4 days prior to a single dose of ramelteon increased the mean area under the plasma concentration-time curve of ramelteon approximately 84%.[1] Pending further data, observe patients receiving ramelteon and ketoconazole for increased ramelteon effect.

RELATED DRUGS: Fluconazole (eg, *Diflucan*) also inhibits the metabolism of ramelteon. Itraconazole (eg, *Sporanox*) and voriconazole (*Vfend*) also are expected to increase the plasma concentrations of ramelteon.

MANAGEMENT OPTIONS:

➡ *Consider Alternative.* Consider using an antifungal that does not affect CYP1A2, CYP3A4, or CYP2C9, such as terbinafine (eg, *Lamisil*), or a sedative that is not metabolized by CYP3A4 or CYP2C9, such as oxazepam (eg, *Serax*) or lorazepam (eg, *Ativan*).

➡ *Monitor.* If ketoconazole and ramelteon are coadministered, monitor patients for increased ramelteon effects, including excess sedation.

REFERENCES:

1. *Rozerem* [package insert]. Otsaka, Japan: Takeda Pharmaceutical Company Limited; 2005.

Ketoconazole (eg, *Nizoral*)

Ranitidine (eg, *Zantac*)

SUMMARY: Ranitidine administration reduces the plasma concentrations of ketoconazole, potentially resulting in loss of antifungal effect.

RISK FACTORS: No specific risk factors are known.

MECHANISM: Ranitidine-induced reduction in gastric acidity reduces the GI absorption of ketoconazole.[1,2]

CLINICAL EVALUATION: Six healthy subjects received ketoconazole 400 mg alone or following ranitidine (150 mg every 12 hours for 2 days before ketoconazole and 150 mg 2 hours before the ketoconazole dose).[1] Pretreatment with ranitidine reduced the ketoconazole area under the concentration-time curve from 37.05 to 1.65 mg•hr/L. The reduction in ketoconazole bioavailability corresponds to an increase in gastric pH and may reduce the antifungal efficacy of ketoconazole.

RELATED DRUGS: Other oral antifungal agents may be affected similarly by ranitidine administration. Other H_2-receptor antagonists (eg, cimetidine [eg, *Tagamet*], nizatidine [eg, *Axid*], famotidine [eg, *Pepcid*]) and proton pump inhibitors (eg, omeprazole [eg, *Prilosec*], lansoprazole [*Prevacid*]) may produce reactions similar to those seen with ketoconazole.

MANAGEMENT OPTIONS:

➡ *Circumvent/Minimize.* Recommendations have been made to avoid this interaction in patients with elevated gastric pH. The product information for ketoconazole suggests that each tablet be dissolved in 4 mL of an aqueous solution of 0.2 N-hydrochloric acid, with the resulting mixture ingested through a straw (to avoid contact with teeth) and followed by a glass of water.[3] An easier and equally effective method is to give 2 capsules of glutamic acid hydrochloride 15 minutes before ketoconazole.[2]

➡ *Monitor.* Until more is known about this interaction, be alert for evidence of reduced ketoconazole effect when ranitidine or other agents that increase gastric pH are coadministered.

REFERENCES:

1. Piscitelli SC, et al. Effects of ranitidine and sucralfate on ketoconazole bioavailability. *Antimicrob Agents Chemother.* 1991;35(9):1765-1771.
2. Lelawongs P, et al. Effect of food and gastric acidity on absorption of orally administered ketoconazole. *Clin Pharm.* 1988;7(3):228-235.
3. *Nizoral* [package insert]. Titusville, NJ: Janssen Pharmaceutica; 1993.

Ketoconazole (eg, *Nizoral*)

Ranolazine (*Ranexa*)

SUMMARY: Ketoconazole increases ranolazine plasma concentrations sufficiently to produce adverse reactions in some patients.

RISK FACTORS: No specific risk factors are known.

MECHANISM: Ketoconazole inhibits CYP3A4, the primary pathway of ranolazine metabolism, reducing first-pass and systemic clearance of ranolazine.

CLINICAL EVALUATION: Sustained-release ranolazine was administered at dosages of 375 or 1,000 mg twice daily alone and concurrently with ketoconazole 200 mg twice daily for 9 doses.[1] During ketoconazole coadministration, the mean area under the plasma concentration-time curve and peak concentration of ranolazine were increased approximately 2.5-fold. Some subjects receiving ranolazine 1,000 mg complained of headache and dizziness. The manufacturer of ranolazine contraindicates its use with CYP3A4 inhibitors.[2]

RELATED DRUGS: Other antifungal agents that inhibit CYP3A4 (eg, itraconazole [eg, *Sporanox*], voriconazole [*Vfend*], fluconazole [eg, *Diflucan*]) are expected to affect ranolazine in a similar manner.

MANAGEMENT OPTIONS:

➥ *Consider Alternative.* Terbinafine (eg, *Lamisil*) may be an alternative antifungal agent because it inhibits CYP2D6 but does not affect CYP3A4 activity. However, limited data suggest that ranolazine plasma concentrations may be increased by CYP2D6 inhibitors.[2]

➥ *Monitor.* Monitor patients taking ranolazine who are coadministered ketoconazole for evidence of ranolazine accumulation (eg, constipation, dizziness, headache, nausea).

REFERENCES:

1. Jerling M, et al. Studies to investigate the pharmacokinetic interactions between ranolazine and ketoconazole, diltiazem, or simvastatin during combined administration in healthy subjects. *J Clin Pharmacol.* 2005;45(4):422-433.

2. *Ranexa* [package insert]. Palo Alto, CA: CV Therapeutics; 2006.

Ketoconazole (eg, *Nizoral*) **4**

Repaglinide (*Prandin*)

SUMMARY: Ketoconazole increases repaglinide plasma concentrations. The effect on glycemic control in patients with diabetes is unknown.

RISK FACTORS: No specific risk factors are known.

MECHANISM: Ketoconazole inhibits the CYP3A4 pathway of repaglinide metabolism.

CLINICAL EVALUATION: Eight subjects received a single dose of repaglinide 2 mg alone or following ketoconazole 200 mg daily for 5 days.[1] Following ketoconazole administration, the mean area under the plasma concentration-time curve of repaglinide increased 15%, and the mean peak repaglinide concentration increased 7%. The half-life of repaglinide was not altered following ketoconazole administration. Larger doses of ketoconazole may produce a greater effect on repaglinide pharmacokinetics. The effect of these changes in repaglinide serum concentrations in patients with diabetes is unknown.

RELATED DRUGS: Itraconazole (eg, *Sporanox*), voriconazole (*Vfend*), and fluconazole (eg, *Diflucan*) also inhibit CYP3A4 and are expected to affect repaglinide in a manner similar to that seen with ketoconazole. Pioglitazone (*Actos*) and nateglinide (*Starlix*) are also partially metabolized by CYP3A4 and could be affected by ketoconazole.

MANAGEMENT OPTIONS:

➡ *Monitor.* Monitor patients requiring ketoconazole and repaglinide for symptoms of hypoglycemia, including tachycardia, tremor, and sweating.

REFERENCES:

1. Hatorp V, et al. Influence of drugs interacting with CYP3A4 on the pharmacokinetics, pharmacodynamics, and safety of the prandial glucose regulator repaglinide. *J Clin Pharmacol*. 2003;43(6):649-660.

Ketoconazole (eg, *Nizoral*)

Rifampin (eg, *Rifadin*)

SUMMARY: Rifampin and isoniazid decrease the plasma concentration of ketoconazole, and ketoconazole appears to decrease the peak plasma concentration of rifampin.

RISK FACTORS: No specific risk factors are known.

MECHANISM: Rifampin appears to increase the metabolism of ketoconazole; the coadministration of isoniazid appears to enhance this response. In addition, ketoconazole reduced the concentration of rifampin when coadministered but not when the doses were separated by 12 hours. This would indicate that ketoconazole probably interferes with rifampin's absorption.

CLINICAL EVALUATION: A child who had a poor clinical response to the coadministration of rifampin, isoniazid, and ketoconazole was studied to determine the effects of various combinations of the 3 drugs.[1] Each combination of drugs was administered for at least 3 days. The addition of rifampin or isoniazid reduced ketoconazole concentrations more than 50%, and the simultaneous administration of both rifampin and isoniazid caused an even greater reduction in the ketoconazole concentrations. Other studies have reported up to an 80% reduction in ketoconazole concentrations following rifampin 600 mg/day.[2-5]

Peak rifampin concentrations produced by a 10 mg/kg dose were reduced from 5 to 2.5 mcg/mL by ketoconazole coadministration; separation of the ketoconazole dose from the rifampin dose by 12 hours eliminated the interaction. Mean rifampin area under the concentration-time curve following 600 mg/day was reduced approximately 20% (not statistically significant) by ketoconazole 200 mg/day for 2 days.[5]

RELATED DRUGS: Rifampin reduces the concentration of fluconazole (eg, *Diflucan*) and itraconazole (eg, *Sporanox*).

MANAGEMENT OPTIONS:

➡ *Circumvent/Minimize.* Separation of the rifampin and ketoconazole doses by 12 hours may prevent depression of rifampin concentrations.

➡ *Monitor.* Monitor patients for therapeutic failure when rifampin or isoniazid are administered with ketoconazole. Likewise, check the response to rifampin when ketoconazole is coadministered.

REFERENCES:

1. Engelhard D, et al. Interaction of ketoconazole with rifampin and isoniazid. *N Engl J Med*. 1984;311(26):1681-1683.

2. Meunier F. Serum fungistatic and fungicidal activity in volunteers receiving antifungal agents. *Eur J Clin Microbiol*. 1986;5(1):103-109.

3. Drouhet E, et al. Laboratory and clinical assessment of ketoconazole in deep-seated mycoses. *Am J Med*. 1983;74(1B):30-47.

4. Brass C, et al. Disposition of ketoconazole, an oral antifungal, in humans. *Antimicrob Agents Chemother*. 1982;21(1):151-158.

5. Doble N, et al. Pharmacokinetic study of the interaction between rifampicin and ketoconazole. *J Antimicrob Chemother*. 1988;21(5):633-635.

Ketoconazole (eg, *Nizoral*)

Ritonavir (*Norvir*)

SUMMARY: Ketoconazole administration increases the plasma concentration of ritonavir; increased side effects could occur in some patients.

RISK FACTORS: No specific risk factors are known.

MECHANISM: Ketoconazole appears to reduce the systemic clearance of ritonavir, probably by inhibiting hepatic CYP3A4. Ketoconazole also appears to inhibit P-glycoprotein, the mechanism probably responsible for the increased cerebrospinal fluid (CSF):plasma ratio of ritonavir observed in this study.

CLINICAL EVALUATION: Twelve patients taking ritonavir 400 mg twice daily and saquinavir 400 mg twice daily were coadministered ketoconazole 200 or 400 mg once daily for 10 days.[1] Ritonavir plasma and CSF samples were collected before and after ketoconazole administration. No differences were observed in ritonavir pharmacokinetics when the 2 doses of ketoconazole were compared, so the results for the 2 dosages were combined. Ketoconazole administration increased the mean area under the concentration-time curve of ritonavir nearly 30% and increased the peak ritonavir concentration 20%. The mean half-life of ritonavir was increased from 3.3 to 4.4 hours following ketoconazole. Ritonavir CSF concentrations were increased 178% during ketoconazole coadministration. A similar increase (181%) was observed in the CSF:plasma unbound ritonavir ratio. The clinical significance of the increase in CSF concentrations is unknown. A prior study of the effect of ketoconazole 200 mg/day on ritonavir 500 mg twice daily demonstrated only an 18% increase in ritonavir concentrations.[2] The reduced effect noted in this study may be a result of the administration of lower ketoconazole doses.

RELATED DRUGS: Ketoconazole has been reported to increase the concentrations of nelfinavir (*Viracept*) and saquinavir (eg, *Fortovase*). Other protease inhibitors such as indinavir (*Crixivan*) may be affected in a similar manner. Itraconazole (*Sporanox*) and fluconazole (eg, *Diflucan*) are inhibitors of CYP3A4 and may reduce the metabolism of ritonavir. Terbinafine (eg, *Lamisil*) does not appear to inhibit CYP3A4 activity and may not increase ritonavir concentrations.

MANAGEMENT OPTIONS:

➡ *Consider Alternative.* Although no data are available, consider terbinafine as an alternative antifungal agent in patients receiving protease inhibitors.

➡ **Monitor.** Monitor patients taking protease inhibitors for increased concentrations and symptoms of toxicity (eg, nausea, vomiting, diarrhea) when ketoconazole is administered.

REFERENCES:

1. Khaliq Y, et al. Effect of ketoconazole on ritonavir and saquinavir concentrations in plasma and cerebrospinal fluid from patients infected with human immunodeficiency virus. *Clin Pharmacol Ther.* 2000;68:637-646.

2. Bertz R, et al. Evaluation of the pharmacokinetics of multiple dose ritonavir and ketoconazole in combination. *Clin Pharmacol Ther.* 1998;63:228.

 Ketoconazole (eg, *Nizoral*)

Rosiglitazone (*Avandia*)

SUMMARY: Ketoconazole increases rosiglitazone plasma concentrations and may increase the hypoglycemic effect of rosiglitazone.

RISK FACTORS: No specific risk factors are known.

MECHANISM: Ketoconazole inhibits the CYP3A4 mediated metabolism of rosiglitazone.

CLINICAL EVALUATION: Ten healthy subjects received a single dose of rosiglitazone 8 mg following 5 days of placebo or ketoconazole 200 mg/day.[1] Compared with placebo, ketoconazole pretreatment increased the mean area under the plasma concentration-time curve of rosiglitazone 47% and its peak concentration 17%. Rosiglitazone's half-life increased from 3.6 to 5.5 hours after ketoconazole. Some patients with diabetes taking rosiglitazone may experience increased hypoglycemic response during ketoconazole coadministration.

RELATED DRUGS: Itraconazole (*Sporanox*), fluconazole (eg, *Diflucan*), and voriconazole (*Vfend*) would be expected to reduce the metabolism of rosiglitazone. Ketoconazole is known to inhibit the metabolism of repaglinide (*Prandin*) and would be expected to reduce the metabolism of pioglitazone (*Actos*).

MANAGEMENT OPTIONS:

➡ **Consider Alternative.** Terbinafine (eg, *Lamisil*) does not inhibit CYP3A4 and would not be expected to interact with rosiglitazone.

➡ **Monitor.** Observe patients taking rosiglitazone for altered glycemic control if ketoconazole is initiated or discontinued.

REFERENCES:

1. Park JY, et al. Effect of ketoconazole on the pharmacokinetics of rosiglitazone in healthy subjects. *Br J Clin Pharmacol.* 2004;58:397-402.

 Ketoconazole (eg, *Nizoral*)

Salmeterol (*Serevent Diskus*)

SUMMARY: Ketoconazole administration increases salmeterol concentrations; some patients may experience toxicity.

RISK FACTORS: No specific risk factors are known.

MECHANISM: Salmeterol metabolism via CYP3A4 is inhibited by ketoconazole.

CLINICAL EVALUATION: While specific data are limited, the manufacturer of salmeterol notes that the coadministration of ketoconazole 400 mg twice daily with salmeterol 50 mcg twice daily for 7 days increased the mean area under the plasma concentration-time curve of salmeterol approximately 16-fold.[1] Pending further data, observe patients receiving salmeterol and ketoconazole for increased salmeterol effect. Several subjects in the study had adverse reactions, including cardiac arrhythmias.

RELATED DRUGS: Fluconazole (eg, *Diflucan*), itraconazole (eg, *Sporanox*), posaconazole (*Noxafil*), and voriconazole (eg, *Vfend*) also inhibit the activity of CYP3A4 and are expected to increase the plasma concentrations of salmeterol.

MANAGEMENT OPTIONS:

➡ *Consider Alternative.* Consider terbinafine (eg, *Lamisil*) as an alternative antifungal agent because it does not affect CYP3A4 activity. Amphotericin (eg, *Amphotec*), caspofungin (*Cancidas*), and anidulafungin (*Eraxis*) do not appear to inhibit CYP3A4.

➡ *Monitor.* Monitor for evidence of salmeterol toxicity (eg, tachycardia and palpitations) if it is administered with ketoconazole or other potent CYP3A4 inhibitors.

REFERENCES:

1. *Serevent Diskus* [package insert]. Research Triangle Park, NC: GlaxoSmithKline; 2008.

Ketoconazole (eg, *Nizoral*)

Saquinavir (*Invirase*)

SUMMARY: Ketoconazole administration can result in a large increase in saquinavir serum concentrations; toxicity may result in some patients.

RISK FACTORS: No specific risk factors are known.

MECHANISM: Ketoconazole appears to inhibit the metabolism (CYP3A4) of saquinavir, resulting in an increase in saquinavir bioavailability and a reduction in its clearance.

CLINICAL EVALUATION: While no published data are available for evaluation, the manufacturer of saquinavir has made available some data on this interaction. The coadministration of ketoconazole 200 mg/day with saquinavir 600 mg 3 times daily resulted in a 3-fold increase in saquinavir concentrations compared with saquinavir alone.[1] Ketoconazole concentrations were unaffected by saquinavir administration. The increased saquinavir concentrations could result in toxicity in some patients.

RELATED DRUGS: Ketoconazole is known to increase the serum concentration of indinavir (*Crixivan*). The effects of other azole antifungal agents (eg, itraconazole [eg, *Sporanox*], fluconazole [eg, *Diflucan*]) that inhibit CYP3A4 metabolism on saquinavir are unknown, but some increase in saquinavir serum concentration is expected. Terbinafine (eg, *Lamisil*) does not appear to inhibit CYP3A4 activity and may not increase saquinavir concentrations.

MANAGEMENT OPTIONS:

➡ ***Consider Alternative.*** Although no specific data are available, terbinafine does not appear to inhibit CYP3A4 activity and might provide an alternative antifungal agent that may not increase saquinavir concentrations.

➡ ***Circumvent/Minimize.*** It may be necessary to reduce the dose of saquinavir when ketoconazole is coadministered.

➡ ***Monitor.*** Pending further information on this interaction, monitor patients for increased saquinavir serum concentrations and abdominal discomfort or diarrhea.

REFERENCES:

1. *Invirase* [package insert]. Nutley, NJ: Hoffman-La Roche; 1995.

3

Ketoconazole (eg, *Nizoral*)

Saxagliptin (*Onglyza*)

SUMMARY: **Saxagliptin plasma concentration and hypoglycemic response may be enhanced during the coadministration of ketoconazole; it is possible some patients will require a dose adjustment.**

RISK FACTORS: No specific risk factors are known.

MECHANISM: Ketoconazole may increase saxagliptin plasma concentrations by inhibition of CYP3A4, P-glycoprotein, or both.

CLINICAL EVALUATION: A single dose of saxagliptin 20 mg was administered alone and following ketoconazole 200 mg twice daily for 7 days.[1] The pretreatment with ketoconazole produced a 3.7-fold increase in the mean area under the concentration-time curve (AUC) of saxagliptin. In another study, ketoconazole 200 mg twice daily for 9 days increased the AUC resulting from a single dose of saxagliptin 100 mg by 2.5-fold. The concentration of saxagliptin's active metabolite was reduced 88% with ketoconazole pretreatment. This magnitude of effect is likely to result in an increased hypoglycemic response.

RELATED DRUGS: Other antifungal agents that inhibit CYP3A4 or P-glycoprotein (eg, itraconazole [eg, *Sporanox*], voriconazole [eg, *Vfend*], posaconazole [*Noxafil*], fluconazole [eg, *Diflucan*]) are expected to affect saxagliptin in a similar manner. While sitagliptin (*Januvia*) is also a P-glycoprotein substrate, the potential for ketoconazole to increase its plasma concentration is unknown.

MANAGEMENT OPTIONS:

➡ ***Consider Alternative.*** Terbinafine (eg, *Lamisil*) could be considered as an alternative antifungal agent because it does not affect CYP3A4 activity. Amphotericin (eg, *Amphotec*), caspofungin (*Cancidas*), and anidulafungin (*Eraxis*) do not appear to inhibit CYP3A4.

➡ ***Monitor.*** Monitor patients stabilized on saxagliptin for changes in their blood glucose levels if ketoconazole is initiated or discontinued from their drug regimen. The manufacturer of saxagliptin recommends reducing the dosage of saxagliptin to 2.5 mg daily during coadministration of ketoconazole.

REFERENCES:

1. *Onglyza* [package insert]. Wilmington, DE: AstraZeneca Pharmaceuticals LP; 2011.

Ketoconazole (eg, *Nizoral*)

Sildenafil (eg, *Viagra*)

SUMMARY: Ketoconazole may produce large increases in sildenafil plasma concentrations; increased sildenafil adverse reactions may occur.

RISK FACTORS: No specific risk factors are known.

MECHANISM: Ketoconazole is known to be a strong inhibitor of CYP3A4, the enzyme primarily responsible for the metabolism of sildenafil.

CLINICAL EVALUATION: While specific data are limited, the manufacturer of sildenafil notes that the coadministration of ketoconazole may produce large increases in the plasma concentration of sildenafil.[1] Other inhibitors of CYP3A4 have increased sildenafil concentrations 2- to 10-fold.[1] Pending further data, observe patients receiving sildenafil and ketoconazole for increased sildenafil adverse reactions, including hypotension, visual disturbances, and dizziness. Sildenafil dose reductions will likely be appropriate in patients taking ketoconazole.

RELATED DRUGS: Fluconazole (eg, *Diflucan*), itraconazole (eg, *Sporanox*), posaconazole (*Noxafil*), and voriconazole (eg, *Vfend*) also inhibit the activity of CYP3A4 and are expected to increase the plasma concentrations of sildenafil. Vardenafil (eg, *Levitra*) and tadalafil (eg, *Cialis*) are also metabolized by CYP3A4 and are expected to interact in a similar manner with ketoconazole.

MANAGEMENT OPTIONS:

➡ **Consider Alternative.** Consider terbinafine (eg, *Lamisil*) as an alternative antifungal agent because it does not affect CYP3A4 activity. Amphotericin (eg, *Amphotec*), caspofungin (*Cancidas*), and anidulafungin (*Eraxis*) do not appear to inhibit CYP3A4.

➡ **Monitor.** Advise patients taking ketoconazole or any other CYP3A4 inhibitor about excessive sildenafil effects.

REFERENCES:

   1. *Viagra* [package insert]. New York, NY: Pfizer Labs; 2008.

Ketoconazole (eg, *Nizoral*)

Silodosin (*Rapaflo*)

SUMMARY: Ketoconazole administration can produce elevated silodosin plasma concentrations; an increase in adverse reactions may occur.

RISK FACTORS: No specific risk factors are known.

MECHANISM: Ketoconazole is known to inhibit the activity of CYP3A4 and P-glycoprotein, both of which contribute to the elimination of silodosin.

CLINICAL EVALUATION: While specific data are limited, the manufacturer of silodosin notes that the coadministration of ketoconazole 400 mg for 4 days prior to a single dose of silodosin 8 mg increased the mean area under the plasma concentration-time curve (AUC) of silodosin 3.2-fold.[1] When ketoconazole was administered at a dosage of 200 mg daily, a single dose of silodosin 4 mg increased the silodosin

AUC 2.9-fold. Pending further data, observe patients receiving silodosin and keto-conazole for increased silodosin effects, including hypotension and dizziness.

RELATED DRUGS: Fluconazole (eg, *Diflucan*), itraconazole (eg, *Sporanox*), posaconazole (*Noxafil*), and voriconazole (eg, *Vfend*) also inhibit the activity of CYP3A4 and are expected to increase the plasma concentrations of silodosin. Tamsulosin (eg, *Flomax*) may interact in a similar manner with ketoconazole.

MANAGEMENT OPTIONS:

➡ *Consider Alternative.* Terbinafine (eg, *Lamisil*) may be considered as an alternative antifungal agent because it does not affect CYP3A4 activity. Amphotericin (eg, *Amphotec*), caspofungin (*Cancidas*), and anidulafungin (*Eraxis*) do not appear to inhibit CYP3A4.

➡ *Monitor.* Observe patients taking silodosin for increased adverse reactions if keto-conazole is coadministered.

REFERENCES:
1. *Rapaflo* [package insert]. Corona, CA: Watson Pharmaceuticals Inc; 2008.

 Ketoconazole (eg, *Nizoral*)

Simvastatin (eg, *Zocor*)

SUMMARY: Ketoconazole can cause elevated simvastatin concentrations leading to myopathy and, potentially, rhabdo-myolysis.

RISK FACTORS: No specific risk factors are known.

MECHANISM: Ketoconazole inhibits the first-pass and systemic CYP3A4-mediated metabolism of simvastatin.

CLINICAL EVALUATION: Several case reports described the development of muscle weak-ness and pain accompanied by elevations of blood creatine phosphokinase con-centrations following the addition of ketoconazole 200 to 400 mg/day for 3 to 4 weeks to simvastatin 20 mg/day.[1] One patient underwent muscle biopsy that showed evidence of muscle fiber necrosis. Both patients recovered following dis-continuation of simvastatin and ketoconazole. These cases are typical of the inter-action expected between ketoconazole and simvastatin.

RELATED DRUGS: Itraconazole (eg, *Sporanox*) and, to a lesser extent, fluconazole (eg, *Diflucan*) and voriconazole (eg, *Vfend*) will reduce the metabolism of simvastatin. The metabolism of lovastatin (eg, *Mevacor*) is markedly reduced by coadministration of ketoconazole. Ketoconazole also reduces the clearance of atorvastatin (*Lipitor*) but to a lesser degree than lovastatin.

MANAGEMENT OPTIONS:

➡ *Use Alternative.* Avoid coadministration of ketoconazole or itraconazole with simva-statin. Use a statin not dependent on CYP3A4 metabolism (eg, fluvastatin [*Lescol*], pravastatin [eg, *Pravachol*]) with ketoconazole. If possible, use an antifungal with-out CYP3A4 inhibition (eg, terbinafine [eg, *Lamisil*]). If a suitable alternative antifungal is not available, withhold statin administration during antifungal therapy. Monitor for evidence of muscle pain or weakness.

REFERENCES:

1. Gilad R, Lampl Y. Rhabdomyolysis induced by simvastatin and ketoconazole treatment. *Clin Neuropharmacol*. 1999;22(5):295-297.

Ketoconazole (eg, *Nizoral*)

Sirolimus (*Rapamune*)

SUMMARY: Ketoconazole produced a marked increase in the plasma concentration of sirolimus. Sirolimus-induced toxicity may result.

RISK FACTORS: No specific risk factors are known.

MECHANISM: Ketoconazole inhibits the first-pass metabolism of sirolimus by reducing CYP3A4 or P-glycoprotein activity. The lack of change in sirolimus half-life indicates a limited effect of ketoconazole on the intrinsic clearance of sirolimus.

CLINICAL EVALUATION: Twenty-three healthy subjects were administered a single dose of sirolimus 5 mg alone and following ketoconazole 200 mg/day for 10 days.[1] Following ketoconazole administration, the area under the concentration-time curve of sirolimus increased 10-fold and its oral clearance was reduced 90%. The half-life of sirolimus was unchanged by pretreatment with ketoconazole. These large increases in sirolimus concentrations may result in toxicity, including elevated lipid concentrations or bone marrow suppression.

RELATED DRUGS: Itraconazole (eg, *Sporanox*) and fluconazole (eg, *Diflucan*) may also increase the bioavailability of orally administered sirolimus. Tacrolimus (*Prograf*) plasma concentrations are also increased by ketoconazole.

MANAGEMENT OPTIONS:

➠ *Consider Alternative.* Consider the use of an antifungal agent that does not inhibit CYP3A4 (eg, terbinafine [eg, *Lamisil*]) in patients stabilized on sirolimus who require antifungal therapy.

➠ *Monitor.* Monitor sirolimus concentrations and adjust the dose as necessary if ketoconazole is added to or discontinued from a patient's regimen. Be alert for signs of sirolimus toxicity, including hyperlipidemia and bone marrow depression.

REFERENCES:

1. Floren LC, et al. Sirolimus oral bioavailability increases ten-fold with concomitant ketoconazole. *Clin Pharmacol Ther*. 1999;65(2):159.

Ketoconazole (eg, *Nizoral*)

Solifenacin (*Vesicare*)

SUMMARY: Ketoconazole increases solifenacin plasma concentrations. Some patients may experience increased solifenacin-induced adverse reactions, such as dry mouth or constipation.

RISK FACTORS: No specific risk factors are known.

MECHANISM: Ketoconazole inhibits the metabolism (CYP3A4) of solifenacin.

CLINICAL EVALUATION: A single dose of solifenacin 10 mg was administered to 17 healthy subjects alone and on day 7 of a 14-day regimen of ketoconazole 200 mg daily.[1] The mean area under the plasma concentration-time curve of solifenacin increased nearly 3-fold, and its half-life was prolonged from 49 to 77 hours following ketoconazole administration. The dose of solifenacin may need to be reduced in patients receiving ketoconazole.

RELATED DRUGS: Other antifungal agents that inhibit CYP3A4 (eg, itraconazole [eg, *Sporanox*], voriconazole [*Vfend*], posaconazole [*Noxafil*], fluconazole [eg, *Diflucan*]) are expected to affect solifenacin in a similar manner.

MANAGEMENT OPTIONS:

➥ *Consider Alternative.* Terbinafine (eg, *Lamisil*) could be considered as an alternative antifungal agent because it does not affect CYP3A4 activity. Amphotericin (eg, *Amphotec*), caspofungin (*Cancidas*), and anidulafungin (*Eraxis*) do not appear to inhibit CYP3A4.

➥ *Monitor.* Carefully monitor patients stabilized on solifenacin for altered drug effect if ketoconazole is added to or removed from their drug regimen.

REFERENCES:

1. Swart PJ, et al. Pharmacokinetic effect of ketoconazole on solifenacin in healthy volunteers. *Basic Clin Pharmacol Toxicol*. 2006;99(1):33-36.

 Ketoconazole (eg, *Nizoral*)

Sucralfate (eg, *Carafate*)

SUMMARY: The coadministration of sucralfate and ketoconazole reduces the plasma concentration of the antifungal agent; the clinical importance of the reduction is unknown.

RISK FACTORS: No specific risk factors are known.

MECHANISM: Not established. Sucralfate may bind to ketoconazole and inhibit its absorption.

CLINICAL EVALUATION: Six healthy subjects received ketoconazole 400 mg alone or with sucralfate 1 g 4 times a day for 2 days before ketoconazole and 5 minutes before the ketoconazole dose.[1] The sucralfate was administered as a suspension in 30 mL of water. The ketoconazole area under the plasma concentration-time curve (AUC) was reduced 21% by the coadministration of sucralfate. A second study reported a 24% reduction in ketoconazole AUC when administered with sucralfate 1 g.[2] The clinical significance of this reduction in ketoconazole bioavailability is unknown but should be limited in most patients.

RELATED DRUGS: No information is available.

MANAGEMENT OPTIONS:

➥ *Circumvent/Minimize.* Administer ketoconazole at least 2 hours before sucralfate to minimize any interaction.

➥ *Monitor.* If ketoconazole and sucralfate are coadministered, monitor for reduced antifungal effects.

REFERENCES:

1. Piscitelli SC, et al. Effects of ranitidine and sucralfate on ketoconazole bioavailability. *Antimicrob Agents Chemother*. 1991;35(9):1765-1771.

2. Carver PL, et al. In vivo interaction of ketoconazole and sucralfate in healthy volunteers. *Antimicrob Agents Chemother.* 1994;38(2):326-329.

Ketoconazole (eg, *Nizoral*)

Sunitinib (*Sutent*)

SUMMARY: Ketoconazole can increase sunitinib plasma concentrations; increased sunitinib adverse reactions may occur.

RISK FACTORS: No specific risk factors are known.

MECHANISM: Ketoconazole is known to inhibit the enzyme (CYP3A4) primarily responsible for sunitinib metabolism.

CLINICAL EVALUATION: While specific data are limited, the manufacturer of sunitinib notes that the coadministration of ketoconazole (dose not reported) prior to a single dose of sunitinib (dose not reported) increased the mean area under the plasma concentration-time curve of sunitinib by about 51%.[1] Pending further data, observe patients receiving sunitinib and ketoconazole for increased sunitinib effect and signs of toxicity.

RELATED DRUGS: Fluconazole (eg, *Diflucan*), itraconazole (eg, *Sporanox*), posaconazole (*Noxafil*), and voriconazole (*Vfend*) also inhibit the activity of CYP3A4 and are expected to increase the plasma concentration of sunitinib.

MANAGEMENT OPTIONS:

➥ *Consider Alternative.* Terbinafine (*Lamisil*) could be considered as an alternative antifungal agent because it does not affect CYP3A4 activity. Amphotericin, caspofungin (*Cancidas*), and anidulafungin (*Eraxis*) do not appear to inhibit CYP3A4.

➥ *Monitor.* Be alert for signs of sunitinib toxicity such as fatigue, diarrhea, nausea, abdominal pain, hypertension, or rash if ketoconazole is coadministered. A reduction in the dose of sunitinib may be indicated.

REFERENCES:

1. *Sutent* [package insert]. New York, NY: Pfizer; 2006.

Ketoconazole (eg, *Nizoral*)

Tacrolimus (eg, *Prograf*)

SUMMARY: Ketoconazole increases the concentration of orally administered tacrolimus; toxicity may result.

RISK FACTORS:

➥ *Route of Administration.* When coadministered with ketoconazole, oral administration of tacrolimus will produce an interaction of greater magnitude than intravenous (IV) tacrolimus.

MECHANISM: It is likely that ketoconazole inhibits the first-pass metabolism of tacrolimus by inhibiting the enzyme CYP3A4 or P-glycoprotein activity in the intestinal mucosa.

CLINICAL EVALUATION: Six healthy subjects received tacrolimus as a single oral dose (0.1 mg/kg) and an IV dose (0.025 mg/kg) separated by 6 days.[1] Ketoconazole 200 mg/day was administered for 12 days and the tacrolimus was given again;

however, doses were reduced to 0.04 mg/kg (oral) and 0.01 mg/kg (IV). Doses of tacrolimus and ketoconazole were separated by 10 hours. The ketoconazole treatment increased mean tacrolimus bioavailability from 14% to 30% and reduced mean tacrolimus oral clearance 65%. The IV clearance and half-life of tacrolimus were not significantly reduced by pretreatment with ketoconazole. The doubling of the bioavailability of tacrolimus could result in increased toxicity (eg, hyperkalemia, hypertension, nephrotoxicity).

RELATED DRUGS: Cyclosporine (eg, *Neoral*) is affected similarly by ketoconazole administration. Other azole antifungal agents (eg, fluconazole [eg, *Diflucan*], itraconazole [eg, *Sporanox*]) are likely to affect orally administered tacrolimus in a similar manner.

MANAGEMENT OPTIONS:

➡ *Consider Alternative.* For patients stabilized on tacrolimus who require antifungal therapy, consider an alternative antifungal agent. Because itraconazole and fluconazole may produce similar effects on the bioavailability of tacrolimus, consider terbinafine (eg, *Lamisil*), which does not appear to reduce CYP3A4 or P-glycoprotein activity.

➡ *Circumvent/Minimize.* Reduce the dose of tacrolimus, based upon blood concentrations, if it is administered with ketoconazole.

➡ *Monitor.* Check tacrolimus blood concentrations during coadministration with ketoconazole.

REFERENCES:
1. Floren LC, et al. Tacrolimus oral bioavailability doubles with coadministration of ketoconazole. *Clin Pharmacol Ther*. 1997;62(1):41-49.

Ketoconazole (eg, *Nizoral*)

Tadalafil (*Cialis*)

SUMMARY: Ketoconazole increases the plasma concentration of tadalafil; increased tadalafil adverse reactions may occur.

RISK FACTORS: No specific risk factors are known.

MECHANISM: Ketoconazole inhibits the metabolism of tadalafil via CYP3A4; increased tadalafil bioavailability and reduced clearance are expected.

CLINICAL EVALUATION: While specific data are limited, the coadministration of ketoconazole 400 mg daily prior to a single dose of tadalafil 20 mg increased the mean area under the plasma concentration-time curve of tadalafil by about 4-fold.[1]

RELATED DRUGS: Other antifungal agents that inhibit CYP3A4 (eg, fluconazole [eg, *Diflucan*], itraconazole [eg, *Sporanox*], posaconazole [*Noxafil*], voriconazole [*Vfend*]) are expected to affect tadalafil in a similar manner. Sildenafil (eg, *Viagra*) and vardenafil (*Levitra*) are likely to be affected in a similar manner by ketoconazole.

MANAGEMENT OPTIONS:

➡ *Consider Alternative.* Terbinafine (eg, *Lamisil*) may be considered as an alternative antifungal agent because it does not affect CYP3A4 activity. Amphotericin, caspofungin (*Cancidas*), and anidulafungin (*Eraxis*) do not appear to inhibit CYP3A4.

➡ *Circumvent/Minimize.* Pending further data, observe patients receiving tadalafil and ketoconazole for increased tadalafil effect, and limit the dosage of tadalafil to 10 mg every 72 hours.[1]

➡ *Monitor.* Be alert for signs of excessive tadalafil effects, such as hypotension, if ketoconazole is coadministered.

REFERENCES:

1. *Cialis* [package insert]. Indianapolis, IN: Eli Lilly and Company; 2003.

Ketoconazole (eg, *Nizoral*)

Tamsulosin (*Flomax*)

SUMMARY: Theoretically, tamsulosin effect may be increased by ketoconazole and other CYP3A4 inhibitors, but the clinical importance of this effect is not established.

RISK FACTORS: No specific risk factors are known.

MECHANISM: Tamsulosin is partially metabolized by CYP3A4 and ketoconazole is a CYP3A4 inhibitor; theoretically, ketoconazole would inhibit tamsulosin metabolism.

CLINICAL EVALUATION: Although the interaction is based on theoretical considerations, tamsulosin should be used with caution with moderate to strong inhibitors of CYP3A4 (eg, ketoconazole).[1]

RELATED DRUGS: Other azole antifungals may also inhibit CYP3A4 (eg, fluconazole [eg, *Diflucan*], itraconazole [eg, *Sporanox*], posaconazole [*Noxafil*], voriconazole [*Vfend*]).

MANAGEMENT OPTIONS: No specific action is required, but be alert for evidence of the interaction.

REFERENCES:

1. *Flomax* [package insert]. Ridgefield, CT: Boehringer Ingelheim; 2009.

Ketoconazole (eg, *Nizoral*)

Telaprevir (*Incivek*)

SUMMARY: The coadministration of ketoconazole increases the plasma concentration of telaprevir; adverse reactions including rash, pruritus, QTc prolongation, and blood dyscrasias may be more likely to occur.

RISK FACTORS: No specific risk factors are known.

MECHANISM: Ketoconazole inhibits the CYP3A4-mediated metabolism of telaprevir as well as telaprevir's P-glycoprotein elimination.

CLINICAL EVALUATION: While specific data are limited, the manufacturer of telaprevir notes that the coadministration of ketoconazole 400 mg as a single dose with a single dose of telaprevir 750 mg increased the mean area under the plasma concentration-time curve (AUC) of telaprevir by approximately 60%.[1] It is likely that long-term dosing will produce an interaction of greater magnitude. Pending further data, observe patients receiving telaprevir and ketoconazole for increased telaprevir adverse reactions. Telaprevir 1,250 mg every 8 hours for 4 doses increased the AUC of a single dose of ketoconazole by 50% to 125%. The clinical significance of this increase is unknown.

RELATED DRUGS: Fluconazole (eg, *Diflucan*), itraconazole (eg, *Sporanox*), posaconazole (*Noxafil*), and voriconazole (eg, *Vfend*) also inhibit the activity of CYP3A4 and are expected to increase the plasma concentrations of telaprevir. Other protease inhibitors that are metabolized by CYP3A4 (eg, atazanavir [*Reyataz*], indinavir [*Crixivan*], nelfinavir [*Viracept*], ritonavir [*Norvir*], saquinavir [*Invirase*]) are likely to interact in a similar manner with ketoconazole.

MANAGEMENT OPTIONS:

➡ *Consider Alternative.* Terbinafine (eg, *Lamisil*) could be considered as an alternative antifungal agent because it does not affect CYP3A4 activity. Amphotericin, caspofungin (*Cancidas*), and anidulafungin (*Eraxis*) do not appear to inhibit CYP3A4.

➡ *Monitor.* Monitor patients stabilized on telaprevir for adverse effects if ketoconazole or other CYP3A4 inhibitors are coadministered.

REFERENCES:

1. *Incivek* [package insert]. Cambridge, MA: Vertex Pharmaceuticals Inc; 2011.

 ## Ketoconazole (eg, *Nizoral*)

AVOID Terfenadine[†]

SUMMARY: Excessive terfenadine concentrations following ketoconazole coadministration may increase the risk of cardiac arrhythmias.

RISK FACTORS:

➡ *Concurrent Diseases.* Preexisting cardiac conduction problems increase the risk for the interaction.

MECHANISM: Ketoconazole inhibits the metabolism (CYP3A4) of terfenadine and its active metabolite.

CLINICAL EVALUATION: A patient taking terfenadine 60 mg twice daily developed episodes of palpitations, dyspnea, diaphoresis, and syncope beginning several days after the addition of ketoconazole 200 mg twice daily to her regimen.[1,2] Polymorphic ventricular tachycardia (torsades de pointes) was diagnosed by electrocardiographic (ECG) monitoring. The patient's symptoms resolved over 2 days, and the ECG abnormalities disappeared over 5 to 7 days. Twelve healthy subjects received a single dose of terfenadine 120 mg alone and following ketoconazole 400 mg/day for 7 days.[3] Terfenadine concentrations peaked at 27 ng/mL following ketoconazole, but were unmeasurable when administered alone. The apparent clearance of the active carboxylic acid metabolite of terfenadine was reduced 30% during ketoconazole coadministration. ECG abnormalities may occur within 5 to 7 days after ketoconazole is started.[4]

RELATED DRUGS: Other oral antifungal agents (eg, itraconazole [eg, *Sporanox*], fluconazole [eg, *Diflucan*]) have been reported to inhibit the metabolism of terfenadine. Astemizole[†] metabolism also has been noted to be reduced during oral antifungal therapy.

MANAGEMENT OPTIONS:

➡ *AVOID COMBINATION.* Until more information on the interaction between ketoconazole and terfenadine is available, avoid coadministration. The use of sedating antihistamines or perhaps cetirizine (eg, *Zyrtec*) or loratadine (eg, *Claritin*) instead of terfenadine is preferred in patients taking ketoconazole or other oral antifungal agents.

REFERENCES:

1. Monahan BP, et al. Torsades de pointes occurring in association with terfenadine use. *JAMA.* 1990;264(21):2788-2790.

2. Zimmermann M, et al. Torsades de pointes after treatment with terfenadine and ketoconazole. *Eur Heart J.* 1992;13(7):1002-1003.

3. Eller MG, et al. Pharmacokinetic interaction between terfenadine and ketoconazole. *Clin Pharmacol Ther.* 1991;49:130.

4. Honig P, et al. The pharmacokinetics and cardiac consequences of the terfenadine-ketoconazole interaction. *Clin Pharmacol Ther.* 1993;53:206.

† Not available in the United States.

Ketoconazole (eg, *Nizoral*)

Theophylline (eg, *Theo-24*)

SUMMARY: Ketoconazole does not appear to alter the pharmacokinetics of theophylline, but may alter the absorption of sustained-release theophylline dosage forms.

RISK FACTORS: No specific risk factors are known.

MECHANISM: Not established.

CLINICAL EVALUATION: Ketoconazole 200 mg/day was reported to decrease theophylline concentrations in a patient receiving sustained-release theophylline twice daily.[1] However, single- or multiple-dose ketoconazole had no effect on intravenous aminophylline in healthy subjects.[2,3] Therefore, it would appear that ketoconazole does not alter the clearance of theophylline. A prospective trial is required to evaluate ketoconazole's potential for altering the absorption of sustained-release theophylline.

RELATED DRUGS: No information is available.

MANAGEMENT OPTIONS: No specific action is required, but be alert for evidence of the interaction.

REFERENCES:

1. Murphy E, et al. Ketoconazole-theophylline interaction. *Irish Med J.* 1987;80(4).123-124.

2. Heusner JJ, et al. Effect of chronically administered ketoconazole on the elimination of theophylline in man. *Drug Intell Clin Pharm.* 1987;21(6):514-517.

3. Brown MW, et al. Effect of ketoconazole on hepatic oxidative drug metabolism. *Clin Pharmacol Ther.* 1985;37(3):290-297.

Ketoconazole (eg, *Nizoral*)

Ticagrelor (*Brilinta*)

SUMMARY: Ketoconazole markedly increases the plasma concentration of ticagrelor and reduces the concentration of its active metabolite; the net effect is likely to be increased antiplatelet effect and risk of bleeding.

RISK FACTORS: No specific risk factors are known.

MECHANISM: Ketoconazole inhibits CYP3A4, the primary enzyme responsible for the metabolism of ticagrelor.

CLINICAL EVALUATION: While specific data are limited, the manufacturer of ticagrelor notes that the coadministration of ketoconazole 200 mg twice daily increased the mean area under the plasma concentration-time curve (AUC) of ticagrelor by 6- to 8-fold.[1] The AUC of ticagrelor's active metabolite was reduced during ketoconazole coadministration. Pending further data, observe patients receiving ticagrelor and ketoconazole for increased ticagrelor effects, including bleeding.

RELATED DRUGS: Fluconazole (eg, *Diflucan*), itraconazole (eg, *Sporanox*), posaconazole (*Noxafil*), and voriconazole (eg, *Vfend*) also inhibit the activity of CYP3A4 and are expected to increase the plasma concentrations of ticagrelor. Ketoconazole causes a significant reduction in the formation of clopidogrel's (*Plavix*) active metabolite, but has minimal effect on the conversion of prasugrel (*Effient*) to its active metabolite.[2]

MANAGEMENT OPTIONS:

➡ **Use Alternative.** Terbinafine (eg, *Lamisil*) could be considered as an alternative antifungal agent because it does not affect CYP3A4 activity. Amphotericin, caspofungin (*Cancidas*), and anidulafungin (*Eraxis*) do not appear to inhibit CYP3A4. Prasugrel may be considered as an alternative to ticagrelor because prasugrel's antiplatelet activity is not altered by ketoconazole.

➡ **Monitor.** If ticagrelor is administered with ketoconazole or other CYP3A4 inhibitors, monitor patients carefully for evidence of excessive antiplatelet effects and consider reducing the ticagrelor dose.

REFERENCES:

1. *Brilinta* [package insert]. Wilmington, DE: AstraZeneca LP; 2011.
2. Farid NA, et al. Cytochrome P450 3A inhibition by ketoconazole affects prasugrel and clopidogrel pharmacokinetics and pharmacodynamics differently. *Clin Pharmacol Ther*. 2007;81(5):735-741.

Ketoconazole (eg, *Nizoral*)

Tolbutamide

SUMMARY: Ketoconazole increased tolbutamide plasma concentrations and its hypoglycemic effect in healthy subjects.

RISK FACTORS: No specific risk factors are known.

MECHANISM: Ketoconazole may inhibit the hydroxylation (CYP2C9) of tolbutamide.

CLINICAL EVALUATION: Seven healthy subjects received a single 500 mg oral dose of tolbutamide before and following 7 days of ketoconazole 200 mg daily.[1] Plasma was only sampled for 12 hours following the tolbutamide doses. Treatment with ketoconazole caused a mean increase in the tolbutamide area under the plasma concentration-time curve from 0 to 12 hours of 76%. The half-life of tolbutamide was reported as 3.7 hours when administered alone and 12.3 hours following ketoconazole coadministration. Several subjects reported symptoms of hypoglycemia during ketoconazole-tolbutamide administration. Blood glucose reduction was greater following tolbutamide and ketoconazole compared with tolbutamide alone. Patients with diabetes mellitus may experience lower blood glucose concentrations during the coadministration of ketoconazole and tolbutamide.

RELATED DRUGS: Fluconazole (eg, *Diflucan*) is known to reduce the clearance of tolbutamide. Voriconazole (eg, *Vfend*) also is likely to reduce tolbutamide metabolism. The effect of ketoconazole on other hypoglycemic agents is unknown.

MANAGEMENT OPTIONS:

➡ *Monitor.* Monitor patients taking tolbutamide for increased hypoglycemic effects during the coadministration of ketoconazole.

REFERENCES:

1. Krishnaiah YS, et al. Interaction between tolbutamide and ketoconazole in healthy subjects. *Br J Clin Pharmacol.* 1994;37(2):205-207.

Ketoconazole (eg, *Nizoral*)

Tolterodine (*Detrol*)

SUMMARY: Ketoconazole moderately increases tolterodine serum concentrations, but it is not known how often this effect will result in adverse outcomes.

RISK FACTORS:

➡ *Pharmacogenetics.* This interaction is likely to be significant only in patients who are deficient in CYP2D6.

MECHANISM: Tolterodine is metabolized by CYP2D6 to an active metabolite, 5-hydroxymethyl tolterodine. Tolterodine is also metabolized by CYP3A4 (normally a minor pathway), but under conditions of CYP2D6 deficiency (genetic or pharmacological), CYP3A4 probably serves a greater role in tolterodine elimination. Therefore, ketoconazole and other potent CYP3A4 inhibitors may increase tolterodine serum concentrations in CYP2D6-deficient patients.

CLINICAL EVALUATION: Eight healthy CYP2D6-deficient subjects received both single- and multiple-dose tolterodine with and without concurrent ketoconazole 200 mg/day.[1] Ketoconazole increased tolterodine area under the serum concentration-time curve more than 2-fold, and it was concluded that the effect may be clinically important in patients lacking in CYP2D6 activity.[1,2]

RELATED DRUGS: Itraconazole (eg, *Sporanox*) is also a potent inhibitor of CYP3A4; fluconazole (eg, *Diflucan*) is somewhat weaker, but in larger doses it also inhibits CYP3A4.

MANAGEMENT OPTIONS:

➡ *Circumvent/Minimize.* The manufacturer recommends patients receiving CYP3A4 inhibitors, such as ketoconazole and itraconazole, not take tolterodine in dosages greater than 1 mg twice daily.

➡ *Monitor.* In patients receiving tolterodine with ketoconazole or other CYP3A4 inhibitors, monitor for excessive antimuscarinic effects (eg, dry mouth, constipation, blurred vision, dry eyes).

REFERENCES:

1. Brynne N, et al. Ketoconazole inhibits the metabolism of tolterodine in subjects with deficient CYP2D6 activity. *Br J Clin Pharmacol.* 1999;48(4):564-572.

2. Short DD. Tolterodine, a new antimuscarinic drug for treatment of bladder overactivity—a comment. *Pharmacotherapy.* 1999;19(10):1188.

Ketoconazole (eg, *Nizoral*)

Tolvaptan (*Samsca*)

SUMMARY: Ketoconazole administration has been reported to markedly increase the plasma concentration of tolvaptan; some patients may experience increased adverse reactions.

RISK FACTORS: No specific risk factors are known.

MECHANISM: Ketoconazole inhibits CYP3A4, the primary enzyme that metabolizes tolvaptan. Ketoconazole-induced inhibition of P-glycoprotein may also contribute to the increased tolvaptan concentrations.

CLINICAL EVALUATION: While specific data are limited, the manufacturer of tolvaptan notes that the coadministration of ketoconazole 200 mg daily prior to tolvaptan increased the mean area under the plasma concentration-time curve of tolvaptan by approximately 5-fold.[1] Pending further data, observe patients receiving tolvaptan and ketoconazole for increased tolvaptan adverse reactions, including constipation, dry mouth, and hyperglycemia.

RELATED DRUGS: Fluconazole (eg, *Diflucan*), itraconazole (eg, *Sporanox*), posaconazole (*Noxafil*), and voriconazole (eg, *Vfend*) also inhibit the activity of CYP3A4 and are expected to increase the plasma concentrations of tolvaptan.

MANAGEMENT OPTIONS:

➡ **Consider Alternative.** Terbinafine (eg, *Lamisil*) could be considered as an alternative antifungal agent because it does not affect CYP3A4 activity. Amphotericin, caspofungin (*Cancidas*), and anidulafungin (*Eraxis*) do not appear to inhibit CYP3A4.

➡ **Monitor.** If ketoconazole is administered with tolvaptan, monitor patients for evidence of tolvaptan toxicity.

REFERENCES:

1. *Samsca* [package insert]. Rockville, MD: Otsuka America Pharmaceutical Inc; 2009.

Ketoconazole (eg, *Nizoral*)

Triazolam (eg, *Halcion*)

SUMMARY: Triazolam plasma concentrations are markedly elevated by the coadministration of ketoconazole; increased toxicity is likely to result.

RISK FACTORS: No specific risk factors are known.

MECHANISM: Ketoconazole inhibits the metabolism of triazolam by the CYP3A4 enzyme. This reduces triazolam's systemic clearance and increases its bioavailability.

CLINICAL EVALUATION: Nine healthy subjects received oral triazolam 0.125 mg preceded 1 and 17 hours earlier by placebo or ketoconazole 200 mg.[1] The average reduction in the oral clearance of triazolam following ketoconazole was 88%. The triazolam peak plasma concentration increased from 1.32 to 3 ng/mL, while its half-life increased from 3.4 to 13.5 hours. These pharmacokinetic changes were accompanied by an increase in the pharmacodynamic effects of triazolam. Another study reported similar changes in triazolam pharmacokinetics following a single dose of triazolam 0.25 mg and a twice-daily dose of ketoconazole 200 mg.[2]

RELATED DRUGS: Itraconazole (eg, *Sporanox*), fluconazole (eg, *Diflucan*), and miconazole (eg, *Monistat*) are likely to reduce triazolam's metabolism. Ketoconazole is likely to inhibit other benzodiazepines that are metabolized by CYP3A4, such as alprazolam (eg, *Xanax*) and oral midazolam. Benzodiazepines not metabolized via the CYP3A4 enzyme (eg, lorazepam [eg, *Ativan*], oxazepam [eg, *Serax*]) are less likely to be affected.

MANAGEMENT OPTIONS:

➡ *Consider Alternative.* Prescribe a benzodiazepine that is not metabolized via the CYP3A4 enzyme to patients maintained on ketoconazole (see Related Drugs). Consider prescribing terbinafine for patients stabilized on triazolam who require antifungal therapy.

➡ *Monitor.* Carefully monitor patients receiving triazolam and ketoconazole for increased sedation and reduced psychomotor performance.

REFERENCES:

1. von Moltke LL, et al. Triazolam biotransformation by human liver microsomes in vitro: effects of metabolic inhibitors and clinical confirmation of a predicted interaction with ketoconazole. *J Pharmacol Exp Ther.* 1996;276(2):370-379.

2. Wright CE, et al. Ketoconazole inhibition of triazolam and alprazolam clearance: differential kinetic and dynamic consequences. *Clin Pharmacol Ther.* 1997;61:183.

Ketoconazole (eg, *Nizoral*)

Vardenafil (*Levitra*)

SUMMARY: Ketoconazole increases the plasma concentration of vardenafil; increased vardenafil adverse reactions may occur.

RISK FACTORS: No specific risk factors are known.

MECHANISM: Ketoconazole inhibits the metabolism of vardenafil via CYP3A4; increased vardenafil bioavailability and reduced clearance are expected.

CLINICAL EVALUATION: While specific data are limited, the coadministration of ketoconazole 200 mg daily prior to a single dose of vardenafil 5 mg increased the mean area under the plasma concentration-time curve of vardenafil by about 10-fold.[1]

RELATED DRUGS: Other antifungal agents that inhibit CYP3A4 (eg, itraconazole [eg, *Sporanox*], voriconazole [*Vfend*], posaconazole [*Noxafil*], fluconazole [eg, *Diflucan*]) are expected to affect vardenafil in a similar manner. Sildenafil (eg, *Viagra*) and tadalafil (*Cialis*) are likely to be affected in a similar manner by ketoconazole.

MANAGEMENT OPTIONS:

➡ *Consider Alternative.* Terbinafine (eg, *Lamisil*) may be considered as an alternative antifungal agent because it does not affect CYP3A4 activity. Amphotericin, caspofungin (*Cancidas*), and anidulafungin (*Eraxis*) do not appear to inhibit CYP3A4.

➡ *Circumvent/Minimize.* Pending further data, observe patients receiving vardenafil and ketoconazole for increased vardenafil effect, and limit the dosage of vardenafil to 5 mg every 24 hours. A 2.5 mg daily limit on vardenafil is suggested for patients taking ketoconazole 400 mg daily.[1]

➡ **Monitor.** Be alert for signs of excessive vardenafil effects, such as hypotension, if ketoconazole is coadministered.

REFERENCES:

1. *Levitra* [package insert]. West Haven, CT: Bayer Pharmaceuticals Corporation; 2008.

Ketoconazole (eg, *Nizoral*)

Venlafaxine (*Effexor*)

SUMMARY: Ketoconazole causes an increase in venlafaxine plasma concentrations; increased adverse reactions may occur during coadministration.

RISK FACTORS:

➡ **Pharmacogenetics.** It appears from this preliminary study that, in patients who are poor metabolizers (PM) of CYP2D6, venlafaxine metabolism may be more dependent on CYP3A4 and thus more affected by CYP3A4 inhibitors such as ketoconazole.

MECHANISM: Ketoconazole appears to inhibit the CYP3A4 pathway of venlafaxine metabolism. Because CYP2D6 is the major pathway for venlafaxine metabolism, the magnitude of the interaction may depend on the patient's CYP2D6 genotype.

CLINICAL EVALUATION: Twenty healthy subjects (14 PMs and 6 extensive metabolizers [EMs] of CYP2D6) were administered a single oral dose of venlafaxine, 25 mg to the PMs and 50 mg to the EMs.[1] The venlafaxine also was administered on the second day of a ketoconazole 100 mg twice-daily regimen. Overall, the mean area under the plasma concentration-time curve of venlafaxine was increased 36% by coadministration of ketoconazole. The effect of ketoconazole was greater in the PMs (mean increase, 70%) than in the EMs (mean increase, 21%). The half-life of venlafaxine was not altered by ketoconazole.

RELATED DRUGS: Itraconazole (eg, *Sporanox*), fluconazole (eg, *Diflucan*), and voriconazole (*Vfend*) also are known to inhibit CYP3A4. Terbinafine (eg, *Lamisil*) is known to inhibit CYP2D6 and is expected to interact with venlafaxine in patients who are EMs for CYP2D6.

MANAGEMENT OPTIONS:

➡ **Consider Alternative.** Use an antidepressant that is not metabolized by CYP3A4 (eg, paroxetine [eg, *Paxil*], sertraline [eg, *Zoloft*]) in patients taking ketoconazole whenever possible.

➡ **Monitor.** Monitor patients for evidence of excessive venlafaxine concentrations such as nausea and vomiting.

REFERENCES:

1. Lindh JD, et al. Effect of ketoconazole on venlafaxine plasma concentrations in extensive and poor metabolisers of debrisoquine. *Eur J Clin Pharmacol.* 2003;59(5-6):401-406.

Ketoconazole (*Nizoral*)

Warfarin (eg, *Coumadin*)

SUMMARY: Isolated case reports, as well as the known interactive properties of the 2 drugs, suggest that ketoconazole increases the hypoprothrombinemic response of warfarin.

RISK FACTORS: No specific risk factors are known.

MECHANISM: Ketoconazole probably inhibits the metabolism of warfarin.

CLINICAL EVALUATION: A 75-year-old woman stabilized on warfarin was given ketoconazole 400 mg/day for a vaginal thrush infection.[1] Although the hypoprothrombinemic response was not prolonged by the second day of ketoconazole therapy, she presented with spontaneous bruising and a markedly enhanced hypoprothrombinemic response after 3 weeks. Her warfarin therapy was later restabilized at previous levels in the absence of ketoconazole. A similar case was reported to the British Committee on the Safety of Medicines, again with a positive dechallenge. Although the clinical evidence of this interaction is limited, the known ability of ketoconazole to act as a potent inhibitor of hepatic microsomal drug metabolism supports the contention that the interaction does occur.

RELATED DRUGS: Other azole antifungal agents such as fluconazole (*Diflucan*), itraconazole (*Sporanox*), and miconazole (eg, *Monistat*) also have been reported to increase the hypoprothrombinemic response to warfarin. The effect of ketoconazole on oral anticoagulants other than warfarin is not established, but an interaction may occur (with the possible exception of phenprocoumon, which is metabolized primarily by glucuronidation).

MANAGEMENT OPTIONS:

➡ **Monitor.** Monitor for altered oral anticoagulant effect if ketoconazole is initiated, discontinued, or changed in dosage. Adjust the anticoagulant dose as needed.

REFERENCES:

1. Smith AG. Potentiation of oral anticoagulants by ketoconazole. *Br Med J.* 1984;288:188-189.

Ketoconazole (*Nizoral*)

Ziprasidone (*Geodon*)

SUMMARY: Ketoconazole administration resulted in a modest increase in ziprasidone plasma concentrations; some increase in side effects might occur.

RISK FACTORS: No specific risk factors are known.

MECHANISM: Ketoconazole appears to inhibit the CYP3A4 metabolism of ziprasidone. More study is needed to determine if this effect is limited to intestinal CYP3A4 or includes a reduction in hepatic ziprasidone metabolism.

CLINICAL EVALUATION: Thirteen healthy subjects received a single oral dose of ziprasidone 40 mg following 6 days of placebo or ketoconazole 400 mg daily.[1] Subjects ate a high-fat meal just prior to drug administration on the days when ziprasidone and ketoconazole were coadministered. Ketoconazole plasma concentrations were twice as high on the day of ziprasidone administration compared with the day prior. The cause of this increase is unknown but may have been caused by the high-fat meal. The mean area under the concentration-time curve for ziprasidone increased 33% and its peak plasma concentration increased 34% following ketoconazole pretreatment. Ziprasidone half-life was not significantly altered by ketoconazole administration; however, the duration of plasma sampling after peak concentrations were obtained may not have been adequate to properly characterize small changes in half-life. The subjects reported some increase in side effects (eg, dizziness, asthenia, somnolence) during combined ketoconazole and ziprasidone administration. Potentially the use of a high-fat meal just prior to administration of ziprasidone and ketoconazole may have exaggerated the effect of ketoconazole on ziprasidone in this study.

RELATED DRUGS: Itraconazole (*Sporanox*) and fluconazole (*Diflucan*) can inhibit CYP3A4 activity and may reduce the metabolism of ziprasidone.

MANAGEMENT OPTIONS:

➡ *Circumvent/Minimize.* Terbinafine (*Lamisil*) does not appear to inhibit CYP3A4 activity and could be considered as an alternative antifungal agent in patients taking ziprasidone.

➡ *Monitor.* Be alert for some increase in side effects including dizziness, asthenia, and somnolence if ketoconazole and ziprasidone are administered concomitantly.

REFERENCES:

1. Miceli JJ, et al. The effects of ketoconazole on ziprasidone pharmacokinetics–a placebo-controlled crossover study in healthy volunteers. *Br J Clin Pharmacol.* 2000;49(suppl 1):71S-76S.

Ketoconazole (eg, *Nizoral*)

Zolpidem (*Ambien*)

SUMMARY: Ketoconazole produces an increase in zolpidem concentrations; increased sedation may occur.

RISK FACTORS: No specific risk factors are known.

MECHANISM: Ketoconazole reduces the clearance of zolpidem, probably by inhibiting the CYP3A4 metabolism of zolpidem.

CLINICAL EVALUATION: Twelve healthy subjects received a single oral dose of zolpidem 5 mg alone and 1 hour after the third of 4 doses of ketoconazole 200 mg twice daily.[1] The ketoconazole treatment increased the area under the concentration-time curve for zolpidem 67% and reduced its apparent oral clearance 40%. Zolpidem's half-life increased from 1.86 hours when administered alone to 2.41 hours when coadministered with ketoconazole. The increase in zolpidem plasma concentrations was accompanied by an increase in the drug's pharmacodynamic effects. Patients taking zolpidem are at risk of suffering increased sedation if ketoconazole is prescribed.

RELATED DRUGS: Itraconazole (*Sporanox*) and fluconazole (*Diflucan*) have been reported to produce a minimal increase in zolpidem plasma concentrations.

MANAGEMENT OPTIONS:

➡ *Consider Alternative.* Because itraconazole and fluconazole produce minimal changes in zolpidem concentrations, they may be safer alternatives to ketoconazole. Terbinafine (*Lamisil*) is not an inhibitor of CYP3A4 and would not be expected to affect zolpidem metabolism. A benzodiazepine that is not a substrate for CYP3A4 (eg, lorazepam [eg, *Ativan*], oxazepam [eg, *Serax*]), could be substituted for zolpidem to avoid an interaction with ketoconazole.

➡ *Monitor.* Observe patients taking ketoconazole and zolpidem for enhanced sedation.

REFERENCES:

1. Greenblatt DJ, et al. Kinetic and dynamic interaction study of zolpidem with ketoconazole, itraconazole, and fluconazole. *Clin Pharmacol Ther.* 1998;64:661–671.

Ketoprofen (eg, *Orudis*)

Methotrexate (eg, *Rheumatrex*)

SUMMARY: Isolated cases indicate that ketoprofen may increase the toxicity of antineoplastic doses of methotrexate.

RISK FACTORS:

➡ *Concurrent Diseases.* Particular caution is suggested in patients with preexisting renal impairment (who may be more susceptible to nonsteroidal anti-inflammatory drug [NSAID]-induced renal failure).

➡ *Dosage Regimen.* The risk of adverse effects from this interaction is primarily in patients receiving antineoplastic doses of methotrexate, rather than the lower doses used to treat rheumatoid arthritis, psoriasis, and related diseases.

MECHANISM: It is widely held that NSAIDs interfere with renal secretion of methotrexate, by inhibiting tubular secretion of methotrexate or by reducing renal blood flow by inhibiting prostaglandin synthesis. Alterations in plasma protein binding have been proposed, but is unlikely to be clinically significant because methotrexate is normally only 50% to 70% bound to plasma proteins. Pharmacokinetic studies involving several different NSAIDs have failed to consistently identify an alteration in methotrexate pharmacokinetics by NSAIDs[1-8]; however, even in studies where methotrexate pharmacokinetics remained unchanged overall, occasional patients appeared to exhibit reduced clearance of methotrexate after NSAID administration.[1,3]

CLINICAL EVALUATION: Following the observation of fatal methotrexate toxicity in 2 patients who also were receiving ketoprofen, a retrospective study was conducted of 118 cycles of high-dose methotrexate therapy in 36 patients.[9] Of the 9 cases of severe methotrexate toxicity found, 4 had received concurrent ketoprofen and 1 other case had received another NSAID, diclofenac (eg, *Voltaren*). When methotrexate was given in combination with ketoprofen, serum methotrexate concentrations were markedly higher than concentrations achieved with methotrexate alone. Although this retrospective study does not constitute proof of an interaction between methotrexate and ketoprofen, the severity of the reaction (death in 3 of 4 patients) dictates that it should not be ignored. Patients on low-dose methotrexate for rheumatoid arthritis frequently receive concurrent NSAIDs and severe methotrexate toxicity in such patients is unusual.[10-12] Although these patients would appear to be at low risk, caution is warranted since NSAID use in patients on low-dose methotrexate is occasionally associated with severe methotrexate toxicity.[13,14]

RELATED DRUGS: Other NSAIDs may interact similarly; however, more information is needed.

MANAGEMENT OPTIONS:

➡ *Avoid Unless Benefit Outweighs Risk.* Until more information is available on this inter-action, it would be prudent to avoid ketoprofen (as well as other NSAIDs) in patients receiving antineoplastic doses of methotrexate. Particular caution is sug-gested in patients with preexisting renal impairment, who may be more suscep-tible to NSAID-induced renal failure.

➡ *Monitor.* If the combination is used, monitor for methotrexate toxicity. Findings in methotrexate toxicity can include stomatitis, severe GI symptoms (eg, nausea, diarrhea, vomiting), bone marrow suppression, fever, bleeding, skin rashes, neph-rotoxicity, and hepatotoxicity. Although decreasing the methotrexate dosage would be expected to reduce the likelihood of toxicity, the magnitude of the required reduction in methotrexate dosage has not been established.

REFERENCES:

1. Ahern AM, et al. Methotrexate kinetics in rheumatoid arthritis: is there an interaction with nonsteroi-dal antiinflammatory drugs? *J Rheumatol.* 1988;15:1356-1360.

2. Furst DE, et al. Effect of aspirin and sulindac on methotrexate clearance. *J Pharm Sci.* 1990;79:782-786.

3. Dupuis LL, et al. Methotrexate-nonsteroidal antiinflammatory drug interaction in children with arthri-tis. *J Rheumatol.* 1990;17:1469-1473.

4. Liegler DG, et al. The effect of organic acids on renal clearance of methotrexate in man. *Clin Pharmacol Ther.* 1969;10:849-857.

5. Skeith KJ, et al. Lack of significant interaction between low dose methotrexate and ibuprofen or flurbiprofen in patients with arthritis. *J Rheumatol.* 1990;17:1008-1010.

6. Stewart CF, et al. Effect of aspirin (ASA) on the disposition of methotrexate (MTX) in patients with rheumatoid arthritis (RA). *Clin Pharmacol Ther.* 1990;47:139.

7. Taylor JR, et al. Effect of sodium salicylate and indomethacin on methotrexate-serum albumin bind-ing. *Arch Dermatol.* 1977;113:588-591.

8. Tracy FS, et al. The effect of NSAIDS on methotrexate disposition in patients with rheumatoid arthri-tis. *Clin Pharmacol Ther.* 1990;47:138.

9. Thyss A, et al. Clinical and pharmacokinetic evidence of a life-threatening interaction between metho-trexate and ketoprofen. *Lancet.* 1986;1:256-258.

10. Boh LE, et al. Low-dose weekly oral methotrexate therapy for inflammatory arthritis. *Clin Pharm.* 1986;5:503.

11. Andersen PA, et al. Weekly pulse methotrexate in rheumatoid arthritis: clinical and immunologic effects in a randomized, double-blind study. *Ann Intern Med.* 1985;103:489-496.

12. Tugwell P, et al. Methotrexate in rheumatoid arthritis: indications, contraindications, efficacy, and safety. *Ann Intern Med.* 1987;107:358-366.

13. Daly HM, et al. Methotrexate toxicity precipitated by azapropazone. *Br J Dermatol.* 1986;114:733.

14. Adams JD, et al. Drug interactions in psoriasis. *Australas J Dermatol.* 1976;17:39-40.

 4   **Ketoprofen (eg, *Orudis*)**

Probenecid

SUMMARY: Probenecid may increase serum ketoprofen concentrations, but the clinical importance of this effect is not established.

RISK FACTORS: No specific risk factors are known.

MECHANISM: Not established. Probenecid probably inhibits the hepatic conjugation of ketoprofen.

CLINICAL EVALUATION: Six healthy subjects were given ketoprofen 50 mg every 6 hours for 13 doses with and without concurrent probenecid 500 mg with every ketoprofen dose plus 500 mg every 6 hours for 3 doses after the last ketoprofen dose.[1] Probenecid decreased total ketoprofen clearance 67%, thus substantially increasing plasma ketoprofen concentrations. The magnitude of change in ketoprofen pharmacokinetics appears to be large enough to cause an increase in the incidence of dose-related ketoprofen adverse effects, but additional studies are needed. Possible adverse effects of increased ketoprofen levels include dizziness, drowsiness, headache, tinnitus, impaired renal function, and possible gastrointestinal symptoms such as dyspepsia, abdominal pain, and diarrhea.

RELATED DRUGS: Probenecid also inhibits the elimination of some other nonsteroidal anti-inflammatory drugs (eg, indomethacin [eg, *Indocin*], naproxen [eg, *Naprosyn*]).

MANAGEMENT OPTIONS: No specific action is required, but be alert for evidence of the interaction.

REFERENCES:
1. Upton RA, et al. Effects of probenecid on ketoprofen kinetics. *Clin Pharmacol Ther.* 1982;31:705.

Ketoprofen (eg, *Orudis*)

Warfarin (eg, *Coumadin*)

SUMMARY: A patient well controlled on chronic warfarin therapy developed excessive hypoprothrombinemia and bleeding after starting ketoprofen therapy. However, this patient may have been particularly predisposed to the interaction, and more study will be needed to determine the incidence and magnitude of the effect.

RISK FACTORS:

➡ **Concurrent Diseases.** Patients with peptic ulcer disease or a history of gastrointestinal (GI) bleeding are probably at greater risk for the interaction.

MECHANISM: Not established.

CLINICAL EVALUATION: A 62-year-old man on chronic warfarin therapy with stable prothrombin times (PTs) was started on ketoprofen 25 mg 3 times a day.[1] One week later, the patient developed bloody stools and vomited bright red blood; his PT was 41 seconds. Other than the ketoprofen therapy, no likely cause for the bleeding and excessive hypoprothrombinemia could be found. However, the patient was receiving allopurinol and verapamil. There is some evidence that allopurinol may impair the hepatic metabolism of oral anticoagulants,[2,3] and verapamil has been shown to inhibit hepatic drug metabolism.[4] Even though the allopurinol and verapamil therapy were presumably constant before and during the ketoprofen therapy, they could have interfered with the compensatory increase in warfarin metabolism that would follow any displacement of warfarin from plasma protein binding sites by ketoprofen. Ketoprofen (100 mg twice daily for 7 days) did not affect the hypoprothrombinemic response to multiple doses of warfarin in healthy subjects.[6] However, as with any nonsteroidal anti-inflammatory drug (NSAID), the possible detrimental effects of ibuprofen on the GI mucosa and platelet function must be considered. In a retrospective cohort study, hospitalizations for hemorrhagic peptic ulcer disease were about 13 times higher in patients receiving warfarin plus an NSAID than in patients receiving neither drug.[5]

RELATED DRUGS: All NSAIDs inhibit platelet function, cause gastric erosions, and probably increase the risk of GI bleeding. Some NSAIDs, however, such as ibuprofen (eg, *Advil*), naproxen (eg, *Naprosyn*), or diclofenac (eg, *Voltaren*), may be less likely to increase oral anticoagulant-induced hypoprothrombinemia than other NSAIDs.

MANAGEMENT OPTIONS:

➡ *Avoid Unless Benefit Outweighs Risk.* Since all NSAIDs probably increase the risk of GI bleeding in patients on oral anticoagulants, use the combination only after careful consideration of the benefit versus risk. If an NSAID must be used with an oral anticoagulant, it would be prudent to use NSAIDs that are unlikely to affect the hypoprothrombinemic response to oral anticoagulants. If the NSAID is being used as an analgesic or antipyretic, acetaminophen (eg, *Tylenol*) probably is safer to use with oral anticoagulants. Nonacetylated salicylates (eg, choline salicylate, magnesium salicylate, salsalate, sodium salicylate) also probably are safer with oral anticoagulants than NSAIDs, since such salicylates have minimal effects on platelet function and the gastric mucosa.

➡ *Monitor.* If any NSAID is used with an oral anticoagulant, one should carefully monitor the prothrombin time and watch for evidence of bleeding, especially from the GI tract.

REFERENCES:
1. Flessner MF, et al. Prolongation of prothrombin time and severe gastrointestinal bleeding associated with combined use of warfarin and ketoprofen. *JAMA.* 1988;259:353.
2. Jahnchen E, et al. Interaction of allopurinol with phenprocoumon in man. *Klin Wschr.* 1977;55:759.
3. McInnes GT, et al. Acute adverse reactions attributed to allopurinol in hospitalized patients. *Ann Rheum Dis.* 1981;40:245.
4. Bach D, et al. The effect of verapamil on antipyrine pharmacokinetics and metabolism in man. *Br J Clin Pharmacol.* 1986;21:655.
5. Shorr RI, et al. Concurrent use of nonsteroidal anti-inflammatory drugs and oral anticoagulants places elderly persons at high risk for hemorrhagic peptic ulcer disease. *Arch Intern Med.* 1993;153:1665.
6. Mieszczak C, et al. Lack of interaction of ketoprofen with warfarin. *Eur J Clin Pharmacol.* 1993;44:205.

Ketorolac (eg, *Toradol*)

Lithium (eg, *Eskalith*)

SUMMARY: A patient receiving lithium developed about a doubling of his lithium serum concentrations after starting ketorolac, but the incidence and magnitude of this interaction is not established.

RISK FACTORS: No specific risk factors are known.

MECHANISM: Although the mechanism of this interaction has not been studied, ketorolac, like many other nonsteroidal anti-inflammatory drugs (NSAIDs), probably inhibits the renal elimination of lithium.

CLINICAL EVALUATION: An 80-year-old man on chronic therapy with lithium (450 mg/day) had stable lithium serum concentrations of 0.5 to 0.7 mEq/L.[1] He also was receiving stable doses of haloperidol (eg, *Haldol*), procyclidine (*Kemadrin*), clonazepam (eg, *Klonopin*), aspirin, and digoxin (eg, *Lanoxin*). One day after he started ketorolac (30 mg/day), his serum lithium concentration was 0.9 mEq/L, and 6 days later it was 1.1 mEq/L. The lithium serum concentration decreased to 0.7 mEq/L after the lithium dose was reduced to 300 mg/day. When the lithium dose was increased to 450 mg/day 8 days later, the lithium concentrations increased to 0.9 mEq/L by the sixth day of the increased dose. Reducing the lithium dose to 300 mg/day brought the lithium concentration back down to 0.8 mEq/L. After the ketorolac was discontinued, he was stabilized again on lithium 450 mg/day with lithium serum concentrations in the range of 0.5 to 0.7 mEq/L. The temporal relationship of the changes in lithium dosage requirements and the administration of ketorolac suggest that an interaction occurred. Moreover, several other NSAIDs have been shown to increase lithium serum concentrations. Nonetheless, additional study is needed to firmly establish that ketorolac and lithium interact.

RELATED DRUGS: Most NSAIDs increase lithium serum concentrations, but sulindac (eg, *Clinoril*) and aspirin appear to have minimal effects.

MANAGEMENT OPTIONS:

➡ *Consider Alternative.* If appropriate for the patient, consider using an anti-inflammatory agent that is less likely to affect lithium, such as sulindac or aspirin.

➡ *Monitor.* If ketorolac therapy is initiated in a patient taking lithium, monitor serum lithium concentrations and look for evidence of lithium toxicity (eg, nausea, vomiting, diarrhea, anorexia, coarse tremor, slurred speech, vertigo, confusion, lethargy; in severe cases, seizures, stupor, coma, cardiovascular collapse). In a patient stabilized on lithium and an NSAID, discontinuation of the NSAID may result in inadequate lithium serum concentrations.

REFERENCES:

1. Langlois R, et al. Increased serum lithium levels due to ketorolac therapy. *CMAJ.* 1994;150:1455-1456.

Lamivudine (*Epivir*)

Trimethoprim-Sulfamethoxazole (eg, *Bactrim*)

SUMMARY: Trimethoprim-sulfamethoxazole (TMP-SMZ) administration increases the serum concentration of lamivudine; the clinical significance appears to be limited.

RISK FACTORS: No specific risk factors are known.

MECHANISM: TMP-SMZ appears to inhibit the renal secretion of lamivudine. In vitro studies demonstrate a competitive inhibition of lamivudine by trimethoprim in the rat kidney.[1]

CLINICAL EVALUATION: Fourteen patients with human immunodeficiency virus received 2 single doses of lamivudine 300 mg orally.[2] The first dose of lamivudine was administered alone, and the second followed 5 days of TMP-SMZ (160/800 mg trimethoprim/sulfamethoxazole). Lamivudine renal clearance decreased 35% and the area under its concentration-time curve increased 43% when administered with TMP-SMZ. Lamivudine did not affect the pharmacokinetics of trimethoprim or sulfamethoxazole. Higher doses of TMP-SMZ (eg, 15 to 20 mg/kg/day) would be expected to increase the magnitude of this interaction; however, no data are available. The potential for TMP-SMZ-induced lamivudine toxicity (ie, headache, nausea, diarrhea, neutropenia) is not known.

RELATED DRUGS: Trimethoprim (eg, *Proloprim*) is known to reduce the renal clearance of zidovudine (eg, *Retrovir*). Cimetidine (eg, *Tagamet*), like trimethoprim, is a basic drug that is secreted renally. Because cimetidine has been shown to inhibit the elimination of zidovudine, it is possible that cimetidine also would inhibit the renal elimination of lamivudine.

MANAGEMENT OPTIONS: No specific action is required, but be alert for evidence of the interaction.

REFERENCES:
1. Sweeney KR, et al. The renal disposition of lamivudine (3TC) in the isolated perfused rat kidney (IPK). *Pharm Res.* 1993;10:S368.
2. Moore KH, et al. Pharmacokinetics of lamivudine administered alone and with trimethoprim-sulfamethoxazole. *Clin Pharmacol Ther.* 1996;59:550-558.

Lamotrigine (*Lamictal*)

Phenytoin (eg, *Dilantin*)

SUMMARY: Phenytoin stimulates the metabolism of lamotrigine, resulting in lower plasma concentrations and decreased elimination half-life.

RISK FACTORS: No specific risk factors are known.

MECHANISM: Lamotrigine is eliminated primarily by hepatic metabolism to a glucuronide conjugate. Drugs that induce uridine diphosphate glucuronyltransferase will stimulate the metabolism of lamotrigine.

CLINICAL EVALUATION: Patients receiving lamotrigine in combination with liver enzyme-inducing antiepileptic drugs (eg, phenytoin, carbamazepine, phenobarbital) have significantly shorter elimination half-lives (14 ± 7 hours)[1,2] than those receiving lamotrigine monotherapy (25 ± 10 hours).[3] Higher fluctuations in lamotrigine plasma concentrations are found in patients on enzyme-inducing drugs.[4]

RELATED DRUGS: The effect of phenobarbital (eg, *Solfoton*) on lamotrigine has not been studied directly. However, the known inducing properties of phenobarbital and carbamazepine would be consistent with decreasing lamotrigine concentrations.

MANAGEMENT OPTIONS:

➡ *Monitor.* In patients stabilized on enzyme-inducing drugs, monitor for the need to use larger than expected doses of lamotrigine. Also be aware that discontinuing phenytoin may affect lamotrigine dosage requirements.

REFERENCES:

1. Binnie CD, et al. Double blind crossover trial of lamotrigine (*Lamictal*) as add-on therapy in intractable epilepsy. *Epilepsy Res.* 1986;4:222.

2. Jawad S, et al. Lamotrigine: single dose pharmacokinetics and initial 1 week experience in refractory epilepsy. *Epilepsy Res.* 1987;1:194.

3. Cohen AF, et al. Lamotrigine, a new anticonvulsant: pharmacokinetics in normal humans. *Clin Pharmacol Ther.* 1987;41:535-541.

4. Wolf P, et al. Lamotrigine: preliminary clinical observations on pharmacokinetics and interactions with traditional antiepileptic drugs. *J Epilepsy.* 1992;5:73.

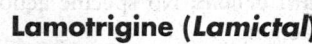

Lamotrigine (*Lamictal*)

Rifampin (eg, *Rifadin*)

SUMMARY: Rifampin reduces the plasma concentration of lamotrigine; reduced antiepileptic efficacy may result.

RISK FACTORS: No specific risk factors are known.

MECHANISM: Rifampin induces the metabolism (glucuronidation) of lamotrigine.

CLINICAL EVALUATION: Ten healthy subjects received a single oral dose of lamotrigine 25 mg after placebo or rifampin 600 mg/day for 5 days.[1] The mean oral clearance of lamotrigine was nearly doubled following rifampin pretreatment. Lamotrigine's mean half-life was reduced from 23.8 to 14.1 hours. Peak plasma lamotrigine concentration was unchanged; however, the mean area under the concentration-time curve for lamotrigine was reduced about 44%. A reduction in the efficacy of lamotrigine, particularly at the end of the dosing interval, may occur when the drug is administered with rifampin.

RELATED DRUGS: Rifampin is known to induce the metabolism of several other antiepileptic agents. While no data are available, rifabutin (*Mycobutin*) also may increase lamotrigine metabolism.

MANAGEMENT OPTIONS:

➡ *Monitor.* Monitor patients receiving lamotrigine and rifampin for reduced lamotrigine plasma concentrations and reduced antiepileptic effect.

REFERENCES:

1. Ebert U, et al. Effects of rifampicin and cimetidine on pharmacokinetics and pharmacodynamics of lamotrigine in healthy subjects. *Eur J Clin Pharmacol.* 2000;56:299-304.

4   Lamotrigine (*Lamictal*)

Sertraline (*Zoloft*)

SUMMARY: Two patients developed lamotrigine toxicity after starting sertraline therapy, but a causal relationship was not established.

RISK FACTORS: No specific risk factors are known.

MECHANISM: Not established. The authors propose that sertraline may have impaired lamotrigine glucuronidation.

CLINICAL EVALUATION: Two epileptic patients maintained on lamotrigine 200 and 450 mg/day, respectively, developed elevated lamotrigine serum concentrations after starting sertraline 25 and 75 mg/day, respectively.[1] Symptoms of lamotrigine toxicity included fatigue, sedation, confusion, and decreased cognition. However, lamotrigine is metabolized primarily by glucuronidation, and sertraline is not known to affect this metabolic pathway.

RELATED DRUGS: The effect of other selective serotonin reuptake inhibitors on lamotrigine is not established.

MANAGEMENT OPTIONS: No specific action is required, but be alert for evidence of the interaction.

REFERENCES:
1. Kaufman KR, et al. Lamotrigine toxicity secondary to sertraline. *Seizure.* 1998;7;163–165.

Lamotrigine (eg, *Lamictal*)

Valproic Acid (eg, *Depakene*)

SUMMARY: Clinical evidence suggests that combined therapy with lamotrigine and valproic acid may increase the risk of toxic epidermal necrolysis, but a causal relationship has not been proved.

RISK FACTORS: No specific risk factors are known.

MECHANISM: Not established. Valproic acid might inhibit the glucuronidation of lamotrigine, thus increasing its toxicity.

CLINICAL EVALUATION: A 54-year-old man developed fatal toxic epidermal necrolysis 4 weeks after lamotrigine was added to his valproic acid therapy.[1] Of the 8 previously reported cases of lamotrigine-associated toxic epidermal necrolysis, 5 were receiving concurrent valproic acid. While the precise role of an interaction between lamotrigine and valproic acid in these reactions is not established, the severity of the adverse outcome dictates caution.

RELATED DRUGS: No information is available.

MANAGEMENT OPTIONS:

➥ *Circumvent/Minimize.* In patients receiving lamotrigine and valproic acid, discontinue lamotrigine immediately if any rash appears.[1]

➡ *Monitor.* Be alert for any evidence of rash.

REFERENCES:
1. Page RL 2nd, et al. Fatal toxic epidermal necrolysis related to lamotrigine administration. *Pharmacotherapy.* 1998;18(2):392-398.

Lansoprazole (*Prevacid*)

Tacrolimus (*Prograf*)

SUMMARY: A patient on tacrolimus developed a substantial increase in tacrolimus blood concentrations after starting lansoprazole, but a causal relationship was not established.

RISK FACTORS:

➡ *Pharmacogenetics.* This patient had a mutation in the gene for CYP2C19 and may have been predisposed to the interaction because of higher lansoprazole serum concentrations.

MECHANISM: Not established.

CLINICAL EVALUATION: A 57-year-old woman was receiving tacrolimus, prednisolone, and mycophenolate mofetil following a renal transplant.[1] Lansoprazole 30 mg/day was started 19 days after transplant, and, 3 days later, her tacrolimus trough levels had increased from around 17 to 27 ng/mL. Substituting famotidine for lansoprazole was followed by a decline in tacrolimus trough levels. Famotidine was then switched to rabeprazole without any increase in tacrolimus trough levels.

RELATED DRUGS: This case suggests that rabeprazole (*Aciphex*) does not affect tacrolimus, but more data are needed.

MANAGEMENT OPTIONS: No specific action is required, but be alert for evidence of the interaction.

REFERENCES:
1. Homma M, et al. Effects of lansoprazole and rabeprazole on tacrolimus blood concentration: case of a renal transplant recipient with CYP2C19 gene mutation. *Transplantation.* 2002;73(2):303-304.

Lapatinib (*Tykerb*)

Colchicine

SUMMARY: Based on the interactive properties of the 2 drugs, it is likely that lapatinib substantially increases colchicine plasma concentrations. Avoid the combination whenever possible.

RISK FACTORS: No specific risk factors are known.

MECHANISM: Colchicine is a P-glycoprotein and CYP3A4 substrate, and lapatinib inhibits both P-glycoprotein and CYP3A4; colchicine plasma concentrations are likely to increase.[1]

CLINICAL EVALUATION: Although the interaction is based primarily on theoretical considerations, it is likely that lapatinib would increase the risk of colchicine toxicity. Given that colchicine toxicity can be fatal, even a theoretical interaction warrants close attention.

RELATED DRUGS: Imatinib (*Gleevec*) inhibits CYP3A4 and may increase colchicine plasma concentrations.

MANAGEMENT OPTIONS:

➥ *Avoid Unless Benefit Outweighs Risk.* Given that colchicine toxicity can be life-threatening, use lapatinib only if it is likely to provide therapeutic benefits that cannot be achieved with noninteracting alternatives.

➥ *Use Alternative.* If possible, use an alternative to lapatinib that does not inhibit P-glycoprotein or CYP3A4, or use an alternative to colchicine.

➥ *Monitor.* If the combination must be used, monitor carefully for colchicine toxicity (eg, abdominal pain, diarrhea, fever, muscle pain, vomiting). Advise the patient to immediately contact a health care provider if any of these symptoms occur. Colchicine-induced pancytopenia can result in infections, bleeding, and anemia, and is often the cause of death in fatal cases.

REFERENCES:
1. Rautio J, et al. In vitro p-glycoprotein inhibition assays for assessment of clinical drug interaction potential of new drug candidates: a recommendation for probe substrates. *Drug Metab Dispos.* 2006;34(5):786-792.

 Levamisole (*Ergamisol*)

Warfarin (eg, *Coumadin*)

SUMMARY: A patient on warfarin developed an increased anticoagulant effect after starting chemotherapy with levamisole and fluorouracil. Although fluorouracil appears more likely to be responsible, one cannot rule out an effect of levamisole.

RISK FACTORS: No specific risk factors are known.

MECHANISM: Not established.

CLINICAL EVALUATION: A 73-year-old man stabilized on warfarin was started on 5-fluorouracil and levamisole for colon cancer.[1] The International Normalized Ratio was 3 prior to chemotherapy, and four weeks later it had increased to almost 40. A positive dechallenge and rechallenge supports a causal relationship between the chemotherapy and the increased warfarin effect. Since fluorouracil and levamisole were used together, it is not possible to determine whether the increased warfarin effect was due to one of the drugs acting alone or a combination of the two. Nonetheless, fluorouracil appears more likely than levamisole to have produced the effect.

RELATED DRUGS: The effect of levamisole on oral anticoagulants other than warfarin is not established.

MANAGEMENT OPTIONS: No specific action is required, but be alert for evidence of the interaction.

REFERENCES:
1. Scarfe MA, et al. Possible drug interaction between warfarin and combination of levamisole and fluorouracil. *Ann Pharmacother.* 1994;28:464.

Levodopa (eg, *Larodopa*)

Methionine

SUMMARY: L-methionine may inhibit the clinical response to levodopa in parkinsonian patients.

RISK FACTORS: No specific risk factors are known.

MECHANISM: Not established.

CLINICAL EVALUATION: Fourteen parkinsonian patients receiving levodopa were placed on a restricted L-methionine diet for 8 days and then given either a placebo (7 patients) or methionine (7 patients) in a dose of 4.5 g/day.[1] Patients receiving a placebo demonstrated little change with some subjective improvement in 3 patients. Five of the seven patients on methionine developed a worsening of their parkinsonism.

RELATED DRUGS: No information is available.

MANAGEMENT OPTIONS:

➡ *Circumvent/Minimize.* Large doses of methionine probably should be avoided in parkinsonian patients receiving levodopa.

➡ *Monitor.* Monitor for reduced levodopa effect if the combination is used.

REFERENCES:

1. Pearce LA, et al. L-methionine: a possible levodopa antagonist. *Neurology.* 1974;24:640.

Levodopa (eg, *Larodopa*)

Methyldopa (eg, *Aldomet*)

SUMMARY: The bulk of evidence indicates that methyldopa may enhance the therapeutic response to levodopa; however, additive hypotensive effects may also occur.

RISK FACTORS: No specific risk factors are known.

MECHANISM: The mechanism for the reported beneficial response to combined use of levodopa and methyldopa in parkinsonism is unknown. The hypotension seen when levodopa is given alone may be additive with that produced by methyldopa. Carbidopa (without levodopa) has been shown to produce a small decrease in the supine diastolic pressure of patients maintained on methyldopa.[8]

CLINICAL EVALUATION: Although methyldopa had been reported to inhibit the antiparkinsonian response to levodopa,[4,7,9] several researchers intentionally have used this combination to advantage, especially in patients with a fluctuating response to levodopa.[2,3,5,6] Thus, it appears that the combination is more likely to have a beneficial than a detrimental effect. Methyldopa and levodopa appear to have additive hypotensive effects although severe hypotensive episodes are unlikely to occur.[1,6]

RELATED DRUGS: No information available.

MANAGEMENT OPTIONS: No specific action is required, but be alert for evidence of the interaction.

REFERENCES:

1. Gibberd FB, et al. Interaction between levodopa and methyldopa. *Br Med J.* 1973;2:90.
2. Fermaglich J, et al. Methyldopa or methyldopa-hydrazine as levodopa synergists. *Lancet.* 1973;1:1261.
3. Mones RJ. Evaluation of alpha methyl dopa and alpha methyl dopa hydrazine with L-dopa therapy. *NY State J Med.* 1974;74:47.
4. Cotzias GC, et al. L-Dopa in Parkinson's syndrome. *N Engl J Med.* 1969;281:272.
5. Sweet RD, et al. Methyldopa as an adjunct to levodopa treatment of Parkinson's disease. *Clin Pharmacol Ther.* 1972;13:23.
6. Fermaglich J, et al. Second generation of L-dopa therapy. *Neurology.* 1971;21:408.
7. Kofman O. Treatment of Parkinson's disease with L-dopa: a current appraisal. *Can Med Assoc J.* 1971;104:483.
8. Kersting F, et al. Clinical and cardiovascular effects of alpha methyldopa in combination with decarboxylase inhibitors. *Clin Pharmacol Ther.* 1977;21:547.
9. Strang RR. Parkinsonism occurring during methyldopa therapy. *Can Med Assoc J.* 1966;95:928.

Levodopa (eg, *Larodopa*)

Moclobemide

SUMMARY: Moclobemide appeared to increase the risk of adverse effects (eg, headache, nausea) in healthy subjects receiving levodopa; but more study is needed.

RISK FACTORS: No specific risk factors are known.

MECHANISM: Not established. Although monoamine oxidase (MAO)-B is more important than MAO-A in the metabolism of dopamine, an MAO-A inhibitor such as moclobemide may have some effect on dopamine response.

CLINICAL EVALUATION: Twelve healthy subjects received a single dose of *Madopar* (levodopa and benserazide) with and without concurrent moclobemide (400 mg/day).[1] The combination was associated with more adverse effects (headache, insomnia, nausea) than with either drug alone. However, it was not clear that the study allowed enough time for the decarboxylase inhibitor (benserazide) to exert full activity. Thus, studies in patients receiving the drugs chronically are needed to assess the clinical importance of this interaction.

RELATED DRUGS: The effect of other MAO-A inhibitors on levodopa is not established.

MANAGEMENT OPTIONS:

➥ *Monitor.* If moclobemide is used in a patient receiving levodopa, one should monitor for the need to adjust the levodopa dosage.

REFERENCES:

1. Dingemanse J. An update of recent moclobemide interaction data. *Int Clin Psychopharmacol.* 1993;7:167.

Levodopa (eg, *Larodopa*)

Phenelzine (*Nardil*)

SUMMARY: The administration of levodopa with nonselective monoamine oxidase inhibitors (MAOIs) may result in a hypertensive response.

RISK FACTORS:

➡ *Other Drugs.* Concurrent use of carbidopa with levodopa appears to minimize the interaction with nonselective MAOIs.

➡ *Dosage Regimen.* One patient receiving phenelzine became hypertensive with a 50 mg dose of levodopa but not with a 25 mg dose.[5]

MECHANISM: Levodopa is the precursor of dopamine, which in turn is converted to norepinephrine. A major pathway of degradation of dopamine involves monoamine oxidase; thus MAOIs decrease dopamine degradation, while levodopa increases dopamine and probably norepinephrine formation. The adverse cardiovascular effects seen with concomitant levodopa and MAOI administration are probably due to increased storage and release of dopamine, norepinephrine, or both.[3,4,7]

CLINICAL EVALUATION: Hypertension, flushing of the face, pounding of the heart, and lightheadedness have been reported with concomitant administration of nialamide and levodopa to normal volunteers.[2] Another patient on phenelzine developed hypertension after taking levodopa.[5] An attempt to use this interaction intentionally was reported in 2 patients with idiopathic orthostatic hypotension who were given levodopa and tranylcypromine (*Parnate*).[1,10] However, 1 patient developed palpitations, a diastolic pressure of 150 mm Hg, and 2 small retinal hemorrhages.[1] One report indicates that carbidopa may inhibit the hypertensive reaction to levodopa in patients receiving an MAOI.[8] Preliminary evidence also indicates that the addition of an MAOI to patients on levodopa may result in worsening of akinesia and tremor.[6] Levodopa can be used with the selective MAO-B inhibitor, selegiline (eg, *Eldepryl*), although the dosage of the levodopa may need to be reduced.[9,11]

RELATED DRUGS: All nonselective MAOIs including isocarboxazid (*Marplan*) and tranylcypromine would be expected to interact with levodopa in the absence of a decarboxylase inhibitor.

MANAGEMENT OPTIONS:

➡ *Circumvent/Minimize.* The use of a decarboxylase inhibitor (eg, carbidopa) with levodopa apparently prevents the hypertensive reactions.

➡ *Monitor.* The use of nonselective MAOIs with levodopa (in the absence of a decarboxylase inhibitor) generally should be avoided. Remember that the effects of nonselective MAOIs should be assumed to persist for 2 weeks after they are discontinued. If they are given concomitantly, blood pressure must be monitored very carefully. If hypertension ensues, the results of 1 case indicate that phentolamine (eg, *Regitine*) may reverse the hypertension.[5]

REFERENCES:

1. Sharpe J, et al. Idiopathic orthostatic hypotension treated with levodopa and MAO inhibitor: a preliminary report. *Can Med Assoc J.* 1972;107:296.
2. Friend DG, et al. The action of 1-dihydroxyphenylalanine in patients receiving nialamide. *Clin Pharmacol Ther.* 1965;6:362.

3. Cotzias GC, et al. L-dopa in Parkinson's syndrome. *N Engl J Med.* 1969;281:272.

4. Cotzias GC. Metabolic modification of some neurologic disorders. *JAMA.* 1969;210:1255.

5. Hunter KR, et al. Monoamine oxidase inhibitors and L-dopa. *Br Med J.* 1970;3:388.

6. Kott E, et al. Excretion of dopa metabolites. *N Engl J Med.* 1971;284:395.

7. Goldberg LI, et al. Cardiovascular effects of levodopa. *Clin Pharmacol Ther.* 1971;12:376.

8. Teychenne PF, et al. Interactions of levodopa with inhibitors of monoamine oxidase and L-aromatic amino acid decarboxylase. *Clin Pharmacol Ther.* 1975;18:273.

9. Birkmayer W et al. Implications of combined treatment with "madopar" and L-Deprenil in Parkinson's disease. *Lancet.* 1977;1:439.

10. Corder CN, et al. Postural hypotension:adrenergic responsivity and levodopa therapy. *Neurology.* 1977;27:921.

11. Collier DS, et al. Parkinsonism treatment: Part III—update. *Ann Pharmacother.* 1992;26:227.

 4 ## Levodopa (eg, *Larodopa*)

Phenylbutazone

SUMMARY: Phenylbutazone appeared to antagonize the therapeutic response to levodopa in 1 patient, but a causal relationship was not established.

RISK FACTORS: No specific risk factors are known.

MECHANISM: Not established.

CLINICAL EVALUATION: The purported interaction between phenylbutazone and levodopa is based on only 1 patient[1]; more information is needed to substantiate this interaction.

RELATED DRUGS: No information is available on the effect of other nonsteroidal anti-inflammatory drugs on levodopa response.

MANAGEMENT OPTIONS: No specific action is required, but be alert for evidence of the interaction.

REFERENCES:
1. Wodak J, et al. Review of 12 months' treatment with L-DOPA in Parkinson's disease, with remarks on unusual side effects. *Med J Aust.* 1972;2:1277.

4 ## Levodopa (eg, *Larodopa*)

Phenylephrine (eg, *Neo-Synephrine*)

SUMMARY: Levodopa may inhibit the response to phenylephrine eyedrops, but the clinical importance of this effect is not established.

RISK FACTORS: No specific risk factors are known.

MECHANISM: Not established. Levodopa or its metabolites may inhibit agents competitively that act on alpha-adrenergic receptors (eg, phenylephrine).

CLINICAL EVALUATION: Levodopa administration reduces the mydriasis following topical phenylephrine.[1] It is not known whether other pharmacologic effects of phenylephrine given by different routes of administration would also be affected by levodopa.

RELATED DRUGS: No information is available.

MANAGEMENT OPTIONS: No specific action is required, but be alert for evidence of the interaction.

REFERENCES:

1. Godwin-Austen RB, et al. Mydriatic responses to sympathomimetic amines in patients treated with L-DOPA. *Lancet.* 1969;2:1043.

Levodopa (eg, *Larodopa*)

Phenytoin (eg, *Dilantin*)

SUMMARY: Preliminary patient data indicate that phenytoin may inhibit the antiparkinsonian effect of levodopa.

RISK FACTORS: No specific risk factors are known.

MECHANISM: Not established.

CLINICAL EVALUATION: In 5 patients with parkinsonism and levodopa-induced dyskinesias, phenytoin not only alleviated the levodopa dyskinesias but also inhibited the therapeutic effect of levodopa.[1] Four of the 5 patients were receiving levodopa/ carbidopa (eg, *Sinemet*), so it is clear that carbidopa does not prevent this interaction.

RELATED DRUGS: No information is available.

MANAGEMENT OPTIONS:

➥ **Consider Alternative.** Although this interaction is based on limited evidence, consider alternatives to phenytoin in parkinsonian patients receiving levodopa.

➥ **Circumvent/Minimize.** If the combination is used, a larger dose of levodopa may be required.

➥ **Monitor.** Be alert for evidence of levodopa's reduced antiparkinson effect if phenytoin is taken concurrently.

REFERENCES:

1. Mendez JS, et al. Diphenylhydantoin blocking of levodopa effects. *Arch Neurol.* 1975;32:44.

Levodopa (eg, *Larodopa*)

Propranolol (eg, *Inderal*)

SUMMARY: The combination of levodopa and propranolol generally is favorable.

RISK FACTORS: No specific risk factors are known.

MECHANISM: The mechanisms for this interaction are: 1) Propranolol may antagonize the beta-adrenergic properties of dopamine, a metabolite of levodopa. 2) Propranolol may enhance the therapeutic effect of levodopa in patients with parkinsonian tremor. 3) Propranolol may enhance levodopa-induced stimulation of growth hormone secretion.[6]

CLINICAL EVALUATION: Limited clinical observations indicate that propranolol may antagonize both the hypotensive[4] and positive inotropic[3] effects of levodopa. Antagonism of the hypotensive effect of levodopa would be considered a favorable interaction in most cases. In one study of 25 patients with Parkinson disease with tremor, propranolol plus levodopa produced better therapeutic results than either drug used alone[1]; however, others have failed to confirm these observations.[7] Propranolol markedly enhances the elevated plasma growth hormone levels produced by levodopa; in some cases these levels were reportedly close to those seen in patients with acromegaly.[2] This combined effect on growth hormone has been used advantageously as a provocative test in children with short stature.[5]

RELATED DRUGS: Other beta blockers may produce similar reactions with levodopa.

MANAGEMENT OPTIONS:

➡ *Monitor.* Most of the consequences of the interaction between levodopa and propranolol appear to be favorable. Patients on combined therapy for prolonged periods should be monitored more closely.

REFERENCES:

1. Kissel P, et al. Levodopa-propranolol therapy in parkinsonian tremor. *Lancet.* 1974;1:403.
2. Camanni F, et al. Enhancement of levodopa-induced growth-hormone stimulation by propranolol. *Lancet.* 1974;1:942.
3. Whitsett TL, et al. Propranolol blockade of positive inotropic effects of L-dopa in dog and man. *The Pharmacologist.* 1970;12:213.
4. Duvoisin RC. Hypotension caused by L-dopa. *Br Med J.* 1970;3:47.
5. Collu R et al. Stimulation of growth hormone secretion by levodopapropranolol in children and adolescents. *Pediatrics.* 1975;56:262.
6. Lotti G, et al. Enhancement of levodopa-induced growth hormone stimulation by practolol. *Lancet.* 1974;2:1329.
7. Sandler M, et al. Oxprenolol and levodopa in parkinsonian patients. *Lancet.* 1975;1:168.

Levodopa (eg, *Larodopa*)

Pyridoxine (Vitamin B₆)

SUMMARY: Pyridoxine inhibits the antiparkinsonian effect of levodopa, but few patients are affected since concurrent use of carbidopa negates the interaction.

RISK FACTORS:

➡ *Other Drugs.* The interaction occurs only in the absence of concurrent therapy with a peripheral decarboxylase inhibitor (eg, carbidopa [*Lodosyn*]).

MECHANISM: Pyridoxine appears to enhance the metabolism of levodopa, thus decreasing the amount available at the site of levodopa action in the brain.

CLINICAL EVALUATION: Doses as small as 10 to 25 mg of pyridoxine may be sufficient to reverse the levodopa-induced improvement in Parkinson's syndrome.[2,3,5-7,10-13] This antagonism apparently does not occur if the patient also is receiving a peripheral decarboxylase inhibitor such as carbidopa.[1,4,8,9]

RELATED DRUGS: No information is available.

MANAGEMENT OPTIONS:

➡ *Circumvent/Minimize.* Pyridoxine and vitamin preparations containing pyridoxine should be avoided in patients receiving levodopa unless a peripheral decarboxylase inhibitor (eg, carbidopa) is also being given.

➥ *Monitor.* Monitor for reduced levodopa response if pyridoxine is used in the absence of a decarboxylase inhibitor.

REFERENCES:

1. Fahn S. "On-off" phenomenon with levodopa therapy in parkinsonism. *Neurology.* 1974;24:431.
2. Bianchine JR, et al. Levodopa and pyridoxine co-administration:differential metabolic effect in parkinsonian and normal subjects. *Ann Intern Med.* 1973;78:830.
3. Carter AB. Pyridoxine and parkinsonism. *Br Med J.* 1973;4:236.
4. Mars H. Levodopa, carbidopa, and pyridoxine in Parkinson disease. Metabolic interactions. *Arch Neurol.* 1974;30:444.
5. Duvoisin RC, et al. Pyridoxine reversal of L-DOPA effects in parkinsonism. *Trans Am Neurol Assoc.* 1969;94:81.
6. Cotzias GC. Metabolic modification of some neurologic disorders. *JAMA.* 1969;210:1255.
7. Leon AS. Pyridoxine antagonism of levodopa in parkinsonism. *JAMA.* 1971;218:1924.
8. Papavasiliou PS, et al. Levodopa in parkinsonism: potentiation of central effects with a peripheral inhibitor. *N Engl J Med.* 1972;286:8.
9. Cotzias GC, et al. Blocking the negative effects of pyridoxine on patients receiving levodopa. *JAMA.* 1971;215:1504.
10. Mims RB et al. Inhibition of L-dopa-induced growth hormone stimulation of pyridoxine and chlorpromazine. *J Clin Endocrinol Metab.* 1975;40:256.
11. Hildick-Smith M. Pyridoxine in parkinsonism. *Lancet.* 1973;2:1029.
12. Jones CJ. Pyridoxine in parkinsonism. *Lancet.* 1973;2:1030.
13. Yahr MD, et al. Pyridoxine and levodopa in the treatment of parkinsonism. *JAMA.* 1972;220:861.

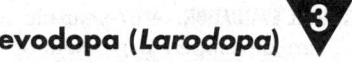

Levodopa (*Larodopa*)

Spiramycin†

SUMMARY: Spiramycin reduces the plasma concentration of levodopa; antiparkinson efficacy may be reduced.

RISK FACTORS: No specific risk factors are known.

MECHANISM: Not established. Spiramycin markedly reduces the concentration of carbidopa and levodopa following administration of the combination product. Inhibition of carbidopa absorption would permit more extensive peripheral metabolism of levodopa by L-amino acid decarboxylase. Because levodopa, and perhaps carbidopa, is absorbed by active transport in the small bowel, the promotility effects of spiramycin may move the levodopa past its absorption sites before complete absorption occurs. The effect also will reduce levodopa plasma concentrations.

CLINICAL EVALUATION: Seven healthy subjects were administered levodopa 250 mg/carbidopa 250 mg alone and following 3 days of spiramycin 1,000 mg twice daily.[1] The area under the plasma concentration-time curve (AUC) of levodopa was reduced 56% during the administration of spiramycin compared with control values. The AUC of carbidopa was reduced 96% after the administration of spiramycin. Accompanying this decrease was a 90% increase in dihydrophenylacetic acid, a metabolite formed following the decarboxylation of levodopa to dopamine. This reduction in levodopa concentration and increase in its peripheral metabolism is expected to decrease levodopa efficacy.

RELATED DRUGS: It is not known whether other macrolide antibiotics (eg, erythromycin [eg, *Ery-Tab*]) that stimulate gastric motility would produce a similar effect.

MANAGEMENT OPTIONS:

➥ **Monitor.** Until studies in patients with Parkinson disease are available, closely observe patients taking levodopa/carbidopa combinations for increased symptoms of Parkinson disease when spiramycin and other macrolide antibiotics that increase GI transit are administered.

REFERENCES:

1. Brion N, et al. Effect of a macrolide (spiramycin) on the pharmacokinetics of L-dopa and carbidopa in healthy volunteers. *Clin Neuropharmacol.* 1992;15(3):229-235.

† Not available in the United States.

Levodopa (*Larodopa*)

Tacrine (*Cognex*)

SUMMARY: Tacrine may inhibit the effect of levodopa in patients with parkinsonism; dosage adjustments of one or both drugs may be required.

RISK FACTORS: No specific risk factors are known.

MECHANISM: Patients with parkinsonism are thought to have an excess of cholinergic activity in the striatum, and the administration of a centrally acting cholinergic agent such as tacrine is expected to worsen the disease.

CLINICAL EVALUATION: A 67-year-old woman with Alzheimer disease and mild parkinsonism developed a worsening of her parkinsonism after her tacrine dosage was increased from 10 mg 4 times daily to 20 mg 4 times daily.[1] Because the tacrine had produced mild improvement in her Alzheimer disease, it was continued, and carbidopa/levodopa was started. The carbidopa/levodopa resulted in prompt improvement of the parkinsonism (eg, tremor, gait instability, rigidity). However, even in the presence of levodopa, she was not able to tolerate a subsequent increase in the dosage of tacrine to 30 mg 4 times daily without recurrence of parkinsonian symptoms.

RELATED DRUGS: No information is available.

MANAGEMENT OPTIONS:

➥ **Consider Alternative.** Before giving tacrine to a patient with parkinsonism (whether on levodopa or not), consider the risk of worsening the parkinsonism.

➥ **Monitor.** If tacrine is used in a patient with parkinsonism, the doses of tacrine and/or the antiparkinson drugs may need to be adjusted.

REFERENCES:

1. Ott BR, et al. Exacerbation of parkinsonism by tacrine. *Clin Neuropharmacol.* 1992;15(4):322-325.

Levodopa (*Larodopa*)

Trihexyphenidyl (eg, *Trihexy-2*)

SUMMARY: Trihexyphenidyl and other anticholinergics may reduce the bioavailability of levodopa in some patients, but the effect is probably clinically unimportant in most patients.

RISK FACTORS: No specific risk factors are known.

MECHANISM: Sufficient doses of anticholinergics may delay gastric emptying, thus increasing the degradation of levodopa in the stomach and decreasing the amount of levodopa delivered to the small intestine for absorption.

CLINICAL EVALUATION: Trihexyphenidyl reduced levodopa bioavailability in a few patients.[1] One patient required large doses of levodopa (7 g/day) while taking homatropine concomitantly.[2] When the homatropine was discontinued, symptoms of levodopa toxicity appeared, and the patient subsequently was stabilized on levodopa 4 g/day. However, anticholinergic agents can relieve some symptoms of parkinsonism, which would tend to offset the reduction in levodopa bioavailability.

RELATED DRUGS: Based on the mechanism, all anticholinergics are expected to interact similarly with levodopa.

MANAGEMENT OPTIONS: No specific action is required, but be alert for evidence of the interaction.

REFERENCES:

1. Algeri S, et al. Effect of anticholinergic drugs on gastrointestinal absorption of L-dopa in rats and in man. *Eur J Pharmacol*. 1976;35(2):293-299.
2. Fermaglich J, et al. Effect of gastric motility on levodopa. *Dis Nerv Syst*. 1972;33(9):624-625.

Levofloxacin (*Levaquin*)

Procainamide (eg, *Procanbid*)

SUMMARY: Levofloxacin administration results in a modest increase in procainamide plasma concentrations; some patients may have an increase in procainamide effect on cardiac conduction.

RISK FACTORS: No specific risk factors are known.

MECHANISM: Levofloxacin reduces the renal elimination of procainamide and its metabolite.

CLINICAL EVALUATION: Ten healthy subjects received procainamide 15 mg/kg intravenously alone and on day 5 of receiving levofloxacin 500 mg daily.[1] Coadministration of levofloxacin resulted in a mean 20% increase in the concentration of procainamide. The mean concentration of the active metabolite of procainamide, N-acetylprocainamide, was increased 16%. Procainamide renal clearance was reduced 35%. These changes in procainamide plasma concentrations could produce an increased risk of adverse reactions in some patients. The administration of ciprofloxacin 500 mg every 12 hours did not significantly alter procainamide concentrations.

RELATED DRUGS: Ofloxacin (eg, *Floxin*) is known to increase procainamide plasma concentrations.

MANAGEMENT OPTIONS:

➡ *Monitor.* Monitor electrocardiogram or procainamide plasma levels when levofloxacin is added to the drug regimen of patients stabilized on procainamide.

REFERENCES:

1. Bauer LA, et al. Levofloxacin and ciprofloxacin decrease procainamide and N-acetylprocainamide renal clearances. *Antimicrob Agents Chemother*. 2005;49(4):1649-1651.

5　Levofloxacin (*Levaquin*)

Theophylline (eg, *Theo-24*)

SUMMARY: No interaction.

RISK FACTORS: No specific risk factors are known.

MECHANISM: No interaction.

CLINICAL EVALUATION: While no specific data have been reported, the manufacturer of levofloxacin has noted that it does not alter theophylline concentrations.[1]

RELATED DRUGS: Some quinolones (eg, ciprofloxacin [eg, *Cipro*], enoxacin[†]) have reduced theophylline metabolism while others (eg, lomefloxacin [*Maxaquin*]) have no effect on theophylline.

MANAGEMENT OPTIONS: No interaction.

REFERENCES:

　　1. *Levaquin* [package insert]. Raritan, NJ: Ortho-McNeil Pharmaceuticals, Inc; 1997.

　　† Not available in the United States.

4　Levofloxacin (*Levaquin*)

Warfarin (eg, *Coumadin*)

SUMMARY: Levofloxacin does not appear to affect warfarin; infections are known to reduce drug metabolism and probably increase the anticoagulant effect of warfarin.

RISK FACTORS: No specific risk factors are known.

MECHANISM: Increased anticoagulation effect, probably caused by inhibition of CYP-450 activity by cytokines induced by infection, resulted in increased catabolism of clotting factors, altered vitamin K intake, or some combination of the two. There is no evidence of a direct effect of levofloxacin on warfarin pharmacokinetics or pharmacodynamics.

CLINICAL EVALUATION: Fifteen healthy subjects received a single dose of warfarin 30 mg on day 4 of a 9-day, multiple-dose regimen of levofloxacin 500 mg twice daily or placebo.[1] The pharmacokinetics of R- and S-warfarin were unchanged by levofloxacin administration. Prothrombin times following the single dose of warfarin were not affected by levofloxacin administration. Several case reports have appeared noting an increase in anticoagulation during the administration of levofloxacin and warfarin.[2-4] Because a prospective study found no interaction, and there does not appear to be a reasonable mechanism for levofloxacin to interact with warfarin, consider other possibilities. One of the primary reasons a patient's sensitivity to warfarin might change is because of concurrent diseases. It has been reported that infection and inflammation can stimulate the release of cytokines that have been shown to inhibit CYP-450 activity, including CYP2C9 and CYP3A4, which are enzymes that metabolize warfarin.[5] Thus, it is not unexpected that patients with infections would have altered warfarin dosage requirements. It remains to be proven if levofloxacin plays any role in the observed changes in warfarin requirements.

RELATED DRUGS: Altered warfarin dosage requirements have been reported with nearly all antibiotics. The most likely cause of many of these changes is the underlying disease being treated with the antibiotic.

MANAGEMENT OPTIONS:

➡ *Monitor.* No special precautions are necessary. Monitor all patients who develop an infection and are receiving warfarin for increased sensitivity to the anticoagulant.

REFERENCES:

1. Liao S, et al. Absence of an effect of levofloxacin on warfarin pharmacokinetics and anticoagulation in male volunteers. *J Clin Pharmacol.* 1996;36(11):1072-1077.
2. Ravnan SL, et al. Levofloxacin and warfarin interaction. *Pharmacotherapy.* 2001;21(7):884-885.
3. Gheno G, et al. Levofloxacin-warfarin interaction. *Eur J Clin Pharmacol.* 2001;57(5):427.
4. Jones CB, et al. Levofloxacin and warfarin interaction. *Ann Pharmacother.* 2002;36(10):1554-1557.
5. Morgan ET. Regulation of cytochrome p450 by inflammatory mediators: why and how? *Drug Metab Dispos.* 2001;29(3):207-212.

Levothyroxine (eg, *Synthroid*)

Aluminum Hydroxide (eg, *Amphojel*)

SUMMARY: Aluminum hydroxide may reduce levothyroxine bioavailability; some patients may develop hypothyroidism.

RISK FACTORS:

➡ *Concurrent Diseases.* Patients with no thyroid function are probably at greater risk because they cannot increase endogenous thyroid output in response to the interaction. Some patients receiving levothyroxine have at least partial thyroid function, and the increased thyrotropin concentrations can increase endogenous thyroid output.

MECHANISM: Aluminum hydroxide appears to bind with levothyroxine in the GI tract, thus reducing levothyroxine bioavailability.

CLINICAL EVALUATION: A patient stabilized on long-term levothyroxine replacement developed elevated thyrotropin serum concentrations while taking an antacid containing aluminum hydroxide.[1] When the aluminum hydroxide was stopped, the thyrotropin concentrations returned to normal. In another study of patients stabilized on levothyroxine, the addition of aluminum hydroxide for 2 to 4 weeks substantially increased the thyrotropin serum concentrations.[2] Another patient on levothyroxine developed a marked increase in thyrotropin after starting aluminum hydroxide, and a subsequent in vitro investigation showed adsorption (binding) of levothyroxine to aluminum hydroxide.[3]

RELATED DRUGS: Aluminum hydroxide is expected to reduce the absorption of other thyroid preparations. Other antacids, such as calcium carbonate (eg, *Os-Cal*), also appear to inhibit absorption of levothyroxine. Limited evidence suggests that magnesium-containing antacids may also interact.

MANAGEMENT OPTIONS:

➡ *Consider Alternative.* In patients receiving levothyroxine, consider using H_2-receptor antagonists or proton pump inhibitors instead of aluminum hydroxide or other antacids.

➡ *Circumvent/Minimize.* If the combination is used, administer levothyroxine or other thyroid preparations no closer than 4 hours before or 6 hours after antacids.

➡ *Monitor.* If the combination is used, monitor thyroid function, particularly thyrotropin concentrations.

REFERENCES:
1. Sperber AD, Liel Y. Evidence for interference with the intestinal absorption of levothyroxine sodium by aluminum hydroxide. *Arch Intern Med.* 1992;152(1):183-184.

2. Liel Y, et al. Nonspecific intestinal adsorption of levothyroxine by aluminum hydroxide. *Am J Med.* 1994;97(4):363-365.

3. Mersebach H, et al. Intestinal adsorption of levothyroxine by antacids and laxatives: case stories and in vitro experiments. *Pharmacol Toxicol.* 1999;84(3):107-109.

Levothyroxine (eg, *Synthroid*)

Caffeine

SUMMARY: Limited clinical evidence suggests that ingestion of coffee may reduce levothyroxine bioavailability.

RISK FACTORS:

➡ *Concurrent Diseases.* Patients with no thyroid function are probably at greater risk because they cannot increase endogenous thyroid output in response to the interaction. Some patients receiving levothyroxine have at least partial thyroid function, and the increased thyrotropin concentrations can increase endogenous thyroid output.

MECHANISM: Not established. Some substance in coffee may bind with levothyroxine in the GI tract, thus reducing levothyroxine bioavailability.

CLINICAL EVALUATION: After the clinical observation of possible reduced levothyroxine effect when taken with coffee or espresso, a study of levothyroxine absorption was done of patients on levothyroxine and healthy subjects.[1] Giving coffee with levothyroxine reduced its absorption, but giving coffee 1 hour after levothyroxine did not. The substance in the coffee that inhibited levothyroxine absorption was not identified; it may not be caffeine.

RELATED DRUGS: Coffee may reduce the absorption of thyroid preparations other than levothyroxine.

MANAGEMENT OPTIONS:

➡ *Circumvent/Minimize.* Based on available evidence, giving levothyroxine 1 hour before drinking coffee eliminates the interaction.

REFERENCES:
1. Benvenga S, et al. Altered intestinal absorption of L-thyroxine caused by coffee. *Thyroid.* 2008;18(3):293-301.

Levothyroxine (eg, *Synthroid*)

Calcium Carbonate (eg, *Os-Cal*)

SUMMARY: Calcium carbonate may reduce levothyroxine bioavailability; some patients may develop hypothyroidism.

RISK FACTORS:

➡ *Concurrent Diseases.* Patients with no thyroid function are probably at greater risk because they cannot increase endogenous thyroid output in response to the interaction.

MECHANISM: Calcium carbonate appears to bind with levothyroxine in the GI tract, thus reducing levothyroxine bioavailability.

CLINICAL EVALUATION: Patients on levothyroxine replacement have developed evidence of hypothyroidism when calcium carbonate was taken concurrently.[1,2] The interaction was confirmed in 20 patients stabilized on chronic levothyroxine therapy who took calcium carbonate (1,200 mg of elemental calcium) with their levothyroxine for 3 months.[3] Thirteen of the 20 patients had an increase in thyrotropin concentrations during the calcium carbonate, and, in 4 patients, it rose above the upper limit of normal. In a study of 7 healthy subjects, levothyroxine 1,000 mcg was given with and without concurrent dose of calcium carbonate 2 g.[4] With levothyroxine alone, 84% of the dose was absorbed, but absorption was only 58% when given with calcium carbonate. In another study of 67 hemodialysis patients on levothyroxine, the effect of adding various phosphate binders on thyrotropin was evaluated.[5] Calcium carbonate was associated with an increase in thyrotropin serum concentrations. It appears that calcium carbonate can substantially reduce levothyroxine absorption. The substantial variability in the 20 patients on levothyroxine[3] is probably because the thyroid glands of some of the patients were at least partially functioning. Accordingly, they were able to release endogenous thyroid hormone in response to decreased circulating thyroid hormones caused by the calcium carbonate.

RELATED DRUGS: Calcium carbonate is expected to reduce the absorption of other thyroid preparations. Other antacids, such as aluminum hydroxide (eg, *Amphojel*), also appear to inhibit absorption of levothyroxine. Limited evidence suggests that magnesium-containing antacids may also interact.

MANAGEMENT OPTIONS:

➡ *Consider Alternative.* In patients receiving levothyroxine, consider using H_2-receptor antagonists or proton pump inhibitors instead of calcium carbonate or other antacids.

➡ *Circumvent/Minimize.* If the combination is used, administer levothyroxine or other thyroid preparations no closer than 4 hours before or 6 hours after antacids.

➡ *Monitor.* If the combination is used, monitor thyroid function, particularly thyrotropin concentrations.

REFERENCES:

1. Schneyer CR. Calcium carbonate and reduction of levothyroxine efficacy. *JAMA.* 1998;279(10):750.
2. Csako G, et al. Exaggerated levothyroxine malabsorption due to calcium carbonate supplementation in gastrointestinal disorders. *Ann Pharmacother.* 2001;35(12):1578-1583.
3. Singh N, et al. Effect of calcium carbonate on the absorption of levothyroxine. *JAMA.* 2000;283(21):2822-2825.

4. Singh N, et al. The acute effect of calcium carbonate on the intestinal absorption of levothyroxine. *Thyroid.* 2001;11(10):967-971.

5. Diskin CJ, et al. Effect of phosphate binders upon TSH and L-thyroxine dose in patients on thyroid replacement. *Int Urol Nephrol.* 2007;39(2):599-602.

Levothyroxine (eg, *Synthroid*)

Ciprofloxacin (eg, *Cipro*)

SUMMARY: Limited clinical evidence suggests that ciprofloxacin may reduce levothyroxine bioavailability.

RISK FACTORS:

➡ *Concurrent Diseases.* Patients with no thyroid function are probably at greater risk because they cannot increase endogenous thyroid output in response to the interaction. Some patients receiving levothyroxine have at least partial thyroid function, and the increased thyrotropin concentrations can increase endogenous thyroid output.

MECHANISM: Not established. Ciprofloxacin may bind with levothyroxine in the GI tract, thus reducing levothyroxine bioavailability.

CLINICAL EVALUATION: Two cases of possible reduced levothyroxine absorption caused by ciprofloxacin have been reported.[1] In an 80-year-old woman stabilized on levothyroxine, 3 weeks of ciprofloxacin therapy was associated with clinical and laboratory evidence of hypothyroidism. Stopping the ciprofloxacin resulted in normalization of thyroid function. In a 79-year-old woman stabilized on levothyroxine, 4 weeks of ciprofloxacin was associated with a substantial increase in thyrotropin serum concentrations. Her thyroid function tests normalized when the levothyroxine and ciprofloxacin doses were separated by 6 hours. Although the ciprofloxacin appeared to reduce levothyroxine absorption in these 2 patients, more data are needed to establish the clinical importance of this interaction.

RELATED DRUGS: Ciprofloxacin may reduce the absorption of other thyroid preparations. The effect of other fluoroquinolones on thyroid hormone absorption is not established.

MANAGEMENT OPTIONS:

➡ *Circumvent/Minimize.* If the combination is used, separate ciprofloxacin doses by 6 or more hours from levothyroxine or other thyroid preparations.

➡ *Monitor.* If the combination is used, monitor thyroid function, particularly thyrotropin concentrations.

REFERENCES:

1. Cooper JG, et al. Ciprofloxacin interacts with thyroid replacement therapy. *BMJ.* 2005;330(7498):1002.

Levothyroxine (eg, *Synthroid*)

Iron (eg, *FeroSul*)

SUMMARY: Iron products may reduce levothyroxine bioavailability; some patients may develop hypothyroidism.

RISK FACTORS:

➥ *Concurrent Diseases.* Patients with no thyroid function are probably at greater risk because they cannot increase endogenous thyroid output in response to the interaction. Some patients receiving levothyroxine have at least partial thyroid function, and the increased thyrotropin concentrations can increase endogenous thyroid output.

MECHANISM: Iron appears to bind with levothyroxine in the GI tract, thus reducing levothyroxine bioavailability.

CLINICAL EVALUATION: A 29-year-old woman stabilized on levothyroxine 150 mcg daily started taking ferrous sulfate after becoming pregnant.[1] Even though she was instructed to take levothyroxine 4 to 6 hours after the ferrous sulfate, her levothyroxine requirements increased to 225 mcg and then 250 mcg daily. Then she became clinically hyperthyroid after she delivered, and the ferrous sulfate was stopped. Her dose of levothyroxine was reduce to 150 mcg daily. Twelve weeks after delivery, she started ferrous sulfate again and became clinically hypothyroid, which was confirmed by thyroid testing. It is probable that ferrous sulfate reduced levothyroxine absorption in this patient. In another study, 14 patients stabilized on levothyroxine took ferrous sulfate 300 mg with their levothyroxine for 12 weeks.[2] Thyrotropin serum concentrations increased substantially, and 9 of the 12 patients developed signs and symptoms of hypothyroidism. In vitro investigation found a poorly soluble purple complex formed when iron was combined with levothyroxine.

RELATED DRUGS: Iron preparations are expected to reduce the absorption of other thyroid preparations.

MANAGEMENT OPTIONS:

➥ *Circumvent/Minimize.* If the combination is used, administer levothyroxine or other thyroid preparations no closer than 4 hours before or 6 hours after iron preparations. If possible, allow an 8- to 12-hour separation.

➥ *Monitor.* If the combination is used, monitor thyroid function, particularly thyrotropin concentrations.

REFERENCES:
1. Shakir KM, et al. Ferrous sulfate-induced increase in requirement for thyroxine in a patient with primary hypothyroidism. *South Med J.* 1997;90(6):637-639.
2. Campbell NR, et al. Ferrous sulfate reduces thyroxine efficacy in patients with hypothyroidism. *Ann Intern Med.* 1992;117(12):1010-1013.

Levothyroxine (eg, *Synthroid*)

Magnesium (eg, *Mag-Ox*)

SUMMARY: Magnesium-containing antacids or laxatives may reduce levothyroxine bioavailability; some patients may develop hypothyroidism.

RISK FACTORS:

➡ ***Concurrent Diseases.*** Patients with no thyroid function are probably at greater risk because they cannot increase endogenous thyroid output in response to the interaction. Some patients receiving levothyroxine have at least partial thyroid function, and the increased thyrotropin concentrations can increase endogenous thyroid output.

MECHANISM: Magnesium-containing products appear to bind with levothyroxine in the GI tract, thus reducing levothyroxine bioavailability.

CLINICAL EVALUATION: A patient stabilized on long-term levothyroxine replacement developed elevated thyrotropin serum concentrations while taking a magnesium-containing laxative.[1] When the magnesium product was stopped, the thyrotropin concentrations returned to normal. Additional in vitro investigation showed adsorption (binding) of levothyroxine to magnesium salts. Although a magnesium-levothyroxine interaction is not nearly as well documented as the interactions of levothyroxine with calcium carbonate or aluminum hydroxide, it would be prudent to assume that magnesium products interact until more data are available.

RELATED DRUGS: Magnesium-containing antacids and laxatives are expected to reduce the absorption of other thyroid preparations. Other antacids (eg, calcium carbonate [eg, *Os-Cal*], aluminum hydroxide [eg, *Amphojel*]) also appear to inhibit absorption of levothyroxine.

MANAGEMENT OPTIONS:

➡ ***Consider Alternative.*** In patients receiving levothyroxine, consider using H_2-receptor antagonists or proton pump inhibitors instead of magnesium antacids or other antacids. If the magnesium product is being used as a laxative, consider alternative laxatives.

➡ ***Circumvent/Minimize.*** If the combination is used, administer levothyroxine or other thyroid preparations no closer than 4 hours before or 6 hours after antacids.

➡ ***Monitor.*** If the combination is used, monitor thyroid function, particularly thyrotropin concentrations.

REFERENCES:

    1. Mersebach H, et al. Intestinal adsorption of levothyroxine by antacids and laxatives: case stories and in vitro experiments. *Pharmacol Toxicol.* 1999;84(3):107-109.

Levothyroxine (eg, *Synthroid*)

Sertraline (eg, *Zoloft*)

SUMMARY: Preliminary evidence suggests that sertraline may reduce levothyroxine effect; more data are needed to assess the clinical importance.

RISK FACTORS: No specific risk factors are known.

MECHANISM: Not established.

CLINICAL EVALUATION: In 11 patients on levothyroxine, addition of sertraline resulted in elevations in thyrotropin.[1] The increases in serum thyrotropin responded to an increase in the dose of levothyroxine.

RELATED DRUGS: The effect of other selective serotonin reuptake inhibitors on levothyroxine is not established.

MANAGEMENT OPTIONS:

➡ *Monitor.* Monitor patients taking levothyroxine for altered thyroid function tests if sertraline is started, stopped, or changed in dosage.

REFERENCES:

1. McCowen KC, et al. Elevated serum thyrotropin in thyroxine-treated patients with hypothyroidism given sertraline. *N Engl J Med.* 1997;337(14):1010-1011.

Levothyroxine (eg, *Synthroid*)

Sevelamer (eg, *Renagel*)

SUMMARY: Sevelamer may reduce levothyroxine bioavailability; some patients may develop hypothyroidism.

RISK FACTORS:

➡ *Concurrent Diseases.* Patients with no thyroid function are probably at greater risk because they cannot increase endogenous thyroid output in response to the interaction. Some patients receiving levothyroxine have at least partial thyroid function, and the increased thyrotropin concentrations can increase endogenous thyroid output.

MECHANISM: Sevelamer appears to bind with levothyroxine in the GI tract, thus reducing levothyroxine bioavailability.

CLINICAL EVALUATION: A 62-year-old woman on hemodialysis receiving sevelamer 3,200 mg daily was hypothyroid and started on levothyroxine.[1] After 3 months of levothyroxine (taken at the same time as the sevelamer), she still had symptoms of hypothyroidism and her thyrotropin remained high. When she was instructed to take the levothyroxine at night (4 hours after any other medication), her symptoms improved and the thyrotropin decreased markedly. Her thyrotropin increased again 9 months later when she was hospitalized and the sevelamer was given with the levothyroxine; separating the doses resulted in normalization of the thyrotropin. In another study of 67 hemodialysis patients on levothyroxine, the effect of adding phosphate binders on thyrotropin was evaluated.[2] Sevelamer was associated with a substantial increase in thyrotropin despite an increased mean dosage requirement of levothyroxine. Patients taking calcium carbonate also had an increase in thyrotropin, but not as large as with sevelamer; in patients on calcium acetate as a phosphate binder there was no effect on thyrotropin, suggesting no interaction with levothyroxine.

RELATED DRUGS: Sevelamer is expected to reduce the absorption of other thyroid preparations. Other phosphate binders (eg, calcium carbonate [eg, *Os-Cal*], aluminum hydroxide [eg, *Amphojel*]) also appear to inhibit absorption of levothyroxine.

MANAGEMENT OPTIONS:

➡ *Consider Alternative.* In patients receiving levothyroxine, consider using calcium acetate as a phosphate binder instead of sevelamer or calcium carbonate.

➡ *Circumvent/Minimize.* If the combination is used, administer levothyroxine or other thyroid preparations no closer than 4 hours before or 6 hours after sevelamer. Because patients on hemodialysis often have gastroparesis, such a separation of doses may not completely avoid the interaction.

➡ *Monitor.* If the combination is used, monitor thyroid function, particularly thyrotropin concentrations.

REFERENCES:

1. Arnadottir M, et al. Phosphate binders and timing of levothyroxine administration. *Nephrol Dial Transplant.* 2008;23(1):420.

2. Diskin CJ, et al. Effect of phosphate binders upon TSH and L-thyroxine dose in patients on thyroid replacement. *Int Urol Nephrol.* 2007;39(2):599-602.

Levothyroxine (eg, *Synthroid*)

Sucralfate (eg, *Carafate*)

SUMMARY: Sucralfate may reduce levothyroxine bioavailability; some patients may develop hypothyroidism.

RISK FACTORS:

➡ *Concurrent Diseases.* Patients with no thyroid function are probably at greater risk because they cannot increase endogenous thyroid output in response to the interaction. Some patients receiving levothyroxine have at least partial thyroid function, and the increased thyrotropin concentrations can increase endogenous thyroid output.

MECHANISM: Sucralfate appears to bind with levothyroxine in the GI tract, thus reducing levothyroxine bioavailability.

CLINICAL EVALUATION: In a study of 5 healthy subjects, levothyroxine was given alone, with concurrent sucralfate, and with sucralfate 8 hours after the levothyroxine.[1] Concurrent sucralfate markedly reduced the bioavailability of levothyroxine, while sucralfate 8 hours after levothyroxine circumvented the interaction. Sucralfate contains a substantial amount of aluminum, a substance known to bind with levothyroxine.

RELATED DRUGS: Sucralfate is expected to reduce the absorption of other thyroid preparations. Antacids (eg, calcium carbonate [eg, *Os-Cal*], aluminum hydroxide [eg, *Amphojel*], magnesium salts [eg, *Mag-Ox*]) also appear to inhibit absorption of levothyroxine.

MANAGEMENT OPTIONS:

➥ *Consider Alternative.* In patients receiving levothyroxine, consider using H_2-receptor antagonists or proton pump inhibitors instead of sucralfate or antacids.

➥ *Circumvent/Minimize.* If the combination is used, administer levothyroxine or other thyroid preparations no closer than 4 hours before or 6 hours after sucralfate.

➥ *Monitor.* If the combination is used, monitor thyroid function, particularly thyrotropin concentrations.

REFERENCES:

1. Sherman SI, et al. Sucralfate causes malabsorption of L-thyroxine. *Am J Med.* 1994;96(6):531-535.

Lidocaine (eg, *Xylocaine*)

Morphine (eg, *Duramorph*)

SUMMARY: A patient who had received morphine and fentanyl (eg, *Sublimaze*) during anesthetic induction developed respiratory depression and lost consciousness after receiving IV lidocaine; carefully monitor patients receiving opioids and lidocaine for excessive opioid effects.

RISK FACTORS:

➥ *Route of Administration.* The observed reaction occurred following IV use of lidocaine. Theoretically, an interaction with opioids would be unlikely to occur with routes of lidocaine administration that do not result in lidocaine reaching the CNS.

MECHANISM: Not established. The authors propose that lidocaine may enhance opioid effects by reducing calcium concentrations in selected CNS sites.

CLINICAL EVALUATION: A 74–year-old man underwent coronary artery bypass surgery with morphine and fentanyl for anesthetic induction.[1] He was transferred to the surgical ICU, breathing spontaneously. He was then administered a lidocaine 200 mg IV bolus and a 2 mg/min infusion for treatment of ventricular tachycardia. During the next 5 minutes, he developed progressive slowing of the respiratory rate, lost consciousness, and required reintubation. Spontaneous ventilation and consciousness returned within 1 to 2 minutes of administering naloxone (eg, *Narcan*) 0.2 mg. The rapid reversal with naloxone is consistent with the authors' contention that lidocaine enhances opioid effects; more study is needed to establish the clinical importance of this interaction.

RELATED DRUGS: Theoretically, lidocaine would enhance the effect of any opioid.

MANAGEMENT OPTIONS:

➥ *Monitor.* If lidocaine is used concurrently with opioids, monitor for excessive opioid effects (eg, respiratory depression, CNS depression). Based on the case reported, administration of an opioid antagonist such as naloxone may be effective in reversing the reaction.

REFERENCES:

1. Jensen E, et al. Potentiation of narcosis after intravenous lidocaine in a patient given spinal opioids. *Anesth Analg.* 1999;89:758–59.

5 Lidocaine (eg, *Xylocaine*)

Omeprazole (*Prilosec*)

SUMMARY: Omeprazole does not alter the pharmacokinetics of lidocaine.

RISK FACTORS: No specific risk factors are known.

MECHANISM: No interaction.

CLINICAL EVALUATION: Ten healthy subjects received 1 mg/kg lidocaine IV alone and following pretreatment with omeprazole 40 mg/day for 7 days.[1] Omeprazole had no effect on the concentrations of lidocaine or its metabolite.

RELATED DRUGS: Lansoprazole (*Prevacid*) is not likely to interact with lidocaine.

MANAGEMENT OPTIONS: No interaction.

REFERENCES:
1. Noble DW, et al. The effect of oral omeprazole on the disposition of lignocaine. *Anaesthesia.* 1994;49:497.

4 Lidocaine (eg, *Xylocaine*)

Phenobarbital

SUMMARY: Barbiturates such as phenobarbital may enhance the metabolism of lidocaine, resulting in a slightly increased dosage requirement.

RISK FACTORS: No specific risk factors are known.

MECHANISM: Barbiturates probably induce hepatic microsomal enzymes that metabolize lidocaine.

CLINICAL EVALUATION: Barbiturates markedly reduce the bioavailability of oral lidocaine,[2,3] but lidocaine seldom is given orally for systemic use. In studies of IV lidocaine administration in humans,[1,2] lidocaine elimination is enhanced slightly by pretreatment with phenobarbital. Since lidocaine is titrated to achieve the desired response, it would be uncommon for patients to be affected adversely by this interaction.

RELATED DRUGS: Other barbiturates also may increase lidocaine's metabolism.

MANAGEMENT OPTIONS: No specific action is required, but be alert for evidence of the interaction.

REFERENCES:
1. Heinonen J et al. Plasma lidocaine levels in patients treated with potential inducers of microsomal enzymes. *Acta Anaesthesiol Scand.* 1970;14:89.
2. Perucca E, et al. Reduction of oral bioavailability of lignocaine by induction of first pass metabolism in epileptic patients. *Br J Clin Pharmacol.* 1979;8:21.
3. Perucca E, et al. Effect of low-dose phenobarbitone on five indirect indices of hepatic microsomal enzyme induction and plasma lipoproteins in normal subjects. *Br J Clin Pharmacol.* 1981;12:592.

Lidocaine (eg, *Xylocaine*) 4

Phenytoin (eg, *Dilantin*)

SUMMARY: Phenytoin can reduce lidocaine serum concentrations while producing an independent additive effect on myocardial tissue.

RISK FACTORS: No specific risk factors are known.

MECHANISM: Phenytoin can enhance the metabolism of lidocaine and add to lidocaine's cardiac depressant effects.[1,2]

CLINICAL EVALUATION: Epileptic patients who are receiving phenytoin and other anticonvulsants eliminate IV lidocaine at an increased rate.[2] In another study, patients taking anticonvulsants tended to have a higher clearance of IV lidocaine than healthy volunteers, but the differences were not clinically significant.[3] The consequence of this interaction on the antiarrhythmic response to lidocaine is unknown, but it is probably small since lidocaine is titrated to effect. Phenytoin appears to substantially reduce the bioavailability of oral lidocaine.[3] The additive depressant effect of lidocaine and IV phenytoin on cardiac pacemaker tissue may have resulted in sinoatrial arrest in 1 patient.[1]

RELATED DRUGS: No information available.

MANAGEMENT OPTIONS: No specific action is required, but be alert for evidence of the interaction.

REFERENCES:
1. Wood RA. Sinoatrial arrest: an interaction between phenytoin and lignocaine. *Br Med J*. 1971;1:645.
2. Heinonen J, et al. Plasma lidocaine levels in patients treated with potential inducers of microsomal enzymes. *Acta Anaesthesiol Scand*. 1970;14:89.
3. Perucca E, et al. Reduction of oral bioavailability of lignocaine by induction of first pass metabolism in epileptic patients. *Br J Clin Pharmacol*. 1979;8:21.

Lidocaine (eg, *Xylocaine*) 4

Procainamide (eg, *Pronestyl*)

SUMMARY: Central nervous system toxicity has been reported in 1 patient receiving both lidocaine and procainamide.

RISK FACTORS: No specific risk factors are known.

MECHANISM: Not established; however, psychiatric side effects possibly could be additive.

CLINICAL EVALUATION: A single case has been reported in which delirium occurred in a patient receiving both lidocaine and procainamide.[1] The authors proposed that procainamide could have precipitated the delirium by adding to the neurotoxic effects of lidocaine.

RELATED DRUGS: No information is available.

MANAGEMENT OPTIONS: No specific action is required, but be alert for evidence of the interaction.

REFERENCES:
1. Ilyas M, et al. Delirium induced by a combination of anti-arrhythmic drugs. *Lancet*. 1969;2:1368.

4　**Lidocaine (eg, *Xylocaine*)**

Propafenone (*Rythmol*)

SUMMARY: Lidocaine administration attenuates some of the electrophysiologic actions of propafenone while enhancing its negative inotropic effects. Propafenone causes a small increase in lidocaine concentrations; the clinical importance of these effects is not established.

RISK FACTORS: No specific risk factors are known.

MECHANISM: Not established. The observed effects probably represent the summation of pharmacodynamic actions of the 2 agents.

CLINICAL EVALUATION: Twenty patients with ventricular arrhythmias underwent electrophysiologic study with 1 or 2 mg/kg propafenone IV either before or after receiving lidocaine (100 mg bolus and a 2 mg/min infusion).[1] Both lidocaine and propafenone exerted an additive negative inotropic effect when administered concurrently. Propafenone increased blood pressure, pulmonary wedge pressure, and right atrial pressure, and these effects were accentuated by lidocaine administration. Prolongation of atrial and ventricular refractoriness induced by propafenone was reversed by the addition of lidocaine. No apparent changes in serum concentrations of either drug were noted. Propafenone 225 mg every 8 hours for 4 days resulted in a small (7%) reduction in the area under the concentration-time curve of lidocaine.[2] The clinical significance of these findings is unknown but likely to be limited.

RELATED DRUGS: No information is available.

MANAGEMENT OPTIONS: No specific action is required, but be alert for evidence of the interaction.

REFERENCES:
1. Feld GK, et al. Hemodynamic and electrophysiologic effects of combined infusion of lidocaine and propafenone in humans. *J Clin Pharmacol.* 1987;27:52.
2. Ujhelyi MR, et al. The pharmacokinetic and pharmacodynamic interaction between propafenone and lidocaine. *Clin Pharmacol Ther.* 1993;53:38.

Lidocaine (eg, *Xylocaine*)

Propranolol (eg, *Inderal*)

SUMMARY: Lidocaine concentrations may become excessive during concomitant propranolol administration.

RISK FACTORS: No specific risk factors are known.

MECHANISM: Propranolol and other beta blockers tend to reduce cardiac output and hepatic blood flow, which in turn reduces lidocaine hepatic metabolism.[6,8] Propranolol also inhibits the activity of hepatic microsomal drug-metabolizing enzymes.[1,4,9,11] Lidocaine may enhance the negative inotropic effect of propranolol (and possibly other beta blockers).[10]

CLINICAL EVALUATION: Propranolol,[1-3,5-8] metoprolol (eg, *Lopressor*),[8] and nadolol (eg, *Corgard*)[3] reduce lidocaine clearance 15% to 45%. The magnitude of the changes in lidocaine disposition found in these studies appears sufficient to increase the risk of lidocaine toxicity, and 2 cases of toxicity that may have been due to this interaction have been reported.[7] The clinical importance of the additive negative inotropic effect of lidocaine and beta blockers is not yet established.[10]

RELATED DRUGS: Metoprolol and nadolol interact similarly with lidocaine. Other beta blockers also may enhance the negative inotropic effects of lidocaine. Pindolol (eg, *Visken*) reportedly has no effect on lidocaine clearance.[2]

MANAGEMENT OPTIONS:

➡ *Monitor.* Patients who receive concurrent therapy with beta blockers and lidocaine should be monitored carefully for increased lidocaine effects. The magnitude of the reduction in lidocaine clearance probably varies with different beta blockers, but no generalizations are possible at this time.

REFERENCES:

1. Bax NDS, et al. The impairment of lidocaine clearance by propranolol—major contribution from enzyme inhibition. *Br J Clin Pharmacol.* 1985;19:597.
2. Svendsen TL, et al. Effects of propranolol and pindolol on plasma lignocaine clearance in man. *Br J Clin Pharmacol.* 1982;13:223S.
3. Schneck DW, et al. Effects of nadolol and propranolol on plasma lidocaine clearance. *Clin Pharmacol Ther.* 1984;36:584.
4. Greenblatt DJ. Impairment of antipyrine clearance in humans by propranolol. *Circulation.* 1978;57:1161.
5. Branch RA, et al. The reduction of lidocaine clearance by dl-propranolol: an example of hemodynamic drug interaction. *J Pharmacol Exp Ther.* 1973;184:515.
6. Ochs HR, et al. Reduction in lidocaine clearance during continuous infusion and by coadministration of propranolol. *N Engl J Med.* 1980;303:373.
7. Graham CF, et al. Lidocaine-propranolol interactions. *N Engl J Med.* 1981;304:1301.
8. Conrad KA, et al. Lidocaine elimination: effects of metoprolol and of propranolol. *Clin Pharmacol Ther.* 1983;33:133.
9. Deacon CS, et al. Inhibition of oxidative drug metabolism by betaadrenoreceptor antagonist is related to their lipid solubility. *Br J Clin Pharmacol.* 1981;12:429.
10. Boudoulas H, et al. Negative inotropic effect of lidocaine in patients with coronary arterial disease and normal subjects. *Chest.* 1977;71:170.
11. Greenblatt DJ, et al. Impairment of antipyrine clearance in humans by propranolol. *Circulation.* 1978;57:1161.

Lidocaine (eg, *Xylocaine*) 4

Ranitidine (eg, *Zantac*)

SUMMARY: Ranitidine has no clinically significant effect on lidocaine concentrations.

RISK FACTORS: No specific risk factors are known.

MECHANISM: Not established.

CLINICAL EVALUATION: Ranitidine 150 mg twice daily for 5 days reduced lidocaine clearance 11% and the volume of distribution at a steady state 15% in healthy subjects.[1] Neither change is likely to result in clinically significant changes in lidocaine concentrations. Other studies found no change in lidocaine disposition after ranitidine treatment (up to 400 mg/day).[2-4]

RELATED DRUGS: Cimetidine (eg, *Tagamet*) is known to decrease lidocaine clearance. It is unlikely that famotidine (eg, *Pepcid*) and nizatidine (eg, *Axid AR*) would alter lidocaine clearance significantly.

MANAGEMENT OPTIONS: No specific action is required, but be alert for evidence of the interaction.

REFERENCES:

1. Robson RA, et al. The effect of ranitidine on the disposition of lignocaine. *Br J Clin Pharmacol.* 1985;20:170.

2. Jackson JE, et al. Effects of histamine-2 receptor blockade on lidocaine kinetics. *Clin Pharmacol Ther.* 1985;37:544.

3. Freely J, et al. Lack of effect of ranitidine on the disposition of lignocaine. *Br J Clin Pharmacol.* 1983;15:378.

4. Jackson JE, et al. The effects of H_2 blockers on lidocaine disposition. *Clin Pharmacol Ther.* 1983;33:255.

4 Lidocaine (eg, *Xylocaine*)

Succinylcholine (eg, *Anectine*)

SUMMARY: Large doses of lidocaine may prolong succinylcholine's duration of action.

RISK FACTORS:

➡ *Dosage Regimen.* Lidocaine doses higher than 3 mg/kg may prolong succinylcholine apnea duration.

MECHANISM: Not established. Lidocaine and other antiarrhythmics may enhance the neuromuscular blockade of skeletal muscle relaxants by impairing transmission of impulses at the motor nerve terminals.[1,2] It has been proposed that lidocaine may displace succinylcholine from plasma protein binding, although this effect would be transient.[3]

CLINICAL EVALUATION: Bolus doses of lidocaine 1 to 16.5 mg/kg prolonged the duration of succinylcholine-induced (0.7 mg/kg) apnea in humans. Lidocaine doses of up to 3.3 mg/kg only modestly increased the duration of apnea. At a dose of lidocaine 5 mg/kg, the duration of succinylcholine apnea was approximately doubled; at lidocaine 16.5 mg/kg, it was approximately 3 times that of the control.[3] Thus, commonly used clinical doses of lidocaine are not likely to have a major effect on the duration of succinylcholine apnea. In another study, bolus intravenous lidocaine 6 mg/kg prevented succinylcholine-induced increases in intragastric pressure.[4]

RELATED DRUGS: Other neuromuscular blockers are likely to be affected similarly by lidocaine.

MANAGEMENT OPTIONS: No specific action is required, but be alert for evidence of the interaction.

REFERENCES:

1. Harrah MD, et al. The interaction of d-tubocurarine with antiarrhythmic drugs. *Anesthesiology.* 1970;33(4):406-410.

2. Brückner J, et al. Neuromuscular drug interactions of clinical importance. *Anesth Analg.* 1980;59(9):678-682.

3. Usubiaga JE, et al. Interaction of intravenously administered procaine, lidocaine and succinylcholine in anesthetized subjects. *Anesth Analg.* 1967;46(1):39-45.

4. Miller RD, et al. Inhibition of succinylcholine-induced increased intragastric pressure by nondepolarizing muscle relaxants and lidocaine. *Anesthesiology.* 1971;34(2):185-188.

Linezolid (*Zyvox*)
Milnacipran (*Savella*)

SUMMARY: Milnacipran is contraindicated with nonselective monoamine oxidase inhibitors (MAOIs) because of the risk of potentially fatal serotonin syndrome. Linezolid is a relatively weak MAOI, but it may interact in some patients.

RISK FACTORS: No specific risk factors are known.

MECHANISM: Milnacipran inhibits the reuptake of both serotonin and norepinephrine, and may have additive serotonergic effects with nonselective MAOIs.

CLINICAL EVALUATION: The combination of serotonin reuptake inhibitors with nonselective MAOIs has resulted in severe (sometimes fatal) serotonin syndrome, and the product information for milnacipran states that concurrent therapy with MAOIs is contraindicated.[1] Linezolid is usually a relatively weak MAOI, and theoretically should be unlikely to interact with serotonin reuptake inhibitors such as milnacipran. However, linezolid has been occasionally associated with serotonin syndrome when combined with serotonin reuptake inhibitors, so it may interact with milnacipran in some people.

RELATED DRUGS: Any serotonergic drug has the potential to interact with linezolid, but the risk of such combinations is not established.

MANAGEMENT OPTIONS:

➡ ***Consider Alternative.*** It would be prudent to use an alternative to one of the drugs, but this may be difficult given the indications for which these drugs are used.

➡ ***Monitor.*** If the combination is used, monitor for evidence of serotonin syndrome, including myoclonus, rigidity, tremor, hyperreflexia, fever, sweating, seizures, confusion, agitation, incoordination, and coma.

REFERENCES:
   1. *Savella* [package insert]. St. Louis, MO: Forest Pharmaceuticals; 2010.

Linezolid (*Zyvox*) ▼3
Paroxetine (eg, *Paxil*)

SUMMARY: A case of possible serotonin syndrome has been reported with concurrent linezolid and paroxetine. Although the incidence of this reaction is not established, the linezolid prescribing information recommends careful monitoring if linezolid is used with drugs that inhibit serotonin uptake.

RISK FACTORS: No specific risk factors are known.

MECHANISM: Linezolid is a weak nonselective monoamine oxidase inhibitor; in some patients, this may increase the risk of serotonin syndrome when combined with serotonergic drugs, such as paroxetine.

CLINICAL EVALUATION: A 56-year-old woman developed evidence of serotonin syndrome when linezolid was started several days after she discontinued taking paroxetine.[1] Because some patients may have delayed paroxetine elimination due to decreased CYP2D6 activity or other factors, it is possible that the serotonin syndrome was caused by a drug interaction between linezolid and paroxetine. Although it appears that most patients who receive linezolid and selective serotonin reuptake inhibitors (SSRIs) do not develop serotonin syndrome,[2] serotonin reuptake inhibitors are contraindicated with linezolid unless the patient can be carefully observed for evidence of serotonin syndrome.[3]

RELATED DRUGS: Other SSRIs may interact similarly, including citalopram (eg, *Celexa*), escitalopram (*Lexapro*), fluoxetine (eg, *Prozac*), fluvoxamine (eg, *Luvox*), and sertraline (eg, *Zoloft*). Selective serotonin-norepinephrine reuptake inhibitors may also interact, including clomipramine (eg, *Anafranil*), desvenlafaxine (*Pristiq*), duloxetine (*Cymbalta*), imipramine (eg, *Tofranil*), and venlafaxine (eg, *Effexor*).

MANAGEMENT OPTIONS:

➡ *Monitor.* Monitor for evidence of serotonin syndrome (eg, agitation, coma, confusion, fever, hyperreflexia, hypomania, incoordination, myoclonus, rigidity, seizures, shivering, sweating, tachycardia, tremor).

REFERENCES:

1. Wigen CL, et al. Serotonin syndrome and linezolid. *Clin Infect Dis.* 2002;34(12):1651-1652.
2. Taylor JJ, et al. Linezolid and serotonergic drug interactions: a retrospective survey. *Clin Infect Dis.* 2006;43(2):180-187.
3. *Zyvox* [package insert]. New York, NY: Pfizer Inc; 2008.

4   Linezolid (*Zyvox*)

Pseudoephedrine (eg, *Sudafed*)

SUMMARY: Linezolid increases pseudoephedrine concentrations and hypertensive effects to a modest degree.

RISK FACTORS: No specific risk factors are known.

MECHANISM: Linezolid appears to reduce the metabolism of pseudoephedrine, perhaps by its limited monoamine oxidase inhibition.

CLINICAL EVALUATION: Two doses of pseudoephedrine 60 mg or placebo were administered 4 hours apart before and following 2 days of linezolid 600 mg daily to 14 healthy subjects.[1] Linezolid administration resulted in a mean increase in the pseudoephedrine area under the plasma concentration-time curve (AUC) of 20%. This increase in pseudoephedrine concentration was accompanied by an increase in systolic blood pressure (32 mm Hg) compared with placebo (11 mm Hg), linezolid (15 mm Hg), or pseudoephedrine (18 mm Hg) administered alone. Diastolic pressure rose about 7 mm Hg more following the coadministration of pseudoephedrine and linezolid than with either drug alone. Pseudoephedrine did not affect the AUC of linezolid compared with placebo. The modest increases in blood pressure would not be expected to produce an adverse outcome for most patients, particularly if they use pseudoephedrine intermittently.

RELATED DRUGS: Other indirect-acting sympathomimetics might be affected in a similar manner if administered with linezolid.

MANAGEMENT OPTIONS:

➡ *Monitor.* Counsel patients stabilized on linezolid to avoid sympathomimetics if possible. Monitor patients with cardiovascular disease, such as hypertension or heart disease, for increased blood pressure and advise them to avoid this combination and sympathomimetics in general.

REFERENCES:

1. Hendershot PE, et al. Linezolid: pharmacokinetic and pharmacodynamic evaluation of coadministration with pseudoephedrine HCl, phenylpropanolamine HCl, and dextromethorphan HBr. *J Clin Pharmacol.* 2001;41(5):563-572.

Linezolid (*Zyvox*)

Rifampin (eg, *Rifadin*)

SUMMARY: Rifampin appears to modestly reduce linezolid plasma concentrations.

RISK FACTORS: No specific risk factors are known.

MECHANISM: Rifampin probably enhances linezolid metabolism.

CLINICAL EVALUATION: Sixteen healthy subjects received linezolid (600 mg twice daily for 6 doses) with and without concurrent rifampin 600 mg/day for 8 days.[1] Rifampin reduced linezolid area under the plasma concentration-time curve by 32%. The clinical importance of this effect is not established, but it is possible that some patients will manifest reduced linezolid antimicrobial effect.

RELATED DRUGS: No information is available.

MANAGEMENT OPTIONS: No specific action is required, but be alert for evidence of the interaction.

REFERENCES:

1. *Zyvox* [package insert]. New York, NY: Pfizer Inc; 2008.

Linezolid (*Zyvox*)

Sertraline (eg, *Zoloft*)

SUMMARY: Cases of possible serotonin syndrome have been reported with concurrent linezolid and sertraline. Although the incidence of this reaction is not established, the linezolid prescribing information recommends careful monitoring if linezolid is used with drugs that inhibit serotonin uptake.

RISK FACTORS: No specific risk factors are known.

MECHANISM: Linezolid is a weak nonselective monoamine oxidase inhibitor; in some patients, the effect may be sufficient to increase the risk of serotonin syndrome when combined with serotonergic drugs, such as sertraline.

CLINICAL EVALUATION: Several cases of serotonin syndrome have been reported in patients receiving linezolid and sertraline concomitantly.[1-4] In some cases, other serotonergic drugs were given concurrently and may have contributed to the reactions. Although it appears that most patients who receive linezolid and selective serotonin reuptake inhibitors (SSRIs) do not develop serotonin syndrome,[4] serotonin reuptake inhibitors are contraindicated with linezolid unless the patient can be carefully observed for evidence of serotonin syndrome.[5]

RELATED DRUGS: Other SSRIs may interact similarly, including citalopram (eg, *Celexa*), escitalopram (*Lexapro*), fluoxetine (eg, *Prozac*), fluvoxamine (eg, *Luvox*), and paroxetine (eg, *Paxil*). Selective serotonin/norepinephrine reuptake inhibitors may also interact, including clomipramine (eg, *Anafranil*), desvenlafaxine (*Pristiq*), duloxetine (*Cymbalta*), imipramine (eg, *Tofranil*), and venlafaxine (eg, *Effexor*).

MANAGEMENT OPTIONS:

➡ ***Monitor.*** Monitor for evidence of serotonin syndrome (eg, agitation, coma, confusion, fever, hyperreflexia, hypomania, incoordination, myoclonus, rigidity, seizures, shivering, sweating, tachycardia, tremor).

REFERENCES:

1. Lavery S, et al. Linezolid and serotonin syndrome. *Psychosomatics.* 2001;42(5):432-434.
2. Hachem RY, et al. Myelosuppression and serotonin syndrome associated with concurrent use of linezolid and selective serotonin reuptake inhibitors in bone marrow transplant patients. *Clin Infect Dis.* 2003;37(1):e8-e11.
3. Clark DB, et al. Drug interactions between linezolid and selective serotonin reuptake inhibitors: case report involving sertraline and review of the literature. *Pharmacotherapy.* 2006;26(2):269-276.
4. Taylor JJ, et al. Linezolid and serotonergic drug interactions: a retrospective survey. *Clin Infect Dis.* 2006;43(2):180-187.
5. *Zyvox* [package insert]. New York, NY: Pfizer Inc; 2008.

 Linezolid (*Zyvox*)

AVOID **Tranylcypromine (eg, *Parnate*)**

SUMMARY: Linezolid is contraindicated with inhibitors of monoamine oxidase type-A (MAO-A) or MAO-B.

RISK FACTORS: No specific risk factors are known.

MECHANISM: Linezolid is a weak nonspecific MAO inhibitor (MAOI); presumably it would have additive effects with other MAOIs.

CLINICAL EVALUATION: This interaction is based on theoretical considerations, but linezolid is contraindicated with all MAOIs.[1]

RELATED DRUGS: Consider linezolid contraindicated with other nonselective MAOIs, such as furazolidone,† isocarboxazid (*Marplan*), and phenelzine (*Nardil*), as well as the MAO-B inhibitors rasagiline (*Azilect*) and selegiline (eg, *Eldepryl*).

MANAGEMENT OPTIONS:

➡ ***AVOID COMBINATION.*** Avoid concurrent use of linezolid and tranylcypromine or other MAOIs, and avoid linezolid within 2 weeks of stopping an MAOI.

REFERENCES:

1. *Zyvox* [package insert]. New York, NY: Pfizer Inc; 2008.

† Not available in the United States.

 Linezolid (*Zyvox*)

Venlafaxine (eg, *Effexor*)

SUMMARY: Isolated cases of possible serotonin syndrome have been reported with concurrent linezolid and venlafaxine. Although the incidence of this reaction is not established, the linezolid prescribing information recommends careful monitoring if linezolid is used with drugs that inhibit serotonin uptake.

RISK FACTORS: No specific risk factors are known.

MECHANISM: Linezolid is a weak nonselective monoamine oxidase inhibitor; in some patients, this may increase the risk of serotonin syndrome when combined with serotonergic drugs, such as venlafaxine.

CLINICAL EVALUATION: An 85-year-old man taking long-term venlafaxine developed evidence of serotonin syndrome after linezolid was started.[1] The symptoms (eg, confusion, disorientation, hyperreflexia, increased muscle tone, myoclonic jerks) supported a diagnosis of serotonin syndrome. A 38-year-old woman developed serotonin syndrome after linezolid was added to her venlafaxine therapy.[2] A 58-year-old woman taking long-term venlafaxine developed disorientation and cerebellar signs 4 days after starting linezolid.[3] The reaction resolved after discontinuation of both drugs. Although the patient was thought to have serotonin syndrome, the diagnosis is difficult to assess from the information provided. Although it appears that most patients who receive linezolid and selective serotonin reuptake inhibitors (SSRIs) do not develop serotonin syndrome,[4] serotonin reuptake inhibitors are contraindicated with linezolid unless the patient can be carefully observed for evidence of serotonin syndrome.[5]

RELATED DRUGS: Other serotonin-norepinephrine reuptake inhibitors may interact similarly, including clomipramine (eg, *Anafranil*), desvenlafaxine (*Pristiq*), duloxetine (*Cymbalta*), and imipramine (eg, *Tofranil*). SSRIs may also interact with linezolid.

MANAGEMENT OPTIONS:

➥ *Monitor.* Monitor for evidence of serotonin syndrome (eg, agitation, coma, confusion, fever, hyperreflexia, hypomania, incoordination, myoclonus, rigidity, seizures, shivering, sweating, tachycardia, tremor).

REFERENCES:

1. Jones SL, et al. Serotonin syndrome due to co-administration of linezolid and venlafaxine. *J Antimicrob Chemother.* 2004;54(1):289-290.

2. Bergeron L, et al. Serotonin toxicity associated with concomitant use of linezolid. *Ann Pharmacother.* 2005;39(5):956-961.

3. Mason LW, et al. Serotonin toxicity as a consequence of linezolid use in revision hip arthroplasty. *Orthopedics.* 2008;31(11):1140.

4. Taylor JJ, et al. Linezolid and serotonergic drug interactions: a retrospective survey. *Clin Infect Dis.* 2006;43(2):180-187.

5. *Zyvox* [package insert]. New York, NY: Pfizer Inc; 2008.

Lisinopril (eg, *Prinivil*)

Lithium

SUMMARY: Several case reports suggest that lisinopril and other angiotensin-converting enzyme (ACE) inhibitors may increase the risk of serious lithium toxicity, but the incidence of this effect is unknown.

RISK FACTORS: No specific risk factors are known.

MECHANISM: Not established. It has been proposed that ACE inhibitor–induced sodium depletion results in more reabsorption of lithium from the renal tubule.[1] The resulting increase in serum lithium concentrations could have the following consequences: diarrhea (leading to volume depletion and further reduction in renal lithium excretion) and a renal concentration deficit (that could lead to further dehydration and lithium toxicity).

CLINICAL EVALUATION: A 65-year-old woman stabilized on lithium 800 mg/day and lisinopril 10 mg/day had serum lithium concentrations that were consistently in the therapeutic range (from 0.5 to 0.7 mmol/L).[2] However, after 4 days of loose stools, she was hospitalized with hypotension, oliguria, hyponatremia, and a lithium concentration that had increased to 2.5 mmol/L. She responded to discontinuation of the medications and 6 L of IV saline 0.9%. In a 49-year-old woman stabilized on lithium 1,500 mg/day, lisinopril 20 mg/day was substituted for clonidine 0.2 mg/day to treat hypertension.[1] Over the next 3 weeks, she developed tremor, fatigue, nausea, diarrhea, and slurred speech. She was hospitalized following the abrupt onset of confusion and agitation; her trough lithium concentration had risen to the toxic level of 3 mmol/L, and later to 3.8 mmol/L. Another case of possible enalapril-induced lithium toxicity was reported in a 61-year-old woman in whom the plasma lithium increased from 0.88 to 3.3 mmol/L.[3] She was later given nifedipine in place of enalapril without recurrence of lithium toxicity. Two additional cases of acute lithium toxicity were reported to occur 3 to 4 weeks after starting lisinopril or enalapril.[4]

RELATED DRUGS: Given the proposed mechanism, it appears likely that all ACE inhibitors (eg, enalapril [eg, *Vasotec*]) have the potential to produce lithium toxicity.

MANAGEMENT OPTIONS:

➡ ***Consider Alternative.*** If possible, avoid the concurrent use of an ACE inhibitor and lithium. Although it appears that patients can be stabilized on the 2 drugs, it is possible that other factors (eg, diarrhea) may unmask the interaction, resulting in lithium toxicity. If an alternative to an ACE inhibitor is used, remember that other antihypertensives, such as thiazides, calcium channel blockers, methyldopa, and possibly propranolol (eg, *Inderal*) and spironolactone (eg, *Aldactone*), also may affect lithium response.

➡ ***Monitor.*** If the combination of an ACE inhibitor and lithium is used, monitor the serum lithium concentration if the ACE inhibitor is initiated, discontinued, or changed in dosage. Monitor the patient for clinical evidence of lithium toxicity (eg, nausea, vomiting, diarrhea, anorexia, coarse tremor, slurred speech, vertigo, confusion, lethargy; in severe cases, seizures, stupor, coma, cardiovascular collapse). Adjust lithium dose as needed.

REFERENCES:

1. Baldwin CM, et al. A case of lisinopril-induced lithium toxicity. *DICP*. 1990;24(10):946-947.

2. Navis GJ, et al. Volume homeostasis, angiotensin converting enzyme inhibition, and lithium therapy. *Am J Med*. 1989;86(5):621.

3. Douste-Blazy P, et al. Angiotensin converting enzyme inhibitors and lithium treatment. *Lancet*. 1986;1(8495):1448.

4. Correa FJ, et al. Angiotensin-converting enzyme inhibitors and lithium toxicity. *Am J Med*. 1992;93(1):108-109.

4 **Lisinopril (eg, *Prinivil*)**

Olanzapine (*Zyprexa*)

SUMMARY: A patient on olanzapine developed pancreatitis 3 months after starting lisinopril, but a causal relationship was not established.

RISK FACTORS: No specific risk factors are known.

MECHANISM: Not established.

CLINICAL EVALUATION: A 69-year-old woman on long-term olanzapine therapy developed pancreatitis 3 months after starting lisinopril, and no other causes of pancreatitis were evident.[1] Olanzapine and lisinopril have been reported to cause pancreatitis, and it is possible that the pancreatitis resulted from the additive effect of the 2 drugs. Nonetheless, the data are also compatible with lisinopril-induced pancreatitis, so it is not possible to conclude that an interaction occurred. This case is rated "doubtful" using the Drug Interaction Probability Scale (DIPS).[2]

RELATED DRUGS: No information is available.

MANAGEMENT OPTIONS: No specific action is required, but be alert for evidence of the interaction.

REFERENCES:

1. Bracamonte JD, et al. Acute pancreatitis associated with lisinopril and olanzapine. *Am J Health Syst Pharm.* 2010;67(3):214-216.

2. Horn JR, et al. Proposal for a new tool to evaluate drug interaction cases. *Ann Pharmacother.* 2007;41(4):674-680.

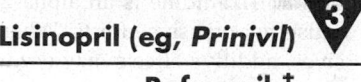

Lisinopril (eg, *Prinivil*)

Rofecoxib†

SUMMARY: Rofecoxib appears to inhibit the antihypertensive effect of lisinopril; monitor blood pressure and adjust lisinopril dosage as needed.

RISK FACTORS: No specific risk factors are known.

MECHANISM: Not established. Rofecoxib-induced inhibition of renal prostaglandins may be involved.

CLINICAL EVALUATION: A 59-year-old man with mild hypertension was successfully treated with lisinopril 10 mg/day.[1] Five weeks after starting rofecoxib 25 mg/day, a routine office visit revealed that his blood pressure had increased substantially to 168/98 mm Hg. Rofecoxib was discontinued, with lisinopril maintained at 10 mg/day. Within 4 days, his blood pressure had returned to prerofecoxib levels: 128/83 mm Hg. Several weeks later, rofecoxib 25 mg/day was again started and the blood pressure rose. However, increasing the lisinopril dose to 20 mg/day succeeded in bringing the blood pressure down to an average of 121/81 mm Hg. Given the positive dechallenge and rechallenge, it is likely that rofecoxib was responsible for the blood pressure changes in this patient. Moreover, these findings are consistent with the known interactive properties of both drugs. Although increasing the lisinopril dose controlled the blood pressure in this patient, other measures may be necessary in patients with more severe hypertension.

RELATED DRUGS: Theoretically, other COX-2 inhibitors such as celecoxib (*Celebrex*) may interact similarly with lisinopril and other ACE inhibitors, but little information is available. Several nonsteroidal anti-inflammatory drugs have been shown to inhibit the antihypertensive effect of ACE inhibitors.

MANAGEMENT OPTIONS:

➡ *Consider Alternative.* Antihypertensive agents other than ACE inhibitors (eg, calcium-channel blockers) may be less affected by COX-2 inhibitors.

➡ **Monitor.** If rofecoxib or other COX-2 inhibitors are used with lisinopril or other ACE inhibitors, monitor blood pressure carefully. Based on limited evidence, increasing the ACE inhibitor dose may circumvent the interaction in patients with mild hypertension.

REFERENCES:
1. Brown CH. Effect of rofecoxib on the antihypertensive activity of lisinopril. *Ann Pharmacother.* 2000;34:1486.

† Not available in the United States.

Lisinopril (eg, *Zestril*)

Tizanidine (eg, *Zanaflex*)

SUMMARY: Case reports and theoretical considerations suggest that tizanidine can result in hypotensive reactions when combined with lisinopril or other ACE inhibitors; monitor blood pressure closely.

RISK FACTORS: No specific risk factors are known.

MECHANISM: Tizanidine is an alpha-2 adrenergic agonist (like clonidine) and thus can cause hypotensive effects. When tizanidine is combined with other antihypertensives, additive effects may occur.

CLINICAL EVALUATION: A 48-year-old woman receiving lisinopril for hypertension following a cerebral hemorrhage developed acute hypotension 2 hours after receiving tizanidine 2 mg.[1] Lisinopril was discontinued, and tizanidine was later used without recurrence of the acute hypotension. A similar hypotensive reaction was reported in a 10-year-old boy on chronic lisinopril therapy who was started on tizanidine for spasticity.[2] Although clinical data are scarce, theoretical considerations strongly suggest that tizanidine would have additive effects with other antihypertensive drugs.

RELATED DRUGS: Other ACE inhibitors are likely to interact similarly with tizanidine, including benazepril (eg, *Lotensin*), captopril (eg, *Capoten*), enalapril (eg, *Vasotec*), fosinopril (eg, *Monopril*), lisinopril (eg, *Zestril*), moexipril (*Univasc*), quinapril (eg, *Accupril*), ramipril (*Altace*), and trandolapril (*Mavik*). Theoretically, tizanidine may also have additive effects with other types of antihypertensive agents, including angiotensin receptor blockers.

MANAGEMENT OPTIONS:

➡ **Monitor.** If tizanidine is used concurrently with ACE inhibitors or other antihypertensive agents, consider the possibility of an acute hypotensive reaction and take appropriate precautions. Monitor blood pressure closely. In patients requiring long-term therapy with tizanidine and antihypertensives, stabilization may be possible with adjustments to the antihypertensive regimen. However, any substantial change in tizanidine dose is likely to necessitate additional adjustments to the antihypertensive therapy.

REFERENCES:
1. Kao CD, et al. Hypotension due to interaction between lisinopril and tizanidine. *Ann Pharmacother.* 2004;38:1840-1843.
2. Johnson TR, et al. Hypotension following the initiation of tizanidine in a patient treated with an angiotensin-converting enzyme inhibitor for chronic hypertension. *J Child Neurol.* 2000;15:818-819.

Lithium (eg, *Eskalith*)

Losartan (*Cozaar*)

SUMMARY: An elderly patient developed lithium toxicity after starting losartan, but more study is needed to establish the clinical importance of this effect.

RISK FACTORS: No specific risk factors are known.

MECHANISM: Not established. Losartan may reduce the renal elimination of lithium.

CLINICAL EVALUATION: A 77-year-old woman stabilized on lithium developed lithium toxicity (eg, ataxia, confusion, dysarthria) 5 weeks after starting losartan 50 mg/day.[1] Plasma lithium increased from 0.63 to 2 mmol/L. She was subsequently stabilized on her previous dose of lithium when losartan was replaced with nicardipine. Although it appears that losartan increased plasma lithium concentrations in this patient, more study is needed to establish the incidence and magnitude of this interaction.

RELATED DRUGS: The effect of angiotensin-2 receptor antagonists other than losartan on lithium is not established; theoretically, they should interact similarly.

MANAGEMENT OPTIONS:

➡ **Monitor.** Be alert for evidence of lithium toxicity (eg, anorexia, coarse tremor, confusion, diarrhea, lethargy, nausea, slurred speech, vomiting, vertigo; in severe cases, cardiovascular collapse, coma, seizures, stupor). Adjust lithium dose as needed.

REFERENCES:

1. Blanche P, et al. Lithium intoxication in an elderly patient after combined treatment with losartan. *Eur J Clin Pharmacol.* 1997;52:501.

Lithium (eg, *Eskalith*)

Mefenamic Acid (*Ponstel*)

SUMMARY: Isolated cases of lithium toxicity have been associated with mefenamic acid therapy.

RISK FACTORS: No specific risk factors are known.

MECHANISM: Mefenamic acid may reduce the renal clearance of lithium. It has been proposed that renal tubular prostaglandins are involved in the excretion of lithium and that the antiprostaglandin effects of nonsteroidal anti-inflammatory drugs (NSAIDs) interfere with renal lithium elimination. More study is needed.

CLINICAL EVALUATION: A 29-year-old woman taking lithium developed a marked reduction in her lithium dosage requirements during therapy with mefenamic acid 500 mg 3 times daily for dysmenorrhea.[1] A subsequent challenge was positive, with symptoms consistent with lithium toxicity (eg, ataxia, disorientation, dysarthria) developing 4 days after mefenamic acid 250 to 500 mg 4 times daily was added to her lithium therapy.[2] Because several other NSAIDs have produced clinical evidence of lithium toxicity, it is reasonable to assume that mefenamic acid is capable of producing lithium toxicity in some patients.

RELATED DRUGS: Most NSAIDs increase lithium serum concentrations, but sulindac (eg, *Clinoril*) and aspirin appear to have minimal effects.

MANAGEMENT OPTIONS:

➡ *Consider Alternative.* If appropriate, consider using an anti-inflammatory agent that is less likely to affect lithium, such as sulindac or aspirin.

➡ *Monitor.* If mefenamic acid therapy is initiated in the presence of lithium therapy, monitor serum lithium concentrations. Be alert for symptoms consistent with lithium toxicity (eg, anorexia, coarse tremor, confusion, diarrhea, lethargy, nausea, slurred speech, vertigo, vomiting; in severe cases, cardiovascular collapse, coma, seizures, stupor). In patients stabilized on lithium and an NSAID, discontinuation of the NSAID may result in inadequate serum lithium concentrations.

REFERENCES:

1. MacDonald J, et al. Toxic interaction of lithium carbonate and mefenamic acid. *BMJ.* 1988;297:1339.
2. Shelley RK. Lithium toxicity and mefenamic acid. A possible interaction and the role of prostaglandin inhibition. *Br J Psychiatry.* 1987;151:847-848.

Lithium (eg, *Eskalith*)

Meloxicam (*Mobic*)

SUMMARY: Meloxicam increases lithium plasma concentrations and may produce lithium toxicity; the magnitude of the effect varies considerably among patients.

RISK FACTORS: No specific risk factors are known.

MECHANISM: Meloxicam probably reduces the renal clearance of lithium.

CLINICAL EVALUATION: Sixteen healthy subjects were given lithium with and without concurrent meloxicam 15 mg/day.[1] Meloxicam was associated with a 21% increase in lithium predose concentrations and lithium area under the plasma concentration-time curve.[1] While the mean increases in lithium plasma concentrations were modest, there was substantial interindividual variation. For example, the range for the changes in lithium predose concentrations was from a 9% decrease to a 59% increase. Thus, it seems likely that some patients would be adversely affected by this interaction.

RELATED DRUGS: Most NSAIDs appear to increase lithium plasma concentrations, and available evidence suggests that COX-2 inhibitors such as celecoxib (*Celebrex*) and rofecoxib (*Vioxx*) do as well. Some evidence suggests that sulindac (eg, *Clinoril*) does not interact with lithium, but isolated cases of increased lithium levels have been reported. Available evidence suggests that aspirin (even large doses) has little effect on lithium.

MANAGEMENT OPTIONS:

➡ *Monitor.* If meloxicam or another NSAID is used with lithium, monitor plasma lithium concentrations for symptoms consistent with lithium toxicity (eg, nausea, vomiting, diarrhea, anorexia, coarse tremor, slurred speech, vertigo, confusion, lethargy; in severe cases, seizures, stupor, coma, and cardiovascular collapse).

REFERENCES:

1. Turck D, et al. Steady-state pharmacokinetics of lithium in healthy volunteers receiving concomitant meloxicam. *Br J Clin Pharmacol.* 2000;50:197-204.

Lithium (eg, *Eskalith*)

Methyldopa (eg, *Aldomet*)

SUMMARY: Methyldopa was associated with evidence of lithium toxicity in several patients, but a causal relationship was not firmly established.

RISK FACTORS: No specific risk factors are known.

MECHANISM: Not established.

CLINICAL EVALUATION: Two patients stabilized on lithium carbonate therapy developed signs of lithium toxicity when methyldopa was added to their therapy.[1,2] Another patient receiving methyldopa developed signs of lithium intoxication after 2 days of lithium therapy.[3] Three healthy subjects developed adverse effects when methyldopa was added to lithium therapy.[4] In all these cases, serum lithium concentrations were within the therapeutic range. Another patient well controlled on lithium presented with signs of lithium toxicity and excessive lithium plasma concentrations 3 days after starting methyldopa.[5] Although these cases do not prove a causal relationship, they are sufficient to warrant caution when methyldopa and lithium are used concurrently.

RELATED DRUGS: No information is available.

MANAGEMENT OPTIONS:

➡ *Consider Alternative.* In patients who need lithium therapy, consider using antihypertensive therapy other than methyldopa.

➡ *Monitor.* If the combination is used, monitor for evidence of lithium intoxication (eg, nausea, vomiting, tremor, confusion, weakness, dizziness, slurred speech). Plasma lithium concentrations may not be useful in detecting this interaction because they may be in the therapeutic range.

REFERENCES:

1. O'Regan JB. Adverse interactions of lithium carbonate and methyldopa. *Can Med Assoc J.* 1976;115:385. Letter.
2. Byrd GJ. Methyldopa and lithium carbonate: suspected interaction. *JAMA.* 1975;233:320. Letter.
3. Osanloo E, et al. Interaction of lithium and methyldopa. *Ann Intern Med.* 1980;92:433.
4. Walker N, et al. Lithium-methyldopa interactions in normal subjects. *DICP.* 1980;14:638.
5. Yassa R. Lithium-methyldopa interaction. *Can Med Assoc J.* 1986;134:141.

Lithium (eg, *Eskalith*) **5**

Moclobemide†

SUMMARY: Preliminary evidence indicates that moclobemide does not interact adversely with lithium.

RISK FACTORS: No specific risk factors are known.

MECHANISM: No interaction.

CLINICAL EVALUATION: Fifty patients stabilized on lithium were given moclobemide 150 to 675 mg/day for 3 to 52 weeks.[1] No difference in adverse effects was noted in the patients receiving lithium plus moclobemide compared with those receiving moclobemide alone. Moreover, combined therapy did not appear to result in changes in vital signs, ECG, or laboratory tests. Although few details of the study are presented, the evidence suggests that moclobemide and lithium do not interact adversely.

RELATED DRUGS: No information is available.

MANAGEMENT OPTIONS: No interaction.

REFERENCES:

1. Amrein R, et al. Interactions of moclobemide with concomitantly administered medication: evidence from pharmacological and clinical studies. *Psychopharmacology*. 1992;106:S24.

† Not available in the United States.

Lithium (eg, *Eskalith*)

Naproxen (eg, *Naprosyn*)

SUMMARY: Naproxen increases lithium serum concentrations and may increase the risk of lithium toxicity; the magnitude of the effect appears to vary considerably from patient to patient.

RISK FACTORS: No specific risk factors are known.

MECHANISM: Naproxen appears to reduce the renal clearance of lithium. It has been proposed that renal tubular prostaglandins are involved in the excretion of lithium and that the antiprostaglandin effects of nonsteroidal anti-inflammatory drugs (NSAIDs) interfere with renal lithium elimination; more study is needed.

CLINICAL EVALUATION: In 7 patients with steady-state lithium serum concentrations, the addition of naproxen 750 mg/day for 6 days resulted in a steady increase in serum lithium concentrations over the 6 day period.[1] Although the mean increase in serum lithium was only 16%, there was marked interpatient variability (range: 0% to 42%). Since several other NSAIDs have produced clinical evidence of lithium toxicity, it is reasonable to assume that naproxen also is capable of doing so in at least some patients.

RELATED DRUGS: Most NSAIDs increase lithium serum concentrations, but sulindac (eg, *Clinoril*) and aspirin appear to have minimal effects.

MANAGEMENT OPTIONS:

➡ **Consider Alternative.** If appropriate for the patient, consider using an anti-inflammatory agent that is less likely to affect lithium, such as sulindac or aspirin.

➡ **Monitor.** If naproxen therapy is initiated in the presence of lithium therapy, monitor serum lithium concentrations and for symptoms consistent with lithium toxicity (eg, nausea, vomiting, diarrhea, anorexia, coarse tremor, slurred speech, vertigo, confusion, lethargy; in severe cases, seizures, stupor, coma, cardiovascular collapse). In a patient stabilized on lithium and an NSAID, discontinuation of the NSAID may result in inadequate serum lithium concentrations.

REFERENCES:

1. Ragheb M, et al. Lithium interaction with sulindac and naproxen. *J Clin Psychopharmacol*. 1986;6:150.

Lithium (eg, *Eskalith*)

Norepinephrine (*Levophed*)

SUMMARY: Lithium may decrease slightly the pressor response to norepinephrine, but the clinical importance of this effect is probably minimal.

RISK FACTORS: No specific risk factors are known.

MECHANISM: Not established.

CLINICAL EVALUATION: Eight patients with manic depressive illness were given norepinephrine before and after 7 to 10 days of lithium carbonate treatment.[1] Lithium decreased the pressor response to norepinephrine 22%. This effect would seem unlikely to cause clinical difficulties.

RELATED DRUGS: No information is available.

MANAGEMENT OPTIONS: No specific action is required, but be alert for evidence of the interaction.

REFERENCES:

1. Fann WE, et al. Effects of lithium on adrenogenic function in man. *Clin Pharmacol Ther.* 1973;13:71.

Lithium (eg, *Eskalith*) 4

Paroxetine (*Paxil*)

SUMMARY: A patient on paroxetine developed symptoms consistent with serotonin syndrome after starting lithium therapy, but a causal relationship was not established.

RISK FACTORS: No specific risk factors are known.

MECHANISM: Not established.

CLINICAL EVALUATION: A 59-year-old woman stabilized on paroxetine developed evidence of serotonin syndrome (ie, shivering, tremor, flushed face, agitation) six days after lithium therapy was started.[1] The paroxetine serum concentration was about six times higher than expected. Another patient on paroxetine alone developed a similar paroxetine serum concentration, but had no adverse effects. The authors propose that some patients develop particularly high serum concentrations of paroxetine, and in such patients lithium therapy may increase the risk of serotonin syndrome through a pharmacodynamic interaction. More study is needed to establish whether lithium increases the risk of serotonin syndrome in patients receiving paroxetine or other selective serotonin reuptake inhibitors.

RELATED DRUGS: Adverse neurological effects have also been noted in several patients when lithium was combined with fluoxetine (*Prozac*) or fluvoxamine (*Luvox*).

MANAGEMENT OPTIONS: No specific action is required, but be alert for evidence of the interaction.

REFERENCES:

1. Sobanski T, et al. Serotonin syndrome after lithium add-on medication to paroxetine. *Pharmacopsychiatry.* 1997;30:106.

Lithium (eg, *Eskalith*)

Phenelzine (*Nardil*)

SUMMARY: Two fatal cases of malignant hyperpyrexia have been reported in patients taking lithium and phenelzine, but a causal relationship was not established.

RISK FACTORS: No specific risk factors are known.

MECHANISM: Not established.

CLINICAL EVALUATION: A patient with a history of depression had been taking phenelzine 15 mg 3 times a day, lithium carbonate 800 mg/day, L-tryptophan 1 g/day, diazepam 2 mg 3 times a day, and triazolam 0.25 mg/day.[1] Six weeks after starting phenelzine, she developed rigidity, hyperthermia, tachycardia, hypotension, and hepatic failure that culminated in her death. A second fatal reaction was reported in a patient taking lithium 800 mg/day, L-tryptophan 6 g/day, and chlorpromazine 300 mg/day.[2] Approximately 1 month later, she developed rigidity, nystagmus, hyperreflexia, hyperthermia, hepatic failure, and eventually cardiac arrest. In both cases, the authors attributed the adverse events to an interaction between lithium and phenelzine. However, both patients were taking L-tryptophan which could have contributed to the reactions.

RELATED DRUGS: Until more information is available, one should assume that other nonselective monoamine oxidase inhibitors (MAOIs) such as isocarboxazid (*Marplan*) and tranylcypromine (*Parnate*) also can interact with lithium.

MANAGEMENT OPTIONS:

➡ *Avoid Unless Benefit Outweighs Risk.* Given the severity of the reported interactions, it would be prudent to avoid concurrent use of lithium with nonselective MAOIs until additional information is available. The effects of nonselective MAOIs should be assumed to persist for 2 weeks after they are discontinued.

➡ *Monitor.* Patients treated with nonselective MAOIs and lithium should be observed closely for evidence of neuroleptic malignant-like syndrome.

REFERENCES:
1. Brennan D, et al. Neuroleptic malignant syndrome without neuroleptics. *Br J Psychiatry*. 1988;152:578.
2. Staufenberg EF, et al. Malignant hyperpyrexia syndrome in combined treatment. *Br J Psychiatry*. 1989;154:577.

 Lithium (eg, *Eskalith*)

Phenylbutazone

SUMMARY: Phenylbutazone appears to increase lithium serum concentrations, but the magnitude of the effect appears to vary considerably from patient to patient. Limited evidence suggests that phenylbutazone may result in adverse psychiatric symptoms in patients receiving lithium.

RISK FACTORS: No specific risk factors are known.

MECHANISM: Phenylbutazone, like other nonsteroidal anti-inflammatory drugs (NSAIDs), probably inhibits the renal clearance of lithium.

CLINICAL EVALUATION: In 5 patients with bipolar affective illness and steady-state lithium serum concentrations, serum lithium concentrations increased only slightly when given phenylbutazone 100 mg 3 times a day for 6 days.[1] However, 1 patient was receiving theophylline, a drug known to enhance renal lithium excretion. Three of the patients developed adverse symptoms after starting the phenylbutazone, including 1 with paranoid delusions and 1 with confusion and disorientation. These symptoms resolved when the phenylbutazone was stopped. The small increases in lithium serum concentrations are in contrast to 2 previous case reports cited by the authors in which lithium levels doubled within 36 hours of starting phenylbutazone 750 mg/day as suppositories. Since several other NSAIDs have produced clinical evidence of lithium toxicity, it is reasonable to assume that phenylbutazone (and oxyphenbutazone) also is capable of doing so in at least some patients.

RELATED DRUGS: Most NSAIDs increase lithium serum concentrations, but sulindac (eg, *Clinoril*) and aspirin appear to have minimal effects.

MANAGEMENT OPTIONS:

➡ *Consider Alternative.* If appropriate for the patient, consider using an anti-inflammatory agent that is less likely to affect lithium, such as sulindac or aspirin.

➡ *Monitor.* Monitor serum lithium concentrations and for symptoms consistent with lithium toxicity (eg, nausea, vomiting, diarrhea, anorexia, coarse tremor, slurred speech, vertigo, confusion, lethargy; in severe cases, seizures, stupor, coma, cardiovascular collapse) when phenylbutazone therapy is initiated. In a patient stabilized on lithium and an NSAID, discontinuation of the NSAID may result in inadequate serum lithium concentrations.

REFERENCES:

1. Ragheb M. The interaction of lithium with phenylbutazone in bipolar affective patients. *J Clin Psycho pharmacol.* 1990;10:149. Letter.

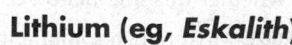

Lithium (eg, *Eskalith*)

Phenytoin (eg, *Dilantin*)

SUMMARY: Some patients have developed lithium intoxication following phenytoin use, but a causal relationship has not been established.

RISK FACTORS: No specific risk factors are known.

MECHANISM: Not established.

CLINICAL EVALUATION: A few cases of possible phenytoin enhanced lithium toxicity have been reported.[1-3] However, it was not clearly established that a lithium-phenytoin interaction was responsible for the effects. The patients developed ataxia,[1] tremor with gastrointestinal symptoms[2] or tremor with polyuria, and increased thirst.[3]

RELATED DRUGS: No information is available.

MANAGEMENT OPTIONS:

➡ *Monitor.* Until more information is available, be alert for evidence of lithium toxicity when phenytoin is given concurrently.

REFERENCES:

1. Salem RB, et al. Ataxia as the primary symptom of lithium toxicity. *Drug Intell Clin Pharm.* 1980;14:621.

2. Spiers J et al. Severe lithium toxicity within normal serum concentrations. *Br Med J.* 1978;1:815.

3. MacCallum WAG. Interaction of lithium and phenytoin. *Br Med J.* 1980;280:610.

Lithium (eg, *Eskalith*)

Piroxicam (eg, *Feldene*)

SUMMARY: Piroxicam was associated with symptoms of lithium toxicity in one well-documented case report, but the incidence of this effect in patients receiving this drug combination is not known.

RISK FACTORS: No specific risk factors are known.

MECHANISM: Not established. Piroxicam-induced prostaglandin inhibition may inhibit renal sodium excretion, leading to increased lithium reabsorption from the renal tubule.

CLINICAL EVALUATION: A 56-year-old woman stabilized on lithium for 10 years developed elevated serum lithium levels and symptoms of lithium toxicity after starting piroxicam therapy.[1] The same patient subsequently was studied under controlled conditions while on lithium 750 mg/day. The serum lithium increased to 1.5 mmol/L (therapeutic range: 0.8 to 1.4 mmol/L) after starting piroxicam 20 mg/day and fell to 1.0 mmol/L a few weeks after discontinuation of piroxicam. Piroxicam probably was responsible for the changes in serum lithium levels in this patient given the temporal relationship and the known effect of other prostaglandin inhibitors on lithium disposition. Additional study is required to determine whether this interaction consistently occurs in patients receiving the 2 drugs.

RELATED DRUGS: Most nonsteroidal anti-inflammatory drugs increase lithium serum concentrations, but sulindac (eg, *Clinoril*) and aspirin appear to have minimal effects.

MANAGEMENT OPTIONS:

➡ *Consider Alternative.* If appropriate for the patient, consider using an anti-inflammatory agent that is less likely to affect lithium, such as sulindac or aspirin.

➡ *Monitor.* Be alert for evidence of increased lithium effect when piroxicam is started or stopped (eg, nausea, vomiting, diarrhea, anorexia, coarse tremor, slurred speech, vertigo, confusion, lethargy; in severe cases, seizures, stupor, coma, cardiovascular collapse). Serum lithium determinations would be useful in monitoring this interaction.

REFERENCES:

1. Kerry RJ, et al. Possible toxic interaction between lithium and piroxicam. *Lancet.* 1983;1:418.

Lithium (eg, *Eskalith*)

Potassium Iodide

SUMMARY: Hypothyroidism may be more likely in patients receiving both lithium and potassium iodide than in those receiving either drug alone, but the degree of increased risk is not established.

RISK FACTORS: No specific risk factors are known.

MECHANISM: Lithium carbonate and iodide preparations may have synergistic hypothyroid activity.

CLINICAL EVALUATION: Either lithium carbonate or iodide alone can produce hypothyroidism. Nevertheless, several patients have been described in whom potassium iodide appeared to act synergistically with lithium carbonate in producing hypothyroidism.[1-4]

RELATED DRUGS: No information is available.

MANAGEMENT OPTIONS:

➡ *Monitor.* If it is necessary to use lithium and iodide concomitantly, monitor the patient for signs of hypothyroidism.

REFERENCES:

1. Shopsin B, et al. Iodine and lithium-induced hypothyroidism: documentation of synergism. *Am J Med.* 1973;55:695.
2. Swedberg K, et al. Heart failure as complication of lithium treatment. *Acta Med Scand.* 1974;196:279.
3. Wiener JD. Lithium carbonate-induced myxedema. *JAMA.* 1972;220:587.
4. Jorgensen JV, et al. Possible synergism between iodine and lithium carbonate. *JAMA.* 1973;223:192.

Lithium (eg, *Eskalith*)

Propranolol (eg, *Inderal*)

SUMMARY: Limited clinical data suggest that propranolol may increase lithium serum concentrations.

RISK FACTORS: No specific risk factors are known.

MECHANISM: Not established. Propranolol may reduce lithium renal clearance.

CLINICAL EVALUATION: Lithium clearance in patients who also were taking propranolol was noted to be approximately 20% lower than in patients not receiving propranolol.[1] No difference in clinical response was reported (nor would it be expected) between the 2 groups of patients. In another report, a patient maintained on chronic lithium therapy developed bradycardia and syncope 6 weeks after propranolol 30 mg/day was prescribed.[2] Both drugs were discontinued; the pulse returned to normal and did not fall in response to lithium rechallenge.

RELATED DRUGS: Other beta blockers may produce similar effects.

MANAGEMENT OPTIONS: No specific action is required, but be alert for evidence of the interaction.

REFERENCES:

1. Schou M, et al. Use of propranolol during lithium treatment: an enquiry and suggestion. *Pharmacopsychiatry.* 1987;20:131.
2. Becker D. Lithium and propranolol: possible synergism? *J Clin Psychiatry.* 1989;50:473.

Lithium (eg, *Eskalith*)

Sibutramine (*Meridia*)

SUMMARY: The risk of serotonin syndrome would theoretically increase when sibutramine is combined with other serotonergic drugs such as lithium.

RISK FACTORS: No specific risk factors are known.

MECHANISM: Sibutramine inhibits serotonin reuptake; additive serotonergic effects may occur with lithium. However, the serotonergic effect of lithium is not well characterized.

CLINICAL EVALUATION: While no published data are available for evaluation, the manufacturer of sibutramine has made available some data on this interaction.[1] Since sibutramine has serotonergic effects, its concurrent use with other serotonergic drugs (eg, lithium) may increase the risk of serotonin syndrome.[1] Although the actual risk of combining sibutramine with serotonergic drugs is unknown, the fact that serotonin syndrome can result in serious or fatal reactions must be considered.

RELATED DRUGS: No information is available.

MANAGEMENT OPTIONS:

➡ *Avoid Unless Benefit Outweighs Risk.* The manufacturer states that sibutramine should not be used with lithium. This is a prudent recommendation until more information is available.

➡ *Monitor.* Serotonin syndrome can result in neurotoxicity (ie, myoclonus, tremors, rigidity, incoordination, restlessness, hyperreflexia, seizures, coma), psychiatric symptoms (ie, agitation, confusion, hypomania), and temperature regulation abnormalities (ie, fever, sweating). Note that mild forms of serotonin syndrome have also been reported, so any combination of the above symptoms should be considered possibly related to excessive serotonin activity.

REFERENCES:

1. Product information. Sibutramine (*Meridia*). Knoll Pharmaceuticals. 1997.
2. Mills KC. Serotonin syndrome: a clinical update. *Crit Care Clin.* 1997;13:763.

 Lithium (eg, *Eskalith*)

Sodium Bicarbonate

SUMMARY: Sodium bicarbonate may lower plasma lithium concentrations.

RISK FACTORS: No specific risk factors are known.

MECHANISM: Sodium bicarbonate appears to increase the renal excretion of lithium.[1] This may be partly due to the sodium content of the sodium bicarbonate.

CLINICAL EVALUATION: Increased lithium excretion by sodium bicarbonate could impair the therapeutic response to lithium carbonate; however, the magnitude of this interaction is not established.

RELATED DRUGS: No information is available.

MANAGEMENT OPTIONS:

➡ **Monitor.** Patients on combined sodium bicarbonate and lithium therapy should be monitored for decreased lithium effect. Lithium blood levels may be helpful in assessing this interaction.

REFERENCES:

1. Thomsen K, et al. Renal lithium excretion in man. *Am J Physiol.* 1968;215:823.

Lithium (eg, *Eskalith*)

Sodium Chloride

SUMMARY: High sodium intake may reduce serum lithium concentrations, while restriction of sodium may increase serum lithium.

RISK FACTORS: No specific risk factors are known.

MECHANISM: Lithium excretion appears to be proportional to the intake of sodium chloride.

CLINICAL EVALUATION: Patients on salt-restricted diets who receive lithium carbonate are prone to developing symptoms of lithium toxicity.[1-4] In contrast, increased sodium intake has been associated with a reduced therapeutic response to lithium as well as a decrease in side effects.[5] Large doses of sodium chloride increase lithium excretion and have been recommended by some for the treatment of lithium intoxication.

RELATED DRUGS: No information is available.

MANAGEMENT OPTIONS:

➡ **Circumvent/Minimize.** Extremely large or small intakes of sodium chloride should be avoided in patients receiving lithium carbonate. Patients on severe salt-restricted diets probably should not be given lithium carbonate.

➡ **Monitor.** Monitor for increased lithium response if sodium intake is reduced and for decreased lithium response if sodium intake is increased.

REFERENCES:

1. Hurtig HI, et al. Lithium toxicity enhanced by diuresis. *N Engl J Med.* 1974;290:748.
2. Platman SR, et al. Lithium retention and excretion. The effect of sodium and fluid intake. *Arch Gen Psychiatry.* 1969;20:285.
3. Bleiweiss H. Salt supplements with lithium. *Lancet.* 1970;1:416. Letter.
4. Levy ST, et al. Lithium-induced diabetes insipidus: manic symptoms, brain and electrolyte correlates, and chlorothiazide treatment. *Am J Psychiatry.* 1973;130:1014.
5. Demers RG, et al. Sodium intake and lithium treatment in mania. *Am J Psychiatry.* 1971;128:1.

Lithium (eg, *Eskalith*)

Spironolactone (eg, *Aldactone*)

SUMMARY: Spironolactone may enhance lithium effects, but the clinical importance is not established.

RISK FACTORS: No specific risk factors are known.

MECHANISM: Not established.

CLINICAL EVALUATION: In several patients with manic depressive illness, spironolactone 100 mg/day was associated with increasing serum lithium concentrations.[2] Another patient has been described in whom spironolactone and lithium act synergistically in the treatment of mania.[1] Studies in additional patients are needed to assess the clinical importance of these findings.

RELATED DRUGS: No information is available.

MANAGEMENT OPTIONS: No specific action is required, but be alert for evidence of the interaction.

REFERENCES:

1. Gillman MA, et al. Synergism of spironolactone and lithium in mania. *Br Med J.* 1986;292;661.
2. Baer L, et al. Mechanisms of renal lithium handling and their relationship to mineralocorticoids: a dissociation between sodium and lithium ions. *J Psychiatr Res.* 1971;8;91.

 Lithium (eg, *Eskalith*)

Succinylcholine (eg, *Anectine*)

SUMMARY: Lithium may prolong the effect of neuromuscular blockers such as succinylcholine, but the clinical importance of this effect is not established.

RISK FACTORS: No specific risk factors are known.

MECHANISM: Not established.

CLINICAL EVALUATION: A patient on chronic lithium carbonate therapy developed a prolonged apnea (4 hours) following the use of succinylcholine during surgery.[3] Some have questioned the clinical importance of this interaction.[4]

RELATED DRUGS: Lithium also has enhanced the neuromuscular blocking activity of pancuronium.[2] Studies in dogs indicate that lithium can prolong the neuromuscular blockade of succinylcholine, decamethonium, and pancuronium (eg, *Pavulon*).[1]

MANAGEMENT OPTIONS: No specific action is required, but be alert for evidence of the interaction.

REFERENCES:

1. Hill GE, et al. Lithium carbonate and neuromuscular blocking agents. *Anesthesiology.* 1977;46:122.
2. Borden H, et al. The use of pancuronium bromide in patients receiving lithium carbonate. *Can Anaesth Soc J.* 1974;21:79.
3. Hill GE, et al. Potentiation of succinylcholine neuromuscular blockade by lithium carbonate. *Anesthesiology.* 1976;44:439.
4. Martin BA, et al. Clinical significance of the interaction between lithium and a neuromuscular blocker. *Am J Psychiatry.* 1982;139:1326.

4 **Lithium (eg, *Eskalith*)**

Sulindac (eg, *Clinoril*)

SUMMARY: Sulindac appears to reduce serum lithium concentrations temporarily, but current evidence suggests that no changes in lithium dose are required.

RISK FACTORS: No specific risk factors are known.

MECHANISM: Not established.

CLINICAL EVALUATION: In 2 patients stabilized on lithium, the administration of sulindac (200 to 400 mg/day) was associated with substantial but temporary *reductions* in serum lithium concentrations.[1] There were no obvious changes in lithium effect. In 6 patients with steady-state lithium serum concentrations, the addition of sulindac 300 mg/day for 6 days appeared to reduce serum lithium somewhat on the third day of sulindac, but by day 6 there was no effect on serum lithium concentrations or lithium clearance.[2] These investigators also described briefly a patient on lithium in whom sulindac was started and stopped on several occasions without any effect on serum lithium concentration or the need to adjust lithium dosage. Another report described 4 patients in whom sulindac had no effect on serum lithium concentrations,[3] but at least some of these patients are the same as those described in the report described above.[2] Nonsteroidal anti-inflammatory drugs (NSAIDs) other than sulindac appear to *increase* serum lithium concentrations.

RELATED DRUGS: Most NSAIDs other than sulindac appear to increase lithium serum concentrations, but aspirin, like sulindac, appears to have minimal effects.

MANAGEMENT OPTIONS: No specific action is required, but be alert for evidence of the interaction.

REFERENCES:
1. Furnell MM, et al. The effect of sulindac on lithium therapy. *DICP.* 1985;19:374.
2. Ragheb M, et al. Lithium interaction with sulindac and naproxen. *J Clin Psychopharmacol.* 1986;6:150.
3. Ragheb M, et al. Failure of sulindac to increase serum lithium levels. *J Clin Psychiatry.* 1986;47:33.

Lithium (eg, *Eskalith*)

Sumatriptan (*Imitrex*)

SUMMARY: A patient on lithium and sumatriptan developed serotonin syndrome, but the patient was also receiving other serotonergic drugs and the role that lithium played in the reaction was not established.

RISK FACTORS: No specific risk factors known.

MECHANISM: Lithium and sumatriptan theoretically may have additive serotonergic effects, but the serotonergic effect of lithium is not well characterized.

CLINICAL EVALUATION: A 44-year-old woman on methysergide, lithium, and sertraline for migraine prophylaxis administered a 6 mg subcutaneous dose of sumatriptan for an acute migraine attack. One hour later she was brought to the emergency room with evidence of serotonin syndrome (ie, weakness, incoordination, myoclonic jerking, hypomania, shivering, and hyperreflexia).[1] Her symptoms resolved over 24 to 48 hours, and she was discharged on prophylaxis with methysergide, sertraline, and sumatriptan for acute attacks. In the next month she used sumatriptan 5 times, and had a similar (but less severe) reaction each time. After discontinuation of sertraline, she used sumatriptan without developing any evidence of serotonin syndrome. Thus, the patient developed severe serotonin syndrome while on 4 serotonergic drugs (methysergide, lithium, sertraline, sumatriptan), mild serotonergic syndrome while on 3 serotonergic drugs (methysergide, sertraline, sumatriptan), and no reaction while on 2 (methysergide, sumatriptan). Other isolated cases of possible serotonin syndrome have been reported in patients receiving sumatriptan and lithium, but some patients have also received the combination with no evidence of excess serotonin activity.

RELATED DRUGS: Little is known regarding concurrent use of zolmitriptan (*Zomig*) and lithium, but it is possible that there may be a small increase in the risk of serotonin syndrome.

MANAGEMENT OPTIONS: No specific action is required, but be alert for evidence of the interaction.

REFERENCES:

1. Mathew NT, et al. Serotonin syndrome complicating migraine pharmacotherapy. *Cephalagia*. 1996;16:323.

2. Gardner DM, et al. Sumatriptan contraindications and the serotonin syndrome. *Ann Pharmacother*. 1998;32:33.

3. Mills KC. Serotonin syndrome: a clinical update. *Crit Care Clin*. 1997;13:763.

 Lithium (eg, *Eskalith*)

Tetracycline (eg, *Achromycin V*)

SUMMARY: In a single case report lithium concentrations increased following tetracycline administration; however, a prospective study found small decreases in lithium concentrations when both drugs were administered.

RISK FACTORS: No specific risk factors are known.

MECHANISM: It has been proposed that tetracycline-induced renal impairment may reduce urinary lithium excretion, but the mechanism is unknown and is likely to be limited.

CLINICAL EVALUATION: A patient's plasma lithium concentration increased from 0.81 mmol/L (0.56 mg/100 mL) to 2.74 mmol/L (1.9 mg/100 mL) 4 days after initiation of tetracycline therapy 750 mg/day.[1] Lithium concentrations fell after discontinuation of both drugs; no rechallenge was attempted. In a study of 13 healthy subjects who received controlled-release lithium 450 mg twice daily alone and with tetracycline 500 mg twice daily for 7 days,[2] lithium concentrations were 8% lower during tetracycline dosing.

RELATED DRUGS: No information is available.

MANAGEMENT OPTIONS: No specific action is required, but be alert for evidence of the interaction.

REFERENCES:

1. McGennis AJ. Lithium carbonate and tetracycline interaction. *Br Med J*. 1978;1:1183.

2. Frankhauser MP, et al. Evaluation of lithium-tetracycline interaction. *Clin Pharm*. 1988;7:314.

 Lithium (eg, *Lithobid*)

Theophylline (eg, *Theo-24*)

SUMMARY: Theophylline appears to increase renal lithium clearance in most patients; the magnitude of the effect probably is sufficient to reduce lithium efficacy in some patients.

RISK FACTORS: No specific risk factors are known.

MECHANISM: Theophylline enhances the renal clearance of lithium, which tends to reduce serum lithium concentrations.[1-3]

CLINICAL EVALUATION: In 5 healthy subjects given lithium carbonate 600 mg with and without administration of oral aminophylline 1 g, renal lithium excretion increased a mean of 58% during aminophylline administration.[1] In another study, theophylline increased renal lithium clearance 30% in 10 healthy subjects given lithium for 3 weeks with concurrent theophylline given during week 2 (mean theophylline serum level 9.2 mcg/mL).[3] A 65-year-old man with chronic obstructive pulmonary disease and mania required an increased lithium dosage when his theophylline dosage was increased.[2]

RELATED DRUGS: No information is available.

MANAGEMENT OPTIONS:

➤ *Circumvent/Minimize.* Avoid intermittent use of theophylline in a patient on chronic lithium because the patient's response to lithium may fluctuate each time the theophylline is started or stopped.

➤ *Monitor.* When initiating theophylline therapy in a patient on chronic lithium, be alert for evidence of reduced lithium response. Discontinuation of theophylline therapy in a patient receiving lithium may result in excessive lithium response. When initiating lithium therapy in a patient on chronic theophylline, lithium dosage requirements may be higher than anticipated. Measurement of serum lithium concentrations would be useful in monitoring this interaction.

REFERENCES:

1. Thomsen K, et al. Renal lithium excretion in man. *Am J Physiol.* 1968;215(4):823-827.
2. Sierles FS, et al. Concurrent use of theophylline and lithium in a patient with chronic obstructive lung disease and bipolar disorder. *Am J Psychiatry.* 1982;139(1):117-118.
3. Cook BL, et al. Theophylline-lithium interaction. *J Clin Psychiatry.* 1985;46(7):278-279.

Lithium (eg, *Lithobid*)

Topiramate (*Topamax*)

SUMMARY: Two cases of lithium toxicity caused by topiramate have been reported, but a causal relationship was not established.

RISK FACTORS: No specific risk factors are known.

MECHANISM: Not established.

CLINICAL EVALUATION: A 26-year-old woman on chronic lithium therapy (900 mg/day), with a lithium concentration of 0.82 mmol/L, was started on topiramate 75 mg/day upon admission.[1] One week later, her lithium concentration had increased to 1.24 mmol/L, and the lithium dose was reduced to 750 mg/day. Four days later, the lithium concentration continued to increase to 1.97 mmol/L, and the lithium was discontinued. After lithium was restarted at 450 mg/day, increasing the dose of topiramate was associated with corresponding increases in lithium concentrations. Another case of lithium toxicity following an increase in topiramate dose has been reported.[2] Additional study is needed to determine whether topiramate increases lithium serum concentrations, and, if so, under which conditions.

RELATED DRUGS: No information is available.

MANAGEMENT OPTIONS: No specific action is required, but be alert for evidence of the interaction.

REFERENCES:
1. Abraham G, et al. Topiramate can cause lithium toxicity. *J Clin Psychopharmacol.* 2004;24(5):565-567.
2. Pinninti NR, et al. Does topiramate elevate serum lithium levels? *J Clin Psychopharmacol.* 2002;22(3):340.

4 Lithium (eg, *Lithobid*)

Urea (*Ureaphil*)

SUMMARY: Urea may reduce serum lithium concentrations.

RISK FACTORS: No specific risk factors are known.

MECHANISM: Urea appears to increase the renal excretion of lithium.

CLINICAL EVALUATION: Single-dose studies in healthy subjects indicate that urea may enhance the renal excretion of lithium.[1] The clinical significance of this finding is unclear.

RELATED DRUGS: No information is available.

MANAGEMENT OPTIONS: No specific action is required, but be alert for evidence of the interaction.

REFERENCES:
1. Thomsen K, et al. Renal lithium excretion in man. *Am J Physiol.* 1968;215(4):823-827.

Lithium (eg, *Lithobid*)

Venlafaxine (*Effexor*)

SUMMARY: A patient on lithium and venlafaxine developed serotonin toxicity, but a causal relationship was not established.

RISK FACTORS: No specific risk factors are known.

MECHANISM: Probable additive serotonergic effects.

CLINICAL EVALUATION: A 71-year-old woman on venlafaxine 150 mg/day and lithium 600 mg/day developed myoclonus, tremor, hyperreflexia, tremor, and confusion.[1] The symptoms clearly supported a diagnosis of serotonin toxicity.[2,3] Both drugs have serotonergic effects, but lithium is generally considered to have a modest effect. Moreover, patients often receive lithium and selective serotonin reuptake inhibitors (SSRIs) concurrently without evidence of serotonin toxicity.

RELATED DRUGS: Theoretically other antidepressants that inhibit serotonin reuptake (clomipramine [eg, *Anafranil*], duloxetine [*Cymbalta*], escitalopram [*Lexapro*], fluoxetine [eg, *Prozac*], fluvoxamine, imipramine [eg, *Tofranil*], paroxetine [eg, *Paxil*], sertraline [eg, *Zoloft*]) may also increase the risk of serotonin toxicity when combined with lithium.

MANAGEMENT OPTIONS:

➡ *Monitor.* If the combination is used, monitor for symptoms of serotonin toxicity, including myoclonus, rigidity, tremor, hyperreflexia, seizures, confusion, agitation, hypomania, incoordination, fever, sweating, shivering, and coma.

REFERENCES:

1. Adan-Manes J, et al. Lithium and venlafaxine interaction: a case of serotonin syndrome. *J Clin Pharm Ther*. 2006;31(4):397-400.

2. Isbister GK, et al. Serotonin toxicity: a practical approach to diagnosis and treatment. *Med J Aust*. 2007;187(6):361-365.

3. Boyer EW, et al. The serotonin syndrome. *N Engl J Med*. 2005;352(11):1112-1120.

Lithium (eg, *Lithobid*)

Verapamil (eg, *Calan*)

SUMMARY: The addition of verapamil or diltiazem (eg, *Cardizem*) to the regimen of patients stabilized on lithium therapy may result in neurotoxicity.

RISK FACTORS: No specific risk factors are known.

MECHANISM: Lithium can decrease the transport of calcium ions into cells and alter neurotransmitter secretion. Calcium channel blocker effects may be additive to that of lithium on transmitter secretion in the CNS.

CLINICAL EVALUATION: A 42-year-old woman with a bipolar disorder developed nausea, vomiting, weakness, tinnitus, and ataxia 9 days after verapamil 80 mg 3 times/day was added to her lithium therapy (900 mg/day).[1] Lithium concentrations before and after the addition of verapamil remained the same (1 to 1.1 mEq/L). The symptoms responded to withdrawal of verapamil but returned when verapamil was readministered. In a similar case, nausea, vomiting, tremors, and ataxia developed after verapamil 80 mg 3 times/day was added to lithium therapy (serum concentration 0.5 to 1.5 mEq/L).[2] Reduction of the lithium dosage to 150 mg twice daily with serum concentrations of 0.3 to 0.5 mEq/L resolved the symptoms. Choreoathetosis also has been reported after verapamil 120 mg 3 times/day was added to the regimen of a patient stabilized on lithium.[3]

RELATED DRUGS: If this interaction is caused by additive effects on cellular calcium transport, other calcium channel blockers might interact in a similar manner. Other case reports describe the development of stiffness and rigidity[4] or psychosis[5] after diltiazem was added to lithium therapy.

MANAGEMENT OPTIONS:

➡ *Monitor.* Begin the use of calcium blockers carefully in the treatment of patients with bipolar disorders who are receiving lithium. Observe for neurotoxic effects. More experience with this interaction is necessary to determine if anticholinergic agents will be useful in controlling some of the symptoms associated with the interaction.

REFERENCES:

1. Price WA, et al. Neurotoxicity caused by lithium-verapamil synergism. *J Clin Pharmacol*. 1986;26(8):717-719.

2. Price WA, et al. Lithium-verapamil toxicity in the elderly. *J Am Geriatr Soc*. 1987;35(2):177-178.

3. Helmuth D, et al. Choreoathetosis induced by verapamil and lithium treatment. *J Clin Psychopharmacol*. 1989;9(6):454-455.

4. Valdiserri EV. A possible interaction between lithium and diltiazem: case report. *J Clin Psychiatry*. 1985;46(12):540-541.

5. Binder EF, et al. Diltiazem-induced psychosis and a possible diltiazem-lithium interaction. *Arch Intern Med*. 1991;151(2):373-374.

4 | Loperamide (eg, *Imodium*)

Quinidine

SUMMARY: Quinidine appears to increase loperamide plasma concentrations and increase the potential for loperamide to suppress ventilatory response to increased carbon dioxide concentrations.

RISK FACTORS: No specific risk factors are known.

MECHANISM: Pending more data, it appears that quinidine inhibits P-glycoprotein transport of loperamide. This would result in increased plasma and possibly CNS concentrations of loperamide.

CLINICAL EVALUATION: Eight healthy subjects received a single dose of loperamide 16 mg preceded 1 hour by placebo or a single dose of quinidine 600 mg.[1] Loperamide plasma concentrations and ventilatory response to increasing carbon dioxide concentrations were compared. The mean loperamide area under the concentration-time curve increased approximately 2.5-fold following quinidine administration compared with placebo. Insufficient plasma sampling prevented an estimation of the effect of quinidine on loperamide half-life. Thus, it is not clear if quinidine affected the absorption and/or elimination of loperamide. Compared with loperamide plus placebo, the preadministration of quinidine impaired the respiratory response to carbon dioxide. This effect appeared to occur prior to quinidine-induced elevation of loperamide plasma concentrations, suggesting that quinidine was affecting the amount of loperamide entering the CNS. Determination of the clinical significance of this interaction awaits further study with conventional doses of loperamide and quinidine. Consider a possible increased risk of respiratory depression when loperamide is combined with quinidine.

RELATED DRUGS: Other opiates may be affected in a similar manner by quinidine coadministration. Other P-glycoprotein inhibitors (eg, amiodarone [eg, *Cordarone*], erythromycin, verapamil [eg, *Calan*]) are expected to affect loperamide plasma and CNS concentrations. Note that some P-glycoprotein inhibitors are also known to inhibit CYP3A4 (eg, erythromycin, verapamil) and may reduce the metabolism of loperamide.

MANAGEMENT OPTIONS:

➥ *Monitor.* Pending further data, monitor patients taking quinidine and loperamide for increased opiate effects. Aluminum hydroxide has been shown to be effective in treating quinidine-induced diarrhea without altering the absorption of quinidine and can be considered as an alternative to loperamide in these patients.[2]

REFERENCES:

1. Sadeque AJ, et al. Increased drug delivery to the brain by P-glycoprotein inhibition. *Clin Pharmacol Ther*. 2000;68:231-237.

2. Mauro VF, et al. Effect of aluminum hydroxide gel on quinidine gluconate absorption. *DICP*. 1990;24:252-254.

Loperamide (eg, *Imodium*) 4

Ritonavir (*Norvir*)

SUMMARY: Ritonavir administration increases plasma concentrations of loperamide; however, no increase in adverse reactions has been observed.

RISK FACTORS: No specific risk factors are known.

MECHANISM: Ritonavir appears to inhibit the metabolism (CYP3A4) of loperamide.

CLINICAL EVALUATION: Twelve healthy subjects received a single dose of loperamide 16 mg immediately following placebo or a single dose of ritonavir 600 mg.[1] Compared with placebo, the coadministration of ritonavir resulted in a nearly 3-fold increase in the mean loperamide area under the concentration-time curve (AUC), a 17% increase in loperamide peak concentration, and no significant change in loperamide half-life. The oral, but not renal, clearance of loperamide was reduced by ritonavir. The peak concentration of the major metabolite of loperamide was increased (32%) but its AUC was unchanged by ritonavir administration. No changes in pupil diameter, pain threshold, or transcutaneous PO_2 or PCO_2 were noted in any subjects.

RELATED DRUGS: Other protease inhibitors such as amprenavir (*Agenerase*), indinavir (*Crixivan*), nelfinavir (*Viracept*), and saquinavir (*Invirase*) are expected to decrease loperamide clearance.

MANAGEMENT OPTIONS:

➡ *Monitor.* Based on limited data, patients requiring both ritonavir and loperamide do not appear to require any special monitoring.

REFERENCES:

1. Tayrouz Y, et al. Ritonavir increases loperamide plasma concentrations without evidence for P-glycoprotein involvement. *Clin Pharmacol Ther.* 2001;70:405-414.

Lopinavir/Ritonavir (*Kaletra*) 1

Disulfiram (*Antabuse*) AVOID

SUMMARY: The oral solution formulation of *Kaletra* contains a considerable amount of alcohol and should not be used by patients taking disulfiram.

RISK FACTORS: No specific risk factors are known.

MECHANISM: Disulfiram inhibits the metabolism of alcohol, resulting in the accumulation of acetaldehyde. *Kaletra* oral solution contains alcohol.

CLINICAL EVALUATION: *Kaletra* oral solution contains 42% alcohol, and thus could cause a disulfiram reaction if used in a patient taking disulfiram.

RELATED DRUGS: All solutions containing alcohol are contraindicated in patients taking disulfiram.[1]

MANAGEMENT OPTIONS:

➡ *AVOID COMBINATION.* Do not use *Kaletra* oral solution in patients taking disulfiram; *Kaletra* capsules can be used.

REFERENCES:

1. *Kaletra* [package insert]. Abbott Park, IL: Abbott Laboratories; 2000.

Lopinavir/Ritonavir (*Kaletra*)

Midazolam

SUMMARY: Lopinavir/ritonavir administration causes an increase in midazolam plasma concentrations; some increase in midazolam adverse reactions is expected.

RISK FACTORS: No specific risk factors are known.

MECHANISM: It appears that lopinavir/ritonavir inhibits the metabolism (CYP3A4 enzyme) of midazolam.

CLINICAL EVALUATION: Fourteen healthy subjects received a single oral dose of midazolam 10 mg and a single intravenous (IV) dose of midazolam 0.025 mg/kg before and after the administration of lopinavir 400 mg/ritonavir 100 mg twice daily for 14 days.[1] The mean oral clearance of midazolam was reduced 92% (range, 89% to 93%) by the administration of lopinavir/ritonavir. The mean IV clearance of midazolam was reduced 77% by lopinavir/ritonavir. This large magnitude of effect is likely to lead to increased adverse reactions in patients receiving both drugs.

RELATED DRUGS: Other benzodiazepines that are substrates of CYP3A4 (eg, alprazolam [eg, *Xanax*], triazolam [eg, *Halcion*], prazepam[†]) will likely be affected in a similar manner by lopinavir/ritonavir administration. Other protease inhibitors such as atazanavir (*Agenerase*), indinavir (*Crixivan*), and nelfinavir (*Viracept*) that are CYP3A4 inhibitors are likely to reduce the metabolism of midazolam.

MANAGEMENT OPTIONS:

➡ *Monitor.* Carefully monitor patients receiving lopinavir/ritonavir plus midazolam for increased midazolam effects, such as sedation.

REFERENCES:

1. Yeh RF, et al. Lopinavir/ritonavir induces the hepatic activity of cytochrome P450 enzymes CYP2C9, CYP2C19, and CYP1A2 but inhibits the hepatic and intestinal activity of CYP3A as measured by a phenotyping drug cocktail in healthy volunteers. *J Acquir Immune Defic Syndr.* 2006;42(1):52-60.

† Not available in the United States.

Lopinavir/Ritonavir (*Kaletra*)

Omeprazole (eg, *Prilosec*)

SUMMARY: Lopinavir/ritonavir administration causes a reduction in the plasma concentration of omeprazole; potential effects on gastric pH are unknown.

RISK FACTORS: No specific risk factors are known.

MECHANISM: It appears that lopinavir/ritonavir increases the metabolism of omeprazole, probably via induction of the CYP2C19 enzyme pathway.

CLINICAL EVALUATION: Fourteen healthy subjects received a single oral dose of omeprazole 40 mg before and after the administration of lopinavir 400 mg/ritonavir 100 mg twice daily for 14 days.[1] The ratio of the concentration of omeprazole to its 5-OH metabolite was reduced by the administration of lopinavir/ritonavir. Because the 5-OH omeprazole metabolite is formed primarily by CYP2C19, a reduction in its formation indicates inhibition of this enzyme. The authors estimated that lopinavir/ritonavir increased CYP2C19 activity approximately 100%. The effect of these changes in omeprazole metabolism on its efficacy is unknown. Lopinavir/ritonavir is known to inhibit the enzyme CYP3A4 that also contributes to the elimination of omeprazole. This effect may partially offset the induction of CYP2C19 caused by lopinavir/ritonavir. In addition, omeprazole is an inhibitor of CYP2C19, and with chronic dosing, some of the induction effect of lopinavir/ritonavir on this enzyme may be reversed.

RELATED DRUGS: The effect of lopinavir/ritonavir on other proton pump inhibitors primarily metabolized by CYP2C19 such as esomeprazole (*Nexium*), pantoprazole (*Protonix*), and lansoprazole (*Prevacid*) would probably be similar.

MANAGEMENT OPTIONS:

➡ *Monitor.* Monitor patients stabilized on omeprazole in whom lopinavir/ritonavir is initiated for adequate GI symptom relief.

REFERENCES:

1. Yeh RF, et al. Lopinavir/ritonavir induces the hepatic activity of cytochrome P450 enzymes CYP2C9, CYP2C19, and CYP1A2 but inhibits the hepatic and intestinal activity of CYP3A as measured by a phenotyping drug cocktail in healthy volunteers. *J Acquir Immune Defic Syndr.* 2006;42(1):52-60.

Lopinavir/Ritonavir (*Kaletra*)

Tipranavir (*Aptivus*)

SUMMARY: Lopinavir plasma concentrations are reduced by coadministration of tipranavir; some reduction in antiviral efficacy may occur.

RISK FACTORS: No specific risk factors are known.

MECHANISM: Unknown.

CLINICAL EVALUATION: While specific data are limited, the manufacturer of tipranavir notes that the coadministration of multiple doses of lopinavir 400 mg/ritonavir 100 mg twice daily with tipranavir 500 mg/ritonavir 200 mg twice daily decreased the mean area under the plasma concentration-time curve of lopinavir about 65% and its trough concentration 70%.[1] Pending further data, observe patients receiving tipranavir and lopinavir for reduced lopinavir efficacy.

RELATED DRUGS: Tipranavir is known to reduce the plasma concentration of amprenavir (*Agenerase*) and saquinavir (*Invirase*).

MANAGEMENT OPTIONS:

➡ *Monitor.* Monitor patients receiving ritonavir-boosted tipranavir and lopinavir for adequate antiviral response.

REFERENCES:

1. *Aptivus* [package insert]. Ridgefield, CT: Boehringer Ingelheim Pharmaceuticals Inc; 2005.

Lopinavir/Ritonavir (*Kaletra*)

Warfarin (eg, *Coumadin*)

SUMMARY: Lopinavir/ritonavir administration causes a modest reduction in warfarin plasma concentrations; some loss of anticoagulant effect may occur.

RISK FACTORS: No specific risk factors are known.

MECHANISM: It appears that lopinavir/ritonavir increases the metabolism of warfarin, probably via induction of the CYP2C9 enzyme pathway.

CLINICAL EVALUATION: Fourteen healthy subjects received a single oral dose of warfarin 10 mg before and after the administration of lopinavir 400 mg/ritonavir 100 mg twice daily for 14 days.[1] The mean area under the plasma concentration-time curve (AUC) of S-warfarin was reduced 29% (range, 17% to 34%) by the administration of lopinavir/ritonavir. R-warfarin AUC was also reduced by a mean of 37%. It is possible that some reduction in international normalized ratio (INR) will be associated with this degree of change in warfarin plasma concentration.

RELATED DRUGS: None known.

MANAGEMENT OPTIONS:

➡ ***Monitor.*** Monitor patients stabilized on warfarin in whom lopinavir/ritonavir is initiated or discontinued for a change in their INR.

REFERENCES:

1. Yeh RF, et al. Lopinavir/ritonavir induces the hepatic activity of cytochrome P450 enzymes CYP2C9, CYP2C19, and CYP1A2 but inhibits the hepatic and intestinal activity of CYP3A as measured by a phenotyping drug cocktail in healthy volunteers. *J Acquir Immune Defic Syndr.* 2006;42(1):52-60.

Loratadine (eg, *Claritin*)

Nefazodone

SUMMARY: Nefazodone increases loratadine serum concentrations, resulting in a modest increase in the QTc interval on the electrocardiogram (ECG), but the clinical importance of this effect is not established.

RISK FACTORS:

➡ ***Hypokalemia.*** The QTc interval on the ECG may be prolonged in patients with hypokalemia, increasing the risk of this interaction.[1]

➡ ***Miscellaneous.*** Other factors that may prolong the QTc interval (eg, bradycardia, hypomagnesemia, hypothyroidism, impaired liver function) also may increase the risk of ventricular arrhythmias.[1]

MECHANISM: Not established. Loratadine is metabolized by CYP3A4 and, to a lesser extent, CYP2D6. Thus, it is possible that nefazodone inhibits the metabolism of loratadine in the gut wall and liver. The role of P-glycoprotein or other ABC transporters in loratadine disposition is disputed, so it is not known if P-glycoprotein is involved in this interaction.

CLINICAL EVALUATION: In a double-blind parallel study, healthy subjects were given loratadine alone (20 mg daily for 15 days) or with nefazodone added on days 8 through 15 (400 to 600 mg/day).[2] Nefazodone moderately increased loratadine area under the plasma concentration-time curve (39%) compared with placebo. Loratadine alone had no effect on the QTc interval of the ECG, but the QTc was 22 msec longer (range, 14 to 29 msec) when nefazodone was given with loratadine. In a patient without predisposing factors, it is unlikely that this magnitude of prolongation of the QT interval is arrhythmogenic.[1] But it is possible that the loratadine-nefazodone interaction may increase the risk of ventricular arrhythmia in a predisposed patient (see Risk Factors).

RELATED DRUGS: Citalopram (eg, *Celexa*), sertraline (eg, *Zoloft*), and venlafaxine (*Effexor*) have little effect on CYP3A4 or CYP2D6, and theoretically are unlikely to interact with loratadine. Cetirizine (*Zyrtec*) and fexofenadine (eg, *Allegra*) do not appear to be metabolized by CYP-450 isozymes, and do not appear to affect the QTc interval. Thus, they theoretically are unlikely to interact with nefazodone.

MANAGEMENT OPTIONS:

➡ *Consider Alternative.* Consider using an alternative antihistamine (eg, fexofenadine, cetirizine) instead of loratadine, or consider an alternative antidepressant (eg, citalopram, sertraline, venlafaxine) in place of nefazodone (see Related Drugs).

➡ *Monitor.* If loratadine and nefazodone are used concurrently, monitor for evidence of arrhythmias (eg, syncope) and for prolonged QT intervals.

REFERENCES:

1. De Ponti F, et al. QT-interval prolongation by non-cardiac drugs: lessons to be learned from recent experience. *Eur J Clin Pharmacol.* 2000;56(1):1-18.
2. Abernethy DR, et al. Loratadine and terfenadine interaction with nefazodone: Both antihistamines are associated with QTc prolongation. *Clin Pharmacol Ther.* 2001;69(3):96-103.

Lorazepam (eg, *Ativan*)

Loxapine (eg, *Loxitane*)

SUMMARY: Isolated cases of respiratory depression, stupor, and hypotension have been observed in patients receiving loxapine and lorazepam, but the role that a drug interaction played in these cases was not established.

RISK FACTORS: No specific risk factors are known.

MECHANISM: Not established.

CLINICAL EVALUATION: A 35-year-old woman given loxapine 25 mg and lorazepam 2 mg orally to treat an acute manic episode developed severe respiratory depression that was thought to result from the combined effects of the 2 drugs. Subsequent use of lorazepam 1 mg in the presence of perphenazine therapy did not produce respiratory depression.[1] In 2 other patients, the combined use of loxapine and lorazepam was associated with prolonged stupor and respiratory depression; one patient also developed hypotension.[2]

RELATED DRUGS: Positive results of combining benzodiazepines and neuroleptics have been reported. Diazepam increased the antipsychotic response to neuroleptic agents in schizophrenic patients,[3] and lorazepam appeared to alleviate auditory hallucinations in a schizophrenic patient receiving chlorpromazine (eg, *Thorazine*) 1 g/day.[4] Other combinations of neuroleptics and benzodiazepines have been used without excessive adverse reactions.

MANAGEMENT OPTIONS:

➡ **Monitor.** Until more information is available, carefully monitor patients receiving loxapine and lorazepam for excessive sedation and respiratory depression. With any other combination of a neuroleptic and a benzodiazepine, consider the possibility of additive sedative effects and monitor patients accordingly.

REFERENCES:

1. Cohen S, et al. Respiratory distress with use of lorazepam in mania. *J Clin Psychopharmacol.* 1987;7(3):199-200.
2. Battaglia J, et al. Loxapine-lorazepam-induced hypotension and stupor. *J Clin Psychopharmacol.* 1989;9(3):227-228.
3. Lingjaerde O, et al. Antipsychotic effect of diazepam when given in addition to neuroleptics in chronic psychotic patients: a double-blind clinical trial. *Curr Ther Res.* 1979;26:505-514.
4. Yassa R, et al. Lorazepam as an adjunct in the treatment of auditory hallucinations in a schizophrenic patient. *J Clin Psychopharmacol.* 1989;9(5):386.

Lorcainide†

Rifampin (eg, *Rifadin*)

SUMMARY: Evidence from one patient suggests that rifampin may decrease lorcainide plasma concentrations.

RISK FACTORS: No specific risk factors are known.

MECHANISM: Rifampin appears to stimulate the metabolism of lorcainide.

CLINICAL EVALUATION: A patient taking rifampin 600 mg/day required approximately 3 times the normal daily lorcainide dose to reach therapeutic plasma concentrations.[1] In addition, an unusually large accumulation of the metabolite of lorcainide was measured in this patient. The use of rifampin may result in a reduction of lorcainide effects.

RELATED DRUGS: No information is available.

MANAGEMENT OPTIONS:

➡ **Monitor.** Patients receiving lorcainide may require increased doses while taking rifampin; be alert for loss of efficacy.

REFERENCES:

1. Mauro VF, et al. Drug interaction between lorcainide and rifampicin. *Eur J Clin Pharmacol.* 1987;31(6):737-738.

† Not available in the United States.

Losartan (*Cozaar*)

Orlistat (*Xenical*)

SUMMARY: Orlistat did not affect losartan pharmacokinetics in healthy subjects.

RISK FACTORS: No specific risk factors are known.

MECHANISM: None (no interaction).

CLINICAL EVALUATION: In a randomized, crossover study in 20 healthy subjects, orlistat 120 mg 3 times daily for 6 days did not affect losartan pharmacokinetics.[1]

RELATED DRUGS: No information is available.

MANAGEMENT OPTIONS: No interaction.

REFERENCES:

1. Zhi J, et al. Pharmacokinetic evaluation of the possible interaction between selected concomitant medications and orlistat at steady-state in healthy subjects. *J Clin Pharmacol.* 2002;42:1011-1019.

Losartan (*Cozaar*)

Rifampin (eg, *Rifadin*)

SUMMARY: Rifampin administration reduces the plasma concentrations of losartan and its active metabolite. A reduction in hypotensive efficacy may occur.

RISK FACTORS: No specific risk factors are known.

MECHANISM: Rifampin induces the metabolism of losartan (CYP2C9) and its metabolite.

CLINICAL EVALUATION: Ten healthy subjects received losartan 50 mg/day for 1 week alone or with 300 mg rifampin twice daily.[1] The coadministration of rifampin reduced the area under the concentration-time curve of losartan and its active metabolite E-3174 35% and 40%, respectively. The half-lives of losartan and its metabolite were reduced approximately 50% during rifampin administration. A reduction in the hypotensive efficacy of losartan may occur during the coadministration of rifampin.

RELATED DRUGS: Eprosartan (*Teveten*), a related angiotensin II receptor inhibitor, is not metabolized by the cytochrome P450 system and is not expected to interact with rifampin. Rifabutin (*Mycobutin*) is expected to have a similar effect on eprosartan.

MANAGEMENT OPTIONS:

➡ **Consider Alternative.** Switch patients stabilized on losartan who require rifampin to an alternative hypotensive agent that does not interact with rifampin, such as an angiotensin-converting enzyme inhibitor.

➡ **Monitor.** Observe patients who receive rifampin and losartan for loss of hypotensive effect.

REFERENCES:

1. Williamson KM, et al. Effects of erythromycin or rifampin on losartan pharmacokinetics in healthy volunteers. *Clin Pharmacol Ther.* 1998;63:316-323.

Lovastatin (eg, *Mevacor*)

Nicotinic Acid (eg, *Niaspan*)

SUMMARY: Isolated cases of myopathy and rhabdomyolysis have occurred in patients receiving lovastatin and niacin, but a causal relationship has not been established.

RISK FACTORS: No specific risk factors are known.

MECHANISM: Lovastatin therapy, alone or combined with other hypolipidemic drugs, has been associated with elevations in creatine kinase with and without symptoms of myopathy.[1-3] It is possible that niacin somehow enhances the propensity of lovastatin to produce myopathy.

CLINICAL EVALUATION: A 43-year-old man with familial hypercholesterolemia received lovastatin for over 2 years without clinical or laboratory evidence of myopathy.[4] Niacin therapy was then added in gradually increasing doses. After the niacin dose had reached 2.5 g/day, he developed pain and stiffness in his back and legs, darkened urine that was positive for myoglobin, and a creatine kinase of 233,000 units/L. The reaction resolved over 2 weeks after all drugs were withdrawn. At least 1 other case of rhabdomyolysis has been reported during combined use of lovastatin, niacin, and cyclosporine (eg, *Sandimmune*).[5] Nonetheless, in a long-term study of 22 patients with familial hypercholesterolemia, combined therapy with lovastatin, niacin, and colestipol (*Colestid*) was well tolerated; 4 patients manifested increases in creatine kinase, but clinical evidence of myopathy was not mentioned.[2] Thus, it is not yet clear whether the cases of myopathy in patients receiving lovastatin and niacin result from the effects of individual drugs or from an interaction between 2 or more drugs.

RELATED DRUGS: Little is known about whether niacin increases the risk of myopathy when it is combined with simvastatin (*Zocor*). Fluvastatin (*Lescol*) does not appear to result in myopathy when combined with niacin. Theoretically, pravastatin (*Pravachol*) also is unlikely to interact with niacin.

MANAGEMENT OPTIONS:

➡ ***Monitor.*** Although the interaction between lovastatin and niacin is not well documented, patients receiving the combination should be alert for muscular symptoms such as pain, tenderness, or weakness; measure creatine kinase in patients with such symptoms. Early recognition of this disorder is important as it may progress to acute renal failure in some patients if the drugs are not discontinued promptly.

REFERENCES:

1. Tobert JA. Rhabdomyolysis in patients receiving lovastatin after cardiac transplantation. *N Engl J Med.* 1988;318:47.
2. Malloy MJ, et al. Complementarity of colestipol, niacin, and lovastatin in treatment of severe familial hypercholesterolemia. *Ann Intern Med.* 1987;107:616.
3. McKenney JM. Lovastatin: a new cholesterol-lowering agent. *Clin Pharm.* 1988;7:21.
4. Reaven P, et al. Lovastatin, nicotinic acid, and rhabdomyolysis. *Ann Intern Med.* 1988;109:597.
5. Norman DJ, et al. Myolysis and acute renal failure in a heart-transplant recipient receiving lovastatin. *N Engl J Med.* 1988;318:46.

Lovastatin (eg, *Mevacor*)

Pectin (eg, *Kapectolin*)

SUMMARY: Preliminary results from a few patients suggest that pectin inhibits the cholesterol-lowering effect of lovastatin; more study is needed to assess the clinical importance.

RISK FACTORS: No specific risk factors are known.

MECHANISM: Not established. Pectin may inhibit the gastrointestinal absorption of lovastatin.

CLINICAL EVALUATION: Three patients receiving lovastatin 80 mg/day developed 12% to 59% increases in low density lipoprotein cholesterol (LDL-C) levels 4 weeks after the addition of pectin 15 g/day.[1] LDL-C levels measured 8 weeks after stopping pectin returned to pre-pectin levels. Although it appears that pectin inhibited the

LDL-C-lowering effect of lovastatin in these patients, more study is needed to determine the incidence and magnitude of this effect.

RELATED DRUGS: The effect of pectin on HMG-CoA reductase inhibitors other than lovastatin is not established.

MANAGEMENT OPTIONS:

➥ *Circumvent/Minimize.* Although it is unknown whether separating the administration of lovastatin and pectin would avoid the interaction, it would be prudent to give lovastatin 2 hours before or 4 hours after pectin.

➥ *Monitor.* Monitor for reduced lovastatin response if the combination is given.

REFERENCES:

1. Richter WO, et al. Interaction between fibre and lovastatin. *Lancet.* 1991;338:706.

Lovastatin (eg, Mevacor)

Posaconazole (*Noxafil*)

SUMMARY: Posaconazole administration is likely to produce an increase in lovastatin plasma concentrations; patients may be more likely to develop lovastatin toxicity.

RISK FACTORS: No specific risk factors are known.

MECHANISM: Posaconazole is likely to inhibit lovastatin elimination via the CYP3A4 pathway, increase lovastatin bioavailability, or both.

CLINICAL EVALUATION: While specific data are limited, the manufacturer of posaconazole cautions that posaconazole oral suspension may increase the mean plasma concentration of lovastatin.[1] Because of the very low bioavailability of lovastatin, large increases in lovastatin plasma concentrations may occur.

RELATED DRUGS: Other antifungal agents that inhibit CYP3A4 (eg, fluconazole [eg, *Diflucan*], itraconazole [eg, *Sporanox*], ketoconazole [eg, *Nizoral*], voriconazole [*Vfend*]) affect lovastatin in a similar manner. Simvastatin (eg, *Zocor*) and, to a lesser degree, atorvastatin (*Lipitor*) may also be affected by posaconazole.

MANAGEMENT OPTIONS:

➥ *Consider Alternative.* Consider terbinafine (*Lamisil*) as an alternative antifungal agent because it does not affect CYP3A4 activity. Theoretically, fluvastatin (*Lescol*), pravastatin (*Pravachol*), and rosuvastatin (*Crestor*) would be less likely to interact with posaconazole.

➥ *Monitor.* Monitor patients taking lovastatin for muscle pain, weakness, and possibly elevated liver enzymes if posaconazole is initiated.

REFERENCES:

1. *Noxafil* [package insert]. Kenilworth, NJ: Schering Corporation; 2006.

4 **Lovastatin (eg, *Mevacor*)**

Propranolol (eg, *Inderal*)

SUMMARY: Propranolol reduces the plasma concentrations of lovastatin and pravastatin; however, the clinical significance of the reduction is unknown.

RISK FACTORS: No specific risk factors are known.

MECHANISM: Not established. Propranolol may increase the first-pass metabolism of lovastatin and pravastatin by reducing liver blood flow.

CLINICAL EVALUATION: Sixteen healthy subjects received a single dose of lovastatin 20 mg or pravastatin (eg, *Pravachol*) 20 mg alone or after 4 doses of propranolol 40 mg administered twice daily.[1] Propranolol administration moderately reduced (approximately 20%) the area under the concentration-time curve of these 2 HMG-CoA reductase inhibitors. Although this degree of reduction in plasma concentration should cause minimal loss of efficacy, larger doses of propranolol might have a greater effect.

RELATED DRUGS: Pravastatin interacts similarly with propranolol. The effect of propranolol and other beta-adrenergic blockers on the concentrations of chronically administered HMG-CoA reductase inhibitors is unknown.

MANAGEMENT OPTIONS: No specific action is required, but be alert for evidence of the interaction.

REFERENCES:
1. Pan HY, et al. Pharmacokinetic interaction between propranolol and the HMG-CoA reductase inhibitors pravastatin and lovastatin. *Br J Clin Pharmacol.* 1991;31:665-670.

2 **Lovastatin (eg, *Mevacor*)**

Telithromycin (*Ketek*)

SUMMARY: Telithromycin is likely to cause a large increase in lovastatin concentrations.

RISK FACTORS: No specific risk factors are known.

MECHANISM: Telithromycin is known to inhibit CYP3A4, the isozyme primarily responsible for the metabolism of lovastatin. Lovastatin's bioavailability will be increased and its systemic clearance decreased by telithromycin administration.

CLINICAL EVALUATION: While published data are limited, the manufacturer reports that telithromycin increased simvastatin area under the plasma concentration-time curve (AUC) nearly 9-fold and the AUC of its active metabolite 12-fold.[1] Because lovastatin's metabolism is similar to simvastatin, a similar increase in lovastatin plasma concentrations is expected. This could cause adverse reactions, including muscle pain and weakness or hepatotoxicity. Based on telithromycin's half-life of 10 hours, it would be appropriate to discontinue lovastatin during telithromycin administration and for 3 to 5 days after discontinuing telithromycin.

RELATED DRUGS: Telithromycin is likely to affect other statins that are CYP3A4 substrates (eg, atorvastatin [*Lipitor*], simvastatin [eg, *Zocor*]).

MANAGEMENT OPTIONS:

➡ **Use Alternative.** Fluvastatin (*Lescol*), pravastatin (eg, *Pravachol*), and rosuvastatin (*Crestor*) are unlikely to be affected by telithromycin.

REFERENCES:

1. *Ketek* [package insert]. Bridgewater, NJ: Aventis Pharmaceuticals, Inc.; 2004.

Lovastatin (eg, *Mevacor*) 4

Thyroid

SUMMARY: One case each of hypothyroidism (well documented) and hyperthyroidism (possible) has been reported in patients on thyroid replacement therapy who received lovastatin, but evidence suggests that such reactions are rare.

RISK FACTORS: No specific risk factors are known.

MECHANISM: Not established.

CLINICAL EVALUATION: An 18-year-old woman with type 1 diabetes and Hashimoto thyroiditis treated with thyroxine developed laboratory evidence of hypothyroidism (borderline free thyroxine index and increased thyroid-stimulating hormone) on 2 occasions when lovastatin was given.[1] In each case, thyroid function tests returned to normal when lovastatin was discontinued. Given the temporal relationship of the lovastatin administration and the altered thyroid function, it seems likely that lovastatin was responsible for the changes.

A 54-year-old man who also had type 1 diabetes and Hashimoto thyroiditis who had been taking levothyroxine chronically and several other drugs was started on lovastatin 20 mg/day.[2] Within 2 or 3 days, he developed weakness and muscle aches. He lost 10% of his body weight over the 27 days of lovastatin therapy, and the serum thyroxine concentration rose from 11.3 to 27.2 mcg/dL. Although the temporal relationship between the lovastatin and the dramatic increase in serum thyroxine concentration suggests a causal relationship, a true dechallenge was not conducted. Thus, additional study is necessary to determine whether lovastatin is likely to affect patient response to thyroid replacement hormones.

In contrast to the previous cases, the manufacturer states that lovastatin had no effect on thyroid function in 22 patients on chronic thyroid replacement. Also, lovastatin had no effect on serum thyroxine concentrations in patients without thyroid disease.[3]

RELATED DRUGS: The effect of lovastatin-like agents such as fluvastatin (*Lescol*), pravastatin (eg, *Pravachol*), or simvastatin (eg, *Zocor*) on thyroid replacement is not established.

MANAGEMENT OPTIONS: No specific action is required, but be alert for evidence of the interaction.

REFERENCES:

1. Demke DM. Drug interaction between thyroxine and lovastatin. *N Engl J Med.* 1989;321:1341-1342.

2. Lustgarten BP. Catabolic response to lovastatin therapy. *Ann Intern Med.* 1988;109:171-172.

3. Gormley GJ, et al. Drug interaction between thyroxine and lovastatin. *N Engl J Med.* 1989;321:1341-1342.

Lovastatin (eg, *Mevacor*)

Warfarin (eg, *Coumadin*)

SUMMARY: Lovastatin has been associated with increased hypoprothrombinemic response to warfarin in a number of patients, but the incidence with magnitude of this effect is not established.

RISK FACTORS: No specific risk factors are known.

MECHANISM: Not established. It has been proposed that lovastatin displaces warfarin from plasma protein binding sites. However, protein binding displacement alone seldom results in clinically important drug interactions, and the time course of the interaction in case reports is not consistent with protein binding as the only mechanism. It is possible that lovastatin also inhibits the hepatic metabolism of warfarin.

CLINICAL EVALUATION: At least 10 patients have developed enhanced hypoprothrombinemic responses to warfarin (some with bleeding) following the use of lovastatin.[1,2,3] A 48-year-old man stabilized on 5 mg/day of warfarin developed bleeding and a marked increase in his hypoprothrombinemic response (to 48 seconds) after starting lovastatin 20 mg/day.[1] A similar increase in hypoprothrombinemic response, along with epistaxis and hematuria, was noted in another patient 10 days after lovastatin 20 mg/day was added to stabilized warfarin therapy. The manufacturer of lovastatin also has received reports of enhanced warfarin hypoprothrombinemic response and/or bleeding in several patients given lovastatin concurrently. In a preliminary report, 8 patients stabilized on warfarin were given lovastatin (40 mg/day), pravastatin (eg, *Pravachol*) (20 mg/day), or placebo for 7 days in a randomized, 3-way, crossover study.[4] Lovastatin increased the international normalized ratios by 17%, but pravastatin had no effect. A small premarketing clinical trial did not show an effect of lovastatin on the hypoprothrombinemic response in patients receiving warfarin.[3] Thus, although case reports and preliminary data from clinical studies suggest that lovastatin can enhance the anticoagulant effect of warfarin, controlled clinical trials in larger numbers of patients are needed to establish the clinical importance of this interaction.

RELATED DRUGS: The effect of lovastatin on oral anticoagulants other than warfarin is unknown, but assume that an interaction occurs until proven otherwise. Fluvastatin (*Lescol*) appears to inhibit CYP2C9, the primary enzyme in the metabolism of warfarin; therefore, expect fluvastatin to increase warfarin response.[5] Simvastatin (eg, *Zocor*) appears to produce a small increase in warfarin effect, while available evidence suggests that pravastatin does not affect warfarin. Clofibrate[+] and gemfibrozil (eg, *Lopid*) may enhance the hypoprothrombinemic response to warfarin, while cholestyramine (eg, *Questran*) and colestipol (eg, *Colestid*) may reduce its effect.

MANAGEMENT OPTIONS:

➥ ***Consider Alternative.*** Pravastatin appears less likely to interact with warfarin, but monitor patients for altered hypoprothrombinemic response.

➡ *Monitor.* If lovastatin is used with oral anticoagulants, monitor for altered hypoprothrombinemic response if lovastatin is initiated, discontinued, or changed in dosage. Adjust the anticoagulant dose as needed.

REFERENCES:

1. Ahmad S. Lovastatin. Warfarin interaction. *Arch Intern Med.* 1990;150(11):2407.
2. Tobert JA, et al. Clinical experience with lovastatin. *Am J Cardiol.* 1990;65(12):23F-26F.
3. *Mevacor* [package insert]. Whitehouse Station, NJ: Merck; 1993.
4. O'Rangers EA, et al. The effect of HMG-CoA reductase inhibitors on the anticoagulant response to
warfarin. *Pharmacotherapy.* 1994;14:349.
5. Transon C, et al. In vivo inhibition profile of cytochrome P450TB (CYP2C9) by (±)-fluvastatin. *Clin
Pharmacol Ther.* 1995;58(4):412-417.

† Not available in the United States.

Loxapine (eg, *Loxitane*)

Phenytoin (eg, *Dilantin*)

SUMMARY: Loxapine appeared to reduce serum phenytoin concentrations in 1 patient; more study is needed.

RISK FACTORS: No specific risk factors are known.

MECHANISM: Loxapine may stimulate phenytoin metabolism.

CLINICAL EVALUATION: In 1 case, loxapine was associated with relatively low serum phenytoin concentrations, and discontinuation of the loxapine was followed by a considerable increase in serum phenytoin.[1] More study is needed to assess the clinical
significance of the possible interaction between these drugs.

RELATED DRUGS: No information is available.

MANAGEMENT OPTIONS: No specific action is required, but be alert for evidence of the
interaction.

REFERENCES:

1. Ryan GM, et al. Phenytoin metabolism stimulated by loxapine. *DICP.* 1977;11:428.

Lurasidone (*Latuda*)

Rifampin (eg, *Rifadin*)

SUMMARY: Rifampin administration produces very large decreases in lurasidone plasma concentrations; avoid coadministration of these drugs.

RISK FACTORS: No specific risk factors are known.

MECHANISM: Rifampin is an inducer of CYP3A4, the primary pathway of elimination
for lurasidone.

CLINICAL EVALUATION: While specific data are limited, the manufacturer of lurasidone
notes that the coadministration of rifampin 600 mg daily for 8 days prior to a
single dose of lurasidone 40 mg decreased the mean area under the plasma
concentration-time curve (AUC) of lurasidone by approximately 80% and the
AUC of its active metabolite by 90%.[1] Pending further data, patients receiving lurasidone should avoid coadministration with rifampin.

RELATED DRUGS: Rifabutin (*Mycobutin*) and rifapentine (*Priftin*) are known to induce
CYP3A4 and would likely affect lurasidone in a similar manner.

MANAGEMENT OPTIONS:

➡ **Use Alternative.** Patients requiring treatment with rifampin should be considered for an alternative antipsychotic drug that is not primarily dependent on CYP3A4 for elimination, such as paliperidone (*Invega*) or risperidone (eg, *Risperdal*).

➡ **Monitor.** If a CYP3A4 inducer is administered with lurasidone, carefully monitor for signs of a lack of antipsychotic efficacy.

REFERENCES:

1. *Latuda* [package insert]. Marlborough, MA: Sunovion Pharmaceuticals Inc; 2010.

Magnesium (eg, *Mag-200*)

Nifedipine (eg, *Procardia*)

SUMMARY: The addition of nifedipine to methyldopa (eg, *Aldomet*) and magnesium sulfate produced transient hypotensive effects.

RISK FACTORS: No specific risk factors are known.

MECHANISM: Nifedipine may produce additive hypotensive effects in patients being treated for preeclampsia. Magnesium inhibits calcium entry into smooth muscle cells and may augment the effects of calcium channel blockers.

CLINICAL EVALUATION: Two women with preeclampsia were treated with methyldopa 2 g and magnesium sulfate 20 mg/day by intravenous infusion.[1] When the combination therapy failed to lower the blood pressure, they were given nifedipine 10 mg orally. Within 1 hour, both patients suffered hypotensive episodes; blood pressure spontaneously returned to previous levels after 30 minutes. No fetal harm was apparent. While either drug could have produced the hypotension, the similar mechanisms of action of magnesium and nifedipine make the combination a likely cause. Further study is needed to determine a causal relationship.

RELATED DRUGS: Other calcium channel blockers are expected to enhance the hypotensive actions of magnesium.

MANAGEMENT OPTIONS:

➥ *Monitor.* Carefully monitor patients receiving magnesium for preeclampsia for hypotension if calcium channel blockers are given concomitantly.

REFERENCES:
1. Waisman GD, et al. Magnesium plus nifedipine: potentiation of hypotensive effect in preeclampsia? *Am J Obstet Gynecol.* 1988;159(2):308-309.

Magnesium (eg, *Mag-200*)

Succinylcholine (eg, *Anectine*)

SUMMARY: Parenteral magnesium salts may enhance the effect of neuromuscular blockers (eg, succinylcholine).

RISK FACTORS: No specific risk factors are known.

MECHANISM: The magnesium ion possesses neuromuscular blocking activity, presumably by decreasing acetylcholine release from motor nerve terminals.[1] Theoretically, this would result in at least additive, and perhaps potentiating, effects with muscle relaxants such as succinylcholine, tubocurarine, and decamethonium.

CLINICAL EVALUATION: In at least 2 reported cases, excessive neuromuscular blockade occurred in patients receiving magnesium sulfate and a neuromuscular blocker.[2] A partially controlled study of patients who had undergone cesarean deliveries indicated that considerably less succinylcholine was required in those patients who also were receiving magnesium sulfate.[3] This effect was not seen in a small number of patients who received tubocurarine instead of succinylcholine. There is also clinical evidence that administration of magnesium sulfate may attenuate succinylcholine-induced hyperkalemia and muscle fasciculations.[4] Further study is needed.

RELATED DRUGS: Tubocurarine does not appear to interact.

MANAGEMENT OPTIONS:

➥ **Monitor.** Monitor for increased effect of succinylcholine (and other neuromuscular blocking agents) if parenteral magnesium is used concurrently. Intravenous administration of calcium may partially ameliorate the excessive neuromuscular blockade that may occur.

REFERENCES:

1. Giesecke AH Jr, et al. Of magnesium, muscle relaxants, toxemic parturients, and cats. *Anesth Analg.* 1968;47(6):689-695.
2. Ghoneim MM, et al. The interaction between magnesium and other neuromuscular blocking agents. *Anesthesiology.* 1970;32(1):23-27.
3. Morris R, et al. Potentiation of muscle relaxants by magnesium sulfate therapy in toxemia of pregnancy. *South Med J.* 1968;61:25-28.
4. Aldrete JA, et al. Prevention of succinylcholine-induced hyperkalaemia by magnesium sulfate. *Can Anaesth Soc J.* 1970;17(5):477-484.

4 Maprotiline

Risperidone (eg, *Risperdal*)

SUMMARY: Three patients on maprotiline developed increased maprotiline plasma concentrations after starting risperidone; further study is needed to establish a causal relationship.

RISK FACTORS: No specific risk factors are known.

MECHANISM: Not established.

CLINICAL EVALUATION: Three patients on maprotiline developed increased maprotiline plasma concentrations after risperidone was added to their therapy.[1] One patient manifested anticholinergic adverse reactions (eg, blurred vision, constipation, dry mouth, urinary retention). Although it appeared that risperidone was responsible for the increased maprotiline concentrations, the patients were receiving other medications. Further study is needed to establish a causal relationship.

RELATED DRUGS: No information is available.

MANAGEMENT OPTIONS: No specific action is required, but be alert for evidence of the interaction.

REFERENCES:

1. Normann C, et al. Increased plasma concentration of maprotiline by coadministration of risperidone. *J Clin Psychopharmacol.* 2002;22(1):92-94.

Maraviroc (*Selzentry*)

Rifampin (eg, *Rifadin*)

SUMMARY: Rifampin administration reduces maraviroc plasma concentrations; a reduction in the antiviral effect of maraviroc is likely to occur.

RISK FACTORS: No specific risk factors are known.

MECHANISM: Rifampin is known to induce CYP3A4 and P-glycoprotein activity, thus decreasing the plasma concentration of maraviroc.

CLINICAL EVALUATION: Twelve healthy subjects received maraviroc 100 mg twice daily for 21 days with either placebo or efavirenz 600 mg daily coadministered on days 8 to 21.[1] The mean area under the concentration-time curve (AUC) of maraviroc was reduced by approximately 50% during efavirenz dosing. Peak maraviroc concentrations were similarly reduced; however, the half-life of maraviroc did not change significantly during rifampin administration. Increasing the maraviroc dosage to 200 mg twice daily during concurrent rifampin therapy returned the maraviroc AUC to values observed with the maraviroc 100 mg twice daily dosage administered without rifampin.

RELATED DRUGS: Rifabutin (*Mycobutin*) and rifapentine (*Priftin*) are known to induce CYP3A4 and would likely affect maraviroc in a similar manner.

MANAGEMENT OPTIONS:

➥ *Monitor.* Monitor for reduced maraviroc efficacy if rifampin is coadministered. A dose increase of maraviroc would likely be needed.

REFERENCES:

1. Abel S, et al. Effects of CYP3A4 inducers with and without CYP3A4 inhibitors on the pharmacokinetics of maraviroc in healthy volunteers. *Br J Clin Pharmacol.* 2008;65(suppl 1):38-46.

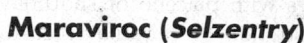

Maraviroc (*Selzentry*)

Ritonavir (*Norvir*)

SUMMARY: The coadministration of ritonavir can increase the concentration of maraviroc; some patients may experience increased adverse reactions.

RISK FACTORS: No specific risk factors are known.

MECHANISM: Ritonavir appears to inhibit the CYP3A4 metabolism of maraviroc, the P-glycoprotein transport of maraviroc, or both.

CLINICAL EVALUATION: Eight healthy subjects received maraviroc 100 mg twice daily alone for 7 days and then with ritonavir 100 mg twice daily, with both drugs administered for another 14 days.[1] The coadministration of ritonavir resulted in a mean increase in the area under the concentration-time curve (AUC) and peak concentration of maraviroc of 261% and 128%, respectively. The combination of lopinavir 400 mg/ritonavir 100 mg (*Kaletra*) twice daily produced a greater increase in maraviroc concentrations than ritonavir alone, with the mean maraviroc AUC increasing by nearly 400%.[1] These increases in maraviroc concentrations are likely to produce an increase in adverse reactions (eg, dizziness, pyrexia, rash) in some patients.

RELATED DRUGS: Amprenavir (*Agenerase*), atazanavir (*Reyataz*), darunavir (*Prezista*), indinavir (*Crixivan*), nelfinavir (*Viracept*), saquinavir (*Invirase*), and fosamprenavir (*Lexiva*) also inhibit the activity of CYP3A4 and are expected to increase the plasma concentrations of maraviroc. Maraviroc doses may require reduction during ritonavir coadministration.

MANAGEMENT OPTIONS:

➡ **Monitor.** Monitor patients taking maraviroc for changing maraviroc response if ritonavir is initiated or discontinued from their drug regimen.

REFERENCES:

1. Abel S, et al. Effects of CYP3A4 inhibitors on the pharmacokinetics of maraviroc in healthy volunteers. *Br J Clin Pharmacol.* 2008;65(suppl 1):27-37.

Maraviroc (*Selzentry*)

Saquinavir (*Invirase*)

SUMMARY: The coadministration of saquinavir can increase the concentration of maraviroc; some patients may experience increased adverse reactions.

RISK FACTORS: No specific risk factors are known.

MECHANISM: Saquinavir appears to inhibit the CYP3A4 metabolism of maraviroc, the P-glycoprotein transport of maraviroc, or both.

CLINICAL EVALUATION: Twelve healthy men received maraviroc 100 mg twice daily for 7 days with placebo or saquinavir 1,200 mg 3 times daily for 9 days.[1] The coadministration of saquinavir resulted in a mean increase in the area under the concentration-time curve (AUC) and peak concentration of maraviroc of 425% and 332%, respectively. The combination of saquinavir 1,000 mg/ritonavir 100 mg twice daily produced a greater increase in maraviroc concentrations than saquinavir alone, with the mean maraviroc AUC increasing by more than 975%.[1] These increases in maraviroc concentrations are likely to produce an increase in adverse reactions (eg, pyrexia, rash, dizziness) in some patients. Maraviroc doses may require reduction.

RELATED DRUGS: Amprenavir (*Agenerase*), atazanavir (*Reyataz*), darunavir (*Prezista*), fosamprenavir (*Lexiva*), indinavir (*Crixivan*), nelfinavir (*Viracept*), and ritonavir (*Norvir*) also inhibit the activity of CYP3A4 and are expected to increase the plasma concentrations of maraviroc.

MANAGEMENT OPTIONS:

➡ **Monitor.** Monitor patients taking maraviroc for changing maraviroc response if saquinavir is initiated or discontinued from their drug regimen.

REFERENCES:

1. Abel S, et al. Effects of CYP3A4 inhibitors on the pharmacokinetics of maraviroc in healthy volunteers. *Br J Clin Pharmacol.* 2008;65(suppl 1):27-37.

Maraviroc (*Selzentry*)

St. John's Wort

SUMMARY: St. John's wort is likely to reduce maraviroc plasma concentrations; loss of antiviral efficacy is expected.

RISK FACTORS: No specific risk factors are known.

MECHANISM: St. John's wort is an inducer of CYP3A4 and P-glycoprotein and is expected to increase maraviroc clearance.

CLINICAL EVALUATION: While specific data are lacking, the prescribing information for maraviroc warns against the coadministration of maraviroc and St. John's wort.[1] In addition to suboptimal concentrations of maraviroc, the coadministration of St. John's wort could lead to the development of a virus that is resistant to maraviroc.

RELATED DRUGS: None known.

MANAGEMENT OPTIONS:

➡ *Avoid Unless Benefit Outweighs Risk.* St. John's wort should not be administered to patients taking maraviroc unless the benefit clearly exceeds the risk of reduced antiviral efficacy.

➡ *Monitor.* If St. John's wort is coadministered with maraviroc, monitor carefully for any loss of antiviral effect.

REFERENCES:

1. *Selzentry* [package insert]. New York, NY: Pfizer Labs; 2008.

Maraviroc (*Selzentry*) 5

Tipranavir (*Aptivus*)

SUMMARY: The coadministration of tipranavir/ritonavir produced only minimal changes in maraviroc plasma concentrations.

RISK FACTORS: No specific risk factors are known.

MECHANISM: No interaction is observed. This may be the result of the combination effects of CYP3A4 inhibition with P-glycoprotein induction that is thought to occur during combination therapy with tipranavir/ritonavir.

CLINICAL EVALUATION: Twelve healthy subjects received maraviroc 150 mg twice daily plus placebo or tipranavir 500 mg/ritonavir 100 mg for 8 days.[1] While the trough maraviroc levels tended to be higher during the first 5 to 6 days of coadministration, the area mean under the concentration-time curve of maraviroc was not significantly increased by administration of tipranavir/ritonavir. No change in clinical response is expected.

RELATED DRUGS: Many other antiviral drugs are known to affect the plasma concentrations of maraviroc.

MANAGEMENT OPTIONS:

➡ *Monitor.* No special precautions appear necessary when tipranavir/ritonavir are coadministered.

REFERENCES:

1. Abel S, et al. Effects of CYP3A4 inhibitors on the pharmacokinetics of maraviroc in healthy volunteers. *Br J Clin Pharmacol.* 2008;65(suppl 1):27-37.

Marijuana

Olanzapine (eg, *Zyprexa*)

SUMMARY: A man taking olanzapine developed extrapyramidal reactions following the use of marijuana, but a causal relationship was not established.

RISK FACTORS: No specific risk factors are known.

MECHANISM: Not established.

CLINICAL EVALUATION: A man 20 years of age with paranoid schizophrenia on olanzapine 30 mg/day and clorazepate 10 to 20 mg/day developed extrapyramidal symptoms (cervical and jaw dystonia, oculogyric crises) several times after high-dose marijuana use.[1] He had previously developed similar reactions to marijuana while receiving risperidone plus clorazepate. When the patient was convinced to limit marijuana use, the extrapyramidal episodes stopped. Additional evidence is needed to assess whether marijuana use increases the risk of extrapyramidal reactions in patients taking olanzapine or risperidone.

RELATED DRUGS: No information is available.

MANAGEMENT OPTIONS: No specific action is required, but be alert for evidence of the interaction.

REFERENCES:
1. Rejón Altable C, et al. Cannabis-induced extrapyramidalism in a patient on neuroleptic treatment. *J Clin Psychopharmacol.* 2005;25(1):91-92.

Marijuana

Propranolol (eg, *Inderal*)

SUMMARY: Propranolol inhibits the increases in heart rate and blood pressure that may accompany marijuana smoking.

RISK FACTORS: No specific risk factors are known.

MECHANISM: Not established. It is proposed that propranolol blocks beta-adrenergic stimulation produced by marijuana.

CLINICAL EVALUATION: In a study of 6 healthy, experienced marijuana smokers, propranolol 120 mg orally inhibited the increase in heart rate and systolic blood pressure that normally follows a marijuana cigarette (10 mg of delta-9-tetrahydrocannabinol).[1] Propranolol also seemed to prevent marijuana learning impairment and reduced marijuana-induced reddening of the eyes. The effects of propranolol on orally ingested marijuana are unknown but could be anticipated to be similar.

RELATED DRUGS: Other beta-blockers may produce similar effects.

MANAGEMENT OPTIONS: No specific action is required, but be alert for evidence of the interaction.

REFERENCES:
1. Sulkowski A, et al. Propranolol effects on acute marijuana intoxication in man. *Psychopharmacology.* 1977;52:47-53.

Marijuana 4

Risperidone (*Risperdal*)

SUMMARY: A man on risperidone developed extrapyramidal reactions following the use of marijuana, but a causal relationship was not established.

RISK FACTORS: No specific risk factors are known.

MECHANISM: Not established.

CLINICAL EVALUATION: A 20-year-old man was diagnosed with paranoid schizophrenia and was controlled in the hospital with risperidone 9 mg/day and clorazepate 10 to 20 mg/day.[1] After discharge, he developed extrapyramidal symptoms (cervical and jaw dystonia, oculogyric crises) several times after high-dose marijuana use. When olanzapine 30 mg/day was substituted for risperidone, the extrapyramidal episodes continued to occur following marijuana use. When the patient was convinced to limit marijuana use, the extrapyramidal episodes stopped. Additional evidence is needed to assess whether marijuana use increases the risk of extrapyramidal reactions in patients on risperidone or olanzapine.

RELATED DRUGS: No information is available.

MANAGEMENT OPTIONS: No specific action is required, but be alert for evidence of the interaction.

REFERENCES:
1. Rejon Altable C, et al. Cannabis-induced extrapyramidalism in a patient on neuroleptic treatment. *J Clin Psychopharmacol.* 2005;25:91-92.

Mebendazole (eg, *Vermox*)

Phenytoin (eg, *Dilantin*)

SUMMARY: In patients receiving high oral doses of mebendazole for *Echinococcus multilocularis* or *Echinococcus granulosus* (hydatid disease), phenytoin has been shown to lower plasma mebendazole concentrations, possibly impairing its therapeutic effect.

RISK FACTORS:

➥ **Concurrent Diseases.** Patients with tissue-dwelling organisms appear to be at greater risk for the interaction than those with intestinal helminths.

MECHANISM: Mebendazole appears to undergo metabolism by hepatic microsomal enzymes.[1,2] Phenytoin, a known hepatic microsomal enzyme inducer, likely enhances mebendazole metabolism.

CLINICAL EVALUATION: When mebendazole is used to treat intestinal helminths such as whipworms or hookworms, the rate of hepatic mebendazole metabolism probably has little bearing on the therapeutic outcome. However, when mebendazole is used to treat tissue-dwelling organisms such as those causing hydatid disease, low plasma mebendazole concentrations caused by enzyme induction could impair the therapeutic response. In a group of patients receiving mebendazole in addition to several other drugs, those patients taking phenytoin or carbamazepine (eg, *Tegretol*) had considerably lower plasma mebendazole concentrations than those who were not taking enzyme inducers.[3] Several patients who could not be adequately treated with mebendazole while on phenytoin or carbamazepine were switched to valproic acid (eg, *Depakene*), which resulted in a therapeutically significant increase in plasma mebendazole concentrations in each case.

RELATED DRUGS: Other enzyme-inducing agents would be expected to produce a similar effect.

MANAGEMENT OPTIONS:

➥ *Avoid Unless Benefit Outweighs Risk.* Avoid using enzyme-inducing drugs in patients receiving mebendazole for tissue-dwelling organisms. No precautions appear necessary during cotherapy with phenytoin in patients receiving mebendazole to treat intestinal helminths. If possible, use valproic acid in place of phenytoin because it does not appear to reduce plasma mebendazole concentrations.

➥ *Monitor.* Be alert for evidence of reduced mebendazole response if phenytoin or other enzyme inducers are used with mebendazole.

REFERENCES:

1. Witassek F, et al. Chemotherapy of larval echinococcus with mebendazole: microsomal liver function and cholestasis as determinants of plasma drug level. *Eur J Clin Pharmacol.* 1983;25:85-90.

2. Bekhti A, et al. A correlation between serum mebendazole concentrations and the aminopyrine breath test. Implications in the treatment of hydatid disease. *Br J Clin Pharmacol.* 1986;21:223-226.

3. Luder PJ, et al. Treatment of hydatid disease with high oral doses of mebendazole. Long-term follow-up of plasma mebendazole levels and drug interactions. *Eur J Clin Pharmacol.* 1986;31:443-448.

 Meclofenamate

Warfarin (eg, *Coumadin*)

SUMMARY: Preliminary evidence indicates that meclofenamate may increase the hypoprothrombinemic response to warfarin; presumably, it also might effect the response to other oral anticoagulants. The possible detrimental effects of meclofenamate on the gastric mucosa and platelet function is another reason to undertake cotherapy with caution.

RISK FACTORS:

➥ *Concurrent Diseases.* Patients with peptic ulcer disease (PUD) or a history of GI bleeding probably are at greater risk for the interaction.

MECHANISM: The mechanism for the possible increased hypoprothrombinemic response as a result of meclofenamate is not established. Meclofenamate-induced gastric erosions and inhibition of platelet function theoretically would increase the risk of bleeding in patients receiving oral anticoagulants.

CLINICAL EVALUATION: The hypoprothrombinemic response to warfarin reportedly has been increased by meclofenamate,[1,2] but details of the studies were not provided. In a retrospective cohort study, hospitalizations for hemorrhagic PUD were about 13 times higher in patients receiving warfarin plus a nonsteroidal anti-inflammatory drug (NSAID) than in patients receiving neither drug.[3]

RELATED DRUGS: All nonsteroidal anti-inflammatory drugs (NSAIDs) inhibit platelet function, cause gastric erosions, and probably increase the risk of GI bleeding. Some NSAIDs; however, such as ibuprofen (eg, *Advil*), naproxen (eg, *Naprosyn*), or diclofenac (eg, *Voltaren*), may be less likely to increase oral anticoagulant-induced hypoprothrombinemia than other NSAIDs.

MANAGEMENT OPTIONS:

➡ *Avoid Unless Benefit Outweighs Risk.* Because all NSAIDs probably increase the risk of GI bleeding in patients on oral anticoagulants, use the combination only after careful consideration of the benefit versus risk. If an NSAID must be used with an oral anticoagulant, it would be prudent to use NSAIDs that are unlikely to affect the hypoprothrombinemic response to oral anticoagulants as mentioned in Related Drugs. If the NSAID is being used as an analgesic or antipyretic, acetaminophen (eg, *Tylenol*) probably is safer to use with oral anticoagulants. Nonacetylated salicylates (eg, choline salicylate, magnesium salicylate, salsalate, sodium salicylate) also probably are safer with oral anticoagulants than NSAIDs, because such salicylates have minimal effects on platelet function and the gastric mucosa.

➡ *Monitor.* If any NSAID is used with an oral anticoagulant, one should carefully monitor the prothrombin time and watch for evidence of bleeding, especially from the GI tract.

REFERENCES:

1. AMA Drug Evaluation. 6th ed. American Medical Association. Chicago; 1986:1066.
2. Product information. Meclofenamate (*Meclomen*). Parke-Davis. 1990.
3. Shorr RI, et al. Concurrent use of nonsteroidal anti-inflammatory drugs and oral anticoagulants places elderly persons at high risk for hemorrhagic peptic ulcer disease. *Arch Intern Med*. 1993;153:1665.

Mefenamic Acid (*Ponstel*)

Warfarin (eg, *Coumadin*)

SUMMARY: Limited clinical evidence indicates that mefenamic acid may produce a small increase in the hypoprothrombinemic response to warfarin and, presumably, other oral anticoagulants. Another reason for caution during cotherapy with these drugs is the possible detrimental effects of mefenamic acid on the gastric mucosa and platelet function.

RISK FACTORS:

➡ *Concurrent Diseases.* Patients with peptic ulcer disease (PUD) or a history of GI bleeding probably are at greater risk for the interaction.

MECHANISM: Although mefenamic acid may displace warfarin from albumin binding sites, the clinical importance of this mechanism is unclear.[3,4] Also, mefenamic acid-induced gastric erosions and inhibition of platelet function theoretically could increase the risk of bleeding in patients receiving oral anticoagulants.

CLINICAL EVALUATION: The hypothesis that mefenamic acid can enhance the response to oral anticoagulants clinically[1] was substantiated by a preliminary clinical study in 12 healthy volunteers.[2] In the study, a small but significant decrease in prothrombin concentration occurred when the warfarin-treated volunteers were given mefenamic acid 500 mg 4 times a day. Although more evidence is needed, mefenamic acid appears to enhance the effect of coumarin anticoagulants. The possibility of mefenamic acid-induced GI hemorrhage also should be kept in mind in patients receiving oral anticoagulants. In a retrospective cohort study, hospitalizations for hemorrhagic PUD were about 13 times higher in patients receiving warfarin plus a nonsteroidal anti-inflammatory drug (NSAID) than in patients receiving neither drug.[5]

RELATED DRUGS: All nonsteroidal anti-inflammatory drugs (NSAIDs) inhibit platelet function, cause gastric erosions, and probably increase the risk of GI bleeding.

Some NSAIDs; however, such as ibuprofen (eg, *Advil*), naproxen (eg, *Naprosyn*), or diclofenac (eg, *Voltaren*), may be less likely to increase oral anticoagulant-induced hypoprothrombinemia than other NSAIDs.

MANAGEMENT OPTIONS:

➥ *Avoid Unless Benefit Outweighs Risk.* Because all NSAIDs probably increase the risk of GI bleeding in patients on oral anticoagulants, use the combination only after careful consideration of the benefit versus risk. If an NSAID must be used with an oral anticoagulant, it would be prudent to use NSAIDs that are unlikely to affect the hypoprothrombinemic response to oral anticoagulants as mentioned in the Related Drugs. If the NSAID is being used as an analgesic or antipyretic, acetaminophen (eg, *Tylenol*) probably is safer to use with oral anticoagulants. Nonacetylated salicylates (eg, choline salicylate, magnesium salicylate, salsalate, sodium salicylate) also probably are safer with oral anticoagulants than NSAIDs, because such salicylates have minimal effects on platelet function and the gastric mucosa.

➥ *Monitor.* If any NSAID is used with an oral anticoagulant, one should carefully monitor the prothrombin time and watch for evidence of bleeding, especially from the GI tract.

REFERENCES:

1. Anon. Today's drugs. Mefenamic acid. *BMJ.* 1966;2:1506.
2. Homes EL. Pharmacology of the fenamates. IV. Toleration by normal human subjects. *Ann Phys Med.* 1967;9(Suppl.):36.
3. Sellers EM, et al. Displacement of warfarin from human albumin by diazoxide and ethacrynic, mefenamic and nalidixic acids. *Clin Pharmacol Ther.* 1970;11:524.
4. Sellers EM, et al. Kinetics and clinical importance of displacement of warfarin from albumin by acidic drugs. *Ann NY Acad Sci.* 1971;179:213.
5. Shorr RI, et al. Concurrent use of nonsteroidal anti-inflammatory drugs and oral anticoagulants places elderly persons at high risk for hemorrhagic peptic ulcer disease. *Arch Intern Med.* 1993;153:1665.

4 Mefloquine (eg, *Lariam*)

Metoclopramide (eg, *Reglan*)

SUMMARY: Mefloquine peak plasma concentrations were increased by the administration of metoclopramide; the clinical significance of this change is unknown.

RISK FACTORS: No specific risk factors are known.

MECHANISM: Metoclopramide-induced increase in gastric emptying could reduce the time required for absorption and perhaps increase peak mefloquine concentrations by increasing the rate of mefloquine delivery to absorption sites in the small intestine.

CLINICAL EVALUATION: Seven volunteers received a single dose of mefloquine 750 mg alone or with metoclopramide 10 mg in a randomized protocol that separated these 2 treatment regimens by at least 12 weeks.[1] The administration of metoclopramide with mefloquine reduced the apparent absorption half-life from 3.2 to 2.4 hours. The peak plasma concentration of mefloquine increased 24%, while the area under the concentration-time curve was unchanged. No subjects experienced adverse reactions. The significance of the increased peak concentration during long-term dosing in patients is unknown. The potential for increased toxicity appears to be limited, but additional study is needed to determine the risk.

RELATED DRUGS: The effects of other prokinetic agents, such as cisapride (available from the manufacturer on a limited-access protocol), are unknown; similar results can be expected.

MANAGEMENT OPTIONS: No specific action is required, but be alert for evidence of the interaction.

REFERENCES:

1. Na Bangchang K, et al. The effect of metoclopramide on mefloquine pharmacokinetics. *Br J Clin Pharmacol.* 1991;32(5):640-641.

Mefloquine (eg, *Lariam*)

Primaquine

SUMMARY: A single dose of mefloquine had no effect on primaquine concentrations.

RISK FACTORS: No specific risk factors are known.

MECHANISM: No interaction.

CLINICAL EVALUATION: Nine healthy subjects received a single oral dose of primaquine 45 mg alone and with a single oral dose of mefloquine 10 mg/kg.[1] No changes in primaquine pharmacokinetics were noted.

RELATED DRUGS: No information is available.

MANAGEMENT OPTIONS: No interaction.

REFERENCES:

1. Edwards G, et al. Interactions among primaquine, malaria infection and other antimalarials in Thai subjects. *Br J Clin Pharmacol.* 1993;35(2):193-198.

Mefloquine (eg, *Lariam*)

Warfarin (eg, *Coumadin*)

SUMMARY: Isolated case reports suggest that mefloquine can increase warfarin effect.

RISK FACTORS: No specific risk factors are known.

MECHANISM: Not established.

CLINICAL EVALUATION: A 66-year-old man on long-term warfarin therapy developed a severe bleeding episode and markedly prolonged prothrombin time after starting on malaria prophylaxis with mefloquine.[1] In another case, a 63-year-old man stabilized on warfarin developed bleeding and a dramatic increase in prothrombin time after starting mefloquine.[1] These cases suggest that mefloquine can increase the anticoagulant response to warfarin, but more study is needed.

RELATED DRUGS: The effect mefloquine on other oral anticoagulants is not established.

MANAGEMENT OPTIONS:

➡ *Monitor.* In patients receiving warfarin, be alert for changes in international normalized ratio if mefloquine is given concurrently.

REFERENCES:

1. Loefler I. Mefloquine and anticoagulant interaction. *J Travel Med.* 2003;10(3):194-195.

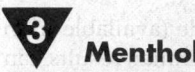

Menthol

Warfarin (eg, *Coumadin*)

SUMMARY: Isolated cases suggest that menthol may reduce warfarin response, but more study is needed.

RISK FACTORS: No specific risk factors known.

MECHANISM: Not established.

CLINICAL EVALUATION: A 57-year-old man stabilized on warfarin 7 mg/day developed a marked drop in his international normalized ratio (INR) after taking menthol cough drops (6 per day for 4 days) for a flu-like illness.[1] He denied missing any warfarin doses, and no other causes for a reduced effect of warfarin were found. In another case, a 46-year-old man stabilized on warfarin developed a marked decrease in his INR after taking menthol cough drops (8 to 10 cough drops daily for 3 weeks).[2] The INR returned to baseline values after the cough drops were stopped, and no other cause for the reduced warfarin effect was found. Both cases are rated "possible" using the Drug Interaction Probability Scale (DIPS),[3] and more study is needed to establish whether menthol interacts with warfarin.

RELATED DRUGS: No information is available.

MANAGEMENT OPTIONS:

➡ **Monitor.** If menthol cough drops are used with warfarin monitor the INR if the cough drops are started, stopped, or changed in dosage.

REFERENCES:

1. Kassebaum PJ, et al. Possible warfarin interaction with menthol cough drops. *Ann Pharmacother*. 2005;39(2):365-367.
2. Coderre K, et al. Probable warfarin interaction with menthol cough drops. *Pharmacotherapy*. 2010;30(1):110.
3. Horn JR, et al. Proposal for a new tool to evaluate drug interaction cases. *Ann Pharmacother*. 2007;41(4):674-680.

5　Meperidine (eg, *Demerol*)

Contraceptives, Oral

SUMMARY: Oral contraceptives do not appear to affect the disposition of meperidine.

RISK FACTORS: No specific risk factors are known.

MECHANISM: No interaction.

CLINICAL EVALUATION: Information from urinary excretion data suggested that subjects on oral contraceptives excreted more unchanged meperidine, while controls tended to excrete more of the demethylated metabolite.[1] However, a subsequent study failed to confirm these findings.[2]

RELATED DRUGS: No information is available.

MANAGEMENT OPTIONS: No interaction.

REFERENCES:

1. Crawford JS, et al. Some alterations in the pattern of drug metabolism associated with pregnancy, oral contraceptives, and the newly-born. *Br J Anaesth*. 1966;38(6):446-454.

2. Stambaugh JE Jr, et al. Drug interactions I: meperidine and combination oral contraceptives. *J Clin Pharmacol.* 1975;15:46.

Meperidine (eg, *Demerol*)

Phenelzine (*Nardil*) AVOID

SUMMARY: Some patients receiving nonselective monoamine oxidase inhibitors (MAOIs) and meperidine have developed life-threatening serotonin syndrome.

RISK FACTORS: No specific risk factors are known.

MECHANISM: Meperidine appears to block the neuronal uptake of serotonin. It has been suggested that the combination of meperidine and MAOIs results in accumulation of CNS serotonin, leading to agitation, blood pressure changes, hyperpyrexia, and convulsions.

CLINICAL EVALUATION: Administration of meperidine to a patient receiving a nonselective MAOI may result in rapid development of serotonin syndrome (agitation, confusion, hypomania, myoclonus, rigidity, hyperreflexia, tremor, incoordination, sweating, shivering, seizures, coma).[1-6] Although several deaths have been attributed to this interaction, not all patients react adversely to the combination.[1]

RELATED DRUGS: Meperidine is contraindicated in patients receiving any nonselective MAOI, including isocarboxazid (*Marplan*) and tranylcypromine (*Parnate*). Morphine (eg, *Roxanol*) does not appear to cause such severe reactions; thus, although it cannot be used with impunity with nonselective MAOIs, it is preferable to meperidine. Epidural fentanyl (eg, *Sublimaze*) has been reported to be an acceptable analgesic for postoperative pain in a patient taking tranylcypromine.[7]

MANAGEMENT OPTIONS:

➡ *AVOID COMBINATION.* Avoid meperidine in patients receiving nonselective MAOIs. Assume the effects of nonselective MAOIs will persist for 2 weeks after they are discontinued. Available evidence suggests that morphine is safer than meperidine in patients receiving nonselective MAOIs.

REFERENCES:

1. Evans-Prosser CD. The use of pethidine and morphine in the presence of monoamine oxidase inhibitors. *Br J Anaesth.* 1968;40:279-282.
2. Browne B, et al. Monoamine oxidase inhibitors and narcotic analgesics. A critical review of the implications for treatment. *Br J Psychiatry.* 1987;151:210-212.
3. Goldberg LI. Monoamine oxidase inhibitors. Adverse reactions and possible mechanism. *JAMA.* 1964;190:456-462.
4. Sjoqvist F. Psychotropic drugs (2). Interaction between monoamine oxidase (MAO) inhibitors and other substances. *Proc R Soc Med.* 1965;58:967-978.
5. Vigran IM. Dangerous potentiation of meperidine hydrochloride by pargyline hydrochloride. *JAMA.* 1964;187:953-954.
6. Analgesics and monoamine oxidase inhibitors. *BMJ.* 1967;4:284.
7. Youssef MS, et al. Epidural fentanyl and monoamine oxidase inhibitors. *Anaesthesia.* 1988;43:210-212.

Meperidine (eg, *Demerol*)

Phenobarbital (eg, *Solfoton*)

SUMMARY: Phenobarbital and meperidine coadministration can result in excessive CNS depression.

RISK FACTORS: No specific risk factors are known.

MECHANISM: Barbiturates purportedly enhance the metabolism of meperidine to the toxic metabolite normeperidine.[1] Also, barbiturates and narcotic analgesics may exhibit additive or synergistic CNS depression.[2]

CLINICAL EVALUATION: A patient who had been receiving phenobarbital developed prolonged sedation when given meperidine,[3] although previous administration of meperidine alone had not resulted in excessive CNS depression. Subsequent study in patients and a healthy volunteer indicated that phenobarbital enhances the demethylation of meperidine to normeperidine. It is not yet clear whether the increased CNS depression observed with combined phenobarbital and meperidine was caused by increased normeperidine levels or simply caused by the combined depressant effects of the drugs.

RELATED DRUGS: Most combinations of barbiturates and narcotic analgesics are expected to exhibit additive CNS depressant effects. Moreover, the metabolism of narcotic analgesics that are converted to inactive products might be increased by barbiturates, thus reducing their effect.

MANAGEMENT OPTIONS:

➡ **Monitor.** Monitor for excessive CNS depression when barbiturates and narcotic analgesics are given concurrently; adjust dosage of 1 or both drugs as needed.

REFERENCES:

1. Stambaugh JE, et al. The effect of phenobarbital on the metabolism of meperidine in normal volunteers. *J Clin Pharmacol*. 1978;18:482-490.
2. Bellville JW, et al. The hypnotic effects of codeine and secobarbital and their interaction in man. *Clin Pharmacol Ther*. 1971;12:607-612.
3. Stambaugh JE, et al. A potentially toxic drug interaction between pethidine (meperidine) and phenobarbitone. *Lancet*. 1977;1:398-399.

Meperidine (eg, *Demerol*)

Phenytoin (eg, *Dilantin*)

SUMMARY: Phenytoin may reduce meperidine serum concentrations, but the clinical importance of this effect is not established.

RISK FACTORS: No specific risk factors are known.

MECHANISM: Phenytoin may enhance the hepatic metabolism of meperidine.

CLINICAL EVALUATION: The pharmacokinetics of meperidine (50 mg IV and 100 mg orally) were studied in 4 healthy subjects before and after the administration of phenytoin 1 g followed by 300 mg/day for 9 days.[1] Phenytoin enhanced the systemic clearance of meperidine and reduced meperidine half-life and bioavailability. The area under the blood concentration-time curve for normeperidine was considerably increased in the presence of phenytoin, indicating enhanced metabolism of merperidine to normeperidine. However, the degree to which phenytoin reduces the analgesic effect of meperidine or increases its toxicity because of increased normeperidine concentrations is not established. Because oral meperidine produces more normeperidine than equianalgesic IV doses of meperidine, parenteral meperidine may be less likely to interact with phenytoin than the oral form[1]; however, this effect has not been tested clinically.

RELATED DRUGS: No information is available.

MANAGEMENT OPTIONS:

➡ *Monitor.* Until more information is available, be alert for evidence of reduced analgesic efficacy or increased toxicity when meperidine is used in patients receiving phenytoin.

REFERENCES:

1. Pond SM, et al. Effect of phenytoin on meperidine clearance and normeperidine formation. *Clin Pharmacol Ther.* 1981;30:680-686.

Meperidine (eg, *Demerol*)

Rasagiline (*Azilect*)

SUMMARY: Concomitant use of rasagiline and meperidine should generally be avoided.

RISK FACTORS: No specific risk factors are known.

MECHANISM: Not established. The combination may have additive serotonergic effects.

CLINICAL EVALUATION: Because severe serotonin syndrome-like reactions (including fatalities) have occurred when meperidine was used in patients on nonselective MAO inhibitors, as well as with selegiline, the product information for rasagiline states that meperidine is contraindicated in patients taking rasagiline.[1,2] Despite its basis on theoretical considerations, the severity of the potential reactions dictates that the combination should generally be avoided.

RELATED DRUGS: Selegiline is also listed in the package insert as contraindicated with meperidine, although the case report that generated the concern was not conclusive.[3] Rasagiline is also identified as contraindicated with other analgesics (eg, methadone, propoxyphene, tramadol [eg, *Ultram*]).

MANAGEMENT OPTIONS:

➡ *Avoid Unless Benefit Outweighs Risk.* Meperidine should generally not be used concomitantly with rasagiline or within 2 weeks of stopping rasagiline.

REFERENCES:

1. *Azilect* [package insert]. North Wales, PA: Teva Neuroscience, Inc.; 2006.
2. Chen JJ, et al. Rasagiline. A second-generation monoamine oxidase type-B inhibitor for the treatment of Parkinson's disease. *Am J Health Syst Pharm.* 2006;63:915-928.
3. Zornberg GL, et al. Severe adverse interaction between pethidine and selegiline. *Lancet.* 1991;337:246.

2 **Meperidine (eg, Demerol)**

Selegiline (eg, Eldepryl)

SUMMARY: A patient on selegiline developed agitation, delirium, rigidity, sweating, and hyperpyrexia after starting meperidine, but it was not established that the reaction resulted from an interaction between selegiline and meperidine.

RISK FACTORS:

➡ **Other Drugs.** The concurrent use of other drugs that inhibit serotonin reuptake may increase the risk.

MECHANISM: Not established. Although selegiline is an MAO-B inhibitor, it also has some inhibitory effect on MAO-A (for which serotonin is a substrate). The patient was also receiving imipramine (eg, Tofranil) and meperidine, both of which can inhibit serotonin uptake.

CLINICAL EVALUATION: A 56-year-old man with Parkinson disease was taking selegiline 5 mg twice daily, pergolide (eg, Permax) 0.75 mg twice daily, levodopa/carbidopa (eg, Sinemet) 10/100 mg 4 times a day, imipramine 175 mg 4 times a day, and desipramine (eg, Norpramin) 25 mg 4 times a day before admission for a surgical procedure.[1] He received meperidine 100 mg on postoperative day 1, 75 mg on postoperative day 2, and 150 mg on postoperative day 3. He became progressively restless on day 2 and was severely agitated and delirious on the fourth postoperative day. He also developed muscular rigidity, sweating, and increased temperature. Selegiline was discontinued on day 5, and 4 days later the reaction had dissipated. The signs and symptoms described are consistent with those of serotonin syndrome. Although the reaction was attributed to an interaction between selegiline and meperidine, it is possible that an imipramine-meperidine interaction also contributed to the reaction. Imipramine is known to inhibit serotonin reuptake, and theoretically could produce serotonin syndrome if combined with meperidine. It seems unlikely that the patient was taking imipramine 175 mg 4 times a day as stated in the case report, as half that amount would be a large dose. Nonetheless, based upon this and other cases, the manufacturer states that meperidine is contraindicated in patients receiving selegiline.[2]

RELATED DRUGS: Theoretically, morphine (eg, Roxanol) is less likely to interact with meperidine, but little is known about other opiates.

MANAGEMENT OPTIONS:

➡ **Use Alternative.** Although it has not been established that the reported reaction resulted from a selegiline-meperidine interaction, the potential severity of the reaction dictates caution. Until more data are available, use analgesics other than meperidine in patients taking selegiline when possible. The manufacturer recommends caution.

REFERENCES:

1. Zornberg GL, et al. Severe adverse interaction between pethidine and selegiline. *Lancet*. 1991;337:246.

2. *Eldepryl* [package insert]. Tampa, FL: Somerset Pharmaceuticals, Inc.; 1996.

Meperidine (eg, *Demerol*)

Sibutramine†

SUMMARY: The risk of serotonin syndrome would theoretically increase when sibutramine is combined with other serotonergic drugs, such as meperidine.

RISK FACTORS: No specific risk factors are known.

MECHANISM: Sibutramine inhibits serotonin reuptake; additive serotonergic effects may occur with meperidine.

CLINICAL EVALUATION: While no published data are available for evaluation, the manufacturer of sibutramine has made some data on this interaction available.[1] Because sibutramine has serotonergic effects, its concurrent use with other serotonergic drugs (eg, meperidine) may increase the risk of serotonin syndrome.[2] Although the actual risk of combining sibutramine with serotonergic drugs is unknown, the fact that serotonin syndrome can result in serious or fatal reactions must be considered.

RELATED DRUGS: Little is known regarding the serotonergic effects of opioids other than meperidine.

MANAGEMENT OPTIONS:

➡ *Avoid Unless Benefit Outweighs Risk.* The manufacturer states that sibutramine should not be used with meperidine. This is recommended until more information is available.

➡ *Monitor.* Serotonin syndrome can result in neurotoxicity (eg, coma, hyperreflexia, incoordination, myoclonus, restlessness, rigidity, seizures, tremors), psychiatric symptoms (eg, agitation, confusion, hypomania), and temperature regulation abnormalities (eg, fever, sweating). Note that mild forms of serotonin syndrome have also been reported; therefore, consider any combination of the above symptoms possibly related to excessive serotonin activity.

REFERENCES:

1. *Meridia* [package insert]. North Chicago, IL: Abbott Laboratories Pharmaceutical Division; 1997.
2. Mills KC. Serotonin syndrome. A clinical update. *Crit Care Clin.* 1997;13(4):763-783.

† Not available in the United States.

Meprobamate (eg, *Miltown*)

Warfarin (eg, *Coumadin*)

SUMMARY: Meprobamate does not appear to affect the hypoprothrombinemic response to oral anticoagulants, such as warfarin.

RISK FACTORS: No specific risk factors are known.

MECHANISM: No interaction.

CLINICAL EVALUATION: Several studies have not shown any clinically significant effect of meprobamate on the hypoprothrombinemic response to oral anticoagulants,[1-3] even at the maximum recommended dose.[2]

RELATED DRUGS: Theoretically, meprobamate is not expected to interact with oral anticoagulants.

MANAGEMENT OPTIONS: No interaction.

REFERENCES:

1. Udall JA. Warfarin therapy not influenced by meprobamate. A controlled study in nine men. *Curr Ther Res Clin Exp.* 1970;12(11):724-728.

2. Gould L, et al. Prothrombin levels maintained with meprobamate and warfarin. A controlled study. *JAMA.* 1972;220(11):1460-1462.

3. DeCarolis PP, et al. Effect of tranquilizers on prothrombin time response to coumarin. *J Clin Pharmacol.* 1975;15:557.

 Mercaptopurine (eg, *Purinethol*)

Infliximab (*Remicade*)

SUMMARY: The combination of mercaptopurine and infliximab may increase the risk of opportunistic infection over either drug alone, especially if corticosteroids are given concurrently. Some evidence suggests that combining infliximab with mercaptopurine or azathioprine may increase the risk of lymphoma.

RISK FACTORS:

➡ **Effects of age.** In patients receiving mercaptopurine or azathioprine concurrently with infliximab, those older than 50 years may be at greater risk of opportunistic infections. [1] Lymphoma has occurred mostly in adolescent or young adult males taking infliximab with azathioprine or mercaptopurine.[2]

MECHANISM: Both mercaptopurine and infliximab can increase the risk of opportunistic infections, and their effects may be additive.

CLINICAL EVALUATION: In a case-control study of patients with inflammatory bowel disease, 100 consecutive patients with opportunistic infections were compared with 200 matched controls. Therapy with mercaptopurine/azathioprine, infliximab, or corticosteroids, were individually associated with increased odds for infection (odds ratios of approximately 3), whereas use of 2 or 3 of these agents concurrently was associated with an odds ratio of almost 15.[1] Also, the product information states that a rare, fatal lymphoma (hepatosplenic T-cell lymphoma) has been reported in younger males with inflammatory bowel disease who received mercaptopurine or azathioprine with infliximab.[2] Make a careful assessment of benefit versus risk before using infliximab with mercaptopurine or azathioprine, particularly if the patient is also taking corticosteroids.

RELATED DRUGS: Azathioprine (eg, *Imuran*) is a prodrug for mercaptopurine, so it is likely to interact with infliximab in the same way as mercaptopurine.

MANAGEMENT OPTIONS:

➡ **Circumvent/Minimize.** If possible, avoid the concurrent use of mercaptopurine or azathioprine with infliximab, particularly if the patient is also receiving corticosteroids.

➡ *Monitor.* If the combination is used, monitor the patient carefully for opportunistic infections and also for evidence of other potential adverse reactions, such as lymphoma.

REFERENCES:

1. Toruner M, et al. Risk factors for opportunistic infections in patients with inflammatory bowel disease. *Gastroenterology.* 2008;134(4):929-936.
2. *Remicade* [package insert]. Horsham, PA: Janssen Biotech, Inc; 2011.

Mercaptopurine (eg, *Purinethol*)

Prednisolone (eg, *Millipred*)

SUMMARY: The combination of mercaptopurine with prednisolone or other corticosteroids appears to substantially increase the risk of opportunistic infection over either drug alone; consider the benefit versus risk of using the combination, particularly in patients with inflammatory bowel disease.

RISK FACTORS:

➡ *Effects of age.* In patients receiving mercaptopurine concurrently with corticosteroids, those older than 50 years may be at greater risk of opportunistic infections.[1]

MECHANISM: Both mercaptopurine and corticosteroids can increase the risk of opportunistic infections, and their effects may be additive.

CLINICAL EVALUATION: In a case-control study of patients with inflammatory bowel disease, 100 consecutive patients with opportunistic infections were compared with 200 matched controls. Therapy with mercaptopurine, azathioprine, or corticosteroids was individually associated with an approximate 3-fold increase in infection, whereas use of azathioprine or mercaptopurine with corticosteroids was associated with an approximate 15-fold increase in infection.[1] A 41-year-old man with ulcerative colitis developed life-threatening infective endocarditis after infliximab was added to his therapy with azathioprine and prednisolone.[2] Thus, the clinical evidence suggests that the combination of mercaptopurine or azathioprine with corticosteroids increases the risk of opportunistic infections.

RELATED DRUGS: Azathioprine (eg, *Imuran*) is metabolized to mercaptopurine, so azathioprine is likely to interact with corticosteroids in the same way as mercaptopurine.

MANAGEMENT OPTIONS:

➡ *Circumvent/Minimize.* Make a careful assessment of benefit versus risk before using any combination of mercaptopurine/azathioprine, corticosteroids, and infliximab.

➡ *Monitor.* If the combination is used, monitor the patient carefully for evidence of opportunistic infections.

REFERENCES:

1. Toruner M, et al. Risk factors for opportunistic infections in patients with inflammatory bowel disease. Gastroenterology. 2008;134(4):929-936.
2. Baumgart DC. How many lives does an ulcerative colitis patient have? *Lancet.* 2010;376(9744):928.

Mercaptopurine (eg, *Purinethol*)

Warfarin (eg, *Coumadin*)

SUMMARY: Mercaptopurine appeared to inhibit the hypoprothrombinemic response to warfarin in one patient, a finding consistent with animal studies. More study is needed to evaluate the incidence and significance of this interaction.

RISK FACTORS: No specific risk factors are known.

MECHANISM: Not established. Animal studies indicate that mercaptopurine increases prothrombin synthesis or activation.[1] If this is the primary mechanism, all oral anticoagulants are expected to interact with mercaptopurine.

CLINICAL EVALUATION: In a patient well controlled on long-term warfarin therapy, the prothrombin time decreased during mercaptopurine therapy.[2] When the mercaptopurine was stopped, the response to warfarin returned to normal; subsequent administration of mercaptopurine produced changes similar to the first episode. Although mercaptopurine most likely caused the reduced hypoprothrombinemic response to warfarin in this patient, it is unknown how frequently this effect may occur in other patients receiving the combination.

RELATED DRUGS: Azathioprine (eg, *Imuran*) is metabolized to mercaptopurine, and also has been reported to inhibit the hypoprothrombinemic response to warfarin. The effect of mercaptopurine on oral anticoagulants other than warfarin is unknown, but be alert for a similar effect with all oral anticoagulants.

MANAGEMENT OPTIONS:

➡ **Monitor.** Monitor for altered oral anticoagulant effect if mercaptopurine is initiated, discontinued, or changed in dosage. Adjust the anticoagulant dose as needed.

REFERENCES:
1. Martini A, Jähnchen E. Studies in rats on the mechanisms by which 6-mercaptopurine inhibits the anticoagulant effect of warfarin. *J Pharmacol Exp Ther.* 1977;201(3):547-553.
2. Spiers AS, et al. Increased warfarin requirement during mercaptopurine therapy: a new drug interaction. *Lancet.* 1974;2(7874):221-222.

Meropenem (*Merrem I.V.*)

Valproic Acid (eg, *Depakene*)

SUMMARY: The administration of meropenem has been associated with a marked reduction in the plasma concentrations of valproic acid; increased seizures may occur.

RISK FACTORS: No specific risk factors are known.

MECHANISM: Unknown. Meropenem may increase the glucuronidation of valproic acid.

CLINICAL EVALUATION: A number of cases of reduced valproic acid plasma concentrations in patients receiving concurrent meropenem have been reported.[1-6] Valproic acid plasma concentrations declined 50% to 80% in most of the cases with increased seizures, which were observed in some patients. For example, in 29 patients receiving meropenem while stabilized on valproic acid, the mean plasma concentration of valproic acid declined from 64.3 to 22.5 mg/L during meropenem coadministration.[1] Several patients received valproic acid dose increases, but plasma concentrations increased accordingly. Valproic acid doses as high as 12 g daily were needed to achieve therapeutic plasma concentrations during meropenem administration.

RELATED DRUGS: A similar case has been reported with imipenem-cilastatin (*Primaxin*).[6]

MANAGEMENT OPTIONS:

➡ *Monitor.* Carefully monitor plasma concentrations in patients stabilized on valproic acid if meropenem is coadministered. Increased valproic acid doses may be necessary to maintain therapeutic plasma concentrations.

REFERENCES:

1. Spriet I, et al. Interaction between valproate and meropenem: a retrospective study. *Ann Pharmacother.* 2007;41(7):1130-1136.

2. Spriet I, et al. Meropenem-valproic acid interaction in patients with cefepime-associated status epilepticus. *Am J Health Syst Pharm.* 2007;64(1):54-58.

3. Fudio S, et al. Epileptic seizures caused by low valproic acid concentrations from an interaction with meropenem. *J Clin Pharm Ther.* 2006;31(4):393-396.

4. Clause D, et al. Pharmacokinetic interaction between valproic acid and meropenem. *Intensive Care Med.* 2005;31(9):1293-1294.

5. Nacarkucuk E, et al. Meropenem decreases serum level of valproic acid. *Pediatr Neurol.* 2004;31(3):232-234.

6. Llinares-Tello F, et al. Pharmacokinetic interaction between valproic acid and carbapenem-like antibiotics: a discussion of three cases. *Farm Hosp.* 2003;27(4):258-263.

Mesalamine (eg, *Asacol*)

Warfarin (eg, *Coumadin*)

SUMMARY: Mesalamine appeared to inhibit the effect of warfarin in one patient, but a causal relationship was not established.

RISK FACTORS: No specific risk factors are known.

MECHANISM: Not established. The possibility that mesalamine inhibits warfarin absorption was not investigated.

CLINICAL EVALUATION: A 51-year-old woman on chronic warfarin 5 mg/day with stable international normalized ratio (INR) values between 2 and 3 was started on mesalamine 800 mg 3 times a day.[1] Four weeks later, she was admitted with acute venous thrombosis; her INR was 0.9, and serum warfarin concentrations were undetectable. No other reasons for the lack of warfarin effect appeared to be involved (eg, noncompliance, other drugs, herbal medications).

RELATED DRUGS: No information is available.

MANAGEMENT OPTIONS:

➡ *Circumvent/Minimize.* If the mesalamine inhibits warfarin absorption, separating the doses might reduce the magnitude of the interaction. However, because the mechanism of this purported interaction is not known, it is premature to make such recommendations. Moreover, because warfarin undergoes enterohepatic circulation, separation of doses of warfarin from binding agents does not completely eliminate such interactions.

➥ **Monitor.** Closely monitor the hypoprothrombinemic response to warfarin if mesalamine is initiated, discontinued, or changed in dosage.

REFERENCES:
1. Marinella MA. Mesalamine and warfarin therapy resulting in decreased warfarin effect. *Ann Pharmacother.* 1998;32(7-8):841-842.

 Metaraminol (*Aramine*)

AVOID **Pargyline**

SUMMARY: Metaraminol administration in patients taking a monoamine oxidase (MAO) inhibitor, such as pargyline, may result in a severe hypertensive response.

RISK FACTORS: No specific risk factors are known.

MECHANISM: Metaraminol is an indirect-acting sympathomimetic producing its pressor effect by releasing norepinephrine, which reacts with the adrenergic receptor. Because MAO inhibitors tend to increase the amount of norepinephrine present in storage sites of the adrenergic neuron, patients taking an MAO inhibitor would be expected to manifest an enhanced response to metaraminol.[1]

CLINICAL EVALUATION: A hypertensive patient who had a hypotensive episode while receiving pargyline was given metaraminol 4 mg intramuscular. Within 10 minutes, his systolic blood pressure was 300 mm Hg; he lost consciousness and developed an irregular cardiac rhythm.[2]

RELATED DRUGS: Metaraminol is contraindicated in patients receiving any nonselective MAO inhibitor, including isocarboxazid (*Marplan*), phenelzine (*Nardil*), and tranylcypromine (*Parnate*). Levarterenol (*Levophed*) is likely to be a safer pressor agent than metaraminol in such patients.

MANAGEMENT OPTIONS:

➥ ***AVOID COMBINATION.*** Avoid metaraminol in patients taking a monoamine inhibitor. Remember that the effects of nonselective monoamine inhibitors should be assumed to persist for 2 weeks after they are discontinued.

REFERENCES:
1. Sjoqvist F. Psychotropic drugs (2). Interaction between monoamine oxidase (MAO) inhibitors and other substances. *Proc R Soc Med.* 1965;58:967-978.
2. Horler AR, et al. Hypertensive crisis due to pargyline and metaraminol. *BMJ.* 1965;3:460.

 Metformin (eg, *Glucophage*)

Orlistat (*Xenical*)

SUMMARY: Orlistat did not affect metformin pharmacokinetics in healthy subjects.

RISK FACTORS: No specific risk factors are known.

MECHANISM: None (no interaction).

CLINICAL EVALUATION: In a randomized, crossover study in 21 healthy subjects, orlistat 120 mg 3 times daily for 6 days did not affect metformin pharmacokinetics.[1]

RELATED DRUGS: No information is available.

MANAGEMENT OPTIONS: No interaction.

REFERENCES:

1. Zhi J, et al. Pharmacokinetic evaluation of the possible interaction between selected concomitant medications and orlistat at steady state in healthy subjects. *J Clin Pharmacol.* 2002;42:1011-1019.

Methadone (eg, *Dolophine*)

Nevirapine (*Viramune*)

SUMMARY: Nevirapine reduces methadone concentrations; methadone withdrawal symptoms may result.

RISK FACTORS: No specific risk factors are known.

MECHANISM: Nevirapine induces the activity of CYP3A4, the enzyme responsible for the metabolism of methadone. Increased first-pass and systemic clearance is likely to result in lower plasma concentrations of methadone.

CLINICAL EVALUATION: Eight patients with HIV who were on stable methadone maintenance therapy had their methadone pharmacokinetics determined on 2 occasions, once while on just methadone and again after 2 weeks of HIV therapy that included nevirapine 200 mg/day in combination with stavudine, zidovudine, lamivudine, or didanosine.[1] The mean area under the concentration-time curve of methadone was decreased in excess of 50% following the nevirapine therapy. Six of the 8 patients complained of methadone withdrawal symptoms following 9 to 12 days of nevirapine coadministration. Several other case reports have noted withdrawal in patients receiving methadone maintenance after the initiation of nevirapine.[2-4]

RELATED DRUGS: Efavirenz (*Sustiva*) has been noted to reduce methadone plasma concentrations.

MANAGEMENT OPTIONS:

→ **Consider Alternative.** Consider the use of an analgesic (eg, morphine, codeine) not metabolized by CYP3A4 in patients taking methadone for its analgesic activity.

→ **Monitor.** Observe patients on methadone maintenance therapy for evidence of withdrawal symptoms if nevirapine is instituted. Methadone dosage may require an increase to prevent withdrawal symptoms. Monitor for excess methadone effect if the nevirapine is discontinued in a patient taking methadone.

REFERENCES:

1. Clarke SM, et al. Pharmacokinetic interactions of nevirapine and methadone and guidelines for use of nevirapine to treat injection drug users. *Clin Infect Dis.* 2001;33:1595-1597.
2. Otero MJ, et al. Nevirapine-induced withdrawal symptoms in HIV patients on methadone maintenance programme: an alert. *AIDS.* 1999;13:1004-1005.
3. Altice FL, et al. Nevirapine-induced opiate withdrawal among injection drug users with HIV infection receiving methadone. *AIDS.* 1999;13:957-962.
4. Heelon MW, et al. Methadone withdrawal when starting an antiretroviral regimen including nevirapine. *Pharmacotherapy.* 1999;19:471-472.

Methadone (eg, *Dolophine*)

Phenobarbital (eg, *Solfoton*)

SUMMARY: Phenobarbital may enhance methadone metabolism, resulting in methadone withdrawal.

RISK FACTORS: No specific risk factors are known.

MECHANISM: Barbiturates probably enhance the hepatic metabolism of methadone.

CLINICAL EVALUATION: A patient on methadone developed withdrawal symptoms after barbiturate therapy.[1] This is consistent with the known ability of other enzyme inducers (eg, phenytoin [*Dilantin*]) to result in methadone withdrawal symptoms.

RELATED DRUGS: All barbiturates would be expected to enhance methadone metabolism.

MANAGEMENT OPTIONS:

➡ ***Monitor.*** Monitor for methadone withdrawal if barbiturates are given concurrently.

REFERENCES:

1. Liu SJ, et al. Case report of barbiturate-induced enhancement of methadone metabolism and withdrawal syndrome. *Am J Psychiatry*. 1984;141:1287-1288.

 Methadone (eg, *Dolophine*)

Phenytoin (eg, *Dilantin-125*)

SUMMARY: Phenytoin may reduce serum methadone concentrations, resulting in symptoms of methadone withdrawal.

RISK FACTORS: No specific risk factors are known.

MECHANISM: Phenytoin may enhance the metabolism of methadone by hepatic microsomal enzymes.

CLINICAL EVALUATION: One case report described a methadone-treated patient who developed signs and symptoms of methadone withdrawal after a few days of phenytoin therapy.[1] These symptoms subsided when phenytoin was stopped and reappeared when the patient was rechallenged with phenytoin. In a study of 5 patients on methadone maintenance, phenytoin therapy induced withdrawal symptoms within 3 or 4 days.[2] These findings are consistent with the established ability of another enzyme inducer, rifampin (eg, *Rifadin*), to reduce the effect of methadone.

RELATED DRUGS: Other enzyme inducers such as barbiturates, carbamazepine (eg, *Tegretol*), primidone (eg, *Mysoline*), and rifampin may also enhance methadone metabolism.

MANAGEMENT OPTIONS:

➡ ***Avoid Unless Benefit Outweighs Risk.*** If possible, avoid using methadone with enzyme inducers such as phenytoin.

➡ ***Monitor.*** If the combination is necessary, monitor for any necessary methadone dose adjustment if phenytoin therapy is initiated, discontinued, or changed in dosage.

REFERENCES:

1. Finelli PF. Letter: Phenytoin and methadone tolerance. *N Engl J Med*. 1976;294:227.
2. Tong TG, et al. Phenytoin-induced methadone withdrawal. *Ann Intern Med*. 1981;94:349-351.

Methadone
Rasagiline (*Azilect*)

SUMMARY: Concomitant use of rasagiline and methadone should generally be avoided, although the risk of the concurrent use is not well established.

RISK FACTORS: No specific risk factors are known.

MECHANISM: Not established.

CLINICAL EVALUATION: The inclusion of methadone as contraindicated with rasagiline in the product information is apparently because related drugs such as meperidine and tramadol have serotonergic effects, resulting in severe serotonin syndrome-like reactions when combined with MAO inhibitors or other serotonergic drugs. Despite its basis on theoretical considerations, because it is contraindicated in the labeling, the combination should generally be avoided.[1]

RELATED DRUGS: Rasagiline is also contraindicated with other analgesics (eg, meperidine, propoxyphene, tramadol). Any interaction between rasagiline and methadone is likely to be similar to the interaction between selegiline and methadone.

MANAGEMENT OPTIONS:

➡ *Avoid Unless Benefit Outweighs Risk.* Methadone should generally not be used concomitantly with rasagiline or within 2 weeks of stopping rasagiline.

REFERENCES:
1. *Azilect* [package insert]. North Wales, PA: Teva Neuroscience, Inc.; 2006.

Methadone (eg, *Dolophine*)
Rifabutin (*Mycobutin*)

SUMMARY: Rifabutin does not appear to affect methadone serum concentrations.

RISK FACTORS: No specific risk factors are known.

MECHANISM: No interaction.

CLINICAL EVALUATION: Twenty-four patients on methadone maintenance had methadone serum and urine concentrations measured before and after 13 days of rifabutin 300 mg/day.[1] The mean pharmacokinetic parameters of methadone were unaffected by rifabutin administration. No changes in patient symptoms could be associated with changes in methadone concentrations.

RELATED DRUGS: Rifampin (eg, *Rifadin*) is known to reduce methadone serum concentrations and precipitate methadone withdrawal.

MANAGEMENT OPTIONS: No interaction.

REFERENCES:
1. Brown LS, et al. Lack of a pharmacologic interaction between rifabutin and methadone in HIV-infected former injecting drug users. *Drug Alcohol Depend.* 1996;43:71-77.

Methadone (eg, *Dolophine*)

Rifampin (eg, *Rifadin*)

SUMMARY: Rifampin can decrease methadone serum concentrations, resulting in withdrawal symptoms.

RISK FACTORS: No specific risk factors are known.

MECHANISM: Rifampin stimulates the hepatic metabolism of methadone.

CLINICAL EVALUATION: Of 30 patients on methadone maintenance given rifampin 600 to 900 mg/day, 21 developed evidence of narcotic withdrawal.[1] In a subsequent study of 6 of these patients, plasma methadone concentrations were considerably lower in the presence of rifampin. Two cases of methadone withdrawal occurring within 5 days of rifampin initiation have also been reported.[2,3] The interval between initiation of rifampin and symptoms of withdrawal is variable, but it usually occurs within the first week.

RELATED DRUGS: No information is available.

MANAGEMENT OPTIONS:

➡ **Monitor.** Observe methadone-treated patients for evidence of methadone withdrawal when they are started on rifampin. If the methadone dose is increased to offset the effect of rifampin, be alert for excessive methadone effect when the rifampin is discontinued.

REFERENCES:

1. Kreek MJ, et al. Rifampin-induced methadone withdrawal. *N Engl J Med.* 1976;294:1104-1106.
2. Bending MR, et al. Rifampicin and methadone withdrawal. *Lancet.* 1977;1:1211.
3. Holmes VE. Rifampin-induced methadone withdrawal in AIDS. *J Clin Psychopharmacol.* 1990;10:443-444.

Methadone (eg, *Dolophine*)

Ritonavir (*Norvir*)

SUMMARY: Ritonavir appears to reduce methadone activity; loss of analgesia or narcotic withdrawal may result.

RISK FACTORS: No specific risk factors are known.

MECHANISM: Methadone is primarily metabolized by CYP3A4. Several other enzymes may also contribute to its metabolism. Ritonavir may induce 1 of these metabolic pathways, resulting in a reduction of methadone plasma concentrations. In addition, ritonavir could affect methadone access to the CNS system by induction of the P-glycoprotein system that pumps drugs out of the CNS.

CLINICAL EVALUATION: A patient maintained for several years on methadone 90 mg/day was being treated for HIV with indinavir (*Crixivan*), zidovudine (eg, *Retrovir*), and lamivudine (eg, *Epivir*). These drugs were discontinued, and ritonavir 400 mg twice daily, saquinavir (eg, *Fortovase*) 400 mg twice daily, and stavudine (*Zerit*) 40 mg twice daily were started.[1] One week later, the patient was admitted with symptoms of narcotic withdrawal. The methadone plasma concentration was 210 ng/mL (usual methadone range, 50 to 1000 ng/mL) on admission; but other methadone concentrations were not reported, making an assessment of the mechanism difficult. The patient was treated with increased methadone doses and stabilized on methadone 130 mg/day.

RELATED DRUGS: While there is no information regarding the potential for other antiviral agents to reduce the concentration of methadone, agents that induce CYP3A4 activity such as nevirapine (*Viramune*) may affect methadone in a similar manner.

MANAGEMENT OPTIONS:

➠ **Monitor.** Observe patients taking methadone for a loss of efficacy during ritonavir administration.

REFERENCES:

1. Geletko SM, et al. Decreased methadone effect after ritonavir initiation. *Pharmacotherapy.* 2000;20:93-94.

Methadone (eg, *Dolophine*)

Somatostatin (*Zecnil*)

SUMMARY: Somatostatin appeared to inhibit the analgesic effect of methadone in 1 patient; the clinical importance of this effect is not established.

RISK FACTORS: No specific risk factors are known.

MECHANISM: Not established.

CLINICAL EVALUATION: A patient with severe cancer pain was well-controlled on oral methadone 4 mg 3 times/day. She developed a marked reduction in methadone analgesia after somatostatin was started, and the pain persisted even after an increase in methadone dose to 10 mg 3 times/day.[1] A switch to morphine (eg, *Roxanol*) was not helpful, but discontinuation of the somatostatin was followed by a substantial increase in morphine analgesia. Morphine was also ineffective in 2 other cancer patients receiving somatostatin.

RELATED DRUGS: It is not known whether the somatostatin analog octreotide (eg, *Sandostatin*) also inhibits methadone analgesia, but be alert for the possibility. Somatostatin has also been reported to inhibit morphine analgesia (see Morphine/Somatostatin), but its effect on other opioids is not established.

MANAGEMENT OPTIONS:

➠ **Monitor.** Watch for evidence of reduced analgesia if somatostatin is used with methadone or other opioid analgesics. If methadone analgesia appears diminished, it would be prudent to stop somatostatin. If somatostatin cannot be stopped, evidence suggests that it may be difficult to achieve adequate analgesia.

REFERENCES:

1. Ripamonti C, et al. Can somatostatin be administered in association with morphine in advanced cancer patients with pain? *Ann Oncol.* 1998;9:921-923.

Methadone (eg, *Dolophine*)

St. John's Wort

SUMMARY: St. John's wort appears to reduce methadone plasma concentrations and may lead to symptoms of methadone withdrawal.

RISK FACTORS: No specific risk factors are known.

MECHANISM: St. John's wort is known to induce both CYP3A4 and P-glycoprotein; it probably reduces the bioavailability and increases the hepatic metabolism and elimination of methadone.

CLINICAL EVALUATION: In 4 patients receiving methadone maintenance therapy, the addition of St. John's wort 900 mg/day resulted in marked reductions in methadone plasma concentrations.[1] Two of the 4 patients developed symptoms consistent with methadone withdrawal. Although the data are from only 4 patients, the results are consistent with the known interactive properties of both methadone and St. John's wort.

RELATED DRUGS: No information is available.

MANAGEMENT OPTIONS:

➡ **Monitor.** Observe methadone-treated patients for evidence of methadone withdrawal if they take St. John's wort concurrently. If the methadone dose is increased to offset the effect of St. John's wort, be alert for excessive methadone effect when rifampin is discontinued.

REFERENCES:

1. Eich-Höchli D, et al. Methadone maintenance treatment and St. John's wort. *Pharmacopsychiatry.* 2003;36:35-37.

4 Methadone (eg, *Dolophine*)

Zidovudine (*Retrovir*)

SUMMARY: Preliminary data suggest that methadone may increase zidovudine concentrations; the clinical significance of this increase is unknown.

RISK FACTORS: No specific risk factors are known.

MECHANISM: Not established.

CLINICAL EVALUATION: Nine patients receiving methadone maintenance therapy were studied before and after the addition of zidovudine.[1] The coadministration of zidovudine had no effect on the pharmacokinetics of methadone. Zidovudine pharmacokinetics in these patients were compared with 5 control patients not taking methadone. The patients taking methadone had zidovudine concentrations 43% higher than controls. The lack of a crossover study design limits the significance of this difference. The potential interaction awaits further controlled studies to define the magnitude and clinical significance of this purported interaction.

RELATED DRUGS: No information is available.

MANAGEMENT OPTIONS: No specific action is required, but be alert for evidence of the interaction.

REFERENCES:
1. Schwartz EL, et al. Pharmacokinetic interactions of zidovudine and methadone in intravenous drug-using patients with HIV infection. *J Acquir Immune Defic Syndr.* 1992;5:619-626.

Methandrostenolone

Tolbutamide (eg, *Orinase*)

SUMMARY: Anabolic steroids may enhance the hypoglycemic effect of tolbutamide and possibly other antidiabetic agents.

RISK FACTORS: No specific risk factors are known.

MECHANISM: Anabolic steroids may decrease blood glucose in some diabetic patients. Normal patients do not appear to be affected. Some have proposed that anabolic steroids also may inhibit the metabolism of oral hypoglycemic agents.[1,2]

CLINICAL EVALUATION: Methandrostenolone enhances the hypoglycemic response to tolbutamide. Anabolic steroids may decrease insulin requirements in diabetics and restore sensitivity in insulin-resistant patients.[3]

RELATED DRUGS: Although some anabolic steroids would be expected to enhance the hypoglycemic response to other antidiabetic drugs, specific data demonstrating this effect on hypoglycemic agents other than tolbutamide are lacking.

MANAGEMENT OPTIONS:

➡ *Consider Alternative.* Nandrolone (eg, *Durabolin*) and methenolone acetate did not appear to affect tolbutamide's hypoglycemic effects.[4]

➡ *Monitor.* If anabolic steroids are added to antidiabetic drug therapy, the patient should be monitored more closely for evidence of hypoglycemia.

REFERENCES:
1. Sotaniemi EA, et al. Drug metabolism and androgen control therapy in prostatic cancer. *Clin Pharmacol Ther.* 1973;14:413.
2. Kontturi M, et al. Estrogen-induced metabolic changes during treatment of prostatic cancer. *Scan J Lab Clin Invest.* 1970;25(Suppl. 113):45.
3. Sachs BA, et al. Effect of oxandrolone on plasma lipids and lipoproteins of patients with disorders of lipid metabolism. *Metabolism.* 1968;17:400.
4. Landon J, et al. The effect of anabolic steroids on blood sugar and plasma insulin levels in man. *Metabolism.* 1963;12:924.

Methenamine

Sodium Bicarbonate

SUMMARY: Sodium bicarbonate administration interferes with the antibacterial activity of methenamine compounds.

RISK FACTORS: No specific risk factors are known.

MECHANISM: Sodium bicarbonate tends to render the urine alkaline. During therapy with methenamine compounds, the urine must be kept at approximately pH 5.5 or lower to effect proper conversion of methenamine to free formaldehyde.

Sodium bicarbonate administration could increase the urine pH and prevent the conversion of methenamine to formaldehyde.

CLINICAL EVALUATION: Although little clinical evidence exists, large doses of sodium bicarbonate can effectively alkalinize the urine and would be expected to inhibit the effect of methenamine compounds that require a urine pH less than 5.5 for optimal effect.[1-3]

RELATED DRUGS: Certain antacids (eg, magnesium, aluminum hydroxides) and acetazolamide (eg, *Diamox*) also may alkalinize the urine somewhat, but it is unknown whether this effect would be sufficient to affect methenamine.

MANAGEMENT OPTIONS:

➡ **Monitor.** If the urine cannot be kept at an approximate pH 5.5 or lower during the use of sodium bicarbonate, methenamine compounds should not be used.

REFERENCES:

1. Product information. Mandelamine. Warner-Chilcott. 1993.
2. Kevorkian CG, et al. Methenamine mandelate with acidification: an effective urinary antiseptic in patients with neurogenic bladder. *Mayo Clin Proc.* 1984;59:523.
3. Pearman JW, et al. The antimicrobial activity of urine of paraplegic patients receiving methenamine mandelate. *Invest Urol.* 1978;16:91.2.

Methenamine

Sulfadiazine

SUMMARY: The combination of methenamine and sulfadiazine may result in crystalluria.

RISK FACTORS: No specific risk factors are known.

MECHANISM: With some sulfonamides, the danger of crystalluria is enhanced in an acid urine. Methenamine compounds require a urine pH of approximately 5.5 or less in order to be active.

CLINICAL EVALUATION: The less soluble sulfonamides are more likely than others to result in crystalluria in an acid urine. This has been well documented in the past but rarely occurs now because more soluble agents such as sulfisoxazole (eg, *Gantrisin*) are more widely used. The concomitant administration of methenamine compounds and sulfamethizole (*Thiosulfil*) frequently results in formation of a precipitate in the urine.[1] Cotherapy with methenamine and sulfathiazole reportedly results in a similar effect.

RELATED DRUGS: Sulfamethizole and sulfathiazole interact similarly with methenamine. However, more soluble agents, such as sulfisoxazole, rarely interact.

MANAGEMENT OPTIONS:

➡ **Consider Alternative.** Methenamine compounds should not be used with sulfonamides that may precipitate in an acid urine. The use of sulfathiazole or sulfamethizole with methenamine compounds should be avoided. If a methenamine product and a sulfonamide are to be used together, it would be preferable to use the more soluble sulfonamides, such as sulfisoxazole.

➡ *Monitor.* Patients receiving methenamine and sulfadiazine should be monitored for crystalluria.

REFERENCES:

1. Mandelamine. Physician's Desk Reference. 47th ed. Oradell: Medical Economics Data; 1993:1780.

Methenamine

Vitamin C

SUMMARY: Vitamin C has minimal effect on the formation of formaldehyde in the urine. The clinical significance of this interaction appears to be limited.

RISK FACTORS: No specific risk factors are known.

MECHANISM: Methenamine's conversion to formaldehyde in the urine is responsible for its antibacterial activity. An acid pH is necessary for this conversion to occur efficiently. Moderate doses of vitamin C do not appear to alter urine pH significantly or enhance the antibacterial efficacy of methenamine.

CLINICAL EVALUATION: In a study of 27 patients with indwelling urinary catheters and chronic bacteriuria, methenamine mandelate 4 g/day was administered alone, with vitamin C 4 g/day, or with vitamin C plus cranberry cocktail 1 L/day.[1] Vitamin C alone or combined with cranberry cocktail had no significant effect on urinary pH. However, vitamin C administration did result in a higher urine concentration of formaldehyde, but urine cultures remained positive in most of the patients. In another study, the urine from 3 healthy subjects was collected before and following 3 days of vitamin C 1 g 4 times daily. Vitamin C 1 g 4 times daily failed to affect the formation rates of formaldehyde from methenamine.[2]

RELATED DRUGS: No information is available.

MANAGEMENT OPTIONS: No specific action is required, but be alert for evidence of the interaction.

REFERENCES:

1. Nahata MC, et al. Effect of urinary acidifiers on formaldehyde concentration and efficacy with methenamine therapy. *Eur J Clin Pharmacol.* 1982;22:281.

2. Strom JG Jr, et al. Effect of urine pH and ascorbic acid on the rate of conversion of methenamine to formaldehyde. *Biopharm Drug Disposit.* 1993;14:61.

Methocarbamol (eg, *Robaxin*)

Pyridostigmine Bromide (eg, *Mestinon*)

SUMMARY: One case report indicated that methocarbamol may inhibit the effect of pyridostigmine, but a causal relationship was not established.

RISK FACTORS: No specific risk factors are known.

MECHANISM: Not established.

CLINICAL EVALUATION: Methocarbamol may have impaired the therapeutic effect of pyridostigmine bromide in 1 patient with myasthenia gravis.[1]

RELATED DRUGS: No information is available.

MANAGEMENT OPTIONS: No specific action is required, but be alert for evidence of the interaction.

REFERENCES:

1. Podrizki A. Methocarbamol and myasthenia gravis. *JAMA*. 1968;205:938.

 Methotrexate (eg, *Rheumatrex*)

Naproxen (eg, *Naprosyn*)

SUMMARY: A patient on chronic methotrexate for arthritis developed evidence of methotrexate toxicity and died after receiving naproxen.

RISK FACTORS:

➥ ***Concurrent Diseases.*** Particular caution is suggested in patients with pre-existing renal impairment (who may be more susceptible to nonsteroidal anti-inflammatory drug [NSAID]-induced renal failure).

➥ ***Dosage Regimen.*** The risk of adverse effects from this interaction is primarily in patients receiving antineoplastic doses of methotrexate, rather than the lower doses used to treat rheumatoid arthritis, psoriasis, and related diseases.

MECHANISM: It is widely held that NSAIDs interfere with renal secretion of methotrexate, either by inhibiting tubular secretion of methotrexate or by reducing renal blood flow by inhibiting prostaglandin synthesis. Alterations in plasma protein binding also have been proposed, but this is unlikely to be clinically significant because methotrexate is normally only 50% to 70% bound to plasma proteins. Pharmacokinetic studies involving several different NSAIDs have failed to consistently identify an alteration in methotrexate pharmacokinetics by NSAIDs[1-8]; however, even in studies where methotrexate pharmacokinetics remained unchanged overall, occasional patients appeared to exhibit reduced clearance of methotrexate after NSAID administration.[1,3]

CLINICAL EVALUATION: A patient receiving methotrexate for rheumatoid arthritis developed fever and diarrhea following administration of naproxen.[14] Over 7 days, the reaction progressed to intractable diarrhea, melena, vomiting, hematemesis, epistaxis, extensive mucosal ulcerations, pyrexia, severe pancytopenia, and death. Although the patient had, by mistake, taken 27. 5 mg of methotrexate during the week instead of the prescribed 7.5 mg, the larger dose should not have produced such a severe reaction. Although the reaction is consistent with naproxen-induced enhancement of methotrexate toxicity, too few details about the case are presented to establish a cause and effect relationship. Patients on low-dose methotrexate for rheumatoid arthritis frequently receive concurrent NSAIDs, and severe methotrexate toxicity in such patients is unusual.[10-12] Although these patients would appear to be at low risk, caution is warranted because NSAID use in patients on low-dose methotrexate occasionally is associated with severe methotrexate toxicity.[9,13]

RELATED DRUGS: See Clinical Evaluation.

MANAGEMENT OPTIONS:

➥ ***Avoid Unless Benefit Outweighs Risk.*** Until more information is available on this interaction, it would be prudent to avoid naproxen (as well as other NSAIDs) in patients receiving antineoplastic doses of methotrexate. Particular caution is suggested in patients with pre-existing renal impairment, who may be more susceptible to NSAID-induced renal failure.

➡ *Monitor.* If the combination is used, monitor for methotrexate toxicity. Findings in methotrexate toxicity can include stomatitis, severe GI symptoms (nausea, diarrhea, vomiting), bone marrow suppression, fever, bleeding, skin rashes, nephrotoxicity, and hepatotoxicity. Although decreasing the methotrexate dosage would be expected to reduce the likelihood of toxicity, the magnitude of the required reduction in methotrexate dosage has not been established.

REFERENCES:

1. Aherene A, et al. Methotrexate kinetics in rheumatoid arthritis: is there an interaction with nonsteroidal antiinflammatory drugs? *J Rheumatol.* 1988;15:1356.

2. Furst DE, et al. Effect of aspirin and sulindac on methotrexate clearance. *J Pharm Sci.* 1990;79:782.

3. Dupuis LL, et al. Methotrexate-nonsteroidal antiinflammatory drug interaction in children with arthritis. *J Rheumatol.* 1990;17:469.

4. Liegler DG, et al. The effect of organic acids on renal clearance of methotrexate in man. *Clin Pharmacol Ther.* 1969;10:849.

5. Skeith KJ, et al. Lack of significant interaction between low dose methotrexate and ibuprofen or flurbiprofen in patients with arthritis. *J Rheumatol.* 1990;17:1008.

6. Stewart CF, et al. Effect of aspirin (ASA) on the disposition of methotrexate (MTX) in patients with rheumatoid arthritis (RA). *Clin Pharmacol Ther.* 1990;47:139. Abstract PP-56.

7. Taylor JR, et al. Effect of sodium salicylate and indomethacin on methotrexate-serum albumin binding. *Arch Dermatol.* 1977;113:588.

8. Tracy FS, et al. The effect of NSAIDS on methotrexate disposition in patients with rheumatoid arthritis. *Clin Pharmacol Ther.* 1990;47:138. Abstract PP-54.

9. Daly HM, et al. Methotrexate toxicity precipitated by azapropazone. *Br J Dermatol.* 1986;114:733.

10. Boh LE, et al. Low-dose weekly oral methotrexate therapy for inflammatory arthritis. *Clin Pharm.* 1986;5:503.

11. Anderson PA, et al. Weekly pulse methotrexate in rheumatoid arthritis: clinical and immunologic effects in a randomized, double-blind study. *Ann Intern Med.* 1985;103:489.

12. Tugwell P, et al. Methotrexate in rheumatoid arthritis: indications, contraindications, efficacy, and safety. *Ann Intern Med.* 1987;107:358.

13. Adams JD, et al. Drug interactions in psoriasis. *Aust J Dermatol.* 1976;17:39.

14. Singh RR, et al. Fatal interaction between methotrexate and naproxen. *Lancet.* 1986;1:1390.

Methotrexate (eg, *Rheumatrex*)

Neomycin (eg, *Neo-fradin*) AVOID

SUMMARY: Oral absorption of methotrexate is decreased by 30% to 50% in patients receiving oral antibiotic mixtures including paromomycin (*Humatin*), neomycin, nystatin (eg, *Mycostatin*), and vancomycin (eg, *Vancocin*).

RISK FACTORS: No specific risk factors are known.

MECHANISM: Not established. Oral nonabsorbable antibiotics may decrease the absorption of methotrexate.

CLINICAL EVALUATION: The pharmacokinetics of methotrexate were studied in 25 men receiving chemotherapy for lung cancer.[1] Patients were randomized into 1 of 3 groups. One group received intensive chemotherapy, were confined to a laminar air flow room, and received prophylactic oral nonabsorbable antibiotics (PNAA) consisting of polymyxin B, paromomycin, nystatin, and vancomycin. Another group received intensive chemotherapy without PNAA and remained on a hospital ward, and the third group received conventional chemotherapy. Half of the patients on PNAA had decreases in oral methotrexate absorption of over 30%. Before the start of PNAA, a mean of 68.72% ± 8.42% of the oral dose of methotrexate was recovered within 72 hours in the urine, compared with 44.4% ± 12.66% while patients were receiving PNAA.

RELATED DRUGS: No information is available.

MANAGEMENT OPTIONS:

➡ **AVOID COMBINATION.** Patients receiving oral methotrexate should not receive oral nonabsorbable antibiotics. It is not known whether this interaction occurs with parenteral methotrexate; however, the possibility cannot be excluded.

REFERENCES:

1. Cohen MH, et al. Effect of oral prophylactic broad spectrum nonabsorbable antibiotics on the gastrointestinal absorption of nutrients and methotrexate in small cell bronchogenic carcinoma patients. *Cancer.* 1976;38:1556–1559.

Methotrexate (eg, *Rheumatrex*)

Omeprazole (*Prilosec*)

SUMMARY: A patient with osteosarcoma developed elevated methotrexate serum concentrations while receiving concurrent omeprazole; more study is needed to establish the clinical importance of this purported interaction.

RISK FACTORS: No specific risk factors are known.

MECHANISM: Not established. Methotrexate undergoes active secretion in the kidney, and it is proposed that omeprazole interferes with the renal H^+, K^+-ATPase that mediates this process.

CLINICAL EVALUATION: A 41-year-old man with osteosarcoma was started on chemotherapy that included methotrexate with leucovorin (eg, *Wellcovorin*) rescue.[1] He was concurrently receiving several other drugs including omeprazole 20 mg/day. During his first course of therapy with methotrexate, his serum methotrexate levels unexpectedly remained elevated for several days. He was aggressively hydrated, his urine was alkalinized, and he received leucovorin for 8 days. Omeprazole was then discontinued, and methotrexate retention was not observed during 3 subsequent cycles of methotrexate. The patient was not rechallenged with the combination, so it is not possible to establish a causal relationship with certainty. Nonetheless, given the potentially serious nature of methotrexate toxicity, consider the possibility of the interaction. The effect of omeprazole on the smaller doses of methotrexate given in the treatment of rheumatoid arthritis and related diseases is not established, but caution is in order.

RELATED DRUGS: Theoretically, H_2-receptor antagonists such as ranitidine (eg, *Zantac*), cimetidine (eg, *Tagamet*), famotidine (eg, *Pepcid*), and nizatidine (*Axid*) would be less likely than omeprazole to interact with methotrexate, but little clinical information is available.

MANAGEMENT OPTIONS:

➡ **Monitor.** Until more data are available, monitor for excessive methotrexate effect if omeprazole is given concurrently.

REFERENCES:

1. Reid T, et al. Impact of omeprazole on the plasma clearance of methotrexate. *Cancer Chemother Pharmacol.* 1993;33:82-84.

Methotrexate (eg, *Rheumatrex*)

Oxacillin (*Bactocill*)

SUMMARY: A patient developed severe methotrexate toxicity following 3 doses of oxacillin.

RISK FACTORS: No specific risk factors are known.

MECHANISM: Oxacillin may interfere with the organic anion active renal secretion of methotrexate.

CLINICAL EVALUATION: A patient with osteosarcoma was treated with methotrexate, 15 g infused over 6 hours.[1] Following the second methotrexate dose 1 week later, an infection was noted and oxacillin 1 g was administered 6, 14, and 23 hours following the end of the methotrexate infusion. Methotrexate concentrations were over 50 times higher 24 hours following the second methotrexate dose than had occurred with the first methotrexate dose. The patient developed acute renal failure, hepatic toxicity, mucitis, and aplastic anemia. Oxacillin was discontinued and treatment included folinic acid and hemodialysis.

RELATED DRUGS: Other penicillins (eg, amoxicillin, piperacillin, mezlocillin) are known to inhibit methotrexate elimination.

MANAGEMENT OPTIONS:

➡ ***Consider Alternative.*** Treat patients receiving methotrexate with alternative antibiotics that do not compete with the renal organic anion transporter.

➡ ***Monitor.*** Watch patients for evidence of enhanced methotrexate effect and possible toxicity when large doses of oxacillin or other penicillins are coadministered.

REFERENCES:

1. Titier K, et al. Pharmacokinetic interaction between high-dose methotrexate and oxacillin. *Ther Drug Monit.* 2002;24:570-572.

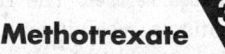

Methotrexate

Pantoprazole (*Protonix*)

SUMMARY: A patient on pantoprazole developed myopathy following low-dose methotrexate. A causal relationship was strong in this case, but it is not known how often the combination would produce adverse outcomes.

RISK FACTORS: Not established.

MECHANISM: Not established. Pantoprazole may interfere with the renal elimination of the primary methotrexate metabolite, 7-hydroxymethotrexate.

CLINICAL EVALUATION: A 59-year-old man with lymphoma on pantoprazole 20 mg/day for Barrett syndrome began receiving low-dose methotrexate (15 mg IM once weekly).[1] Within hours of the first injection of methotrexate, he developed severe myalgia and bone pain. The symptoms resolved when pantoprazole was replaced by ranitidine. Eight weeks later a rechallenge with pantoprazole plus methotrexate produced the symptoms again, associated with a 70% elevation in 7-hydroxymethotrexate concentrations compared with methotrexate alone. It is highly likely that the reaction was due to a drug interaction between methotrexate and pantoprazole in this patient, given a positive dechallenge, positive rechallenge, and the fact that the neither drug alone produced the effect. Also, another proton pump inhibitor, omeprazole, has been associated with methotrexate toxicity.[2,3]

RELATED DRUGS: Omeprazole (eg, *Prilosec*) also has been associated with methotrexate toxicity, so it is possible that other proton pump inhibitors also would interact with methotrexate.

MANAGEMENT OPTIONS:

➡ *Monitor.* In patients receiving methotrexate, one should be particularly alert for evidence of methotrexate toxicity if pantoprazole, omeprazole, or other proton pump inhibitor is given concurrently.

REFERENCES:

1. Troger U, et al. Severe myalgia from an interaction between treatments with pantoprazole and methotrexate. *BMJ.* 2002;324:1497.

2. Beorlegui B, et al. Potential interaction between methotrexate and omeprazole. *Ann Pharmacother.* 2000;34:1024-1027.

3. Reid T, et al. Impact of omeprazole on the plasma clearance of methotrexate. *Cancer Chemother Pharmacol.* 1993;33:82-84.

 Methotrexate (eg, *Rheumatrex*)

Phenylbutazone

SUMMARY: Two patients on methotrexate developed evidence of severe methotrexate toxicity after starting phenylbutazone; 1 patient died.

RISK FACTORS:

➡ *Concurrent Diseases.* Particular caution is suggested in patients with pre-existing renal impairment (who may be more susceptible to nonsteroidal anti-inflammatory drug [NSAID]-induced renal failure).

➡ *Dosage Regimen.* The risk of adverse effects from this interaction is primarily in patients receiving antineoplastic doses of methotrexate, rather than the lower doses used to treat rheumatoid arthritis, psoriasis, and related diseases.

MECHANISM: It is widely held that NSAIDs interfere with renal secretion of methotrexate, either by inhibiting tubular secretion of methotrexate or by reducing renal blood flow by inhibiting prostaglandin synthesis. Alterations in plasma protein binding also have been proposed, but this is unlikely to be clinically significant because methotrexate is normally only 50% to 70% bound to plasma proteins. Pharmacokinetic studies involving several different NSAIDs have failed to consistently identify an alteration in methotrexate pharmacokinetics by NSAIDs[1-8]; however, even in studies in which methotrexate pharmacokinetics remained unchanged overall, occasional patients appeared to exhibit reduced clearance of methotrexate after NSAID administration.[1,3] The ability of phenylbutazone and other NSAIDs to produce acute renal failure[9] also might result in accumulation of methotrexate.

CLINICAL EVALUATION: A 65-year-old man with psoriasis had been receiving low-dose methotrexate 15 mg/week with minimal toxicity for several years.[10] Following addition of phenylbutazone 200 mg/day for 2 days (supplied by a neighbor), he developed widespread skin erosions, oral ulcerations, and fever. He recovered with supportive therapy. Another patient, a 61-year-old woman, developed cutaneous and oral ulcerations, fever, severe bone marrow suppression, and fatal septicemia after 6 days of combined therapy with methotrexate 2.5 mg/day and phenylbutazone 600 mg/day.[9] Although one cannot be certain that the phenylbutazone was responsible for the methotrexate toxicity, a cause and effect relationship is supported by the relatively low doses of methotrexate, the temporal relationship of the reaction and the phenylbutazone therapy, and the known properties of phenylbutazone (eg, interference with active renal tubular secretion and avid binding to plasma proteins).

RELATED DRUGS: Oxyphenbutazone also would be expected to enhance methotrexate toxicity, but clinical data are lacking.

MANAGEMENT OPTIONS:

➡ *Avoid Unless Benefit Outweighs Risk.* Although only limited clinical evidence exists, it would be prudent to avoid phenylbutazone (as well as other NSAIDs) in patients receiving antineoplastic doses of methotrexate. Particular caution is suggested in patients with preexisting renal impairment who may be more susceptible to NSAID-induced renal failure.

➡ *Monitor.* If the combination is used, monitor for methotrexate toxicity. Findings in methotrexate toxicity can include stomatitis, severe GI symptoms (eg, nausea, diarrhea, vomiting), bone marrow suppression, fever, bleeding, skin rashes, nephrotoxicity, and hepatotoxicity. Although decreasing the methotrexate dosage would be expected to reduce the likelihood of toxicity, the magnitude of the required reduction in methotrexate dosage has not been established.

REFERENCES:

1. Ahern M, et al. Methotrexate kinetics in rheumatoid arthritis: is there an interaction with nonsteroidal anti-inflammatory drugs? *J Rheumatol.* 1988;15:1356-1360.
2. Furst DE, et al. Effect of aspirin and sulindac on methotrexate clearance. *J Pharm Sci.* 1990;79:782-786.
3. Dupuis LL, et al. Methotrexate-nonsteroidal anti-iflammatory drug interaction in children with arthritis. *J Rheumatol.* 1990;17:1469-1473.
4. Liegler DG, et al. The effect of organic acids on renal clearance of methotrexate in man. *Clin Pharmacol Ther.* 1969;10:849-857.
5. Skeith KJ, et al. Lack of significant interaction between low dose methotrexate and ibuprofen or flurbiprofen in patients with arthritis. *J Rheumatol.* 1990;17:1008-1010.
6. Stewart CF, et al. Effect of aspirin (ASA) on the disposition of methotrexate (MTX) in patients with rheumatoid arthritis (RA). *Clin Pharmacol Ther.* 1990;47:139.
7. Taylor JR, et al. Effect of sodium salicylate and indomethacin on methotrexate-serum albumin binding. *Arch Dermatol.* 1977;113:588-591.
8. Tracy FS, et al. The effect of NSAIDs on methotrexate disposition in patients with rheumatoid arthritis. *Clin Pharmacol Ther.* 1990;47:138.
9. Greenstone M, et al. Acute nephrotic syndrome with reversible renal failure after phenylbutazone. *Br Med J.* 1981;282:950-951.
10. Adams JD, et al. Drug interaction in psoriasis. *Australas J Dermatol.* 1976;17:39-40.

Methotrexate (eg, *Rheumatrex*)

Polio Vaccine AVOID

SUMMARY: Administration of live-virus vaccines such as oral polio vaccine (OPV) to immunosuppressed patients, including those undergoing cytotoxic chemotherapy, may result in infection by the live virus.

RISK FACTORS: No specific risk factors are known.

MECHANISM: While patients are receiving immunosuppressive antineoplastic drugs, they may lack the immunologic function required to keep live vaccines from producing infection.

CLINICAL EVALUATION: Immunization of patients with measles-virus vaccine, oral polio vaccine, and smallpox vaccine have resulted in fatal infections in immunocompromised patients, including patients receiving chemotherapy. In 1 case, a patient developed disseminated vaccinia infection after receiving smallpox vaccine while on methotrexate.[1] In another case, fatal giant-cell pneumonia developed in a pediatric patient with acute leukemia after receiving attenuated measles-virus vaccine.[2] Immunization with inactivated vaccines such as influenza vaccine and pneumococcal vaccine are not contraindicated but may not induce the same levels of protective antibodies in patients receiving chemotherapy as in the general population.[3]

RELATED DRUGS: Other vaccines that may result in infections in immunocompromised patients include BCG vaccine, typhoid vaccine, measles vaccine, mumps vaccine, rubella vaccine, or yellow fever vaccine.

MANAGEMENT OPTIONS:

➠ *AVOID COMBINATION.* Current recommendations state that patients with leukemia in remission should not receive live vaccines until at least 3 months have passed since the completion of all chemotherapy.[3,4] Similar guidelines should be followed for patients receiving chemotherapy for other malignancies.

REFERENCES:

1. Allison J. Methotrexate and smallpox vaccination. *Lancet.* 1968;2:1250. Letter.
2. Mitus A, et al. Attenuated measles vaccine in children with acute leukemia. *Am J Dis Child.* 1962;103:243.
3. Pizzo PA, et al. Infections in the cancer patient. In: DeVita VT et al., eds. Cancer: principles and practice of oncology. 4th ed. Philadelphia: J. B. Lippincott; 1993:2292.
4. Immunization Practices Advisory Committee. Update on adult immunization. Recommendations of the Immunization practices advisory committee (ACIP). *MMWR.* 1991;40(RR-12):1.

 Methotrexate (eg, *Rheumatrex*)

Probenecid

SUMMARY: Probenecid markedly increases serum methotrexate concentrations and would be expected to increase both the therapeutic effect and toxicity of methotrexate.

RISK FACTORS: No specific risk factors are known.

MECHANISM: Probenecid appears to inhibit the active renal tubular secretion of methotrexate.

CLINICAL EVALUATION: Serum concentrations of methotrexate were considerably higher in 4 patients given probenecid (various doses) plus methotrexate (200 mg/m^2 by IV bolus) than in 4 similar patients receiving methotrexate alone.[1] In a crossover study of 4 patients, serum methotrexate concentrations were approximately 300% higher when probenecid (1.7 g/m^2) was given with methotrexate as compared with methotrexate alone.[4] In another study of 20 patients, treatment with probenecid (500 mg every 6 hours for 5 doses) doubled serum methotrexate concentrations.[2] The magnitude and predictability of the increases in serum methotrexate indicate that toxicity could occur if the interaction were not anticipated. Although probenecid inhibits the transfer of methotrexate from the cerebrospinal fluid in dogs,[3] this effect was not seen in a study of 4 patients.[4]

RELATED DRUGS: Sulfinpyrazone (eg, *Anturane*) would be expected to produce a similar effect on methotrexate.

MANAGEMENT OPTIONS:

➡ *Avoid Unless Benefit Outweighs Risk.* Probenecid and sulfinpyrazone generally should be avoided in patients receiving methotrexate.

➡ *Monitor.* If the combination is used, one should anticipate that a reduction in methotrexate dosage may be required. Serum methotrexate determinations would be helpful, and one also should monitor for excessive methotrexate effect (eg, gastrointestinal toxicity, stomatitis, bone marrow suppression, hepatotoxicity, infection).

REFERENCES:

1. Aherne GW, et al. Prolongation and enhancement of serum methotrexate concentrations by probenecid. *BMJ.* 978;1:1097.
2. Lilly MB, et al. Clinical pharmacology of oral intermediate-dose methotrexate with or without probenecid. *Cancer Chemother Pharmacol.* 1985;15:220.
3. Ramu A, et al. Probenecid inhibition of methotrexate excretion from cerebrospinal fluid in dogs. *J Pharmacokinet Biopharm.* 1978;6:389.
4. Howell SB, et al. Effect of probenecid on cerebrospinal fluid methotrexate kinetics. *Clin Pharmacol Ther.* 1979;26:641.

Methotrexate (eg, *Rheumatrex*) 4

Theophylline (eg, *Theolair*)

SUMMARY: Weekly IM injections of methotrexate increase serum theophylline concentrations, but the clinical importance is not established.

RISK FACTORS: No specific risk factors are known.

MECHANISM: Not established.

CLINICAL EVALUATION: Fifteen steroid-dependent patients with asthma were treated with methotrexate 15 mg/kg IM weekly or placebo for 6 weeks.[1] Theophylline pharmacokinetics were determined following a single oral dose before and after methotrexate treatment. Theophylline clearance after oral administration was significantly reduced (19%) by methotrexate administration. The clinical significance of this interaction requires additional study with multiple-dose theophylline administration. Larger doses of methotrexate might be expected to increase the magnitude of this interaction.

RELATED DRUGS: No information is available.

MANAGEMENT OPTIONS: No specific action is required, but be alert for evidence of the interaction.

REFERENCES:

1. Glynn-Barnhart, A et al. Effect of methotrexate on prednisolone and theophylline pharmacokinetics. *Clin Pharmacol Ther.* 1990;47:130. Abstract.

Methotrexate (eg, *Rheumatrex*)

Thiazides

SUMMARY: Thiazides may increase bone marrow suppression in patients on chemotherapy, possibly by increasing the effect of methotrexate.

RISK FACTORS: No specific risk factors are known.

MECHANISM: Not established. Theoretically, thiazides could reduce the renal elimination of methotrexate.

CLINICAL EVALUATION: In 14 women with breast cancer who were receiving chemotherapy (cyclophosphamide [eg, *Cytoxan*], methotrexate, and fluorouracil [eg, *Adrucil*]), thiazide therapy appeared to enhance the myelosuppressive effect.[1] This interaction, if real, may result from an effect of thiazides on 1 of the components (eg, methotrexate) rather than on cytotoxic agents in general.

RELATED DRUGS: No information is available.

MANAGEMENT OPTIONS:

➡ **Monitor.** Patients should be monitored for enhanced bone marrow suppression when thiazides are used with methotrexate (or other cytotoxic agents). Adjust cytotoxic drug dosage as needed.

REFERENCES:

1. Orr LE. Potentiation of myelosuppression from cancer chemotherapy and thiazide diuretics. *Drug Intell Clin Pharm.* 1981;15:967.

Methotrexate (eg, *Rheumatrex*)

Trimethoprim (eg, *Bactrim*)

SUMMARY: The administration of trimethoprim and methotrexate has resulted in severe methotrexate toxicity.

RISK FACTORS:

➡ **Concurrent Diseases.** Preexisting renal disease will reduce methotrexate elimination.

MECHANISM: Trimethoprim appears to increase the free fraction of methotrexate by displacing it from protein binding sites and inhibits the renal tubular elimination of methotrexate.[1]

CLINICAL EVALUATION: Nine children with leukemia demonstrated an average 40% reduction in the clearance of unbound methotrexate when trimethoprim and sulfamethoxazole were coadministered.[1] The renal clearance of methotrexate was reduced about 54% during the antibiotic administration. Several case reports have noted myelosuppression in patients taking methotrexate who were treated with trimethoprim or combinations of trimethoprim and sulfamethoxazole.[2-5]

RELATED DRUGS: None known.

MANAGEMENT OPTIONS:

➡ *Use Alternative.* Do not administer trimethoprim to patients taking methotrexate. Choose an alternative antibiotic. Avoid penicillins because they can have a similar effect on methotrexate renal elimination.

REFERENCES:

1. Ferrazzini G, et al. Interaction between trimethoprim-sulfamethoxazole and methotrexate in children with leukemia. *J Pediatr.* 1990;117:823-826.
2. Govert JA, et al. Pancytopenia from using trimethoprim and methotrexate. *Ann Intern Med.* 1992;117:877-878.
3. Groenendal H, et al. Methotrexate and trimethoprim-sulphamethoxazole—a potentially hazardous combination. *Clin Exper Derm.* 1990;15:358-360.
4. Steuer A, et al. Methotrexate and trimethoprim: a fatal interaction. *Br J Rheumatol.* 1998;37:105-106.
5. Saravana S, et al. Myelotoxicity due to methotrexate - an iatrogenic cause. *Eur J Haematol.* 2003;71:315-316.

Methotrexate (eg, *Rheumatrex*)

Vancomycin (eg, *Vancocin*)

SUMMARY: Methotrexate serum concentrations can be reduced by oral vancomycin and aminoglycosides.

RISK FACTORS: No specific risk factors are known.

MECHANISM: Oral aminoglycosides may reduce absorption of oral methotrexate.

CLINICAL EVALUATION: Methotrexate absorption in 10 patients with bronchogenic carcinoma was reduced 36% during the administration of a group of oral antibiotics (paromomycin [*Humatin*], polymyxin B, nystatin [eg, *Mycostatin*], vancomycin).[1] It is not possible to determine the relative contribution of the various antibiotics administered. More study is needed to define the incidence and significance of this interaction.

RELATED DRUGS: No information is available.

MANAGEMENT OPTIONS:

➡ *Monitor.* Watch for decreased methotrexate response if oral aminoglycosides are administered.

REFERENCES:

1. Cohen MH, et al. Effect of oral prophylactic broad spectrum nonabsorbable antibiotics on the gastro-intestinal absorption of nutrients and methotrexate in small cell bronchogenic carcinoma patients. *Cancer.* 1976;38:1556-1559.

Methotrimeprazine

Pargyline　AVOID

SUMMARY: Coadministration of pargyline and methotrimeprazine was associated with fatality in 1 reported case.

RISK FACTORS: No specific risk factors are known.

MECHANISM: Not established.

CLINICAL EVALUATION: A fatal reaction occurred in a patient receiving pargyline and methotrimeprazine, but a drug interaction was not unequivocally established as the cause.[1,2]

RELATED DRUGS: All nonselective monoamine oxidase (MAO) inhibitors, including iso-carboxazid (*Marplan*), phenelzine (*Nardil*), and tranylcypromine (*Parnate*), should be considered contraindicated with methotrimeprazine.

MANAGEMENT OPTIONS:

➡ *AVOID COMBINATION.* Although the interaction between methotrimeprazine and MAO inhibitors is not well documented, the possibility of a fatal reaction contra-indicates concomitant use of these drugs. Remember that the effects of nonselec-tive MAO inhibitors should be assumed to persist for 2 weeks after they are discontinued.

REFERENCES:

1. Sjoqvist F. Psychotropic drugs (2). Interaction between monoamine oxidase (MAO) inhibitors and other substances. *Proc R Soc Med.* 1965;58(11 pt 2):967-978.

2. Barsa JA, et la. A comparative study of tranylcypromine and paragyline. *Psychopharmacologia.* 1964;6:295-298.

Methoxyflurane (*Penthrane*)

Secobarbital

SUMMARY: Barbiturates like secobarbital may enhance the nephrotoxic effect of methoxyflurane.

RISK FACTORS: No specific risk factors are known.

MECHANISM: Induction of hepatic microsomal enzymes by barbiturates may stimulate the metabolism of methoxyflurane to nephrotoxic metabolites.

CLINICAL EVALUATION: In a study of the effects of methoxyflurane on renal function in 13 patients, 1 patient had been receiving an enzyme inducer, secobarbital 100 mg/day.[1] The secobarbital-treated patient developed nonoliguric renal insufficiency; serum inorganic fluoride levels were considerably higher than the mean of the other 12 patients. The proposal that the barbiturate may have predisposed this patient to methoxyflurane nephrotoxicity is consistent with previous studies in animals. Another patient has been described who also may have represented an example of this interaction.[2]

RELATED DRUGS: Based upon the mechanism, one would expect all barbiturates to inter-act similarly with methoxyflurane.

MANAGEMENT OPTIONS:

➡ *Consider Alternative.* Consider anesthetics other than methoxyflurane in patients who are receiving enzyme inducers such as barbiturates. Remember that enzyme induction dissipates slowly following discontinuation of the inducing agent, so the enhanced metabolic activity usually returns to normal within 2 to 3 weeks.

➡ *Monitor.* Monitor for nephrotoxicity if the combination is given.

REFERENCES:

1. Churchill D, et al. Toxic nephropathy after low-dose methoxyflurane anesthesia: drug interaction with secobarbital? *Can Med Assoc J.* 1976;114:326-328,333.

2. Cousins MJ, et al. Methoxyflurane nephrotoxicity. A study of dose response in man. *JAMA.* 1973;225:1611-1616.

Methoxyflurane (*Penthrane*)

Tetracycline

SUMMARY: Patients receiving methoxyflurane anesthesia appear to be at increased risk of developing renal toxicity if they are treated with tetracycline.

RISK FACTORS: No specific risk factors are known.

MECHANISM: Not established. A combined nephrotoxic action appears to be involved.

CLINICAL EVALUATION: Five of 7 patients who received tetracycline in addition to methoxyflurane anesthesia developed signs of nephrotoxicity, and 3 of the patients died[1] Additional cases have appeared in which the combined use of methoxyflurane and tetracycline seemed to cause renal damage.[2-6] Methoxyflurane is known to have some nephrotoxic potential,[7] and tetracycline is known to be hazardous in patients with renal malfunction. The 2 drugs together appear to be a dangerous combination, although more information is needed to unequivocally establish the relationship of drug interaction to renal failure.

RELATED DRUGS: Other antibiotics, including kanamycin (eg, *Kantrex*) and gentamicin (eg, *Garamycin*), have been implicated in similar nephrotoxic effects in patients who receive methoxyflurane.[8]

MANAGEMENT OPTIONS:

➡ *Use Alternative.* The severe consequences of this possible interaction warrant great caution in administering tetracycline (and perhaps other nephrotoxic antibiotics) to patients who will soon undergo or have recently undergone methoxyflurane anesthesia. Avoid the use of tetracycline with methoxyflurane.

REFERENCES:

1. Kuzucu EY. Methoxyflurane, tetracycline, and renal failure. *JAMA.* 1970;211:1162.
2. Churchill D. Persisting renal insufficiency after methoxyflurane anesthesia. Report of two cases and review of literature. *Am J Med.* 1974;56:575.
3. Dryden GE. Incidence of tubular degeneration with microlithiasis following methoxyflurane compared with other anesthetic agents. *Anesth Analg.* 1974;53:383.
4. Stoelting RK, et al. Effect of tetracycline therapy on renal function after methoxyflurane anesthesia. *Anesth Analg.* 1973;52:431.
5. Albers DD, et al. Renal failure following prostatovesiculectomy related to methoxyflurane anesthesia and tetracycline complicated by candida infection. *J Urol.* 1971;106:348.
6. Proctor EA, et al. Polyuric acute renal failure after methoxyflurane and tetracycline. *BMJ.* 1971;4:661.
7. Mazze RI, et al. Renal dysfunction associated with methoxyflurane anesthesia. A randomized, prospective clinical evaluation. *JAMA.* 1971;216:278.
8. Cousins MJ. Tetracycline, methoxyflurane anesthesia, and renal dysfunction. *Lancet.* 1972;1:751.

Methyldopa (eg, *Aldomet*)

Norepinephrine (Levarterenol; *Levophed*)

SUMMARY: Methyldopa therapy may prolong the pressor response to norepinephrine.

RISK FACTORS: No specific risk factors are known.

MECHANISM: Not established.

CLINICAL EVALUATION: Norepinephrine 1 to 8 mcg was administered rapidly IV to 10 hypertensive patients before and after methyldopa therapy. A slight increase in the pressor response to norepinephrine was seen following methyldopa, and the duration of the pressor response was considerably prolonged.[1,2]

RELATED DRUGS: No information is available.

MANAGEMENT OPTIONS:

➡ **Monitor.** Monitor for increased blood pressure response to norepinephrine in patients receiving methyldopa.

REFERENCES:

1. Dollery CT. Physiological and pharmacological interactions of antihypertensive drugs. *Proc R Soc Med.* 1965;58:983.
2. Dollery CT, et al. Haemodynamic studies with methyldopa: effect on cardiac output and response to pressor amines. *Br Heart J.* 1963;25:670.

 Methyldopa (eg, *Aldomet*)

Pargyline

SUMMARY: One patient developed hallucinations while on pargyline and methyldopa, but a causal relationship was not established.

RISK FACTORS: No specific risk factors are known.

MECHANISM: Not established.

CLINICAL EVALUATION: A single case report, supported by animal studies, has appeared describing a possible interaction between methyldopa and monoamine oxidase inhibitors (MAOIs).[1,2] The patient developed hallucinations while receiving methyldopa and pargyline, although a causal relationship was not established.[1] Further, others have reported the combination to be safe.[3]

RELATED DRUGS: The effect of combining methyldopa with other nonselective MAOIs such as isocarboxazid (*Marplan*), phenelzine (*Nardil*), and tranylcypromine (*Parnate*) is unknown.

MANAGEMENT OPTIONS: No specific action is required, but be alert for evidence of the interaction.

REFERENCES:

1. Paykel ES. Hallucinosis on combined methyldopa and pargyline. *BMJ.* 1966;1:803.
2. Van Rossum JM. Potential dangers of monoamine oxidase inhibitors and alpha-methyldopa. *Lancet.* 1963;1:950.
3. Herting RL. Monoamine oxidase inhibitors. *Lancet.* 1965;1:1324.

 Methyldopa (eg, *Aldomet*)

Phenobarbital (eg, *Solfoton*)

SUMMARY: Phenobarbital does not appear to affect the disposition of methyldopa.

RISK FACTORS: No specific risk factors are known.

MECHANISM: No interaction.

CLINICAL EVALUATION: Although evidence was presented that phenobarbital may reduce methyldopa blood levels,[1] others could not confirm these findings using a more specific assay for methyldopa.[2,3]

RELATED DRUGS: No information is available.

MANAGEMENT OPTIONS: No interaction.

REFERENCES:

1. Kaldor A, et al. Enhancement of methyldopa metabolism with barbiturate. *BMJ.* 1971;3:518.
2. Kristensen M, et al. Barbiturates and methyldopa metabolism. *BMJ.* 1973;1:49.
3. Kristensen M, et al. Plasma concentration of alphamethyldopa and its main metabolite, methyldopa-O-sulfate during long-term treatment with alfamethyldopa, with special reference to possible interaction with other drugs given simultaneously. *Clin Pharmacol Ther.* 1973;14:139.

Methyldopa (eg, *Aldomet*)

Propranolol (eg, *Inderal*)

SUMMARY: Some evidence indicates that patients receiving propranolol and methyldopa may develop hypertension when there is a release of catecholamines.

RISK FACTORS: No specific risk factors are known.

MECHANISM: The following mechanism for the interaction between a beta-blocker and methyldopa has been proposed.[1] Methyldopa results in accumulation of alpha-methylnorepinephrine in storage sites of the adrenergic neuron. Because alpha-methylnorepinephrine has a greater beta-adrenergic (vasodilating) activity than norepinephrine, it is a less potent pressor agent. If propranolol is administered, the beta-adrenergic stimulation of alpha-methylnorepinephrine is inhibited, resulting in unopposed alpha-adrenergic stimulation and increased pressor response.

CLINICAL EVALUATION: One case report describes a patient 36 years of age with hypertension taking methyldopa and hydralazine (eg, *Apresoline*) who developed an increasing blood pressure following propranolol 5 mg by slow intravenous injection.[1] However, 2 subsequent patients taking methyldopa did not manifest a hypertensive reaction following propranolol. In a similar case subsequently described, administration of neostigmine (eg, *Prostigmin*) to a patient who had received methyldopa, atropine, and practolol was followed by a hypertensive reaction (260/140 mm Hg).[2] It also should be noted that paradoxical hypertension following methyldopa has been observed in the absence of beta-blockers.[3] More data are needed to establish causation.

RELATED DRUGS: Other beta-blockers may produce similar effects.

MANAGEMENT OPTIONS: No specific action is required, but be alert for evidence of the interaction.

REFERENCES:

1. Nies AS, et al. Hypertensive response to propranolol in a patient treated with methyldopa—a proposed mechanism. *Clin Pharmacol Ther.* 1973;14(5):823-826.
2. Palmer RF. Pharmacological autopsy of anesthetic death after aortography for aortic dissection (Question and Answer). *JAMA.* 1975;232:1281.
3. Zehnle CG. Paradoxical hypertension experienced during methyldopa therapy. *Am J Hosp Pharm.* 1981;38(11):1774-1775.

Methyldopa (eg, *Aldomet*)

Tolbutamide (eg, *Orinase*)

SUMMARY: Methyldopa administration may cause a small increase in tolbutamide concentrations, but the clinical importance of this effect is probably minimal.

RISK FACTORS: No specific risk factors are known.

MECHANISM: Not established. Methyldopa may inhibit the metabolism of tolbutamide.

CLINICAL EVALUATION: In 10 patients, the half-life and apparent clearance of a single dose of tolbutamide 3 g were determined before and after the administration of methyldopa 1 g/day for 7 days.[1] The half-life increased an average of 24%, while the apparent clearance was reduced by 16%. While no data on glucose or insulin concentrations were presented, these changes are not likely to result in altered glycemic control in most diabetic patients taking tolbutamide.

RELATED DRUGS: Methyldopa may exert a similar effect on other sulfonylureas.

MANAGEMENT OPTIONS: No specific action is required, but be alert for evidence of the interaction.

REFERENCES:

1. Gachályi B, et al. Effect of alphamethyldopa on the half-lives of antipyrine, tolbutamide and D-glucaric acid excretion in man. *Int J Clin Pharmacol Ther Toxicol.* 1980;18(3):133-135.

4   **Methyldopa (eg, *Aldomet*)**

Trifluoperazine

SUMMARY: One patient taking trifluoperazine developed a hypertensive reaction following methyldopa, but a causal relationship was not established.

RISK FACTORS: No specific risk factors are known.

MECHANISM: It has been proposed that neuroleptics can block the reuptake of the methyldopa metabolite, alpha-methylnorepinephrine, into the adrenergic neuron, resulting in a paradoxical hypertensive response to methyldopa.[1,2]

CLINICAL EVALUATION: The blood pressure of a woman 23 years of age with systemic lupus erythematosus and renal disease increased when methyldopa was added to her trifluoperazine therapy.[1] This response was attributed to excess alpha-methylnorepinephrine concentrations resulting from neuroleptic-induced inhibition of uptake and diminished excretion as a result of the renal disease. However, previously, hypertensive reactions had been associated with methyldopa in a patient who was not receiving neuroleptics.[2]

RELATED DRUGS: The effect of other phenothiazines on methyldopa response is not established.

MANAGEMENT OPTIONS: No specific action is required, but be alert for evidence of the interaction.

REFERENCES:

1. Westervelt FB Jr, et al. Letter: methyldopa-induced hypertension. *JAMA.* 1974;227(5):557.
2. Levine RJ, et al. Hypertensive responses to methyldopa. *N Engl J Med.* 1966;275(17):946-948.

Methylene Blue

Paroxetine (eg, *Paxil*) `AVOID`

SUMMARY: Giving methylene blue to patients receiving paroxetine or other serotonergic drugs may result in serotonin syndrome; the combination is best avoided.

RISK FACTORS: No specific risk factors are known.

MECHANISM: Methylene blue appears to be a strong inhibitor of monoamine oxidase type A (MAO-A) and a weak inhibitor of MAO-B.[1,2] Selective serotonin reuptake inhibitors (SSRIs), such as paroxetine, and selective serotonin-norepinephrine reuptake inhibitors (SNRIs) may cause severe serotonin syndrome when combined with MAO inhibitors (MAOIs).

CLINICAL EVALUATION: Several patients on long-term paroxetine therapy who were given methylene blue developed evidence of serotonin syndrome (eg, agitation, disorientation, fever, hyperreflexia, muscle rigidity, clonus).[1,3-5] In 1 case, a very small dose of methylene blue was used (1 mg/kg).[5] Virtually all cases of serotonin syndrome following methylene blue have occurred in patients receiving SSRIs or SNRIs, which is consistent with the view that a drug interaction is involved. (SSRIs and SNRIs given alone rarely produce serious serotonin toxicity, even when taken in overdose.)

RELATED DRUGS: Methylene blue has been associated with serotonin syndrome in patients receiving other SSRIs, such as citalopram (eg, *Celexa*) and fluoxetine (eg, *Prozac*), and also in patients receiving SNRIs, such as clomipramine (eg, *Anafranil*) and venlafaxine (eg, *Effexor*). Methylene blue is likely to also interact with other SSRIs such as escitalopram (*Lexapro*), fluvoxamine, and sertraline (eg, *Zoloft*), and other SNRIs, such as desvenlafaxine (*Pristiq*), duloxetine (*Cymbalta*), and imipramine (eg, *Tofranil*).

MANAGEMENT OPTIONS:

➡ *AVOID COMBINATION.* Given that serotonin syndrome can be life-threatening, it is prudent to avoid the combination.[6] Stopping paroxetine or other SSRIs or SNRIs for 2 weeks before using methylene blue would minimize the risk, except for fluoxetine, where 5 weeks should elapse before using an MAOI, such as methylene blue. Available evidence suggests that the interaction cannot be avoided by decreasing the dose of methylene blue.[1,5]

REFERENCES:

1. Stanford SC, et al. Risk of severe serotonin toxicity following co-administration of methylene blue and serotonin reuptake inhibitors: an update on a case report of post-operative delirium [published online ahead of print May 7, 2009]. *J Psychopharmacol.* doi:10.1177/0269881109105450.

2. Ramsay RR, et al. Methylene blue and serotonin toxicity: inhibition of monoamine oxidase A (MAO A) confirms a theoretical prediction. *Br J Pharmacol.* 2007;152(6):946-951.

3. Ng BK, et al. Serotonin syndrome following methylene blue infusion during parathyroidectomy: a case report and literature review. *Can J Anaesth.* 2008;55(1):36-41.

4. Bach KK, et al. Prolonged postoperative disorientation after methylene blue infusion during parathyroidectomy. *Anesth Analg.* 2004;99(5):1573-1574.

5. Schwiebert C, et al. Small doses of methylene blue, previously considered safe, can precipitate serotonin toxicity. *Anaesthesia.* 2009;64(8):924.

6. Pollack G, et al. Parathyroid surgery and methylene blue: a review with guidelines for safe intraoperative use [published online ahead of print May 13, 2009]. *Laryngoscope.* doi:10.1002/lary.20581.

Methylene Blue

AVOID **Venlafaxine (eg, *Effexor*)**

SUMMARY: Giving methylene blue to patients receiving venlafaxine or other serotonergic drugs may result in serotonin syndrome; the combination is best avoided.

RISK FACTORS: No specific risk factors are known.

MECHANISM: Methylene blue appears to be a strong inhibitor of monoamine oxidase type A (MAO-A) and a weak inhibitor of MAO-B.[1,2] Selective serotonin-norepinephrine reuptake inhibitors (SNRIs), such as venlafaxine, and selective serotonin reuptake inhibitors (SSRIs) may cause severe serotonin syndrome when combined with MAO inhibitors (MAOIs).

CLINICAL EVALUATION: Several cases of neurological toxicity have occurred when methylene blue was given to patients on long-term venlafaxine therapy.[3,4] The symptoms reported were consistent with serotonin syndrome, but not unequivocal. Nonetheless, given the known serotonergic effects of venlafaxine, one would expect that it would increase the risk of serotonin syndrome when combined with methylene blue. Virtually all cases of serotonin syndrome following methylene blue have occurred in patients receiving SNRIs or SSRIs, which is consistent with the view that a drug interaction is involved. (SNRIs or SSRIs given alone rarely produce serious serotonin toxicity, even when taken in overdose.)

RELATED DRUGS: Methylene blue has been associated with serotonin syndrome in patients receiving other SSRIs, such as citalopram (eg, *Celexa*), fluoxetine (eg, *Prozac*), and paroxetine (eg, *Paxil*), and also in patients receiving SNRIs, such as clomipramine (eg, *Anafranil*). Methylene blue is likely to also interact with other SSRIs, such as escitalopram (*Lexapro*), fluvoxamine, and sertraline (eg, *Zoloft*), and other SNRIs, such as desvenlafaxine (*Pristiq*), duloxetine (*Cymbalta*), and imipramine (eg, *Tofranil*).

MANAGEMENT OPTIONS:

➡ ***AVOID COMBINATION.*** Given that serotonin syndrome can be life-threatening, it is prudent to avoid the combination.[5] Stopping clomipramine or other SSRIs or SNRIs for 2 weeks before using methylene blue would minimize the risk, except for fluoxetine, where 5 weeks should elapse before using an MAOI such as methylene blue. Available evidence suggests that the interaction cannot be avoided by decreasing the dose of methylene blue.[1,6]

REFERENCES:

1. Stanford SC, et al. Risk of severe serotonin toxicity following co-administration of methylene blue and serotonin reuptake inhibitors: an update on a case report of post-operative delirium [published online ahead of print May 7, 2009]. *J Psychopharmacol.* doi:10.1177/0269881109105450.

2. Ramsay RR, et al. Methylene blue and serotonin toxicity: inhibition of monoamine oxidase A (MAO A) confirms a theoretical prediction. *Br J Pharmacol.* 2007;152(6):946-951.

3. Majithia A, et al. Methylene blue toxicity following infusion to localize parathyroid adenoma. *J Laryngol Otol.* 2006;120(2):138-140.

4. Sweet G, et al. Methylene-blue-associated encephalopathy. *J Am Coll Surg.* 2007;204(3):454-458.

5. Pollack G, et al. Parathyroid surgery and methylene blue: a review with guidelines for safe intraoperative use [published online ahead of print May 13, 2009]. *Laryngoscope.* doi:10.1002/lary.20581.

6. Schwiebert C, et al. Small doses of methylene blue, previously considered safe, can precipitate serotonin toxicity. *Anaesthesia.* 2009;64(8):924.

Methylphenidate (eg, *Ritalin*) 4

Phenytoin (eg, *Dilantin*)

SUMMARY: Methylphenidate has been associated with isolated cases of phenytoin intoxication, although most patients do not appear to be affected.

RISK FACTORS: No specific risk factors are known.

MECHANISM: Methylphenidate may inhibit the metabolism of phenytoin,[1] but there is debate about the significance of this effect.

CLINICAL EVALUATION: One patient in whom an interaction between phenytoin and methylphenidate reportedly occurred was receiving relatively large doses of phenytoin.[1] In another patient, increasing plasma phenytoin concentrations followed the administration of methylphenidate on one occasion, but not on another. It is interesting that, in this patient, phenytoin concentrations increased following discontinuation of amphetamine therapy[2]; animal studies have indicated that amphetamine impairs GI absorption of phenytoin.[3] In another study of 11 patients, methylphenidate had no effect on phenytoin plasma concentrations.[4] One clinician cites experience with more than 100 patients who received concomitant phenytoin and methylphenidate without any obvious complications.[5] Thus, the interaction between these drugs may be manifested only in those patients who are receiving doses of phenytoin large enough to nearly saturate the hepatic enzymes responsible for its metabolism or in patients with some other predisposing factors.

RELATED DRUGS: No information is available.

MANAGEMENT OPTIONS: No specific action is required, but be alert for evidence of the interaction.

REFERENCES:

1. Garrettson LK, et al. Methylphenidate interaction with both anticonvulsants and ethyl biscoumacetate. *JAMA*. 1969;207(11):2053-2056.
2. Mirkin BL, et al. Drug interactions: effect of methylphenidate on the disposition of diphenylhydantoin in man. *Neurology*. 1971;21(11):1123-1128.
3. Frey HH, et al. Interaction of amphetamine with anticonvulsant drugs. II. Effect of amphetamine on the absorption of anticonvulsant drugs. *Acta Pharmacol Toxicol (Copenh)*. 1966;24(4):310-316.
4. Kupferberg HJ, et al. Effect of methylphenidate on plasma anticonvulsant levels. *Clin Pharmacol Ther*. 1972;13(2):201-204.
5. Oettinger L. Interaction of methylphenidate and diphenylhydantoin (questions and answers). *Drug Ther*. 1976;5:107.

Methylprednisolone (eg, *Medrol*)

Troleandomycin†

SUMMARY: Troleandomycin markedly enhances methylprednisolone effects and may enhance prednisolone effects in some patients.

RISK FACTORS: No specific risk factors are known.

MECHANISM: Troleandomycin probably inhibits hepatic metabolism of methylprednisolone and possibly some other corticosteroids.

CLINICAL EVALUATION: Troleandomycin can considerably reduce the elimination and dosage requirement of methylprednisolone.[1-3]

RELATED DRUGS: Although prednisolone (eg, *Prelone*) disposition was not affected by troleandomycin in 3 steroid-dependent patients with asthma, troleandomycin slightly reduced prednisolone elimination in the presence of phenobarbital (eg, *Solfoton*).[4] Little is known regarding the effect of troleandomycin on other corticosteroids in humans. Erythromycin (eg, *Ery-Tab*) and clarithromycin (eg, *Biaxin*) are likely to produce a similar effect on methylprednisolone. Azithromycin (eg, *Zithromax*) and dirithromycin[†] would be unlikely to enhance the effects of methylprednisolone.

MANAGEMENT OPTIONS:

➡ *Monitor.* A considerable reduction in methylprednisolone dosage requirement is likely in the presence of troleandomycin. Monitor patients on other corticosteroids for possible corticosteroid dosage adjustments when troleandomycin is started or stopped.

REFERENCES:

1. Szefler SJ, et al. The effect of troleandomycin on methylprednisolone elimination. *J Allergy Clin Immunol.* 1980;66:447-451.

2. Selenke W, et al. Nonantibiotic effects of macrolide antibiotics of the oleandomycin-erythromycin group with special reference to their "steroid-sparing" effects. *J Allergy Clin Immunol.* 1980;65:454-464.

3. Nelson HS, et al. A double-blind study of troleandomycin and methylprednisolone in asthmatic subjects who require daily corticosteroids. *Am Rev Respir Dis.* 1993;147:398-404.

4. Szefler SJ, et al. Steroid-specific and anticonvulsant interaction aspects of troleandomycin-steroid therapy. *J Allergy Clin Immunol.* 1982;69:455-460.

† Not available in the United States.

 Methysergide†

AVOID **Sumatriptan (*Imitrex*)**

SUMMARY: Do not administer sumatriptan or other triptans within 24 hours of methysergide.

RISK FACTORS: No specific risk factors are known.

MECHANISM: Additive pharmacodynamic effects.

CLINICAL EVALUATION: The product information for *Imitrex* (sumatriptan) states that it should not be used within 24 hours of methysergide because excessive (additive) vasoconstriction may occur.[1] Although this is based primarily on theoretical considerations, the adverse effect could be severe, and concurrent use may present medicolegal risks.

RELATED DRUGS: All other triptans such as almotriptan (*Axert*), eletriptan (*Relpax*), frovatriptan (*Frova*), naratriptan (*Amerge*), rizatriptan (*Maxalt*), and zolmitriptan (*Zomig*) also are contraindicated within 24 hours of taking methysergide or other ergot alkaloids.

MANAGEMENT OPTIONS:

➡ *AVOID COMBINATION.* Do not use sumatriptan and other triptans within 24 hours of methysergide or other ergot alkaloids.

REFERENCES:

1. *Imitrex* [package insert]. Research Triangle Park, NC: GlaxoSmithKline; 2006.

† Not available in the United States.

Metoclopramide (eg, *Reglan*) 5

Propranolol (eg, *Inderal*)

SUMMARY: Metoclopramide does not interact with long-acting propranolol.

RISK FACTORS: No specific risk factors are known.

MECHANISM: No interaction.

CLINICAL EVALUATION: In 12 healthy subjects, pretreatment with oral metoclopramide 20 mg did not affect the serum concentrations of long-acting oral propranolol 160 mg.[1] It is not known if metoclopramide interacts with an immediate-release propranolol preparation.

RELATED DRUGS: No information is available.

MANAGEMENT OPTIONS: No interaction.

REFERENCES:
1. Charles BG, et al. Effect of metoclopramide on the bioavailability of long-acting propranolol. *Br J Clin Pharmacol.* 1981;11:517-518.

Metoclopramide (eg, *Reglan*) 4

Sertraline (*Zoloft*)

SUMMARY: A case of extrapyramidal symptoms, possibly caused by cotherapy with metoclopramide and sertraline, has been reported, but a causal relationship was not established.

RISK FACTORS: No specific risk factors are known.

MECHANISM: Not established.

CLINICAL EVALUATION: A 23-year-old woman taking metoclopramide 15 mg 4 times daily for gastroesophageal reflux disease was admitted for an acute depressive episode.[1] After 2 doses of sertraline 50 mg/day, she developed extrapyramidal symptoms (eg, grinding of teeth, jaw tightness, periauricular pain). The patient's symptoms were relieved with diphenhydramine 50 mg. The next day, she experienced similar symptoms about 8 hours after taking sertraline; the symptoms abated with benztropine (eg, *Cogentin*) 2 mg. Sertraline was then discontinued, and the symptoms did not recur. It was proposed that combined therapy with metoclopramide and sertraline may have produced the extrapyramidal symptoms, but a causal relationship was not established.

RELATED DRUGS: The effect of combining metoclopramide with selective serotonin reuptake inhibitors other than sertraline has not been established.

MANAGEMENT OPTIONS: No specific action is required, but be alert for evidence of the interaction.

REFERENCES:
1. Christensen RC, Byerly MJ. Mandibular dystonia associated with the combination of sertraline and metoclopramide. *J Clin Psychiatry.* 1996;57:596.

Metoclopramide (eg, *Reglan*)

Tacrolimus (eg, *Prograf*)

SUMMARY: A patient on tacrolimus developed elevated tacrolimus concentrations and toxicity after metoclopramide was added; monitor tacrolimus concentrations and clinical status.

RISK FACTORS:

➡ *Concurrent Diseases.* If the proposed mechanism is correct, the interaction would be most marked in patients with diseases and/or taking drugs that slow GI motility.

MECHANISM: In patients with slow gastric motility, it is proposed that metoclopramide, by speeding gastric emptying, can facilitate delivery of tacrolimus to sites of absorption in the small intestine.

CLINICAL EVALUATION: A 52-year-old woman taking tacrolimus following a liver transplant had undetectable tacrolimus concentrations, even with concurrent ketoconazole (eg, *Nizoral*).[1] Following the addition of metoclopramide 10 mg 4 times daily to improve gastric motility, she developed elevated tacrolimus concentrations and evidence of tacrolimus nephrotoxicity and neurotoxicity.

RELATED DRUGS: Metoclopramide also has been reported to increase cyclosporine (eg, *Neoral*) serum concentrations.

MANAGEMENT OPTIONS: No specific action is required, but be alert for evidence of the interaction.

REFERENCES:
1. Prescott WA Jr, et al. Tacrolimus toxicity associated with concomitant metoclopramide therapy. *Pharmacotherapy.* 2004;24:532-537.

Metoclopramide (eg, *Reglan*)

Venlafaxine (*Effexor*)

SUMMARY: A patient developed symptoms of serotonin syndrome after concurrent use of venlafaxine and metoclopramide, but more data are needed to establish a causal relationship.

RISK FACTORS: No specific risk factors are known.

MECHANISM: Not established.

CLINICAL EVALUATION: A 32-year-old woman stabilized on venlafaxine 225 mg/day developed evidence of serotonin syndrome (eg, agitation, confusion, diaphoresis, muscle rigidity, myoclonus) after receiving 2 doses of metoclopramide 10 mg IV.[1] She improved with administration of diazepam (eg, *Valium*) and discontinuation of venlafaxine and metoclopramide. She was later restarted on the previous dose of venlafaxine with no recurrence of adverse effects.

RELATED DRUGS: The combination of sertraline (eg, *Zoloft*) and metoclopramide caused extrapyramidal symptoms in 1 patient, but little is known about the combination of metoclopramide with other selective serotonin reuptake inhibitors.

MANAGEMENT OPTIONS: No specific action is required, but be alert for evidence of the interaction.

REFERENCES:

1. Fisher AA, Davis MW. Serotonin syndrome caused by selective serotonin reuptake-inhibitors-metoclopramide interaction. *Ann Pharmacother.* 2002;36:67-71.

Metoprolol (eg, *Lopressor*)

Paroxetine (eg, *Paxil*)

SUMMARY: Paroxetine increases the plasma concentration of metoprolol; hypotension or bradycardia may occur.

RISK FACTORS:

➡ **Pharmacogenetics.** Only patients who are extensive metabolizers of CYP2D6 are susceptible to the interaction.

MECHANISM: Paroxetine inhibits the activity of the enzyme CYP2D6 that is responsible for a majority of the metabolism of metoprolol.

CLINICAL EVALUATION: In a study of 8 healthy subjects, pretreatment with paroxetine 20 mg/day for 6 days increased the mean area under the concentration-time curve (AUC) of the beta-blocking enantiomer (S-)metoprolol by about 5-fold.[1] Its half-life was doubled. A similar increase in metoprolol AUC was noted in patients with acute myocardial infarctions who received paroxetine 20 mg/day.[2] Heart rate was significantly reduced and hypotension was noted in several of the patients. A case report of complete atrioventricular block was noted in a patient receiving paroxetine 20 mg/day 2 weeks after metoprolol 50 mg/day was added.[3] The heart block resolved after discontinuation of the paroxetine and metoprolol. Rechallenge with metoprolol and paroxetine monotherapy did not reproduce the arrhythmia.

RELATED DRUGS: Propranolol (eg, *Inderal*), timolol (eg, *Blocadren*), carvedilol (eg, *Coreg*), and nebivolol (*Bystolic*) are at least partially metabolized by CYP2D6 and would be expected to have some increased plasma concentration if administered with paroxetine. Citalopram (eg, *Celexa*) and escitalopram (*Lexapro*) are known to increase metoprolol concentrations. Other antidepressants that inhibit CYP2D6 (eg, fluoxetine [eg, *Prozac*], duloxetine [*Cymbalta*]) are expected to increase metoprolol's plasma concentrations.

MANAGEMENT OPTIONS:

➡ **Consider Alternative.** Consider administering a beta-blocker that is not metabolized by CYP2D6, such as atenolol (eg, *Tenormin*), or an antidepressant that does not inhibit CYP2D6 (eg, trazodone).

➡ **Monitor.** Monitor patients requiring metoprolol and paroxetine for bradycardia and hypotension.

REFERENCES:

1. Hemeryck A, et al. Paroxetine affects metoprolol pharmacokinetics and pharmacodynamics in healthy volunteers. *Clin Pharmacol Ther.* 2000;67(3):283-291.

2. Goryachkina K, et al. Inhibition of metoprolol metabolism and potentiation of its effects by paroxetine in routinely treated patients with acute myocardial infarction (AMI). *Eur J Clin Pharmacol.* 2008,64(3):275-282.

3. Onalan O, et al. Complete atrioventricular block associated with concomitant use of metoprolol and paroxetine. *Mayo Clin Proc.* 2008;83(5):595-599.

Metoprolol (eg, *Lopressor*)

Propafenone (eg, *Rythmol*)

SUMMARY: Metoprolol or propranolol (eg, *Inderal*) concentrations may significantly increase after administration of propafenone.

RISK FACTORS: No specific risk factors are known.

MECHANISM: Propafenone inhibits the metabolic clearance of metoprolol and propranolol.

CLINICAL EVALUATION: The effects of propafenone and metoprolol coadministration were studied in healthy subjects (single-dose study) and patients being treated for arrhythmias (multiple-dose study).[1] Propafenone decreased the clearance of metoprolol 65% to 80% and increased metoprolol concentrations 2 to 5 times compared with the controls. In contrast, metoprolol did not alter the pharmacokinetics of propafenone. Two of the patients developed beta-blocker adverse reactions (eg, bradycardia, heart failure, hypotension) during administration of both drugs.

RELATED DRUGS: Propafenone 225 mg every 8 hours for 7 days in healthy subjects resulted in an 83% and 213% increase in propranolol peak and steady-state serum concentrations, respectively.[2] Beta-blocking effects were minimally enhanced during combination therapy. Beta-blockers that are renally eliminated, such as atenolol (eg, *Tenormin*) or nadolol (eg, *Corgard*), are unlikely to be affected by propafenone.

MANAGEMENT OPTIONS:

➡ **Monitor.** Monitor patients receiving metoprolol or propranolol for increased beta-blockade (eg, bradycardia, heart failure, hypotension) when propafenone is added to their therapy and for a reduced effect when it is withdrawn.

REFERENCES:

1. Wagner F, et al. Drug interaction between propafenone and metoprolol. *Br J Clin Pharmacol.* 1987;24(2):213-220.
2. Kowey PR, et al. Interaction between propranolol and propafenone in healthy volunteers. *J Clin Pharmacol.* 1989;29(6):512-517.

Metoprolol (eg, *Lopressor*)

Propoxyphene (eg, *Darvon*)

SUMMARY: Propoxyphene may increase the plasma concentration of highly metabolized beta blockers such as metoprolol; increased beta blocker effects may occur.

RISK FACTORS: No specific risk factors are known.

MECHANISM: Propoxyphene may inhibit the metabolism of beta blockers that undergo significant hepatic elimination, such as propranolol (eg, *Inderal*) and metoprolol.

CLINICAL EVALUATION: In a study of healthy subjects, propoxyphene increased the bioavailability of metoprolol (100 mg orally) 3-fold and reduced metoprolol total body clearance by approximately 20%.[1] The bioavailability of propranolol 40 mg orally was increased by approximately 70%. While little clinical data are available, changes of this magnitude are likely to produce enhanced beta blocker effects including bradycardia or hypotension.

RELATED DRUGS: Propranolol interacts similarly with propoxyphene. It is unlikely that beta blockers excreted primarily by the kidneys (eg, atenolol [eg, *Tenormin*], nadolol [eg, *Corgard*], and sotalol [eg, *Betapace*]) would be affected by propoxyphene.

MANAGEMENT OPTIONS:

➡ *Monitor.* Until more information is available, be aware of increased response to metoprolol and propranolol when propoxyphene is initiated and a decreased response when it is discontinued.

REFERENCES:

1. Lundborg P, et al. The effect of propoxyphene pretreatment on the disposition of metoprolol and propranolol. *Clin Pharmacol Ther.* 1981;29:263.

Metoprolol (eg, *Lopressor*)

Quinidine

SUMMARY: Quinidine may increase the plasma concentration of metoprolol, but the incidence of adverse effects due to the interactions is unknown.

RISK FACTORS:

➡ *Pharmacogenetics.* Patients who are rapid metabolizers of metoprolol are at increased risk for the interaction.

MECHANISM: Quinidine decreases the metabolism of metoprolol, and both quinidine and beta blockers exert a negative inotropic action on the heart.

CLINICAL EVALUATION: After receiving quinidine 50 mg (a dose known to inhibit CYP2D6), patients who rapidly metabolize metoprolol had an 85% increase in their metoprolol concentrations 3 hours after a 100 mg dose.[1] Quinidine inhibits the metabolism of both enantiomers of metoprolol.[2] Changes in metoprolol pharmacokinetics are reflected in increased magnitude and duration of metoprolol effect on heart rate.[3]

RELATED DRUGS: Quinidine also decreases the metabolism of propranolol (eg, *Inderal*), and timolol (eg, *Blocadren*). Preliminary evidence suggests that quinidine has no effect on labetalol (eg, *Normodyne*) pharmacokinetics or pharmacodynamics.[4] Atenolol (eg, *Tenormin*) and other renally excreted beta blockers are less likely to interact.

MANAGEMENT OPTIONS:

➡ *Consider Alternative.* Renally excreted beta blockers (eg, atenolol [eg, *Tenormin*]) should be less likely to interact with quinidine, because their clearance is unlikely to be affected by quinidine. Nevertheless, additive cardiac depressant effects cannot be overlooked.

➡ *Monitor.* Concomitant use of quinidine and metoprolol should be undertaken with careful monitoring. Watch for bradycardia, heart failure, and arrhythmias.

REFERENCES:

1. Leeman NT, et al. Single dose quinidine treatment inhibits metoprolol oxidation in extensive metabolizers. *Eur J Clin Pharmacol.* 1986;29:739.

2. Schlanz KD, et al. Loss of stereoselective metoprolol metabolism following quinidine inhibition of P450IID6. *Pharmacotherapy*. 1991;11:271.

3. Schlanz KD, et al. Metoprolol pharmacodynamics and quinidine-induced inhibition of polymorphic drug metabolism. *Pharmacotherapy*. 1990;10:232.

4. Gearhart MO, et al. Lack of effects on labetalol pharmacodynamics with quinidine inhibition of P450IID6. *Pharmacotherapy*. 1991;11:P-36.

Metoprolol (eg, *Lopressor*)

Rifampin (eg, *Rifadin*)

SUMMARY: Plasma concentrations of beta-blockers that are metabolized in the liver, such as metoprolol, may decline with concomitant rifampin therapy.

RISK FACTORS: No specific risk factors are known.

MECHANISM: Rifampin enhances the hepatic metabolism of propranolol (eg, *Inderal*), metoprolol, and bisoprolol (*Zebeta*).

CLINICAL EVALUATION: Rifampin 600 mg/day reduced the bioavailability of metoprolol 33% and increased the clearance of propranolol 4-fold.[1,2] Rifampin increased the total clearance of bisoprolol 51%.[3] The magnitude of these changes seems large enough to reduce beta-blocker effects, but the degree to which rifampin inhibits the therapeutic response to beta-blockers is not established.

RELATED DRUGS: Rifampin is likely to increase the clearance of all beta-blockers that are oxidatively metabolized by the liver, such as propranolol and bisprolol. Atenolol (eg, *Tenormin*) and other renally excreted beta-blockers are less likely to interact.

MANAGEMENT OPTIONS:

➡ **Consider Alternative.** Beta-adrenergic blockers that are primarily eliminated by the kidneys, such as atenolol, could be used.

➡ **Circumvent/Minimize.** Beta-blocker dosages may need to be increased when rifampin therapy is initiated and decreased when rifampin is discontinued.

➡ **Monitor.** Watch for reduced beta-adrenergic effects if rifampin is administered with beta-adrenergic blockers that are eliminated by hepatic metabolism.

REFERENCES:

1. Shaheen O, et al. Effect of debrisoquine phenotype on the inducibility of propranolol metabolism. *Clin Pharmacol Ther*. 1989;45:439.

2. Bennett PN, et al. Effects of rifampin on metoprolol and antipyrine kinetics. *Br J Clin Pharmacol*. 1982;13:387.

3. Kirch W, et al. Interaction of bisoprolol with cimetidine and rifampicin. *Eur J Clin Pharmacol*. 1986;31:59.

Metoprolol (eg, *Lopressor*)

Terbutaline (eg, *Brethaire*)

SUMMARY: Beta-blocker–induced bronchoconstriction may antagonize the bronchodilating effect of beta-agonists; metoprolol increases terbutaline serum concentrations. The use of $beta_1$-selective beta-blockers is preferable in asthmatics receiving beta-agonists.

RISK FACTORS:

→ **Pharmacogenetics.** Patients who are slow metoprolol metabolizers are at increased risk for the interaction.

MECHANISM: Metoprolol appears to inhibit the metabolism of terbutaline. Nonselective beta-blockers would be expected to antagonize the beta-agonist–induced bronchodilation produced by terbutaline.

CLINICAL EVALUATION: The administration of 150 mg of metoprolol increased the area under the serum concentration-time curve of terbutaline 67% and 20%, respectively, in slow and fast metabolizers of metoprolol.[2] The clinical effects of these changes are unknown; the increase in terbutaline concentration may partially off set the pharmacodynamic interaction between the 2 drugs. In a group of 29 patients with chronic bronchial asthma, practolol did not appear to impair the bronchodilator activity of terbutaline.[1] It appears that cardioselective beta-blockers may be used more safely in asthmatics if a $beta_2$-stimulating drug, such as terbutaline or metaproterenol (eg, *Alupent*), is given concurrently.

RELATED DRUGS: Nonspecific beta-blockers, such as propranolol (eg, *Inderal*), would appear more likely to antagonize bronchodilators, such as terbutaline. Practolol does not appear to impair the bronchodilator activity of terbutaline.

MANAGEMENT OPTIONS:

→ **Use Alternative.** If possible, beta-blockers should be avoided in patients receiving beta-agonists or theophylline for bronchospastic pulmonary disease. If beta-blockers are required, cardioselective agents are preferable. If a cardioselective beta-blocker is administered to a patient with asthma taking a beta-agonist, observe the patient for worsening asthma.

REFERENCES:

1. Formgren H, et al. Effects of practolol in combination with terbutaline in the treatment of hypertension and arrhythmics in asthmatic patients. *Scand J Respir Dis.* 1975;56:217.
2. Jonkers RE, et al. Debrisoquine phenotype and the pharmacokinetics and beta-2 receptor pharmacodynamics of metoprolol and its enantiomers. *J Pharmacol Exp Ther.* 1991;256:959.

Metronidazole (eg, *Flagyl*)

Phenobarbital (eg, *Solfoton*)

SUMMARY: Preliminary evidence suggests that phenobarbital administration may reduce the serum concentration of metronidazole.

RISK FACTORS: No specific risk factors are known.

MECHANISM: Barbiturates may enhance the hepatic metabolism of metronidazole.

CLINICAL EVALUATION: A woman with vaginal trichomoniasis failed to respond to metronidazole while on phenobarbital 100 mg/day but did respond when the dose of metronidazole was doubled to 500 mg/day for 7 days.[1] Pharmacokinetic studies in this patient indicated that she eliminated metronidazole very rapidly.

RELATED DRUGS: Other barbiturates may affect metronidazole in a similar manner.

MANAGEMENT OPTIONS: No specific action is required, but be alert for evidence of the interaction.

REFERENCES:
1. Mead PB, et al. Possible alteration of metronidazole metabolism by phenobarbital. *N Engl J Med.* 1982;306:1490.

Metronidazole (eg, *Flagyl*)

Phenytoin (*Dilantin*)

SUMMARY: Metronidazole may moderately increase phenytoin serum concentrations.

RISK FACTORS: No specific risk factors are known.

MECHANISM: Metronidazole appears to inhibit the metabolism of phenytoin.

CLINICAL EVALUATION: Phenytoin clearance was reduced 15% by metronidazole treatment, 250 mg 3 times daily for 4 days before and 3 days after a single dose of phenytoin.[1] The small change in phenytoin clearance observed in this study would not cause toxicity in most patients.

RELATED DRUGS: No information is available.

MANAGEMENT OPTIONS:

➡ **Monitor.** Patients who have serum phenytoin concentrations near the upper limit of the therapeutic range should be monitored more carefully for increased phenytoin effect when metronidazole is added to their therapy.

REFERENCES:
1. Blyden GT, et al. Metronidazole impairs clearance of phenytoin but not alprazolam or lorazepam. *J Clin Pharmacol.* 1988;28:240.

Metronidazole (eg, *Flagyl*)

Trimethoprim-Sulfamethoxazole (eg, *Bactrim*)

SUMMARY: Metronidazole may produce a disulfiram-like reaction when administered with IV trimethoprim-sulfamethoxazole (TMP-SMX).

RISK FACTORS:

➡ **Route of Administration.** Administration of IV TMP-SMX increases the risk for the interaction.

MECHANISM: Metronidazole is known to produce disulfiram-like reactions when administered with ethanol. Intravenous TMP-SMX contains 10% ethanol as a solubilizing agent, and this may be a sufficient amount to cause the reaction in some patients.

CLINICAL EVALUATION: Following 2 doses of IV TMP-SMX and metronidazole, a patient vomited and complained of feeling hot and flushed.[1] The symptoms continued until oral TMP-SMX was substituted for the IV product. A repeat course of IV TMP-SMX without metronidazole was well tolerated.

RELATED DRUGS: The coadministration of metronidazole and IV drugs containing ethanol (eg, phenytoin [*Dilantin*], phenobarbital [eg, *Solfoton*], diazepam [eg, *Valium*], and nitroglycerin [eg, *Tridil*]) may result in flushing and vomiting. Disulfiram (eg, *Antabuse*) may react with IV TMP-SMX.

MANAGEMENT OPTIONS:

➡ *Circumvent/Minimize.* The use of oral dosage forms of these agents will prevent this interaction.

➡ *Monitor.* Watch for signs of disulfiram-like reaction when metronidazole is administered with IV drugs containing ethanol.

REFERENCES:
1. Edwards DL, et al. Disulfiram-like reaction associated with intravenous trimethoprim-sulfamethoxazole and metronidazole. *Clin Pharm.* 1986;5:999.

Metronidazole (eg, *Flagyl*)

Warfarin (eg, *Coumadin*)

SUMMARY: Metronidazole increases the hypoprothrombinemic response to warfarin, and bleeding has occurred in some patients receiving both drugs. Adjustments in warfarin dosage may be needed during cotherapy.

RISK FACTORS: No specific risk factors are known.

MECHANISM: Metronidazole appears to inhibit the metabolism of the more active S-isomer of warfarin, but has no effect on the R-isomer.[1] Because commercially available warfarin consists of both the S- and R-isomers, metronidazole enhances the hypoprothrombinemic effect.

CLINICAL EVALUATION: In 8 healthy subjects, a single dose of warfarin (1.5 mg/kg body weight) was given with and without pretreatment with metronidazole 750 mg/day for 7 days.[1] Metronidazole markedly increased the hypoprothrombinemic response and plasma warfarin concentrations. Clinical reports indicate that patients on chronic warfarin therapy may develop prolonged prothrombin times and bleeding episodes after receiving metronidazole.[2,3]

RELATED DRUGS: No information is available.

MANAGEMENT OPTIONS:

➡ *Avoid Unless Benefit Outweighs Risk.* Concomitant use of metronidazole and oral anticoagulants should be avoided if possible.

➡ *Monitor.* Patients receiving oral anticoagulants should be monitored for an increased anticoagulant effect when metronidazole is started and the converse when it is stopped. If oral anticoagulant therapy is begun in a patient receiving metronidazole, use conservative doses until the maintenance dose is established.

REFERENCES:
1. O'Reilly RA. The stereoselective interaction of warfarin and metronidazole in man. *N Engl J Med.* 1976;295:354.

2. Kazmier FJ. A significant interaction between metronidazole and warfarin. *Mayo Clin Proc.* 1976;51:782.

3. Dean RP, et al. Bleeding associated with concurrent warfarin and metronidazole therapy. *Drug Intell Clin Pharm.* 1980;14:864.

Metyrapone (*Metopirone*)

Phenytoin (*Dilantin*)

SUMMARY: Phenytoin lowers blood metyrapone concentrations and invalidates the metyrapone test.

RISK FACTORS: No specific risk factors are known.

MECHANISM: Phenytoin probably enhances the metabolism of orally administered metyrapone on its first pass through the liver. An inhibitory effect of phenytoin on the GI absorption of metyrapone also is possible, but not as likely as enhanced metabolism.

CLINICAL EVALUATION: Oral metyrapone administration in patients receiving chronic phenytoin therapy results in inadequate metyrapone blood concentrations[1] and invalidates the metyrapone test.[1,2] Doubling the metyrapone dose or giving the metyrapone IV circumvented the interfering effect of phenytoin as reflected by normal plasma ACTH and corticosteroid responses.[1]

RELATED DRUGS: Other enzyme inducers also may interfere with metyrapone tests.

MANAGEMENT OPTIONS:

➡ *Circumvent/Minimize.* The standard oral metyrapone test will be invalid in patients receiving chronic phenytoin therapy. Doubling the oral metyrapone dose in such patients may produce valid results.[1,2]

➡ *Monitor.* Be alert for evidence of invalid metyrapone tests if phenytoin or other enzyme inducers are used.

REFERENCES:

1. Meikle AW, et al. Effect of diphenylhydantoin on the metabolism of metyrapone and release of ACTH in man. *J Clin Endocrinol Metab.* 1969;29:1553.

2. Werk EE, Jr et al. Failure of metyrapone to inhibit 11-hydroxylation of 11-deoxycortisol during drug therapy. *J Clin Endocrinol Metab.* 1967;27:1358.

Mexiletine (eg, *Mexitil*)

Phenytoin (eg, *Dilantin*)

SUMMARY: A study in healthy subjects suggests that phenytoin substantially reduces mexiletine concentrations.

RISK FACTORS: No specific risk factors are known.

MECHANISM: Phenytoin enhances the hepatic metabolism of mexiletine.

CLINICAL EVALUATION: The pharmacokinetics of mexiletine in 6 healthy, nonsmoking subjects were measured before and after 1 week of phenytoin 300 mg/day.[1] The mean area under the concentration-time curve (AUC) was reduced 54% and the half-life declined 51% (from 17. 2 to 8.4 hours). Assuming no significant changes in protein binding occurred, the reduction in AUC approximates the increase in mexiletine's systemic clearance after the administration of phenytoin. This may result in a significant decline in mexiletine plasma concentrations and efficacy.

RELATED DRUGS: No information is available.

MANAGEMENT OPTIONS:

➡ *Circumvent/Minimize.* Mexiletine dosage requirements are likely to increase when phenytoin is administered and decrease when it is discontinued.

➡ *Monitor.* Measure mexiletine concentrations to ensure that dosage adjustments are adequate. Monitor patients for a decreased therapeutic response when phenytoin is used concurrently and an increased response if phenytoin is discontinued.

REFERENCES:

1. Begg EJ, et al. Enhanced metabolism of mexiletine after phenytoin administration. *Br J Clin Pharmacol.* 1982;14(2):219-223.

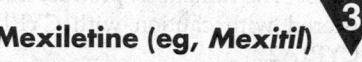

Mexiletine (eg, *Mexitil*)

Quinidine

SUMMARY: Quinidine administration increases the concentrations and antiarrhythmic effects of mexiletine.

RISK FACTORS:

➡ *Pharmacogenetics.* Patients who are extensive mexiletine metabolizers are at increased risk for the interaction.

MECHANISM: Quinidine reduces the metabolism of mexiletine in extensive mexiletine metabolizers; it has little effect in slow metabolizers of mexiletine. The electrophysiologic effects of mexiletine and quinidine appear to potentiate the antiarrhythmic activity of both drugs.

CLINICAL EVALUATION: Fourteen healthy subjects received a single dose of mexiletine 200 mg alone and after 2 days of quinidine 50 mg 4 times daily.[1] Total mexiletine clearance was reduced 24%, while nonrenal clearance declined 31% following quinidine coadministration. Mexiletine half-life increased from 8.9 to 10.6 hours. Quinidine had no effect on mexiletine kinetics in slow mexiletine metabolizers. The combination of quinidine and mexiletine has been demonstrated to enhance the antiarrhythmic activity of either drug used alone because of their complementary effects on cardiac conduction.[2-4]

RELATED DRUGS: No information is available.

MANAGEMENT OPTIONS:

➡ *Monitor.* Monitor patients stabilized on mexiletine for increased serum concentrations and electrophysiologic effects of mexiletine when quinidine is administered.

REFERENCES:

1. Turgeon J, et al. Influence of debrisoquine phenotype and of quinidine on mexiletine disposition in man. *J Pharmacol Exp Ther.* 1991;259(2):789-798.

2. Duff HJ, et al. Role of quinidine in the mexiletine-quinidine interaction: electrophysiologic correlates of enhanced antiarrhythmic efficacy. *J Cardiovasc Pharmacol.* 1990;16(5):685-692.

3. Duff HJ, et al. Electropharmacologic synergism with mexiletine and quinidine. *J Cardiovasc Pharmacol.* 1986;8(4):840-846.

4. Duff HJ, et al. Mexiletine/quinidine combination therapy: electrophysiologic correlates of antiarrhythmic efficacy. *Clin Invest Med.* 1991;14(5):476-483.

Mexiletine (eg, *Mexitil*)

Ramelteon (*Rozerem*)

SUMMARY: Ramelteon is very sensitive to inhibition of CYP1A2; theoretically, mexiletine increases ramelteon plasma concentrations.

RISK FACTORS: No specific risk factors are known.

MECHANISM: Ramelteon is metabolized primarily by CYP1A2, and mexiletine is a CYP1A2 inhibitor.

CLINICAL EVALUATION: In healthy subjects, the potent CYP1A2 inhibitor fluvoxamine (100 mg twice daily for 3 days) produced a 190-fold increase in ramelteon plasma concentrations and a 70-fold increase in the ramelteon maximal plasma concentrations.[1] The ramelteon product information states that ramelteon should be administered with caution with CYP1A2 inhibitors[1]; mexiletine is known to inhibit CYP1A2.

RELATED DRUGS: No information is available.

MANAGEMENT OPTIONS:

➤ **Monitor.** Monitor for excessive ramelteon effects if mexiletine and ramelteon are used concurrently.

REFERENCES:

1. *Rozerem* [package insert]. Lincolnshire, IL: Takeda Pharmaceuticals; 2006.

Mexiletine (eg, *Mexitil*)

Rifampin (eg, *Rifadin*)

SUMMARY: Rifampin may reduce mexiletine concentrations and inhibit mexiletine efficacy.

RISK FACTORS: No specific risk factors are known.

MECHANISM: Probable increase in mexiletine metabolism.

CLINICAL EVALUATION: Eight healthy subjects received a single oral dose of mexiletine with and without rifampin pretreatment (300 mg twice daily for 10 days).[1] Rifampin substantially reduced the mexiletine half-life and correspondingly increased its nonrenal clearance. The interaction appears to reduce mexiletine efficacy in some patients.

RELATED DRUGS: Theoretically, other enzyme inducers, including barbiturates, carbamazepine (eg, *Tegretol*), efavirenz (*Sustiva*), nafcillin, nevirapine (*Viramune*), oxcarbazepine (*Trileptal*), primidone (*Mysoline*), phenytoin (eg, *Dilantin*), rifabutin (*Mycobutin*), rifapentine (*Priftin*), and St. John's wort, may interact similarly with mexiletine.

MANAGEMENT OPTIONS:

➡ *Monitor.* Monitor for altered mexiletine effect if rifampin is started or stopped, or if the dosage is changed. Note that rifampin enzyme induction is gradual; it may take several days to a week or more for maximal effects to occur.

REFERENCES:

1. Pentikäinen PJ, et al. Effect of rifampicin treatment on the kinetics of mexiletine. *Eur J Clin Pharmacol.* 1982;23(3):261-266.

Mexiletine (eg, *Mexitil*)

Sodium Bicarbonate

SUMMARY: An increase in urine pH may result in clinically significant increases in mexiletine concentrations.

RISK FACTORS: No specific risk factors are known.

MECHANISM: Because mexiletine is a weak base, its renal clearance depends upon urine pH. Acidification of the urine will increase its excretion, while alkalinization will retard its elimination.[1]

CLINICAL EVALUATION: When mexiletine was administered with sodium bicarbonate to maintain the urine pH between 7 and 8, mexiletine's half-life averaged 17.2 hours compared with a typical half-life of 9 to 12 hours.[2,3] The renal clearance of mexiletine decreased from more than 200 mL/min at a pH less than 6 to less than 5 mL/min at a pH greater than 8.2. The renal clearance of mexiletine usually is only 10% of the total body clearance, whereas in patients with a low urine pH, it may represent 40% to 50% of the total clearance. In this situation, urine alkalinization with large doses of sodium bicarbonate or with drugs such as acetazolamide (eg, *Diamox*) may lead to significant accumulation of mexiletine and possibly toxic plasma concentrations.

RELATED DRUGS: Other agents that alkalinize the urine (eg, acetazolamide) are expected to produce a similar interaction with mexiletine.

MANAGEMENT OPTIONS:

➡ *Monitor.* Monitor patients receiving mexiletine who have large changes in urine pH as a result of concurrent drug therapy for changes in mexiletine plasma concentration.

REFERENCES:

1. Kiddie MA, et al. The influence of urinary pH on the elimination of mexiletine. *Br J Clin Pharmacol.* 1974;1:229.
2. Begg EJ, et al. Enhanced metabolism of mexiletine after phenytoin administration. *Br J Clin Pharmacol.* 1982;14(2):219-223.
3. Pentikäinen PJ, et al. Effect of rifampicin treatment on the kinetics of mexiletine. *Eur J Clin Pharmacol.* 1982;23(3):261-266.

Mexiletine (eg, *Mexitil*)

Theophylline (eg, *Theochron*)

SUMMARY: Patients maintained on theophylline may develop elevated theophylline serum concentrations and toxicity after concomitant mexiletine therapy is initiated.

RISK FACTORS: No specific risk factors are known.

MECHANISM: Mexiletine inhibits the metabolism of theophylline.

CLINICAL EVALUATION: A 74-year-old patient taking sustained-release theophylline 300 mg twice daily was given mexiletine 200 mg 3 times daily.[1] His steady-state trough serum theophylline concentration increased from 15.3 to 25 mcg/mL, and he developed symptoms of theophylline toxicity (including anorexia, nausea, and vomiting). The patient's symptoms resolved when the theophylline dosage was reduced to 100 mg twice daily. Additional case reports of elevated theophylline concentrations accompanied by toxicity have been published.[2-4] Fifteen healthy subjects received mexiletine 200 mg 3 times daily for 5 days.[5] Theophylline 5 mg/kg was administered intravenously over 30 minutes before and after mexiletine treatment. The mean theophylline clearance was reduced more than 40% and its half-life increased approximately 80%. Similar changes have been reported by other authors.[6,7] These changes are likely to produce theophylline toxicity in some patients receiving both drugs.

RELATED DRUGS: No information is available.

MANAGEMENT OPTIONS:

➥ *Use Alternative.* Avoid theophylline administration in patients taking mexiletine; consider the use of a beta-agonist or steroid. Consider an alternative to mexiletine in patients receiving theophylline. Carefully monitor patients who are stabilized on theophylline and receive mexiletine for increased theophylline concentrations and potentially toxic symptoms, including arrhythmias, GI upset, seizures, and tachycardia.

REFERENCES:

1. Katz A, et al. Oral mexiletine-theophylline interaction. *Int J Cardiol.* 1987;17(2):227-228.

2. Stanley R, et al. Mexiletine-theophylline interaction. *Am J Med.* 1989;86(6 pt 1):733-734.

3. Kessler KM, et al. Proarrhythmia related to a kinetic and dynamic interaction of mexiletine and theophylline. *Am Heart J.* 1989;117(4):964-966.

4. Kendall JD, et al. Theophylline-mexiletine interaction: a case report. *Pharmacotherapy.* 1992;12(5):416-418.

5. Loi CM, et al. Effect of mexiletine on theophylline metabolism [abstract]. *Clin Pharmacol Ther.* 1990;47:130.

6. Hurwitz A, et al. Mexiletine effects on theophylline disposition. *Clin Pharmacol Ther.* 1991;50(3):299-307.

7. Stoysich AM, et al. Influence of mexiletine on the pharmacokinetics of theophylline in healthy volunteers. *J Clin Pharmacol.* 1991;31(4):354-357.

Mexiletine (eg, *Mexitil*)

Tizanidine (eg, *Zanaflex*)

SUMMARY: Mexiletine administration increases the plasma concentration of tizanidine and enhances its hypotensive effects.

RISK FACTORS: No specific risk factors are known.

MECHANISM: Mexiletine inhibits the activity of CYP1A2, the enzyme known to metabolize tizanidine.

CLINICAL EVALUATION: Twelve healthy subjects received a single dose of tizanidine 2 mg alone and following pretreatment with mexiletine 50 mg three times a day for 2 days.[1] Compared with tizanidine alone, the coadministration of mexiletine increased the mean peak concentration and area under the concentration-time curve of tizanidine 3.1- and 3.6-fold, respectively. The half-life of tizanidine was increased from 1.3 to 1.8 hours by mexiletine administration. The hypotensive effect of tizanidine was significantly increased following the coadministration of mexiletine. Because the usual therapeutic dose of mexiletine is 4 to 6 times greater than the dose used in this study, it is possible that a larger magnitude interaction will occur.

RELATED DRUGS: None known.

MANAGEMENT OPTIONS:

➡ **Consider Alternative.** Consider other spasmolytic drugs that are not metabolized by CYP1A2 (eg, diazepam [eg, *Valium*], baclofen [eg, *Lioresal*]) as alternatives if mexiletine is required.

➡ **Monitor.** Carefully monitor patients receiving tizanidine and mexiletine for evidence of enhanced tizanidine effects, including hypotension, sedation, and dry mouth.

REFERENCES:

1. Momo K et al. Effects of mexiletine, a CYP1A2 inhibitor, on tizanidine pharmacokinetics and pharmacodynamics. *J Clin Pharmacol.* 2010;50(3):331-337.

Micafungin (*Mycamine*)

Nifedipine (eg, *Procardia*)

SUMMARY: Micafungin administration has been reported to modestly increase the plasma concentration of nifedipine; however, increased nifedipine effect is unlikely.

RISK FACTORS: No specific risk factors are known.

MECHANISM: Unknown.

CLINICAL EVALUATION: While no specific details are currently available, the manufacturer of micafungin notes that the mean area under the plasma concentration-time curve of nifedipine was increased 18% during chronic micafungin dosing compared with nifedipine administered alone.[1] The mean peak nifedipine concentration increased 42%. Nifedipine does not affect micafungin plasma concentrations.[1] Monitor patients receiving nifedipine and micafungin as usual for signs of excess vasodilatation such as hypotension or headache.

RELATED DRUGS: The effect of micafungin on other calcium channel blockers is unknown.

MANAGEMENT OPTIONS:

➡ **Monitor.** Observe patients receiving nifedipine and micafungin for evidence of increased nifedipine effect, including hypotension, headache, or tachycardia.

REFERENCES:

1. *Mycamine* [package insert]. Deerfield, IL: Fujisawa Healthcare, Inc.; 2005.

 Micafungin (*Mycamine*)

Sirolimus (*Rapamune*)

SUMMARY: Micafungin administration has been reported to modestly increase the plasma concentration of sirolimus; some patients may be at increased risk for sirolimus adverse effects.

RISK FACTORS: No specific risk factors are known.

MECHANISM: Unknown.

CLINICAL EVALUATION: While no specific details are currently available, the manufacturer of micafungin notes that the mean area under the plasma concentration-time curve of sirolimus was increased 21% during chronic micafungin dosing compared with sirolimus administered alone.[1] No change in the peak sirolimus concentration was noted. Sirolimus does not affect micafungin plasma concentrations.[1] Pending further data, monitor patients receiving this combination for increased sirolimus concentrations.

RELATED DRUGS: Micafungin does not appear to alter the plasma concentrations of tacrolimus (*Prograf*) but may increase cyclosporine (eg, *Neoral*) plasma concentrations. Ketoconazole (eg, *Nizoral*), itraconazole (eg, *Sporanox*), voriconazole (*Vfend*), and fluconazole (*Diflucan*) may increase sirolimus concentrations.

MANAGEMENT OPTIONS:

➡ **Monitor.** Monitor patients receiving sirolimus and micafungin for increased sirolimus plasma concentrations.

REFERENCES:

1. *Mycamine* [package insert]. Deerfield, IL: Fujisawa Healthcare, Inc.; 2005.

 Miconazole (eg, *Monistat*)

Tobramycin (eg, *Nebcin*)

SUMMARY: Miconazole reduces tobramycin peak serum concentrations; dosage adjustments may be required to maintain adequate serum concentrations.

RISK FACTORS: No specific risk factors are known.

MECHANISM: Not established.

CLINICAL EVALUATION: Eight patients undergoing bone marrow transplants received intravenous (IV) tobramycin, IV ticarcillin (*Ticar*) 3 g every 4 hours, IV vancomycin (eg, *Vancocin*), and IV miconazole 10 mg/kg every 6 hours for febrile episodes.[1] During miconazole administration, tobramycin volume of distribution and clearance increased, resulting in significant reductions in peak tobramycin concentrations.

Pharmacokinetic parameters returned to baseline in 4 patients in whom amphotericin B (eg, *Fungizone*) was substituted for miconazole.

RELATED DRUGS: Other aminoglycosides may be affected similarly by miconazole or related azole antifungals such as ketoconazole (eg, *Nizoral*) or itraconazole (*Sporanox*).

MANAGEMENT OPTIONS:

➥ *Consider Alternative.* Choose an alternative antifungal agent. Note that amphotericin can produce increased nephrotoxicity when administered with aminoglycosides. The effects of other antifungal agents on aminoglycoside pharmacokinetics are unknown.

➥ *Monitor.* Monitor aminoglycoside concentrations in patients receiving miconazole and aminoglycosides.

REFERENCES:

1. Hatfield SM, et al. Miconazole-induced alteration in tobramycin pharmacokinetics. *Clin Pharm.* 1986;5:415.

Miconazole (eg, *Monistat*) ▼3

Warfarin (eg, *Coumadin*)

SUMMARY: Miconazole given systemically and as an oral gel has been associated with enhanced hypoprothrombinemia and bleeding in some patients receiving oral anticoagulants.

RISK FACTORS: No specific risk factors are known.

MECHANISM: Miconazole inhibits the hepatic metabolism of warfarin.

CLINICAL EVALUATION: Several patients have developed an enhanced hypoprothrombinemic response to warfarin following systemic or topical (oral gel) miconazole therapy.[1-5] At least 2 of the patients responded similarly when they were rechallenged. Although miconazole likely was responsible for the excessive anticoagulation in these patients, the general incidence of this interaction in patients receiving both drugs is not known. The likelihood of a clinically important interaction probably depends upon the serum concentration of miconazole. Although the oral gel has been associated with increased warfarin effect, it is not clear whether other topical forms of miconazole (eg, vaginal, dermatological) can result in high enough serum miconazole concentrations to interact.

RELATED DRUGS: The effect of miconazole on oral anticoagulants other than warfarin is not known, but be alert for a similar effect with all oral anticoagulants until information to the contrary is available.

MANAGEMENT OPTIONS:

➥ *Monitor.* Monitor for altered oral anticoagulant effect if miconazole is initiated, discontinued, or changed in dosage. Adjust the anticoagulant dose as needed.

REFERENCES:

1. Watson PG, et al. Drug interaction with coumarin derivative anticoagulants. *Br Med J.* 1982;285:1045-1046.

2. Goenen M, et al. A case of *Candida albicans* endocarditis 3 years after an aortic valve replacement. Successful combined medical and surgical therapy. *J Cardiovasc Surg.* 1977;18:391-396.

3. Deresinski SC, et al. Miconazole treatment of human coccidioidomycosis: status report. In: Ajello L, ed. Coccidioidomycosis: Current Clinical and Diagnostic Status. Vol 1. Miami, FL: Symposia Specialists; 1977:267-292.

4. Colquhoun MC, et al. Interaction between warfarin and miconazole oral gel. *Lancet*. 1987;1:695.

5. Shenfield GM, et al. Potentiation of warfarin action by miconazole oral gel. *Aust N Z J Med*. 1991;21:928.

Midazolam

Phenytoin (eg, *Dilantin*)

SUMMARY: Phenytoin markedly reduces the effect of oral midazolam, but parenteral midazolam is less likely to be affected.

RISK FACTORS:

➡ **Route of Administration.** Because the majority of the interaction is likely caused by increased presystemic metabolism of oral midazolam by the gut wall and liver, parenteral midazolam is much less likely to be affected.

MECHANISM: Phenytoin appears to enhance the presystemic metabolism of oral midazolam in the gut wall and liver by CYP3A4, thus reducing midazolam bioavailability. The subsequent hepatic metabolism of midazolam by CYP3A4 also may be increased.

CLINICAL EVALUATION: The pharmacokinetics and pharmacodynamics of a single oral dose of midazolam 15 mg were compared in patients receiving phenytoin (150 to 300 mg/day) or carbamazepine versus healthy subjects not receiving enzyme inducers.[1] The midazolam area under the plasma concentration-time curve was dramatically lower in those receiving phenytoin or carbamazepine (7% of value in control subjects); midazolam half-life also was substantially lower. The pharmacodynamic response to midazolam was reduced markedly as measured by various objective and subjective methods. Because the majority of the interaction likely is caused by increased presystemic metabolism of oral midazolam by the gut wall and liver, parenteral midazolam is much less likely to be affected. Nonetheless, if parenteral midazolam is given in multiple doses or continuously to patients on enzyme inducers, larger midazolam doses may be required because of enhanced hepatic metabolism.

RELATED DRUGS: Carbamazepine (eg, *Tegretol*) interacts similarly with midazolam. Alprazolam (eg, *Xanax*), triazolam (eg, *Halcion*), and, to some extent, diazepam (eg, *Valium*) also are metabolized by CYP3A4 and are expected to interact with enzyme inducers in a manner similar to midazolam.

MANAGEMENT OPTIONS:

➡ **Consider Alternative.** When midazolam is used orally as a sedative-hypnotic (as it is in several countries), patients receiving enzyme inducers such as phenytoin are unlikely to respond unless very large doses of midazolam are used. Thus, it may be preferable to use alternative sedative-hypnotics in these patients.

➡ *Monitor.* Although parenteral midazolam is much less likely to be affected, monitor for inadequate midazolam effect and increase its dose if needed.

REFERENCES:

1. Backman JT, et al. Concentrations and effects of oral midazolam are greatly reduced in patients treated with carbamazepine or phenytoin. *Epilepsia.* 1996;37(3):253-257.

Midazolam
Posaconazole (*Noxafil*)

SUMMARY: Midazolam plasma concentrations following intravenous (IV) administration were nearly doubled by posaconazole; some patients may experience increased sedation.

RISK FACTORS: No specific risk factors are known.

MECHANISM: Posaconazole appears to reduce the activity of CYP3A4, resulting in a reduced systemic clearance of midazolam.

CLINICAL EVALUATION: A single dose of midazolam 0.05 mg/kg IV was administered over 30 minutes to 12 subjects alone and following posaconazole 200 mg tablets once daily for 10 days.[1] The mean area under the plasma concentration-time curve of midazolam was increased 83%. The effect of posaconazole on the oral clearance of midazolam was not studied. Because of the apparent decrease in CYP3A activity by posaconazole, drugs undergoing first-pass metabolism via CYP3A are expected to have increased bioavailability as well as reduced systemic clearance when coadministered with posaconazole.

RELATED DRUGS: Other benzodiazepines metabolized by CYP3A4 (eg, alprazolam [eg, *Xanax*], triazolam [eg, *Halcion*]) are likely to be affected in a similar manner by posaconazole. Antifungal agents that inhibit CYP3A4 (eg, fluconazole [eg, *Diflucan*], itraconazole [eg, *Sporanox*], ketoconazole [eg, *Nizoral*], voriconazole [*Vfend*]) are expected to affect midazolam systemic clearance in a similar manner.

MANAGEMENT OPTIONS:

➡ *Consider Alternative.* Consider terbinafine (eg, *Lamisil*) as an alternative antifungal agent because it does not affect CYP3A4 activity. The metabolism of benzodiazepines that are not CYP3A4 substrates (eg, lorazepam, oxazepam, temazepam) is unlikely to be affected by posaconazole administration.

➡ *Monitor.* Be alert for increased sedation in patients receiving posaconazole and midazolam.

REFERENCES:

1. Wexler D, et al. Effect of posaconazole on cytochrome P450 enzymes: a randomized, open-label, two-way crossover study. *Eur J Pharm Sci.* 2004;21(5):645-653.

Midazolam
Rifampin (eg, *Rifadin*)

SUMMARY: Rifampin administration results in a marked reduction in midazolam plasma concentrations; loss of efficacy may occur.

RISK FACTORS: No specific risk factors are known.

MECHANISM: Rifampin induces the first-pass and systemic metabolism (via CYP3A4) of midazolam.

CLINICAL EVALUATION: Ten healthy subjects took rifampin 600 mg or placebo daily for 5 days.[1] On day 6, a single dose of midazolam 15 mg was administered 17 hours after the last dose of rifampin. The mean area under the concentration-time curve of midazolam was reduced 96% following pretreatment with rifampin. Midazolam half-life fell from 3.1 to 1.3 hours after rifampin. Mean peak midazolam concentrations were reduced from 55 to 3.5 ng/mL with rifampin pretreatment. A second study administered midazolam intravenously and orally alone and after rifampin 600 mg daily for 7 days.[2] The mean oral clearance of midazolam increased 16- and 30-fold in women and men, respectively, following rifampin administration. Systemic clearance was increased by rifampin from 2- to 2.3-fold. The magnitude of these changes suggests that a marked reduction in midazolam efficacy can be expected in patients receiving rifampin.

RELATED DRUGS: Rifampin will affect other benzodiazepines undergoing high first-pass metabolism via CYP3A4 such as triazolam (eg, *Halcion*) and diazepam (eg, *Valium*). Rifabutin (*Mycobutin*) is likely to interact in a similar manner with midazolam.

MANAGEMENT OPTIONS:

➥ *Consider Alternative.* Avoid the interaction with the selection of a benzodiazepine that is not a CYP3A4 substrate, such as temazepam (eg, *Restoril*) or oxazepam.

➥ *Monitor.* Monitor patients receiving rifampin for reduced midazolam efficacy. If rifampin is discontinued in a patient receiving both agents, the dose of midazolam will require reduction during the following 7 to 10 days to avoid excess sedation.

REFERENCES:

1. Backman JT, et al. Rifampin drastically reduces plasma concentrations and effects of oral midazolam. *Clin Pharmacol Ther.* 1996;59(1):7-13.
2. Gorski JC, et al. The effect of rifampin on intestinal and hepatic CYP3A activity. *Clin Pharmacol Ther.* 2000;67:133.

Midazolam

Ritonavir (*Norvir*)

SUMMARY: Ritonavir administration produces a marked increase in midazolam plasma concentrations; increased and prolonged sedation is expected to occur.

RISK FACTORS:

➥ *Route of Administration.* The magnitude of the interaction will be greater in patients taking oral midazolam compared with intravenous dosing.

MECHANISM: Ritonavir reduces the first-pass and systemic metabolism of midazolam by inhibiting CYP3A4.

CLINICAL EVALUATION: Thirteen healthy men were administered midazolam 3 mg orally with the second dose of either placebo or ritonavir 100 mg given 3 times with approximately 12 hours between doses.[1] The mean area under the concentration-time curve (AUC) of midazolam was increased nearly 30-fold by ritonavir coadministration. The half-life of midazolam increased from 2 to 18 hours with ritonavir. In a second study of 18 healthy subjects, a single oral dose of midazolam 7.5 mg was administered alone and following 14 days of saquinavir 1,000 mg/ritonavir 100 mg twice daily.[2] With saquinavir/ritonavir pretreatment, the AUC of midazolam increased 12.4-fold and its half-life increased from 4.7 to 14.9 hours. The clearance of intravenous (IV) and oral midazolam was compared in 16 HIV-positive men taking ritonavir (at least 100 mg daily) and 10 HIV-positive men not taking ritonavir.[3] The mean midazolam clearance in patients not taking ritonavir was approximately 5.5- and 17-fold higher for IV and oral midazolam, respectively, compared with the patients receiving concurrent ritonavir. The bio-availability of midazolam was increased approximately 3-fold and its half-life increased from less than 3 hours to more than 13 hours in patients taking ritonavir.

RELATED DRUGS: Other benzodiazepines metabolized by CYP3A4 (eg, alprazolam [eg, *Xanax*], triazolam [eg, *Halcion*]) are likely to be affected in a similar manner by ritonavir. Atazanavir (*Reyataz*), darunavir (*Prezista*), fosamprenavir (*Lexiva*), indinavir (*Crixivan*), nelfinavir (*Viracept*), and saquinavir (*Invirase*) also inhibit the activity of CYP3A4 and can be expected to increase the plasma concentrations of midazolam.

MANAGEMENT OPTIONS:

➥ *Consider Alternative.* Other benzodiazepines (eg, lorazepam [eg, *Ativan*], oxazepam) that are not metabolized by CYP3A4 are unlikely to be affected by ritonavir.

➥ *Monitor.* If midazolam is administered to patients taking ritonavir, monitor for increased extent and duration of sedation.

REFERENCES:

1. Greenblatt DJ, et al. Inhibition of oral midazolam clearance by boosting doses of ritonavir, and by 4,4-dimethyl-benziso-(2H)-selenazine (ALT-2074), an experimental catalytic mimic of glutathione oxidase. *Br J Clin Pharmacol.* 2009;68(6):920-927.
2. Schmitt C, et al. Effect of saquinavir-ritonavir on cytochrome P450 3A4 activity in healthy volunteers using midazolam as a probe. *Pharmacotherapy.* 2009;29(10):1175-1181.
3. Knox TA, et al. Ritonavir greatly impairs CYP3A activity in HIV infection with chronic viral hepatitis. *J Acquir Immune Defic Syndr.* 2008;49(4):358-368.

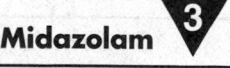

Midazolam

Saquinavir (*Invirase*)

SUMMARY: Saquinavir increases midazolam concentrations, particularly following oral midazolam. Increased midazolam-induced sedation is likely to result.

RISK FACTORS:

➥ *Route of Administration.* The effect of saquinavir on midazolam clearance is increased when midazolam is administered orally.

MECHANISM: Saquinavir inhibits the first-pass and systemic clearance of midazolam by reducing the CYP3A4 metabolism of midazolam.

CLINICAL EVALUATION: Twelve healthy subjects received placebo or saquinavir 400 mg 3 times daily for 5 days and on the morning of study day 6.[1] On study day 3, each subject was administered midazolam 7.5 mg orally or 0.05 mg/kg IV as a single dose 2 hours after the dose of saquinavir. Coadministration of saquinavir reduced the systemic clearance of midazolam 56% and prolonged its half-life from 4.1 to 9.5 hours. The area under the plasma concentration-time curve (AUC) of midazolam following IV dosing was increased more than 2-fold by pretreatment with saquinavir. The AUC of midazolam following oral dosing increased more than 5-fold, while the half-life of oral midazolam increased from 4.3 to 10.9 hours by pretreatment with saquinavir. The bioavailability of midazolam increased from 41% to 90% during saquinavir coadministration. The combined administration of saquinavir and midazolam produced significant sedation (especially following oral midazolam) compared with the administration of midazolam alone. A case report of prolonged sedation following IV midazolam in a patient receiving saquinavir has been published.[2]

RELATED DRUGS: Benzodiazepines such as triazolam (eg, *Halcion*) or zolpidem (*Ambien*) that are metabolized by CYP3A4 are expected to interact with saquinavir in a similar manner. Other protease inhibitors that have been reported to inhibit CYP3A4 (eg, ritonavir [*Norvir*], nelfinavir [*Viracept*], amprenavir [*Agenerase*], indinavir [*Crixivan*]) are expected to inhibit the metabolism of midazolam.

MANAGEMENT OPTIONS:

➡ **Consider Alternative.** Consider an anxiolytic that is not metabolized by CYP3A4, such as oxazepam (eg, *Serax*) or lorazepam (eg, *Ativan*), as an alternative to midazolam for some indications.

➡ **Monitor.** Patients who are receiving saquinavir will probably require lower doses of oral or IV midazolam and may remain sedated for a longer period of time following a single dose of midazolam or the discontinuation of chronic midazolam therapy.

REFERENCES:

1. Palkama VJ, et al. Effect of saquinavir on the pharmacokinetics and pharmacodynamics of oral and intravenous midazolam. *Clin Pharmacol Ther.* 1999;66:33-39.
2. Merry C, et al. Saquinavir interaction with midazolam: pharmacokinetic considerations when prescribing protease inhibitors for patients with HIV disease. *AIDS.* 1997;11:268-269.

Midazolam

St. John's Wort

SUMMARY: Some St. John's wort products may substantially reduce the effect of oral midazolam, but parenteral midazolam is likely to be less affected.

RISK FACTORS:

➡ **Route of Administration.** Because the majority of the interaction is likely caused by increased presystemic metabolism of oral midazolam by the gut wall and liver, parenteral midazolam is likely to be much less affected.

MECHANISM: St. John's wort appears to enhance the presystemic metabolism of oral midazolam in the gut wall and liver by CYP3A4, thus reducing midazolam bioavailability. The subsequent hepatic metabolism of midazolam by CYP3A4 may also be increased.

CLINICAL EVALUATION: In a randomized study of 42 healthy subjects, single oral doses of midazolam were given alone and following pretreatment with 14 days of various St. John's wort products.[1] One St. John's wort preparation reduced midazolam area under the plasma concentration-time curve (AUC) almost 80%, while another preparation reduced midazolam AUC only 21%. The effect of other St. John's wort preparations on midazolam AUC was intermediate between these 2 extremes. The magnitude of the reduction in midazolam AUC was proportional to the amount of hyperforin in the daily dose of St. John's wort. Theoretically, the effect on parenteral midazolam by St. John's wort administration should only be minimal.

RELATED DRUGS: St. John's wort would also be expected to reduce plasma concentrations of other benzodiazepines that are metabolized by CYP3A4, such as triazolam (eg, *Halcion*), alprazolam (eg, *Xanax*), and, to some extent, diazepam (eg, *Valium*).

MANAGEMENT OPTIONS:

➥ *Monitor.* Monitor for reduced oral midazolam effect in patients taking St. John's wort.

REFERENCES:

1. Mueller SC, et al. The extent of induction of CYP3A4 by St. John's wort varies among products and is linked to hyperforin dose. *Eur J Clin Pharmacol.* 2006;62:29-36.

Midazolam

Tacrolimus (*Prograf*)

SUMMARY: Drug interaction studies using human liver microsomes in vitro suggest that midazolam inhibits the metabolism of tacrolimus; watch for excessive tacrolimus concentrations if the drugs are used concurrently.

RISK FACTORS:

➥ *Route of Administration.* Theoretically, one would expect multiple oral doses of midazolam to be more likely to affect tacrolimus than parenteral use of midazolam during procedures.

MECHANISM: Tacrolimus is metabolized by cytochrome P450 3A4 (CYP3A4), and it appears to inhibit this process.

CLINICAL EVALUATION: Thirty-four drugs were tested for interactions with tacrolimus using in vitro human liver microsomal preparations.[1] Midazolam was found to inhibit tacrolimus metabolism. Although the clinical importance of this finding is not established, in vitro human microsomal studies have been remarkably accurate in predicting which drugs will interact in the clinical setting.

RELATED DRUGS: The effect of midazolam on cyclosporine (eg, *Neoral*) is not established, but cyclosporine and tacrolimus tend to have similar drug interactions.

MANAGEMENT OPTIONS: No specific action is required, but be alert for evidence of the interaction.

REFERENCES:

1. Christians U, et al. Identification of drugs inhibiting the in vitro metabolism of tacrolimus by human liver microsomes. *Br J Clin Pharmacol.* 1996;41:187-190.

Midazolam

Telaprevir (*Incivek*)

SUMMARY: The coadministration of telaprevir increases the plasma concentration of midazolam; adverse reactions including sedation, ataxia, or respiratory depression may be more likely to occur.

RISK FACTORS: No specific risk factors are known.

MECHANISM: Telaprevir inhibits the CYP3A4-mediated metabolism of midazolam.

CLINICAL EVALUATION: While specific data are limited, the manufacturer of telaprevir notes that the coadministration of telaprevir 750 mg every 8 hours for 9 to 11 days increased the mean area under the plasma concentration-time curve (AUC) of oral midazolam nearly 9-fold and the AUC of intravenous midazolam 3.5-fold.[1] Pending further data, observe patients receiving telaprevir and midazolam for increased midazolam response.

RELATED DRUGS: Boceprevir (*Victrelis*) also inhibits midazolam metabolism. Atazanavir (*Reyataz*), darunavir (*Prezista*), fosamprenavir (*Lexiva*), indinavir (*Crixivan*), nelfinavir (*Viracept*), ritonavir (*Norvir*), and saquinavir (*Invirase*) also inhibit the activity of CYP3A4 and would be expected to increase the plasma concentration of midazolam. The elimination of other benzodiazepines metabolized by CYP3A4 (eg, alprazolam [eg, *Xanax*], triazolam [eg, *Halcion*]) are likely to be affected in a similar manner by telaprevir.

MANAGEMENT OPTIONS:

➡ **Monitor.** Monitor patients receiving midazolam for adverse reactions if telaprevir is coadministered; midazolam doses may need to be reduced.

REFERENCES:
1. *Incivek* [package insert]. Cambridge, MA: Vertex Pharmaceuticals Inc; 2011.

Midazolam

Telithromycin (*Ketek*)

SUMMARY: Telithromycin causes a large increase in midazolam concentrations.

RISK FACTORS:

➡ **Route of Administration.** The oral administration of midazolam will increase the risk of this interaction.

MECHANISM: Telithromycin is known to inhibit CYP3A4, the isozyme primarily responsible for the metabolism of midazolam. Midazolam's bioavailability will be increased and systemic clearance decreased by telithromycin administration.

CLINICAL EVALUATION: While published data are limited, the manufacturer reports that telithromycin increased midazolam area under the plasma concentration-time curve 6- and 2-fold following oral and intravenous midazolam administration, respectively.[1] This magnitude of increase in midazolam plasma concentration could cause adverse reactions, including excess sedation, respiratory depression, and confusion.

RELATED DRUGS: Telithromycin is likely to affect other benzodiazepines that are CYP3A4 substrates (eg, diazepam [eg, *Valium*], alprazolam [eg, *Xanax*]).

MANAGEMENT OPTIONS:

➡ **Consider Alternative.** Temazepam (eg, *Restoril*), lorazepam (eg, *Ativan*), and oxazepam are not likely to interact with telithromycin.

➡ *Monitor.* Monitor patients taking midazolam for increased sedation during the administration of telithromycin.

REFERENCES:

1. *Ketek* [package insert]. Bridgewater, NJ: Aventis Pharmaceuticals, Inc; 2004.

Midazolam

Terbinafine (eg, *Lamisil*)

SUMMARY: Terbinafine did not affect the serum concentrations of midazolam.

RISK FACTORS: No specific risk factors are known.

MECHANISM: No interaction.

CLINICAL EVALUATION: Twelve healthy subjects took terbinafine 250 mg/day or placebo for 4 days.[1] On day 4, midazolam 7.5 mg was taken orally. Compared with placebo, terbinafine administration produced no significant change in any pharmacokinetic parameter of midazolam.

RELATED DRUGS: Terbinafine is unlikely to affect other benzodiazepines that undergo CYP3A4 metabolism (eg, triazolam [eg, *Halcion*], alprazolam [eg, *Xanax*]).

MANAGEMENT OPTIONS: No interaction.

REFERENCES:

1. Ahonen J, et al. Effect of itraconazole and terbinafine on the pharmacokinetics and pharmacodynamics of midazolam in healthy volunteers. *Br J Clin Pharmacol.* 1995;40(3):270-272.

Midazolam

Troleandomycin†

SUMMARY: Troleandomycin increases midazolam concentrations; excess sedation may result, particularly if midazolam is administered orally.

RISK FACTORS:

➡ *Route of Administration.* The oral administration of midazolam increases the risk of this interaction.

MECHANISM: Troleandomycin inhibits CYP3A4, the enzyme known to metabolize midazolam. This increases the bioavailability of orally administered midazolam and reduces its systemic clearance, resulting in increased midazolam plasma concentrations.

CLINICAL EVALUATION: Midazolam 1 mg intravenous (IV) was administered to 12 healthy subjects before and after troleandomycin 500 mg every 12 hours for 3 days.[1] The mean clearance of midazolam was reduced 62% by troleandomycin pretreatment. Mean midazolam half-life increased from 2.5 to 4.5 hours. Increased midazolam effect should be expected if troleandomycin is coadministered. In 2 other studies, troleandomycin reduced the clearance of IV midazolam approximately 75%.[2,3] Troleandomycin reduced the clearance of a single oral dose of midazolam 3 mg 94% and prolonged its half-life from 2.3 to 11.8 hours.[3]

RELATED DRUGS: Erythromycin (eg, *Ery-Tab*), clarithromycin (eg, *Biaxin*), and roxithromycin† also are known to inhibit midazolam metabolism.

MANAGEMENT OPTIONS:

➡ *Consider Alternative.* Azithromycin (eg, *Zithromax*) and dirithromycin do not inhibit CYP3A4 and are not expected to affect midazolam metabolism. Other benzodiazepines such as diazepam (eg, *Valium*) and triazolam (eg, *Halcion*) that are metabolized by CYP3A4 are likely to be affected in a similar manner by troleandomycin. Lorazepam (eg, *Ativan*) and oxazepam are benzodiazepines that are not metabolized by CYP3A4 and are not expected to interact with troleandomycin.

➡ *Monitor.* Watch for excess sedation in patients administered midazolam during therapy with troleandomycin.

REFERENCES:

1. Kharasch ED, et al. Role of hepatic and intestinal cytochrome P450 3A and 2B6 in the metabolism, disposition, and miotic effects of methadone. *Clin Pharmacol Ther.* 2004;76(3):250-269.

2. Kharasch ED, et al. The role of cytochrome P450 3A4 in alfentanil clearance. Implications for interindividual variability in disposition and perioperative drug interactions. *Anesthesiology.* 1997;87(1):36-50.

3. Kharasch ED, et al. Intravenous and oral alfentanil as in vivo probes for hepatic and first-pass cytochrome P450 3A activity: noninvasive assessment by use of pupillary miosis. *Clin Pharmacol Ther.* 2004;76(5):452-466.

† Not available in the United States.

Midazolam

Voriconazole (eg, *Vfend*)

SUMMARY: Voriconazole increases the plasma concentration of midazolam; be alert for increased level and duration of sedation.

RISK FACTORS:

➡ *Route of Administration.* Midazolam administered orally will be affected to a greater extent by voriconazole than intravenous (IV) midazolam.

MECHANISM: Voriconazole inhibits the first-pass and systemic metabolism of midazolam by CYP3A4.

CLINICAL EVALUATION: Ten healthy subjects received placebo or voriconazole 400 mg twice daily for one day and 200 mg twice daily on the second day.[1] Midazolam 0.05 mg/kg IV or 7.5 mg orally was administered 1 hour after the last voriconazole dose. Following IV midazolam, the mean area under the concentration-time curve (AUC) increased nearly 260% and the midazolam half-life increased from 2.8 to 8.3 hours. The AUC of oral midazolam increased approximately 840% with a half-life increase similar to that seen during the IV midazolam administration. Marked increases in sedative effects were observed following the coadministration of midazolam and voriconazole. Also observe patients for prolonged sedation if voriconazole and midazolam are coadministered.

RELATED DRUGS: Alprazolam (eg, *Xanax*), diazepam (eg, *Valium*), and triazolam (eg, *Halcion*) are also metabolized by CYP3A4 and are likely affected by voriconazole. Other antifungal agents that inhibit CYP3A4 (eg, itraconazole [eg, *Sporanox*], ketoconazole [eg, *Nizoral*], fluconazole [eg, *Diflucan*]) are known to affect midazolam in a similar manner.

MANAGEMENT OPTIONS:

➡ *Consider Alternative.* Other benzodiazepines (eg, lorazepam [eg, *Ativan*], oxazepam) that are not metabolized by CYP3A4 are unlikely to be affected by voriconazole. Terbinafine (eg, *Lamisil*) may be considered as an alternative antifungal agent because it does not affect CYP3A4 activity. Because of the large magnitude of the interaction, avoid oral midazolam in patients taking CYP3A4 inhibitors.

➡ *Circumvent/Minimize.* If IV midazolam is administered to patients taking voriconazole, consider reducing the dose.

➡ *Monitor.* Monitor for increased magnitude and duration of sedation in patients receiving voriconazole and midazolam.

REFERENCES:

1. Saari TI, et al. Effect of voriconazole on the pharmacokinetics and pharmacodynamics of intravenous and oral midazolam. *Clin Pharmacol Ther*. 2006;79(4):362-370.

Milnacipran (*Savella*)

Lithium (eg, *Lithobid*)

SUMMARY: Theoretically, combining milnacipran with lithium may increase the risk of serotonin syndrome.

RISK FACTORS: No specific risk factors are known.

MECHANISM: Milnacipran inhibits the reuptake of serotonin and norepinephrine and may have additive serotonergic effects with lithium.

CLINICAL EVALUATION: The manufacturer advises caution in using this combination.[1] This interaction is based largely on theoretical considerations, and it is not known how often adverse outcomes would be observed. Lithium is a relatively weak serotonergic agent, so frequent problems are not expected.

RELATED DRUGS: There have been occasional reports of serotonin toxicity when lithium was combined with selective serotonin reuptake inhibitors or other serotonin-norepinephrine reuptake inhibitors.

MANAGEMENT OPTIONS:

➡ *Consider Alternative.* If possible, use an alternative to one of the drugs.

➡ *Monitor.* If the combination is used, monitor for evidence of serotonin syndrome, including agitation, coma, confusion, fever, hyperreflexia, incoordination, myoclonus, rigidity, seizures, sweating, and tremor.

REFERENCES:

1. *Savella* [package insert]. St. Louis, MO: Forest Pharmaceuticals; 2010.

Milnacipran (*Savella*)

Paroxetine (eg, *Paxil*)

SUMMARY: Theoretically, combining milnacipran with selective serotonin reuptake inhibitors (SSRIs) may increase the risk of serotonin syndrome.

RISK FACTORS: No specific risk factors are known.

MECHANISM: Milnacipran inhibits the reuptake of serotonin and norepinephrine and may have additive serotonergic effects with SSRIs.

CLINICAL EVALUATION: The manufacturer states that combined use of milnacipran and SSRIs is not recommended.[1] The interaction is based largely on theoretical considerations, but it is reasonable given the pharmacodynamic effects of the drugs. Theoretically, it may be possible to use both drugs by adjusting the dose of one or both drugs, but the medicolegal implications should be considered.

RELATED DRUGS: All SSRIs are expected to interact similarly with milnacipran, including citalopram (eg, *Celexa*), escitalopram (*Lexapro*), fluoxetine (eg, *Prozac*), fluvoxamine (eg, *Luvox*), and sertraline (eg, *Zoloft*).

MANAGEMENT OPTIONS:

➡ *Consider Alternative.* If possible, use an alternative to one of the drugs.

➡ *Monitor.* If the combination is used, monitor for evidence of serotonin syndrome, including agitation, coma, confusion, fever, hyperreflexia, incoordination, myoclonus, rigidity, seizures, sweating, and tremor.

REFERENCES:

1. *Savella* [package insert]. St. Louis, MO: Forest Pharmaceuticals; 2010.

 Milnacipran (*Savella*)

Selegiline (eg, *Eldepryl*)

SUMMARY: Milnacipran is contraindicated with nonselective monoamine oxidase inhibitors (MAOIs) because of the risk of potentially fatal serotonin syndrome; although selegiline is a selective monoamine oxidase type B (MAO-B) inhibitor, it may interact in some patients.

RISK FACTORS: No specific risk factors are known.

MECHANISM: Milnacipran inhibits the reuptake of serotonin and norepinephrine and may have additive serotonergic effects with nonselective MAOIs.

CLINICAL EVALUATION: The combination of serotonin reuptake inhibitors with nonselective MAOIs has resulted in severe (sometimes fatal) serotonin syndrome. The product information for milnacipran states that concurrent therapy with MAOIs is contraindicated.[1] Selegiline is a selective MAO-B inhibitor, and theoretically is unlikely to interact with serotonin reuptake inhibitors, such as milnacipran. However, some patients appear to develop nonselective MAO inhibition following selegiline, so it is possible that it interacts with milnacipran under some circumstances.

RELATED DRUGS: Like selegiline, rasagiline (*Azilect*) is a selective MAO-B inhibitor that may become nonselective in some patients, so it may also interact with milnacipran.

MANAGEMENT OPTIONS:

➡ *Consider Alternative.* It is recommended to use an alternative to one of the drugs, but this may be difficult given the indications for which these drugs are used.

➡ *Monitor.* If the combination is used, monitor for evidence of serotonin syndrome, including agitation, coma, confusion, fever, hyperreflexia, incoordination, myoclonus, rigidity, seizures, sweating, and tremor.

REFERENCES:

1. *Savella* [package insert]. St. Louis, MO: Forest Pharmaceuticals; 2010.

Milnacipran (*Savella*)

Sumatriptan (eg, *Imitrex*)

SUMMARY: Theoretically, combining milnacipran with sumatriptan or other triptans may increase the risk of serotonin syndrome.

RISK FACTORS: No specific risk factors are known.

MECHANISM: Milnacipran inhibits the reuptake of serotonin and norepinephrine and may have additive serotonergic effects with triptans.

CLINICAL EVALUATION: The manufacturer advises caution in using this combination.[1] The interaction is based largely on theoretical considerations, and it is not known how often adverse outcomes would be observed.

RELATED DRUGS: All triptans are expected to interact similarly with milnacipran, including almotriptan (*Axert*), eletriptan (*Relpax*), frovatriptan (*Frova*), naratriptan (eg, *Amerge*), rizatriptan (*Maxalt*), and zolmitriptan (*Zomig*).

MANAGEMENT OPTIONS:

➡ *Consider Alternative.* If possible, use an alternative to one of the drugs.

➡ *Monitor.* If the combination is used, monitor for evidence of serotonin syndrome, including agitation, coma, confusion, fever, hyperreflexia, incoordination, myoclonus, rigidity, seizures, sweating, and tremor.

REFERENCES:

1. *Savella* [package insert]. St. Louis, MO: Forest Pharmaceuticals; 2010.

Milnacipran (*Savella*)

Tranylcypromine (eg, *Parnate*)   AVOID

SUMMARY: Milnacipran is contraindicated with nonselective monoamine oxidase inhibitors (MAOIs) because of the risk of potentially fatal serotonin syndrome.

RISK FACTORS: No specific risk factors are known.

MECHANISM: Milnacipran inhibits the reuptake of serotonin and norepinephrine and may have additive serotonergic effects with nonselective MAOIs.

CLINICAL EVALUATION: The combination of serotonin reuptake inhibitors with nonselective MAOIs has resulted in severe (sometimes fatal) serotonin syndrome. The product information for milnacipran states that concurrent therapy with MAOIs is contraindicated.[1] Symptoms of serotonin syndrome include agitation, coma, confusion, fever, hyperreflexia, incoordination, myoclonus, rigidity, seizures, sweating, and tremor.

RELATED DRUGS: Milnacipran is also contraindicated with other nonselective MAOI antidepressants, such as phenelzine (eg, *Nardil*) and isocarboxazid (*Marplan*). Furazolidone⁺ and methylene blue can act as nonselective MAOIs and are also contraindicated with milnacipran.

MANAGEMENT OPTIONS:

➡ *AVOID COMBINATION.* Avoid concurrent use of milnacipran with nonselective MAOIs.

REFERENCES:

1. *Savella* [package insert]. St. Louis, MO: Forest Pharmaceuticals; 2010.

† Not available in the United States.

Milnacipran (*Savella*)

Tryptophan†

SUMMARY: Theoretically, combining milnacipran with tryptophan may increase the risk of serotonin syndrome.

RISK FACTORS: No specific risk factors are known.

MECHANISM: Milnacipran inhibits the reuptake of serotonin and norepinephrine and may have additive serotonergic effects with tryptophan.

CLINICAL EVALUATION: The manufacturer states that combined use of milnacipran and tryptophan is not recommended.[1] This interaction is based largely on theoretical considerations, and it is not known how often adverse outcomes would be observed.

RELATED DRUGS: Tryptophan may also interact with other serotonin-norepinephrine reuptake inhibitors, such as clomipramine (eg, *Anafranil*), desvenlafaxine (*Pristiq*), duloxetine (*Cymbalta*), imipramine (eg, *Tofranil*), venlafaxine (eg, *Effexor XR*), or selective serotonin reuptake inhibitors, such as citalopram (eg, *Celexa*), escitalopram (*Lexapro*), fluoxetine (eg, *Prozac*), fluvoxamine (eg, *Luvox*), paroxetine (eg, *Paxil*), and sertraline (eg, *Zoloft*).

MANAGEMENT OPTIONS:

➡ *Consider Alternative.* If possible, use an alternative to one of the drugs.

➡ *Monitor.* If the combination is used, monitor for evidence of serotonin syndrome, including agitation, coma, confusion, fever, hyperreflexia, incoordination, myoclonus, rigidity, seizures, sweating, and tremor.

REFERENCES:

1. *Savella* [package insert]. St. Louis, MO: Forest Pharmaceuticals; 2010.

† Not available in the United States.

Milnacipran (*Savella*)

Venlafaxine (eg, *Effexor XR*)

SUMMARY: Theoretically, combining milnacipran with other serotonin-norepinephrine reuptake inhibitors (SNRIs) may increase the risk of serotonin syndrome.

RISK FACTORS: No specific risk factors are known.

MECHANISM: Milnacipran is an SNRI that inhibits the reuptake of serotonin and norepinephrine and may have additive serotonergic effects with other SNRIs.

CLINICAL EVALUATION: The manufacturer states that combined use of milnacipran and SNRIs is not recommended.[1] The interaction is based largely on theoretical considerations, but it is reasonable given the pharmacodynamic effects of the drugs. Theoretically, it may be possible to use both drugs by adjusting the dose of one or both drugs, but the medicolegal implications should be considered.

RELATED DRUGS: All SNRIs are expected to interact similarly with milnacipran, including clomipramine (eg, *Anafranil*), desvenlafaxine (*Pristiq*), duloxetine (*Cymbalta*), and imipramine (eg, *Tofranil*). One patient on clomipramine developed euphoria and postural hypotension after being switched to milnacipran.

MANAGEMENT OPTIONS:

➡ *Consider Alternative.* If possible, use an alternative to one of the drugs.

➡ *Monitor.* If the combination is used, monitor for evidence of serotonin syndrome, including agitation, coma, confusion, fever, hyperreflexia, incoordination, myoclonus, rigidity, seizures, sweating, and tremor.

REFERENCES:

1. *Savella* [package insert]. St. Louis, MO: Forest Pharmaceuticals; 2010.

Mineral Oil

Contraceptives, Oral (eg, *Ortho-Novum*)

SUMMARY: Uncontrolled clinical impressions indicate that mineral oil may reduce the therapeutic effect of estrogen, but a causal relationship is not established.

RISK FACTORS: No specific risk factors are known.

MECHANISM: Theoretically, mineral oil could impair the absorption of estrogens and oral contraceptives, thus reducing their effect.

CLINICAL EVALUATION: Not established. Some patients receiving oral estrogens for prostatic carcinoma have had exacerbations when mineral oil was taken.[1] Whether the mineral oil was responsible or whether the action of oral contraceptives could be affected remains to be established.

RELATED DRUGS: No information is available.

MANAGEMENT OPTIONS: No specific action is required, but be alert for evidence of the interaction.

REFERENCES:

1. Swyer GI. Liquid paraffin and oral contraception. *Practitioner.* 1969;202:592.

Mineral Oil

Vitamin A

SUMMARY: Mineral oil reportedly inhibits vitamin A absorption, but clinical evidence of this effect is lacking.

RISK FACTORS: No specific risk factors are known.

MECHANISM: Not established.

CLINICAL EVALUATION: Although many feel that vitamin A absorption is affected by mineral oil, a review of the literature failed to reveal evidence for such an effect.[1]

RELATED DRUGS: No information is available.

MANAGEMENT OPTIONS: No interaction.

REFERENCES:

1. Cohen H. Mineral oil, vitamin A, and carotene. Genesis and correction of a common misconception. *J Med Soc N J.* 1970;67:111-115.

Mineral Oil

Warfarin (eg, *Coumadin*)

SUMMARY: Although mineral oil theoretically could interact with oral anticoagulants such as warfarin, clinical evidence is lacking.

RISK FACTORS: No specific risk factors are known.

MECHANISM: Mineral oil is said to reduce the absorption of fat-soluble nutrients such as vitamin K. Such a decrease could enhance the hypoprothrombinemia produced by oral anticoagulants. However, there is little supporting clinical evidence.

CLINICAL EVALUATION: Not established. Little clinical information is available on either of the 2 possible mechanisms mentioned.[1-3]

RELATED DRUGS: Other anticoagulants theoretically could interact similarly.

MANAGEMENT OPTIONS: No specific action is required, but be alert for evidence of the interaction.

REFERENCES:

1. Becker GL. The case against mineral oil. *Am J Dig Dis.* 1952;19:344-348.
2. Morowitz DA. Complications of long-term mineral oil intake. *JAMA.* 1968;204:937.
3. O'Reilly RA, et al. Determinants of the response to oral anticoagulant drugs in man. *Pharmacol Rev.* 1970;22:35-96.

Mirtazapine

Rasagiline (*Azilect*)

SUMMARY: Concomitant use of rasagiline and mirtazapine should generally be avoided.

RISK FACTORS: No specific risk factors are known.

MECHANISM: Not established. The combination may have additive serotonergic effects.

CLINICAL EVALUATION: Mirtazapine has serotonergic effects and may increase the risk of serotonin syndrome when combined with other serotonergic drugs or MAO inhibitors. Mirtazapine is contraindicated in rasagiline product information.[1]

RELATED DRUGS: Any interaction between mirtazapine and rasagiline is likely to be similar to the interaction between mirtazapine and selegiline.

MANAGEMENT OPTIONS:

➧ ***Avoid Unless Benefit Outweighs Risk.*** Mirtazapine should generally not be used concomitantly with rasagiline or within 2 weeks of stopping rasagiline.

REFERENCES:

1. *Azilect* [package insert]. North Wales, PA: Teva Neuroscience, Inc.; 2006.

Mirtazapine (eg, *Remeron*)
Venlafaxine (*Effexor*)

SUMMARY: A man developed hypertension after receiving mirtazapine and venlafaxine, but a causal relationship was not established.

RISK FACTORS: No specific risk factors are known.

MECHANISM: Not established. Additive noradrenergic activity was proposed.

CLINICAL EVALUATION: In a 36-year-old man on mirtazapine 60 mg/day, the addition of venlafaxine was followed by hypertension and mydriasis.[1] The reaction may have resulted from a combined effect of the 2 drugs, but an effect from venlafaxine alone cannot be ruled out.

RELATED DRUGS: No information is available.

MANAGEMENT OPTIONS: No specific action is required, but be alert for evidence of the interaction.

REFERENCES:

1. Zullino DF, Cucchia G. Mydriasis, hypertension, and tachycardia possibly associated with venlafaxine augmentation of mirtazapine. *J Pharm Technol.* 2004;20:334-335.

Misoprostol (eg, *Cytotec*) ▼3
Phenylbutazone†

SUMMARY: The combined use of phenylbutazone and misoprostol has been associated with adverse effects (eg, dizziness, headache, hot flushes, nausea, tingling) in some patients, but a causal relationship has not been established.

RISK FACTORS: No specific risk factors are known.

MECHANISM: Not established.

CLINICAL EVALUATION: A 29-year-old woman on phenylbutazone developed dizziness, hot flushes, nausea, and tingling 5 days after starting misoprostol 800 mcg/day.[1] Phenylbutazone was stopped, and the symptoms disappeared within 3 days. The fact that the symptoms did not occur with either drug alone supports the possibility that a drug interaction was involved. A later challenge with naproxen (eg, *Naprosyn*) 1,100 mg/day while the patient was still taking misoprostol did not produce any symptoms. Similar cases of neurosensory disturbances (eg, ambulatory instability, diplopia, dizziness, headaches, tingling) have been observed in 2 other patients receiving phenylbutazone and misoprostol concurrently.[2] In both cases, either drug alone did not produce symptoms. Challenge with etodolac (eg, *Lodine*) 400 mg/day plus misoprostol in 1 of the patients did not produce a recurrence of the reaction.

RELATED DRUGS: Naproxen and etodolac do not appear to affect misoprostol. The effect of other nonsteroidal anti-inflammatory drugs on misoprostol is not established.

MANAGEMENT OPTIONS:

➡ ***Monitor.*** Until more information is available, be alert for adverse effects such as dizziness, headache, hot flushes, nausea, and tingling when misoprostol is used in patients receiving phenylbutazone.

REFERENCES:

1. Chassagne P, et al. Neurosensory adverse effects after combined phenylbutazone and misoprostol. *Br J Rheumatol.* 1991;30:392.

2. Jacquemier JM, et al. Neurosensory adverse effects after phenylbutazone and misoprostol combined treatment. *Lancet.* 1989;2:1283.

† Not available in the United States.

 Mitomycin (*Mutamycin*)

Vinblastine (eg, *Velban*)

SUMMARY: Administration of vinblastine following treatment with mitomycin has been associated with acute broncho-spasm and dyspnea.

RISK FACTORS: No specific risk factors are known.

MECHANISM: Not established. Mitomycin is known to cause pulmonary toxicity; however, the reaction that occurs with vinblastine and mitomycin is much more abrupt than is typical of mitomycin pulmonary toxicity.

CLINICAL EVALUATION: Numerous cases of acute respiratory distress developing 30 minutes to 3 hours following a dose of vinblastine have been reported in patients receiving combination regimens containing mitomycin and vinblastine.[1-7] The incidence of this syndrome is not known, although in a clinical trial of this combination involving 90 patients, the incidence of acute respiratory distress was approxmately 3%.[4] Patients who develop this syndrome frequently complain of shortness of breath and are found to be hypoxic with evidence of pulmonary edema on chest X-ray. Interventions such as oxygen, bronchodilators, steroids, or intubation may be required depending on the severity of symptoms. Despite these measures, several patients have died from respiratory failure. The process appears to resolve over 2 to 3 days; but when rechallenged with vinblastine, reports suggest that the syndrome may recur.[2,4]

RELATED DRUGS: No information is available.

MANAGEMENT OPTIONS:

➡ ***Avoid Unless Benefit Outweighs Risk.*** Although most patients do not appear to develop pulmonary toxicity, the severity of the reaction dictates that the combination generally should be avoided.

➡ ***Monitor.*** In instances where the combination is felt to be necessary, advise patients to contact their physician or go to the emergency room immediately if they develop difficulty in breathing. Both drugs should be discontinued immediately at the first sign of respiratory compromise. Avoid further therapy with this combination in patients who experience dyspnea, as it appears to recur upon repeated administration.

REFERENCES:

1. Israel RH, et al. Pulmonary edema associated with intravenous vinblastine. *JAMA.* 1978;240:1585.

2. Konits PH, et al. Possible pulmonary toxicity secondary to vinblastine. *Cancer.* 1982;50:277.

3. Ozols RF, et al. MVP (mitomycin, vinblastine, and progesterone): a second-line regimen in ovarian cancer with a high incidence of pulmonary toxicity. *Cancer Treat Rep*. 1983;67:721.

4. Dyke RW. Acute bronchospasm after vinca alkaloid in patients previously treated with mitomycin. *N Engl J Med*. 1984;310:389.

5. Kris MG, et al. Dyspnea following vinblastine or vindesine administration in patients receiving mitomycin plus vinca alkaloid combination therapy. *Cancer Treat Rep*. 1984;68:1029.

6. Rao SX, et al. Fatal acute respiratory failure after vinblastine-mitomycin therapy in lung carcinoma. *Arch Intern Med*. 1985;145:1905.

7. Hoelzer KL. Vinblastine-associated pulmonary toxicity in patients receiving combination therapy with mitomycin and cisplatin. *Drug Intell Clin Pharm*. 1986;20:287.

Mitotane (*Lysodren*)

Spironolactone (eg, *Aldactone*) AVOID

SUMMARY: Spironolactone may antagonize the activity of mitotane.

RISK FACTORS: No specific risk factors are known.

MECHANISM: Studies in dogs have shown that destruction of adrenocortical tissue by mitotane was not achieved when the animals were pretreated with spironolactone.[1]

CLINICAL EVALUATION: A 65-year-old woman with Cushing's syndrome was treated with spironolactone 50 mg 4 times daily to combat hypokalemia due to mineralocorticoid excess.[1] The patient was later started on mitotane; but she exhibited none of the side effects of mitotane and had persistently elevated morning serum cortisol levels. In view of information in animals that spironolactone antagonizes the activity of mitotane, spironolactone therapy was stopped. Within 24 to 48 hours the patient began to experience nausea and severe diarrhea, normal side effects of mitotane. The patient never was able to tolerate mitotane, so it was not possible to determine whether a suppression of cortisol could be achieved without spironolactone.

RELATED DRUGS: No information is available.

MANAGEMENT OPTIONS:

➡ **AVOID COMBINATION.** Patients on mitotane should not receive concurrent spironolactone.

REFERENCES:

1. Wortsman J, et al. Mitotane Spironolactone antagonism in Cushing's syndrome. *JAMA*. 1977;238:2527.

Mitotane (*Lysodren*)

Warfarin (eg, *Coumadin*)

SUMMARY: Mitotane appears to inhibit the hypoprothrombinemic response to warfarin and probably other oral anticoagulants as well. Oral anticoagulant dose requirements may be increased in patients taking both drugs.

RISK FACTORS: No specific risk factors are known.

MECHANISM: Mitotane probably enhances the metabolism of warfarin by inducing hepatic microsomal enzymes. Mitotane induces enzymes in animals, and it is structurally similar to insecticides that induce hepatic metabolism in humans.

CLINICAL EVALUATION: In a 58-year-old woman warfarin requirements increased when mitotane was given concurrently.[1] She initially was maintained on a warfarin dose of 3.75 mg/day, but over 6 weeks of mitotane therapy her warfarin requirement increased to 12.5 mg/day. Although there was no apparent cause for the decreasing warfarin response other than the mitotane, controlled studies will be required to assess the incidence and magnitude of this interaction.

RELATED DRUGS: The effect of mitotane on oral anticoagulants other than warfarin is not known, but be alert for a similar effect with all oral anticoagulants until information to the contrary is available.

MANAGEMENT OPTIONS:

➡ *Monitor.* Monitor for altered oral anticoagulant effect if mitotane is initiated, discontinued, or changed in dosage. Adjust the anticoagulant dose as needed.

REFERENCES:
1. Cuddy PG, et al. Influence of mitotane on the hypoprothrombinemic effect of warfarin. *South Med J.* 1986;79:387.

 Moclobemide†

Rizatriptan (*Maxalt*)

SUMMARY: Moclobemide substantially increases plasma concentrations of rizatriptan and its active metabolite; concurrent use is generally not recommended, although adverse clinical outcomes have not been reported.

RISK FACTORS: No specific risk factors are known.

MECHANISM: Rizatriptan is metabolized primarily by monoamine oxidase-A (MAO-A), and moclobemide is an MAO-A inhibitor. Therefore, moclobemide probably decreases the metabolism of rizatriptan and its active metabolite.

CLINICAL EVALUATION: In a randomized, crossover study, 12 healthy subjects took a single oral 10 mg dose of rizatriptan with and without pretreatment with moclobemide 150 mg twice daily for 4 days.[1] Moclobemide increased the area under the plasma concentration-time curve for rizatriptan and its active metabolite by 2.2- and 5.3-fold, respectively. Because the rizatriptan metabolite is approximately twice as potent as the parent drug, this interaction would be expected to substantially increase the effect of administered rizatriptan, leading the authors to recommend that rizatriptan not be used with moclobemide. Although the concern about this interaction is based primarily on theoretical considerations rather than actual observations of adverse consequences, the manufacturer of rizatriptan lists MAO-A inhibitors and nonselective MAO inhibitors as contraindicated with rizatriptan.

RELATED DRUGS: Theoretically, any selective MAO-A inhibitor or nonselective MAO-A/MAO-B inhibitor such as phenelzine (*Nardil*) or tranylcypromine (*Parnate*) would also substantially increase rizatriptan plasma concentrations. Sumatriptan (*Imitrex*) and zolmitriptan (*Zomig*), like rizatriptan, are metabolized by MAO-A. They would be expected to interact similarly with MAO-A inhibitors such as moclobemide or nonselective MAO-A/MAO-B inhibitors such as phenelzine or tranylcypromine.

MANAGEMENT OPTIONS:

➡ *Use Alternative.* Use an alternative to moclobemide (ie, a non-MAO-A inhibitor) or rizatriptan (ie, a non-MAO-A substrate). Naratriptan (*Amerge*) is predominantly eliminated in the urine, and theoretically would be less likely than other "triptans" to interact with moclobemide or nonselective MAO inhibitors.

➡ *Monitor.* Theoretically, the combination of moclobemide and rizatriptan could result in excessive vasoconstriction. If the combination is used, monitor for increased blood pressure and other evidence of vasoconstriction.

REFERENCES:

1. van Haarst AD, et al. The effects of moclobemide on the pharmacokinetics of the 5-HT$_{1B/1D}$ agonist rizatriptan in healthy volunteers. *Br J Clin Pharmacol.* 1999;48:190-96

† Not available in the United States.

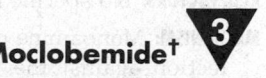

Moclobemide†

Selegiline (eg, *Eldepryl*)

SUMMARY: Combined use of selegiline and moclobemide substantially increases the pressor effect of tyramine over either drug used alone.

RISK FACTORS: No specific risk factors are known.

MECHANISM: Selegiline is a selective monoamine oxidase (MAO)-B inhibitor. Combined therapy of selegiline with a selective MAO-A inhibitor such as moclobemide would be expected to result in MAO inhibition similar to that seen with nonselective MAOIs such as phenelzine (*Nardil*) and tranylcypromine (*Parnate*).

CLINICAL EVALUATION: Twelve healthy subjects received moclobemide 400 mg/day for 18 days with either selegiline 10 mg/day or a placebo added for the last 10 days in a parallel study.[1] Twelve other healthy subjects received selegiline 10 mg/day for 18 days with moclobemide 400 mg/day or a placebo added for the last 10 days. IV tyramine tests were conducted at baseline, with monotherapy on either drug, and with combined therapy. Selegiline alone increased the pressor response to IV tyramine only slightly, while moclobemide increased it moderately. However, the 2 drugs together markedly increased the pressor response to tyramine.

RELATED DRUGS: This interaction is likely to occur with any combination of an MAO-B and MAO-A inhibitor.

MANAGEMENT OPTIONS:

➡ *Consider Alternative.* Given the likely increase in risk of adverse drug or food interactions, consider using an antidepressant other than moclobemide in patients receiving MAO-B inhibitors such as selegiline.

➡ *Circumvent/Minimize.* Until more data are available, give patients receiving combined therapy with moclobemide and selegiline (or any other combination of an MAO-A and MAO-B inhibitor) the same dietary and drug interaction instructions as patients receiving nonselective MAOI such as phenelzine or tranylcypromine.

➥ *Monitor.* Monitor for evidence of tyramine-induced hypertension if the combination is used.

REFERENCES:

1. Dingemanse J. An update of recent moclobemide interaction data. *Int Clin Psychopharmacol.* 1993;7:167.

† Not available in the United States.

Moclobemide†

Tyramine

SUMMARY: Moclobemide may increase the pressor response to large amounts of tyramine; avoid high-tyramine foods (eg, aged cheese).

RISK FACTORS: No specific risk factors are known.

MECHANISM: Monoamine oxidase (MAO)-A in the intestine and liver is important protection against the pressor response to dietary tyramine. However, because MAO-B also is involved in tyramine metabolism, selective inhibitors of MAO-A such as moclobemide would not be expected to enhance the pressor response to tyramine as much as nonselective monoamine oxidase MAOIs.

CLINICAL EVALUATION: Twelve healthy subjects received IV tyramine tests before and after treatment with moclobemide 400 mg/day for 8 days.[1] The "tyramine sensitivity factor" during moclobemide was about 2.5. In other words, it took about 2.5 times more tyramine to increase systolic blood pressure by 30 mm Hg at baseline vs post-moclobemide. In another study of 8 healthy subjects who took moclobemide 450 mg/day for 28 days, the mean dose of oral tyramine needed to increase systolic blood pressure by 30 mm Hg was 240 mg. However, 3 subjects had an increase in systolic blood pressure over 100 mm Hg following only 160 mg oral tyramine. No subject on moclobemide responded to a tyramine dose below 160 mg/day. This is in contrast to nonselective MAOIs such as phenelzine, where as little as 10 mg of tyramine may produce a substantial increase in blood pressure.[2] One would not expect the tyramine content of a typical meal to interact significantly with moclobemide, but high-tyramine foods may be a problem. The potentiating effect of moclobemide is rapidly reversible; another tyramine test was performed on day 31 of the study (after 2 days of no moclobemide), and the effect of moclobemide on the pressor response to tyramine had dissipated in all of the subjects.

RELATED DRUGS: Other MAO-A inhibitors may interact similarly with tyramine.

MANAGEMENT OPTIONS:

➥ *Circumvent/Minimize.* Although moclobemide appears much less likely to interact with dietary tyramine than nonselective MAOIs, it would be prudent to avoid foods with high tyramine content. It also has been suggested that moclobemide be taken after meals to minimize the interaction,[3] but more study is needed to assess the value of this precaution.

➥ *Monitor.* Monitor blood pressure if the interaction is suspected.

REFERENCES:

1. Dingemanse J. An update of recent moclobemide interaction data. *Int Clin Psychopharmacol.* 1993;7:167.
2. Simpson GM, et al. Comparison of the pressor effect of tyramine after treatment with phenelzine and moclobemide in healthy male volunteers. *Clin Pharmacol Ther.* 1992;52:286.
3. Freeman H. Moclobemide. *Lancet.* 1993;342:1528.

† Not available in the United States.

Modafinil (*Provigil*)

Contraceptives, Oral (eg, *Ortho-Novum*)

SUMMARY: Modafinil appears to modestly reduce ethinyl estradiol plasma concentrations; reduced contraceptive efficacy may occur in some patients.

RISK FACTORS: No specific risk factors are known.

MECHANISM: Modafinil appears to induce CYP3A4, and may enhance the metabolism of ethinyl estradiol.

CLINICAL EVALUATION: In a placebo-controlled study of 41 women taking an oral contraceptive (ethinyl estradiol 0.035 mg plus norgestimate 0.180 to 0.250 mg), ethinyl estradiol pharmacokinetics were measured before and after modafinil (200 mg/day for 7 days, then 400 mg/day for 21 days).[1] Modafinil was associated with a 18% decrease in ethinyl estradiol area under the plasma concentration-time curve. The magnitude of this effect could be enough to increase the risk of unintended pregnancy in at least some patients.

RELATED DRUGS: No information is available.

MANAGEMENT OPTIONS:

➡ ***Consider Alternative.*** In patients on modafinil, consider using contraceptive methods other than oral contraceptives.

➡ ***Circumvent/Minimize.*** If oral contraceptives are used in conjunction with modafinil therapy, it would be prudent to use additional methods of contraceptive during and for 1 month after stopping modafinil.

➡ ***Monitor.*** If oral contraceptives are used in conjunction with modafinil therapy, be alert for evidence of reduced contraceptive effect such as menstrual irregularities (eg, spotting, breakthrough bleeding).

REFERENCES:

1. Robertson P, et al. Effect of modafinil on the pharmacokinetics of ethinyl estradiol and triazolam in healthy volunteers. *Clin Pharmacol Ther.* 2002;71:46-56.

Modafinil (*Provigil*)

Triazolam (*Halcion*)

SUMMARY: Modafinil appears to substantially reduce triazolam plasma concentrations, and may reduce its hypnotic effect.

RISK FACTORS: No specific risk factors are known.

MECHANISM: Modafinil appears to induce CYP3A4, with most of the effect being on intestinal CYP3A4 rather than hepatic CYP3A4. Triazolam undergoes extensive presystemic metabolism by intestinal CYP3A4, which is probably increased by modafinil.

CLINICAL EVALUATION: In a placebo-controlled study of 41 women taking an oral contraceptive, a single oral dose of triazolam (0.125 mg) was given before and after modafinil (200 mg/day for 7 days, then 400 mg/day for 21 days).[1] Modafinil was associated with a substantial (59%) decrease in triazolam area under the plasma concentration-time curve, while there was an 8% increase with placebo. The magnitude of this effect would be expected to reduce the pharmacodynamic effect of triazolam in at least some patients.

RELATED DRUGS: No information is available.

MANAGEMENT OPTIONS:

➡️ *Monitor.* Be alert for evidence of reduced triazolam effect if modafinil is given concurrently. A larger dose of triazolam may be needed.

REFERENCES:

1. Robertson P, et al. Effect of modafinil on the pharmacokinetics of ethinyl estradiol and triazolam in healthy volunteers. *Clin Pharmacol Ther*. 2002;71:46-56.

Montelukast (*Singulair*)

Prednisone (eg, *Deltasone*)

SUMMARY: A patient developed edema after receiving concurrent montelukast and prednisone, but a causal relationship was not established.

RISK FACTORS: No specific risk factors are known.

MECHANISM: Not established.

CLINICAL EVALUATION: A 23-year-old man on montelukast 10 mg/day developed severe peripheral edema 10 days after starting prednisone 40 to 60 mg/day.[1] He had received montelukast and prednisone alone without developing edema. Nonetheless, more information is needed to establish a causal relationship.

RELATED DRUGS: No information is available.

MANAGEMENT OPTIONS: No specific action is required, but be alert for evidence of the interaction.

REFERENCES:

1. Geller M. Marked peripheral edema associated with montelukast and prednisone. *Ann Intern Med*. 2000;132:924.

Moricizine (*Ethmozine*)

Theophylline (eg, *Theolair*)

SUMMARY: Moricizine reduces theophylline serum concentrations; the clinical effects of this pharmacokinetic interaction have not been described.

RISK FACTORS: No specific risk factors are known.

MECHANISM: Moricizine appears to increase the metabolism of theophylline.

CLINICAL EVALUATION: Moricizine 250 mg every 8 hours was administered to 12 healthy subjects for 13 days.[1] Subjects received a single dose of immediate-release theophylline and a single dose of sustained-release theophylline before and after moricizine. The area under the theophylline concentration-time curve was reduced 32% and 36% for the immediate- and sustained-release theophylline formulations, respectively. The half-life of both theophylline products was reduced significantly, and the peak theophylline concentrations produced by the sustained-release theophylline product were decreased. The magnitude of change in theophylline concentrations would be expected to reduce its clinical effects in some patients.

RELATED DRUGS: No information is available.

MANAGEMENT OPTIONS:

➡ *Monitor.* Monitor patients taking theophylline for reduced theophylline concentrations and potential loss of effect when moricizine is added to their therapy.

REFERENCES:

1. Pieniaszek HJ, et al. Effect of moricizine on the pharmacokinetics of single-dose theophylline in healthy subjects. *Ther Drug Monit.* 1993;15:199.

Moricizine (*Ethmozine*) 5

Warfarin (eg, *Coumadin*)

SUMMARY: Moricizine did not affect the pharmacokinetics or pharmacodynamics after a single dose of warfarin.

RISK FACTORS: No specific risk factors are known.

MECHANISM: No interaction.

CLINICAL EVALUATION: A single dose of warfarin was administered alone and following moricizine 250 mg every 8 hours for 14 days.[1] No significant changes in warfarin pharmacokinetics or anticoagulation were noted.

RELATED DRUGS: No information is available.

MANAGEMENT OPTIONS: No interaction.

REFERENCES:

1. Benedek IH, et al. Effect of moricizine on the pharmacokinetics and pharmacodynamics of warfarin in healthy volunteers. *J Clin Pharmacol.* 1992;32:558.

Morphine (eg, *Roxanol*) 4

Nifedipine (eg, *Procardia*)

SUMMARY: Nifedipine administration appears to increase the analgesic effect of morphine; the clinical significance is unclear.

RISK FACTORS: No specific risk factors are known.

MECHANISM: Not established.

CLINICAL EVALUATION: Twenty-six postoperative patients randomly were assigned to receive 20 mg slow-release nifedipine or a placebo for 3 doses before surgery.[1] Morphine 5 mg was administered 10 to 20 minutes after surgery to conscious patients. The percentage decrease in pain was greater in the patients receiving nifedipine compared with the placebo. Nifedipine-treated patients had lower systolic blood pressures during surgery, but respiratory parameters were similar in both groups. Plasma morphine concentrations obtained at 0.5 and 1 hour after the dose were not different between the 2 patient groups. Nifedipine 10 mg has been noted to prolong and enhance the analgesia following epidural morphine.[2] The significance of this interaction and its potential to increase other effects of morphine require more study.

RELATED DRUGS: No information is available.

MANAGEMENT OPTIONS: No specific action is required, but be alert for evidence of the interaction.

REFERENCES:

1. Carta F, et al. Effect of nifedipine on morphine-induced analgesia. *Anesth Analg.* 1990;70:493.
2. Pereira IT, et al. Enhancement of the epidural morphine-induced analgesia by systemic nifedipine. *Pain.* 1993;53:341.

Morphine (eg, *Roxanol*)

Ranitidine (eg, *Zantac*)

SUMMARY: The combination of ranitidine and morphine appeared to result in confusion and disorientation in 1 patient, but the clinical importance of this interaction is not established.

RISK FACTORS: No specific risk factors are known.

MECHANISM: Not established.

CLINICAL EVALUATION: A 42-year-old man with terminal cancer of the larynx was receiving IV ranitidine 150 mg every 8 hours.[1] After a morphine infusion was begun (50 mg/day IV), administration of ranitidine was associated with confusion, agitation, and disorientation; on 3 occasions the symptoms improved when the ranitidine was stopped. The positive challenges and dechallenges suggest that an interaction occurred in this patient, but confirmation is needed.

RELATED DRUGS: Little is known regarding the effect of ranitidine on narcotic analgesics other than morphine. The relative ability of H_2-receptor antagonists to interact with narcotic analgesics is unknown, but available evidence indicates that cimetidine (eg, *Tagamet*) would be the most likely to interact. Cimetidine may impair the metabolism of some narcotic analgesics such as meperidine (eg, *Demerol*)[2-4] although it did not affect morphine metabolism in 1 study of healthy subjects.[5]

MANAGEMENT OPTIONS: No specific action is required, but be alert for evidence of the interaction.

REFERENCES:

1. Martinez-Abad M, et al. Ranitidine-induced confusion with concomitant morphine. *DICP.* 1988;22:914.
2. Guay DRP, et al. Cimetidine alters pethidine disposition in man. *Br J Clin Pharmacol.* 1984;18:907.
3. Fine A, et al. Potentially lethal interaction of cimetidine and morphine. *Can Med Assoc J.* 1981;124:1434.
4. Lam AM, et al. Cimetidine and prolonged post-operative somnolence. *Can Anaesth Soc J.* 1981;28:450.
5. Mojaverian P, et al. Cimetidine does not alter morphine disposition in man. *Br J Clin Pharmacol.* 1982;14:809.

Morphine (eg, *Roxanol*)

Rifampin (eg, *Rifadin*)

SUMMARY: Rifampin administration reduces the concentrations of morphine and 2 of its metabolites, as well as its analgesic efficacy.

RISK FACTORS: No specific risk factors are known.

MECHANISM: Unknown. Rifampin may increase the metabolism of morphine to unknown metabolites or increase the elimination of morphine into the bile or bowel lumen via P-glycoprotein induction.

CLINICAL EVALUATION: Ten healthy subjects received 10 mg of morphine orally alone and following 13 days of rifampin 600 mg/day.[1] Following rifampin treatment, the oral clearance of morphine was increased by over 50%. The areas under the concentration-time curves for the 2 major morphine metabolites, morphine-3-glucuronide and morphine-6-glucuronide, were reduced approximately 20% following rifampin dosing. These changes in morphine concentrations were accompanied by a significant reduction in the analgesic efficacy of morphine as measured by the cold pressor test. It is likely that the administration of rifampin with morphine would result in a reduction of analgesic efficacy.

RELATED DRUGS: Rifampin also reduces the plasma concentrations of methadone (eg, *Dolophine*). Rifabutin (*Mycobutin*) does not appear to affect methadone pharmacokinetics. Its effects on morphine are unknown.

MANAGEMENT OPTIONS:

➥ *Circumvent/Minimize.* Increased doses of morphine are likely to be required during coadministration of rifampin. Adjustments in morphine doses should be anticipated. Patients receiving morphine and rifampin should have their morphine doses adjusted based upon analgesic response when rifampin is added or removed from their drug regimen.

➥ *Monitor.* Until specific analgesics that are not affected by rifampin are identified, patients taking rifampin and narcotic analgesics should be monitored for adequate analgesic effect.

REFERENCES:

1. Fromm MF, et al. Loss of analgesic effect of morphine due to coadministration of rifampin. *Pain.* 1997;72:261.

Morphine (eg, *Roxanol*)

Somatostatin†

SUMMARY: Limited clinical evidence suggests that somatostatin inhibits the analgesic effect of morphine.

RISK FACTORS: No specific risk factors are known.

MECHANISM: Not established.

CLINICAL EVALUATION: Three patients with severe cancer pain developed a marked reduction in morphine analgesia when somatostatin was given.[1] In 1 case, discontinuation of the somatostatin was followed by a substantial increase in morphine analgesia. The other 2 patients refused discontinuation of the somatostatin, and morphine analgesia continued to be inadequate. All 3 patients failed to manifest typical morphine effects (eg, myosis, sedation) while taking somatostatin.

RELATED DRUGS: It is not known whether the somatostatin analog octreotide (eg, *Sandostatin*) also inhibits morphine analgesia, but be alert to the possibility. Somatostatin has also been reported to inhibit methadone analgesia (see Methadone/Somatostatin), but its effect on other opioids is not established

MANAGEMENT OPTIONS:

➥ *Monitor.* Monitor for evidence of reduced analgesia if somatostatin is used with morphine or other opioid analgesics. If morphine analgesia appears diminished, consider discontinuing somatostatin. If somatostatin cannot be discontinued, current evidence suggests that it may be difficult to achieve adequate analgesia.

REFERENCES:

1. Ripamonti C, et al. Can somatostatin be administered in association with morphine in advanced cancer patients with pain? *Ann Oncol.* 1998;9(8):921-923.

† Not available in the United States.

 Morphine (eg, *Roxanol*)

Tramadol (eg, *Ultram*)

SUMMARY: A patient taking morphine and tramadol developed serotonin toxicity, but a causal relationship was not established.

RISK FACTORS: No information is available.

MECHANISM: The proposed mechanism was additive serotonergic effects, but there is little evidence to suggest that morphine is serotonergic.

CLINICAL EVALUATION: A 49-year-old man admitted for a broken leg was given morphine 30 mg and tramadol 100 mg. He then developed a generalized tonic-clonic seizure, profuse diaphoresis, flushing, and tachycardia.[1] Although these symptoms support a diagnosis of serotonin toxicity using standard diagnostic methods,[2,3] it is not clear that the serotonin toxicity was caused by a drug interaction. Although other opiates such as meperidine and fentanyl have been associated with increased serotonin activity, it is not clear that morphine has a similar effect.

RELATED DRUGS: Combining tramadol with meperidine (eg, *Demerol*) or fentanyl (eg, *Fentora*) theoretically may increase the risk of serotonin toxicity.

MANAGEMENT OPTIONS: No specific action is required, but be alert for evidence of the interaction. Symptoms of serotonin toxicity include myoclonus, rigidity, tremor, hyperreflexia, seizures, confusion, agitation, hypomania, incoordination, fever, sweating, shivering, and coma.

REFERENCES:

1. Vizcaychipi MP, et al. Serotonin syndrome triggered by tramadol. *Br J Anaesth.* 2007;99(6):919.
2. Isbister GK, et al. Serotonin toxicity: a practical approach to diagnosis and treatment. *Med J Aust.* 2007;187(6):361-365.
3. Boyer EW, et al. The serotonin syndrome. *N Engl J Med.* 2005;352(11):1112-1120.

 Morphine (eg, *Roxanol*)

Trovafloxacin†

SUMMARY: Intravenous (IV) morphine reduces the serum concentration of orally administered trovafloxacin. Reduced antibiotic efficacy may result.

RISK FACTORS:

➡ ***Route of Administration.*** This interaction has only been reported to occur with IV morphine and oral trovafloxacin.

MECHANISM: Unknown.

CLINICAL EVALUATION: While no published data are available for evaluation, the manufacturer of trovafloxacin has made available some data on this interaction.[1] The IV administration of morphine 0.15 mg/kg with oral trovafloxacin 200 mg decreased the area under the concentration-time curve of trovafloxacin 36% and its peak concentration 46%. A reduction in the antibiotic efficacy may result.

RELATED DRUGS: No information is available regarding the interaction of other quinolones with morphine.

MANAGEMENT OPTIONS:

➡ *Monitor.* Monitor patients receiving trovafloxacin and IV morphine for possible reduced trovafloxacin efficacy.

REFERENCES:

1. *Trovan* [package insert]. New York, NY: Pfizer, Inc; 1998.

† Not available in the United States.

Moxalactam†

Warfarin (eg, *Coumadin*)

SUMMARY: Moxalactam may produce hypoprothrombinemia and thus may enhance the anticoagulant effect of warfarin and other oral anticoagulants.

RISK FACTORS:

➡ *Concurrent Diseases.* Renal dysfunction, hepatic dysfunction, and reduced dietary vitamin K can increase the risk of interaction.

MECHANISM: Cephalosporins with a methylthiotetrazole ring appear to inhibit the production of vitamin K–dependent clotting factors, perhaps by a direct effect on synthesis.

CLINICAL EVALUATION: Cephalosporins with a methylthiotetrazole ring (eg, cefmetazole, cefotetan [eg, *Cefotan*], moxalactam) and have been associated with prolonged prothrombin times and bleeding.[1-4] Evidence from patients undergoing cardiac valve replacement suggests that cefamandole and, to a lesser extent, cefazolin enhance the hypoprothrombinemic response to warfarin.[5] Other reports of cephalosporin-induced coagulopathy with cefoxitin (eg, *Mefoxin*), ceftriaxone (eg, *Rocephin*), and cefazolin have appeared, but the incidence of these reactions is unknown.[1,6]

RELATED DRUGS: Intravenous cefonicid† 2 mg/day for 7 days did not affect the hypoprothrombinemic response.[7]

MANAGEMENT OPTIONS:

➡ *Use Alternative.* If possible, avoid cefmetazole, cefotetan, and moxalactam in patients taking warfarin.

REFERENCES:

1. Brown RB, et al. Enhanced bleeding with cefoxitin or moxalactam. Statistical analysis within a defined population of 1493 patients. *Arch Intern Med.* 1986;146(11):2159-2164.
2. Freedy HR Jr, et al. Cefoperazone-induced coagulopathy. *Drug Intell Clin Pharm.* 1986;20(4):281-283.
3. Rymer W, et al. Hypoprothrombinemia associated with cefamandole. *Drug Intell Clin Pharm.* 1980;14:780-783.
4. Conjura A, et al. Cefotetan and hypoprothrombinemia. *Ann Intern Med.* 1988;108(4):643.

5. Angaran DM, et al. The comparative influence of prophylactic antibiotics on the prothrombin response to warfarin in the postoperative prosthetic cardiac valve patient. Cefamandole, cefazolin, vancomycin. *Ann Surg.* 1987;206(2):155-161.

6. Dupuis LL, et al. Cefazolin-induced coagulopathy. *Clin Pharmacol Ther.* 1984;35:237.

7. Anagaran DM, et al. Effect of cefonicid (CN) on prothrombin time (PT) in outpatients (OP) receiving warfarin (W) therapy. *Pharmacotherapy.* 1988;8:120.

† Not available in the United States.

5 Moxifloxacin (*Avelox*)

Ranitidine (*Zantac*)

SUMMARY: No interaction.

RISK FACTORS: No specific risk factors are known.

MECHANISM: No interaction.

CLINICAL EVALUATION: Ten healthy subjects received ranitidine 150 mg twice daily for 3 days and a single dose the morning of day 4 together with a single 400 mg dose of moxifloxacin.[1] The administration of ranitidine for 3 days prior to moxifloxacin administration had no effect on moxifloxacin pharmacokinetics compared with moxifloxacin administered without ranitidine.

RELATED DRUGS: Ranitidine and other H_2-receptor antagonists would not be expected to affect the kinetics of other quinolone antibiotics.

MANAGEMENT OPTIONS: No interaction.

REFERENCES:
1. Stass H, et al. Evaluation of the influence of antacids and H_2 antagonists on the absorption of moxifloxacin after oral administration of a 400 mg dose to health volunteers. *Clin Pharmacokinet.* 2001;40(suppl 1):39.

Moxifloxacin (*Avelox*)

Sucralfate (*Carafate*)

SUMMARY: Sucralfate reduces the plasma concentrations of moxifloxacin; a reduction in moxifloxacin efficacy is likely to occur in some patients.

RISK FACTORS: No specific risk factors are known.

MECHANISM: Sucralfate appears to bind moxifloxacin (via aluminum cations) and reduce its absorption or its GI circulation.

CLINICAL EVALUATION: Twelve healthy subjects were administered a single oral dose of moxifloxacin 400 mg alone and with sucralfate 190 mg that was administered just before and at 5, 10, 15, and 24 hours after moxifloxacin.[1] Compared with moxifloxacin administration alone, the coadministration of sucralfate reduced the area under the concentration-time curve of moxifloxacin 60%, its peak concentration 71% but had no effect on the half-life of moxifloxacin. The antibiotic efficacy of moxifloxacin would likely be inhibited by coadministration with sucralfate.

RELATED DRUGS: Other quinolone antibiotics such as ciprofloxacin (*Cipro*) and ofloxacin (*Floxin*) are affected in a similar manner by sucralfate.

MANAGEMENT OPTIONS:

➡ **Consider Alternative.** Because it may be difficult to separate the doses of sucralfate and moxifloxacin sufficiently to prevent the interaction, consider using H_2-receptor antagonists or proton pump inhibitors in patients requiring gastric acid suppression.

➡ **Circumvent/Minimize.** Pending further information, avoid the coadministration of sucralfate and moxifloxacin. Administer moxifloxacin several hours before sucralfate; however, some degree of reduction in moxifloxacin plasma concentration may still occur.

➡ **Monitor.** Watch for reduced antibiotic efficacy if moxifloxacin and antacids are coadministered.

REFERENCES:

1. Stass H, et al. Effects of sucralfate on the oral bioavailability of moxifloxacin, a novel 8-methoxyfluoroquinolone, in healthy volunteers. *Clin Pharmacokinet.* 2001;40(suppl 1):49.

Moxifloxacin (*Avelox*)

Ziprasidone (*Geodon*)

SUMMARY: Ziprasidone and moxifloxacin can prolong the corrected QT (QTc) interval on the electrocardiogram (ECG). Theoretically, this could increase the risk of ventricular arrhythmias such as torsades de pointes.

RISK FACTORS:

➡ **Hypokalemia.** The QTc on the ECG may be prolonged in patients with hypokalemia, increasing the risk of this interaction.[1]

➡ **Miscellaneous.** Other factors that may prolong the QTc interval (eg, hypomagnesemia, bradycardia, impaired liver function, hypothyroidism) also may increase the risk of ventricular arrhythmias.[1]

MECHANISM: Possible additive prolongation of the QTc interval.

CLINICAL EVALUATION: In initial controlled trials, ziprasidone increased the QTc interval approximately 10 msec at the highest recommended dose of 160 mg/day. But because of concern that the QTc measurements were done when ziprasidone serum concentrations were low, the FDA recommended additional study.[2,3] In a subsequent study in patients with psychotic disorders, the QTc interval was measured following administration of several antipsychotic drugs (eg, ziprasidone, thioridazine, quetiapine, risperidone, haloperidol, olanzapine) when the antipsychotic drug concentrations were calculated to be at their peak. Ziprasidone increased the QTc by a mean of approximately 21 msec, which was less than thioridazine (36 msec) but about twice that of the other antipsychotics. Theoretically, the ability of moxifloxacin to prolong the QTc would be additive with ziprasidone, but the extent to which this would increase the risk of ventricular arrhythmias, such as torsades de pointes, is not known.

RELATED DRUGS: Available data suggest that ziprasidone produces less QTc prolongation than thioridazine (*Mellaril*) but about twice that of quetiapine (*Seroquel*), risperidone (*Risperdal*), haloperidol (*Haldol*), and olanzapine (*Zyprexa*). Sparfloxacin (*Zagam*), like moxifloxacin, can prolong the QTc interval substantially, but other fluoroquinolones such as levofloxacin (*Levaquin*), ofloxacin (*Floxin*), gatifloxacin (*Tequin*), and ciprofloxacin (*Cipro*) usually produce only minimal effects.

MANAGEMENT OPTIONS:

➡ *Use Alternative.* Given the theoretical risk and the fact that moxifloxacin is listed in the ziprasidone product information as "contraindicated," it would be prudent to use an alternative to one of the drugs (see Related Drugs).

➡ *Monitor.* If moxifloxacin and ziprasidone are used concurrently, monitor for evidence of arrhythmias (eg, syncope) and for prolonged QT intervals.

REFERENCES:

1. De Ponti F, et al. QT-interval prolongation by non-cardiac drugs: lessons to be learned from recent experience. *Eur J Clin Pharmacol.* 2000;56:1.

2. *Geodon* [package insert]. New York, NY: Pfizer Pharmaceuticals; 2001.

3. Briefing Information, Psychopharmacological Drugs Advisory Committee, U.S. Food and Drug Administration, July 19, 2000.

Nabumetone

Warfarin (eg, *Coumadin*)

SUMMARY: Preliminary data suggest that nabumetone does not affect the hypoprothrombinemic response to warfarin, but cotherapy requires caution because of possible detrimental effects of nabumetone on the gastric mucosa and platelet function.

RISK FACTORS:

➡ **Concurrent Diseases.** Patients with peptic ulcer disease (PUD) or a history of GI bleeding are probably at greater risk.

MECHANISM: Although preliminary evidence suggests that nabumetone does not enhance the hypoprothrombinemic response to oral anticoagulants, ibuprofen-induced gastric erosions and inhibition of platelet function could theoretically increase the risk of bleeding in anticoagulated patients.

CLINICAL EVALUATION: In a preliminary report, nabumetone did not affect warfarin hypoprothrombinemic response in 58 patients on chronic warfarin therapy.[1] Nevertheless, any nonsteroidal anti-inflammatory drug (NSAID) should be used cautiously in anticoagulated patients because NSAID-induced gastric erosions and possible platelet inhibition may lead to bleeding. In a retrospective cohort study, hospitalizations for hemorrhagic PUD were about 13 times higher in patients receiving warfarin plus an NSAID than in patients receiving neither drug.[2]

RELATED DRUGS: All NSAIDs inhibit platelet function, cause gastric erosions, and probably increase the risk of GI bleeding.

MANAGEMENT OPTIONS:

➡ **Avoid Unless Benefit Outweighs Risk.** Because all NSAIDs probably increase the risk of GI bleeding in patients on oral anticoagulants, use the combination only after careful consideration of the benefit versus risk. If the NSAID is being used as an analgesic or antipyretic, acetaminophen is likely to be safer to use with oral anticoagulants. Nonacetylated salicylates (eg, choline salicylate, magnesium salicylate, salsalate, sodium salicylate) also are likely to be safer with oral anticoagulants than NSAIDs because they have minimal effects on platelet function and the gastric mucosa.

➡ **Monitor.** If any NSAID is used with an oral anticoagulant, carefully monitor the prothrombin time and watch for evidence of bleeding, especially from the GI tract.

REFERENCES:

1. Hilleman DE, et al. Hypoprothrombinemic effect of nabumetone in warfarin-treated patients [abstract]. *Pharmacotherapy.* 1993;13:270.
2. Shorr RI, et al. Concurrent use of nonsteroidal anti-inflammatory drugs and oral anticoagulants places elderly persons at high risk for hemorrhagic peptic ulcer disease. *Arch Intern Med.* 1993;153:1665-1670.

4 Nadolol (eg, *Corgard*)

Neomycin (eg, *Neo-Fradin*)

SUMMARY: Antibiotics that reduce bowel flora may increase peak nadolol concentrations and reduce its half-life, but the clinical importance of these findings is not established.

RISK FACTORS:

➡ **Route of Administration.** Antibiotics administered orally may increase nadolol concentrations.

MECHANISM: Not established. Reduction of GI flora may increase the bioavailability of nadolol while reducing its enterohepatic reabsorption.

CLINICAL EVALUATION: In 8 healthy subjects, administration of oral erythromycin 0.5 g 4 times daily and oral neomycin 0.5 g 4 times daily for 2 days more than doubled the mean peak plasma concentration of nadolol following a single oral dose of 80 mg.[1] However, nadolol half-life was reduced from 17.3 to 11.6 hours in the presence of the antibiotics. The clinical significance of this interaction is likely limited.

RELATED DRUGS: Other orally administered broad-spectrum antibiotics also may affect nadolol serum concentrations.

MANAGEMENT OPTIONS: No specific action is required, but be alert for evidence of the interaction.

REFERENCES:
1. du Souich P, et al. Enhancement of nadolol elimination by activated charcoal and antibiotics. *Clin Pharmacol Ther.* 1983;33:585-590.

4 Nadolol (eg, *Corgard*)

Phenelzine (*Nardil*)

SUMMARY: There is little evidence to substantiate an interaction between monoamine oxidase inhibitors (MAOIs) such as phenelzine and beta-blockers such as nadolol.

RISK FACTORS: No specific risk factors are known.

MECHANISM: Not established.

CLINICAL EVALUATION: Some studies indicate that propranolol is contraindicated in patients receiving an MAOI and in those who may still be affected by previous MAOI administration (eg, within 2 weeks).[1] Two patients taking the beta-blockers nadolol or metoprolol (eg, *Lopressor*) developed bradycardia when phenelzine was added to their therapy.[2] The beta-blocker sotalol (eg, *Betapace*) appears to inhibit tranylcypromine-induced insulin secretion, but the effect of propranolol (eg, *Inderal*) on tranylcypromine (eg, *Parnate*) was not studied.[3] Determining the actual clinical manifestations of concomitant MAOI and propranolol administration awaits additional study.

RELATED DRUGS: Other beta-blockers are expected to interact in a similar manner.

MANAGEMENT OPTIONS:

➡ *Monitor.* No specific action is required, but be alert for evidence of the interaction.

REFERENCES:

1. Frieden J. Propranolol as an antiarrhythmic agent. *Am Heart J.* 1967;74:283-285.
2. Reggev A, et al. Bradycardia induced by an interaction between phenelzine and beta blockers. *Psychosomatics.* 1989;30:106-108.
3. Bressler R, et al. Tranylcypromine: a potent insulin secretagogue and hypoglycemic agent. *Diabetes.* 1968;17:617-624.

Nafcillin (eg, *Unipen*)

Nifedipine (*Procardia*)

SUMMARY: Nafcillin administration results in a large reduction in the plasma concentration of nifedipine; loss of efficacy is likely to result.

RISK FACTORS:

➡ *Route of Administration.* The administration of nafcillin or the calcium channel blocker, nifedipine, orally would increase the magnitude of this interaction.

MECHANISM: Nafcillin appears to be an inducer of CYP3A4, the enzyme responsible for the metabolism of nifedipine. This would increase the first-pass metabolism as well as the systemic metabolism of nifedipine following oral administration.

CLINICAL EVALUATION: Nine healthy subjects received a single oral dose of 10 mg nifedipine before and after 5 days of nafcillin 500 mg 4 times daily orally for 5 days.[1] The area under the concentration-time curve of nifedipine was reduced by 72% and its oral clearance increased 115% following pretreatment with nafcillin. This degree of reduction in nifedipine's plasma concentration is likely to result in a reduction in its efficacy.

RELATED DRUGS: Nafcillin would be expected to reduce the plasma concentrations of other calcium channel blockers including felodipine (*Plendil*), nicardipine (eg, *Cardene*), verapamil (eg, *Calan*), and diltiazem (eg, *Cardizem*). There is no evidence that other penicillins affect nifedipine.

MANAGEMENT OPTIONS:

➡ *Avoid Unless Benefit Outweighs Risk.* The combination of nafcillin and nifedipine, or other calcium channel blockers, should be avoided. Selection of an alternative antibiotic should be considered.

➡ *Monitor.* Patients stabilized on nifedipine or other calcium channel blockers should be monitored for loss of efficacy during the administration of nafcillin.

REFERENCES:

1. Jamal SK, et al. Nafcillin is a potent inducer of cytochrome P4503A activity in humans. *Clin Pharmacol Ther.* 1998;63:151. Abstract.

Nafcillin (eg, *Unipen*)

Warfarin (eg, *Coumadin*)

SUMMARY: Several case reports suggest that nafcillin may inhibit the hypoprothrombinemic response to warfarin.

RISK FACTORS: No specific risk factors are known.

MECHANISM: It has been proposed that nafcillin and perhaps other penicillinase-resistant penicillins may enhance the hepatic metabolism of warfarin, but this mechanism has not been studied rigorously.

CLINICAL EVALUATION: Several patients had increased requirements for warfarin following the addition of nafcillin to their therapy.[1-4] The warfarin resistance dissipated slowly after discontinuation of the nafcillin. In a subsequent study in 1 patient, warfarin half-life was 5.3 hours during nafcillin treatment and 14.5 hours 2 weeks after nafcillin was discontinued.[3]

RELATED DRUGS: Dicloxacillin (eg, *Dynapen*) also may inhibit the hypoprothrombinemic response to warfarin, but data are limited.

MANAGEMENT OPTIONS:

➡ ***Monitor.*** In patients receiving warfarin or other oral anticoagulants, monitor for a decreased hypoprothrombinemic response whenever nafcillin or other penicillinase-resistant penicillins are given. Available evidence suggests that the onset of the interaction is delayed for several days after starting the penicillin, and the effect may persist for weeks after the penicillin is discontinued.

REFERENCES:

1. Qureshi GD, et al. Warfarin resistance with nafcillin therapy. *Ann Intern Med.* 1984;100:527.
2. Fraser GL, et al. Warfarin resistance associated with nafcillin therapy. *Am J Med.* 1989;87:237.
3. Davis RL, et al. Warfarin-nafcillin interaction. *J Pediatr.* 1991;118:300.
4. Shovick VA, et al. Decreased hypoprothrombinemic response to warfarin secondary to the warfarin-nafcillin interaction. *DICP.* 1991;25:598.

4 Nalidixic Acid (*NegGram*)

Probenecid (*Benemid*)

SUMMARY: Probenecid may increase the serum concentration of nalidixic acid.

RISK FACTORS: No specific risk factors are known.

MECHANISM: Probenecid reduces the renal excretion of nalidixic acid and its metabolite.

CLINICAL EVALUATION: Extremely high serum nalidixic acid concentrations were noted in a patient who had apparently taken an overdose of a number of drugs, including nalidixic acid and probenecid.[1] In studies of 3 normal subjects, probenecid increased the serum concentration of nalidixic acid and of its active metabolite.[1,2]

RELATED DRUGS: No information is available.

MANAGEMENT OPTIONS: No specific action is required, but be alert for evidence of the interaction.

REFERENCES:

1. Rowe JW, et al. Severe metabolic acidosis associated with nalidixic acid overdose. *Ann Intern Med.* 1976;84:570.

2. Vree TB, et al. Probenecid inhibits the renal clearance and renal glucuronidation of nalidixic acid. *Pharm World Sci.* 1993;15:165.

Nalidixic Acid (*NegGram*)

Warfarin (eg, *Coumadin*)

SUMMARY: Isolated case reports indicate that nalidixic acid enhances the hypoprothrombinemic response to warfarin and acenocoumarol,[†] but the incidence of this interaction in patients receiving the combination is unknown.

RISK FACTORS:

➥ *Concurrent Diseases.* Patients with fever or low albumin concentrations are at risk.

MECHANISM: Nalidixic acid has been shown to displace warfarin from human albumin binding sites in vitro,[1] but the sustained nature of the interaction raises the possibility that nalidixic acid inhibits the hepatic metabolism of oral anticoagulants as well. Fever also may enhance the elimination of clotting factors.[2] Thus, the infection for which the nalidixic acid is used theoretically could enhance oral anticoagulant hypoprothrombinemia, an effect that should dissipate as nalidixic acid lowers the fever.

CLINICAL EVALUATION: Several patients stabilized on warfarin developed excessive hypoprothrombinemia, purpura, and bruising a few days after nalidixic acid was started.[3-5]

RELATED DRUGS: Acenocoumarol[†] interacts similarly with nalidixic acid. Little is known regarding the effect of nalidixic acid on other anticoagulants, but assume that an interaction may occur with all oral anticoagulants until evidence to the contrary is available.

MANAGEMENT OPTIONS:

➥ *Monitor.* Monitor patients for an altered hypoprothrombinemic response when nalidixic acid therapy is started or stopped in patients receiving oral anticoagulants.

REFERENCES:

1. Sellers EM, et al. Displacement of warfarin from human albumin by diazoxide and ethacrynic, mefenamic and nalidixic acids. *Clin Pharmacol Ther.* 1970;11:524.
2. Loeliger EA, et al. The biological disappearance rate of prothrombin and factors VII, IX and X from plasma in hypothyroidism, hyperthyroidism and during fever. *Thromb Diath Haemorrh.* 1964;10:267.
3. Hoffbrand BI. Interaction of nalidixic acid and warfarin. *BMJ.* 1974;2:666. Letter.
4. Potasman I, et al. Nicoumalone and nalidixic acid interaction. *Ann Intern Med.* 1980;92:572.
5. Leor J, et al. Interaction between nalidixic acid and warfarin. *Ann Intern Med.* 1987;107:601.

† Not available in the United States.

Naproxen (eg, *Naprosyn*)

Probenecid

SUMMARY: Probenecid may increase plasma naproxen concentrations, but the clinical importance of this effect is not established.

RISK FACTORS: No specific risk factors are known.

MECHANISM: Probenecid may inhibit the renal excretion and hepatic metabolism of naproxen.

CLINICAL EVALUATION: In a study of 6 healthy subjects given naproxen 500 mg orally with and without probenecid pretreatment, probenecid increased plasma naproxen levels 50%.[1] The degree to which this interaction would increase naproxen toxicity or efficacy has not been established.

RELATED DRUGS: Probenecid also inhibits the elimination of some other nonsteroidal anti-inflammatory drugs (eg, indomethacin [eg, *Indocin*], ketoprofen).

MANAGEMENT OPTIONS: No specific action is required, but be alert for evidence of the interaction.

REFERENCES:

1. Runkel R, et al. Naproxen-probenecid interaction. *Clin Pharmacol Ther.* 1978;24(6):706-713.

 Naproxen (eg, *Naprosyn*)

Warfarin (eg, *Coumadin*)

SUMMARY: Naproxen does not appear to affect the hypoprothrombinemic response to warfarin in most patients; however, use naproxen cautiously because of its possible detrimental effects on gastric mucosa and platelet function.

RISK FACTORS:

➡ **Concurrent Diseases.** Patients with peptic ulcer disease or a history of GI bleeding are likely at greater risk.

MECHANISM: Because the anticoagulant response to warfarin generally is not affected by naproxen, a clinically significant pharmacokinetic mechanism is unlikely. Naproxen-induced gastric erosions and inhibition of platelet function theoretically could increase the risk of bleeding in patients receiving oral anticoagulants.

CLINICAL EVALUATION: When 10 healthy subjects taking oral warfarin for 25 days were given naproxen 375 mg twice daily from day 11 to day 20, they did not manifest changes in the disposition of warfarin or its hypoprothrombinemic effect.[1] In another study, naproxen 375 mg twice daily for 17 days did not affect the pharmacokinetics or anticoagulant effect of a single dose of warfarin 50 mg.[2] Thus, the available evidence indicates that naproxen has minimal effects on oral anticoagulants in healthy subjects. Nonetheless, an occasional anticoagulated patient might manifest an enhanced anticoagulant response when naproxen is coadministered. In addition, naproxen-induced GI bleeding and impaired platelet function may cause problems in such patients. In a retrospective cohort study, hospitalizations for hemorrhagic peptic ulcer disease were approximately 13 times higher in patients receiving warfarin plus a nonsteroidal anti-inflammatory drug (NSAID) than in patients receiving neither drug.[3]

RELATED DRUGS: All NSAIDs inhibit platelet function, cause gastric erosions, and probably increase the risk of GI bleeding.

MANAGEMENT OPTIONS:

➡ **Avoid Unless Benefit Outweighs Risk.** Because all NSAIDs probably increase the risk of GI bleeding in patients taking oral anticoagulants, use the combination only after careful consideration of the benefits and risks. If the NSAID is being used as an analgesic or antipyretic, acetaminophen may be safer to use with oral anticoagulants. Nonacetylated salicylates (eg, choline salicylate, magnesium salicylate, salsalate, sodium salicylate) also are likely to be safer with oral anticoagulants than NSAIDs because they have minimal effects on platelet function and the gastric mucosa.

➥ **Monitor.** If any NSAID is used with an oral anticoagulant, carefully monitor the prothrombin time and watch for evidence of bleeding, especially from the GI tract.

REFERENCES:

1. Jain A, et al. Effect of naproxen on the steady-state serum concentration and anticoagulant activity of warfarin. *Clin Pharmacol Ther*. 1979;25(1):61-66.
2. Slattery JT, et al. Effect of naproxen on the kinetics of elimination and anticoagulant activity of a single dose or warfarin. *Clin Pharmacol Ther*. 1979;25(1):51-60.
3. Shorr RI, et al. Concurrent use of nonsteroidal anti-inflammatory drugs and oral anticoagulants places elderly persons at high risk for hemorrhagic peptic ulcer disease. *Arch Intern Med*. 1993;153(14):1665-1670.

Naproxen (eg, *Naprosyn*) | 5

Zidovudine (eg, *Retrovir*)

SUMMARY: Naproxen does not appear to alter zidovudine serum concentrations.

RISK FACTORS: No specific risk factors are known.

MECHANISM: No interaction.

CLINICAL EVALUATION: Although naproxen inhibits the glucuronidation of zidovudine in vitro,[1] naproxen 250 to 500 mg every 12 hours had no effect on zidovudine pharmacokinetics in patients with HIV.[2,3] No change was noted in zidovudine peak serum concentrations, half-life, or area under the concentration-time curve following coadministration of naproxen.

RELATED DRUGS: The effect of other naproxen dosage regimens is unknown, but a clinically significant interaction seems unlikely. In addition, indomethacin (eg, *Indocin*) had no effect on zidovudine pharmacokinetics.[3]

MANAGEMENT OPTIONS: No interaction.

REFERENCES:

1. Sim SM, et al. The effect of various drugs on the glucuronidation of zidovudine (azidothymidine; AZT) by human liver microsomes. *Br J Clin Pharmacol*. 1991;32(1):17 21.
2. Sahai J, et al. Evaluation of the in vitro effect of naproxen on zidovudine pharmacokinetics in patients infected with human immunodeficiency virus. *Clin Pharmacol Ther*. 1992;52(5):464-470.
3. Barry M, et al. The effects of indomethacin and naproxen on zidovudine pharmacokinetics. *Br J Clin Pharmacol*. 1993;36(1):82-85.

Nateglinide (eg, *Starlix*) | 4

Rifampin (eg, *Rifadin*)

SUMMARY: Rifampin administration produces a modest reduction in nateglinide plasma concentrations; some patients may have a reduced hypoglycemic response to nateglinide.

RISK FACTORS: No specific risk factors are known.

MECHANISM: Rifampin-induced induction of CYP2C9 and/or CYP3A4 would lead to a reduction in nateglinide plasma concentration.

CLINICAL EVALUATION: Ten subjects were administered placebo or rifampin 600 mg once daily for 10 days.[1] On day 6, a single oral dose of nateglinide 60 mg was given. Treatment with rifampin reduced the area under the concentration-time curve of nateglinide 24% (range, 5% to 53%) and shortened its half-life from 1.6 to 1.3 hours. The pretreatment with rifampin did not affect the glucose-reducing effect of nateglinide in these healthy subjects. While the magnitude of this interaction appears to be modest, patients with diabetes may be at greater risk of developing hyperglycemia during rifampin coadministration.

RELATED DRUGS: Rifampin has been demonstrated to reduce the plasma concentration of other oral hypoglycemic drugs, including glyburide (*DiaBeta*) and repaglinide (*Prandin*). Rifabutin (*Mycobutin*) and rifapentine (*Priftin*) are known to induce CYP3A4 and may affect nateglinide in a similar manner.

MANAGEMENT OPTIONS:

➥ *Monitor.* Monitor patients taking nateglinide for altered glucose response if rifampin is initiated or discontinued from their dosage regimen.

REFERENCES:
1. Niemi M, et al. Effect of rifampicin on the pharmacokinetics and pharmacodynamics of nateglinide in healthy subjects. *Br J Clin Pharmacol.* 2003;56(4):427-432.

Nebivolol (*Bystolic*)

Quinidine

SUMMARY: Quinidine is expected to increase the plasma concentration of nebivolol; excess beta-blockade may occur.

RISK FACTORS:

➥ *Pharmacogenetics.* Rapid metabolizers of nebivolol via CYP2D6 will be at an increased risk of developing the interaction.

MECHANISM: Quinidine is a potent inhibitor of CYP2D6, one of the pathways of metabolism for nebivolol. In addition, quinidine and nebivolol may reduce cardiac conduction, increasing the potential for cardiac arrhythmias to occur.

CLINICAL EVALUATION: While specific data are not provided, the manufacturer of nebivolol recommends using caution if quinidine is coadministered.[1] Pending further data, observe patients receiving nebivolol and quinidine for increased beta-blockade, including bradycardia and hypotension.

RELATED DRUGS: Other beta-blockers that are metabolized by CYP2D6, including propranolol (eg, *Inderal*), timolol, metoprolol (eg, *Lopressor*), and carvedilol (eg, *Coreg*), may be affected in a similar manner by quinidine.

MANAGEMENT OPTIONS:

➥ *Consider Alternative.* Consider beta-blockers that are not metabolized by CYP2D6, such as atenolol (eg, *Tenormin*) or acebutolol (eg, *Sectral*), in patients requiring quinidine administration.

➥ *Monitor.* Monitor patients receiving both nebivolol and quinidine for evidence of excess beta-blockade.

REFERENCES:
1. *Bystolic* [package insert]. St. Louis, MO: Forest Pharmaceuticals; 2007.

Nebivolol (*Bystolic*)

Verapamil (eg, *Calan*)

SUMMARY: Verapamil and nebivolol both reduce myocardial conduction; cardiac arrhythmias may occur.

RISK FACTORS: No specific risk factors are known.

MECHANISM: Both verapamil and nebivolol slow cardiac conduction.

CLINICAL EVALUATION: While specific data are not provided, the manufacturer of nebivolol recommends using caution if verapamil is coadministered.[1] Pending further data, observe patients receiving nebivolol and verapamil for slowed cardiac conduction and reduced myocardial inotropic activity. The combination may intentionally be used in some patients to control heart rate or blood pressure.[1]

RELATED DRUGS: Other beta-blockers interact in a similar manner with verapamil. Diltiazem (eg, *Cardizem*) is also expected to slow cardiac conduction when administered with nebivolol.

MANAGEMENT OPTIONS:

➡ ***Monitor.*** Monitor patients receiving both nebivolol and verapamil for evidence of cardiac conduction disturbances and reduced cardiac output.

REFERENCES:

1. *Bystolic* [package insert]. St. Louis, MO: Forest Pharmaceuticals; 2007.

Nefazodone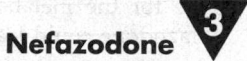

Paroxetine (eg, *Paxil*)

SUMMARY: A patient developed evidence of serotonin syndrome when paroxetine therapy was started soon after discontinuation of nefazodone.

RISK FACTORS: No specific risk factors are known.

MECHANISM: Probably additive. Both nefazodone and paroxetine inhibit the reuptake of serotonin.

CLINICAL EVALUATION: In a 51-year-old woman on chronic nefazodone therapy, the drug was tapered and stopped.[1] One day later, she was started on paroxetine 20 mg/day and quickly developed diaphoresis, muscle rigidity, and hyponatremia, and became unresponsive. This case qualifies as serotonin syndrome according to Sternbach's criteria.[2] She was brought to the emergency room and responded well to supportive treatment. Seven days later, a challenge with paroxetine did not result in a recurrence of the symptoms of serotonin syndrome. This reaction appears to have resulted from the combined effects of nefazodone and paroxetine, but it is unknown how often patients on this combination would develop such symptoms.

RELATED DRUGS: Theoretically, combined therapy of nefazodone with other selective serotonin reuptake inhibitors (SSRIs), such as fluoxetine (eg, *Prozac*), sertraline (eg, *Zoloft*), fluvoxamine, and citalopram (eg, *Celexa*) may also result in serotonin syndrome, but reports of such interactions are lacking.

MANAGEMENT OPTIONS:

➡ *Circumvent/Minimize.* When switching from nefazodone to an SSRI or visa versa, begin the new agent with conservative doses, if possible, to avoid excessive serotonergic effects.

➡ *Monitor.* In patients receiving nefazodone and paroxetine (or other SSRIs), be alert for evidence of serotonin syndrome. Serotonin syndrome can result in neurotoxicity (eg, myoclonus, tremors, rigidity, incoordination, hyperreflexia, seizures, coma), psychiatric symptoms (eg, agitation, confusion, hypomania, restlessness), and autonomic dysfunction (eg, fever, sweating, tachycardia, hypertension).

REFERENCES:

1. John L, et al. Serotonin syndrome associated with nefazodone and paroxetine. *Ann Emerg Med.* 1997;29(2):287-289.

2. Sternbach H. The serotonin syndrome. *Am J Psychiatry.* 1991;148(6):705-713.

 Nefazodone

Pimozide (*Orap*)

SUMMARY: Elevated pimozide concentrations and cardiac arrhythmias may occur if pimozide and nefazodone are coadministered.

RISK FACTORS: No specific risk factors are known.

MECHANISM: Nefazodone is known to be an inhibitor of CYP3A4, the enzyme responsible for the metabolism of pimozide. The coadministration of pimozide and nefazodone could lead to ventricular arrhythmias, including torsades de pointes.

CLINICAL EVALUATION: While specific data are lacking, the manufacturer of pimozide contraindicates the coadministration of pimozide and nefazodone.[1] Patients with bradycardia, hypokalemia, or hypomagnesemia may be at increased risk to develop torsades de pointes.

RELATED DRUGS: In vitro studies indicate that paroxetine (eg, *Paxil*), fluoxetine (eg, *Prozac*), and fluvoxamine do not inhibit the metabolism of pimozide.[2] However, fluvoxamine is known to produce some inhibition of CYP3A4 and CYP1A2, a lesser pathway of pimozide metabolism. Pending in vivo studies, avoid coadministration of pimozide and fluvoxamine.

MANAGEMENT OPTIONS:

➡ *Use Alternative.* Do not administer nefazodone to patients receiving pimozide. Consider other selective serotonin reuptake inhibitor antidepressants that do not affect CYP3A4, but avoid fluvoxamine.

➡ *Monitor.* If nefazodone is coadministered with pimozide, monitor the electrocardiogram for evidence of QTc prolongation.

REFERENCES:

1. *Orap* [package insert]. North Wales, PA: Gate Pharmaceuticals; 1999.

2. Desta Z, et al. In vitro inhibition of pimozide N-dealkylation by selective serotonin reuptake inhibitors and azithromycin. *J Clin Psychopharmacol.* 2002;22(2):162-168.

Nefazodone

Simvastatin (eg, *Zocor*)

SUMMARY: A patient taking simvastatin developed muscle damage (myositis and rhabdomyolysis) after starting nefazodone therapy.

RISK FACTORS:

➡ ***Dosage Regimen.*** The ability of simvastatin to produce damage to skeletal muscle appears to be dose related. Thus, the risk of combined therapy with nefazodone is probably higher in patients taking larger doses of simvastatin.

MECHANISM: Nefazodone probably inhibits the metabolism of simvastatin by CYP3A4. The resultant increase in simvastatin serum concentrations damages skeletal muscle.

CLINICAL EVALUATION: A 44-year-old man taking simvastatin 40 mg/day for several months was started on nefazodone 100 mg twice daily.[1] One month later, he returned to his physician with "tea-colored" urine; he was treated for a urinary tract infection. A month later, his urine was still dark, and he also had developed severe leg pain and weakness. The rhabdomyolysis and myositis resolved with discontinuation of simvastatin and nefazodone along with hydration. Although this interaction is not well established, it is consistent with the known properties of simvastatin and nefazodone.

RELATED DRUGS: Lovastatin (eg, *Mevacor*) is also known to result in muscle damage when given with CYP3A4 inhibitors; pravastatin (eg, *Pravachol*), fluvastatin (*Lescol*), and atorvastatin (*Lipitor*) may be less likely to do so. Fluoxetine (eg, *Prozac*) may inhibit CYP3A4 to a lesser extent than nefazodone.

MANAGEMENT OPTIONS:

➡ ***Use Alternative.*** The use of an HMG-CoA reductase inhibitor other than simvastatin or lovastatin is likely to reduce the risk. Nefazodone is a potent CYP3A4 inhibitor, so using an alternative antidepressant may reduce the interaction. Fluoxetine also may inhibit CYP3A4, but to a lesser extent than nefazodone. If the combination is used, be alert for evidence of muscle damage (eg, muscle pain, weakness, darkened urine, elevated muscle enzymes such as creatine kinase). Use conservative doses of simvastatin or lovastatin when used with a CYP3A4 inhibitor such as nefazodone.

REFERENCES:

1. Jacobson RH, et al. Myositis and rhabdomyolysis associated with concurrent use of simvastatin and nefazodone. *JAMA.* 1997;277(4):296-297.

Nefazodone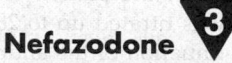

Tacrolimus (*Prograf*)

SUMMARY: A patient taking tacrolimus developed evidence of nephrotoxicity and neurotoxicity 1 week after nefazodone was started.

RISK FACTORS: No specific risk factors are known.

MECHANISM: Nefazodone probably inhibits the metabolism of tacrolimus.

CLINICAL EVALUATION: A 57-year-old woman received a renal transplant and was stabilized on tacrolimus, prednisone (eg, *Sterapred*), and azathioprine (eg, *Imuran*).[1] Two years after the transplant, she was switched from sertraline to nefazodone 50 mg twice daily for depression. Within 1 week, she developed headache, confusion, and "gray areas" in her vision. Her serum creatinine concentration increased from 1.5 to 2.2 mg/dL, and her trough tacrolimus concentration increased more than 3-fold (to greater than 30 ng/mL). Given the temporal relationship of the reaction and the known inhibitory effect of nefazodone on CYP3A4, it appears likely that the reaction was caused by the addition of nefazodone.

RELATED DRUGS: Nefazodone probably also inhibits the metabolism of cyclosporine (eg, *Neoral*) because the latter drug is also metabolized by CYP3A4. Most selective serotonin reuptake inhibitors (eg, citalopram [eg, *Celexa*], paroxetine [eg, *Paxil*], sertraline [eg, *Zoloft*]) have little or no effect on CYP3A4. Fluoxetine (eg, *Prozac*) is a weak inhibitor of CYP3A4 and is expected to have only a small effect on tacrolimus, but fluvoxamine appears to be a moderate inhibitor of CYP3A4 and might interact with tacrolimus to some degree.

MANAGEMENT OPTIONS:

➡ *Consider Alternative.* In patients receiving tacrolimus (or cyclosporine), it is preferable to use an antidepressant that has little or no effect on CYP3A4 (see Related Drugs).

➡ *Monitor.* Be alert for altered tacrolimus effect if nefazodone is initiated, discontinued, or changed in dosage. Possible evidence of tacrolimus toxicity includes decreased renal function, headache, confusion, and visual disturbances.

REFERENCES:

1. Olyaei AJ, et al. Interaction between tacrolimus and nefazodone in a stable renal transplant recipient. *Pharmacotherapy.* 1998;18(6):1356-1359.

 Nelfinavir (*Viracept*)

Methadone (eg, *Dolophine*)

SUMMARY: Nelfinavir appears to reduce methadone concentrations; methadone withdrawal or loss of analgesic effect may occur.

RISK FACTORS: No specific risk factors are known.

MECHANISM: Nelfinavir may increase the elimination of methadone.

CLINICAL EVALUATION: A patient stabilized on methadone 100 mg daily was also receiving indinavir (*Crixivan*) 800 mg 3 times daily and zalcitabine 0.75 mg 3 times daily.[1] Within 6 weeks of the addition of stavudine (*Zerit*) and nelfinavir 750 mg 3 times daily, the patient complained of opiate withdrawal symptoms. The methadone was titrated up to 285 mg daily. The methadone dose was reduced upon discontinuation of the antiretroviral therapy.

RELATED DRUGS: Ritonavir (*Norvir*) has also been reported to reduce methadone plasma concentrations.

MANAGEMENT OPTIONS:

➡ *Consider Alternative.* An analgesic that is eliminated differently than methadone (eg, codeine, morphine) may be a suitable alternative. However, the effect of nelfinavir on other analgesics is unknown.

➡ **Monitor.** Be alert for reduced methadone effect during nelfinavir coadministration. Methadone dosage may have to be increased.

REFERENCES:

1. McCance-Katz EF, et al. Decrease in methadone levels with nelfinavir mesylate. *Am J Psychiatry.* 2000;157(3):481.

Nelfinavir (*Viracept*)

Nevirapine (*Viramune*)

SUMMARY: Nevirapine administration reduces the concentration of nelfinavir; reduction in antiviral activity may result.

RISK FACTORS: No specific risk factors are known.

MECHANISM: Nevirapine is known to be an inducer of CYP3A4, the primary metabolic pathway for nelfinavir.

CLINICAL EVALUATION: Seven patients with HIV were administered nelfinavir 750 mg 3 times daily for 2 weeks.[1] Following 3 days of nelfinavir, nevirapine 200 mg daily for 2 weeks then 200 mg twice daily for 1 week was added to their therapy. Blood samples were obtained on day 3 of nelfinavir and at the end of the week of therapy with nevirapine 200 mg twice daily. The area under the concentration-time curve of nelfinavir was reduced 50%, while its peak concentration was reduced 57% following 2 weeks of nevirapine treatment. The reduction in nelfinavir concentrations observed in this study could produce subtherapeutic concentrations of nelfinavir in some patients. Nelfinavir dosage may need to be increased when nevirapine is coadministered.

RELATED DRUGS: Nevirapine may produce similar effects on other protease inhibitors (eg, indinavir [*Crixivan*], ritonavir [*Norvir*], saquinavir [eg, *Invirase*]). Delavirdine (*Rescriptor*) is an inhibitor of CYP3A4 and, if it has any effect on nelfinavir, it is expected to increase nelfinavir concentrations.

MANAGEMENT OPTIONS:

➡ **Monitor.** When nevirapine is started or discontinued in a patient taking nelfinavir, monitor serum concentrations of nelfinavir to ensure they are maintained in the therapeutic range.

REFERENCES:

1. Merry C, et al. The pharmacokinetics of combination therapy with nelfinavir plus nevirapine. *AIDS.* 1998;12(10):1163-1167.

Nelfinavir (*Viracept*)

Omeprazole (eg, *Prilosec*)

SUMMARY: The coadministration of omeprazole and nelfinavir may reduce the antiviral effectiveness of nelfinavir.

RISK FACTORS: No specific risk factors are known.

MECHANISM: Unknown. Omeprazole may reduce the absorption of nelfinavir by increasing gastric pH and reducing the solubility of nelfinavir. Omeprazole inhibits CYP2C19, which is the enzyme that converts nelfinavir to its active metabolite.

CLINICAL EVALUATION: Nineteen healthy subjects received nelfinavir 1,250 mg every 12 hours for 4 days alone and with omeprazole 40 mg daily.[1] The mean area under the plasma concentration-time curve (AUC) of nelfinavir was reduced about 30% during omeprazole coadministration. In 3 of the subjects, nelfinavir AUC increased with omeprazole. The mean AUC of nelfinavir's active metabolite was reduced 70% with omeprazole. All subjects had a reduction in the concentration of the metabolite and it was undetectable in 4 subjects during omeprazole administration.

RELATED DRUGS: Esomeprazole (*Nexium*) is expected to affect nelfinavir in a similar manner. If increased gastric pH is partially responsible for the changes in nelfinavir pharmacokinetics, other proton pump inhibitors (PPIs) will likely have an effect on nelfinavir plasma concentrations. The plasma concentrations of protease inhibitors such as atazanavir (*Reyataz*) and indinavir (*Crixivan*) are reduced by omeprazole.

MANAGEMENT OPTIONS:

➡ *Consider Alternative.* PPIs that do not inhibit CYP2C19 (eg, lansoprazole [eg, *Prilosec*], pantoprazole [eg, *Protonix*], rabeprazole [*Aciphex*]) may have less effect on nelfinavir and its active metabolite.

➡ *Monitor.* Carefully monitor patients taking nelfinavir who require acid suppression therapy for adequate antiviral effect.

REFERENCES:

1. Fang AF, et al. Significant decrease in nelfinavir systemic exposure after omeprazole coadministration in healthy subjects. *Pharmacotherapy.* 2008;28(1):42-50.

 Nelfinavir (*Viracept*)

Rifampin (eg, *Rifadin*)

SUMMARY: Rifampin increases nelfinavir clearance; loss of efficacy is likely to result.

RISK FACTORS: No specific risk factors are known.

MECHANISM: Rifampin is known to induce CYP3A4, the enzyme responsible for a majority of the nelfinavir metabolism.

CLINICAL EVALUATION: Nelfinavir 750 mg every 8 hours was administered orally for 5 days alone and in combination with rifampin 600 mg/day for 7 days to 12 healthy subjects.[1] The oral clearance of nelfinavir increased from 37.4 L/hr when administered alone to 212 L/hr during rifampin coadministration. This increase in oral clearance would likely result in a loss of nelfinavir efficacy.

RELATED DRUGS: Rifampin increases the clearance of ritonavir (*Norvir*), indinavir (*Crixivan*), and saquinavir (eg, *Fortovase*). Rifabutin (*Mycobutin*) would be expected to have a similar affect on nelfinavir clearance.

MANAGEMENT OPTIONS:

➡ *Use Alternative.* Based on the magnitude of this interaction, it would be difficult to administer an effective dose of nelfinavir. Because other protease inhibitors are also likely to be affected, consider an alternative to rifampin.

REFERENCES:

1. Yuen GJ, et al. The pharmacokinetics of nelfinavir administration alone and with rifampin in healthy volunteers [abstract]. *Clin Pharmacol Ther.* 1997;61:147.

Nelfinavir (*Viracept*)

Saquinavir (eg, *Fortovase*)

SUMMARY: Nelfinavir appears to cause a large increase in saquinavir plasma concentrations; increased saquinavir toxicity may occur.

RISK FACTORS: No specific risk factors are known.

MECHANISM: Nelfinavir appears to reduce the metabolism of saquinavir, probably via inhibition of the CYP3A4 isozyme.

CLINICAL EVALUATION: While no published data are available for evaluation, the manufacturer of nelfinavir has made available some data on this interaction.[1] The administration of nelfinavir 750 mg 3 times/day for 4 days to 14 subjects resulted in a mean increase in the area under the plasma saquinavir concentration-time curve of 392% following a single, 1,200 mg saquinavir dose. Based on these data, some patients taking the combination of nelfinavir and saquinavir are likely to develop saquinavir-induced adverse effects, such as abdominal discomfort and diarrhea.

RELATED DRUGS: Nelfinavir may increase the concentrations of other protease inhibitors that undergo CYP3A4 mediated metabolism, such as indinavir or ritonavir.

MANAGEMENT OPTIONS:

➡ *Monitor.* Pending further information on this interaction, carefully monitor patients taking saquinavir when nelfinavir is initiated or discontinued from the antiretroviral drug regimen.

REFERENCES:

1. *Viracept* [package insert]. La Jolla, CA: Agouron Pharmaceuticals, Inc.; 2001.

Nelfinavir (*Viracept*)

Sildenafil (*Viagra*)

SUMMARY: Nelfinavir may increase sildenafil plasma concentrations; increased sildenafil toxicity may occur. Sildenafil does not affect nelfinavir plasma concentrations.

RISK FACTORS: No specific risk factors are known.

MECHANISM: Nelfinavir appears to inhibit the activity of CYP3A4, the enzyme known to metabolize sildenafil. Sildenafil does not appear to alter the metabolism of nelfinavir.

CLINICAL EVALUATION: While no published data are available for evaluation, the manufacturer of nelfinavir has noted that nelfinavir may reduce the metabolism of sildenafil.[1] Increased sildenafil concentrations may occur and result in hypotension, visual disturbances, or tachycardia. In 5 patients taking nelfinavir and other antiretroviral medications including zidovudine and lamivudine, the administration of sildenafil 25 mg produced no change in nelfinavir plasma concentrations.[2]

RELATED DRUGS: Other protease inhibitors that inhibit CYP3A4 such as ritonavir may increase sildenafil concentrations.

MANAGEMENT OPTIONS:

➡ *Monitor.* Pending further information on this interaction, carefully monitor patients taking nelfinavir and sildenafil for increased sildenafil response.

REFERENCES:

1. *Nelfinavir* [package insert]. La Jolla, CA: Agouron Pharmaceuticals, Inc.; 2001.
2. Bratt G, et al. Sildenafil does not alter nelfinavir pharmacokinetics. *Ther Drug Monit.* 2003;25:240-242.

 Nelfinavir (*Viracept*)

Simvastatin (*Zocor*)

SUMMARY: Nelfinavir administration markedly increases simvastatin concentrations; some patients may experience increased side effects.

RISK FACTORS: No specific risk factors are known.

MECHANISM: Nelfinavir may inhibit the activity of CYP3A4 or P-glycoprotein, resulting in a decrease in the clearance of simvastatin.

CLINICAL EVALUATION: Sixteen healthy subjects received simvastatin 20 mg/day for 14 days. Nelfinavir 1,250 mg twice daily was then added, and both drugs were taken for an additional 14 days.[1] The coadministration of nelfinavir resulted in a mean increase in the simvastatin area under the concentration-time curve of 505% (range, 145% to 1,524%) and a mean increase in simvastatin's peak concentration of 517%. No significant changes in the cholesterol-lowering effects of simvastatin were noted during the 2-week coadministration of nelfinavir. While no subjects experienced side effects thought to be related to increased simvastatin concentrations, some patients might be at increased risk for myopathy.

RELATED DRUGS: Other protease inhibitors such as ritonavir (*Norvir*), amprenavir (*Agenerase*), indinavir (*Crixivan*), and saquinavir (eg, *Invirase*) would be expected to affect simvastatin in a similar manner. The clearance of other statins that are metabolized by CYP3A4 would likely be reduced by nelfinavir. Lovastatin (eg, *Mevacor*) is likely to be affected to a similar degree as simvastatin by nelfinavir.

MANAGEMENT OPTIONS:

➡ *Use Alternative.* Because pravastatin (*Pravachol*) and fluvastatin (*Lescol*) are not metabolized by CYP3A4, consider using 1 of these agents in patients taking protease inhibitors. The affect of nelfinavir on atorvastatin (*Lipitor*) is less than that observed with simvastatin; low doses of atorvastatin with close monitoring could be considered in patients taking nelfinavir.

➡ *Monitor.* Monitor patients taking any statin that is metabolized by CYP3A4 and a protease inhibitor for side effects, including myopathy and myoglobinuria.

REFERENCES:

1. Hsyu PH, et al. Pharmacokinetic interactions between nelfinavir and 3-hydroxy-3-methylglutaryl coenzyme A reductase inhibitors atorvastatin and simvastatin. *Antimicrob Agents Chemother.* 2001;45:3445-3450.

Nelfinavir (*Viracept*)

Zidovudine (eg, *Retrovir*)

SUMMARY: Nelfinavir administration modestly reduces zidovudine plasma concentrations; some reduction in antiviral effect is possible.

RISK FACTORS: No specific risk factors are known.

MECHANISM: Unknown.

CLINICAL EVALUATION: While specific data are limited, the manufacturer of nelfinavir reported that nelfinavir 750 mg every 8 hours for 7 to 10 days reduced the mean area under the plasma concentration-time curve 35% following a single dose of zidovudine 200 mg, compared with zidovudine alone.[1] It is possible that some patients may experience a limited reduction in the antiviral effectiveness of zidovudine.

RELATED DRUGS: Tipranavir/ritonavir combination therapy has been noted to reduce zidovudine plasma concentrations.

MANAGEMENT OPTIONS:

➡ *Monitor.* Monitor patients taking zidovudine for reduce antiviral effect if nelfinavir is coadministered.

REFERENCES:

1. *Viracept* [package insert]. La Jolla, CA: Agouron Pharmaceuticals, Inc; 2006.

Neomycin (eg, *Neo-fradin*)

Penicillin V (eg, *Veetids*)

SUMMARY: Neomycin reduces the serum concentration of penicillin V and may reduce its efficacy.

RISK FACTORS: No specific risk factors are known.

MECHANISM: Oral neomycin can decrease penicillin V absorption, presumably because of the production of a malabsorption syndrome.

CLINICAL EVALUATION: Oral neomycin 3 g 4 times/day reduced serum concentrations of penicillin V more than 50% compared with control values.[1]

RELATED DRUGS: Penicillin G (eg, *Pfizerpen*) may be affected similarly by neomycin.

MANAGEMENT OPTIONS:

➡ *Circumvent/Minimize.* Administer the penicillin parenterally to avoid this interaction or select an alternative oral antibiotic.

➡ *Monitor.* Monitor patients taking oral neomycin and oral penicillin for reduced penicillin effect.

REFERENCES:

1. Cheng SH, et al. Effect of orally administered neomycin on the absorption of penicillin V. *N Engl J Med.* 1962;267:1296-1297.

4   Neomycin (eg, *Neo-fradin*)

Vitamin B$_{12}$ (Cyanocobalamin)

SUMMARY: Neomycin administration is unlikely to result in vitamin B$_{12}$ deficiency.

RISK FACTORS:

➡ **Concurrent Diseases.** Colchicine administration may increase neomycin-induced malabsorption of vitamin B$_{12}$.[1]

MECHANISM: The GI absorption of vitamin B$_{12}$ can be decreased considerably by oral neomycin.

CLINICAL EVALUATION: Prolonged administration of large doses of neomycin would be necessary to induce vitamin B$_{12}$ deficiency anemia.[2] This interaction is not likely to be important in patients who are being treated for vitamin B$_{12}$ deficiency anemia because B$_{12}$ is generally given parenterally. However, Schilling tests of vitamin B$_{12}$ absorption may be affected.

RELATED DRUGS: No information is available.

MANAGEMENT OPTIONS: No specific action is required, but be alert for evidence of the interaction.

REFERENCES:

1. Faloon WW, et al. Vitamin B$_{12}$ absorption studies using colchicine, neomycin and continuous ^{57}CO B$_{12}$ administration. *Gastroenterology.* 1969;56:1251.
2. Jacobson ED, et al. An experimental malabsorption syndrome induced by neomycin. *Am J Med.* 1960;28:524-533.

3   Neomycin (eg, *Neo-Tabs*)

Warfarin (eg, *Coumadin*)

SUMMARY: Oral administration of aminoglycosides like neomycin appears to enhance the hypoprothrombinemic response to oral anticoagulants like warfarin in certain predisposed patients.

RISK FACTORS:

➡ **Concurrent Diseases.** Deficiency of dietary vitamin K and impaired liver function place a patient at greater risk.

➡ **Dosage Regimen.** Large oral aminoglycoside doses produce a greater risk.

MECHANISM: The mechanism for this interaction is not established; several possibilities exist. Aminoglycosides may reduce vitamin K production by GI bacteria, thus enhancing the hypoprothrombinemic response to oral anticoagulants.[3,5,7,8] Impaired vitamin K absorption due to oral neomycin also has been proposed. Streptomycin has been implicated in the production of a factor V inhibitor in several patients,[1] which would add theoretically to the anticoagulant effect of oral anticoagulants. Animal studies indicate that oral neomycin may inhibit the enterohepatic circulation of warfarin, thus reducing plasma warfarin concentrations.[2]

CLINICAL EVALUATION: In patients with sufficient dietary vitamin K, the reduction of bacterial vitamin K by orally administered neomycin is probably of minor significance. However, in some predisposed patients the combination is more likely to produce or enhance hypoprothrombinemia.[4] Studies of patients on warfarin have demonstrated both increased prothrombin times[4] and no change in anticoagulant requirements[6] with oral neomycin treatment. The association of streptomycin therapy with a factor V inhibitor has been reported several times, but the nature of the association and its incidence are not clear.

RELATED DRUGS: Other orally administered aminoglycosides may increase hypopro-thrombinemic response to warfarin.

MANAGEMENT OPTIONS:

➡ *Monitor.* Careful monitoring of hypoprothrombinemia appears warranted when an oral aminoglycoside is coadministered for more than 1 to 2 days, particularly when a patient is predisposed to a dietary vitamin K deficiency.

REFERENCES:

1. Stenbjerg S, et al. A circulating factor V inhibitor: possible side effect of treatment with streptomycin. *Scand J Haematol.* 1975;14:280.
2. Remmel RP, et al. The effect of broad-spectrum antibiotics on warfarin excretion and metabolism in the rat. *Res Commun Chem Pathol Pharmacol.* 1981;34:503.
3. Rodriguez-Erdmann F, et al. Interaction of antibiotics with vitamin K. *JAMA.* 1981;246:937.
4. Schade RWB, et al. A comparative study of the effects of cholestyramine and neomycin in the treatment of type II hyperlipoproteinaemia. *Acta Med Scand.* 1976;199:175.
5. Kippel AP, et al. Hypoprothrombinemia secondary to antibiotic therapy and manifested by massive gastrointestinal hemorrhage. Report of three cases. *Arch Surg.* 1968;96:266.
6. Udall JA. Drug interference with warfarin therapy. *Clin Med.* 1970;77:20.
7. Finegold SM. Interaction of antimicrobial therapy and intestinal flora. *Am J Clin Nutr.* 1970;23:1466.
8. Messinger WJ, et al. The effect of a bowel sterilizing antibiotic on blood coagulation mechanisms. *Angiology.* 1965;16:29.

Neostigmine (eg, *Prostigmin*)

Procainamide (eg, *Procan*)

SUMMARY: In patients receiving cholinergic agents for myasthenia gravis, symptoms may be exacerbated by procain-amide administration.

RISK FACTORS: No specific risk factors are known.

MECHANISM: Procainamide has neuromuscular blocking properties and can antagonize the effect of cholinergic drugs on skeletal muscles.

CLINICAL EVALUATION: The cholinergic treatment of myasthenia gravis may be antagonized by procainamide. Isolated cases of worsened myasthenic symptoms have been reported several days after starting procainamide therapy.[2] Also, edrophonium (eg, *Tensilon*) tests may be unreliable in procainamide-treated patients.[2]

RELATED DRUGS: Although lidocaine (eg, *Xylocaine*) and propranolol (eg, *Inderal*) also might be expected to worsen myasthesia,[1] limited use of lidocaine in 2 myasthenic patients did not result in aggravation of symptoms.[2]

MANAGEMENT OPTIONS:

➡ *Monitor.* Watch for increased weakness in patients with myasthenia gravis if procainamide is coadministered.

REFERENCES:

1. Flacke W. Treatment of myasthenia gravis. *N Engl J Med.* 1973; 288:27.
2. Kornfeld P, et al. Myasthenia gravis unmasked by antiarrhythmic agents. *Mt Sinai J Med.* 1976;43:10.

Neostigmine (eg, *Prostigmin*)

Propranolol (eg, *Inderal*)

SUMMARY: Both neostigmine and beta-adrenergic blockers, such as propranolol, can slow the heart rate; additive bradycardia would be expected, but the risk of adverse consequences from the combination is not known.

RISK FACTORS: No specific risk factors are known.

MECHANISM: Both cholinergic stimulation and beta blockade can slow the heart rate, and the effects may be additive.

CLINICAL EVALUATION: Prolonged and severe bradycardia has been reported in patients receiving cholinergic agents such as neostigmine or physostigmine (*Antilirium*) concurrently with beta-adrenergic blockers such as atenolol (eg, *Tenormin*), nadolol (eg, *Corgard*), or propranolol.[1-4]

RELATED DRUGS: Other beta-blockers (eg, atenolol, nadolol) may produce similar effects. Physostigmine affects propranolol similarly.

MANAGEMENT OPTIONS:

➡ **Monitor.** Monitor for excessive bradycardia in patients receiving beta-adrenergic blockers concurrently with neostigmine or other cholinergic agents.

REFERENCES:

1. Sprague DH. Severe bradycardia after neostigmine in a patient taking propranolol to control paroxysmal atrial tachycardia. *Anesthesiology*. 1975;42:208.
2. Seidl DC, Martin DE. Prolonged bradycardia after neostigmine administration in a patient taking nadolol. *Anesth Analg*. 1984;63:365.
3. Baraka A, Dajani A. Severe bradycardia following physostigmine in the presence of beta-adrenergic blockade. *Middle East J Anesthesiol*. 1984;7:291.
4. Eldor J, et al. Prolonged bradycardia and hypotension after neostigmine administration in a patient receiving atenolol. *Anesthesia*. 1987;42:1294.

Neostigmine (eg, *Prostigmin*)

Quinidine

SUMMARY: Quinidine may block the therapeutic effects of cholinergic drugs.

RISK FACTORS: No specific risk factors are known.

MECHANISM: Quinidine has anticholinergic properties and may antagonize the effects of cholinergic drugs.

CLINICAL EVALUATION: Quinidine tends to prevent the cardiac slowing produced by neostigmine and other cholinergic drugs. Thus, in patients receiving quinidine, cholinergic drugs may fail to terminate paroxysmal supraventricular tachycardia. Quinidine also may antagonize the effects of neostigmine and edrophonium (eg, *Tensilon*) in the treatment of myasthenia gravis.[1,2] This interaction has been used to clinical advantage in cases of delirium caused by the combination of quinidine and other anticholinergic agents. Physostigmine, a cholinergic drug, has been used successfully to counteract this delirium.[3]

RELATED DRUGS: Edrophonium (eg, *Tensilon*) may interact similarly with quinidine.

MANAGEMENT OPTIONS: No specific action is required, but be alert for evidence of the interaction.

REFERENCES:

1. Flacke W. Treatment of myasthenia gravis. *N Engl J Med.* 1973;288:27-31.

2. Kornfeld P, et al. Myasthenia gravis unmasked by antiarrhythmic agents. *Mt Sinai J Med.* 1976;43:10-14.

3. Summers WK, et al. Does physostigmine reverse quinidine delirium? *West J Med.* 1981;135:411-414.

Nevirapine (*Viramune*)

Rifampin (eg, *Rifadin*)

SUMMARY: Rifampin administration can result in a reduction in nevirapine plasma concentrations; some reduction in antiretroviral efficacy may occur.

RISK FACTORS: No specific risk factors are known.

MECHANISM: Nevirapine is metabolized by CYP3A4 and CYP2B6. Rifampin is known to induce the activity of several cytochrome P450 enzymes and probably caused an increase in the first-pass and/or systemic clearance of nevirapine.

CLINICAL EVALUATION: Five HIV-infected patients taking nevirapine 200 mg twice daily were treated for tuberculosis with rifampin 600 mg twice daily, isoniazid, pyrazinamide, and ethambutol.[1] Following at least 12 days of rifampin therapy, the mean area under the concentration-time curve of nevirapine was reduced 31% by concurrent rifampin administration. It is possible that this degree of reduction in nevirapine plasma concentration would reduce its antiretroviral efficacy in some patients. In 3 of the 5 patients completing antituberculosis therapy, no diminution in antiviral activity was observed. A prior study found that rifampin administration twice weekly had no effect on the trough plasma concentration of nevirapine.[2] Rifampin concentrations in the 5 patients taking rifampin and nevirapine were not different from the rifampin concentrations in 5 other patients taking rifampin without nevirapine.[1]

RELATED DRUGS: Rifabutin may also cause a modest reduction in the plasma concentration of nevirapine.

MANAGEMENT OPTIONS:

➡ *Monitor.* Be alert for reduced nevirapine antiretroviral activity and lower plasma concentrations during coadministration with rifampin.

REFERENCES:

1. Ribera E, et al. Pharmacokinetic interaction between nevirapine and rifampicin in HIV-infected patients with tuberculosis. *J Acquir Immune Defic Syndr.* 2001;28:450-453.

2. Deal GL, et al. Effect of tuberculosis therapy on nevirapine trough plasma concentrations. *AIDS.* 1999;13:2489-2490.

Nicardipine (eg, *Cardene*)

Propranolol (eg, *Inderal*)

SUMMARY: Nicardipine administration increases propranolol concentrations; an increase in beta-blocker effect may occur in some patients.

RISK FACTORS: No specific risk factors are known.

MECHANISM: Dihydropyridine calcium channel blockers (eg, nifedipine, nicardipine, felodipine [*Plendil*], isradipine, nisoldipine) may increase the bioavailability of beta-blockers (perhaps by increasing liver blood flow)[1] or reduce their clearance. Additive hemodynamic effects may result from the combination of beta-blockers and calcium channel blockers.

CLINICAL EVALUATION: A single 30 mg dose of nicardipine increased the area under the concentration-time curve (AUC) of propranolol 47% and its peak concentration 80% following an 80 mg dose of propranolol. Nicardipine clearance was reduced by 30% in patients taking propranolol 160 to 480 mg/day[2] but was unaffected by metoprolol.[3] The combination of a beta-blocker and calcium channel blocker may be of benefit in certain situations, although some patients have developed marked hypotension.[4,5]

RELATED DRUGS: A single dose of nicardipine 30 mg had no effect on the pharmacokinetics of atenolol (eg, *Tenormin*).[6] Nicardipine increased metoprolol (eg, *Lopressor*) concentration by approximately 25%.[3] Nimodipine (*Nimotop*) and propranolol had minimal effect on each other's plasma concentrations.[7] Nisoldipine (*Sular*) and nifedipine (eg, *Procardia*) increased the AUC of propranolol.[1,8] Conversely, nisoldipine AUC and peak serum concentrations were increased 30% and 57%, respectively, by propranolol. Others found no change in drug concentrations during chronic nisoldipine and propranolol dosing.[9] Propranolol also blunted the increase in cardiac output observed following nisoldipine alone. Isradipine (*DynaCirc*) 10 mg increased the AUC of propranolol 28% and its peak concentration 60%.[10]

MANAGEMENT OPTIONS:

➡ ***Monitor.*** Monitor patients receiving combined therapy with propranolol and nicardipine for enhanced effects resulting from pharmacokinetic or pharmacodynamic interactions.

REFERENCES:

1. Levine MA, et al. Pharmacokinetic and pharmacodynamic interactions between nisoldipine and propranolol. *Clin Pharmacol Ther*. 1988;43:39-48.
2. Rocha P, et al. Kinetics and hemodynamic effects of intravenous nicardipine modified by previous propranolol oral treatment. *Cardiovasc Drugs Ther*. 1990;4:1525-1532.
3. Funck-Brentano C, et al. Influence of CYP2D6-dependent metabolism on the steady-state pharmacokinetics and pharmacodynamics of metoprolol and nicardipine, alone and in combination. *Br J Clin Pharmacol*. 1993;36:531.
4. Packer M, et al. Hemodynamic consequences of combined beta-adrenergic and slow calcium channel blockade in man. *Circulation*. 1982;65:660-668.
5. Winniford MD, et al. Hemodynamic and electrophysiologic effects of verapamil and nifedipine in patients on propranolol. *Am J Cardiol*. 1982;50:704-710.
6. Vercruysse I, et al. Nicardipine does not influence the pharmacokinetics and pharmacodynamics of atenolol. *Br J Clin Pharmacol*. 1990;30:499-500.

7. Breuel HP, et al. Chronic administration of nimodipine and propranolol in elderly normotensive subjects—an interaction study. *Int J Clin Pharmacol Ther.* 1995;33:103-108.

8. Vinceneux PH, et al. Pharmacokinetic and pharmacodynamic interactions between nifedipine and propranolol or betaxolol. *Int J Clin Pharmacol Ther Toxicol.* 1986;24:153-158.

9. Shaw-Stiffel TA, et al. Pharmacokinetic and pharmacodynamic interactions during multiple-dose administration of nisoldipine and propranolol. *Clin Pharmacol Ther.* 1994;55:661-669.

10. Rosenkranz B, et al. Interaction between nifedipine and atenolol: pharmacokinetics and pharmacodynamics in normotensive volunteers. *J Cardiovasc Pharmacol.* 1986;8:943-949.

Nifedipine (eg, *Procardia*)

Omeprazole (*Prilosec*)

SUMMARY: Multiple dose omeprazole modestly increases nifedipine plasma concentrations; the clinical significance of these changes is likely to be limited.

RISK FACTORS: No specific risk factors are known.

MECHANISM: While the exact mechanism of this interaction is unknown, omeprazole appears to increase the bioavailability of nifedipine perhaps by increasing gastric pH.

CLINICAL EVALUATION: Ten healthy subjects were administered one 10 mg nifedipine capsule after a placebo, after a single 20 mg dose of omeprazole or after omeprazole 20 mg/day for 8 days.[1] The mean area under the concentration-time curve of nifedipine was increased 26% during multiple dose omeprazole compared with placebo. The mean nifedipine half-life, peak concentration, and time-to-peak concentration were not affected by omeprazole administration. Nifedipine-induced changes in heart rate and blood pressure were not altered significantly by omeprazole pretreatment. The clinical significance of this interaction in patients with hypertension or angina or in those receiving larger omeprazole dosages is unknown but probably would be limited.

RELATED DRUGS: Other drugs that increase gastric pH (eg, cimetidine [eg, *Tagamet*], ranitidine [eg, *Zantac*], famotidine [eg, *Pepcid*], nizatidine [*Axid*], lansoprazole [*Prevacid*]) also increase nifedipine absorption. Other dihydropyridine calcium blockers (eg, felodipine [*Plendil*], nicardipine [eg, *Cardene*]) may be affected similarly.

MANAGEMENT OPTIONS: No specific action is required, but be alert for evidence of the interaction.

REFERENCES:
1. Soons PA, et al. Influence of single-and multiple-dose omeprazole treatment on nifedipine pharmacokinetics and effects in healthy subjects. *Eur J Clin Pharmacol.* 1992;42:319.

Nifedipine (eg, *Procardia*)

Orlistat (*Xenical*)

SUMMARY: The administration of nifedipine with orlistat had only a minor effect on the pharmacokinetics of nifedipine resulting in a delay in reaching peak serum concentrations.

RISK FACTORS: No specific risk factors known.

MECHANISM: Not established.

CLINICAL EVALUATION: A single 20 mg dose of nifedipine-sustained release (*Adalat*) was administered alone and after 7 days of orlistat 50 mg 3 times daily to 8 healthy subjects.[1] The orlistat was taken during meals. During the coadministration of orlistat, the peak concentration of nifedipine occurred at 2.1 hours after the dose compared to 1.3 hours when the nifedipine was administered alone. This degree of change should not be clinically significant. No changes were observed in nifedipine peak concentration, half-life, or area under the concentration-time curve during orlistat administration. No change in blood pressure, pulse rate, or electrocardiogram was noted.

RELATED DRUGS: The effect of orlistat on other calcium channel blockers is unknown.

MANAGEMENT OPTIONS:

➥ *Monitor.* No specific action is required, but be alert for evidence of the interaction.

REFERENCES:

1. Weber C, et al. Effect of the lipase inhibitor orlistat on the pharmacokinetics of four different antihypertensive drugs in healthy volunteers. *Eur J Clin Pharmacol.* 1996;51:87.

Nifedipine (eg, *Procardia*)

Phenobarbital (eg, *Solfoton*)

SUMMARY: Phenobarbital substantially reduces the plasma concentrations of nifedipine.

RISK FACTORS: No specific risk factors are known.

MECHANISM: Phenobarbital appears to enhance the metabolism of nifedipine probably by increasing hepatic enzyme (CYP3A4) activity.

CLINICAL EVALUATION: Fifteen healthy subjects received a single 20 mg oral dose of nifedipine before and following 2 weeks of phenobarbital 100 mg/day.[1] Phenobarbital increased the clearance of nifedipine from 1,088 mL/min to 2,981 mL/min and decreased the nifedipine area under the concentration-time curve 61%.

RELATED DRUGS: Phenobarbital also increases the metabolism of verapamil (eg, *Calan*). Other calcium channel blockers may be affected similarly by phenobarbital.

MANAGEMENT OPTIONS:

➥ *Circumvent/Minimize.* Patients receiving phenobarbital may require higher than usual doses of nifedipine.

➥ *Monitor.* Patients stabilized on nifedipine should be monitored for the possibility of decreased effectiveness when phenobarbital is administered concomitantly.

REFERENCES:

1. Schellens JHM, et al. Influence of enzyme induction and inhibition on the oxidation of nifedipine, sparteine, mephenytoin and antipyrine in humans as assessed by a cocktail study design. *J Pharmacol Exp Ther.* 1989;249:638.

Nifedipine (eg, *Procardia*)

Phenytoin (eg, *Dilantin*)

SUMMARY: Nifedipine was associated with increased plasma phenytoin concentration in 1 case; more study is needed.

RISK FACTORS: No specific risk factors are known.

MECHANISM: Not established, but nifedipine may reduce the metabolism of phenytoin. Theoretically phenytoin may enhance the hepatic metabolism of nifedipine.

CLINICAL EVALUATION: A patient stabilized on phenytoin 300 mg/day was started on nifedipine 30 mg/day. After 4 weeks of therapy the patient developed headaches, nystagmus, tremors, slurred speech, ataxia, and depression. The phenytoin concentration was 30.4 mcg/mL and declined, after discontinuation of nifedipine, to 10.5 mcg/mL after 2 weeks.[1] Although nifedipine appeared to interact with phenytoin in this case, most evidence suggests that nifedipine is unlikely to inhibit hepatic drug metabolism.

RELATED DRUGS: The bioavailability of most calcium channel blockers appears to be reduced by enzyme inducers such as phenytoin.

MANAGEMENT OPTIONS:

➡ *Monitor.* Until more information regarding this potential interaction is available, patients receiving phenytoin should be monitored carefully when nifedipine or diltiazem is added to or removed from their regimen.

REFERENCES:

1. Ahmad S. Nifedipine-phenytoin interaction. *J Am Coll Cardiol.* 1984;3:1581.

Nifedipine (eg, *Procardia*)

Propranolol (eg, *Inderal*)

SUMMARY: The combination of nifedipine and propranolol may result in hypotension; nifedipine can increase propranolol concentrations.

RISK FACTORS: No specific risk factors are known.

MECHANISM: Dihydropyridine calcium channel blockers (nifedipine, felodipine, isradipine, nisoldipine) may increase the bioavailability of beta-blockers (perhaps by increasing liver blood flow)[1,15] or reduce their clearance. Propranolol may increase the bioavailability of nifedipine and reduce its clearance. Additive hemodynamic effects may result from the combination of beta-blockers and calcium channel blockers.

CLINICAL EVALUATION: The combination of nifedipine and beta-blockers may produce positive clinical effects in the treatment of angina or hypertension.[2-4] However, several cases of severe hypotension or cardiac failure associated with the combination have been reported.[5,6] A 23% increase in the area under the concentration-time curve (AUC) was reported for propranolol after 2 days of therapy with nifedipine 10 mg 3 times daily,[7] but others found no change in the pharmacokinetics of propranolol, metoprolol (eg, *Lopressor*), or atenolol (eg, *Tenormin*)[8,9,14] following nifedipine administration. Propranolol increased the bioavailability of nifedipine and reduced its systemic clearance while nifedipine increased the clearance of propranolol in 1 study.[10]

RELATED DRUGS: Atenolol (eg, *Tenormin*) and metoprolol may interact similarly with nifedipine. Felodipine (*Plendil*) 10 mg twice daily increased the AUC of metoprolol 31%,[11] but the AUC of felodipine was not altered by chronic metoprolol or atenolol therapy.[13] Nisoldipine (*Sular*) 20 mg increased the propranolol AUC by approximately 50%.[1,15] Conversely, nisoldipine AUC and peak serum concentrations were increased 30% and 57%, respectively, by propranolol. Propranolol also blunted the increase in cardiac output observed following nisoldipine alone. Isradipine (*DynaCirc*) 10 mg increased the AUC of propranolol 28% and its peak concentration 60%.[12]

MANAGEMENT OPTIONS:

➡ **Monitor.** Patients receiving combined therapy with propranolol and nifedipine should be monitored for enhanced effects resulting from pharmacokinetic or pharmacodynamic interactions.

REFERENCES:

1. Levine MAH, et al. Pharmacokinetic and pharmacodynamic interactions between nisoldipine and propranolol. *Clin Pharmacol Ther.* 1988;43:39.

2. Dargie HJ, et al. Nifedipine and propranolol: a beneficial drug interaction. *Am J Med.* 1981;71:676.

3. Pfisterer M, et al. Combined acebutolol/nifedipine therapy in patients with chronic coronary artery disease: additional improvement of ischemia-induced left ventricular dysfunction. *Am J Cardiol.* 1982;49:1259.

4. Eggertsen R, et al. Effects of treatment with nifedipine and metoprolol in essential hypertension. *Eur J Clin Pharmacol.* 1982;21:389.

5. Robson RH, et al. Nifedipine and beta-blockade as a cause of cardiac failure. *BMJ.* 1982;284:104.

6. Anastassiades CJ. Nifedipine and beta blocker drugs. *BMJ.* 1980;281:1251.

7. Vinceneux PH, et al. Pharmacokinetic and pharmacodynamic interactions between nifedipine and propranolol or betaxolol. *Int J Clin Pharmacol Ther Toxicol.* 1986;24:153.

8. Gangji D, et al. Study of the influence of nifedipine on the pharmacokinetics and pharmacodynamics of propranolol, metoprolol and atenolol. *Br J Clin Pharmacol.* 1984;17:29S.

9. Rosenkranz B, et al. Interaction between nifedipine and atenolol: pharmacokinetics and pharmacodynamics in normotensive volunteers. *J Cardiovasc Pharmacol.* 1986;8:943.

10. Kleinbloesem CH, et al. Pharmacokinetic and haemodynamic interaction between nifedipine and propranolol. *Br J Clin Pharmacol.* 1985;19:537.

11. Smith SR, et al. Pharmacokinetic interactions between felodipine and metoprolol. *Eur J Clin Pharmacol.* 1987;31:575.

12. Shepherd AMM, et al. Pharmacokinetic interaction between isradipine and propranolol. *Clin Pharmacol Ther.* 1988;43:194. Abstract.

13. Bengtsson-Hasselgren B, et al. Haemodynamic effects and pharmacokinetics of felodipine at rest and during exercise in hypertensive patients treated with metoprolol. *Eur J Clin Pharmacol.* 1989;37:459.

14. Bauer LA, et al. Influence of nifedipine therapy on indocyanine green and oral propranolol pharmacokinetics. *Eur J Clin Pharmacol.* 1989;37:257.

15. Elliott HL, et al. The interactions between nisoldipine and two betaadrenoceptor antagonists-atenolol and propranolol. *Br J Clin Pharmacol.* 1991;32:379.

Nifedipine (eg, *Procardia*)

Quinidine (eg, *Quinora*)

SUMMARY: Nifedipine appears to reduce the serum concentrations of quinidine, and quinidine appears to increase the serum concentration of nifedipine.

RISK FACTORS: No specific risk factors are known.

MECHANISM: Quinidine may inhibit the metabolism of nifedipine, and quinidine clearance appears to increase following nifedipine administration.

CLINICAL EVALUATION: Nifedipine can decrease the quinidine serum concentration 20% to 40%,[1-4] although no effect was noted by 1 study.[8] Quinidine sulfate 200 mg doubled the area under the concentration-time curve (AUC) and the half-life of nifedipine (5 mg administered 15 minutes after the quinidine).[5] When nifedipine 20 mg was administered after quinidine sulfate 200 mg every 8 hours for 4 doses, the AUC of nifedipine increased 36% following quinidine administration compared with nifedipine AUC when administered alone.[8] In contrast nifedipine serum concentration was unchanged by the administration of 200 mg of quinidine 1 hour before nifedipine.[6] Likewise, nifedipine did not appear to have any effect on quinidine concentrations.[6,9] The disparity in the results of the studies cited above may be based upon differences in the protocols. More studies in patients are needed to evaluate the significance of this interaction.

RELATED DRUGS: Verapamil (eg, *Calan*) increases quinidine concentrations. Diltiazem (eg, *Cardizem*) 120 mg/day had no effect on quinidine concentrations.[7]

MANAGEMENT OPTIONS:

➡ *Circumvent/Minimize.* Quinidine doses may require upward adjustment when nifedipine is added or downward adjustment if quinidine is discontinued.

➡ *Monitor.* Nifedipine and quinidine coadministration may reduce quinidine concentration and increase nifedipine concentration; monitor patients carefully.

REFERENCES:

1. Farringer JA, et al. Nifedipine-induced alterations in serum quinidine concentrations. *Am Heart J.* 1984;108:1570.

2. Van Lith RM, et al. Quinidine-nifedipine interaction. *Drug Intell Clin Pharm.* 1985;19:829.

3. Green JA, et al. Nifedipine-quinidine interaction. *Clin Pharm.* 1983;2:461.

4. Munger MA, et al. Elucidation of the nifedipine-quinidine interaction. *Clin Pharmacol Ther.* 1989;45:411.

5. Oates NS, et al. Influence of quinidine on nifedipine plasma pharmacokinetics. *Br J Clin Pharmacol.* 1988;25:675.

6. Schellens JHM, et al. Differential effects of quinidine on the disposition of nifedipine, sparteine, and mephenytoin in humans. *Clin Pharmacol Ther.* 1991;50:520.

7. Matera MG, et al. Quinidine-diltiazem: pharmacokinetic interaction in humans. *Curr Ther Res.* 1986;40:653.

8. Bowles SK, et al. Evaluation of the pharmacokinetic and pharmacodynamic interaction between quinidine and nifedipine. *J Clin Pharmacol.* 1993;33:727.

9. Bailey DG, et al. Quinidine interaction with nifedipine and felodipine: pharmacokinetic and pharmacodynamic evaluation. *Clin Pharmacol Ther.* 1993;53:354.

Nifedipine (eg, *Procardia*)

Quinupristin/Dalfopristin (*Synercid*)

SUMMARY: The plasma concentration of nifedipine is increased by the coadministration of quinupristin/dalfopristin; reduced doses of nifedipine may be necessary.

RISK FACTORS: No specific risk factors are known.

MECHANISM: Nifedipine metabolism (CYP3A4) is inhibited by quinupristin/dalfopristin.

CLINICAL EVALUATION: Although published data are lacking, the manufacturer of quinupristin/dalfopristin reports a 44% increase in the area under the concentration-time curve of nifedipine following multiple doses of quinupristin/dalfopristin.[1] An increase in the hypotensive effect of nifedipine would be expected.

RELATED DRUGS: The metabolism of other calcium channel blockers, all of which are metabolized by CYP3A4, would likely be reduced by quinupristin/dalfopristin.

MANAGEMENT OPTIONS:

➡ ***Consider Alternative.*** If appropriate for the disease being treated, consider a noncalcium channel blocker for patients taking quinupristin/dalfopristin. In patients requiring calcium channel blockers, consider an alternative antibiotic that does not affect CYP3A4 activity.

➡ ***Monitor.*** Carefully monitor patients stabilized on nifedipine for increasing nifedipine response, such as hypotension, when quinupristin/dalfopristin is added.

REFERENCES:

1. *Synercid* [package insert]. Collegeville, PA: Rhone-Poulenc Rorer; 1999.

 Nifedipine (eg, *Procardia*)

Rifampin (eg, *Rifadin*)

SUMMARY: Rifampin decreases nifedipine plasma concentrations; loss of therapeutic effect may result.

RISK FACTORS: No specific risk factors are known.

MECHANISM: Rifampin appears to induce the metabolism (CYP3A4) of nifedipine.

CLINICAL EVALUATION: A patient with angina taking nifedipine, isosorbide dinitrate (eg, *Isordil*), and nicorandil[†] experienced increased chest pain during treatment with rifampin 450 mg daily.[1] The interaction appeared to be confirmed by a rifampin dechallenge and rechallenge. The area under the concentration-time curve and peak serum concentration of nifedipine were reduced approximately 50% during rifampin therapy. Another patient's nifedipine concentration was reduced 40% after taking rifampin 450 mg daily.[2] Blood pressure increased during rifampin dosing and declined when rifampin was discontinued.

RELATED DRUGS: Rifampin probably affects other calcium channel blockers in a similar manner. Rifabutin (*Mycobutin*) can be expected to affect nifedipine in a similar manner.

MANAGEMENT OPTIONS:

➥ *Consider Alternative.* Because this interaction is likely to reduce the efficacy of nifedipine, consider an alternative agent for nifedipine. Other calcium channel blockers also may be affected; a therapeutic substitution to a different class of agent may be required.

➥ *Circumvent/Minimize.* Larger doses of calcium channel blockers (particularly those administered orally) may be required when rifampin is coadministered.

➥ *Monitor.* Monitor patients taking calcium channel blockers for a reduction in efficacy when rifampin is given.

REFERENCES:

1. Tsuchihashi K, et al. A case of variant angina exacerbated by administration of rifampicin. *Heart Vessels.* 1987;3:214-217.

2. Tada Y, et al. Case report: nifedipine-rifampicin interaction attenuates the effect on blood pressure in a patient with essential hypertension. *Am J Med Sci.* 1992;303:25-27.

† Not available in the United States.

Nifedipine (eg, *Procardia*)

Rosiglitazone (*Avandia*)

SUMMARY: Rosiglitazone caused a slight reduction in nifedipine plasma concentrations; no special precautions are necessary.

RISK FACTORS: No specific risk factors are known.

MECHANISM: Unknown.

CLINICAL EVALUATION: A single, 20 mg oral dose of immediate-release nifedipine was administered to 26 subjects alone and following rosiglitazone 8 mg for 14 days.[1] The mean plasma nifedipine area under the plasma concentration-time curve (AUC) was reduced 13% (range, 56% to 51%). The response was variable, with 9 of the subjects demonstrating an increase in nifedipine AUC following rosiglitazone. These limited changes in nifedipine plasma concentrations are unlikely to produce any change in patient response.

RELATED DRUGS: It is possible that the plasma concentration of other calcium channel blockers would also be affected by rosiglitazone.

MANAGEMENT OPTIONS:

➥ *Monitor.* Because of the minimal magnitude of this interaction, no specific monitoring appears to be necessary.

REFERENCES:

1. Harris RZ, et al. Rosiglitazone has no clinically significant effect on nifedipine pharmacokinetics. *J Clin Pharmacol.* 1999;39:1189-1194.

Nifedipine (eg, *Procardia*)

St. John's Wort

SUMMARY: St. John's wort reduces the plasma concentration of nifedipine; some loss of efficacy is likely to result.

RISK FACTORS: No specific risk factors are known.

MECHANISM: St. John's wort is known to induce CYP3A4, the enzyme responsible for the metabolism of nifedipine.

CLINICAL EVALUATION: Twenty-two subjects received nifedipine 10 mg alone and after 18 days of St. John's wort 900 mg daily.[1] Nifedipine plasma concentration was sampled 0.5 hours after its administration. St. John's wort administration reduced the nifedipine concentration 53%. While no data on nifedipine area under the concentration-time curve or clinical effect were provided, a reduction of nifedipine concentration of this magnitude can be expected to reduce its efficacy in some patients.

RELATED DRUGS: St. John's wort is likely to increase the metabolism of other calcium channel blockers because all are metabolized by CYP3A4.

MANAGEMENT OPTIONS:

➡ ***Monitor.*** Pending more complete data on this interaction, monitor patients for reduction in nifedipine effect if St. John's wort is coadministered.

REFERENCES:

1. Smith M, et al. An open trial of nifedipine-herb interactions: nifedipine with St. John's wort, ginseng or *Ginkgo biloba. Clin Pharmacol Ther.* 2001;69:P86.

Nifedipine (eg, *Procardia*)

Tacrolimus (eg, *Prograf*)

SUMMARY: Nifedipine administration reduced the dosage requirements of tacrolimus; tacrolimus dosage adjustments may be required.

RISK FACTORS: No specific risk factors are known.

MECHANISM: Unknown. It is suggested that nifedipine may inhibit the metabolism of tacrolimus, because both are substrates for CYP3A4. A nifedipine-induced increase in hepatic blood flow may also increase the concentration of tacrolimus by reducing its first-pass metabolism.

CLINICAL EVALUATION: The effect of nifedipine administration on tacrolimus dosing requirements was evaluated in a retrospective study.[1] Fifty patients who had undergone orthotopic liver transplants and were receiving tacrolimus were evaluated. Twenty-two patients were treated with nifedipine for hypertension, while the remaining patients did not receive nifedipine. The average dose of tacrolimus at 3, 6, and 12 months after initiation of nifedipine was recorded. In the group receiving nifedipine, the dose of tacrolimus was 26% to 38% less than that taken by patients not receiving nifedipine. Both groups had similar tacrolimus blood concentrations following dose adjustments at 1 month after the initiation of nifedipine. The study suggests that nifedipine administration reduces the dosage requirement of tacrolimus.

RELATED DRUGS: Other calcium channel blocking drugs may affect tacrolimus in a similar manner. Nifedipine appears to have limited effect on cyclosporine (eg, *Neoral*) concentrations.

MANAGEMENT OPTIONS:

➡ *Monitor.* Pending further study of this interaction, observe patients receiving tacrolimus and nifedipine for reduced tacrolimus dose requirements.

REFERENCES:

1. Seifeldin RA, et al. Nifedipine interaction with tacrolimus in liver transplant recipients. *Ann Pharmacother.* 1997;31(5):571-575.

Nifedipine (eg, *Procardia*)

Tamsulosin (*Flomax*)

SUMMARY: Tamsulosin does not appear to affect the antihypertensive response to nifedipine.

RISK FACTORS: No specific risk factors are known.

MECHANISM: Theoretically, additive hypotension could occur, but does not appear to be a problem clinically.

CLINICAL EVALUATION: Eight hypertensive subjects stabilized on nifedipine for at least 3 months were given tamsulosin 0.4 mg/day for 7 days followed by 0.8 mg/day for 7 days.[1] Tamsulosin did not produce any clinically significant effects on blood pressure or pulse rate compared with placebo.

RELATED DRUGS: Tamsulosin also did not affect the hypotensive response to atenolol (eg, *Tenormin*) or enalapril (eg, *Vasotec*).

MANAGEMENT OPTIONS: No specific action is required, but be alert for evidence of the interaction.

REFERENCES:

1. *Flomax* [package insert]. Ridgefield, CT: Boehringer Ingelheim; 2009.

Nifedipine (eg, *Procardia*)

Vincristine (eg, *Vincasar*)

SUMMARY: Nifedipine appeared to markedly increase the half-life of vincristine; the clinical significance is unknown.

RISK FACTORS: No specific risk factors are known.

MECHANISM: Not established. In vitro studies indicate that calcium channel blockers may inhibit the outward transport of intracellular vincristine.[1] Because nifedipine and vincristine are metabolized by CYP3A4, it is also possible that nifedipine inhibits vincristine metabolism.

CLINICAL EVALUATION: Fourteen control patients with solid tumors received vincristine 2 mg intravenously; 12 other patients received nifedipine 10 mg 3 times daily for 3 days before and 7 days after an equal dose of vincristine.[2] The half-life of vincristine was prolonged from 21.7 hours in the control patients to 85.5 hours in the patients treated with nifedipine and vincristine. The vincristine area under the concentration-time curve was 240% higher in the patients receiving nifedipine. The urinary excretion of vincristine was reduced by nifedipine during the first 24 hours after vincristine administration. No adverse reactions were noted in either group of patients.

RELATED DRUGS: Little is known regarding the effect of other calcium channel blockers on vincristine, but consider the possibility that they also interact.

MANAGEMENT OPTIONS:

➡ *Monitor.* Until further information is available, monitor patients receiving vincristine and nifedipine concomitantly for enhanced pharmacodynamic effects of vincristine. It may be necessary to adjust vincristine dose.

REFERENCES:

1. Tsuruo T, et al. Potentiation of vincristine and adriamycin effects in human hemopoietic tumor cell lines by calcium antagonists and calmodulin inhibitors. *Cancer Res.* 1983;43(5):2267-2272.

2. Fedeli L, et al. Pharmacokinetics of vincristine in cancer patients treated with nifedipine. *Cancer.* 1989;64(9):1805-1811.

Nifedipine (eg, *Procardia*)

Voriconazole (*Vfend*)

SUMMARY: Voriconazole increases the hypotensive effects of nifedipine.

RISK FACTORS: No specific risk factors are known.

MECHANISM: Voriconazole inhibits the activity of CYP3A4, an enzyme that metabolizes both nifedipine and eplerenone.

CLINICAL EVALUATION: A patient with hypertension taking nifedipine 40 mg daily, candesartan (*Atacand*) 8 mg daily, and eplerenone (eg, *Inspra*) 50 mg daily underwent a bone marrow transplantation.[1] Cyclosporine (eg, *Neoral*) and methylprednisolone were administered for graft-verses-host disease. Voriconazole was begun at 6 mg/kg intravenously every 12 hours for 2 doses then dosed at 4 mg/kg every 12 hours. Within 1 day of starting the voriconazole, the patient became hypotensive. Hypotensive medications were held for 5 days. Candesartan and nifedipine (20 mg daily) were restarted with appropriate blood pressure control.

RELATED DRUGS: Ketoconazole (eg, *Nizoral*), fluconazole (eg, *Diflucan*), itraconazole (eg, *Sporanox*), and posaconazole (*Noxafil*) also inhibit the activity of CYP3A4 and are expected to increase the plasma concentrations of nifedipine and eplerenone. All calcium channel blockers are metabolized by CYP3A4 and would likely interact with voriconazole.

MANAGEMENT OPTIONS:

➡ *Consider Alternative.* Amphotericin B (*Abelcet*), caspofungin (*Cancidas*), and anidulafungin (*Eraxis*) do not appear to inhibit CYP3A4. Antihypertensive drugs that are not substrates for CYP3A4, including angiotensin-converting enzyme inhibitors, beta-blockers, or alpha-blockers, could be considered in patients requiring voriconazole.

➡ *Monitor.* If voriconazole is coadministered with calcium channel blockers, monitor the patient carefully for hypotension.

REFERENCES:

1. Kato J, et al. Hypotension due to the drug interaction of voriconazole with eplerenone and nifedipine. *Eur J Clin Pharmacol.* 2009;65(3):323-324.

Nilotinib (*Tasigna*)

Rifampin (eg, *Rifadin*)

SUMMARY: Rifampin administration will decrease the plasma concentration of nilotinib; loss of nilotinib efficacy is likely to occur in some patients

RISK FACTORS: No specific risk factors are known.

MECHANISM: Rifampin induces the CYP3A4 metabolism of nilotinib.

CLINICAL EVALUATION: While specific data are limited, the manufacturer of nilotinib notes that the coadministration of ritonavir 600 mg daily for 12 days decreased the mean area under the plasma concentration-time curve of nilotinib by about 80%.[1] Pending further data, observe patients receiving nilotinib and rifampin for diminished nilotinib efficacy.

RELATED DRUGS: Rifabutin (*Mycobutin*) and rifapentine (*Priftin*) are likely to induce the metabolism of nilotinib in a similar manner. The metabolism of dasatinib (*Sprycel*) is also known to be induced by rifampin.

MANAGEMENT OPTIONS:

➡ *Monitor.* If nilotinib is coadministered with rifampin, monitor for signs of reduced efficacy. An increase in the dosage of nilotinib is likely to be required if rifampin is coadministered.

REFERENCES:

1. *Tasigna* [package insert]. East Hanover, NJ: Novartis Pharmaceuticals Corporation; 2007.

Nimodipine

Valproic Acid (eg, *Depakene*)

SUMMARY: Valproic acid increases the area under the plasma concentration-time curve of nimodipine with no effect on the elimination half-life.

RISK FACTORS: No specific risk factors are known.

MECHANISM: Valproic acid appears to inhibit the first-pass metabolism of nimodipine and increases the oral bioavailability.

CLINICAL EVALUATION: Single-dose pharmacokinetic studies of oral nimodipine were done in 3 groups of 8 subjects: healthy control subjects; patients receiving enzyme-induced anticonvulsants (phenobarbital, phenytoin [eg, *Dilantin*], and carbamazepine [eg, *Tegretol*]); and patients receiving valproic acid. The area under the plasma nimodipine concentration-time curve was 7-fold lower in patients taking enzyme-induced anticonvulsants and 50% higher in patients taking valproic acid, compared with healthy controls. The mean elimination half-lives in the control group and in the patients receiving valproic acid were about the same (9.1 vs 8.2 hours); however, the half-life was significantly shorter in the patients receiving the enzyme-inducing anticonvulsants (3.9 hours).[1]

RELATED DRUGS: No information is available.

MANAGEMENT OPTIONS:

➡ *Monitor.* Monitor patients receiving nimodipine and valproic acid for altered nimodipine effect if valproic acid is initiated, discontinued, or changed in dosage.

REFERENCES:

   1. Tartara A, et al. Differential effects of valproic acid and enzyme-inducing anticonvulsants on nimodipine pharmacokinetics in epileptic patients. *Br J Clin Pharmacol.* 1991;32(3):335-340.

5   Nitrazepam

Warfarin (eg, *Coumadin*)

SUMMARY: Nitrazepam does not appear to interact with oral anticoagulants like warfarin.

RISK FACTORS: No specific risk factors are known.

MECHANISM: No interaction.

CLINICAL EVALUATION: In a double-blind study of 22 volunteers, nitrazepam had no significant effect on long-term anticoagulant therapy with phenprocoumon.[†1] One patient on long-term warfarin therapy did not manifest changes in plasma warfarin levels when nitrazepam was given.[2]

RELATED DRUGS: Phenprocoumon is not affected by nitrazepam. Other benzodiazepines probably also have little or no effect on oral anticoagulants.

MANAGEMENT OPTIONS: No interaction.

REFERENCES:

   1. Bieger R, et al. Influence of nitrazepam on oral anticoagulation with phenprocoumon. *Clin Pharmacol Ther.* 1972;13:361-365.

   2. Whitfield JB, et al. Changes in plasma gamma-glutamyl transpeptidase activity associated with alterations in drug metabolism in man. *Br Med J.* 1973;1:316-318.

   † Not available in the United States.

4   Nitrofurantoin (eg, *Macrodantin*)

Phenytoin (eg, *Dilantin*)

SUMMARY: In 1 patient plasma phenytoin concentrations decreased and seizures developed during nitrofurantoin therapy; more study is needed.

RISK FACTORS: No specific risk factors are known.

MECHANISM: Not established.

CLINICAL EVALUATION: In a patient on chronic phenytoin therapy, the plasma phenytoin concentration fell and seizures developed following the initiation of nitrofurantoin therapy.[1] Phenytoin dosage requirements increased during nitrofurantoin treatment and then returned to normal when the nitrofurantoin was stopped. The nitrofurantoin appeared to be responsible for the change in phenytoin concentrations in this patient, but it is not known how commonly this effect occurs in other people.

RELATED DRUGS: No information is available.

MANAGEMENT OPTIONS: No specific action is required, but be alert for evidence of the interaction.

REFERENCES:

1. Heipertz R, et al. Interaction of nitrofurantoin with diphenylhydantoin. *J Neurol.* 1978;218:297-301.

Nitrofurantoin (eg, *Macrodantin*)

Propantheline (eg, *Pro-Banthine*)

SUMMARY: Anticholinergics like propantheline may increase the serum concentration of nitrofurantoin to a limited degree.

RISK FACTORS: No specific risk factors are known.

MECHANISM: Anticholinergic agents may enhance nitrofurantoin bioavailability by slowing GI motility, thus allowing increased dissolution of nitrofurantoin before its arrival in the small intestine where absorption occurs.

CLINICAL EVALUATION: Cumulative urinary excretion of nitrofurantoin in 6 healthy subjects was increased 68% with propantheline 30 mg pretreatment.[1] The clinical significance of these findings is probably limited, but an increase in both therapeutic efficacy and dose-related adverse effects of nitrofurantoin may occur when anticholinergics are coadministered.

RELATED DRUGS: Other anticholinergics may interact similarly.

MANAGEMENT OPTIONS: No specific action is required, but be alert for evidence of the interaction.

REFERENCES:

1. Jaffe JM. Effect of propantheline on nitrofurantoin absorption. *J Pharm Sci.* 1975;64:1729-1730.

Nitroglycerin (eg, *Nitrostat*)

Tadalafil (*Cialis*) `AVOID`

SUMMARY: Blood pressure may be markedly reduced when nitrates are used with tadalafil.

RISK FACTORS: No specific risk factors are known.

MECHANISM: Additive hypotensive effects.

CLINICAL EVALUATION: Phosphodiesterase 5 (PDE5) inhibitors such as sildenafil have resulted in severe hypotensive episodes when combined with nitrates.[1] All PDE5 inhibitors, including tadalafil, can be expected to interact similarly with nitrates. In a controlled study of 150 men, the additive hypotensive effect of tadalafil lasted 24 hours after tadalafil was given, but was not seen 48 hours after tadalafil.[2]

RELATED DRUGS: Tadalafil and other PDE5 inhibitors such as sildenafil (*Viagra*) and vardenafil (*Levitra*) are contraindicated with all nitrates including nitroglycerin, isosorbide mononitrate (eg, *ISMO*), and isosorbide dinitrate (eg, *Isordil*).

MANAGEMENT OPTIONS:

➥ **AVOID COMBINATION.** Tadalafil and nitrates should not be used concurrently.

REFERENCES:

1. *Cialis* [package insert]. Indianapolis, IN: Eli Lilly and Co.; 2004.
2. Kloner RA, et al. Time course of the interaction between tadalafil and nitrates. *J Am Coll Cardiol.* 2003;42:1855-1860.

Nitroglycerin (eg, *Nitrostat*)

AVOID **Vardenafil (*Levitra*)**

SUMMARY: Blood pressure may be markedly reduced when nitrates are used with vardenafil.

RISK FACTORS: No specific risk factors are known.

MECHANISM: Additive hypotensive effects.

CLINICAL EVALUATION: Phosphodiesterase 5 (PDE5) inhibitors such as sildenafil have resulted in severe hypotensive episodes when combined with nitrates.[1] All PDE5 inhibitors, including vardenafil, can be expected to interact similarly with nitrates.

RELATED DRUGS: Vardenafil and other PDE5 inhibitors such as sildenafil (*Viagra*) and tadalafil (*Cialis*) are contraindicated with all nitrates including nitroglycerin, isosorbide mononitrate (eg, *ISMO*), and isosorbide dinitrate (eg, *Isordil*).

MANAGEMENT OPTIONS:

➥ *AVOID COMBINATION.* Vardenafil and nitrates should not be used concurrently.

REFERENCES:

1. *Levitra* [package insert]. Westhaven, CT: Bayer Pharmaceuticals Corp.; 2004.

 Norepinephrine (eg, *Levophed*)

Phenelzine (*Nardil*)

SUMMARY: Monoamine oxidase (MAO) inhibitors may slightly increase the pressor response to norepinephrine.

RISK FACTORS: No specific risk factors are known.

MECHANISM: Catechol-o-methyltransferase appears to be much more important in the metabolism of exogenous norepinephrine than is MAO. Thus, administered norepinephrine should not be affected appreciably by MAO inhibitors. The small enhancement of norepinephrine that occasionally occurs when an MAO inhibitor is coadministered may result from denervation supersensitivity induced by the MAO inhibitor.[1-4]

CLINICAL EVALUATION: In a study in 4 healthy subjects (2 receiving phenelzine and 2 receiving tranylcypromine [*Parnate*]), the administration of norepinephrine did not affect heart rate or blood pressure significantly.[5] Only patients with decreased blood pressure from the MAO inhibitor have manifested a somewhat increased response to norepinephrine.

RELATED DRUGS: Theoretically other nonselective MAO inhibitors, including isocarboxazid (*Marplan*), would interact with norepinephrine in a similar manner.

MANAGEMENT OPTIONS:

➥ *Monitor.* Monitor blood pressure carefully if patients on nonselective MAO inhibitors receive norepinephrine. Remember that the effects of nonselective MAO inhibitors should be assumed to persist for 2 weeks after they are discontinued.

REFERENCES:

1. Boakes AJ. Sympathomimetic amines and antidepressant agents. *Br Med J.* 1973;2:114.

2. Goldberg LI. Monoamine oxidase inhibitors: adverse reactions and possible mechanisms. *JAMA.* 1964;190:456-462.

3. Sjoqvist F. Psychotropic drugs (2). Interaction between monoamine oxidase (MAO) inhibitors and other substances. *Proc R Soc Med.* 1965;58(11 pt 2)):967-978.

4. Ellis J, et al. Modification by monoamine oxidase inhibitors of the effect of some sympathomimetics on blood pressure. *Br Med J.* 1967;2:75.

5. Boakes AJ, et al. Interactions between sympathomimetic amines and antidepressant agents in man. *Br Med J.* 1973;1:311-315.

Norfloxacin (*Noroxin*)

Probenecid

SUMMARY: Probenecid may increase the serum concentration of some quinolones; the clinical significance of this appears to be limited.

RISK FACTORS: No specific risk factors are known.

MECHANISM: Probenecid inhibits the renal tubular secretion of norfloxacin.

CLINICAL EVALUATION: Five healthy subjects received norfloxacin 200 mg alone and with probenecid 1 g.[1] The urinary recovery of norfloxacin was reduced from 28% to 14% of the dose. Because this represents a relatively small portion of the total elimination of norfloxacin, no significant change in serum concentrations was seen. The clinical significance of this interaction is likely to be greater in quinolones when renal elimination comprises most of the body clearance (eg, ofloxacin).

RELATED DRUGS: Other quinolones that are renally eliminated (eg, ofloxacin [eg, *Floxin*]) may be affected by probenecid.

MANAGEMENT OPTIONS: No specific action is required, but be alert for evidence of the interaction.

REFERENCES:
1. Shimada J, et al. Mechanism of renal excretion of AM-715, a new quinolonecarboxylic acid derivative, in rabbits, dogs, and humans. *Antimicrob Agents Chemother.* 1983;23:1-7.

Norfloxacin (*Noroxin*)

Sucralfate (eg, *Carafate*)

SUMMARY: The administration of sucralfate markedly reduces the serum and urine concentrations of norfloxacin and may reduce its clinical efficacy.

RISK FACTORS: No specific risk factors are known.

MECHANISM: Aluminum atoms released from sucralfate in the GI tract bind to norfloxacin and inhibit its absorption.

CLINICAL EVALUATION: Compared with norfloxacin taken alone, the relative bioavailability of norfloxacin was 56.6% when taken 2 hours after sucralfate and 1.8% when taken concomitantly with sucralfate.[1] The mean 12-hour urine norfloxacin concentration was 118.9 mg/L following norfloxacin alone and 6.8 mg/L when sucralfate was administered concomitantly. This marked decrease in bioavailability also was reported by Lehto, et al.[2] and would likely result in subtherapeutic norfloxacin concentrations.

RELATED DRUGS: Aluminum-containing antacids also reduce the absorption of norfloxacin. Sucralfate inhibits the absorption of ciprofloxacin (*Cipro*), fleroxacin,[†] and ofloxacin (*Floxin*).

MANAGEMENT OPTIONS:

➡ *Consider Alternative.* If dosage separation is not possible, an alternative to sucralfate (eg, H₂-receptor antagonist, omeprazole [*Prilosec*], but not an antacid) should be considered.

➡ *Circumvent/Minimize.* Until further information is available, the coadministration of norfloxacin and sucralfate should be avoided. Norfloxacin should be administered several hours before sucralfate.

➡ *Monitor.* If sucralfate and a quinolone are coadministered, monitor the patient for reduced antibiotic efficacy.

REFERENCES:

1. Parpia SH, et al. Sucralfate reduces the gastrointestinal absorption of norfloxacin. *Antimicrob Agents Chemother.* 1989;33:99.

2. Lehto P, et al. Effect of sucralfate on absorption of norfloxacin and ofloxacin. *Antimicrob Agents Chemother.* 1994;38:248.

† Not available in the United States.

Norfloxacin (*Noroxin*)

Theophylline (eg, *Theolair*)

SUMMARY: Norfloxacin may increase the serum concentration of theophylline; however, the increase is unlikely to result in the development of theophylline toxicity in most patients.

RISK FACTORS: No specific risk factors are known.

MECHANISM: The quinolone purportedly is responsible for inhibiting the N-demethylation of theophylline.

CLINICAL EVALUATION: Theophylline clearance usually is reduced minimally (10% to 15%) by the coadministration of norfloxacin (600 to 800 mg/day).[1-5] Norfloxacin appears to have less effect on theophylline concentrations then enoxacin or ciprofloxacin.

RELATED DRUGS: Quinolones reported to inhibit the metabolism of drugs include ciprofloxacin (*Cipro*), enoxacin (*Penetrex*), pipemidic acid, and pefloxacin.[†]

MANAGEMENT OPTIONS:

➡ *Consider Alternative.* Quinolones reported to produce no or minor changes in theophylline pharmacokinetics include fleroxacin,[†] lomefloxacin (*Maxaquin*), ofloxacin (*Floxin*), rufloxacin,[†] and sparfloxacin, (*Zagam*).

➡ *Monitor.* Patients maintained on theophylline are at limited risk to develop theophylline toxicity (palpitations, tachycardia, nausea, tremor) during concomitant administrations of norfloxacin.

REFERENCES:

1. Bowles SK, et al. Effect of norfloxacin on theophylline pharmacokinetics at steady state. *Antimicrob Agents Chemother.* 1988;32:510.

2. Ho G, et al. Evaluation of the effect of norfloxacin on the pharmacokinetics of theophylline. *Clin Pharmacol Ther.* 1989;44:35.

3. Prince RA, et al. The effect of quinolone antibiotics on theophylline pharmacokinetics. *J Clin Pharmacol.* 1989;20:650.

4. Davis RL, et al. The effect of norfloxacin on theophylline metabolism. *Antimicrob Agents Chemother.* 1989;33:212.

5. Sano M, et al. Comparative pharmacokinetics of theophylline following two fluoroquinolones co-administration. *Eur J Clin Pharmacol.* 1987;32:431.

† Not available in the United States.

Norfloxacin (*Noroxin*)

Warfarin (eg, *Coumadin*)

SUMMARY: A patient on chronic warfarin therapy developed excessive hypoprothrombinemia and fatal hemorrhage during therapy with norfloxacin, but a study in healthy subjects suggests that norfloxacin does not affect warfarin response.

RISK FACTORS:

➡ *Concurrent Diseases.* Fever may place a patient at increased risk.

MECHANISM: Not established. There is evidence that norfloxacin is a mild inhibitor of hepatic drug metabolism, and it is possible that warfarin is affected.

CLINICAL EVALUATION: A 91-year-old woman on chronic warfarin therapy and relatively stable prothrombin times was admitted with a brain hemorrhage and excessive hypoprothrombinemia 5 days after she started "full dose" norfloxacin therapy.[1] Although the norfloxacin therapy appears to be the most likely explanation for the excessive warfarin effect, other factors might have contributed to the reaction. For example, it was not stated whether the patient was febrile or whether the patient had stopped taking trimethoprim-sulfamethoxazole (eg, *Bactrim*), a drug known to increase the hypoprothrombinemic response to warfarin. Moreover, in a randomized crossover study, norfloxacin 400 mg/day did not affect the hypoprothrombinemic response to single 30 mg doses of warfarin in 10 healthy men.[2]

RELATED DRUGS: Ciprofloxacin (*Cipro*) and ofloxacin (*Floxin*) have been noted to increase INRs in a few case reports.

MANAGEMENT OPTIONS:

➡ *Monitor.* Until additional information is available, monitor the prothrombin time carefully if norfloxacin therapy is initiated or discontinued in a patient receiving warfarin or other anticoagulants.

REFERENCES:

1. Linville T, et al. Norfloxacin and warfarin. *Ann Intern Med.* 1989;110:751. Letter.

2. Vlasses PH, et al. Warfarin in healthy men. *Pharmacotherapy.* 1988;8:120. Abstract.

Nortriptyline (eg, *Pamelor*)

Pentobarbital (eg, *Nembutal*)

SUMMARY: Pentobarbital may substantially reduce nortriptyline serum concentrations, and probably reduces its therapeutic response.

RISK FACTORS: No specific risk factors are known.

MECHANISM: Pentobarbital probably stimulates the metabolism of nortriptyline.

CLINICAL EVALUATION: Six healthy subjects received nortriptyline (10 mg 3 times daily for 4 weeks) with pentobarbital (200 mg/day) added during weeks 2 and 3.[1] Nortriptyline serum concentrations decreased markedly in all subjects within a few days of the addition of pentobarbital, and the maximal decrease occurred after about 10 days of pentobarbital. The dissipation of the effect appeared somewhat more gradual. The magnitude of the reductions in nortriptyline serum concentrations would be expected to reduce its therapeutic response.

RELATED DRUGS: Other barbiturates probably have a similar effect on nortriptyline. Other tricyclic antidepressants have also been shown to interact with various barbiturates, and one should assume that all barbiturates reduce serum concentrations of all tricyclic antidepressants until proved otherwise.

MANAGEMENT OPTIONS:

➡ **Monitor.** Monitor for altered nortriptyline effect if pentobarbital is initiated, discontinued, or changed in dosage. The same precautions apply to any other combination of a tricyclic antidepressant and a barbiturate.

REFERENCES:

1. von Bahr C, et al. Time course of enzyme induction in humans: effect of pentobarbital on nortriptyline metabolism. *Clin Pharmacol Ther.* 1998;64:18.

Nortriptyline (eg, *Pamelor*)

Rifampin (eg, *Rifadin*)

SUMMARY: Rifampin and isoniazid (eg, *Rifater*) administration appeared to decrease nortriptyline concentrations in 1 patient; the significance of this interaction is not known.

RISK FACTORS: No specific risk factors are known.

MECHANISM: Rifampin appears to increase the metabolism of nortriptyline.

CLINICAL EVALUATION: A 51-year-old man with pulmonary tuberculosis was treated with isoniazid 300 mg/day, rifampin 600 mg/day, pyrazinamide 500 mg 3 times daily, and pyridoxine (eg, *Nestrex*) 25 mg/day.[1] Nortriptyline was initiated for depression; doses slowly were increased to 175 mg/day to produce a serum concentration of 193 nmol/L (therapeutic range: 150 to 500 nmol/L). Pyrazinamide was stopped, but this had no effect on the nortriptyline concentration. Three weeks after the discontinuation of isoniazid and rifampin, the patient complained of drowsiness, and the nortriptyline concentration had risen to 671 nmol/L. The nortriptyline dose was reduced to 75 mg/day and serum concentrations decreased to within the usual therapeutic range. The effect of rifampin on other cyclic antidepressants is unknown.

RELATED DRUGS: If this interaction is confirmed, other cyclic antidepressants also may be affected by rifampin administration.

MANAGEMENT OPTIONS:

➡ *Circumvent/Minimize.* The dose of nortriptyline may have to be adjusted when rifampin is started or discontinued.

➡ *Monitor.* Until information is available, patients taking both nortriptyline and rifampin should be monitored for reduced nortriptyline concentration and effect. Discontinuation of rifampin may result in toxic antidepressant concentrations.

REFERENCES:

1. Bebchuk JM, et al. Drug interaction between rifampin and nortriptyline: a case report. *Int J Psychiatry Med.* 1991;21:183.

Ofloxacin (*Floxin*)

Procainamide (eg, *Procanbid*)

SUMMARY: Ofloxacin administration increases procainamide concentrations; it is possible that some patients may experience clinically significant increases in procainamide effects.

RISK FACTORS: No specific risk factors are known.

MECHANISM: Procainamide is partially eliminated by active renal tubular secretion via the organic cationic transport system. A portion of ofloxacin's renal elimination is also by this system. Ofloxacin appears to be capable of competing with procainamide for renal tubular secretion, resulting in an inhibition of the renal clearance of procainamide.

CLINICAL EVALUATION: Nine healthy subjects received a single oral dose of 1 g procainamide alone and with the fifth dose of ofloxacin 400 mg administered twice daily.[1] Compared with procainamide alone, the administration of ofloxacin resulted in a 30% reduction in the mean renal clearance and a 22% reduction in the mean total clearance of procainamide. N-acetyl procainamide (NAPA) concentrations were not altered by ofloxacin coadministration. No changes in the pharmacodynamics of procainamide were noted by electrocardiographic analysis. Chronic administration of ofloxacin with procainamide could result in an increased procainamide effect in some patients. The effect of procainamide on ofloxacin renal clearance was not assessed.

RELATED DRUGS: Lomefloxacin (*Maxaquin*) also is partially eliminated by the organic cationic transport system and may affect procainamide renal clearance to some degree.[2] The effects of other quinolone antibiotics on procainamide renal clearance are unknown.

MANAGEMENT OPTIONS:

➡ **Monitor.** Patients stabilized on procainamide therapy should have procainamide plasma concentrations monitored during coadministration of ofloxacin. Electrocardiogram monitoring for widened QRS and QTc intervals would be warranted.

REFERENCES:

1. Martin DE, et al. Effects of ofloxacin on the pharmacokinetics and pharmacodynamics of procainamide. *J Clin Pharmacol*. 1996;36:85-91.
2. Hoffler D, et al. Pharmacokinetics of lomefloxacin in normal and impaired renal function. *Acta Ther*. 1989;15:321.

Ofloxacin (*Floxin*)

Sucralfate (*Carafate*)

SUMMARY: The cadministration of sucralfate with ofloxacin results in a marked reduction in ofloxacin serum concentrations and potentially reduced clinical efficacy.

RISK FACTORS: No specific risk factors are known.

MECHANISM: Aluminum atoms released from sucralfate in the GI tract bind to ofloxacin and prevent its absorption.

CLINICAL EVALUATION: Eight healthy subjects received ofloxacin 400 mg on the following 3 occasions: with only water, with 1 g sucralfate, and with 1 g of sucralfate administered 2 hours after the ofloxacin. The mean area under the concentration-time curve (AUC) of ofloxacin was reduced 61% and the peak concentration fell 70% during concomitant sucralfate dosing.[1] This degree of reduction in ofloxacin absorption is likely to reduce its efficacy. Similar effects of sucralfate on ofloxacin have been described; sucralfate administration with food may produce a lesser effect (40% reduction in ofloxacin AUC).[2] Because most of an ofloxacin dose will be absorbed from the GI tract within 2 hours, administering the ofloxacin 2 hours before the sucralfate avoids the interaction.

RELATED DRUGS: Sucralfate also inhibits the absorption of ciprofloxacin (*Cipro*), fleroxacin,[†] and norfloxacin (*Noroxin*). Aluminum-containing antacids also reduce ofloxacin absorption.

MANAGEMENT OPTIONS:

➡ **Consider Alternative.** If dosage separation is not possible, consider an alternative to sucralfate (eg, H_2-receptor antagonist, omeprazole [*Prilosec*], but not an antacid).

➡ **Circumvent/Minimize.** Patients prescribed sucralfate and ofloxacin should avoid coadministration of the 2 agents. To avoid the interaction, the ofloxacin should be taken 2 hours before the sucralfate dose.

➡ **Monitor.** If sucralfate and a quinolone are coadministered, monitor the patient for reduced antibiotic efficacy.

REFERENCES:

1. Lehto P, et al. Effect of sucralfate on absorption of norfloxacin and ofloxacin. *Antimicrob Agents Chemother.* 1994;38:248-251.

2. Kawakami J, et al. The effect of food on the interaction of ofloxacin with sucralfate in healthy volunteers. *Eur J Clin Pharmacol.* 1994;47:67-69.

† Not available in the United States.

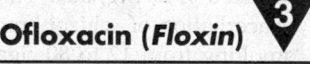

Ofloxacin (*Floxin*)

Warfarin (eg, *Coumadin*)

SUMMARY: Ofloxacin therapy was associated with an increased hypoprothrombinemic response to warfarin in 2 patients, but a causal relationship was not established.

RISK FACTORS:

➡ **Concurrent Diseases.** Fever may place a patient at increased risk.

MECHANISM: Not established.

CLINICAL EVALUATION: Two patients receiving warfarin and other drugs began ofloxacin 600 to 800 mg/day.[1,2] Over the following week, their hypoprothrombinemic response had increased considerably. Warfarin and ofloxacin were stopped, and the hypoprothrombinemic response returned to normal. Although the temporal relationship of the reaction suggests that ofloxacin increased warfarin response, there was no dechallenge or rechallenge with ofloxacin. Confirmation of these reports is needed.

RELATED DRUGS: Ciprofloxacin (*Cipro*) and norfloxacin (*Noroxin*) have been noted to increase international normalized ratios in a few case reports.

MANAGEMENT OPTIONS:

➡ *Monitor.* Until more information is available, monitor patients for an altered hypo-prothrombinemic response to warfarin if ofloxacin is initiated, discontinued, or changed in dosage.

REFERENCES:

1. Leor J, et al. Ofloxacin and warfarin. *Ann Intern Med.* 1988;109:761.
2. Baciewicz AM, et al. Interaction of ofloxacin and warfarin. *Ann Intern Med.* 1993;119:1223.

Olanzapine (eg, *Zyprexa*)

Cigarette Smoking

SUMMARY: Smoking tends to reduce olanzapine plasma concentrations, and smoking cessation may increase the risk of olanzapine toxicity.

RISK FACTORS: No specific risk factors are known.

MECHANISM: Cigarette smoking may induce the metabolism of olanzapine, probably by CYP1A2; discontinuation of smoking results in reduction in CYP1A2 activity and increased olanzapine serum concentrations. The reduction in CYP1A2 activity following cessation of smoking appears quickly, with a half-life decrease in CYP1A2 activity of about 40 hours in 1 study.[1]

CLINICAL EVALUATION: In a study of 19 patients on olanzapine, smokers had about a 5-fold lower concentration-to-dose ratio compared with nonsmokers, suggesting that smoking substantially reduces olanzapine serum concentrations.[2] Another study of 250 patients on olanzapine therapy found dose-adjusted olanzapine concentrations substantially lower in smokers.[3] A 25-year-old man on olanzapine 30 mg/day developed extrapyramidal symptoms after reducing his smoking from 40 to 10 cigarettes per day. His symptoms improved when his olanzapine dose was reduced to 20 mg/day.[4] Another patient taking olanzapine 15 mg/day developed exacerbation of schizophrenic symptoms when he rapidly increased his cigarette smoking from 12 to 80 cigarettes per day.[5] Thus, it appears that smoking affects olanzapine response, and smoking status must be considered in patients on olanzapine.

RELATED DRUGS: Smoking is known to reduce concentrations of clozapine (eg, *Clozaril*), and possibly also thioridazine and chlorpromazine (eg, *Thorazine*).

MANAGEMENT OPTIONS:

➡ *Monitor.* Carefully monitor patients receiving olanzapine for elevated olanzapine concentrations if they stop smoking cigarettes. Patients on olanzapine therapy who start smoking or increase their cigarettes per day are likely to need an increase in olanzapine dosage. Indeed, any change in cigarette smoking may affect olanzapine dosage requirements; monitor patients accordingly.

REFERENCES:

1. Faber MS, Fuhr U. Time response of cytochrome P450 1A2 activity on cessation of heavy smoking. *Clin Pharmacol Ther.* 2004;76:178-184.
2. Carrillo JA, et al. Role of the smoking-induced cytochrome P450 (CYP)1A2 and polymorphic CYP2D6 in steady-state concentration of olanzapine. *J Clin Psychopharmacol.* 2003;23:119-127.
3. Gex-Fabry M, et al. Therapeutic drug monitoring of olanzapine: the combined effect of age, gender, smoking, and comedication. *Ther Drug Monit.* 2003;25:46-53.

4. Zullino DF, et al. Tobacco and cannabis smoking cessation can lead to intoxication with clozapine or olanzapine. *Int Clin Psychopharmacol.* 2002;17:141-143.

5. Chiu CC, et al. Heavy smoking, reduced olanzapine levels, and treatment effects: a case report. *Ther Drug Monit.* 2004;26:579-581.

Olanzapine (eg, *Zyprexa*)

Ritonavir (*Norvir*)

SUMMARY: Ritonavir may reduce olanzapine serum concentrations, but it is not known how often this effect reduces the therapeutic effect of olanzapine.

RISK FACTORS: No specific risk factors are known.

MECHANISM: Not established. It is possible that ritonavir increases the metabolism of olanzapine via CYP1A2 or glucuronide conjugation.

CLINICAL EVALUATION: Fourteen healthy subjects were given a single oral dose of olanzapine with and without pretreatment with ritonavir 600 to 1,000 mg/day for 11 days.[1] Ritonavir was associated with a 53% reduction in the olanzapine area under the plasma concentration-time curve. The magnitude of this effect appears sufficient to reduce the therapeutic response to olanzapine in at least some patients.

RELATED DRUGS: No information is available.

MANAGEMENT OPTIONS:

➡ *Monitor.* If ritonavir and olanzapine are used concurrently, monitor for reduced olanzapine effect and adjust olanzapine dose as needed.

REFERENCES:

1. Penzak SR, et al. Influence of ritonavir on olanzapine pharmacokinetics in healthy volunteers. *J Clin Psychopharmacol.* 2002;22:366-370.

Olanzapine (eg, *Zyprexa*)

Sertraline (*Zoloft*)

SUMMARY: Sertraline does not appear to affect the metabolism of olanzapine.

RISK FACTORS: No specific risk factors are known.

MECHANISM: No interaction.

CLINICAL EVALUATION: The olanzapine serum concentration/daily dose ratio was not different in patients taking olanzapine plus sertraline (n = 21) compared with patients receiving olanzapine without sertraline (n = 134).[1]

RELATED DRUGS: Fluvoxamine is a potent inhibitor of CYP1A2 and has been shown to substantially increase olanzapine serum concentrations. Other selective serotonin reuptake inhibitors such as fluoxetine (eg, *Prozac*), paroxetine (eg, *Paxil*), and citalopram (eg, *Celexa*) are not known to be significant inhibitors of CYP1A2 and theoretically are not expected to interact to the same degree.

MANAGEMENT OPTIONS: No interaction.

REFERENCES:
1. Weigmann H, et al. Fluvoxamine but not sertraline inhibits the metabolism of olanzapine: evidence from a therapeutic drug monitoring service. *Ther Drug Monit.* 2001;23:410-413.

5 | Olanzapine (*Zyprexa*)

Theophylline (eg, *Theolair*)

SUMMARY: Olanzapine does not appear to affect theophylline pharmacokinetics.

RISK FACTORS: No specific risk factors are known.

MECHANISM: No interaction.

CLINICAL EVALUATION: In a randomized, crossover study, 12 healthy subjects received a single intravenous dose of aminophylline 350 mg with and without pretreatment with olanzapine for 9 days (10 mg/day for the last 7 days).[1] Olanzapine had no effect on the pharmacokinetics of theophylline. As a positive control, a similar study of theophylline pharmacokinetics was performed in another group of 7 healthy subjects, but the subjects received cimetidine 1,200 mg/day instead of olanzapine. As expected, cimetidine (eg, *Tagamet*) reduced theophylline clearance 25% and increased the theophylline area under the serum concentration-time curve 46%.

RELATED DRUGS: No information is available.

MANAGEMENT OPTIONS: No interaction.

REFERENCES:
1. Macias WL, et al. Lack of effect of olanzapine on the pharmacokinetics of a single aminophylline dose in healthy men. *Pharmacotherapy.* 1998;18:1237-1248.

Omeprazole (eg, *Prilosec*)

Phenytoin (eg, *Dilantin*)

SUMMARY: Omeprazole modestly increased plasma phenytoin concentrations in healthy subjects given single oral or intravenous (IV) doses of phenytoin. The importance of the interaction in patients on long-term phenytoin therapy has not been established.

RISK FACTORS:

➡ *Dosage Regimen.* Omeprazole dosages of 40 mg/day or more may inhibit phenytoin metabolism.

MECHANISM: Omeprazole may inhibit the hepatic metabolism of phenytoin. Studies of omeprazole with human liver microsomes suggest that omeprazole inhibits the cytochrome P450 (CYP-450) subfamily 2C, which is responsible for the metabolism of phenytoin.[1,2]

CLINICAL EVALUATION: Eight healthy subjects were given a single IV dose of phenytoin 250 mg before and after omeprazole 40 mg/day for 7 days.[3] Omeprazole reduced the plasma clearance of phenytoin 15%. In another study, a single oral dose of phenytoin 300 mg was given before and after omeprazole 40 mg/day for 7 days.[4] The phenytoin area under the concentration-time curve (AUC) increased 25% in the presence of omeprazole. There was considerable intersubject variation in the response, with one subject manifesting a more than 100% increase in the AUC and another manifesting a small decrease. If similar changes in phenytoin pharmacokinetics occur when omeprazole is given to patients on long-term phenytoin therapy, there may be a risk of phenytoin toxicity.

RELATED DRUGS: The effect of lansoprazole (eg, *Prevacid*) on phenytoin is not established, but lansoprazole is less likely to inhibit drug metabolism than omeprazole.

MANAGEMENT OPTIONS:

➡ *Monitor.* Until data on long-term phenytoin therapy are available, monitor for an excessive phenytoin response when omeprazole is started and a reduced phenytoin response when omeprazole is stopped. It may be necessary to adjust the phenytoin dose in some cases.

REFERENCES:

1. Andersson T, et al. Identification of human liver cytochrome P450 isoforms mediating secondary omeprazole metabolism. *Br J Clin Pharmacol.* 1994;37(6):597-604.
2. Andersson T. Omeprazole drug interaction studies. *Clin Pharmacokinet.* 1991;21(3):195-212.
3. Gugler R, et al. Omeprazole inhibits oxidative drug metabolism. Studies with diazepam and phenytoin in vivo and 7-ethoxycoumarin in vitro. *Gastroenterology.* 1985;89(6):1235-1241.
4. Prichard PJ, et al. Oral phenytoin pharmacokinetics during omeprazole therapy. *Br J Clin Pharmacol.* 1987;24(4):543-545.

Omeprazole (eg, *Prilosec*)
Posaconazole (*Noxafil*)

SUMMARY: Omeprazole may reduce the plasma concentration of posaconazole; some loss of antifungal efficacy may be expected.

RISK FACTORS: No specific risk factors are known.

MECHANISM: Elevated gastric pH may reduce posaconazole absorption.

CLINICAL EVALUATION: A patient receiving posaconazole suspension for a fungal infection appeared to have stable plasma posaconazole concentrations.[1] Omeprazole 40 mg was added to his regimen for 3 days. During this time, the patient's posaconazole concentration decreased approximately 50%. Following withdrawal of omeprazole, the posaconazole concentration returned to pre-omeprazole values over the following 20 days. The effect of long-term omeprazole administration on posaconazole is unknown. The posaconazole package insert notes proton pump inhibitors have no clinically relevant effect on posaconazole plasma concentrations, but it does not provide any data in support of this assertion.[2] More data are needed to assess the potential interaction between posaconazole and drugs that increase gastric pH.

RELATED DRUGS: Pending additional data, assume other drugs that lower gastric acidity may also reduce posaconazole plasma concentrations. The bioavailability of ketoconazole (eg, *Nizoral*) and itraconazole (eg, *Sporanox*) is reduced by drugs that increase gastric pH.

MANAGEMENT OPTIONS:

➡ *Consider Alternative.* Oral antifungal agents that are not affected by changes in gastric pH include voriconazole (*Vfend*), terbinafine (eg, *Lamisil*), and fluconazole (eg, *Diflucan*).

➡ *Monitor.* Be alert for reduced antifungal efficacy if posaconazole is coadministered with omeprazole.

REFERENCES:

1. Alffenaar JW, et al.. Omeprazole significantly reduces posaconazole serum trough level. *Clin Infect Dis.* 2009;48(6):839.

2. *Noxafil* [package insert]. Kenilworth, NJ: Schering Corporation; 2008.

Omeprazole (eg, *Prilosec*)

Raltegravir (*Isentress*)

SUMMARY: Omeprazole administration has been reported to increase the concentration of raltegravir; the clinical significance is unknown, but some patients might experience raltegravir adverse reactions with concurrent omeprazole.

RISK FACTORS: No specific risk factors are known.

MECHANISM: Not known; it appears that omeprazole-induced elevation of gastric pH increases the absorption of raltegravir.

CLINICAL EVALUATION: Fourteen healthy subjects received a single dose of raltegravir 400 mg alone and following 4 days of omeprazole 20 mg daily.[1] The mean area under the concentration-time curve and peak concentration of raltegravir were increased by approximately 3- and 4-fold, respectively, following omeprazole pretreatment. The raltegravir half-life was not altered by omeprazole pretreatment. Pending further study, patients receiving raltegravir and omeprazole should be observed for increased raltegravir effect.

RELATED DRUGS: If increased gastric pH is responsible for the observed increase in raltegravir concentrations, other proton pump inhibitors, including esomeprazole (*Nexium*), pantoprazole (eg, *Protonix*), rabeprazole (*AcipHex*), and lansoprazole (eg, *Prevacid*), would be expected to interact with raltegravir in a similar manner. H_2-receptor antagonists (cimetidine [eg, *Tagamet*], ranitidine [eg, *Zantac*]) may also increase raltegravir concentrations.

MANAGEMENT OPTIONS:

➡ *Monitor.* Monitor patients receiving raltegravir and omeprazole for increased raltegravir adverse reactions, such as asthenia, fatigue, headache, insomnia, and nausea.

REFERENCES:

1. Iwamoto M, et al. Effects of omeprazole on plasma levels of raltegravir. *Clin Infect Dis.* 2009;48(4):489-492.

Omeprazole (eg, *Prilosec*)

Saquinavir (*Invirase*)

SUMMARY: Omeprazole administration increases the plasma concentrations of saquinavir. Some patients may experience increased adverse reactions.

RISK FACTORS: No significant risk factors are known.

MECHANISM: Unknown. Omeprazole may increase saquinavir absorption and plasma concentrations by affecting transporters of saquinavir or increasing gastric pH.

CLINICAL EVALUATION: Eighteen healthy subjects received oral tablets containing saquinavir 1,000 mg and ritonavir 100 mg twice daily for 15 days.[1] On days 11 to 16, omeprazole 40 mg was administered once daily. The coadministration of omeprazole resulted in a mean increase in saquinavir plasma area under the concentration-time curve of 82%.

RELATED DRUGS: Other formulations of saquinavir (eg, saquinavir hard capsules) may be affected in a similar manner. Other drugs increasing gastric pH (eg, ranitidine [eg, *Zantac*]) have been reported to increase saquinavir concentrations.[2] Other proton pump inhibitors may also increase saquinavir plasma concentrations.

MANAGEMENT OPTIONS:

➡ ***Monitor.*** Monitor patients receiving omeprazole and saquinavir for elevated saquinavir plasma concentrations and signs of toxicity (eg, fatigue, GI complaints, and hyperglycemia).

REFERENCES:

1. Winston A, et al. Effect of omeprazole on the pharmacokinetics of saquinavir-500 mg formulation with ritonavir in healthy male and female volunteers. *AIDS*. 2006;20(10):1401-1406.
2. *Invirase* [package insert]. Nutley, NJ: Roche Laboratories Inc; 2007.

Omeprazole (eg, *Prilosec*)

St. John's Wort

SUMMARY: St. John's wort substantially reduced omeprazole plasma concentrations in healthy subjects, but the clinical importance of this effect is not established.

RISK FACTORS:

➡ ***Pharmacogenetics.*** The reduction in omeprazole plasma concentrations was slightly greater in extensive metabolizers (EMs) of CYP2C19 (44% decrease) compared with poor metabolizers (PMs) of CYP2C19 (38% decrease). The difference in peak plasma concentrations was also larger in EMs, with a 50% decrease in EMs and 38% decrease in PMs.

MECHANISM: St. John's wort appeared to enhance the metabolism of omeprazole by CYP2C19 and CYP3A4.

CLINICAL EVALUATION: In healthy subjects taking St. John's wort for 14 days, omeprazole area under the plasma concentration-time curve was reduced 44% in EMs of CYP2C19.[1] The magnitude of this effect may be sufficient to reduce omeprazole efficacy, but additional study is needed. Because herbal medications are generally not standardized, individual brands may interact differently because of varying amounts of active ingredient, additional ingredients not on the label, and, in some cases, no active ingredients at all. Moreover, different lots of the same brand may vary substantially.

RELATED DRUGS: The effect of St. John's wort on other proton pump inhibitors is not established, but some are also metabolized by cytochrome P450 isozymes.

MANAGEMENT OPTIONS:

➡ *Monitor.* Monitor for reduced omeprazole response when St. John's wort is taken concurrently.

REFERENCES:
1. Wang LS, et al. St. John's wort induces both cytochrome P450 3A4-catalyzed suloxidation and 2C19-dependent hydroxylation of omeprazole. *Clin Pharmacol Ther.* 2004;75(3):191-197.

Omeprazole (eg, *Prilosec*)

Tacrolimus (*Prograf*)

SUMMARY: Drug interaction studies using human liver microsomes in vitro suggest that omeprazole inhibits the metabolism of tacrolimus. Watch for excessive tacrolimus levels if the drugs are used concurrently.

RISK FACTORS: No specific risk factors are known.

MECHANISM: Tacrolimus is metabolized by CYP3A4; omeprazole appears to inhibit this process.

CLINICAL EVALUATION: Thirty-four drugs were tested for interactions with tacrolimus using in vitro human liver microsomal preparations.[1] Omeprazole was found to inhibit tacrolimus metabolism. Although the clinical importance of this finding is not established, in vitro human microsomal studies have been remarkably accurate in predicting which drugs will interact in the clinical setting.

RELATED DRUGS: The effect of omeprazole on cyclosporine (eg, *Neoral*) is not established, but cyclosporine and tacrolimus tend to have similar interactions.

MANAGEMENT OPTIONS: No specific action is required, but be alert for evidence of the interaction.

REFERENCES:
1. Christians U, et al. Identification of drugs inhibiting the in vitro metabolism of tacrolimus by human liver microsomes. *Br J Clin Pharmacol.* 1996;41(3):187-190.

Omeprazole (eg, *Prilosec*)

Tolbutamide (eg, *Orinase*)

SUMMARY: Omeprazole causes a small increase in tolbutamide concentrations; the clinical significance of this change is likely to be limited.

RISK FACTORS: No specific risk factors are known.

MECHANISM: Not established. Omeprazole may inhibit the metabolism of tolbutamide to a small extent.

CLINICAL EVALUATION: Sixteen healthy subjects received a single dose of tolbutamide 500 mg alone and after 7 days of omeprazole 40 mg/day.[1] The coadministration of omeprazole increased the area under the plasma concentration-time curve of tolbutamide 10%.

RELATED DRUGS: Omeprazole could affect other sulfonylureas in a similar manner.

MANAGEMENT OPTIONS: No specific action is required, but be alert for evidence of the interaction.

REFERENCES:

1. Toon S, et al. Effects of cimetidine, ranitidine and omeprazole on tolbutamide pharmacokinetics. *J Pharm Pharmacol.* 1995;47:85.

Omeprazole (eg, *Prilosec*)

Trovafloxacin†

SUMMARY: Omeprazole administration modestly reduces the plasma concentrations of trovafloxacin; the clinical significance may be greater with chronic omeprazole administration.

RISK FACTORS:

➥ *Pharmacogenetics.* Patients who are slow metabolizers of omeprazole will have greater acid suppression and would likely demonstrate a more profound reduction in trovafloxacin absorption.

MECHANISM: Trovafloxacin absorption may be reduced by the suppression of gastric acid.

CLINICAL EVALUATION: Twelve healthy subjects received trovafloxacin 300 mg with water and following omeprazole 20 mg administered the night prior to and 2 hours before the trovafloxacin dose.[1] The mean area under the concentration-time curve of trovafloxacin was reduced 18%, and peak trovafloxacin concentrations fell more than 30% following the 2 doses of omeprazole compared with administration with water. Because omeprazole requires up to 5 days to reach maximal acid suppression, the effect of omeprazole on trovafloxacin demonstrated in this study is likely to understate the effect observed in clinical situations.

RELATED DRUGS: The effect of omeprazole on other fluoroquinolone antibiotics is unknown. If the mechanism of this interaction involves the reduction of gastric acid, other proton pump inhibitors (eg, esomeprazole [*Nexium*], lansoprazole [*Prevacid*], pantoprazole [*Protonix*], rabeprazole [*Aciphex*]) are likely to affect trovafloxacin in a similar manner. H_2-receptor antagonists such as cimetidine (eg, *Tagamet*) or ranitidine (eg, *Zantac*) also may reduce trovafloxacin absorption.

MANAGEMENT OPTIONS:

➥ *Monitor.* Pending further information on this interaction, monitor for adequate antibiotic response when trovafloxacin is coadministered with acid suppression therapy.

REFERENCES:

1. Teng R, et al. Effect of *Maalox* and omeprazole on the bioavailability of trovafloxacin. *J Antimicrob Chemother.* 1997;39(suppl B):93-97.

† No longer available in the United States.

Omeprazole (eg, _Prilosec_)

Voriconazole (_Vfend_)

SUMMARY: Voriconazole increases omeprazole plasma concentrations; some increase in side effects may be expected.

RISK FACTORS:

➡ **_Pharmacogenetics._** Patients who are poor metabolizers for CYP2C19 will have higher voriconazole and omeprazole concentrations, and thus are likely to have an interaction of larger magnitude.

MECHANISM: Omeprazole is primarily metabolized by CYP2C19, with CYP3A4 contributing to its elimination. Voriconazole inhibits both of these pathways, resulting in a marked increase in omeprazole plasma concentrations.

CLINICAL EVALUATION: Based on limited information provided by the manufacturer, voriconazole (200 mg every 12 hours for 7 days) increased the area under the concentration-time curve and peak concentration of omeprazole (40 mg/day for 7 days) nearly 4- and 2-fold, respectively.[1] Some patients may experience an increase in omeprazole-induced adverse effects during voriconazole coadministration.

RELATED DRUGS: Esomeprazole (_Nexium_), lansoprazole (_Prevacid_), and pantoprazole (_Protonix_) are also metabolized by CYP2C19 and CYP3A4 and probably are affected by voriconazole in a similar manner. Rabeprazole (_Aciphex_) has minimal dependence on CYP2C19 and CYP3A4 for its metabolism and may be less affected by voriconazole coadministration. Ketoconazole (eg, _Nizoral_), itraconazole (eg, _Sporanox_), and fluconazole (eg, _Diflucan_) may increase omeprazole plasma concentrations.

MANAGEMENT OPTIONS:

➡ **_Circumvent/Minimize._** Reduction of the dose of the proton pump inhibitors (PPIs) may be necessary. The use of rabeprazole may lessen the likelihood of adverse effects during voriconazole coadministration.

➡ **_Monitor._** While PPIs are generally well tolerated, be alert for increased side effects (eg, diarrhea, headache) if voriconazole is coadministered with PPIs metabolized by CYP2C19 or CYP3A4.

REFERENCES:

1. _Vfend_ [package insert]. New York, NY: Pfizer, Inc.; 2002.

 Omeprazole (_Prilosec_)

Warfarin (eg, _Coumadin_)

SUMMARY: Omeprazole slightly increases the hypoprothrombinemic response to warfarin in healthy subjects, but the frequency with which there would be a clinically important increase in warfarin response in patients is not established.

RISK FACTORS:

➡ **_Dosage Regimen._** The ability of omeprazole to inhibit CYP2C9 is probably dose related with 20 mg/day producing only minor inhibition in most patients.

MECHANISM: Omeprazole probably inhibits the hepatic metabolism of warfarin. In vitro studies have shown that omeprazole, like cimetidine (eg, *Tagamet*), inhibits the metabolism of another coumarin, 7-ethoxycoumarin.[1,2]

CLINICAL EVALUATION: Twenty-one healthy subjects were given warfarin for 3 weeks in doses sufficient to reduce their vitamin K-dependent clotting factors 10% to 20% of normal.[3] Warfarin was continued for an additional 2 weeks with addition of placebo or omeprazole 20 mg/day in a randomized, crossover manner. Omeprazole produced a slight (12%) increase in the mean plasma concentration of the less potent warfarin enantiomer, R-warfarin, but did not significantly affect the more active S-warfarin. The Thrombotest values decreased 11%, indicating that omeprazole produced a slight increase in the hypoprothrombinemic response to warfarin. In a randomized, crossover study of 35 patients on chronic warfarin, omeprazole (20 mg/day) had no effect on the hypoprothrombinemic response.[4] Although these results suggest that omeprazole has minimal effects on the hypoprothrombinemic response to warfarin, the results cannot automatically be extended to doses of omeprazole more than 20 mg/day. A 78-year-old woman on acenocoumarol developed hematuria and a marked increase in her INR 5 days after starting omeprazole. Although there was a positive dechallenge, a causal relationship was not established conclusively.[5] Nonetheless, it seems likely that at least an occasional patient on warfarin will manifest a clinically important increase in hypoprothrombinemic response because of the interaction with omeprazole.

RELATED DRUGS: The effect of omeprazole on oral anticoagulants other than warfarin and acenocoumarol is not established.

MANAGEMENT OPTIONS: No specific action is required, but be alert for evidence of the interaction.

REFERENCES:
1. Jensen JC, et al. Inhibition of human liver cytochrome P-450 by omeprazole. *Br J Clin Pharmacol.* 1986;21:328-330.
2. Gugler R, et al. Omeprazole inhibits oxidative drug metabolism: studies with diazepam and phenytoin in vivo and 7-ethoxycoumarin in vitro. *Gastroenterology.* 1985;89:1235-1241.
3. Sutfin T, et al. Stereoselective interaction omeprazole with warfarin in healthy men. *Ther Drug Monit.* 1989;11:176-184.
4. Unge P, et al. A study of the interaction of omeprazole and warfarin in anticoagulated patients. *Br J Clin Pharmacol.* 1992;34:509.
5. Garcia B, et al. Possible potentiation of anticoagulant effect of acenocoumarol by omeprazole. *Pharm World Sci.* 1994;16:231.

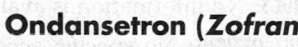

Ondansetron (*Zofran*)

Rifampin (eg, *Rifadin*)

SUMMARY: Rifampin increases the metabolism of ondansetron; a loss of antiemetic activity may result.

RISK FACTORS: No specific risk factors are known.

MECHANISM: Rifampin increases the metabolism and reduces the bioavailability of ondansetron, probably by inducing the activity of CYP3A4 and CYP1A2, enzymes known to metabolize ondansetron.

CLINICAL EVALUATION: Ten healthy subjects were administered oral or IV ondansetron following 5 days of pretreatment with placebo or rifampin 600 mg once daily.[1] Compared with placebo, the area under the concentration-time curve (AUC) of orally administered ondansetron was reduced 65% following rifampin. Ondansetron bioavailability was reduced from 60% to 40% following rifampin pretreatment. Rifampin increased the systemic clearance of IV ondansetron 83% and reduced its AUC 48%. The half-life of IV ondansetron was reduced 46% following rifampin. A reduction in the antiemetic effect of ondansetron is likely to occur during the coadministration of rifampin.

RELATED DRUGS: Rifabutin (*Mycobutin*) would be likely to affect ondansetron in a similar manner.

MANAGEMENT OPTIONS:

➡ *Monitor.* Observe patients receiving ondansetron and rifampin or other potent inducers of CYP3A4 or CYP1A2 for reduced antiemetic effect. Increased ondansetron doses may be required for effective antiemetic control.

REFERENCES:

1. Villikka K, et al. The effect of rifampin on the pharmacokinetics of oral and intravenous ondansetron. *Clin Pharmacol Ther*. 1999;65:377-381.

 Ondansetron (eg, *Zofran*)

Tramadol (*Ultram*)

SUMMARY: In a study of patients undergoing lumbar surgery, ondansetron appeared to reduce the analgesic effect of tramadol.

RISK FACTORS: No specific risk factors are known.

MECHANISM: Not established. Part of the analgesic effect of tramadol is caused by inhibition of serotonin (5-HT) reuptake, and it is possible that ondansetron-induced antagonism of 5-HT$_3$ receptors may inhibit this action of tramadol.

CLINICAL EVALUATION: In a randomized, double-blind study, 40 patients undergoing lumbar laminectomy were given ondansetron 4 mg or saline immediately prior to anesthesia.[1] After the procedure, patients who had been given ondansetron prior to surgery required somewhat more tramadol than control patients given saline, suggesting that the ondansetron reduced the analgesic efficacy of tramadol. Also, ondansetron did not reduce the incidence of postoperative nausea and vomiting during the 24 hours after surgery. More study is needed to determine the clinical importance of this interaction.

RELATED DRUGS: No information is available.

MANAGEMENT OPTIONS: No specific action is required, but be alert for evidence of the interaction.

REFERENCES:

1. De Witte JL, et al. The analgesic efficacy of tramadol is impaired by concurrent administration of ondansetron. *Anesth Analg*. 2001;92:1319-1321.

Orange Juice

Fexofenadine (*Allegra*)

SUMMARY: Ingestion of large amounts of orange juice reduces the absorption of fexofenadine, and may reduce fexofenadine efficacy.

RISK FACTORS: No specific risk factors are known.

MECHANISM: In vitro studies suggest that orange juice inhibits organic anion transporting polypeptide (OATP), a transporter involved in the intestinal absorption of fexofenadine.

CLINICAL EVALUATION: In a randomized, crossover study in 10 healthy subjects, a single oral 120 mg dose of fexofenadine was given with water and with orange juice (1.2 L over 3 hours).[1] Orange juice was associated with a 63% reduction in fexofenadine plasma concentrations. The magnitude of this effect appears sufficient to reduce the efficacy of fexofenadine in at least some patients. However, the amount of orange juice used in this study was larger than most people consume, and smaller amounts of orange juice would probably have less effect.

RELATED DRUGS: Apple juice and grapefruit juice also appear to reduce fexofenadine bioavailability.

MANAGEMENT OPTIONS:

➡ **Circumvent/Minimize.** Until more data are available, take fexofenadine with water rather than orange juice or other fruit juices.

REFERENCES:

1. Dresser GK, et al. Fruit juices inhibit organic anion transporting polypeptide-mediated drug uptake to decrease the oral availability of fexofenadine. *Clin Pharmacol Ther.* 2002;71:11-20.

Orlistat (*Xenical*) **4**

Amiodarone (eg, *Cordarone*)

SUMMARY: Orlistat modestly reduced amiodarone serum concentrations, but the clinical importance of this effect is not established.

RISK FACTORS: No specific risk factors are known.

MECHANISM: Orlistat appears to reduce the bioavailability of amiodarone.

CLINICAL EVALUATION: In a double-blind, randomized parallel study 16 healthy subjects received a single 1,200 mg dose of amiodarone after several days of orlistat 120 mg 3 times/day, and 16 other subjects received amiodarone with placebo in the same manner.[1] Amiodarone area under the concentration-time curve was 27% lower in the subjects receiving orlistat than in those receiving placebo. The clinical importance of this effect is not clear because the effect appears to be modest. It is possible that initiation of orlistat in a patient stabilized on amiodarone could result in reduced amiodarone efficacy.

RELATED DRUGS: No information is available.

MANAGEMENT OPTIONS: No specific action is required, but be alert for evidence of the interaction.

REFERENCES:

1. Zhi J, et al. Effects of orlistat, a lipase inhibitor, on the pharmacokinetics of three highly lipophilic drugs (amiodarone, fluoxetine, and simvastatin) in healthy volunteers. *J Clin Pharmacol*. 2003;43:428-435.

 Orlistat (*Xenical*)

Cyclosporine (eg, *Neoral*)

SUMMARY: Pharmacokinetic studies and case reports suggest that orlistat can reduce cyclosporine blood concentrations; avoid concurrent therapy.

RISK FACTORS: No specific risk factors are known.

MECHANISM: Not established.

CLINICAL EVALUATION: In a randomized, crossover study of 30 healthy subjects, orlistat (120 mg 3 times/day for 6 days) reduced cyclosporine blood concentrations by approximately 30%.[1] The cyclosporine was given as *Neoral* in a dose of 50 mg twice daily. In a third arm of the study, orlistat was given 3 hours before the cyclosporine instead of concurrently, but the interaction still occurred. Given that orlistat generally is given 3 times/day, it would be difficult to space doses of the drugs enough to avoid the interaction. The FDA received several reports of sub-therapeutic cyclosporine blood concentrations occurring after initiation of orlistat therapy.[2] The details of these cases have not been published, but they are consistent with the pharmacokinetic results.

RELATED DRUGS: The effect of orlistat on tacrolimus (*Prograf*) and sirolimus (*Rapamune*) is not established.

MANAGEMENT OPTIONS:

➡ ***Avoid Unless Benefit Outweighs Risk.*** Because alterations in cyclosporine blood concentrations can have serious consequences, it would be best to avoid this combination.

➡ ***Monitor.*** If the combination is used, monitor cyclosporine blood concentrations carefully and adjust cyclosporine dosage as needed.

REFERENCES:

1. Zhi J, et al. Pharmacokinetic evaluation of the possible interaction between selected concomitant medications and orlistat at steady state in healthy subjects. *J Clin Pharmacol*. 2002;42:1011-1019.

2. Colman E, et al. Reduction in blood cyclosporine concentrations by orlistat. *N Engl J Med*. 2000;342:1141-1142.

5 **Orlistat (*Xenical*)**

Fluoxetine (eg, *Prozac*)

SUMMARY: Orlistat does not appear to affect the pharmacokinetics of fluoxetine.

RISK FACTORS: None (no interaction).

MECHANISM: None (no interaction).

CLINICAL EVALUATION: In a double-blind, randomized, crossover study, 24 healthy subjects received a single 40 mg dose of fluoxetine with and without pretreatment with several days of orlistat 120 mg 3 times/day.[1] Fluoxetine pharmacokinetics were not significantly affected by orlistat.

RELATED DRUGS: No information is available.

MANAGEMENT OPTIONS: No interaction.

REFERENCES:
1. Zhi J, et al. Effects of orlistat, a lipase inhibitor, on the pharmacokinetics of three highly lipophilic drugs (amiodarone, fluoxetine, and simvastatin) in healthy volunteers. *J Clin Pharmacol.* 2003;43:428-435.

Orlistat (*Xenical*) 5

Phentermine (eg, *Ionamin*)

SUMMARY: Orlistat did not affect phentermine pharmacokinetics in healthy subjects.

RISK FACTORS: No specific risk factors are known.

MECHANISM: None (no interaction).

CLINICAL EVALUATION: In a randomized, crossover study in 20 healthy subjects, orlistat (120 mg 3 times/day for 7 days) did not affect phentermine pharmacokinetics.[1]

RELATED DRUGS: No information is available.

MANAGEMENT OPTIONS: No interaction.

REFERENCES:
1. Zhi J, et al. Pharmacokinetic evaluation of the possible interaction between selected concomitant medications and orlistat at steady state in healthy subjects. *J Clin Pharmacol.* 2002;42:1011-1019.

Orlistat (*Xenical*) 5

Simvastatin (*Zocor*)

SUMMARY: Orlistat does not appear to affect the pharmacokinetics of simvastatin.

RISK FACTORS: None (no interaction).

MECHANISM: None (no interaction).

CLINICAL EVALUATION: In a double-blind, randomized crossover study, 29 healthy subjects received a single 80 mg dose of simvastatin with and without pretreatment with several days of orlistat 120 mg 3 times/day.[1] Simvastatin pharmacokinetics were not significantly affected by orlistat.

RELATED DRUGS: No information is available.

MANAGEMENT OPTIONS: No interaction.

REFERENCES:
1. Zhi J, et al. Effects of orlistat, a lipase inhibitor, on the pharmacokinetics of three highly lipophilic drugs (amiodarone, fluoxetine, and simvastatin) in healthy volunteers. *J Clin Pharmacol.* 2003;43:428-435.

Orlistat (*Xenical*)

Warfarin (eg, *Coumadin*)

SUMMARY: A patient developed increased warfarin response after starting orlistat, but a causal relationship was not established.

RISK FACTORS: No specific risk factors are known.

MECHANISM: Not established. It is possible that orlistat reduced vitamin K absorption in this patient.

CLINICAL EVALUATION: A 66-year-old man on chronic warfarin therapy was found to have an increased INR (4.7) 18 days after starting orlistat therapy (120 mg 3 times/day).[1] He was eventually stabilized on a lower dose of warfarin. A previous study found no effect of orlistat on warfarin response after single doses of warfarin in healthy subjects,[2] but these findings do not rule out an effect in patients receiving chronic doses of warfarin. More data are needed to establish the clinical importance of this purported interaction.

RELATED DRUGS: No information is available.

MANAGEMENT OPTIONS: No specific action is required, but be alert for evidence of the interaction.

REFERENCES:
1. MacWalter RS, et al. Orlistat enhances warfarin effect. *Ann Pharmacother*. 2003;37:510-512.
2. Zhi J, et al. The effect of orlistat on the pharmacokinetics and pharmacodynamics of warfarin in healthy volunteers. *J Clin Pharmacol*. 1996;36:659-656.

4 **Orphenadrine (eg, *Norflex*)**

Propoxyphene (eg, *Darvon*)

SUMMARY: Isolated reports of mental confusion, anxiety, and tremors in patients on propoxyphene and orphenadrine have been published, but a causal relationship is not established.

RISK FACTORS: No specific risk factors are known.

MECHANISM: Not established. If an interaction between propoxyphene and orphenadrine exists, it may be caused by an undefined combined effect on the CNS. Another possible mechanism is the production of hypoglycemia, as hypoglycemic activity has been attributed to propoxyphene[1] and orphenadrine[2]; furthermore, the symptoms attributed to this interaction are similar to those that may occur during a hypoglycemic episode. Another possibility is that propoxyphene impairs the hepatic metabolism of orphenadrine.

CLINICAL EVALUATION: Not established. Although the manufacturer of *Norflex* warns about an interaction with propoxyphene,[3] communications with health care providers from the manufacturers of *Norflex* and *Darvon* indicate that evidence for an interaction is not impressive.[4,5] The warning is apparently based on a few reports of reactions following the use of both drugs.[5] There is little doubt that many patients have received these 2 drugs concomitantly with no apparent adverse effects, and it may be that if the interaction occurs, it is only in an occasional predisposed patient.

RELATED DRUGS: No information is available.

MANAGEMENT OPTIONS: No specific action is required, but be alert for evidence of the interaction.

REFERENCES:
1. Wiederholt IC, et al. Recurrent episodes of hypoglycemia induced by propoxyphene. *Neurology.* 1967;17:703-706.
2. Buckle RM, et al. Hypoglyceamic coma occurring during treatment with chlorpromazine and orphenadrine. *Br Med J.* 1967;4:599-600.
3. Product information. Orphenadrine (*Norflex*). 3M Pharmaceuticals. 1992.
4. Maxwell SB. Personal communication. March 31, 1970.
5. Silverglade A. Personal communication. April 10, 1970.

Oxacillin (eg, *Bactocill*) **4**

Sulfamethoxypyridazine

SUMMARY: Oxacillin serum concentrations may be reduced by some sulfonamides (eg, sulfamethoxypyridazine), but the clinical significance of this effect is unknown.

RISK FACTORS: No specific risk factors are known.

MECHANISM: Some sulfonamides appear to inhibit the gastrointestinal absorption of oxacillin; others may reduce the elimination of penicillin G.

CLINICAL EVALUATION: In 1 study, sulfamethoxypyridazine and sulfaethidole given in conjunction with oxacillin resulted in decreased oxacillin serum concentrations and urinary recovery.[1] However, the doses of both the oxacillin and the sulfonamides were higher than normal, and the significance of these findings for patients on multiple-dosing schedules with standard doses has not been established. In another report preliminary evidence was presented that sulfaphenazole (but not sulfamethizole or sulfamethoxypyridazine) prolonged the half-life of penicillin G.[2]

RELATED DRUGS: Some sulfonamides may reduce oxacillin serum concentrations.

MANAGEMENT OPTIONS: No specific action is required, but be alert for evidence of the interaction.

REFERENCES:
1. Kunin CM. Clinical pharmacology of the new penicillins. II. Effect of drugs which interfere with binding to serum proteins. *Clin Pharmacol Ther.* 1966;7:180.
2. Kampmann J, et al. Effect of some drugs on penicillin half-life in blood. *Clin Pharmacol Ther.* 1972;13:516.

Oxazepam (eg, *Serax*) **4**

Paroxetine (*Paxil*)

SUMMARY: Paroxetine appears to have mixed effects on oxazepam-induced psychomotor impairment, but the overall effect is probably of minimal clinical importance.

RISK FACTORS: No specific risk factors are known.

MECHANISM: Not established.

CLINICAL EVALUATION: Eleven healthy subjects were given single oral 30 mg doses of oxazepam with and without pretreatment with paroxetine 30 mg/day.[1] Paroxetine actually tended to antagonize oxazepam-induced impairment of certain psycho-motor tests, but the subjective assessment of sedation was somewhat higher with oxazepam plus paroxetine than with oxazepam alone. A subsequent report apparently was based on the same data.[2] In 6 healthy subjects oxazepam did not affect the pharmacokinetics of paroxetine, but few details of the study were presented.[3]

RELATED DRUGS: The effect of selective serotonin reuptake inhibitors other than paroxetine on oxazepam is not established.

MANAGEMENT OPTIONS: No specific action is required, but be alert for evidence of the interaction.

REFERENCES:

1. McClelland GR, et al. Paroxetine and oxazepam: effects on psychomotor performance. *Br J Clin Pharmacol.* 1986;23:117P. Abstract.

2. Cooper SM, et al. The psychomotor effects of paroxetine alone and in combination with haloperidol, amylobarbitone, oxazepam, or alcohol. *Acta Psychiatr Scand.* 1989;80(suppl 350):53.

3. Kaye CM, et al. A review of the metabolism and pharmacokinetics of paroxetine in man. *Acta Psychiatr Scand.* 1989;80(suppl 350):60.

---

4   Oxazepam (eg, *Serax*)

Zidovudine (eg, *Retrovir*)

SUMMARY: The combined administration of oxazepam and zidovudine has minimal effects on the pharmacokinetics of the drugs, but increased headaches have been reported.

RISK FACTORS: No specific risk factors are known.

MECHANISM: Not established.

CLINICAL EVALUATION: Six patients with human immunodeficiency virus were studied after oral zidovudine alone (100 mg every 4 hours for 12 hours) and after coadministration of oxazepam (15 mg every 8 hours for 48 hours). Single 30 mg doses of oxazepam and 70 mg doses of zidovudine IV were also administered.[1] Oxazepam administration had no significant effect on zidovudine pharmacokinetics, although the bioavailability of zidovudine was increased 23%. Headaches were more frequent when both drugs were taken concomitantly. Zidovudine administration increased oxazepam clearance after oral administration 14%. It is unlikely that this degree of change will result in any clinically important change in response to oxazepam.

RELATED DRUGS: No information is available.

MANAGEMENT OPTIONS: No specific action is required, but be alert for evidence of the interaction.

REFERENCES:

1. Mole L, et al. Pharmacokinetics of zidovudine alone and in combination with oxazepam in the HIV infected patient. *J Acquir Immune Defic Syndr.* 1993;6:56.

Oxycodone (eg, *Oxycontin*)

Rifampin (eg, *Rifadin*)

SUMMARY: Oxycodone concentrations are reduced during rifampin coadministration; loss of analgesic effect may occur.

RISK FACTORS: No specific risk factors are known.

MECHANISM: Rifampin increases the metabolism of oxycodone via the CYP3A4 pathway.

CLINICAL EVALUATION: Twelve subjects received either placebo or rifampin 600 mg daily for 7 days.[1] Oxycodone was administered on 2 separate occasions (a 0.1 mg/kg intravenous [IV] dose or a 15 mg oral dose) on day 6 of rifampin dosing. Rifampin treatment reduced the mean area under the concentration-time curve (AUC) of IV oxycodone 53% and the AUC of oral oxycodone 86%. The half-life of oxycodone was reduced approximately 40% by pretreatment with rifampin. This magnitude of reduction in oxycodone concentration is likely to result in a diminution of oxycodone's analgesic efficacy and its adverse reactions.

RELATED DRUGS: Rifabutin (*Mycobutin*) and rifapentine (*Priftin*) are known to induce CYP3A4 and are likely to affect oxycodone in a similar manner as rifampin.

MANAGEMENT OPTIONS:

➡ *Monitor.* Monitor patients taking oxycodone for reduced analgesic effect if rifampin is coadministered.

REFERENCES:
1. Nieminen TH, et al. Rifampin greatly reduces the plasma concentrations of intravenous and oral oxycodone. *Anesthesiology.* 2009;110(6):1371-1378.

Oxycodone (eg, *Percodan*)

Ritonavir (*Norvir*)

SUMMARY: Ritonavir increases the plasma concentration of oxycodone; subjects reported an increase in the subjective effects of oxycodone during ritonavir coadministration.

RISK FACTORS: No specific risk factors are known.

MECHANISM: Ritonavir inhibits CYP3A4.

CLINICAL EVALUATION: Twelve subjects were administered ritonavir 300 mg, lopinavir 400 mg/ritonavir 100 mg, or placebo twice daily for 4 days.[1] On the third day of each regimen, a single dose of oxycodone 10 mg was given orally. The concurrent dosing of ritonavir and lopinavir/ritonavir increased oxycodone's mean area under the concentration-time curve 3- and 2.5-fold, respectively. The conversion of oxycodone to oxymorphone was also increased. Studies of this interaction during long-term dosing are needed to assess the potential for adverse outcomes in patients.

RELATED DRUGS: Atazanavir (*Reyataz*), darunavir (*Prezista*), fosamprenavir (*Lexiva*), indinavir (*Crixivan*), nelfinavir (*Viracept*), and saquinavir (*Invirase*) also inhibit the activity of CYP3A4 and are expected to increase the plasma concentrations of oxycodone. Other analgesics (eg, fentanyl) that are metabolized by CYP3A4 are affected in a similar manner by ritonavir.

MANAGEMENT OPTIONS:

➡ **Monitor.** Carefully monitor patients requiring oxycodone and ritonavir for excessive narcotic effects, including dizziness, respiratory depression, and sedation.

REFERENCES:

1. Nieminen TH, et al. Oxycodone concentrations are greatly increased by the concomitant use of ritonavir or lopinavir/ritonavir. *Eur J Clin Pharmacol.* 2010;66(10):977-985.

Oxycodone (eg, *OxyContin*)

Sertraline (eg, *Zoloft*)

SUMMARY: Isolated case reports suggest that concurrent therapy with oxycodone and sertraline (or other selective serotonin reuptake inhibitors [SSRIs]) may increase the risk of serotonin syndrome, but more information is needed to establish a causal relationship.

RISK FACTORS: No specific risk factors are known.

MECHANISM: Not established. Initial therapy with or increasing doses of oxycodone might result in release of serotonin, resulting in additive effects with SSRIs.

CLINICAL EVALUATION: A 34-year-old man stabilized on sertraline and cyclosporine (eg, *Neoral*) developed visual hallucinations and severe tremors after substantially increasing his dose of oxycodone.[1] Another case of classic serotonin syndrome occurred in a woman taking fluvoxamine (eg, *Luvox*) who started taking oxycodone.[2] The combination of escitalopram (*Lexapro*) and oxycodone reportedly also has caused serotonin syndrome.[3] Because SSRIs and oxycodone are widely used, it is likely that many patients have received them concurrently. Thus, the lack of reports may signal that adverse drug interactions in patients receiving these combinations are not common.

RELATED DRUGS: If the interaction is real, oxycodone is expected to interact with other SSRIs, such as citalopram (eg, *Celexa*), escitalopram, fluvoxamine, fluoxetine (eg, *Prozac*), and paroxetine (eg, *Paxil*), as well as serotonin-norepinephrine reuptake inhibitors (SNRIs), such as clomipramine (eg, *Anafranil*), duloxetine (*Cymbalta*), imipramine (eg, *Tofranil*), and venlafaxine (eg, *Effexor*).

MANAGEMENT OPTIONS:

➡ **Monitor.** Advise patients receiving sertraline (or other SSRIs or SNRIs) to monitor for evidence of serotonin syndrome if oxycodone is also taken. Symptoms of serotonin syndrome include agitation, coma, confusion, fever, hyperreflexia, hypomania, incoordination, myoclonus, rigidity, seizures, shivering, sweating, and tremor.

REFERENCES:

1. Rosebraugh CJ, et al. Visual hallucination and tremor induced by sertraline and oxycodone in a bone marrow transplant patient. *J Clin Pharmacol.* 2001;41(2):224-227.

2. Karunatilake H, et al. Serotonin syndrome induced by fluvoxamine and oxycodone. *Ann Pharmacother.* 2006;40(1):155-157.

3. Gnanadesigan N, et al. Interaction of serotonergic antidepressants and opioid analgesics: Is serotonin syndrome going undetected? *J Am Med Dir Assoc.* 2005;6(4):265-269.

Oxycodone (eg, *Oxycontin*)

Telithromycin (*Ketek*)

SUMMARY: Oxycodone plasma concentrations were increased by coadministration of telithromycin; increased opioid effects may occur.

RISK FACTORS: No specific risk factors are known.

MECHANISM: Telithromycin inhibits the activity of CYP3A4, the enzyme thought to be primarily responsible for the metabolism of oxycodone.

CLINICAL EVALUATION: Eleven healthy subjects received a single dose of oxycodone 10 mg after 3 days of telithromycin 800 mg daily or placebo.[1] Compared with placebo, the pretreatment with telithromycin resulted in an increase in the mean area under the concentration-time curve of oxycodone of nearly 80%. The half-life of oxycodone was increased from 3.4 to 3.9 hours. Coadministration of telithromycin increased the pharmacodynamic effects (eg, pupil size) of oxycodone to a modest degree. It is likely that long-term dosing of oxycodone in the presence of telithromycin would increase the pharmacodynamic response to oxycodone.

RELATED DRUGS: Fentanyl (eg, *Duragesic*) and sufentanil (eg, *Sufenta*) are likely to be affected in a similar manner by telithromycin. Clarithromycin (eg, *Biaxin*), erythromycin (eg, *Ery-Tab*), and troleandomycin[†] also are likely to inhibit the metabolism of oxycodone.

MANAGEMENT OPTIONS:

➡ *Consider Alternative.* Azithromycin (eg, *Zithromax*) does not inhibit CYP3A4 and may be considered as an alternative to telithromycin in patients receiving oxycodone. Other analgesics not metabolized by CYP3A4 (eg, hydrocodone, morphine) may be considered.

➡ *Monitor.* Observe patients receiving oxycodone and telithromycin concurrently for excessive opioid effects, such as respiratory depression and sedation.

REFERENCES:

1. Grönlund J, et al. Effect of telithromycin on the pharmacokinetics and pharmacodynamics of oral oxycodone. *J Clin Pharmacol*. 2010;50(1):101-108.

† Not available in the United States.

Oxycodone (eg, *Oxycontin*)

Voriconazole (*Vfend*)

SUMMARY: Voriconazole administration resulted in an increase in oxycodone plasma concentrations; some patients may experience increased oxycodone effects.

RISK FACTORS: No specific risk factors are known.

MECHANISM: Voriconazole appears to inhibit the CYP3A4-mediated metabolism of oxycodone, resulting in decreased first-pass and systemic metabolism via CYP3A4.

CLINICAL EVALUATION: Twelve subjects took placebo or 2 doses of voriconazole 400 mg 12 hours apart and then 200 mg twice daily for an additional 3 days.[1] A single dose of oxycodone 10 mg was administered orally on day 3. The mean area under the concentration-time curve (AUC) of oxycodone was increased 3.6-fold, and its half-life increased 2-fold following voriconazole dosing. The AUC of the oxycodone CYP3A4 metabolite noroxycodone was reduced 66%, while the AUC of the metabolite formed by CYP2D6 (oxymorphone) increased 2-fold. While some pharmacodynamic changes were noted in this study, a complete pharmacodynamic assessment will require studies using long-term dosing.

RELATED DRUGS: Ketoconazole (eg, *Nizoral*), fluconazole (eg, *Diflucan*), itraconazole (eg, *Sporanox*), and posaconazole (*Noxafil*) also inhibit the activity of CYP3A4 and are expected to increase the plasma concentrations of oxycodone.

MANAGEMENT OPTIONS:

➡ *Consider Alternative.* Consider narcotic analgesics (eg, codeine, meperidine, morphine) as a substitute for oxycodone. Terbinafine (eg, *Lamisil*) may be an alternative antifungal agent because it does not affect CYP3A4 activity. Amphotericin (eg, *Abelcet*), caspofungin (*Cancidas*), and anidulafungin (*Eraxis*) do not appear to inhibit CYP3A4.

➡ *Monitor.* Monitor patients taking oxycodone for increased narcotic effect if voriconazole is coadministered.

REFERENCES:
   1. Hagelberg NM, et al. Voriconazole drastically increases exposure to oral oxycodone. *Eur J Clin Pharmacol.* 2009;65(3):263-271.

 Oxymetholone (*Anadrol*)

Warfarin (eg, *Coumadin*)

SUMMARY: Several anabolic steroids have been shown to enhance the hypoprothrombinemic response to oral anticoagulants; bleeding episodes have been reported in some cases.

RISK FACTORS: No specific risk factors are known.

MECHANISM: Not established. Anabolic steroids may decrease the formation or increase the degradation of clotting factors. The fibrinolytic activity of anabolic steroids may be involved in patients who develop hemorrhages.

CLINICAL EVALUATION: A number of patients receiving both oral anticoagulants and anabolic steroids have developed excessive hypoprothrombinemia and hemorrhages.[1-12] One case of enhanced warfarin hypoprothrombinemia following a 2% testosterone propionate ointment also has been reported.[1] Based on the available case reports and clinical studies, the magnitude of this interaction appears to be large enough to increase the risk of bleeding in most patients rather than just in certain predisposed individuals.

RELATED DRUGS: Some evidence indicates that 17-alpha-alkylated anabolic steroids such as methandrostenolone (*Dianabol*), norethandrolone, methyltestosterone (*Metandren*), and stanozolol (*Winstrol*) are more likely to potentiate oral anticoagulants than anabolic steroids that are not so substituted. Testosterone also interacts with warfarin.

MANAGEMENT OPTIONS:

➡ *Avoid Unless Benefit Outweighs Risk.* Concomitant use of oral anticoagulants and anabolic steroids should be avoided if possible.

➥ *Monitor.* If the combination is necessary, monitor patients carefully for altered anticoagulant response when the anabolic steroid is initiated, discontinued, or changed in dosage.

REFERENCES:

1. Lorentz SM, et al. Potentiation of warfarin anticoagulation by topical testosterone ointment. *Clin Pharm.* 1985;4:333.

2. Murakami M, et al. Effects of anabolic steroids on anticoagulant requirements. *Jpn Circ J.* 1965;29:243.

3. Schrogie JJ, et al. The anticoagulant response to bishydroxycoumarin II: the effect of D-thyroxine, clofibrate, and norethandrolone. *Clin Pharmacol Ther.* 1967;8:70.

4. Dresdale FC, et al. Potential dangers in the combined use of methandrostenolone and sodium warfarin. *J Med Soc NJ.* 1967;64:609.

5. Robinson BHB, et al. Decreased anticoagulant tolerance with oxymetholone. *Lancet.* 1971;1:1356. Letter.

6. Longridge RGM, et al. Decreased anticoagulant tolerance with oxymetholone. *Lancet.* 1971;2:90. Letter.

7. Edwards MS, et al. Decreased anticoagulant tolerance with oxymetholone. *Lancet.* 1971;2:221. Letter.

8. De Oya JC, et al. Decreased anticoagulant tolerance with oxymetholone in paroxysmal nocturnal haemoglobinuria. *Lancet.* 1971;2:259. Letter.

9. Husted S, et al. Increased sensitivity to phenprocoumon during methyltestosterone therapy. *Eur J Clin Pharmacol.* 1976;10:209.

10. Acomb C, et al. A significant interaction between warfarin and stanozolol. *Pharmaceutical J.* 1985;234;73.

11. McLaughlin GE, et al. Hemarthrosis complicating anticoagulant therapy: report of three cases. *JAMA.* 1966;196:1020.

12. Shaw PW, et al. Possible interaction of warfarin and stanozolol. *Clin Pharm.* 1987;6:500.

Oxytetracycline (eg, *Terramycin*)

Tolbutamide (eg, *Orinase*)

SUMMARY: Oxytetracycline may increase the hypoglycemic effects of insulin or tolbutamide.

RISK FACTORS: No specific risk factors are known.

MECHANISM: Not established. Animal studies indicate that oxytetracycline enhances the hypoglycemic effect of insulin.[2]

CLINICAL EVALUATION: Oxytetracycline has been reported to reduce insulin requirements and increase the hypoglycemic effect of tolbutamide.[1,2] Tetracycline may contribute to lactic acidosis in patients receiving phenformin.[3]

RELATED DRUGS: Oxytetracycline has been reported to reduce insulin requirements. The effect of other combinations of tetracyclines and sulfonylureas is unknown.

MANAGEMENT OPTIONS: No specific action is required, but be alert for evidence of the interaction.

REFERENCES:

1. Miller JB. Hypoglycemic effect of oxytetracycline. *BMJ.* 1966;2:1007. Letter.

2. Hiatt N, et al. Insulin response in pancreatectomized dogs treated with oxytetracycline. *Diabetes.* 1970;19:307.

3. Philips PJ, et al. Phenformin, tetracycline and lactic acidosis. *Ann Intern Med.* 1977;86:111. Letter.

Paclitaxel (eg, *Taxol*)

Saquinavir (eg, *Fortovase*)

SUMMARY: Two patients on combined therapy with saquinavir and delavirdine (*Rescriptor*) developed unexpectedly severe paclitaxel toxicity, but a causal relationship was not established.

RISK FACTORS: No specific risk factors are known.

MECHANISM: Not established. Saquinavir and delavirdine may inhibit the metabolism of paclitaxel by CYP3A4.

CLINICAL EVALUATION: Two patients on combination antiretroviral therapy with saquinavir, delavirdine, and didansosine (*Videx*) developed severe paclitaxel toxicity (eg, mucositis, neutropenia, alopecia). One of the patients also received fluconazole (*Diflucan*), a known CYP3A4 inhibitor. Both patients had tolerated numerous previous cycles of paclitaxel therapy with only relatively mild toxicity (eg, nausea, alopecia). During the previous paclitaxel courses, the patients received various combinations of antiretroviral drugs, such as zidovudine (*Retrovir*), zalcitabine (*Hivid*), lamivudine (*Epivir*), stavudine (*Zerit*), and indinavir (*Crixivan*). Although the findings in these patients are consistent with an interaction between paclitaxel and saquinavir/delvirdine, a causal relationship was not established. Additional study is needed for confirmation.

RELATED DRUGS: Little is known about the effect of other antiretroviral agents on paclitaxel toxicity. Theoretically, any antiretroviral agents that inhibit CYP2A4 may be expected to increase paclitaxel serum concentrations, including ritonavir (*Norvir*), indinavir, nelfinavir (*Viracept*), and amprenavir (*Agenerase*).

MANAGEMENT OPTIONS:

➡ **Monitor.** Monitor patients on saquinavir or other antiretroviral agents that inhibit CYP3A4 and may be expected to increase paclitaxel toxicity, and reduce paclitaxel doses if necessary.

REFERENCES:
1. Schwartz JD, et al. Potential interaction of antiretroviral therapy with paclitaxel in patients with AIDS-related Kaposi's sarcoma. *AIDS*. 1999;13:283.

Pancuronium (*Pavulon*)

Polymyxin

SUMMARY: Polymyxin may prolong apnea following the use of muscle relaxants such as pancuronium.

RISK FACTORS: No specific risk factors are known.

MECHANISM: Both polymyxin B and colistin (*Coly-Mycin S*) can produce neuromuscular blockade, which may enhance the blockade of muscle relaxants.

CLINICAL EVALUATION: Several cases have been reported in which patients receiving polymyxin alone or in combination with surgical neuromuscular blockers experienced respiratory paralysis.[1-4] It has been proposed that this neuromuscular blockade may be enhanced by either an intracellular potassium deficit or a low serum ionized calcium concentration.

RELATED DRUGS: Other neuromuscular blockers may interact with polymyxin.

MANAGEMENT OPTIONS:

➡ *Avoid Unless Benefit Outweighs Risk.* Only give polymyxin with caution during surgery or in the postoperative period.

➡ *Monitor.* If the polymyxin and neuromuscular blocking drugs are used together, monitor the patient carefully for enhanced neuromuscular blockade.

REFERENCES:

1. Pohlmann G. Respiratory arrest associated with intravenous administration of polymyxin B sulfate. *JAMA.* 1966;196:181.
2. Levi RA, et al. Polymyxin B-induced respiratory paralysis reversed by intravenous calcium chloride. *J Mt Sinai Hosp.* 1969;36:380.
3. Pittinger CB, et al. Antibiotic-induced paralysis. *Anesth Analg.* 1970;49:487.
4. Fogdall RP, et al. Prolongation of a pancuronium-induced neuronmuscular blockade by polymyxin B. *Anesthesiology.* 1974;40:84.

Pantoprazole (*Protonix*) 5

Phenytoin (eg, *Dilantin*)

SUMMARY: Pantoprazole does not appear to affect the pharmacokinetics of phenytoin.

RISK FACTORS: No specific risk factors are known.

MECHANISM: No interaction.

CLINICAL EVALUATION: A randomized, crossover study in healthy subjects suggests that pantoprazole does not affect the absorption or elimination of phenytoin.[1]

RELATED DRUGS: Omeprazole (*Prilosec*) can produce a small increase in phenytoin serum concentrations, probably because of its ability to inhibit CYP2C19 (a minor pathway for phenytoin metabolism). Little is known regarding the effect of lansoprazole (*Prevacid*) on phenytoin metabolism, but the manufacturer states that no clinically significant interaction exists.

MANAGEMENT OPTIONS: No interaction.

REFERENCES:

1. Middle MV, et al. No influence of pantoprazole on the pharmacokinetics of phenytoin. *Int J Clin Pharmacol Ther.* 1995;33:304.

Para-Aminobenzoic Acid (*Potaba*) 4

Procainamide (eg, *Pronestyl*)

SUMMARY: In 1 patient the administration of para-aminobenzoic acid (PABA) increased the serum procainamide concentrations and reduced the N-acetylprocainamide (NAPA) concentrations; the clinical importance of this effect is unknown.

RISK FACTORS:

➡ *Pharmacogenetics.* Rapid acetylators of procainamide are at increased risk for this interaction.

MECHANISM: PABA is an inhibitor of acetylation, the major route of hepatic metabolism for procainamide.

CLINICAL EVALUATION: A 61-year-old patient had multiple episodes of ventricular tachycardia that responded to procainamide.[1] A high ratio of NAPA to procainamide (including a rapid rate of metabolism by acetylation of procainamide) was noted in this patient. On several occasions, he was given PABA 1.5 g every 6 hours while taking procainamide. PABA decreases the metabolism of procainamide to NAPA, thus increasing the procainamide concentration and reducing NAPA concentration (NAPA/procainamide ratio is decreased). Theoretically, this might be useful in patients who are responsive to procainamide but who develop NAPA toxicity at high doses. However, PABA also reduces the renal elimination of NAPA.[2] The effect of PABA administration on the procainamide clearance of a slow procainamide acetylator is unknown but would likely be minimal.

RELATED DRUGS: No information is available.

MANAGEMENT OPTIONS: No specific action is required, but be alert for evidence of the interaction.

REFERENCES:
1. Nylen ES, et al. Reduced acetylation of procainamide by para-aminobenzoic acid. *J Am Coll Cardiol.* 1986;7:185.
2. Tisdale JE, et al. Inhibition of procainamide N-acetylation by para-aminobenzoic acid. *Clin Pharmacol Ther.* 1995;57:184.

 Para-Aminobenzoic Acid (eg, *Potaba*)

Sulfamethoxazole

SUMMARY: Para-aminobenzoic acid (PABA) may interfere with the antibacterial activity of sulfonamides.

RISK FACTORS: No specific risk factors are known.

MECHANISM: Because sulfonamides act by competitive inhibition of PABA in microorganisms, PABA administration in sufficient doses antagonizes the antibacterial effect of sulfamethoxazole and other sulfonamides.

CLINICAL EVALUATION: This interaction has been well documented in the past.[1] It should be remembered that PABA may be found in some vitamin supplements.

RELATED DRUGS: Do not administer PABA to patients receiving antibacterial sulfonamides.

MANAGEMENT OPTIONS:

➥ *Use Alternative.* Do not administer PABA to patients receiving antibacterial sulfonamides.

REFERENCES:
1. Mandell GL, et al. Antimicrobial agents. Sulfonamides, trimethoprim-sulfamethoxazole, quinolones, and agents for urinary tract infections. In: Gilman AG, et al., eds. *Goodman and Gilman's The Pharmacological Basis of Therapeutics.* 8th ed. New York: Pergamon; 1990:1048.

 Paroxetine (eg, *Paxil*)

Phenobarbital (eg, *Solfoton*)

SUMMARY: In a preliminary study in healthy subjects, phenobarbital tended to reduce paroxetine serum concentrations, but additional study is needed to determine the magnitude of this effect.

RISK FACTORS: No specific risk factors are known.

MECHANISM: Not established. It is possible that barbiturates enhance the hepatic metabolism of paroxetine.

CLINICAL EVALUATION: Ten healthy subjects received a single oral dose of paroxetine 30 mg with and without pretreatment with phenobarbital 100 mg at bedtime for 14 days.[1] The phenobarbital pretreatment was associated with a 25% decrease in area under the paroxetine serum concentration-time curve and a 38% increase in the paroxetine half-life. Neither change was statistically significant; however, 1 subject had a substantial increase in both parameters in the presence of phenobarbital. Moreover, data for paroxetine alone were missing for 3 of the 10 subjects and for paroxetine plus phenobarbital for 1 subject. Thus, it is possible that additional investigation would demonstrate an effect of phenobarbital on paroxetine pharmacokinetics. In another study, paroxetine did not affect amobarbital-induced sedation or impairment of psychomotor function.[2] This is consistent with the lack of additive effects of selective serotonin reuptake inhibitors (SSRIs) with other CNS depressants (eg, alcohol, benzodiazepines).

RELATED DRUGS: Other SSRIs are also metabolized by the liver and also may interact with barbiturates and alcohol.

MANAGEMENT OPTIONS: No specific action is required, but be alert for evidence of the interaction.

REFERENCES:
1. Greb WH, et al. The effect of liver enzyme inhibition by cimetidine and enzyme induction by phenobarbitone on the pharmacokinetics of paroxetine. *Acta Psychiatr Scand Suppl.* 1989;350:95-98.
2. Cooper SM, et al. The psychomotor effects of paroxetine alone and in combination with haloperidol, amylobarbitone, oxazepam, or alcohol. *Acta Psychiatr Scand Suppl.* 1989;350:53-55.

Paroxetine (eg, *Paxil*)

Pimozide (*Orap*) AVOID

SUMMARY: Paroxetine may increase pimozide plasma concentrations; given the potential risk of ventricular arrhythmias, the combination is contraindicated.

RISK FACTORS: No specific risk factors are known.

MECHANISM: Not established. Paroxetine does not appear to be a CYP3A4 inhibitor, so it is possible that drug transporters may be involved.

CLINICAL EVALUATION: The manufacturer reports a study in healthy subjects in which paroxetine 60 mg daily resulted in a 151% increase in pimozide area under the plasma concentration-time curve after a single dose of pimozide 2 mg.[1] Given the potential for pimozide-induced QTc prolongation leading to cardiac arrhythmias, such as torsade de pointes, the combination is contraindicated.

RELATED DRUGS: Sertraline (*Zoloft*) also increases pimozide plasma concentrations, and combined use of sertraline and pimozide also is contraindicated. Little is known about the effect of other selective serotonin reuptake inhibitors on pimozide; theoretically, fluvoxamine (a moderate CYP3A4 inhibitor) would increase pimozide concentrations. Pending additional information, avoid coadministration of fluvoxamine and pimozide. Also, some evidence suggests that fluoxetine (eg, *Prozac*) can be a modest inhibitor of CYP3A4, but little is known regarding a possible effect on pimozide.

MANAGEMENT OPTIONS:

➥ *AVOID COMBINATION.* Avoid concurrent use of pimozide and paroxetine.

REFERENCES:

1. *Paxil* [package insert]. Research Triangle Park, NC: GlaxoSmithKline; 2005.

Paroxetine (eg, *Paxil*)

Sumatriptan (eg, *Imitrex*)

SUMMARY: The risk of serotonin syndrome may be increased when paroxetine is used with sumatriptan or other triptans.

RISK FACTORS: No specific risk factors are known.

MECHANISM: Not established. It has been proposed that triptans may have additive serotonergic effects with selective serotonin reuptake inhibitors (SSRIs) or serotonin-norepinephrine reuptake inhibitors (SNRIs).

CLINICAL EVALUATION: A 65-year-old woman developed confusion, fever, tachycardia, hypertension, and strange behavior after receiving concomitant therapy with paroxetine and sumatriptan.[1] Although these symptoms are consistent with a diagnosis of serotonin syndrome, they were relatively nonspecific, and some of the symptoms could have been caused by sumatriptan alone. Classic symptoms of serotonin syndrome (eg, hyperreflexia, myoclonus, rigidity) were absent. However, it is possible that the reaction resulted from combined serotonergic effects of paroxetine and sumatriptan. Other cases of possible serotonin syndrome have occasionally been reported with combined use of triptans and SSRIs.[2]

These cases notwithstanding, clinical studies of the combined use of triptans with SSRIs generally have found little evidence of an increased risk of serotonin syndrome. In a prospective study of 12,339 patients who received sumatriptan for migraine, evidence of serotonin syndrome was not seen in the 485 patients receiving paroxetine concurrently.[3] In a randomized, double-blind, crossover study of 20 healthy subjects, fluoxetine (eg, *Prozac*) did not affect the pharmacokinetics, pharmacodynamics, or adverse reactions of zolmitriptan (*Zomig*).[4] In another randomized, double-blind, crossover study of 12 healthy subjects, paroxetine did not affect the pharmacokinetics, pharmacodynamics, or adverse reactions of rizatriptan (*Maxalt*).[5] Taken together, this information suggests that combined use of triptans and SSRIs usually does not result in adverse drug interactions, but it is possible that serotonin syndrome occurs in certain susceptible individuals.

However, in July 2006, the Food and Drug Administration issued a public health advisory stating that new information suggests combined use of triptans with SSRIs or SNRIs can result in serotonin syndrome.[6] Few details were presented on the nature of the information that led to this advisory.

RELATED DRUGS: Theoretically, the risk of serotonin syndrome may be increased by any combination of a triptan (eg, almotriptan [*Axert*], eletriptan [*Relpax*], frovatriptan [*Frova*], naratriptan [*Amerge*], rizatriptan [*Maxalt*], zolmitriptan [*Zomig*]) with an SSRI (eg, citalopram [eg, *Celexa*], escitalopram [*Lexapro*], fluoxetine, fluvoxamine [eg, *Luvox*], paroxetine, sertraline [eg, *Zoloft*]) or an SNRI (eg, clomipramine [eg, *Anafranil*], duloxetine [*Cymbalta*], imipramine [eg, *Tofranil*], venlafaxine [*Effexor*]).

MANAGEMENT OPTIONS:

➡ *Monitor.* Monitor patients receiving paroxetine (or other SSRIs or SNRIs) for evidence of serotonin syndrome if they take sumatriptan or other triptans. Symptoms of serotonin syndrome include agitation, coma, confusion, fever, hyperreflexia, hypomania, incoordination, myoclonus, rigidity, seizures, shivering, sweating, and tremor. Advise patients to contact their health care provider if any of these symptoms occur.

REFERENCES:

1. Hendrix Y, et al. Serotonin syndrome as a result of concomitant use of paroxetine and sumatriptan [in Dutch]. *Ned Tijdschr Geneeskd.* 2005;149(16):888-890.

2. Mathew NT, et al. Serotonin syndrome complicating migraine pharmacotherapy. *Cephalalgia.* 1996;16(5):323-327.

3. Putnam GP, et al. Migraine polypharmacy and the tolerability of sumatriptan: a large-scale, prospective study. *Cephalalgia.* 1999;19(7):668-675.

4. Smith DA, et al. Zolmitriptan (311C90) does not interact with fluoxetine in healthy volunteers. *Int J Clin Pharmacol Ther.* 1998;36(6):301-305.

5. Goldberg MR, et al. Lack of pharmacokinetic and pharmacodynamic interaction between rizatriptan and paroxetine. *J Clin Pharmacol.* 1999;39(2):192-199.

6. FDA Public Health Advisory. Combined Use of 5-Hydroxytryptamine Receptor Agonists (Triptans), Selective Serotonin Reuptake Inhibitors (SSRIs) or Selective Serotonin/Norepinephrine Reuptake Inhibitors (SNRIs) May Result in Life-threatening Serotonin Syndrome. Center for Drug Evaluation and Research (CDER), U.S. Food and Drug Administration. http://www.fda.gov/CDER/DRUG/advisory/SSRI_SS200607.htm. Published July 19, 2006. Updated November 24, 2006. Accessed May 29, 2008.

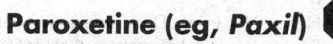

Paroxetine (eg, *Paxil*)

Tamoxifen (eg, *Soltamox*)

SUMMARY: CYP2D6 inhibitors such as paroxetine appear to reduce the efficacy of tamoxifen in the treatment of breast cancer.

RISK FACTORS: No specific risk factors are known.

MECHANISM: Tamoxifen is metabolized to 2 active metabolites by CYP2D6, the most important of which is endoxifen. By reducing endoxifen formation, CYP2D6 inhibitors such as paroxetine may reduce tamoxifen efficacy.[1-5]

CLINICAL EVALUATION: In a preliminary study of 12 women on tamoxifen, the addition of paroxetine (10 mg/day for 4 weeks) resulted in a 56% decrease in endoxifen plasma concentrations.[6] A subsequent study in 80 patients starting tamoxifen therapy found that those on CYP2D6 inhibitor antidepressants had substantially lower endoxifen concentrations.[7] The reduction in endoxifen was greatest with paroxetine, intermediate with sertraline, and minimal with venlafaxine. Another study in patients with breast cancer found substantial reductions in endoxifen plasma concentrations in patients taking potent CYP2D6 inhibitors, such as paroxetine and fluoxetine, while weak inhibitors, such as sertraline and citalopram, produced only small reductions.[8] Venlafaxine had no effect on endoxifen concentrations. Another tamoxifen study found a nearly 2-fold increase the in risk of breast cancer relapse in women with low CYP2D6 activity, either due to CYP2D6-inhibiting drugs or genetic deficiency.[9] Taken together, these results strongly suggest that CYP2D6 inhibitors reduce the efficacy of tamoxifen in the treatment of breast cancer.

RELATED DRUGS: Fluoxetine (eg, *Prozac*), like paroxetine, is a potent CYP2D6 inhibitor; duloxetine (*Cymbalta*) and bupropion (eg, *Wellbutrin*) also inhibit CYP2D6. Weaker inhibitors of CYP2D6 include citalopram (eg, *Celexa*), escitalopram (*Lexapro*), desvenlafaxine (*Pristiq*), and sertraline (eg, *Zoloft*). Venlafaxine (*Effexor*) and mirtazapine (eg, *Remeron*) appear to have little or no effect on CYP2D6, and are unlikely to interact.

MANAGEMENT OPTIONS:

➡ *Use Alternative.* Paroxetine, fluoxetine, duloxetine, and bupropion are best avoided in patients on tamoxifen. Although other SSRIs such as citalopram and sertraline are weaker inhibitors of CYP2D6, they can reduce endoxifen concentrations somewhat and may reduce tamoxifen efficacy in some patients. Available evidence suggests that venlafaxine does not affect endoxifen concentrations, so it may be preferable. Mirtazapine has been used effectively for hot flashes in breast cancer survivors, and theoretically is unlikely to interact with tamoxifen.[10]

➡ *Monitor.* If a CYP2D6 inhibitor such as paroxetine is used with tamoxifen, cancer recurrence may be an indication that tamoxifen efficacy has been reduced. If this happens, consider discontinuing the CYP2D6 inhibitor.

REFERENCES:

1. Dezentje VO, et al. Clinical implications of CYP2D6 genotyping in tamoxifen treatment for breast cancer. *Clin Cancer Res.* 2009;15(1):15-21.

2. Tan SH, et al. Pharmacogenetics in breast cancer therapy. *Clin Cancer Res.* 2008;14(24):8027-8041.

3. Newman WG, et al. Impaired tamoxifen metabolism reduces survival in familial breast cancer patients. *Clin Cancer Res.* 2008;14(18):5913-5918.

4. Henry NL, et al. Drug interactions and pharmacogenomics in the treatment of breast cancer and depression. *Am J Psychiatry.* 2008;165(10):1251-1255.

5. Algeciras-Schimnich A, et al. Pharmacogenomics of tamoxifen and irinotecan therapies. *Clin Lab Med.* 2008;28(4):553-567.

6. Stearns V, et al. Active tamoxifen metabolite plasma concentrations after coadministration of tamoxifen and the selective serotonin reuptake inhibitor paroxetine. *J Natl Cancer Inst.* 2003;95(23):1758-1764.

7. Jin Y, et al. CYP2D6 genotype, antidepressant use, and tamoxifen metabolism during adjuvant breast cancer treatment. *J Natl Can Inst.* 2005;97(1):30-39.

8. Borges S, et al. Quantitative effect of CYP2D6 genotype and inhibitors on tamoxifen metabolism: implication for optimization of breast cancer treatment. *Clin Pharmacol Ther.* 2006;80(1):61-74.

9. Goetz MP, et al. The impact of cytochrome P450 2D6 metabolism in women receiving adjuvant tamoxifen. *Breast Cancer Res Treat.* 2007;101(1):113-121.

10. Biglia N, et al. Mirtazapine for the treatment of hot flushes in breast cancer survivors: a prospective pilot trial. *Breast J.* 2007;13(5):490-495.

Paroxetine (eg, *Paxil*)

Tetrabenazine (*Xenazine*)

SUMMARY: Paroxetine has been shown to produce marked increases in the plasma concentrations of the 2 active metabolites of tetrabenazine.

RISK FACTORS: No specific risk factors are known.

MECHANISM: The 2 active metabolites of tetrabenazine are both metabolized by CYP2D6, and paroxetine is a potent inhibitor of CYP2D6.

CLINICAL EVALUATION: The manufacturer reports a study in 25 healthy subjects in which paroxetine (20 mg/day for 10 days) produced about a 3-fold increase in one active metabolite and a 9-fold increase in the other.[1] An interaction of this magnitude is expected to increase the risk of tetrabenazine toxicity.

RELATED DRUGS: Fluoxetine (eg, *Prozac*) also inhibits CYP2D6, and it is likely to increase tetrabenazine serum concentrations. Theoretically, other CYP2D6-inhibitor antidepressants, such as bupropion (eg, *Wellbutrin*) and duloxetine (*Cymbalta*), are expected to have a similar effect.

MANAGEMENT OPTIONS:

➡ *Use Alternative.* If possible, use an alternative antidepressant; agents with generally weak inhibitory effects on CYP2D6 include citalopram (eg, *Celexa*), desvenlafaxine (*Pristiq*), escitalopram (*Lexapro*), and sertraline (eg, *Zoloft*). Venlafaxine (eg, *Effexor*) and mirtazapine (eg, *Remeron*) have little or no effect on CYP2D6 and are unlikely to interact with tetrabenazine.

➡ *Circumvent/Minimize.* The *Xenazine* product information states that the dose of tetrabenazine should be reduced to one-half the normal dose if it is used with CYP2D6 inhibitors, such as fluoxetine.[1]

➡ *Monitor.* If the combination is used, monitor for altered tetrabenazine effect if paroxetine or other CYP2D6 inhibitors are started, stopped, or changed in dosage. Dose-dependent adverse effects of tetrabenazine may include akathisia, depression, fatigue, insomnia, parkinsonism, and sedation.

REFERENCES:

1. *Xenazine* [package insert]. Deerfield, IL: Lundbeck Inc; 2010.

Paroxetine (eg, *Paxil*)

Thiazides

SUMMARY: The combined use of paroxetine and a thiazide diuretic has been noted to increase the risk of hyponatremia and its associated symptoms (eg, confusion, disorientation, weakness).

RISK FACTORS:

➡ *Effects of Age.* Elderly patients appear to be at greater risk; lower body weight may play a role, as well as diseases and changes in kidney function that may predispose to hyponatremia.

➡ *Gender.* The majority of case reports involve women, although it is not clear that female gender is an independent risk factor.

MECHANISM: Selective serotonin reuptake inhibitors (SSRIs) and selective serotonin-norepinephrine reuptake inhibitors (SNRIs) can produce the syndrome of inappropriate antidiuretic hormone, resulting in hyponatremia. The natriuretic effect of thiazide diuretics can result in additive hyponatremia.

CLINICAL EVALUATION: Cases of hyponatremia have been reported following combined use of paroxetine and thiazides.[1,2] Paroxetine alone has been associated with hyponatremia,[3,4] but it is likely that thiazide diuretics increase the risk. Numerous cases of hyponatremia have been reported with other SSRIs, both alone and combined with diuretics.[5-11]

RELATED DRUGS: Most other SSRIs have also been associated with hyponatremia, including citalopram (eg, *Celexa*), escitalopram (*Lexapro*), fluoxetine (eg, *Prozac*), fluvoxamine (eg, *Luvox*), and sertraline (eg, *Zoloft*). The following SNRIs may also interact: clomipramine (eg, *Anafranil*), duloxetine (*Cymbalta*), imipramine (eg, *Tofranil*), and venlafaxine (*Effexor*).

MANAGEMENT OPTIONS:

➡ *Consider Alternative.* Mirtazapine (eg, *Remeron*) may be less likely to cause hyponatremia than SSRIs or SNRIs. In 1 case of citalopram-induced hyponatremia, mirtazapine was substituted for the citalopram without a recurrence of hyponatremia.[10] Mirtazapine has been associated with hyponatremia in isolated case reports; therefore, exercise caution.[11,12]

➡ *Monitor.* Hyponatremia usually occurs in the first 2 to 3 weeks after starting therapy with the second drug (SSRI, SNRI, or the diuretic). Monitor for symptoms of hyponatremia (eg, anorexia, confusion, disorientation, fatigue, headache, muscle cramps, nausea, weakness); in severe cases, seizures, coma, and death can occur. In predisposed patients, such as elderly patients who are taking diuretics (especially women), measure serum sodium at baseline and again 7 to 10 days after starting the second drug.

REFERENCES:

1. Rosner MH. Severe hyponatremia associated with the combined use of thiazide diuretics and selective serotonin reuptake inhibitors. *Am J Med Sci.* 2004;327(2):109-111.

2. Strachan J, et al. Hyponatraemia associated with the use of selective serotonin re-uptake inhibitors. *Aust NZ J Psychiatry.* 1998;32(2):295-298.

3. Fabian TJ, et al. Paroxetine-induced hyponatremia in older adults: a 12-week prospective study. *Arch Intern Med.* 2004;164(3):327-332.

4. Leung VP, et al. Hyponatremia associated with paroxetine. *Pharmacopsychiatry.* 1998;31(1):32-34.

5. Wright SK, et al. Hyponatremia as a complication of selective serotonin reuptake inhibitors. *J Am Acad Nurse Pract.* 2008;20(1):47-51.

6. Romero S, et al. Syndrome of inappropriate secretion of antidiuretic hormone due to citalopram and venlafaxine. *Gen Hosp Psychiatry.* 2007;29(1):81-84.

7. Flores G, et al. Severe symptomatic hyponatremia during citalopram therapy—a case report. *BMC Nephrol.* 2004;5:2.

8. Jacob S, et al. Hyponatremia associated with selective serotonin-reuptake inhibitors in older adults. *Ann Pharmacother.* 2006;40(9):1618-1622.

9. Fitzgerald MA. Hyponatremia associated with SSRI use in a 65-year-old woman. *Nurse Pract.* 2008;33(2):11-12.

10. Jagsch C, et al. Successful mirtazapine treatment of an 81-year-old patient with syndrome of inappropriate antidiuretic hormone secretion. *Pharmacopsychiatry.* 2007;40(3):129-131.

11. Bavbek N, et al. Recurrent hyponatremia associated with citalopram and mirtazapine. *Am J Kidney Dis.* 2006;48(4):e61-e62.

12. Ladino M, et al. Mirtazapine-induced hyponatremia in an elderly hospice patient. *J Palliat Med.* 2006;9(2):258-260.

Paroxetine (eg, *Paxil*)

Thioridazine

SUMMARY: Paroxetine may increase thioridazine serum concentrations, and thus may increase the risk of ventricular arrhythmias; avoid concurrent use.

RISK FACTORS:

➡ ***Pharmacogenetics.*** Only patients with the extensive metabolizer CYP2D6 phenotype are expected to experience this interaction. Poor metabolizers do not have the gene for production of CYP2D6 and likely already have high serum concentrations of thioridazine. Approximately 8% of white patients are deficient in CYP2D6, but the deficiency is rare in Asian patients (usually 1% or less).

➡ ***Hypokalemia.*** The corrected QT interval (QTc) may be prolonged in patients with hypokalemia, therefore increasing the risk of this interaction. Any other factor that may prolong the QTc interval also would increase the risk of this interaction.

MECHANISM: Paroxetine probably inhibits the hepatic metabolism of thioridazine by CYP2D6.

CLINICAL EVALUATION: In a double-blind, randomized, crossover study of the pharmaco-dynamic effects of thioridazine alone, single oral doses of thioridazine 10 and 50 mg in 9 healthy subjects were compared with placebo.[1] The dose of thioridazine 50 mg increased QTc on the electrocardiogram (ECG) 23 msec, and the 10 mg dose increased QTc 9 msec. These results suggest that thioridazine produces a dose-related slowing of cardiac repolarization. Thus, drugs such as paroxetine that inhibit CYP2D6 can be expected to reduce the metabolism of thioridazine and increase the risk of excessive prolongation of the QTc and ventricular arrhythmias. Although this interaction is based primarily on theoretical considerations, the potential severity of the interaction suggests that the combination should be avoided. Moreover, the manufacturer's product information for *Mellaril*[+] (thioridazine) states that combined use of thioridazine and paroxetine is contraindicated[2]; therefore, medicolegal issues also must be considered.

RELATED DRUGS: Fluoxetine (eg, *Prozac*), like paroxetine, is a potent inhibitor of CYP2D6 and inhibits CYP2C19, and is also expected to increase the risk of arrhythmias. Fluvoxamine, although not a significant CYP2D6 inhibitor, also increases thioridazine serum concentrations, possibly by inhibiting CYP2C19 and CYP1A2. Other selective serotonin reuptake inhibitors, such as citalopram (eg, *Celexa*) and sertraline (eg, *Zoloft*), are less likely to significantly inhibit CYP2D6, CYP2C19, or CYP1A2. Theoretically, they are less likely to interact with thioridazine, but little clinical information is available. Although a number of antipsychotic drugs, like thioridazine, prolong the QT interval, clinical evidence suggests that thioridazine may produce the greatest risk.

MANAGEMENT OPTIONS:

➡ ***Use Alternative.*** Although the risk of this combination is not well established, use alternatives for one of the drugs (see Related Drugs).

➥ **Monitor.** If the combination must be used, monitor the ECG for evidence of QT prolongation, and monitor for clinical evidence of arrhythmias (eg, syncope).

REFERENCES:
1. Hartigan-Go K, et al. Concentration-related pharmacodynamic effects of thioridazine and its metabolites in humans. *Clin Pharmacol Ther.* 1996;60(5):543-553.
2. "Dear Doctor or Pharmacist" [letter]. East Hanover, NJ: Novartis Pharmaceuticals; July 7, 2000. Available at http://www.fda.gov/medwatch/safety/2000/mellar.htm. Accessed May 29, 2008.

† Not available in the United States.

Paroxetine (*Paxil*)

Tramadol (*Ultram*)

SUMMARY: A patient on paroxetine and tramadol developed serotonin syndrome, but it is unknown how often this occurs in patients receiving the combination. Theoretically, paroxetine would partially inhibit the analgesic effect of tramadol.

RISK FACTORS: No specific risk factors are known.

MECHANISM: Probably additive. Both paroxetine and tramadol have serotonergic effects. Also, tramadol is converted to an active metabolite by CYP2D6, and the ability of paroxetine to inhibit this enzyme would theoretically reduce tramadol analgesia.

CLINICAL EVALUATION: A 47-year-old man on paroxetine 20 mg/day started therapy with tramadol 100 mg/day for joint pain.[1] Twelve hours after the first dose of tramadol he developed shivering, sweating, myoclonus, and became semicomatose. After the tramadol was discontinued and the paroxetine dose was halved, the symptoms dissipated over the next week. This case would qualify as serotonin syndrome by Sternbach's criteria,[2] and the temporal relationship of the reaction is consistent with an interaction between paroxetine and tramadol. Moreover, the patient received both drugs alone without developing serotonin syndrome. But it is not clear what predisposed this patient to develop serotonin syndrome, while many other patients have received this combination without problems. It also should be noted that the analgesic effect of tramadol appears to be partially dependent upon the patient's CYP2D6 activity.[3] Accordingly, potent inhibitors of CYP2D6 such as paroxetine (and also fluoxetine [eg, *Prozac*]) would theoretically inhibit the analgesic effect of tramadol.

RELATED DRUGS: The combination of sertraline (*Zoloft*) and tramadol also has been reported to produce serotonin syndrome. It is possible that other selective serotonin reuptake inhibitors such as fluoxetine, fluvoxamine (*Luvox*), and citalopram (*Celexa*) also may increase the risk of serotonin syndrome if combined with tramadol. However, inhibition of tramadol analgesia caused by inhibition of CYP2D6 would likely apply only to fluoxetine and paroxetine because the other selective serotonin reuptake inhibitors have only minimal effects of CYP2D6. Meperidine (eg, *Demerol*) may interact similarly with the SSRIs.

MANAGEMENT OPTIONS:

➥ **Consider Alternative.** In patients on paroxetine or other selective serotonin reuptake inhibitors, consider the use of an analgesic that is not serotonergic (eg, an agent other than tramadol or meperidine) to minimize the risk of serotonin syndrome. To avoid the possibility of reduced tramadol analgesia caused by inhibition of

CYP2D6, consider the use of fluvoxamine or sertraline in place of paroxetine or fluoxetine.

➡ *Monitor.* In patients receiving tramadol and paroxetine (or other SSRIs) be alert for evidence of serotonin syndrome. Serotonin syndrome can result in neurotoxicity (myoclonus, tremors, rigidity, incoordination, hyperreflexia, seizures, coma), psychiatric symptoms (agitation, confusion, hypomania, restlessness), and autonomic dysfunction (fever, sweating, tachycardia, hypertension). If the SSRI used is paroxetine or fluoxetine, monitor for reduced tramadol analgesia.

REFERENCES:

1. Egberts AC, et al. Serotonin syndrome attributed to tramadol addition to paroxetine therapy. *Int Clin Psychopharmacol.* 1997;12:181-82.

2. Sternbach H. The serotonin syndrome. *Am J Psychiatry.* 1991;148:705-13.

3. Poulsen L, et al. The hypoalgesic effect of tramadol in relation to CYP2D6. *Clin Pharmacol Ther.* 1996;60:636-44.

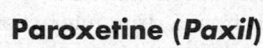

Paroxetine (*Paxil*)

Warfarin (eg, *Coumadin*)

SUMMARY: Although paroxetine does not appear to affect the hypoprothrombinemic response to warfarin in most people, the combination may increase the risk of bleeding.

RISK FACTORS: No specific risk factors are known.

MECHANISM: Not established.

CLINICAL EVALUATION: In 27 healthy subjects, warfarin 5 mg/day and paroxetine 30 mg/day were given alone and in combination in a multiple-dose study.[1] Although paroxetine did not affect the mean hypoprothrombinemic response to warfarin, 5 of the 27 subjects had clinically significant bleeding after several days of combined treatment with paroxetine and warfarin. Three of the subjects were withdrawn from the study because of either increased prothrombin time or bleeding. The absence of such bleeding with either drug alone suggests that the combination was responsible, but additional study is needed to establish a causal relationship.

RELATED DRUGS: The effect of paroxetine on the response to other oral anticoagulants is not established, but the same precautions would apply until data are available. Data are insufficient to determine the relative risk of paroxetine versus other selective serotonin reuptake inhibitors (SSRIs) in anticoagulated patients.

MANAGEMENT OPTIONS:

➡ *Consider Alternative.* Although the ability of paroxetine to increase the risk of bleeding in patients on warfarin is not well established, it would be prudent to avoid the combination when possible. The use of an SSRI other than paroxetine may or may not reduce the risk.

➡ *Monitor.* If the combination is used, monitor for altered hypoprothrombinemic response to warfarin if paroxetine is initiated, discontinued, or changed in dosage. Note an increased bleeding risk may occur in the absence of excessive hypoprothrombinemia.

REFERENCES:

1. Bannister SJ, et al. Evaluation of the potential for interactions of paroxetine with diazepam, cimetidine, warfarin, and digoxin. *Acta Psychiatr Scand.* 1989;80(Suppl. 350):102.

Paroxetine (*Paxil*)

Zolpidem (*Ambien*)

SUMMARY: A patient developed delirium after taking paroxetine and zolpidem, but a causal relationship was not established.

RISK FACTORS: No specific risk factors are known.

MECHANISM: Not established.

CLINICAL EVALUATION: A 16-year-old girl began paroxetine 20 mg/day for depression, and on the third day took zolpidem 10 mg at night.[1] One hour later she developed hallucinations and disorientation. The delirium lasted 4 hours and resolved spontaneously. The author asked some of his other patients on this combination about adverse effects, and some of them reported transient visual hallucinations. Nonetheless, additional study is needed to determine whether or not these findings result from a drug interaction between paroxetine and zolpidem.

RELATED DRUGS: No information is available.

MANAGEMENT OPTIONS: No specific action is required, but be alert for evidence of the interaction.

REFERENCES:
1. Katz SE. Possible paroxetine-zolpidem interaction. *Am J Psychiatry*. 1995;152:1689. Letter.

 ## Pefloxacin

Rifampin (eg, *Rifadin*)

SUMMARY: Pefloxacin serum concentrations are reduced by coadministration of rifampin; the clinical significance of this interaction probably is limited.

RISK FACTORS: No specific risk factors are known.

MECHANISM: Rifampin increases the nonrenal clearance of pefloxacin, probably by enhancing its hepatic metabolism.

CLINICAL EVALUATION: Eight healthy subjects received pefloxacin 400 mg orally twice daily for 3 days followed by a single 400 mg IV dose alone and after 10 days administration of rifampin 900 mg/day.[1] Rifampin administration increased the plasma clearance (approximately 75% metabolic) of pefloxacin by 35% and reduced pefloxacin half-life by a similar amount. Pefloxacin renal clearance was not altered by rifampin administration. The clinical significance of this interaction probably will be limited in most patients; however, reduced serum concentrations should be expected.

RELATED DRUGS: Rifampin also reduces the concentration of fleroxacin and may affect other quinolones in a similar manner.

MANAGEMENT OPTIONS: No specific action is required, but be alert for evidence of the interaction.

REFERENCES:
1. Humbert G, et al. Influence of rifampin on the pharmacokinetics of pefloxacin. *Clin Pharmacol Ther*. 1991;50:682.

Pefloxacin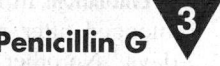

Theophylline

SUMMARY: Pefloxacin increases the serum concentration of theophylline; this may result in the development of theophylline toxicity.

RISK FACTORS: No specific risk factors are known.

MECHANISM: The quinolone purportedly is responsible for inhibiting the N-demethylation by CYP1A2 of theophylline.

CLINICAL EVALUATION: Pefloxacin 400 mg twice daily reduced theophylline clearance 30% in patients maintained on theophylline, an effect of about the same magnitude as that seen after ciprofloxacin in these patients.[1] Theophylline does not alter pefloxacin serum concentrations.[2]

RELATED DRUGS: Quinolones reported to inhibit the metabolism of drugs include ciprofloxacin (*Cipro*), enoxacin (*Penetrex*), norfloxacin (*Noroxin*), pipemidic acid, and pefloxacin. Quinolones reported to produce no or minor changes in theophylline pharmacokinetics include fleroxacin, flosequinan, lomefloxacin (*Maxaquin*), ofloxacin (*Floxin*), rufloxacin, sparfloxacin, and temafloxacin.

MANAGEMENT OPTIONS:

➡ *Consider Alternative.* Consider using a quinolone which does not produce changes in theophylline metabolism (eg, fleroxacin, flosequinan, lomefloxacin, ofloxacin, rufloxacin, sparfloxacin, temafloxacin).

➡ *Monitor.* Monitor patients maintained on theophylline for elevated theophylline concentrations and signs of toxicity (eg, palpitations, tachycardia, nausea, tremor) during coadministration of pefloxacin.

REFERENCES:

1. Wijnands WJA, et al. The influence of quinolone derivatives of theophylline clearance. *Br J Clin Pharmacol.* 1986;22:677.

2. Wijnands WJA, et al. Steady-state kinetics of the quinolone derivatives ofloxacin, enoxacin, ciprofloxacin, and pefloxacin during maintenance treatment with theophylline. *Drugs.* 1987;34(Suppl. 1):159.

Penicillin G ▼

Tetracycline

SUMMARY: Tetracycline administration may impair the efficacy of penicillin (eg, penicillin G) therapy.

RISK FACTORS: No specific risk factors are known.

MECHANISM: Since penicillin, a bactericidal agent, acts by inhibiting cell wall synthesis, bacteriostatic agents, such as tetracycline, which inhibit protein synthesis could antagonize the bactericidal effect of penicillin.

CLINICAL EVALUATION: Some have suggested that antibiotic antagonism occurs only under specific conditions, such as dose and order of therapy, and thus probably plays a minor role in clinical medicine. However, clinical examples of possible tetracycline antagonism of penicillin in the treatment of pneumococcal meningitis and streptococcal pharyngitis have been reported.[1-6] Some manufacturers' product information contains warnings against using tetracyclines and penicillins concomitantly.

Such warning statements could have medicolegal implications should a patient experience difficulty while taking such a combination.

RELATED DRUGS: Other penicillins may interact similarly.

MANAGEMENT OPTIONS:

➡ *Circumvent/Minimize.* When a penicillin is used with a tetracycline, be certain that adequate amounts of each agent are given because antagonism is most likely to occur when minimal doses of each agent are administered. If possible, begin penicillin administration a few hours before tetracycline administration.

➡ *Monitor.* If penicillin and tetracycline are coadministered, watch for reduced antibiotic efficacy.

REFERENCES:

1. Garrod LP. Causes of failure in antibiotic treatment. *BMJ.* 1972;4:441.
2. Kabins SA. Interactions among antibiotics and other drugs. *JAMA.* 1972;219:206.
3. Jawetz E. The use of combinations of antimicrobial drugs. *Ann Rev Pharmacol.* 1968;8:151.
4. Mills J, et al. Clinical use of antimicrobials. In: Katzung BG. Basic and Clinical Pharmacology. 4th ed. Los Altos: Lange Medical Publications; 1989:624.
5. Jawetz E. Synergism and antagonism among antimicrobial drugs, a personal perspective. *West J Med.* 1975;123:87.
6. Olsson RA, et al. Pneumococcal meningitis in the adult. *Ann Intern Med.* 1961;55:545.

4   Penicillin G

Warfarin (eg, *Coumadin*)

SUMMARY: One warfarin-treated patient developed an increased hypoprothrombinemic response following high doses of IV penicillin G, but more information is needed to establish a causal relationship.

RISK FACTORS: No specific risk factors are known.

MECHANISM: Not established. Large IV doses of penicillin G, as well as extended-spectrum penicillins such as carbenicillin (*Geocillin*) and ticarcillin (*Ticar*), may produce impaired platelet function and prolong bleeding times. In an *in vitro* study, penicillin G did not displace warfarin from plasma protein-binding sites.[2]

CLINICAL EVALUATION: In 1 patient on chronic warfarin therapy, the prothrombin time was prolonged after receiving high-dose IV penicillin G 24 million units/day for 7 days.[1] No other cause for the increased hypoprothrombinemia was found, and his warfarin response returned to prepenicillin levels after the penicillin G was discontinued. If high-dose IV penicillin G increased the effect of warfarin in this patient, the results cannot necessarily be extrapolated to smaller parenteral doses or oral administration of penicillin G.

RELATED DRUGS: No information is available.

MANAGEMENT OPTIONS: No specific action is required, but be alert for evidence of the interaction.

REFERENCES:

1. Brown MA, et al. Interaction of penicillin-G and warfarin? *Can J Hosp Pharm.* 1979;32:18.
2. Wallace SM, et al. Interaction of penicillin-G and warfarin: a followup. *Can J Hosp Pharm.* 1979;32:78.

Pentoxifylline (eg, *Trental*)

Theophylline

SUMMARY: Pentoxifylline increased plasma theophylline concentrations in healthy subjects; theophylline toxicity may be increased in patients receiving the combination, but more study is needed.

RISK FACTORS: No specific risk factors are known.

MECHANISM: Not established. Pentoxifylline may inhibit the hepatic metabolism of theophylline, but the studies were not designed to assess this possibility.

CLINICAL EVALUATION: Nine healthy subjects randomly received all 3 of the following treatments in 7-day courses: Sustained-release theophylline 300 mg twice daily; pentoxifylline 400 mg 3 times daily; and both drugs in the same respective doses. The mean theophylline serum concentration increased 30% in the presence of pentoxifylline, but the increases were highly variable ranging from no change in some subjects approximately 100% in others.[1] Studies of the use of pentoxifylline in patients receiving theophylline are needed to confirm these findings. Theophylline serum concentrations were undetectable during the use of pentoxifylline alone, suggesting that the increased theophylline concentrations were not caused by assay interference. Other studies, although limited, also suggest a lack of interference of pentoxifylline on various types of theophylline assays.[2,3]

RELATED DRUGS: Whether other forms of theophylline would be affected similarly by pentoxifylline is unknown. If the mechanism of the interaction is inhibition of theophylline elimination, the interaction is likely to be similar with all forms of theophylline. If another mechanism is involved (eg, increased theophylline absorption), the interaction may or may not be similar for other theophylline dosage forms.

MANAGEMENT OPTIONS:

➥ *Monitor.* Monitor for evidence of altered theophylline effect if pentoxifylline therapy is initiated and for decreased theophylline effect if it is discontinued. Alteration of theophylline dose may be needed.

REFERENCES:

1. Ellison MJ, et al. Influence of pentoxifylline on steady-state theophylline serum concentrations from sustained-release formulation. *Pharmacotherapy*. 1990;10:383.
2. Cummings DM, et al. Interference potential of pentoxifylline and its major metabolite with theophylline assays. *Am J Hosp Pharm*. 1985;42:2717.
3. Cohen IA, et al. Effect of pentoxifylline and its metabolites on three theophylline assays. *Clin Pharm*. 1988;7:457.

Phenelzine (*Nardil*)

Phenylephrine (*Neo-Synephrine*) AVOID

SUMMARY: Monoamine oxidase (MAO) inhibitors such as phenelzine enhance the effects of phenylephrine, especially when it is administered orally. Concomitant use of these drugs may result in hypertensive reactions.

RISK FACTORS:

➥ *Route of Administration.* The interaction is likely to be much greater with oral than with parenteral phenylephrine.

MECHANISM: Phenylephrine appears to act primarily by direct action on adrenergic receptors, with relatively little indirect activity. Because phenylephrine is metabolized by monoamine oxidase in the intestine and liver, normal oral doses of phenylephrine would be expected to have a markedly enhanced effect in the presence of an MAO inhibitor. Parenteral doses of phenylephrine would not be expected to be appreciably affected because much smaller doses are used and less exposure to intestinal and hepatic monoamine oxidase occurs.

CLINICAL EVALUATION: In 1 clinical study, MAO inhibitors markedly enhanced the hypertensive response to oral phenylephrine[1]; on 3 occasions, it was necessary to use phentolamine (eg, *Regitine*) to abate the severe hypertension. As expected from the preceding discussion of mechanisms, MAO inhibitors caused only a moderate potentiation of the pressor response to parenteral (in this case IV) phenylephrine. In a subsequent study in 4 healthy subjects, pretreatment with an MAO inhibitor resulted in a 2- to 2.5-fold increase in the pressor response to oral phenylephrine.[2] In another study of 4 patients with hypotension, phenylephrine produced a pronounced pressor effect when it was combined with an MAO inhibitor.[3] Another patient on phenelzine developed a severe headache, palpitations, and a blood pressure of 240/120 mm Hg after taking 2 teaspoons of phenylephrine-containing cough syrup.[4] Thus, the evidence is convincing that a significant interaction occurs between MAO inhibitors and phenylephrine.

RELATED DRUGS: All nonselective MAO inhibitors including isocarboxazid (*Marplan*) and tranylcypromine (*Parnate*) would be expected to interact with phenylephrine.

MANAGEMENT OPTIONS:

➥ *AVOID COMBINATION.* Avoid oral phenylephrine in patients taking an MAO inhibitor. Note that phenylephrine is found in many OTC cold remedies. Use parenteral phenylephrine with great care in patients on an MAO inhibitor. The effect of phenylephrine-containing nasal sprays in those taking an MAO inhibitor has not been studied, but avoid them until information on their safety is available. Remember that effects of nonselective MAO inhibitors should be assumed to persist for 2 weeks after they are discontinued.

REFERENCES:
1. Elis J, et al. Modification by monoamine oxidase inhibitors of the effect of some sympathomimetics on blood pressure. *BMJ*. 1967;2:75-78.
2. Boakes AJ, et al. Interactions between sympathomimetic amines and antidepressant agents in man. *BMJ*. 1973;1:311-315.
3. Davies B, et al. Pressor amines and monoamine-oxidase inhibitors for treatment of postural hypotension in autonomic failure. Limitations and hazards. *Lancet*. 1978;1:172-175.
4. Harrison WM, et al. MAOIs and hypertensive crises: the role of OTC drugs. *J Clin Psychiatry*. 1989;50:64-65.

 Phenelzine (*Nardil*)

AVOID **Pseudoephedrine (eg, *Sudafed*)**

SUMMARY: Indirect-acting sympathomimetics, such as pseudoephedrine, may produce severe hypertension when administered to patients receiving a monoamine oxidase (MAO) inhibitor such as phenelzine.

RISK FACTORS: No specific risk factors are known.

MECHANISM: MAO inhibitors tend to increase the amount of norepinephrine in storage sites of the adrenergic neuron. Subsequent displacement of these increased stores of norepinephrine by indirect-acting sympathomimetics (eg, pseudoephedrine) can result in an exaggerated response.

CLINICAL EVALUATION: A patient on MAO inhibitor therapy died following ingestion of a single dose of pseudoephedrine but no details were given.[1] Another patient on phenelzine developed a hypertensive crisis and intracerebral bleeding after taking 2 tablets of a product containing pseudoephedrine and dextromethorphan.[2] (Note that dextromethorphan also is contraindicated in patients on nonselective MAO inhibitors because of the risk of serotonin syndrome.)

RELATED DRUGS: All nonselective MAO inhibitors including isocarboxazid (*Marplan*) and tranylcypromine (*Parnate*) would be expected to interact with pseudoephedrine (as well as other indirect-acting sympathomimetics and phenylephrine [*Neo-Synephrine*]).

MANAGEMENT OPTIONS:

➡ **AVOID COMBINATION.** Do not give pseudoephedrine to patients receiving nonselective MAO inhibitors. Remember that the effects of nonselective MAO inhibitors should be assumed to persist for 2 weeks after they are discontinued.

REFERENCES:

1. Wright SP. Hazards with monoamine-oxidase inhibitors: a persistent problem. *Lancet.* 1978;1:284-285.
2. Harrison WM, et al. MAOIs and hypertensive crises: the role of OTC drugs. *J Clin Psychiatry.* 1989;50:64-65.

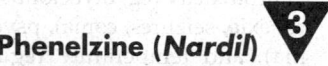

Phenelzine (*Nardil*)

Reserpine (*Serpalan*)

SUMMARY: Reserpine reportedly may cause a hypertensive reaction in patients receiving a monoamine oxidase inhibitor (MAOI) like phenelzine, but supporting clinical evidence is scanty.

RISK FACTORS:

➡ **Order of Drug Administration.** Theoretically, this interaction is most likely to occur in a patient who has been taking nonselective MAOIs who then is started on reserpine (rather than the reverse order of administration).

MECHANISM: Nonselective MAOIs cause accumulation of norepinephrine in storage sites within the adrenergic neuron. If reserpine is subsequently given, the reserpine-induced release of norepinephrine may result in an exaggerated response caused by the increased quantity of neurotransmitter present at the adrenergic receptor. Other factors also may be involved.

CLINICAL EVALUATION: Excitation and hypertension may occur if reserpine is given to a patient receiving an MAOI,[1] but clinical reports describing this interaction are lacking.

RELATED DRUGS: Theoretically, all nonselective MAOIs including isocarboxazid (*Marplan*) and tranylcypromine (*Parnate*) would be expected to interact with reserpine.

MANAGEMENT OPTIONS:

➡ **Consider Alternative.** Although more clinical information is needed to clarify this interaction, it would be prudent to consider antihypertensive therapy other than reserpine in patients on nonselective MAOIs. Remember that the effects of nonselective MAOIs should be assumed to persist for 2 weeks after they are discontinued.

➡ *Monitor.* Monitor for evidence of hypertensive reaction if the combination is given.

REFERENCES:
1. Goldberg LI. Monoamine oxidase inhibitors. Adverse reactions and possible mechanisms. *JAMA*. 1964;190:456.

 Phenelzine (*Nardil*)

AVOID **Sibutramine (*Meridia*)**

SUMMARY: Given the theoretical risk of serotonin syndrome, sibutramine should not be given concurrently with monoamine oxidase inhibitors (MAOIs).

RISK FACTORS: No specific risk factors are known.

MECHANISM: Possible additive serotonergic effects.

CLINICAL EVALUATION: While no published data are available for evaluation, the manufacturer of sibutramine has made available some data on this interaction.[1] The manufacturer states that sibutramine is contraindicated in combination with MAOIs, given the potential risk of serotonin syndrome.[1] Serotonin syndrome can result in neurotoxicity (eg, myoclonus, tremors, rigidity, incoordination, restlessness, hyperreflexia, seizures, coma), psychiatric symptoms (eg, agitation, confusion, hypomania), and temperature regulation abnormalities (eg, fever, sweating). Severe serotonin syndrome can be fatal. Although the caution against concurrent use of sibutramine and MAOIs is based upon theoretical considerations, the contraindication appears reasonable given the potential severity of serotonin syndrome.

RELATED DRUGS: Avoid sibutramine with other MAOIs such as tranylcypromine (*Parnate*) and selegiline (*Eldepryl*).

MANAGEMENT OPTIONS:

➡ *AVOID COMBINATION.* Do not give sibutramine concurrently with MAOIs.

REFERENCES:
1. Knoll Pharmaceuticals. *Meridia* product information. Mount Olive, NJ. 1997.
2. Mills KC. Serotonin syndrome: a clinical update. *Crit Care Clin*. 1997;13:763.

 Phenelzine (*Nardil*)

Succinylcholine (eg, *Anectine*)

SUMMARY: Phenelzine may prolong the muscle relaxation caused by succinylcholine administration.

RISK FACTORS: No specific risk factors are known.

MECHANISM: A preliminary report indicates that phenelzine may decrease plasma pseudocholinesterase to the subnormal range. Thus, succinylcholine, which is metabolized by pseudocholinesterase, may have an enhanced effect in patients on phenelzine.

CLINICAL EVALUATION: One case report describes a patient on phenelzine who developed prolonged apnea following administration of succinylcholine. This patient and 3 others taking phenelzine were shown to have decreased pseudocholinesterase levels.

RELATED DRUGS: Based upon information from this preliminary study, other monoamine oxidase inhibitors do not appear to affect pseudocholinesterase.[1]

MANAGEMENT OPTIONS:

➡ *Monitor.* Monitor for prolonged succinylcholine effect in patients receiving phenelzine. Remember that the effects of phenelzine should be assumed to persist for 2 weeks after it is discontinued.

REFERENCES:
1. Bodley PO, et al. Low serum pseudocholinesterase levels complicating treatment with phenelzine. *BMJ.* 1969;3:510.

Phenelzine (*Nardil*)

Venlafaxine (*Effexor*) `AVOID`

SUMMARY: Severe serotonin syndrome can occur when venlafaxine is used with or within 2 weeks of discontinuation of phenelzine or other nonselective monoamine oxidase inhibitors (MAOIs). Strictly avoid the combination.

RISK FACTORS: No specific risk factors are known.

MECHANISM: Additive. Phenelzine, a nonselective MAOI, inhibits serotonin metabolism, and venlafaxine is a potent inhibitor of serotonin reuptake.

CLINICAL EVALUATION: A number of patients have developed severe serotonin syndrome with combined use of phenelzine and venlafaxine.[1-4] In most cases, the reaction occurred during a transition from phenelzine to venlafaxine, with insufficient washout time (ie, less than 2 weeks).

RELATED DRUGS: All nonselective MAOIs should be expected to result in serotonin syndrome if combined with venlafaxine. This would include tranylcypromine (*Parnate*) and isocarboxazid (*Marplan*); selegiline (*Eldepryl*) can act as a nonselective MAOI in some patients, especially if large doses are used.

MANAGEMENT OPTIONS:

➡ *AVOID COMBINATION.* Avoid combined use of venlafaxine with phenelzine (or any other nonselective MAOIs). This would include the use of venlafaxine within 2 weeks of discontinuation of a MAOI.

REFERENCES:
1. Weiner LA, et al. Serotonin syndrome secondary to phenelzine-venlafaxine interaction. *Pharmacotherapy.* 1998;18:399.
2. Diamond S, et al. Serotonin syndrome induced by transitioning from phenelzine to venlafaxine: four patient reports. *Neurology.* 1998;51:274.
3. Heisler MA, et al. Serotonin syndrome induced by administration of venlafaxine and phenelzine. *Ann Pharmacother.* 1996;30:84. Letter.
4. Phillips SD, Ringo P. Phenelzine and venlafaxine interaction. *Am J Psychiatry.* 1995;152:1400. Letter.

4 Phenformin

Warfarin (eg, *Coumadin*)

SUMMARY: One case report and theoretical considerations suggest that phenformin may increase the hypoprothrombinemic response to oral anticoagulants; more study is needed to evaluate the incidence and significance of this effect.

RISK FACTORS: No specific risk factors are known.

MECHANISM: The phenformin-induced increase in fibrinolytic activity may produce a tendency to hemorrhage in patients receiving oral anticoagulants, even in the absence of excessively prolonged prothrombin times.

CLINICAL EVALUATION: Not established. A single case has been reported in which a patient on warfarin therapy developed severe hematuria 3 months after initiation of phenformin therapy.[1] Coagulation tests were within the therapeutic range, but there was evidence of increased fibrinolytic activity.

RELATED DRUGS: It does not seem likely that oral anticoagulants would interact with insulin.

MANAGEMENT OPTIONS:

→ *Monitor.* Although this interaction is poorly documented, monitor for increased bleeding tendency if phenformin is used with oral anticoagulants. Theoretically, any interaction would not be detected by monitoring the hypoprothrombinemic response, since increased fibrinolytic activity would not be detected.

REFERENCES:

1. Hamblin TJ. Interaction between warfarin and phenformin. *Lancet.* 1971;2:1323. Letter.

4 Phenobarbital

Phenylbutazone (*Butazolidin*)

SUMMARY: Phenobarbital may reduce serum phenylbutazone concentrations, but the clinical importance of this effect is not established.

RISK FACTORS: No specific risk factors are known.

MECHANISM: Phenobarbital appears to stimulate the metabolism of phenylbutazone through induction of hepatic microsomal enzymes.

CLINICAL EVALUATION: In studies with a large number of healthy subjects[1] and patients with sickle cell anemia,[2] phenobarbital reduced the half-life of phenylbutazone. This effect seemed to be most marked in those who had longer phenylbutazone half-lives before eg, phenobarbital.[1] The effect of the reduced half-life on the therapeutic response to phenylbutazone has not been established.

RELATED DRUGS: Barbiturates other than phenobarbital also would be expected to enhance phenylbutazone hepatic metabolism.

MANAGEMENT OPTIONS: No specific action is required, but be alert for evidence of the interaction.

REFERENCES:

1. Whittaker JA, et al. Genetic control of phenylbutazone metabolism in man. *BMJ.* 1970;4:323.

2. Anderson KE, et al. Oxidative drug metabolism and inducibility by phenobarbital in sickle cell anemia. *Clin Pharmacol Ther.* 1977;22:580.

Phenobarbital

Phenytoin (eg, *Dilantin*)

SUMMARY: Phenobarbital tends to decrease serum phenytoin concentrations; it occasionally does not change and sometimes even increases the serum phenytoin concentration. Combined use of barbiturates and phenytoin can be beneficial in many patients; however, the phenytoin serum concentration can be affected when phenobarbital is started or stopped.

RISK FACTORS: No specific risk factors are known.

MECHANISM: Phenobarbital can induce hepatic microsomal enzymes and increase phenytoin metabolism; however, phenobarbital also appears to competitively inhibit the metabolism of phenytoin.[1-19] Therapeutic doses of phenobarbital usually are associated with hepatic enzyme induction and enhanced phenytoin metabolism; competitive inhibition usually would be negligible. Large doses of phenobarbital, however, may increase serum phenytoin concentrations.

CLINICAL EVALUATION: Phenytoin serum concentrations can be decreased by concomitant phenobarbital administration, and phenytoin serum concentrations can be increased to toxic levels following discontinuation of phenobarbital.[11,16] In some patients, phenytoin serum concentrations are not affected by phenobarbital or may even be increased. Patients whose phenytoin-metabolizing enzymes are relatively *saturated* may be more likely to develop increased serum phenytoin concentrations following barbiturate administration. The ability of phenobarbital to inhibit phenytoin competitively would depend upon the dose of phenobarbital, with average doses having a minimal inhibiting effect. Conversely, phenytoin can increase phenobarbital plasma concentrations.[16,19] Finally, the combination of phenytoin and phenobarbital may be more likely to cause osteomalacia than either agent alone.[4] A preliminary report suggests that determination of free phenytoin concentrations may be much more useful in patients receiving concurrent phenobarbital.[20] In some patients receiving phenytoin as an antiarrhythmic, clinically significant decreases in serum phenytoin when given barbiturates could be observed, but this remains to be established.

RELATED DRUGS: Little is known regarding the effect of barbiturates other than phenobarbital on phenytoin, but they probably will reduce phenytoin serum concentrations.

MANAGEMENT OPTIONS:

➡ *Circumvent/Minimize.* Avoid large doses of phenobarbital probably in patients with high blood levels of phenytoin because of the potential for competitive inhibition of phenytoin metabolism.

➡ *Monitor.* Observe patients maintained on phenytoin and a barbiturate for signs of phenytoin intoxication if the barbiturate therapy is stopped. Epileptic patients who manifest decreases in phenytoin blood concentrations caused by phenobarbital administration do not appear to be adversely affected clinically, and no action is required.

REFERENCES:

1. Gallagher BB, et al. Primidone, diphenylhydantoin and phenobarbital. Aspects of acute and chronic toxicity. *Neurology*. 1973;23:145.

2. Garrettson LK, et al. Disappearance of phenobarbital and diphenylhydantoin from serum of children. *Clin Pharmacol Ther*. 1970;11:674.

3. Buchanan RA, et al. Diphenylhydantoin and phenobarbital blood levels of epileptic children. *Neurology*. 1971;21:866.

4. Hahn TJ, et al. Effect of chronic anticonvulsant therapy on serum 25-hydroxy calciferol levels in adults. *N Engl J Med*. 1972;287:900.

5. Hansten PD. Interactions between anticonvulsant drugs: primidone, diphenylhydantoin and phenobarbital. *Northwest Med J*. 1974;1:17.

6. Cucinell SA, et al. Drug interactions in man. I. Lowering effect of phenobarbital on plasma levels of bishydroxycoumarin (*Dicumarol*) and diphenylhydantoin (*Dilantin*). *Clin Pharmacol Ther*. 1965;6:420.

7. Kutt H, et al. The effect of phenobarbital on plasma diphenylhydantoin level and metabolism in man and in rat liver microsomes. *Neurology*. 1969;19:611.

8. Buchanan RA, et al. The effect of phenobarbital on diphenylhydantoin metabolism in children. *Pediatrics*. 1969;43:114.

9. Kutt H, et al. The effect of phenobarbital upon diphenylhydantoin metabolism in man. *Neurology*. 1965;15:274. Abstract.

10. Kokenge R, et al. Neurological sequelae following *Dilantin* overdose in a patient and in experimental animals. *Neurology*. 1965;15:823.

11. Tudhope GR. Advances in medicine. *Practitioner*. 1969;203:405.

12. Diamond WD, et al. A clinical study of the effect of phenobarbital on diphenylhydantoin plasma levels. *J Clin Pharmacol*. 1970;10:306.

13. Sotaniemi E, et al. The clinical significance of microsomal enzyme induction in the therapy of epileptic patients. *Ann Clin Res*. 1970;2:223.

14. Booker HE, et al. Concurrent administration of phenobarbital and diphenylhydantoin: lack of an interference effect. *Neurology*. 1971;21:383.

15. Buchthal F, et al. Serum concentrations of diphenylhydantoin (phenytoin) and phenobarbital and their relation to therapeutic and toxic effects. *Psychiatr Neurol Neurochir*. 1971;74:117.

16. Morselli PL, et al. Interaction between phenobarbital and diphenylhydantoin in animals and in epileptic patients. *Ann NY Acad Sci*. 1971;179:88.

17. Rizzo M, et al. Further observations on the interactions between phenobarbital and diphenylhydantoin during chronic treatment in the rat. *Biochem Pharmacol*. 1972;21:449.

18. Callaghan N, et al. The effect of anticonvulsant drugs which induce liver enzymes on derived and ingested phenobarbitone levels. *Acta Neurol Scand*. 1977;56:1.

19. Lambie DG, et al. Therapeutic and pharmacokinetic effects of increasing phenytoin in chronic epileptics on multiple drug therapy. *Lancet*. 1976;2:386.

20. Cuzzolin L, et al. Phenytoin-phenobarbital interaction: importance of free plasma phenytoin monitoring. *Pharmacol Res Commun*. 1988;20:627.

Phenobarbital (eg, *Bellatal*)

Prednisone (eg, *Deltasone*)

SUMMARY: Barbiturates may reduce serum concentrations of prednisone and other corticosteroids sufficiently to impair their therapeutic effect.

RISK FACTORS: No specific risk factors are known.

MECHANISM: Barbiturates appear to enhance the metabolism of corticosteroids, probably by inducing hepatic microsomal enzymes.[1-4]

CLINICAL EVALUATION: Three prednisone-dependent asthmatic patients developed worsening of their asthma following initiation of phenobarbital.[5] This reversed when the phenobarbital was withdrawn. Results of subsequent pharmacokinetic studies in several patients using phenobarbital and dexamethasone (*Decadron*) were consistent with the view that phenobarbital enhances corticosteroid metabolism by enzyme induction. In another study, renal transplant patients receiving phenobarbital or phenytoin eliminated prednisolone (*Prelone*) more rapidly than 12 control patients who were not receiving these drugs.[6] Another report describes a decrease in the renal allograft survival in patients receiving phenobarbital. This was presumably caused by phenobarbital-induced increases in prednisone disposition with a resultant reduction in immunosuppression.[7] Phenobarbital has been shown to reduce the half-life of methylprednisolone (*Medrol*).[8] Thus, there is substantial evidence that barbiturates can reduce the effects of corticosteroids.

RELATED DRUGS: Dexamethasone, prednisolone, and methylprednisolone interact similarly with phenobarbital. Assume that all combinations of barbiturates and corticosteroids interact until proven otherwise.

MANAGEMENT OPTIONS:

➡ *Consider Alternative.* If appropriate, consider possible alternatives to barbiturates (eg, benzodiazepines).

➡ *Monitor.* Monitor for altered corticosteroid effect if a barbiturate is initiated, discontinued, or changed in dosage; substantial adjustments in corticosteroid dosage may be needed.

REFERENCES:

1. Falliers CJ. Corticosteroids and phenobarbital in asthma. *N Engl J Med*. 1972;287:201.
2. Berman ML, et al. Acute stimulation of cortisol metabolism by pentobarbital in man. *Anesthesiology*. 1971;34:365.
3. Southren AL, et al. Effect of N-phenylbarbital (phetharbital) on the metabolism of testosterone and cortisol in man. *J Clin Endocrinol Metab*. 1969;29:251.
4. Brooks PM, et al. Effects of enzyme induction on metabolism of prednisolone. Clinical and laboratory study. *Ann Rheum Dis*. 1976;35:339.
5. Brooks SM, et al. Adverse effects of phenobarbital on corticosteroid metabolism in patients with bronchial asthma. *N Engl J Med*. 1972;286:1125.
6. Gambertoglio J, et al. Enhancement of prednisolone elimination by anticonvulsants in renal transplant recipients. *Clin Pharmacol Ther*. 1982;31:228.
7. Wassner SJ, et al. The adverse effect of anticonvulsant therapy on renal allograft survival. *J Pediatr*. 1976;88:134.
8. Stjernholm MR, et al. Effects of diphenylhydantoin, phenobarbital, and diazepam on the metabolism of methylprednisolone and its sodium succinate. *J Clin Endocrinol Metab*. 1975;41:887.

Phenobarbital (eg, *Bellatal*)

Primidone (*Mysoline*)

SUMMARY: The combination of primidone and phenobarbital may result in excessive serum phenobarbital concentrations.

RISK FACTORS: No specific risk factors are known.

MECHANISM: A considerable portion of primidone is converted to phenobarbital in the body. Thus, coadministration of primidone and phenobarbital may result in excessive serum phenobarbital concentrations.

CLINICAL EVALUATION: Excessive serum concentrations of phenobarbital have been found in patients receiving primidone plus phenobarbital[1] or primidone plus phenobarbital and phenytoin.[2] Thus, the propriety of adding phenobarbital to a regimen that already includes primidone has been questioned. This would be especially true in patients also receiving phenytoin, because it seems to promote the conversion of primidone to phenobarbital.[2-4]

RELATED DRUGS: No information is available.

MANAGEMENT OPTIONS:

➥ *Consider Alternative.* For most patients, do not use primidone and phenobarbital concomitantly.

➥ *Monitor.* If the combination is used, monitor the patient for excessive phenobarbital serum concentrations.

REFERENCES:

1. Griffin GD, et al. Primidone-phenobarbital intoxication. *Drug Ther.* 1976;60:76.
2. Fincham RW, et al. The influence of diphenylhydantoin on primidone metabolism. *Arch Neurol.* 1974;30:259.
3. Wilson JT, et al. Chronic and severe phenobarbital intoxication in a child treated with primidone and diphenylhydantoin. *J Pediatr.* 1973;83:484.
4. Gallagher BB, et al. Primidone, diphenylhydantoin and phenobarbital. Aspects of acute and chronic toxicity. *Neurology.* 1973;23:145.

Phenobarbital (eg, *Bellatal*)

Propafenone (*Rythmol*)

SUMMARY: Phenobarbital increases the metabolism of propafenone and reduces its plasma concentrations in healthy subjects; the clinical importance of this interaction is not established.

RISK FACTORS: No specific risk factors are known.

MECHANISM: Phenobarbital is known to stimulate hepatic enzymes and appears to increase the clearance of propafenone.

CLINICAL EVALUATION: Seven healthy subjects took a single 300 mg dose orally of propafenone before and after a 3-week period during which they received phenobarbital 100 mg/day HS.[1] The peak serum concentration of propafenone and the area under its serum concentration-time curve decreased significantly. The clearance after oral administration of propafenone was increased 11% to 849% in the subjects. These changes could lead to loss of antiarrhythmic efficacy in some patients.

RELATED DRUGS: No information is available.

MANAGEMENT OPTIONS:

➥ *Monitor.* Until this interaction is studied in patients receiving chronic propafenone and phenobarbital, monitor patients for diminished propafenone efficacy and toxicity when phenobarbital is added to or removed from the drug regimen.

REFERENCES:

1. Chan GL-Y, et al. The effect of phenobarbital on the pharmacokinetics of propafenone in man. *Pharm Res.* 1988;5:S-153.

Phenobarbital

Propoxyphene (eg, *Darvocet-N*)

SUMMARY: Preliminary clinical evidence indicates that propoxyphene slightly increases serum phenobarbital concentrations, but the clinical importance of this effect is not established.

RISK FACTORS: No specific risk factors are known.

MECHANISM: Not established. Propoxyphene might inhibit the hepatic metabolism of phenobarbital.

CLINICAL EVALUATION: In 4 epileptic patients on chronic phenobarbital propoxyphene 65 mg 3 times daily increased mean phenobarbital levels by 20% after 1 week.[1] The effect of propoxyphene on other barbiturates is not established.

RELATED DRUGS: The effect of propoxyphene on barbiturates other than phenobarbital is not established.

MANAGEMENT OPTIONS: No specific action is required, but be alert for evidence of the interaction.

REFERENCES:

1. Hansen BS, et al. Influence of dextropropoxyphene on steady state serum levels and protein binding of three antiepileptic drugs in man. *Acta Neurol Scand.* 1980;61:357.

Phenobarbital

Protriptyline (eg, *Vivactil*)

SUMMARY: Phenobarbital and other barbiturates may reduce serum concentrations of protriptyline and other tricyclic antidepressants (TCAs); the therapeutic response to the antidepressants probably is reduced in some patients.

RISK FACTORS:

➥ *Dosage Regimen.* Barbiturate-induced enzyme induction is known to be dose related; small or occasional doses are unlikely to significantly affect drug metabolism. Depending upon the barbiturate, it may take 1 to 2 weeks or more for the maximal reduction in serum concentrations of the affected drug.

MECHANISM: Barbiturates appear to stimulate the metabolism of TCAs and may decrease their blood levels. Barbiturates also may potentiate the effects of toxic doses of TCAs (eg, respiratory depression).

CLINICAL EVALUATION: Several reports have described individual patients whose serum concentrations of TCAs decreased in the presence of a barbiturate. Subsequent study in patients receiving protriptyline confirmed that TCA serum concentrations may be lower in the presence of barbiturate therapy.[1,3-11]

RELATED DRUGS: Other barbiturates may reduce serum concentrations of protriptyline and other TCAs. Unlike barbiturates, benzodiazepines do not appear likely to affect TCA serum concentrations.

MANAGEMENT OPTIONS:

➥ *Consider Alternative.* Patients on TCAs probably respond better without barbiturates, and it has been recommended that barbiturates be avoided in such patients.[2]

➡ *Monitor.* Monitor for altered TCA effect if barbiturate therapy is initiated, discontinued, or changed in dosage; adjust tricyclic antidepressant dose as needed.

REFERENCES:

1. Moody JP, et al. Pharmacokinetic aspects of protriptyline plasma levels. *Eur J Clin Pharmacol.* 1977;11:51.
2. Burrows GD, et al. Antidepressants and barbiturates. *BMJ.* 1971;4:113. Letter.
3. Silverman G, et al. Interaction of benzodiazepines with tricyclic antidepressants. *BMJ.* 1972;4:111. Letter.
4. Borden EC, et al. Recovery from massive amitriptyline overdosage. *Lancet.* 1968;1:1256. Letter.
5. Alexanderson B, et al. Steady state plasma levels of nortriptyline in twins: influence of genetic factors and drug therapy. *BMJ.* 1969;4:764.
6. Crocker, et al. Tricyclic (antidepressant) drug toxicity. *Clin Toxicol.* 1969;2:397.
7. Noble, et al. Acute poisoning by tricyclic antidepressants: clinical features and management of 100 patients. *Clin Toxicol.* 1969;2:403.
8. Sjoqvist F, et al. Plasma level of monomethylated tricyclic antidepressants and side-effects in man. In: Toxicity and Side-Effects of Psychotropic Drugs. Amsterdam: Excerpta Medica Foundation; 1968:246–57.
9. Hammer W, et al. A comparative study of the metabolism of desmethylimipramine, nortriptyline, and oxyphenbutazone in man. *Clin Pharmacol Ther.* 1969;10:44.
10. Metabolism of drugs. *BMJ.* 1970;1:767.
11. Royds R, et al. Tricyclic antidepressant poisoning. *Practitioner.* 1970;204:282.

 4   Phenobarbital

Pyridoxine (*Vitamin B₆*)

SUMMARY: Preliminary clinical data from a few patients indicate that large doses of pyridoxine reduce serum phenobarbital concentrations, but a causal relationship was not established.

RISK FACTORS:

➡ *Dosage Regimen.* Large doses of pyridoxine appear to be required; it is unlikely that vitamin supplements containing pyridoxine would affect phenobarbital.

MECHANISM: Not established. Pyridoxine administration might enhance the activity of pyridoxal phosphate-dependent enzymes,[1] thus enhancing phenobarbital metabolism.

CLINICAL EVALUATION: Reductions in serum phenobarbital concentrations were noted in several epileptic patients who were given pyridoxine 200 mg/day for 4 weeks.[1] Confirmation of this finding is needed, but high-dose pyridoxine should be considered in the differential diagnosis of inadequate response to phenobarbital.

RELATED DRUGS: The effect of pyridoxine on other barbiturates is not known, nor is the effect of smaller doses of pyridoxine on phenobarbital.

MANAGEMENT OPTIONS: No specific action is required, but be alert for evidence of the interaction.

REFERENCES:

1. Hansson O, et al. Pyridoxine and serum concentrations of phenytoin and phenobarbitone. *Lancet.* 1976;1:256. Letter.

Phenobarbital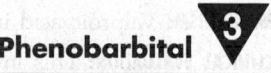

Quinidine

SUMMARY: Barbiturates can reduce quinidine plasma concentrations; loss of efficacy could result.

RISK FACTORS: No specific risk factors are known.

MECHANISM: Phenobarbital appears to enhance the hepatic metabolism of quinidine.

CLINICAL EVALUATION: In several cases barbiturate or phenytoin (*Dilantin*) therapy was associated with low plasma quinidine concentrations.[1-3] A study of normal subjects confirmed that phenobarbital can considerably increase the elimination of quinidine.[1]

RELATED DRUGS: Other barbiturates would be expected to produce a similar response.

MANAGEMENT OPTIONS:

➡ *Circumvent/Minimize.* Initiation or discontinuation of phenobarbital therapy in patients taking quinidine may necessitate a change in quinidine dosage.

➡ *Monitor.* Quinidine response and plasma concentrations may be reduced when barbiturates are added or increased when phenobarbital is discontinued.

REFERENCES:
1. Data JL, et al. Interaction of quinidine with anticonvulsant drugs. *N Engl J Med.* 1976;294:699.
2. Chapron DJ, et al. Apparent quinidine-induced digoxin toxicity after withdrawal of pentobarbital. A case of sequential drug interactions. *Arch Intern Med.* 1979;139:363.
3. Kroboth FJ, et al. Phenytoin-theophylline-quinidine interaction. *N Engl J Med.* 1983;308:725. Letter.

Phenobarbital

Theophylline

SUMMARY: Barbiturates like phenobarbital may reduce serum theophylline concentrations; in some patients, the effect may be large enough to reduce the therapeutic response to theophylline.

RISK FACTORS: No specific risk factors are known.

MECHANISM: Barbiturates probably enhance the metabolism of theophylline by inducing hepatic microsomal enzymes, primarily CYP1A2.

CLINICAL EVALUATION: In 6 healthy subjects, phenobarbital 90 mg/day for 4 weeks enhanced the clearance of theophylline.[4] Large IV doses of pentobarbital (*Nembutal*) markedly increased the clearance of theophylline in one patient.[1] In contrast, another study in 12 healthy men indicated that phenobarbital 1.5 mg/kg/day for 2 weeks only slightly increased the clearance of IV theophylline 4.5 mg/kg,[3] but the duration of phenobarbital administration (2 weeks) in this study may have been insufficient to produce maximal enzyme induction. In another report, secobarbital (*Seconal*) appears to have increased the clearance of theophylline in an infant.[2] Taking all of the evidence together, expect that some patients receiving chronic theophylline therapy will develop impaired control of their asthma if barbiturates are added. Recognition of the interaction between barbiturates and theophylline has caused some to question the logic of products containing both drugs (eg, *Tedral*). Whether the maximum daily dose of phenobarbital contained in such preparations is sufficient to enhance theophylline metabolism and reduce its effect is not established, but it seems likely that at least some patients would be so affected.

RELATED DRUGS: Pentobarbital and secobarbital interact similarly with theophylline. All barbiturates probably have a similar effect on theophylline.

MANAGEMENT OPTIONS:

➥ *Monitor.* Monitor patients receiving chronic theophylline therapy for altered theophylline effect when barbiturate therapy is started or stopped.

REFERENCES:

1. Gibson GA, et al. Influence of high-dose pentobarbital theophylline pharmacokinetics: a case study. *Ther Drug Monit.* 1985;7:181.

2. Paladino JA, et al. Effect of secobarbital on theophylline clearance. *Ther Drug Monit.* 1983;5:135.

3. Piafsky KM, et al. Effect of phenobarbital on the disposition of intravenous theophylline. *Clin Pharmacol Ther.* 1977;22:336.

4. Landay RA, et al. Effect of phenobarbital on theophylline disposition. *J Allergy Clin Immunol.* 1978;62:27.

Phenobarbital

Valproic Acid (eg, *Depakene*)

SUMMARY: Valproic acid increases serum phenobarbital concentrations; phenobarbital intoxication may occur in some patients.

RISK FACTORS: No specific risk factors are known.

MECHANISM: Valproic acid inhibits the hepatic metabolism of phenobarbital.

CLINICAL EVALUATION: This interaction is well documented. Several studies have shown that phenobarbital elimination is reduced substantially by valproic acid.[1-3] The magnitude of the interaction is large enough to cause symptoms of phenobarbital toxicity (eg, excessive sedation) in some patients.

RELATED DRUGS: No information is available.

MANAGEMENT OPTIONS:

➥ *Monitor.* Monitor for excessive phenobarbital effect when valproic acid is given concurrently; reductions in the phenobarbital dose may be necessary for many patients.

REFERENCES:

1. Wilder BJ, et al. Valproic acid: interaction with other anticonvulsant drugs. *Neurology.* 1978;28:892.

2. Patel IH, et al. Phenobarbital-valproic acid interaction. *Clin Pharmacol Ther.* 1980;27:515.

3. Bruni J, et al. Valproic acid and plasma levels of phenobarbital. *Neurology.* 1980;30:94.

Phenobarbital ▼ 3

Verapamil (eg, *Calan*)

SUMMARY: Phenobarbital substantially reduces the plasma concentrations of verapamil, especially when verapamil is given orally.

RISK FACTORS:

➡ *Route of Administration.* Oral verapamil dosing can increase the risk of interaction.

MECHANISM: Phenobarbital appears to enhance the metabolism of verapamil probably by increasing hepatic enzyme (CYP3A4) activity.

CLINICAL EVALUATION: Verapamil pharmacokinetics were evaluated in 7 healthy subjects before and after 21 days of treatment with phenobarbital 100 mg/day.[1] Each subject received verapamil as single 80 mg orally and 0.15 mg/day IV doses as well as 80 mg oral doses every 6 hours for 5 days. Phenobarbital administration increased the clearance after oral administration of verapamil 4- to 5-fold and decreased the verapamil area under the concentration-time curve 3- to 4-fold. The apparent bioavailability of chronically administered verapamil was reduced from 0.6 to 0.2 during phenobarbital dosing. The clearance following IV verapamil was approximately doubled by phenobarbital pretreatment. Phenobarbital also increased the free fraction of verapamil 25%.

RELATED DRUGS: Phenobarbital also increases the metabolism of nifedipine (eg, *Procardia*). Other calcium channel blockers may be similarly affected by phenobarbital and other barbiturates.

MANAGEMENT OPTIONS:

➡ *Circumvent/Minimize.* Patients receiving phenobarbital may require higher than usual doses of verapamil, especially if the verapamil is administered orally.

➡ *Monitor.* Monitor patients stabilized on verapamil (especially if taken orally) for the possibility of decreased effectiveness when phenobarbital is administered concomitantly.

REFERENCES:

1. Rutledge DR, et al. Effects of chronic phenobarbital on verapamil disposition in humans. *J Pharmacol Exp Ther.* 1988;246:7.

2 Phenobarbital

Warfarin (eg, *Coumadin*)

SUMMARY: Barbiturates inhibit the hypoprothrombinemic response to oral anticoagulants like warfarin. Fatal bleeding episodes have occurred when barbiturates were discontinued in patients stabilized on an anticoagulant.

RISK FACTORS:

➥ **Dosage Regimen.** The effect of barbiturates on anticoagulants may be dose related. For example, plasma warfarin did not change in 1 patient when 100 mg/day of secobarbital was given, but it decreased considerably when the dosage was increased to 200 mg/day.[3] However, in 6 healthy subjects, 100 mg/day of secobarbital was sufficient to enhance warfarin metabolism.[4] A decrease in the anticoagulant response usually develops gradually after a barbiturate is initiated, with maximal effects occurring at about 2 weeks. The time course following discontinuation of the barbiturate is similar; the results of enzyme induction usually begin to diminish within a week, with little induction remaining by 2 to 3 weeks. Note that the onset and offset of enzyme induction by barbiturates will vary depending upon the half-life of the specific barbiturate.

MECHANISM: Barbiturates induce hepatic microsomal enzymes, resulting in an increased metabolism of coumarin anticoagulants.[6-14,16-20] Barbiturates may decrease the gastrointestinal absorption of dicumarol,[1,2] but they are not likely to significantly affect the absorption of warfarin.

CLINICAL EVALUATION: The interaction between barbiturates and anticoagulants is well documented. A patient on an oral anticoagulants who starts taking a barbiturate may become underanticoagulated. A patient on both barbiturate and oral anticoagulant therapy who stops taking the barbiturate runs the risk of hemorrhage if his anticoagulant dosage is not readjusted.

RELATED DRUGS: Phenobarbital (eg, *Solfoton*), butabarbital (eg, *Butisol*), heptabarbital, pentobarbital (eg, *Nembutal*), secobarbital (*Seconal*), and amobarbital (*Amytal*) have all been shown to decrease the response to coumarin anticoagulants. Most barbiturates (including primidone [eg, *Mysoline*], which is metabolized to phenobarbital) probably have this ability. Most of the interaction studies have involved warfarin or dicumarol, but barbiturates also appear to increase the metabolism of other anticoagulants such as phenprocoumon,[15] acenocoumarol,[21,22] and ethyl biscoumacetate.[21]

MANAGEMENT OPTIONS:

➥ **Avoid Unless Benefit Outweighs Risk.** If the barbiturate is being used as a sedative/hypnotic, its use with an oral anticoagulant generally should be avoided. Alternative sedative/hypnotic drugs unlikely to interact with oral anticoagulants include flurazepam (*Dalmane*), chlordiazepoxide (*Librium*), diazepam (eg, *Valium*), or diphenhydramine (eg, *Benadryl*). Nonetheless, the consistent use of stable doses of barbiturates, as in epileptic patients, does not appear to interfere significantly with anticoagulant control.[5]

➥ **Monitor.** If a barbiturate is used in a patient receiving an oral anticoagulant, monitor for altered hypoprothrombinemic response if the barbiturate is initiated, discontinued, or changed in dosage. Moreover, advise patients stabilized on a barbiturate and an oral anticoagulant not to stop taking the barbiturate or change its dosage without consulting with their physician for careful monitoring of their anticoagulant response.

REFERENCES:

1. Aggeler PM, et al. Effect of heptabarbital on the response to bishydroxycoumarin in man. *J Lab Clin Med.* 1969;74:229.

2. Lewis RJ. Effect of barbiturates on anticoagulant therapy. *N Engl J Med.* 1966;274:110. Letter.

3. Whitfield JB, et al. Changes in plasma gamma-glutamyl transpeptidase activity associated with alterations in drug metabolism in man. *BMJ.* 1973;1:316.

4. O'Reilly RA, et al. Interaction of secobarbital with warfarin pseudoracemates. *Clin Pharmacol Ther.* 1980;28:187.

5. Williams JRB, et al. Effect of concomitantly administered drugs on the control of long term anticoagulant therapy. *Q J Med.* 1976;45:63.

6. Starr KJ, et al. Drug interactions in patients on long term oral anticoagulant and antihypertensive adrenergic neuron-blocking drugs. *BMJ.* 1972;4:133.

7. Zaroslinski J, et al. Effect of subacute administration of methaqualone, phenobarbital and glutethimide on plasma levels of bishydroxycoumarin. *Arch Int Pharmacodyn Ther.* 1972;195:185.

8. Therapeutic conferences. Drug interaction. *BMJ.* 1971;1:389.

9. Breckenridge A, et al. Dose-dependent enzyme induction. *Clin Pharmacol Ther.* 1973;14:514.

10. Cucinell SA, et al. Drug interactions in man. I. Lowering effect of phenobarbital on plasma levels of bishydroxycoumarin (*Dicumarol*) and diphenylhydantoin (*Dilantin*). *Clin Pharmacol Ther.* 1965;6:420.

11. Corn M. Effect of phenobarbital and glutethimide on biological halflife of warfarin. *Thromb Diath Haemorrh.* 1966;16:606.

12. Robinson DS, et al. The effect of phenobarbital administration on the control of coagulation achieved during warfarin therapy in man. *J Pharmacol Exp Ther.* 1966;153:250.

13. Robinson DS, et al. Interaction of commonly prescribed drugs and warfarin. *Ann Intern Med.* 1970;72:853.

14. Hunninghake DB, et al. Drug interactions with warfarin. *Arch Intern Med.* 1968;121:349.

15. Antlitz AM, et al. Effect of butabarbital on orally administered anticoagulants. *Curr Ther Res.* 1968;10:70.

16. MacDonald MG, et al. Clinical observations of possible barbiturate interference with anticoagulation. *JAMA.* 1968;204:97.

17. MacDonald MG, et al. The effects of phenobarbital, chloral betaine, and glutethimide administration on warfarin plasma levels and hypoprothrombinemic responses in man. *Clin Pharmacol Ther.* 1969;10:80.

18. Goss JE, et al. Increased bishydroxycoumarin requirements in patients receiving phenobarbital. *N Engl J Med.* 1965;273:1094.

19. Levy G, et al. Pharmacokinetic analysis of the effect of barbiturate on the anticoagulant action of warfarin in man. *Clin Pharmacol Ther.* 1970;11:372.

20. Udall JA. Clinical implications of warfarin interactions with five sedatives. *Am J Cardiol.* 1975;35:67.

21. Dayton PG, et al. The influence of barbiturates on coumarin plasma levels and prothrombin response. *J Clin Invest.* 1961;40:1797.

22. Kroon C, et al. Interaction between single dose acenocoumarol and cimetidine or pentobarbitone: validation of a single dose model to predict interactions in steady state. *Br J Clin Pharmacol.* 1990;29:643P.

Phenylbutazone (*Butazolidin*)

Phenytoin (eg, *Dilantin*)

SUMMARY: Phenylbutazone appears to increase serum phenytoin concentrations, but the incidence of phenytoin intoxication in patients on this combination is unknown.

RISK FACTORS: No specific risk factors are known.

MECHANISM: Phenylbutazone and its metabolite oxyphenbutazone may inhibit the hepatic metabolism of phenytoin.[1] In addition, *in vitro* studies have shown that phenylbutazone can displace phenytoin from plasma protein-binding sites.[4,5]

CLINICAL EVALUATION: In a study of 14 pairs of healthy twins, phenylbutazone increased the half-life of IV phenytoin,[1] lending support to earlier undocumented statements that a significant interaction occurs between phenylbutazone and phenytoin.[2,3] In a subsequent study of 6 patients stabilized on phenytoin, phenylbutazone decreased serum phenytoin levels after 2 days; this was followed by increasing levels over the next 12 days. This biphasic effect on serum phenytoin concentrations is consistent with phenylbutazone-induced displacement of phenytoin and inhibition of hepatic phenytoin metabolism.[6] One patient developed evidence of phenytoin toxicity.

RELATED DRUGS: Although oxyphenbutazone probably interacts with phenytoin in a similar manner, the effect of other nonsteroidal anti-inflammatory drugs is not established.

MANAGEMENT OPTIONS:

➥ *Consider Alternative. Butazolidin* is no longer available for human use in the United States, so alternative NSAIDs would be used in any case.

➥ *Monitor.* Closely watch patients receiving both phenylbutazone and phenytoin for signs of phenytoin intoxication (eg, ataxia, nystagmus, mental impairment, involuntary muscular movements, seizures). Serum phenytoin determinations may be useful for monitoring this interaction, but any given total phenytoin concentration may correspond to a higher-than-normal free serum phenytoin level when phenylbutazone is given concurrently (caused by possible displacement of phenytoin from plasma protein binding).

REFERENCES:

1. Andreasen PB, et al. Diphenylhydantoin half life in man and its inhibition by phenylbutazone: the role of genetic factors. *Acta Med Scand.* 1973;193:561.
2. Hansen JM, et al. Dicumarol-induced diphenylhydantoin intoxication. *Lancet.* 1966;2:265.
3. Lucas BG. "*Dilantin*" overdosage. *Med J Aust.* 1968;2:639. Letter.
4. Lunde PKM, et al. Plasma protein binding of diphenylhydantoin in man. Interaction with other drugs and the effect of temperature and plasma dilution. *Clin Pharmacol Ther.* 1970;11:846.
5. Lunde PKM. Plasma protein binding of diphenylhydantoin in man. *Acta Pharmacol Toxicol.* 1971;29:152.
6. Neuvonen PJ, et al. Antipyretic analgesics in patients on antiepileptic drug therapy. *Eur J Clin Pharmacol.* 1979;15:263.

 Phenylbutazone (*Butazolidin*)

Tolbutamide (*Orinase*)

SUMMARY: Phenylbutazone increases the serum concentrations of tolbutamide and several other oral hypoglycemic drugs and may increase their hypoglycemic action.

RISK FACTORS: No specific risk factors are known.

MECHANISM: Phenylbutazone administration prolongs the half-life of the active metabolite of acetohexamide (hydroxyhexamide).[1] The half-life of acetohexamide itself was not affected. The increased serum tolbutamide concentrations that are found following phenylbutazone administration are probably because of inhibition of tolbutamide metabolism.[5] Displacement of tolbutamide from plasm protein binding by phenylbutazone also may be involved in the enhanced hypoglycemic effect of tolbutamide.

CLINICAL EVALUATION: Enhanced hypoglycemic responses to acetohexamide (*Dymelor*), tolbutamide, and perhaps other sulfonylurea hypoglycemic drugs should be anticipated following phenylbutazone administration. Several cases of severe hypoglycemia caused by phenylbutazone-acetohexamide and phenylbutazone-tolbutamide interactions have been reported.[1-4] Studies in normal volunteers have found that phenylbutazone and oxyphenbutazone considerably prolong tolbutamide half-life.[5] Phenylbutazone reportedly potentiates the action of insulin and chlorpropamide (*Diabinese*). The hypoglycemic effects of glyburide (*DiaBeta*) were increased by coadministration of a single dose and 7 days of piroxicam (*Feldene*) 10 mg/day.[10] Pirprofen had no influence on glyburide pharmacokinetics of pharmacodynamics.[6] Tolmetin (*Tolectin*) and naproxen (*Naprosyn*) appear to have no effect on tolbutamide effects[8] while tenoxicam has been shown not to interact with glibornuride[7] or tolbutamide.[9]

RELATED DRUGS: See Clinical Evaluation. It is not known whether other oral hypoglycemics are affected by phenylbutazone. Other nonsteroidal anti-inflammatory drugs appear to be safer than phenylbutazone to use with hypoglycemic drugs.

MANAGEMENT OPTIONS:

➡ *Use Alternative.* Do not administer phenylbutazone to patients taking oral hypoglycemic agents. Other nonsteroidal anti-inflammatory drugs appear to be acceptable alternatives.

REFERENCES:

1. Field JB, et al. Potentiation of acetohexamide hypoglycemia by phenylbutazone. *N Engl J Med.* 1967;277:889.
2. Slade IH, et al. Fatal hypoglycemic coma from the use of tolbutamide in elderly patients: report of two cases. *J Am Geriatr Soc.* 1967;15:948.
3. Harris EL. Adverse reactions to oral antidiabetic agents. *BMJ.* 1971;3:29.
4. Metz R. Bulletin of the Mason Clinic (Case Notes). 1976;30:38.
5. Pond SM, et al. Mechanisms of inhibition of tolbutamide metabolism: phenylbutazone, oxyphenbutazone, sulfaphenazole. *Clin Pharmacol Ther.* 1977;22:573.
6. Morrison PJ, et al. Effect of pirprofen on glibenclamide kinetics and response. *Br J Clin Pharmacol.* 1982;14:123.
7. Stoeckel K, et al. Lack of effect of tenoxicam on glibornuride kinetics and response. *Br J Clin Pharmacol.* 1985;19:249.
8. Verbeeck RK, et al. Clinical pharmacokinetics of nonsteroidal anti-inflammatory drugs. *Clin Pharmacokin.* 1983;8:297.
9. Day RO, et al. The effect of tenoxicam on tolbutamide pharmacokinetics and glucose concentrations in healthy volunteers. *Int J Clin Pharmacol Ther.* 1995;33:308.
10. Diwan PV, et al. Potentiation of hypoglycemic response of glibenclamide by piroxicam in rats and humans. *Indian J Exp Biol.* 1992;30:317.

1 Phenylbutazone (*Butazolidin*)

AVOID **Warfarin (eg, *Coumadin*)**

SUMMARY: Phenylbutazone dramatically enhances the hypoprothrombinemic response to warfarin, leading to severe bleeding in some patients. Avoid this combination.

RISK FACTORS:

➡ *Concurrent Diseases.* Patients with peptic ulcer disease (PUD) or a history of GI bleeding are probably at greater risk.

MECHANISM: Phenylbutazone and oxyphenbutazone appear to inhibit the metabolism of the more potent S-isomer of warfarin and also may displace warfarin from plasma protein-binding sites. Phenylbutazone-induced gastric erosions and inhibition of platelet function could theoretically increase the risk of bleeding in patients receiving oral anticoagulants.

CLINICAL EVALUATION: The interaction between phenylbutazone and warfarin is probably the most critical of all interactions involving coumarin anticoagulants. The enhanced anticoagulant response is marked and occurs in nearly all patients treated with both drugs.[1-16] In patients stabilized on oral anticoagulants, enhanced hypoprothrombinemia may occur as early as 1 to 2 days after phenylbutazone therapy is started. In 1 study,[5] all 10 patients on warfarin therapy exhibited increased prothrombin times (mean increase: 14.4 seconds) with phenylbutazone administration 300 mg/day for 2 weeks. A number of bleeding episodes have occurred in patients receiving both oral anticoagulants and phenylbutazone or oxyphenbutazone. Possible phenylbutazone-induced peptic ulcers and impaired platelet function are added hazards to the patient receiving anticoagulants. In a retrospective cohort study, hospitalizations for hemorrhagic PUD were approximately 13 times higher in patients receiving warfarin plus a nonsteroidal anti-inflammatory drug (NSAID) than in patients receiving either drug.[17]

RELATED DRUGS: All NSAIDs inhibit platelet function, cause gastric erosions, and probably increase the risk of GI bleeding. However, some NSAIDs such as ibuprofen (eg, *Motrin*), naproxen (eg, *Naprosyn*), or diclofenac (*Voltaren*) may be less likely to increase oral anticoagulant-induced hypoprothrombinemia than other NSAIDs.

MANAGEMENT OPTIONS:

➡ *AVOID COMBINATION.* Avoid phenylbutazone in patients receiving oral anticoagulants. Probably no condition exists in which the benefit of phenylbutazone therapy outweighs the serious risk of concomitant therapy with oral anticoagulants. It would be prudent to use NSAIDs that are unlikely to affect the hypoprothrombinemic response to oral anticoagulants. If the NSAID is being used as an analgesic or antipyretic, acetaminophen is probably safer to use with oral anticoagulants. Nonacetylated salicylates (eg, choline salicylate, magnesium salicylate, salsalate, sodium salicylate) probably also are safer with oral anticoagulants than NSAIDs because such salicylates have minimal effects on platelet function and the gastric mucosa. If any NSAID is used with an oral anticoagulant, carefully monitor the prothrombin time and watch for evidence of bleeding, especially from the GI tract.

REFERENCES:
    1. Udall JA. Drug interference with warfarin therapy. *Clin Med*. 1970;77:20.
    2. Brozovic M, et al. Prothrombin during warfarin treatment. *Br J Haematol*. 1973;24:579.

3. Packham MA, et al. Alteration of the response of platelets to surface stimuli by pyrazole compounds. *J Exp Med*. 1967;126:171.

4. Wosilait WD, et al. The effect of oxyphenbutazone on the excretion of 14 C-warfarin in the bile of rat. *Res Commun Chem Pathol Pharmacol*. 1972;4:413.

5. Weiner M, et al. Drug interactions: the effect of combined administration of the half-life of coumarin and pyrazolone drugs in man. *Fed Proc*. 165;24:153.

6. O'Reilly RA. The binding of sodium warfarin to plasma albumin and its displacement by phenylbutazone. *Ann NY Acad Sci*. 1973;226:293.

7. Aggeler PM, et al. Potentiation of anticoagulant effect of warfarin by phenylbutazone. *N Engl J Med*. 1967;276:496.

8. Hoffbrand BI, et al. Potentiation of anticoagulants. *BMJ*. 1967;2:838. Letter.

9. Kleinman PD, et al. Studies of the epidemiology of anticoagulant-drug interactions. *Arch Intern Med*. 1970;126:522.

10. Zucker MB, et al. Effect of acetylsalicylic acid, other nonsteroidal antiinflammatory agents, and dipyridamole on human blood platelets. *J Lab Clin Med*. 1970;76:66.

11. Lewis RJ, et al. Warfarin. Stereochemical aspects of its metabolism and the interaction with phenylbutazone. *J Clin Invest*. 1974;53:1607.

12. Bull J, et al. Phenylbutazone and anticoagulant control. *Practitioner*. 1975;215:767.

13. Chierichetti S, et al. Comparison of feprazone and phenylbutazone interaction with warfarin in man. *Curr Ther Res*. 1975;18:568.

14. O'Reilly RA. Phenylbutazone and sulfinpyrazone interaction with oral anticoagulant phenprocoumon. *Arch Int Med*. 1982;142:1634.

15. O'Reilly RA, et al. Comparative interaction of sulfinpyrazone and phenylbutazone with racemic warfarin: alteration in vivo of free fraction of plasma warfarin. *J Pharmacol Exp Ther*. 1981;219:691.

16. O'Reilly RA, et al. Stereoselective interaction of phenylbutazone with 12 C/ 13C warfarin pseudoracemates in man. *J Clin Invest*. 1980;68:746.

17. Shorr RI, et al. Concurrent use of nonsteroidal anti-inflammatory drugs and oral anticoagulants places elderly persons at high risk for hemorrhagic peptic ulcer disease. *Arch Intern Med*. 1993;153:1665.

Phenylephrine (*Neo-Synephrine*)

Propranolol (eg, *Inderal*)

SUMMARY: Very limited evidence suggests that propranolol may predispose patients to acute hypertensive episodes when phenylephrine is administered.

RISK FACTORS:

➡ **Dosage Regimen.** IV or intraocularly administered phenylephrine increases the risk of interaction.

MECHANISM: While phenylephrine is predominantly an alpha-receptor stimulant with less beta-receptor agonism, beta-blockers may enhance the pressor response to phenylephrine by blocking its beta-agonist activity.

CLINICAL EVALUATION: A fatal intracerebral hemorrhage occurred in a 55-year-old woman who was taking chronic propranolol 160 mg/day after she received 1 drop of phenylephrine 10% in each eye.[1] Presumably, the hemorrhage resulted from an acute hypertensive episode; previous administration of phenylephrine eyedrops to this patient in the absence of propranolol produced no apparent ill effects. However, because phenylephrine 10% eyedrops have occasionally produced acute hypertensive episodes in the absence of propranolol,[2,3] the role of a drug interaction in this case is not established. Eight subjects received increasing IV infusions of phenylephrine, with and without pretreatment with propranolol plus atropine. The infusion rate of phenylephrine needed to increase the diastolic blood pressure

20 mm Hg decreased 77% with propranolol plus atropine.[4] Intranasal phenyl-ephrine in 14 hypertensive patients taking metoprolol (eg, *Lopressor*) did not increase blood pressure.[5]

RELATED DRUGS: If the interaction between beta-blockers and phenylephrine occurs, it is likely to be most important with nonselective beta-blockers, such as propranolol, nadolol (eg, *Corgard*), timolol (eg, *Blocadren*), or pindolol (eg, *Visken*). Metoprolol does not interact.

MANAGEMENT OPTIONS:

➡ *Consider Alternative.* The use of cardioselective beta-blockers (eg, metoprolol) may minimize the risk of this interaction.

➡ *Monitor.* Until this potential interaction is substantiated or disproved, carefully monitor blood pressure when phenylephrine is coadministered with beta-blockers, particularly when the phenylephrine is administered IV or intraocularly.

REFERENCES:

1. Cass E, et al. Hazards of phenylephrine topical medication in persons taking propranolol. *Can Med Assoc J.* 1979;120:1261-1262.
2. Brown MM, et al. Lack of side effects from topically administered 10% phenylephrine eyedrops. A controlled study. *Arch Ophthalmol.* 1980;98:487-489.
3. Adler AG, et al. Systemic effects of eye drops. *Arch Intern Med.* 1982;142:2293-2294.
4. Shephard AM, et al. Dependence of phenylephrine dose/blood responses on autonomic activity in humans. *Clin Pharmacol Ther.* 1989;45:168.
5. Myers MG, et al. Intranasally administered phenylephrine and blood pressure. *Can Med Assoc J.* 1982;127:365-368.

Phenytoin (eg, *Dilantin*)

Posaconazole (*Noxafil*)

SUMMARY: Phenytoin reduces posaconazole plasma concentrations by about one half; diminution of antifungal efficacy may occur. Posaconazole administration produced a small increase in phenytoin plasma concentrations.

RISK FACTORS: No specific risk factors are known.

MECHANISM: Phenytoin appears to induce the metabolism of posaconazole via the uridine disphosphate glucuronidation pathway. Posaconazole appears to inhibit the metabolism of phenytoin via CYP3A4.

CLINICAL EVALUATION: Although data are limited, the manufacturer of posaconazole has noted that administration of posaconazole 200 mg daily with phenytoin 200 mg daily results in a mean decrease in the posaconazole area under the plasma concentration-time curve of 50%.[1] The manufacturer has recommended that coadministration of phenytoin generally be avoided in patients taking posaconazole. Posaconazole administration increased phenytoin concentrations a modest 16%.[1]

RELATED DRUGS: Posaconazole also may inhibit the metabolism of other anticonvulsant drugs that undergo CYP3A4 metabolism, including carbamazepine (eg, *Tegretol*), tiagabine (*Gabitril*), and zonisamide (eg, *Zonegran*).

MANAGEMENT OPTIONS:

➡ *Consider Alternative.* Consider alternative antifungal therapies; however, because phenytoin is metabolized by CYP2C9, the substitution of some antifungals (eg, fluconazole [eg, *Diflucan*], voriconazole [*Vfend*]) might lead to elevated phenytoin concentrations. Itraconazole (eg, *Sporanox*), ketoconazole (eg, *Nizoral*), and terbinafine (*Lamisil*) do not appear to affect phenytoin metabolism and could be considered in a patient taking phenytoin. However, phenytoin may reduce the plasma concentrations of other antifungal agents.

➥ **Monitor.** Monitor for reduction of antifungal efficacy when phenytoin and posaconazole are coadministered.

REFERENCES:

1. *Noxafil* [package insert]. Kenilworth, NJ: Schering Corporation; 2006.

Phenytoin (eg, *Dilantin*)

Primidone (eg, *Mysoline*)

SUMMARY: Phenytoin may enhance the conversion of primidone to phenobarbital. Excessive phenobarbital serum concentrations may occur in some patients.

RISK FACTORS:

➥ **Other Drugs.** Concurrent therapy with phenobarbital or carbamazepine can increase the magnitude of this interaction.

MECHANISM: A considerable amount of primidone is converted to phenobarbital in humans. The addition of phenytoin to primidone therapy increases phenobarbital serum concentrations, probably by stimulating the conversion of primidone to phenobarbital.[1] Phenytoin-induced competitive inhibition of phenobarbital metabolism may contribute.

CLINICAL EVALUATION: Serum phenobarbital concentrations are considerably higher in patients receiving primidone plus phenytoin than in patients receiving primidone alone.[2,3] In another study, serum phenobarbital concentrations were consistently higher in patients receiving primidone plus phenytoin than in patients receiving phenobarbital plus phenytoin.[4] Finally, an infant developed extremely high phenobarbital concentrations (202 mcg/mL) following the use of phenytoin and primidone in recommended doses.[5] Although the preceding reports offer good evidence that phenytoin promotes the formation of phenobarbital from primidone, this may be a favorable interaction in most epileptic patients treated with the combination. Only an occasional susceptible patient may be adversely affected.

RELATED DRUGS: No information is available.

MANAGEMENT OPTIONS:

➥ **Monitor.** No special precautions are necessary with the concomitant use of phenytoin and primidone, although relatively high concentrations of phenobarbital can be generated. The presence of supratherapeutic phenobarbital concentrations in patients receiving phenytoin, primidone, and phenobarbital[2] sheds doubt on the advantage of adding phenobarbital to the regimen.

REFERENCES:

1. Windorfer A. Drug interaction during anticonvulsive therapy. *Int J Clin Pharmacol.* 1976;14:236.

2. Fincham RW, et al. The influence of diphenylhydantoin on primidone metabolism. *Arch Neurol.* 1974;30:259-262.

3. Callaghan N, et al. The effect of anticonvulsant drugs which induce liver microsomal enzymes on derived and ingested phenobarbitone levels. *Acta Neurol Scand.* 1977;56:1-6.

4. Gallagher BB, et al. Primidone, diphenylhydantoin and phenobarbital. Aspects of acute and chronic toxicity. *Neurology.* 1973;23:145-149.

5. Wilson JT, et al. Chronic and severe phenobarbital intoxication in a child treated with primidone and diphenylhydantoin. *J Pediatr.* 1973;83:484-489.

Phenytoin (eg, *Dilantin*)

Pyridoxine (eg, Vitamin B₆)

SUMMARY: There is limited evidence that large doses of pyridoxine may reduce phenytoin serum concentrations.

RISK FACTORS:

➥ *Dosage Regimen.* The potential effect was seen with very large doses of pyridoxine; smaller doses, such as in multivitamins, probably have a minimal effect.

MECHANISM: Pyridoxine administration may enhance the activity of phenytoin-metabolizing enzymes in the liver.

CLINICAL EVALUATION: A preliminary study of patients with seizure disorders indicated that pyridoxine 200 mg/day for 4 weeks was associated with decreased phenytoin serum concentrations.[1] Although phenytoin concentrations were reduced to approximately 50% in several patients, others were not affected by pyridoxine therapy. The effect of pyridoxine doses less than 200 mg/day on serum phenytoin is unknown.

RELATED DRUGS: No information is available.

MANAGEMENT OPTIONS:

➥ *Monitor.* No special precautions appear necessary when small doses of pyridoxine (as in multivitamins) are coadministered with phenytoin. Monitor for reduced serum phenytoin concentrations if large doses of pyridoxine are used.

REFERENCES:

1. Hansson O, et al. Pyridoxine and serum concentration of phenytoin and phenobarbitone. *Lancet.* 1976;1:256.

Phenytoin (eg, *Dilantin*)

Quetiapine (*Seroquel*)

SUMMARY: Preliminary results suggest that phenytoin substantially increases the elimination of quetiapine; reduced quetiapine effect would be expected, but more study is needed.

RISK FACTORS: No specific risk factors are known.

MECHANISM: Not established. Phenytoin probably increases the metabolism of quetiapine.

CLINICAL EVALUATION: While no published data are available for evaluation, the manufacturer of quetiapine has made available some data on this interaction.[1] Phenytoin 100 mg 3 times daily produced a 5-fold increase in quetiapine oral clearance.[1] Because the details of the study were not presented, its validity cannot be assessed. Nonetheless, quetiapine appears to be metabolized largely by CYP34A, and phenytoin is a known inducer of this isozyme. Thus, a substantial reduction in quetiapine serum concentrations caused by phenytoin is expected on theoretical grounds.

RELATED DRUGS: No information is available.

MANAGEMENT OPTIONS:

➡ *Monitor.* Monitor for altered quetiapine response if phenytoin is initiated, discontinued, or changed in dosage.

REFERENCES:
1. *Seroquel* [package insert]. Wilmington, DE: AstraZeneca LP; 1997.

Phenytoin (eg, *Dilantin*)

Quinidine

SUMMARY: Phenytoin may substantially decrease quinidine serum concentrations.

RISK FACTORS: No specific risk factors are known.

MECHANISM: Phenytoin appears to enhance the hepatic metabolism of quinidine.

CLINICAL EVALUATION: In a few cases, phenytoin or phenobarbital therapy has been associated with low quinidine plasma concentrations.[1,2] A study of healthy subjects confirmed that phenytoin can considerably enhance the disposition of quinidine.[3] Some patients receiving phenytoin and quinidine develop subtherapeutic quinidine plasma concentrations.

RELATED DRUGS: No information is available.

MANAGEMENT OPTIONS:

➡ *Monitor.* Starting or stopping phenytoin therapy in patients receiving quinidine may necessitate a change in quinidine dosage.

REFERENCES:
1. Data JL, et al. Interaction of quinidine with anticonvulsant drugs. *N Engl J Med*. 1976;294:699-702.
2. Urbano AM. Phenytoin-quinidine interaction in a patient with recurrent ventricular tachyarrhythmias. *N Engl J Med*. 1982;308:225.
3. Kroboth FJ, et al. Phenytoin-theophylline-quinidine interaction. *N Engl J Med*. 1983;308:725.

Phenytoin (eg, *Dilantin*)

Rifampin (eg, *Rifadin*)

SUMMARY: Pharmacokinetic data and a case report indicate that rifampin decreases serum phenytoin concentrations; adjustments in the phenytoin dose may be needed.

RISK FACTORS: No specific risk factors are known.

MECHANISM: Rifampin appears to stimulate the hepatic metabolism of phenytoin.

CLINICAL EVALUATION: After rifampin 300 to 450 mg/day, phenytoin clearance was more than doubled and phenytoin half-life was halved, even when isoniazid and ethambutol were administered in addition to the rifampin.[1] Thus, the known ability of isoniazid to inhibit the hepatic metabolism of phenytoin appears to be overwhelmed by the potent enzyme-inducing abilities of rifampin. A 65-year-old man on chronic phenytoin therapy developed seizures 3 days after rifampin was started at a dosage of 600 mg/day. His serum phenytoin concentration fell from 16.2 to 5.1 mcg/mL over the 3-day period.[2] Controlled studies involving multiple doses of phenytoin will be required to ascertain the clinical significance of this interaction.

RELATED DRUGS: No information is available.

MANAGEMENT OPTIONS:

➡ *Circumvent/Minimize.* The phenytoin dose may require adjustment if rifampin is added or removed from a patient's regimen.

➡ *Monitor.* Carefully monitor patients on phenytoin therapy who receive rifampin for reduced serum phenytoin concentrations.

REFERENCES:

1. Kay L, et al. Influence of rifampicin and isoniazid on the kinetics of phenytoin. *Br J Clin Pharmacol.* 1985;20:323-326.

2. Wagner JC. Rifampin-phenytoin drug interaction. *Drug Intell Clin Pharm.* 1984;18:497.

 Phenytoin (eg, *Dilantin*)

Sertraline (*Zoloft*)

SUMMARY: Isolated cases of increased phenytoin serum concentrations have occurred after starting sertraline, but a causal relationship was not established.

RISK FACTORS: No specific risk factors are known.

MECHANISM: Not established.

CLINICAL EVALUATION: Two patients on phenytoin developed increased phenytoin serum concentration after starting sertraline therapy.[1] A 78-year-old man developed an extremely high phenytoin serum concentration (48 mcg/mL, corrected for serum albumin) but manifested no clinical evidence of phenytoin toxicity. This represented almost a 4-fold increase in the phenytoin serum concentration, which would suggest that sertraline is an inhibitor of CYP2C9, the primary metabolizing enzyme for phenytoin. However, sertraline has only minimal effects on the pharmacokinetics of warfarin, another CYP2C9 substrate. The other patient, an 85-year-old man, developed only a small increase in phenytoin serum concentrations (from 15.6 to 20 mcg/mL). Taking into consideration the normal variation in laboratory results and the normal day-to-day variation in phenytoin concentrations, this increase may or may not have resulted from sertraline. Thus, additional study is needed to determine whether sertraline affects phenytoin pharmacokinetics.

RELATED DRUGS: Fluoxetine (*Prozac*) has been associated with increased phenytoin serum concentrations and phenytoin toxicity.

MANAGEMENT OPTIONS: No specific action is required, but be alert for evidence of the interaction.

REFERENCES:

1. Haselberger MB, et al. Elevated serum phenytoin concentrations associated with coadministration of sertraline. *J Clin Psychopharmacol.* 1997;17:107-109.

Phenytoin (eg, *Dilantin***)**

Simvastatin (*Zocor*)

SUMMARY: A woman on simvastatin developed increased total cholesterol after phenytoin was added to her therapy. Although the effect is consistent with the known interactive properties of the drugs, additional information is needed to determine the clinical importance of this interaction.

RISK FACTORS: No specific risk factors are known.

MECHANISM: Probably enzyme induction. Simvastatin is metabolized extensively in the gut wall and liver by CYP3A4, and phenytoin is known to enhance CYP3A4 activity. Enhanced P-glycoprotein activity in the gut wall may also be involved.

CLINICAL EVALUATION: A 50-year-old woman on simvastatin 10 mg/day developed a 70% increase in her total cholesterol after she was started on phenytoin 325 mg/day.[1] When the simvastatin dose was increased to 40 mg/day, her cholesterol was still 28% higher than before phenytoin therapy. Fluvastatin (*Lescol*) 40 mg/day was also relatively ineffective in the presence of phenytoin. Her total cholesterol returned to baseline when the phenytoin dose was decreased to 225 mg/day and the patient was placed on atorvastatin (*Lipitor*) 80 mg/day. A further 34% decrease in total cholesterol occurred when phenytoin was discontinued in the presence of atorvastatin 80 mg/day. It is difficult to evaluate the effect of phenytoin on atorvastatin, because the phenytoin dose was decreased when the atorvastatin was started. Nonetheless, the effect of atorvastatin may have been somewhat reduced by phenytoin.

RELATED DRUGS: Like simvastatin, lovastatin (*Mevacor*) is extensively metabolized by CYP3A4, and would be expected to interact with phenytoin in a similar manner. Atorvastatin does not undergo as much first pass metabolism by CYP3A4 as simvastatin or lovastatin, and would not be expected to interact to the same degree. Fluvastatin is metabolized primarily by CYP2A9, an isozyme which, like CYP3A4, is susceptible to enzyme induction. Pravastatin (*Pravachol*) is not metabolized to a clinically important extent by cytochrome P450 isozymes, and would not be expected to interact with phenytoin or other enzyme inducers.

MANAGEMENT OPTIONS:

➡ *Consider Alternative.* If phenytoin or another enzyme inducer appears to be inhibiting the effect of simvastatin or lovastatin, consider using pravastatin as an alternative. Theoretically, enzyme inducers would not affect pravastatin. The effect of atorvastatin may be reduced by enzyme inducers, but probably to a lesser extent than simvastatin and lovastatin.

➡ *Monitor.* Monitor patients receiving simvastatin or lovastatin with phenytoin or other enzyme inducers for reduced cholesterol-lowering effect.

REFERENCES:

1. Murphy MJ, et al. Efficacy of statin therapy: possible effect of phenytoin. *Postgrad Med J.* 1999;75;359-360.

Phenytoin (eg, *Dilantin*)

Sucralfate (*Carafate*)

SUMMARY: Sucralfate modestly reduces the GI absorption of phenytoin, but the clinical importance of this effect is not established.

RISK FACTORS: No specific risk factors are known.

MECHANISM: The mechanism by which sucralfate reduces phenytoin absorption has not been established.

CLINICAL EVALUATION: In a double-blind crossover study, oral phenytoin 300 mg was given to 8 healthy subjects, with and without coadministration of 1 g of sucralfate; sucralfate reduced phenytoin bioavailability 20%.[1] In a similar study of 9 healthy subjects, 500 mg of phenytoin was given orally with and without sucralfate 1 g 4 times daily for 2 days; sucralfate reduced phenytoin bioavailability less than 10%.[2] The magnitude of the reductions in phenytoin absorption observed in these studies is not large, but an occasional patient may become unresponsive to phenytoin.

RELATED DRUGS: No information is available.

MANAGEMENT OPTIONS:

➥ *Circumvent/Minimize.* Although any reduction in phenytoin absorption is likely to be modest, it would be prudent to give phenytoin 2 hours before or 6 hours after sucralfate and keep the interval between the drugs as constant as possible.

➥ *Monitor.* Monitor for altered phenytoin response if sucralfate is initiated, discontinued, or if the interval between the drugs is changed.

REFERENCES:

1. Smart HL, et al. The effects of sucralfate upon phenytoin absorption in man. *Br J Clin Pharmacol.* 1985;20:238-240.

2. Hall TG, et al. Effect of sucralfate on phenytoin bioavailability. *Drug Intell Clin Pharm.* 1986;20:607–611.

 Phenytoin (eg, *Dilantin*)

Sulfaphenazole

SUMMARY: Some sulfonamides, including sulfaphenazole, appears to increase serum phenytoin concentrations; adjustment of the phenytoin dose may be required.

RISK FACTORS: No specific risk factors are known.

MECHANISM: Sulfamethizole and sulfaphenazole may inhibit the metabolism of phenytoin.[1,3,5] Sulfisoxazole has been shown to displace phenytoin from plasma protein-binding sites *in vitro*.[4]

CLINICAL EVALUATION: Sulfaphenazole and sulfamethizole (*Thiosulfil*) have been noted to inhibit phenytoin metabolism in patients.[1-3,5]

RELATED DRUGS: Sulfamethoxazole (*Gantanol*) appears to increase phenytoin half-life only modestly.[6] Phenytoin half-life increased from an average of 11.3 hours before, to 20.5 hours after, sulfamethizole administration (4 g/day for 7 days). Sulfamethizole also inhibits phenytoin metabolism. Sulfisoxazole, sulfadimethoxine, and sulfamethoxypyridazine do not appear to inhibit phenytoin metabolism.[1]

MANAGEMENT OPTIONS:

➟ **Consider Alternative.** Consider using a sulfonamide that does not inhibit phenytoin metabolism.

➟ **Monitor.** Monitor patients for increased phenytoin serum concentrations and signs of phenytoin toxicity (eg, ataxia, nystagmus, mental impairment) when sulfamethizole or sulfaphenazole is started. Stopping these sulfonamides may cause a fall in serum phenytoin concentrations.

REFERENCES:

1. Siersbaek-Nielsen K, et al. Sulfamethizole-induced inhibition of diphenylhydantoin and tolbutamide metabolism in man. *Clin Pharmacol Ther.* 1973;14:148. Abstract.
2. Hansen JM, et al. Dicumarol-induced diphenylhydantoin intoxication. *Lancet.* 1966;2:265.
3. Christensen LK, et al. Inhibition of drug metabolism by chloramphenicol. *Lancet.* 1969;2:1397.
4. Lunde PKM, et al. Plasma protein binding of diphenylhydantoin in man. Interaction with other drugs and the effect of temperature and plasma dilution. *Clin Pharmacol Ther.* 1970;11:846.
5. Lumholtz B, et al. Sulfamethizole-induced inhibition of diphenylhydantoin, tolbutamide, and warfarin metabolism. *Clin Pharmacol Ther.* 1975;17:731.
6. Hansen JM, et al. The effect of different sulfonamides on phenytoin metabolism in man. *Acta Med Scand.* 1979;624(Suppl.):106.

Phenytoin (eg, *Dilantin*)

Sulthiame (*Ospolot*)

SUMMARY: Sulthiame may increase serum phenytoin concentrations; phenytoin intoxication has occurred in some patients receiving both drugs.

RISK FACTORS: No specific risk factors are known.

MECHANISM: Sulthiame probably inhibits the metabolism of phenytoin by the liver.[1,2]

CLINICAL EVALUATION: In one study of 8 patients, sulthiame increased phenytoin serum concentrations considerably and prolonged its half-life.[3] Another group found toxic phenytoin concentrations in 8 of 20 patients receiving phenytoin plus sulthiame and in only 15 of 116 patients receiving phenytoin without sulthiame.[5] Another report mentions 5 patients with high serum phenytoin concentrations, presumably because of an interaction with sulthiame.[4]

RELATED DRUGS: No information is available.

MANAGEMENT OPTIONS:

➟ **Monitor.** Monitor patients receiving both sulthiame and phenytoin for signs of phenytoin intoxication (eg, ataxia, nystagmus, mental impairment, involuntary muscular movements, seizures); reduce the phenytoin dose if necessary.

REFERENCES:

1. Richens A, et al. Phenytoin intoxication caused by sulthiame. *Lancet.* 1973;2:1442. Letter.
2. Morselli PL, et al. Effect of sulthiame on blood and brain levels of diphenylhydantoin in the rat. *Biochem Pharmacol.* 1970;19:1846.
3. Hansen JM, et al. Sulthiame (*Ospolot*) as inhibitor of diphenylhydantoin metabolism. *Epilepsia.* 1968;9:17.

4. Kariks J, et al. Serum folic acid and phenytoin levels in permanently hospitalized epileptic patients receiving anticonvulsant drug therapy. *Med J Aust.* 1971;2:368.

5. Houghton GW, et al. Phenytoin intoxication induced by sulthiame in epileptic patients. *J Neurol Neurosurg Psychiatry.* 1974;37:275.

Phenytoin (eg, *Dilantin*)

Tacrolimus (*Prograf*)

SUMMARY: Phenytoin probably reduces tacrolimus blood concentrations; increased tacrolimus dosage may be needed.

RISK FACTORS: No specific risk factors are known.

MECHANISM: Tacrolimus is metabolized by CYP3A4, an isozyme that is induced by phenytoin. Thus, it appears likely that phenytoin enhances the metabolism of tacrolimus in the gut wall and liver.

CLINICAL EVALUATION: A 46-year-old man on phenytoin and tacrolimus required increasing doses of tacrolimus because of low blood concentrations.[1] Although it is not possible to establish a causal relationship between the low tacrolimus concentrations and the phenytoin therapy, the findings are consistent with the known interactive properties of both drugs.

RELATED DRUGS: Other enzyme inducers such as aminoglutethimide (*Cytadren*), barbiturates, carbamazepine (eg, *Tegretol*), glutethimide (*Doriden*), primidone (eg, *Mysoline*), rifabutin (*Mycobutin*), and rifampin (eg, *Rifadin*) also may reduce tacrolimus blood concentrations.

MANAGEMENT OPTIONS:

➡ **Monitor.** Monitor for subtherapeutic tacrolimus blood concentrations if phenytoin or other enzyme inducers are used concurrently.

REFERENCES:
1. Thompson PA, et al. Tacrolimus-phenytoin interaction. *Ann Pharmacother.* 1996;30:544. Letter.

Phenytoin (eg, *Dilantin*)

Teniposide (*Vumon*)

SUMMARY: Phenytoin substantially increased the systemic clearance of teniposide and may reduce teniposide's efficacy.

RISK FACTORS: No specific risk factors are known.

MECHANISM: This interaction is consistent with phenytoin stimulating the hepatic metabolism of teniposide.

CLINICAL EVALUATION: The systemic clearance of teniposide was compared in 6 pediatric patients receiving anticonvulsants (phenytoin or phenobarbital) and 6 age, sex, and race matched control patients. Phenytoin increased the systemic clearance of teniposide 2- to 3-fold.[1] These limited data suggest that patients receiving teniposide chemotherapy concurrent with phenytoin will have decreased teniposide plasma concentrations and may experience reduce teniposide efficacy.

RELATED DRUGS: No information is available.

MANAGEMENT OPTIONS:

➡ *Monitor.* Monitor for altered teniposide effect if phenytoin is initiated, discontinued, or changed in dosage; adjust teniposide dose as needed.

REFERENCES:

1. Baker, et al. Increased teniposide clearance with concomitant anticonvulsant therapy. *J Clin Oncol.* 1992;10:311.

Phenytoin (eg, *Dilantin*)

Terfenadine (*Seldane*)

SUMMARY: A study in patients with seizure disorders indicates that terfenadine does not affect the pharmacokinetics of phenytoin, but the effect of phenytoin on terfenadine was not studied.

RISK FACTORS: No specific risk factors are known.

MECHANISM: No interaction.

CLINICAL EVALUATION: Twelve epileptic patients with stable phenytoin serum concentrations were given terfenadine 60 mg twice daily for 14 days.[1] Terfenadine did not affect any of the following: Total or free serum phenytoin concentrations, area under the phenytoin concentration-time curve, maximum serum concentrations, or urinary excretion of HPPH (a phenytoin metabolite).

RELATED DRUGS: No information is available.

MANAGEMENT OPTIONS: No interaction.

REFERENCES:

1. Coniglio AA, et al. Effect of acute and chronic terfenadine on free and total serum phenytoin concentrations in epileptic patients. *Epilepsia.* 1989;30:611.

Phenytoin (eg, *Dilantin*)

Theophylline (eg, *Theo-Dur*)

SUMMARY: Phenytoin reduces serum theophylline concentrations and may increase theophylline dosage requirements. Also, theophylline may decrease serum phenytoin concentrations, but the clinical importance of this latter effect is not established.

RISK FACTORS: No specific risk factors are known.

MECHANISM: Phenytoin probably enhances the hepatic metabolism of theophylline.[1] The mechanism for the reduction in serum phenytoin concentrations because of theophylline is not established.

CLINICAL EVALUATION: In one case report, a patient on long-term phenytoin 400 mg/day did not respond adequately to large doses of sustained-release theophylline (eg, *Theo-Dur*). Subsequently, 10 healthy subjects were given aminophylline (5.6 mg/kg body weight IV over 30 minutes) with and without phenytoin pretreatment (300 to 400 mg/day for 10 to 15 days).[2] The theophylline half-life was shorter (5.2 hours versus 10.1 hours) and theophylline clearance was higher (more than 5.5 mL/hr/kg versus 43.7 mL/hr/kg) following phenytoin therapy. Additional case reports and controlled studies have confirmed that phenytoin can reduce the serum concentrations and the therapeutic effect of theophylline.[4,5] Furthermore, a single study of 14 volunteers indicates that theophylline may reduce phenytoin serum concentrations somewhat.[3] Thus, combined therapy may result in lowered serum concentrations of both theophylline and phenytoin.

RELATED DRUGS: Other enzyme inducers also are likely to enhance theophylline metabolism.

MANAGEMENT OPTIONS:

➡ *Monitor.* Be alert for the need to increase the theophylline dose when phenytoin is started and decrease the dose when phenytoin is stopped. Patients on chronic phenytoin therapy may require larger-than-expected theophylline doses. Also monitor for a reduced phenytoin response in patients receiving theophylline.

REFERENCES:
1. Miller M, et al. Influence of phenytoin on theophylline clearance. *Clin Pharmacol Ther*. 1984;35:666.
2. Marquis JF, et al. Phenytoin-theophylline interaction. *N Engl J Med*. 1982;307:1189.
3. Taylor JW, et al. The interaction of phenytoin and theophylline. *Drug Intell Clin Pharm*. 1980;14:638.
4. Reed RC, et al. Phenytoin-theophylline-quinidine interaction. *N Engl J Med*. 1983;308:724.
5. Sklar SJ, et al. Enhanced theophylline clearance secondary to phenytoin therapy. *Drug Intell Clin Pharm*. 1985;19:34.

Phenytoin (eg, *Dilantin*)

Thyroid

SUMMARY: Limited evidence indicates phenytoin may increase thyroid replacement dose requirements in some patients.

RISK FACTORS: No specific risk factors are known.

MECHANISM: Phenytoin appears to enhance the metabolism of thyroid hormones and also may displace thyroxine from plasma protein-binding sites.

CLINICAL EVALUATION: In patients without an intact pituitary-thyroid axis, phenytoin-induced increases in the metabolism of thyroid may increase thyroid replacement dose requirements. This has been reported in 1 case.[2] Other enzyme inducers might produce a similar effect. Also, a case has been reported in which a patient with atrial flutter on thyroid replacement therapy developed supraventricular tachycardia when he was given IV phenytoin.[1] The tachycardia might have been because of phenytoin-induced displacement of thyroxine from plasma protein-binding sites, but a causal relationship was not established.

RELATED DRUGS: No information is available.

MANAGEMENT OPTIONS:

➡ *Monitor.* In patients on thyroid replacement, starting or stopping phenytoin therapy may increase or decrease thyroid dose requirements, respectively. Also, give patients requiring thyroid replacement therapy IV phenytoin with caution, especially if they also have a cardiac disease.

REFERENCES:
1. Fulop M, et al. Possible diphenylhydantoin-induced arrhythmia in hypothyroidism. *JAMA*. 1966;196:454.
2. Blackshear JL, et al. Thyroxine replacement requirements in hypothyroid patients receiving phenytoin. *Ann Intern Med*. 1983;99:341.

Phenytoin (eg, *Dilantin*)

Ticlopidine (*Ticlid*)

SUMMARY: Patients have developed phenytoin toxicity after ticlopidine was added to their therapy; it may be necessary to reduce phenytoin dose in the presence of ticlopidine.

RISK FACTORS: No specific risk factors are known.

MECHANISM: Not established. The most likely explanation is ticlopidine-induced inhibition of phenytoin metabolism by CYP2C9.

CLINICAL EVALUATION: Cases of apparent ticlopidine-induced phenytoin toxicity have been reported.[1-3] the phenytoin serum concentration approximately doubled in each case and was associated with clinical evidence of phenytoin toxicity (eg, dizziness, ataxia, drowsiness). In 2 of the 3 cases, phenytoin toxicity occurred several weeks after the ticlopidine was started,[1,2] but in the other case, toxicity appeared after only a week.[3]

RELATED DRUGS: No information is available.

MANAGEMENT OPTIONS:

➡ ***Monitor.*** Monitor for altered phenytoin effect if ticlopidine is initiated, discontinued, or changed in dosage; adjust phenytoin dose as needed. If phenytoin is initiated in the presence of ticlopidine therapy, it would be prudent to begin with conservative doses of phenytoin.

REFERENCES:
1. Rindone JP, et al. Phenytoin toxicity associated with ticlopidine administration. *Arch Intern Med.* 1996;156:1113. Letter.
2. Privitera M, et al. Axute phenytoin toxicity followed by seizure break-though from a ticlopidine-phenytoin interaction. *Arch Neurol.* 1996;53:1191.
3. Riva R, et al. Ticlopidine impairs phenytoin clearance: a case report. *Neurology.* 1996;46:1172.

Phenytoin (eg, *Dilantin*)

Tolbutamide (eg, *Orinase*)

SUMMARY: Although excessive phenytoin doses may result in hyperglycemia, alteration in glucose tolerance appears unlikely in patients with free serum phenytoin concentrations within the usual therapeutic range. Tolbutamide may transiently increase free serum phenytoin concentrations, but the incidence of toxicity from this effect is unknown.

RISK FACTORS: No specific risk factors are known.

MECHANISM: Phenytoin appears to inhibit insulin release. Tolbutamide appears to displace phenytoin from plasma protein binding.

CLINICAL EVALUATION: Patients with excessive serum phenytoin concentrations may manifest hyperglycemia[1-7]; however, hyperglycemia is unlikely to develop in nondiabetics receiving therapeutic doses of phenytoin. Therapeutic doses of phenytoin purportedly seldom increase insulin requirements in insulindependent diabetics.[8] In 17 epileptic patients on phenytoin, the addition of tolbutamide 500 mg twice daily or 3 times daily was followed by a decrease in total plasma phenytoin and an increase in phenytoin plasma free fraction, both of which are consistent with tolbutamide-induced displacement of phenytoin from plasma protein binding.[9] None of the patients manifested evidence of phenytoin toxicity during the 4 days that the phenytoin plasma free fraction was increased. A 48-year-old woman stabilized on phenytoin therapy was started on tolbutamide 500 mg 3 times daily for 5 days, followed by 1 g 3 times daily.[10] Within 48 hours of increasing the tolbutamide dose, she developed evidence of phenytoin toxicity (eg, ataxia, nystagmus, nausea, headache). The symptoms resolved when the tolbutamide was stopped and the phenytoin dose was reduced. Although tolbutamide can precipitate phenytoin toxicity, it is likely to be limited to only the first few days of tolbutamide therapy.

RELATED DRUGS: The effect of other sulfonylureas on phenytoin is not well established, although one possible case of tolazamide (eg, *Tolinase*)-induced phenytoin toxicity has been reported.[10]

MANAGEMENT OPTIONS:

➡ *Monitor.* Monitor for alterations in antidiabetic drug requirements if phenytoin therapy is started, stopped, or changed in dosage. Warn patients stabilized on phenytoin of the possibility of transient phenytoin toxicity (eg, ataxia, dizziness, nausea, headache) when tolbutamide therapy is begun.

REFERENCES:

1. Klein JP. Diphenylhydantoin intoxication associated with hyperglycemia. *J Pediatr.* 1966;69:463.
2. Dahl JR. Diphenylhydantoin toxic psychosis with associated hyperglycemia. *Calif Med.* 1967;107:345.
3. Peters BH, et al. Hyperglycemia with relative hypoinsulinemia in diphenylhydantoin toxicity. *N Engl J Med.* 1969;281:91.
4. Sanbar SS, et al. Diabetogenic effect of *Dilantin* (diphenylhydantoin). *Diabetes.* 1967;16:533.
5. Fariss BL, et al. Diphenylhydantoin-induced hyperglycemia and impaired insulin release. *Diabetes.* 1971;20:177.
6. Malherbe C, et al. Effect of diphenylhydantoin on insulin secretion in man. *N Engl J Med.* 1972;286:339.
7. Saudek CD, et al. Phenytoin in the treatment of diabetic symmetrical polyneuropathy. *Clin Pharmacol Ther.* 1977;22:196.
8. Millichap JG. Hyperglycemic effect of diphenylhydantoin. *N Engl J Med.* 1969;281:447.
9. Wesseling H, et al. Diphenylhydantoin (DPH) and tolbutamide in man. *Eur J Clin Pharmacol.* 1975;8:75.
10. Beech E, et al. Phenytoin toxicity produced by tolbutamide. *BMJ.* 1988;297:1613.

Phenytoin (eg, *Dilantin*)

Trimethoprim (eg, *Proloprim*)

SUMMARY: Trimethoprim may increase serum phenytoin concentrations; phenytoin toxicity may occur in some patients.

RISK FACTORS: No specific risk factors are known.

MECHANISM: Trimethoprim appears to inhibit the hepatic metabolism of phenytoin.

CLINICAL EVALUATION: In 7 subjects given phenytoin 100 mg IV with and without pretreatment with trimethoprim 320 mg/day for 7 days, trimethoprim increased the phenytoin half-life approximately 50%.[1] Some patients may experience phenytoin toxicity.

RELATED DRUGS: Phenytoin half-life was similarly prolonged by trimethoprim-sulfamethoxazole (eg, *Bactrim*), but sulfamethoxazole (*Gantanol*) alone produced only a small increase in phenytoin half-life.

MANAGEMENT OPTIONS:

➡ *Monitor.* Monitor for signs of phenytoin toxicity (eg, nystagmus, ataxia, mental impairment) when trimethoprim is given concurrently with phenytoin. Serum phenytoin determinations would be useful if the interaction is suspected.

REFERENCES:

1. Hansen JM, et al. The effect of different sulfonamides on phenytoin metabolism in man. *Acta Med Scand.* 1979;624(Suppl.):106.

Phenytoin (eg, *Dilantin*)

Valproic Acid (eg, *Depakene*)

SUMMARY: Valproic acid can increase, decrease, or have no effect on total phenytoin plasma concentrations. Phenytoin may decrease serum valproic acid concentrations.

RISK FACTORS: No specific risk factors are known.

MECHANISM: Valproic acid appears to displace phenytoin from plasma protein-binding sites[3,10]; it also may inhibit the hepatic metabolism of phenytoin. Phenytoin may stimulate valproic acid metabolism.[1-10]

CLINICAL EVALUATION: In patients taking phenytoin, valproic acid lowers total plasma phenytoin concentrations by approximately 30% during the first several weeks of therapy. Although total serum phenytoin concentrations are depressed, the percentage of unbound serum phenytoin rises concomitantly. Thus, the concentration of the active, free-form of phenytoin in the serum usually is not appreciably changed in the presence of valproic acid. Nevertheless, an occasional patient with serum phenytoin concentrations close to the toxic range might develop phenytoin intoxication as a result of the initial displacement of phenytoin from plasma protein-binding sites by valproic acid. Impaired phenytoin metabolism also may contribute. Although the half-life of phenytoin tends to be shortened during the first several weeks of valproic acid therapy, a prolongation of phenytoin half-life has been noted after several more weeks on valproic acid.

The effect of phenytoin on valproic acid concentrations also has been studied. Serum valproic acid concentrations tend to be lower in patients on phenytoin concurrently than in patients receiving valproic acid alone; the clinical importance of this finding is unclear. Some patients have developed an increase in seizure frequency when valproic acid was added to phenytoin therapy, but this is uncommon; the relationship of this clinical observation to the interaction between these 2 drugs is unknown.

RELATED DRUGS: No information is available.

MANAGEMENT OPTIONS:

➡ *Monitor.* Patients receiving phenytoin may not require an alteration in the dose of phenytoin when valproic acid therapy is initiated because the free serum concentration of phenytoin may not change. Nevertheless, watch for signs of phenytoin toxicity (eg, ataxia, nystagmus, mental impairment, involuntary muscular movements, seizures) when valproic acid is used concurrently. The decreased total serum phenytoin concentrations seen during the first few weeks of valproic acid therapy should not prompt an increase in phenytoin dose unless poor seizure control occurs concurrently. Free phenytoin in plasma concentrations should be followed whenever possible because total phenytoin concentrations may be altered without a change in the free phenytoin plasma concentration.

REFERENCES:

1. Bardy A, et al. Valproate may lower serum-phenytoin. *Lancet.* 1976;2:1297. Letter.
2. Patsalos PN, et al. Valproate may lower serum-phenytoin. *Lancet.* 1977;1:50. Letter.
3. Patsalos PN, et al. Effect of sodium valproate on plasma protein binding of diphenylhydantoin. *J Neurol Neurosurg Psychiatr.* 1977;40:570.
4. Windorfer A, et al. Elevation of diphenylhydantoin and primidone serum concentration by addition of dipropylacetate, a new anticonvulsant drug. *Acta Paediatr Scand.* 1975;64:771.
5. Reunanen MI, et al. Low serum valproic acid concentrations in epileptic patients on combination therapy. *Curr Ther Res.* 1980;28:456.
6. Dahlqvist R, et al. Decreased plasma protein binding of phenytoin in patients on valproic acid. *Br J Clin Pharmacol.* 1979;8:547.
7. Sansom LN, et al. Interaction between phenytoin and valproate. *Med J Aust.* 1980;2:212.
8. Monks A, et al. Effect of single doses of sodium valproate on serum phenytoin levels and protein binding in epileptic patients. *Clin Pharmacol Ther.* 1980;27:89.
9. Bruni J, et al. Interactions of valproic acid with phenytoin. *Neurology.* 1980;30:1233.
10. Miles MV, et al. Predictability of unbound antiepileptic drug concentrations in children treated with valproic acid and phenytoin. *Clin Pharm.* 1988;7:688.

Phenytoin (eg, *Dilantin*)

Vigabatrin (*Sabril*)

SUMMARY: Vigabatrin has been found to decrease the serum concentrations of phenytoin 20% to 30%.

RISK FACTORS: No specific risk factors are known.

MECHANISM: At this time, it is unclear what the mechanism of the interaction is. Vigabatrin has not been shown to stimulate the metabolism of any other antiepileptic drugs.

CLINICAL EVALUATION: In clinical trials evaluating the efficacy of vigabatrin, phenytoin concentrations decreased 20% to 30% after addition of vigabatrin.[1,2] In a study in 8 patients with epilepsy treated with phenytoin, vigabatrin 3 g/day given for 4 weeks resulted in a 23% decrease in phenytoin concentrations. However, there was no change in the urinary ratio of the major metabolite of phenytoin (parahydroxyphenytoin) to phenytoin.[3] A further study in 21 patients with epilepsy comparing intravenous and oral phenytoin with and without vigabatrin found similar decreases in phenytoin concentrations. A significant decrease in phenytoin plasma concentrations of phenytoin was observed in a subgroup of only 7 patients. In the other 14 patients, concentrations decreased an average of less than 15%. The study comparing oral and intravenous phenytoin concluded that decreased oral bioavailability of phenytoin could not explain the decreased oral clearance of phenytoin.[4]

RELATED DRUGS: No information is available.

MANAGEMENT OPTIONS:

➡ *Monitor.* Monitor phenytoin plasma concentrations for 1 month after initiation or removal of vigabatrin therapy. Patients receiving phenytoin may require an increase in the dose of phenytoin when vigabatrin therapy is initiated.

REFERENCES:

1. Rimmer EM, et al. Double blind study of gamma-vinyl-GABA in patients with refractory epilepsy. *Lancet.* 1984;i:189.

2. Tartara A, et al. Vigabatrin in the treatment of epilepsy: a long-term follow-up study. *J Neurol Neurosurg Psych.* 1989;52:467.

3. Rimmer EM, et al. Interaction between vigabatrin and phenytoin. *Br J Clin Pharmacol.* 1989;27(Suppl. 1):S27.

4. Gatti G, et al. Vigabatrin induced decrease in serum phenytoin concentration does not involve a change in phenytoin bioavailability. *Br J Clin Pharmacol.* 1993;35:603.

Phenytoin (eg, *Dilantin*)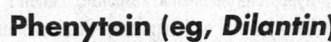

Voriconazole (*Vfend*)

SUMMARY: Voriconazole increases phenytoin concentrations; toxicity may result. Phenytoin reduces voriconazole concentrations.

RISK FACTORS: No specific risk factors are known.

MECHANISM: Voriconazole inhibits the metabolism of phenytoin while phenytoin induces the metabolism of voriconazole.

CLINICAL EVALUATION: Ten volunteers took 200 mg voriconazole twice daily for 7 days followed by placebo or phenytoin 300 mg daily for 2 weeks.[1] Phenytoin administration reduced the area under the plasma concentration-time curve (AUC) of voriconazole 65%. In a separate study, the subjects were given a loading dose of phenytoin followed by 300 mg daily for 17 days. Starting on day 8 of phenytoin administration, placebo or voriconazole 400 mg twice daily was administered. The addition of voriconazole increased the mean AUC of phenytoin 85% compared with placebo. Phenytoin toxicity including dizziness, visual changes, or nausea may occur if voriconazole is administered to patients stabilized on phenytoin. The dose of voriconazole may need to be increased to provide adequate antifungal concentrations during phenytoin coadministration.

RELATED DRUGS: Fosphenytoin (*Cerebyx*) would be expected to interact in a similar manner with voriconazole. Fluconazole (*Diflucan*) is known to inhibit phenytoin's metabolism.

MANAGEMENT OPTIONS:

➡ *Consider Alternative.* Consider antiepileptic agents that do not undergo metabolism by CYP2C9, CYP2C19, or CYP3A4 as an alternative to phenytoin in patients requiring voriconazole. Antifungal agents with similar indications that do not affect CYP2C9 could be considered as an alternative for voriconazole.

➡ *Monitor.* Monitor phenytoin concentrations whenever voriconazole therapy is initiated, discontinued, or the dose of voriconazole is changed. Be alert for reduced antifungal efficacy when voriconazole is coadministered with phenytoin.

REFERENCES:
1. Purkins L, et al. Coadministration of voriconazole and phenytoin: pharmacokinetic interaction, safety, and toleration. *Br J Clin Pharmacol.* 2003;56:37-44.

Phenytoin (eg, *Dilantin*)

Warfarin (eg, *Coumadin*)

SUMMARY: Initiation of phenytoin therapy may transiently increase the hypoprothrombinemic response to warfarin (and probably other oral anticoagulants). This is followed within 1 to 2 weeks by an inhibition of the hypoprothrombinemic response. Patients on chronic phenytoin therapy may require larger-than-expected doses of oral anticoagulants. Dicumarol and phenprocoumon may increase serum phenytoin concentrations, whereas warfarin does not appear to do so.

RISK FACTORS: No specific risk factors are known.

MECHANISM: The interactions between phenytoin and oral anticoagulants are complex. The following mechanisms appear to be involved: 1) Phenytoin may stimulate metabolism of oral anticoagulants through enzyme induction. 2) Phenytoin may displace oral anticoagulants from plasma protein-binding sites. 3) Phenytoin alone may prolong the prothrombin time in some patients.[1,2] 4) Dicumarol, and probably phenprocoumon, inhibit the parahydroxylation of phenytoin in the liver. Note that phenytoin and S-warfarin are metabolized primarily by CYP2C9. The overall effect of these (and perhaps other) mechanisms on the half-life, blood concentration, and therapeutic effect of the 2 drugs will require much more study.

CLINICAL EVALUATION: On the basis of current knowledge, the following clinical effects may be expected: 1) When phenytoin is given to a patient maintained on oral anticoagulants, a transient increase in anticoagulant effect may occur initially as a result of displacement of a protein-bound oral anticoagulant; isolated cases have been reported.[3,4] One of these case reports described a 74-year-old man receiving warfarin 6 mg/day who developed a fatal retroperitoneal hemorrhage 1 week after starting phenytoin 300 mg/day. His INR increased from 2.4 to 10.4. If a patient does not have a bleeding episode during the first week and is continued on phenytoin therapy, expect that the enhanced hypoprothrombinemic response will initially fall back toward the prephenytoin levels and eventually decline to below the prephenytoin levels. This would occur because of the transient nature of protein-binding displacement interactions and the enzyme-inducing effect of phenytoin. 2) When dicumarol or phenprocoumon is given to a patient maintained on phenytoin, serum concentrations of phenytoin are likely to increase, perhaps to a level at which signs of phenytoin toxicity will occur.[5-7] Warfarin does not appear to increase serum phenytoin levels.[8] In such patients, higher-than-normal doses of anticoagulant might be required, but this has not yet been documented clinically.

RELATED DRUGS: Interactions of phenytoin with oral anticoagulants other than warfarin, dicumarol, and phenprocoumon are not established.

MANAGEMENT OPTIONS:

➥ *Consider Alternative.* Warfarin is preferable to dicumarol in patients receiving phenytoin because warfarin does not appear to affect phenytoin serum concentrations.

➥ *Monitor.* Monitor for altered oral anticoagulant effect if phenytoin is initiated, discontinued, or changed in dosage. Adjust the anticoagulant dose as needed. If an oral anticoagulant is started in the presence of phenytoin therapy, remember that the anticoagulant dosage requirements may be greater than usual.

REFERENCES:

1. Andreasen PB, et al. Abnormalities in liver function tests during long-term diphenylhydantoin therapy in epileptic outpatients. *Acta Med Scand*. 1973;194:261-264.
2. Solomon GE, et al. Coagulation defects caused by diphenylhydantoin. *Neurology*. 1972;22:1165-1171.
3. Nappi JM. Warfarin and phenytoin interaction. *Ann Intern Med*. 1979;90:852.
4. Taylor JW, et al. Oral anticoagulant-phenytoin interactions. *Drug Intell Clin Pharm*. 1980;14:669.
5. Hansen JM, et al. Dicumarol-induced diphenylhydantoin intoxication. *Lancet*. 1966;2:265-266.
6. Hansen JM, et al. Effect of diphenylhydantoin on the metabolism of dicumarol in man. *Acta Med Scand*. 1971;189:15-19.
7. Rothermich NO. Diphenylhydantoin intoxication. *Lancet*. 1966;2:640.
8. Skovsted L, et al. The effect of different oral anticoagulants on diphenylhydantoin (DPH) and tolbutamide metabolism. *Acta Med Scand*. 1976;199:513-515.

Phenytoin (eg, *Dilantin*)   4
Zidovudine (*Retrovir*)

SUMMARY: Zidovudine probably does not alter the oral pharmacokinetics of phenytoin in asymptomatic HIV-positive patients.

RISK FACTORS: No specific risk factors are known.

MECHANISM: Zidovudine does not appear to affect phenytoin plasma concentrations, but phenytoin would theoretically enhance zidovudine metabolism.

CLINICAL EVALUATION: Twelve asymptomatic HIV-positive patients received a single dose of oral phenytoin with and without zidovudine 200 mg every 4 hours. There were no significant differences between areas under the phenytoin plasma concentration-time curves, C_{max}, or T_{max}.[1] Zidovudine metabolism is susceptible to enzyme induction, so phenytoin would theoretically enhance zidovudine metabolism.

RELATED DRUGS: No information is available.

MANAGEMENT OPTIONS: No specific action is required, but be alert for evidence of the interaction.

REFERENCES:

1. Sarver P, et al. Effect of zidovudine on the pharmacokinetic disposition of phenytoin in HIV positive asymptomatic patients. *Pharmacotherapy*. 1991;11:108.

Pimozide (*Orap*)

Ritonavir (*Norvir*)

SUMMARY: Elevated pimozide concentrations and cardiac arrhythmias may occur if pimozide and ritonavir are coadministered.

RISK FACTORS: No specific risk factors are known.

MECHANISM: Ritonavir is known to be an inhibitor of CYP3A4, the enzyme responsible for the metabolism of pimozide. The coadministration of pimozide and ritonavir can lead to ventricular arrhythmias, including torsades de pointes.

CLINICAL EVALUATION: While specific data are lacking, the manufacturer of pimozide contraindicates the coadministration of pimozide and ritonavir.[1] Patients with bradycardia, hypokalemia, or hypomagnesemia may be at increased risk to develop torsades de pointes.

RELATED DRUGS: Avoid other antiviral agents that inhibit CYP3A4 (eg, amprenavir [*Agenerase*], delavirdine [*Rescriptor*], indinavir [*Crixivan*], nelfinavir [*Viracept*], saquinavir [eg, *Fortovase*]) in patients taking pimozide.

MANAGEMENT OPTIONS:

➥ *Use Alternative.* Do not administer ritonavir or other antiviral agents that inhibit CYP3A4 to patients receiving pimozide.

➥ *Monitor.* If ritonavir is coadministered with pimozide, monitor the electrocardiogram for evidence of corrected QT interval prolongation.

REFERENCES:
   1. *Orap* [package insert]. North Wales, PA: Gate Pharmaceuticals; 1999.

 Pimozide (*Orap*)

AVOID Sertraline (*Zoloft*)

SUMMARY: Preliminary pharmacokinetic evidence suggests that sertraline may increase pimozide plasma concentrations; given that elevated pimozide concentrations can be life-threatening, the combination is contraindicated.

RISK FACTORS: No specific risk factors are known.

MECHANISM: Not established.

CLINICAL EVALUATION: A single dose of sertraline 200 mg increased the plasma concentrations of a single dose of pimozide 2 mg about 40%.[1] There were no changes in the electrocardiogram, but given the potential for pimozide to cause life-threatening ventricular arrhythmias, the product labeling for sertraline states that concurrent use with pimozide is contraindicated.

RELATED DRUGS: Paroxetine (eg, *Paxil*) also has been shown to increase pimozide plasma concentrations, and this combination is contraindicated as well. Little is known about the effect of other selective serotonin reuptake inhibitors on pimozide; theoretically, fluvoxamine (a moderate CYP3A4 inhibitor) would increase pimozide concentrations. Pending additional information, avoid coadministration of fluvoxamine and pimozide.

MANAGEMENT OPTIONS:

➡ *AVOID COMBINATION.* Although this interaction is based on limited clinical data, the potential adverse outcome could be life-threatening. The product information states that the combination is contraindicated.

REFERENCES:

1. Alderman J. Coadministration of sertraline with cisapride or pimozide: an open-label, nonrandomized examination of pharmacokinetics and corrected QT intervals in healthy adult volunteers. *Clin Ther.* 2005;27:1050-1063.

Pimozide (*Orap*)

Thioridazine AVOID

SUMMARY: Pimozide may produce additive prolongation of the QT interval with thioridazine and, therefore, may increase the risk of ventricular arrhythmias; avoid concurrent use.

RISK FACTORS:

➡ *Hypokalemia.* The corrected QT interval (QTc) may be prolonged in patients with hypokalemia, increasing the risk of this interaction. Any other factor that may prolong the QTc interval also increases the risk of this interaction.

MECHANISM: Thioridazine and pimozide can prolong the QT interval; additive effects may be seen.

CLINICAL EVALUATION: In a double-blind, randomized, crossover study of the pharmaco-dynamic effects of thioridazine alone, 9 healthy subjects received single oral doses of thioridazine 10 and 50 mg compared with placebo.[1] The thioridazine 50 mg dose increased the QTc on the electrocardiogram 23 msec, and the 10 mg dose increased the QTc 9 msec. These results suggest that thioridazine produces a dose-related slowing of cardiac repolarization. Thus, drugs such as pimozide that can independently prolong the QT interval may increase the risk of ventricular arrhythmias in patients taking thioridazine. Although this interaction is based primarily on theoretical considerations, its potential severity dictates avoiding the combination. Moreover, the manufacturer's product information for *Mellaril* (not available in the United States) states that combined use of thioridazine with other drugs that are known to prolong the QT interval is contraindicated[2]; thus, also consider medicolegal issues.

RELATED DRUGS: Several phenothiazines have been associated with prolongation of the QT interval, but clinical evidence suggests that the risk of excessive prolongation is greater with thioridazine than with other phenothiazines.

MANAGEMENT OPTIONS:

➡ *AVOID COMBINATION.* Although the risk of this combination is not well established, avoid concurrent use.

REFERENCES:

1. Hartigan-Go K, et al. Concentration-related pharmacodynamic effects of thioridazine and its metabolites in humans. *Clin Pharmacol Ther.* 1996;60:543-553.

2. "Dear Doctor or Pharmacist" Letter, Novartis Pharmaceuticals, July 7, 2000. FDA Web site. MedWatch. Available at: http://www.fda.gov/medwatch/safety/2000/mellar.htm. Accessed June 9, 2005.

2　Pimozide (*Orap*)

Verapamil (eg, *Calan*)

SUMMARY: Elevated pimozide concentrations and cardiac arrhythmias may occur if pimozide and verapamil are coadministered.

RISK FACTORS: No specific risk factors are known.

MECHANISM: Verapamil is known to be an inhibitor of CYP3A4, the enzyme responsible for the metabolism of pimozide.[1]

CLINICAL EVALUATION: While specific data are lacking, the coadministration of pimozide and verapamil could lead to ventricular arrhythmias, including torsades de pointes.[1] Patients with bradycardia, hypokalemia, or hypomagnesemia may be at an increased risk of developing torsades de pointes.

RELATED DRUGS: Diltiazem (eg, *Cardizem*) also inhibits CYP3A4; avoid diltiazem in patients taking pimozide. The dihydropyridine calcium channel blockers do not appear to inhibit CYP3A4.

MANAGEMENT OPTIONS:

➡ ***Use Alternative.*** Treat patients receiving pimozide who require treatment with a calcium channel blocker with a dihydropyridine calcium channel blocker such as amlodipine (eg, *Norvasc*) or felodipine (*Plendil*).

➡ ***Monitor.*** If verapamil or diltiazem is coadministered with pimozide, monitor the electrocardiogram for evidence of corrected QT interval prolongation.

REFERENCES:
　　1. *Orap* [package insert]. North Wales, PA: Gate Pharmaceuticals; 1999.

2　Pimozide (*Orap*)

Voriconazole (*Vfend*)

SUMMARY: Elevated pimozide concentrations and cardiac arrhythmias may occur if pimozide and voriconazole are coadministered.

RISK FACTORS: No specific risk factors are known.

MECHANISM: Voriconazole is known to be an inhibitor of CYP3A4, the enzyme responsible for the metabolism of pimozide. The coadministration of pimozide and voriconazole may lead to ventricular arrhythmias, including torsades de pointes.

CLINICAL EVALUATION: While specific data are lacking, the manufacturer of voriconazole contraindicates the coadministration of pimozide and voriconazole.[1] Patients with bradycardia, hypokalemia, or hypomagnesemia may be at increased risk of developing torsades de pointes.

RELATED DRUGS: Itraconazole (eg, *Sporanox*), ketoconazole (eg, *Nizoral*), and fluconazole (eg, *Diflucan*) also would be likely to produce increased pimozide plasma concentrations and thus increase the risk of corrected QT interval (QTc) prolongation.

MANAGEMENT OPTIONS:

➡️ *Use Alternative.* Do not administer voriconazole or any antifungal agent known to inhibit CYP3A4 to patients receiving pimozide. Consider terbinafine (*Lamisil*) as an alternative because it does not affect CYP3A4 activity.

➡️ *Monitor.* If voriconazole is coadministered with pimozide, monitor the electrocardiogram for evidence of QTc prolongation.

REFERENCES:

1. *Vfend* [package insert]. New York, NY: Pfizer, Inc.; 2003.
2. Boucher HW, et al. Newer systemic antifungal agents: pharmacokinetics, safety and efficacy. *Drugs.* 2004;64:1997-2020.

Pimozide (*Orap*)

Ziprasidone (*Geodon*)

SUMMARY: Ziprasidone and pimozide can prolong the corrected QT interval (QTc) on the electrocardiogram (ECG), theoretically increasing the risk of ventricular arrhythmias such as torsades de pointes.

RISK FACTORS:

➡️ *Hypokalemia.* The QTc on the ECG may be prolonged in patients with hypokalemia, increasing the risk of this interaction.[1]

➡️ *Miscellaneous.* Other factors that may prolong the QTc interval (eg, bradycardia, hypomagnesemia, hypothyroidism, impaired liver function) also may increase the risk of ventricular arrhythmias.[1]

MECHANISM: Possible additive prolongation of the QTc interval.

CLINICAL EVALUATION: In initial controlled trials, ziprasidone increased the QTc interval approximately 10 msec at the highest recommended dose of 160 mg/day. But because of concern that the QTc measurements were done when ziprasidone serum concentrations were low, the FDA recommended additional study.[2,3] In a subsequent study in patients with psychotic disorders, the QTc interval was measured following administration of several antipsychotic drugs (haloperidol, olanzapine, quetiapine, risperidone, thioridazine, ziprasidone) when the concentrations were calculated to be at their peak. Ziprasidone increased the QTc by a mean of approximately 21 msec, which was less than thioridazine (36 msec) but about twice that of the other antipsychotics. Theoretically, the ability of pimozide to prolong the QTc would be additive with ziprasidone, but the extent to which this would increase the risk of ventricular arrhythmias, such as torsades de pointes, is not known.

RELATED DRUGS: Available data suggest that ziprasidone produces less QTc prolongation than thioridazine, but about twice that of quetiapine (*Seroquel*), risperidone (*Risperdal*), haloperidol (eg, *Haldol*), and olanzapine (*Zyprexa*).

MANAGEMENT OPTIONS:

➡️ *Use Alternative.* Given the theoretical risk and the fact that pimozide is listed in the ziprasidone product information as contraindicated, it would be prudent to use an alternative to 1 of the drugs (see Related Drugs).

➡ **Monitor.** If pimozide and ziprasidone are used concurrently, monitor for evidence of arrhythmias (eg, syncope) and for prolonged QT intervals.

REFERENCES:
1. De Ponti F, et al. QT-interval prolongation by non-cardiac drugs: lessons to be learned from recent experience. *Eur J Clin Pharmacol.* 2000;56:1-18.
2. *Geodon* [package insert]. New York, NY: Pfizer, Inc.; 2001.
3. *Office of Drug Safety Annual Report.* Center for Drug Evaluation and Research. FDA Web site. Available at: www.fda.gov/cder/Offices/ODS/AnnRep2001/annualreport2001.htm. Accessed June 9, 2005.

4   Pindolol (eg, *Visken*)

Trimethoprim (eg, *Proloprim*)

SUMMARY: The plasma concentration of pindolol is increased to a small degree by trimethoprim administration; no adverse effects are likely to be seen.

RISK FACTORS: No specific risk factors are known.

MECHANISM: Trimethoprim inhibits the renal elimination of pindolol.

CLINICAL EVALUATION: Eight young (22 to 33 years of age) and 7 elderly men (62 to 79 years of age) received oral pindolol 10 mg twice daily alone and with trimethoprim 200 mg every day for 3 days.[1] Trimethoprim reduced the renal clearance of both isomers of pindolol 25% to 35% in young and elderly subjects. Trimethoprim had no effect on the nonrenal clearance of pindolol in either group of subjects. The limited effects of trimethoprim on pindolol elimination are unlikely to have a significant effect on pindolol's beta-blocking activity. No dose adjustments appear to be necessary.

RELATED DRUGS: No information is available.

MANAGEMENT OPTIONS: No specific action is required, but be alert for evidence of the interaction.

REFERENCES:
1. Ujhelyi MR, et al. Aging effects on the organic base transporter and stereoselective renal clearance. *Clin Pharmacol Ther.* 1997;62:117-128.

3   Pioglitazone (*Actos*)

Rifampin (eg, *Rifadin*)

SUMMARY: Rifampin reduced the plasma concentrations of pioglitazone; a decrease in glycemic control could occur in some patients.

RISK FACTORS: No specific risk factors are known.

MECHANISM: Rifampin induces the activity of CYP2C8, the enzyme primarily responsible for the metabolism of pioglitazone.

CLINICAL EVALUATION: Following 6 days of rifampin 600 mg or placebo once daily, 10 healthy subjects received a single dose of pioglitazone 30 mg.[1] Rifampin administration reduced the mean area under the plasma concentration-time curve of pioglitazone 54% and shortened its half-life from 4.9 to 2.3 hours. It is possible that some diabetic patients could experience some loss of glycemic control if rifampin is added to their regimen.

RELATED DRUGS: Rifampin has been shown to reduce the concentrations of rosiglitazone (*Avandia*), repaglinide (*Prandin*), nateglinide (*Starlix*), and sulfonylurea hypoglycemic agents. Rifabutin (*Mycobutin*) may affect pioglitazone in a similar manner.

MANAGEMENT OPTIONS:

➡ *Monitor.* Patients taking pioglitazone should monitor their blood glucose whenever rifampin is added to or removed from their drug regimen.

REFERENCES:

1. Jaakkola T, et al. Effect of rifampicin on the pharmacokinetics of pioglitazone. *Br J Clin Pharmacol.* 2005;61:70-78.

Piroxicam (eg, *Feldene*)

Warfarin (eg, *Coumadin*)

SUMMARY: Preliminary clinical evidence indicates that piroxicam may increase the hypoprothrombinemic response to acenocoumarol,[†] warfarin, and possibly other oral anticoagulants.

RISK FACTORS:

➡ *Concurrent Diseases.* Patients with peptic ulcer disease or a history of GI bleeding are probably at greater risk.

MECHANISM: The mechanism for piroxicam-induced increases in hypoprothrombinemia is not established. Piroxicam-induced gastric erosions and inhibition of platelet function theoretically may increase the risk of bleeding in patients receiving oral anticoagulants.

CLINICAL EVALUATION: In one study, a slight increase in the hypoprothrombinemic response was noted in 4 of 10 subjects given piroxicam 20 mg/day in addition to acenocoumarol.[1] On 2 occasions, a 60-year-old man stabilized on warfarin developed increased hypoprothrombinemia after starting piroxicam and decreased hypoprothrombinemia upon stopping piroxicam.[2] The ability of piroxicam to produce GI bleeding and to inhibit platelet function also must be considered when anticoagulants are coadministered.[1,3] In a retrospective cohort study, hospitalizations for hemorrhagic peptic ulcer disease were approximately 13 times higher in patients receiving warfarin plus a nonsteroidal anti-inflammatory drug (NSAID) than in patients receiving neither drug.[4]

RELATED DRUGS: All NSAIDs inhibit platelet function, cause gastric erosions, and probably increase the risk of GI bleeding. However, some NSAIDs, such as ibuprofen (eg, *Advil*), naproxen (eg, *Naprosyn*), or diclofenac (eg, *Voltaren*), may be less likely to increase oral anticoagulant-induced hypoprothrombinemia than other NSAIDs.

MANAGEMENT OPTIONS:

➡ *Avoid Unless Benefit Outweighs Risk.* Because all NSAIDs probably increase the risk of GI bleeding in patients taking oral anticoagulants, use the combination only after careful consideration of benefit versus risk. If NSAIDs must be used with an oral anticoagulant, use those unlikely to affect the hypoprothrombinemic response to oral anticoagulants (see Related Drugs). If an NSAID is used as an analgesic or antipyretic, acetaminophen (eg, *Tylenol*) is probably safest with oral anticoagulants. Nonacetylated salicylates (eg, choline salicylate, magnesium salicylate, salsalate, sodium salicylate) are probably also safer with oral anticoagulants because of their minimal effects on platelet function and gastric mucosa.

➡ **Monitor.** If any NSAID is used with an oral anticoagulant, monitor the prothrombin time carefully and watch for evidence of bleeding, especially from the GI tract.

REFERENCES:

1. Dahl SL, et al. Pharmacology, clinical efficacy, and adverse effects of piroxicam, a new nonsteroidal anti-inflammatory agent. *Pharmacotherapy*. 1982;2(2):80-90.

2. Rhodes RS, et al. A warfarin-piroxicam drug interaction. *Drug Intell Clin Pharm*. 1985;19(7-8):556-558.

3. Emery P, et al. Gastrointestinal blood loss and piroxicam. *Lancet*. 1982;1(8284):1302-1303.

4. Shorr RI, et al. Concurrent use of nonsteroidal anti-inflammatory drugs and oral anticoagulants places elderly persons at high risk for hemorrhagic peptic ulcer disease. *Arch Intern Med*. 1993;153(14):1665-1670.

† Not available in the United States.

Pitavastatin (*Livalo*)

Rifampin (eg, *Rifadin*)

SUMMARY: Rifampin has been reported to increase the concentrations of pitavastatin; increased adverse reactions may occur in some patients.

RISK FACTORS: No specific risk factors are known.

MECHANISM: Unknown. Pitavastatin is a substrate for the organic anion-transporting polypeptide (OATP) and rifampin is known to inhibit this transporter. Inhibition of OATP reduces the uptake of pitavastatin into hepatocytes where it is metabolized. Rifampin may also induce the glucuronidation of pitavastatin; in response, pitavastatin plasma concentrations tend to be reduced.

CLINICAL EVALUATION: While specific data are limited, the manufacturer of pitavastatin notes that the coadministration of rifampin 600 mg daily for 5 days prior to a single dose of pitavastatin 4 mg increased the mean area under the plasma concentration-time curve (AUC) of pitavastatin by approximately 30% and increased its peak concentration by 2-fold.[1] Pending further data, observe patients receiving pitavastatin and rifampin for increased pitavastatin effect. Pitavastatin labeling recommends limiting the dosage of pitavastatin to 2 mg daily during rifampin coadministration.

RELATED DRUGS: Rifabutin (*Mycobutin*) may produce a similar effect on pitavastatin. Rifampin is known to reduce the plasma concentrations of many other statins.

MANAGEMENT OPTIONS:

➡ **Monitor.** Monitor patients receiving pitavastatin who require rifampin for signs of pitavastatin toxicity, including muscle weakness and myalgia.

REFERENCES:

1. *Livalo* [package insert]. Montgomery, AL: Kowa Pharmaceuticals America Inc; 2009.

Posaconazole (*Noxafil*)

Rifabutin (*Mycobutin*)

SUMMARY: Rifabutin reduces posaconazole plasma concentrations by approximately 50%; diminution of antifungal efficacy may occur. Posaconazole increased rifabutin concentrations more than 70%; some patients may experience rifabutin-induced adverse reactions.

RISK FACTORS: No specific risk factors are known.

MECHANISM: Rifabutin may induce the metabolism of posaconazole via the uridine diphosphate glucuronidation pathway. Posaconazole appears to inhibit the metabolism of rifabutin via CYP3A4.

CLINICAL EVALUATION: Although data are limited, the manufacturer states that the administration of posaconazole 200 mg daily with rifabutin 300 mg daily resulted in a mean decrease in the posaconazole area under the plasma concentration-time curve of 49%.[1] The manufacturer recommends that coadministration of rifabutin in patients taking posaconazole generally be avoided. Posaconazole administration increased rifabutin concentrations 72%.[1]

RELATED DRUGS: Rifampin (eg, *Rifadin*) may affect posaconazole in a similar manner.

MANAGEMENT OPTIONS:

➡ **Consider Alternative.** Consider alternative antifungal therapies; however, because rifabutin is metabolized by CYP3A4, the substitution of some antifungals (eg, itraconazole [eg, *Sporanox*], ketoconazole [eg, *Nizoral*], fluconazole [eg, *Diflucan*], voriconazole [*Vfend*]) might lead to elevated rifabutin concentrations. Terbinafine (eg, *Lamisil*) does not appear to affect CYP3A4 activity and may be coadministered with rifabutin.

➡ **Monitor.** Monitor for reduction of antifungal efficacy and increased rifabutin adverse reactions when rifabutin and posaconazole are coadministered.

REFERENCES:

1. *Noxafil* [package insert]. Kenilworth, NJ: Schering Corporation; 2006.

Posaconazole (*Noxafil*)

Rifampin (eg, *Rifadin*)

SUMMARY: The addition of rifampin produced a marked reduction in the plasma concentration of posaconazole in a patient; loss of antifungal efficacy may occur.

RISK FACTORS: No specific risk factors are known.

MECHANISM: Rifampin appears to increase the metabolism of posaconazole via the uridine diphosphate glucuronidation pathway.

CLINICAL EVALUATION: A patient receiving posaconazole 200 mg 4 times daily for a pulmonary fungal infection was started on rifampin (dose not stated) for methicillin-resistant *Staphylococcus aureus*.[1] Posaconazole plasma concentration was reduced by 80% following 3 weeks of rifampin therapy. Loss of antifungal efficacy may require alternative antifungal therapy if rifampin is coadministered with posaconazole.

RELATED DRUGS: Rifabutin (*Mycobutin*) is known to reduce the concentration of posaconazole. Rifampin may have similar effects on other antifungal agents that are metabolized by CYP3A4, including itraconazole (eg, *Sporanox*) and ketoconazole (eg, *Nizoral*).

MANAGEMENT OPTIONS:

➡ *Consider Alternative.* Based on the fungal infection being treated, consider an antifungal agent that is not metabolized by CYP3A4 or uridine diphosphate glucuronidation in patients requiring rifampin coadministration.

➡ *Monitor.* If posaconazole and rifampin are coadministered, monitor posaconazole plasma concentrations to avoid subtherapeutic plasma concentrations.

REFERENCES:
1. Hohmann C, et al. Rifampin and posaconazole coadministration leads to decreased serum posaconazole concentrations. *Clin Infect Dis.* 2010;50(6):939-940.

Posaconazole (*Noxafil*)

Simvastatin (eg, *Zocor*)

SUMMARY: Posaconazole administration is likely to produce an increase in simvastatin plasma concentrations; patients may be more likely to develop simvastatin toxicity.

RISK FACTORS: No specific risk factors are known.

MECHANISM: Posaconazole is likely to inhibit simvastatin elimination via the CYP3A4 pathway, increase simvastatin bioavailability, or both.

CLINICAL EVALUATION: While specific data are limited, the manufacturer of posaconazole cautions that posaconazole oral suspension may increase the mean plasma concentration of simvastatin.[1] Because of the very low bioavailability of simvastatin, large increases in simvastatin plasma concentrations may occur.

RELATED DRUGS: Other antifungal agents that inhibit CYP3A4 (eg, itraconazole [eg, *Sporanox*], ketoconazole [eg, *Nizoral*], voriconazole [*Vfend*], fluconazole [eg, *Diflucan*]) affect simvastatin in a similar manner. Lovastatin (eg, *Mevacor*) and, to a lesser degree, atorvastatin (*Lipitor*) may also be affected by posaconazole.

MANAGEMENT OPTIONS:

➡ *Consider Alternative.* Consider terbinafine (eg, *Lamisil*) as an alternative antifungal agent because it does not affect CYP3A4 activity. Theoretically, pravastatin (eg, *Pravachol*), rosuvastatin (*Crestor*), and fluvastatin (*Lescol*) are less likely to interact with posaconazole.

➡ *Monitor.* If posaconazole is initiated, monitor patients taking simvastatin for muscle pain, weakness, and possibly elevated liver enzymes.

REFERENCES:
1. *Noxafil* [package insert]. Kenilworth, NJ: Schering Corporation; 2006.

Posaconazole (*Noxafil*)

Vincristine (*Oncovin*)

SUMMARY: Posaconazole inhibits the metabolism of vincristine; some patients may experience severe vincristine-induced neurotoxicity.

RISK FACTORS: No specific risk factors are known.

MECHANISM: Posaconazole inhibits the CYP3A4 metabolism of vincristine. Posaconazole-induced reduction in P-glycoprotein activity may also contribute to reduced clearance of vincristine.

CLINICAL EVALUATION: Two cases of severe neurotoxicity associated with the concurrent use of posaconazole and vincristine have been reported.[1,2] In 1 case, the peripheral neuropathy did not resolve following discontinuation of the posaconazole and vincristine. Patients receiving vincristine should not be treated with posaconazole without careful assessment of risk and potential benefit.

RELATED DRUGS: Ketoconazole (eg, *Nizoral*), fluconazole (eg, *Diflucan*), itraconazole (eg, *Sporanox*), and voriconazole (*Vfend*) also inhibit the activity of CYP3A4 and would be expected to increase the plasma concentrations of vincristine. Vinblastine and vinorelbine (eg, *Navelbine*) are also CYP3A4 substrates and would likely interact with posaconazole.

MANAGEMENT OPTIONS:

➡ **Consider Alternative.** Consider terbinafine (eg, *Lamisil*) as an alternative antifungal agent because it does not affect CYP3A4 activity. Amphotericin, caspofungin (*Cancidas*), and anidulafungin (*Eraxis*) do not appear to inhibit CYP3A4.

➡ **Monitor.** If posaconazole is coadministered with vincristine, carefully monitor patients for any evidence of neurotoxicity.

REFERENCES:

1. Eiden C, et al. Posaconazole-increased vincristine neurotoxicity in a child: a case report. *J Pediatr Hematol Oncol.* 2009;31(4):292-295.

2. Mantadakis E, et al. Possible increase of the neurotoxicity of vincristine by the concurrent use of posaconazole in a young adult with leukemia. *J Pediatr Hematol Oncol.* 2007;29(2):130.

2 **Potassium**

Spironolactone (eg, *Aldactone*)

SUMMARY: Coadministration of potassium supplements and spironolactone may result in severe hyperkalemia.

RISK FACTORS:

➡ ***Other Drugs.*** Coadministration of angiotensin-converting enzyme inhibitors may enhance the risk.

➡ ***Concurrent Diseases.*** Patients with impaired renal function or severe diabetes may be at greater risk. Patients with diet-controlled diabetes do not appear to be particularly predisposed to potassium-sparing, diuretic-induced hyperkalemia if no other predisposing factors are present.[1]

➡ ***Effects of Age.*** The elderly may be at a greater risk.

➡ ***Diet/Food.*** A high-potassium diet (including salt substitutes) may enhance the risk of hyperkalemia.

MECHANISM: Because spironolactone conserves potassium, hyperkalemia may result when potassium supplements are given concurrently.

CLINICAL EVALUATION: Severe or fatal hyperkalemia has been reported in patients receiving concomitant spironolactone and potassium chloride.[2-5] In 1 study of patients with severe azotemia who were receiving spironolactone plus potassium chloride, the incidence of hyperkalemia was 42%.[5] In another study, the combined use of spironolactone and oral potassium chloride in at least 104 patients during a 2-year period in 1 hospital revealed after chart review that 13 of 25 patients (52%) developed hyperkalemia.[6] Nonetheless, the combination of spironolactone and potassium chloride has been used successfully to treat severe potassium depletion with close monitoring.

RELATED DRUGS: Amiloride (*Midamor*) and triamterene (*Dyrenium*) also can result in hyperkalemia when combined with potassium supplements.

MANAGEMENT OPTIONS:

➡ ***Avoid Unless Benefit Outweighs Risk.*** Use the combination of potassium-sparing diuretics and potassium supplementation only for severe or refractory hypokalemia. Particular caution is needed in predisposed patients (eg, elderly diabetic patients with impaired renal function).

➡ ***Monitor.*** Carefully monitor serum potassium concentrations if this combination is used.

REFERENCES:

1. Lowenthal DT, et al. Effects of amiloride on oral glucose loading, serum potassium, renin, and aldosterone in diet-controlled diabetes. *Clin Pharmacol Ther.* 1980;27:671-676.
2. Mashford ML, et al. Spironolactone and ammonium and potassium chloride. *Br Med J.* 1972;4:298-299.
3. Kalbian VV. Iatrogenic hyperkalemic paralysis with electrocardiographic changes. *South Med J.* 1974;67:342-345.
4. Shapiro S, et al. Fatal drug reactions among medical inpatients. *JAMA.* 1971;216:467-472.
5. Greenblatt DJ, et al. Adverse reactions to spironolactone. A report from the Boston Collaborative Drug Surveillance Program. *JAMA.* 1973;225:40-43.
6. Simborg DW. Medication prescribing on a university medical service—the incidence of drug combinations with potential adverse interactions. *Johns Hopkins Med J.* 1976;139:23-26.

Potassium

Triamterene (*Dyrenium*)

SUMMARY: Potassium supplementation in patients taking triamterene may result in severe hyperkalemia.

RISK FACTORS:

➡ *Other Drugs.* Coadministration of angiotensin-converting enzyme inhibitors may increase the risk.

➡ *Concurrent Diseases.* Patients with impaired renal function or severe diabetes may be at a greater risk. Patients with diet-controlled diabetes do not appear to be particularly predisposed to potassium-sparing, diuretic-induced hyperkalemia if no other predisposing factors are present.[1]

➡ *Effects of Age.* Elderly patients may be at a greater risk.

➡ *Diet/Food.* A high-potassium diet (including salt substitutes) may place a patient at greater risk.

MECHANISM: Because triamterene conserves potassium, hyperkalemia may result when potassium supplements also are given.

CLINICAL EVALUATION: Severe hyperkalemia occasionally has resulted from triamterene administration, and the addition of potassium supplements increases the likelihood of this adverse reaction. One reported case of pacemaker failure caused by hyperkalemia resulted from the combined administration of potassium and a preparation containing triamterene and hydrochlorothiazide (eg, *Dyazide*).[2] Patients with azotemia probably are predisposed to hyperkalemia during combined use of triamterene and potassium salts.

RELATED DRUGS: Amiloride (*Midamor*) and spironolactone (eg, *Aldactone*) also can result in hyperkalemia when combined with potassium supplements.

MANAGEMENT OPTIONS:

➡ *Avoid Unless Benefit Outweighs Risk.* Use the combination of potassium-sparing diuretics and potassium supplementation only for severe or refractory hypokalemia. Particular caution is needed in predisposed patients (eg, elderly diabetic patients with impaired renal function).

➡ *Monitor.* If the combination is used, monitor serum potassium concentrations carefully.

REFERENCES:

1. Lowenthal DT, et al. Effects of amiloride on oral glucose loading, serum potassium, renin, and aldosterone in diet-controlled diabetes. *Clin Pharmacol Ther.* 1980;27:671-676.
2. O'Reilly MV, et al. Transvenous pacemaker failure induced by hyperkalemia. *JAMA.* 1974;228:336-337.

Pravastatin (*Pravachol*)

Rifampin (eg, *Rifadin*)

SUMMARY: Rifampin administration results in a modest reduction in pravastatin plasma concentrations; limited effect on pravastatin lipid-lowering efficacy would be expected.

RISK FACTORS: No specific risk factors are known.

MECHANISM: Unknown. Rifampin may increase the activity of an active efflux transporter (eg, organic anion transporter) of pravastatin in the small intestine.

CLINICAL EVALUATION: Ten healthy subjects received a single 40 mg dose of pravastatin alone and following 6 days of rifampin 600 mg daily.[1] Rifampin administration resulted in a mean reduction in the pravastatin area under the plasma concentration-time curve of 31%. Pravastatin half-life and renal clearance were unchanged. This degree of change in pravastatin plasma concentrations could result in a modest reduction in its efficacy.

RELATED DRUGS: Rifampin is known to reduce the plasma concentration of other statins. It is unknown if rifabutin (*Mycobutin*) increases pravastatin elimination. However, pending further study, monitor for reduced lipid-lowering effect in patients administered pravastatin and rifabutin.

MANAGEMENT OPTIONS:

➡ *Monitor.* Patients taking pravastatin who require rifampin should be monitored for any loss of lipid-lowering efficacy.

REFERENCES:

1. Kyrklund C, et al. Effect of rifampicin on pravastatin pharmacokinetics in healthy subjects. *Br J Clin Pharmacol*. 2004;57:181-187.

---

5 Pravastatin (*Pravachol*)

St. John's Wort
___

SUMMARY: St. John's wort does not appear to affect the pharmacokinetics of pravastatin.

RISK FACTORS: No specific risk factors are known.

MECHANISM: No interaction.

CLINICAL EVALUATION: In a double-blind crossover study, 8 healthy subjects took a single oral dose of pravastatin 20 mg with and without pretreatment with St. John's wort (900 mg daily for 14 days).[1] St. John's wort did not affect plasma pravastatin concentrations.

RELATED DRUGS: St. John's wort substantially reduces simvastatin serum concentrations.[1] Theoretically, lovastatin (eg, *Mevacor*) would interact with St. John's wort in a manner similar to simvastatin. Atorvastatin (*Lipitor*) also may interact, but probably to a lesser degree.

MANAGEMENT OPTIONS: No interaction.

REFERENCES:

1. Sugimoto K, et al. Different effects of St. John's wort on the pharmacokinetics of simvastatin and pravastatin. *Clin Pharmacol Ther*. 2001;70:518-524.

---

5 Pravastatin (*Pravachol*)

Warfarin (eg, *Coumadin*)
___

SUMMARY: Preliminary evidence from patients and healthy subjects suggests that pravastatin does not affect the anticoagulant response of warfarin.

RISK FACTORS: No specific risk factors are known.

MECHANISM: No interaction.

CLINICAL EVALUATION: In a 6-day study of the combined use of pravastatin and warfarin in healthy subjects, there was no effect on the hypoprothrombinemic response to warfarin or on the bioavailability of pravastatin.[1] Pravastatin also did not affect warfarin binding to plasma proteins,[1] which is consistent with the modest (55% to 60%) binding of pravastatin to plasma proteins.[2] One controlled clinical trial of patients receiving warfarin found pravastatin did not affect the hypoprothrombinemic response.[2] In a preliminary report, 8 patients stabilized on warfarin were given lovastatin 40 mg/day, pravastatin 20 mg/day, or placebo for 7 days in a randomized, 3-way, crossover study.[3] Pravastatin had no effect on warfarin response. Thus, it does not appear that pravastatin interacts with warfarin.

RELATED DRUGS: The effect of pravastatin on other oral anticoagulants is not established. Fluvastatin (eg, *Lescol*) appears to inhibit CYP2C9, the primary enzyme in the metabolism of S-warfarin; thus, fluvastatin is expected to increase warfarin response.[4] Simvastatin (*Zocor*) appears to produce a small increase in warfarin effect. Clofibrate† and gemfibrozil (eg, *Lopid*) may enhance the hypoprothrombinemic response to warfarin, while cholestyramine (eg, *Questran*) and colestipol (*Colestid*) may reduce its effect.

MANAGEMENT OPTIONS: No interaction.

REFERENCES:

1. Pan HY. Clinical pharmacology of pravastatin, a selective inhibitor of HMG-CoA reductase. *Eur J Clin Pharmacol.* 1991;40(suppl 1):S15-S18.
2. Jungnickel PW, et al. Pravastatin: a new drug for the treatment of hypercholesterolemia. *Clin Pharm.* 1992;11:677-689.
3. O'Rangers EA, et al. The effect of HMG CoA reductase inhibitors on the anticoagulant response to warfarin. *Pharmacotherapy.* 1994;14:349.
4. Transon C, et al. In vivo inhibition profile of cytochrome P450TB (CYP2C9) by (±)-fluvastatin. *Clin Pharmacol Ther.* 1995;58:412-417.

† Not available in the United States.

Praziquantel (*Biltricide*)
Rifampin (eg, *Rifadin*)

SUMMARY: Rifampin markedly reduces praziquantel plasma concentrations; loss of therapeutic effect may occur.

RISK FACTORS: No specific risk factors are known.

MECHANISM: Rifampin induces the CYP3A4-mediated metabolism of praziquantel.

CLINICAL EVALUATION: Ten healthy subjects received a single dose of praziquantel 40 mg/kg and 3 doses of praziquantel 25 mg/kg.[1] Both doses were administered with water and again following 5 days of rifampin 600 mg/day. Following the single-dose study, praziquantel plasma concentrations were undetectable in 7 of the subjects following rifampin pretreatment. With multiple doses of praziquantel, rifampin pretreatment prevented the measurement of praziquantel in 5 of the subjects. In the remaining subjects, rifampin pretreatment reduced the mean area under the concentration-time curve of praziquantel 80%. Rifampin administration with praziquantel likely will eliminate the anthelmintic activity of praziquantel.

RELATED DRUGS: Rifabutin (*Mycobutin*) also is an inducer of CYP3A4 and could cause a similar interaction with praziquantel. Other inducers of CYP3A4 are expected to reduce praziquantel bioavailability and plasma concentrations.

MANAGEMENT OPTIONS:

➡ *Use Alternative.* Avoid the use of praziquantel in patients taking rifampin or in patients who have discontinued rifampin within 14 days.

REFERENCES:

1. Ridtitid W, et al. Rifampin markedly decreases plasma concentrations of praziquantel in healthy volunteers. *Clin Pharmacol Ther*. 2002;72:505-513.

 Prazosin (eg, *Minipress*)

Propranolol (eg, *Inderal*)

SUMMARY: The first-dose syncopal response to prazosin may be enhanced by beta-blockade.

RISK FACTORS: No specific risk factors are known.

MECHANISM: Beta-blockers may inhibit the compensatory cardiovascular responses (ie, increases in heart rate and cardiac output) that normally would follow prazosin-induced hypotension. Neither propranolol nor alprenolol appear to affect prazosin pharmacokinetics.[1,2]

CLINICAL EVALUATION: The acute postural hypotension that may occur following the first dose of prazosin appears to be enhanced in hypertensive patients taking propranolol[3] and in healthy subjects who were given prazosin 1 mg orally with or without propranolol or primidolol, a cardioselective beta-blocker.[4]

RELATED DRUGS: A similar increase in the incidence of first-dose hypotensive reaction was observed with combined use of prazosin and alprenolol in hypertensive patients.[3] The combination of other beta-blockers and alpha-blockers (eg, terazosin [eg, *Hytrin*]) may produce acute postural hypotension.

MANAGEMENT OPTIONS:

➡ *Circumvent/Minimize.* The addition of propranolol to patients stabilized on prazosin will lessen the likelihood of a syncopal episode. However, monitor for orthostatic blood pressure changes.

➡ *Monitor.* In patients receiving beta-blockers, initiate prazosin therapy with caution and with conservative doses (eg, 50% of normal). Taking the initial prazosin dose at bedtime would be prudent.

REFERENCES:

1. Seideman P, et al. Prazosin first dose phenomenon during combined treatment with a beta-adrenoceptor in hypertensive patients. *Br J Clin Pharmacol*. 1982;13:865-870.

2. Rubin P, et al. Studies on the clinical pharmacology of prazosin. II: The influence of indomethacin and of propranolol on the action and disposition of prazosin. *Br J Clin Pharmacol*. 1980;10:33-39.

3. Graham RM, et al. Prazosin: the first-dose phenomenon. *Br Med J*. 1976;4:1293-1294.

4. Elliott HL, et al. Immediate cardiovascular responses to oral prazosin–effects of concurrent beta-blockers. *Clin Pharmacol Ther*. 1981;29:303-309.

Prazosin (eg, *Minipress*)

Verapamil (eg, *Calan*)

SUMMARY: The combination of verapamil with prazosin can enhance hypotensive effects.

RISK FACTORS: No specific risk factors are known.

MECHANISM: Verapamil increases prazosin plasma concentrations probably by decreasing the first-pass clearance of prazosin. A pharmacodynamic interaction also is likely since verapamil reduces the reflex increase in heart rate that occurs after prazosin is administered.

CLINICAL EVALUATION: Eight normotensive subjects received a single dose of prazosin 1 mg, verapamil 160 mg or placebo alone and in combination.[1] Mean peak prazosin plasma concentrations increased from 5.2 ng/mL when administered alone to 9.6 ng/mL with concomitant verapamil administration. The area under the prazosin concentration-time curve increased 62% when verapamil was coadministered. Prazosin half-life did not change. Although neither drug alone altered supine blood pressure, the combination significantly reduced both supine and standing pressure. Mean standing pressure reached a nadir of 89/60 mm Hg 2.5 hours after the drugs were administered. Episodes of orthostatic hypotension increased with the coadministration of prazosin and verapamil. The effects of this combination on blood pressure and pharmacokinetics have been affirmed.[2,5]

RELATED DRUGS: The combination of verapamil and terazosin (*Hytrin*) also has been noted to produce increased pharmacodynamic effect. Verapamil apparently reduces the first-pass metabolism of terazosin.[3,4] Other calcium channel blockers may have additive hypotensive effects when administered with prazosin, terazosin, or doxazosin (*Cardura*).

MANAGEMENT OPTIONS:

➥ *Circumvent/Minimize.* Smaller doses of prazosin may be indicated when verapamil is coadministered.

➥ *Monitor.* The combination of verapamil and prazosin appears to produce a potent antihypertensive effect. Carefully monitor patients stabilized on one of these drugs for hypotension during the institution of the second drug.

REFERENCES:

1. Pasanisi F, et al. Combined alpha-adrenoceptor antagonism and calcium channel blockade in normal subjects. *Clin Pharmacol Ther.* 1984;36:716.

2. Elliott HL, et al. Verapamil and prazosin in essential hypertension: evidence of synergistic combination? *J Cardiovasc Pharmacol.* 1987;10(Suppl. 10):108.

3. Lenz M, et al. Combined terazosin and verapamil therapy in essential hypertension; haemodynamic interactions. *Clin Pharmacol Ther.* 1991;49:146. Abstract.

4. Varghese A, et al. Combined terazosin and verapamil therapy in essential hypertension; pharmacokinetic interactions. *Clin Pharmacol Ther.* 1991;49:130. Abstract.

5. Meredith PA, et al. An additive or synergistic drug interaction: application of concentration-effect modeling. *Clin Pharmacol Ther.* 1992;51:708.

Prednisolone

Rifampin (eg, *Rifadin*)

SUMMARY: Rifampin appears to reduce the effect of corticosteroids like prednisolone significantly in some patients.

RISK FACTORS: No specific risk factors are known.

MECHANISM: Rifampin appears to stimulate the metabolism of corticosteroids.

CLINICAL EVALUATION: Rifampin administration has been associated with a shortened cortisol half-life, increased requirements for replacement therapy with cortisone, increased urinary 6-betahydroxycortisol excretion, and diminished therapeutic response to prednisolone.[1-6]

RELATED DRUGS: It is likely that most corticosteroids would be affected similarly by rifampin.

MANAGEMENT OPTIONS:

➡ *Circumvent/Minimize.* The dose of corticosteroid may require an increase.

➡ *Monitor.* It does not seem necessary to avoid concomitant use of corticosteroids and rifampin, but be alert for evidence of reduced corticosteroid effect.

REFERENCES:

1. Maisey DN, et al. Rifampicin and cortisone replacement therapy. *Lancet.* 1974;2:896.
2. Yamada S, et al. Induction of hepatic cortisol-6-hydroxylase by rifampicin. *Lancet.* 1976;2:366.
3. Edwards OM, et al. Changes in cortisol metabolism following rifampicin therapy. *Lancet.* 1974;2:549.
4. Buffington GA, et al. Interaction of rifampin and glucocorticoids. *JAMA.* 1976;236:1958.
5. van Marle W, et al. Concurrent steroid and rifampicin therapy. *BMJ.* 1979;1:1029.
6. Carrie F, et al. Rifampin-induced nonresponsiveness of giant cell arteritis to prednisone treatment. *Arch Intern Med.* 1994;154:1521.

 Prednisone

Warfarin (eg, *Coumadin*)

SUMMARY: Corticosteroids like prednisone have been reported both to increase oral anticoagulant dosage requirements and, paradoxically, to increase the likelihood of bleeding; data to support either effect are limited.

RISK FACTORS: No specific risk factors are known.

MECHANISM: Corticosteroids have been shown to produce hypercoagulability of the blood.[1] Thus, the possibility exists that the effects of anticoagulants could be antagonized by corticosteroids. Conversely, some have proposed an adverse effect of corticosteroids on vascular integrity, which could increase the danger of hemorrhage at a given level of anticoagulation.[2,3] Theoretically, the ulcerogenic potential of corticosteroids could predispose an anticoagulated patient to bleeding.

CLINICAL EVALUATION: Some investigators have reported that corticosteroids or corticotropin may increase oral anticoagulant requirements,[4] while others have reported hemorrhage as a result of combined corticotropin (eg, *Acthar*) and ethyl biscoumacetate therapy[3] and increased warfarin sensitivity in a patient receiving prednisone.[5] These studies were limited, and the results are not necessarily contradictory; that is, corticosteroids may both antagonize the hypoprothrombinemic effect of oral anticoagulants and increase the risk of hemorrhage in some patients because of their vascular effects. More study is needed.

RELATED DRUGS: Other corticosteroids and oral anticoagulants may interact similarly.

MANAGEMENT OPTIONS: No specific action is required, but be alert for evidence of the interaction.

REFERENCES:

1. Wadman B, et al. Thromboembolic complications during corticosteroid treatment of temporal arteritis. *Lancet.* 1972;1:907. Letter.
2. Hamblin TJ. Interaction between warfarin and phenformin. *Lancet.* 1971;2:1323. Letter.
3. Van Cauwenberge H, et al. Hemorrhagic effect of ACTH with anticoagulants. *Can Med Assoc J.* 1958;79:536.
4. Chatterjea JB, et al. Antagonistic effect of ACTH and cortisone on the anticoagulant activity of ethyl biscoumacetate. *BMJ.* 1954;2:790.
5. Brozovic M, et al. Prothrombin during warfarin treatment. *Br J Haematol.* 1973;24:579.

Primidone (*Mysoline*)

Valproic Acid (*Depakene*)

SUMMARY: Valproic acid may increase serum concentrations of the phenobarbital that is produced from primidone; excessive phenobarbital response may occur.

RISK FACTORS: No specific risk factors are known.

MECHANISM: Valproic acid inhibits the hepatic metabolism of phenobarbital.

CLINICAL EVALUATION: A considerable percentage of primidone is metabolized to phenobarbital, and valproic acid is known to inhibit phenobarbital metabolism. Thus, valproic acid would be expected to increase the risk of phenobarbital intoxication in patients receiving primidone. Valproic acid also may increase serum primidone initially followed by a return to normal with continued valproate therapy,[1] but confirmation of this effect is needed.

RELATED DRUGS: No information is available.

MANAGEMENT OPTIONS:

➥ *Monitor.* Monitor patients receiving primidone for signs of phenobarbital toxicity when valproate is given concomitantly.

REFERENCES:

1. Windorfer A, et al. Elevation of diphenylhydantoin and primidone serum concentration by addition of dipropylacetate, a new anticonvulsant drug. *Acta Paediatr Scand.* 1975;64:771.

Probenecid (*Benemid*)

Rifampin (eg, *Rifadin*)

SUMMARY: Probenecid appears to increase rifampin serum concentrations in some patients.

RISK FACTORS: No specific risk factors are known.

MECHANISM: It has been proposed that probenecid competes with rifampin for hepatic uptake, resulting in higher rifampin blood concentrations.[1]

CLINICAL EVALUATION: An initial study in normal subjects indicated that probenecid resulted in considerable increases in rifampin serum concentrations[1]; however, subsequent studies have indicated that this effect is not consistent.[2,3] In some cases, increased serum rifampin concentrations may be desirable.

RELATED DRUGS: No information is available.

MANAGEMENT OPTIONS: No specific action is required, but be alert for evidence of the interaction.

REFERENCES:
1. Kenwright S, et al. Impairment of hepatic uptake of rifamycin antibiotics by probenecid, and its therapeutic implications. *Lancet.* 1973;21:1401.
2. Allen BW, et al. Probenecid and serum-rifampicin. *Lancet.* 1975;2:1309. Letter.
3. Fallon RJ, et al. Probenecid and rifampicin serum levels. *Lancet.* 1975;2:792.

Probenecid (*Benemid*)

Sulfinpyrazone (eg, *Anturane*)

SUMMARY: Probenecid may increase serum sulfinpyrazone concentrations, but the clinical importance of this effect is unknown.

RISK FACTORS: No specific risk factors are known.

MECHANISM: Probenecid markedly inhibits the renal tubular secretion of sulfinpyrazone and its major metabolite.

CLINICAL EVALUATION: Not established. In 1 study, no additive uricosuric activity was noted.[1] The possibility of increased sulfinpyrazone toxicity in the presence of probenecid needs further study.

RELATED DRUGS: No information is available.

MANAGEMENT OPTIONS: No specific action is required, but be alert for evidence of the interaction.

REFERENCES:
1. Perel JM, et al. Studies of interactions among drugs in man at the renal level: probenecid and sulfinpyrazone. *Clin Pharmacol Ther.* 1969;10:834.

Probenecid (*Benemid*)

Thiopental (eg, *Pentothal*)

SUMMARY: Probenecid may prolong thiopental anesthesia.

RISK FACTORS: No specific risk factors are known.

MECHANISM: Not established.

CLINICAL EVALUATION: A single 0.5 to 1 g dose of probenecid prolonged thiopental anesthesia in a placebo-controlled study of 86 patients.[1]

RELATED DRUGS: No information is available.

MANAGEMENT OPTIONS:

➠ *Monitor.* Monitor for prolonged anesthesia in patients receiving probenecid.

REFERENCES:

1. Kaukinen S, et al. Prolongation of thiopentone anaesthesia by probenecid. *Br J Anæsth*. 1980;52:603.

Probenecid (eg, *Benemid*)

Zidovudine (*Retrovir*)

SUMMARY: Probenecid increases the plasma concentration of zidovudine and may allow zidovudine to be administered less frequently and in lower doses.

RISK FACTORS: No specific risk factors are known.

MECHANISM: Probenecid appears to inhibit the metabolism and renal excretion of zidovudine as well as the renal clearance of the metabolite zidovudine glucuronide.

CLINICAL EVALUATION: Probenecid 500 mg every 6 to 8 hours increases the area under the concentration-time curve of zidovudine 75% to 115%.[1-4] A higher incidence of rash has been noted with the combination of zidovudine and probenecid[2,5] although some have reported good results with the combination.[6]

RELATED DRUGS: No information is available.

MANAGEMENT OPTIONS:

➠ *Circumvent/Minimize.* Reduce the dose of zidovudine when probenecid is administered concomitantly. The coadministration of probenecid with zidovudine may enable every 8 hours dosing of zidovudine that would be more convenient than taking zidovudine every 4 hours. The decreased total daily dose of zidovudine also would decrease the financial expenditure for this costly medication.

➠ *Monitor.* Observe patients for rash and other side effects when both agents are administered.

REFERENCES:

1. Hedaya MA, et al. Probenecid inhibits the metabolic and renal clearances of zidovudine (AZT) in human volunteers. *Pharm Res*. 1990;7:411.
2. Kornhauser DM, et al. Probenecid and zidovudine metabolism. *Lancet*. 1989;2:473.
3. de Mirande P, et al. Alterations of zidovudine pharmacokinetics by probenecid in patients with AIDS or AIDS-related complex. *Clin Pharmacol Ther*. 1989;46:494.
4. Campion JJ, et al. Effect of probenecid on the pharmacokinetics of zidovudine and zidovudine glucuronide. *Pharmacotherapy*. 1990;10:235. Abstract.
5. Petty BG, et al. Zidovudine with probenecid: a warning. *Lancet*. 1990;335:1044.
6. Duckworth AS, et al. Zidovudine with probenecid. *Lancet*. 1990;336:441. Letter.

Procainamide (eg, *Procan SR*)

Propranolol (eg, *Inderal*)

SUMMARY: One study suggested that propranolol may increase procainamide concentrations; the clinical significance of the purported interaction is unknown.

RISK FACTORS: No specific risk factors are known.

MECHANISM: Not established.

CLINICAL EVALUATION: In 1 study, 6 healthy subjects received oral procainamide with and without long-term propranolol pretreatment.[1] Procainamide elimination half-life increased approximately 50% and procainamide plasma clearance decreased 16% in the presence of propranolol. It is unlikely that this small change in clearance would affect a patient's response to procainamide. However, in a subsequent study of 8 subjects neither propranolol 240 mg/day nor metoprolol (*Lopressor*) 200 mg/day affected the pharmacokinetics of a single procainamide dose 500 mg IV.[2]

RELATED DRUGS: Metoprolol does not appear to interact.

MANAGEMENT OPTIONS: No specific action is required, but be alert for evidence of the interaction.

REFERENCES:
1. Weidler DJ, et al. The effect of long-term propranolol administration on the pharmacokinetics of procainamide in humans. *Clin Pharmacol Ther*. 1981;29:289. Abstract.
2. Ochs HR, et al. Do beta blockers alter the kinetics of procainamide? *Clin Pharmacol Ther*. 1983;33:209.

Procainamide (eg, *Procan SR*)

Quinidine

SUMMARY: Quinidine markedly increased procainamide serum concentrations in 1 patient; more study is needed.

RISK FACTORS: No specific risk factors are known.

MECHANISM: The mechanism of this interaction is unknown, but quinidine may reduce the renal clearance of procainamide.

CLINICAL EVALUATION: A 53-year-old patient with sustained ventricular tachycardia responded to therapy with sustained-release procainamide 3 g every 6 hours.[1] Quinidine gluconate (*Quinaglute*) 324 mg every 8 hours was added and the procainamide dose was reduced to 2 g every 6 hours. After the addition of quinidine, procainamide concentrations rose 70% and the half-life of procainamide nearly doubled. Electrocardiographic changes in the QRS and QTc intervals reflected the increased serum concentrations.

RELATED DRUGS: No information is available.

MANAGEMENT OPTIONS:

➡ *Circumvent/Minimize.* Until further data are available, avoid the concomitant use of procainamide and quinidine.

➡ *Monitor.* Monitor patients receiving procainamide for antiarrhythmic therapy for an increased response, increased serum concentrations, and toxicity (wide QRS, QT interval) when quinidine is added to their drug regimens. Discontinuing quinidine may reduce the serum concentration and efficacy of coadministered procainamide.

REFERENCES:
1. Hughes B, et al. Increased procainamide plasma concentrations caused by quinidine: a new drug interaction. *Am Heart J*. 1987;114:908.

Procainamide (eg, *Procan SR*)   **4**

Ranitidine (eg, *Zantac*)

SUMMARY: Ranitidine causes a small increase in procainamide plasma concentration in some patients.

RISK FACTORS:

➡ **Dosage Regimen.** Ranitidine doses higher than 300 mg daily may produce a greater risk.

MECHANISM: Ranitidine interferes with the renal tubular secretion of procainamide and may reduce its bioavailability as well.

CLINICAL EVALUATION: Ranitidine (150 mg twice daily initiated 13 hours before 1 g oral procainamide) increased the procainamide area under the concentration-time curve (AUC) 13.7% and decreased its renal clearance 18%. N-acetylprocainamide (NAPA) AUC was increased 13%, and its renal clearance decreased 10%.[1] The absorption of procainamide appeared to be reduced 10%. A higher dose of ranitidine (750 mg over 12 hours) increased the procainamide AUC 20.8%, reduced its renal clearance 35%, and reduced its apparent absorption 24%. In another study, ranitidine 150 mg twice daily for 4 days had no effect on the nonrenal or renal clearance of procainamide or NAPA.[3] However, in subjects with high renal clearance, ranitidine tended to reduce renal and increase nonrenal clearance. The opposite effects were seen in patients with low basal renal procainamide clearance. Usual doses of ranitidine are unlikely to cause procainamide toxicity, particularly when procainamide is administered orally.

RELATED DRUGS: Cimetidine (eg, *Tagamet*) produces a greater inhibition in procainamide renal clearance. Famotidine (eg, *Pepcid*) does not appear to alter the half-life or renal clearance of procainamide or NAPA.[2] Although no data exist, the proton pump inhibitors (eg, omeprazole [*Prilosec*], lansoprazole [*Prevacid*]) would be unlikely to alter procainamide clearance.

MANAGEMENT OPTIONS: No specific action is required, but be alert for evidence of the interaction.

REFERENCES:

1. Somogyi A, et al. Dose and concentration dependent effect of ranitidine on procainamide disposition and renal clearance in man. *Br J Clin Pharmacol*. 1984;18:175.
2. Klotz U, et al. Interaction study of diazepam and procainamide with the new H$_2$-receptor antagonist famotidine. *Clin Pharmacol Ther*. 1985;37:205.
3. Rocci ML, et al. Ranitidine-induced changes in the renal and hepatic clearances of procainamide are correlated. *J Pharmacol Exp Ther*. 1989;248:923.

Procainamide (*Procan SR*)   **5**

Sodium Bicarbonate

SUMMARY: Sodium bicarbonate does not alter procainamide elimination.

RISK FACTORS: No specific risk factors are known.

MECHANISM: Procainamide renal clearance is not influenced by sodium bicarbonate.

CLINICAL EVALUATION: Several studies show that alkalinization of the urine does not alter the renal clearance of procainamide.[1-3]

RELATED DRUGS: No information is available.

MANAGEMENT OPTIONS: No interaction.

REFERENCES:

1. Galeazzi RL, et al. The renal elimination of procainamide. *Clin Pharmacol Ther.* 1976; 19:55.

2. Meyer N, et al. A study of the influence of pH on the buccal absorption and renal excretion of procainamide. *Eur J Clin Pharmacol.* 1974;7:287.

3. Reidenberg MM, et al. Polymorphic acetylation of procainamide in man. *Clin Pharmacol Ther.* 1975;17:722.

---

5   Procainamide (eg, *Procan SR*)

Sucralfate (eg, *Carafate*)

SUMMARY: Sucralfate appears to have minimal effect on procainamide serum concentrations.

RISK FACTORS: No specific risk factors are known.

MECHANISM: Not established. Sucralfate appears to reduce the absorption of procainamide slightly.

CLINICAL EVALUATION: Four healthy subjects took a single dose of procainamide 250 mg alone or half hour after a 1 g dose of sucralfate.[1] Procainamide peak concentration declined approximately 5%, and the area under the concentration-time curve fell 11%; neither were statistically significant. These changes would not be expected to alter the response to procainamide. The effect of multiple doses of sucralfate, separating the doses of the 2 drugs by more than half hour, or the use of sustained-release procainamide on the outcome of this interaction is unknown.

RELATED DRUGS: No information is available.

MANAGEMENT OPTIONS: No interaction.

REFERENCES:

1. Abdulghafoot AA, et al. Effect of sucralfate on procainamide absorption. *Int J Pharmaceut.* 1990;59:R1.

 Procainamide (eg, *Pronestyl*)

Thioridazine (eg, *Mellaril*)

SUMMARY: Procainamide may produce additive prolongation of the QT interval with thioridazine, and thus may increase the risk of ventricular arrhythmias; avoid concurrent use.

RISK FACTORS:

➠ *Hypokalemia.* The corrected QT interval (QTc) may be prolonged in patients with hypokalemia, thus increasing the risk of this interaction. Any other factor that may prolong the QTc interval would also increase the risk of this interaction.

MECHANISM: Thioridazine and procainamide can prolong the QT interval; additive effects may be seen.

CLINICAL EVALUATION: In a double-blind, randomized, crossover study of the pharmacodynamic effects of thioridazine alone, 9 healthy subjects received single oral doses of thioridazine (10 and 50 mg) compared with placebo.[1] The 50 mg dose of thioridazine increased the QTc on the ECG by 23 msec, and the 10 mg dose increased QTc by 9 msec. These results suggest that thioridazine produces a dose-related slowing of cardiac repolarization. Thus, drugs such as procainamide that can independently prolong the QT interval may increase the risk of ventricular arrhythmias in patients taking thioridazine. Although this interaction is based primarily on theoretical considerations, the potential severity of the interaction suggests that the combination should be avoided. Moreover, the manufacturer's product information for *Mellaril* states that combined use of thioridazine with other drugs that are known to prolong the QT interval is contraindicated[2]; thus, medicolegal issues must also be considered.

RELATED DRUGS: Other antiarrhythmics such as amiodarone (eg, *Cordarone*), disopyramide (eg, *Norpace*), and quinidine can also increase the QT interval, and may increase the risk of arrhythmias. Also, amiodarone, propafenone (*Rythmol*), and quinidine are known inhibitors of CYP2D6, and may increase thioridazine serum concentrations. Although a number of antipsychotic drugs have, like thioridazine, have shown to prolong the QT interval, clinical evidence suggests that thioridazine may produce the greatest risk.

MANAGEMENT OPTIONS:

➡ *Use Alternative.* Although the risk of this combination is not well established, it would be prudent to use alternatives for 1 of the drugs (see Related Drugs).

➡ *Monitor.* If the combination must be used, monitor the ECG for evidence of QT prolongation, and monitor for clinical evidence of arrhythmias (eg, syncope).

REFERENCES:

1. Hartigan-Go K, et al. Concentration-related pharmacodynamic effects of thioridazine and its metabolites in humans. *Clin Pharmacol Ther.* 1996;60:543-53.
2. "Dear Doctor or Pharmacist" Letter, Novartis Pharmaceuticals, July 7, 2000.

Procainamide (eg, *Pronestyl*)

Trimethoprim (eg, *Proloprim*)

SUMMARY: Trimethoprim significantly increases serum concentrations of procainamide and N-acetylprocainamide (NAPA); cardiac toxicity may result.

RISK FACTORS: No specific risk factors are known.

MECHANISM: Trimethoprim and procainamide are weak bases that are actively secreted by the renal tubules. Trimethoprim competes with the renal secretion of procainamide and NAPA. It inhibits the metabolism of procainamide, probably by inhibiting hepatocyte uptake of procainamide.

CLINICAL EVALUATION: The pharmacokinetics of procainamide sustained-release (500 mg every 6 hours) and its metabolite, NAPA, were determined in 8 healthy subjects before and after 4 days of trimethoprim 200 mg/day.[1] The procainamide area under the concentration-time curve was increased 63%, and its total clearance and renal clearance were reduced 42% and 47%, respectively, by trimethoprim administration. The net effect was a 69% increase in the steady-state serum concentrations of procainamide. NAPA concentrations increased 50% because of a 13% reduction in NAPA clearance and an increase in serum procainamide concentrations. Similar results were reported in a second study.[2] Subjects with the highest baseline clearances had the largest decreases in clearance following trimethoprim administration.

RELATED DRUGS: No information is available.

MANAGEMENT OPTIONS:

➡ **Monitor.** Monitor serum procainamide and NAPA concentrations. Observe patients for procainamide toxicity (wide QRS, QT interval) when trimethoprim is coadministered.

REFERENCES:

1. Kosoglou T, et al. Trimethoprim alters the disposition of procainamide and N-acetylprocainamide. *Clin Pharmacol Ther*. 1988;44:467.

2. Vlasses PH, et al. Trimethoprim inhibition of the renal clearance of procainamide and N-acetylprocainamide. *Arch Intern Med*. 1989;149:1350.

Procarbazine (*Matulane*)

Prochlorperazine (eg, *Compazine*)

SUMMARY: Use of phenothiazines in patients receiving procarbazine has been associated with increased sedation and possibly with increased severity of extrapyramidal symptoms.

RISK FACTORS: No specific risk factors are known.

MECHANISM: Procarbazine appears to be a weak inhibitor of monoamine oxidase (MAO). Potentiation of the sedative effects of phenothiazines, narcotics, and barbiturates is known to occur with other MAO inhibitors.

CLINICAL EVALUATION: Potentiation of sedation associated with phenothiazines has been reported with procarbazine.[1-3] Three patients taking procarbazine became stuporous with diffusely abnormal electroencephalograms after receiving phenothiazines.[1] Some patients appear to have tolerated low doses of phenothiazines, but when larger doses were administered, "semicoma" followed.[3,4] Increased extrapyramidal symptoms also have been reported in a patient receiving prochlorperazine while being treated with procarbazine,[5] but it is not possible to tell whether procarbazine contributed to this effect.

RELATED DRUGS: Procarbazine purportedly can increase sedation from opiates and barbiturates, but cases in humans are lacking.[6]

MANAGEMENT OPTIONS:

➡ **Monitor.** Instruct patients and families to watch for increased sedation and changes in extrapyramidal symptoms if phenothiazines are used with procarbazine.

REFERENCES:

1. Brunner KW, et al. A methylhydrazine derivative in Hodgkin's disease and other malignant neoplasms. Therapeutic and toxic effects studied in 51 patients. *Ann Int Med*. 1965;63:69-86.

2. Sicher K, et al. Experiences with methylhydrazine. *Br Med J*. 1965;1(5438):858-859.

3. Sicher K, et al. Methyl-hydrazine in malignant disease. *Lancet*. 1963;2(7320):1278-1279.

4. Todd ID. Natulan in management of late Hodgkin's disease, other lymphoreticular neoplasms, and malignant melanoma. *Br Med J*. 1965;1(5435):628-631.

5. Poster DS. Procarbazine-prochlorperazine interaction: an underreported phenomenon. *J Med*. 1978;9(6):519-524.

6. Weiss HD, et al. Neurotoxicity of commonly used antineoplastic agents (second of two parts). *N Engl J Med*. 1974;291(3):127-133.

Progestins 4

Warfarin (eg, *Coumadin*)

SUMMARY: A patient on warfarin developed a substantial increase in her INR when given levonorgestrel for emergency contraception, but a causal relationship was not established.

RISK FACTORS: No specific risk factors are known.

MECHANISM: Not established.

CLINICAL EVALUATION: A 35-year-old woman on warfarin developed a dramatic increase in her INR (from 2.1 to 8.1) 3 days after emergency contraception with levonorgestrel (2 doses of 0.75 mg, 12 hours apart).[1] More study is needed to establish whether levonorgestrel or other progestins can increase warfarin response.

RELATED DRUGS: No information is available.

MANAGEMENT OPTIONS: No specific action is required, but be alert for evidence of the interaction.

REFERENCES:

1. Ellison J, et al. Drug Points: Apparent interaction between warfarin and levonorgestrel used for emergency contraception. *BMJ*. 2000;321(7273):1382.

Propafenone (eg, *Rythmol*)

Colchicine

SUMMARY: Based on the interactive properties of the 2 drugs, it is likely that propafenone substantially increases colchicine plasma concentrations. Avoid the combination whenever possible.

RISK FACTORS: No specific risk factors are known.

MECHANISM: Colchicine is a P-glycoprotein substrate, and propafenone is a P-glycoprotein inhibitor, so colchicine plasma concentrations are likely to increase.[1,2]

CLINICAL EVALUATION: Although the interaction is based primarily on theoretical considerations, it is likely that propafenone would increase the risk of colchicine toxicity. Given that colchicine toxicity can be fatal, even a theoretical interaction warrants close attention.

RELATED DRUGS: Other antiarrhythmic agents and cardiovascular drugs that inhibit P-glycoprotein include amiodarone (eg, *Cordarone*), quinidine, and the calcium channel blockers diltiazem (eg, *Cardizem*), nicardipine (eg, *Cardene*), and verapamil (eg, *Calan*).

MANAGEMENT OPTIONS:

➡ **Avoid Unless Benefit Outweighs Risk.** Given that colchicine toxicity can be life-threatening, use propafenone only if it is likely to provide therapeutic benefits that cannot be achieved with noninteracting alternatives.

➡ **Use Alternative.** If possible, use an alternative to propafenone that does not inhibit P-glycoprotein, or use an alternative to colchicine.

➡ **Monitor.** If the combination must be used, monitor carefully for colchicine toxicity, (eg, abdominal pain, diarrhea, fever, muscle pain, vomiting). Advise the patient to immediately contact a health care provider if any of these symptoms occur. Colchicine-induced pancytopenia can result in infections, bleeding, and anemia, and is often the cause of death in fatal cases.

REFERENCES:

1. Rautio J, et al. In vitro p-glycoprotein inhibition assays for assessment of clinical drug interaction potential of new drug candidates: a recommendation for probe substrates. *Drug Metab Dispos.* 2006;34(5):786-792.

2. Cramer J, et al. Multispecificity of drug transporters: probing inhibitor selectivity for the human drug efflux transporters ABCB1 and ABCG2. *ChemMedChem.* 2007;2(12):1783-1788.

Propafenone (eg, *Rythmol*)

Quinidine

SUMMARY: Quinidine increases propafenone serum concentrations and reduces the serum concentrations of its active metabolite. The result may be no net change in response.

RISK FACTORS:

➡ *Pharmacogenetics.* Rapid propafenone metabolizers may be at increased risk for the interaction.

MECHANISM: Quinidine is a potent inhibitor of CYP2D6, the enzyme responsible for the metabolism of propafenone to its active metabolite, 5-hydroxypropafenone. This results in an accumulation of propafenone and a reduction in its metabolite concentration.

CLINICAL EVALUATION: In 9 patients taking propafenone for ventricular arrhythmias, the dosage was decreased to 150 mg every 8 hours for 4 days before the addition of quinidine 50 mg every 8 hours.[1] After 4 days of drug coadministration, propafenone pharmacokinetic parameters were studied and compared with prequinidine values. Quinidine reduced propafenone clearance 58% in the extensive metabolizers but had no effect on slow propafenone metabolizers.[2] No changes in propafenone pharmacodynamic effects were observed based on electrocardiogram analysis. This finding may be explained by the quinidine-induced fall (48%) in the concentration of 5-hydroxypropafenone, which has equivalent antiarrhythmic activity to propafenone. Quinidine appears to inhibit the metabolism of both of propafenone's enantiomers.[3]

RELATED DRUGS: No information is available.

MANAGEMENT OPTIONS:

➡ *Circumvent/Minimize.* Note that, in this group of patients, doses of propafenone were reduced an average of 45% before quinidine was initiated. In all likelihood, this attenuated the increase in propafenone concentration and the potential for toxicity to occur. Prophylactic reduction of the propafenone dose may be the most judicious approach.

➡ *Monitor.* Until more data are available, carefully monitor patients stabilized on propafenone for toxicity when quinidine is added.

REFERENCES:

1. Funck-Brentano C, et al. Genetically-determined interaction between propafenone and low dose quinidine: role of active metabolites in modulating net drug effect. *Br J Clin Pharmacol.* 1989;27(4):435-444.

2. Siddoway LA, et al. Polymorphism of propafenone metabolism and disposition in man: clinical and pharmacokinetic consequences. *Circulation*. 1987;75(4):785-791.

3. Mörike KE, et al. Quinidine-enhanced beta-blockade during treatment with propafenone in extensive metabolizer human subjects. *Clin Pharmacol Ther*. 1994;55(1):28-34.

Propafenone (eg, *Rythmol*)

Rifampin (eg, *Rifadin*)

SUMMARY: Rifampin significantly reduces propafenone plasma concentrations; loss of antiarrhythmic activity may occur.

RISK FACTORS: No specific risk factors are known.

MECHANISM: Rifampin induces the metabolism of propafenone via several pathways including CYP3A4, CYP1A2, and glucuronidation.

CLINICAL EVALUATION: Twelve subjects (6 extensive [EM] and 6 poor [PM] metabolizers for CYP2D6) took 600 mg rifampin once daily for 9 days.[1] Before and at the end of rifampin administration, each subject received an oral (300 mg) and IV (140 mg deuterated) dose of propafenone. Following IV propafenone dosing, rifampin administration produced no significant changes in the pharmacokinetic parameters of propafenone in the EM patients. The PMs had a 2-fold increase in the systemic clearance of propafenone after rifampin treatment. Propafenone half-life was reduced from 12.6 to 8.3 hours by rifampin pretreatment in the PMs. The bioavailability of propafenone was reduced 67% and 41% following rifampin in the EM and PM patients, respectively. In EM and PM patients, the area under the concentration-time curve after oral propafenone administration was reduced approximately 70% by rifampin pretreatment. A reduction in propafenone pharmacodynamic effect (QRS prolongation) was observed following rifampin pretreatment. These changes could result in a loss of antiarrhythmic control in patients stabilized on propafenone who are coadministered rifampin. In 1 case report, a patient stabilized on propafenone was administered rifampin 450 mg twice daily.[2] Nine days later his propafenone plasma concentrations had declined approximately 80% and his arrhythmias returned. Two weeks following discontinuation of the rifampin his arrhythmia was again controlled.

RELATED DRUGS: Rifabutin (*Mycobutin*) may not be as potent an inducer as rifampin and would be less likely to produce a large reduction in propafenone concentrations.

MANAGEMENT OPTIONS:

➡ ***Monitor.*** Monitor propafenone plasma concentrations in patients when rifampin is initiated or discontinued. Up to 2 weeks may be required to observe the maximum change in propafenone concentration after rifampin is initiated or discontinued.

REFERENCES:

1. Dilger K, et al. Consequences of rifampicin on propafenone disposition in extensive and poor metabolizers of CYP2D6. *Pharmacogenetics*. 1999;9:551.

2. Castel JM, et al. Rifampicin lowers plasma concentrations of propafenone and its antiarrhythmic effect. *Br J Clin Pharmacol*. 1990,30:155.

Propafenone (eg, *Rythmol*)

Theophylline (eg, *Theochron*)

SUMMARY: Case reports suggest that propafenone elevates theophylline plasma concentrations and may produce symptoms of theophylline toxicity.

RISK FACTORS: No specific risk factors are known.

MECHANISM: Not established; propafenone appears to reduce the clearance of theophylline.

CLINICAL EVALUATION: A 71-year-old man with chronic obstructive pulmonary disease was taking theophylline 300 mg twice daily and his serum theophylline concentrations were between 10 and 13 mcg/mL.[1] Six weeks after starting propafenone 150 mg 3 times daily, the theophylline concentration was 19 mcg/mL, and the patient complained of anorexia. The propafenone was discontinued, and 1 day later the theophylline concentration was 10.8 mcg/mL. A retrial of propafenone 150 mg 3 times daily increased theophylline concentrations from 12.8 to 17.5 mcg/mL 1 week later. In a second case, theophylline clearance in a 63-year-old patient was reduced approximately 70% following the addition of propafenone at doses up to 300 mg every 8 hours.[2]

RELATED DRUGS: No information is available.

MANAGEMENT OPTIONS:

➡ ***Circumvent/Minimize.*** Theophylline doses may require reduction following the addition of propafenone.

➡ ***Monitor.*** Monitor patients stabilized on theophylline for elevated theophylline concentrations and signs of theophylline toxicity (eg, anorexia, nausea, tachycardia, tremor) if propafenone therapy is added. Discontinuing propafenone may result in subtherapeutic theophylline concentrations.

REFERENCES:

1. Lee BL, et al. Theophylline toxicity after propafenone treatment: evidence for drug interaction. *Clin Pharmacol Ther*. 1992;51:353-355.

2. Spinler SA, et al. Propafenone-theophylline interaction. *Pharmacotherapy*. 1993;13:68-71.

Propafenone (eg, *Rythmol*)

Thioridazine

SUMMARY: Propafenone may increase thioridazine serum concentrations, and thus may increase the risk of ventricular arrhythmias; avoid concurrent use.

RISK FACTORS:

➥ *Pharmacogenetics.* Patients with the extensive metabolizer CYP2D6 phenotype (EMs) are expected to experience this interaction. Poor metabolizers (PMs) do not have the gene for production of CYP2D6, and likely already have high serum concentrations of thioridazine. Approximately 8% of white patients are deficient in CYP2D6, but the deficiency is rare in Asian patients, usually 1% or less.

➥ *Hypokalemia.* The corrected QT interval (QTc) may be prolonged in patients with hypokalemia, thus increasing the risk of this interaction. Any other factor that may prolong the QTc interval also may increase the risk of this interaction.

MECHANISM: Propafenone probably inhibits the hepatic metabolism of thioridazine by CYP2D6.

CLINICAL EVALUATION: In 1 study of the pharmacodynamic effects of thioridazine alone, 9 healthy subjects received single oral doses of thioridazine (10 and 50 mg) compared with placebo.[1] The dose of thioridazine 50 mg increased the QTc on the ECG 23 msec; the 10 mg dose increased QTc 9 msec. These results suggest thioridazine produces a dose-related slowing of cardiac repolarization. Thus, drugs such as propafenone that inhibit CYP2D6 may reduce the metabolism of thioridazine and increase the risk of excessive prolongation of the QTc and ventricular arrhythmias. Although this interaction is based primarily on theoretical considerations, the potential severity of the interaction suggests the combination should be avoided. The manufacturer's product information states that combined use of thioridazine and CYP2D6 inhibitors is contraindicated[2]; thus, consider medicolegal issues.

RELATED DRUGS: Antiarrhythmics such as amiodarone (eg, *Cordarone*), disopyramide (eg, *Norpace*), procainamide (eg, *Procanbid*), and quinidine can increase the QT interval, and may also increase the risk of arrhythmias. Amiodarone and quinidine, known inhibitors of CYP2D6, may increase thioridazine serum concentrations. Although a number of antipsychotic drugs have, like thioridazine, been shown to prolong the QT interval, clinical evidence suggests that thioridazine may produce the greatest risk.

MANAGEMENT OPTIONS:

➥ *Use Alternative.* Although the risk of this combination is not well established, use alternatives for 1 of the drugs when possible (see Related Drugs).

➥ *Monitor.* If the combination must be used, monitor the ECG for evidence of QT prolongation, and monitor for clinical evidence of arrhythmias (eg, syncope).

REFERENCES:

1. Hartigan-Go K, et al. Concentration-related pharmacodynamic effects of thioridazine and its metabolites in humans. *Clin Pharmacol Ther.* 1996;60:543-553.
2. 'Dear Doctor or Pharmacist' Letter. East Hanover, NJ: Novartis Pharmaceuticals; July 7, 2000.

Propafenone (eg, *Rythmol*)

Warfarin (eg, *Coumadin*)

SUMMARY: Propafenone increases warfarin serum concentrations and prolongs the prothrombin time in subjects taking low doses of both drugs.

RISK FACTORS: No specific risk factors are known.

MECHANISM: While the mechanism of this interaction is unknown, propafenone probably inhibits the oxidative metabolism of warfarin.

CLINICAL EVALUATION: Eight healthy subjects received propafenone 225 mg 3 times daily for 8 days, warfarin 5 mg/day for 7 days, and both drugs concurrently for 7 days.[1] The coadministration of propafenone and warfarin resulted in a 39% increase in the mean steady-state warfarin plasma concentration compared with warfarin alone. Prothrombin times also were increased significantly during combined therapy. Warfarin protein binding was not affected by propafenone, and warfarin had no effect on propafenone pharmacokinetics.

RELATED DRUGS: In a case report, a similar enhancement of anticoagulant effect was noted in a patient taking phenprocoumon and propafenone.[2]

MANAGEMENT OPTIONS:

➡ *Monitor.* Although data from therapeutically anticoagulated patients are limited, the administration of propafenone in antiarrhythmic doses may enhance the anticoagulation effect of warfarin significantly. Monitor patients stabilized on warfarin if propafenone is added or withdrawn from therapy.

REFERENCES:

1. Kates RE, et al. Interaction between warfarin and propafenone in healthy volunteer subjects. *Clin Pharmacol Ther*. 1987;42:305-311.
2. Korst HA, et al. Beware: propafenon potentiates the effect of oral anticoagulants [in German]. *Med Klin*. 1981;76:349-350.

 Propoxyphene (eg, *Darvon*)

Rasagiline (*Azilect*)

SUMMARY: Concomitant use of rasagiline and propoxyphene should generally be avoided.

RISK FACTORS: No specific risk factors are known.

MECHANISM: Not established.

CLINICAL EVALUATION: Inclusion of propoxyphene as contraindicated with rasagiline in the product information is apparently because related drugs such as meperidine and tramadol have serotonergic effects, resulting in severe serotonin syndrome-like reactions when combined with MAO inhibitors or other serotonergic drugs. Even though the interaction is based on questionable theoretical considerations, the labeling contraindication dictates that the combination should generally be avoided.[1]

RELATED DRUGS: Rasagiline also is contraindicated with some other analgesics (eg, meperidine [eg, *Demerol*], methadone [eg, *Dolophine*], tramadol [eg, *Ultram*]). Any interaction between rasagiline and propoxyphene is likely similar to that of selegiline (eg, *Eldepryl*) and propoxyphene.

MANAGEMENT OPTIONS:

➡ **Avoid Unless Benefit Outweighs Risk.** In general, do not use propoxyphene concomitantly with rasagiline or within 2 weeks of stopping rasagiline.

REFERENCES:

1. *Azilect* [package insert]. Kansas City, MO: Teva Neuroscience, Inc.; 2006.

Propoxyphene (eg, *Darvon*)

Spironolactone (eg, *Aldactone*)

SUMMARY: The development of gynecomastia has been reported following the coadministration of propoxyphene and spironolactone, but a causal relationship was not established.

RISK FACTORS: No specific risk factors are known.

MECHANISM: Propoxyphene has been shown to inhibit the metabolism of some drugs and may increase serum concentrations of spironolactone, which can produce gynecomastia when administered alone. The mechanism of these effects is not established.

CLINICAL EVALUATION: A patient who had been receiving spironolactone for 4 years with no evidence of gynecomastia was given *Darvon Compound* (propoxyphene, aspirin, caffeine, and phenacetin).[1] Two weeks later, the patient complained of swollen, tender breasts and a pruritic rash, both of which resolved when spironolactone and *Darvon Compound* were discontinued. Challenge with *Darvon Compound* alone resulted in reappearance of the rash, and the drug was discontinued. Readministration of the spironolactone alone did not produce breast changes, but both gynecomastia and the rash reappeared when *Darvon Compound* was added to the spironolactone. Although the combination may have caused gynecomastia in this patient, few conclusions can be drawn until additional studies are done.

RELATED DRUGS: No information is available.

MANAGEMENT OPTIONS: No specific action is required, but be alert for evidence of the interaction.

REFERENCES:

1. Licata AA, et al. Spironolactone-induced gynaecomastia related to allergic reaction to "Darvon compound." *Lancet.* 1976;2(7991):905.

Propoxyphene (eg, *Darvon*)

Tamoxifen (eg, *Soltamox*)

SUMMARY: Theoretically, propoxyphene may reduce the efficacy of tamoxifen in the treatment of breast cancer.

RISK FACTORS: No specific risk factors are known.

MECHANISM: Tamoxifen is metabolized to 2 active metabolites by CYP2D6, the most important of which is endoxifen. By reducing endoxifen formation, CYP2D6 inhibitors such as propoxyphene may reduce tamoxifen efficacy.[1-3]

CLINICAL EVALUATION: A study in patients with breast cancer found substantial reductions in endoxifen plasma concentrations in patients taking potent CYP2D6 inhibitors such as fluoxetine and paroxetine.[4] Another tamoxifen study found a nearly 2-fold increase in the risk of breast cancer relapse in women with low CYP2D6 activity, either due to CYP2D6-inhibiting drugs or genetic deficiency.[5] Taken together, these and other results strongly suggest that CYP2D6 inhibitors reduce the efficacy of tamoxifen in the treatment of breast cancer. Propoxyphene is a CYP2D6 inhibitor, and may inhibit the anticancer effects of tamoxifen.

RELATED DRUGS: Most other analgesics are probably less likely than propoxyphene to inhibit CYP2D6.

MANAGEMENT OPTIONS:

➥ **Consider Alternative.** If possible, use an alternative to propoxyphene. It is of questionable efficacy as an analgesic, and should generally be avoided in any case.

➥ **Monitor.** If a CYP2D6 inhibitor such as propoxyphene is used with tamoxifen, cancer recurrence may be an indication that tamoxifen efficacy has been reduced. If this happens, consider discontinuing the CYP2D6 inhibitor.

REFERENCES:

1. Dezentjé VO, et al. Clinical implications of CYP2D6 genotyping in tamoxifen treatment for breast cancer. *Clin Cancer Res*. 2009;15(1):15-21.
2. Tan SH, et al. Pharmacogenetics in breast cancer therapy. *Clin Cancer Res*. 2008;14(24):8027-8041.
3. Newman WG, et al. Impaired tamoxifen metabolism reduces survival in familial breast cancer patients. *Clin Cancer Res*. 2008;14(18):5913-5918.
4. Borges S, et al. Quantitative effect of CYP2D6 genotype and inhibitors on tamoxifen metabolism: implication for optimization of breast cancer treatment. *Clin Pharmacol Ther*. 2006;80(1):61-74.
5. Goetz MP, et al. The impact of cytochrome P450 2D6 metabolism in women receiving adjuvant tamoxifen. *Breast Cancer Res Treat*. 2007;101(1):113-121.

Propoxyphene (eg, *Darvon*)

Warfarin (eg, *Coumadin*)

SUMMARY: Several cases of enhanced hypoprothrombinemic response to warfarin have been reported during the use of a propoxyphene-acetaminophen preparation, but an effect of propoxyphene alone on oral anticoagulant response has not been documented.

RISK FACTORS: No specific risk factors are known.

MECHANISM: It has been proposed that propoxyphene inhibits the metabolism of warfarin. Although propoxyphene has been shown to inhibit the metabolism of drugs metabolized by CYP3A4 (eg, carbamazepine [eg, *Tegretol*]), there is no direct evidence that it inhibits CYP2C9, the isozyme that metabolizes S-warfarin.

CLINICAL EVALUATION: Several patients stabilized on warfarin developed bleeding episodes following administration of a preparation containing propoxyphene and acetaminophen.[1-4] In one 53-year-old man, the prothrombin time increased to 80 seconds 3 days after he started taking acetaminophen with propoxyphene 32 mg (2 to 4 times daily).[3] After discontinuation of the acetaminophen-propoxyphene preparation, the warfarin dosage requirement returned to the pre-analgesic therapy level. Because the product involved in these cases also contained acetaminophen, it is not possible to determine which drug was primarily responsible for the interaction.

RELATED DRUGS: No information is available.

MANAGEMENT OPTIONS:

➡ *Monitor.* Although this interaction is not well established, monitor for altered oral anticoagulant effect if propoxyphene is initiated, discontinued, or changed in dosage. Adjust the anticoagulant dose as needed.

REFERENCES:

1. Orme M, et al. Warfarin and distalgesic interaction. *Br Med J.* 1976;1(6003):200.
2. Jones RV. Letter: Warfarin and distalgesic interaction. *Br Med J.* 1976;1(6007):460.
3. Smith R, et al. Propoxyphene and warfarin interaction. *Drug Intell Clin Pharm.* 1984;18(10):822.
4. Justice JL, et al. Analgesics and warfarin. A case that brings up questions and cautions. *Postgrad Med.* 1988;83(5):217-218, 220.

Propranolol (eg, *Inderal*)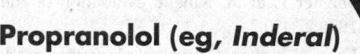

Quinidine

SUMMARY: Quinidine may increase the plasma concentration of propranolol, but the incidence of adverse effects caused by these interactions is unknown. Propranolol does not affect quinidine kinetics.

RISK FACTORS:

➡ *Pharmacogenetics.* Rapid metabolizers of propranolol may be at increased risk to develop the interaction.

MECHANISM: Quinidine decreases the metabolism of some beta-blockers, including metoprolol, propranolol, and timolol. Both quinidine and beta-blockers exert a negative inotropic action on the heart.

CLINICAL EVALUATION: Although 1 study found that patients on propranolol had a lower quinidine clearance than patients not on propranolol,[5] subsequent crossover studies showed that propranolol does not affect the pharmacokinetics of quinidine.[3,6] Two reports described a 2- to 3-fold increase in propranolol area under the concentration-time curve following a single 50 to 200 mg dose of quinidine.[8,9] Quinidine had the greatest effect on the clearance of ± propranolol, the least active enantiomer.[9] Nevertheless, enhanced reductions in exercise-induced tachycardia and PR intervals also were noted. Because of the possibility of combined cardiac depressant effects, caution has been recommended in the concurrent use of quinidine and propranolol[1,2,7]; however, combination therapy has been used advantageously in the treatment of various cardiac arrhythmias.[4]

RELATED DRUGS: Quinidine decreases the metabolism of metoprolol (*Lopressor*), and timolol (eg, *Blocadren*).

MANAGEMENT OPTIONS:

➡ *Consider Alternative.* Preliminary evidence suggests no effect of quinidine on labetalol pharmacokinetics or pharmacodynamics.[10] Renally excreted beta-blockers (eg, atenolol [*Tenormin*]) should be less likely to interact with quinidine because their metabolism is unlikely to be affected by quinidine. Nevertheless, additive cardiac depressant effects cannot be overlooked.

➥ *Monitor.* Carefully monitor concomitant use of quinidine and propranolol. Watch for bradycardia, heart failure, and arrhythmias.

REFERENCES:
1. Dreifus LS, et al. Propranolol and quinidine in the management of ventricular tachycardia. *JAMA.* 1986;204:736.
2. Hillestad L, et al. Conversion of chronic atrial fibrillation to sinus rhythm with combined propranolol and quinidine treatment. *Am Heart J.* 1969;77:137.
3. Kates RE, et al. Disposition kinetics of oral quinidine when administered concurrently with propranolol. *J Clin Pharmacol.* 1979;19:378.
4. Fors WJ, et al. Evaluation of propranolol and quinidine in the treatment of quinidine-resistant arrhythmias. *Am J Cardiol.* 1971;27:190.
5. Kessler KM, et al. Quinidine pharmacokinetics in patients with cirrhosis or receiving propranolol. *Am Heart J.* 1978;96:627.
6. Fenster P, et al. Kinetic evaluation of the propranolol-quinidine combination. *Clin Pharmacol Ther.* 1980;27:450.
7. Loon NR, et al. Orthostatic hypotension due to quinidine and propranolol. *Am J Med.* 1986;81:1101.
8. Yasuhara M, et al. Alteration of propranolol pharmacokinetics and pharmacodynamics by quinidine in man. *J Pharmacobiodyn.* 1990;13:681.
9. Zhou H-H, et al. Quinidine reduces clearance of ± propranolol more than ± propranolol through marked reduction in 4-hydroxylation. *Clin Pharmacol Ther.* 1990;47:686.
10. Gearhart MO, et al. Lack of effects on labetalol pharmacodynamics with quinidine inhibition of P450IID6. *Pharmacotherapy.* 1991;11:P36. Abstract.

5 | Propranolol (eg, *Inderal*)

Ranitidine (eg, *Zantac*)

SUMMARY: Ranitidine does not appear to affect propranolol or atenolol disposition and probably has little effect on other beta-blockers. There is some evidence that metoprolol pharmacokinetics may be altered by ranitidine, but confirmation of this unexpected effect is needed.

RISK FACTORS: No specific risk factors are known.

MECHANISM: Not established.

CLINICAL EVALUATION: Ranitidine did not affect single-dose or steady-state plasma propranolol concentrations.[3,4] In other studies cimetidine, but not ranitidine, reduced propranolol clearance.[5,6] In a study of healthy subjects, ranitidine 300 mg/day substantially increased plasma concentrations produced by metoprolol (*Lopressor*) 200 mg/day for 1 week.[7] In 2 additional studies, metoprolol peak plasma concentrations were increased by ranitidine without changes in clearance, possibly indicating changes in absorption of metoprolol.[1,2] The disposition of atenolol (*Tenormin*) does not appear to be affected by ranitidine 300 mg/day in healthy subjects.[2,7]

RELATED DRUGS: Cimetidine (eg, *Tagamet*) and etinidine also inhibit metoprolol and labetalol (*DynaCirc*) metabolism. Nizatidine (*Axid*) and famotidine (eg, *Pepcid*) would not be expected to alter propranolol elimination.

MANAGEMENT OPTIONS: No interaction.

REFERENCES:
1. Kelly JG, et al. Effects of ranitidine on the disposition of metoprolol. *Br J Clin Pharmacol.* 1985;19:219.
2. Mutschler E, et al. The interaction between H₂-receptor antagonists and beta-adrenoceptor blockers. *Br J Clin Pharmacol.* 1984;17:51S.

3. Reimann IW, et al. Effects of cimetidine and ranitidine on steady-state propranolol kinetics and dynamics. *Clin Pharmacol Ther.* 1982;32:749.

4. Heagerty AM, et al. Failure of ranitidine to interact with propranolol. *BMJ.* 1982;284:1304.

5. Heagerty AM, et al. The influence of histamine (H_2) antagonists on propranolol pharmacokinetics. *Int J Clin Pharmacol Res.* 1982;2:203.

6. Patel L, et al. Effect of cimetidine and ranitidine on propranolol clearance. *Br J Clin Pharmacol.* 1983;15:152P.

7. Spahn H, et al. Influence of ranitidine on plasma metoprolol and atenolol concentrations. *BMJ.* 1983;286:1546.

Propranolol (*Inderal*)

Rizatriptan (*Maxalt*)

SUMMARY: Propranolol increases the plasma concentration of rizatriptan.

RISK FACTORS: No specific risk factors are known.

MECHANISM: Unknown. Propranolol may competitively inhibit the first-pass metabolism (by monoamine oxidase A) of rizatriptan.

CLINICAL EVALUATION: While no published data are available for evaluation, the manufacturer of rizatriptan has made available some data on this interaction.[1] Eleven healthy subjects received a single oral dose of rizatriptan 10 mg alone and concurrently with propranolol 240 mg/day. The duration of propranolol therapy was not noted. During the coadministration of propranolol, the area under the concentration-time curve of rizatriptan was increased 70%.

RELATED DRUGS: Metoprolol (*Lopressor*) 100 mg every 12 hours and nadolol (*Corgard*) 80 mg every 12 hours did not interact with rizatriptan.[1] In vitro studies suggest that timolol (*Blocadren*) and atenolol (*Tenormin*) will not interact with rizatriptan. Propranolol has been reported to have no interaction with sumatriptan (*Imitrex*).[2] The effects of other 5-HT agonists and propranolol are not known.

MANAGEMENT OPTIONS:

➡ **Consider Alternative.** The use of metoprolol or nadolol could be considered for patients taking rizatriptan.

➡ **Circumvent/Minimize.** Reduce the dose of rizatriptan to 5 mg for patients receiving propranolol.

➡ **Monitor.** Be alert for increased myocardial ischemia, vasospasms, elevated blood pressure, or dizziness when propranolol and rizatriptan are coadministered.

REFERENCES:

1. Product information. Rixaptriptan (*Maxalt*). Merck & Co., Inc. 1998.

2. Scott AK, et al. Lack of an interaction between propranolol and sumatriptan. *Br J Clin Pharmacol.* 1991;32:581.

Propranolol (eg, *Inderal*)

Sumatriptan (*Imitrex*)

SUMMARY: Sumatriptan and propranolol do not interact and may be used in combination for migraine therapy.

RISK FACTORS: No specific risk factors are known.

MECHANISM: No interaction.

CLINICAL EVALUATION: Ten healthy subjects received sumatriptan 300 mg alone and after 7 days of propranolol 80 mg twice daily.[1] Propranolol had no effect on sumatriptan pharmacokinetics or pharmacodynamics.

RELATED DRUGS: No information is available.

MANAGEMENT OPTIONS: No interaction.

REFERENCES:

1. Scott AK, et al. Lack of an interaction between propranolol and sumatriptan. *Br J Clin Pharmacol.* 1991;32:581-584.

Propranolol (eg, *Inderal*)

Tacrine (*Cognex*)

SUMMARY: Both tacrine and propranolol can slow the heart rate. Additive bradycardia would be expected, but the risk of adverse consequences from the combination is not known.

RISK FACTORS: No specific risk factors are known.

MECHANISM: Both cholinergic stimulation and beta-blockade can slow the heart rate, and the effects may be additive.

CLINICAL EVALUATION: Prolonged and severe bradycardia has been reported in a few patients receiving cholinergic agents such as neostigmine or physostigmine concurrently with propranolol or other beta-adrenergic blockers such as atenolol (*Tenormin*) and nadolol (*Corgard*).[1-4] Because tacrine can produce bradycardia,[5,6] one would expect that it also would result in additive bradycardia with beta-blockers. However, it is not known how often this interaction would produce adverse effects.

RELATED DRUGS: Other beta-blockers (eg, atenolol, nadolol) may produce similar additive bradycardia.

MANAGEMENT OPTIONS:

➥ *Monitor.* Monitor for excessive bradycardia in patients receiving beta-adrenergic blockers concurrently with tacrine or other cholinergic agents.

REFERENCES:

1. Sprague DH. Severe bradycardia after neostigmine in a patient taking propranolol to control paroxysmal atrial tachycardia. *Anesthesiology.* 1975;42:208-210.

2. Seidl DC, et al. Prolonged bradycardia after neostigmine administration in a patient taking nadolol. *Anesth Analg.* 1984;63:365-367.

3. Baraka A, et al. Severe bradycardia following physostigmine in the presence of beta-adrenergic blockade — a case report. *Middle East J Anesthesiol.* 1984;7:291-293.

4. Eldor J, et al. Prolonged bradycardia and hypotension after neostigmine administration in a patient receiving atenolol. *Anaesthesia.* 1987;42:1294-1297.

5. Taylor P. Agents acting at the neuromuscular junction and autonomic ganglia. In: Gilman AG, Rall TW, Nies AS, Taylor P, eds. The Pharmacological Basis of Therapeutics. 8th ed. New York: Pergamon Press; 1990:166-186.

6. Hartvig P, et al. Pharmacokinetics and effects of 9-amino-1,2,3,4-tetrahydroacridine in the immediate postoperative period in neurosurgical patients. *J Clin Anesth.* 1991;3:137-142.

Propranolol (eg, *Inderal*)

Tetracaine (*Pontocaine*)

SUMMARY: The use of propranolol with tetracaine or other local anesthetics, particularly those containing epinephrine, may enhance sympathomimetic side effects resulting in hypertensive reactions. Acute discontinuation of beta-blockers before local anesthesia may increase the risk of side effects caused by the anesthetic.

RISK FACTORS:

➥ **Anesthetic Combinations.** Local anesthetics containing epinephrine may be at risk for hypertensive reactions.

MECHANISM: Patients taking beta-blockers and given local anesthetics containing epinephrine may experience hypertensive reactions. These reactions are caused by unopposed alpha-receptor stimulation in the presence of beta-receptor blockade.

CLINICAL EVALUATION: Patients whose chronic beta-blocker therapy was discontinued before surgery had more side effects after spinal anesthesia with tetracaine (including arrhythmias and angina) than those whose beta blocker therapy was continued.[1] Similar results were obtained in patients receiving bupivacaine (eg, *Marcaine*) for intercostal nerve blockade; however, bupivacaine can produce cardiodepression and heart block in the presence of beta-blockade.[2,3] beta-blockade therapy combined with local anesthesia using large amounts of lidocaine (eg, *Xylocaine*) and epinephrine resulted in severe hypertension.[4] Conversely, in 10 patients on propranolol who received small doses of local anesthetic plus epinephrine (eg, *Adrenalin*) (mean epinephrine dose approximately equal to 0.03 mg), no hypertensive reactions were noted.[5]

RELATED DRUGS: Bupivacaine and lidocaine appear to interact similarly with propranolol. Cardioselective beta-blocker (eg, metoprolol [*Lopressor*], acebutolol [*Sectral*], atenolol [*Tenormin*]) are probably less likely to predispose patients to epinephrine-induced hypertension.

MANAGEMENT OPTIONS:

➥ **Consider Alternative.** If possible, avoid local anesthetics containing epinephrine in patients receiving propranolol or other nonselective beta-blockers, such as nadolol, pindolol, or timolol.

➥ **Circumvent/Minimize.** These studies indicate that chronic beta-blocker therapy should not be discontinued before the use of local anesthetics such as tetracaine or bupivacaine, although be alert for evidence of cardiodepression.

➥ **Monitor.** If local anesthetics and beta-blockers are coadministered, monitor for hypertensive or cardiotoxic reactions.

REFERENCES:

1. Ponten J, et al. Beta-receptor blockade and spinal anesthesia. Withdrawal versus continuation of long-term therapy. *Acta Anesthesiol Scand*. 1982;76:62-69.
2. Ponten J, et al. Bupivacaine for intercostal nerve blockade in patients on long-term beta-receptor blocking therapy. *Acta Anesthesiol Scand. Suppl*. 1982;76:70-77.
3. Roitman K, et al. Enhancement of bupivacaine cardiotoxicity with cardiac glycosides and beta-adrenergic blockers: a case report. *Anesth Analg*. 1993;76:658-661.
4. Foster CA, et al. Propranolol-epinephrine interaction: a potential disaster. *Plast Reconstr Surg*. 1983;72:74-78.

5. Dzubow LM. The interaction between propranolol and epinephrine as observed in patients undergoing Mohs'surgery. *J Am Acad Dermatol.* 1986;15:71-75.

 Propranolol (eg, *Inderal*)

Theophylline

SUMMARY: Propranolol increases theophylline serum concentrations in a dose-dependent manner. Theophylline and beta-blockers have antagonistic pharmacodynamic effects.

RISK FACTORS:

➡ ***Dosage Regimen.*** Higher doses of propranolol may reduce theophylline clearance.

MECHANISM: Beta-blockers inhibit hepatic microsomal drug metabolism,[3,4,7,8] in particular the demethylation of theophylline.[1] Also, beta-blockers (especially nonselective ones) may antagonize the bronchodilation produced by theophylline.

CLINICAL EVALUATION: In 9 healthy subjects, propranolol 40 mg every 6 hours and, to a lesser extent, metoprolol (*Lopressor*) 50 mg every 6 hours reduced the clearance of theophylline.[5] The effect was most pronounced in subjects whose theophylline metabolism was enhanced by cigarette smoking. Theophylline clearance decreased 30% and 52% after propranolol doses of 120 and 720 mg/day, respectively.[1] A 38% reduction in theophylline clearance was reported after propranolol 180 mg/day.[2] The mild inotropic effect of theophylline in healthy subjects is blocked by pretreatment with propranolol or metoprolol.[6]

RELATED DRUGS: Metoprolol appears to interact similarly with theophylline. Atenolol (*Tenormin*) and nadolol (*Corgard*) do not appear to alter the theophylline pharmacokinetics but may interact pharmacodynamically.[9,10] Other beta-blockers may produce similar antagonistic effects with theophylline.

MANAGEMENT OPTIONS:

➡ ***Use Alternative.*** If possible, avoid beta-blockers in patients receiving theophylline for bronchospastic pulmonary disease. If beta-blockers are required, cardioselective agents are preferable.

➡ ***Monitor.*** If cardioselective beta-blockers are administered to asthmatics, monitor carefully for reduced bronchodilator response.

REFERENCES:

1. Miners JO, et al. Selectivity and dose-dependency of the inhibitory effect of propranolol on theophylline. *Br J Clin Pharmacol.* 1985;20:219.
2. Lombardi TP, et al. The effects of a beta$_2$ agonist and a nonselective beta antagonist on theophylline clearance. *Drug Intell Clin Pharm.* 1986;20:455.
3. Deacon CS, et al. Inhibition of oxidative drug metabolism by betaadrenoreceptor antagonists is related to their lipid solubility. *Br J Clin Pharmacol.* 1981;12:429.
4. Greenblatt DJ, et al. Impairment of antipyrine clearance in humans by propranolol. *Circulation.* 1978;57:1161.
5. Conrad KA, et al. Effects of metoprolol and propranolol on theophylline elimination. *Clin Pharmacol Ther.* 1980;28:463.
6. Conrad KA, et al. Cardiovascular effects of theophylline. Partial attenuation by beta-blockade. *Eur J Clin Pharmacol.* 1981;21:109.
7. Bax NDS, et al. Inhibition of antipyrine metabolism by beta-adrenoceptor antagonists. *Br J Clin Pharmacol.* 1981;12:779.
8. Daneshmend TK, et al. The short term effects of propranolol, atenolol, and labetalol on antipyrine kinetics in normal subjects. *Br J Clin Pharmacol.* 1982;13:817.

9. Cerasa LA, et al. Lack of effect of atenolol on the pharmacokinetics of theophylline. *Br J Clin Pharmacol.* 1988;26:800.

10. Corsi CM, et al. Lack of effect of atenolol and nadolol on the metabolism of theophylline. *Br J Clin Pharmacol.* 1990;29:265.

Propranolol (eg, *Inderal*)

Thiazides

SUMMARY: The combination of a thiazide and propranolol increases blood glucose and triglyceride concentrations.

RISK FACTORS:

➡ *Concurrent Diseases.* Patients with diabetes mellitus are at particular risk.

MECHANISM: Not established.

CLINICAL EVALUATION: Fifteen hypertensive patients with type 2 diabetes mellitus were treated for 3 weeks with hydrochlorothiazide (HCTZ), propranolol or a combination of the 2.[1] Fasting glucose was increased 9% by propranolol, 31% by HCTZ, and 53% by the combination. Patients with hypertension were treated for 3 years with HCTZ alone or in combination with either methyldopa or propranolol.[2] HCTZ produced a small increase in triglycerides and uric acid, while the HCTZ-propranolol combination resulted in a 31% increase in triglycerides and a 19% increase in uric acid. Cholesterol concentrations were unchanged in all groups. Another study found that the HCTZ-propranolol combination resulted in a 50% increase in triglycerides compared with no drug therapy in a group of patients during 1 year of therapy following a myocardial infarction.[3] The clinical significance of these changes is unknown.

RELATED DRUGS: Other beta-blockers may produce similar effects, although the degree of effect may differ.

MANAGEMENT OPTIONS: No specific action is required, but be alert for evidence of the interaction.

REFERENCES:

1. Dornhorst A, et al. Aggravation by propranolol of hyperglycemic effect of hydrochlorothiazide in type II diabetics without alteration of insulin secretion. *Lancet.* 1985;1:123.

2. Helgelan A. The impact on serum lipids of combinations of diuretics and beta blockers and of beta blockers alone. *J Cardiovasc Pharmacol.* 1986;6:S474.

3. Hietanen E, et al. Beta blockers, diuretics and physical fitness as determinants of serum lipids in myocardial infarction patients. *Scand J Clin Lab Invest.* 1986;46:97.

Propranolol (eg, *Inderal*)

Tubocurarine

SUMMARY: Propranolol may prolong the effects of tubocurarine.

RISK FACTORS: No specific risk factors are known.

MECHANISM: Propranolol may enhance the neuromuscular blockade of tubocurarine by impairing transmission of impulses at the motor nerve terminals.

CLINICAL EVALUATION: Two patients with thyrotoxicosis who received propranolol 120 mg/day before surgery appeared to have manifested an increase in the duration of action of tubocurarine.[1] Beta-adrenergic blockers also have been associated with symptoms of myasthenia gravis[2] which is further evidence of a neuromuscular blocking action.

RELATED DRUGS: Combinations of other beta-blockers and neuromuscular blockers may produce similar effects.

MANAGEMENT OPTIONS: No specific action is required, but be alert for evidence of the interaction.

REFERENCES:

1. Rozen MS, et al. Prolonged curarization associated with propranolol. *Med J Aust.* 1972;1:467.
2. Herishanu Y, et al. Beta blockers and myasthenia gravis. *Ann Intern Med.* 1975;83:834.

Propranolol (eg, *Inderal*)

Verapamil (eg, *Calan*)

SUMMARY: Propranolol serum concentrations may be increased by verapamil; beta-blocker and verapamil combinations may result in a greater risk of bradycardia or hypotension than when either is used alone.

RISK FACTORS: No specific risk factors are known.

MECHANISM: Calcium channel blockers inhibit the hepatic metabolism of some beta-blockers.[1,2] Verapamil and diltiazem may add to the effects of beta-blockers on cardiac conduction (slowing atrioventricular conduction) and the hypotensive effects of beta-blockade.

CLINICAL EVALUATION: *Effect of Verapamil on the Pharmacokinetics of Beta-Blockers.* Verapamil 360 mg daily increased the area under the concentration-time curve (AUC) of propranolol 30% to 60%[3,10] and reduced propranolol clearance.[11,13] The combination has been associated with significant reduction in inotropic, chronotropic, and dromotropic effects during exercise. Verapamil has been reported to increase significantly (up to 300%) the serum concentration of metoprolol (*Lopressor*) in a patient with hypertension[1] and in patients with angina pectoris.[2] Verapamil also has been reported to reduce the renal clearance of atenolol (*Tenormin*) in 2 patients.[9]

Effect of Beta-Blockers on the Pharmacokinetics of Verapamil. A single 80 mg dose of propranolol reduced the AUC of verapamil 32%[3]; propranolol 80 mg every 6 hours reduced the AUC of oral verapamil 37%.[11] However, other studies did not observe alteration of verapamil kinetics following the administration of propranolol or metoprolol.[4,12] The reason for these disparate observations is unclear.

Additive Pharmacodynamic Effects. The combination of a beta-blocker and a calcium channel blocker may be of benefit in certain situations although some patients have developed marked bradycardia and hypotension.[6-8,10,14] A patient being treated with timolol (*Timoptic*) eyedrops developed bradycardia after verapamil 160 mg/day was added[5]; substitution of nifedipine reversed the interaction.

RELATED DRUGS: Atenolol, metoprolol, and timolol appear to interact similarly with verapamil. Diltiazem (eg, *Cardizem*) reduces the metabolism of several beta-blockers. (Also see Clinical Evaluation.)

MANAGEMENT OPTIONS:

➡ *Circumvent/Minimize.* The use of beta-blockers that are not metabolized (eg, atenolol) should minimize pharmacokinetic (but not pharmacodynamic) interactions with verapamil.

➡ **Monitor.** Monitor patients receiving therapy with beta-blockers and verapamil for enhanced effects, particularly atrioventricular conduction slowing, resulting from pharmacokinetic or pharmacodynamic interactions.

REFERENCES:

1. McLean AJ, et al. Clearance-based oral drug interaction between verapamil and metoprolol and comparison with atenolol. *Am J Cardiol.* 1985;55:1628.

2. Keech AC, et al. Pharmacokinetic interaction between oral metoprolol and verapamil for angina pectoris. *Am J Cardiol.* 1986;58:551.

3. Carruthers SG, et al. Synergistic adverse hemodynamic interaction between oral verapamil and propranolol. *Clin Pharmacol Ther.* 1989;46:469.

4. Warrington SJ, et al. Pharmacokinetics and pharmacodynamics of verapamil in combination with atenolol, metoprolol and propranolol. *Br J Clin Pharmacol.* 1984;17:37S.

5. Pringle SD, et al. Severe bradycardia due to interaction of timolol eye drops and verapamil. *BMJ.* 1987;294:155.

6. Packer M, et al. Hemodynamic and clinical effects of combined verapamil and propranolol therapy in angina pectoris. *Am J Cardiol.* 1982;50:903.

7. Winniford MD, et al. Randomized, double-blind comparison of propranolol alone and a propranolol-verapamil combination in patients with severe angina of effort. *J Am Coll Cardiol.* 1983;1:492.

8. Winniford MD, et al. Hemodynamic and electrophysiologic effects of verapamil and nifedipine in patients on propranolol. *Am J Cardiol.* 1982;50:704.

9. Keech AC, et al. Extent and pharmacokinetic mechanisms of oral atenolol-verapamil interaction in man. *Eur J Clin Pharmacol.* 1988;35:363.

10. McCourty JC, et al. The effect of combined therapy on the pharmacokinetics and pharmacodynamics of verapamil and propranolol in patients with angina pectoris. *Br J Clin Pharmacol.* 1988;25:349.

11. Pieper JA, et al. Pharmacokinetic interaction between verapamil and propranolol. *Drug Intell Clin Pharm.* 1987;21:16A. Abstract.

12. Murdoch DL, et al. Evaluation of potential pharmacodynamic and pharmacokinetic interactions between verapamil and propranolol in normal subjects. *Br J Clin Pharmacol.* 1991;31:323.

13. Hunt BA, et al. Effects of calcium channel blockers on the pharmacokinetics of propranolol stereoisomers. *Clin Pharmacol Ther.* 1990;47:584.

14. Bailey DG, et al. Interaction between oral verapamil and beta-blockers during submaximal exercise: relevance of ancillary properties. *Clin Pharmacol Ther.* 1991;49:370.

Propranolol (eg, *Inderal*) 4

Warfarin (eg, *Coumadin*)

SUMMARY: Propranolol increases the serum concentration of warfarin slightly; its effect on hypoprothrombinemic response to warfarin in anticoagulated patients is unknown but is probably minimal in most patients.

RISK FACTORS: No specific risk factors are known.

MECHANISM: Not established. Propranolol may inhibit the metabolism of warfarin.

CLINICAL EVALUATION: In 6 healthy subjects, single 15 mg doses of warfarin were administered alone or after 3 days of propranolol 80 mg twice daily.[1] Propranolol increased the mean warfarin area under the concentration-time curve 17% and increased peak warfarin concentration 25%. In another study, propranolol 80 mg twice daily for 2 weeks significantly increased warfarin serum concentrations 15% in 6 healthy subjects who had received an average of 3.2 mg/day of warfarin for several weeks.[2] It is difficult to determine whether this interaction is of potential clinical importance since the hypoprothrombinemic response of warfarin was not measured.

RELATED DRUGS: Atenolol (*Tenormin*), bisoprolol (*Zebeta*), and metoprolol (*Lopressor*) appear to have no effect on the response to warfarin or acenocoumarol, but little is known about other combinations of beta-adrenergic blockers and oral anticoagulants.

MANAGEMENT OPTIONS: No specific action is required, but be alert for evidence of the interaction.

REFERENCES:

1. Bax NDS, et al. The effect of beta-adrenoceptor antagonists on the pharmacokinetics and pharmacodynamics of warfarin. *Br J Clin Pharmacol.* 1984;17:85S.

2. Scott AK, et al. Interaction between warfarin and propranolol. *Br J Clin Pharmacol.* 1984;17:86S.

Propylthiouracil

Warfarin (eg, *Coumadin*)

SUMMARY: A reduction in thyrometabolic status caused by antithyroid drugs, such as propylthiouracil (PTU) and methimazole, or any other factor tends to reduce the hypoprothrombinemic response to oral anticoagulants.

RISK FACTORS: No specific risk factors are known.

MECHANISM: In clinically hyperthyroid patients, the catabolism of vitamin K-dependent clotting factors tends to increase, resulting in increased sensitivity to the hypoprothrombinemic effect of oral anticoagulants.[1-4] By reducing the degree of hyperthyroidism, the administration of antithyroid drugs tends to attenuate the rapid catabolism of clotting factors, which in turn tends to decrease the hypoprothrombinemic response to oral anticoagulants. Also, an effect of alteration in thyroid function on the GI absorption of oral anticoagulants has not been ruled out. A detailed discussion of these mechanisms has been published.[5]

CLINICAL EVALUATION: It is well established that the response to oral anticoagulants increases as the thyrometabolic status increases, and decreases as the thyrometabolic status decreases.[1-7] Thus, to the extent that antithyroid drugs reverse the hyperthyroid state in any given patient, the hypoprothrombinemic response to oral anticoagulants will correspondingly be reduced. Also, propylthiouracil alone has been reported to produce hypoprothrombinemia, although the reaction appears to be rare.[8-11]

RELATED DRUGS: In 1 patient receiving warfarin, the discontinuation of methimazole (eg, *Tapazole*) resulted in a return of thyrotoxicosis and a marked increase in prothrombin time on 2 occasions.[2] Any agent that reduces thyrometabolic status would be expected to reduce the hypoprothrombinemic response to any oral anticoagulant.

MANAGEMENT OPTIONS:

➥ *Monitor.* Be alert for evidence of an altered hypoprothrombinemic response to oral anticoagulants when antithyroid drugs are initiated, discontinued, or changed in dosage. Monitor prothrombin time carefully and adjust the oral anticoagulant dose as needed.

REFERENCES:

1. Loeliger EA, et al. The biological disappearance rate of prothrombin, factors VII, IX and X from plasma in hypothyroidism, hyperthyroidism, and during fever. *Thromb Diath Haemorrh.* 1964;10:267-277.

2. Vagenakis AG, et al. Enhancement of warfarin-induced hypoprothrombinemia by thyrotoxicosis. *Johns Hopkins Med J*. 1972;131:69-73.

3. McIntosh TJ, et al. Increased sensitivity to warfarin in thyrotoxicosis. *J Clin Invest*. 1970;49:63a.

4. Self T, et al. Warfarin-induced hypoprothrombinemia. Potentiation by hyperthyroidism. *JAMA*. 1975;231:1165-1166.

5. Hansten PD. Oral anticoagulants and drugs which alter thyroid function. *Drug Intell Clin Pharm*. 1980;14:331.

6. Walters MB. The relationship between thyroid function and anticoagulant therapy. *Am J Cardiol*. 1963;11:112-114.

7. Rice AJ, et al. Decreased sensitivity to warfarin in patients with myxedema. *Am J Med Sci*. 1971;262:211-215.

8. Naeye RL, et al. Hemorrhagic state after therapy with propylthiouracil. *Am J Clin Path*. 1960;34:254.

9. Gotta AW, et al. Prolonged intraoperative bleeding caused by propylthiouracil-induced hypoprothrombinemia. *Anesthesiology*. 1972;37:562-563.

10. D'Angelo G, et al. Severe hypoprothrombinaemia after propylthiouracil therapy. *Can Med Assoc J*. 1959;81:479.

11. Greenstein RH. Hypoprothrombinemia due to propylthiouracil therapy. *JAMA*. 1960;173:1014-1015.

Pseudoephedrine (eg, *Sudafed*)

Rasagiline (*Azilect*)

SUMMARY: Avoid concomitant use of rasagiline and pseudoephedrine when possible.

RISK FACTORS: No specific risk factors are known.

MECHANISM: Nonselective monoamine oxidase (MAO) inhibitors tend to increase the amount of norepinephrine in adrenergic neuron storage sites. Subsequent displacement of these increased stores of norepinephrine by indirect-acting sympathomimetics (eg, pseudoephedrine) can result in an exaggerated response.

CLINICAL EVALUATION: When combined with nonselective MAO inhibitors, pseudoephedrine can produce a life-threatening hypertensive crisis. Hypertensive crisis also has been reported in at least 1 patient who received ephedrine with the selective MAO-B inhibitor selegiline.[1] Because rasagiline may become a nonselective MAO inhibitor in some patients, avoid the use of pseudoephedrine and other indirect-acting sympathomimetics in patients receiving rasagiline.

RELATED DRUGS: Avoid using other indirect-acting sympathomimetics (eg, amphetamines, cocaine, ephedrine, isometheptene, methylphenidate, phenylpropanolamine) in patients taking rasagiline. Phenylephrine is largely a direct-acting sympathomimetic, but it is contraindicated with rasagiline because it is a substrate for MAO. Rasagiline and selegiline are likely to interact similarly with pseudoephedrine.

MANAGEMENT OPTIONS:

➡ *Avoid Unless Benefit Outweighs Risk.* In general, do not give pseudoephedrine and related sympathomimetics concurrently with rasagiline or within 2 weeks of stopping rasagiline. Advise patients taking rasagiline that many nonprescription cough and cold products contain decongestant sympathomimetics such as phenylephrine and pseudoephedrine.

REFERENCES:

1. *Azilect* [package insert]. Kansas City, MO: Teva Neuroscience, Inc.; 2006.

5   Psyllium (eg, *Metamucil*)

Warfarin (eg, *Coumadin*)

SUMMARY: Psyllium does not appear to affect warfarin absorption or the hypoprothrombinemic response.

RISK FACTORS: No specific risk factors are known.

MECHANISM: No interaction.

CLINICAL EVALUATION: In 6 healthy subjects, psyllium (as *Metamucil*) did not affect the plasma concentrations or the hypoprothrombinemic effect of coadministered warfarin.[1]

RELATED DRUGS: The effect of psyllium on other oral anticoagulants is not known.

MANAGEMENT OPTIONS: No interaction.

REFERENCES:
1. Robinson DS, et al. Interaction of warfarin and nonsystemic gastrointestinal drugs. *Clin Pharmacol Ther*. 1971;12:491-495.

Quetiapine (*Seroquel*)

Ritonavir (*Norvir*)

SUMMARY: Ritonavir administration may result in elevated quetiapine concentrations and increased adverse reactions.

RISK FACTORS: No specific risk factors are known.

MECHANISM: Ritonavir and atazanavir (*Reyataz*) have been reported to inhibit CYP3A4, the enzyme that metabolizes quetiapine.

CLINICAL EVALUATION: There have been 2 reported cases of patients developing quetiapine adverse reactions (eg, confusion, sedation, weight gain) following the coadministration of quetiapine and atazanavir-ritonavir.[1] In both cases, the adverse reactions appeared to be temporally related to the administration of atazanavir-ritonavir and resolved after the drugs were no longer coadministered. Case reports of prolonged quetiapine elimination in an overdose patient taking ritonavir-atazanavir and priapism following lopinavir-ritonavir plus quetiapine and perphenazine have also been reported.[2,3]

RELATED DRUGS: Amprenavir,[†] darunavir (*Prezista*), fosamprenavir (*Lexiva*), indinavir (*Crixivan*), nelfinavir (*Viracept*), and saquinavir (*Invirase*) also inhibit the activity of CYP3A4 and are expected to increase the plasma concentrations of quetiapine.

MANAGEMENT OPTIONS:

➡ *Monitor.* Monitor patients receiving quetiapine and protease inhibitors that inhibit CYP3A4 for increased quetiapine plasma concentrations and adverse reactions.

REFERENCES:

1. Pollack TM, et al. Clinically significant adverse events from a drug interaction between quetiapine and atazanavir-ritonavir in two patients. *Pharmacotherapy*. 2009;29(11):1386-1391.
2. Hantson P, et al. Toxicokinetic interaction between quetiapine and antiretroviral therapy following quetiapine overdose. *Drug Metab Lett*. 2010;4(1):7-8.
3. Geraci MJ, et al. Antipsychotic-induced priapism in an HIV patient: a cytochrome P450-mediated drug interaction. *Int J Emerg Med*. 2010;3(2):81-84.

† Not available in the United States.

Quetiapine (*Seroquel*)

Thioridazine

SUMMARY: Preliminary results suggest that thioridazine increases the elimination of quetiapine, but the clinical importance of this effect is not established.

RISK FACTORS: No specific risk factors are known.

MECHANISM: Not established.

CLINICAL EVALUATION: While no published data are available for evaluation, there is some data on this interaction from the quetiapine manufacturer.[1] Thioridazine 200 mg twice daily increased quetiapine oral clearance 65%.[1] Because the details of the study were not presented, it is not possible to assess validity.

RELATED DRUGS: No information is available.

MANAGEMENT OPTIONS: No specific action is required, but be alert for evidence of the interaction.

REFERENCES:
1. *Seroquel* [package insert]. Wilmington, DE: AstraZeneca; 1997.

Quilinggao

Warfarin (eg, *Coumadin*)

SUMMARY: A patient on warfarin developed increased warfarin response on 2 occasions after starting a quilinggao product, but the clinical importance of this purported effect is not established.

RISK FACTORS: No specific risk factors are known.

MECHANISM: Not established.

CLINICAL EVALUATION: A 61-year-old man stabilized on chronic warfarin therapy switched from one brand to another of the herbal product quilinggao (essence of tortoise shell).[1] Five days later he developed bleeding gums, epistaxis, and bruising with an INR greater than 6. He later took a third brand of quilinggao, and 3 days later his INR was 5.2. Although a causal relationship was not established, the lack of evidence for efficacy of quilinggao suggests that it should be avoided in patients on warfarin. Herbal medications are not standardized; herbal brands may interact differently because of varying amounts of active ingredient or additional ingredients not listed on the label (and in some cases no active ingredients at all). Moreover, different lots of the same brand may vary substantially.

RELATED DRUGS: No information is available.

MANAGEMENT OPTIONS:

➡ *Circumvent/Minimize.* Advise patients on warfarin to avoid quilinggao and other herbal products, unless there is a compelling reason to use them and the warfarin response can be closely monitored.

➡ *Monitor.* If patients on warfarin take quilinggao, monitor for altered warfarin response when quilinggao is started, stopped, or changed in dosage.

REFERENCES:
1. Wong AL, et al. Interaction between warfarin and the herbal product quilinggao. *Ann Pharmacother.* 2003:37(6):836-838.

Quinidine

Colchicine

SUMMARY: Based on the interactive properties of the 2 drugs, it is likely that quinidine would substantially increase colchicine plasma concentrations.

RISK FACTORS: No specific risk factors are known.

MECHANISM: Colchicine is a P-glycoprotein substrate, and quinidine is a P-glycoprotein inhibitor; therefore, colchicine plasma concentrations are likely to increase.[1,2]

CLINICAL EVALUATION: Although the interaction is based primarily on theoretical considerations, it is likely that quinidine would increase the risk of colchicine toxicity.

Given that colchicine toxicity can be fatal, even a theoretical interaction warrants close attention.

RELATED DRUGS: Other antiarrhythmic agents and cardiovascular drugs that inhibit P-glycoprotein include amiodarone (eg, *Cordarone*), propafenone (eg, *Rythmol*), and the calcium channel blockers diltiazem (eg, *Cardizem*), nicardipine (eg, *Cardene*), and verapamil (eg, *Calan*).

MANAGEMENT OPTIONS:

➥ *Avoid Unless Benefit Outweighs Risk.* Given that colchicine toxicity can be life-threatening, use quinidine only if it is likely to provide therapeutic benefits that cannot be achieved with noninteracting alternatives.

➥ *Use Alternative.* If possible, use an alternative to quinidine that does not inhibit P-glycoprotein, or use an alternative to colchicine.

➥ *Monitor.* If the combination must be used, monitor carefully for colchicine toxicity such as diarrhea, vomiting, fever, abdominal pain, and muscle pain. Advise the patient to immediately contact a health care provider if any of these symptoms occur. Colchicine-induced pancytopenia can result in infections, bleeding, and anemia, and is often the cause of death in fatal cases.

REFERENCES:

1. Rautio J, et al. In vitro p-glycoprotein inhibition assays for assessment of clinical drug interaction potential of new drug candidates: a recommendation for probe substrates. *Drug Metab Dispos.* 2006;34(5):786-792.

2. Keogh JP, Kunta JR. Development, validation and utility of an in vitro technique for assessment of potential clinical drug-drug interactions involving P-glycoprotein. *Eur J Pharm Sci.* 2006;27(5):543-554.

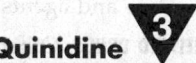

Quinidine

Rifampin (eg, *Rifadin*)

SUMMARY: Rifampin markedly reduces quinidine plasma concentrations.

RISK FACTORS: No specific risk factors are known.

MECHANISM: Rifampin stimulates the hepatic metabolism of quinidine.

CLINICAL EVALUATION: A patient whose ventricular arrhythmia responded to quinidine developed a recurrence after rifampin therapy was added.[1] Additional case reports support the occurrence of this interaction.[2,3] Eight healthy subjects were given oral or intravenous (IV) quinidine (6 mg/kg as a single dose) with and without rifampin pretreatment (600 mg/day for 7 days).[4] Rifampin reduced the elimination half-life of oral quinidine approximately 6-fold. The disposition of IV quinidine was affected similarly by rifampin pretreatment. The magnitude of these changes indicates that rifampin is likely to reduce quinidine plasma concentrations in a majority of patients.

RELATED DRUGS: Theoretically, rifabutin (*Mycobutin*) may affect quinidine in a similar manner.

MANAGEMENT OPTIONS:

➥ *Circumvent/Minimize.* In patients receiving rifampin, the quinidine dose may have to be increased substantially to maintain therapeutic efficacy. Discontinuation of rifampin will result in increased quinidine concentrations.

➡ **Monitor.** Plasma quinidine determinations can be used to achieve the optimal dose of quinidine in the presence of rifampin. Carefully observe patients for changes in quinidine response for several days to 2 weeks following the addition or discontinuation of rifampin therapy.

REFERENCES:

1. Ahmad D, et al. Rifampicin-quinidine interaction. *Br J Dis Chest*. 1979;73(4):409–411.

2. Schwartz A, et al. Quinidine-rifampin interaction. *Am Heart J*. 1984;107(4):789–790.

3. Bussey HI, et al. Influence of rifampin on quinidine and digoxin. *Arch Intern Med*. 1984;144(5):1021–1023.

4. Twum-Barima Y, et al. Quinidine-rifampin interaction. *N Engl J Med*. 1981;304(24):1466–1469.

Quinidine

Sodium Bicarbonate

SUMMARY: Sodium bicarbonate can increase quinidine concentrations; toxicity may result.

RISK FACTORS: No specific risk factors are known.

MECHANISM: Sodium bicarbonate tends to alkalinize the urine, resulting in an increased proportion of non-ionized quinidine. Thus, renal tubular reabsorption of quinidine is increased, and serum concentrations may be increased.

CLINICAL EVALUATION: In a study of 4 subjects, the average quinidine urine concentration was 115 mg/L when urine pH was lower than 6, and 13 mg/L when urine pH was higher than 7.5. Quinidine toxicity may result from the coadministration of quinidine and agents that increase urine pH.[1,2]

RELATED DRUGS: Other agents that alkalinize the urine (eg, antacids, acetazolamide [eg, *Diamox*]) are expected to produce similar results.

MANAGEMENT OPTIONS:

➡ **Monitor.** When a urinary alkalizer such as sodium bicarbonate is initiated, the quinidine dose may have to be reduced to avoid toxicity.

REFERENCES:

1. Knouss RF, et al. Variation in quinidine excretion with changing urine pH. *Ann Intern Med*. 1968;68(5):1157.

2. Milne MD. Influence of acid-base balance on efficacy and toxicity of drugs. *Proc R Soc Med*. 1965;58(11 pt 2):961–963.

Quinidine

Tacrine (*Cognex*)

SUMMARY: Quinidine does not appear to affect the pharmacokinetics of tacrine.

RISK FACTORS: No specific risk factors are known.

MECHANISM: No interaction.

CLINICAL EVALUATION: Eleven healthy subjects received a single oral dose of tacrine 40 mg with and without concurrent treatment with quinidine 83 mg every 8 hours.[1] Quinidine did not affect the pharmacokinetics of tacrine. This finding suggests that CYP2D6 is not important in tacrine metabolism.

RELATED DRUGS: No information is available.

MANAGEMENT OPTIONS: No interaction.

REFERENCES:
1. de Vries TM, et al. Effect of cimetidine and low-dose quinidine on tacrine pharmacokinetics in humans. *Pharm Res*. 1993;10:S337.

Quinidine

Tamoxifen (eg, *Soltamox*)

SUMMARY: Theoretically, quinidine is likely to reduce the efficacy of tamoxifen in the treatment of breast cancer.

RISK FACTORS: No specific risk factors are known.

MECHANISM: Tamoxifen is metabolized to 2 active metabolites by CYP2D6, the most important of which is endoxifen. By reducing endoxifen formation, CYP2D6 inhibitors such as quinidine may reduce tamoxifen efficacy.[1-3]

CLINICAL EVALUATION: A study in patients with breast cancer found substantial reductions in endoxifen plasma concentrations in patients taking potent CYP2D6 inhibitors such as fluoxetine and paroxetine.[4] Another tamoxifen study found a nearly 2-fold increase in the risk of breast cancer relapse in women with low CYP2D6 activity, either due to CYP2D6-inhibiting drugs or genetic deficiency.[5] Taken together, these and other results strongly suggest that CYP2D6 inhibitors reduce the efficacy of tamoxifen in the treatment of breast cancer. Quinidine is a potent CYP2D6 inhibitor, and would be expected to inhibit the anticancer effects of tamoxifen.

RELATED DRUGS: Other antiarrhythmics that substantially inhibit CYP2D6 include amiodarone (eg, *Cordarone*) and propafenone (eg, *Rythmol*).

MANAGEMENT OPTIONS:

➡ *Use Alternative.* If possible, use an antiarrhythmic other than quinidine, amiodarone, or propafenone.

➡ *Monitor.* If a CYP2D6 inhibitor such as quinidine is used with tamoxifen, cancer recurrence may be an indication that tamoxifen efficacy has been reduced. If this happens, consider discontinuing the CYP2D6 inhibitor.

REFERENCES:
1. Dezentjé VO, et al. Clinical implications of CYP2D6 genotyping in tamoxifen treatment for breast cancer. *Clin Cancer Res*. 2009;15(1):15-21.
2. Tan SH, et al. Pharmacogenetics in breast cancer therapy. *Clin Cancer Res*. 2008;14(24):8027-8041.
3. Newman WG, et al. Impaired tamoxifen metabolism reduces survival in familial breast cancer patients. *Clin Cancer Res*. 2008;14(18):5913-5918.
4. Borges S, et al. Quantitative effect of CYP2D6 genotype and inhibitors on tamoxifen metabolism: implication for optimization of breast cancer treatment. *Clin Pharmacol Ther*. 2006;80(1):61-74.
5. Goetz MP, et al. The impact of cytochrome P450 2D6 metabolism in women receiving adjuvant tamoxifen. *Breast Cancer Res Treat*. 2007;101(1):113-121.

Quinidine

Tetrabenazine (*Xenazine*)

SUMMARY: Quinidine is likely to produce marked increases in the plasma concentrations of the 2 active metabolites of tetrabenazine.

RISK FACTORS: No specific risk factors are known.

MECHANISM: The 2 active metabolites of tetrabenazine are both metabolized by CYP2D6, and quinidine is a potent inhibitor of CYP2D6.

CLINICAL EVALUATION: The manufacturer reports a study in 25 healthy subjects in which another potent CYP2D6 inhibitor (paroxetine) produced about a 3-fold increase in one active metabolite of tetrabenazine and a 9-fold increase in the other active metabolite.[1] Quinidine is also a potent CYP2D6 inhibitor, and is likely to produce similar increases in the plasma concentrations of the active metabolites of tetrabenazine. An interaction of this magnitude is expected to increase the risk of tetrabenazine toxicity.

RELATED DRUGS: Other antiarrhythmic agents that are known to inhibit CYP2D6 include amiodarone (eg, *Cordarone*) and propafenone (eg, *Rythmol*); theoretically, they would also substantially increase tetrabenazine serum concentrations.

MANAGEMENT OPTIONS:

➡ **Circumvent/Minimize.** The *Xenazine* product information states that the dose of tetrabenazine should be reduced to one-half the normal dose if it is used with CYP2D6 inhibitors, such as quinidine.[1]

➡ **Monitor.** If the combination is used, monitor for altered tetrabenazine effect if paroxetine or other CYP2D6 inhibitors are started, stopped, or changed in dosage. Dose-dependent adverse reactions of tetrabenazine may include depression, fatigue, insomnia, sedation, parkinsonism, and akathisia.

REFERENCES:
   1. *Xenazine* [package insert]. Deerfield, IL: Lundbeck Inc; 2010.

 Quinidine

AVOID **Thioridazine**

SUMMARY: Quinidine may increase thioridazine serum concentrations and also may produce additive prolongation of the QT interval, thus increasing the risk of ventricular arrhythmias. Avoid concurrent use.

RISK FACTORS:

➡ **Pharmacogenetics.** Only patients with the extensive metabolizer CYP2D6 phenotype are expected to experience increased thioridazine serum concentrations. Poor metabolizers do not have the gene for production of CYP2D6, and would likely already have high serum concentrations of thioridazine. Approximately 8% of white patients are deficient in CYP2D6, but the deficiency is rare in Asian patients, usually 1% or less.

➡ **Hypokalemia:.** The corrected QT interval (QTc) may be prolonged in patients with hypokalemia, thus increasing the risk of this interaction. Any other factor that may prolong the QTc interval may also increase the risk of this interaction.

MECHANISM: Quinidine is a potent inhibitor of CYP2D6, and probably inhibits the hepatic metabolism of thioridazine. Also, both quinidine and thioridazine prolong the QT interval, and additive effects may be seen.

CLINICAL EVALUATION: In a double-blind, randomized, crossover study of the pharmacodynamic effects of thioridazine alone, 9 healthy subjects received single oral doses of thioridazine (10 and 50 mg) compared with placebo.[1] The 50 mg dose of thioridazine increased the QTc on the electrocardiogram (ECG) by 23 msec, and the 10 mg dose increased QTc by 9 msec. These results suggest that thioridazine produces a dose-related slowing of cardiac repolarization. Thus, drugs such as quinidine that inhibit CYP2D6 are expected to reduce the metabolism of thioridazine and increase the risk of excessive prolongation of the QTc and ventricular arrhythmias. Although this interaction is based primarily on theoretical considerations, the potential severity of the interaction dictates that the combination should be avoided. Moreover, the manufacturer's product information for thioridazine states that combined use of thioridazine with CYP2D6 inhibitors or with drugs that prolong the QT interval is contraindicated.[2] Quinidine does both, and is therefore contraindicated based on the product information.

RELATED DRUGS: Other antiarrhythmics such as amiodarone (eg, *Cordarone*), disopyramide (eg, *Norpace*), and procainamide (eg, *Procanbid*) can also increase the QT interval and may increase the risk of arrhythmias. Also, amiodarone and propafenone (eg, *Rythmol*) are known inhibitors of CYP2D6 and may increase thioridazine serum concentrations. Although a number of antipsychotic drugs have been shown to prolong the QT interval, clinical evidence suggests that thioridazine may produce the greatest risk.

MANAGEMENT OPTIONS:

➥ *AVOID COMBINATION.* Although the risk of this combination is not well established, avoid concurrent use when possible.

REFERENCES:

1. Hartigan-Go K, et al. Concentration-related pharmacodynamic effects of thioridazine and its metabolites in humans. *Clin Pharmacol Ther*. 1996;60(5):543-553.
2. "Dear Doctor or Pharmacist" [letter]. East Hanover, NJ: Novartis Pharmaceuticals; July 7, 2000.

Quinidine (eg, *Quinora*)

Timolol (eg, *Blocadren*)

SUMMARY: Quinidine may increase the plasma concentration of timolol, but the incidence of adverse effects due to these interactions is unknown.

RISK FACTORS:

➥ *Pharmacogenetics.* Patients who are rapid metabolizers of timolol are at increased risk for the interaction.

MECHANISM: Quinidine decreases the metabolism of some beta-blockers, including metoprolol, propranolol, and timolol. Both quinidine and beta-blockers exert a negative inotropic action on the heart.

CLINICAL EVALUATION: A patient taking timolol eyedrops (eg, *Timoptic*) developed bradycardia after the addition of quinidine bisulfate 500 mg 3 times daily to his therapy.[1] The bradycardia responded to quinidine dechallenge and rechallenge. In a study of 6 healthy subjects administered 0.25 mg timolol (the amount in 1 drop of Timoptic) IV alone and following a single dose of quinidine 100 mg, timolol concentrations and the dose response to isoproterenol infusion were significantly (up to 40%) increased.[2] The magnitude of this interaction may be greater following oral timolol administration since IV dosing avoids first-pass metabolism. The latter may be markedly reduced by quinidine administration.

RELATED DRUGS: Quinidine also decreases the metabolism of metoprolol (eg, *Lopressor*) and propranolol (eg, *Inderal*). It would not likely affect renally eliminated beta-blockers such as atenolol (eg, *Tenormin*). Preliminary evidence suggests no effect of quinidine on labetalol (eg, *Normodyne*) pharmacokinetics or pharmacodynamics.[3]

MANAGEMENT OPTIONS:

➥ *Consider Alternative.* Renally excreted beta-blockers (eg, atenolol) should be less likely to interact with quinidine, since their metabolism is unlikely to be affected by quinidine. Nevertheless, additive cardiac depressant effects cannot be overlooked.

➥ *Monitor.* Concomitant use of quinidine and timolol should be undertaken with careful monitoring. Watch for bradycardia, heart failure, and arrhythmias.

REFERENCES:

1. Dinai Y, et al. Bradycardia induced by interaction between quinidine and ophthalmic timolol. *Ann Intern Med.* 1985;103:890.
2. Kaila T, et al. Beta blocking effects of timolol at low plasma concentrations. *Clin Pharmacol Ther.* 1991;49:53.
3. Gearhart MO, et al. Lack of effects on labetalol pharmacodynamics with quinidine inhibition of P450IID6. *Pharmacotherapy.* 1991;11:P36. Abstract.

Quinidine (eg, *Quinora*)

Tubocurarine

SUMMARY: Quinidine administration may enhance the effects of tubocurarine and other neuromuscular blockers.

RISK FACTORS: No specific risk factors are known.

MECHANISM: Quinidine appears to potentiate both nondepolarizing and depolarizing muscle relaxants. This effect is mediated by a curare-like action on the myoneural junction, depression of the muscle action potential, and inhibition of cholinesterase activity.

CLINICAL EVALUATION: Quinidine administration in patients who are recovering from the effects of tubocurarine may result in recurarization, leading to unresponsiveness and apnea.[1] Quinidine also has been associated with prolonged neuromuscular blockade in a patient receiving tubocurarine and succinylcholine (eg, *Anectine*).[4] Quinidine depressed plasma cholinesterase activity by approximately 70%. Neostigmine (eg, *Prostigmin*) did not appear to reverse the effects of this interaction.

RELATED DRUGS: A similar effect might be seen with other neuromuscular blockers (eg, succinylcholine).[2,3]

MANAGEMENT OPTIONS:

➡ *Monitor.* If possible, quinidine should be avoided in the immediate postoperative period when the effects of muscle relaxants still may be present. If quinidine must be used, the need for respiratory support should be anticipated.

REFERENCES:

1. Way WL, et al. Recurarization with quinidine. *JAMA.* 1967;200:153.
2. Schmidt JL, et al. The effect of quinidine on the action of muscle relaxants. *JAMA.* 1963;183:669.
3. Cuthbert MF. The effect of quinidine and procainamide on the neuromuscular blocking action of suxamethonium. *Br J Anaesth.* 1966;38:775.
4. Kambam JR, et al. Effect of quinidine on plasma cholinesterase activity and succinylcholine neuromuscular blockade. *Anesthesiology.* 1987;67:858.

Quinidine (eg, *Quinora*)

Valproic Acid (eg, *Depakene*)

SUMMARY: Small doses of quinidine did not alter valproic acid metabolism.

RISK FACTORS: No specific risk factors are known.

MECHANISM: No interaction.

CLINICAL EVALUATION: Eight healthy subjects received a single dose of valproic acid 250 mg and with quinidine 50 mg/day for 2 days.[1] Quinidine did not alter the pharmacokinetics of valproic acid. The effects of larger, multiple doses of quinidine are not known, but quinidine inhibition of drug metabolism (CYP2D6) has been noted following single 50 mg doses.

RELATED DRUGS: No information is available.

MANAGEMENT OPTIONS: No interaction.

REFERENCES:

1. Bottorff MB, et al. Valproic acid pharmacokinetics are not altered following CYP2D6 inhibition with quinidine. *Clin Pharmacol Ther.* 1993;53:177. Abstract.

Quinidine (eg, *Quinora*)

Verapamil (eg, *Calan*)

SUMMARY: Verapamil administration with quinidine increases quinidine concentrations and may result in quinidine toxicity.

RISK FACTORS: No specific risk factors are known.

MECHANISM: Verapamil inhibits the metabolism of quinidine, increases quinidine concentrations, and increases the potential for quinidine toxicity.

CLINICAL EVALUATION: Verapamil 80 mg every 8 hours reduced the clearance of quinidine in a patient taking quinidine gluconate 648 mg every 6 hours.[1] The serum concentration of quinidine increased over 1 week and was accompanied by hypotension, blurred vision, and complete atrioventricular heart block. During a trial of quinidine gluconate 648 mg every 8 hours and verapamil 80 mg every 6 hours, quinidine clearance after oral administration decreased from 15.5 mL/min/kg to 7.6 mL/min/kg after verapamil and quinidine half-life increased from 2.9 hours to

5.3 hours. In another study, 6 subjects received a single 400 mg dose of quinidine before and after 3 days of verapamil 80 mg 3 times daily or 120 mg 3 times daily.[2] Quinidine half-life was prolonged from 6.9 hours to approximately 9 hours, and quinidine clearance was reduced by approximately 35% after both dosage regimens. No changes in protein binding were observed, but the metabolism of quinidine to 3-hydroxyquinidine was reduced.

RELATED DRUGS: Nifedipine (eg, *Procardia*) reduces quinidine concentrations. Diltiazem (eg, *Cardizem*) 120 mg/day had no effect on quinidine concentrations.[3]

MANAGEMENT OPTIONS:

➡ *Circumvent/Minimize.* The addition of verapamil to quinidine therapy may necessitate a reduction in the dose of quinidine.

➡ *Monitor.* If quinidine and verapamil are coadministered, monitor for quinidine toxicity including hypotension, arrhythmia, and heart block.

REFERENCES:

1. Trohman RG, et al. Increased quinidine plasma concentrations during administration of verapamil: a new quinidine-verapamil interaction. *Am J Cardiol*. 1986;57:706.
2. Edwards DJ, et al. The effect of co-administration of verapamil on the pharmacokinetics and metabolism of quinidine. *Clin Pharmacol Ther*. 1987;41:68.
3. Matera MG, et al. Quinidine-diltiazem: pharmacokinetic interaction in humans. *Curr Ther Res*. 1986;40:653.

 Quinidine

Voriconazole (*Vfend*)

SUMMARY: Elevated quinidine concentrations and cardiac arrhythmias may occur if voriconazole and quinidine are coadministered.

RISK FACTORS: No specific risk factors are known.

MECHANISM: Voriconazole is known to be an inhibitor of CYP3A4, the enzyme responsible for the metabolism of quinidine.

CLINICAL EVALUATION: While specific data are lacking, the manufacturer of voriconazole contraindicates the coadministration of quinidine and voriconazole.[1]

RELATED DRUGS: Itraconazole (eg, *Sporanox*), ketoconazole (eg, *Nizoral*), and fluconazole (eg, *Diflucan*) also are likely to produce increased quinidine plasma concentrations and thus increase the risk of toxicity, including prolongation of the corrected QT interval (QTc) on the electrocardiogram.

MANAGEMENT OPTIONS:

➡ *Use Alternative.* Do not administer voriconazole or any antifungal agent that is known to inhibit CYP3A4 to patients receiving quinidine. Consider terbinafine (*Lamisil*) as an alternative because it does not affect CYP3A4 activity.

➡ *Monitor.* If voriconazole is coadministered with quinidine, monitor the patient for evidence of excess QTc prolongation and possible cardiac arrhythmias.

REFERENCES:

1. *Vfend* [package insert]. New York, NY: Pfizer, Inc.; 2003.
2. Boucher HW, et al. Newer systemic antifungal agents: pharmacokinetics, safety and efficacy. *Drugs*. 2004;64:1997-2020.

Quinidine

Warfarin (eg, *Coumadin*)

SUMMARY: A few patients experienced enhanced anticoagulation after quinidine was added to warfarin therapy. Prospective studies do not indicate that the interaction is widespread or of substantial magnitude.

RISK FACTORS: No specific risk factors are known.

MECHANISM: Quinidine may produce additive hypoprothrombinemic effects with coumarin anticoagulants in an occasional patient.

CLINICAL EVALUATION: Quinidine appears to have resulted in hemorrhage in a few patients taking warfarin.[1,2] Another patient receiving quinidine and warfarin developed corpus luteum hemorrhage, although the authors did not mention the possibility of drug interaction.[3] However, in 10 patients on chronic warfarin therapy, quinidine 800 mg/day did not alter the hypoprothrombinemic response.[4] Thus, it appears that quinidine may enhance warfarin hypoprothrombinemia, but only in occasional predisposed patients.

RELATED DRUGS: Theoretically, the same effect could be seen with other oral anticoagulants.

MANAGEMENT OPTIONS:

➡ *Monitor.* Closely observe patients on oral anticoagulants who subsequently receive quinidine for prolonged prothrombin times and signs of bleeding.

REFERENCES:

1. Koch-Weser J. Quinidine-induced hypoprothrombinemic hemorrhage in patients on chronic warfarin therapy. *Ann Intern Med*. 1968;68:511-517.
2. Gazzaniga AB, et al. Possible quinidine-induced hemorrhage in a patient on warfarin sodium. *N Engl J Med*. 1969;280:711-712.
3. Sopher IM, et al. Fatal corpus luteum hemorrhage during anticoagulant therapy. *Obstet Gynecol*. 1971;37:695-697.
4. Udall JA. Drug interference with warfarin therapy. *Clin Med*. 1970;77:20.

Quinidine ②

Ziprasidone (*Geodon*)

SUMMARY: Both ziprasidone and quinidine can prolong the corrected QT interval (QTc) on the electrocardiogram (ECG). Theoretically, this could increase the risk of ventricular arrhythmias such as torsades de pointes.

RISK FACTORS:

➡ *Hypokalemia.* The QTc on the ECG may be prolonged in patients with hypokalemia, increasing the risk of this interaction.[1]

➡ *Miscellaneous.* Other factors that may prolong the QTc interval (eg, hypomagnesemia, bradycardia, impaired liver function, hypothyroidism) also may increase the risk of ventricular arrhythmias.[1]

MECHANISM: Possible additive prolongation of the QTc interval.

CLINICAL EVALUATION: In initial controlled trials, ziprasidone increased the QTc interval approximately 10 msec at the highest recommended dose of 160 mg/day. But because of concern that the QTc measurements were done when ziprasidone serum concentrations were low, the FDA recommended additional study.[2,3] In a subsequent study in patients with psychotic disorders, the QTc interval was measured following administration of several antipsychotic drugs (ziprasidone, thioridazine, quetiapine, risperidone, haloperidol, olanzapine) when the antipsychotic drug concentrations were calculated to be at their peak. Ziprasidone increased the QTc by a mean of approximately 21 msec, which was less than thioridazine (36 msec) but about twice that of the other antipsychotics. Theoretically, the ability of quinidine to prolong the QTc would be additive with ziprasidone, but the extent to which this could increase the risk of ventricular arrhythmias, such as torsades de pointes, is not known.

RELATED DRUGS: Available data suggest that ziprasidone produces less QTc prolongation than thioridazine, but about twice that of quetiapine (*Seroquel*), risperidone (*Risperdal*), haloperidol (eg, *Haldol*), and olanzapine (*Zyprexa*).

MANAGEMENT OPTIONS:

➡ *Use Alternative.* Given the theoretical risk and the fact that quinidine is listed in the ziprasidone product information as "contraindicated," it would be prudent to use an alternative to 1 of the drugs (see Related Drugs).

➡ *Monitor.* If quinidine and ziprasidone are used concurrently, monitor for evidence of arrhythmias (eg, syncope) and for prolonged QT intervals.

REFERENCES:

1. De Ponti F, et al. QT-interval prolongation by non-cardiac drugs: lessons to be learned from recent experience. *Eur J Clin Pharmacol.* 2000;56:1-18.
2. *Geodon* [package insert]. New York, NY: Pfizer Inc.; 2001.
3. Office of Drug Safety Annual Report. Center for Drug Evaluation and Research. FDA Web site. Available at: www.fda.gov/cder/Offices/ODS/AnnRep2001/annualreport2001.htm. Accessed June 9, 2005.

4 Quinine

Sodium Bicarbonate

SUMMARY: Sodium bicarbonate may increase serum quinine concentrations.

RISK FACTORS: No specific risk factors are known.

MECHANISM: The urinary alkalinization produced by sodium bicarbonate may increase the proportion of quinine present in the unionized form, thus promoting renal tubular reabsorption of the quinine.

CLINICAL EVALUATION: Alkalinization of the urine has been shown to reduce the urinary output of quinine from 17.4% of the administered dose (with acid urine) to 8.9% (with alkaline urine).[1] It is unknown whether the increased quinine blood concentration expected to accompany the decreased urinary excretion would increase the therapeutic efficacy of quinine or its dose-related adverse effects.

RELATED DRUGS: Other drugs that alkalinize the urine (eg, acetazolamide [eg, *Diamox*]) will produce similar effects on quinine elimination.

MANAGEMENT OPTIONS: No specific action is required, but be alert for evidence of the interaction.

REFERENCES:

1. Haag HB, et al. The effect of urinary pH on the elimination of quinine in man. *J Pharmacol.* 1943;79:136.

Radioactive Iodine (I^{131})

Theophylline (eg, *Theo-24*)

SUMMARY: A patient developed theophylline toxicity following I^{131} therapy for thyrotoxicosis; this response is consistent with the known effect of thyroid function on theophylline elimination.

RISK FACTORS:

➥ ***Concurrent Diseases.*** Patients who develop hypothyroidism following I^{131} are at increased risk for the interaction.

MECHANISM: The rate of theophylline elimination tends to be increased in hyperthyroidism and reduced in hypothyroidism. Therefore, I^{131} treatment of hyperthyroidism may result in increased serum theophylline concentrations, especially if the I^{131} therapy results in hypothyroidism.

CLINICAL EVALUATION: An asthmatic patient on long-term therapy with theophylline 400 mg 4 times/day and with therapeutic serum theophylline concentrations was given I^{131} treatment for newly diagnosed hyperthyroidism.[1] Three months later, the patient developed clinical and laboratory evidence of hypothyroidism, accompanied by a doubling of his theophylline half-life (to 10 hours) and his serum theophylline concentrations (to 30.9 mcg/mL). He also had a 2-week history of symptoms consistent with theophylline toxicity (eg, cramping, diarrhea, nausea), which resolved when the theophylline dose was reduced. Thyroid replacement with levothyroxine was started, and 2 months later his theophylline half-life and serum concentration had returned to approximately pre-I^{131} levels.

RELATED DRUGS: Theoretically, antithyroid drugs, such as methimazole (eg, *Tapazole*) and propylthiouracil, would produce an effect similar to that of I^{131} (an increase in serum theophylline concentrations).

MANAGEMENT OPTIONS:

➥ ***Monitor.*** Monitor for theophylline toxicity in patients receiving I^{131} therapy for hyperthyroidism. Although hypothyroidism following I^{131} therapy is not unusual, it may take months or years to occur; therefore, the timing of any increase in serum theophylline concentrations is highly variable.

REFERENCES:

1. Johnson CE, et al. Theophylline toxicity after iodine 131 treatment for hyperthyroidism. *Clin Pharm.* 1988;7(8):620-622.

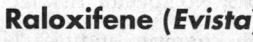

Raloxifene (*Evista*)

Levothyroxine (eg, *Synthroid*)

SUMMARY: Two patients taking levothyroxine developed increased thyroid requirements after starting raloxifene; the incidence and magnitude of the interaction have not been established.

RISK FACTORS: No specific risk factors are known.

MECHANISM: Raloxifene appears to reduce the bioavailability of levothyroxine, but the mechanism of the reduction has not been established.

CLINICAL EVALUATION: A 79-year-old woman on long-term thyroid replacement therapy developed gradually increasing levothyroxine requirements after starting raloxifene (given at the same time as levothyroxine).[1] When the administration of raloxifene and levothyroxine was separated by 12 hours during two 6- to 8-week periods, levothyroxine regained most of its effect. A levothyroxine absorption test also showed reduced serum thyroxine concentrations when raloxifene and levothyroxine were given together, compared with levothyroxine given alone. A 47-year-old woman stabilized on levothyroxine developed increasing levothyroxine requirements after raloxifene was started.[2] Separating the doses by 12 hours appeared to mitigate the interaction. Raloxifene resulted in a clinically important reduction in levothyroxine effect in this patient, but more data are needed to establish the incidence and magnitude of the interaction.

RELATED DRUGS: Until additional information is available, assume that all thyroid replacement agents will interact in a similar manner.

MANAGEMENT OPTIONS:

➡ *Circumvent/Minimize.* Pending additional information, separate doses of levothyroxine (or other thyroid replacement) from raloxifene by as much time as possible. Keep the interval between doses of levothyroxine and raloxifene as consistent as possible to minimize fluctuation in levothyroxine response.

➡ *Monitor.* Monitor thyroid function and adjust the levothyroxine dose as needed in patients taking raloxifene and levothyroxine (or other thyroid replacement). Monitoring is especially important when the dose of raloxifene is started, stopped, or changed, or if the interval between administration of levothyroxine and raloxifene is changed. Note that changes in levothyroxine effect are likely to be gradual and may take place over many weeks.

REFERENCES:

1. Siraj ES, et al. Raloxifene causing malabsorption of levothyroxine. *Arch Intern Med.* 2003;163(11):1367-1370.

2. Garwood CL, et al. Increased thyroid-stimulating hormone levels associated with concomitant administration of levothyroxine and raloxifene. *Pharmacotherapy.* 2006;26(6):881-885.

Raltegravir (*Isentress*)

Rifampin (eg, *Rifadin*)

SUMMARY: Rifampin administration reduces the plasma concentration of raltegravir; reduced antiviral effect may occur.

RISK FACTORS: No specific risk factors are known.

MECHANISM: Rifampin induces UDP-glucuronosyltransferase (UGT1A1), the primary pathway of raltegravir metabolism.

CLINICAL EVALUATION: Nine healthy subjects received a single oral dose of raltegravir 400 mg alone and following 14 days of rifampin 600 mg daily.[1] The mean area under the concentration-time curve (AUC) of raltegravir was reduced by 40% during rifampin coadministration while the trough raltegravir concentration was reduced 60%. In a second study, increasing the dosage of raltegravir to 800 mg twice daily during rifampin coadministration resulted in an AUC similar to that observed following raltegravir 400 mg twice daily administered alone. Raltegravir peak concentration was higher (62%) and its trough lower (50%) with rifampin plus raltegravir 800 mg twice daily. Some increase in the raltegravir dosage may be needed during rifampin administration; current labeling recommends raltegravir 800 mg twice daily.

RELATED DRUGS: Rifampin is known to reduce the plasma concentrations of many antiretroviral drugs, such as ritonavir (*Norvir*), indinavir (*Crixivan*), atazanavir (*Reyataz*), and saquinavir (*Invirase*).

MANAGEMENT OPTIONS:

➡ **Monitor.** Monitor patients taking raltegravir for reduced antiviral effect during rifampin coadministration.

REFERENCES:

1. Wenning LA, et al. Effect of rifampin, a potent inducer of drug-metabolizing enzymes, on the pharmacokinetics of raltegravir. *Antimicrob Agents Chemother.* 2009;53(7):2852-2856.

Ramelteon (*Rozerem*)

Rifampin (eg, *Rifadin*)

SUMMARY: Rifampin reduces ramelteon plasma concentrations; a reduction of ramelteon's efficacy may occur in some patients.

RISK FACTORS: No specific risk factors are known.

MECHANISM: Rifampin is known to induce CYP3A4, an enzyme partially responsible for the metabolism of ramelteon.

CLINICAL EVALUATION: While specific data are limited, administration of rifampin 600 mg once daily for 11 days prior to a single dose of ramelteon reduced the mean area under the plasma concentration-time curve of ramelteon approximately 80%.[1] Pending further data, observe patients receiving ramelteon and rifampin for reduced ramelteon efficacy.

RELATED DRUGS: Rifabutin (*Mycobutin*) may affect ramelteon in a similar manner.

MANAGEMENT OPTIONS:

➡ **Monitor.** If rifampin and ramelteon are coadministered, monitor patients for a reduction in ramelteon's efficacy.

REFERENCES:

1. *Rozerem* [package insert]. Lincolnshire, IL: Takeda Pharmaceuticals; 2005.

Ramelteon (*Rozerem*)

Tacrine (*Cognex*)

SUMMARY: Ramelteon is very sensitive to inhibition of CYP1A2; theoretically, tacrine would increase ramelteon plasma concentrations.

RISK FACTORS: No specific risk factors are known.

MECHANISM: Ramelteon is metabolized primarily by CYP1A2, and tacrine is a CYP1A2 inhibitor.

CLINICAL EVALUATION: In healthy subjects, the potent CYP1A2 inhibitor fluvoxamine (100 mg twice daily for 3 days) produced a 190-fold increase in ramelteon plasma concentrations and a 70-fold increase in the ramelteon maximal plasma concentrations.[1] Administer ramelteon with caution with CYP1A2 inhibitors[1]; tacrine is known to inhibit CYP1A2.

RELATED DRUGS: No information is available.

MANAGEMENT OPTIONS:

➥ *Monitor.* If tacrine and ramelteon are used concurrently, monitor for excessive ramelteon effects.

REFERENCES:

   1. *Rozerem* [package insert]. Lincolnshire, IL: Takeda Pharmaceuticals; 2006.

Ramelteon (*Rozerem*)

Thiabendazole (*Mintezol*)

SUMMARY: Ramelteon is very sensitive to inhibition of CYP1A2; theoretically, thiabendazole would increase ramelteon plasma concentrations.

RISK FACTORS: No specific risk factors are known.

MECHANISM: Ramelteon is metabolized primarily by CYP1A2, and thiabendazole is a CYP1A2 inhibitor.

CLINICAL EVALUATION: In healthy subjects, the potent CYP1A2 inhibitor fluvoxamine (100 mg twice daily for 3 days) produced a 190-fold increase in ramelteon plasma concentrations and a 70-fold increase in the ramelteon maximal plasma concentrations.[1] Administer ramelteon with caution with CYP1A2 inhibitors[1]; thiabendazole is known to inhibit CYP1A2.

RELATED DRUGS: No information is available.

MANAGEMENT OPTIONS:

➥ *Monitor.* If thiabendazole and ramelteon are used concurrently, monitor for excessive ramelteon effects.

REFERENCES:

   1. *Rozerem* [package insert]. Lincolnshire, IL: Takeda Pharmaceuticals; 2006.

Ramelteon (*Rozerem*)

Zileuton (*Zyflo*)

SUMMARY: Ramelteon is very sensitive to inhibition of CYP1A2; theoretically, zileuton would increase ramelteon plasma concentrations.

RISK FACTORS: No specific risk factors are known.

MECHANISM: Ramelteon is metabolized primarily by CYP1A2, and zileuton is a CYP1A2 inhibitor.

CLINICAL EVALUATION: In healthy subjects, the potent CYP1A2 inhibitor fluvoxamine (100 mg twice daily for 3 days) produced a 190-fold increase in ramelteon plasma concentrations and a 70-fold increase in the ramelteon maximal plasma concentrations.[1] Administer ramelteon with caution with CYP1A2 inhibitors[1]; zileuton is known to inhibit CYP1A2.

RELATED DRUGS: No information is available.

MANAGEMENT OPTIONS:

➡ *Monitor.* If zileuton and ramelteon are used concurrently, monitor for excessive ramelteon effects.

REFERENCES:

1. *Rozerem* [package insert]. Lincolnshire, IL: Takeda Pharmaceuticals; 2006.

Ranitidine (eg, *Zantac*)

Saquinavir (*Invirase*)

SUMMARY: The administration of ranitidine to patients taking saquinavir with food appears to increase saquinavir plasma concentrations.

RISK FACTORS: No specific risk factors are known.

MECHANISM: Unknown.

CLINICAL EVALUATION: Twelve healthy men received 3 capsules of saquinavir mesylate 200 mg on 3 different occasions: once with food (treatment A), once fasting 1 hour after the second of 2 doses of ranitidine 150 mg administered 12 hours apart (treatment B), and finally with both food and ranitidine pretreatment (treatment C).[1] The mean areas under the plasma concentration-time curve (AUCs) of saquinavir were 164, 34.5, and 306 ng/h/mL for treatment A, B, and C, respectively. Mean maximum gastric pH measurements were 4.8, 7.4, and 6.5 following treatment A, B, and C, respectively. The plasma concentration of saquinavir administered without food but with ranitidine was very low. Ranitidine added to food increased the AUC of saquinavir 85% compared with saquinavir administered with food alone.

RELATED DRUGS: Other H_2-receptor antagonists (eg, cimetidine [eg, *Tagamet*], famotidine [eg, *Pepcid*], nizatidine [eg, *Axid*]), and proton pump inhibitors also may increase saquinavir plasma concentrations.

MANAGEMENT OPTIONS:

➡ *Monitor.* Monitor patients receiving saquinavir for evidence of elevated plasma concentrations if ranitidine is added to their regimen.

REFERENCES:

1. Kakuda TN, et al. Effect of food and ranitidine on saquinavir pharmacokinetics and gastric pH in healthy volunteers. *Pharmacotherapy.* 2006;26(8):1060-1068.

Ranitidine (eg, *Zantac*)

Sucralfate (eg, *Carafate*)

SUMMARY: The combined use of ranitidine and sucralfate has not been any more effective than either drug alone; concurrent use increases cost and the risk of adverse reactions without proven benefit.

RISK FACTORS: No specific risk factors are known.

MECHANISM: No interaction.

CLINICAL EVALUATION: In a single-dose, crossover study, ranitidine 150 mg was given orally to 6 healthy subjects with and without concurrent sucralfate 1 g orally.[1] Sucralfate slowed the absorption rate of ranitidine but did not affect its bioavailability. Preliminary results of a similar study in 12 healthy subjects indicated that sucralfate 2 g reduced the bioavailability of ranitidine 150 mg 29%.[2] The clinical importance of these findings has not been established, but it is not likely to be great.

RELATED DRUGS: Cimetidine (eg, *Tagamet*) does not appear to reduce the efficacy of sucralfate. In a double-blind study of 61 patients with duodenal ulcer, sucralfate, cimetidine, and a combination of the 2 were equally effective in ulcer healing.[3] It is unlikely that the action of any H_2-receptor antagonist would be affected by the concurrent use of sucralfate.

MANAGEMENT OPTIONS: No interaction.

REFERENCES:
1. Mullersman G, et al. Lack of clinically significant in vitro and in vivo interactions between ranitidine and sucralfate. *J Pharm Sci*. 1986;75(10):995-998.
2. Maconochie JG, et al. Ranitidine sucralfate interaction study. *Clin Pharmacol Ther*. 1987;41:205.
3. Van Deventer G, et al. Comparison of sucralfate and cimetidine taken alone and in combination for treatment of active duodenal ulcer (DU). *Gastroenterology*. 1984;86:1287.

5 Ranitidine (eg, *Zantac*)

Theophylline (eg, *Theolair*)

SUMMARY: Although there have been a few case reports purporting to represent ranitidine-induced theophylline toxicity, several controlled studies have shown that ranitidine has minimal effects on the elimination of theophylline.

RISK FACTORS: No specific risk factors are known.

MECHANISM: No interaction.

CLINICAL EVALUATION: Although ranitidine was thought to have increased plasma theophylline levels in a few cases,[1,2] subsequent analysis of the cases shed doubt on ranitidine as a cause.[3,4] Further, several clinical studies in healthy subjects failed to find an effect of ranitidine on theophylline disposition.[5-8] In a study of 30 adults receiving theophylline for chronic obstructive pulmonary disease, ranitidine 150 mg twice daily for 7 days did not affect plasma theophylline concentrations, while cimetidine 400 mg twice daily increased plasma theophylline concentrations 32%.[9] In a study of 12 subjects, large doses of ranitidine (4,200 mg/day) did not affect theophylline disposition.

RELATED DRUGS: Cimetidine (eg, *Tagamet*) can inhibit theophylline elimination, but other H_2-receptor antagonists such as famotidine (eg, *Pepcid*) and nizatidine (eg, *Axid*) are unlikely to do so.

MANAGEMENT OPTIONS: No interaction.

REFERENCES:
1. Fernandes E, et al. Ranitidine and theophylline. *Ann Intern Med*. 1984;100:459.
2. Roy AK, et al. Induction of theophylline toxicity and inhibition of clearance rates by ranitidine. *Am J Med*. 1988;85:525-527.
3. Dobbs JH, et al. Ranitidine and theophylline. *Ann Intern Med*. 1984;100:769.

4. Muir JG, et al. Induction of theophylline toxicity and inhibition of clearance rates by ranitidine. *Am J Med*. 1989;86:513.

5. Breen KJ, et al. Effects of cimetidine and ranitidine on hepatic drug metabolism. *Clin Pharmacol Ther*. 1982;31:297-300.

6. Rogers JF, et al. The influence of cimetidine versus ranitidine on theophylline pharmacokinetics. *Clin Pharmacol Ther*. 1982;21:261.

7. Ruff E. Drug interferences with theophylline. Absence of interaction between theophylline and ranitidine [in French]. *Nouv Presse Med*. 1982;11:3512.

8. Kelly HW, et al. Ranitidine at very large doses does not inhibit theophylline elimination. *Clin Pharmacol Ther*. 1986;39:577-581.

9. Boehning W. Effect of cimetidine and ranitidine on plasma theophylline in patients with chronic obstructive airways disease treated with theophylline and corticosteroids. *Eur J Clin Pharmacol*. 1990;38:43-45.

Ranitidine (eg, *Zantac*)

Triamterene (*Dyrenium*)

SUMMARY: Ranitidine may slightly decrease the diuretic response to triamterene, but it does not appear to affect the potassium-sparing ability of triamterene.

RISK FACTORS: No specific risk factors are known.

MECHANISM: Ranitidine reduces the renal and metabolic clearance of triamterene, which would be expected to increase plasma triamterene concentrations. However, ranitidine also appears to reduce the absorption of triamterene, which results in a decrease in the plasma triamterene concentration. These effects may be caused by ranitidine-induced reduction in triamterene metabolism, inhibition of renal and hepatic transport, and a reduced solubility of triamterene in a relatively alkaline stomach following ranitidine administration.

CLINICAL EVALUATION: The clinical significance of this interaction is unknown. Eight healthy subjects received in random order triamterene 100 mg, ranitidine 150 mg twice daily, or both drugs in combination for 4 days.[1] The coadministration of ranitidine and triamterene resulted in a 51% reduction in the renal clearance of triamterene. Ranitidine also reduced the hepatic metabolism of triamterene 21%. Despite these reductions in triamterene clearances, the area under the triamterene concentration-time curve was reduced an average of 24%. The urinary recovery of triamterene and its metabolite was reduced 52% with the addition of ranitidine, probably caused by the reduction in triamterene absorption. The net effect was a lower triamterene plasma concentration, which, in turn, was associated with a small reduction in urinary sodium excretion. The combination did not alter triamterene's effect on potassium excretion. Triamterene administration also reduced the renal clearance of ranitidine 14%.

RELATED DRUGS: If an increased gastric pH reduces the absorption of triamterene, other H_2-receptor antagonists (eg, famotidine [eg, *Pepcid*], nizatidine [eg, *Axid*]) also may reduce the concentration of triamterene. Cimetidine (eg, *Tagamet*) has been reported to reduce the renal and metabolic clearances of triamterene.[2]

MANAGEMENT OPTIONS: No specific action is required, but be alert for evidence of the interaction.

REFERENCES:

1. Muirhead M, et al. Pharmacokinetic drug interactions between triamterene and ranitidine in humans: alterations in renal and hepatic clearances and GI absorption. *J Pharmacol Exp Ther*. 1988;244:734-739.

2. Muirhead M, et al. Effect of cimetidine on renal and hepatic drug elimination: studies with triamterene. *Clin Pharmacol Ther.* 1986;40:400-407.

 Ranitidine (eg, *Zantac*)

Voriconazole (*Vfend*)

SUMMARY: No interaction.

RISK FACTORS: No specific risk factors are known.

MECHANISM: No interaction.

CLINICAL EVALUATION: Twelve healthy subjects received voriconazole 200 mg twice daily alone and concurrently with ranitidine 150 mg twice daily for 8 days.[1] The mean voriconazole plasma area under the plasma concentration-time curve was increased about 4% during ranitidine coadministration. Voriconazole half-life was unchanged by ranitidine administration. None of these changes was statistically or clinically significant.

RELATED DRUGS: Cimetidine has been demonstrated to produce a small increase in voriconazole plasma concentrations. Other H_2-receptor antagonists would be unlikely to interact with voriconazole. Ranitidine administration does not affect fluconazole (eg, *Diflucan*) but does reduce the absorption of ketoconazole (eg, *Nizoral*) and itraconazole (*Sporanox*) by increasing gastric pH.

MANAGEMENT OPTIONS: No interaction.

REFERENCES:
1. Purkins L, et al. Histamine H2-receptor antagonists have no clinically significant effect on the steady-state pharmacokinetics of voriconazole. *J Clin Pharmacol.* 2003;56:51-55.

 Ranitidine (eg, *Zantac*)

Warfarin (eg, *Coumadin*)

SUMMARY: Ranitidine does not appear to affect the hypoprothrombinemic response to warfarin in the majority of patients; whether isolated patients may manifest an increased anticoagulant response remains to be established.

RISK FACTORS: No specific risk factors are known.

MECHANISM: No interaction.

CLINICAL EVALUATION: Ranitidine did not affect the hypoprothrombinemic response to warfarin in 3 studies involving healthy subjects.[1-3] In another study of 5 healthy subjects, ranitidine 150 mg twice daily for 5 days reduced warfarin clearance 26%, but the hypoprothrombinemic response was not measured.[4] The results of the latter study, however, do not necessarily conflict with the others. Commercially available warfarin is a racemic mixture (the S-enantiomer being several times more potent than the R-enantiomer), and interacting drugs are known to selectively affect the metabolism of 1 enantiomer. Thus, warfarin interaction studies that measure neither the hypoprothrombinemic response nor warfarin enantiomers cannot determine whether or not a drug affects the anticoagulant response to warfarin.

A 65-year-old woman with recurrent deep vein thrombosis and recurrent GI bleeding was discharged on warfarin 5 mg/day, ranitidine 300 mg twice daily, sucralfate slurry 1 g 4 times daily, ferrous sulfate 325 mg 3 times daily, and amitriptyline 25 mg/day.[5] The ranitidine dose had been increased from 300 to 600 mg/day 4 days before discharge. Her prothrombin time at discharge was 17.6 seconds (control, 10.8 to 12.4 seconds), but 1 week after discharge she was admitted with hematemesis and a prothrombin time of 36.7 seconds. She later was stabilized on warfarin 5 mg/day and ranitidine 300 mg/day with a prothrombin time of 19 to 20 seconds. The authors propose that 600 mg/day of ranitidine increased the warfarin response, while the smaller dose of 300 mg/day did not. Possible explanations for these findings include: 1) Ranitidine in large doses increased the hypoprothrombinemic response to warfarin in this patient. 2) There was a change in warfarin compliance upon discharge. 3) The patient stopped or reduced the intake of the sucralfate slurry upon discharge (some evidence suggests that sucralfate may bind with warfarin in some patients).[6] 4) Some other change at discharge altered warfarin response. It is curious that no interaction was detected after 4 days of ranitidine at 600 mg/day. If ranitidine reduced warfarin metabolism, one would expect to see some effect on warfarin response by this time.

RELATED DRUGS: Cimetidine (eg, *Tagamet*) increased the hypoprothrombinemic response to warfarin, while famotidine (eg, *Pepcid*) and probably nizatidine (*Axid*) are unlikely to do so. Omeprazole (eg, *Prilosec*), at least in doses of 20 mg/day, appears to produce a small increase in the hypoprothrombinemic response to warfarin.

MANAGEMENT OPTIONS: No interaction.

REFERENCES:

1. Serlin MJ, et al. Lack of effect of ranitidine on warfarin action. *Br J Clin Pharmacol.* 1981;12:791-794.
2. O'Reilly R. Comparative interaction of cimetidine and ranitidine with racemic warfarin in man. *Arch Intern Med.* 1984;144:989-991.
3. Toon S, et al. Comparative effects of ranitidine and cimetidine on the pharmacokinetics and pharmacodynamics of warfarin in man. *Eur J Clin Pharmacol.* 1987;32:165-172.
4. Desmond PV, et al. Decreased oral warfarin clearance after ranitidine and cimetidine. *Clin Pharmacol Ther.* 1984;35:338-341.
5. Baciewicz AM, et al. Ranitidine-warfarin interaction. *Ann Intern Med.* 1991;112:76-77.
6. Mungall D, et al. Sucralfate and warfarin. *Ann Intern Med.* 1983;98:557.

Ranitidine (eg, *Zantac*)

Zidovudine (eg, *Retrovir*)

SUMMARY: Ranitidine did not affect zidovudine serum concentrations.

RISK FACTORS: No specific risk factors are known.

MECHANISM: No interaction.

CLINICAL EVALUATION: Six subjects infected with HIV received 3 regimens: zidovudine 600 mg/day alone, zidovudine with cimetidine 1,200 mg/day, and zidovudine with ranitidine 300 mg/day.[1] Each dosage regimen was administered for 7 days. Zidovudine pharmacokinetics were unaltered during ranitidine administration.

RELATED DRUGS: Cimetidine (eg, *Tagamet*) appears to reduce the renal secretion of zidovudine, but serum concentrations are not significantly increased. Other H₂-receptor antagonists (eg, nizatidine [eg, *Axid*], famotidine [eg, *Pepcid*]) are not expected to alter zidovudine renal elimination. The effect of ranitidine on the renal excretion of other antiviral agents is unknown.

MANAGEMENT OPTIONS: No interaction.

REFERENCES:

1. Fletcher CV, et al. The effect of cimetidine and ranitidine administration with zidovudine. *Pharmacotherapy*. 1995;15(6):701-708.

Ranolazine (*Ranexa*)

Rifampin (eg, *Rifadin*)

SUMMARY: Rifampin reduces the plasma concentration of ranolazine; some loss of ranolazine's therapeutic efficacy is likely to occur.

RISK FACTORS: No specific risk factors are known.

MECHANISM: Rifampin is known to induce CYP3A4 and P-glycoprotein; ranolazine is a substrate for both.

CLINICAL EVALUATION: While specific data are limited, the manufacturer of ranolazine notes that the coadministration of rifampin 600 mg daily reduced the plasma concentration of ranolazine by approximately 95%.[1] Pending further data, observe patients receiving ranolazine and rifampin for reduced ranolazine antianginal effect.

RELATED DRUGS: Rifabutin (*Mycobutin*) and rifapentine (*Priftin*) are known to induce CYP3A4 and would likely affect ranolazine in a similar manner.

MANAGEMENT OPTIONS:

➡ **Monitor.** Carefully monitor patients stabilized on ranolazine if rifampin is added to or discontinued from their medication regimen.

REFERENCES:

1. *Ranexa* [package insert]. Palo Alto, CA: CV Therapeutics Inc; 2009.

Ranolazine (*Ranexa*)

Simvastatin (eg, *Zocor*)

SUMMARY: Ranolazine produces a modest increase in simvastatin plasma concentration; some patients may experience myopathy from the combination.

RISK FACTORS: No specific risk factors are known.

MECHANISM: Ranolazine is a weak inhibitor of CYP3A4, the enzyme known to metabolize simvastatin.

CLINICAL EVALUATION: Seventeen healthy subjects received a single dose of simvastatin 80 mg alone, and then on days 4 to 7 of a 7-day regimen of ranolazine 1,000 mg twice daily following an initial dose of 1,750 mg.[1] The pharmacokinetics of simvastatin and its metabolites were measured on day 1 and the last day of ranolazine administration. The coadministration of ranolazine increased the mean area under the concentration-time curve of simvastatin and its metabolites by less than 20%. In another report, a patient taking simvastatin 80 mg daily and extended release ranolazine 500 mg daily developed symptoms of rhabdomyolysis approximately 7 days after starting ranolazine.[2] Rhabdomyolysis was also reported in a patient taking simvastatin 40 mg daily after extended-release ranolazine 500 mg twice daily and diltiazem 60 mg twice daily were initiated.[3] Although the likelihood of developing this interaction is modest, alternative therapies are available to reduce patient risk of harm.

RELATED DRUGS: Lovastatin (eg, *Mevacor*) and atorvastatin (*Lipitor*) are also metabolized by CYP3A4, and may also interact with ranolazine; however, the magnitude of the interaction is expected to be less with atorvastatin.

MANAGEMENT OPTIONS:

➡ *Consider Alternative.* Pravastatin (*Pravachol*), fluvastatin (*Lescol*), and rosuvastatin (*Crestor*) are unlikely to be affected by ranolazine.

➡ *Monitor.* Observe patients taking simvastatin for signs of muscle pain or weakness if ranolazine is coadministered.

REFERENCES:

1. Jerling M, et al. Studies to investigate the pharmacokinetic interactions between ranolazine and keto-conazole, diltiazem, or simvastatin during combined administration in healthy subjects. *J Clin Pharmacol.* 2005;45(4):422-433.

2. Hylton AC, et al. Rhabdomyolysis in a patient receiving ranolazine and simvastatin. *Am J Health Syst Pharm.* 2010;67(21):1829-1831.

3. Rifkin SI. Multiple drug interactions in a renal transplant patient leading to simvastatin-induced rhabdomyolysis: a case report. *Medscape J Med.* 2008;10(11):264.

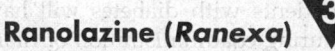

Ranolazine (*Ranexa*)

Verapamil (eg, *Calan*)

SUMMARY: Verapamil produces a modest increase in ranolazine plasma concentrations; some patients may experience adverse reactions as a result of this interaction.

RISK FACTORS: No specific risk factors are known.

MECHANISM: Verapamil is an inhibitor of CYP3A4, one of the enzymes known to metabolize ranolazine. Verapamil also inhibits P-glycoprotein, which is known to be a transporter of ranolazine.

CLINICAL EVALUATION: Fifteen healthy subjects received a single dose of ranolazine 1,125 mg, followed by 750 mg twice daily for 8 days.[1] Verapamil 120 mg 3 times daily was administered on days 4 to 8 of ranitidine dosing. The coadministration of verapamil increased the area under the concentration-time curve of ranolazine by more than 2-fold.

RELATED DRUGS: Diltiazem (eg, *Cardizem*) is known to affect ranolazine in a similar manner.

MANAGEMENT OPTIONS:

➡ *Consider Alternative.* Consider calcium channel blockers that do not inhibit CYP3A4 or P-glycoprotein (eg, amlodipine [eg, *Norvasc*], nifedipine [eg, *Procardia*], felodipine) for patients taking ranolazine.

➡ **Monitor.** Monitor patients receiving verapamil and ranolazine for evidence of QT prolongation, such as fainting or palpitations.

REFERENCES:
1. Jerling M. Clinical pharmacokinetics of ranolazine. *Clin Pharmacokinet.* 2006;45(5):469-491.

Repaglinide (*Prandin*)

Rifampin (eg, *Rimactane*)

SUMMARY: Rifampin reduces repaglinide plasma concentrations and its glucose-lowering effect.

RISK FACTORS: No specific risk factors are known.

MECHANISM: Rifampin reduces the plasma concentrations of repaglinide probably by increasing its first-pass and systemic CYP3A4 metabolism.

CLINICAL EVALUATION: Nine healthy subjects were administered rifampin 600 mg or placebo daily for 5 days.[1] On day 6, a single dose of repaglinide 0.5 mg was given about 12 hours after the last rifampin dose. The mean area under the concentration-time curve (AUC) of repaglinide was reduced 57% following rifampin treatment. The mean half-life of repaglinide was reduced from 1.5 to 1.1 hours, and the peak concentration of repaglinide fell more than 40% with rifampin pretreatment. Repaglinide-induced reduction in blood glucose was decreased by rifampin. Long-term rifampin administration may produce a larger effect on repaglinide concentrations. Based on limited data from a second study, a single dose of repaglinide 4 mg was administered following 6 days of rifampin 600 mg or placebo daily.[2] Rifampin pretreatment resulted in a mean decrease in repaglinide AUC and peak plasma concentration of 32% and 26%, respectively. It is likely that patients with diabetes will have a reduced hypoglycemic effect of repaglinide during coadministration of rifampin.

RELATED DRUGS: Rifabutin (*Mycobutin*) is likely to reduce the concentrations of repaglinide. Rifampin coadministration may reduce the efficacy of other oral hypoglycemic drugs that are metabolized by CYP3A4 or CYP2C9 (eg, glimepiride [eg, *Amaryl*], glipizide [eg, *Glucotrol*], nateglinide [*Starlix*], tolbutamide [eg, *Orinase*]).

MANAGEMENT OPTIONS:

➡ **Circumvent/Minimize.** Patients stabilized on repaglinide who initiate rifampin may require increased repaglinide doses. Adjust repaglinide doses based on blood glucose response.

➡ **Monitor.** Monitor blood glucose concentrations in patients maintained on repaglinide for several weeks after starting or stopping rifampin or other inducers of CYP3A4 to determine if a repaglinide dose adjustment is necessary.

REFERENCES:
1. Niemi M, et al. Rifampin decreases the plasma concentrations and effects of repaglinide. *Clin Pharmacol Ther.* 2000;68(5):495-500.
2. *Prandin* [package insert]. Princeton, NJ: Novo Nordisk Pharmaceuticals Inc; 2002.

Repaglinide (*Prandin*)

Trimethoprim (eg, *Proloprim*)

SUMMARY: Trimethoprim increases the plasma concentration of repaglinide. Monitor patients with diabetes for altered blood glucose control.

RISK FACTORS: No specific risk factors are known.

MECHANISM: Trimethoprim appears to reduce the metabolism of repaglinide by inhibiting CYP2C8 activity.

CLINICAL EVALUATION: Trimethoprim 160 mg or placebo was administered daily for 3 days to 9 healthy subjects.[1] On the third day, 1 hour after the last dose of trimethoprim, a single oral dose of repaglinide 0.25 mg was administered. The mean area under the plasma concentration-time curve of repaglinide was increased 61% (range, 30% to 117%) following trimethoprim. The half-life of repaglinide increased from 0.9 to 1.1 hours after trimethoprim administration. No changes in the blood glucose were noted in these healthy subjects. This degree of change in plasma repaglinide concentrations is expected to increase the hypoglycemic response to repaglinide in some patients with diabetes.

RELATED DRUGS: Pioglitazone (*Actos*) and rosiglitazone (*Avandia*) are also partially metabolized by CYP2C8 and are expected to interact with trimethoprim.

MANAGEMENT OPTIONS:

➡ **Consider Alternative.** Other antibiotics that do not inhibit CYP2C8 may be selected to treat infections in patients taking repaglinide. Do not administer other oral hypoglycemic agents, except pioglitazone and rosiglitazone, with trimethoprim.

➡ **Monitor.** Advise patients stabilized on repaglinide to monitor blood glucose concentrations closely during coadministration of trimethoprim.

REFERENCES:
1. Niemi M, et al. The CYP2C8 inhibitor trimethoprim increases the plasma concentrations of repaglinide in healthy subjects. *Br J Clin Pharmacol.* 2004;57(4):441-447.

Reserpine

Tetrabenazine (*Xenazine*) AVOID

SUMMARY: Tetrabenazine is contraindicated with reserpine, based largely on theoretical considerations.

RISK FACTORS: No specific risk factors are known.

MECHANISM: Tetrabenazine binds reversibly to human vesicular monoamine transporter type 2 (VMAT2), and reserpine binds irreversibly to VMAT2; theoretically, the two drugs would have additive effects on VMAT2.

CLINICAL EVALUATION: Clinical evidence of an interaction between tetrabenazine and reserpine is lacking, but theoretically the combination could result in serious depletion of serotonin and norepinephrine in the CNS. Thus, the combination is considered contraindicated.[1]

RELATED DRUGS: No information is available.

MANAGEMENT OPTIONS: Avoid the combination of tetrabenazine with reserpine. Given that reserpine is an irreversible inhibitor of VMAT2, wait at least 20 days after stopping reserpine before starting tetrabenazine. After stopping reserpine, the manufacturer recommends waiting until after chorea re-emerges before giving tetrabenazine.

REFERENCES:

1. *Xenazine* [package insert]. Deerfield, IL: Lundbeck Inc; 2010.

 Reserpine

Warfarin (eg, *Coumadin*)

SUMMARY: Little evidence is available to indicate that reserpine affects the hypoprothrombinemic response to warfarin or other oral anticoagulants.

RISK FACTORS: No specific risk factors are known.

MECHANISM: Not established.

CLINICAL EVALUATION: Although it has been suggested that long-term reserpine therapy may enhance the effect of oral anticoagulants, convincing evidence of such an interaction in humans is lacking.[1]

RELATED DRUGS: In rats, short-term therapy has been shown to inhibit the hypoprothrombinemic response to ethylbiscoumacetate.[2]

MANAGEMENT OPTIONS: No specific action is required, but be alert for evidence of the interaction.

REFERENCES:

1. Weiner M. Effect of centrally active drugs on the action of coumarin anticoagulants. *Nature.* 1966;212:1599.

2. Hrdina P, et al. Effect of reserpine and some adrenolytics on the anticoagulant activity of pelentan (ethylbiscoumacetate). *Thromb Diath Haemorrh.* 1967;18(3-4):759-765.

 Ribavirin (eg, *Rebetol*)

Warfarin (eg, *Coumadin*)

SUMMARY: A patient on warfarin developed reduced anticoagulant effect when ribavirin was added. Although a causal relationship was well established in this case, it is not known how often other patients would be similarly affected.

RISK FACTORS: No specific risk factors are known.

MECHANISM: Not established.

CLINICAL EVALUATION: A 61-year-old man on chronic warfarin therapy developed a 40% increase in warfarin dosage requirements when ribavirin and interferon were given for hepatitis C.[1] When ribavirin and interferon were stopped, the warfarin requirements returned to baseline over about 3 weeks. A rechallenge with ribavirin 1 year later reduced the warfarin effect again; the warfarin response returned upon discontinuation of ribavirin. Given a positive dechallenge, rechallenge, and another dechallenge, it is highly probable that ribavirin was responsible for the inhibition of warfarin response in this patient. However, the incidence and magnitude of this interaction cannot be predicted from a single case. It is unlikely that the interferon was responsible for the reduced warfarin effect because interferon is an inhibitor of the CYP-450 isozymes. Moreover, the positive rechallenge and subsequent dechallenge involved only ribavirin.

RELATED DRUGS: No information is available.

MANAGEMENT OPTIONS:

➡ **Monitor.** Monitor for altered anticoagulant effect of warfarin if ribavirin dosage is initiated, discontinued, or changed. Adjust warfarin dose as needed.

REFERENCES:

1. Schulman S. Inhibition of warfarin activity by ribavirin. *Ann Pharmacother.* 2002;36(1):72-74.

Rifabutin (*Mycobutin*)
Ritonavir (*Norvir*)

SUMMARY: Ritonavir administration produces marked increases in rifabutin concentrations; rifabutin toxicity may result.

RISK FACTORS: No specific risk factors are known.

MECHANISM: Ritonavir inhibits the enzyme CYP3A4 that metabolizes rifabutin.

CLINICAL EVALUATION: While no published data are available for evaluation, the manufacturer of ritonavir has made available some data on this interaction. In 5 subjects who received rifabutin 150 mg/day for 16 days, the coadministration of ritonavir 500 mg twice daily for 10 days resulted in 4-fold higher rifabutin concentrations compared with 11 subjects receiving rifabutin alone.[1] Peak rifabutin concentrations were 2.5-fold higher than in the control subjects. Because ritonavir has been noted to induce its own metabolism, discontinuation of ritonavir may result in an increased metabolism of rifabutin, resulting in reduced rifabutin concentrations. The effects of rifabutin (a CYP3A4 inducer) on ritonavir metabolism were not reported. However, rifabutin may reduce ritonavir plasma concentrations.

RELATED DRUGS: Indinavir (*Crixivan*) also inhibits the metabolism of rifabutin. Rifabutin decreases the area under the concentration-time curve of saquinavir (*Invirase*). The effects of saquinavir and nelfinavir (*Viracept*) on rifabutin are unknown.

MANAGEMENT OPTIONS:

➡ **Consider Alternative.** If monotherapy for *Mycobacterium avium* complex is required, consider azithromycin (eg, *Zithromax*) or clarithromycin (eg, *Biaxin*). Note that ritonavir inhibits the metabolism of clarithromycin; lower doses of clarithromycin may be required.

➡ **Circumvent/Minimize.** Pending further information on this interaction, avoid the combined use of ritonavir and rifabutin, if possible. Rifabutin dose and frequency may require reduction during coadministration with ritonavir.

➡ **Monitor.** If ritonavir and rifabutin are coadministered, watch for signs of rifabutin toxicity, including arthralgia, dyspepsia, anemia, and skin discoloration. Be alert for subtherapeutic rifabutin concentrations when ritonavir is discontinued.

REFERENCES:

1. *Norvir* [package insert]. Abbott Park, IL: Abbott Laboratories; 1996.

Rifabutin (*Mycobutin*)

Saquinavir (*Invirase*)

SUMMARY: Rifabutin markedly reduces the serum concentration of saquinavir; loss of efficacy or development of resistant organisms may result.

RISK FACTORS: No specific risk factors are known.

MECHANISM: Rifabutin is known to induce CYP3A4, the enzyme responsible for the metabolism of saquinavir.

CLINICAL EVALUATION: While no published data are available for evaluation, the manufacturer of saquinavir has made available some data on this interaction. The administration of saquinavir 600 mg 3 times/day with rifabutin 300 mg/day to 12 patients reduced the that area under the concentration-time curve of saquinavir at steady state 40%.[1] It is likely that the efficacy of saquinavir will be reduced and that the development of resistant strains of HIV will be encouraged by this interaction.

RELATED DRUGS: Rifabutin reduces the concentrations of other protease inhibitors, including ritonavir (*Norvir*), indinavir (*Crixivan*), and probably nelfinavir (*Viracept*). Rifampin (eg, *Rifadin*) also reduces saquinavir serum concentrations.

MANAGEMENT OPTIONS:

➠ *Circumvent/Minimize.* The dose of saquinavir may require a substantial increase to produce therapeutic serum concentrations. If possible, monitor saquinavir serum concentrations when dosage adjustments are attempted.

➠ *Monitor.* Watch for loss of saquinavir efficacy during rifabutin coadministration.

REFERENCES:

1. *Invirase* [package insert]. Nutley, NJ: Roche Pharmaceuticals; 1995.

5 | Rifabutin (*Mycobutin*)

Theophylline (eg, *Uniphyl*)

SUMMARY: Rifabutin does not significantly alter theophylline plasma concentrations.

RISK FACTORS: No specific risk factors are known.

MECHANISM: No interaction.

CLINICAL EVALUATION: Eleven healthy subjects received a single, oral dose of theophylline 5 mg/kg before and following 15 days of rifabutin 300 mg/day.[1] Theophylline area under the concentration-time curve was reduced by a mean of 5% following rifabutin. No change in theophylline half-life occurred. No significant change in patient response would be expected.

RELATED DRUGS: Rifampin (eg, *Rifadin*) is known to increase the metabolism of theophylline.

MANAGEMENT OPTIONS: No interaction.

REFERENCES:

1. Gillum JG, et al. Induction of theophylline clearance by rifampin and rifabutin in healthy male volunteers. *Antimicrob Agents Chemother.* 1996;40(8):1866-1869.

Rifabutin (*Mycobutin*)

Tipranavir (*Aptivus*)

SUMMARY: Tipranavir/ritonavir combinations may markedly increase rifabutin plasma concentrations; toxicity is likely to occur in some patients.

RISK FACTORS: No specific risk factors are known.

MECHANISM: It is possible that the combination of tipranavir and ritonavir inhibited the CYP3A4 metabolism of rifabutin.

CLINICAL EVALUATION: While specific data are limited, the manufacturer of tipranavir notes that the mean area under the plasma concentration-time curve following a single dose of rifabutin 150 mg administered alone, or after 10 days of tipranavir 500 mg and ritonavir 200 mg twice daily, was increased by nearly 3-fold.[1] This degree of increase in rifabutin plasma concentrations could increase the risk of developing adverse reactions. The single dose of rifabutin did not affect the plasma concentrations of tipranavir. It is possible that multiple doses of rifabutin could exert an effect on tipranavir.

RELATED DRUGS: Other protease inhibitors that inhibit CYP3A4, such as indinavir (*Crixivan*) and saquinavir (*Invirase*), produce a similar increase in rifabutin plasma concentrations.

MANAGEMENT OPTIONS:

➥ **Monitor.** Carefully monitor patients administered rifabutin and tipranavir/ritonavir for signs of rifabutin toxicity such as uveitis and hepatic or hematologic toxicity.

REFERENCES:
1. *Aptivus* [package insert]. Ridgefield, CT: Boehringer Ingelheim Pharmaceuticals, Inc; 2007.

Rifabutin (*Mycobutin*)

Voriconazole (*Vfend*)

SUMMARY: Rifabutin reduces the plasma concentration of voriconazole; a loss of antifungal activity may result. Voriconazole increases the concentration of rifabutin; watch for evidence of rifabutin toxicity.

RISK FACTORS:

➥ **Pharmacogenetics.** Patients who are poor metabolizers for CYP2C19 will have higher voriconazole concentrations, and, therefore, are likely to have an interaction of larger magnitude.

MECHANISM: Rifabutin increases the activity of CYP3A4 and perhaps other enzymes responsible for voriconazole metabolism. Voriconazole inhibits the activity of CYP3A4, the enzyme that metabolizes rifabutin.

CLINICAL EVALUATION: Based on limited information, rifabutin 300 mg/day for 23 days decreased the mean area under the concentration-time curve (AUC) and peak concentration of voriconazole (200 mg every 12 hours for 14 days) 79% and 67%, respectively.[1] The study was done in healthy subjects. The reduction in voriconazole concentrations during rifabutin coadministration is likely to result in a loss of antifungal activity. When the dosage of voriconazole was increased to 350 mg every 12 hours for 7 days, the coadministration of rifabutin (300 mg/day) produced a 32% and 4% reduction in voriconazole AUC and peak plasma concentration, respectively. In a second study, voriconazole 400 mg every 12 hours was administered with rifabutin 300 mg every 12 hours for 14 days.[1] Compared with rifabutin alone, coadministration of voriconazole increased the mean rifabutin AUC and peak concentration by 4- and 3-fold, respectively. It is unknown how much effect smaller doses of voriconazole would have on rifabutin concentrations because of the 2-way interaction.

RELATED DRUGS: Rifampin (eg, *Rifadin*) is known to be an inducer of CYP-450 enzymes and also reduces the plasma concentration of voriconazole. Rifabutin may also reduce the concentrations of ketoconazole (eg, *Nizoral*), fluconazole (eg, *Diflucan*), and itraconazole (eg, *Sporanox*) in a similar manner.

MANAGEMENT OPTIONS:

➡ *Circumvent/Minimize.* The dose of voriconazole may need to be increased substantially when rifabutin is coadministered. Rifabutin doses may need to be reduced during voriconazole coadministration.

➡ *Monitor.* It will be difficult to predict the outcome of this drug combination. Careful monitoring for decreased voriconazole efficacy and rifabutin toxicity (eg, uveitis, bone marrow depression) is necessary if voriconazole and rifabutin are coadministered.

REFERENCES:
1. *Vfend* [package insert]. New York, NY: Pfizer, Inc; 2002.

 Rifabutin (*Mycobutin*)

Zidovudine (*Retrovir*)

SUMMARY: Rifabutin does not appear to significantly alter zidovudine serum concentrations.

RISK FACTORS: No specific risk factors are known.

MECHANISM: Not established.

CLINICAL EVALUATION: A population pharmacokinetic study was conducted on 128 patients enrolled in phase 3 studies.[1] The apparent clearance of zidovudine in patients taking it alone was compared with its clearance in patients concomitantly taking rifabutin. No significant increase in zidovudine clearance was noted between the 2 patient groups. Further details of the study were not provided. The clinical significance of this interaction is unknown. A prospective trial is needed to evaluate this potential interaction.

RELATED DRUGS: Rifampin (eg, *Rifadin*) is known to induce the metabolism of zidovudine.

MANAGEMENT OPTIONS: No specific action is required, but be alert for evidence of the interaction.

REFERENCES:
1. Narang PK, et al. Population based assessment of rifabutin effect on zidovudine disposition in AIDS patients. *Clin Pharmacol Ther.* 1993;53:219.

Rifampin (eg, *Rifadin*)

Ritonavir (*Norvir*)

SUMMARY: Rifampin appears to reduce ritonavir plasma concentrations; loss of antiviral efficacy may result.

RISK FACTORS: No specific risk factors are known.

MECHANISM: Rifampin is known to induce CYP3A4, an enzyme responsible for the metabolism of ritonavir.

CLINICAL EVALUATION: While no published data are available for evaluation, the manufacturer of ritonavir has made available some data on this interaction. In a study of 7 patients taking rifampin 300 or 600 mg/day for 10 days with ritonavir 500 mg/day for 20 days, the area under the concentration-time curve of ritonavir was 35% lower compared with 9 controls receiving only ritonavir.[1] The peak ritonavir plasma concentration was reduced 25% in the combination therapy group. A reduction in the efficacy of ritonavir may occur in some patients, and reduced concentrations of ritonavir may lead to the emergence of resistant organisms. However, because a metabolite of ritonavir has antiviral activity, the clinical significance of this interaction may be diminished.

RELATED DRUGS: Rifabutin (*Mycobutin*) also may reduce the concentrations of ritonavir. Other protease inhibitors such as indinavir (*Crixivan*), saquinavir (eg, *Invirase*), and nelfinavir (*Viracept*) may be affected by rifampin in a similar manner.

MANAGEMENT OPTIONS:

➡ *Circumvent/Minimize.* Pending further clinical data, consider increasing the dosage of ritonavir during coadministration of rifampin.

➡ *Monitor.* Monitor for reduced ritonavir efficacy.

REFERENCES:
1. *Norvir* [package insert]. Abbott Park, IL: Abbott Laboratories; 1996.

Rifampin (eg, *Rifadin*)

Ropivacaine (*Naropin*)

SUMMARY: Rifampin increased the metabolism of ropivacaine; a reduction in anesthetic effect may occur in some patients.

RISK FACTORS: No specific risk factors are known.

MECHANISM: Rifampin induction of CYP3A4 and CYP1A2, enzymes known to metabolize ropivacaine, increased the plasma clearance of ropivacaine.

CLINICAL EVALUATION: Eighteen subjects were administered rifampin 600 mg/day or placebo for 5 days.[1] On the sixth day, ropivacaine was administered IV as a single dose of 0.6 mg/kg. Compared with placebo, rifampin pretreatment reduced the mean area under the concentration-time curve of ropivacaine 52% and 38% in the nonsmokers and smokers, respectively. Ropivacaine clearance was increased 93% and 47% in nonsmokers and smokers, respectively. The half-life of ropivacaine was reduced in smokers and nonsmokers. The reduced effect of rifampin in smokers is probably caused by the partial induction of ropivacaine metabolism caused by smoking. In most patients requiring ropivacaine for local anesthesia, little change in efficacy will be likely to occur.

RELATED DRUGS: While no data are available, rifabutin (*Mycobutin*) also may increase the metabolism of ropivacaine.

MANAGEMENT OPTIONS:

➡ *Monitor.* Monitor patients taking rifampin for a potential reduction in anesthetic effect if ropivacaine is used for local anesthesia.

REFERENCES:

1. Jokinen MJ, et al. Effect of rifampin and tobacco smoking on the pharmacokinetics of ropivacaine. *Clin Pharmacol Ther.* 2001;70:344-350.

Rifampin (eg, *Rifadin*)

Rosiglitazone (*Avandia*)

SUMMARY: Rifampin reduces the plasma concentration of rosiglitazone; reduction of hypoglycemic effect may occur.

RISK FACTORS: No specific risk factors are known.

MECHANISM: Rifampin induces the metabolism of rosiglitazone via CYP2C8 and perhaps CYP2C9.

CLINICAL EVALUATION: Ten healthy subjects received a single 8 mg dose of rosiglitazone following 6 days of rifampin 600 mg once daily or placebo.[1] The administration of rifampin reduced the mean area under the concentration-time curve of rosiglitazone 65%. The half-life of rosiglitazone was reduced from 3.9 hours to 1.5 hours, and the mean oral clearance of rosiglitazone increased 3-fold (range, 2.4- to 4.6-fold). The effect of rosiglitazone on blood glucose was not determined in this study. However, this degree of reduction in rosiglitazone concentration would be expected to reduce its hypoglycemic efficacy.

RELATED DRUGS: Rifabutin (*Mycobutin*) is likely to produce a similar increase in the metabolism of rosiglitazone. Because of the broad cytochrome P450 induction attributed to rifampin, expect all oral hypoglycemic agents, except metformin (eg, *Glucophage*), which is renally eliminated, to have increased metabolism during rifampin administration.

MANAGEMENT OPTIONS:

➡ *Monitor.* Monitor patients stabilized on rosiglitazone for altered blood glucose levels if concurrent rifampin is initiated or discontinued.

REFERENCES:

1. Park JY, et al. Effect of rifampin on the pharmacokinetics of rosiglitazone in healthy subjects. *Clin Pharmacol Ther.* 2004;75:157-162.

Rifampin (eg, *Rifadin*)

Saquinavir (*Invirase*)

SUMMARY: Rifampin markedly reduces the serum concentration of saquinavir; loss of efficacy or development of resistant organisms may result.

RISK FACTORS: No specific risk factors are known.

MECHANISM: Rifampin is known to induce CYP3A4, the enzyme responsible for the metabolism of saquinavir.

CLINICAL EVALUATION: While no published data are available for evaluation, the manufacturer of saquinavir has made available some data on this interaction. The administration of saquinavir 600 mg 3 times/day with rifampin 600 mg/day to 12 subjects reduced the area under the concentration-time curve of saquinavir at steady state by 80%.[1] It is likely that the efficacy of saquinavir will be severely reduced, and the development of resistant strains of HIV may be encouraged by this interaction.

RELATED DRUGS: Rifampin reduces the concentrations of other protease inhibitors, including ritonavir (*Norvir*), indinavir (*Crixivan*), and nelfinavir (*Viracept*). Rifabutin (*Mycobutin*) also reduces saquinavir serum concentrations.

MANAGEMENT OPTIONS:

➡ *Use Alternative.* Based on the magnitude of this interaction, it would be difficult to administer an effective dose of saquinavir. Because other protease inhibitors also are likely to be affected, consider an alternative to rifampin.

REFERENCES:
1. *Invirase* [package insert]. Nutley, NJ: Hoffman-La Roche, Inc; 1995.

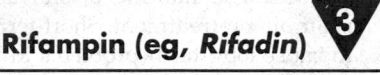

Rifampin (eg, *Rifadin*)
Saxagliptin (*Onglyza*)

SUMMARY: Saxagliptin plasma concentration and hypoglycemic response may be reduced during the coadministration of rifampin; it is possible some patients will require a dose adjustment.

RISK FACTORS: No specific risk factors are known.

MECHANISM: Rifampin may reduce saxagliptin plasma concentrations by the induction of CYP3A4, P-glycoprotein, or both.

CLINICAL EVALUATION: In a study of 14 healthy subjects, a single dose of saxagliptin 5 mg was administered alone and following rifampin 600 mg daily for 6 days.[1] The pretreatment with rifampin produced a 76% decrease in the mean area under the plasma concentration-time curve (AUC) of saxagliptin. The half-life of saxagliptin was reduced from 3 to 1.7 hours following rifampin dosing. The concentration of saxagliptin's active metabolite was unchanged with rifampin pretreatment. This magnitude of change in saxagliptin pharmacokinetics may result in a reduced hypoglycemic response in some patients; however, the effect of saxagliptin on dipeptidyl peptidase-4 (DPP-4) was not significantly altered by rifampin exposure.

RELATED DRUGS: Rifabutin (*Mycobutin*) and rifapentine (*Priftin*) may also reduce the AUC of saxagliptin.

MANAGEMENT OPTIONS:

➡ *Monitor.* Monitor patients stabilized on saxagliptin for changes in their blood glucose levels if rifampin is initiated or discontinued from their drug regimen.

REFERENCES:
1. *Onglyza* [package insert]. Princeton, NJ: Bristol-Meyers Squibb; 2011.

2 Rifampin (eg, *Rifadin*)

Simvastatin (eg, *Zocor*)

SUMMARY: Rifampin produces a profound reduction in simvastatin and simvastatin acid plasma concentrations; therapeutic failure is likely to occur.

RISK FACTORS: No specific risk factors are known.

MECHANISM: Rifampin appears to increase the metabolism of simvastatin and simvastatin acid, most likely by induction of CYP3A4 enzymes. Induction of P-glycoprotein by rifampin also may contribute to the magnitude of this interaction.

CLINICAL EVALUATION: Ten healthy subjects received 5 days of rifampin 600 mg/day or placebo.[1] On the sixth day, a single dose of simvastatin 40 mg was administered. Following rifampin pretreatment, the mean peak concentration (C_{max}) and area under the plasma concentration-time curve (AUC) of simvastatin were reduced 90% and 87%, respectively, compared with placebo. The C_{max} and AUC of simvastatin acid were reduced 90% and 93%, respectively. The effect of rifampin on simvastatin acid AUC was nearly uniform, ranging from 82% to 97% in the 10 subjects. The half-life of simvastatin and simvastatin acid were unchanged by rifampin pretreatment. Short-term (less than 2 weeks) rifampin therapy is unlikely to cause long-term problems in patients taking simvastatin, but long-term rifampin therapy would likely eliminate the efficacy of simvastatin.

RELATED DRUGS: Lovastatin (eg, *Mevacor*), because of its similar metabolism to simvastatin, is expected to display a similar interaction with rifampin. Other statins that are metabolized by CYP3A4 or CYP2C9 (eg, atorvastatin [*Lipitor*], fluvastatin [*Lescol*]) are likely to be affected by rifampin, but perhaps to a lesser extent. Because pravastatin (eg, *Pravachol*) is not a CYP3A4 substrate, rifampin may have limited effect on its pharmacokinetics. Rifabutin (*Mycobutin*) also is known to induce CYP3A4 and is expected to reduce simvastatin concentrations, although perhaps to a lesser extent.

MANAGEMENT OPTIONS:

➥ *Use Alternative.* For patients taking rifampin, select cholesterol-lowering drugs that are not dependent on CYP3A4 or CYP2C9 for their metabolism.

➥ *Monitor.* Monitor serum cholesterol in patients taking statins when rifampin is administered for more than a few weeks.

REFERENCES:

1. Kyrklund C, et al. Rifampin greatly reduces plasma simvastatin and simvastatin acid concentrations. *Clin Pharmacol Ther.* 2000;68(6):592-597.

 Rifampin (eg, *Rifadin*)

Sulfasalazine (eg, *Azulfidine*)

SUMMARY: Rifampin appears to reduce the serum concentrations of sulfapyridine in patients taking sulfasalazine.

RISK FACTORS: No specific risk factors are known.

MECHANISM: Sulfasalazine is converted by bacteria in the large bowel to sulfapyridine and aminosalicylic acid. Rifampin either increases the metabolism of sulfapyridine or reduces the bacterial conversion of sulfasalazine to sulfapyridine and aminosalicylic acid.

CLINICAL EVALUATION: Eleven patients with Crohn disease who were taking sulfasalazine 2 to 4 g/day were given either rifampin 10 mg/kg/day combined with ethambutol 15 mg/kg/day or placebo for 1 year.[1] Rifampin reduced the sulfapyridine concentrations nearly 60% in 10 of the 11 patients. The clinical significance of this reduction was not reported. The role of ethambutol in this report is unknown.

RELATED DRUGS: No information is available.

MANAGEMENT OPTIONS: No specific action is required, but be alert for evidence of the interaction.

REFERENCES:

1. Shaffer JL, Houston JB. The effect of rifampicin on sulfapyridine plasma concentrations following sulphasalazine administration. *Br J Clin Pharmacol.* 1985;19(4):526-528.

Rifampin (eg, *Rifadin*)

Sunitinib (*Sutent*)

SUMMARY: Rifampin administration can reduce sunitinib plasma concentrations; some loss of antitumor efficacy may occur.

RISK FACTORS: No specific risk factors are known.

MECHANISM: Rifampin is an inducer of CYP3A4, the enzyme primarily responsible for sunitinib metabolism.

CLINICAL EVALUATION: While specific data are limited, coadministration of rifampin (dose not reported) prior to a single dose of sunitinib (dose not reported) decreased the mean area under the plasma concentration-time curve of sunitinib and its active metabolite by 46%.[1] Pending further data, observe patients receiving sunitinib and rifampin for reduced sunitinib efficacy. Patients taking rifampin, or other inducers of CYP3A4, may require an increase in their sunitinib dose.

RELATED DRUGS: Rifabutin (*Mycobutin*) may also increase the metabolism of sunitinib.

MANAGEMENT OPTIONS:

➡ **Monitor.** Carefully monitor patients receiving sunitinib and rifampin for the expected response to sunitinib. Dose adjustment of sunitinib may be required.

REFERENCES:

1. *Sutent* [package insert]. New York, NY: Pfizer; 2006.

Rifampin (eg, *Rifadin*)

Tacrolimus (*Prograf*)

SUMMARY: Rifampin sufficiently decreased tacrolimus plasma concentrations to reduce the immunosuppressive efficacy of tacrolimus.

RISK FACTORS: No specific risk factors are known.

MECHANISM: Rifampin appears to induce CYP3A4 or P-glycoprotein activity, which may increase the metabolism of tacrolimus.

CLINICAL EVALUATION: Six healthy subjects received a single dose of tacrolimus 0.1 mg/kg orally or 0.025 mg/kg intravenously alone and after 7 to 14 days of rifampin 600 mg/day.[1] The clearance of tacrolimus increased 46% (range, 6.4% to 203%), and its bioavailability was reduced from 14.4% to 7% following rifampin pretreatment. Much of the reduction in the bioavailability was caused by increased presystemic metabolism in the small intestine. This study is consistent with a case report that noted a reduction of tacrolimus concentration following rifampin administration.[2] The magnitude of this interaction is likely to reduce the immunosuppressant effect of tacrolimus.

RELATED DRUGS: Rifampin is known to increase the metabolism of cyclosporine (eg, *Neoral*). Sirolimus (*Rapamune*) may be affected in a similar manner. Rifabutin (*Mycobutin*) would probably reduce the concentration of tacrolimus.

MANAGEMENT OPTIONS:

➡ *Monitor.* If rifampin is started or stopped, monitor patients taking tacrolimus for altered tacrolimus concentrations.

REFERENCES:

1. Hebert MF, et al. Effects of rifampin on tacrolimus pharmacokinetics in healthy volunteers. *J Clin Pharmacol.* 1999;39(1):91-96.

2. Furlan V, et al. Interactions between FK506 and rifampicin or erythromycin in pediatric liver recipients. *Transplantation.* 1995;59(8):1217-1218.

Rifampin (eg, *Rifadin*)

Tadalafil (*Cialis*)

SUMMARY: Rifampin reduces the plasma concentrations of tadalafil; reduced tadalafil efficacy may result.

RISK FACTORS: No specific risk factors are known.

MECHANISM: Rifampin is known to induce CYP3A4, the primary enzyme pathway for tadalafil metabolism.

CLINICAL EVALUATION: While specific data are limited, coadministration of rifampin 600 mg daily prior to a single dose of tadalafil 10 mg decreased the mean area under the plasma concentration time-curve of tadalafil by about 88%.[1] Pending further data, observe patients receiving tadalafil and rifampin for increased tadalafil effect.

RELATED DRUGS: Rifabutin (*Mycobutin*) and rifapentine (*Priftin*) are likely to reduce tadalafil plasma concentrations. Sildenafil (eg, *Viagra*) and vardenafil (*Levitra*) are likely to be affected in a similar manner by rifampin.

MANAGEMENT OPTIONS:

➡ *Monitor.* Observe patients taking tadalafil for reduced effect if rifampin is being coadministered.

REFERENCES:

1. *Cialis* [package insert]. Indianapolis, IN: Eli Lilly and Company; 2003.

Rifampin (eg, *Rifadin*)

Tamoxifen

SUMMARY: Rifampin administration markedly reduces tamoxifen plasma concentrations; loss of tamoxifen's antiestrogenic effect is likely.

RISK FACTORS: No specific risk factors are known.

MECHANISM: Rifampin is known to induce the activity of CYP3A4, the isozyme that metabolizes tamoxifen. Rifampin appears to increase the first-pass and systemic clearance of tamoxifen.

CLINICAL EVALUATION: Ten healthy subjects took either rifampin 600 mg or placebo daily for 5 days.[1] On day 6, a single oral dose of tamoxifen 80 mg was administered 17 hours after the last rifampin dose. The administration of rifampin reduced the area under the plasma concentration-time curve (AUC) of tamoxifen 86% and its peak concentration 55%. The half-life of tamoxifen was reduced from 118 to 68 hours following rifampin dosing. Rifampin increased the metabolism of toremifene (*Fareston*), a derivative of tamoxifen, by a similar amount (87% reduction in AUC). The effect of long-term rifampin therapy on tamoxifen is unknown, but the magnitude of the interaction may be greater than that observed in this study.

RELATED DRUGS: Rifabutin (*Mycobutin*) is likely to affect tamoxifen and toremifene metabolism similarly.

MANAGEMENT OPTIONS:

➡ *Monitor.* Monitor patients taking tamoxifen for loss of efficacy if rifampin is coadministered. The dosage of tamoxifen may need to be increased.

REFERENCES:

1. Kivistö KT, et al. Tamoxifen and toremifene concentrations in plasma are greatly decreased by rifampin. *Clin Pharmacol Ther.* 1998;64(6):648-654.

Rifampin (eg, *Rifadin*)

Tamsulosin (eg, *Flomax*)

SUMMARY: Theoretically, tamsulosin's effect may be reduced by rifampin and other CYP3A4 inducers, but the clinical importance has not been established.

RISK FACTORS: No specific risk factors are known.

MECHANISM: Tamsulosin is metabolized by CYP3A4 and rifampin is a CYP3A4 inducer; theoretically, rifampin increases tamsulosin metabolism.

CLINICAL EVALUATION: Although the interaction is based on theoretical considerations, caution is recommended when tamsulosin is taken with drugs that may affect tamsulosin metabolism.[1]

RELATED DRUGS: Rifabutin and rifapentine also induce enzymes and may increase tamsulosin metabolism.

MANAGEMENT OPTIONS: No specific action is required, but be alert for evidence of the interaction.

REFERENCES:

1. *Flomax* [package insert]. Ridgefield, CT: Boehringer Ingelheim; 2009.

 Rifampin (eg, *Rifadin*)

Telaprevir (*Incivek*)

SUMMARY: The coadministration of rifampin decreases the plasma concentration of telaprevir; loss of antiviral efficacy is likely to occur.

RISK FACTORS: No specific risk factors are known.

MECHANISM: Rifampin induces the CYP3A4-mediated metabolism and P-glycoprotein elimination of telaprevir, resulting in reduced telaprevir plasma concentrations.

CLINICAL EVALUATION: While specific data are limited, the manufacturer of telaprevir notes that the coadministration of rifampin 600 mg daily for 8 days reduced the mean area under the plasma concentration-time curve of a single dose of telaprevir 750 mg by approximately 90%.[1] This large reduction in the concentration of telaprevir is expected to eliminate the antiviral activity of telaprevir.

RELATED DRUGS: Rifabutin (*Mycobutin*) and rifapentine (*Priftin*) are known to induce CYP3A4 and are likely to reduce the plasma concentration of telaprevir. Other protease inhibitors that are metabolized by CYP3A4 (eg, atazanavir [*Reyataz*], indinavir [*Crixivan*], nelfinavir [*Viracept*], ritonavir [*Norvir*], saquinavir [*Invirase*]) are likely to interact in a similar manner with telaprevir.

MANAGEMENT OPTIONS:

➠ *Avoid Unless Benefit Outweighs Risk.* The coadministration of rifampin and telaprevir should generally be avoided.

➠ *Monitor.* Carefully monitor patients stabilized on telaprevir for loss of efficacy if rifampin is coadministered. Consider measuring telaprevir plasma concentrations during concurrent rifampin treatment.

REFERENCES:

1. *Incivek* [package insert]. Cambridge, MA: Vertex Pharmaceuticals Inc; 2011.

 Rifampin (eg, *Rifadin*)

Theophylline (eg, *Theochron*)

SUMMARY: Rifampin lowers the plasma concentration of theophylline; a reduction of theophylline efficacy may result.

RISK FACTORS: No specific risk factors are known.

MECHANISM: Rifampin increases the metabolic clearance of theophylline.

CLINICAL EVALUATION: In 4 studies involving healthy subjects, rifampin 600 mg/day for 6 to 14 days increased the plasma theophylline clearance 25%.[1-4] In a 15-month-old patient, theophylline half-life fell from 3.7 to 1.9 hours 3 days after rifampin 20 mg/kg/day was started.[5] Symptoms of wheezing worsened during rifampin administration, resulting in a theophylline dosage increase of 26%.

RELATED DRUGS: No information is available.

MANAGEMENT OPTIONS:

➡ *Monitor.* Be alert for the need to adjust the theophylline dose when rifampin therapy is started or stopped. The theophylline dose requirement may be higher in patients receiving rifampin.

REFERENCES:

1. Robson RA, et al. Theophylline-rifampicin interaction: non-selective induction of theophylline metabolic pathways. *Br J Clin Pharmacol.* 1984;18(3):445-448.
2. Hauser AR, et al. The effect of rifampin on theophylline disposition. *Clin Pharmacol Ther.* 1983;33(2):254.
3. Straughn AB, et al. Effect of rifampin on theophylline disposition. *Ther Drug Monit.* 1984;6(2):153-156.
4. Boyce EG, et al. The effect of rifampin on theophylline kinetics. *J Clin Pharmacol.* 1986;26(8):696-699.
5. Brocks DR, et al. Theophylline-rifampin interaction in a pediatric patient. *Clin Pharm.* 1986;5(7):602-604.

Rifampin (eg, *Rifadin*)
Ticagrelor (*Brilinta*)

SUMMARY: Rifampin decreases the plasma concentration of ticagrelor and reduces the concentration of its active metabolite; the net effect is likely to be decreased antiplatelet activity.

RISK FACTORS: No specific risk factors are known.

MECHANISM: Rifampin induces the activity of CYP3A4, the primary enzyme responsible for the metabolism of ticagrelor.

CLINICAL EVALUATION: While specific data are limited, the manufacturer of ticagrelor notes that the coadministration of rifampin 600 mg once daily decreased the mean area under the plasma concentration-time curve (AUC) of ticagrelor.[1] The AUC of ticagrelor's active metabolite was also reduced during rifampin coadministration. Pending further data, observe patients receiving ticagrelor and rifampin for decreased ticagrelor effects.

RELATED DRUGS: Rifabutin (*Mycobutin*) and rifapentine (*Priftin*) are known to induce CYP3A4 and are likely to affect ticagrelor in a similar manner. Rifampin has been noted to cause a modest reduction in the antiplatelet activity of prasugrel (*Effient*)[2] but may increase the activity of clopidogrel (*Plavix*).[3]

MANAGEMENT OPTIONS:

➡ *Monitor.* Monitor patients stabilized on ticagrelor for altered antiplatelet effects if rifampin is initiated or discontinued.

REFERENCES:

1. *Brilinta* [package insert]. Wilmington, DE: AstraZeneca LP; 2011.
2. Farid NA, et al. Effect of rifampin on the pharmacokinetics and pharmacodynamics of prasugrel in healthy male subjects. *Curr Med Res Opin.* 2009;25(8):1821-1829.
3. Lau WC, et al. Atorvastatin reduces the ability of clopidogrel to inhibit platelet aggregation: a new drug-drug interaction. *Circulation.* 2003;107(1):32-37.

Rifampin (eg, *Rifadin*)

Tocainide†

SUMMARY: Rifampin administration to healthy subjects reduces tocainide serum concentrations considerably. A loss of efficacy resulting from diminished tocainide concentrations may occur.

RISK FACTORS: No specific risk factors are known.

MECHANISM: Rifampin appears to enhance the hepatic metabolism of tocainide, thereby increasing its clearance and reducing its half-life.

CLINICAL EVALUATION: An oral dose of tocainide 600 mg was given alone and following 5 days of pretreatment with rifampin 300 mg every 12 hours to 8 healthy subjects.[1] Pretreatment with rifampin resulted in a significant reduction in the half-life and area under the serum concentration-time curve (both approximately 50%) and a 30% increase in the clearance. No significant changes in tocainide renal clearance or volume of distribution were noted. Tocainide is available in the racemic form; the R-tocainide isomer has a half-life of approximately 10 hours, while that of the S-tocainide isomer is 16 hours.[2,3] The effects of rifampin on the metabolism of tocainide isomers and tocainide's pharmacodynamic parameters were not measured.

RELATED DRUGS: No information is available.

MANAGEMENT OPTIONS:

➡ *Monitor.* Monitor patients stabilized on tocainide for decreased response and serum concentrations if rifampin is started. Discontinuing concomitant rifampin therapy could result in an increased tocainide concentration and effect.

REFERENCES:

1. Rice TL, et al. Influence of rifampin on tocainide pharmacokinetics in humans. *Clin Pharm.* 1989;8(3):200-205.
2. Edgar B, et al. The pharmacokinetics of R- and S-tocainide in healthy subjects. *Br J Clin Pharmacol.* 1984;17:216P.
3. Hoffmann KJ, et al. Stereoselective disposition of RS-tocainide in man. *Eur J Drug Metab Pharmacokinet.* 1984;9(3):215-222.

† Not available in the United States.

Rifampin (eg, *Rifadin*)

Tolbutamide (eg, *Orinase*)

SUMMARY: Rifampin reduces tolbutamide and glyburide serum concentrations and may reduce hypoglycemic activity.

RISK FACTORS: No specific risk factors are known.

MECHANISM: Rifampin appears to stimulate the hepatic metabolism of tolbutamide and glyburide.

CLINICAL EVALUATION: Rifampin enhances the clearance of tolbutamide after oral administration in patients and healthy volunteers.[1-3] The magnitude of the decreases in tolbutamide half-life caused by the concurrent use of rifampin indicates that it may impair the hypoglycemic response to tolbutamide.

RELATED DRUGS: A 67-year-old patient taking rifampin 600 mg/day and glyburide (eg, *DiaBeta*) 15 mg/day had glyburide concentrations between 30 and 40 ng/mL.[4] After cessation of the rifampin therapy, the glyburide concentrations increased more than 160 ng/mL. Blood glucose concentrations did not appear to be altered by the change in glyburide concentrations. Little is known concerning the effect of rifampin on other oral antidiabetic drugs, but their metabolism also might be enhanced by rifampin. Rifabutin (*Mycobutin*) might affect tolbutamide in a similar manner.

MANAGEMENT OPTIONS:

➡ *Monitor.* When rifampin is coadministered with tolbutamide or glyburide and possibly other sulfonylureas, be alert for the potential for diminished hypoglycemic activity. Discontinuation of rifampin could result in hypoglycemia.

REFERENCES:

1. Zilly W, et al. Induction of drug metabolism in man after rifampicin treatment measured by increased hexobarbital and tolbutamide clearance. *Eur J Clin Pharmacol.* 1975;9(2-3):219-227.

2. Syvälahti E, et al. Effect of tuberculostatic agents on the response of serum growth hormone and immunoreactive insulin to intravenous tolbutamide, and on the half-life of tolbutamide. *Int J Clin Pharmacol Biopharm.* 1976;13(2):83-89.

3. Zilly W, et al. Stimulation of drug metabolism by rifampicin in patients with cirrhosis or cholestasis measured by increased hexobarbital and tolbutamide clearance. *Eur J Clin Pharmacol.* 1977;11(4):287-293.

4. Self TH, et al. Interaction of rifampin and glyburide. *Chest.* 1989;96(6):1443-1444.

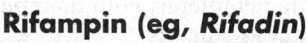

Rifampin (eg, *Rifadin*)

Tolvaptan (*Samsca*)

SUMMARY: Rifampin administration has been noted to markedly reduce the plasma concentration of tolvaptan.

RISK FACTORS: No specific risk factors are known.

MECHANISM: Rifampin induces CYP3A4, the primary enzyme that metabolizes tolvaptan. Rifampin induction of P-glycoprotein may also contribute to the decreased tolvaptan concentrations.

CLINICAL EVALUATION: While specific data are limited, the manufacturer of tolvaptan notes that the coadministration of rifampin (dose not stated) with tolvaptan decreased the exposure to tolvaptan approximately 85%.[1] Pending further data, observe patients receiving tolvaptan and rifampin for loss of tolvaptan efficacy. Tolvaptan doses will likely need to be increased if coadministered with rifampin.

RELATED DRUGS: Rifabutin (*Mycobutin*) and rifapentine (*Priftin*) are known to induce CYP3A4 and would likely affect tolvaptan in a similar manner.

MANAGEMENT OPTIONS:

➡ *Monitor.* Monitor patients stabilized on tolvaptan for altered response if rifampin is added or discontinued.

REFERENCES:

1. *Samsca* [package insert]. Rockville, MD: Otsuka America Pharmaceutical, Inc; 2009.

Rifampin (eg, *Rifadin*)

Triazolam (eg, *Halcion*)

SUMMARY: Rifampin markedly reduces the plasma concentrations of triazolam; loss of triazolam effect is likely to occur during coadministration.

RISK FACTORS: No specific risk factors are known.

MECHANISM: Rifampin induces CYP3A4, the enzyme responsible for the metabolism of triazolam. This results in a reduction in the bioavailability of triazolam and an increase in its systemic clearance.

CLINICAL EVALUATION: Ten healthy subjects received placebo or rifampin 600 mg/day for 5 days.[1] On day 6, each subject was administered a single oral dose of triazolam 0.5 mg approximately 17 hours after the last rifampin dose. Following rifampin administration, the mean triazolam area under the concentration-time curve was reduced 95% compared with placebo. Mean peak triazolam concentrations fell from 2.9 to 0.36 ng/mL, and the half-life of triazolam was reduced from 2.8 to 1.3 hours. The effects of triazolam on psychomotor tests were abolished by pre-treatment with rifampin.

RELATED DRUGS: Rifabutin (*Mycobutin*) is likely to produce a similar effect on triazolam pharmacokinetics. Rifampin is known to increase the elimination of other benzo-diazepines, including midazolam and diazepam (eg, *Valium*). Benzodiazepines that do not interact with rifampin include temazepam (eg, *Restoril*) and oxazepam.

MANAGEMENT OPTIONS:

➡ *Consider Alternative.* Select a benzodiazepine that does not interact with rifampin when possible to avoid the interaction (see Related Drugs).

➡ *Monitor.* Monitor patients receiving rifampin for reduced triazolam efficacy. If rifampin is discontinued in a patient receiving both agents, the dose of triazolam may require reduction during the 1 to 2 weeks to avoid excess sedation.

REFERENCES:
1. Villikka K, et al. Triazolam is ineffective in patients taking rifampin. *Clin Pharmacol Ther*. 1997;61(1):8-14.

Rifampin (eg, *Rifadin*)

Trimethoprim/Sulfamethoxazole (eg, *Bactrim*)

SUMMARY: Rifampin reduces trimethoprim-sulfamethoxazole (TMP-SMZ) plasma concentrations; a reduction in antimicrobial efficacy is possible. TMP-SMZ modestly increases the concentration of rifampin.

RISK FACTORS: No specific risk factors are known.

MECHANISM: Rifampin appears to induce the metabolism of TMP and SMZ, by induction of CYP2C9, CYP3A4, and perhaps other elimination pathways.

CLINICAL EVALUATION: Ten HIV-positive patients receiving TMP-SMZ (TMP 160 mg and SMZ 800 mg daily) for pneumocystis prophylaxis were treated for tuberculosis with rifampin 600 mg/day, isoniazid 300 mg/day, pyrazinamide 30 mg/kg/day, and ethambutol 25 mg/kg/day.[1] Serum concentrations of TMP and SMZ were measured prior to and after at least 12 days of antituberculosis treatment. Following rifampin coadministration, the mean TMP area under the concentration-time curve (AUC) was reduced 47% and SMZ AUC was reduced 23%. It is unknown if this degree of reduction in TMP-SMZ concentration will reduce its efficacy; however, rifampin has been reported to reduce the efficacy of TMP-SMZ in the prevention of toxoplasmic encephalitis.[2] The effect of TMP-SMZ on rifampin pharmacokinetics has also been studied. The coadministration of TMP-SMZ (TMP 320 mg, SMZ 800 mg) for 5 to 10 days to 15 patients taking rifampin increased the mean AUC of rifampin 60% and the mean peak rifampin concentration 31%.[3] None of the patients developed evidence of rifampin toxicity.

RELATED DRUGS: Rifabutin (*Mycobutin*) may affect TMP-SMZ in a similar manner, although the magnitude of effect is likely to be less.

MANAGEMENT OPTIONS:

➡ *Monitor.* Patients taking TMP-SMZ who are coadministered rifampin may be at risk for loss of efficacy. If possible, monitor TMP-SMZ concentrations and administer larger doses if necessary.

REFERENCES:

1. Ribera E, et al. Rifampin reduces concentrations of trimethoprim and sulfamethoxazole in serum in human immunodeficiency virus-infected patients. *Antimicrob Agents Chemother.* 2001;45(11):3238-3241.

2. Ribera E, et al. Comparison of high and low doses of trimethoprim-sulfamethoxazole for primary prevention of toxoplasmic encephalitis in human immunodeficiency virus-infected patients. *Clin Infect Dis.* 1999;29(6):1461-1466.

3. Bhatia RS, et al. Drug interaction between rifampicin and cotrimoxazole in patients with tuberculosis. *Hum Exp Toxicol.* 1991;10(6):419-421.

Rifampin (eg, *Rifadin*)

Verapamil (eg, *Calan*)

SUMMARY: Rifampin decreases verapamil plasma concentrations; loss of therapeutic effect may result.

RISK FACTORS:

➡ *Route of Administration.* Administration of verapamil orally increases the magnitude of this interaction.

MECHANISM: Rifampin induces the metabolism (CYP3A), reduces the bioavailability, increases the hepatic clearance, and reduces the protein binding of verapamil.

CLINICAL EVALUATION: In 1 report, 3 of 4 patients receiving rifampin had unmeasurable verapamil concentrations following a single 40 mg dose.[1] Other reports have found a large increase in verapamil clearance following the coadministration of rifampin.[2,3,4] The protein binding of verapamil decreased 30% in the presence of rifampin.[5] The magnitude of the reduction in verapamil serum concentration is much larger after oral verapamil compared with IV administration and is likely to result in a reduction of efficacy.

RELATED DRUGS: Rifampin is likely to affect other calcium channel blockers in a similar manner. Rifabutin (*Mycobutin*) might affect verapamil similarly.

MANAGEMENT OPTIONS:

➡ *Consider Alternative.* Because this interaction is likely to reduce the efficacy of verapamil, consider an alternative agent for verapamil. Other calcium channel blockers also may be affected; a therapeutic substitution to a different class of agent may be required.

➡️ *Circumvent/Minimize.* Larger doses of calcium channel blockers (particularly those administered orally) may be required when rifampin is coadministered.

➡️ *Monitor.* Monitor patients taking calcium channel blockers for a reduction in efficacy when rifampin is given.

REFERENCES:

1. Rahn KH, et al. Reduction of bioavailability of verapamil by rifampin. *N Engl J Med.* 1985;312:920-921.
2. Barbarash RA. Verapamil-rifampin interaction. *Drug Intell Clin Pharm.* 1985;19:559-560.
3. Barbarash RA, et al. Near-total reduction in verapamil bioavailability by rifampin. *Chest.* 1988;94:954-959.
4. Mooy J, et al. The influence of antituberculosis drugs on the plasma level of verapamil. *Eur J Clin Pharmacol.* 1987;32:107-109.
5. Pieper JA, et al. Rifampin alters serum albumin concentrations and verapamil protein binding. *Clin Pharmacol Ther.* 1988;43:146.

 Rifampin (eg, *Rifadin*)

Voriconazole (*Vfend*)

SUMMARY: Do not administer rifampin with voriconazole; a loss of antifungal efficacy is likely to result.

RISK FACTORS: No specific risk factors are known.

MECHANISM: Rifampin induces several cytochrome P450 enzymes that are known to metabolize voriconazole including CYP3A4, CYP2C9, and CYP2C19. The result is a marked increase in voriconazole clearance and reduction in its plasma concentration.

CLINICAL EVALUATION: In a study done in healthy subjects, the administration of rifampin 600 mg/day for 23 days reduced the area under the concentration-time curve (AUC) of voriconazole (200 mg twice daily for 14 days) by an average of 96%.[1] When the dose of voriconazole was increased to 400 mg every 12 hours for 7 days, the AUC of voriconazole was reduced an average of 81% by rifampin coadministration. While data are limited, a doubling of the voriconazole dose in the presence of rifampin did not result in adequate antifungal voriconazole plasma concentrations. It is likely that rifampin administration will result in a loss of voriconazole antifungal activity.

RELATED DRUGS: Rifabutin (*Mycobutin*) is known to be an inducer of cytochrome P450 enzymes and also reduces the plasma concentration of voriconazole. Although data are limited, rifampin reduces the concentrations of ketoconazole (eg, *Nizoral*), fluconazole (*Diflucan*), and itraconazole (eg, *Sporanox*) in a similar manner.

MANAGEMENT OPTIONS:

➡️ *Use Alternative.* If possible, avoid coadministration of voriconazole and rifampin. It is likely to be very difficult to obtain adequate antifungal concentrations of voriconazole in patients taking rifampin.

➡️ *Monitor.* If rifampin and voriconazole are coadministered, voriconazole doses may have to be increased several fold. Monitor for lack of antifungal effect.

REFERENCES:

1. Product information. Voriconazole (*Vfend*). Pfizer, Inc. 2002.

Rifampin (eg, *Rifadin*)

Warfarin (eg, *Coumadin*)

SUMMARY: Rifampin reduces the hypoprothrombinemic effect of warfarin and other oral anticoagulants in most patients to a clinically significant extent; anticoagulant dosage adjustments are likely to be necessary during cotherapy with these drugs.

RISK FACTORS: No specific risk factors are known.

MECHANISM: Rifampin stimulates the metabolism of warfarin and other oral anticoagulants.[1] Also, as rifampin decreases fever which enhances the catabolism of clotting factors, the hypoprothrombinemic response could be further reduced.

CLINICAL EVALUATION: In a study of 10 healthy subjects, the elimination of a single dose of warfarin was increased considerably and the hypoprothrombinemic effect was decreased by rifampin.[2] A similar decrease in the hypoprothrombinemic effect of warfarin,[3-5] phenprocoumon,[6] and acenocoumarol (*Sintrom*) has been noted. Dose adjustments of at least 50% or more may be required in some patients. Based upon studies to date, rifampin-induced inhibition of warfarin hypoprothrombinemia is maximal 5 to 10 days after starting rifampin; it probably dissipates over a similar time period when rifampin is discontinued.

RELATED DRUGS: Phenprocoumon and acenocoumarol interact similarly with rifampin.

MANAGEMENT OPTIONS:

➡ ***Avoid Unless Benefit Outweighs Risk.*** Do not coadminister rifampin and oral anticoagulants unless no alternative is available.

➡ ***Monitor.*** If rifampin is administered to patients requiring warfarin, evaluate the patient's anticoagulant response carefully and readjust the anticoagulant dose as needed when rifampin is started, stopped, or changed in dosage.

REFERENCES:

1. Heimark LD, et al. The mechanism of the warfarin-rifampin drug interaction in humans. *Clin Pharmacol Ther.* 1987;42:388-394.
2. O'Reilly RA. Interaction of sodium warfarin and rifampin. Studies in man. *Ann Intern Med.* 1974;81:337-340.
3. O'Reilly RA. Interaction of chronic daily warfarin therapy and rifampin. *Ann Intern Med.* 1975;83:506-508.
4. Self TH, et al. Interaction of rifampin and warfarin. *Chest.* 1975;67:490-491.
5. Romankiewicz JA, et al. Rifampin and warfarin: a drug interaction. *Ann Intern Med.* 1975;82:224-225.
6. Boekhout-Mussert RJ, et al. Inhibition by rifampicin of the anticoagulant effect of phenprocoumon. *JAMA.* 1974;229:1903-1904.

Rifampin (eg, *Rifadin*)

Zaleplon (*Sonata*)

SUMMARY: Rifampin reduced the concentration of zaleplon to the point that loss of efficacy can result.

RISK FACTORS: No specific risk factors are known.

MECHANISM: Rifampin appears to induce the metabolism of zaleplon via CYP3A4.

CLINICAL EVALUATION: While no published data are available, the manufacturer of zaleplon has provided some information regarding the interaction between zaleplon and rifampin. Rifampin 600 mg/day for 14 days reduced the area under the concentration curve of zaleplon 80%. The magnitude of this interaction would be expected to reduce the efficacy of zaleplon.[1]

RELATED DRUGS: Rifabutin (*Mycobutin*) may have a similar effect on zaleplon.

MANAGEMENT OPTIONS:

➡ **Monitor.** Expect patients taking zaleplon and rifampin to demonstrate a reduced response to zaleplon. When rifampin is discontinued in patients receiving zaleplon, monitor for increased zaleplon effects, including sedation.

REFERENCES:

1. Product information. Zaleplon (*Sonata*). Wyeth-Ayerst Laboratories. 1999.

 Rifampin (eg, *Rifadin*)

Zidovudine (eg, *Retrovir*)

SUMMARY: Zidovudine plasma concentrations are reduced by the coadministration of rifampin; loss of efficacy could result.

RISK FACTORS: No specific risk factors are known.

MECHANISM: Rifampin apparently induces the metabolism of zidovudine and may reduce zidovudine's bioavailability by increasing its first-pass elimination.

CLINICAL EVALUATION: The pharmacokinetics of zidovudine in 4 patients also taking rifampin 600 mg/day were compared with data obtained from nearly 70 patients taking zidovudine without rifampin.[1] Each of the 4 patients was taking rifampin as well as a variety of other antibiotics and antifungal agents. Nevertheless, the patients taking rifampin had significantly reduced zidovudine concentrations, and their clearance after oral administration of zidovudine during rifampin averaged about 2.5 times the clearance after oral administration in patients not taking rifampin. Following discontinuation of rifampin in one of the patients, the zidovudine concentration normalized.

RELATED DRUGS: No information is available.

MANAGEMENT OPTIONS:

➡ **Monitor.** Monitor zidovudine plasma concentrations of patients taking zidovudine and watch for a change in zidovudine response if rifampin therapy is added or discontinued. Zidovudine dose adjustments are likely to be necessary.

REFERENCES:

1. Burger DM, et al. Pharmacokinetic interaction between rifampin and zidovudine. *Antimicrob Agents Chemother.* 1993;37(7):1426-1431.

Rifampin (eg, *Rifadin*)
Zolmitriptan (*Zomig*)

SUMMARY: Rifampin administration produces a small reduction in the concentration of zolmitriptan and its active metabolite; changes in clinical response are not likely to occur.

RISK FACTORS: No specific risk factors are known.

MECHANISM: While the metabolic fate of zolmitriptan is not well defined, it would appear that rifampin induction of cytochrome P450 enzymes might be responsible for increased metabolism of zolmitriptan and its N-desmethyl metabolite.

CLINICAL EVALUATION: A single dose of zolmitriptan 5 mg was administered to 14 subjects alone and following 8 days of rifampin 600 mg/day.[1] The area under the concentration-time curve and peak plasma concentration of zolmitriptan were reduced 18% and 15%, respectively, following rifampin administration. The half-life of zolmitriptan was reduced from 2.7 to 2.4 hours. The concentration of an active metabolite of zolmitriptan also was reduced by rifampin administration. These changes in zolmitriptan plasma concentrations are not likely to result in a clinically significant change in patient response to zolmitriptan.

RELATED DRUGS: Rifabutin (*Mycobutin*) does not appear to be as potent an inducer as rifampin and is less likely to produce a reduction in zolmitriptan concentrations.

MANAGEMENT OPTIONS:

➡ ***Monitor.*** Patients taking zolmitriptan for migraine are unlikely to experience a reduced therapeutic response if rifampin is administered. Nevertheless, be alert for reduced zolmitriptan effect.

REFERENCES:
1. Dixon R, et al. The metabolism of zolmitriptan: effects of an inducer and an inhibitor of cytochrome p450 on its pharmacokinetics in healthy volunteers. *Clin Drug Investig.* 1998;15(6):515-522.

Rifampin (eg, *Rifadin*)
Zolpidem (eg, *Ambien*)

SUMMARY: Rifampin reduced the plasma concentration of zolpidem; loss of efficacy may occur in some patients.

RISK FACTORS: No specific risk factors are known.

MECHANISM: Rifampin is an inducer of CYP3A4, the enzyme that appears to metabolize zolpidem.

CLINICAL EVALUATION: Eight healthy subjects received a single dose of zolpidem 20 mg following 5 days of rifampin 600 mg daily or placebo.[1] The mean area under the concentration-time curve of zolpidem was reduced by 73%, while its peak concentration declined nearly 60% following rifampin pretreatment. Zolpidem half-life was reduced from 2.5 to 1.6 hours following rifampin. The reduction in zolpidem plasma concentration was accompanied by a reduced pharmacologic effect as measured by psychomotor testing. The hypnotic effects of zolpidem are likely to be reduced in patients taking rifampin.

LATED DRUGS: Rifabutin (*Mycobutin*) and rifapentine (*Priftin*) are likely to reduce zolpidem plasma concentrations. Other benzodiazepines metabolized by CYP3A4 (eg, alprazolam [eg, *Xanax*], midazolam, triazolam [eg, *Halcion*]) are likely to be affected in a similar manner.

MANAGEMENT OPTIONS:

➥ **Consider Alternative.** Rifampin does not appear to alter the elimination of temazepam (eg, *Restoril*).

➥ **Monitor.** Observe patients receiving rifampin for reduced hypnotic effects when zolpidem is administered.

REFERENCES:

1. Villikka K, et al. Rifampin reduces plasma concentrations and effects of zolpidem. *Clin Pharmacol Ther.* 1997;62(6):629-634.

 Rifampin (eg, *Rifadin*)

Zopiclone

SUMMARY: Rifampin reduced the plasma concentration of zopiclone; loss of efficacy may occur in some patients.

RISK FACTORS: No specific risk factors are known.

MECHANISM: Rifampin is an inducer of CYP3A4, the enzyme that appears to metabolize zopiclone.

CLINICAL EVALUATION: Eight healthy subjects received a single dose of zopiclone 10 mg following 5 days of rifampin 600 mg daily or placebo.[1] The mean area under the concentration-time curve of zopiclone was reduced by more than 80%, while its peak concentration declined 70% following rifampin pretreatment. Zopiclone half-life was reduced from 3.8 to 2.3 hours following rifampin. The reduction in zopiclone plasma concentration was accompanied by a reduced pharmacologic effect as measured by psychomotor testing. The hypnotic effects of zopiclone are likely to be reduced in patients taking rifampin.

RELATED DRUGS: Rifabutin (*Mycobutin*) and rifapentine (*Priftin*) are likely to reduce zopiclone plasma concentrations. Other benzodiazepines metabolized by CYP3A4 (eg, alprazolam [eg, *Xanax*], midazolam, eszopiclone [*Lunesta*], triazolam [eg, *Halcion*]) are likely to be affected in a similar manner.

MANAGEMENT OPTIONS:

➥ **Consider Alternative.** Rifampin does not appear to alter the elimination of temazepam (eg, *Restoril*).

➥ **Monitor.** Observe patients receiving rifampin for reduced hypnotic effects when zopiclone is administered.

REFERENCES:

1. Villikka K, et al. Concentrations and effects of zopiclone are greatly reduced by rifampicin. *Br J Clin Pharmacol.* 1997;43(5):471-474.

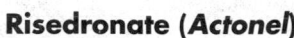

Risedronate (*Actonel*)

Antacids

SUMMARY: Antacids containing aluminum, magnesium, or calcium reduce risedronate bioavailability; doses need to be separated.

RISK FACTORS: No specific risk factors are known.

MECHANISM: Cations bind with risedronate in the GI tract.

CLINICAL EVALUATION: The cations in antacids bind with risedronate in the GI tract and can markedly reduce risedronate bioavailability.[1]

RELATED DRUGS: Antacids also reduce the bioavailability of other bisphosphonates, such as alendronate (*Fosamax*), etidronate (eg, *Didronel*), ibandronate (*Boniva*), and tiludronate (*Skelid*).

MANAGEMENT OPTIONS:

➡ ***Circumvent/Minimize.*** Because risedronate is taken in the morning, instruct the patient to avoid antacids and other drugs or foods for at least 30 minutes after taking risedronate or other bisphosphonates.

REFERENCES:

1. *Actonel* [package insert]. Bridgewater, NJ: Aventis Pharmaceuticals; 2004.

Risedronate (*Actonel*)

Calcium

SUMMARY: Calcium reduces risedronate bioavailability; doses need to be separated.

RISK FACTORS: No specific risk factors are known.

MECHANISM: Calcium binds with risedronate in the GI tract.

CLINICAL EVALUATION: Calcium supplements or calcium antacids bind with risedronate in the GI tract and can markedly reduce risedronate bioavailability. Because patients on risedronate and other bisphosphonates are generally taking calcium supplements, it is important they avoid taking the drugs too closely together.[1]

RELATED DRUGS: Calcium also reduces the bioavailability of other bisphosphonates, such as alendronate (*Fosamax*), etidronate (eg, *Didronel*), ibandronate (*Boniva*), and tiludronate (*Skelid*). Other cations, such as aluminum and magnesium, also inhibit risedronate absorption.

MANAGEMENT OPTIONS:

➡ ***Circumvent/Minimize.*** Because risedronate is taken in the morning, instruct the patient to avoid calcium and other drugs or foods within 30 minutes of taking risedronate or other bisphosphonates.

REFERENCES:

1. *Actonel* [package insert]. Bridgewater, NJ: Aventis Pharmaceuticals; 2004.

4 Risperidone (*Risperdal*)

Valproic Acid (eg, *Depakote*)

SUMMARY: A patient taking risperidone and valproic acid developed generalized edema, but a causal relationship was not established.

RISK FACTORS: No specific risk factors are known.

MECHANISM: Not established. Valproic acid alone is known to cause edema, but it is not known if risperidone contributed to the effect.

CLINICAL EVALUATION: A 35-year-old man taking clorazepate and valproic acid (in the form of divalproex) reported generalized edema 2.5 weeks after risperidone was added for mania.[1] The edema responded to diuretic therapy, and he continued taking both risperidone and the diuretic. Although it is possible that the edema resulted from the combined effects of valproic acid and risperidone, a causal relationship was not established.

RELATED DRUGS: No information is available.

MANAGEMENT OPTIONS: No specific action is required, but be alert for evidence of the interaction.

REFERENCES:

1. Baldassano CF, et al. Generalized edema with risperidone: divalproex sodium treatment. *J Clin Psychiatry.* 1996;57:422.

Ritonavir (*Norvir*)

Saquinavir (*Invirase*)

SUMMARY: Ritonavir increases saquinavir plasma concentrations; saquinavir toxicity may result.

RISK FACTORS: No specific risk factors are known.

MECHANISM: Ritonavir inhibits the metabolism of saquinavir via the CYP3A4 enzyme, resulting in an increase in saquinavir bioavailability and a reduction in its clearance.

CLINICAL EVALUATION: While no published data are available for evaluation, the manufacturer of ritonavir has made available some data on this interaction.[1] Saquinavir undergoes extensive first-pass metabolism and is reported to have a bioavailability of only 4%.[2] Because saquinavir is metabolized by the enzyme CYP3A4 that is found in the intestinal wall and liver, inhibition of CYP3A4 by ritonavir is expected to markedly increase the plasma concentration of saquinavir. It is possible that this interaction could be used to enhance the plasma concentrations of saquinavir.

RELATED DRUGS: Other protease inhibitors, such as indinavir (*Crixivan*) and nelfinavir (*Viracept*), may affect saquinavir metabolism in a similar manner, although the magnitude of the inhibition may be less than that observed with ritonavir. Ritonavir may inhibit the metabolism of other protease inhibitors, such as indinavir and nelfinavir.

MANAGEMENT OPTIONS:

➡ **Consider Alternative.** Using another protease inhibitor instead of ritonavir may reduce, but not eliminate, the interaction. Be alert for evidence of increased saquinavir plasma concentrations.

➡ **Circumvent/Minimize.** Reduction of the saquinavir dose may be necessary to avoid toxic symptoms such as GI upset and increased liver function tests (LFTs).

➡ **Monitor.** Monitor for GI upset and elevated LFTs when saquinavir is administered with ritonavir.

REFERENCES:
1. *Norvir* [package insert]. Abbott Park, IL: Abbott Laboratories; 1996.
2. *Invirase* [package insert]. Nutley, NJ: Hoffman-La Roche, Inc.; 1996.

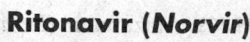

Ritonavir (*Norvir*)
Sildenafil (eg, *Viagra*)

SUMMARY: Ritonavir administration increases sildenafil plasma concentrations; observe patients for side effects.

RISK FACTORS: No specific risk factors are known.

MECHANISM: Ritonavir appears to reduce the metabolism of sildenafil by CYP3A4 (and perhaps CYP2C9), resulting in a reduction of first-pass metabolism and intrinsic clearance of sildenafil.

CLINICAL EVALUATION: Twenty-seven healthy men took a single dose of sildenafil 100 mg followed by placebo or ritonavir 300, 400, and 500 mg twice daily on days 2, 3, and 4 through 8 after the sildenafil.[1] Another single dose of sildenafil 100 mg was administered following the placebo or ritonavir administration. The mean area under the concentration-time curve of sildenafil was increased 11-fold; its peak plasma concentration increased 3.9-fold following ritonavir administration. The half-life of sildenafil increased from 3.7 to 5.4 hours after ritonavir pretreatment. The single dose of sildenafil did not alter the concentrations of ritonavir. Although no increase in adverse effects was noted in this study, the magnitude of the interaction suggests the need to carefully monitor patients when coadministering sildenafil and ritonavir.

RELATED DRUGS: Other protease inhibitors such as indinavir (*Crixivan*), saquinavir (*Invirase*), amprenavir (*Agenerase*), and nelfinavir (*Viracept*) are known to inhibit CYP3A4 and are expected to interact with sildenafil.

MANAGEMENT OPTIONS:

➡ **Circumvent/Minimize.** Because of the potential for serious side effects, counsel patients taking protease inhibitors that are CYP3A4 inhibitors to avoid concurrent sildenafil administration. If sildenafil is coadministered to patients taking ritonavir, it would be prudent to use a starting dose of 25 mg.

➡ **Monitor.** Carefully monitor patients for side effects (eg, headache, flushing, hypotension, abnormal vision) if sildenafil and ritonavir are coadministered.

REFERENCES:
1. Muirhead GJ, et al. Pharmacokinetic interactions between sildenafil and saquinavir/ritonavir. *Br J Clin Pharmacol.* 2000;50:99-107.

Ritonavir (*Norvir*)

Tadalafil (eg, *Cialis*)

SUMMARY: Ritonavir increases the plasma concentration of tadalafil; increased tadalafil adverse reactions may occur.

RISK FACTORS: No specific risk factors are known.

MECHANISM: Ritonavir inhibits the metabolism of tadalafil via CYP3A4; increased tadalafil bioavailability and reduced clearance are expected.

CLINICAL EVALUATION: While specific data are limited, coadministration of ritonavir 200 mg twice daily prior to a single dose of tadalafil 20 mg increased the mean area under the plasma concentration-time curve of tadalafil by approximately 124%.[1]

RELATED DRUGS: Atazanavir (*Reyataz*), darunavir (*Prezista*), indinavir (*Crixivan*), nelfinavir (*Viracept*), and saquinavir (*Invirase*) also inhibit the activity of CYP3A4 and are expected to increase the plasma concentrations of tadalafil. Sildenafil (eg, *Viagra*) and vardenafil (eg, *Levitra*) are likely to be affected in a similar manner by ritonavir.

MANAGEMENT OPTIONS:

➡ **Circumvent/Minimize.** Pending further data, observe patients receiving tadalafil and ritonavir for increased tadalafil effect and limit the dosage of tadalafil to 10 mg every 72 hours.[1]

➡ **Monitor.** Be alert for signs of excessive tadalafil effects, such as hypotension, if ritonavir is coadministered.

REFERENCES:

1. *Cialis* [package insert]. Indianapolis, IN: Eli Lilly and Company; 2003.

 Ritonavir (*Norvir*)

Telaprevir (*Incivek*)

SUMMARY: The coadministration of ritonavir may initially increase, and then reduce, the plasma concentration of telaprevir; some patients may experience a transient increase in adverse reactions.

RISK FACTORS: No specific risk factors are known.

MECHANISM: Acute ritonavir administration inhibits the CYP3A4-mediated metabolism of telaprevir, but long-term ritonavir administration results in an increase in telaprevir metabolism.

CLINICAL EVALUATION: While specific data are limited, the manufacturer of telaprevir notes that the coadministration of ritonavir 100 mg as a single dose with a single dose of telaprevir 750 mg increased the mean area under the plasma concentration-time curve (AUC) of telaprevir approximately 2-fold.[1] However, with ritonavir administered as 100 mg every 12 hours for 14 days, the mean AUC of telaprevir was reduced 25%. The clinical significance of this reduction in telaprevir plasma concentration is likely to be limited. Telaprevir labeling also notes that long-term administration of ritonavir combined with darunavir, fosamprenavir, or lopinavir results in a reduction in the AUC of telaprevir.

RELATED DRUGS: Atazanavir (*Reyataz*), darunavir (*Prezista*), fosamprenavir (*Lexiva*), indinavir (*Crixivan*), nelfinavir (*Viracept*), and saquinavir (*Invirase*) also inhibit the activity of CYP3A4 and are expected to increase the plasma concentrations of telaprevir.

MANAGEMENT OPTIONS:

➥ *Monitor.* Monitor patients stabilized on telaprevir for adverse reactions shortly after ritonavir is initiated and for possible reduced efficacy if ritonavir is administered long-term.

REFERENCES:

1. *Incivek* [package insert]. Cambridge, MA: Vertex Pharmaceuticals Inc; 2011.

Ritonavir (*Norvir*)

Theophylline (eg, *Theochron*)

SUMMARY: Ritonavir reduces theophylline plasma concentrations; a reduction in theophylline efficacy may result.

RISK FACTORS: No specific risk factors are known.

MECHANISM: It appears that ritonavir increases theophylline metabolism, perhaps by induction of CYP1A2.

CLINICAL EVALUATION: While no published data are available for evaluation, there are some data on this interaction from the ritonavir manufacturer. Twenty-seven subjects received theophylline alone for 5 days followed by 10 days of coadministration with ritonavir 500 mg twice daily.[1] The mean area under the concentration-time curve of theophylline was reduced 43% and the peak concentration was decreased 32% during ritonavir administration. Changes of this magnitude could result in a reduction in theophylline efficacy.

RELATED DRUGS: The effect of other protease inhibitors, such as indinavir (*Crixivan*), saquinavir (*Invirase*), and nelfinavir (*Viracept*), on theophylline metabolism is unknown.

MANAGEMENT OPTIONS:

➥ *Consider Alternative.* While specific information is not available, avoid the interaction by using other protease inhibitors with theophylline.

➥ *Circumvent/Minimize.* The coadministration of theophylline and ritonavir may require increasing the dose of theophylline to maintain therapeutic concentrations.

➥ *Monitor.* Monitor theophylline concentrations to ensure adequate plasma levels during ritonavir administration. Watch for inadequate theophylline response, such as bronchospasm or wheezing.

REFERENCES:

1. *Norvir* [package insert]. Abbott Park, IL: Abbott Laboratories; 1996.

4 Ritonavir (*Norvir*)

Tipranavir (*Aptivus*)

SUMMARY: Ritonavir increases the plasma concentration of tipranavir; this interaction is useful to ensure adequate antiviral concentrations of tipranavir.

RISK FACTORS: No specific risk factors are known.

MECHANISM: Ritonavir inhibits the metabolism (CYP3A4) of tipranavir, increasing its bioavailability and plasma concentrations.

CLINICAL EVALUATION: While specific data are limited, coadministration of ritonavir 200 mg with tipranavir 500 mg twice daily increased the mean steady-state trough concentration of tipranavir approximately 29-fold, compared with tipranavir administered without ritonavir.[1] Because the absorption of tipranavir without ritonavir is very limited, the combination of tipranavir and ritonavir is recommended to achieve adequate tipranavir plasma concentrations.

RELATED DRUGS: Other protease inhibitors that inhibit CYP3A4, such as atazanavir (*Reyataz*), indinavir (*Crixivan*), or saquinavir (*Invirase*), are likely to inhibit the metabolism of tipranavir.

MANAGEMENT OPTIONS:

➡ *Monitor.* Patients receiving tipranavir will usually be administered ritonavir. If additional antiviral agents that inhibit CYP3A4 are coadministered, watch for signs of tipranavir toxicity, such as hepatic impairment or bleeding.

REFERENCES:
1. *Aptivus* [package insert]. Ridgefield, CT: Boehringer Ingelheim Pharmaceuticals, Inc; 2007.

4 Ritonavir (*Norvir*)

Trimethoprim/Sulfamethoxazole (eg, *Bactrim*)

SUMMARY: Ritonavir administration produces limited changes in sulfamethoxazole and trimethoprim plasma concentrations. Limited clinical effect is expected.

RISK FACTORS: No specific risk factors are known.

MECHANISM: Not established.

CLINICAL EVALUATION: While no published data are available for evaluation, there are some data on this interaction from the ritonavir manufacturer. In a noncrossover study, 15 subjects received the combination of sulfamethoxazole 800 mg and trimethoprim 160 mg as a single dose alone or during concomitant therapy with ritonavir 500 mg twice daily for 12 days.[1] The area under the concentration-time curve (AUC) of sulfamethoxazole was reduced 20%, while the AUC of trimethoprim was increased 20% during ritonavir administration. The effects of trimethoprim/sulfamethoxazole on ritonavir concentrations are unknown.

RELATED DRUGS: Indinavir (*Crixivan*) is known to increase the AUC of trimethoprim. It does not appear to affect sulfamethoxazole concentrations. The effects of other protease inhibitors, such as saquinavir (*Invirase*) and nelfinavir (*Viracept*), on trimethoprim/sulfamethoxazole are unknown.

MANAGEMENT OPTIONS: No specific action is required, but be alert for evidence of the interaction.

REFERENCES:

1. *Norvir* [package insert]. Abbott Park, IL: Abbott Laboratories; 1996.

Ritonavir (*Norvir*)

Vardenafil (eg, *Levitra*)

SUMMARY: Ritonavir increases the plasma concentration of vardenafil; increased vardenafil adverse reactions may occur.

RISK FACTORS: No specific risk factors are known.

MECHANISM: Ritonavir inhibits the metabolism of vardenafil via CYP3A4; increased vardenafil bioavailability and reduced clearance are expected.

CLINICAL EVALUATION: While specific data are limited, coadministration of ritonavir 600 mg 3 times daily prior to a single dose of vardenafil 5 mg increased the mean area under the plasma concentration-time curve of vardenafil approximately 49-fold.[1] Pending further data, observe patients receiving vardenafil and ritonavir for increased vardenafil effect and limit the dosage of vardenafil to 2.5 mg every 72 hours.

RELATED DRUGS: Atazanavir (*Reyataz*), darunavir (*Prezista*), indinavir (*Crixivan*), nelfinavir (*Viracept*), and saquinavir (*Invirase*) also inhibit the activity of CYP3A4 and are expected to increase the plasma concentrations of vardenafil. Sildenafil (eg, *Viagra*) and tadalafil (eg, *Cialis*) are likely to be affected in a similar manner by ritonavir.

MANAGEMENT OPTIONS:

➥ *Circumvent/Minimize.* Pending further data, observe patients receiving vardenafil and ritonavir for increased vardenafil effect and limit the dosage of vardenafil to 2.5 mg every 72 hours.

➥ *Monitor.* Be alert for signs of excessive vardenafil effects, such as hypotension, if ritonavir is coadministered.

REFERENCES:

1. *Levitra* [package insert]. West Haven, CT: Bayer Pharmaceuticals Corporation; 2008.

Ritonavir (*Norvir*)

Vincristine (eg, *Vincasar*)

SUMMARY: The coadministration of ritonavir and vincristine has been reported to produce paralytic ileus.

RISK FACTORS: No specific risk factors are known.

MECHANISM: Ritonavir appears to inhibit the CYP3A and P-glycoprotein elimination of vincristine.

CLINICAL EVALUATION: A patient with HIV was being treated with abacavir, lamivudine, ritonavir, lopinavir, co-trimoxazole, and valacyclovir.[1] Following a diagnosis of Burkitt lymphoma, cyclophosphamide, doxorubicin, methotrexate, cytarabine, and vincristine were added. After 2 doses of vincristine 7 days apart, the patient developed constipation, and paralytic ileus was diagnosed. Vincristine was discontinued and the patient recovered over the next 10 days.

RELATED DRUGS: Other protease inhibitors, including atazanavir (*Reyataz*), darunavir (*Prezista*), fosamprenavir (*Lexiva*), indinavir (*Crixivan*), nelfinavir (*Viracept*), and saquinavir (*Invirase*), also inhibit the activity of CYP3A and are expected to increase the plasma concentration of vincristine. Vinblastine and vinorelbine (eg, *Navelbine*) are also substrates of CYP3A and may be inhibited by ritonavir.

MANAGEMENT OPTIONS:

➡ *Monitor.* Carefully monitor patients taking vincristine and ritonavir for signs of neurotoxicity, including paralytic ileus.

REFERENCES:

1. Levêque D, et al. Paralytic ileus possibly associated with interaction between ritonavir/lopinavir and vincristine. *Pharm World Sci.* 2009;31(6):619-621.

---

4 **Ritonavir (*Norvir*)**

Zidovudine (eg, *Retrovir*)

SUMMARY: Zidovudine does not affect ritonavir concentrations. Ritonavir appears to reduce the plasma concentrations of zidovudine approximately 25%.

RISK FACTORS: No specific risk factors are known.

MECHANISM: Ritonavir may decrease the bioavailability of zidovudine.

CLINICAL EVALUATION: While no published data are available for evaluation, the manufacturer of ritonavir has made available some data on this interaction. Ten men received ritonavir 300 mg 4 times daily alone and in combination with zidovudine 200 mg 3 times daily for 4 days.[1] During coadministration, drug administration was separated by at least 2 hours. Ritonavir concentrations were not affected by zidovudine coadministration. Zidovudine's peak concentration and area under the concentration-time curve was reduced 25% during ritonavir administration. Because the half-life of zidovudine was not affected by ritonavir, the reduction in zidovudine plasma concentration is thought to be caused by a reduction in zidovudine bioavailability.

RELATED DRUGS: Other protease inhibitors such as indinavir (*Crixivan*), saquinavir (*Invirase*), and nelfinavir (*Viracept*) may affect zidovudine in a similar manner.

MANAGEMENT OPTIONS: No specific action is required, but be alert for evidence of the interaction.

REFERENCES:

1. *Norvir* [package insert]. Abbott Park, IL: Abbott Laboratories; 1996.

 Rofecoxib (*Vioxx*)†

Lithium (eg, *Lithobid*)

SUMMARY: Rofecoxib has been associated with elevated lithium serum concentrations; monitor for lithium toxicity.

RISK FACTORS: No specific risk factors are known.

MECHANISM: Rofecoxib probably reduces renal lithium clearance, presumably through inhibition of cyclooxygenase (COX)-2.

CLINICAL EVALUATION: A number of cases of lithium toxicity have been reported following the use of rofecoxib, including more than a dozen reported to the FDA.[1,2] Given the nature of the case reports, a causal relationship cannot be established. Nonetheless, the fact that nonsteroidal anti-inflammatory drugs (inhibitors of COX-1 and COX-2) are known to cause lithium toxicity suggests that COX-2 inhibitors may produce a similar effect.

RELATED DRUGS: All COX-2 inhibitors, including celecoxib (*Celebrex*) and valdecoxib (*Bextra*), appear to increase lithium serum concentrations. Some evidence suggests that rofecoxib produces the largest increases, but confirmation is needed.

MANAGEMENT OPTIONS:

➡ *Monitor.* If rofecoxib is initiated in patients receiving lithium, monitor lithium concentrations and for evidence of lithium toxicity (eg, nausea, vomiting, diarrhea, anorexia, coarse tremor, slurred speech, vertigo, confusion, lethargy; in severe cases, seizures, stupor, coma, cardiovascular collapse).

REFERENCES:

1. Lundmark J, et al. A possible interaction between lithium and rofecoxib [letter]. *Br J Clin Pharmacol.* 2002;53:403-404.

2. Phelan KM, et al. Lithium interaction with the cyclooxygenase 2 inhibitors rofecoxib and celecoxib and other nonsteroidal anti-inflammatory drugs. *J Clin Psychiatry.* 2003;64:1328-1334.

† Withdrawn from the market.

Rofecoxib (*Vioxx*)† **4**

Tizanidine (eg, *Zanaflex*)

SUMMARY: Limited evidence suggests that rofecoxib may increase the risk of tizanidine toxicity.

RISK FACTORS: No specific risk factors are known.

MECHANISM: Not established. Rofecoxib might inhibit the metabolism of tizanidine by CYP1A2.

CLINICAL EVALUATION: The manufacturer of tizanidine has received case reports of tizanidine toxicity (eg, hypotension, bradycardia, CNS depression) following concurrent use of rofecoxib, but a causal relationship has not been established.[1]

RELATED DRUGS: No information is available.

MANAGEMENT OPTIONS: No specific action is required, but be alert for evidence of the interaction.

REFERENCES:

1. *Zanaflex* [package insert]. San Francisco, CA: Elan Pharmaceuticals; 2004.

† Withdrawn from the market.

Rofecoxib (Vioxx)†

Warfarin (eg, Coumadin)

SUMMARY: Rofecoxib appears to slightly increase the hypoprothrombinemic response to warfarin.

RISK FACTORS: No specific risk factors are known.

MECHANISM: Not established.

CLINICAL EVALUATION: Single- and multiple-dose studies in healthy subjects have found an approximate 10% increase in international normalized ratio (INR) when rofecoxib 25 mg/day is given concurrently.[1] The effect on the INR is not likely to be clinically significant in most patients. Rofecoxib and celecoxib appear to increase the risk of GI bleeding, albeit to a lesser extent than standard NSAIDs, but the extent to which this increases the risk of bleeding in patients on warfarin is not established.

RELATED DRUGS: Celecoxib (Celebrex) is like rofecoxib in that it does not affect platelets and appears less likely than standard NSAIDs to adversely affect the GI tract. Hence, both COX-2 inhibitors are probably safer than standard NSAIDs in patients on oral anticoagulants.

MANAGEMENT OPTIONS: No special precautions appear necessary, but it is prudent to monitor for altered hypoprothrombinemic response and bleeding when any drug is added to warfarin therapy.

REFERENCES:

1. Schwartz JI, et al. The effect of rofecoxib on the pharmacodynamics and pharmacokinetics of warfarin. *Clin Pharmacol Ther.* 2000;68:626-636.

† Withdrawn from the market.

Rosiglitazone (Avandia)

Trimethoprim (eg, Proloprim)

SUMMARY: Trimethoprim administration produces a modest increase in rosiglitazone plasma concentrations; some patients may have enhanced hypoglycemic effect with coadministration of rosiglitazone and trimethoprim.

RISK FACTORS: No specific risk factors are known.

MECHANISM: Trimethoprim appears to inhibit the metabolism of rosiglitazone, possibly by inhibition of CYP2C8.

CLINICAL EVALUATION: Ten healthy subjects were administered trimethoprim 160 mg or placebo twice daily for 4 days.[1] On the third day, each was given a single dose of rosiglitazone 4 mg. The mean area under the plasma concentration-time curve of rosiglitazone increased 37% (range, 16% to 51%) following trimethoprim administration. The mean half-life of rosiglitazone was increased from 3.8 to 4.8 hours.

RELATED DRUGS: Repaglinide (Prandin) is partially metabolized by CYP2C8. Trimethoprim would likely cause some inhibition of the metabolism of repaglinide.

MANAGEMENT OPTIONS:

➡ *Monitor.* Observe patients stabilized on rosiglitazone for enhanced hypoglycemic response when trimethoprim is coadministered.

REFERENCES:

1. Niemi M, et al. Effects of trimethoprim and rifampin on the pharmacokinetics of the cytochrome P450 2C8 substrate rosiglitazone. *Clin Pharmacol Ther*. 2004;76:239-249.

Roxithromycin†

Theophylline (eg, *Theolair*)

SUMMARY: Roxithromycin administration produces small increases in theophylline serum concentrations; the clinical significance of these changes is limited.

RISK FACTORS: No specific risk factors are known.

MECHANISM: Roxithromycin appears to inhibit the metabolism of theophylline.

CLINICAL EVALUATION: Twelve healthy subjects received theophylline 200 mg 3 times daily alone and concurrently with roxithromycin 150 mg twice daily.[1] The area under the theophylline concentration-time curve increased 16% during roxithromycin administration. A second study found no effect of roxithromycin 300 mg twice daily for 5 days on theophylline concentrations.[2] The magnitude of this interaction indicates that few patients will be at risk of developing theophylline toxicity during roxithromycin theophylline administration.

RELATED DRUGS: Other macrolides (eg, erythromycin [eg, *E-Mycin*], clarithromycin [eg, *Biaxin*]) also inhibit theophylline metabolism.

MANAGEMENT OPTIONS: No specific action is required, but be alert for evidence of the interaction.

REFERENCES:

1. Saint-Salvi B, et al. A study of the interaction of roxithromycin with theophylline and carbamazepine. *J Antimicrob Chemother*. 1987;20(suppl B):121-129.

2. Hashiguchi K, et al. Roxithromycin does not raise serum theophylline levels. *Chest*. 1992;102:653-654.

† Not available in the United States.

Saquinavir (*Invirase*)

Sildenafil (eg, *Viagra*)

SUMMARY: Saquinavir administration increases sildenafil plasma concentrations. Observe patients for adverse reactions.

RISK FACTORS: No specific risk factors are known.

MECHANISM: Saquinavir appears to reduce the metabolism of sildenafil by CYP3A4, resulting in a reduction of first-pass metabolism as well as intrinsic clearance of sildenafil.

CLINICAL EVALUATION: Twenty-seven healthy men took a single dose of sildenafil 100 mg followed by placebo or saquinavir 1,200 mg 3 times daily on days 2 through 8 after the sildenafil.[1] Another single dose of sildenafil 100 mg was administered following the placebo or saquinavir administration. The mean area under the plasma concentration-time curve of sildenafil was increased 3.1-fold; its peak plasma concentration increased 2.4-fold following saquinavir administration. The half-life of sildenafil increased from 3.3 to 4.4 hours after saquinavir pretreatment. The single dose of sildenafil did not alter the concentrations of saquinavir. Although no increase in adverse reactions was noted in this study, the magnitude of the interaction suggests that patients be carefully monitored if sildenafil and saquinavir are coadministered.

RELATED DRUGS: Other protease inhibitors, such as indinavir (*Crixivan*), ritonavir (*Norvir*), amprenavir (*Agenerase*), and nelfinavir (*Viracept*), are known to inhibit CYP3A4 and are expected to interact with sildenafil.

MANAGEMENT OPTIONS:

➡ ***Circumvent/Minimize.*** Because of the potential for serious adverse reactions, counsel patients taking protease inhibitors that are CYP3A4 inhibitors to avoid sildenafil coadministration. If sildenafil is coadministered to patients taking saquinavir, start dosing with sildenafil 25 mg.

➡ ***Monitor.*** Carefully monitor patients treated with sildenafil for adverse reactions (eg, headache, flushing, hypotension, abnormal vision) if saquinavir is prescribed.

REFERENCES:

1. Muirhead GJ, et al. Pharmacokinetic interactions between sildenafil and saquinavir/ritonavir. *Br J Clin Pharmacol*. 2000;50(2):99-107.

 Saquinavir (*Invirase*)

Tipranavir (*Aptivus*)

SUMMARY: Coadministration of saquinavir with tipranavir/ritonavir may result in lower plasma concentrations of saquinavir and less antiviral effect.

RISK FACTORS: No specific risk factors are known.

MECHANISM: Unknown. Saquinavir is considered to be a substrate of both CYP3A4 and P-glycoprotein. The combination of tipranavir/ritonavir has been shown to inhibit CYP3A4 and induce P-glycoprotein. These offsetting effects may account for the reduction in saquinavir plasma concentrations, possibly by reducing its bioavailability via P-glycoprotein induction.

CLINICAL EVALUATION: While specific data are limited, the manufacturer of tipranavir notes that coadministration of tipranavir 500 mg with ritonavir 200 mg twice daily and saquinavir 600 mg with ritonavir 100 mg twice daily decreased the mean area under the plasma concentration-time curve of saquinavir 76% compared with administration of the combination of saquinavir/ritonavir alone.[1]

RELATED DRUGS: Tipranavir/ritonavir also has been reported to reduce the plasma concentrations of lopinavir (*Kaletra*) and amprenavir (*Agenerase*).

MANAGEMENT OPTIONS:

➡ *Monitor.* Carefully monitor patients being treated with tipranavir/ritonavir and saquinavir for any change in antiviral efficacy.

REFERENCES:

1. *Aptivus* [package insert]. Ridgefield, CT: Boehringer Ingelheim Pharmaceuticals, Inc; 2007.

Selegiline (eg, *Eldepryl*) 5

Tacrine (*Cognex*)

SUMMARY: The combination of tacrine or physostigmine (eg, *Antilirium*) with selegiline did not result in adverse reactions in a study of patients with Alzheimer disease.

RISK FACTORS: No specific risk factors are known.

MECHANISM: No interaction.

CLINICAL EVALUATION: Ten patients with Alzheimer disease receiving cholinesterase inhibitor therapy (7 on tacrine, 3 on physostigmine) were given the monoamine oxidase (MAO)-B inhibitor selegiline (5 mg twice daily for 4 weeks) in a randomized, double-blind, crossover study.[1] Selegiline appeared to somewhat improve the therapeutic effect of the cholinesterase inhibitors without increasing adverse effects. Although the study involved a small number of patients, it does suggest that tacrine and selegiline (10 mg/day) do not interact adversely. Little is known about the use of tacrine with larger doses of selegiline (in which it may lose some of its MAO-B selectivity) or with other types of MAO inhibitors (nonselective or MAO-A selective).

RELATED DRUGS: Little is known about the use of selegiline with other MAO inhibitors.

MANAGEMENT OPTIONS: No interaction.

REFERENCES:

1. Schneider LS, et al. A double-blind crossover pilot study of I-deprenyl (selegiline) combined with cholinesterase inhibitor in Alzheimer's disease. *Am J Psychiatry*. 1993;150:321-323.

Selegiline (eg, *Eldepryl*)

Tyramine

SUMMARY: Selegiline may increase the pressor response to food or drink containing tyramine, but the effect usually is not significant.

RISK FACTORS:

➤ ***Dosage Regimen.*** Selegiline doses of up to 10 mg/day usually have only a small inhibitory effect on monoamine oxidase (MAO)-A, but larger doses can have a clinically important effect.

MECHANISM: Tyramine in foods is normally metabolized by MAO in the intestinal wall (MAO-A) and liver (MAO-A and MAO-B) before reaching the systemic circulation. Inhibition of MAO-A or MAO-B can increase the amount of tyramine reaching the systemic circulation, resulting in an increased pressor response. Because MAO-A is more important than MAO-B in the presystemic metabolism of tyramine, selegiline would be expected to have less effect on the pressor response to tyramine than nonselective MAO inhibitors or MAO-A inhibitors.

CLINICAL EVALUATION: Selegiline can enhance the pressor effect of tyramine, but to a lesser extent than nonselective or type A MAO inhibitors. The enhancement was greater with larger doses of selegiline and following the oral administration of tyramine.[1,2]

RELATED DRUGS: Mofegiline, another MAO-B inhibitor, does not appear to lose its MAO-B selectivity when large doses are used.

MANAGEMENT OPTIONS:

➤ ***Circumvent/Minimize.*** Although strict avoidance of tyramine-containing foods is not necessary, it would be prudent to avoid high-tyramine foods, especially if the patient is taking more than of selegiline 10 mg/day.

➤ ***Monitor.*** Monitor for evidence of tyramine-induced hypertension.

REFERENCES:

1. Elsworth JD, et al. Deprenyl administration in man: a selective monoamine oxidase B inhibitor without the "cheese effect." *Psychopharmacology*. 1978;57:33-38.
2. Schulz R, et al. Tyramine kinetics and pressor sensitivity during monoamine oxidase inhibition by selegiline. *Clin Pharmacol Ther*. 1989;46:528-536.

Sertraline (*Zoloft*)

Sumatriptan (*Imitrex*)

SUMMARY: The risk of serotonin syndrome may be increased when sertraline is used with sumatriptan or other triptans.

RISK FACTORS: No specific risk factors are known.

MECHANISM: Not established. It has been proposed that triptans may have additive serotonergic effects with selective serotonin reuptake inhibitors (SSRIs) or serotonin/norepinephrine reuptake inhibitors (SNRIs).

CLINICAL EVALUATION: Cases of possible serotonin syndrome occasionally have been reported with combined use of triptans and SSRIs such as fluoxetine (eg, *Prozac*) and paroxetine (eg, *Paxil*).[1,2] These cases notwithstanding, clinical studies of the combined use of triptans with SSRIs generally have found little evidence of an increased risk of serotonin syndrome. In a prospective study of 12,339 patients who received sumatriptan for migraine, evidence of serotonin syndrome was not observed in the 676 patients receiving sertraline concurrently.[3] In a randomized, double-blind, crossover study of 20 healthy subjects, fluoxetine did not affect the pharmacokinetics, pharmacodynamics, or side effects of zolmitriptan (*Zomig*).[4] In another randomized, double-blind, crossover study of 12 healthy subjects, paroxetine did not affect the pharmacokinetics, pharmacodynamics, or side effects of rizatriptan (*Maxalt*).[5] Taken together, this information suggests that combined use of triptans and SSRIs usually does not result in adverse drug interactions, but that it is possible that serotonin syndrome occurs in certain susceptible individuals.

In July 2006, however, the FDA issued a public health advisory stating that new information suggests that combined use of triptans with SSRIs or SNRIs can result in serotonin syndrome.[6] Few details were presented on the nature of the information that led to this advisory.

RELATED DRUGS: Theoretically, the risk of serotonin syndrome may be increased by any combination of a triptan (almotriptan [*Axert*], eletriptan [*Relpax*], frovatriptan [*Frova*], naratriptan [*Amerge*], rizatriptan, sumatriptan, zolmitriptan) with an SSRI (citalopram [eg, *Celexa*], escitalopram [*Lexapro*], fluoxetine, fluvoxamine, paroxetine, sertraline) or an SNRI (clomipramine [eg, *Anafranil*], duloxetine [*Cymbalta*], imipramine [eg, *Tofranil*], venlafaxine [*Effexor*]).

MANAGEMENT OPTIONS:

➡ *Monitor.* Patients receiving sertraline (or other SSRIs or SNRIs) should be alert for evidence of serotonin syndrome if they take sumatriptan (or other triptans). Symptoms of serotonin syndrome include agitation, coma, confusion, fever, hyperreflexia, hypomania, incoordination, myoclonus, rigidity, seizures, shivering, sweating, and tremor. Advise patients to contact their health care provider if any of these symptoms occur.

REFERENCES:

1. Hendrix Y, van Zagten MS. Serotonin syndrome as a result of concomitant use of paroxetine and sumatriptan. *Ned Tijdschr Geneeskd.* 2005;149:888-890.
2. Mathew NT, et al. Serotonin syndrome complicating migraine pharmacotherapy. *Cephalalgia.* 1996;16:323-327.
3. Putnam GP, et al. Migraine polypharmacy and the tolerability of sumatriptan: a large-scale, prospective study. *Cephalalgia.* 1999;19:668-675.
4. Smith DA, et al. Zolmitriptan (311C90) does not interact with fluoxetine in healthy volunteers. *Int J Clin Pharmacol Ther.* 1998;36:301-305.
5. Goldberg MR, et al. Lack of pharmacokinetic and pharmacodynamic interaction between rizatriptan and paroxetine. *J Clin Pharmacol.* 1999;39:192-199.
6. FDA Public Health Advisory. Combined Use of 5-Hydroxytryptamine Receptor Agonists (Triptans), Selective Serotonin Reuptake Inhibitors (SSRIs) or Selective Serotonin/Norepinephrine Reuptake Inhibitors (SNRIs) May Result in Life-threatening Serotonin Syndrome. Center for Drug Evaluation and Research (CDER), U.S. Food and Drug Administration. July 19, 2006. Available at http://www.fda.gov/CDER/DRUG/advisory/SSRI_SS200607.htm. Accessed September 6, 2006.

Sertraline (eg, *Zoloft*)

Tamoxifen (eg, *Soltamox*)

SUMMARY: It appears that CYP2D6 inhibitors reduce the efficacy of tamoxifen in the treatment of breast cancer, but the effect of modest inhibitors of CYP2D6 such as sertraline is not established.

RISK FACTORS: No specific risk factors are known.

MECHANISM: Tamoxifen is metabolized to 2 active metabolites by CYP2D6, the most important of which is endoxifen. By reducing endoxifen formation, CYP2D6 inhibitors such as sertraline may reduce tamoxifen efficacy.[1-4]

CLINICAL EVALUATION: A study in patients with breast cancer found endoxifen plasma concentrations in patients taking weak CYP2D6 inhibitors such as sertraline and citalopram were lower than in patients not taking CYP2D6 inhibitors.[5] Endoxifen concentrations were substantially lower in patients receiving potent CYP2D6 inhibitors such as fluoxetine and paroxetine. A subsequent study in 80 patients starting tamoxifen therapy found that those on CYP2D6 inhibitor antidepressants had substantially lower endoxifen concentrations.[6] The reduction in endoxifen was greatest with paroxetine, intermediate with sertraline, and minimal with venlafaxine. Venlafaxine had no effect on endoxifen concentrations. Another tamoxifen study found a nearly 2-fold increase in the risk of breast cancer relapse in women with low CYP2D6 activity, either due to CYP2D6-inhibiting drugs or genetic deficiency.[7] Taken together, these results strongly suggest that CYP2D6 inhibitors reduce the efficacy of tamoxifen in the treatment of breast cancer.

RELATED DRUGS: Other selective serotonin reuptake inhibitors (SSRIs) that, like sertraline, are also modest inhibitors of CYP2D6 include citalopram (eg, *Celexa*), escitalopram (*Lexapro*), and desvenlafaxine (*Pristiq*). They are likely to interact similarly with tamoxifen. Paroxetine (eg, *Paxil*) and fluoxetine (eg, *Prozac*) are potent CYP2D6 inhibitors, while duloxetine (*Cymbalta*) and bupropion (eg, *Wellbutrin*) also substantially inhibit CYP2D6. They are likely to inhibit tamoxifen more than sertraline. Venlafaxine (*Effexor*) and mirtazapine (eg, *Remeron*) appear to have little or no effect on CYP2D6, and are unlikely to interact.

MANAGEMENT OPTIONS:

➡ **Consider Alternative.** Fluoxetine, paroxetine, duloxetine, and bupropion are best avoided in patients on tamoxifen. Although other SSRIs such as citalopram and sertraline are weaker inhibitors of CYP2D6, they can reduce endoxifen concentrations somewhat and may reduce tamoxifen efficacy in some patients. Available evidence suggests that venlafaxine does not affect endoxifen concentrations, so it may be preferable. Mirtazapine has been used effectively for hot flashes in breast cancer survivors, and theoretically is unlikely to interact with tamoxifen.[8]

➡ **Monitor.** If a CYP2D6 inhibitor such as fluoxetine is used with tamoxifen, cancer recurrence may be an indication that tamoxifen efficacy has been reduced. If this happens, consider discontinuing the CYP2D6 inhibitor.

REFERENCES:

1. Dezentje VO, et al. Clinical implications of CYP2D6 genotyping in tamoxifen treatment for breast cancer. *Clin Cancer Res.* 2009;15(1):15-21.
2. Tan SH, et al. Pharmacogenetics in breast cancer therapy. *Clin Cancer Res.* 2008;14(24):8027-8041.

3. Newman WG, et al. Impaired tamoxifen metabolism reduces survival in familial breast cancer patients. *Clin Cancer Res*. 2008;14(18):5913-5918.

4. Henry NL, et al. Drug interactions and pharmacogenomics in the treatment of breast cancer and depression. *Am J Psychiatry*. 2008;165(10):1251-1255.

5. Borges S, et al. Quantitative effect of CYP2D6 genotype and inhibitors on tamoxifen metabolism: implication for optimization of breast cancer treatment. *Clin Pharmacol Ther*. 2006;80(1):61-74.

6. Jin Y, et al. CYP2D6 genotype, antidepressant use, and tamoxifen metabolism during adjuvant breast cancer treatment. *J Natl Can Inst*. 2005;97(1):30-39.

7. Goetz MP, et al. The impact of cytochrome P450 2D6 metabolism in women receiving adjuvant tamoxifen. *Breast Cancer Res Treat*. 2007;101(1):113-121.

8. Biglia N, et al. Mirtazapine for the treatment of hot flushes in breast cancer survivors: a prospective pilot trial. *Breast J*. 2007;13(5):490-495.

Sertraline (eg, *Zoloft*)

Tolbutamide (eg, *Orinase*)

SUMMARY: Sertraline appears to cause a small reduction in the clearance of tolbutamide; no change in hypoglycemic response is expected.

RISK FACTORS: No specific risk factors are known.

MECHANISM: Unknown.

CLINICAL EVALUATION: Twenty-three healthy subjects received a single intravenous dose of tolbutamide 1,000 mg on day 1 and following 20 days of placebo (12 subjects) or sertraline (11 subjects) in a parallel study design. The sertraline dose was initiated at 50 mg and increased by 50 mg every 3 days until 200 mg daily was reached. This dose was continued for the remainder of the study period. There was a mean reduction in tolbutamide clearance of 16% in the subjects taking sertraline compared with the placebo group. Sertraline increased the half-life of tolbutamide from 6.9 to 8.6 hours.[1] The sertraline-induced changes in tolbutamide clearance are unlikely to result in a change in glycemic response to tolbutamide in patients with diabetes mellitus.

RELATED DRUGS: No information is available.

MANAGEMENT OPTIONS:

➡ **Monitor.** No specific monitoring appears to be required beyond the usual blood glucose monitoring.

REFERENCES:

1. Tremaine LM, et al. A study of the potential effect of sertraline on the pharmacokinetics and protein binding of tolbutamide. *Clin Pharmacokinet*. 1997;32(suppl 1):31-36.

Sertraline (eg, *Zoloft*)

Tramadol (eg, *Ultram*)

SUMMARY: A patient on sertraline and tramadol developed serotonin syndrome, but it is unknown how often this occurs in patients receiving the combination.

RISK FACTORS: No specific risk factors are known.

MECHANISM: Probably additive. Both sertraline and tramadol have serotonergic effects.

CLINICAL EVALUATION: A 42-year-old woman taking sertraline 100 mg/day developed confusion, psychosis, agitation, diaphoresis, and tremor after starting tramadol.[1] This case would qualify as serotonin syndrome by Sternbach criteria,[2] and the temporal relationship of the reaction is consistent with an interaction between sertraline and tramadol. It is not clear what predisposed this patient to develop serotonin syndrome, as many other patients have received this combination without problems. The patient also was receiving theophylline (eg, *Theochron*), and it has been proposed that theophylline may contribute to serotonin syndrome. However, any role of theophylline is unproven.

RELATED DRUGS: The combination of paroxetine (eg, *Paxil*) and tramadol also has been reported to produce serotonin syndrome. It is possible that other selective serotonin reuptake inhibitors (SSRIs), such as fluoxetine (eg, *Prozac*), fluvoxamine, and citalopram (eg, *Celexa*), may increase the risk of serotonin syndrome if combined with tramadol. Meperidine (eg, *Demerol*) may interact similarly with SSRIs.

MANAGEMENT OPTIONS:

➡ *Consider Alternative.* In patients taking sertraline or other SSRIs, consider the use of an analgesic that is not serotonergic (eg, an agent other than tramadol or meperidine) to minimize the risk of serotonin syndrome.

➡ *Monitor.* In patients receiving tramadol and sertraline (or other SSRIs), be alert for evidence of serotonin syndrome. Serotonin syndrome can result in neurotoxicity (eg, coma, hyperreflexia, incoordination, myoclonus, rigidity, seizures, tremors), psychiatric symptoms (eg, agitation, confusion, hypomania, restlessness), and autonomic dysfunction (eg, fever, hypertension, sweating, tachycardia).

REFERENCES:

1. Mason BJ, et al. Possible serotonin syndrome associated with tramadol and sertraline coadministration. *Ann Pharmacother.* 1997;31(2):175-177.

2. Sternbach H. The serotonin syndrome. *Am J Psychiatry.* 1991;148(6):705-713.

Sertraline (eg, *Zoloft*)

Warfarin (eg, *Coumadin*)

SUMMARY: A preliminary report suggests that sertraline may slightly increase the hypoprothrombinemic response to warfarin.

RISK FACTORS: No specific risk factors are known.

MECHANISM: Not established.

CLINICAL EVALUATION: Twelve healthy subjects received a single oral dose of warfarin 7.5 mg/kg with and without 22 days of pretreatment with sertraline 50 mg/day titrated up to a dose of 200 mg/day.[1] Sertraline produced a small increase in the prothrombin time and slightly delayed the normalization of the prothrombin time following warfarin. The degree to which this effect may increase the risk of bleeding is not established.

RELATED DRUGS: Some selective serotonin reuptake inhibitors (SSRIs) (eg, fluoxetine [eg, *Prozac*], paroxetine [eg, *Paxil*]) have been reported to have an intrinsic inhibitory effect on hemostasis, but it is not known if sertraline has a similar effect. The effect of sertraline on oral anticoagulants other than warfarin is not established.

MANAGEMENT OPTIONS:

➡ *Monitor.* Although data are sparse, be alert for evidence of an altered hypoprothrombinemic response to warfarin (or other anticoagulants) if sertraline is initiated, discontinued, or changed in dose. Although not reported for sertraline, some SSRIs may impair hemostasis; thus, be alert for evidence of bleeding even if the hypoprothrombinemic response is in the desired range.

REFERENCES:

1. Wilner KD, et al. The effects of sertraline on the pharmacodynamics of warfarin in healthy volunteers. *Biol Psychiatry.* 1991;29(suppl):333S-355S.

Sertraline (eg, *Zoloft*)

Zolpidem (eg, *Ambien*)

SUMMARY: Preliminary evidence suggests that sertraline may speed the onset of hypnosis with zolpidem, but it seems unlikely that this would result in adverse reactions.

RISK FACTORS: No specific risk factors are known.

MECHANISM: Not established.

CLINICAL EVALUATION: In a preliminary study, 28 healthy subjects were given zolpidem 10 mg at night with and without pretreatment with sertraline 50 mg/day.[1] Sertraline was associated with higher and more rapid peak plasma concentrations of zolpidem, but the combination was well tolerated. It is possible that patients on sertraline would achieve an earlier onset of effect from zolpidem; however, based on this study, it seems unlikely that this would result in adverse consequences.

RELATED DRUGS: No information is available.

MANAGEMENT OPTIONS: No specific action is required, but be alert for evidence of the interaction.

REFERENCES:

1. Allard S, et al. Coadministration of short-term zolpidem with sertraline in healthy women. *J Clin Pharmacol.* 1999;32(2):184-191.

Sibutramine†

Sumatriptan (eg, *Imitrex*)

SUMMARY: The risk of serotonin syndrome would theoretically increase when sibutramine is combined with other serotonergic drugs, such as sumatriptan.

RISK FACTORS: No specific risk factors are known.

MECHANISM: Sibutramine inhibits serotonin reuptake; additive serotonergic effects may occur with sumatriptan.

CLINICAL EVALUATION: While no published data are available for evaluation, the manufacturer of sibutramine has some data on this interaction.[1] Because sibutramine has serotonergic effects, its concurrent use with other serotonergic drugs (eg, sumatriptan) may increase the risk of serotonin syndrome.[2] Although the actual risk of combining sibutramine with serotonergic drugs is unknown, serotonin syndrome can result in serious or fatal reactions.

RELATED DRUGS: Little is known regarding concurrent use of zolmitriptan (*Zomig*) and sibutramine, but it is possible that there may be an increase in the risk of serotonin syndrome.

MANAGEMENT OPTIONS:

➡ *Avoid Unless Benefit Outweighs Risk.* The manufacturer states that sibutramine should not be used with sumatriptan. This is a prudent recommendation until more information is available.

➡ *Monitor.* Serotonin syndrome can result in neurotoxicity (eg, coma, hyperreflexia, incoordination, myoclonus, restlessness, rigidity, seizures, tremors), psychiatric symptoms (eg, agitation, confusion, hypomania), and temperature regulation abnormalities (eg, fever, sweating). Note that mild forms of serotonin syndrome also have been reported; consider any combination of the above symptoms possibly related to excessive serotonin activity.

REFERENCES:

1. *Meridia* [package insert]. Abbott, IL: Knoll Pharmaceuticals; 1997.
2. Mills KC. Serotonin syndrome. A clinical update. *Crit Care Clin*. 1997;13(4):763-783.

† Not available in the United States.

 Sibutramine†

Tryptophan†

SUMMARY: The risk of serotonin syndrome would theoretically increase when sibutramine is combined with other serotonergic drugs, such as tryptophan.

RISK FACTORS: No specific risk factors are known.

MECHANISM: Sibutramine inhibits serotonin reuptake; additive serotonergic effects may occur with sumatriptan.

CLINICAL EVALUATION: While no published data are available for evaluation, the manufacturer of sibutramine has some data on this interaction.[1] Because sibutramine has serotonergic effects, its concurrent use with other serotonergic drugs (eg, tryptophan) may increase the risk of serotonin syndrome.[2] Although the actual risk of combining sibutramine with serotonergic drugs is unknown, serotonin syndrome can result in serious or fatal reactions.

RELATED DRUGS: No information is available.

MANAGEMENT OPTIONS:

➡ *Avoid Unless Benefit Outweighs Risk.* The manufacturer states that sibutramine should not be used with tryptophan. This is a prudent recommendation until more information is available.

➡ *Monitor.* Serotonin syndrome can result in neurotoxicity (eg, coma, hyperreflexia, incoordination, myoclonus, restlessness, rigidity, seizures, tremors), psychiatric symptoms (eg, agitation, confusion, hypomania), and temperature regulation abnormalities (eg, fever, sweating). Note that mild forms of serotonin syndrome have also been reported; consider any combination of the above symptoms to possibly be related to excessive serotonin activity.

REFERENCES:

1. *Meridia* [package insert]. Abbott, IL: Knoll Pharmaceuticals; 1997.
2. Mills KC. Serotonin syndrome. A clinical update. *Crit Care Clin*. 1997;13(4):763-783.

† Not available in the United States.

Sildenafil (eg, *Viagra*) | 4

Simvastatin (eg, *Zocor*)

SUMMARY: A patient taking simvastatin developed severe muscle pain after a single dose of sildenafil, but a causal relationship was not established.

RISK FACTORS: No specific risk factors are known.

MECHANISM: Not established. Sildenafil and simvastatin are metabolized by CYP3A4, so it is possible that sildenafil competes with simvastatin for metabolism. Nonetheless, it is not known whether sildenafil is capable of inhibiting CYP3A4.

CLINICAL EVALUATION: A 76-year-old man stabilized on simvastatin 10 mg/day was prescribed sildenafil 50 mg prior to sexual activity.[1] He developed severe muscle aches 8 to 10 hours after taking his first dose of sildenafil. When he presented to the clinic 3 days after the reaction, he was asymptomatic and his creatine phosphokinase level was mildly elevated at 406 units/L. Other causes of myopathy did not appear to be present. More data are needed to establish a causal relationship.

RELATED DRUGS: No information is available.

MANAGEMENT OPTIONS: No specific action is required, but be alert for evidence of the interaction.

REFERENCES:
1. Gutierrez CA. Sildenafil-simvastatin interaction: possible cause of rhabdomyolysis? *Am Fam Physician.* 2001;63(4):636-637.

Sildenafil (eg, *Viagra*)

Telaprevir (*Incivek*)

SUMMARY: The coadministration of telaprevir and sildenafil is expected to markedly increase the plasma concentration of sildenafil; adverse reactions, including hypotension, prolonged erection, or syncope, may be more likely to occur.

RISK FACTORS: No specific risk factors are known.

MECHANISM: Telaprevir inhibits the CYP3A4-mediated metabolism of sildenafil.

CLINICAL EVALUATION: While specific data are limited, the manufacturer of telaprevir notes that the coadministration of telaprevir and sildenafil should be avoided if possible.[1] Pending further data, observe patients receiving telaprevir and sildenafil for sildenafil adverse reactions.

RELATED DRUGS: Atazanavir (*Reyataz*), darunavir (*Prezista*), fosamprenavir (*Staxyn*), indinavir (*Crixivan*), nelfinavir (*Viracept*), and saquinavir (*Invirase*) also inhibit the activity of CYP3A4 and are expected to increase the plasma concentrations of sildenafil. Tadalafil (eg, *Adcirca*) and vardenafil (*Levitra*) would likely be affected in a similar manner by telaprevir.

MANAGEMENT OPTIONS:

➡ *Avoid Unless Benefit Outweighs Risk.* Avoid coadministration of telaprevir with sildenafil.

➥ **Monitor.** Monitor patients stabilized on sildenafil for adverse reactions if telaprevir is coadministered. The telaprevir package insert recommends limiting the dose of sildenafil for patients taking telaprevir; however, no data are provided to support the recommendation.

REFERENCES:
    1. *Incivek* [package insert]. Cambridge, MA: Vertex Pharmaceuticals Inc; 2011.

Sildenafil (eg, *Viagra*)

Tolbutamide

SUMMARY: A single dose of sildenafil did not produce a change in tolbutamide plasma concentrations.

RISK FACTORS: No specific risk factors are known.

MECHANISM: No interaction.

CLINICAL EVALUATION: While no published data are available for evaluation, the manufacturer of sildenafil has some data on this interaction. Twelve healthy men received single oral doses of tolbutamide 250 mg with sildenafil 50 mg or placebo.[1] Sildenafil had no effect on tolbutamide plasma concentrations or on the concentration of tolbutamide metabolites. The effect of a dose of sildenafil 100 mg was not evaluated, but little effect on tolbutamide is expected.

RELATED DRUGS: The effect of sildenafil on other oral hypoglycemic agents is unknown, but it is expected to be similar to tolbutamide.

MANAGEMENT OPTIONS: No interaction.

REFERENCES:
    1. *Viagra* [package insert]. New York, NY: Pfizer Pharmaceuticals; 1998.

Simethicone (eg, *Mylicon*)

Warfarin (eg, *Coumadin*)

SUMMARY: Simethicone in a food product purportedly reduced the hypoprothrombinemic response to oral anticoagulants in a few patients, but whether simethicone used as a drug would have any effect is unknown.

RISK FACTORS: No specific risk factors are known.

MECHANISM: It has been proposed that simethicone impairs absorption of oral anticoagulants.

CLINICAL EVALUATION: Several patients who had eaten potato chips cooked in an oil containing methyl polysiloxane (simethicone) manifested a decreased hypoprothrombinemic response to warfarin or phenindione; a causal relationship was not established in this study.[1]

RELATED DRUGS: Phenindione† is affected similarly by simethicone.

MANAGEMENT OPTIONS: No specific action is required, but be alert for evidence of the interaction.

REFERENCES:
    1. Talbot JM, et al. Effect of silicones on the absorption of anticoagulant drugs. *Lancet*. 1971;1(7712):1292.

† Not available in the United States.

Simvastatin (eg, Zocor)

Ritonavir (Norvir)

SUMMARY: Ritonavir administration appears to increase the risk of serious toxicity in patients taking simvastatin.

RISK FACTORS: No specific risk factors are known.

MECHANISM: Ritonavir is a potent inhibitor of CYP3A4, the enzyme that metabolizes simvastatin. The addition of ritonavir may precipitate simvastatin toxicity. Indinavir (*Crixivan*) also inhibits CYP3A4 activity and may have contributed to the interaction with simvastatin observed in this patient.

CLINICAL EVALUATION: A patient with a history of HIV, diabetes mellitus, gastroesophageal reflux disease, and hypercholesterolemia was stabilized on zidovudine (eg, *Retrovir*) 200 mg 3 times daily, lamivudine (*Epivir*) 150 mg twice daily, indinavir 800 mg twice daily, simvastatin 20 mg twice daily, omeprazole (eg, *Prilosec*) 30 mg/day, insulin, and metformin (eg, *Glucophage*) 1,000 mg twice daily.[1] She had tolerated the regimen for more than 2 years. One week prior to developing muscle weakness and body aches, ritonavir 100 mg twice daily was added to her regimen. In addition to pain and weakness, the patient's creatine kinase peaked at more than 23,000 units/L (normal less than 195 units/L). A diagnosis of rhabdomyolysis was made and all drugs except insulin and omeprazole were discontinued. After 10 days, the patient made a full recovery. The potential for indinavir to inhibit the metabolism of simvastatin may have been decreased by the administration of omeprazole because indinavir plasma concentrations can be reduced by omeprazole.[2]

RELATED DRUGS: The clearance of other statins that are metabolized by CYP3A4 (eg, atorvastatin [*Lipitor*], lovastatin [eg, *Mevacor*]) would likely be reduced by ritonavir. Other protease inhibitors, such as amprenavir,† indinavir, nelfinavir (*Viracept*), and saquinavir (*Invirase*), are expected to decrease simvastatin clearance.

MANAGEMENT OPTIONS:

➡ **Use Alternative.** Because pravastatin (eg, *Pravachol*) and fluvastatin (*Lescol*) are not metabolized by CYP3A4, consider using one of these agents in patients taking protease inhibitors.

➡ **Monitor.** Monitor patients taking statins that are metabolized by CYP3A4 and a protease inhibitor for adverse reactions, including myopathy and myoglobinemia.

REFERENCES:

1. Cheng CH, et al. Rhabdomyolysis due to probable interaction between simvastatin and ritonavir. *Am J Health Syst Pharm.* 2002;59(8):728-730.
2. Burger DM, et al. Pharmacokinetic interaction between the proton pump inhibitor omeprazole and the HIV protease inhibitor indinavir. *AIDS.* 1998;12(15):2080-2082.

† Not available in the United States.

Simvastatin (eg, Zocor)

St. John's Wort

SUMMARY: St. John's wort appears to substantially lower simvastatin plasma concentrations; consider using pravastatin as an alternative.

RISK FACTORS: No specific risk factors are known.

MECHANISM: St. John's wort probably enhances the first-pass metabolism of simvastatin by CYP3A4. Enhanced P-glycoprotein activity also may be involved.

CLINICAL EVALUATION: In a double-blind, crossover study, 8 healthy subjects took a single oral dose of simvastatin 10 mg with and without pretreatment with St. John's wort (900 mg/day for 14 days).[1] St. John's wort reduced the simvastatin acid area under the plasma concentration-time curve 62%. The magnitude of this effect is likely to reduce the hypolipidemic response to simvastatin.

RELATED DRUGS: Theoretically, lovastatin (eg, *Mevacor*) would interact with St. John's wort in a manner similar to simvastatin. Atorvastatin (*Lipitor*) also may interact, but probably to a lesser degree. Pravastatin (eg, *Pravachol*) pharmacokinetics were not affected by St. John's wort.[1]

MANAGEMENT OPTIONS:

➠ **Consider Alternative.** Pravastatin does not appear to interact with St. John's wort and would be preferable to simvastatin or lovastatin. Consider an alternative antidepressant to St. John's wort, but nefazodone would not be a good choice with any HMG-CoA reductase inhibitor that is metabolized by CYP3A4 (eg, atorvastatin, lovastatin, simvastatin).

➠ **Monitor.** If St. John's wort is used with simvastatin, lovastatin, or atorvastatin, monitor serum lipid concentrations for evidence of reduced effect.

REFERENCES:
   1. Sugimoto K, et al. Different effects of St John's wort on the pharmacokinetics of simvastatin and pravastatin. *Clin Pharmacol Ther.* 2001;70(6):518-524.

 Simvastatin (eg, Zocor)

Tacrolimus (eg, *Prograf*)

SUMMARY: A patient on tacrolimus developed rhabdomyolysis after simvastatin was added, but a causal relationship was not established.

RISK FACTORS: No specific risk factors are known.

MECHANISM: Not established. Simvastatin is metabolized by CYP3A4, and the authors propose that tacrolimus may be a CYP3A4 inhibitor. However, tacrolimus is not well established as a CYP3A4 inhibitor, and it would be unusual for a drug with such a low dosage (2 mg/day in this patient) to act as a CYP3A4 inhibitor.

CLINICAL EVALUATION: A 51-year-old woman stabilized on tacrolimus after a renal transplant developed rhabdomyolysis approximately 6 weeks after her simvastatin dosage was increased from 10 to 20 mg/day.[1] Although a tacrolimus-simvastatin interaction appears to be the most plausible explanation for the rhabdomyolysis, the patient was also started on fusidic acid (500 mg 3 times daily) 10 days after the simvastatin dose was increased. Isolated cases of rhabdomyolysis after simvastatin and fusidic acid coadministration have been reported; therefore, fusidic acid cannot be ruled out of the reaction.

RELATED DRUGS: Theoretically, other statins metabolized by CYP3A4, such as atorvastatin (*Lipitor*) and lovastatin (eg, *Mevacor*), would also interact with tacrolimus. Numerous cases of myopathy and rhabdomyolysis have been reported with concurrent use of simvastatin or lovastatin with cyclosporine (eg, *Neoral*), and isolated cases have been reported with atorvastatin and cyclosporine. However, pravastatin (eg, *Pravachol*) and fluvastatin (*Lescol*) do not appear to interact with CYP3A4 inhibitors such as cyclosporine and probably would not interact with tacrolimus.

MANAGEMENT OPTIONS:

➡ *Consider Alternative.* Although this interaction is not well documented, until more data are available, avoid simvastatin, lovastatin, or atorvastatin in patients receiving tacrolimus. Pravastatin and fluvastatin are unlikely to interact with tacrolimus and are preferred.

➡ *Monitor.* If simvastatin, lovastatin, or atorvastatin are used with tacrolimus, advise patients to monitor for evidence of myopathy (eg, muscle pain or weakness, dark urine). Elevated creatine kinase levels are another indication of possible myopathy.

REFERENCES:
1. Kotanko P, et al. Rhabdomyolysis and acute renal graft impairment in a patient treated with simvastatin, tacrolimus, and fusidic acid. *Nephron*. 2002;90(2):234-235.

Simvastatin (eg, *Zocor*)

Telithromycin (*Ketek*)

SUMMARY: Telithromycin causes a large increase in simvastatin concentrations.

RISK FACTORS: No specific risk factors are known.

MECHANISM: Telithromycin is known to inhibit CYP3A4, the isozyme primarily responsible for the metabolism of simvastatin. Simvastatin's bioavailability will be increased and its systemic clearance decreased by telithromycin administration.

CLINICAL EVALUATION: While published data are limited, the manufacturer reports that telithromycin increased simvastatin area under the plasma concentration-time curve (AUC) nearly 9-fold and the AUC of its active metabolite 12-fold.[1] This magnitude of increase in simvastatin plasma concentration could cause adverse reactions, including muscle or hepatic toxicity. Based on telithromycin's half-life of 10 hours, discontinue simvastatin during telithromycin administration and for 3 to 5 days after discontinuing telithromycin.

RELATED DRUGS: Telithromycin is likely to affect other statins that are CYP3A4 substrates (eg, lovastatin [eg, *Mevacor*], atorvastatin [*Lipitor*]).

MANAGEMENT OPTIONS:

➡ *Use Alternative.* Pravastatin (eg, *Pravachol*), fluvastatin (*Lescol*), and rosuvastatin (*Crestor*) are unlikely to be affected by telithromycin.

REFERENCES:
1. *Ketek* [package insert]. Bridgewater, NJ: Aventis Pharmaceuticals Inc; 2004.

Simvastatin (eg, *Zocor*)

Ticagrelor (*Brilinta*)

SUMMARY: Ticagrelor modestly increases the plasma concentration of simvastatin; an increased risk of simvastatin adverse reactions is possible.

RISK FACTORS: No specific risk factors are known.

MECHANISM: Ticagrelor appears to modestly inhibit CYP3A4, the primary enzyme responsible for the metabolism of simvastatin.

CLINICAL EVALUATION: While specific data are limited, the manufacturer of ticagrelor notes that the coadministration of ticagrelor 180 mg twice daily increased the mean area under the plasma concentration-time curve of simvastatin 1.5- to 2-fold.[1] Pending further data, observe patients receiving ticagrelor and simvastatin for increased simvastatin adverse reactions, including myopathy and weakness. The manufacturer recommends a maximum simvastatin dose of 40 mg daily during ticagrelor coadministration.

RELATED DRUGS: Lovastatin (eg, *Mevacor*) and atorvastatin (*Lipitor*) are also metabolized by CYP3A4 and expected to interact with ticagrelor.

MANAGEMENT OPTIONS:

➡ *Consider Alternative.* Pravastatin (eg, *Pravachol*), fluvastatin (*Lescol*), and rosuvastatin (*Crestor*) are unlikely to be affected by ticagrelor.

➡ *Monitor.* Monitor patients stabilized on simvastatin for adverse reactions if ticagrelor is initiated.

REFERENCES:
1. *Brilinta* [package insert]. Wilmington, DE: AstraZeneca LP; 2011.

 5

Simvastatin (eg, *Zocor*)

Tolbutamide

SUMMARY: Simvastatin administration produces a minor change in tolbutamide concentrations; patient hypoglycemic response would not be affected.

RISK FACTORS: No specific risk factors are known.

MECHANISM: No interaction.

CLINICAL EVALUATION: Sixteen healthy subjects received simvastatin 20 mg/day for 15 days.[1] A single oral dose of tolbutamide 1 g was administered on days 1 and 15 of simvastatin dosing. The area under the concentration-time curve and peak concentration of tolbutamide were increased less than 10% by simvastatin administration. Oral glucose tolerance tests administered 1.5 hours after tolbutamide administration were not changed by simvastatin coadministration. Tolbutamide administration did not alter simvastatin concentrations. The changes in tolbutamide concentrations are not likely to affect glucose control.

RELATED DRUGS: Fluvastatin (*Lescol*) produces a greater but mild increase in tolbutamide concentrations. The effect of other HMG-CoA inhibitors on tolbutamide is unknown. Simvastatin produced a moderate increase in glyburide (eg, *DiaBeta*) concentrations.

MANAGEMENT OPTIONS: No interaction.

REFERENCES:

1. Appel S, et al. Lack of interaction between fluvastatin and oral hypoglycemic agents in healthy subjects and in patients with non-insulin-dependent diabetes mellitus. *Am J Cardiol.* 1995;76(2):29A-32A.

Simvastatin (*Zocor*)
Verapamil (eg, *Calan*)

SUMMARY: Verapamil administration may increase simvastatin concentrations markedly; avoid using the drugs together for the risk of increased side effects.

RISK FACTORS: No specific risk factors are known.

MECHANISM: Verapamil reduces the intrinsic and first-pass metabolism of simvastatin by inhibition of CYP3A4, the enzyme responsible for simvastatin's metabolism in the intestinal wall and liver.

CLINICAL EVALUATION: A single dose of simvastatin 40 mg was administered to 12 healthy subjects after 2 days of placebo or verapamil 80 mg 3 times/day.[1] The area under the concentration-time curve of simvastatin and its active metabolite, simvastatin acid, were increased 4.6- and 2.8-fold, respectively, by verapamil pretreatment. The half-life of simvastatin increased from 1.2 hours during placebo to 2 hours following verapamil. The increase was not statistically significant, although only 4 subjects in the control phase had half-life determinations. A longer duration of therapy with verapamil may result in an increased magnitude of the effect on simvastatin pharmacokinetics. These verapamil-induced increases in simvastatin concentrations could increase the potential for side effects including myalgias and rhabdomyolysis.

RELATED DRUGS: Diltiazem (eg, *Cardizem*) may affect simvastatin metabolism in a similar manner. The effect of other calcium channel blockers on simvastatin metabolism is unknown but would not be expected to be significant. Verapamil will likely produce a similar increase in lovastatin (*Mevacor*) plasma concentrations. While no data are available, verapamil also may increase the plasma concentration of atorvastatin (*Lipitor*). The metabolism of pravastatin (*Pravachol*) and fluvastatin (*Lescol*) would not be expected to be affected by verapamil.

MANAGEMENT OPTIONS:

➡ *Use Alternative.* Consider the use of an HMG-CoA reductase inhibitor other than simvastatin or lovastatin for patients receiving verapamil. Atorvastatin and cerivastatin plasma concentrations are likely to be increased by a smaller amount during verapamil coadministration. Do not alter pravastatin and fluvastatin metabolism by verapamil.

REFERENCES:

1. Kantola T, et al. Erythromycin and verapamil considerably increase serum simvastatin and simvastatin acid concentrations. *Clin Pharmacol Ther.* 1998;64:177-182.

4   Simvastatin (eg, *Zocor*)

Warfarin (eg, *Coumadin*)

SUMMARY: Preliminary evidence from healthy subjects suggests that simvastatin slightly increases the hypoprothrombinemic response to warfarin, but the clinical importance of this interaction is not established.

RISK FACTORS: No specific risk factors are known.

MECHANISM: Not established. Simvastatin is highly bound to plasma proteins, and it is possible that displacement of warfarin from protein binding would produce a transient increase in hypoprothrombinemic response.

CLINICAL EVALUATION: The manufacturer states that simvastatin increased the prothrombin time approximately 2 seconds in healthy subjects.[1] A 59-year-old woman stabilized on long-term warfarin therapy started simvastatin 10 mg/day for 3 weeks followed by 20 mg/day thereafter.[2] The international normalized ratio remained stable during the simvastatin therapy. Controlled trials in an adequate number of patients receiving warfarin are needed to establish what effect simvastatin has on warfarin response. Although available evidence suggests that simvastatin has only a small effect on warfarin, the possibility that an occasional patient would have a clinically important increase in warfarin response cannot be ruled out.

RELATED DRUGS: Little is known regarding the effect of simvastatin on other oral anticoagulants. Fluvastatin (*Lescol*) appears to inhibit CYP2C9, the primary enzyme in the metabolism of S-warfarin; thus, expect fluvastatin to increase warfarin response. Lovastatin (eg, *Mevacor*) appears to increase warfarin effect, while available evidence suggests that pravastatin (eg, *Pravachol*) does not affect warfarin. Clofibrate[†] and gemfibrozil (eg, *Lopid*) may enhance the hypoprothrombinemic response to warfarin, while cholestyramine (eg, *Questran*) and colestipol (eg, *Colestid*) may reduce its effect.

MANAGEMENT OPTIONS: No specific action is required, but be alert for evidence of the interaction.

REFERENCES:
1. *Zocor* [package insert]. Whitehouse, NJ: Merck; 1993.
2. Gaw A, Wosornu D. Simvastatin during warfarin therapy in hyperlipoproteinaemia. *Lancet.* 1992;340(8825):979-980.

† Not available in the United States.

Sirolimus (*Rapamune*)

Rifampin (eg, *Rifadin*)

SUMMARY: Rifampin administration may markedly reduce sirolimus plasma concentrations; reduction of immunosuppressive effect is likely to occur.

RISK FACTORS: No specific risk factors are known.

MECHANISM: Rifampin is an inducer of the enzyme CYP3A4, which is known to metabolize sirolimus. Rifampin-induced P-glycoprotein activity may also contribute to this interaction by lowering sirolimus plasma concentrations.

CLINICAL EVALUATION: A renal transplant patient was stabilized on sirolimus 4 mg daily. In response to a sputum positive for mycobacterium, rifampin, isoniazid, pyrazinamide, and ethambutol were initiated.[1] The patient's sirolimus dose was raised to 30 mg daily to maintain therapeutic sirolimus concentrations. In a second case, a patient maintained on sirolimus required a 5-fold increase in dose following the initiation of rifampin therapy.[1] While data are limited, the large dose increase of sirolimus required in these cases implies that this interaction is likely to place many patients at risk for subtherapeutic sirolimus concentrations.

RELATED DRUGS: The metabolism of tacrolimus (eg, *Prograf*) is also increased by rifampin. Rifabutin (*Mycobutin*) and rifapentine (*Priftin*) are known to induce CYP3A4 and affect sirolimus in a similar manner.

MANAGEMENT OPTIONS:

➥ *Monitor.* Carefully monitor patients taking sirolimus and monitor plasma sirolimus concentrations when rifampin is initiated and again when it is discontinued.

REFERENCES:

1. Ngo BT, et al. Drug interaction between rifampicin and sirolimus in transplant patients. *Saudi J Kidney Dis Transpl.* 2011;22(1):112-115.

Sirolimus (*Rapamune*)

Voriconazole (eg, *Vfend*)

SUMMARY: Voriconazole administration with sirolimus causes a marked increase in sirolimus plasma concentrations, which are likely to result in toxicity such as bone marrow suppression.

RISK FACTORS:

➥ *Pharmacogenetics.* Patients who are poor metabolizers for CYP2C19 will have higher voriconazole concentrations, and thus are likely to have an interaction of larger magnitude.

MECHANISM: Voriconazole appears to inhibit the metabolism of sirolimus by CYP3A4.

CLINICAL EVALUATION: Based on limited information provided by the manufacturer, a single oral dose of sirolimus 2 mg was administered alone and following voriconazole dosing in healthy subjects.[1] Voriconazole was administered in a dosage of 400 mg every 12 hours for the first day and then 200 mg every 12 hours for 8 days. Following voriconazole dosing, the mean area under the concentration-time curve and peak concentration of sirolimus were increased 11- and 7-fold, respectively. While data are limited, it appears that sirolimus concentrations could frequently be elevated to toxic levels.

RELATED DRUGS: Tacrolimus (eg, *Prograf*) and cyclosporine (eg, *Neoral*) metabolism is reduced by voriconazole administration. The metabolism of other immunosuppressants, such as everolimus (eg, *Afinitor*), is likely to be decreased by voriconazole. Other azole antifungal agents, including ketoconazole (eg, *Nizoral*) and itraconazole (eg, *Sporanox*), are known to reduce the metabolism of sirolimus. Fluconazole (eg, *Diflucan*) also may reduce the metabolism of sirolimus.

MANAGEMENT OPTIONS:

➥ *Use Alternative.* If possible, avoid the coadministration of voriconazole and sirolimus.

REFERENCES:

1. *Vfend* [package insert]. New York, NY: Pfizer Inc; 2002.

Sotalol (eg, *Betapace*)

Ziprasidone (*Geodon*)

SUMMARY: Ziprasidone and sotalol can prolong the QTc interval on the electrocardiogram (ECG). Theoretically, this could increase the risk of ventricular arrhythmias, such as torsades de pointes.

RISK FACTORS:

➡ *Hypokalemia.* The QTc interval on the ECG may be prolonged in patients with hypokalemia, increasing the risk of this interaction.[1]

➡ *Miscellaneous.* Other factors that may prolong the QTc interval (eg, hypomagnesemia, bradycardia, impaired liver function, hypothyroidism) also may increase the risk of ventricular arrhythmias.[1]

MECHANISM: Possible additive prolongation of the QTc interval.

CLINICAL EVALUATION: In initial controlled trials, ziprasidone increased the QTc interval by about 10 msec at the highest recommended dosage of 160 mg/day. However, because of concern that the QTc measurements were done when ziprasidone serum concentrations were low, the Food and Drug Administration recommended additional study.[2,3] In a subsequent study in patients with psychotic disorders, the QTc interval was measured following administration of several antipsychotic drugs (ziprasidone, thioridazine, quetiapine, risperidone, haloperidol, olanzapine) when the antipsychotic drug concentrations were calculated to be at their peak. Ziprasidone increased the QTc by a mean of about 21 msec, which was less than thioridazine (36 msec) but about twice that of the other antipsychotics. Theoretically, the ability of sotalol to prolong the QTc would be additive with ziprasidone, but the extent to which this would increase the risk of ventricular arrhythmias, such as torsades de pointes, is not known.

RELATED DRUGS: Available data suggest that ziprasidone produces less QTc prolongation than thioridazine, but about twice that of quetiapine (*Seroquel*), risperidone (eg, *Risperdal*), haloperidol (eg, *Haldol*), and olanzapine (*Zyprexa*).

MANAGEMENT OPTIONS:

➡ *Use Alternative.* Given the theoretical risk and the fact that sotalol is listed in the ziprasidone prescribing information as "contraindicated," it would be prudent to use an alternative to one of the drugs (see Related Drugs).

➡ *Monitor.* If sotalol and ziprasidone are used concurrently, monitor for evidence of arrhythmias (eg, syncope) and for prolonged QT intervals.

REFERENCES:

1. De Ponti F, et al. QT-interval prolongation by non-cardiac drugs: lessons to be learned from recent experience. *Eur J Clin Pharmacol.* 2000;56(1):1-18.

2. *Geodon* [package insert]. New York, NY: Pfizer; 2001.

3. FDA Psychopharmacological Drugs Advisory Committee. Briefing Document for *Zeldox* Capsules (Ziprasidone HCl). http://www.fda.gov/ohrms/dockets/ac/00/backgrd/3619b1a.pdf. Published July 19, 2000. Accessed June 1, 2011.

Sparfloxacin†

Sucralfate (eg, *Carafate*)

SUMMARY: Sucralfate reduces the plasma concentration of sparfloxacin; loss of efficacy may occur.

RISK FACTORS: No specific risk factors are known.

MECHANISM: It appears that aluminum ions contained in sucralfate may bind to the antibiotic and inhibit its absorption.

CLINICAL EVALUATION: Fifteen healthy subjects received sparfloxacin 400 mg as a single oral dose alone and after 2 days of sucralfate 1 g 4 times daily.[1] Compared with sparfloxacin administered alone, administration with sucralfate resulted in a 39% decrease in the mean peak sparfloxacin concentration. The area under the plasma concentration-time curve of sparfloxacin was reduced 47% by sucralfate preadministration. This reduction in sparfloxacin concentrations could reduce the efficacy of the antibiotic.

RELATED DRUGS: Aluminum-containing antacids (eg, *Maalox*) may produce a similar change in the absorption of sparfloxacin. Sucralfate is known to reduce the absorption of other quinolone antibiotics, such as ciprofloxacin (*Cipro*) and ofloxacin (eg, *Floxin*).

MANAGEMENT OPTIONS:

➡ *Circumvent/Minimize.* While there are no direct data to support separating the doses of sparfloxacin and sucralfate, administration of sparfloxacin 2 to 3 hours prior to sucralfate dosing may minimize the interaction.

➡ *Monitor.* Monitor patients receiving sparfloxacin for reduction in antibiotic efficacy if sucralfate is coadministered.

REFERENCES:

1. Zix JA, et al. Pharmacokinetics of sparfloxacin and interaction with cisapride and sucralfate. *Antimicrob Agents Chemother.* 1997;41(8):1668-1672.

† Not available in the United States.

Sparfloxacin (*Zagam*) 2

Ziprasidone (*Geodon*)

SUMMARY: Ziprasidone and sparfloxacin can prolong the corrected QT interval (QTc) interval on the electrocardiogram (ECG). Theoretically, this can increase the risk of ventricular arrhythmias such as torsades de pointes.

RISK FACTORS:

➡ *Hypokalemia.* The QTc on the ECG may be prolonged in patients with hypokalemia, increasing the risk of this interaction.[1]

➡ *Miscellaneous.* Other factors that may prolong the QTc interval (eg, hypomagnesemia, bradycardia, impaired liver function, hypothyroidism) may also increase the risk of ventricular arrhythmias.[1]

MECHANISM: Possible additive prolongation of the QTc interval.

CLINICAL EVALUATION: In initial controlled trials, ziprasidone increased the QTc interval by approximately 10 msec at the highest recommended dose of 160 mg/day. Because of concern that the QTc measurements were done when ziprasidone serum concentrations were low, the FDA recommended additional study.[2,3] In a subsequent study in patients with psychotic disorders, the QTc interval was measured following administration of several antipsychotic drugs (ziprasidone, thioridazine, quetiapine, risperidone, haloperidol, olanzapine) when the antipsychotic drug concentrations were calculated to be at their peak. Ziprasidone increased the QTc a mean of approximately 21 msec, which was less than thioridazine (36 msec) but about twice that of the other antipsychotics. Theoretically, the ability of sparfloxacin to prolong the QTc would be additive with ziprasidone, but the extent to which this would increase the risk of ventricular arrhythmias, such as torsades de pointes, is not known.

RELATED DRUGS: Available data suggest that ziprasidone produces less QTc prolongation than thioridazine (eg, *Mellaril*), but about twice that of quetiapine (*Seroquel*), risperidone (eg, *Risperdal*), haloperidol (eg, *Haldol*), and olanzapine (eg, *Zyprexa*). Moxifloxacin (eg, *Avelox*), like sparfloxacin, can prolong the QTc interval substantially, but other fluoroquinolones such as levofloxacin (*Levaquin*), ofloxacin (eg, *Floxin*), gatifloxacin (*Tequin*), and ciprofloxacin (eg, *Cipro*) usually produce only minimal effects.

MANAGEMENT OPTIONS:

➡ *Use Alternative.* Given the theoretical risk and the fact that sparfloxacin is listed in the ziprasidone product information as contraindicated, it would be prudent to use an alternative to one of the drugs (see Related Drugs).

➡ *Monitor.* If sparfloxacin and ziprasidone are used concurrently, monitor for evidence of arrhythmias (eg, syncope) and for prolonged QT intervals.

REFERENCES:

1. De Ponti F, et al. QT-interval prolongation by non-cardiac drugs: lessons to be learned from recent experience. *Eur J Clin Pharmacol.* 2000;56:1-18.

2. Product information. Ziprasidone (*Geodon*). Pfizer Pharmaceuticals. 2001.

3. Briefing Information, Psychopharmacological Drugs Advisory Committee, U.S. Food and Drug Administration, July 19, 2000.

Spironolactone (eg, *Aldactone*)

Candesartan (*Atacand*)

SUMMARY: Combining spironolactone with candesartan or other angiotensin II receptor blockers (ARBs) increases the risk of hyperkalemia, especially in patients with 1 or more risk factors.

RISK FACTORS:

➥ *Other Drugs.* In patients taking spironolactone and ARBs, the addition of other hyperkalemic drugs can increase the risk. Such drugs include potassium supplements, nonselective beta-adrenergic blockers, cyclosporine, tacrolimus, NSAIDs, COX-2 inhibitors, trimethoprim, and pentamidine.

➥ *Concurrent Diseases.* Diseases that increase the risk of hyperkalemia for this interaction include diabetes and significant renal impairment.

➥ *Dosage Regimen.* Patients receiving spironolactone in doses of 50 mg/day or more are at greater risk of hyperkalemia from this interaction.

➥ *Effects of Age.* Most of the patients who have developed hyperkalemia from this interaction have been elderly.

➥ *Diet/Food.* A diet high in potassium may increase the risk of hyperkalemia from this interaction. Some salt substitutes contain potassium.

MECHANISM: Both spironolactone and ARBs tend to increase serum potassium, and their effects are additive.

CLINICAL EVALUATION: Wrenger et al describe 44 cases of life-threatening hyperkalemia in patients receiving either ARBs or ACE inhibitors in combination with spironolactone.[1] Numerous other cases have been reported of severe and fatal hyperkalemia following concurrent use of spironolactone and ACE inhibitors.[2-5] It is likely that ARBs also increase the risk of spironolactone-induced hyperkalemia, especially in patients with 1 or more risk factors. Concurrent use of spironolactone and ARBs can be very effective, but without careful patient selection and monitoring, severe hyperkalemia can occur.

RELATED DRUGS: Spironolactone would be expected to interact with other ARBs, including eprosartan (*Teveten*), irbesartan (*Avapro*), losartan (*Cozaar*), telmisartan (*Micardis*), and valsartan (*Diovan*).

MANAGEMENT OPTIONS:

➥ *Circumvent/Minimize.* Use the minimum effective dose of spironolactone; 25 mg/day may be enough for many patients.

➥ *Monitor.* In patients receiving spironolactone and an ARB, monitor serum potassium and renal function, particularly if the patient has 1 or more of the risk factors listed above.

REFERENCES:

1. Wrenger E, et al. Interaction of spironolactone with ACE inhibitors or antiogensin receptor blockers: analysis of 44 cases. *BMJ.* 2003;327:147-149.

2. Schepkens H, et al. Life-threatening hyperkalemia during combined therapy with angiotensin-converting enzyme inhibitors and spironolactone: an analysis of 25 cases. *Am J Med.* 2001;110:438-441.

3. Berry C, et al. Life-threatening hyperkalemia during combined therapy with angiotensin-converting enzyme inhibitors and spironolactone. *Am J Med.* 2001;111:587.

4. Blaustein DA, et al. Estimation of glomerular filtration rate to prevent life-threatening hyperkalemia due to combined therapy with spironolactone and angiotensin-converting enzyme inhibition or angiotensin receptor blockade. *Am J Cardiol*. 2002;90:662-663.

5. Weber EW, et al. Incidence of hyperkalemia in chronic heart failure patients taking spironolactone in a VA medical center. *Pharmacotherapy*. 2003;23:391.

Spironolactone (eg, *Aldactone*)

Enalapril (eg, *Vasotec*)

SUMMARY: Combining spironolactone with enalapril or other ACE inhibitors increases the risk of hyperkalemia, especially in patients with 1 or more risk factors.

RISK FACTORS:

➥ *Other Drugs.* In patients taking spironolactone and ACE inhibitors, the addition of other hyperkalemic drugs can increase the risk. Such drugs include potassium supplements, nonselective beta-adrenergic blockers, cyclosporine, tacrolimus, NSAIDs, COX-2 inhibitors, trimethoprim, and pentamidine.

➥ *Concurrent Diseases.* Diseases that increase the risk of hyperkalemia for this interaction include diabetes and significant renal impairment.

➥ *Dosage Regimen.* Patients receiving spironolactone in doses of 50 mg/day or more are at greater risk of hyperkalemia from this interaction.

➥ *Effects of Age.* Most of the patients who have developed hyperkalemia from this interaction have been elderly.

➥ *Diet/Food.* A diet high in potassium may increase the risk of hyperkalemia from this interaction. Some salt substitutes contain potassium.

MECHANISM: Both spironolactone and ACE inhibitors tend to increase serum potassium, and their effects are additive.

CLINICAL EVALUATION: Following the publication of the RALES study[1] the concurrent use of spironolactone and ACE inhibitors has become commonplace. But while the RALES study found only a 2% risk of hyperkalemia, reports of severe and fatal hyperkalemia have started to appear, especially in patients with risk factors.[2-6] The difference is likely caused by the fact that patients in the RALES study were more carefully monitored and received lower doses of spironolactone. The recommended dose of spironolactone in the RALES study was 25 mg/day. Concurrent use of spironolactone and ACE inhibitors can be very effective, but without careful patient selection and monitoring, life-threatening hyperkalemia can occur.

RELATED DRUGS: Spironolactone would be expected to interact with other ACE inhibitors, including benazepril (*Lotensin*), captopril (eg, *Capoten*), fosinopril (*Monopril*), lisinopril (eg, *Prinivil*), moexipril (eg, *Univasc*), quinapril (*Accupril*), ramipril (*Altace*), and trandolapril (*Mavik*).

MANAGEMENT OPTIONS:

➥ *Circumvent/Minimize.* Use the minimum effective dose of spironolactone; 25 mg/day may be enough for many patients.

➡ **Monitor.** In patients receiving spironolactone and an ACE inhibitor, monitor serum potassium and renal function, particularly if the patient has 1 or more of the risk factors listed above.

REFERENCES:
1. Pitt B, et al. The effect of spironolactone on morbidity and mortality in patients with severe heart failure. Randomized *Aldactone* Evaluation Study Investigators. *New Engl J Med.* 1999;341:709-717.
2. Schepkens H, et al. Life-threatening hyperkalemia during combined therapy with angiotensin-converting enzyme inhibitors and spironolactone. *Am J Med.* 2001;110:438-441.
3. Berry C, et al. Life-threatening hyperkalemia during combined therapy with angiotensin-converting enzyme inhibitors and spironolactone. *Am J Med.* 2001;111:587.
4. Blaustein DA, et al. Estimation of glomerular filtration rate to prevent life-threatening hyperkalemia due to combined therapy with spironolactone and angiotensin-converting enzyme inhibition or angiotensin receptor blockade. *Am J Cardiol.* 2002;90:662-663.
5. Wrenger E, et al. Interaction of spironolactone with ACE inhibitors or angiotensin receptor blockers: analysis of 44 cases. *BMJ.* 2003;327:147-149.
6. Weber EW, et al. Incidence of hyperkalemia in chronic heart failure patients taking spironolactone in a VA medical center. *Pharmacotherapy.* 2003;23:391.

Spironolactone (eg, *Aldactone*)

Warfarin (eg, *Coumadin*)

SUMMARY: Spironolactone reduced the hypoprothrombinemic response to warfarin in healthy subjects, but it is not known whether this effect would be significant under clinical conditions.

RISK FACTORS: No specific risk factors are known.

MECHANISM: Spironolactone diuresis probably increases the concentration of clotting factors in the blood.

CLINICAL EVALUATION: In 9 healthy subjects, spironolactone 200 mg/day for 7 days reduced the hypoprothrombinemic response to a single dose of warfarin (1.5 mg/kg body weight).[1] The plasma warfarin concentration was not changed, but the hematocrit was increased, indicating that the interaction was caused by diuresis and the resultant concentration of clotting factors. This study involved healthy subjects and does not indicate whether the interaction would have been observed in volume-overloaded patients who needed a diuretic. Furthermore, because therapy with spironolactone was short term, this study does not provide evidence about whether this drug interaction would be clinically significant if spironolactone therapy had been initiated well before the anticoagulant or continued chronically.

RELATED DRUGS: The effect of other potassium-sparing diuretics (eg, amiloride [*Midamor*], triamterene [*Dyrenium*]) on oral anticoagulant response is not established.

MANAGEMENT OPTIONS: No specific action is required, but be alert for evidence of the interaction.

REFERENCES:
1. O'Reilly RA. Spironolactone and warfarin interaction. *Clin Pharmacol Ther.* 1980;27:198-201.

5   St. John's Wort

Mycophenolate Mofetil (*CellCept*)

SUMMARY: Preliminary clinical evidence suggests that St. John's wort does not affect the pharmacokinetics of mycophenolate.

RISK FACTORS: None (no interaction).

MECHANISM: None (no interaction).

CLINICAL EVALUATION: In a preliminary open-label study, St. John's wort extract (600 mg for 14 days) was given to renal transplant patients taking mycophenolate and other immunosuppressive agents.[1] Mycophenolate area under the concentration-time curve was unaffected by St. John's wort.

RELATED DRUGS: It is well documented that St. John's wort reduces serum concentrations of cyclosporine and can lead to organ transplant rejection. Preliminary clinical evidence suggests that tacrolimus (*Prograf*) is similarly affected.[1] Theoretically, St. John's wort would also reduce plasma concentrations of sirolimus (*Rapamune*).

MANAGEMENT OPTIONS: No interaction.

REFERENCES:
1. Bauer S, et al. The influence of St. John's wort extract on blood concentrations of cyclosporine A, tacrolimus and mycophenolic acid in renal transplant patients. *Ther Drug Monit*. 2003;25:511.

  St. John's Wort

Rasagiline (*Azilect*)

SUMMARY: Avoid concomitant use of rasagiline and St. John's wort when possible.

RISK FACTORS: No specific risk factors are known.

MECHANISM: Not established. The combination may have additive serotonergic effects.

CLINICAL EVALUATION: St. John's wort reportedly has serotonergic effects and may produce serotonin syndrome when combined with other serotonergic drugs or monoamine oxidase inhibitors, but this effect is not well documented.[1] Nonetheless, the combination is contraindicated in the rasagiline product information, and it would be prudent to follow this advice.

RELATED DRUGS: Any interaction between St. John's wort and rasagiline is likely to be similar with selegiline (eg, *Eldepryl*) and St. John's wort.

MANAGEMENT OPTIONS:

➡ *Avoid Unless Benefit Outweighs Risk.* Avoid concomitant use of St. John's wort with rasagiline or within 2 weeks of stopping rasagiline when possible.

REFERENCES:
1. *Azilect* [package insert]. North Wales, PA: Teva Neuroscience, Inc.; 2006.

St. John's Wort

Tacrolimus (*Prograf*)

SUMMARY: Preliminary clinical evidence suggests that St. John's wort substantially reduces tacrolimus plasma concentrations; avoid the combination.

RISK FACTORS: No specific risk factors are known.

MECHANISM: St. John's wort is known to be a CYP3A4 inducer, the primary isozyme in the metabolism of tacrolimus. It appears likely that St. John's wort reduces the bioavailability and increases the metabolic elimination of tacrolimus.

CLINICAL EVALUATION: In a preliminary open-label study, St. John's wort extract (600 mg for 14 days) was given to renal transplant patients taking tacrolimus and other immunosuppressive agents.[1] The tacrolimus area under the concentration-time curve decreased 58%. The magnitude of this interaction is likely to reduce the efficacy of tacrolimus, increasing the risk of transplant rejection.

RELATED DRUGS: It is well documented that St. John's wort reduces serum concentrations of cyclosporine and can lead to organ transplant rejection. Theoretically, St. John's wort would also reduce plasma concentrations of sirolimus (*Rapamune*).

MANAGEMENT OPTIONS:

➡ *Use Alternative.* In patients receiving tacrolimus, cyclosporine, and probably sirolimus, use antidepressant agents other than St. John's wort when possible. Selective serotonin reuptake inhibitors (SSRIs) and related antidepressants (eg, paroxetine [eg, *Paxil*], sertraline [*Zoloft*], citalopram [eg, *Celexa*], venlafaxine [*Effexor*]) are not known to induce or inhibit CYP3A4 to a clinically important extent. Fluoxetine (eg, *Prozac*) appears to be a weak inhibitor of CYP3A4. Fluvoxamine is a moderate CYP3A4 inhibitor and nefazodone is a potent inhibitor of CYP3A4.

➡ *Monitor.* If St. John's wort is used with tacrolimus, cyclosporine, or sirolimus, monitor for reduced immunosuppressant effect.

REFERENCES:
1. Bauer S, et al. The influence of St. John's wort extract on blood concentrations of cyclosporine A, tacrolimus and mycophenolic acid in renal transplant patients. *Ther Drug Monit*. 2003;25:511.

St. John's Wort

Theophylline (eg, *Theocron*)

SUMMARY: A patient developed decreased theophylline serum concentrations after starting St. John's wort, but a causal relationship was not established.

RISK FACTORS: No specific risk factors are known.

MECHANISM: Not established. The authors propose that the hypericin in St. John's wort may have increased theophylline metabolism.

CLINICAL EVALUATION: A 42-year-old woman developed increasing dosing requirements for theophylline, eventually leading to a dose of 800 mg twice daily with a steady-state theophylline serum concentration of 9.2 mcg/mL.[1] Because St. John's wort was the only agent added during this time, it was discontinued. Seven days later, the theophylline concentration had increased to 19.6 mcg/mL. Although the temporal relationship of the changes in theophylline concentration with the starting and stopping of St. John's wort suggests that an interaction occurred, confirmation is needed.

RELATED DRUGS: No information is available.

MANAGEMENT OPTIONS: No specific action is required, but be alert for evidence of the interaction.

REFERENCES:

1. Nebel A, et al. Potential metabolic interaction between St. John's wort and theophylline. *Ann Pharmacother.* 1999;33:502.

St. John's Wort

Warfarin (eg, *Coumadin*)

SUMMARY: Several cases of reduced warfarin response have been reported with the use of St. John's wort. Although a causal relationship has not been conclusively established, it would be prudent to carefully monitor a patient's warfarin response carefully if St. John's wort is used concurrently.

RISK FACTORS: No specific risk factors are known.

MECHANISM: Not established. Evidence suggests that St. John's wort may act as an enzyme inducer.[1,2] Therefore, it is possible that St. John's wort enhances the hepatic metabolism of warfarin.

CLINICAL EVALUATION: The Swedish Medical Products Agency has received 7 case reports of reduced warfarin effect following the use of St. John's wort.[3,4] In 4 of the cases, the warfarin response returned to baseline after the St. John's wort was discontinued. Although few details of the cases were presented, the evidence suggests that St. John's wort reduces the hyperprothrombinemic response to warfarin.

RELATED DRUGS: Theoretically, acenocoumarol (not available in the US) would interact similarly with St. John's wort, but data are lacking. Phenprocoumon (not available in the US) is metabolized primarily by glucuronide conjugation, a process that may be enhanced by enzyme induction.

MANAGEMENT OPTIONS:

➡ *Consider Alternative.* In patients receiving oral anticoagulants, consider using alternative antidepressants. Selective serotonin reuptake inhibitors (SSRIs) (eg, fluoxetine [eg, *Prozac*], paroxetine [*Paxil*], sertraline [*Zoloft*], citalopram [*Celexa*]) are not known to inhibit CYP2C9, the isozyme primarily responsible for the metabolism of S-warfarin. However, some SSRIs have been reported to increase the risk of bleeding in anticoagulated patients in the absence of an increase in the INR.

➡ *Monitor.* Monitor patients taking warfarin or other oral anticoagulants for altered hypoprothrombinemic response if St. John's wort is started, stopped, or changed in dosage.

REFERENCES:

1. Ruschitzka F, et al. Acute heart transplant rejection due to Saint John's wort. *Lancet.* 2000;355:548.
2. Piscitelli SC, et al. Indinavir concentrations and St. John's wort. *Lancet.* 2000;355:547.
3. Yue QY, et al. Safety of St. John's wort (*Hypericum perforatum*). *Lancet.* 2000;355(9203):576-77.
4. De Smet PA, et al. Safety of St. John's wort (*Hypericum perforatum*). *Lancet.* 2000;355:575.

Succinylcholine (eg, *Anectine*)

Tacrine (*Cognex*)

SUMMARY: Tacrine may prolong the effect of depolarizing neuromuscular blockers such as succinylcholine and theoretically would antagonize the effect of nondepolarizing agents such as curare.

RISK FACTORS: No specific risk factors are known.

MECHANISM: Cholinesterase inhibitors such as tacrine increase the concentration of acetylcholine (*Miochol*) at motor end plates and would be expected to enhance the effect of depolarizing neuromuscular blockers such as succinylcholine. Moreover, succinylcholine is metabolized by plasma acetylcholinesterase, the activity of which is reduced for several hours after tacrine is given.[1-3] Unlike depolarizing neuromuscular blockers, nondepolarizing neuromuscular blockers, such as tubocurarine, tend to be inhibited by cholinesterase inhibitors.

CLINICAL EVALUATION: Based upon the pharmacology and metabolism of tacrine and succinylcholine, it seems quite likely that they would exhibit additive neuromuscular blockade. Although clinical information suggesting adverse consequences from the interaction appears to be lacking, the enhanced neuromuscular blockade could cause difficulties if it is not anticipated. In 1 study of 20 women undergoing laparoscopy, tacrine was combined with succinylcholine intentionally with apparently good results.[4]

RELATED DRUGS: Theoretically, tacrine should antagonize the neuromuscular blockade of nondepolarizing neuromuscular blockers such as tubocurarine, although clinical evidence of the interaction appears to be lacking.[5]

MANAGEMENT OPTIONS:

➡ *Circumvent/Minimize.* Because of the short half-life of tacrine, it should not be difficult to avoid tacrine interactions with neuromuscular blockers. Theoretically, the effect of tacrine should be minimal 10 to 12 hours after the last dose.

➡ *Monitor.* Be alert for altered neuromuscular blockade if tacrine has been given within the previous 24 hours.

REFERENCES:

1. Moriearty PL, et al. Estimation of plasma tacrine concentrations using an *in vitro* cholinesterase inhibition assay. *Alzheimer Dis Assoc Discord.* 1989;3:143.

2. Eldon MA, et al. Investigation of the central and peripheral cholinomimetic effects and plasma cholinesterase inhibition of tacrine. *Clin Pharmacol Ther.* 1992;51:175.

3. Ford JM, et al. Serum concentrations of tacrine hydrochloride predict its adverse effects in Alzheimer's disease. *Clin Pharmacol Ther.* 1993;53:691.

4. Oberoi GS et al. The use of tacrine (THA) and succinylcholine compared with alcuronium during laparoscopy. *P N G Med J.* 1990;33:25.

5. Taylor P. Agents acting at the neuromuscular junction and autonomic ganglia. In: Gilman AG, et al., eds. *The Pharmacological Basis of Therapeutics.* 8th ed. New York, NY: Pergamon Press; 1990:166.

Sucralfate (eg, *Carafate*)

Theophylline (eg, *Theolair*)

SUMMARY: Sucralfate does not affect the bioavailability of nonsustained-release theophylline.

RISK FACTORS: No specific risk factors are known.

MECHANISM: Not established.

CLINICAL EVALUATION: Eight healthy men received a single 5 mg/kg dose of nonsustained-release theophylline with and without sucralfate in a randomized crossover study.[1] Sucralfate was given as 1 g tablets twice daily for 2 days before the theophylline, 1 tablet with the theophylline dose, and 1 tablet 6 hours after the dose. Although sucralfate was associated with a slight reduction in theophylline bioavailability, the effect was not large enough to be clinically important. Nevertheless, the results of this study do not necessarily apply to patients receiving multiple doses of both drugs or to sustained-release theophylline products.

RELATED DRUGS: No information is available.

MANAGEMENT OPTIONS: No specific action is required, but be alert for evidence of the interaction.

REFERENCES:
1. Cantral KA, et al. Effect of sucralfate on theophylline absorption in healthy volunteers. *Clin Pharm.* 1988;7:58.

 Sucralfate (eg, *Carafate*)

Trovafloxacin (*Trovan*)

SUMMARY: Sucralfate reduces the bioavailability of trovafloxacin; a loss of therapeutic efficacy may occur in some patients.

RISK FACTORS: No specific risk factors are known.

MECHANISM: Sucralfate releases aluminum ions when administered. These aluminum ions reduce the bioavailability of trovafloxacin.

CLINICAL EVALUATION: While no published data are available for evaluation, the manufacturer of trovafloxacin has made available some data on this interaction.[1] Like other quinolone antibiotics, the absorption of trovafloxacin is reduced when administered with sucralfate. The area under the concentration-time curve of trovafloxacin administered with sucralfate 1 g was reduced 70%. A reduction of antibiotic efficacy would be expected.

RELATED DRUGS: Sucralfate similarly affects other quinolones such as ciprofloxacin (*Cipro*) and ofloxacin (*Floxin*).

MANAGEMENT OPTIONS:

➥ *Consider Alternative.* The use of H_2-receptor antagonists in place of sucralfate should be considered when trovafloxacin is being administered.

➥ *Circumvent/Minimize.* Administer the antibiotic at least 2 hours before the sucralfate.

➡ *Monitor.* Observe patients receiving trovafloxacin who are administered sucralfate for reduced antibiotic effect.

REFERENCES:

1. Product information. Trovafloxacin (*Trovan*). Pfizer Pharmaceuticals. 1998.

Sucralfate (eg, *Carafate*)

Warfarin (eg, *Coumadin*)

SUMMARY: In isolated cases, sucralfate appeared to inhibit the effect of warfarin, but subsequent studies have failed to demonstrate an interaction.

RISK FACTORS: No specific risk factors are known.

MECHANISM: Not established. If an interaction between sucralfate and warfarin occurs at all, the most likely mechanism would be inhibition of the absorption of warfarin since sucralfate has minimal systemic effects.

CLINICAL EVALUATION: When a 59-year-old man on chronic warfarin therapy (prothrombin times of 26 to 29 seconds) developed upper GI bleeding, the warfarin was stopped and sucralfate started.[1] When the warfarin was restarted and given at the same time as the sucralfate, the prothrombin time was subtherapeutic (12.5 to 14.5 seconds). Discontinuation of the sucralfate was accompanied by a return of the previous hypoprothrombinemic response to warfarin. Sucralfate also was associated with a reduction in the hypoprothrombinemic response to warfarin in a 71-year-old woman, an effect that reversed when the sucralfate was discontinued.[4] In 2 other patients (a 62-year-old woman and 55-year-old man) sucralfate also was associated with reduced hypoprothrombinemic response to warfarin.[5,6] Although it appeared that the sucralfate reduced the effect of warfarin in these patients, 2 subsequent studies in patients stabilized on chronic warfarin therapy failed to demonstrate any effect of sucralfate on plasma warfarin concentrations or hypoprothrombinemic response.[2,3] Thus, it is possible that only certain predisposed patients are affected.

RELATED DRUGS: The effect of sucralfate on oral anticoagulants other than warfarin is not established. Ranitidine (eg, *Zantac*) and famotidine (eg, *Pepcid*) do not interact.

MANAGEMENT OPTIONS:

➡ *Consider Alternative.* Consider using a noninteracting H_2-receptor antagonist, such as ranitidine (*Zantac*) or famotidine (*Pepcid*).

➡ *Circumvent/Minimize.* Take oral anticoagulants at least 2 hours before or 6 hours after sucralfate and try to maintain a relatively constant interval and sequence of administration of the 2 drugs.

➡ *Monitor.* Although this interaction is not well established, monitor for altered oral anticoagulant effect if sucralfate is initiated, discontinued, or changed in dosage. Adjust the anticoagulant dose as needed.

REFERENCES:

1. Mungall D, et al. Sucralfate and warfarin. *Ann Intern Med*. 1983;98:557.

2. Talbert RL, et al. Effect of sucralfate on plasma warfarin concentration in patients requiring chronic warfarin therapy. *Drug Intell Clin Pharm*. 1985;19:456.

3. Neuvonen PJ, et al. Clinically significant sucralfate-warfarin interaction is not likely. *Br J Clin Pharmacol*. 1985;20:178.

4. Rey AM, et al. Altered absorption of digoxin, sustained-release quinidine, and warfarin with sucralfate administration. *DICP*. 1991;25:745.

5. Braverman SE, et al. Sucralfate-warfarin interaction. *Drug Intell Clin Pharm*. 1988;22:913. Letter.

6. Parrish RH, et al. Sucralfate-warfarin interaction. *Ann Pharmacother*. 1992;26:1015. Letter.

Sulfasalazine (eg, *Azulfidine*)

Talinolol

SUMMARY: Serum concentrations of the selective beta-blocker, talinolol, are markedly reduced by the coadministration of sulfasalazine; reduced clinical efficacy is likely to result.

RISK FACTORS: No specific risk factors are known.

MECHANISM: Not established. Sulfasalazine may adsorb talinolol in the gastrointestinal (GI) tract and inhibit the absorption of this beta-blocker or increase talinolol metabolism.

CLINICAL EVALUATION: Eleven healthy subjects were administered 50 mg of talinolol alone or with 4 g sulfasalazine.[1] Following coadministration with sulfasalazine, talinolol was detectable in only 3 of the 11 subjects. The sulfasalazine administration resulted in a dramatic decrease in talinolol concentrations. This interaction is likely to reduce efficacy of talinolol.

RELATED DRUGS: Other beta-blockers may be similarly affected by sulfasalazine administration.

MANAGEMENT OPTIONS:

➡ *Circumvent/Minimize.* If binding in the GI tract is the mechanism for this interaction, giving the talinolol several hours before the sulfasalazine would minimize the interaction. Talinolol and, pending further studies, other beta-blockers should be administered 2 to 3 hours before doses of sulfasalazine.

➡ *Monitor.* If talinolol and sulfasalazine are coadministered, be alert for a reduction in beta-blocker activity.

REFERENCES:

1. Terhaag B, et al. Interaction of talinolol and sulfasalazine in the human GI tract. *Eur J Clin Pharmacol*. 1992;42:461.

Sulfinpyrazone (eg, *Anturane*)

Sulfisoxazole (eg, *Gantrisin*)

SUMMARY: Sulfinpyrazone administration may result in some increase in sulfonamide concentrations, but this increase is unlikely to be clinically significant.

RISK FACTORS: No specific risk factors are known.

MECHANISM: Sulfinpyrazone may displace some sulfonamides from plasma protein binding, resulting in more active (free) drug in the plasma. However, clearance also would increase in this situation, resulting in maintenance of the active drug concentration. Sulfinpyrazone also may affect renal excretion of sulfonamides, which could increase their steady-state concentrations.

CLINICAL EVALUATION: Not established. The action of sulfadiazine and sulfisoxazole reportedly are enhanced by concomitant sulfinpyrazone administration.[1]

RELATED DRUGS: Sulfadiazine is similarly affected by sulfinpyrazone.

MANAGEMENT OPTIONS: No specific action is required, but be alert for evidence of the interaction.

REFERENCES:
1. Anton AH. The effect of disease, drugs, and dilution on the binding of sulfonamides in human plasma. *Clin Pharmacol Ther*. 1968;9:561.

Sulfinpyrazone (eg, *Anturane*)

Tolbutamide (eg, *Orinase*)

SUMMARY: Sulfinpyrazone may increase the hypoglycemic effects of tolbutamide.

RISK FACTORS: No specific risk factors are known.

MECHANISM: Sulfinpyrazone appears to inhibit the metabolism of tolbutamide.

CLINICAL EVALUATION: Six healthy subjects received an IV infusion of 500 mg tolbutamide alone, 30 minutes after a single 400 mg dose of sulfinpyrazone, and 24 hours after the completion of a 7-day course of sulfinpyrazone 200 mg every 6 hours.[1] Tolbutamide clearance was reduced 40% following the single-dose study. Tolbutamide clearance still was 30% below baseline 24 hours after the sulfinpyrazone multiple-dose study despite undetectable sulfinpyrazone plasma concentrations. The changes in tolbutamide clearance induced by sulfinpyrazone are likely to alter the glycemic control of diabetic patients taking tolbutamide. Determination of the effects of chronic sulfinpyrazone (administered at typical dosages) on tolbutamide pharmacokinetics awaits further testing.

RELATED DRUGS: Sulfinpyrazone could potentially affect other sulfonylureas.

MANAGEMENT OPTIONS:

➡ *Monitor.* Diabetic patients receiving tolbutamide may require dosage adjustments when therapy with sulfinpyrazone is initiated or withdrawn. Monitor blood glucose and watch for symptoms of hypoglycemia if sulfinpyrazone is initiated or hyperglycemia if it is withdrawn.

REFERENCES:
1. Miners JO. The effect of sulfinpyrazone on oxidative drug metabolism in man: inhibition of tolbutamide elimination. *Eur J Clin Pharmacol*. 1982;22:321.

Sulfinpyrazone (eg, *Anturane*)

Warfarin (eg, *Coumadin*)

SUMMARY: Sulfinpyrazone markedly increases the hypoprothrombinemic response to warfarin, acenocoumarol, and possibly other oral anticoagulants. If the combination must be used, monitor carefully for excessive hypoprothrombinemia and clinical evidence of bleeding.

RISK FACTORS: No specific risk factors are known.

MECHANISM: The primary mechanism of the sulfinpyrazone-warfarin interaction is inhibition of hepatic warfarin metabolism, although sulfinpyrazone-induced platelet inhibition and protein-binding competition with warfarin also may be involved.

CLINICAL EVALUATION: Numerous cases have been reported of substantial increases in the hypoprothrombinemic response to warfarin following sulfinpyrazone.[1-7] Bleeding occurred in several patients. Controlled studies have confirmed that warfarin and acenocoumarol (*Sintrom*) response is enhanced by sulfinpyrazone.[8-10]

RELATED DRUGS: Acenocoumarol is affected similarly by sulfinpyrazone. Phenprocoumon does not appear to interact with sulfinpyrazone.[11] The effect of sulfinpyrazone on other oral anticoagulants is unknown, but assume that they interact until proven otherwise.

MANAGEMENT OPTIONS:

➥ *Avoid Unless Benefit Outweighs Risk.* Do not use sulfinpyrazone in anticoagulated patients unless the potential benefit clearly outweighs the substantial risk.

➥ *Monitor.* If sulfinpyrazone is used, closely monitor the hypoprothrombinemic response. When warfarin therapy is initiated in patients receiving sulfinpyrazone, increased sensitivity to warfarin's hypoprothrombinemic effect may occur.

REFERENCES:

1. Weiss M. Potentiation of coumarin effect by sulfinpyrazone. *Lancet.* 1979;1:609.
2. Jamil A, et al. Interaction between sulfinpyrazone and warfarin. *Chest.* 1981;79:373.
3. Bailey RR, et al. Potentiation of warfarin action by sulfinpyrazone. *Lancet.* 1980;1:254.
4. Davis JW, et al. Possible interaction of sulfinpyrazone with coumarins. *N Engl J Med.* 1978;299:955.
5. Gallus A, et al. Sulfinpyrazone and warfarin: a probable drug interaction. *Lancet.* 1980;1:535.
6. Thompson PL, et al. Potentially serious interaction of warfarin with sulfinpyrazone. *Med J Aust.* 1981;1:41.
7. Nenci GG, et al. Biphasic sulfinpyrazone-warfarin interaction. *BMJ.* 1981;282:1361.
8. O'Reilly RA. Stereoselective interaction of sulfinpyrazone with racemic warfarin and its separated enantiomorphs in man. *Circulation.* 1982;65:202.
9. Girolami A, et al. Potentiation of anticoagulated response to warfarin by sulfinpyrazone: a double-blind study in patients with prosthetic heart values. *Clin Lab Haematol.* 1982;4:23.
10. Michot F, et al. Uber die Beeiflussung der Gerinnungshemmenden Wirkung von Acenocoumarol durch Sulfinpyrazon. *Schweiz Med Wochenschr.* 1981;111:255.
11. O'Reilly RA. Phenylbutazone and sulfinpyrazone interaction with oral anticoagulant phenprocoumon. *Arch Intern Med.* 1982;142:1634.

4 **Sulfisoxazole (eg, *Gantrisin*)**

Thiopental (eg, *Pentothal*)

SUMMARY: Limited data suggest that sulfisoxazole can potentiate the effects of thiopental.

RISK FACTORS: No specific risk factors are known.

MECHANISM: Some have proposed that sulfisoxazole competes with thiopental for plasma protein-binding, resulting in a temporary reduction in thiopental dosage requirements until plasma clearance increases.[2,3] Phenobarbital may increase the biliary excretion of sulfasalazine, which forms sulfapyridine and 5-aminosalicylic acid in the colon.[1] Also, the hydroxylation of sulfapyridine was increased and its acetylation decreased following phenobarbital administration.[1]

CLINICAL EVALUATION: In 1 study involving 48 patients, IV sulfisoxazole reduced the amount of thiopental required for anesthesia.[3] It is not known whether chronic oral doses of sulfisoxazole would have a similar effect. In a study of 26 healthy subjects and 19 patients with colitis, phenobarbital decreased serum or urine concentrations of sulfasalazine (eg, *Azulfidine*) and some of its metabolites.[1] None of the observed changes seem likely to affect the therapeutic effect of sulfasalazine or increase its toxicity. In a study conducted in children, phenobarbital did not affect the disposition of sulfisoxazole or sulfisomidine.[4]

RELATED DRUGS: Phenobarbital and sulfasalazine interact similarly. Sulfisomidine does not interact with phenobarbital.

MANAGEMENT OPTIONS: No specific action is required, but be alert for evidence of the interaction.

REFERENCES:
1. Schroder H, et al. Metabolism of salicylazosulfapyridine in healthy subjects and in patients with ulcerative colitis. Effects of colectomy and of phenobarbital. *Clin Pharmacol Ther.* 1973;14:802.
2. Csogor SI, et al. Competition between sulphonamides and thiopental for the binding sites of plasma proteins. *Arzneimittelforsch.* 1970;20:1925.
3. Csogor SI, et al. Enhancement of thiopentone anesthesia by sulphafurazole. *Br J Anaesth.* 1970;42:988.
4. Krauer B. Comparative investigations of elimination kinetics of two sulfonamides in children with and without phenobarbital administration. *Schweiz Med Wochenschr.* 1971;101:668. (*Abstract: JAMA.* 1971;216:1888.)

Sulindac (eg, *Clinoril*) **5**

Tolbutamide (eg, *Orinase*)

SUMMARY: No interaction occurs between sulindac and tolbutamide.

RISK FACTORS: No specific risk factors are known.

MECHANISM: No interaction.

CLINICAL EVALUATION: Twelve diabetics stabilized on tolbutamide were given sulindac 400 mg/day for 1 week.[1] No significant changes were noted in tolbutamide plasma concentrations or half-life.

RELATED DRUGS: Phenylbutazone (eg, *Butazolidin*) and aspirin may increase tolbutamide hypoglycemic effects.

MANAGEMENT OPTIONS: No interaction.

REFERENCES:
1. Ryan JR, et al. On the question of an interaction between sulindac and tolbutamide in the control of diabetes. *Clin Pharmacol Ther.* 1977;21:231.

Sulindac (eg, *Clinoril*)

Warfarin (eg, *Coumadin*)

SUMMARY: Although sulindac did not affect the response to warfarin in healthy subjects, several patients receiving warfarin have developed excessive hypoprothrombinemia following sulindac therapy.

RISK FACTORS:

➡ **Concurrent Diseases.** Patients with peptic ulcer disease (PUD) or a history of GI bleeding probably are at a greater risk.

MECHANISM: The mechanism for the enhanced hypoprothrombinemic effect induced by sulindac is not established. Sulindac-induced gastric erosions and inhibition of platelet function theoretically could increase the risk of bleeding in patients receiving oral anticoagulants.

CLINICAL EVALUATION: The hypoprothrombinemic response to chronic warfarin was not significantly different in 10 subjects on sulindac 400 mg/day for 10 days than in 9 control subjects on placebo.[1] However, several cases have been reported describing enhanced hypoprothrombinemia and bleeding when sulindac was added to warfarin therapy.[1-3] Thus, in occasional patients, warfarin and sulindac may interact, but the factors that predispose patients to this interaction have not been established. In a retrospective cohort study, hospitalizations for hemorrhagic PUD were approximately 13 times higher in patients receiving warfarin plus a nonsteroidal anti-inflammatory drug (NSAID) than in patients receiving either drug alone.[4]

RELATED DRUGS: All NSAIDs inhibit platelet function, cause gastric erosions, and probably increase the risk of GI bleeding. However, some NSAIDs such as ibuprofen (eg, *Advil*), naproxen (eg, *Naprosyn*), or diclofenac (eg, *Voltaren*) may be less likely to increase oral anticoagulant–induced hypoprothrombinemia than other NSAIDs.

MANAGEMENT OPTIONS:

➡ **Avoid Unless Benefit Outweighs Risk.** Because all NSAIDs probably increase the risk of GI bleeding in patients on oral anticoagulants, use the combination only after careful consideration of the benefit versus risk. If an NSAID must be used with an oral anticoagulant, it would be prudent to use NSAIDs that are unlikely to affect the hypoprothrombinemic response to oral anticoagulants. If the NSAID is being used as an analgesic or antipyretic, acetaminophen (eg, *Tylenol*) is probably safer to use with oral anticoagulants. Nonacetylated salicylates (eg, choline salicylate, magnesium salicylate, salsalate, sodium salicylate) probably also are safer with oral anticoagulants than NSAIDs, because such salicylates have minimal effects on platelet function and the gastric mucosa.

➡ **Monitor.** If any NSAID is used with an oral anticoagulant, carefully monitor the prothrombin time and watch for evidence of bleeding, especially from the GI tract.

REFERENCES:

1. Loftin JP, Vesell ES. Interaction between sulindac and warfarin: different results in normal subjects and in an unusual patient with a potassium-losing renal tubular defect. *J Clin Pharmacol.* 1979;19:733-742.

2. Ross JR, Beeley L. Sulindac, prothrombin time, and anticoagulants. *Lancet.* 1979;2:1075.

3. Carter SA. Potential effect of sulindac on response of prothrombin-time to oral anticoagulants. *Lancet.* 1979;2:698-699.

4. Shorr RI, et al. Concurrent use of nonsteroidal anti-inflammatory drugs and oral anticoagulants places elderly persons at high risk for hemorrhagic peptic ulcer disease. *Arch Intern Med.* 1993;153:1665-1670.

Sumatriptan (*Imitrex*)

Venlafaxine (*Effexor*)

SUMMARY: The risk of serotonin syndrome may be increased when venlafaxine is used with sumatriptan or other triptans.

RISK FACTORS: No specific risk factors are known.

MECHANISM: Not established. It has been proposed that triptans may have additive serotonergic effects with serotonin/norepinephrine reuptake inhibitors (SNRIs) such as venlafaxine or selective serotonin reuptake inhibitors (SSRIs).

CLINICAL EVALUATION: Cases of possible serotonin syndrome have occasionally been reported with combined use of triptans and SSRIs such as fluoxetine (eg, *Prozac*) and paroxetine (eg, *Paxil*).[1,2] These cases notwithstanding, clinical studies of the combined use of triptans with SNRIs or SSRIs have generally found little evidence of an increased risk of serotonin syndrome. In a prospective study of 12,339 patients who received sumatriptan for migraine, evidence of serotonin syndrome was not seen in the 211 patients receiving venlafaxine concurrently.[3] In a randomized, double-blind, crossover study of 20 healthy subjects, fluoxetine did not affect the pharmacokinetics, pharmacodynamics, or side effects of zolmitriptan (*Zomig*).[4] In another randomized, double-blind, crossover study of 12 healthy subjects, paroxetine did not affect the pharmacokinetics, pharmacodynamics, or side effects of rizatriptan (*Maxalt*).[5] Taken together, this information suggests that combined use of triptans with SNRIs or SSRIs usually does not result in adverse drug interactions, but it is possible that serotonin syndrome occurs in certain susceptible individuals.

In July 2006, however, the FDA issued a public health advisory stating that new information suggests that combined use of triptans with SSRIs or SNRIs can result in serotonin syndrome.[6] Few details were presented on the nature of the information that led to this advisory.

RELATED DRUGS: Theoretically, the risk of serotonin syndrome may be increased by any combination of a triptan (almotriptan [*Axert*], eletriptan [*Relpax*], frovatriptan [*Frova*], naratriptan [*Amerge*], rizatriptan, sumatriptan, zolmitriptan) with an SSRI (citalopram [eg, *Celexa*], escitalopram [*Lexapro*], fluoxetine, fluvoxamine, paroxetine, sertraline [*Zoloft*]) or an SNRI (clomipramine [eg, *Anafranil*], duloxetine [*Cymbalta*], imipramine [eg, *Tofranil*], venlafaxine).

MANAGEMENT OPTIONS: Patients receiving venlafaxine (or other SNRIs or SSRIs) should be alert for evidence of serotonin syndrome if they take sumatriptan or other triptans. Symptoms of serotonin syndrome include agitation, coma, confusion, fever, hyperreflexia, hypomania, incoordination, myoclonus, rigidity, seizures, tremor, shivering, and sweating. Advise patients to contact their health care provider if any of these symptoms occur.

REFERENCES:

1. Hendrix Y, van Zagten MS. Serotonin syndrome as a result of concomitant use of paroxetine and sumatriptan. *Ned Tijdschr Geneeskd.* 2005;149:888-890.
2. Mathew NT, et al. Serotonin syndrome complicating migraine pharmacotherapy. *Cephalalgia.* 1996;16:323-327.
3. Putnam GP, et al. Migraine polypharmacy and the tolerability of sumatriptan: a large-scale, prospective study. *Cephalalgia.* 1999;19:668-675.

4. Smith DA, et al. Zolmitriptan (311C90) does not interact with fluoxetine in healthy volunteers. *Int J Clin Pharmacol Ther.* 1998;36:301-305.

5. Goldberg MR, et al. Lack of pharmacokinetic and pharmacodynamic interaction between rizatriptan and paroxetine. *J Clin Pharmacol.* 1999;39:192-199.

6. FDA Public Health Advisory. Combined Use of 5-Hydroxytryptamine Receptor Agonists (Triptans), Selective Serotonin Reuptake Inhibitors (SSRIs) or Selective Serotonin/Norepinephrine Reuptake Inhibitors (SNRIs) May Result in Life-threatening Serotonin Syndrome. Center for Drug Evaluation and Research (CDER), U.S. Food and Drug Administration. July 19, 2006. Available at http://www.fda.gov/CDER/DRUG/advisory/SSRI_SS200607.htm. Accessed September 6, 2006.

Tacrine (*Cognex*)

Theophylline

SUMMARY: Tacrine can substantially increase theophylline plasma concentrations; reductions in theophylline dosage are likely to be necessary.

RISK FACTORS: No specific risk factors are known.

MECHANISM: Tacrine probably inhibits the hepatic metabolism of theophylline. Tacrine appears to be metabolized by cytochrome P450 1A2,[1] the same isozyme that metabolizes theophylline. Thus, it is possible that tacrine competitively inhibits theophylline metabolism.

CLINICAL EVALUATION: Twelve healthy subjects (older than 50 years of age) took a single oral 158 mg dose of theophylline with and without concurrent multiple dose tacrine (20 mg every 6 hours).[2] Theophylline clearance after oral administration and elimination rate constant were reduced 50% in the presence of tacrine. The manufacturer states that mean plasma theophylline concentrations increase 2-fold in the presence of tacrine.[3] The magnitude of these changes appears sufficient to produce theophylline toxicity in a significant proportion of patients receiving the combination. The effect of theophylline on tacrine plasma concentrations, if any, is unknown.

RELATED DRUGS: No information is available.

MANAGEMENT OPTIONS:

➥ *Consider Alternative.* In patients already receiving tacrine who are being started on theophylline, consider using alternatives to theophylline. If theophylline is used, it would be prudent to begin with smaller than usual doses until the response is determined.

➥ *Circumvent/Minimize.* Given the potential magnitude of the interaction, it may be prudent to adjust theophylline dosage prophylactically in patients at higher risk (eg, those with high pre-existing theophylline plasma concentrations).

➥ *Monitor.* In patients receiving theophylline, monitor clinical status and theophylline plasma concentrations if tacrine is initiated, discontinued, or changed in dosage.

REFERENCES:

1. Madden S, et al. An investigation into the formation of stable, proteinreactive and cytotoxic metabolites from tacrine *in vitro*: studies with human and rat liver microsomes. *Biochem Pharmacol*. 1993;46:13.
2. de Vries TM, et al. Effect of multiple-dose tacrine administration on single-dose pharmacokinetics of digoxin, diazepam, and theophylline. *Pharm Res*. 1993;10:S333. Abstract.
3. Product information. Tacrine (*Cognex*). Parke-Davis. 1993.

Tacrine (*Cognex*) ▼

Trihexyphenidyl (*Artane*)

SUMMARY: Tacrine may inhibit the therapeutic effect of anticholinergic agents such as trihexyphenidyl, and centrally acting anticholinergics may inhibit the therapeutic effect of tacrine.

RISK FACTORS: No specific risk factors are known.

MECHANISM: Tacrine (a cholinergic agent) and anticholinergic agents have mutually antagonistic pharmacologic effects.

CLINICAL EVALUATION: Since tacrine and anticholinergic agents may be mutually inhibitory, the 2 situations will be considered separately.

Effect of Tacrine on Anticholinergic Agents. Tacrine would be expected to inhibit the effect of anticholinergic agents. The effect could be positive if the anticholinergic effect is an unwanted side effect (eg, tricyclic antidepressants, antihistamines, disopryramide [Norpace], phenothiazines). However, when the anticholinergic effect is desired (eg, for Parkinson's disease, GI diseases) the addition of tacrine would be expected to reduce the therapeutic response. Indeed, tacrine has been reported to worsen parkinsonism in at least 1 patient; the worsening responded to the addition of levodopa.[1]

Effect of Anticholinergic Agents on Tacrine. Centrally acting anticholinergics would be expected to inhibit the favorable effect of tacrine on Alzheimer's disease, but little clinical information is available on this point. Peripherally acting anticholinergics would be expected to inhibit the adverse cholinergic effects on tacrine without affecting the therapeutic effect. Indeed, 1 early study of tacrine in a small group of patients with Alzheimer's disease used concurrent therapy with a peripherally acting anticholinergic, glycopyrrolate (*Robinul*), to reduce the incidence of tacrine-induced nausea and vomiting.[2]

RELATED DRUGS: Although more study is needed, one would expect all centrally acting anticholinergic agents to inhibit tacrine response. Tacrine may inhibit the therapeutic effect of anticholinergics.

MANAGEMENT OPTIONS:

➡ **Consider Alternative.** It would be prudent to avoid centrally acting anticholinergic agents in patients receiving tacrine, because they would be expected to antagonize the favorable effects of tacrine in Alzheimer disease.

➡ **Monitor.** If the combination is used, monitor for reduced tacrine response.

REFERENCES:

1. Ott BR, et al. Exacerbation of Parkinsonism by tacrine. *Clin Neuropharmacol.* 1992;15:322.
2. Summers WK, et al. Use of THA in treatment of Alzheimer-like dementia: pilot study in twelve patients. *Biol Psychiatry.* 1981;16:145.

 Tacrine(*Cognex*)

Warfarin (eg, *Coumadin*)

SUMMARY: Tacrine does not appear to affect the anticoagulant response to warfarin.

RISK FACTORS: No specific risk factors are known.

MECHANISM: No interaction.

CLINICAL EVALUATION: Tacrine (20 mg 4 times daily for 5 days) did not affect the hypoprothrombinemic response to warfarin in 13 patients on chronic warfarin therapy.[1]

RELATED DRUGS: No information is available.

MANAGEMENT OPTIONS: No interaction.

REFERENCES:

1. Reece PA, et al. Lack of effect of tacrine administration on the anticoagulant activity of warfarin. *J Clin Pharmacol*. 1995;35:526.

Tacrolimus (*Prograf*)

Posaconazole (*Noxafil*)

SUMMARY: Posaconazole administration results in elevated tacrolimus plasma concentrations; tacrolimus toxicity could result.

RISK FACTORS: No specific risk factors are known.

MECHANISM: Posaconazole is known to inhibit CYP3A4, the primary metabolic pathway for tacrolimus.

CLINICAL EVALUATION: Thirty-six healthy subjects received posaconazole 400 mg twice daily for 8 days.[1] A single oral dose of tacrolimus was administered before and on the eighth day of posaconazole administration. The apparent clearance of tacrolimus was reduced approximately 80% during posaconazole administration. The mean tacrolimus area under the plasma concentration-time curve increased 358% following posaconazole dosing. The occurrence of adverse reactions, including paresthesia, headache, and dizziness, was greater during the posaconazole-tacrolimus coadministration.

RELATED DRUGS: Ketoconazole (eg, *Nizoral*), fluconazole (eg, *Diflucan*), itraconazole (eg, *Sporanox*), and voriconazole (eg, *Vfend*) also inhibit the activity of CYP3A4 and are expected to increase the plasma concentrations of tacrolimus. Posaconazole also reduced the clearance of cyclosporine (eg, *Neoral*) and is expected to affect sirolimus (*Rapamune*) in a similar manner.

MANAGEMENT OPTIONS:

➡ ***Consider Alternative.*** Terbinafine (eg, *Lamisil*) may be considered as an alternative antifungal agent because it does not affect CYP3A4 activity. Amphotericin (eg, *Amphotec*), caspofungin (*Cancidas*), and anidulafungin (*Eraxis*) do not appear to inhibit CYP3A4.

➡ ***Monitor.*** Monitor patients stabilized on tacrolimus for altered tacrolimus dose requirements if posaconazole is added to or discontinued from their drug regimen.

REFERENCES:

1. Sansone-Parsons A, et al. Effect of oral posaconazole on the pharmacokinetics of cyclosporine and tacrolimus. *Pharmacotherapy*. 2007;27(6):825-834.

Tacrolimus (eg, *Prograf*) 4

Tamoxifen (eg, *Soltamox*)

SUMMARY: Drug interaction studies using human liver microsomes in vitro suggest that tamoxifen inhibits the metabolism of tacrolimus; watch for excessive tacrolimus effects if the drugs are used concurrently.

RISK FACTORS: No specific risk factors are known.

MECHANISM: Tacrolimus is metabolized by CYP3A4 and appears to inhibit this process.

CLINICAL EVALUATION: Thirty-four drugs were tested for interactions with tacrolimus using in vitro human liver microsomal preparations.[1] Tamoxifen was found to inhibit tacrolimus metabolism. Although the clinical importance of this finding is not established, in vitro human microsomal studies have been remarkably accurate in predicting which drugs will interact in the clinical setting.

RELATED DRUGS: The effect of tamoxifen on cyclosporine (eg, *Sandimmune*) is not established, but cyclosporine and tacrolimus tend to have similar drug interactions.

MANAGEMENT OPTIONS: No specific action is required, but be alert for evidence of the interaction.

REFERENCES:

1. Christians U, et al. Identification of drugs inhibiting the in vitro metabolism of tacrolimus by human liver microsomes. *Br J Clin Pharmacol.* 1996;41(3):187-190.

 Tacrolimus (eg, *Prograf*)

Telaprevir (*Incivek*)

SUMMARY: The coadministration of telaprevir increases the plasma concentration of tacrolimus; adverse reactions including renal dysfunction may be more likely to occur.

RISK FACTORS: No specific risk factors are known.

MECHANISM: Telaprevir inhibits the CYP3A4-mediated metabolism and P-glycoprotein elimination of tacrolimus.

CLINICAL EVALUATION: While specific data are limited, the manufacturer of telaprevir notes that the coadministration of telaprevir 750 mg every 8 hours for 13 days increased the mean area under the plasma concentration-time curve of tacrolimus by approximately 70-fold.[1] Pending further data, observe patients receiving telaprevir and tacrolimus for increased tacrolimus plasma concentrations and adverse reactions.

RELATED DRUGS: Atazanavir (*Reyataz*), darunavir (*Prezista*), fosamprenavir (*Lexiva*), indinavir (*Crixivan*), nelfinavir (*Viracept*), and saquinavir (*Invirase*) also inhibit the activity of CYP3A4 and are expected to increase the plasma concentrations of tacrolimus. Telaprevir markedly increases the plasma concentration of cyclosporine (eg, *Neoral*); sirolimus (*Rapamune*) may be affected in a similar manner.

MANAGEMENT OPTIONS:

➡ *Avoid Unless Benefit Outweighs Risk.* Generally avoid the coadministration of tacrolimus and telaprevir.

➡ *Monitor.* Monitor patients stabilized on tacrolimus for adverse reactions if telaprevir is coadministered.

REFERENCES:

1. *Incivek* [package insert]. Cambridge, MA: Vertex Pharmaceuticals; 2011.

Tacrolimus (eg, *Prograf*)

Voriconazole (eg, *Vfend*)

SUMMARY: Voriconazole administration increases tacrolimus concentrations; increased adverse reactions may occur in some patients.

RISK FACTORS:

➡ ***Pharmacogenetics.*** Patients who are poor CYP2C19 metabolizers will have higher voriconazole concentrations and, thus, are likely to have an interaction of larger magnitude.

MECHANISM: Voriconazole inhibits the metabolism (CYP3A4) of tacrolimus.

CLINICAL EVALUATION: Based on limited data, voriconazole 400 mg every 12 hours for 1 day followed by 200 mg every 12 hours for 6 days increased the mean area under the concentration-time curve of tacrolimus (0.1 mg/kg orally as a single dose) 3-fold.[1] The mean peak tacrolimus concentration was increased 2-fold. It is likely that some patients may experience tacrolimus toxicity if voriconazole is coadministered.

RELATED DRUGS: The metabolism of sirolimus (*Rapamune*) and cyclosporine (eg, *Neoral*) is reduced by voriconazole administration. The metabolism of other immunosuppressants, such as everolimus (eg, *Afinitor*), is likely to be decreased by voriconazole. Other azole antifungal agents, including ketoconazole (eg, *Nizoral*), fluconazole (eg, *Diflucan*), and itraconazole (eg, *Sporanox*), are known to reduce the metabolism of tacrolimus.

MANAGEMENT OPTIONS:

➡ ***Circumvent/Minimize.*** A reduction in the dose of tacrolimus may be required during coadministration of voriconazole.

➡ ***Monitor.*** Monitor tacrolimus plasma concentrations if voriconazole is prescribed concomitantly. When voriconazole is discontinued, monitor for decreasing tacrolimus concentrations.

REFERENCES:

1. *Vfend* [package insert]. New York, NY: Pfizer Inc; 2002.

Tadalafil (eg, *Cialis*)

Doxazosin (eg, *Cardura*)

SUMMARY: Patients taking doxazosin and tadalafil may have an increased risk of hypotension.

RISK FACTORS: No specific risk factors are known.

MECHANISM: Additive hypotensive effects.

CLINICAL EVALUATION: In a randomized, double-blind, crossover study, 18 healthy subjects received doxazosin 8 mg daily for 7 days followed by tadalafil 20 mg.[1] Tadalafil increased the hypotensive effect of doxazosin, and 5 of the subjects developed systolic blood pressures lower than 85 mm Hg. In another randomized, double-blind, crossover study, 45 healthy men received tadalafil 5 mg daily for 28 days with increasing doses of doxazosin (1, 2, and 4 mg daily) during the last 21 days.[2]

A systolic blood pressure lower than 85 mm Hg was observed in 1 of the 18 men. It appeared that tadalafil produced a low incidence of hypotensive reactions when given with doxazosin.

RELATED DRUGS: Other combinations of alpha-blockers and phosphodiesterase inhibitors may also result in hypotension, but tamsulosin appears to be less likely to interact.

MANAGEMENT OPTIONS:

➡ *Monitor.* If tadalafil or other phosphodiesterase inhibitors are used in patients receiving doxazosin, monitor for evidence of hypotensive reactions.

REFERENCES:

1. Kloner RA, et al. Interaction between the phosphodiesterase 5 inhibitor, tadalafil and 2 alpha-blockers, doxazosin and tamsulosin in healthy normotensive men. *J Urol.* 2004;172(5, pt 1):1935-1940.

2. Guillaume M, et al. Hemodynamic interaction between a daily dosed phosphodiesterase 5 inhibitor, tadalafil, and the alpha-adrenergic blockers, doxazosin and tamsulosin, in middle-aged healthy male subjects. *J Clin Pharmacol.* 2007;47(10):1303-1310.

Tadalafil (eg, *Cialis*)

Tamsulosin (eg, *Flomax*)

SUMMARY: Studies in healthy subjects suggest that tamsulosin does not produce hypotension when combined with tadalafil.

RISK FACTORS: No specific risk factors are known.

MECHANISM: Theoretically, additive hypotension could occur, but it does not appear to be a problem clinically.

CLINICAL EVALUATION: In a randomized, double-blind, crossover study, 18 healthy subjects received tamsulosin 0.4 mg daily for 7 days followed by tadalafil 10 or 20 mg.[1] Additive hypotensive effects were not observed. In another randomized, double-blind, crossover study, 39 healthy men received tadalafil 5 mg daily for 14 days with tamsulosin 0.4 mg daily during the last 21 days. Again, hypotension did not occur.[2]

RELATED DRUGS: Vardenafil (eg, *Levitra*) also does not appear to interact with tamsulosin in producing hypotension.[3] Other combinations of alpha-blockers and phosphodiesterase inhibitors may result in hypotension, but tamsulosin appears to be unlikely to interact.

MANAGEMENT OPTIONS: No specific action is required, but be alert for evidence of hypotensive reactions.

REFERENCES:

1. Kloner RA, et al. Interaction between the phosphodiesterase 5 inhibitor, tadalafil and 2 alpha-blockers, doxazosin and tamsulosin in healthy normotensive men. *J Urol.* 2004;172(5, pt 1):1935-1940.

2. Guillaume M, et al. Hemodynamic interaction between a daily dosed phosphodiesterase 5 inhibitor, tadalafil, and the alpha-adrenergic blockers, doxazosin and tamsulosin, in middle-aged healthy male subjects. *J Clin Pharmacol.* 2007;47(10):1303-1310.

3. Auerbach SM, et al. Simultaneous administration of vardenafil and tamsulosin does not induce clinically significant hypotension in patients with benign prostatic hyperplasia. *Urology.* 2004;64(5):998-1003; discussion 1003-1004.

Tamoxifen (eg, *Soltamox*)

Colchicine (eg, *Colcrys*)

SUMMARY: Based on the interactive properties of the 2 drugs, it is likely that tamoxifen substantially increases colchicine plasma concentrations. Avoid the combination when possible.

RISK FACTORS: No specific risk factors are known.

MECHANISM: Colchicine is a P-glycoprotein and CYP3A4 substrate, and tamoxifen inhibits both P-glycoprotein and CYP3A4; therefore, colchicine plasma concentrations are likely to increase.[1]

CLINICAL EVALUATION: Although the interaction is based primarily on theoretical considerations, it is likely that tamoxifen would increase the risk of colchicine toxicity. Given that colchicine toxicity can be fatal, even a theoretical interaction warrants close attention.

RELATED DRUGS: No information is available.

MANAGEMENT OPTIONS:

➥ *Avoid Unless Benefit Outweighs Risk.* Considering that colchicine toxicity can be life-threatening, use the combination only if it is likely to provide therapeutic benefits that cannot be achieved with noninteracting alternatives.

➥ *Use Alternative.* If possible, avoid colchicine in patients receiving tamoxifen.

➥ *Monitor.* If the combination must be used, monitor carefully for colchicine toxicity (eg, abdominal pain, diarrhea, fever, muscle pain, vomiting). Advise patients to immediately contact their health care provider if any of these symptoms occur. Colchicine-induced pancytopenia can result in infections, bleeding, and anemia, and is often the cause of death in fatal cases.

REFERENCES:

1. Rautio J, et al. In vitro p-glycoprotein inhibition assays for assessment of clinical drug interaction potential of new drug candidates: a recommendation for probe substrates. *Drug Metab Dispos.* 2006;34(5):786-792.

Tapentadol (*Nucynta*)

Almotriptan (*Axert*)

SUMMARY: Theoretically, combined use of tapentadol and triptans such as almotriptan could increase the risk of serotonin syndrome, but the clinical importance of this effect is not established.

RISK FACTORS: No specific risk factors are known.

MECHANISM: Tapentalol may inhibit serotonin and norepinephrine reuptake, and theoretically might have additive serotonergic effects when combined with other serotonergic drugs.

CLINICAL EVALUATION: This interaction is based primarily on theoretical considerations, and reports of serotonin syndrome appear to be lacking. Nonetheless, life-threatening serotonin syndrome is theoretically possible.[1]

RELATED DRUGS: Theoretically, any triptan could interact with tapentadol, including eletriptan (*Relpax*), frovatriptan (*Frova*), naratriptan (*Amerge*), rizatriptan (*Maxalt*), sumatriptan (eg, *Imitrex*), and zolmitriptan (*Zomig*).

MANAGEMENT OPTIONS:

➡ *Monitor.* Monitor for evidence of serotonin syndrome (eg, agitation, coma, confusion, fever, hyperreflexia, hypomania, incoordination, myoclonus, rigidity, seizures, shivering, sweating, tremor).

REFERENCES:

1. *Nucynta* [package insert]. Raritan, NJ: Ortho-McNeil Janssen; 2009.

Tapentadol (*Nucynta*)

Clomipramine (eg, *Anafranil*)

SUMMARY: Theoretically, combined use of tapentadol and selective serotonin/norepinephrine reuptake inhibitors (SNRIs) such as clomipramine could increase the risk of serotonin syndrome, but the clinical importance of this effect is not established.

RISK FACTORS: No specific risk factors are known.

MECHANISM: Tapentalol may inhibit serotonin and norepinephrine reuptake, and theoretically might have additive serotonergic effects when combined with other serotonergic drugs.

CLINICAL EVALUATION: This interaction is based primarily on theoretical considerations, and even though a number of patients have received tapentadol with SNRIs, reports of serotonin syndrome appear to be lacking. Nonetheless, life-threatening serotonin syndrome is theoretically possible.[1]

RELATED DRUGS: Theoretically, any SNRI could interact with tapentadol, including desvenlafaxine (*Pristiq*), duloxetine (*Cymbalta*), imipramine (eg, *Tofranil*), and venlafaxine (eg, *Effexor*). Theoretically, selective serotonin reuptake inhibitors could also interact with tapentadol.

MANAGEMENT OPTIONS:

➡ *Monitor.* Monitor for evidence of serotonin syndrome (eg, agitation, coma, confusion, fever, hyperreflexia, hypomania, incoordination, myoclonus, rigidity, seizures, shivering, sweating, tremor).

REFERENCES:

1. *Nucynta* [package insert]. Raritan, NJ: Ortho-McNeil Janssen; 2009.

Tapentadol (*Nucynta*)

Fluoxetine (eg, *Prozac*)

SUMMARY: Theoretically, the combined use of tapentadol and selective serotonin reuptake inhibitors (SSRIs) such as fluoxetine could increase the risk of serotonin syndrome, but the clinical importance of this effect is not established.

RISK FACTORS: No specific risk factors are known.

MECHANISM: Tapentalol may inhibit serotonin and norepinephrine reuptake, and thus theoretically might have additive serotonergic effects when combined with other serotonergic drugs.

CLINICAL EVALUATION: This interaction is based primarily on theoretical considerations, and even though a number of patients have received tapentadol with SSRIs, reports of serotonin syndrome appear to be lacking. Nonetheless, life-threatening serotonin syndrome is theoretically possible.[1]

RELATED DRUGS: Theoretically, any SSRI could interact with tapentadol, including citalopram (eg, *Celexa*), escitalopram (*Lexapro*), fluvoxamine (eg, *Luvox*), paroxetine (eg, *Paxil*), and sertraline (eg, *Zoloft*). Theoretically, serotonin/norepinephrine reuptake inhibitors could also interact with tapentadol.

MANAGEMENT OPTIONS:

➡ **Monitor.** Monitor for evidence of serotonin syndrome (eg, agitation, coma, confusion, fever, hyperreflexia, hypomania, incoordination, myoclonus, rigidity, seizures, shivering, sweating, tremor).

REFERENCES:

1. *Nucynta* [package insert]. Raritan, NJ: Ortho-McNeil Janssen; 2009.

Tapentadol (*Nucynta*)

Tranylcypromine (eg, *Parnate*) AVOID

SUMMARY: Theoretically, combined use of tapentadol and monoamine oxidase inhibitors (MAOIs) such as tranylcypromine could result in severe cardiovascular reactions.

RISK FACTORS: No specific risk factors are known.

MECHANISM: Tapentalol may inhibit norepinephrine reuptake, and thus produce additive cardiovascular effects with nonselective MAOIs.

CLINICAL EVALUATION: This interaction is based primarily on theoretical considerations, but the reaction is potentially life-threatening. Reactions could include hypertension, seizures, and arrhythmias.[1]

RELATED DRUGS: Expect all nonselective MAOIs to interact similarly with tapentadol. This includes phenelzine (*Nardil*) and isocarboxazid; MAO-B inhibitors such as rasagiline (*Azilect*) and selegiline (eg, *Eldepryl*) may act as nonselective MAOIs in some patients, especially if large doses are used.

MANAGEMENT OPTIONS:

➡ **AVOID COMBINATION.** Avoid giving tapentadol to patients taking MAOIs or within 14 days of stopping an MAOI.

REFERENCES:

1. *Nucynta* [package insert]. Raritan, NJ: Ortho-McNeil Janssen; 2009.

4 Telithromycin (*Ketek*)

Sotalol (eg, *Betapace*)

SUMMARY: Coadministration of telithromycin and sotalol reduces the plasma concentration of sotalol; some patients may have a reduced therapeutic response to sotalol.

RISK FACTORS: No specific risk factors are known.

MECHANISM: Unknown. It appears that coadministration of telithromycin with sotalol reduces the absorption of sotalol.

CLINICAL EVALUATION: Twenty-four healthy women received a single dose of telithromycin 800 mg or placebo with a single dose of sotalol 160 mg.[1] During telithromycin coadministration, the mean area under the plasma concentration-time curve and peak plasma concentration of sotalol was reduced 34% and 20%, respectively. The mean half-life of sotalol was increased 30% by telithromycin coadministration; however, blood sampling time was less than 3 half-lives. The QTc interval was reduced by 15 to 20 msec during telithromycin coadministration compared with sotalol alone. The effect of telithromycin on sotalol when the drugs are not administered at the same time is unknown.

RELATED DRUGS: None known.

MANAGEMENT OPTIONS:

➥ **Monitor.** Monitor the patient's antiarrhythmic response to sotalol if telithromycin is coadministered. Dose adjustments of sotalol may be necessary when telithromycin is initiated or discontinued.

REFERENCES:
1. Démolis JL, et al. Assessment of the effect of a single oral dose of telithromycin on sotalol-induced QT interval prolongation in healthy women. *Br J Clin Pharmacol*. 2005;60(2):120-127.

4 Telithromycin (*Ketek*)

Warfarin (eg, *Coumadin*)

SUMMARY: Telithromycin did not affect warfarin pharmacokinetics in healthy subjects; patients with infections may be more susceptible to alterations in their INR.

RISK FACTORS: No specific risk factors are known.

MECHANISM: Telithromycin does not inhibit CYP2C9, the isoenzyme primarily responsible for the metabolism of warfarin. It is not known if telithromycin's inhibition of CYP3A4 may have contributed to, or if other factors caused, the elevated INR in the patient discussed in the case report.

CLINICAL EVALUATION: In a study of healthy subjects, telithromycin 800 mg daily for 5 days produced no effect on the pharmacokinetics of a single dose of warfarin.[1] A case has been reported of a patient with an elevated INR following 5 days of telithromycin administration for cough and dyspnea.[2] Other factors may have contributed to the increased INR in this patient.

RELATED DRUGS: No information is available.

MANAGEMENT OPTIONS:

➡ *Monitor.* Monitor patients taking warfarin for altered INR during any acute illness, including infections treated with antibiotics.

REFERENCES:

1. *Ketek* [package insert]. Bridgewater, NJ: Aventis Pharmaceuticals, Inc; 2004.

2. Kolilekas L, et al. Potential interaction between telithromycin and warfarin. *Ann Pharmacother.* 2004;38(9):1424-1427.

Temafloxacin†

Warfarin (eg, *Coumadin*)

SUMMARY: Temafloxacin appears to have little or no effect on the hypoprothrombinemic effects of warfarin.

RISK FACTORS: No specific risk factors are known.

MECHANISM: Not established.

CLINICAL EVALUATION: In 10 healthy men receiving warfarin, temafloxacin 600 mg twice daily tended to decrease international normalized ratio (INR) during dosing but not significantly.[1] Mean S-warfarin (the active enantiomer) concentration fell from 0.33 mg/L on day 12 to 0.2 mg/L on day 16. Temafloxacin does not appear to cause a significant alteration in the response to warfarin.

RELATED DRUGS: Ciprofloxacin (eg, *Cipro*), norfloxacin (*Noroxin*), and other quinolones have been noted to increase the response to warfarin.

MANAGEMENT OPTIONS: No specific action is required, but be alert for evidence of the interaction.

REFERENCES:

1. Millar E, et al. Temafloxacin does not potentiate the anticoagulant effect of warfarin in healthy subjects. *Clin Pharmacokinet.* 1992;22(suppl 1):102-106.

† Not available in the United States.

Terbinafine (eg, *Lamisil*)

Tamoxifen (eg, *Soltamox*)

SUMMARY: Theoretically, terbinafine may reduce the efficacy of tamoxifen in the treatment of breast cancer.

RISK FACTORS: No specific risk factors are known.

MECHANISM: Tamoxifen is metabolized to 2 active metabolites by CYP2D6, the most important of which is endoxifen. By reducing endoxifen formation, CYP2D6 inhibitors such as terbinafine may reduce tamoxifen efficacy.[1-3]

CLINICAL EVALUATION: A study in patients with breast cancer found substantial reductions in endoxifen plasma concentrations in patients taking potent CYP2D6 inhibitors such as fluoxetine and paroxetine.[4] Another tamoxifen study found a nearly 2-fold increase in the risk of breast cancer relapse in women with low CYP2D6 activity, either due to CYP2D6-inhibiting drugs or genetic deficiency.[5] Taken together, these (and other) results strongly suggest that CYP2D6 inhibitors reduce the efficacy of tamoxifen in the treatment of breast cancer. Terbinafine is a CYP2D6 inhibitor, and may inhibit the anticancer effects of tamoxifen.

RELATED DRUGS: No information is available.

MANAGEMENT OPTIONS:

➡ **Consider Alternative.** Azole antifungal agents may be less likely to inhibit CYP2D6; check current CYP-450 information and use alternative if possible.

➡ **Monitor.** If a CYP2D6 inhibitor such as terbinafine is used with tamoxifen, cancer recurrence may be an indication that tamoxifen efficacy has been reduced. If this happens, consider discontinuing the CYP2D6 inhibitor.

REFERENCES:
1. Dezentjé VO, et al. Clinical implications of CYP2D6 genotyping in tamoxifen treatment for breast cancer. *Clin Cancer Res*. 2009;15(1):15-21.
2. Tan SH, et al. Pharmacogenetics in breast cancer therapy. *Clin Cancer Res*. 2008;14(24):8027-8041.
3. Newman WG, et al. Impaired tamoxifen metabolism reduces survival in familial breast cancer patients. *Clin Cancer Res*. 2008;14(18):5913-5918.
4. Borges S, et al. Quantitative effect of CYP2D6 genotype and inhibitors on tamoxifen metabolism: implication for optimization of breast cancer treatment. *Clin Pharmacol Ther*. 2006;80(1):61-74.
5. Goetz MP, et al. The impact of cytochrome P450 2D6 metabolism in women receiving adjuvant tamoxifen. *Breast Cancer Res Treat*. 2007;101(1):113-121.

Terbinafine (eg, *Lamisil*)

Triazolam (eg, *Halcion*)

SUMMARY: Terbinafine had no effect on triazolam serum concentrations.

RISK FACTORS: No specific risk factors are known.

MECHANISM: No interaction.

CLINICAL EVALUATION: Twelve healthy subjects received placebo or terbinafine 250 mg/day for 4 days.[1] A single dose of triazolam 0.25 mg was administered on day 4. No significant differences in triazolam pharmacokinetics or pharmacodynamics were noted following terbinafine compared with placebo.

RELATED DRUGS: Other antifungal agents, including ketoconazole (eg, *Nizoral*) and itraconazole (eg, *Sporanox*), are known to inhibit the metabolism of triazolam. Terbinafine is not expected to alter the metabolism of other benzodiazepines, such as diazepam (eg, *Valium*) or midazolam.

MANAGEMENT OPTIONS: No interaction.

REFERENCES:
1. Varhe A, et al. Fluconazole, but not terbinafine, enhances the effect of triazolam by inhibiting its metabolism. *Br J Clin Pharmacol*. 1996;41(4):319-323.

---

5 Terfenadine†

Theophylline (eg, *Uniphyl*)

SUMMARY: Terfenadine does not affect the pharmacokinetics of theophylline in healthy subjects.

RISK FACTORS: No specific risk factors are known.

MECHANISM: No interaction.

CLINICAL EVALUATION: After a case of possible terfenadine-induced theophylline toxicity was reported, 17 healthy subjects were given theophylline 4 mg/kg as immediate-release tablets every 8 hours for 15 days with and without concomitant treatment with terfenadine 60 mg twice daily.[1] Terfenadine was not associated with changes in any of the following theophylline parameters: elimination rate constant, area under the theophylline concentration-time curve, maximum serum concentration, or time to maximum serum concentration.

RELATED DRUGS: No information is available.

MANAGEMENT OPTIONS: No interaction.

REFERENCES:

1. Luskin SS, et al. Pharmacokinetic evaluation of the terfenadine-theophylline interaction. *J Allergy Clin Immunol.* 1989;83(2 pt 1):406-411.

† Not available in the United States.

Terfenadine†

Troleandomycin†

SUMMARY: The administration of troleandomycin with terfenadine may lead to arrhythmias.

RISK FACTORS: No specific risk factors are known.

MECHANISM: Troleandomycin probably inhibits the activity of CYP3A4, the hepatic enzyme responsible for the metabolism of terfenadine. Higher levels of unchanged terfenadine are cardiotoxic.

CLINICAL EVALUATION: A 79-year-old woman was taking terfenadine 60 mg 3 times daily.[1] Troleandomycin 500 mg 3 times daily was added to her therapy for pulmonary infection. Two weeks later, the patient was admitted with torsades de pointes rhythm and a prolonged QTc on the electrocardiogram (ECG). Her ECG returned to normal 3 days after discontinuation of both drugs. A rechallenge with both terfenadine 60 mg 3 times daily and troleandomycin 500 mg 3 times daily again produced prolongation of her QTc. The administration of terfenadine or troleandomycin alone did not produce any change in the ECG.

RELATED DRUGS: Erythromycin (eg, *Ery-Tab*) and clarithromycin (eg, *Biaxin*) inhibit terfenadine metabolism. Astemizole† metabolism may be inhibited by troleandomycin. Azithromycin (eg, *Zithromax*) and dirithromycin† do not alter terfenadine concentrations.

MANAGEMENT OPTIONS:

➡ *Use Alternative.* Avoid taking terfenadine and troleandomycin because of the risk of arrhythmias. Astemizole may not be a safe alternative to terfenadine because it has been associated with arrhythmias when administered with drugs that inhibit its metabolism. The use of sedating antihistamines, cetirizine (eg, *Zyrtec*) or loratadine (eg, *Claritin*), may be preferable in patients who require antihistamine therapy during troleandomycin treatment.

REFERENCES:

1. Fournier P, et al. A new cause of torsades de pointes: combination of terfenadine and troleandomycin [in French]. *Ann Cardiol Angeiol* (Paris). 1993;42(5):249-252.

† Not available in the United States.

Terfenadine (*Seldane*)

Zafirlukast (*Accolate*)

SUMMARY: Studies in healthy subjects suggest that terfenadine substantially reduces the plasma concentrations of zafirlukast, but the degree to which this reduces the therapeutic response of zafirlukast in asthmatic patients is not established.

RISK FACTORS: No specific risk factors are known.

MECHANISM: Not established.

CLINICAL EVALUATION: In 16 healthy subjects, dosing of both zafirlukast 320 mg/day and terfenadine 60 mg twice daily to steady state resulted in a 54% reduction in the zafirlukast area under the plasma concentration-time curve compared with zafirlukast alone.[1] However, there was no effect of zafirlukast on terfenadine plasma concentrations or changes in the electrocardiogram (eg, prolongation of the QTc interval). Because the details of this study were not presented, it is not possible to assess its validity. Nonetheless, the magnitude of the reduction in zafirlukast plasma concentration is expected to reduce its therapeutic effect. Studies in asthmatic patients are needed to assess this possibility.

RELATED DRUGS: The effect of other antihistamines on zafirlukast pharmacokinetics is not established. Because astemizole† has interactive properties similar to terfenadine, it may interact with zafirlukast in a similar manner. However, no information is available.

MANAGEMENT OPTIONS:

➡ **Consider Alternative.** In patients on zafirlukast, consider using antihistamines with fewer interactive properties than terfenadine or astemizole.

➡ **Monitor.** If the combination is used, monitor for reduced zafirlukast response (ie, uncontrolled asthma).

REFERENCES:

1. *Accolate* [package insert]. Wilmington, DE: AstraZeneca LP; 1996.

Tetrabenazine (*Xenazine*)

AVOID Tranylcypromine (eg, *Parnate*)

SUMMARY: Tetrabenazine is contraindicated with monoamine oxidase inhibitors (MAOIs), such as tranylcypromine.

RISK FACTORS: No specific risk factors are known.

MECHANISM: Not established. The interaction is based primarily on theoretical considerations.

CLINICAL EVALUATION: Clinical evidence of an interaction between tetrabenazine and MAOIs is lacking, but given tetrabenazine's effects on monoamine transporters, the combination is contraindicated.[1]

RELATED DRUGS: Other nonselective MAOIs are also contraindicated with tetrabenazine, including furazolidone, isocarboxazid (*Marplan*), methylene blue (eg, *Urolene Blue*), and phenelzine (*Nardil*). The effect of selective MAO-A or selective MAO-B inhibitors is not established.

MANAGEMENT OPTIONS: Avoid the combination of tetrabenazine with MAOIs. Wait at least 2 weeks after stopping the MAOI before starting tetrabenazine.

REFERENCES:

1. *Xenazine* [package insert]. Deerfield, IL: Lundbeck Inc; 2010.

Tetracycline (eg, *Sumycin*)

Theophylline (eg, *Theochron*)

SUMMARY: Case reports have noted that tetracycline increased theophylline plasma concentrations. Prospective studies have not demonstrated a consistent effect.

RISK FACTORS: No specific risk factors are known.

MECHANISM: Not established.

CLINICAL EVALUATION: A patient had been maintained on sustained-release theophylline 300 mg 3 times daily.[1] Her theophylline concentration was 11.7 to 13 mg/L before starting the tetracycline. After 10 days of tetracycline therapy, the patient complained of nausea, vomiting, and tremors, and her theophylline concentration was 30.8 mg/L. Thirty-six hours after discontinuing theophylline and tetracycline, her theophylline concentration was 4.1 mg/L, and theophylline was restarted at a dosage of 300 mg twice daily. Tetracycline was administered again, and her theophylline concentration increased from 9.7 to 14.4 mg/L over the following 6 days. However, 2 prior studies involving patients[2,3] and 1 involving healthy subjects[4] failed to find a statistically significant decrease in theophylline clearance. The duration of tetracycline administration, however, was less (2 to 7 days), and theophylline clearance was reduced more than 20% in some subjects.

RELATED DRUGS: Minocycline (eg, *Minocin*) also has been noted in case reports to increase theophylline concentrations.[5,6] Doxycycline (eg, *Vibramycin*) 100 mg/day produced no effects on theophylline pharmacokinetics.[7]

MANAGEMENT OPTIONS: No specific action is required, but be alert for evidence of the interaction.

REFERENCES:

1. McCormack JP, et al. Theophylline toxicity induced by tetracycline. *Clin Pharm.* 1990;9(7):546-549.
2. Gotz VP, et al. Evaluation of tetracycline on theophylline disposition in patients with chronic obstructive airways disease. *Drug Intell Clin Pharm.* 1986;20(9):694-697.
3. Pfeifer HJ, et al. Effects of three antibiotics on theophylline kinetics. *Clin Pharmacol Ther.* 1979;26(1):36-40.
4. Mathis JW, et al. Effect of tetracycline hydrochloride on theophylline kinetics. *Clin Pharm.* 1982;1(5):446-448.
5. Ueno K, et al. Interaction between theophylline and minocycline. *Jpn J Ther Drug Monit.* 1991;7:140-143.
6. Kawai M, et al. Possible theophylline-minocycline interaction. *Ann Pharmacother.* 1992;26(10):1300-1301.
7. Jonkman JH, et al. No influence of doxycycline on theophylline pharmacokinetics. *Ther Drug Monit.* 1985;7(1):92-94.

4   Tetracycline (eg, *Sumycin*)

Thiazides

SUMMARY: The combined use of tetracyclines and thiazides may result in elevated blood urea nitrogen (BUN) levels.

RISK FACTORS:

➡ *Concurrent Disease: Preexisting Renal Disease.* Patients with preexisting renal disease are at increased risk.

MECHANISM: Both tetracyclines and diuretics have independently been reported to elevate BUN levels. The tetracycline effect probably is caused by its antianabolic action.

CLINICAL EVALUATION: Analysis of data from an epidemiological study has revealed that concomitant therapy with tetracycline and diuretics tends to result in elevated BUN levels.[1,2] The clinical consequences of this effect were not detailed in the report, but it is reasonable to assume that this effect would be undesirable in patients with previous renal impairment. The specific diuretics involved were not specified.

RELATED DRUGS: None known.

MANAGEMENT OPTIONS:

➡ *Monitor.* No specific action is required, but be alert for evidence of the interaction.

REFERENCES:

1. Boston Collaborative Drug Surveillance Program. Tetracycline and drug-attributed rises in blood urea nitrogen. *JAMA.* 1972;220(3):377-379.
2. [No authors listed]. Tetracycline and rises in urea nitrogen. *JAMA.* 1972;221(7):713-714.

3   Tetracycline (eg, *Sumycin*)

Zinc

SUMMARY: Zinc may reduce the serum concentration of tetracycline enough to reduce its antibacterial efficacy.

RISK FACTORS: No specific risk factors are known.

MECHANISM: Zinc appears to impair the GI absorption of tetracycline, possibly by chelation.

CLINICAL EVALUATION: Zinc sulfate 200 to 220 mg decreases both the serum concentrations[1,2] and total urinary excretion of tetracycline.[3] The magnitude of these decreases appears large enough to impair the therapeutic response to tetracycline.

RELATED DRUGS: Doxycycline (eg, *Vibramycin*) absorption was not significantly affected by zinc coadministration.[1]

MANAGEMENT OPTIONS:

➡ *Consider Alternative.* Doxycycline may be considered as an alternative.

➡ *Circumvent/Minimize.* When patients are receiving both tetracycline and zinc sulfate, administer the drugs as far apart as possible to minimize mixing in the GI tract. Tetracycline should be taken 2 to 3 hours before zinc.

➡ *Monitor.* If tetracycline and foods or dairy products containing large amounts of cations are coadministered, be alert for reduced antibiotic effects.

REFERENCES:

1. Penttilä O, et al. Effect of zinc sulphate on the absorption of tetracycline and doxycycline in man. *Eur J Clin Pharmacol.* 1975;9(2-3):131-134.
2. Andersson KE, et al. Inhibition of tetracycline absorption by zinc. *Eur J Clin Pharmacol.* 1976;10:59.
3. Mapp RK, et al. The effect of zinc sulphate and of bicitropeptide on tetracycline absorption. *S Afr Med J.* 1976;50(45):1829-1830.

Theophylline (eg, *Theochron*) **5**
Tamsulosin (*Flomax*)

SUMMARY: Tamsulosin does not appear to affect the pharmacokinetics of theophylline.

RISK FACTORS: No specific risk factors are known.

MECHANISM: None (no interaction).

CLINICAL EVALUATION: Ten healthy subjects received intravenous theophylline 5 mg/kg with or without pretreatment with tamsulosin for 7 to 10 days.[1] There was no effect on the pharmacokinetics of theophylline.

RELATED DRUGS: No information is available.

MANAGEMENT OPTIONS: No interaction.

REFERENCES:

1. Miyazawa Y, et al. Effects of the concomitant administration of tamsulosin (0.8 mg/day) on the pharmacokinetic and safety profile of theophylline (5 mg/kg): a placebo-controlled evaluation. *J Int Med Res.* 2002;30(1):34-43.

Theophylline **3**
Thiabendazole (*Mintezol*)

SUMMARY: Case reports suggest that thiabendazole can substantially increase serum theophylline concentrations; theophylline toxicity may result.

RISK FACTORS: No specific risk factors are known.

MECHANISM: Not established. It appears that thiabendazole inhibits the metabolism of theophylline.

CLINICAL EVALUATION: A 71-year-old man maintained on IV aminophylline 45 mg/hr had a serum concentration of 21 mg/mL.[1] The patient was diagnosed as having strongyloides infestation and was treated with thiabendazole 4g/day for 5 days. His theophylline concentration increased to 46 mg/mL during thiabendazole administration and was accompanied by nausea, lethargy, and malaise. After the thiabendazole was discontinued, his theophylline concentration decreased to 16 mg/mL. A second case report involved a 49-year-old man taking 300 mg twice daily of sustained-release theophylline.[2] Thiabendazole 1.8 g twice daily was initiated and his theophylline dosage was reduced to 200 mg twice daily; however, his theophylline concentration increased from 15 mg/mL to 22 mg/mL. The theophylline concentration fell to 12 mg/mL 2 days after thiabendazole was discontinued. Six healthy subjects received a 6 mg/kg aminophylline infusion alone and following 3 days pretreatment with thiabendazole 1.5 g every 12 hours or mebendazole 100 mg every 12 hours.[3] Thiabendazole decreased theophylline clearance 13%, but mebendazole (eg, *Vermox*) had no effect.

RELATED DRUGS: Mebendazole does not interact.

MANAGEMENT OPTIONS:

➡ *Circumvent/Minimize.* Reduce theophylline dosages in patients who must take thiabendazole with theophylline. Consider alternative drugs for theophylline (eg, beta-agonists, steroids) during thiabendazole treatment.

➡ *Monitor.* Carefully monitor patients taking theophylline for increased theophylline concentrations and manifestations of theophylline toxicity (eg, tachycardia, nervousness, nausea) if they require a course of thiabendazole therapy.

REFERENCES:

1. Sugar AM, et al. Possible thiabendazole-induced theophylline toxicity. *Am Rev Respir Dis.* 1980;122:501.

2. Lew G, et al. Theophylline-thiabendazole drug interaction. *Clin Pharm.* 1989;8:225.

3. Schneider D, et al. Theophylline and antiparasitic drug interactions. A case report and study of the influence of thiabendazole and mebendazole on theophylline pharmacokinetics in adults. *Chest.* 1990;97:84.

Theophylline

Thyroid

SUMMARY: Initiation of thyroid replacement therapy in patients receiving theophylline may reduce serum theophylline concentrations.

RISK FACTORS:

➡ *Order of Drug Administration.* Patients on theophylline therapy who are started on thyroid replacement are at increased risk for the interaction. (Patients stabilized on thyroid replacement before theophylline therapy is started probably are at minimal risk for the interaction.)

MECHANISM: The rate of theophylline elimination tends to increase in hyperthyroid patients and decrease in those who are hypothyroid. Thus, thyroid hormone replacement in a clinically hypothyroid patient may increase theophylline elimination.

CLINICAL EVALUATION: A patient on chronic theophylline therapy developed theophylline toxicity as well as clinical and laboratory evidence of hypothyroidism 3 months after receiving iodine 131 (I^{131}) treatment for hyperthyroidism.[1] When thyroid replacement with levothyroxine was begun, the clinical evidence of theophylline toxicity resolved, and 2 months later his theophylline half-life and serum concentration had returned to pre-I^{131} levels.

RELATED DRUGS: No information is available.

MANAGEMENT OPTIONS:

➠ **Monitor.** Monitor patients for a reduced theophylline response when thyroid replacement therapy is initiated for hypothyroidism.

REFERENCES:

1. Johnson CE, et al. Theophylline toxicity after iodine 131 treatment for hyperthyroidism. *Clin Pharm.* 1988;7:620.

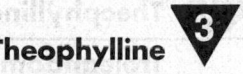

Theophylline

Ticlopidine (eg, *Ticlid*)

SUMMARY: Ticlopidine substantially increased plasma theophylline concentrations in healthy subjects and may increase the risk of theophylline toxicity in patients.

RISK FACTORS: No specific risk factors are known.

MECHANISM: Ticlopidine probably inhibits the hepatic metabolism of theophylline.

CLINICAL EVALUATION: A patient receiving theophylline 500 mg/day and ticlopidine 500 mg/day was noted to have high serum theophylline concentrations and a very low theophylline clearance.[1] In order to study the potential interaction under controlled conditions, 10 healthy subjects then received a single oral dose of theophylline (5 mg/kg) with and without pretreatment with ticlopidine 250 mg twice daily for 10 days. Ticlopidine pretreatment was associated with a 37% reduction in theophylline clearance and a 42% increase in theophylline half-life. If a similar effect is seen in patients receiving these drugs, one would expect to see some cases of theophylline toxicity.

RELATED DRUGS: No information is available.

MANAGEMENT OPTIONS:

➠ **Monitor.** Monitor for altered theophylline effect if ticlopidine therapy is initiated, discontinued, or changed in dosage; adjustments in theophylline dosage may be needed.

REFERENCES:

1. Colli A, et al. Ticlopidine-theophylline interaction. *Clin Pharmacol Ther.* 1987;41:358.

Theophylline

Tocainide (*Tonocard*)

SUMMARY: Tocainide appears to cause a small increase in theophylline serum concentrations; the clinical significance is unknown but is likely to be limited.

RISK FACTORS: No information is available.

MECHANISM: Tocainide reduces the metabolism of theophylline.

CLINICAL EVALUATION: Eight healthy subjects received theophylline 5 mg/kg IV before and after 5 days of tocainide 400 mg every 8 hours.[1] Theophylline clearance was decreased by 10% following tocainide pretreatment. While the clinical significance of this interaction appears limited, additional studies in patients are needed to verify this. Subjects with higher theophylline clearances may react with a greater reduction in clearance following tocainide.

RELATED DRUGS: No information is available.

MANAGEMENT OPTIONS: No specific action is required, but be alert for evidence of the interaction.

REFERENCES:

1. Loi CM, et al. Effect of tocainide on theophylline elimination. *Br J Clin Pharmacol.* 1993;35:437.

 Theophylline

Troleandomycin (*Tao*)

SUMMARY: Troleandomycin may increase theophylline serum concentrations and the potential for theophylline toxicity.

RISK FACTORS:

➡ **Dosage Regimen.** Troleandomycin doses greater than 250 mg/day increases the risk for the interaction.

MECHANISM: Troleandomycin probably impairs the hepatic metabolism of theophylline.

CLINICAL EVALUATION: Theophylline elimination was measured before and after at least 10 days of troleandomycin 250 mg/day in 8 patients with chronic asthma.[1] Troleandomycin was associated with a 50% decrease in the theophylline clearance from serum. There were corresponding increases in serum theophylline concentrations. In 11 patients with asthma, troleandomycin 250 mg/day or every other day reduced the theophylline clearance 24% and the average theophylline dosage 13%.[2] Patients taking higher doses of troleandomycin will be at increased risk of developing elevated theophylline concentrations.

RELATED DRUGS: Erythromycin and clarithromycin (*Biaxin*) will inhibit theophylline metabolism. Azithromycin (*Zithromax*) has been shown to have no effect on theophylline metabolism.

MANAGEMENT OPTIONS:

➡ **Use Alternative.** Patients should avoid theophylline and troleandomycin administration. Azithromycin may be an alternative.

REFERENCES:

1. Weinberger M, et al. Inhibition of theophylline clearance by troleandomycin. *J Allergy Clin Immunol.* 1977;59:228.
2. Kamada AK, et al. Effect of low-dose troleandomycin on theophylline clearance: implications for therapeutic drug monitoring. *Pharmacotherapy.* 1992;12:98.

5 Theophylline

Trovafloxacin (*Trovan*)

SUMMARY: Trovafloxacin does not alter theophylline serum concentration.

RISK FACTORS: No specific risk factors are known.

MECHANISM: No interaction.

CLINICAL EVALUATION: While no published data are available for evaluation, the manufacturer of trovafloxacin has made available some data on this interaction.[1] Trovafloxacin 200 mg/day for 7 days did not alter steady-state theophylline serum concentrations.

RELATED DRUGS: Other quinolones such as lomefloxacin (*Maxaquin*), ofloxacin (*Floxin*), and sparfloxacin (*Zagam*) produced no change in theophylline metabolism. The area under the concentration-time curve of caffeine, which, like theophylline, is metabolized CYP1A2, was increased 17% following trovafloxacin 200 mg administration.[1] This increase in unlikely to cause any change in clinical response to caffeine.

MANAGEMENT OPTIONS: No interaction.

REFERENCES:

1. Pfizer Inc. Trovafloxacin (*Trovan*) product information. New York, NY. 1998.

Theophylline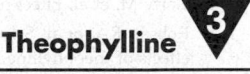

Verapamil (eg, *Calan*)

SUMMARY: Verapamil appears to increase plasma concentrations of theophylline. In some patients, the increases may be large enough to result in theophylline toxicity.

RISK FACTORS:

➡ **Pharmacogenetics.** Children and cigarette smokers are at increased risk for the interaction.

MECHANISM: Verapamil inhibits the metabolism of theophylline, presumably through an effect on hepatic microsomal enzymes. Diltiazem and nifedipine appear to have less consistent and less potent effects on theophylline metabolism.

CLINICAL EVALUATION: In a case report, verapamil 120 mg every 8 hours approximately doubled the patient's theophylline concentrations.[1] A study in healthy subjects found that verapamil 120 mg every 8 hours reduced the mean clearance after oral administration of theophylline 18%.[4] In other studies of healthy subjects, theophylline clearance was reduced 12% to 30% following verapamil 80 to 120 mg every 8 hours.[9-11,14] Patients with elevated baseline theophylline clearances (eg, children, smokers) may be at increased risk. The effect of verapamil on theophylline clearance appears to be dose related.[15]

RELATED DRUGS: The clearance of theophylline was decreased approximately 20%[5,17] or not affected by diltiazem (eg, *Cardizem*).[4,6-9,14,16] Diltiazem attenuated rifampin (*Rifadin*)-induced theophylline clearance[12] but not smoking-induced clearance.[5] Theophylline absorption was noted to be moderately reduced following felodipine (*Plendil*) administration.[13] Additional study is needed to substantiate these findings and establish clinical significance. Isradipine (*DynaCirc*)[17] and nifedipine (eg, *Procardia*) appear to have no[4,6-9,14,16] or minimal[23] effect on theophylline pharmacokinetics.

MANAGEMENT OPTIONS:

➡ **Consider Alternative.** Isradipine and nifedipine may be alternatives to verapamil.

➡ **Monitor.** Carefully monitor patients receiving verapamil and perhaps diltiazem for evidence of theophylline toxicity (eg, tachycardia, tremor, GI upset). Theophylline plasma concentration determinations may be helpful.

REFERENCES:

1. Burnakis TG, et al. Increased serum theophylline concentrations secondary to oral verapamil. *Clin Pharmacol.* 1983;2:458.

2. Parrillo SJ, et al. Elevated theophylline blood levels from institution of nifedipine therapy. *Ann Emerg Med*. 1984;13:216.

3. Harrod CS. Theophylline toxicity and nifedipine. *Ann Intern Med*. 1987;106:480.

4. Sirmans S, et al. Effect of calcium channel blockers on theophylline disposition. *Clin Pharmacol Ther*. 1988;44:29.

5. Nafziger AN, et al. Inhibition of theophylline elimination by diltiazem therapy. *J Clin Pharmacol*. 1987;27:862.

6. Jackson SHD, et al. The interaction between IV theophylline and chronic oral dosing with slow-release nifedipine in volunteers. *Br J Clin Pharmacol*. 1986;21:389.

7. Christopher MA, et al. Clinical relevance of the interaction of theophylline with diltiazem or nifedipine. *Chest*. 1989;95:309.

8. Garty M, et al. Effect of nifedipine and theophylline in asthma. *Clin Pharmacol Ther*. 1986;40:195.

9. Robson RA, et al. Selective inhibitory effects of nifedipine and verapamil on oxidative metabolism: effects of theophylline. *Br J Clin Pharmacol*. 1988;25:397.

10. Nielsen-Kudsk JE, et al. Verapamil-induced inhibition of theophylline elimination in healthy humans. *Pharmacol Toxicol*. 1990;66:101.

11. Gin AS, et al. The effect of verapamil on the pharmacokinetic disposition of theophylline in cigarette smokers. *J Clin Pharmacol*. 1989;29:728.

12. Adebayo GI, et al. Attenuation of rifampicin-induced theophylline metabolism by dilitiazem/rifampicin coadministration in healthy volunteers. *Eur J Clin Pharmacol*. 1989;37:127.

13. Bratel T, et al. Felodipine reduces the absorption of theophylline in man. *Eur J Clin Pharmacol*. 1989;36:481.

14. Abernethy DR, et al. Substrate-selective inhibition by verapamil and diltiazem: differential disposition of antipyrine and theophylline in humans. *J Pharmacol Exp Ther*. 1989;244:994.

15. Stringer KA, et al. The effect of three different oral doses of verapamil on the disposition of theophylline. *Eur J Clin Pharmacol*. 1992;43:35.

16. Yilmaz E, et al. Nifedipine alters serum theophylline levels in asthmatic patients with hypertension. *Fundam Clin Pharmacol*. 1991;5:341.

17. Perreault M, et al. The effect of isradipine on theophylline pharmacokinetics in healthy volunteers. *Pharmacotherapy*. 1993;13:149.

4   Theophylline

Vidarabine (*Vira-A*)

SUMMARY: Vidarabine administration was associated with elevated theophylline serum concentrations in 1 patient, but a causal relationship was not established.

RISK FACTORS: No specific risk factors are known.

MECHANISM: Not established. Vidarabine purportedly inhibits the metabolism of theophylline.

CLINICAL EVALUATION: A woman with a history of congestive heart failure and chronic obstructive pulmonary disease developed increased serum theophylline concentrations 4 days after beginning therapy with vidarabine for diffuse cutaneous herpes zoster.[1] The half-life of theophylline appeared to be prolonged in the presence of vidarabine. The authors ruled out several other obvious causes of altered theophylline disposition, but the patient was acutely ill and received theophylline in varying doses, routes, and formulations during her hospital stay. In view of reports of possible inhibition of theophylline metabolism by various viral infections,[2] the diffuse herpes zoster infection itself may have affected theophylline metabolism in this case. More study is needed to determine the validity of the purported interaction between vidarabine and theophylline.

RELATED DRUGS: No information is available.

MANAGEMENT OPTIONS: No specific action is required, but be alert for evidence of the interaction.

REFERENCES:
1. Gannon R, et al. Possible interaction between vidarabine and theophylline. *Ann Intern Med.* 1984;101:148.
2. Hendeles L, et al. Theophylline: a "state of the art" review. *Pharmacotherapy.* 1983;3:2.

Theophylline ▼ 3

Zafirlukast (*Accolate*)

SUMMARY: The manufacturer reports that theophylline can decrease plasma concentrations of zafirlukast; adjustments in zafirlukast dose may be needed.

RISK FACTORS: No specific risk factors are known.

MECHANISM: Not established.

CLINICAL EVALUATION: In 13 asthmatic patients, concomitant administration of multiple doses of zafirlukast (80 mg/day) with a single dose of theophylline (6 mg/kg) resulted in approximately 30% decrease in zafirlukast mean plasma concentrations. The clinical importance of a reduction in zafirlukast plasma concentrations of this magnitude is not clear, particularly since a reduction in the therapeutic effect of zafirlukast would theoretically be offset by the positive effect of theophylline.[1]

RELATED DRUGS: No information is available.

MANAGEMENT OPTIONS:

➥ *Monitor.* Monitor for altered zafirlukast effect if theophylline is initiated, discontinued, or changed in dosage.

REFERENCES:
1. *Accolate* [package insert]. Wilmington, DE: AstraZeneca; 1997.

Thiazides 5

Valacyclovir (*Valtrex*)

SUMMARY: Patients taking thiazides had similar acyclovir pharmacokinetic parameters as a group of subjects receiving valacyclovir without thiazides.

RISK FACTORS: No specific risk factors are known.

MECHANISM: No interaction.

CLINICAL EVALUATION: The pharmacokinetics of acyclovir (*Zovirax*) was studied in 11 subjects following valacyclovir 500 mg (a prodrug for acyclovir) daily for 8 days.[1] Nine other patients with hypertension taking thiazides (12.5 to 100 mg/day) received similar doses of valacyclovir. The age of the 2 groups of patients was similar. Acyclovir plasma concentrations were similar in the 2 groups. The administration of thiazides does not appear to affect the pharmacokinetics of valacyclovir or acyclovir.

RELATED DRUGS: Acyclovir does not interact with the thiazides. The effect of thiazides on other antiviral agents such as famciclovir (*Famvir*) or ganciclovir (*Cytovene*) is unknown.

MANAGEMENT OPTIONS: No interaction.

REFERENCES:

1. Wang LH, et al. Pharmacokinetics and safety of multiple-dose valaciclovir in geriatric volunteers with and without concomitant diuretic therapy. *Antimicrob Agents Chemother*. 1996;40:80.

 4   Thiazides

Warfarin (eg, *Coumadin*)

SUMMARY: Thiazides and related agents, such as chlorthalidone, indapamide, metolazone, and quinethazone, may be associated with minor changes in anticoagulant response to warfarin, but the effects are probably clinically unimportant.

RISK FACTORS: No specific risk factors are known.

MECHANISM: Some have proposed that thiazides may antagonize the effect of oral anti-coagulants by concentrating circulating clotting factors. Diuretics also may increase clotting factor synthesis by improving hepatic function through a reduction in hepatic congestion.

CLINICAL EVALUATION: In one study of 6 subjects, chlorthalidone (*Dygroton*) reduced the hypoprothrombinemic response to a single dose of warfarin (1.5 mg/kg body weight) compared with the same dose of warfarin given alone.[1] In another study of 8 subjects, treatment with chlorothiazide (eg, *Diuril*) 1 g/day for 21 days did not alter the hypoprothrombinemia or plasma warfarin concentration following single doses of warfarin.[2] However, studies of thiazide-type diuretics in patients taking chronic oral anticoagulants are lacking.

RELATED DRUGS: Chlorthalidone and chlorothiazide may interact similarly with warfarin.

MANAGEMENT OPTIONS: No specific action is required, but be alert for evidence of the interaction.

REFERENCES:

1. O'Reilly RA, et al. Impact of aspirin and chlorthalidone on the pharmacodynamics of oral anticoagulant drugs in man. *Ann NY Acad Sci*. 1971;179:173.
2. Robinson DS, et al. Interaction of commonly prescribed drugs and warfarin. *Ann Intern Med*. 1970;72:853.
3. Koch-Weser J, et al. Drug interactions with coumarin anticoagulants (Second of 2 parts). *N Engl J Med*. 1971;285:547.

Thioridazine (*Mellaril*)

Ziprasidone (*Geodon*)

SUMMARY: Ziprasidone and thioridazine can prolong the QTc interval on the electrocardiogram (ECG). Theoretically, this could increase the risk of ventricular arrhythmias such as torsades de pointes.

RISK FACTORS:

➡ *Hypokalemia.* The corrected QT interval (QTc) on the ECG may be prolonged in patients with hypokalemia, increasing the risk of this interaction.[1]

➡ *Miscellaneous.* Other factors that may prolong the QTc interval (eg, hypomagnesemia, bradycardia, impaired liver function, hypothyroidism) also may increase the risk of ventricular arrhythmias.[1]

MECHANISM: Possible additive prolongation of the QTc interval.

CLINICAL EVALUATION: In initial controlled trials, ziprasidone increased the QTc interval by approximately 10 msec at the highest recommended dose of 160 mg/day. But because of concern that the QTc measurements were done when ziprasidone serum concentrations were low, the FDA recommended additional study.[2,3] In a subsequent study in patients with psychotic disorders, the QTc interval was measured following administration of several antipsychotic drugs (ziprasidone, thioridazine, quetiapine, risperidone, haloperidol, olanzapine) when the antipsychotic drug concentrations were calculated to be at their peak. Ziprasidone increased the QTc by a mean of approximately 21 msec, which was less than thioridazine (36 msec) but about twice that of the other antipsychotics. Theoretically, the ability of thioridazine to prolong the QTc would be additive with ziprasidone, but the extent to which this would increase the risk of ventricular arrhythmias, such as torsades de pointes, is not known.

RELATED DRUGS: Available data suggest that the QTc prolongation following ziprasidone is about twice that of quetiapine (*Seroquel*), risperidone (*Risperdal*), haloperidol (*Haldol*), and olanzapine (*Zyprexa*).

MANAGEMENT OPTIONS:

➡ *Use Alternative.* Given the theoretical risk and the fact that thioridazine is listed in the ziprasidone product information as "contraindicated," it would be prudent to use an alternative to one of the drugs (see Related Drugs).

➡ *Monitor.* If thioridazine and ziprasidone are used concurrently, monitor for evidence of arrhythmias (eg, syncope) and for prolonged QT intervals.

REFERENCES:

1. De Ponti F, et al. QT-interval prolongation by non-cardiac drugs: lessons to be learned from recent experience. *Eur J Clin Pharmacol.* 2000;56:1-18.
2. Product information. Ziprasidone (*Geodon*). Pfizer Pharmaceuticals. 2001.
3. Briefing Information, Psychopharmacological Drugs Advisory Committee, U.S. Food and Drug Administration, July 19, 2000.

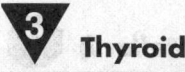

Thyroid

Warfarin (eg, *Coumadin*)

SUMMARY: The hypoprothrombinemic response to oral anticoagulants is altered by changes in clinical thyroid status; adjustments in anticoagulant dosage are likely to be required if the thyrometabolic status changes.

RISK FACTORS:

➡ **Order of Drug Administration.** The primary risk is in starting thyroid replacement therapy in the presence of chronic oral anticoagulants. The risk appears small if the oral anticoagulant is started in the presence of chronic thyroid therapy.

MECHANISM: Thyroid appears to increase catabolism of vitamin K-dependent clotting factors; thus, an increase or decrease in clinical thyroid status will increase or decrease the hypoprothrombinemic response to oral anticoagulants.[1-7] A detailed description of the proposed mechanisms has been presented.[8]

CLINICAL EVALUATION: Patients with hypothyroidism usually are resistant to warfarin and require larger doses to achieve therapeutic levels of anticoagulation. Subsequent thyroid replacement therapy in such patients increases clotting factor catabolism without affecting clotting factor synthesis (suppressed by warfarin), resulting in excessive anticoagulation and possibly a hemorrhagic episode. Reduced oral anticoagulant dose requirements and severe bleeding episodes have been observed when thyroid replacement therapy was started in patients receiving chronic oral anticoagulant therapy.[9,10] On the other hand, a patient rendered euthyroid by maintenance thyroid replacement therapy will respond like any other euthyroid patient to the initiation of oral anticoagulant therapy. Thus, changes in the thyrometabolic status of the patient may cause changes in anticoagulant requirements.[11] This should be considered when evaluating this interaction in specific patients.

RELATED DRUGS: Given the mechanism, it is likely that all oral anticoagulants are affected by all types of thyroid replacement.

MANAGEMENT OPTIONS:

➡ **Monitor.** Monitor for altered oral anticoagulant effect if thyroid replacement therapy is initiated, discontinued, or changed in dosage. Adjust the anticoagulant dose as needed. No special precautions appear necessary when oral anticoagulant therapy is begun in a patient already stabilized on maintenance thyroid replacement therapy.

REFERENCES:

1. Vagenakis AG, et al. Enhancement of warfarin-induced hypoprothrombinemia by thyrotoxicosis. *Johns Hopkins Med J.* 1972;131:69-73.
2. McIntosh TJ, et al. Increased sensitivity to warfarin in thyrotoxicosis. *J Clin Invest.* 1970;49:63a.
3. Rice AJ, et al. Decreased sensitivity to warfarin in patients with myxedema. *Am J Med Sci.* 1971;262:211-215.
4. Self T, et al. Warfarin-induced hypoprothrombinemia. Potentiation by hyperthyroidism. *JAMA.* 1975;231:1165-1166.
5. Edson JR, et al. Low platelet adhesiveness and other hemostatic abnormalities in hypothyroidism. *Ann Intern Med.* 1975;82:342-346.
6. Self TH, et al. Effect of hyperthyroidism on hypoprothrombinemic response to warfarin. *Am J Hosp Pharm.* 1976;33:387-389.
7. Van Dosterom AT, et al. The influence of the thyroid function on the metabolic rate of prothrombin, factor VII, and factor X in the rat. *Thromb Haemost.* 1976;3:607.

8. Hansten PD. Oral anticoagulants and drugs which alter thyroid function. *Drug Intell Clin Pharm.* 1980;14:331.

9. Walters MB. The relationship between thyroid function and anticoagulant therapy. *Am J Cardiol.* 1963;11:112-114.

10. Costigan DC, et al. Potentiation of oral anticoagulant effect by L-thyroxine. *Clin Pediatr.* 1984;23:172-174.

11. Loeliger EA, et al. The biological disappearance rate of prothrombin, factors VII, IX and X from plasma in hypothyroidism, hyperthyroidism and during fever. *Thromb Diath Haemorrh.* 1964;10:267-277.

Ticlopidine (eg, *Ticlid*)

Warfarin (eg, *Coumadin*)

SUMMARY: Ticlopidine may increase the hypoprothrombinemic response to warfarin in some patients, but the clinical importance of this effect is not established.

RISK FACTORS: No specific risk factors are known.

MECHANISM: Not established. Ticlopidine may inhibit the hepatic metabolism of R-warfarin.

CLINICAL EVALUATION: Nine elderly men on chronic warfarin therapy were given ticlopidine 250 mg twice daily for 14 days.[1] Ticlopidine increased R-warfarin plasma concentrations approximately 26%; S-warfarin was not affected. The slight increase in international normalized ratio values was not significant, but there was considerable variation from patient to patient. Thus, it is possible for the occasional patient to manifest a clinically important increase in the hypoprothrombinemic response to warfarin.

RELATED DRUGS: No information is available.

MANAGEMENT OPTIONS: No specific action is required, but be alert for evidence of the interaction.

REFERENCES:

1. Gidal BE, et al. Evaluation of a potential enantioselective interaction between ticlopidine and warfarin in chronically anticoagulated patients. *Ther Drug Monit.* 1995;17:33-38.

Tigecycline (*Tygacil*)

Warfarin (eg, *Coumadin*)

SUMMARY: Tigecycline modestly increases warfarin plasma concentrations; some patients may demonstrate increased international normalized ratios (INRs) during coadministration.

RISK FACTORS: No specific risk factors are known.

MECHANISM: Unknown.

CLINICAL EVALUATION: While data on this interaction is limited, the manufacturer reported the effects of tigecycline 100 mg followed by 50 mg every 12 hours intravenously to healthy subjects on the clearance of a single dose of warfarin 25 mg.[1] Tigecycline reduced the clearance of S-warfarin and R-warfarin 23% and 40%, respectively. However, the INR was not altered by the coadministration of tigecycline. The effect of this modest change in warfarin metabolism on INRs in patients with infections has not been reported. Pending further data, monitor for altered warfarin response.

RELATED DRUGS: None known.

MANAGEMENT OPTIONS:

➡ *Monitor.* Patients stabilized on warfarin should be observed for increased INRs if tigecycline is added to the drug regimen.

REFERENCES:

1. *Tygacil* [package insert]. Philadelphia, PA: Wyeth Pharmaceuticals, Inc.; 2005.

Tipranavir (*Aptivus*)

Vitamin E

SUMMARY: Vitamin E administered with tipranavir has been shown to increase the risk of bleeding.

RISK FACTORS: No specific risk factors are known.

MECHANISM: Unknown. In vitro data indicate that tipranavir inhibits platelet aggregation.

CLINICAL EVALUATION: While specific data are limited, the manufacturer of tipranavir notes that coadministration of vitamin E (alpha-tocopherol polyethylene glycol 1,000 succinate) increases bleeding events and may lead to increased mortality.[1]

RELATED DRUGS: The administration of tipranavir with antiplatelet drugs such as aspirin, nonsteroidal anti-inflammatory drugs, and clopidogrel (eg, *Plavix*) or anticoagulant drugs such as heparin, enoxaparin (*Lovenox*), or warfarin (eg, *Coumadin*) may lead to an increased risk of bleeding.

MANAGEMENT OPTIONS:

➡ *Monitor.* Carefully monitor patients receiving tipranavir and any drug that inhibits platelets or the normal clotting cascade for evidence of bleeding.

REFERENCES:

1. *Aptivus* [package insert]. Ridgefield, CT: Boehringer Ingelheim Pharmaceuticals, Inc; 2007.

Tipranavir (*Aptivus*)

Zidovudine (eg, *Retrovir*)

SUMMARY: Coadministration of zidovudine with tipranavir/ritonavir may result in lower plasma concentrations of zidovudine and reduced antiviral effect.

RISK FACTORS: No specific risk factors are known.

MECHANISM: Tipranavir has been noted to induce glucuronidation, the primary pathway for zidovudine metabolism.

CLINICAL EVALUATION: While specific data are limited, the manufacturer of tipranavir notes that the coadministration of tipranavir 250 to 1,250 mg with ritonavir 100 to 200 mg twice daily and zidovudine 300 mg twice daily decreased the mean area under the plasma concentration-time curve of zidovudine 46% to 51%, compared with the administration of zidovudine alone. Zidovudine administration produced minimal changes in tipranavir plasma concentrations.[1]

RELATED DRUGS: Nelfinavir (*Viracept*) has also been noted to reduce zidovudine plasma concentrations.

MANAGEMENT OPTIONS:

➡ *Monitor.* Carefully monitor patients being treated with tipranavir/ritonavir and zidovudine for any change in antiviral efficacy.

REFERENCES:

1. *Aptivus* [package insert]. Ridgefield, CT: Boehringer Ingelheim Pharmaceuticals, Inc; 2007.

Tolbutamide (eg, *Orinase*)

Trimethoprim/Sulfamethoxazole (eg, *Bactrim*)

SUMMARY: Several sulfonamides, such as trimethoprim/sulfamethoxazole (TMP-SMZ), can increase plasma concentration of oral antidiabetic agents, such as tolbutamide, and enhance their hypoglycemic effects.

RISK FACTORS: No specific risk factors are known.

MECHANISM: More than one mechanism may be involved in the effect of sulfonamides on antidiabetic agents. It has been proposed that sulfaphenazole[1] and sulfamethizole inhibit the hydroxylation of tolbutamide. Displacement of tolbutamide from plasma protein binding also may be partially involved in the potentiation by sulfaphenazole.

CLINICAL EVALUATION: TMP-SMZ reduces the metabolism of tolbutamide[2] and possibly glipizide (eg, *Glucotrol*).[3] The serum concentration, half-life, and hypoglycemic effects of tolbutamide, glyburide (eg, *DiaBeta*), and chlorpropamide (eg, *Diabinese*) have been increased by various sulfonamide antibiotics, including sulfamethizole, sulfaphenazole, and sulfisoxazole (eg, *Gantrisin*).[1-8]

RELATED DRUGS: Glipizide, glyburide, and chlorpropamide are affected similarly by sulfonamides such as TMP-SMZ, sulfamethizole, sulfaphenazole, and sulfisoxazole. Sulfonamides have not been reported to affect the response to insulin.

MANAGEMENT OPTIONS:

➡ *Monitor.* Enhanced hypoglycemic effects may occur with TMP-SMZ and tolbutamide coadministration. Sulfadiazine and sulfadimethoxine do not appear to have this effect.

REFERENCES:

1. Christensen LK, et al. Sulfaphenazole-induced hypoglycaemic attacks in tolbutamide-treated diabetics. *Lancet*. 1963;2:1298-1301.

2. Wing LM, et al. Cotrimoxazole as an inhibitor of oxidative drug metabolism: effects of trimethoprim and sulphamethoxazole separately and combined on tolbutamide disposition. *Br J Clin Pharmacol*. 1985;20(5):482-485.

3. Johnson JF, et al. Symptomatic hypoglycemia secondary to a glipizide-trimethoprim/sulfamethoxazole drug interaction. *DICP*. 1990;24(3):250-251.

4. Soeldner JS, et al. Hypoglycemia in tolbutamide-treated diabetes; report of two cases with measurement of serum insulin. *JAMA*. 1965;193:398-399.

5. Dall JL, et al. Hypoglycaemia due to chlorpropamide. *Scott Med J*. 1967;12(11):403-404.

6. Mihic M, et al. Effect of trimethoprim-sulfamethoxazole on blood insulin and glucose concentrations of diabetics. *Can Med Assoc J*. 1975;112(13 Spec No):80-82.

7. Asplund K, et al. Glibenclamide-associated hypoglycaemia: a report on 57 cases. *Diabetologia*. 1983;24(6):412-417.

8. Baciewicz AM, et al. Hypoglycemia induced by the interaction of chlorpropamide and co-trimoxazole. *Drug Intell Clin Pharm*. 1984;18(4):309-310.

 Tolmetin (eg, *Tolectin*)

Warfarin (eg, *Coumadin*)

SUMMARY: Tolmetin does not appear to affect the hypoprothrombinemic response to warfarin, but caution during cotherapy is indicated because of possible detrimental effects of tolmetin on the gastric mucosa and platelet function.

RISK FACTORS:

➡ ***Concurrent Diseases.*** Patients with peptic ulcer disease (PUD) or a history of GI bleeding probably are at greater risk for the interaction.

MECHANISM: Tolmetin-induced gastric erosions and inhibition of platelet function theoretically could increase the risk of bleeding in patients receiving oral anticoagulants.

CLINICAL EVALUATION: In doses of 800 to 1200 mg/day, tolmetin does not appear to affect the hypoprothrombinemic response to warfarin.[1] However, the limited available evidence does not preclude the possibility that an occasional predisposed patient might manifest an interaction. In a retrospective cohort study, hospitalizations for hemorrhagic PUD were approximately 13 times higher in patients receiving warfarin plus a nonsteroidal anti-inflammatory drug (NSAID) than in patients receiving either drug.[2]

RELATED DRUGS: All NSAIDs inhibit platelet function, cause gastric erosions, and probably increase the risk of GI bleeding.

MANAGEMENT OPTIONS:

➡ ***Avoid Unless Benefit Outweighs Risk.*** Because all NSAIDs probably increase the risk of GI bleeding in patients on oral anticoagulants, use the combination only after careful consideration of the benefit vs risk. If the NSAID is being used as an analgesic or antipyretic, acetaminophen (eg, *Tylenol*) probably is safer to use with oral anticoagulants. Nonacetylated salicylates (eg, choline salicylate, magnesium salicylate, salsalate, sodium salicylate) probably also are safer with oral anticoagulants than NSAIDs since they have minimal effects on platelet function and the gastric mucosa.

➡ ***Monitor.*** If any NSAID is used with an oral anticoagulant, carefully monitor the prothrombin time and watch for evidence of bleeding, especially from the GI tract.

REFERENCES:

1. Pullar T. Interaction between oral anti-coagulant drugs and nonsteroidal anti-inflammatory agents: a review. *Scott Med J*. 1983;28:42.

2. Shorr RI, et al. Concurrent use of nonsteroidal anti-inflammatory drugs and oral anticoagulants places elderly persons at high risk for hemorrhagic peptic ulcer disease. *Arch Intern Med*. 1993;153:1665.

Toloxatone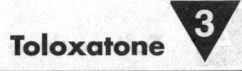

Tyramine

SUMMARY: Large doses of toloxatone (a selective monoamine oxidase [MAO]-A inhibitor) may increase the pressor response to large amounts of tyramine; avoid high tyramine foods (eg, aged cheese).

RISK FACTORS: No specific risk factors are known.

MECHANISM: MAO-A in the intestine and liver is important protection against the pressor response to dietary tyramine. However, since MAO-B is involved in tyramine metabolism, selective inhibitors of MAO-A such as toloxatone would not be expected to enhance the pressor response to tyramine as much as nonselective MAOIs.

CLINICAL EVALUATION: In a 3-way crossover study, 8 healthy subjects received oral tyramine tests after 3 to 5 days of the usual dose of toloxatone (600 mg/day), high dose toloxatone (1,200 mg/day), or a placebo.[1] The tyramine was mixed with stewed apples and given after a standard meal. With placebo pretreatment, the 200 mg dose of tyramine produced only a minimal (approximately 10 mm Hg) increase in systolic blood pressure, and this was not affected by either dose of toloxatone. Similarly, the 400 mg dose of tyramine had minimal effects on systolic blood pressure when given with the placebo or toloxatone 600 mg/day. When 1,200 mg/day of toloxatone was used, tyramine 400 mg resulted in a mean increase in systolic blood pressure of 23 mm Hg. With tyramine 800 mg, the increase in systolic blood pressure after placebo, toloxatone 600 mg/day, and toloxatone 1,200 mg/day was 32, 42, and 57 mm Hg, respectively. A typical European meal reportedly contains less than 40 mg of tyramine,[2] and one would not expect toloxatone to result in adverse effects with such low doses of tyramine. Another selective MAO-A inhibitor, moclobemide, appeared to have a much larger potentiating effect than toloxatone on the pressor response to tyramine,[3] but in that study the tyramine was given after an overnight fast. Thus, it is possible that a greater potentiating effect is seen when a food or drink high in tyramine is taken on an empty stomach rather than as part of a meal. In the latter case, the tyramine may be absorbed more gradually, resulting in lower peak serum concentrations than under fasting conditions.

RELATED DRUGS: Other MAO-A inhibitors, such as moclobemide, may interact similarly with tyramine.

MANAGEMENT OPTIONS:

➥ *Circumvent/Minimize.* Although toloxatone appears less likely to interact with dietary tyramine than nonselective MAOIs, it would be prudent to avoid foods with a high tyramine content.

➥ *Monitor.* Monitor blood pressure if the interaction is suspected.

REFERENCES:

1. Provost JC, et al. Pharmacokinetic and pharmacodynamic interaction between toloxatone, a new reversible monoamine oxidase-A inhibitor, and oral tyramine in healthy subjects. *Clin Pharmacol Ther.* 1992;52:384.
2. Freeman H. Moclobemide. *Lancet.* 1993;342:1528.
3. Simpson GM, et al. Comparison of the pressor effect of tyramine aftertreatment with phenelzine and moclobemide in healthy male volunteers. *Clin Pharmacol Ther.* 1992;52:286.

Tolterodine (*Detrol*)

Warfarin (eg, *Coumadin*)

SUMMARY: Isolated cases of increased warfarin effect have been reported following tolterodine therapy, but a causal relationship has not been established.

RISK FACTORS: No specific risk factors are known.

MECHANISM: Not established. Tolterodine is metabolized primarily by CYP2D6 and (in CYP2D6 deficient patients) by CYP3A4.[1] Neither of these cytochrome P-450 isozymes is important for the metabolism of S-warfarin, so a metabolic interaction seems unlikely.

CLINICAL EVALUATION: Two cases of a possible tolterodine-induced increase in warfarin effect have been reported.[2] Although the temporal relationship and the lack of other causes for the increased international normalized ratio suggest that tolterodine was responsible, more information is needed to determine the clinical importance of this interaction.

RELATED DRUGS: No information is available.

MANAGEMENT OPTIONS: No specific action is required, but be alert for evidence of the interaction.

REFERENCES:
1. Brynne N, et al. Ketoconazole inhibits the metabolism of tolterodine in subjects with deficient CYP2D6 activity. *Br J Clin Pharmacol.* 1999;48:564-572.
2. Colucci VJ, et al. Tolterodine-warfarin drug interaction. *Ann Pharmacother.* 1999;33:1173-1176.

 Tramadol (eg, *Ultram*)

Mirtazapine (eg, *Remeron*)

SUMMARY: A patient developed serotonin syndrome after taking tramadol, mirtazapine, and venlafaxine.

RISK FACTORS: No specific risk factors are known.

MECHANISM: Additive serotonergic effects.

CLINICAL EVALUATION: A 47-year-old man receiving mirtazapine developed clear evidence of serotonin syndrome after tramadol was added to his therapy.[1] The patient was also receiving venlafaxine, which has serotonergic effects as well. It is likely that the serotonin syndrome resulted from the combined serotonergic effects of tramadol, mirtazapine, and venlafaxine.

RELATED DRUGS: The combination of tramadol with other selective serotonin reuptake inhibitors (SSRIs) also appears to increase the risk of serotonin syndrome. SSRIs and related drugs with serotonergic effects include citalopram (eg, *Celexa*), escitalopram (*Lexapro*), fluoxetine (eg, *Prozac*), paroxetine (eg, *Paxil*), sertraline (eg, *Zoloft*), fluvoxamine, trazodone, and venlafaxine (*Effexor*). Some tricyclic antidepressants also have serotonergic effects, especially clomipramine (eg, *Anafranil*) and imipramine (eg, *Tofranil*).

MANAGEMENT OPTIONS:

➡ *Consider Alternative.* In patients taking mirtazapine or other serotonergic antidepressants, consider the use of an analgesic that is not serotonergic (eg, an agent other than tramadol or meperidine) to minimize the risk of serotonin syndrome.

➡ *Monitor.* In patients receiving tramadol and mirtazapine (or other SSRIs), be alert for evidence of serotonin syndrome. Serotonin syndrome can result in neurotoxicity (eg, coma, hyperreflexia, incoordination, myoclonus, rigidity, seizures, tremors), psychiatric symptoms (eg, agitation, confusion, hypomania, restlessness), and autonomic dysfunction (eg, fever, hypertension, sweating, tachycardia).

REFERENCES:
> 1. Houlihan DJ. Serotonin syndrome resulting from coadministration of tramadol, venlafaxine, and mirtazapine. *Ann Pharmacother*. 2004;38:411-413.

Tramadol (eg, *Ultram*)

Rasagiline (*Azilect*)

SUMMARY: Avoid concomitant use of rasagiline and tramadol when possible.

RISK FACTORS: No specific risk factors are known.

MECHANISM: Not established. The combination may have additive serotonergic effects.

CLINICAL EVALUATION: Because severe serotonin syndrome-like reactions have occurred in patients receiving tramadol, the product information for rasagiline states that tramadol is contraindicated in patients taking rasagiline.[1] Even though the interaction is based on theoretical considerations, the severity of the potential reaction suggests that the combination should generally be avoided.

RELATED DRUGS: Rasagiline is also contraindicated with some other analgesics (eg, meperidine [eg, *Demerol*], methadone [eg, *Dolophine*], propoxyphene [eg, *Darvon*]). Any interaction between rasagiline and tramadol is likely to be similar to that of selegiline and tramadol.

MANAGEMENT OPTIONS:

➡ *Avoid Unless Benefit Outweighs Risk.* Avoid concomitant use of tramadol with rasagiline or within 2 weeks of stopping rasagiline when possible.

REFERENCES:
> 1. *Azilect* [package insert]. North Wales, PA: Teva Neuroscience, Inc.; 2006.

Tramadol (eg, *Ultram*)

Tranylcypromine (eg, *Parnate*)

SUMMARY: Tramadol theoretically increases the risk of seizures and serotonin syndrome in patients taking monoamine oxidase (MAO) inhibitors.

RISK FACTORS: No specific risk factors are known.

MECHANISM: Not established. Tramadol inhibits the reuptake of norepinephrine and serotonin. In the presence of MAO inhibitor therapy, these effects would theoretically increase the risk of hypertensive reactions and serotonin syndrome, respectively. Also, seizures have occurred during tramadol therapy, and MAO inhibitors reportedly can increase the risk.

CLINICAL EVALUATION: The manufacturer of tramadol warns that combined use of tramadol and MAO inhibitors may increase the risk of seizures, but no supporting data is presented. It is also stated that the combination increased deaths in animals.[1] In the absence of supporting data, it is difficult to assess the clinical importance of this interaction. Nonetheless, the combination theoretically could increase the risk of serotonin syndrome, a potentially life-threatening reaction. Moreover, the product information states that tramadol should be used only with "great caution" in patients taking MAO inhibitors.

RELATED DRUGS: Until clinical data are available, consider all MAO inhibitors, including phenelzine (*Nardil*) and isocarboxazid (*Marplan*), to be equally likely to interact with tramadol.

MANAGEMENT OPTIONS:

➥ *Avoid Unless Benefit Outweighs Risk.* Although published clinical information is lacking, theoretical and medicolegal considerations suggest that the combination should generally be avoided.

➥ *Monitor.* If the combination is used, monitor for seizures and early evidence of serotonin syndrome. Serotonin syndrome can result in neurotoxicity (eg, coma, hyperreflexia, incoordination, myoclonus, restlessness, rigidity, seizures, tremors), psychiatric symptoms (eg, agitation, confusion, hypomania), and temperature regulation abnormalities (eg, fever, sweating).

REFERENCES:

1. *Ultram* [package insert]. Rariton, NJ: McNeil Pharmaceutical; 1997.

Tramadol (eg, *Ultram*)

Venlafaxine (*Effexor*)

SUMMARY: A patient developed serotonin syndrome after taking tramadol, venlafaxine, and mirtazapine.

RISK FACTORS: No specific risk factors are known.

MECHANISM: Additive serotonergic effects.

CLINICAL EVALUATION: A 47-year-old man receiving venlafaxine developed clear evidence of serotonin syndrome after tramadol was added to his therapy.[1] The patient was also receiving mirtazapine, which has serotonergic effects as well. It is likely that the serotonin syndrome resulted from the combined serotonergic effects of tramadol, venlafaxine, and mirtazapine.

RELATED DRUGS: The combination of tramadol with other selective serotonin reuptake inhibitors (SSRIs) also appears to increase the risk of serotonin syndrome. SSRIs and related drugs with serotonergic effects include citalopram (eg, *Celexa*), escitalopram (*Lexapro*), fluoxetine (eg, *Prozac*), fluvoxamine, mirtazapine (eg, *Remeron*), paroxetine (eg, *Paxil*), sertraline (*Zoloft*), and trazodone. Some tricyclic antidepressants also have serotonergic effects, especially clomipramine (eg, *Anafranil*) and imipramine (eg, *Tofranil*).

MANAGEMENT OPTIONS:

➡ *Consider Alternative.* In patients taking venlafaxine or other serotonergic antidepressants, consider the use of an analgesic that is not serotonergic (eg, an agent other than tramadol or meperidine) to minimize the risk of serotonin syndrome.

➡ *Monitor.* In patients receiving tramadol and venlafaxine (or other SSRIs), be alert for evidence of serotonin syndrome. Serotonin syndrome can result in neurotoxicity (eg, coma, hyperreflexia, incoordination, myoclonus, rigidity, seizures, tremors), psychiatric symptoms (eg, agitation, confusion, hypomania, restlessness), and autonomic dysfunction (eg, fever, hypertension, sweating, tachycardia).

REFERENCES:

1. Houlihan, DJ. Serotonin syndrome resulting from coadministration of tramadol, venlafaxine, and mirtazapine. *Ann Pharmacother.* 2004;38:411-413.

Tranylcypromine (eg, *Parnate*)

Rasagiline (*Azilect*) `AVOID`

SUMMARY: Tranylcypromine and other monoamine oxidase (MAO) inhibitors are contraindicated with rasagiline.

RISK FACTORS: No specific risk factors are known.

MECHANISM: Possible additive effects.

CLINICAL EVALUATION: The rasagiline product information states that concurrent use of rasagiline and other MAO inhibitors is contraindicated.[1] This contraindication is based on theoretical considerations.

RELATED DRUGS: Based on the contraindication in the labeling, avoid rasagiline with all MAO inhibitors, including phenelzine (*Nardil*), isocarboxazid (*Marplan*), and selegiline (eg, *Eldepryl*).

MANAGEMENT OPTIONS:

➡ *AVOID COMBINATION.* Do not use rasagiline and other MAO inhibitors concurrently.

REFERENCES:

1. *Azilect* [package insert]. North Wales, PA: Teva Neuroscience, Inc.; 2006.

Tranylcypromine (eg, *Parnate*)

Tyramine `AVOID`

SUMMARY: The consumption of foods containing large amounts of tyramine can result in hypertensive reactions in patients taking monoamine oxidase (MAO) inhibitors.

RISK FACTORS: No specific risk factors are known.

MECHANISM: Tyramine in foods is normally metabolized by MAO in the GI wall and liver before reaching the systemic circulation. In the presence of an MAO inhibitor, excessive amounts of tyramine may reach the systemic circulation, resulting in an intense pressor response.[1-3] This pressor response can occur following a single dose of an MAO inhibitor.[4]

CLINICAL EVALUATION: Blackwell described 11 tranylcypromine-treated patients who experienced hypertensive crises following ingestion of cheddar cheese (raw or cooked) and, in 1 case, marmite (a yeast extract that reportedly contains tyramine 1.5 mg).[1,5]

The food products were eaten 0.5 to 2 hours before the attack, and in some instances as little as 22 g of cheese were ingested. The ingestion of chicken livers was associated with severe hypertensive crises in 6 patients receiving tranylcypromine,[6] although it has been questioned whether fresh chicken or beef liver contains enough tyramine to cause problems.[7] A similar type of hypertensive crisis occurred when a patient ate pickled herring while taking tranylcypromine.[8] Marked potentiation of the pressor effects of tyramine hydrochloride occurred in 7 hospitalized patients receiving an MAO inhibitor; as little as tyramine 6 mg given orally produced hypertension.[9] Ingestion of whole broad beans (*Vicia fava*) has been associated with hypertensive crisis in several patients; this reaction presumably was attributable to the dopa content of the beans.

RELATED DRUGS: One patient receiving phenelzine (*Nardil*) developed a hypertensive reaction and headache following ingestion of a cup of miso soup.[10] All nonselective MAO inhibitors including isocarboxazid (*Marplan*) interact with tyramine-containing foods.

MANAGEMENT OPTIONS:

➡ *AVOID COMBINATION.* Patients taking MAO inhibitors should avoid foods that may have a high tyramine content. Effects of nonselective MAO inhibitors should be assumed to persist for 2 weeks after they are discontinued. Estimates of the tyramine content of various foods and beverages have been published.[11-13] Foods to be avoided include cheeses (especially aged), red wines, caviar, herring (dried or pickled), canned figs, fermented or spoiled meat (including salami, pepperoni, summer sausage), fava beans, yeast extracts, miso soup, and avocados (especially if overripe).

REFERENCES:
1. Blackwell B. Hypertensive crisis due to monoamine-oxidase inhibitors. *Lancet.* 1963;38:849-850.
2. Cuthill JM, et al. Death associated with tranylcypromine and cheese. *Lancet.* 1964;13:1076-1077.
3. Marley E, et al. Interactions of monoamine oxidase inhibitors, amines, foodstuffs. *Adv Pharmacol Chemother.* 1970;8:185-349.
4. Peet M, et al. The interaction of tyramine with a single dose of tranylcypromine in healthy volunteers. *Br J Clin Pharmacol.* 1981;11:212-214.
5. Blackwell B, et al. Effects of yeast extract after monoamine oxidase inhibition. *Lancet.* 1965;1:940-943.
6. Hedberg DL, et al. Six cases of hypertensive crisis in patients on tranylcypromine after eating chicken livers. *Am J Psychiatry.* 1966;122:933-937.
7. Brown C, et al. The monoamine oxidase inhibitor-tyramine interaction. *J Clin Pharmacol.* 1989;29:529-532.
8. Nuessle WF, et al. Pickled herring and tranylcypromine reaction. *JAMA.* 1965;192:726-727.
9. Tedeschi DH, et al. Monoamine oxidase inhibitors: augmentation of pressor effects of peroral tyramine. *Science.* 1964;144:1225-1226.
10. Mesmer RE. Don't mix miso with MAOIs. *JAMA.* 1987;258:3515.
11. Shullman KI, et al. Dietary restriction, tyramine, and the use of monoamine oxidase inhibitors. *J Clin Psychopharmacol.* 1989;9:397.
12. Sen NP. Analysis and significance of tyramine in foods. *J Food Sci.* 1969;34:22.
13. Monoamine oxidase inhibitors for depression. *Med Lett Drugs Ther.* 1980;22:58-60.

Tranylcypromine (*Parnate*)

Venlafaxine (*Effexor*) AVOID

SUMMARY: Severe serotonin syndrome can occur when venlafaxine is used with or within 2 weeks of discontinuation of tranylcypromine or other nonselective monoamine oxidase inhibitors (MAOIs). Avoid the combination.

RISK FACTORS: No specific risk factors are known.

MECHANISM: Additive. Tranylcypromine, a nonselective MAOI, inhibits serotonin metabolism, and venlafaxine is a potent inhibitor of serotonin reuptake.

CLINICAL EVALUATION: Patients have developed severe serotonin syndrome with combined use of tranylcypromine and venlafaxine.[1,2] A single dose of venlafaxine has been sufficient to produce the reaction.

RELATED DRUGS: Expect all nonselective MAOIs to result in serotonin syndrome if combined with venlafaxine. This would include phenelzine (*Nardil*) and isocarboxazid (*Marplan*); selegiline (*Eldepryl*) can act as a nonselective MAOI in some patients, especially if large doses are used.

MANAGEMENT OPTIONS:

➥ *AVOID COMBINATION.* Avoid combined use of venlafaxine with tranylcypromine (or any other nonselective MAOI). This would include the use of venlafaxine within 2 weeks of discontinuation of an MAOI.

REFERENCES:

1. Brubacher JR, et al. Serotonin syndrome from venlafaxine-tranylcypromine interaction. *Vet Hum Toxicol.* 1996;38:358–361.
2. Hodgman MJ, et al. Serotonin syndrome due to venlafaxine and maintenance tranylcypromine therapy. *Hum Exp Toxicol.* 1997;16:14–17.

Trazodone (eg, *Desyrel*)

Tryptophan

SUMMARY: One patient stopped eating and developed psychiatric symptoms when given trazodone plus tryptophan, but most patients appear to tolerate the combination without serious problems.

RISK FACTORS: No specific risk factors are known.

MECHANISM: Not established. Increased serotonin effect may be involved.

CLINICAL EVALUATION: The combination of trazodone and tryptophan has been used with good results in patients with aggressive behaviors.[1,2] A 29-year-old woman with schizophrenia and mental retardation receiving clonazepam (up to 10.5 mg/day) developed improvement in her aggressive behavior when trazodone 100 mg plus tryptophan 500 mg were given 3 times a week.[3] However, within 2 weeks she stopped eating, developed symptoms of psychosis or hypomania, and became drowsy and withdrawn. Although the reaction may have been caused by the combination of trazodone and tryptophan, one cannot rule out the possibility that clonazepam contributed to the problem (clonazepam concentrations were elevated during the reaction).

RELATED DRUGS: No information is available.

MANAGEMENT OPTIONS: No specific action is required, but be alert for evidence of the interaction.

REFERENCES:

1. Simpson DM, et al. Improvement in organically disturbed behavior with trazodone treatment. *J Clin Psychiatry.* 1986;47:191-193.

2. Pinner E, et al. Effects of trazodone on aggressive behavior in seven patients with organic mental disorders. *Am J Psychiatry.* 1988;145:1295-1296.

3. Patterson BD, et al. Severe anorexia and possible psychosis or hypomania after trazodone-tryptophan treatment of aggression. *Lancet.* 1989;1:1017.

Trazodone (*Desyrel*)

Venlafaxine (*Effexor*)

SUMMARY: A patient on trazodone and venlafaxine developed serotonin syndrome, but it is not clear how often this combination results in adverse effects.

RISK FACTORS: No specific risk factors known.

MECHANISM: Not established. Both trazodone and venlafaxine have serotonergic effects, and it is possible that they are additive.

CLINICAL EVALUATION: A 50-year-old man with depression developed symptoms of serotonin syndrome (eg, myoclonic jerking, diaphoresis, tremor, disorientation) after he was started on venlafaxine and trazodone.[1] The reaction resolved when the medications were discontinued. More clinical data are needed to establish the clinical importance of this purported interaction.

RELATED DRUGS: No information available.

MANAGEMENT OPTIONS: No specific action is required, but be alert for evidence of the interaction.

REFERENCES:

1. McCue RE, et al. Venlafaxine- and trazodone-induced serotonin syndrome. *Am J Psychiatry.* 2001;158:2088-2089.

Trazodone (eg, *Desyrel*)

Warfarin (eg, *Coumadin*)

SUMMARY: A patient developed inhibition of the hypoprothrombinemic response to warfarin following the initiation of trazodone therapy, but a causal relationship was not established.

RISK FACTORS: No specific risk factors are known.

MECHANISM: Not established.

CLINICAL EVALUATION: A 40-year-old woman stabilized on warfarin therapy following a mitral valve replacement developed a 30% reduction in prothrombin time after 5 weeks on trazodone (dosage gradually increased to 300 mg/day).[1] When trazodone was discontinued, the warfarin dose requirement fell to the pre-trazodone levels. Although the temporal relationship is consistent with trazodone-induced inhibition of the hypoprothrombinemic response to warfarin, more study will be required to establish a causal relationship.

RELATED DRUGS: No information is available.

MANAGEMENT OPTIONS: No specific action is required, but be alert for evidence of the interaction.

REFERENCES:

1. Hardy JL, et al. Reduction of prothrombin and partial thromboplastin times with trazodone. *CMAJ.* 1986;135:1372.

Triamterene (*Dyrenium*)

Candesartan (*Atacand*)

SUMMARY: Combining triamterene with candesartan or other angiotensin II receptor blockers (ARBs) may increase the risk of hyperkalemia, especially in patients with 1 or more risk factors.

RISK FACTORS:

➤ *Other Drugs.* The addition of other hyperkalemic drugs may increase the risk of hyperkalemia in patients taking triamterene and ARBs. Hyperkalemic drugs include ACE inhibitors, potassium supplements, cyclosporine, tacrolimus, NSAIDs, COX-2 inhibitors, nonselective beta-adrenergic blockers, trimethoprim, and pentamidine.

➤ *Concurrent Diseases.* Diseases that increase the risk of hyperkalemia for this interaction include diabetes and significant renal impairment.

➤ *Diet/Food.* A diet high in potassium may increase the risk of hyperkalemia from this interaction. Salt substitutes may contain potassium.

MECHANISM: Both triamterene and ARBs tend to increase serum potassium, and their effects are additive.

CLINICAL EVALUATION: Wrenger et al describe 44 cases of life-threatening hyperkalemia in patients receiving either ARBs or ACE inhibitors in combination with spirono-lactone.[1] It is likely that triamterene would also increase the risk of hyperkalemia when combined with ARBs or ACE inhibitors, especially in patients with 1 or more risk factors.

RELATED DRUGS: Triamterene would be expected to increase the risk of hyperkalemia when combined with other ARBs, including eprosartan (*Teveten*), irbesartan (*Avapro*), losartan (*Cozaar*), telmisartan (*Micardis*), and valsartan (*Diovan*).

MANAGEMENT OPTIONS:

➤ *Monitor.* In patients receiving triamterene and an ARB, monitor serum potassium and renal function, particularly if the patient has 1 or more of the risk factors listed before.

REFERENCES:

1. Wrenger E, et al. Interaction of spironolactone with ACE inhibitors or antiogensin receptor blockers: analysis of 44 cases. *BMJ.* 2003;327:147-149.

Triamterene (Dyrenium)

Enalapril (eg, Vasotec)

SUMMARY: Combining triamterene with enalapril or other ACE inhibitors increases the risk of hyperkalemia, especially in patients with 1 or more risk factors.

RISK FACTORS:

➡ **Other Drugs.** In patients taking triamterene and ACE inhibitors, the addition of other hyperkalemic drugs can increase the risk. Such drugs include potassium supplements, nonselective beta-adrenergic blockers, cyclosporine, tacrolimus, NSAIDs, COX-2 inhibitors, trimethoprim, and pentamidine.

➡ **Concurrent Diseases.** Diseases that increase the risk of hyperkalemia for this interaction include diabetes and significant renal impairment.

➡ **Diet/Food.** A diet high in potassium may increase the risk of hyperkalemia from this interaction. Some salt substitutes contain potassium.

MECHANISM: Both triamterene and ACE inhibitors tend to increase serum potassium, and their effects are additive.

CLINICAL EVALUATION: Most of the cases of hyperkalemia in patients receiving concurrent therapy with potassium-sparing diuretics and ACE inhibitors have involved spironolactone. The RALES study, which involved the use of spironolactone and ACE inhibitors, found only a 2% risk of hyperkalemia.[1] But reports of severe and fatal hyperkalemia have started to appear, especially in patients with risk factors.[2-6] The difference is likely caused by the fact that patients in the RALES study were much more carefully monitored and received lower doses of spironolactone. There is not as much information on concurrent use of triamterene and ACE inhibitors, but it is likely that such combinations also increase the risk of hyperkalemia in predisposed patients.

RELATED DRUGS: Triamterene would also be expected to interact with other ACE inhibitors, including benazepril (*Lotensin*), captopril (eg, *Capoten*), fosinopril (*Monopril*), lisinopril (eg, *Prinivil*), moexipril (eg, *Univasc*), quinapril (*Accupril*), ramipril (*Altace*), and trandolapril (*Mavik*).

MANAGEMENT OPTIONS:

➡ **Monitor.** In patients receiving triamterene and an ACE inhibitor, monitor serum potassium and renal function, particularly if the patient has 1 or more of the risk factors listed above.

REFERENCES:

1. Pitt B, et al. The effect of spironolactone on morbidity and mortality in patients with severe heart failure. Randomized *Aldactone* Evaluation Study Investigators. *New Engl J Med*. 1999;341:709-717.
2. Schepkens H, et al. Life-threatening hyperkalemia during combined therapy with angiotensin-converting enzyme inhibitors and spironolactone: an analysis of 25 cases. *Am J Med*. 2001;110:438-441.
3. Berry C, et al. Life-threatening hyperkalemia during combined therapy with angiotensin-converting enzyme inhibitors and spironolactone. *Am J Med*. 2001;111:587.
4. Blaustein DA, et al. Estimation of glomerular filtration rate to prevent life-threatening hyperkalemia due to combined therapy with spironolactone and angiotensin-converting enzyme inhibition or angiotensin receptor blockade. *Am J Cardiol*. 2002;90:662-663.
5. Wrenger E, et al. Interaction of spironolactone with ACE inhibitors or angiotensin receptor blockers: analysis of 44 cases. *BMJ*. 2003;327:147-149.

6. Weber EW, et al. Incidence of hyperkalemia in chronic heart failure patients taking spironolactone in a VA medical center. *Pharmacotherapy.* 2003;23:391.

Triazolam (eg, *Halcion*)

Troleandomycin (*Tao*)

SUMMARY: Troleandomycin causes considerable increase in triazolam serum concentrations and increased sedation may result.

RISK FACTORS: No specific risk factors are known.

MECHANISM: Troleandomycin appears to inhibit the CYP3A4 metabolism of triazolam, reducing its systemic clearance. Triazolam's first-pass clearance also may be reduced, resulting in increased bioavailability. These changes probably are responsible for the marked increases in triazolam concentrations that have been reported.

CLINICAL EVALUATION: Following troleandomycin administration (1 g twice daily for 7 days), the half-life of triazolam increased from 1.8 to 6.5 hours, the apparent clearance was reduced from 60.7 to 15.5 L/hr, and the peak plasma concentration increased more than 100%.[1] Psychomotor impairment, memory dysfunction, and drowsiness were increased when triazolam serum concentrations were increased.

RELATED DRUGS: Erythromycin and clarithromycin (eg, *Biaxin*) may inhibit the metabolism of triazolam. Azithromycin (*Zithromax*) would not be expected to affect triazolam. Other benzodiazepines metabolized by CYP3A4 (eg, alprazolam [eg, *Xanax*], midazolam [eg, *Versed*], diazepam [eg, *Valium*]) may be inhibited similarly by troleandomycin.

MANAGEMENT OPTIONS:

➡ *Monitor.* Carefully observe patients receiving triazolam who are prescribed troleandomycin for enhanced triazolam effects. Several days may be required for the maximum effect of troleandomycin to become evident, and triazolam dosages may require adjustment after addition of the antibiotic and again when it is discontinued.

REFERENCES:
1. Warot D, et al. Troleandomycin-induced interaction in healthy volunteers: pharmacokinetic and psychometric evaluation. *Eur J Clin Pharmacol.* 1987;32:389-393.

Triclofos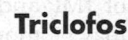

Warfarin (eg, *Coumadin*)

SUMMARY: Because triclofos transiently increases the hypoprothrombinemic response to warfarin, alternative hypnotics are preferable in patients on oral anticoagulants.

RISK FACTORS: No specific risk factors are known.

MECHANISM: A metabolite of triclofos (trichloroacetic acid) may displace warfarin or dicumarol from plasma protein binding sites.[1]

CLINICAL EVALUATION: In a study involving 7 healthy subjects stabilized on warfarin, triclofos considerably increased the hypoprothrombinemic response initially; this effect gradually diminished after the first week.[2] The authors proposed that patients receiving chronic oral anticoagulant therapy who are started on triclofos are only at risk of hemorrhage during the first 2 weeks of combined therapy.

RELATED DRUGS: Alternative sedative/hypnotic drugs unlikely to interact with oral anticoagulants include flurazepam (eg, *Dalmane*), chlordiazepoxide (eg, *Librium*), diazepam (eg, *Valium*), or diphenhydramine (eg, *Benadryl*).

MANAGEMENT OPTIONS:

➡ *Consider Alternative.* Consider an alternative sedative/hypnotic which is unlikely to interact, such as flurazepam, chlordiazepoxide, diazepam, or diphenhydramine.

➡ *Monitor.* If triclofos is used, monitor for altered oral anticoagulant effect when triclofos is initiated, discontinued, or changed in dosage. Adjust the anticoagulant dose as needed.

REFERENCES:

1. Beliles RP, et al. Interaction of bishydroxycoumarin with chloral hydrate and trichloroethyl phosphate. *Toxicol Appl Pharmacol.* 1974;27:225.

2. Sellers EM, et al. Enhancement of warfarin-induced hypoprothrombinemia by triclofos. *Clin Pharmacol Ther.* 1972;13:911.

  Trimethoprim (eg, *Proloprim*)

Zidovudine (*Retrovir*)

SUMMARY: Trimethoprim (TMP) administration tends to increase the serum concentration of zidovudine; the clinical significance appears to be limited.

RISK FACTORS:

➡ *Concurrent Diseases.* Patients with hepatic disease are at greater risk for this interaction.

MECHANISM: TMP reduces the renal clearance of zidovudine and its glucuronide metabolite.

CLINICAL EVALUATION: Seven patients with HIV were administered zidovudine, TMP, and dapsone alone and in combination.[1] Compared with zidovudine administered alone, the addition of TMP significantly (63%) reduced the renal clearance of zidovudine. However, the area under the concentration-time curve of zidovudine was increased only 23%. This effect is limited because renal clearance accounts for only 12% of zidovudine's total clearance. Similar results were noted after the combination of TMP and sulfamethoxazole (SMZ) (TMP-SMZ [eg, *Bactrim*]).[2] This interaction may be more significant in patients with liver failure since the elimination of zidovudine will be primarily via the kidney.

RELATED DRUGS: TMP-SMZ interacts similarly with zidovudine.

MANAGEMENT OPTIONS: No specific action is required, but be alert for evidence of the interaction.

REFERENCES:

1. Lee BL, et al. Trimethoprim decreases the renal clearance of zidovudine. *Clin Pharmacol Ther.* 1992;51:183.

2. Chatton JY, et al. Trimethoprim, alone or in combination with sulphamethoxazole, decreases the renal excretion of zidovudine and its glucuronide. *Br J Clin Pharmacol.* 1992;34:551.

Trimethoprim-Sulfamethoxazole (eg, *Bactrim*)

Warfarin (eg, *Coumadin*)

SUMMARY: Trimethoprim-sulfamethoxazole (TMP-SMZ) increases the hypoprothrombinemic response to warfarin; adjustments in warfarin dose may be required during cotherapy. Oral anticoagulants and other sulfonamides may also interact, but supporting evidence is limited.

RISK FACTORS:

➡ **Concurrent Diseases.** Fever may enhance the catabolism of clotting factors, thus increasing the interaction.

MECHANISM: Some sulfonamides (eg, sulfamethoxazole) appear to impair the hepatic metabolism of oral anticoagulants. Competition for plasma protein binding sites may play an additional role. Although sulfonamides reportedly decrease vitamin K production by GI bacteria, evidence for such an effect is lacking. Fever has been shown to enhance the catabolism of clotting factors.[1] Thus, the infection for which the sulfonamide is used, theoretically could enhance oral anticoagulant hypoprothrombinemia, an effect that would dissipate as the sulfonamide lowers the fever.

CLINICAL EVALUATION: Several reports have described an enhanced hypoprothrombinemic response to warfarin when SMZ (in combination with TMP) was added to the patient's therapy.[2-5] The pharmacokinetic studies in healthy subjects confirmed that TMP-SMZ enhances the hypoprothrombinemic response to warfarin in most people.[6,7] Although the SMZ seems more likely to have been responsible than the TMP, a TMP effect cannot be ruled out.

RELATED DRUGS: Preliminary clinical evidence indicates that sulfamethizole (*Thiosulfil*) inhibits warfarin metabolism[8] and that sulfaphenazole (*Thiosulf*) enhances the hypoprothrombinemic response to phenindione.[9] The effect on phenindione appeared to be more pronounced in patients with hypoalbuminemia.

MANAGEMENT OPTIONS:

➡ **Consider Alternative.** If possible, do not use TMP-SMZ in patients anticoagulated with oral agents. Consider a noninteracting antibiotic or heparin anticoagulation.

➡ **Monitor.** If the combination is used, monitor the patient carefully for an increased hypoprothrombinemic response and risk of bleeding during initiation and decreased effects upon discontinuation of TMP-SMZ.

REFERENCES:

1. Loeliger EA, et al. The biological disappearance rate of prothrombin and factors VII, IX and X from plasma in hypothyroidism, hyperthyroidism and during fever [in German]. *Thromb Diath Haemorrh Suppl.* 1964;10:267.

2. Tilstone WJ, et al. Interaction between warfarin and sulfamethoxazole. *Postgrad Med J.* 1977;53:388.

3. Kaufman JM, et al. Potentiation of warfarin by trimethoprim-sulfamethoxazole. *Urology.* 1980;16:601.

4. Errick JK, et al. Co-trimoxazole and warfarin: case report of an interaction. *Am J Hosp Pharm.* 1978;35:1399.

5. Greenlaw CW. Drug interaction between co-trimoxazole and warfarin. *Am J Hosp Pharm.* 1979;36:1155.

6. O'Reilly RA, et al. Racemic warfarin trimethoprim-sulfamethoxazole interaction in humans. *Ann Intern Med.* 1979;91:34.

7. O'Reilly RA. Stereoselective interaction of trimethoprim-sulfamethoxazole with the separated enantiomorphs of racemic warfarin in man. *N Engl J Med.* 1980;302:33.

8. Lumholtz B, et al. Sulfamethizole-induced inhibition of diphenylhydantoin, tolbutamite, and warfarin metabolsim. *Clin Pharmacol Ther.* 1975;17:731.

9. Varma DL, et al. Prothrombin response to phenindione during hypoalbuminaemia. *Br J Clin Pharmacol.* 1975;2:467.

4 **Trimipramine (eg, *Surmontil*)**

Venlafaxine (*Effexor*)

SUMMARY: A patient on venlafaxine and trimipramine developed seizures, but a causal relationship was not established.

RISK FACTORS: No specific risk factors are known.

MECHANISM: Not established. Venlafaxine appears to modestly inhibit CYP2D6,[1] and theoretically may inhibit the metabolism of trimipramine. It is also possible that the 2 drugs have additive epileptogenic effects.

CLINICAL EVALUATION: A 25-year-old woman receiving venlafaxine 150 mg/day developed seizures 11 days after her trimipramine dose was increased from 50 to 100 mg/day.[2] Although the seizures may have resulted from the combined effects of the 2 drugs, one cannot rule out that the effect resulted from the trimipramine alone. Moreover, because the patient's CYP2D6 genotype was not assessed, a possible role of high trimipramine serum concentrations caused by CYP2D6 deficiency could not be ruled out.

RELATED DRUGS: Venlafaxine also appears to inhibit imipramine (eg, *Tofranil*) metabolism. Theoretically, other tricyclic antidepressants that are metabolized by CYP2D6 (eg, desipramine [eg, *Norpramin*]) would be similarly affected.

MANAGEMENT OPTIONS: No specific action is required, but be alert for evidence of the interaction.

REFERENCES:
1. Albers LJ, et al. Effect of venlafaxine on imipramine metabolism. *Psychiatry Res.* 2000;96:235-243.
2. Schlienger RG, et al. Seizures associated with therapeutic doses of venlafaxine and trimipramine. *Ann Pharmacother.* 2000;34:1402-1405.

 Troleandomycin (*TAO*)

Clopidogrel (*Plavix*)

SUMMARY: Troleandomycin appears to inhibit the antiplatelet effects of clopidogrel, but the extent to which the therapeutic effects of clopidogrel are reduced is not known.

RISK FACTORS: No specific risk factors are known.

MECHANISM: Clopidogrel is a prodrug, and CYP3A4 appears to be the primary isozyme involved in formation of the active metabolite.[1] Troleandomycin is a CYP3A4 inhibitor, and probably inhibits the conversion of clopidogrel to its active metabolite.

CLINICAL EVALUATION: Eight healthy subjects were given a single 450 mg dose of clopidogrel with and without pretreatment with a single dose of 500 mg troleandomycin.[2] Troleandomycin was associated with a reduction in the ability of clopidogrel to inhibit platelet aggregation. With clopidogrel alone, platelet aggregation was 45%, but with concurrent troleandomycin, platelet aggregation increased to 78% of control. It is not known if this modest inhibition of clopidogrel effect would reduce the therapeutic effects of clopidogrel.

RELATED DRUGS: Erythromycin (*TAO*) also appears to inhibit the antiplatelet effects of clopidogrel. Clarithromycin (*Biaxin*) is also an inhibitor of CYP3A4 and would theoretically interact with clopidogrel in a similar manner.

MANAGEMENT OPTIONS:

➡ *Consider Alternative.* Theoretically, azithromycin (*Zithromax*) and dirithromycin (*Dynabac*) would be unlikely to interact with clopidogrel since they do not inhibit CYP3A4.

➡ *Monitor.* Consider monitoring platelet function if troleandomycin is initiated or discontinued. Adjustments in clopidogrel dose may be needed.

REFERENCES:

1. Clarke TA, et al. The metabolism of clopidogrel is catalyzed by human cytochrome P450 3A and is inhibited by atorvastatin. *Drug Metab Dispos.* 2003;31:53-59.

2. Lau WC, et al. Atorvastatin reduces the ability of clopidogrel to inhibit platelet aggregation: a new drug-drug interaction. *Circulation.* 2003;107:32-37.

Valdecoxib (*Bextra*)

Lithium (eg, *Eskalith*)

SUMMARY: Valdecoxib may increase lithium serum concentrations; monitor for lithium toxicity.

RISK FACTORS: No specific risk factors are known.

MECHANISM: Valdecoxib probably reduces renal lithium clearance, presumably through inhibition of COX-2.

CLINICAL EVALUATION: The manufacturer of valdecoxib reports a 34% increase in serum lithium following valdecoxib 40 mg twice daily for 7 days.[1] It is not known how often lithium toxicity occurs, but numerous cases of lithium toxicity have been reported following concurrent use of other COX-2 inhibitors and also nonsteroidal anti-inflammatory drugs (inhibitors of COX-1 and COX-2).[2]

RELATED DRUGS: All COX-2 inhibitors, including celecoxib (*Celebrex*) and rofecoxib (*Vioxx*), appear to increase lithium serum concentrations. Some evidence suggests that rofecoxib produces the largest increases, but confirmation is needed.

MANAGEMENT OPTIONS:

➡ **Monitor.** If valdecoxib is initiated in patients receiving lithium, monitor lithium concentrations and for evidence of lithium toxicity (nausea, vomiting, diarrhea, anorexia, coarse tremor, slurred speech, vertigo, confusion, lethargy; in severe cases, seizures, stupor, coma, cardiovascular collapse).

REFERENCES:

1. *Bextra* [package insert]. New York, NY: Pfizer Pharmaceuticals; 2004.
2. Phelan KM, et al. Lithium interaction with the cyclooxygenase 2 inhibitors rofecoxib and celecoxib and other nonsteroidal anti-inflammatory drugs. *J Clin Psychiatry*. 2003;64:1328-1334.

Vancomycin (eg, *Vancocin*)

Vecuronium (eg, *Norcuron*)

SUMMARY: A case report noted an increased degree and prolonged response to vecuronium in a patient receiving intraoperative vancomycin.

RISK FACTORS: No specific risk factors are known.

MECHANISM: Vancomycin appears to enhance the action of vecuronium.

CLINICAL EVALUATION: A 21-year-old woman was anesthetized for exploratory laparoscopy.[1] Vecuronium 4 mg was administered to assist intubation. Twenty-five minutes after induction, the electromyographic (EMG) response to ulnar nerve stimulation demonstrated a normal recovery to about 35% of control. An infusion of vancomycin 1 g was then given over 35 minutes. The EMG response decreased and slowly began to recover after the vancomycin infusion ended. The vancomycin serum concentration was 70 mcg/mL near the end of the infusion. Neuromuscular function showed delayed recovery following 35 mg edrophonium. Further study is needed to establish the causation, dose response relationship, and clinical significance of this interaction.

RELATED DRUGS: Other neuromuscular blockers may be affected similarly by vancomycin.

MANAGEMENT OPTIONS: No specific action is required, but be alert for evidence of the interaction.

REFERENCES:

1. Huang KC, et al. Vancomycin enhances the neuromuscular blockade of vecuronium. *Anesth Analg.* 1990;71:194-196.

Vecuronium (eg, *Norcuron*)

Verapamil (eg, *Calan*)

SUMMARY: Verapamil (and perhaps other calcium channel blocking drugs) appears to prolong the neuromuscular blockade of nondepolarizing neuromuscular blockers such as vecuronium and pancuronium (*Pavulon*).

RISK FACTORS: No specific risk factors are known.

MECHANISM: Calcium channel blockers may interfere with the release of neurotransmitter (acetylcholine) from prejunctional nerve terminals. Chronic calcium channel blocker administration reduces the concentration of intracellular calcium ions, diminishes the release of acetylcholine, and augments the effect of a neuromuscular blocker. In addition, verapamil may reduce the hepatic metabolism of some neuromuscular blockers.

CLINICAL EVALUATION: A patient receiving IV verapamil 5 mg 3 times a day for supraventricular tachycardia was given vecuronium for muscle relaxation during abdominal surgery.[1] Vecuronium 11 mg was administered during the 2.5-hour operation. Over the next 40 minutes, 6 mg neostigmine (eg, *Prostigmin*) was administered without reversal of the muscle relaxation. In a similar case, a patient was paralyzed with 2 mg pancuronium and 5 mg tubocurarine for a cholecystectomy.[2] At the end of the 2.5-hour operation, 2.5 mg neostigmine failed to reverse the neuromuscular blockade. Edrophonium (eg, *Tensilon*) 28 mg achieved prompt reversal of the muscle paralysis. In both cases, normal doses of muscle relaxants produced prolonged paralysis that did not respond to neostigmine reversal. The dose of vecuronium required to produce muscle relaxation was reduced up to 53% during IV nicardipine (eg, *Cardene*) infusions; higher nicardipine rates had a greater effect on vecuronium-induced muscle relaxation.[3] Nicardipine infusion reduced vecuronium clearance approximately 25%. Diltiazem (eg, *Cardizem*) infusion during surgery reduced the dosage requirements of vecuronium approximately 50% without changing its clearance.[4] It is possible a similar effect could occur following oral doses of nicardipine or diltiazem.

RELATED DRUGS: Other calcium channel blockers (eg, nicardipine, diltiazem) may produce similar interactions with vecuronium and other neuromuscular blockers (eg, pancuronium).

MANAGEMENT OPTIONS:

➡ *Circumvent/Minimize.* Reduction in the dose of muscle relaxant may be needed. Edrophonium may be required to reverse the muscle blockade.

➡ *Monitor.* Until additional information is available, carefully observe patients receiving verapamil or other calcium channel blockers for prolongation of neuromuscular blockade.

REFERENCES:

1. van Poorten JF, et al. Verapamil and reversal of vecuronium neuromuscular blockade. *Anesth Analg.* 1984;63:155-157.
2. Jones RM, et al. Verapamil potentiation of neuromuscular blockade: failure of reversal with neostigmine but prompt reversal with edrophonium. *Anesth Analg.* 1985;64:1021-1025.
3. Kawabata K, et al. Decrease in vecuronium infusion dose requirements by nicardipine in humans. *Anesth Analg.* 1994;79:1159-1164.
4. Sumikawa K, et al. Reduction in vecuronium infusion dose requirements by diltiazem in humans [abstract]. *Anesthesiology.* 1992;77:A939.

Verapamil (eg, *Calan*)

Cigarette Smoking

SUMMARY: Patients who smoke will have a modest reduction in verapamil concentrations; little effect on clinical efficacy is expected.

RISK FACTORS: No specific risk factors are known.

MECHANISM: A portion of verapamil is metabolized by CYP1A2. Smoking is known to induce the activity of this enzyme and may enhance the elimination of verapamil.

CLINICAL EVALUATION: The pharmacokinetics of verapamil following the administration of a 120 mg prolonged-release formulation every 12 hours for 7 days were compared between 12 healthy nonsmokers and 12 smokers.[1] The smokers had verapamil plasma concentrations that were about 20% less than the nonsmoking subjects.

RELATED DRUGS: Other calcium channel blockers are primarily metabolized by CYP3A4 and are not expected to interact in a clinically significant manner with cigarette smoking.

MANAGEMENT OPTIONS:

➡ *Monitor.* Monitor patients taking verapamil for efficacy and adverse reactions regardless of smoking status.

REFERENCES:

1. Fuhr U, et al. Effects of grapefruit juice and smoking on verapamil concentrations in steady state. *Eur J Clin Pharmacol.* 2002;58(1):45-53.

Verapamil (eg, *Calan*)

Colchicine (eg, *Colcrys*)

SUMMARY: A patient taking verapamil developed severe colchicine toxicity. Based on the interactive properties of the 2 drugs, it is likely that verapamil substantially increases colchicine plasma concentrations. Avoid the combination when possible.

RISK FACTORS: No specific risk factors are known.

MECHANISM: Colchicine is a P-glycoprotein substrate, and verapamil is a P-glycoprotein inhibitor; therefore, colchicine plasma concentrations are likely to increase.[1,2] Verapamil is also a CYP3A4 inhibitor and may inhibit the CYP3A4 metabolism of colchicine.

CLINICAL EVALUATION: An 83-year-old man on verapamil 120 mg/day took colchicine for an acute attack of gout.[3] He soon developed severe muscle weakness, and 4 days later, he became immobile and was hospitalized. Colchicine concentrations in the serum and cerebrospinal fluid were very high, and the colchicine half-life was about 8 times longer than expected. Given the interactive properties of the drugs, it is likely that verapamil increases the risk of colchicine toxicity. Colchicine toxicity can be fatal.

RELATED DRUGS: Diltiazem (eg, *Cardizem*) and nicardipine (eg, *Cardene*) also inhibit P-glycoprotein, and are expected to interact with colchicine. Other antiarrhythmic agents and cardiovascular drugs that inhibit P-glycoprotein include propafenone (eg, *Rythmol*) and quinidine.

MANAGEMENT OPTIONS:

➡ *Avoid Unless Benefit Outweighs Risk.* Given that colchicine toxicity can be life-threatening, use verapamil only if it is likely to provide therapeutic benefits that cannot be achieved with noninteracting alternatives.

➡ *Use Alternative.* If possible, use an alternative to verapamil that does not inhibit P-glycoprotein, or use an alternative to colchicine.

➡ *Monitor.* If the combination must be used, monitor carefully for colchicine toxicity (eg, abdominal pain, diarrhea, fever, muscle pain, vomiting). Advise patients to immediately contact their health care provider if any of these symptoms occur. Colchicine-induced pancytopenia can result in infections, bleeding, and anemia, and is often the cause of death in fatal cases.

REFERENCES:

1. Rautio J, et al. In vitro p-glycoprotein inhibition assays for assessment of clinical drug interaction potential of new drug candidates: a recommendation for probe substrates. *Drug Metab Dispos.* 2006;34(5):786-792.
2. Keogh JP, et al. Development, validation and utility of an in vitro technique for assessment of potential clinical drug-drug interactions involving P-glycoprotein. *Eur J Pharm Sci.* 2006;27(5):543-554.
3. Tröger U, et al. Tetraparesis associated with colchicine is probably due to inhibition by verapamil of the P-glycoprotein efflux pump in the blood-brain barrier. *BMJ.* 2005;331(7517):613.

Vincristine (eg, *Vincasar*)

Voriconazole (*Vfend*)

SUMMARY: Coadministration of voriconazole and vincristine may lead to the development of vincristine toxicity in some patients.

RISK FACTORS: No specific risk factors are known.

MECHANISM: Voriconazole is an inhibitor of CYP3A4, the enzyme known to metabolize vincristine.

CLINICAL EVALUATION: A child receiving vincristine as treatment for acute lymphoblastic leukemia was treated with voriconazole and levofloxacin (doses not provided) for febrile neutropenia.[1] The patient received 2 doses of vincristine (doses not provided) separated by a week while taking voriconazole. The patient was noted to have peripheral neuropathy about 3 weeks following the second dose of vincristine. The peripheral neuropathy resolved about 4 months after voriconazole and vincristine were withheld. Vincristine was again administered without voriconazole and there was no recurrence of the neuropathy. While details on this interaction are limited, it would be expected to occur based on the properties of the drugs.

RELATED DRUGS: Ketoconazole (eg, *Nizoral*), fluconazole (eg, *Diflucan*), itraconazole (eg, *Sporanox*), and posaconazole (*Noxafil*) also inhibit the activity of CYP3A4 and are expected to increase the plasma concentrations of vincristine. Vinblastine (eg, *Velban*) and vinorelbine (eg, *Navelbine*) are also CYP3A4 substrates and are likely to interact with voriconazole.

MANAGEMENT OPTIONS:

➡ *Consider Alternative.* Consider terbinafine (eg, *Lamisil*) as an alternative antifungal agent because it does not affect CYP3A4 activity. Amphotericin (eg, *Ambisome*), caspofungin (*Cancidas*), and anidulafungin (*Eraxis*) do not appear to inhibit CYP3A4.

➡ *Monitor.* If voriconazole is coadministered with vincristine, carefully monitor patients for evidence of neurotoxicity.

REFERENCES:

1. Porter CC, et al. Vincristine induced peripheral neuropathy potentiated by voriconazole in a patient with previously undiagnosed CMT1X. *Pediatr Blood Cancer.* 2009;52(2):298-300.

Vitamin C

Warfarin (eg, *Coumadin*)

SUMMARY: Isolated cases of impaired warfarin response associated with large doses of vitamin C have been reported, but this effect has not been confirmed.

RISK FACTORS: No specific risk factors are known.

MECHANISM: Not established. It has been proposed that very large doses of vitamin C (eg, at least 10 g/day) may impair GI absorption of warfarin as a result of the diarrhea produced,[1] but supporting evidence is lacking.

CLINICAL EVALUATION: In 2 case reports, vitamin C impaired the response to warfarin.[2,3] In a subsequent study involving 19 patients, 3, 5, or 10 g/day of ascorbic acid failed to produce a clinically significant effect on the hypoprothrombinemic response to warfarin[1] although plasma warfarin decreased slightly. Others also failed to find an interaction between warfarin and vitamin C.[4,5]

RELATED DRUGS: The effect of vitamin C on oral anticoagulants other than warfarin is not established.

MANAGEMENT OPTIONS: No specific action is required, but be alert for evidence of the interaction.

REFERENCES:

1. Feetam CL, et al. Lack of a clinically important interaction between warfarin and ascorbic acid. *Toxicol Appl Pharmacol.* 1975;31:544-547.

2. Rosenthal G. Interaction of ascorbic acid and warfarin. *JAMA.* 1971;215:1671.

3. Smith EC, et al. Interaction of ascorbic acid and warfarin. *JAMA.* 1972;221:1166.

4. Hume R, et al. Interaction of ascorbic acid and warfarin. *JAMA.* 1972;219:1479.

5. Weintraub M, et al. Warfarin and ascorbic acid: lack of evidence for a drug interaction. *Toxicol Appl Parmacol.* 1974;28:53-56.

Vitamin E

Warfarin (eg, *Coumadin*)

SUMMARY: Vitamin E may increase the hypoprothrombinemic response to warfarin and other oral anticoagulants. Although the incidence of this interaction in patients receiving the combination is not known, avoid vitamin E in anticoagulated patients.

RISK FACTORS:

➡ **Dosage Regimen.** The risk is probably greater with large doses of vitamin E than the small amounts normally present in multivitamin preparations.

MECHANISM: Not established. Some have proposed that vitamin E may interfere with the effects of vitamin K in the production of clotting factors.[1]

CLINICAL EVALUATION: Vitamin E 800 units/day appeared to enhance the hypoprothrombinemic response to warfarin in 1 patient.[1] In a subsequent case, vitamin E (up to 1,200 units/day) was associated with an excessive hypoprothrombinemic response to warfarin and bleeding; there was a positive challenge and dechallenge under controlled conditions in this case.[2] Vitamin E probably can increase the hypoprothrombinemic response to oral anticoagulants in some patients. Experiments in rats also indicated that vitamin E administration can enhance the anticoagulant response to warfarin.[3]

RELATED DRUGS: Three healthy subjects showed a mild increase in hypoprothrombinemic response to dicumarol 150 mg when they were given vitamin E 42 units/day for 30 days.[3]

MANAGEMENT OPTIONS:

➡ **Monitor.** Monitor for altered oral anticoagulant effect if vitamin E is initiated, discontinued, or changed in dosage. Adjust the anticoagulant dose as needed.

REFERENCES:

1. Corrigan JJ, et al. Coagulopathy associated with vitamin E ingestion. *JAMA.* 1974;230:1300-1301.
2. Vitamin K, vitamin E and the coumarin drugs. *Nutr Rev.* 1982;40:180-182.
3. Schrogie JJ, et al. Letter: coagulopathy and fat-soluble vitamins. *JAMA.* 1975;232:19.

Vitamin K

Warfarin (eg, *Coumadin*)

SUMMARY: Ingestion of large amounts of foods high in vitamin K may antagonize the hypoprothrombinemic effect of oral anticoagulants.

RISK FACTORS: No specific risk factors are known.

MECHANISM: Excessive dietary intake of vitamin K could offset oral anticoagulant-induced depression of clotting factor synthesis.

CLINICAL EVALUATION: Inhibition of the hypoprothrombinemic response to oral anticoagulants may occur with excessive intake of foods with a high vitamin K content (eg, asparagus, broccoli, cabbage, lettuce, turnip greens, beef liver, green tea, spinach, watercress, tomato).[1,2] In a study of 21 patients stabilized on warfarin, ingestion of 250 g spinach or 250 g broccoli for 1 day resulted in a small, transient reduction in hypoprothrombinemia, while daily ingestion for 7 days markedly reduced the effect of warfarin.[3] Two additional case reports of warfarin resistance have been reported in patients ingesting large amounts of broccoli.[4] A 50-year-old man receiving an oral anticoagulant developed a marked increase in hypoprothrombinemic response and bruising after he stopped eating porcine livers, while a 42-year-old woman developed inhibition of anticoagulant response and thrombus formation approximately 4 weeks after she started eating broccoli and porcine liver.[5] Case reports suggest that in at least some patients, multivitamin supplements containing vitamin K_1 25 mcg can inhibit warfarin response. It is possible that inhibition of warfarin with this small amount of vitamin K_1 occurs only in the occasional patient who has vitamin K_1 deficiency.[6]

RELATED DRUGS: All oral anticoagulants would be similarly affected by vitamin K.

MANAGEMENT OPTIONS:

➡ *Circumvent/Minimize.* Patients on oral anticoagulants should avoid sudden increases in their intake of leafy vegetables or other foods high in vitamin K content. However, warfarin requirements should not change if patients are consistent in their intake of these foods.

➡ *Monitor.* Monitor for altered hypoprothrombinemic response if vitamin K intake changes substantially.

REFERENCES:

1. Quick A. Leafy vegetables in diet alter prothrombin time in patients taking anticoagulant drugs. *JAMA.* 1987;187:27.
2. Fletcher DC. Do clotting factors in vitamin K-rich vegetables hinder anticoagulant therapy? *JAMA.* 1977;237:1871.
3. Karlson B, et al. On the influence of vitamin K-rich vegetables and wine on the effectiveness of warfarin treatment. *Acta Med Scand.* 1986;220:347-350.
4. Kempin SJ. Warfarin resistance caused by broccoli. *N Engl J Med.* 1983;308:1229-1230.
5. Chow WH, et al. Anticoagulation instability with life-threatening complication after dietary modification. *Postgrad Med J.* 1990;66:855-857.
6. Kurnik D, et al. Multivitamin supplements may affect warfarin anticoagulation in susceptible patients. *Ann Pharmacother.* 2003; 37:1603-1606.

Voriconazole (*Vfend*)

Warfarin (eg, *Coumadin*)

SUMMARY: Warfarin activity will be increased when voriconazole is added to a patient's drug regimen; excessive anticoagulation and increased risk of bleeding may occur.

RISK FACTORS:

➡ *Pharmacogenetics.* Patients who are poor metabolizers for CYP2C19 will have higher voriconazole concentrations, and they are likely to have an interaction of larger magnitude.

MECHANISM: Voriconazole is known to inhibit the activity of CYP-450 enzymes (CYP2C9, CYP2C19, and CYP3A4) responsible for the metabolism of warfarin.

CLINICAL EVALUATION: Based on limited data provided by the manufacturer, the coadministration of voriconazole 300 mg every 12 hours for 12 days and a single dose of warfarin 30 mg resulted in an approximate doubling of the maximum prothrombin time compared with placebo.[1] The study was conducted using healthy subjects. It is likely that some patients receiving warfarin and voriconazole will require an adjustment in their warfarin dosage. Depending on the dosage regimen selected, up to 7 days may be required for steady-state voriconazole concentrations to occur. The maximum effect of voriconazole on warfarin may be delayed.

RELATED DRUGS: All other antifungal agents except terbinafine (*Lamisil*) have been reported to increase the effect of warfarin.

MANAGEMENT OPTIONS:

➡ *Monitor.* Carefully monitor patients stabilized on warfarin for increased anticoagulant effect when voriconazole is initiated. Depending on the dosage regimen, 7 to 14 days may be required to observe the maximum change in the international normalized ratio. Discontinuation of voriconazole is likely to result in decreased anticoagulant effect, and warfarin doses may need to be increased.

REFERENCES:

1. *Vfend* [package insert]. New York, NY: Pfizer, Inc; 2002.

Voriconazole (*Vfend*)
Zolpidem (eg, *Ambien*)

SUMMARY: Voriconazole increases the plasma concentration of zolpidem; some patients may experience increased adverse reactions.

RISK FACTORS: No specific risk factors are known.

MECHANISM: Voriconazole inhibits the CYP3A4-dependent metabolism of zolpidem.

CLINICAL EVALUATION: Ten healthy subjects received a dose of zolpidem 10 mg alone and following voriconazole 400 mg twice daily for 1 day and then 200 mg twice daily for a second day.[1] Zolpidem was administered 1 hour after the last voriconazole dose. Following voriconazole, the mean area under the plasma concentration-time curve of zolpidem increased 40%, and its half-life increased 28%. Some patients may experience increased sedation if voriconazole is coprescribed with zolpidem.

RELATED DRUGS: Other antifungal agents that inhibit CYP3A4 (eg, itraconazole [eg, *Sporanox*], ketoconazole [eg, *Nizoral*], posaconazole [*Noxafil*], and fluconazole [eg, *Diflucan*]) are expected to affect zolpidem in a similar manner.

MANAGEMENT OPTIONS:

➡ *Consider Alternative.* Terbinafine (*Lamisil*) can be considered as an alternative antifungal agent because it does not affect CYP3A4 activity. Amphotericin (eg, *Amphotec*), caspofungin (*Cancidas*), and anidulafungin (*Eraxis*) do not appear to inhibit CYP3A4.

➡ *Monitor.* Be alert for increased sedation in patients taking voriconazole and zolpidem concurrently.

REFERENCES:

1. Saari TI, et al. Effect of voriconazole on the pharmacokinetics and pharmacodynamics of zolpidem in healthy subjects. *Br J Clin Pharmacol*. 2007;63(1):116-120.

Warfarin (eg, *Coumadin*)

Zafirlukast (*Accolate*)

SUMMARY: Zafirlukast appears to increase the hypoprothrombinemic response to warfarin; adjustments in warfarin dosage may be necessary.

RISK FACTORS: No specific risk factors are known.

MECHANISM: Since S-warfarin is metabolized primarily by CYP2C9, it seems likely that zafirlukast inhibits this isozyme.

CLINICAL EVALUATION: Sixteen healthy subjects received a single oral 25 mg dose of warfarin with and without pretreatment with zafirlukast (160 mg/day until steady state). Zafirlukast increased S-warfarin area under the concentration-time curve by 63% and the prothrombin time by 35%.[1] Since the details of this study were not presented, it is possible to assess its validity. Nonetheless, if confirmed, an interaction of this magnitude is likely to require a change in warfarin dose.

RELATED DRUGS: The effect of zafirlukast on oral anticoagulants other than warfarin is not established. If the mechanism of the interaction is inhibition of CYP2C9, phenprocoumon (which is metabolized primarily by glucuronide conjugation) theoretically would be less likely to interact with zafirlukast than warfarin.

MANAGEMENT OPTIONS:

➡ *Consider Alternative.* Given the substantial effect of zafirlukast on warfarin response, consider using alternative antiasthmatic medications. In countries where phenprocoumon is available, consider it as an alternative to warfarin, which (theoretically) would be less likely to interact.

➡ *Monitor.* Monitor for altered hypoprothrombinemic response to warfarin if zafirlukast is initiated, discontinued, or changed in dosage; adjust warfarin dose as needed.

REFERENCES:

1. Product information. Zafirlukast (*Accolate*). Zeneca Pharmaceuticals. 1996.

General Index

The key to the effective use of *Hansten and Horn's Drug Interactions Analysis and Management* is the index. The drug interaction monographs are listed in alphabetical order beginning on page 1.

All drug interaction monographs are listed by generic name except for combination products (eg, antacids, oral contraceptives) and drugs that interact equally within the class (eg, thyroid hormones, thiazide diuretics). The term "homogeneous interactions" is used within the text to refer to drug interactions that apply to all drugs equally within a pharmacological class.

The manufacturer's data for many drugs newly approved for use in the United States have included cautions on possible drug interactions. Although the potential for a drug interaction exists with some of these drugs, the scientific literature may, in the opinion of Drs. Hansten and Horn, be insufficient at the time of publication to warrant an in-depth drug-drug interaction monograph.

Descriptions of intervention categories can be found on each monograph page and are provided below as well.

5-FU
  see Fluorouracil

Abilify
  see Aripiprazole

Acarbose
  4 acetaminophen, 1

Accolate
  see Zafirlukast

Accutane
  see Isotretinoin

Acenocoumarol
  4 chlorpromazine, 1

Acetaminophen
  4 acarbose, 1
  5 amantadine, 2
  4 aspirin, 2
  4 chloramphenicol, 3
  3 cholestyramine, 3
  4 cimetidine, 4
  4 contraceptives, oral, 5
  4 diazepam, 6
  3 ethanol, 6
  4 exenatide, 8
  5 interferon alfa-2a, 8
  3 isoniazid, 9
  4 metoclopramide, 10
  3 phenobarbital, 10
  3 phenytoin, 12
  4 propantheline, 13
  4 propranolol, 13
  5 ranitidine, 14
  5 sucralfate, 15
  3 warfarin, 15
  4 zidovudine, 17

Acetazolamide
  2 aspirin, 18
  4 cyclosporine, 18
  3 methenamine, 19
  3 phenytoin, 20
  3 primidone, 20
  5 procainamide, 21
  3 quinidine, 21
  4 quinine, 22

Acetohexamide
  3 potassium, 22

Acetylcysteine
  4 nitroglycerin, 23

N-Acetylprocainamide
  4 procainamide, 24

Acitretin
  1 ethanol, 25
  2 methotrexate, 25
  1 norethindrone, 26
  3 vitamin A, 26

Actiq
  see Fentanyl

Actonel
  see Risedronate

Actos
  see Pioglitazone

Acyclovir
  4 cimetidine, 27
  4 probenecid, 27
  4 zidovudine, 28

Adenocard
  see Adenosine

Adenosine
  4 caffeine, 29
  3 dipyridamole, 29

Adenosine *(cont.)*
  3 nicotine, 30
  3 theophylline, 31

Adrenalin
  see Epinephrine

Adriamycin
  see Doxorubicin

Adrucil
  see Fluorouracil

Advil
  see Ibuprofen

Agenerase
  see Amprenavir

Albuterol
  4 digoxin, 32

Alcohol
  see Ethanol

Aldactone
  see Spironolactone

Aldomet
  see Methyldopa

Alendronate
  3 naproxen, 32
  2 parathyroid hormone, 34

Alfenta
  see Alfentanil

Alfentanil
  3 cimetidine, 34
  3 diltiazem, 35
  3 erythromycin, 35
  3 fluconazole, 36
  3 rifampin, 37
  3 troleandomycin, 38

1 = Avoid Combination   **2** = Usually Avoid Combination   **3** = Minimize Risk
4 = No Action Needed   **5** = No Interaction

Alfuzosin
  3 atenolol, 38
  4 cimetidine, 39
  3 diltiazem, 39
  1 doxazosin, 40
  3 ketoconazole, 40
  1 ritonavir, 41
  5 warfarin, 41
Aliskiren
  4 amlodipine, 42
  3 itraconazole, 42
  3 ketoconazole, 43
  3 rifampin, 44
  4 valsartan, 44
  4 verapamil, 45
Alkeran
  see Melphalan
Allegra
  see Fexofenadine
Allopurinol
  4 ampicillin, 45
  3 antacids, 46
  5 atenolol, 47
  2 azathioprine, 47
  2 captopril, 48
  4 chlorpropamide, 49
  3 cyclophosphamide, 50
  3 cyclosporine, 51
  3 mercaptopurine, 51
  4 phenytoin, 52
  4 probenecid, 53
  3 theophylline, 54
  3 vidarabine, 55
  3 warfarin, 55
Almotriptan
  3 ketoconazole, 56
  3 tapentadol, 1811
  4 verapamil, 57
Alprazolam
  4 contraceptives, oral, 58
  3 digoxin, 59
  3 erythromycin, 60
  3 fluoxetine, 60
  3 fluvoxamine, 61
  3 itraconazole, 62
  4 kava, 63
  4 lithium, 63
  4 St. John's wort, 64
Alprenolol
  3 pentobarbital, 64
Altretamine
  3 imipramine, 65
Aluminum
  3 cyclosporine, 66
Aluminum Hydroxide
  3 levothyroxine, 1393
Amantadine
  5 acetaminophen, 2

Amantadine *(cont.)*
  3 bupropion, 67
  5 cigarette smoking, 67
  4 quinidine, 68
  4 quinine, 68
  3 triamterene, 69
  3 trihexyphenidyl, 70
  4 trimethoprim/
    sulfamethoxazole, 70
Amaryl
  see Glimepiride
Ambien
  see Zolpidem
Ambrisentan
  4 ketoconazole, 71
Amidate
  see Etomidate
Amiloride
  3 candesartan, 72
  4 cimetidine, 72
  4 digoxin, 73
  3 enalapril, 74
  3 quinidine, 75
Aminoglutethimide
  3 dexamethasone, 75
  3 digitoxin, 76
  3 medroxyprogesterone,
    77
  2 tamoxifen, 78
  3 theophylline, 78
  3 warfarin, 79
Aminosalicylic Acid
  4 digoxin, 80
  4 diphenhydramine, 80
  4 phenytoin, 81
  3 rifampin, 81
  4 vitamin B_{12}, 82
  4 warfarin, 82
Amiodarone
  3 aprindine, 83
  2 aripiprazole, 83
  3 carvedilol, 84
  3 cholestyramine, 85
  3 cimetidine, 85
  4 clonazepam, 86
  4 codeine, 87
  2 colchicine, 88
  3 cyclophosphamide, 89
  3 cyclosporine, 89
  4 dextromethorphan, 90
  3 digoxin, 90
  3 diltiazem, 91
  4 disopyramide, 92
  3 donepezil, 92
  4 fentanyl, 93
  3 flecainide, 94
  3 grapefruit juice, 94
  3 indinavir, 95

Amiodarone *(cont.)*
  3 iohexol, 96
  4 lidocaine, 96
  4 methotrexate, 97
  3 metoprolol, 97
  4 orlistat, 1599
  3 phenytoin, 98
  3 procainamide, 99
  3 quinidine, 100
  3 rifampin, 100
  2 simvastatin, 101
  3 sotalol, 102
  3 theophylline, 103
  1 thioridazine, 103
  3 warfarin, 104
Amitriptyline
  2 bethanidine, 105
  4 chlordiazepoxide, 106
  4 cigarette smoking, 107
  4 disulfiram, 107
  3 donepezil, 108
  3 ethanol, 109
  3 fluconazole, 110
  3 fluoxetine, 111
  3 guanfacine, 112
  3 isoproterenol, 113
  3 lithium, 113
  3 methyldopa, 114
  5 orlistat, 115
  3 propantheline, 116
  4 St. John's wort, 117
  3 tramadol, 117
  4 warfarin, 118
Amlodipine
  4 aliskiren, 42
  4 benazepril, 119
  4 conivaptan, 668
  3 diltiazem, 119
  3 erythromycin, 120
  4 grapefruit juice, 121
  5 ibuprofen, 121
  5 indomethacin, 122
  3 telaprevir, 122
Ammonium Chloride
  4 aspirin, 123
  4 chlorpropamide, 123
  4 ephedrine, 124
  4 methadone, 124
  5 procainamide, 125
  4 pseudoephedrine, 125
  3 spironolactone, 126
Amobarbital
  4 phenmetrazine, 126
  3 tranylcypromine, 127
Amoxicillin
  4 nifedipine, 127
Amoxil
  see Amoxicillin

1 = Avoid Combination   **2** = Usually Avoid Combination   **3** = Minimize Risk
4 = No Action Needed   **5** = No Interaction

Amphojel
see Aluminum Hydroxide
Amphotericin B
3 cyclosporine, 128
3 digoxin, 129
3 gentamicin, 129
3 succinylcholine, 130
Ampicillin
4 allopurinol, 45
3 atenolol, 130
3 contraceptives, oral,
131
4 probenecid, 132
Amprenavir
3 atorvastatin, 132
3 delavirdine, 133
3 ketoconazole, 134
4 methadone, 135
3 rifabutin, 135
3 rifampin, 136
3 tipranavir, 137
Amygdalin
1 vitamin C, 137
Amytal
see Amobarbital
Anadrol
see Oxymetholone
Anafranil
see Clomipramine
Anectine
see Succinylcholine
Ansaid
see Flurbiprofen
Antabuse
see Disulfiram
Antacids
3 allopurinol, 46
3 aspirin, 138
3 atenolol, 139
3 atevirdine, 140
3 cefpodoxime proxetil,
140
4 chlordiazepoxide, 141
4 chloroquine, 141
4 chlorpromazine, 142
4 cimetidine, 143
3 ciprofloxacin, 143
3 dextroamphetamine,
145
4 dicumarol, 145
4 diflunisal, 146
3 enoxacin, 147
3 ephedrine, 147
4 erythromycin, 148
4 famotidine, 149
3 fleroxacin, 150
5 fluconazole, 150

Antacids *(cont.)*
3 gatifloxacin, 151
3 gemifloxacin, 152
3 glipizide, 152
3 glyburide, 153
3 halofantrine, 154
4 indomethacin, 155
3 iron, 155
3 isoniazid, 156
3 itraconazole, 157
3 ketoconazole, 157
5 ketorolac, 158
4 levodopa, 159
3 levofloxacin, 159
5 lithium, 160
3 lomefloxacin, 160
4 metoprolol, 161
4 metronidazole, 161
3 moxifloxacin, 162
4 naproxen, 163
3 norfloxacin, 163
3 ofloxacin, 164
5 paroxetine, 165
3 pefloxacin, 166
3 penicillamine, 167
4 phenytoin, 167
4 prednisone, 168
4 propranolol, 168
3 pseudoephedrine, 169
3 quinidine, 170
4 ranitidine, 171
3 risedronate, 1757
3 sodium polystyrene
sulfonate resin, 172
3 tetracycline, 173
4 ticlopidine, 174
4 tipranavir, 174
4 tocainide, 175
3 trovafloxacin, 175
3 vitamin C, 176
Antibiotics
see also Quinolones
Antipyrine
3 ciprofloxacin, 177
4 ethanol, 177
4 fusidic acid, 178
4 moricizine, 178
4 omeprazole, 179
4 phenobarbital, 180
3 propranolol, 180
3 verapamil, 181
Anturane
see Sulfinpyrazone
Apple Juice
3 fexofenadine, 182
Aprepitant
2 cisapride, 183
3 contraceptives, oral,
183

Aprepitant *(cont.)*
3 dexamethasone, 184
3 diltiazem, 184
3 ketoconazole, 185
3 methylprednisolone,
186
3 midazolam, 186
4 paroxetine, 187
2 pimozide, 187
3 rifampin, 188
4 tolbutamide, 188
3 warfarin, 189
Apresoline
see Hydralazine
Aprindine
3 amiodarone, 83
Aprotinin
4 succinylcholine, 189
Aptivus
see Tipranavir
Aralen
see Chloroquine
Aramine
see Metaraminol
Aripiprazole
2 amiodarone, 83
3 carbamazepine, 190
4 clozapine, 191
4 escitalopram, 191
3 fluoxetine, 192
3 itraconazole, 193
3 ketoconazole, 194
4 lorazepam, 195
3 paroxetine, 195
3 quinidine, 196
4 sertraline, 197
5 venlafaxine, 197
Aromasin
see Exemestane
Artane
see Trihexyphenidyl
Arthropan
see Choline Salicylate
Asacol
see Mesalamine
Ascorbic Acid
see Vitamin C
Aspirin
4 acetaminophen, 2
2 acetazolamide, 18
4 ammonium chloride,
123
3 antacids, 138
4 caffeine, 198
3 captopril, 199
3 chlorpropamide, 200
4 cimetidine, 201

❶ = Avoid Combination ❷ = Usually Avoid Combination ▼❸ = Minimize Risk
4 = No Action Needed **5** = No Interaction

Aspirin *(cont.)*
4 diclofenac, 202
4 diflunisal, 202
3 diltiazem, 203
3 ethanol, 204
4 fenoprofen, 205
3 fluoxetine, 206
4 flurbiprofen, 207
2 ginkgo, 208
4 gold, 208
3 griseofulvin, 209
2 ibuprofen, 209
4 imipramine, 210
4 indomethacin, 211
3 intrauterine contracep-
   tive devices, 212
4 kaolin-pectin, 213
4 ketoprofen, 213
4 levamisole, 214
5 lithium, 214
4 meclofenamate, 215
2 methotrexate, 216
4 metoprolol, 217
4 midazolam, 217
3 milnacipran, 218
4 naproxen, 218
4 nicotinic acid, 219
4 nitroglycerin, 220
4 omeprazole, 220
4 para-aminobenzoic
   acid, 221
3 pentazocine, 221
5 piroxicam, 222
3 prednisone, 223
3 probenecid, 224
4 spironolactone, 224
5 sucralfate, 225
3 sulfinpyrazone, 225
4 sulindac, 226
4 tenoxicam, 227
4 tolmetin, 227
2 warfarin, 228
3 zafirlukast, 230
Astemizole
1 erythromycin, 230
1 fluvoxamine, 231
1 ketoconazole, 232
1 mibefradil, 232
Atacand
   see Candesartan
Atarax
   see Hydroxyzine
Atazanavir
3 clarithromycin, 233
3 diltiazem, 234
3 efavirenz, 234
2 ergotamine, 235
3 erlotinib, 975
2 esomeprazole, 235

Atazanavir *(cont.)*
3 etravirine, 236
4 famotidine, 237
2 lansoprazole, 238
2 lovastatin, 239
3 maraviroc, 239
3 nevirapine, 240
2 omeprazole, 240
3 raltegravir, 241
3 ramelteon, 242
3 rifabutin, 242
2 rifampin, 243
2 simvastatin, 243
4 tenofovir, 244
Atenolol
3 alfuzosin, 38
5 allopurinol, 47
3 ampicillin, 130
3 antacids, 139
3 dipyridamole, 245
3 fingolimod, 245
5 orlistat, 246
4 propantheline, 246
4 rifampin, 247
3 rivastigmine, 247
4 tamsulosin, 248
2 valsartan, 249
5 warfarin, 249
Atevirdine
3 antacids, 140
3 fluconazole, 250
Ativan
   see Lorazepam
Atomoxetine
1 tranylcypromine, 251
Atorvastatin
3 amprenavir, 132
5 azithromycin, 251
5 cimetidine, 252
3 clarithromycin, 252
4 clopidogrel, 253
3 colchicine, 645
3 conivaptan, 669
4 cyclosporine, 254
4 digoxin, 255
3 efavirenz, 255
3 erythromycin, 256
3 etravirine, 257
3 ezetimibe, 1045
3 gemfibrozil, 257
3 itraconazole, 258
4 midazolam, 259
3 nelfinavir, 259
5 orlistat, 260
3 rifampin, 260
2 telaprevir, 261
3 tipranavir, 262
3 verapamil, 262

Atovaquone
4 zidovudine, 263
Atracurium
4 clindamycin, 264
2 gentamicin, 265
Atromid-S
   see Clofibrate
Attapulgite
3 promazine, 265
Avandia
   see Rosiglitazone
Avapro
   see Irbesartan
Axert
   see Almotriptan
Axid
   see Nizatidine
Azapropazone
2 methotrexate, 266
2 warfarin, 267
Azathioprine
2 allopurinol, 47
3 captopril, 268
4 cyclophosphamide, 269
1 febuxostat, 270
2 infliximab, 271
3 mesalamine, 272
3 phenprocoumon, 273
3 prednisolone, 273
2 ribavirin, 274
3 warfarin, 275
Azilect
   see Rasagiline
Azithromycin
5 atorvastatin, 251
5 carbamazepine, 275
5 cimetidine, 275
4 digoxin, 276
5 sildenafil, 277
5 terfenadine, 277
5 theophylline, 278
5 triazolam, 278
5 warfarin, 279
5 zidovudine, 279
Azlin
   see Azlocillin
Azlocillin
4 ciprofloxacin, 280
Azulfidine
   see Sulfasalazine

Bactocill
   see Oxacillin
Bactrim
   see Trimethoprim/
      Sulfamethoxazole

❶ = Avoid Combination ❷ = Usually Avoid Combination ▼³ = Minimize Risk
❹ = No Action Needed ❺ = No Interaction

Baicalin
   4 bupropion, 281

Baypress
   see Nitrendipine

Bellatal
   see Phenobarbital

Benadryl
   see Diphenhydramine

Benazepril
   4 amlodipine, 119

Benemid
   see Probenecid

Benylin DM
   see Dextromethorphan

Benztropine
   3 donepezil, 281
   3 haloperidol, 282

Bepridil
   3 digoxin, 283

Belupace
   see Sotalol

Betaseron
   see Interferon

Bethanechol
   3 tacrine, 284

Bethanidine
   2 amitriptyline, 105

Bezafibrate
   3 dicumarol, 285
   3 warfarin, 285

Biaxin
   see Clarithromycin

BiCNU
   see Carmustine

Bile Salts
   4 cyclosporine, 286

Biltricide
   see Praziquantel

Bismuth
   2 doxycycline, 287
   4 omeprazole, 287
   2 tetracycline, 288

Bitolterol
   2 entacapone, 959

Blocadren
   see Timolol

Bortezomib
   3 itraconazole, 288
   4 ketoconazole, 289

Bosentan
   4 ketoconazole, 290
   3 tadalafil, 290
   3 warfarin, 291

Brethaire
   see Terbutaline

Bromazepam
   5 itraconazole, 291

Bromfenac
   4 cimetidine, 292
   3 lithium, 292
   3 phenytoin, 293
   2 warfarin, 294

Bromocriptine
   3 erythromycin, 294
   4 ethanol, 295
   1 isometheptene, 295
   4 lansoprazole, 296
   4 tacrolimus, 297
   3 thioridazine, 297

Budesonide
   3 grapefruit juice, 298
   3 itraconazole, 299
   3 ketoconazole, 300
   3 ritonavir, 301

Bumetanide
   3 indomethacin, 302
   4 probenecid, 302
   5 warfarin, 303

Bumex
   see Bumetanide

Bunazosin
   3 enalapril, 303

Bupivacaine
   4 itraconazole, 304

Bupropion
   3 amantadine, 67
   4 baicalin, 281
   3 clopidogrel, 304
   4 cyclosporine, 305
   3 desipramine, 305
   3 dextromethorphan, 306
   3 efavirenz, 307
   3 flecainide, 308
   4 guanfacine, 308
   4 levodopa, 309
   4 metoprolol, 309
   3 mexiletine, 310
   4 nelfinavir, 310
   4 nortriptyline, 311
   1 phenelzine, 312
   4 prasugrel, 312
   3 propafenone, 313
   3 rifampin, 313
   4 ritonavir, 314
   4 sertraline, 314
   3 ticlopidine, 315
   4 venlafaxine, 316

Buspar
   see Buspirone

Buspirone
   4 cimetidine, 317
   3 citalopram, 317

Buspirone *(cont.)*
   3 diltiazem, 318
   3 erythromycin, 319
   3 fluoxetine, 320
   4 fluvoxamine, 321
   3 grapefruit juice, 321
   3 itraconazole, 322
   3 rifampin, 323
   3 ritonavir, 323
   3 trazodone, 324
   3 verapamil, 325

Busulfan (Busulphan)
   5 fluconazole, 326
   4 itraconazole, 326

Butazolidin
   see Phenylbutazone

Byetta
   see Exenatide

Bystolic
   see Nebivolol

Cabergoline
   3 clarithromycin, 328
   3 itraconazole, 328

Caffeine
   4 adenosine, 29
   4 aspirin, 198
   4 cimetidine, 329
   3 ciprofloxacin, 330
   4 clozapine, 331
   4 contraceptives, oral, 332
   3 enoxacin, 332
   4 ephedrine, 333
   4 ethanol, 333
   3 fluconazole, 334
   3 levothyroxine, 1394
   4 melatonin, 334
   4 menthol, 335
   3 methotrexate, 335
   4 nifedipine, 336
   3 norfloxacin, 337
   3 pipemidic acid, 337

Calan
   see Verapamil

Calcimar
   see Calcitonin

Calcitonin
   4 lithium, 338

Calcium
   3 digoxin, 339
   3 risedronate, 1757
   3 thiazides, 339
   3 verapamil, 340

Calcium Carbonate
   3 levothyroxine, 1395

Camptosar
   see Irinotecan

1 = Avoid Combination   **2** = Usually Avoid Combination   **3** = Minimize Risk
4 = No Action Needed   **5** = No Interaction

Candesartan
   3 amiloride, 72
   3 eplerenone, 969
   3 lithium, 341
   3 spironolactone, 1789
   3 triamterene, 1843
Capecitabine
   3 phenytoin, 342
   3 warfarin, 342
Capoten
   see Captopril
Captopril
   2 allopurinol, 48
   3 aspirin, 199
   3 azathioprine, 268
   5 digitoxin, 343
   3 insulin, 344
Carafate
   see Sucralfate
Carbamazepine
   3 aripiprazole, 190
   5 azithromycin, 275
   3 cimetidine, 345
   3 ciprofloxacin, 346
   3 citalopram, 347
   3 clarithromycin, 347
   5 clonazepam, 348
   3 clozapine, 349
   4 colestipol, 349
   3 contraceptives, oral, 350
   3 cyclosporine, 351
   2 danazol, 352
   3 darunavir, 353
   2 diltiazem, 353
   3 doxycycline, 354
   3 erlotinib, 976
   3 erythromycin, 355
   3 exemestane, 1041
   3 felbamate, 356
   2 felodipine, 357
   3 fexofenadine, 358
   3 fluconazole, 358
   3 fluoxetine, 359
   3 fluvoxamine, 360
   3 grapefruit juice, 361
   3 haloperidol, 362
   3 imipramine, 363
   2 irinotecan, 364
   3 isoniazid, 365
   3 isotretinoin, 365
   3 ketoconazole, 366
   3 lamotrigine, 367
   3 lapatinib, 368
   3 lithium, 368
   3 mebendazole, 369
   3 methadone, 370
   3 methylphenidate, 371
   3 metronidazole, 371

Carbamazepine *(cont.)*
   3 midazolam, 372
   4 nifedipine, 373
   3 omeprazole, 374
   3 oxybutynin, 374
   5 paroxetine, 375
   5 phenelzine, 375
   4 phenobarbital, 376
   3 phenytoin, 377
   2 propoxyphene, 378
   3 quinidine, 379
   3 risperidone, 379
   3 ritonavir, 380
   3 simvastatin, 381
   3 theophylline, 381
   5 thioridazine, 382
   3 thyroid, 382
   3 troleandomycin, 383
   3 valproic acid, 384
   2 verapamil, 385
   3 warfarin, 386
   3 ziprasidone, 387
Carbenicillin
   3 gentamicin, 387
   3 methotrexate, 388
   3 tobramycin, 389
Carbenoxolone
   3 chlorthalidone, 390
Carboplatin
   3 gentamicin, 391
Cardene
   see Nicardipine
Cardizem
   see Diltiazem
Cardura
   see Doxazosin
Carisoprodol
   3 oxycodone, 391
Carmustine
   3 cimetidine, 392
Carvedilol
   3 amiodarone, 84
   4 cimetidine, 393
   3 cyclosporine, 393
   3 digoxin, 394
   3 fluoxetine, 395
   4 rifampin, 396
Caspofungin
   3 cyclosporine, 397
   3 rifampin, 397
   3 tacrolimus, 398
Catapres
   see Clonidine
Cefamandole
   3 ethanol, 398
Cefixime
   4 nifedipine, 399

Cefizox
   see Ceftizoxime
Cefobid
   see Cefoperazone
Cefpodoxime Proxetil
   3 antacids, 140
   3 ranitidine, 399
Cefprozil
   4 metoclopramide, 400
   4 propantheline, 401
Ceftazidime
   3 chloramphenicol, 401
Ceftin
   see Cefuroxime
Ceftizoxime
   4 probenecid, 402
Ceftriaxone
   4 diclofenac, 402
   4 verapamil, 403
Cefuroxime
   3 ranitidine, 404
Cefzil
   see Cefprozil
Celebrex
   see Celecoxib
Celecoxib
   4 clopidogrel, 405
   3 lithium, 405
   4 rifampin, 406
   4 warfarin, 406
Celexa
   see Citalopram
CellCept
   see Mycophenolate Mofetil
Charcoal
   2 digoxin, 407
Chitosan
   3 valproic acid, 408
   3 warfarin, 408
Chlor-Trimeton
   see Chlorpheniramine
Chloral Hydrate
   3 ethanol, 409
   3 warfarin, 410
Chloramphenicol
   4 acetaminophen, 3
   3 ceftazidime, 401
   3 chlorpropamide, 411
   4 cyclophosphamide, 411
   2 dicumarol, 412
   4 iron, 413
   3 penicillin G, 413
   3 phenobarbital, 414
   3 phenytoin, 415
   3 rifampin, 415

1 = Avoid Combination **2** = Usually Avoid Combination **3** = Minimize Risk
4 = No Action Needed **5** = No Interaction

Chlordiazepoxide
4 amitriptyline, 106
4 antacids, 141
3 ketoconazole, 416
4 phenelzine, 417
5 warfarin, 417

Chlormethiazole
3 cimetidine, 418
5 ranitidine, 418

Chloromycetin
see Chloramphenicol

Chloroquine
4 antacids, 141
3 chlorpromazine, 419
4 cimetidine, 419
4 codeine, 420
3 cyclosporine, 421
5 imipramine, 422
4 kaolin-pectin, 422
3 methotrexate, 422
4 metronidazole, 423
3 praziquantel, 424
3 tamoxifen, 424

Chlorpheniramine
4 phenytoin, 425

Chlorphentermine
4 chlorpromazine, 425

Chlorpromazine
4 acenocoumarol, 1
4 antacids, 142
3 chloroquine, 419
4 chlorphentermine, 426
3 cigarette smoking, 426
4 cimetidine, 427
3 clonidine, 427
4 contraceptives, oral, 428
4 dextroamphetamine, 429
4 diazoxide, 429
3 donepezil, 430
3 epinephrine, 431
3 ethanol, 432
3 guanethidine, 433
4 hydroxyzine, 433
4 insulin, 434
2 levodopa, 434
3 lithium, 435
3 meperidine, 436
3 orphenadrine, 437
4 phenmetrazine, 438
3 phenobarbital, 438
3 propranolol, 439
4 tranylcypromine, 440
3 trazodone, 441

Chlorpropamide
4 allopurinol, 49

Chlorpropamide *(cont.)*
4 ammonium chloride, 123
3 aspirin, 200
3 chloramphenicol, 411
3 clofibrate, 441
4 dicumarol, 442
3 erythromycin, 443
1 ethanol, 443
5 lovastatin, 444
4 probenecid, 445
4 sucralfate, 445

Chlorthalidone
3 carbenoxolone, 390

Cholestyramine
3 acetaminophen, 3
3 amiodarone, 85
3 diclofenac, 446
3 digoxin, 447
3 furosemide, 448
4 glipizide, 448
3 hydrocortisone, 449
3 imipramine, 450
4 iron, 450
4 loperamide, 451
4 lorazepam, 451
3 methotrexate, 452
3 metronidazole, 453
3 piroxicam, 453
3 pravastatin, 454
5 propranolol, 455
3 thyroid, 455
3 valproic acid, 456
3 warfarin, 457

Choline Salicylate
5 vitamin C, 458

Choloxin
see Dextrothyroxine

Cialis
see Tadalafil

Cifenline
4 cimetidine, 458
5 ranitidine, 459

Cigarette Smoking
5 amantadine, 67
4 amitriptyline, 107
3 chlorpromazine, 426
2 clozapine, 623
1 contraceptives, oral, 459
4 diazepam, 460
4 flecainide, 461
4 glutethimide, 461
3 insulin, 462
4 lidocaine, 462
4 olanzapine, 1588
4 pentazocine, 463
4 propoxyphene, 463

Cigarette Smoking *(cont.)*
3 quinine, 464
3 tacrine, 464
3 theophylline, 465
3 thioridazine, 466
4 verapamil, 1852
4 warfarin, 466

Cilostazol
4 diltiazem, 467
3 erythromycin, 467
3 ketoconazole, 468
4 omeprazole, 468

Cimetidine
4 acetaminophen, 4
4 acyclovir, 27
3 alfentanil, 34
4 alfuzosin, 39
4 amiloride, 72
3 amiodarone, 85
4 antacids, 143
4 aspirin, 201
5 atorvastatin, 252
5 azithromycin, 275
4 bromfenac, 292
4 buspirone, 317
4 caffeine, 329
3 carbamazepine, 345
3 carmustine, 392
4 carvedilol, 393
3 chlormethiazole, 418
4 chloroquine, 419
4 chlorpromazine, 427
4 cifenline, 458
4 ciprofloxacin, 469
3 cisapride, 469
3 citalopram, 470
3 clozapine, 471
4 cyclosporine, 472
4 dapsone, 473
3 desipramine, 473
3 diazepam, 474
4 digoxin, 475
3 diltiazem, 476
5 disopyramide, 477
3 dofetilide, 477
3 doxepin, 478
4 enoxacin, 479
4 ethanol, 480
3 femoxetine, 481
3 flecainide, 482
4 fluconazole, 482
4 fluorouracil, 483
3 imipramine, 484
5 indinavir, 485
3 itraconazole, 485
3 ketoconazole, 486
3 lidocaine, 487
4 loratadine, 488
4 mebendazole, 489

1 = Avoid Combination **2** = Usually Avoid Combination **3** = Minimize Risk

4 = No Action Needed **5** = No Interaction

Cimetidine *(cont.)*
4 mefloquine, 489
3 melphalan, 490
3 meperidine, 490
3 metformin, 491
4 metronidazole, 492
5 mexiletine, 493
4 moclobemide, 493
3 moricizine, 494
4 nebivolol, 494
3 nicotine, 495
3 nifedipine, 496
3 nimodipine, 497
3 nisoldipine, 497
3 nitrendipine, 498
3 nortriptyline, 499
3 paroxetine, 500
4 phenobarbital, 501
3 phenytoin, 501
3 posaconazole, 502
3 praziquantel, 503
3 procainamide, 504
3 propafenone, 505
3 propranolol, 506
3 quinidine, 507
5 repaglinide, 508
4 rimantadine, 508
3 sildenafil, 509
5 sucralfate, 509
3 tacrine, 510
3 tamoxifen, 511
3 tamsulosin, 512
4 temafloxacin, 513
5 terfenadine, 513
3 theophylline, 514
3 tizanidine, 515
4 tocainide, 516
3 tolbutamide, 516
4 triamterene, 518
3 verapamil, 518
4 voriconazole, 519
2 warfarin, 520
4 zidovudine, 521
Cinacalcet
3 desipramine, 521
3 ketoconazole, 522
3 tamoxifen, 523
3 thioridazine, 523
Cipralan
see Cifenline
Cipro
see Ciprofloxacin
Ciprofloxacin
3 antacids, 143
3 antipyrine, 177
4 azlocillin, 280
3 caffeine, 330
3 carbamazepine, 346
4 cimetidine, 469

Ciprofloxacin *(cont.)*
3 clozapine, 524
4 cyclophosphamide, 525
4 cyclosporine, 525
3 diazepam, 526
3 didanosine, 527
3 duloxetine, 928
3 erlotinib, 527
5 ethanol, 528
3 food, 528
3 foscarnet, 529
3 glyburide, 530
3 iron, 531
3 levothyroxine, 1396
3 metoprolol, 531
4 mexiletine, 532
3 olanzapine, 533
3 pentoxifylline, 533
3 phenytoin, 534
4 probenecid, 534
5 quinidine, 535
2 ramelteon, 535
3 rasagiline, 536
5 rifampin, 537
3 ropinirole, 537
3 ropivacaine, 538
3 sildenafil, 538
3 sucralfate, 539
3 tamoxifen,
3 theophylline, 540
2 tizanidine, 541
3 warfarin, 541
3 zinc, 542
Cisapride
2 aprepitant, 183
3 cimetidine, 469
2 clarithromycin, 543
5 digoxin, 544
4 disopyramide, 544
2 erythromycin, 545
2 grapefruit juice, 546
2 indinavir, 546
2 itraconazole, 547
2 ketoconazole, 548
2 mibefradil, 549
2 miconazole, 549
2 nefazodone, 550
2 ritonavir, 551
3 sertraline, 551
3 simvastatin, 552
4 sparfloxacin, 553
2 troleandomycin, 554
4 warfarin, 554
4 wine, 555
Cisplatin
3 diazoxide, 555
2 ethacrynic acid, 556
3 gentamicin, 557
4 lithium, 557

Cisplatin *(cont.)*
4 ondansetron, 558
3 phenytoin, 559
3 valproic acid, 560
Citalopram
3 buspirone, 317
3 carbamazepine, 347
3 cimetidine, 470
4 clozapine, 560
3 fentanyl, 561
4 irinotecan, 562
3 linezolid, 562
3 meperidine, 563
1 methylene blue, 564
4 metoprolol, 565
2 moclobemide, 565
3 quetiapine, 566
3 thiazides, 567
3 tramadol, 568
Clarithromycin
3 atazanavir, 233
3 atorvastatin, 252
3 cabergoline, 328
3 carbamazepine, 347
2 cisapride, 543
1 colchicine, 569
2 conivaptan, 670
3 cyclosporine, 570
3 digoxin, 571
3 disopyramide, 890
2 ergotamine, 572
3 erlotinib, 976
3 etravirine, 572
3 fentanyl, 573
4 fluconazole, 574
3 glyburide, 574
3 indinavir, 575
3 itraconazole, 576
3 lansoprazole, 577
3 midazolam, 578
4 nifedipine, 579
4 omeprazole, 579
3 oxycodone, 580
2 pimozide, 581
3 prednisone, 582
3 repaglinide, 583
1 rifabutin, 583
3 rifampin, 584
4 ritonavir, 585
3 sildenafil, 586
2 simvastatin, 586
3 sirolimus, 587
3 tacrolimus, 588
2 terfenadine, 589
4 theophylline, 589
3 tipranavir, 590
3 triazolam, 591
3 verapamil, 591
2 vinorelbine, 592

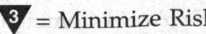

❶ = Avoid Combination ❷ = Usually Avoid Combination ▼❸ = Minimize Risk
❹ = No Action Needed ❺ = No Interaction

Clarithromycin *(cont.)*
3 warfarin, 593
4 zidovudine, 594
Claritin
see Loratadine
Cleocin
see Clindamycin
Clinafloxacin
3 theophylline, 594
Clindamycin
4 atracurium, 264
4 gentamicin, 595
Clinoril
see Sulindac
Clobazam
3 phenytoin, 596
Clofibrate
3 chlorpropamide, 441
4 contraceptives, oral,
596
3 furosemide, 597
3 rifampin, 598
2 warfarin, 598
Clomipramine
3 fluvoxamine, 599
3 grapefruit juice, 600
3 ibuprofen, 600
1 methylene blue, 602
2 moclobemide, 603
3 olanzapine, 604
4 oxybutynin, 604
1 phenelzine, 605
2 rasagiline, 606
3 tapentadol, 1812
Clonazepam
4 amiodarone, 86
5 carbamazepine, 348
4 clozapine, 607
5 fluoxetine, 607
4 phenobarbital, 608
4 phenytoin, 608
4 primidone, 609
3 valproic acid, 609
Clonidine
3 chlorpromazine, 427
3 cyclosporine, 610
2 desipramine, 611
3 insulin, 612
4 levodopa, 613
3 milnacipran, 613
2 mirtazapine, 614
3 nitroprusside, 615
4 piribedil, 615
4 propranolol, 616
4 verapamil, 617
Clopidogrel
4 atorvastatin, 253

Clopidogrel *(cont.)*
3 bupropion, 304
4 celecoxib, 405
3 erythromycin, 981
3 itraconazole, 617
3 ketoconazole, 618
3 omeprazole, 619
3 rifampin, 620
3 troleandomycin, 1848
Clorazepate
4 omeprazole, 620
4 primidone, 621
Clotrimazole
3 midazolam, 621
3 tacrolimus, 622
Clozapine
4 aripiprazole, 191
4 caffeine, 331
3 carbamazepine, 349
2 cigarette smoking, 623
3 cimetidine, 471
3 ciprofloxacin, 524
4 citalopram, 560
4 clonazepam, 607
3 diazepam, 624
2 erythromycin, 625
2 fluvoxamine, 625
4 haloperidol, 626
4 lithium, 627
4 loperamide, 627
3 lorazepam, 628
4 modafinil, 629
4 nefazodone, 629
4 omeprazole, 630
4 risperidone, 630
4 sertraline, 631
3 troleandomycin, 1848
3 valproic acid, 631
Clozaril
see Clozapine
Co-Trimoxazole
see Trimethoprim/
Sulfamethoxazole
Cocaine
3 disulfiram, 632
3 propranolol, 633
Codeine
4 amiodarone, 87
4 chloroquine, 420
4 fluoxetine, 633
4 haloperidol, 634
4 mibefradil, 635
4 paroxetine, 636
4 perphenazine, 637
4 propafenone, 638
4 propoxyphene, 639
4 quinacrine, 640
2 quinidine, 641

Codeine *(cont.)*
3 rifampin, 643
4 thioridazine, 644
Cogentin
see Benztropine
Cognex
see Tacrine
Colchicine
2 amiodarone, 88
3 atorvastatin, 645
1 clarithromycin, 569
2 conivaptan, 670
3 cyclosporine, 646
2 diltiazem, 647
4 disulfiram, 648
1 erythromycin, 649
5 febuxostat, 1047
3 fluvastatin, 649
4 gemfibrozil, 650
1 grapefruit, 651
3 hydroxychloroquine,
652
2 indinavir, 1260
2 itraconazole, 1309
2 ketoconazole, 653
2 lapatinib, 1381
3 lovastatin, 654
3 pravastatin, 655
2 propafenone, 1689
2 quinidine, 1710
2 ritonavir, 656
3 simvastatin, 657
2 tamoxifen, 1811
2 telaprevir, 658
2 verapamil, 1852
Colesevelam
3 contraceptives, oral,
659
3 cyclosporine, 660
4 glyburide, 660
3 levothyroxine, 661
3 phenytoin, 662
4 verapamil, 662
3 warfarin, 663
Colestid
see Colestipol
Colestipol
4 carbamazepine, 349
3 diclofenac, 664
4 digitoxin, 664
4 digoxin, 665
3 furosemide, 666
3 gemfibrozil, 666
3 tetracycline, 667
3 thiazides, 668
Compazine
see Prochlorperazine

1 = Avoid Combination 2 = Usually Avoid Combination 3 = Minimize Risk
4 = No Action Needed 5 = No Interaction

Comtan
  see Entacapone
Conivaptan
  4 amlodipine, 668
  3 atorvastatin, 669
  2 clarithromycin, 670
  2 colchicine, 670
  3 digoxin, 671
  2 ketoconazole, 671
  2 lovastatin, 672
  3 midazolam, 673
  2 ritonavir, 673
  2 simvastatin, 674
  5 warfarin, 675
Contraceptives, Oral
  4 acetaminophen, 5
  4 alprazolam, 58
  3 ampicillin, 131
  4 aprepitant, 183
  4 caffeine, 332
  3 carbamazepine, 350
  4 chlorpromazine, 428
  1 cigarette smoking, 459
  4 clofibrate, 596
  3 colesevelam, 659
  3 cyclosporine, 704
  4 ethanol, 1007
  3 felbamate, 675
  5 fluconazole, 1073
  5 gabapentin, 676
  3 griseofulvin, 1221
  4 imipramine, 1253
  4 insulin, 1282
  3 lamotrigine, 676
  3 meperidine, 1458
  4 mineral oil, 1527
  3 modafinil, 1535
  4 nefazodone, 677
  3 oxcarbazepine, 678
  3 oxybutynin, 679
  3 phenobarbital, 679
  3 phenytoin, 680
  3 prednisolone, 681
  4 prochlorperazine, 682
  3 rifabutin, 682
  3 rifampin, 683
  3 ritonavir, 684
  3 selegiline, 685
  3 St. John's wort, 686
  3 tetracycline, 687
  5 thalidomide, 688
  4 theophylline, 688
  4 thyroid, 689
  3 tizanidine, 690
  3 topiramate, 690
  5 vigabatrin, 691
  2 warfarin, 692
Contrast Media
  3 propranolol, 693

Cordarone
  see Amiodarone
Coreg
  see Carvedilol
Corgard
  see Nadolol
Cortef
  see Hydrocortisone
Coumadin
  see Warfarin
Cozaar
  see Losartan
Cranberry Juice
  4 warfarin, 693
Crixivan
  see Indinavir
Cromolyn
  4 dexamethasone, 694
  5 ethanol, 694
Crystodigin
  see Digitoxin
Cuprimine
  see Penicillamine
Cyanocobalamin
  see Vitamin B_{12}
Cyclizine
  3 donepezil, 695
Cyclobenzaprine
  3 donepezil, 696
  3 droperidol, 697
  2 duloxetine, 697
  3 fluoxetine, 698
  3 phenelzine, 699
  2 rasagiline, 699
Cyclophosphamide
  3 allopurinol, 50
  3 amiodarone, 89
  4 azathioprine, 269
  4 chloramphenicol, 411
  4 ciprofloxacin, 525
  3 digoxin, 700
  4 ondansetron, 701
  4 phenobarbital, 701
  4 phenytoin, 702
  4 prednisone, 702
  3 succinylcholine, 703
  3 warfarin, 703
Cycloserine
  3 isoniazid, 704
Cyclosporine
  4 acetazolamide, 18
  3 allopurinol, 51
  3 aluminum, 66
  3 amiodarone, 89
  3 amphotericin B, 128
  4 atorvastatin, 254

Cyclosporine *(cont.)*
  4 bile salts, 286
  4 bupropion, 305
  3 carbamazepine, 351
  3 carvedilol, 393
  3 caspofungin, 397
  3 chloroquine, 421
  4 cimetidine, 472
  4 ciprofloxacin, 525
  3 clarithromycin, 570
  3 clonidine, 610
  3 colchicine, 646
  3 colesevelam, 660
  3 contraceptives, oral, 704
  2 danazol, 705
  3 diclofenac, 707
  3 digoxin, 708
  3 diltiazem, 708
  3 doxorubicin, 709
  3 droperidol,
  3 enalapril, 710
  3 erythromycin, 711
  4 ethanol, 712
  3 etoposide, 712
  3 felodipine, 713
  3 fluconazole, 714
  4 fluvastatin, 715
  3 gentamicin, 715
  3 glipizide, 716
  3 grapefruit juice, 717
  3 griseofulvin, 718
  3 imipenem, 718
  3 indomethacin, 719
  4 isotretinoin, 720
  3 itraconazole, 720
  3 josamycin, 721
  3 ketoconazole, 722
  3 ketoprofen, 723
  5 levofloxacin, 723
  3 levothyroxine, 724
  3 lovastatin, 724
  3 mefenamic acid, 725
  3 melphalan, 726
  3 methotrexate, 726
  4 methylphenidate, 727
  3 metoclopramide, 727
  4 metronidazole, 728
  3 miconazole, 729
  3 modafinil, 730
  3 nafcillin, 730
  3 naproxen, 731
  3 nicardipine, 732
  4 nifedipine, 732
  4 norfloxacin, 733
  5 ofloxacin, 733
  4 omeprazole, 734
  2 orlistat, 1600
  5 oxybutynin, 734

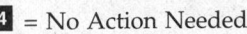 ❶ = Avoid Combination   ❷ = Usually Avoid Combination   ▼❸ = Minimize Risk
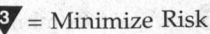 ❹ = No Action Needed   ❺ = No Interaction

Cyclosporine (cont.)
  5 pefloxacin, 735
  3 phenobarbital, 735
  3 phenytoin, 736
  2 pitavastatin, 737
  3 posaconazole, 738
  4 pravastatin, 738
  3 prednisolone, 739
  3 probucol, 740
  4 propafenone, 740
  4 pyrazinamide, 741
  3 quinupristin/
     dalfopristin, 742
  5 ranitidine, 742
  3 repaglinide, 743
  2 rifampin, 744
  4 rosuvastatin, 745
  3 roxithromycin, 745
  4 sertraline, 746
  3 simvastatin, 746
  2 St. John's wort, 747
  3 sulindac, 748
  3 sulphadimidine, 749
  2 telaprevir, 750
  3 ticlopidine, 751
  4 trimethoprim/
     sulfamethoxazole,
     751
  3 verapamil, 752
  3 voriconazole, 753
  4 warfarin, 753
  3 wine, red, 754
Cymbalta
  see Duloxetine
Cyproheptadine
  3 fluoxetine, 755
  4 phenelzine, 756
Cytadren
  see Aminoglutethimide
Cytotec
  see Misoprostol
Cytovene
  see Ganciclovir
Cytoxan
  see Cyclophosphamide

Dalmane
  see Flurazepam
Danazol
  2 carbamazepine, 352
  2 cyclosporine, 705
  3 lovastatin, 757
  2 warfarin, 757
Danocrine
  see Danazol
Danshen
  3 warfarin, 758

Dantrium
  see Dantrolene
Dantrolene
  4 verapamil, 759
Dapsone
  4 cimetidine, 473
  3 didanosine, 760
  3 probenecid, 760
  3 rifampin, 761
  3 trimethoprim, 761
  4 zalcitabine, 762
  5 zidovudine, 762
Daraprim
  see Pyrimethamine
Darunavir
  3 carbamazepine, 353
  4 etravirine, 763
  3 ketoconazole, 764
Darvocet-N
  see Propoxyphene
Darvon
  see Propoxyphene
Dasatinib
  3 famotidine, 764
  3 ketoconazole, 765
  3 rifampin, 766
Debrisoquin
  3 desipramine, 766
Decadron
  see Dexamethasone
Deferasirox
  3 repaglinide, 767
  3 rifampin, 768
Delavirdine
  3 amprenavir, 133
  3 omeprazole, 768
  3 paclitaxel, 769
  3 rifabutin, 770
  3 rifampin, 770
Deltasone
  see Prednisone
Demerol
  see Meperidine
Depakene
  see Valproic Acid
Desflurane
  4 dobutamine, 771
  4 dopamine, 772
Desipramine
  3 bupropion, 305
  3 cimetidine, 473
  3 cinacalcet, 521
  2 clonidine, 611
  3 debrisoquin, 766
  4 duloxetine, 928
  3 fluoxetine, 772

Desipramine (cont.)
  3 guanethidine, 774
  4 ibuprofen, 775
  5 ketoconazole, 776
  4 phenylbutazone, 776
  3 ritonavir, 777
  3 venlafaxine, 777
Desyrel
  see Trazodone
Detrol
  see Tolterodine
Dexamethasone
  3 aminoglutethimide, 75
  3 aprepitant, 184
  4 cromolyn, 694
  4 ephedrine, 778
Dexedrine
  see Dextroamphetamine
Dexfenfluramine
  2 fluoxetine, 778
  1 phenelzine, 779
Dextroamphetamine
  3 antacids, 145
  4 chlorpromazine, 429
  3 furazolidone, 780
  3 guanethidine, 781
  3 imipramine, 781
  4 norepinephrine, 782
  1 tranylcypromine, 782
Dextromethorphan
  4 amiodarone, 90
  3 bupropion, 306
  3 fluoxetine, 784
  4 linezolid, 785
  1 moclobemide, 785
  1 phenelzine, 786
  4 propoxyphene, 787
  3 quinidine, 788
  2 rasagiline, 788
  2 selegiline, 789
  2 sibutramine, 790
  3 terbinafine, 790
Dextrostat
  see Dextroamphetamine
Dextrothyroxine
  2 warfarin, 791
DHEA
  4 triazolam, 792
DiaBeta
  see Glyburide
Diabinese
  see Chlorpropamide
Diamox
  see Acetazolamide
Diasorb
  see Attapulgite

1 = Avoid Combination **2** = Usually Avoid Combination **3** = Minimize Risk
4 = No Action Needed **5** = No Interaction

Diazepam
  4 acetaminophen, 6
  4 cigarette smoking, 460
  3 cimetidine, 474
  3 ciprofloxacin, 526
  3 clozapine, 624
  4 digoxin, 792
  4 diltiazem, 793
  3 disulfiram, 793
  3 ethanol, 794
  5 felodipine, 796
  3 fluconazole, 796
  3 fluoxetine, 797
  4 gallamine, 798
  4 haloperidol, 799
  3 isoniazid, 799
  3 itraconazole, 800
  3 levodopa, 800
  4 lithium, 801
  3 metoprolol, 802
  5 naproxen, 802
  3 omeprazole, 803
  5 paroxetine, 804
  4 propranolol, 804
  3 rifampin, 805
  4 sertraline, 805
  4 succinylcholine, 806
  5 tacrine, 807
  4 valproic acid, 807
  3 voriconazole, 808
  5 warfarin, 808
Diazoxide
  4 chlorpromazine, 429
  3 cisplatin, 555
  3 hydralazine, 809
  3 phenytoin, 809
  3 thiazides, 810
  4 warfarin, 810
Diclofenac
  4 aspirin, 202
  4 ceftriaxone, 402
  3 cholestyramine, 446
  3 colestipol, 664
  3 cyclosporine, 707
  3 lithium, 811
  2 methotrexate, 812
  3 verapamil, 813
  2 warfarin, 814
Dicloxacillin
  4 warfarin, 815
Dicumarol
  4 antacids, 145
  3 bezafibrate, 285
  2 chloramphenicol, 412
  4 chlorpropamide, 442
  3 ethchlorvynol, 815
  3 tolbutamide, 816
Dicyclomine
  3 donepezil, 817

Didanosine
  3 ciprofloxacin, 527
  3 dapsone, 760
  5 fluconazole, 818
  3 food, 818
  5 foscarnet, 819
  3 ganciclovir, 820
  3 indinavir, 820
  3 itraconazole, 821
  3 ketoconazole, 822
  4 ranitidine, 823
  4 rifabutin, 823
  4 ritonavir, 824
  5 stavudine, 824
  3 tenofovir, 825
  4 zidovudine, 826
Diethylpropion
  5 guanethidine, 826
  5 methyldopa, 827
Diflucan
  see Fluconazole
Diflunisal
  4 antacids, 146
  4 aspirin, 202
  2 warfarin, 827
Digitoxin
  3 aminoglutethimide, 76
  5 captopril, 343
  4 colestipol, 664
  3 phenobarbital, 828
  4 phenylbutazone, 829
  3 rifampin, 830
Digoxin
  4 albuterol, 32
  3 alprazolam, 59
  4 amiloride, 73
  4 aminosalicylic acid, 80
  3 amiodarone, 90
  3 amphotericin B, 129
  4 atorvastatin, 255
  4 azithromycin, 276
  3 bepridil, 283
  3 calcium, 339
  3 carvedilol, 394
  2 charcoal, 407
  3 cholestyramine, 447
  4 cimetidine, 475
  5 cisapride, 544
  3 clarithromycin, 571
  4 colestipol, 665
  3 conivaptan, 671
  3 cyclophosphamide, 700
  3 cyclosporine, 708
  4 diazepam, 792
  3 diltiazem, 830
  4 dipyridamole, 831
  4 disopyramide, 832
  5 dofetilide, 906
  2 donepezil, 908

Digoxin *(cont.)*
  3 dronedarone, 833
  4 edrophonium, 833
  3 erythromycin, 834
  4 exenatide, 834
  4 famciclovir, 835
  4 flecainide, 835
  4 grapefruit juice, 837
  3 hydroxychloroquine,
    838
  3 itraconazole, 838
  3 kaolin-pectin, 839
  5 lidocaine, 840
  3 metoclopramide, 840
  3 mibefradil, 841
  4 moricizine, 842
  3 nebivolol, 843
  3 nefazodone, 843
  3 neomycin, 844
  4 nitrendipine, 844
  3 omeprazole, 845
  3 penicillamine, 846
  4 pirmenol, 846
  4 pravastatin, 847
  3 propafenone, 847
  3 propantheline, 848
  3 propranolol, 849
  3 quinidine, 850
  3 quinine, 851
  3 ranolazine, 852
  3 rifampin, 852
  3 ritonavir, 853
  5 ropinirole, 854
  4 Siberian ginseng, 854
  5 silodosin, 855
  3 spironolactone, 855
  3 St. John's wort, 856
  3 succinylcholine, 857
  4 sucralfate, 858
  3 sulfasalazine, 858
  4 tacrine, 859
  5 tamsulosin, 859
  3 telaprevir, 860
  3 telithromycin, 860
  3 telmisartan, 861
  5 tenidap, 861
  5 terbinafine, 862
  3 tetracycline, 862
  4 ticagrelor, 863
  4 ticlopidine, 863
  4 tolvaptan, 864
  4 trimethoprim, 864
  3 verapamil, 865
  5 voriconazole, 866
Dihydrocodeine
  4 sildenafil, 867
Dihydroergotamine
  2 sibutramine, 867

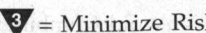

❶ = Avoid Combination   **❷** = Usually Avoid Combination   **▼3** = Minimize Risk
4 = No Action Needed   **5** = No Interaction

Dihydroergotamine (*cont.*)
  1 sumatriptan, 868
Dilantin
  see Phenytoin
Diltiazem
  3 alfentanil, 35
  3 alfuzosin, 39
  3 amiodarone, 91
  3 amlodipine, 119
  3 aprepitant, 184
  3 aspirin, 203
  3 atazanavir, 234
  3 buspirone, 318
  2 carbamazepine, 353
  4 cilostazol, 467
  3 cimetidine, 476
  2 colchicine, 647
  3 cyclosporine, 708
  4 diazepam, 793
  3 digoxin, 830
  3 encainide, 868
  3 fentanyl, 869
  4 grapefruit juice, 870
  3 lovastatin, 870
  3 methylprednisolone,
      871
  3 midazolam, 872
  3 nifedipine, 873
  3 nitroprusside, 874
  4 phenytoin, 874
  5 pravastatin, 875
  3 propranolol, 875
  3 quinidine, 876
  3 ranolazine, 877
  3 rifampin, 878
  3 saxagliptin, 878
  3 sildenafil, 879
  3 sirolimus, 880
  3 tacrolimus, 880
  3 ticagrelor, 881
  4 tolbutamide, 882
  3 triazolam, 882
  4 warfarin, 883
Diphenhydramine
  4 aminosalicylic acid, 80
  3 donepezil, 883
  3 metoprolol, 884
  3 tamoxifen, 885
  2 thioridazine, 886
  4 venlafaxine, 887
  5 warfarin, 888
Diphenoxylate
  4 quinidine, 888
Diprivan
  see Propofol
Dipyridamole
  3 adenosine, 29
  3 atenolol, 245

Dipyridamole (*cont.*)
  4 digoxin, 831
Dirithromycin
  5 terfenadine, 888
  4 theophylline, 889
Disopyramide
  4 amiodarone, 92
  5 cimetidine, 477
  4 cisapride, 544
  3 clarithromycin, 890
  4 digoxin, 832
  3 donepezil, 891
  3 erythromycin, 891
  4 insulin, 892
  3 lidocaine, 893
  4 mexiletine, 893
  3 phenobarbital, 894
  3 phenytoin, 894
  3 potassium, 895
  3 practolol, 896
  4 quinidine, 897
  3 rifampin, 897
  2 thioridazine, 898
  4 warfarin, 899
Disulfiram
  4 amitriptyline, 107
  3 cocaine, 632
  4 colchicine, 648
  3 diazepam, 793
  1 ethanol, 899
  2 isoniazid, 900
  1 lopinavir/ritonavir,
      1433
  3 metronidazole, 901
  4 omeprazole, 901
  5 phenobarbital, 902
  3 phenytoin, 902
  3 theophylline, 903
  5 tolbutamide, 904
  3 tranylcypromine, 904
  4 venlafaxine, 905
  2 warfarin, 905
Ditropan
  see Oxybutynin
Diuretic, Herbal
  4 lithium, 906
Diuretics
  see also Thiazides
Dobutamine
  4 desflurane, 771
  2 entacapone, 960
Dobutrex
  see Dobutamine
Dofetilide
  3 cimetidine, 477
  5 digoxin, 906
  5 warfarin, 907
  2 ziprasidone, 907

Dolobid
  see Diflunisal
Dolophine
  see Methadone
Donepezil
  3 amiodarone, 92
  3 amitrityline, 108
  3 benztropine, 281
  3 chlorpromazine, 430
  3 cyclizine, 695
  3 cyclobenzaprine, 696
  3 dicyclomine, 817
  2 digoxin, 908
  3 diphenhydramine, 883
  3 disopyramide, 891
  4 ketoconazole, 909
Dopamine
  4 desflurane, 772
  3 ergonovine, 910
  4 metoprolol, 910
  3 phenytoin, 911
Dopram
  see Doxapram
Doxapram
  4 phenelzine, 911
Doxazosin
  1 alfuzosin, 40
  3 nifedipine, 912
  3 tadalafil, 1809
Doxepin
  3 cimetidine, 478
  5 crythromycin, 912
  3 propoxyphene, 913
  3 tolazamide, 913
Doxorubicin
  3 cyclosporine, 709
  4 phenobarbital, 914
  3 verapamil, 915
Doxycycline
  2 bismuth, 287
  3 carbamazepine, 354
  3 ethanol, 915
  3 methotrexate, 916
  3 phenobarbital, 916
  3 phenytoin, 917
  3 warfarin, 918
Dronedarone
  3 digoxin, 833
  3 grapefruit juice, 918
  2 ketoconazole, 919
  3 metoprolol, 920
  3 propranolol, 920
  3 rifampin, 921
  3 simvastatin, 922
  3 sirolimus, 922
  3 verapamil, 923
Droperidol
  3 cyclobenzaprine, 697

1 = Avoid Combination   **2** = Usually Avoid Combination   **3** = Minimize Risk
4 = No Action Needed   **5** = No Interaction

Droperidol *(cont.)*
   4 thioridazine, 924

Drospirenone
   3 enalapril, 924
   3 heparin, 925
   3 ibuprofen, 925
   3 losartan, 926
   3 potassium, 927
   3 triamterene, 927

Duloxetine
   3 ciprofloxacin, 928
   2 cyclobenzaprine, 697
   4 desipramine, 928
   4 flecainide, 929
   2 fluvoxamine, 929
   3 lithium, 930
   2 paroxetine, 931
   4 propafenone, 931
   3 quinidine, 932
   3 St. John's wort, 932
   1 thioridazine, 933
   3 tramadol, 933
   1 tranylcypromine, 934
   3 tryptophan, 934

Duramorph
   see Morphine

Dymelor
   see Acetohexamide

Dynabac
   see Dirithromycin

DynaCirc
   see Isradipine

Dynapen
   see Dicloxacillin

Dyphylline
   3 probenecid, 935

Dyrenium
   see Triamterene

E-*Mycin*
   see Erythromycin

Echinacea
   4 midazolam, 936

Echothiophate Iodide
   2 succinylcholine, 936

Edecrin
   see Ethacrynic Acid

Edrophonium
   4 digoxin, 833

Efavirenz
   3 atazanavir, 234
   3 atorvastatin, 255
   3 bupropion, 307
   3 indinavir, 937
   3 ketoconazole, 938
   3 maraviroc, 938
   3 methadone, 939

Efavirenz *(cont.)*
   3 pravastatin, 940
   3 proguanil, 940
   3 raltegravir, 941
   3 rifabutin, 941
   3 rifampin, 942
   3 ritonavir, 943
   3 saquinavir, 943
   3 simvastatin, 944
   3 tipranavir, 945
   3 voriconazole, 945

Effexor
   see Venlafaxine

Elavil
   see Amitriptyline

Eldepryl
   see Selegiline

Eletriptan
   2 erythromycin, 946
   3 fluconazole, 947
   2 ketoconazole, 947
   3 verapamil, 948

Emcyt
   see Estramustine

Emend
   see Aprepitant

Enable
   see Tenidap

Enalapril
   3 amiloride, 74
   3 bunazosin, 303
   3 cyclosporine, 710
   3 drospirenone, 924
   3 eplerenone, 970
   3 furosemide, 949
   3 indomethacin, 950
   3 iron, 951
   3 rofecoxib, 951
   3 spironolactone, 1790
   4 tamsulosin, 952
   3 triamterene, 1844
   3 trimethoprim/
       sulfamethoxazole,
       953

Encainide
   3 diltiazem, 868
   3 quinidine, 953

Enkaid
   see Encainide

Enoxacin
   3 antacids, 147
   3 caffeine, 332
   4 cimetidine, 479
   3 fenbufen, 954
   4 probenecid, 955
   2 ramelteon, 956
   3 ranitidine, 956

Enoxacin *(cont.)*
   3 tacrine, 957
   2 theophylline, 958

Enprostil
   3 ethanol, 959

Entacapone
   2 bitolterol, 959
   2 dobutamine, 960
   2 ephedrine, 960
   2 epinephrine, 961
   2 isoproterenol, 961
   3 methyldopa, 962
   2 phenelzine, 962

Entocort EC
   see Budesonide

Ephedrine
   4 ammonium chloride,
       124
   3 antacids, 147
   4 caffeine, 333
   4 dexamethasone, 778
   2 entacapone, 960
   3 guanethidine, 963
   4 methyldopa, 963
   2 moclobemide, 964
   4 reserpine, 965
   4 theophylline, 965

Epinephrine
   3 chlorpromazine, 431
   2 entacapone, 961
   2 imipramine, 966
   4 phenelzine, 967
   3 propranolol, 967

Epivir
   see Lamivudine

Eplerenone
   3 candesartan, 969
   3 enalapril, 970

Eprosartan
   5 fluconazole, 971

Equanil
   see Meprobamate

Ergamisol
   see Levamisole

Ergomar
   see Ergotamine

Ergonovine
   3 dopamine, 910

Ergostat
   see Ergotamine

Ergotamine
   2 atazanavir, 235
   2 clarithromycin, 572
   2 indinavir, 971
   2 nitroglycerin, 972
   4 propranolol, 972
   2 ritonavir, 973

❶ = Avoid Combination   ❷ = Usually Avoid Combination   ▼ = Minimize Risk
❹ = No Action Needed   ❺ = No Interaction

Ergotamine *(cont.)*
  1 sumatriptan, 974
  4 tacrolimus, 974
  2 voriconazole, 975
Erlotinib
  3 atazanavir, 975
  3 carbamazepine, 976
  3 ciprofloxacin, 527
  3 clarithromycin, 976
  3 grapefruit juice, 977
  3 ketoconazole, 977
  3 nefazodone, 978
  3 omeprazole, 978
  3 rifampin, 979
  3 St. John's wort, 979
Ertapenem
  3 valproic acid, 980
Ery-Tab
  see Erythromycin
EryPed
  see Erythromycin
Erythrocin
  see Erythromycin
Erythromycin
  3 alfentanil, 35
  3 alprazolam, 60
  3 amlodipine, 120
  4 antacids, 148
  1 astemizole, 230
  3 atorvastatin, 256
  3 bromocriptine, 294
  3 buspirone, 319
  3 carbamazepine, 355
  3 chlorpropamide, 443
  3 cilostazol, 467
  2 cisapride, 545
  3 clopidogrel, 981
  2 clozapine, 625
  1 colchicine, 649
  3 cyclosporine, 711
  3 digoxin, 834
  3 disopyramide, 891
  5 doxepin, 912
  2 eletriptan, 946
  3 ethanol, 982
  3 everolimus, 1038
  5 felbamate, 982
  3 felodipine, 983
  3 fentanyl, 983
  3 food, 984
  4 loratadine, 985
  5 losartan, 986
  2 lovastatin, 986
  3 midazolam, 987
  4 nadolol, 988
  3 penicillin G, 988
  3 pitavastatin, 989
  5 pravastatin, 990

Erythromycin *(cont.)*
  3 quetiapine, 990
  3 quinidine, 991
  3 ritonavir, 992
  4 sertindole, 992
  3 sertraline, 993
  3 sildenafil, 994
  2 simvastatin, 995
  5 sufentanil, 995
  3 tacrolimus, 996
  4 tamsulosin, 997
  5 temazepam, 997
  1 terfenadine, 998
  3 theophylline, 998
  3 triazolam, 999
  3 valproic acid, 1000
  3 vardenafil, 1001
  3 verapamil, 1001
  3 warfarin, 1002
  3 zafirlukast, 1003
  3 zopiclone, 1004
Escitalopram
  4 aripiprazole, 191
  4 metoprolol, 1004
Eskalith
  see Lithium
Esomeprazole
  2 atazanavir, 235
Estramustine
  3 food, 1005
Ethacrynic Acid
  2 cisplatin, 556
  2 gentamicin, 1005
  4 lithium, 1006
  4 warfarin, 1007
Ethanol
  3 acetaminophen, 6
  1 acitretin, 25
  3 amitriptyline, 109
  4 antipyrine, 177
  4 aspirin, 204
  4 bromocriptine, 295
  4 caffeine, 333
  3 cefamandole, 398
  3 chloral hydrate, 409
  3 chlorpromazine, 432
  1 chlorpropamide, 443
  4 cimetidine, 480
  5 ciprofloxacin, 528
  4 contraceptives, oral, 1007
  5 cromolyn, 694
  4 cyclosporine, 712
  3 diazepam, 794
  1 disulfiram, 899
  3 doxycycline, 915
  3 enprostil, 959
  3 erythromycin, 982

Ethanol *(cont.)*
  5 famotidine, 1008
  5 fluoxetine, 1009
  5 fluvoxamine, 1009
  3 furazolidone, 1010
  3 glutethimide, 1011
  3 isoniazid, 1011
  3 ketoconazole, 1012
  3 meperidine, 1012
  3 meprobamate, 1013
  1 methotrexate, 1014
  3 metoclopramide, 1014
  3 metronidazole, 1015
  4 nicotinic acid, 1015
  3 nitroglycerin, 1016
  4 nizatidine, 1017
  5 omeprazole, 1018
  5 orlistat, 1018
  4 paroxetine, 1019
  1 phenelzine, 1019
  3 phenobarbital, 1020
  3 phenytoin, 1021
  3 prazosin, 1022
  4 procainamide, 1023
  1 procarbazine, 1023
  4 propofol, 1024
  3 propoxyphene, 1024
  4 propranolol, 1025
  3 quetiapine, 1025
  2 ramelteon, 1026
  5 sertraline, 1026
  3 tacrolimus, 1027
  3 tinidazole, 1027
  3 tizanidine, 1028
  1 tolbutamide, 1028
  2 verapamil, 1029
  4 vitamin C, 1030
  3 warfarin, 1031
Ethchlorvynol
  3 dicumarol, 815
Ethinyl Estradiol
  3 grapefruit juice, 1032
  4 indinavir, 1033
  3 tipranavir, 1033
Ethmozine
  see Moricizine
Ethyl Alcohol
  see Ethanol
Ethyl Biscoumacetate
  5 methylphenidate, 1034
Etintidine
  3 propranolol, 1034
Etodolac
  2 warfarin, 1035
Etomidate
  4 verapamil, 1036
Etoposide
  3 cyclosporine, 712

❶ = Avoid Combination   **❷** = Usually Avoid Combination   **❸** = Minimize Risk

❹ = No Action Needed   **❺** = No Interaction

Etravirine
3 atazanavir, 236
3 atorvastatin, 257
3 clarithromycin, 572
4 darunavir, 763
3 omeprazole, 1036
3 sildenafil, 1037
3 tipranavir, 1038
Everolimus
3 erythromycin, 1038
2 ketoconazole, 1039
3 rifampin, 1040
3 verapamil, 1040
Evista
see Raloxifene
Exemestane
3 carbamazepine, 1041
3 nevirapine, 1042
3 phenobarbital, 1042
3 phenytoin, 1043
3 primidone, 1043
3 rifampin, 1044
3 St. John's wort, 1044
Exenatide
4 acetaminophen, 8
4 digoxin, 834
4 lovastatin, 1045
Ezetimibe
4 atorvastatin, 1045
4 fluvastatin, 1046

Famciclovir
4 digoxin, 835
Famotidine
4 antacids, 149
4 atazanavir, 237
3 dasatinib, 764
5 ethanol, 1008
4 probenecid, 1047
Famvir
see Famciclovir
Febuxostat
1 azathioprine, 270
5 colchicine, 1047
5 indomethacin, 1048
1 mercaptopurine, 1048
4 naproxen, 1049
2 theophylline, 1049
5 warfarin, 1050
Felbamate
3 carbamazepine, 356
3 contraceptives, oral, 675
5 erythromycin, 982
3 phenobarbital, 1050
3 phenytoin, 1051
3 valproic acid, 1052
4 warfarin, 1052

Felbatol
see Felbamate
Feldene
see Piroxicam
Felodipine
2 carbamazepine, 357
3 cyclosporine, 713
5 diazepam, 796
3 erythromycin, 983
3 grapefruit juice, 1201
3 itraconazole, 1053
4 menthol, 1054
3 nelfinavir, 1054
5 warfarin, 1055
Femoxetine
3 cimetidine, 481
Fenbufen
3 enoxacin, 954
Fenfluramine
2 fluoxetine, 1055
4 insulin, 1056
1 phenelzine, 1057
Fenofibrate
5 rosuvastatin, 1058
3 warfarin, 1058
Fenoprofen
4 aspirin, 205
2 warfarin, 1059
Fentanyl
4 amiodarone, 93
3 citalopram, 561
3 clarithromycin, 573
3 diltiazem, 869
3 erythromycin, 983
3 fluconazole, 1060
5 grapefruit juice, 1202
3 itraconazole, 1310
3 lidocaine, 1060
3 quinidine, 1061
3 rifampin, 1062
3 ritonavir, 1062
3 troleandomycin, 1063
Feosol
see Ferrous Sulfate
FeroSul
see Iron
Ferrous Sulfate
3 trovafloxacin, 1064
Fesoterodine
3 ketoconazole, 1064
3 rifampin, 1065
Fexofenadine
3 apple juice, 182
3 carbamazepine, 358
3 grapefruit juice, 1203
4 itraconazole, 1066
3 orange juice, 1599

Fexofenadine *(cont.)*
4 rifampin, 1066
4 verapamil, 1067
Fibocil
see Aprindine
Fingolimod
3 atenolol, 245
3 ketoconazole, 1067
Fish Oil
4 warfarin, 1068
Flagyl
see Metronidazole
Flecainide
3 amiodarone, 94
3 bupropion, 308
4 cigarette smoking, 461
3 cimetidine, 482
4 digoxin, 835
4 duloxetine, 929
3 paroxetine, 1068
3 propranolol, 1069
4 quinidine sulfate, 1070
4 quinine, 1071
3 sodium bicarbonate, 1071
3 sotalol, 1072
4 verapamil, 1072
Fleroxacin
3 antacids, 150
Flexeril
see Cyclobenzaprine
Floxin
see Ofloxacin
Floxyfral
see Ethanol
Fluconazole
3 alfentanil, 36
3 amitriptyline, 110
5 antacids, 150
3 atevirdine, 250
5 busulfan, 326
3 caffeine, 334
3 carbamazepine, 358
4 cimetidine, 482
4 clarithromycin, 574
5 contraceptives, oral, 1073
3 cyclosporine, 714
3 diazepam, 796
5 didanosine, 818
3 eletriptan, 947
5 eprosartan, 971
3 fentanyl, 1060
4 flurbiprofen, 1074
3 fluvastatin, 1074
5 food, 1075
3 glimepiride, 1075

Fluconazole *(cont.)*
3 glipizide, 1076
3 glyburide, 1077
3 halofantrine, 1077
3 ibuprofen, 1244
4 indinavir, 1078
4 irbesartan, 1292
3 losartan, 1078
3 methadone, 1079
3 midazolam, 1080
3 nateglinide, 1080
3 nevirapine, 1081
3 phenytoin, 1082
5 pravastatin, 1083
3 ramelteon, 1083
3 rifabutin, 1084
3 rifampin, 1085
4 ritonavir, 1085
4 saquinavir, 1086
3 simvastatin, 1087
3 sirolimus, 1087
4 sulfamethoxazole, 1088
3 tacrolimus, 1089
3 terfenadine, 1090
4 testosterone, 1091
5 theophylline, 1091
3 tipranavir, 1092
3 tolbutamide, 1092
2 triazolam, 1093
3 warfarin, 1094
4 zidovudine, 1095
4 zolpidem, 1095

Flumadine
see Rimantadine

Fluorouracil
4 cimetidine, 483
2 metronidazole, 1096
3 phenytoin, 1096
3 warfarin, 1097

Fluothane
see Halothane

Fluoxetine
3 alprazolam, 60
3 amitriptyline, 111
3 aripiprazole, 192
3 aspirin, 206
3 buspirone, 320
3 carbamazepine, 359
3 carvedilol, 395
5 clonazepam, 607
4 codeine, 633
3 cyclobenzaprine, 698
3 cyproheptadine, 755
3 desipramine, 772
2 dexfenfluramine, 778
3 dextromethorphan, 784
3 diazepam, 797
5 ethanol, 1009
2 fenfluramine, 1055

Fluoxetine *(cont.)*
3 furosemide, 1098
4 grapefruit juice, 1099
3 haloperidol, 1099
3 ibuprofen, 1100
3 linezolid, 1102
3 lithium, 1102
3 meperidine, 1103
1 methylene blue, 1104
4 midazolam, 1105
4 moclobemide, 1106
3 nefazodone, 1107
4 nifedipine, 1107
5 orlistat, 1600
4 pentazocine, 1108
3 phenytoin, 1108
3 propafenone, 1109
3 propranolol, 1110
2 rasagiline, 1111
4 risperidone, 1112
4 ritonavir, 1112
2 selegiline, 1113
2 sibutramine, 1113
3 sumatriptan, 1114
2 tamoxifen, 1115
4 tamsulosin, 1117
4 tapentadol, 1812
2 terfenadine, 1117
2 thioridazine, 1118
4 tolterodine, 1119
3 tramadol, 1120
1 tranylcypromine, 1121
4 trazodone, 1121
5 triazolam, 1122
2 tryptophan, 1122
3 warfarin, 1123

Fluphenazine
4 olanzapine, 1126

Fluphenazine Decanoate
3 imipramine, 1125

Flurazepam
5 warfarin, 1127

Flurbiprofen
4 aspirin, 207
4 fluconazole, 1074
3 methotrexate, 1127
2 phenprocoumon, 1128

Fluticasone
3 itraconazole, 1129
4 ketoconazole, 1130
3 ritonavir, 1130

Fluvastatin
3 colchicine, 649
4 cyclosporine, 715
4 ezetimibe, 1046
3 fluconazole, 1074
4 glyburide, 1131
5 itraconazole, 1132

Fluvastatin *(cont.)*
3 rifampin, 1132
4 tolbutamide, 1133

Fluvoxamine
3 alprazolam, 61
1 astemizole, 231
3 buspirone, 321
3 carbamazepine, 360
3 clomipramine, 599
2 clozapine, 625
2 duloxetine, 929
5 ethanol, 1009
4 lansoprazole, 1134
3 lithium, 1134
3 methadone, 1135
3 mexiletine, 1136
4 moclobemide, 1136
3 olanzapine, 1137
4 omeprazole, 1138
3 oxycodone, 1139
3 phenytoin, 1140
3 quinidine, 1140
1 ramelteon, 1141
1 rasagiline, 1141
3 sildenafil, 1142
2 tacrine, 1143
1 terfenadine, 1143
2 theophylline, 1144
2 thioridazine, 1145
2 tizanidine, 1146
3 warfarin, 1147

Folic Acid
3 phenytoin, 1148
2 pyrimethamine, 1149

Folvite
see Folic Acid

Food
3 ciprofloxacin, 528
3 didanosine, 818
3 erythromycin, 984
3 estramustine, 1005
5 fluconazole, 1075
4 gatifloxacin, 1150
4 griseofulvin, 1151
3 indinavir, 1151
3 isoniazid, 1152
3 itraconazole, 1152
3 levodopa, 1153
3 lincomycin, 1154
3 melphalan, 1154
3 nifedipine, 1155
3 nilotinib, 1156
4 ofloxacin, 1156
3 propafenone, 1157
4 stavudine, 1157
3 tetracycline, 1158
3 zidovudine, 1159

Fortaz
see Ceftazidime

❶ = Avoid Combination ❷ = Usually Avoid Combination ❸ = Minimize Risk
❹ = No Action Needed ❺ = No Interaction

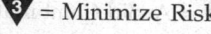

Fortovase
  see Saquinavir
Fosamprenavir
  4 ranitidine, 1160
  see also Amprenavir
Foscarnet
  3 ciprofloxacin, 529
  5 didanosine, 819
  5 ganciclovir, 1161
  5 zalcitabine, 1161
  5 zidovudine, 1161
Foscavir
  see Foscarnet
Frisium
  see Clobazam
Fungizone
  see Amphotericin B
Furazolidone
  3 dextroamphetamine,
    780
  3 ethanol, 1010
Furosemide
  3 cholestyramine, 448
  3 clofibrate, 597
  3 colestipol, 666
  3 digoxin, 836
  3 enalapril, 949
  3 fluoxetine, 1098
  4 gentamicin, 1162
  4 ginseng, 1163
  3 indomethacin, 1163
  4 lithium, 1165
  4 lomefloxacin, 1165
  3 oxcarbazepine, 1166
  3 phenytoin, 1167
  4 probenecid, 1167
  4 propranolol, 1168
  3 terbutaline, 1169
  4 theophylline, 1170
  3 tubocurarine, 1170
  5 warfarin, 1171
Furoxone
  see Furazolidone
Fusidic Acid
  4 antipyrine, 178

Gabapentin
  5 contraceptives, oral,
    676
Gallamine
  4 diazepam, 798
Gamma Globulin
  3 phenytoin, 1172
Ganciclovir
  3 didanosine, 820
  5 foscarnet, 1161
  1 zidovudine, 1172

Gantanol
  see Sulfamethoxazole
Gantrisin
  see Sulfisoxazole
Garamycin
  see Gentamicin
Garlic
  3 saquinavir, 1173
  4 warfarin, 1174
Gatifloxacin
  3 antacids, 151
  4 food, 1150
  3 glyburide, 1175
Gefitinib
  3 itraconazole, 1175
  4 metoprolol, 1176
  4 ranitidine, 1177
  3 rifampin, 1177
Gemcitabine
  3 warfarin, 1178
Gemfibrozil
  3 atorvastatin, 257
  4 colchicine, 650
  3 colestipol, 666
  4 glimepiride, 1178
  3 glyburide, 1179
  2 lovastatin, 1180
  3 montelukast, 1181
  3 pioglitazone, 1182
  3 pravastatin, 1182
  3 repaglinide, 1183
  2 warfarin, 1184
Gemifloxacin
  3 antacids, 152
  4 iron, 1294
  4 probenecid, 1185
Gemzar
  see Gemcitabine
Gentamicin
  3 amphotericin B, 129
  2 atracurium, 265
  3 carbenicillin, 387
  3 carboplatin, 391
  3 cisplatin, 557
  4 clindamycin, 595
  3 cyclosporine, 715
  2 ethacrynic acid, 1005
  4 furosemide, 1162
  3 indomethacin, 1186
  3 methoxyflurane, 1186
  3 vancomycin, 1187
Geocillin
  see Carbenicillin
Gilenya
  see Fingolimod
Ginger
  4 warfarin, 1188

Ginkgo biloba
  2 aspirin, 208
  4 nifedipine, 1189
  2 warfarin, 1189
Ginseng
  4 furosemide, 1163
  4 nifedipine, 1190
  3 warfarin, 1190
Glimepiride
  3 fluconazole, 1075
  4 gemfibrozil, 1178
  4 propranolol, 1192
  4 rifampin, 1192
Glipizide
  3 antacids, 152
  4 cholestyramine, 448
  3 cyclosporine, 716
  3 fluconazole, 1076
  3 ranitidine, 1193
  4 rifampin, 1194
  4 trimethoprim/
    sulfamethoxazole,
    1194
Glucagon
  4 propranolol, 1195
  3 warfarin, 1196
Glucophage
  see Metformin
Glucotrol
  see Glipizide
Glutethimide
  4 cigarette smoking, 461
  3 ethanol, 1011
  2 warfarin, 1196
Glyburide
  3 antacids, 153
  3 ciprofloxacin, 530
  3 clarithromycin, 574
  4 colesevelam, 660
  3 fluconazole, 1077
  4 fluvastatin, 1131
  3 gatifloxacin, 1175
  3 gemfibrozil, 1179
  5 orlistat, 1197
  3 rifampin, 1197
  4 simvastatin, 1198
  3 trimethoprim/
    sulfamethoxazole,
    1199
  3 warfarin, 1199
Glycopyrrolate
  4 potassium, 1200
Glycyrrhizin
  4 prednisolone, 1201
Gold
  4 aspirin, 208
Grapefruit
  1 colchicine, 651

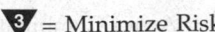 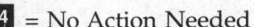 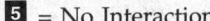

❶ = Avoid Combination   **❷** = Usually Avoid Combination   **▼❸** = Minimize Risk
❹ = No Action Needed   **❺** = No Interaction

Grapefruit Juice
3 amiodarone, 94
4 amlodipine, 121
3 budesonide, 298
3 buspirone, 321
3 carbamazepine, 361
2 cisapride, 546
3 clomipramine, 600
3 cyclosporine, 717
4 digoxin, 837
4 diltiazem, 870
3 dronedarone, 918
3 erlotinib, 977
3 ethinyl estradiol, 1032
3 felodipine, 1201
5 fentanyl, 1202
3 fexofenadine, 1203
4 fluoxetine, 1099
2 halofantrine, 1203
4 indinavir, 1204
3 itraconazole, 1205
4 levothyroxine, 1205
3 lovastatin, 1206
3 methadone, 1207
3 methylprednisolone, 1207
3 midazolam, 1208
4 nicardipine, 1209
3 nifedipine, 1210
3 nilotinib, 1211
3 nimodipine, 1212
3 nisoldipine, 1212
4 primaquine, 1213
4 quinidine, 1214
4 repaglinide, 1214
3 saquinavir, 1215
3 sildenafil, 1216
3 simvastatin, 1216
3 terfenadine, 1217
4 tolvaptan, 1218
3 triazolam, 1219
4 verapamil, 1220
5 warfarin, 1221

Grisactin
see Griseofulvin
Griseofulvin
3 aspirin, 209
3 contraceptives, oral, 1221
3 cyclosporine, 718
4 food, 1151
3 phenobarbital, 1222
3 warfarin, 1222
Guanethidine
3 chlorpromazine, 433
3 desipramine, 774
3 dextroamphetamine, 781
5 diethylpropion, 826

Guanethidine *(cont.)*
3 ephedrine, 963
3 haloperidol, 1223
4 levodopa, 1224
3 methylphenidate, 1224
3 norepinephrine, 1225
3 phenelzine, 1225
3 phenylephrine, 1226
3 thiothixene, 1227
Guanfacine
3 amitriptyline, 112
4 bupropion, 308
3 ketoconazole, 1227

Halcion
see Triazolam
Haldol
see Haloperidol
Halfan
see Halofantrine
Halofantrine
3 antacids, 154
3 fluconazole, 1077
2 grapefruit juice, 1203
Halofenate
4 propranolol, 1229
3 tolbutamide, 1229
Haloperidol
3 benztropine, 282
3 carbamazepine, 362
4 clozapine, 626
4 codeine, 634
4 diazepam, 799
3 fluoxetine, 1099
3 guanethidine, 1223
4 imipramine, 1230
3 indomethacin, 1230
3 itraconazole, 1311
3 lithium, 1231
4 methyldopa, 1232
4 olanzapine, 1233
4 phenindione, 1233
3 quinidine, 1234
4 rifampin, 1234
4 sertraline, 1235
4 tacrine, 1236
3 tamoxifen, 1236
Halothane
4 phenytoin, 1237
4 rifampin, 1237
Heparin
3 drospirenone, 925
4 streptokinase, 1238
3 warfarin, 1238
Hexalen
see Altretamine
Hexobarbital
3 rifampin, 1239

Hismanal
see Astemizole
Hivid
see Zalcitabine
Hycort
see Hydrocortisone
Hydralazine
3 diazoxide, 809
3 indomethacin, 1240
4 propranolol, 1240
Hydrocortisone
3 cholestyramine, 449
4 theophylline, 1241
Hydroxychloroquine
3 colchicine, 652
3 digoxin, 838
3 methotrexate, 1242
4 metoprolol, 1243
Hydroxyzine
4 chlorpromazine, 433
Hygroton
see Chlorthalidone
Hyperstat
see Diazoxide

Ibuprofen
4 amlodipine, 121
2 aspirin, 209
3 clomipramine, 600
4 desipramine, 775
3 drospirenone, 925
3 fluconazole, 1244
3 fluoxetine, 1100
3 lithium, 1244
3 methotrexate, 1245
3 milnacipran, 1246
5 sucralfate, 1247
4 tacrine, 1247
3 voriconazole, 1248
2 warfarin, 1249
Imatinib
4 lansoprazole, 1250
3 levothyroxine, 1250
3 rifampin, 1251
2 St. John's wort, 1251
3 tamoxifen, 1252
Imipenem
3 cyclosporine, 718
3 theophylline, 1253
Imipramine
3 altretamine, 65
4 aspirin, 210
3 carbamazepine, 363
5 chloroquine, 422
3 cholestyramine, 450
3 cimetidine, 484
4 contraceptives, oral, 1253

---

1 = Avoid Combination   **2** = Usually Avoid Combination   **3** = Minimize Risk
4 = No Action Needed   **5** = No Interaction

Imipramine *(cont.)*
3 dextroamphetamine, 781
2 epinephrine, 966
3 fluphenazine decanoate, 1125
4 haloperidol, 1230
4 ketoconazole, 1254
4 labetalol, 1254
4 levodopa, 1255
4 methylphenidate, 1255
2 norepinephrine, 1256
2 phenelzine, 1257
3 phenylephrine, 1258
3 quinidine, 1259
3 venlafaxine, 1259
3 verapamil, 1260

Imitrex
see Sumatriptan

Imodium
see Loperamide

Imuran
see Azathioprine

Inapsine
see Droperidol

Inderal
see Propranolol

Indinavir
3 amiodarone, 95
5 cimetidine, 485
2 cisapride, 546
3 clarithromycin, 575
3 colchicine, 1260
3 didanosine, 820
3 efavirenz, 937
2 ergotamine, 971
4 ethinyl estradiol, 1033
4 fluconazole, 1078
3 food, 1151
4 grapefruit juice, 1204
3 ketoconazole, 1261
5 methadone, 1262
4 nelfinavir, 1262
3 omeprazole, 1263
3 rifabutin, 1264
3 rifapentine, 1265
3 ritonavir, 1265
3 sildenafil, 1266
1 St. John's wort, 1267
3 vardenafil, 1267
4 zidovudine, 1268

Indocin
see Indomethacin

Indomethacin
5 amlodipine, 122
4 antacids, 155
4 aspirin, 211
3 bumetanide, 302

Indomethacin *(cont.)*
3 cyclosporine, 719
3 enalapril, 950
5 febuxostat, 1048
3 furosemide, 1163
3 gentamicin, 1186
3 haloperidol, 1230
3 hydralazine, 1240
3 lithium, 1269
2 methotrexate, 1269
3 nifedipine, 1271
3 prazosin, 1272
3 prednisone, 1272
4 probenecid, 1273
3 propranolol, 1274
4 thiazides, 1275
3 triamterene, 1276
3 vancomycin, 1277
2 warfarin, 1277

Infliximab
2 azathioprine, 271
2 mercaptopurine, 1464

Influenza Vaccine
3 phenytoin, 1279
4 theophylline, 1280
4 warfarin, 1281

INH
see Isoniazid

Inspra
see Eplerenone

Insulin
3 captopril, 344
4 chlorpromazine, 434
3 cigarette smoking, 462
3 clonidine, 612
4 contraceptives, oral, 1282
4 disopyramide, 892
4 fenfluramine, 1056
3 marijuana, 1283
4 nifedipine, 1283
3 prednisone, 1284
3 propranolol, 1285
3 thiazides, 1287
3 tranylcypromine, 1287

Intal
see Cromolyn

Intelence
see Etravirine

Interferon
4 melphalan, 1288
4 prednisone, 1289
3 theophylline, 1289
3 zidovudine, 1290

Interferon Alfa-2a
5 acetaminophen, 8

Intrauterine Contraceptive Devices
3 aspirin, 212

Intrauterine Progesterone System (IUDs)
3 prednisone, 1291

Intropin
see Dopamine

Invirase
see Saquinavir

Iohexol
3 amiodarone, 96

Ionamin
see Phentermine

Irbesartan
4 fluconazole, 1292

Irinotecan
2 carbamazepine, 364
4 citalopram, 562
2 phenytoin, 1292
1 St. John's wort, 1293

Iron
3 antacids, 155
4 chloramphenicol, 413
4 cholestyramine, 450
3 ciprofloxacin, 531
3 enalapril, 951
4 gemifloxacin, 1294
3 levodopa, 1294
3 levothyroxine, 1397
3 methyldopa, 1295
3 moxifloxacin, 1296
2 mycophenolate mofetil, 1296
3 norfloxacin, 1297
4 ofloxacin, 1298
4 pancreatic extracts, 1298
3 penicillamine, 1299
3 tetracycline, 1299
3 vitamin E, 1300

Ismelin
see Guanethidine

ISMO
see Isosorbide Mononitrate

Isocarboxazid
1 venlafaxine, 1301

Isometheptene
1 bromocriptine, 295

Isoniazid
3 acetaminophen, 9
3 antacids, 156
3 carbamazepine, 365
3 cycloserine, 704
3 diazepam, 799
2 disulfiram, 900

1 = Avoid Combination   **2** = Usually Avoid Combination   **▼3** = Minimize Risk

4 = No Action Needed   **5** = No Interaction

Isoniazid *(cont.)*
3 ethanol, 1011
3 food, 1152
3 phenytoin, 1301
3 prednisolone, 1302
4 primidone, 1303
4 procainamide, 1303
3 rifampin, 1304
3 theophylline, 1304
3 triazolam, 1305
3 valproic acid, 1306
3 warfarin, 306

Isoproterenol
3 amitriptyline, 113
2 entacapone, 961
3 propranolol, 1307

Isosorbide Mononitrate
1 sildenafil, 1308

Isotretinoin
3 carbamazepine, 365
4 cyclosporine, 720
4 warfarin, 1308

Isradipine
3 lovastatin, 1309

Isuprel
see Isoproterenol

Itraconazole
3 aliskiren, 42
3 alprazolam, 62
3 antacids, 157
3 aripiprazole, 193
3 atorvastatin, 258
3 bortezomib, 288
5 bromazepam, 291
3 budesonide, 299
4 bupivacaine, 304
3 buspirone, 322
4 busulfan, 326
3 cabergoline, 328
3 cimetidine, 485
2 cisapride, 547
3 clarithromycin, 576
3 clopidogrel, 617
2 colchicine, 1309
3 cyclosporine, 720
3 diazepam, 800
3 didanosine, 821
3 digoxin, 838
3 felodipine, 1053
3 fentanyl, 1310
4 fexofenadine, 1066
3 fluticasone, 1129
5 fluvastatin, 1132
3 food, 1152
3 gefitinib, 1175
3 grapefruit juice, 1205
3 haloperidol, 1311
2 lovastatin, 1312

Itraconazole *(cont.)*
3 methylprednisolone, 1313
3 midazolam, 1314
3 nifedipine, 1315
3 omeprazole, 1316
4 oxybutynin, 1317
3 oxycodone, 1317
2 phenytoin, 1318
5 pioglitazone, 1318
5 pravastatin, 1319
3 quinidine, 1319
3 ranitidine, 1320
3 repaglinide, 1321
3 rifampin, 1322
3 risperidone, 1322
2 simvastatin, 1323
3 sirolimus, 1324
3 tacrolimus, 1324
4 temazepam, 1325
1 terfenadine, 1326
2 triazolam, 1327
3 vincristine, 1327
2 vinorelbine, 1328
3 warfarin, 1329
5 zidovudine, 1330
4 zolpidem, 1330

IUDs
see Intrauterine Contraceptive Devices; Intrauterine Progesterone System

Ixabepilone
3 ketoconazole, 1331
2 St. John's wort, 1331

Josamycin
3 cyclosporine, 721

Kaletra
see Lopinavir/Ritonavir
Kao-Spen
see Kaolin-Pectin

Kaolin-Pectin
4 aspirin, 213
4 chloroquine, 422
3 digoxin, 839
2 lincomycin, 1333
4 pseudoephedrine, 1333
3 quinidine, 1334

Kapectolin
see Pectin
Kava
4 alprazolam, 63
4 levodopa, 1334
Kayexalate
see Sodium Polystyrene Sulfonate Resin

Ketalar
see Ketamine
Ketamine
4 thyroid, 1335
Ketek
see Telithromycin
Ketoconazole
3 alfuzosin, 40
3 aliskiren, 43
3 almotriptan, 56
4 ambrisentan, 71
3 amprenavir, 134
3 antacids, 157
3 aprepitant, 185
3 aripiprazole, 194
1 astemizole, 232
4 bortezomib, 289
4 bosentan, 290
3 budesonide, 300
3 carbamazepine, 366
3 chlordiazepoxide, 416
3 cilostazol, 468
3 cimetidine, 486
3 cinacalcet, 522
2 cisapride, 548
3 clopidogrel, 618
2 colchicine, 653
2 conivaptan, 671
3 cyclosporine, 722
3 darunavir, 764
3 dasatinib, 765
5 desipramine, 776
3 didanosine, 822
4 donepezil, 909
2 dronedarone, 919
3 efavirenz, 938
2 eletriptan, 947
3 erlotinib, 977
3 ethanol, 1012
2 everolimus, 1039
3 fesoterodine, 1064
3 fingolimod, 1067
4 fluticasone, 1130
3 guanfacine, 1227
4 imipramine, 1254
3 indinavir, 1261
3 ixabepilone, 1331
3 lapatinib, 1335
3 loratadine, 1336
5 losartan, 1336
2 lovastatin, 1337
2 lurasidone, 1338
2 maraviroc, 1338
3 mefloquine, 1339
3 methylprednisolone, 1340
3 midazolam, 1340
4 nelfinavir, 1341
3 nilotinib, 1342

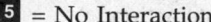

1 = Avoid Combination **2** = Usually Avoid Combination **3** = Minimize Risk
4 = No Action Needed **5** = No Interaction

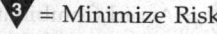

Ketoconazole *(cont.)*
3 nisoldipine, 1342
3 omeprazole, 1343
3 paricalcitol, 1344
5 phenytoin, 1345
2 pimozide, 1345
4 pioglitazone, 1346
4 prednisolone, 1346
3 quetiapine, 1347
3 quinidine, 1348
4 quinine, 1348
3 ramelteon, 1349
3 ranitidine, 1350
3 ranolazine, 1350
4 repaglinide, 1351
3 rifampin, 1352
3 ritonavir, 1353
3 rosiglitazone, 1354
3 salmeterol, 1354
3 saquinavir, 1355
3 saxagliptin, 1356
3 sildenafil, 1357
3 silodosin, 1357
2 simvastatin, 1358
3 sirolimus, 1359
3 solifenacin, 1359
3 sucralfate, 1360
3 sunitinib, 1361
3 tacrolimus, 1361
3 tadalafil, 1362
4 tamsulosin, 1363
3 telaprevir, 1363
1 terfenadine, 1364
4 theophylline, 1365
2 ticagrelor, 1365
3 tolbutamide, 1366
3 tolterodine, 1367
3 tolvaptan, 1368
3 triazolam, 1368
3 vardenafil, 1369
3 venlafaxine, 1370
3 warfarin, 1371
3 ziprasidone, 1371
3 zolpidem, 1372
Ketoprofen
4 aspirin, 213
3 cyclosporine, 723
2 methotrexate, 1373
4 probenecid, 1374
2 warfarin, 1375
Ketorolac
5 antacids, 158
3 lithium, 1376
Klonopin
see Clonazepam
Labetalol
4 imipramine, 1254

Lamictal
see Lamotrigine
Lamisil
see Terbinafine
Lamivudine
4 trimethoprim/
sulfamethoxazole,
1378
Lamotrigine
3 carbamazepine, 367
3 contraceptives, oral,
676
3 phenytoin, 1378
3 rifampin, 1379
4 sertraline, 1380
3 valproic acid, 1380
Laniazid
see Isoniazid
Lanoxin
see Digoxin
Lansoprazole
2 atazanavir, 238
4 bromocriptine, 296
3 clarithromycin, 577
4 fluvoxamine, 1134
4 imatinib, 1250
4 tacrolimus, 1381
Lapatinib
3 carbamazepine, 368
2 colchicine, 1381
3 ketoconazole, 1335
Lariam
see Mefloquine
Larodopa
see Levodopa
Lasix
see Furosemide
Lescol
see Fluvastatin
Levamisole
4 aspirin, 214
4 warfarin, 1382
Levaquin
see Levofloxacin
Levarterenol
see Norepinephrine
Levodopa
4 antacids, 159
4 bupropion, 309
2 chlorpromazine, 434
4 clonidine, 613
3 diazepam, 800
3 food, 1153
4 guanethidine, 1224
4 imipramine, 1255
3 iron, 1294
4 kava, 1334

Levodopa *(cont.)*
3 methionine, 1383
4 methyldopa, 1383
3 moclobemide, 1384
3 phenelzine, 1385
4 phenylbutazone, 1386
4 phenylephrine, 1386
3 phenytoin, 1387
4 propranolol, 1387
3 pyridoxine, 1388
3 spiramycin, 1389
3 tacrine, 1390
4 trihexyphenidyl, 1390
Levofloxacin
3 antacids, 159
5 cyclosporine, 723
4 procainamide, 1391
5 theophylline, 1392
4 warfarin, 1392
Levophed
see Norepinephrine
Levoprome
see Methotrimeprazine
Levothyroxine
3 aluminum hydroxide,
1393
3 caffeine, 1394
3 calcium carbonate, 1395
3 ciprofloxacin, 1396
3 colesevelam, 661
3 cyclosporine, 724
4 grapefruit juice, 1205
3 imatinib, 1250
3 iron, 1397
3 magnesium, 1398
3 raloxifene, 1721
3 sertraline, 1399
3 sevelamer, 1399
3 sucralfate, 1400
see also Thyroid
Lexapro
see Escitalopram
Lexiva
see Fosamprenavir
Librium
see Chlordiazepoxide
Lidocaine
4 amiodarone, 96
4 cigarette smoking, 462
3 cimetidine, 487
5 digoxin, 840
3 disopyramide, 893
3 fentanyl, 1060
3 morphine, 1401
5 omeprazole, 1402
3 phenobarbital, 1402
4 phenytoin, 1403
4 procainamide, 1403

1 = Avoid Combination **2** = Usually Avoid Combination **3** = Minimize Risk
4 = No Action Needed **5** = No Interaction

Lidocaine *(cont.)*
4 propafenone, 1404
3 propranolol, 1404
4 ranitidine, 1405
4 succinylcholine, 1406

Lincocin
see Lincomycin

Lincomycin
3 food, 1154
2 kaolin-pectin, 1333

Linezolid
3 citalopram, 562
4 dextromethorphan, 785
3 fluoxetine, 1102
2 milnacipran, 1407
3 paroxetine, 1407
4 pseudoephedrine, 1408
4 rifampin, 1409
3 sertraline, 1409
1 tranylcypromine, 1410
3 venlafaxine, 1410

Lipitor
see Atorvastatin

Lisinopril
3 lithium, 1411
4 olanzapine, 1412
3 rofecoxib, 1413
3 tizanidine, 1414

Lithium
4 alprazolam, 63
3 amitriptyline, 113
5 antacids, 160
5 aspirin, 214
3 bromfenac, 292
4 calcitonin, 338
3 candesartan, 341
3 carbamazepine, 368
3 celecoxib, 405
3 chlorpromazine, 435
4 cisplatin, 557
4 clozapine, 627
4 diazepam, 801
3 diclofenac, 811
4 diuretic, herbal, 906
3 duloxetine, 930
4 ethacrynic acid, 1006
3 fluoxetine, 1102
3 fluvoxamine, 1134
4 furosemide, 1165
3 haloperidol, 1231
3 ibuprofen, 1244
3 indomethacin, 1269
3 ketorolac, 1376
3 lisinopril, 1411
3 losartan, 1415
3 mefenamic acid, 1415
3 meloxicam, 1416
3 methyldopa, 1417

Lithium *(cont.)*
3 milnacipran, 1523
5 moclobemide, 1417
3 naproxen, 1418
4 norepinephrine, 1419
4 paroxetine, 1419
2 phenelzine, 1420
3 phenylbutazone, 1420
3 phenytoin, 1421
3 piroxicam, 1422
3 potassium iodide, 1423
4 propranolol, 1423
3 rofecoxib, 1764
2 sibutramine, 1424
3 sodium bicarbonate, 1424
3 sodium chloride, 1425
4 spironolactone, 1425
4 succinylcholine, 1426
4 sulindac, 1426
4 sumatriptan, 1427
4 tetracycline, 1428
3 theophylline, 1428
4 topiramate, 1429
4 urea, 1430
3 valdecoxib, 1850
3 venlafaxine, 1430
3 verapamil, 1431

Lodine
see Etodolac

Lomefloxacin
3 antacids, 160
4 furosemide, 1165

Lomotil
see Diphenoxylate

Loperamide
4 cholestyramine, 451
4 clozapine, 627
4 quinidine, 1432
4 ritonavir, 1433

Lopid
see Gemfibrozil

Lopinavir/Ritonavir
1 disulfiram, 1433
3 midazolam, 1434
4 omeprazole, 1434
3 tipranavir, 1435
3 warfarin, 1436

Lopressor
see Metoprolol

Loratadine
4 cimetidine, 488
4 erythromycin, 985
3 ketoconazole, 1336
3 nefazodone, 1436

Lorazepam
4 aripiprazole, 195
4 cholestyramine, 451

Lorazepam *(cont.)*
3 clozapine, 628
3 loxapine, 1437

Lorcainide
3 rifampin, 1438

Losartan
3 drospirenone, 926
5 erythromycin, 986
3 fluconazole, 1078
5 ketoconazole, 1336
3 lithium, 1415
5 orlistat, 1438
3 rifampin, 1439

Lotensin
see Benazepril

Lovastatin
2 atazanavir, 239
5 chlorpropamide, 444
3 colchicine, 654
2 conivaptan, 672
3 cyclosporine, 724
3 danazol, 757
3 diltiazem, 870
2 erythromycin, 986
4 exenatide, 1045
2 gemfibrozil, 1180
3 grapefruit juice, 1206
3 isradipine, 1309
2 itraconazole, 1312
2 ketoconazole, 1337
3 nicotinic acid, 1439
3 pectin, 1440
3 posaconazole, 1441
4 propranolol, 1442
2 telithromycin, 1442
4 thyroid, 1443
3 warfarin, 1444

Loxapine
3 lorazepam, 1437
4 phenytoin, 1445

Loxitane
see Loxapine

Ludiomil
see Maprotiline

Lufyllin
see Dyphylline

Lurasidone
2 ketoconazole, 1338
2 rifampin, 1445

Luvox
see Fluvoxamine

Lysodren
see Mitotane

Maalox
see Antacids

Macrodantin
see Nitrofurantoin

1 = Avoid Combination   **2** = Usually Avoid Combination   **3** = Minimize Risk
4 = No Action Needed   **5** = No Interaction

Mag-Ox
   see Magnesium
Magnesium
   3 levothyroxine, 1398
   3 nifedipine, 1447
   3 succinylcholine, 1447
Mandol
   see Cefamandole
Maprotiline
   4 risperidone, 1448
Maraviroc
   3 atazanavir, 239
   3 efavirenz, 938
   3 ketoconazole, 1338
   3 rifampin, 1448
   3 ritonavir, 1449
   3 saquinavir, 1450
   2 St. John's wort, 1450
   5 tipranavir, 1451
Marblen
   see Antacids
Marijuana
   3 insulin, 1283
   4 olanzapine, 1452
   4 propranolol, 1452
   4 risperidone, 1453
Marplan
   see Isocarboxazid
Matulane
   see Procarbazine
Maxalt
   see Rizatriptan
Maxaquin
   see Lomefloxacin
Mebendazole
   3 carbamazepine, 369
   4 cimetidine, 489
   2 phenytoin, 1453
Meclofenamate
   4 aspirin, 215
   2 warfarin, 1454
Meclomen
   see Meclofenamate
Medrol
   see Methylprednisolone
Medroxyprogesterone
   3 aminoglutethimide, 77
Mefenamic Acid
   3 cyclosporine, 725
   3 lithium, 1415
   2 warfarin, 1455
Mefloquine
   4 cimetidine, 489
   3 ketoconazole, 1339
   4 metoclopramide, 1456
   5 primaquine, 1457

Mefloquine *(cont.)*
   3 warfarin, 1457
Melatonin
   4 caffeine, 334
Mellaril
   see Thioridazine
Meloxicam
   3 lithium, 1416
Melphalan
   3 cimetidine, 490
   3 cyclosporine, 726
   3 food, 1154
   4 interferon, 1288
Menthol
   4 caffeine, 335
   4 felodipine, 1054
   3 warfarin, 1458
Meperidine
   3 chlorpromazine, 436
   3 cimetidine, 490
   3 citalopram, 563
   5 contraceptives, oral,
      1458
   3 ethanol, 1012
   3 fluoxetine, 1103
   1 phenelzine, 1459
   3 phenobarbital, 1460
   3 phenytoin, 1460
   2 rasagiline, 1461
   2 selegiline, 1462
   2 sibutramine, 1463
Meprobamate
   3 ethanol, 1013
   5 warfarin, 1463
Mepron
   see Atovaquone
Mercaptopurine
   2 allopurinol, 51
   1 febuxostat, 1048
   2 infliximab, 1464
   3 prednisolone, 1465
   3 warfarin, 1466
Meridia
   see Sibutramine
Meropenem
   3 valproic acid, 1466
Mesalamine
   3 azathioprine, 272
   3 warfarin, 1467
Mestinon
   see Pyridostigmine Bro-
      mide
Metandren
   see Methyltestosterone
Metaraminol
   1 pargyline, 1468

Metformin
   3 cimetidine, 491
   5 orlistat, 1468
Methadone
   4 ammonium chloride,
      124
   4 amprenavir, 135
   3 carbamazepine, 370
   3 efavirenz, 939
   3 fluconazole, 1079
   3 fluvoxamine, 1135
   3 grapefruit juice, 1207
   5 indinavir, 1262
   3 nelfinavir, 1556
   3 nevirapine, 1469
   3 phenobarbital, 1470
   2 phenytoin, 1470
   2 rasagiline, 1471
   5 rifabutin, 1471
   3 rifampin, 1472
   3 ritonavir, 1472
   3 somatostatin, 1473
   3 St. John's wort, 1474
   4 zidovudine, 1474
Methadose
   see Methadone
Methandrostenolone
   3 tolbutamide, 1475
Methenamine
   3 acetazolamide, 19
   3 sodium bicarbonate,
      1475
   3 sulfadiazine, 1476
   4 vitamin C, 1477
Methionine
   3 levodopa, 1383
Methocarbamol
   4 pyridostigmine bro-
      mide, 1477
Methotrexate
   2 acitretin, 25
   4 amiodarone, 97
   2 aspirin, 216
   2 azapropazone, 266
   3 caffeine, 335
   3 carbenicillin, 388
   3 chloroquine, 422
   3 cholestyramine, 452
   3 cyclosporine, 726
   2 diclofenac, 812
   3 doxycycline, 916
   1 ethanol, 1014
   3 flurbiprofen, 1127
   3 hydroxychloroquine,
      1242
   3 ibuprofen, 1245
   2 indomethacin, 1269
   2 ketoprofen, 1373

1 = Avoid Combination   **2** = Usually Avoid Combination   **3** = Minimize Risk
4 = No Action Needed   **5** = No Interaction

Methotrexate *(cont.)*
2 naproxen, 1478
1 neomycin, 1479
3 omeprazole, 1480
3 oxacillin, 1481
3 pantoprazole, 1481
2 phenylbutazone, 1482
1 polio vaccine, 1483
2 probenecid, 1484
4 theophylline, 1485
3 thiazides, 1486
2 trimethoprim, 1486
3 vancomycin, 1487

Methotrimeprazine
1 pargyline, 1487

Methoxyflurane
3 gentamicin, 1186
3 secobarbital, 1488
2 tetracycline, 1489

Methyldopa
4 amitriptyline, 114
5 diethylpropion, 827
3 entacapone, 962
4 ephedrine, 963
4 haloperidol, 1232
3 iron, 1295
4 levodopa, 1383
3 lithium, 1417
3 norepinephrine, 1489
4 pargyline, 1490
5 phenobarbital, 1490
4 propranolol, 1491
4 tolbutamide, 1492
4 trifluoperazine, 1492

Methylene Blue
1 citalopram, 564
1 clomipramine, 602
1 fluoxetine, 1104
1 paroxetine, 1493
1 venlafaxine, 1494

Methylphenidate
3 carbamazepine, 371
4 cyclosporine, 727
5 ethyl biscoumacetate, 1034
3 guanethidine, 1224
4 imipramine, 1255
3 norepinephrine,
4 phenytoin, 1495

Methylprednisolone
3 aprepitant, 186
3 diltiazem, 871
3 grapefruit juice, 1207
3 itraconazole, 1313
3 ketoconazole, 1340
3 troleandomycin, 1495

Methysergide
1 sumatriptan, 1496

Meticorten
see Prednisone
Metoclopramide
4 acetaminophen, 10
4 cefprozil, 400
3 cyclosporine, 727
3 digoxin, 840
3 ethanol, 1014
4 mefloquine, 1456
5 propranolol, 1497
4 sertraline, 1497
4 tacrolimus, 1498
4 venlafaxine, 1498

Metopirone
see Metyrapone
Metoprolol
3 amiodarone, 97
4 antacids, 161
4 aspirin, 217
4 bupropion, 309
3 ciprofloxacin, 531
4 citalopram, 565
3 diazepam, 802
3 diphenhydramine, 884
4 dopamine, 910
3 dronedarone, 920
4 escitalopram, 1004
4 gefitinib, 1176
4 hydroxychloroquine, 1243
3 paroxetine, 1499
3 propafenone, 1500
3 propoxyphene, 1500
3 quinidine, 1501
3 rifampin, 1502
2 terbutaline, 1503

Metronidazole
4 antacids, 161
3 carbamazepine, 371
4 chloroquine, 423
3 cholestyramine, 453
4 cimetidine, 492
4 cyclosporine, 728
3 disulfiram, 901
3 ethanol, 1015
2 fluorouracil, 1096
4 phenobarbital, 1503
3 phenytoin, 1504
3 trimethoprim/
sulfamethoxazole, 1504
2 warfarin, 1505

Metyrapone
3 phenytoin, 1506

Mevacor
see Lovastatin
Mexate
see Methotrexate

Mexiletine
3 bupropion, 310
5 cimetidine, 493
4 ciprofloxacin, 532
4 disopyramide, 893
3 fluvoxamine, 1136
3 phenytoin, 1506
3 quinidine, 1507
3 ramelteon, 1508
3 rifampin, 1508
3 sodium bicarbonate, 1509
2 theophylline, 1510
3 tizanidine, 1511

Mexitil
see Mexiletine
Mibefradil
2 astemizole, 232
2 cisapride, 549
4 codeine, 635
3 digoxin, 841

Micafungin
4 nifedipine, 1511
4 sirolimus, 1512

Micardis
see Telmisartan
Miconazole
2 cisapride, 549
3 cyclosporine, 729
3 tobramycin, 1512
3 warfarin, 1513

Micronor
see Norethindrone
Midamor
see Amiloride
Midazolam
3 aprepitant, 186
4 aspirin, 217
4 atorvastatin, 259
3 carbamazepine, 372
3 clarithromycin, 578
3 clotrimazole, 621
3 conivaptan, 673
3 diltiazem, 872
4 echinacea, 936
3 erythromycin, 987
3 fluconazole, 1080
4 fluoxetine, 1105
3 grapefruit juice, 1208
3 itraconazole, 1314
3 ketoconazole, 1340
3 lopinavir/ritonavir, 1434
3 phenytoin, 1514
3 posaconazole, 1515
3 rifampin, 1515
3 ritonavir, 1516
3 saquinavir, 1517

1 = Avoid Combination **2** = Usually Avoid Combination **3** = Minimize Risk
4 = No Action Needed **5** = No Interaction

Midazolam *(cont.)*
3 St. John's wort, 1518
4 tacrolimus, 1519
3 telaprevir, 1519
3 telithromycin, 1520
5 terbinafine, 1521
3 troleandomycin, 1521
3 voriconazole, 1522
Midrin
see Isometheptene
Milnacipran
3 aspirin, 218
3 clonidine, 613
3 ibuprofen, 1246
2 linezolid, 1407
3 lithium, 1523
3 paroxetine, 1523
2 selegiline, 1524
3 sumatriptan, 1525
1 tranylcypromine, 1525
2 tryptophan, 1526
3 venlafaxine, 1526
Mineral Oil
4 contraceptives, oral, 1527
5 vitamin A, 1527
4 warfarin, 1528
Minipress
see Prazosin
Mintezol
see Thiabendazole
Mirtazapine
2 clonidine, 614
2 rasagiline, 1528
3 tramadol, 1836
4 venlafaxine, 1529
Misoprostol
3 phenylbutazone, 1529
Mitomycin
2 vinblastine, 1530
Mitotane
1 spironolactone, 1531
3 warfarin, 1531
Mobic
see Meloxicam
Moclobemide
4 cimetidine, 493
2 citalopram, 565
2 clomipramine, 603
1 dextromethorphan, 785
2 ephedrine, 964
4 fluoxetine, 1106
4 fluvoxamine, 1136
3 levodopa, 1384
5 lithium, 1417
2 rizatriptan, 1532
3 selegiline, 1533

Moclobemide *(cont.)*
3 tyramine, 1534
Modafinil
4 clozapine, 629
3 contraceptives, oral, 1535
3 cyclosporine, 730
3 triazolam, 1535
Mogadon
see Nitrazepam
Monistat
see Miconazole
Montelukast
3 gemfibrozil, 1181
4 prednisone, 1536
Moricizine
4 antipyrine, 178
3 cimetidine, 494
4 digoxin, 842
3 theophylline, 1536
5 warfarin, 1537
Morphine
3 lidocaine, 1401
4 nifedipine, 1537
4 ranitidine, 1538
3 rifampin, 1538
3 somatostatin, 1539
4 tramadol, 1540
3 trovafloxacin, 1540
Motrin
see Ibuprofen
Moxalactam
2 warfarin, 1541
Moxifloxacin
3 antacids, 162
3 iron, 1296
5 ranitidine, 1542
3 sucralfate, 1542
2 ziprasidone, 1543
Mucomyst
see Acetylcysteine
Mutamycin
see Mitomycin
Mycamine
see Micafungin
Mycelex
see Clotrimazole
Mycobutin
see Rifabutin
Mycophenolate Mofetil
2 iron, 1296
5 St. John's wort, 1792
Myochrysine
see Gold
Mysoline
see Primidone

Nabumetone
2 warfarin, 1545
Nadolol
4 erythromycin, 988
4 neomycin, 1546
4 phenelzine, 1546
Nafcillin
3 cyclosporine, 730
2 nifedipine, 1547
3 warfarin, 1548
Nalfon
see Fenoprofen
Nalidixic Acid
4 probenecid, 1548
3 warfarin, 1549
NAPA
see N-Acetyl-Procainamide
Naprosyn
see Naproxen
Naproxen
3 alendronate, 32
4 antacids, 163
4 aspirin, 218
3 cyclosporine, 731
5 diazepam, 802
4 febuxostat, 1049
3 lithium, 1418
2 methotrexate, 1478
4 probenecid, 1549
2 warfarin, 1550
5 zidovudine, 1551
Nardil
see Phenelzine
Nateglinide
3 fluconazole, 1080
4 rifampin, 1551
Navane
see Thiothixene
Nebcin
see Tobramycin
Nebivolol
4 cimetidine, 494
3 digoxin, 843
3 quinidine, 1552
3 verapamil, 1553
Nefazodone
2 cisapride, 550
4 clozapine, 629
4 contraceptives, oral, 677
3 digoxin, 843
3 erlotinib, 978
3 fluoxetine, 1107
3 loratadine, 1436
3 paroxetine, 1553

1 = Avoid Combination　**2** = Usually Avoid Combination　**3** = Minimize Risk
4 = No Action Needed　**5** = No Interaction

Nefazodone *(cont.)*
  2 pimozide, 1554
  2 simvastatin, 1555
  3 tacrolimus, 1555
NegGram
  see Nalidixic Acid
Nelfinavir
  3 atorvastatin, 259
  4 bupropion, 310
  3 felodipine, 1054
  4 indinavir, 1262
  4 ketoconazole, 1341
  3 methadone, 1556
  3 nevirapine, 1557
  3 omeprazole, 1557
  2 rifampin, 1558
  3 saquinavir, 1559
  3 sildenafil, 1559
  2 simvastatin, 1560
  4 zidovudine, 1561
Nembutal
  see Pentobarbital
Neo-Fradin
  see Neomycin
Neo-Synephrine
  see Phenylephrine
Neo-Tabs
  see Neomycin
Neomycin
  3 digoxin, 844
  1 methotrexate, 1479
  4 nadolol, 1546
  3 penicillin V, 1561
  4 vitamin B$_{12}$, 1562
  3 warfarin, 1562
Neoral
  see Cyclosporine
Neostigmine
  3 procainamide, 1563
  3 propranolol, 1564
  4 quinidine, 1564
Neurontin
  see Gabapentin
Nevirapine
  3 atazanavir, 240
  3 exemestane, 1042
  3 fluconazole, 1081
  3 methadone, 1469
  3 nelfinavir, 1557
  4 rifampin, 1565
Nexium
  see Esomeprazole
Niacin
  see Nicotinic Acid
Nicardipine
  3 cyclosporine, 732
  4 grapefruit juice, 1209

Nicardipine *(cont.)*
  3 propranolol, 1566
Nicorette
  see Nicotine
Nicotine
  3 adenosine, 30
  3 cimetidine, 495
Nicotinic Acid
  4 aspirin, 219
  4 ethanol, 1015
  3 lovastatin, 1439
Nifedipine
  4 amoxicillin, 127
  4 caffeine, 336
  4 carbamazepine, 373
  4 cefixime, 399
  3 cimetidine, 496
  4 clarithromycin, 579
  4 cyclosporine, 732
  3 diltiazem, 873
  3 doxazosin, 912
  4 fluoxetine, 1107
  3 food, 1155
  4 *Ginkgo biloba*, 1189
  4 ginseng, 1190
  3 grapefruit juice, 1210
  5 indomethacin, 1271
  4 insulin, 1283
  3 itraconazole, 1315
  3 magnesium, 1447
  4 micafungin, 1511
  4 morphine, 1537
  2 nafcillin, 1547
  4 omeprazole, 1567
  4 orlistat, 1567
  3 phenobarbital, 1568
  3 phenytoin, 1569
  3 propranolol, 1569
  3 quinidine, 1571
  3 quinupristin/
     dalfopristin, 1572
  3 rifampin, 1572
  4 rosiglitazone, 1573
  3 St. John's wort, 1573
  3 tacrolimus, 1574
  4 tamsulosin, 1575
  3 vincristine, 1575
  3 voriconazole, 1576
Nilotinib
  3 food, 1156
  3 grapefruit juice, 1211
  3 ketoconazole, 1342
  3 rifampin, 1577
Nimodipine
  3 cimetidine, 497
  3 grapefruit juice, 1212
  3 valproic acid, 1577

Nimotop
  see Nimodipine
Nipride
  see Nitroprusside
Nisoldipine
  3 cimetidine, 497
  3 grapefruit juice, 1212
  3 ketoconazole, 1342
Nitrazepam
  5 warfarin, 1578
Nitrendipine
  3 cimetidine, 498
  4 digoxin, 844
Nitrofurantoin
  4 phenytoin, 1578
  4 propantheline, 1579
Nitroglycerin
  4 acetylcysteine, 23
  4 aspirin, 220
  2 ergotamine, 972
  3 ethanol, 1016
  1 tadalafil, 1579
  1 vardenafil, 1580
Nitroprusside
  3 clonidine, 615
  3 diltiazem, 874
Nizatidine
  4 ethanol, 1017
Nizoral
  see Ketoconazole
Nolvadex
  see Tamoxifen
Nordette-28
  see Contraceptives, Oral
Norepinephrine
  4 dextroamphetamine,
     782
  3 guanethidine, 1225
  2 imipramine, 1256
  4 lithium, 1419
  3 methyldopa, 1489
  3 phenelzine, 1580
Norethindrone
  1 acitretin, 26
Norflex
  see Orphenadrine
Norfloxacin
  3 antacids, 163
  3 caffeine, 337
  4 cyclosporine, 733
  3 iron, 1297
  4 probenecid, 1581
  3 sucralfate, 1581
  3 theophylline, 1582
  3 warfarin, 1583
Normodyne
  see Labetalol

① = Avoid Combination   ② = Usually Avoid Combination   ▼③ = Minimize Risk
④ = No Action Needed   ⑤ = No Interaction

Noroxin
  see Norfloxacin

Norpace
  see Disopyramide

Norpramin
  see Desipramine

Nortriptyline
  4 bupropion, 311
  3 cimetidine, 499
  3 pentobarbital, 1584
  3 rifampin, 1584

Norvasc
  see Amlodipine

Norvir
  see Ritonavir

Nydrazid
  see Isoniazid

Ofloxacin
  3 antacids, 164
  5 cyclosporine, 733
  4 food, 1156
  4 iron, 1298
  3 procainamide, 1586
  3 sucralfate, 1586
  3 warfarin, 1587

Olanzapine
  3 cigarette smoking, 1588
  3 ciprofloxacin, 533
  3 clomipramine, 604
  4 fluphenazine, 1126
  3 fluvoxamine, 1137
  4 haloperidol, 1233
  4 lisinopril, 1412
  4 marijuana, 1452
  3 ritonavir, 1589
  5 sertraline, 1589
  5 theophylline, 1590

Omeprazole
  4 antipyrine, 179
  4 aspirin, 220
  2 atazanavir, 240
  4 bismuth, 287
  3 carbamazepine, 374
  4 cilostazol, 468
  4 clarithromycin, 579
  3 clopidogrel, 619
  4 clorazepate, 620
  4 clozapine, 630
  4 cyclosporine, 734
  4 delavirdine, 768
  3 diazepam, 803
  3 digoxin, 845
  4 disulfiram, 901
  3 erlotinib, 978
  5 ethanol, 1018
  3 etravirine, 1036
  4 fluvoxamine, 1138

Omeprazole (cont.)
  3 indinavir, 1263
  3 itraconazole, 1316
  4 ketoconazole, 1343
  5 lidocaine, 1402
  4 lopinavir/ritonavir,
    1434
  3 methotrexate, 1480
  3 nelfinavir, 1557
  4 nifedipine, 1567
  3 phenytoin, 1590
  3 posaconazole, 1591
  3 raltegravir, 1592
  3 saquinavir, 1593
  3 St. John's wort, 1593
  4 tacrolimus, 1594
  4 tolbutamide, 1594
  4 trovafloxacin, 1595
  3 voriconazole, 1596
  4 warfarin, 1596

Omnipen-N
  see Ampicillin

Oncovin
  see Vincristine

Ondansetron
  4 cisplatin, 558
  4 cyclophosphamide, 701
  3 rifampin, 1597
  4 tramadol, 1598

Orange Juice
  3 fexofenadine, 1599

Orap
  see Pimozide

Orinase
  see Tolbutamide

Orlistat
  4 amiodarone, 1599
  5 amitriptyline, 115
  5 atenolol, 246
  5 atorvastatin, 260
  2 cyclosporine, 1600
  5 ethanol, 1018
  5 fluoxetine, 1600
  5 glyburide, 1197
  5 losartan, 1438
  5 metformin, 1468
  5 nifedipine, 1567
  5 phentermine, 1601
  5 simvastatin, 1601
  4 warfarin, 1602

Orphenadrine
  3 chlorpromazine, 437
  4 propoxyphene, 1602

Ortho-Novum
  see Contraceptives, Oral

Ortho-Novum 1/35
  see Ethinyl Estradiol

Orudis
  see Ketoprofen

Oruvail
  see Ketoprofen

Os-Cal
  see Calcium Carbonate

Ospolot
  see Sulthiame

Oxacillin
  3 methotrexate, 1481
  4 sulfamethoxy-
    pyridazine, 1603

Oxazepam
  4 paroxetine, 1603
  4 zidovudine, 1604

Oxcarbazepine
  3 contraceptives, oral,
    678
  3 furosemide, 1166

Oxybutynin
  3 carbamazepine, 374
  4 clomipramine, 604
  5 contraceptives, oral,
    679
  5 cyclosporine, 734
  4 itraconazole, 1317

Oxycodone
  3 carisoprodol, 391
  3 clarithromycin, 580
  3 fluvoxamine, 1139
  3 itraconazole, 1317
  3 rifampin, 1605
  3 ritonavir, 1605
  3 sertraline, 1606
  3 telithromycin, 1607
  3 voriconazole, 1607

Oxycontin
  see Oxycodone

Oxymetholone
  2 warfarin, 1608

Oxytetracycline
  4 tolbutamide, 1609

PABA
  see Para-Aminobenzoic
    Acid

Paclitaxel
  3 delavirdine, 769
  3 saquinavir, 1610

Pamelor
  see Nortriptyline

Pancreatic Extracts
  4 iron, 1298

Pancuronium
  2 polymyxin, 1610

Pantoprazole
  3 methotrexate, 1481

1 = Avoid Combination **2** = Usually Avoid Combination **3** = Minimize Risk

4 = No Action Needed **5** = No Interaction

Pantoprazole *(cont.)*
  5 phenytoin, 1611
Para-Aminobenzoic Acid
  (PABA)
  4 aspirin, 221
  4 procainamide, 1611
  2 sulfamethoxazole, 1612
Paraplatin
  see Carboplatin
Parathyroid Hormone
  2 alendronate, 34
Pargyline
  1 metaraminol, 1468
  1 methotrimeprazine,
    1487
  4 methyldopa, 1490
Paricalcitol
  3 ketoconazole, 1344
Parlodel
  see Bromocriptine
Parnate
  see Tranylcypromine
Paroxetine
  5 antacids, 165
  4 aprepitant, 187
  3 aripiprazole, 195
  5 carbamazepine, 375
  3 cimetidine, 500
  4 codeine, 636
  5 diazepam, 804
  2 duloxetine, 931
  4 ethanol, 1019
  3 flecainide, 1068
  3 linezolid, 1407
  4 lithium, 1419
  1 methylene blue, 1493
  3 metoprolol, 1499
  3 milnacipran, 1523
  3 nefazodone, 1553
  4 oxazepam, 1603
  4 phenobarbital, 1612
  1 pimozide, 1613
  3 sumatriptan, 1614
  2 tamoxifen, 1615
  3 tetrabenazine. 1616
  3 thiazides, 1617
  2 thioridazine, 1619
  3 tramadol, 1620
  3 warfarin, 1621
  4 zolpidem, 1622
PAS
  see Aminosalicylic Acid
Pavulon
  see Pancuronium
Paxil
  see Paroxetine
Pectin
  3 lovastatin, 1440

Pefloxacin
  3 antacids, 166
  5 cyclosporine, 735
  4 rifampin, 1622
  3 theophylline, 1623
Pen-Vee
  see Penicillin V
Penetrex
  see Enoxacin
Penicillamine
  3 antacids, 167
  3 digoxin, 846
  3 iron, 1299
Penicillin G
  3 chloramphenicol, 413
  3 erythromycin, 988
  3 tetracycline, 1623
  4 warfarin, 1624
Penicillin V
  3 neomycin, 1561
Pentazocine
  3 aspirin, 221
  4 cigarette smoking, 463
  4 fluoxetine, 1108
Penthrane
  see Methoxyflurane
Pentobarbital
  3 alprenolol, 64
  3 nortriptyline, 1584
Pentothal
  see Thiopental
Pentoxifylline
  3 ciprofloxacin, 533
  3 theophylline, 1625
Pepcid
  see Famotidine
Pepto-Bismol
  see Bismuth
Periactin
  see Cyproheptadine
Perphenazine
  4 codeine, 637
Persantine
  see Dipyridamole
Phenelzine
  1 bupropion, 312
  5 carbamazepine, 375
  4 chlordiazepoxide, 417
  1 clomipramine, 605
  3 cyclobenzaprine, 699
  4 cyproheptadine, 756
  1 dexfenfluramine, 779
  1 dextromethorphan, 786
  4 doxapram, 911
  4 epinephrine, 967

Phenelzine *(cont.)*
  1 ethanol, 1019
  1 fenfluramine, 1057
  3 guanethidine, 1225
  2 imipramine, 1257
  3 levodopa, 1385
  2 lithium, 1420
  1 meperidine, 1459
  4 nadolol, 1546
  3 norepinephrine, 1580
  1 phenylephrine, 1625
  1 pseudoephedrine, 1626
  3 reserpine, 1627
  1 sibutramine, 1628
  3 succinylcholine, 1628
  1 venlafaxine, 1629
Phenformin
  4 warfarin, 1630
Phenindione
  4 haloperidol, 1233
Phenmetrazine
  4 amobarbital, 126
  4 chlorpromazine, 438
Phenobarbital
  3 acetaminophen, 10
  4 antipyrine, 180
  4 carbamazepine, 376
  3 chloramphenicol, 414
  3 chlorpromazine, 438
  4 cimetidine, 501
  4 clonazepam, 608
  3 contraceptives, oral,
    679
  4 cyclophosphamide, 701
  3 cyclosporine, 735
  3 digitoxin, 828
  3 disopyramide, 894
  5 disulfiram, 902
  4 doxorubicin, 914
  3 doxycycline, 916
  3 ethanol, 1020
  3 exemestane, 1042
  3 felbamate, 1050
  3 griseofulvin, 1222
  4 lidocaine, 1402
  3 meperidine, 1460
  3 methadone, 1470
  5 methyldopa, 1490
  4 metronidazole, 1503
  3 nifedipine, 1568
  4 paroxetine, 1612
  4 phenylbutazone, 1630
  3 phenytoin, 1631
  3 prednisone, 1632
  3 primidone, 1633
  3 propafenone, 1634
  4 propoxyphene, 1635
  3 protriptyline, 1635
  4 pyridoxine, 1636

❶ = Avoid Combination ❷ = Usually Avoid Combination ▼❸ = Minimize Risk
❹ = No Action Needed ❺ = No Interaction

Phenobarbital *(cont.)*
  3 quinidine, 1637
  3 theophylline, 1637
  3 valproic acid, 1638
  3 verapamil, 1639
  2 warfarin, 1640
Phenprocoumon
  3 azathioprine, 273
  2 flurbiprofen, 1128
Phentermine
  5 orlistat, 1601
Phenylbutazone
  4 desipramine, 779
  4 digitoxin, 829
  4 levodopa, 1386
  3 lithium, 1420
  2 methotrexate, 1482
  3 misoprostol, 1529
  4 phenobarbital, 1630
  3 phenytoin, 1641
  2 tolbutamide, 1642
  1 warfarin, 1644
Phenylephrine
  3 guanethidine, 1226
  3 imipramine, 1258
  4 levodopa, 1386
  1 phenelzine, 1625
  3 propranolol, 1645
Phenytoin
  3 acetaminophen, 12
  3 acetazolamide, 20
  4 allopurinol, 52
  4 aminosalicylic acid, 81
  3 amiodarone, 98
  4 antacids, 167
  3 bromfenac, 293
  3 capecitabine, 342
  3 carbamazepine, 377
  3 chloramphenicol, 415
  4 chlorpheniramine, 425
  3 cimetidine, 501
  3 ciprofloxacin, 534
  3 cisplatin, 559
  3 clobazam, 596
  4 clonazepam, 608
  3 colesevelam, 662
  3 contraceptives, oral,
      680
  4 cyclophosphamide, 702
  3 cyclosporine, 736
  3 diazoxide, 809
  4 diltiazem, 874
  3 disopyramide, 894
  3 disulfiram, 902
  3 dopamine, 911
  3 doxycycline, 916
  3 ethanol, 1021
  3 exemestane, 1043
  3 felbamate, 1051

Phenytoin *(cont.)*
  3 fluconazole, 1082
  3 fluorouracil, 1096
  3 fluoxetine, 1108
  3 fluvoxamine, 1140
  3 folic acid, 1148
  3 furosemide, 1167
  3 gamma globulin, 1172
  4 halothane, 1237
  3 influenza vaccine, 1279
  2 irinotecan, 1292
  3 isoniazid, 1301
  2 itraconazole, 1318
  5 ketoconazole, 1345
  3 lamotrigine, 1378
  3 levodopa, 1387
  4 lidocaine, 1403
  3 lithium, 1421
  4 loxapine, 1445
  2 mebendazole, 1453
  3 meperidine, 1460
  2 methadone, 1470
  4 methylphenidate, 1495
  3 metronidazole, 1504
  3 metyrapone, 1506
  3 mexiletine, 1506
  3 midazolam, 1514
  3 nifedipine, 1569
  4 nitrofurantoin, 1578
  3 omeprazole, 1590
  5 pantoprazole, 1611
  3 phenobarbital, 1631
  3 phenylbutazone, 1641
  3 posaconazole, 1646
  3 primidone, 1647
  3 pyridoxine, 1648
  3 quetiapine, 1648
  3 quinidine, 1649
  3 rifampin, 1649
  4 sertraline, 1650
  3 simvastatin, 1651
  3 sucralfate, 1652
  3 sulfaphenazole, 1652
  3 sulthiame, 1653
  3 tacrolimus, 1654
  3 teniposide, 1654
  5 terfenadine, 1655
  3 theophylline, 1655
  3 thyroid, 1656
  3 ticlopidine, 1657
  3 tolbutamide, 1657
  3 trimethoprim, 1658
  3 valproic acid, 1659
  3 vigabatrin, 1660
  3 voriconazole, 1661
  3 warfarin, 1662
  4 zidovudine, 1663
Phosphate Iodide
  see Echothiophate Iodide

Pimozide
  2 aprepitant, 187
  2 clarithromycin, 581
  2 ketoconazole, 1345
  2 nefazodone, 1554
  1 paroxetine, 1613
  2 ritonavir, 1664
  1 sertraline, 1664
  1 thioridazine, 1665
  2 verapamil, 1666
  2 voriconazole, 1666
  2 ziprasidone, 1667
Pindolol
  4 trimethoprim, 1668
Pioglitazone
  3 gemfibrozil, 1182
  5 itraconazole, 1318
  4 ketoconazole, 1346
  3 rifampin, 1668
Pipemidic Acid
  3 caffeine, 337
Piribedil
  4 clonidine, 615
Pirmenol
  4 digoxin, 846
Piroxicam
  5 aspirin, 222
  3 cholestyramine, 453
  3 lithium, 1422
  2 warfarin, 1669
Pitavastatin
  2 cyclosporine, 737
  3 erythromycin, 989
  3 rifampin, 1670
Placidyl
  see Ethchlorvynol
Plaquenil
  see Hydroxychloroquine
Platinol-AQ
  see Cisplatin
Plavix
  see Clopidogrel
Plendil
  see Felodipine
Polio Vaccine
  1 methotrexate, 1483
Polymyxin
  2 pancuronium, 1610
Pondimin
  see Fenfluramine
Ponstel
  see Mefenamic Acid
Pontocaine
  see Tetracaine
Posaconazole
  3 cimetidine, 502

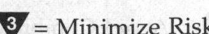

❶ = Avoid Combination   ❷ = Usually Avoid Combination   ▼❸ = Minimize Risk
❹ = No Action Needed   ❺ = No Interaction

Posaconazole *(cont.)*
  3 cyclosporine, 738
  3 lovastatin, 1441
  3 midazolam, 1515
  3 omeprazole, 1591
  3 phenytoin, 1646
  3 rifabutin, 1671
  3 rifampin, 1671
  3 simvastatin, 1672
  3 tacrolimus, 1807
  3 vincristine, 1673
Posicor
  see Mibefradil
Potaba
  see Para-Aminobenzoic
    Acid
Potassium
  3 acetohexamide, 22
  3 disopyramide, 895
  3 drospirenone, 927
  4 glycopyrrolate, 1200
  2 spironolactone, 1674
  2 triamterene, 1675
Potassium Iodide
  3 lithium, 1423
Practolol
  3 disopyramide, 896
Prandin
  see Repaglinide
Prasugrel
  4 bupropion, 312
Pravachol
  see Pravastatin
Pravastatin
  3 cholestyramine, 454
  3 colchicine, 655
  4 cyclosporine, 738
  4 digoxin, 847
  5 diltiazem, 875
  3 efavirenz, 940
  5 erythromycin, 990
  5 fluconazole, 1083
  3 gemfibrozil, 1182
  5 itraconazole, 1319
  4 rifampin, 1675
  5 St. John's wort, 1676
  5 warfarin, 1676
Praziquantel
  3 chloroquine, 424
  3 cimetidine, 503
  2 rifampin, 1677
Prazosin
  3 ethanol, 1022
  3 indomethacin, 1272
  3 propranolol, 1678
  3 verapamil, 1679
Precose
  see Acarbose

Prednisolone
  3 azathioprine, 273
  3 contraceptives, oral,
    681
  3 cyclosporine, 739
  4 glycyrrhizin, 1201
  3 isoniazid, 1302
  4 ketoconazole, 1346
  3 mercaptopurine, 1465
  3 rifampin, 1680
Prednisone
  4 antacids, 168
  3 aspirin, 223
  3 clarithromycin, 582
  4 cyclophosphamide, 702
  3 indomethacin, 1272
  3 insulin, 1284
  4 interferon, 1289
  3 intrauterine proges-
    terone system, 1291
  4 montelukast, 1536
  3 phenobarbital, 1632
  4 warfarin, 1680
Prelone
  see Prednisolone
Preludin
  see Phenmetrazine
Prevacid
  see Lansoprazole
Priftin
  see Rifapentine
Prilosec
  see Omeprazole
Primaquine
  4 grapefruit juice, 1213
  5 mefloquine, 1457
Primaxin
  see Imipenem
Primidone
  3 acetazolamide, 20
  4 clonazepam, 609
  4 clorazepate, 621
  3 exemestane, 1043
  4 isoniazid, 1303
  3 phenobarbital, 1633
  3 phenytoin, 1647
  3 valproic acid, 1681
Principen
  see Ampicillin
Prinivil
  see Lisinopril
Pro-Banthine
  see Propantheline
Probenecid
  4 acyclovir, 27
  4 allopurinol, 53
  4 ampicillin, 132

Probenecid *(cont.)*
  3 aspirin, 224
  4 bumetanide, 302
  4 ceftizoxime, 402
  4 chlorpropamide, 445
  4 ciprofloxacin, 534
  3 dapsone, 760
  3 dyphylline, 935
  4 enoxacin, 955
  4 famotidine, 1047
  4 furosemide, 1167
  4 gemifloxacin, 1185
  4 indomethacin, 1273
  4 ketoprofen, 1374
  2 methotrexate, 1484
  4 nalidixic acid, 1548
  4 naproxen, 1549
  4 norfloxacin, 1581
  4 rifampin, 1681
  4 sulfinpyrazone, 1682
  3 thiopental, 1682
  3 zidovudine, 1683
Probucol
  3 cyclosporine, 740
Procainamide
  5 acetazolamide, 21
  4 N-acetylprocainamide,
    24
  3 amiodarone, 99
  5 ammonium chloride,
    125
  3 cimetidine, 504
  4 ethanol, 1023
  4 isoniazid, 1303
  4 levofloxacin, 1391
  4 lidocaine, 1403
  3 neostigmine, 1563
  3 ofloxacin, 1586
  4 para-aminobenzoic
    acid, 1611
  4 propranolol, 1683
  3 quinidine, 1684
  4 ranitidine, 1685
  5 sodium bicarbonate,
    1685
  5 sucralfate, 1686
  2 thioridazine, 1686
  3 trimethoprim, 1687
Procan SR
  see Procainamide
Procarbazine
  1 ethanol, 1023
  3 prochlorperazine, 1688
Procardia
  see Nifedipine
Prochlorperazine
  4 contraceptives, oral,
    682

1 = Avoid Combination   **2** = Usually Avoid Combination   **3** = Minimize Risk
4 = No Action Needed   **5** = No Interaction

Prochlorperazine *(cont.)*
  3 procarbazine, 1688
Progestasert
  see Intrauterine Proges-
    terone System (IUDs)
Progestins
  4 warfarin, 1689
Prograf
  see Tacrolimus
Proguanil
  3 efavirenz, 940
Prolixin
  see Fluphenazine Decano-
    ate
Proloprim
  see Trimethoprim
Promazine
  3 attapulgite, 265
Pronestyl
  see Procainamide
Propafenone
  3 bupropion, 313
  3 cimetidine, 505
  4 codeine, 638
  2 colchicine, 1689
  4 cyclosporine, 740
  3 digoxin, 847
  4 duloxetine, 931
  3 fluoxetine, 1109
  3 food, 1157
  4 lidocaine, 1404
  3 metoprolol, 1500
  3 phenobarbital, 1634
  3 quinidine, 1690
  3 rifampin, 1691
  3 theophylline, 1692
  2 thioridazine, 1693
  3 warfarin, 1694
Propantheline
  4 acetaminophen, 13
  3 amitriptyline, 116
  4 atenolol, 246
  4 cefprozil, 401
  5 digoxin, 848
  4 nitrofurantoin, 1579
Propofol
  4 ethanol, 1024
Propoxyphene
  2 carbamazepine, 378
  4 cigarette smoking, 463
  4 codeine, 639
  3 contrast media,
  4 dextromethorphan, 787
  3 doxepin, 913
  3 ethanol, 1024
  3 metoprolol, 1500
  4 orphenadrine, 1602

Propoxyphene *(cont.)*
  4 phenobarbital, 1635
  2 rasagiline, 1694
  4 spironolactone, 1695
  3 tamoxifen, 1695
  3 warfarin, 1696
Propranolol
  4 acetaminophen, 13
  4 antacids, 168
  3 antipyrine, 180
  3 chlorpromazine, 439
  5 cholestyramine, 455
  3 cimetidine, 506
  3 clonidine, 616
  3 cocaine, 633
  3 contrast media, 693
  4 diazepam, 804
  3 digoxin, 849
  3 diltiazem, 875
  3 dronedarone, 920
  3 epinephrine, 967
  4 ergotamine, 972
  4 ethanol, 1025
  3 etintidine, 1034
  3 flecainide, 1069
  3 fluoxetine, 1110
  4 furosemide, 1168
  4 glimepiride, 1192
  4 glucagon, 1195
  4 halofenate, 1229
  4 hydralazine, 1240
  3 indomethacin, 1274
  3 insulin, 1285
  3 isoproterenol, 1307
  4 levodopa, 1387
  3 lidocaine, 1404
  4 lithium, 1423
  4 lovastatin, 1442
  4 marijuana, 1452
  4 methyldopa, 1491
  5 metoclopramide, 1497
  3 neostigmine, 1564
  3 nicardipine, 1566
  3 nifedipine, 1569
  3 phenylephrine, 1645
  3 prazosin, 1678
  4 procainamide, 1683
  3 quinidine, 1697
  5 ranitidine, 1698
  3 rizatriptan, 1699
  5 sumatriptan, 1699
  3 tacrine, 1700
  4 tetracaine, 1701
  2 theophylline, 1702
  4 thiazides, 1703
  4 tubocurarine, 1703
  3 verapamil, 1704
  4 warfarin, 1705

Propulsid
  see Cisapride
Propylthiouracil
  3 warfarin, 1706
Prostigmin
  see Neostigmine
Protonix
  see Pantoprazole
Protriptyline
  3 phenobarbital, 1635
Proventil
  see Albuterol
Provera
  see Medroxyprogesterone
Provigil
  see Modafinil
Prozac
  see Fluoxetine
Pseudoephedrine
  4 ammonium chloride,
    125
  3 antacids, 169
  4 kaolin-pectin, 1333
  4 linezolid, 1408
  1 phenelzine,
  2 rasagiline, 1707
Psyllium
  5 warfarin, 1708
Purinethol
  see Mercaptopurine
Pyrazinamide
  3 cyclosporine, 741
Pyridostigmine Bromide
  4 methocarbamol, 1477
Pyridoxine (Vitamin B$_6$)
  3 levodopa, 1388
  4 phenobarbital, 1636
  3 phenytoin, 1648
Pyrimethamine
  2 folic acid, 1149

Questran
  see Cholestyramine
Quetiapine
  3 citalopram, 566
  3 erythromycin, 990
  3 ethanol, 1025
  3 ketoconazole, 1347
  3 phenytoin, 1648
  3 ritonavir, 1709
  4 thioridazine, 1709
Quilinggao
  3 warfarin, 1710
Quinacrine
  4 codeine, 640

1 = Avoid Combination   **2** = Usually Avoid Combination   **3** = Minimize Risk

4 = No Action Needed   **5** = No Interaction

Quinidex
see Quinidine
Quinidine
3 acetazolamide, 21
4 amantadine, 68
3 amiloride, 75
3 amiodarone, 100
3 antacids, 170
3 aripiprazole, 196
3 carbamazepine, 379
3 cimetidine, 507
5 ciprofloxacin, 535
2 codeine, 641
2 colchicine, 1710
3 dextromethorphan, 788
3 digoxin, 850
3 diltiazem, 876
4 diphenoxylate, 888
4 disopyramide, 897
3 duloxetine, 932
3 encainide, 953
3 erythromycin, 991
3 fentanyl, 1061
3 fluvoxamine, 1140
4 grapefruit juice, 1214
3 haloperidol, 1234
3 imipramine, 1259
3 itraconazole, 1319
3 kaolin-pectin, 1334
3 ketoconazole, 1348
4 loperamide, 1432
3 metoprolol, 1501
3 mexiletine, 1507
3 nebivolol, 1552
4 neostigmine, 1564
3 nifedipine, 1571
3 phenobarbital, 1637
3 phenytoin, 1649
3 procainamide, 1684
3 propafenone, 1690
3 propranolol, 1697
3 rifampin, 1711
3 sodium bicarbonate, 1712
5 tacrine, 1712
2 tamoxifen, 1713
3 tetrabenazine, 1714
1 thioridazine, 1714
3 timolol, 1715
3 tubocurarine, 1716
5 valproic acid, 1717
3 verapamil, 1717
2 voriconazole, 1718
3 warfarin, 1719
2 ziprasidone, 1719
Quinidine Sulfate
4 flecainide, 1070
Quinine
4 acetazolamide, 22

Quinine (cont.)
4 amantadine, 68
3 cigarette smoking, 464
3 digoxin, 851
4 flecainide, 1071
4 ketoconazole, 1348
4 sodium bicarbonate, 1720
Quinora
see Quinidine
Quinupristin/Dalfopristin
3 cyclosporine, 742
3 nifedipine, 1572

Radioactive Iodine
3 theophylline, 1721
Raloxifene
3 levothyroxine, 1721
Raltegravir
3 atazanavir, 241
3 efavirenz, 941
3 omeprazole, 1592
3 rifampin, 1722
Ramelteon
3 atazanavir, 242
2 ciprofloxacin, 535
2 enoxacin, 956
2 ethanol, 1026
3 fluconazole, 1083
1 fluvoxamine, 1141
3 ketoconazole, 1349
3 mexiletine, 1508
3 rifampin, 1723
3 tacrine, 1723
3 thiabendazole, 1724
3 zileuton, 1724
Ranexa
see Ranolazine
Ranitidine
5 acetaminophen, 14
4 antacids, 171
3 cefpodoxime proxetil, 399
3 cefuroxime, 404
5 chlormethiazole, 418
5 cifenline, 459
5 cyclosporine, 742
4 didanosine, 823
3 enoxacin, 956
4 fosamprenavir, 1160
4 gefitinib, 1177
3 glipizide, 1193
3 itraconazole, 1320
3 ketoconazole, 1350
4 lidocaine, 1405
4 morphine, 1538
5 moxifloxacin, 1542
4 procainamide, 1685

Ranitidine (cont.)
5 propranolol, 1698
4 saquinavir, 1725
5 sucralfate, 1725
5 theophylline, 1726
4 triamterene, 1727
5 voriconazole, 1728
5 warfarin, 1728
5 zidovudine, 1729
Ranolazine
3 digoxin, 852
3 diltiazem, 877
3 ketoconazole, 1350
3 rifampin, 1730
3 simvastatin, 1730
3 verapamil, 1731
Rapamune
see Sirolimus
Rasagiline
3 ciprofloxacin, 536
2 clomipramine, 606
2 cyclobenzaprine, 699
2 dextromethorphan, 788
2 fluoxetine, 1111
1 fluvoxamine, 1141
2 meperidine, 1461
2 methadone, 1471
2 mirtazapine, 1528
2 propoxyphene, 1694
2 pseudoephedrine, 1707
2 St. John's wort, 1792
2 tramadol, 1837
1 tranylcypromine, 1839
Rebetol
see Ribavirin
Reglan
see Metoclopramide
Relafen
see Nabumetone
Relpax
see Eletriptan
Remeron
see Mirtazapine
Renagel
see Sevelamer
Repaglinide
5 cimetidine, 508
3 clarithromycin, 583
3 cyclosporine, 743
3 deferasirox, 767
3 gemfibrozil, 1183
4 grapefruit juice, 1214
3 itraconazole, 1321
4 ketoconazole, 1351
3 rifampin, 1732
3 trimethoprim, 1733
Requip
see Ropinirole

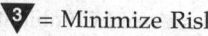

Rescriptor
see Delavirdine
Reserpine
4 ephedrine, 965
3 phenelzine, 1627
1 tetrabenazine, 1733
4 warfarin, 1734
Restoril
see Temazepam
Retrovir
see Zidovudine
Reyataz
see Atazanavir
Rheumatrex
see Methotrexate
Rhinocort
see Budesonide
Ribavirin
3 azathioprine, 274
3 warfarin, 1734
Rifabutin
3 amprenavir, 135
3 atazanavir, 242
1 clarithromycin, 583
3 contraceptives, oral, 682
3 delavirdine, 770
4 didanosine, 823
3 efavirenz, 941
3 fluconazole, 1084
3 indinavir, 1264
5 methadone, 1471
3 posaconazole, 1671
3 ritonavir, 1735
3 saquinavir, 1736
5 theophylline, 1736
3 tipranavir, 1737
3 voriconazole, 1737
4 zidovudine, 1738
Rifadin
see Rifampin
Rifampin
3 alfentanil, 37
3 aliskiren, 44
3 aminosalicylic acid, 81
3 amiodarone, 100
3 amprenavir, 136
3 aprepitant, 188
2 atazanavir, 243
4 atenolol, 247
3 atorvastatin, 260
3 bupropion, 313
3 buspirone, 323
4 carvedilol, 396
3 caspofungin, 397
4 celecoxib, 406
3 chloramphenicol, 415

Rifampin *(cont.)*
5 ciprofloxacin, 537
3 clarithromycin, 584
3 clofibrate, 598
3 clopidogrel, 620
3 codeine, 643
3 contraceptives, oral, 683
2 cyclosporine, 744
3 dapsone, 761
3 dasatinib, 766
3 deferasirox, 768
3 delavirdine, 770
3 diazepam, 805
3 digitoxin, 830
3 digoxin, 852
3 diltiazem, 878
3 disopyramide, 897
3 dronedarone, 921
3 efavirenz, 942
3 erlotinib, 979
3 everolimus, 1040
3 exemestane, 1044
3 fentanyl, 1062
3 fesoterodine, 1065
4 fexofenadine, 1066
3 fluconazole, 1085
3 fluvastatin, 1132
3 gefitinib, 1177
4 glimepiride, 1192
4 glipizide, 1194
3 glyburide, 1197
4 haloperidol, 1234
4 halothane, 1237
3 hexobarbital, 1239
3 imatinib, 1251
3 isoniazid, 1304
3 itraconazole, 1322
3 ketoconazole, 1352
3 lamotrigine, 1379
4 linezolid, 1409
3 lorcainide, 1438
3 losartan, 1439
2 lurasidone, 1445
3 maraviroc, 1448
3 methadone, 1472
3 metoprolol, 1502
3 mexiletine, 1508
3 midazolam, 1515
3 morphine, 1538
4 nateglinide, 1551
2 nelfinavir, 1558
4 nevirapine, 1565
3 nifedipine, 1572
3 nilotinib, 1577
3 nortriptyline, 1584
3 ondansetron, 1597
3 oxycodone, 1605
4 pefloxacin, 1622

Rifampin *(cont.)*
3 phenytoin, 1649
3 pioglitazone, 1668
3 pitavastatin, 1670
3 posaconazole, 1671
4 pravastatin, 1675
2 praziquantel, 1677
3 prednisolone, 1680
4 probenecid, 1681
3 propafenone, 1691
3 quinidine, 1711
3 raltegravir, 1722
3 ramelteon, 1723
3 ranolazine, 1730
3 repaglinide, 1732
3 ritonavir, 1739
3 ropivacaine, 1739
3 rosiglitazone, 1740
2 saquinavir, 1740
3 saxagliptin, 1741
2 simvastatin, 1742
3 sirolimus, 1784
4 sulfasalazine, 1742
3 sunitinib, 1743
3 tacrolimus, 1743
3 tadalafil, 1744
3 tamoxifen, 1745
4 tamsulosin, 1745
2 telaprevir, 1746
3 theophylline, 1746
3 ticagrelor, 1747
3 tocainide, 1748
3 tolbutamide, 1748
3 tolvaptan, 1749
3 triazolam, 1750
4 trimethoprim/
sulfamethoxazole,
1750
3 verapamil, 1751
2 voriconazole, 1752
2 warfarin, 1753
3 zaleplon, 1753
3 zidovudine, 1754
4 zolmitriptan, 1755
3 zolpidem, 1755
3 zopiclone, 1756
Rifapentine
3 indinavir, 1265
Rimactane
see Rifampin
Rimantadine
4 cimetidine, 508
3 contraceptives, oral,
Risedronate
3 antacids, 1757
3 calcium, 1757
Risperdal
see Risperidone

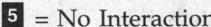 = Avoid Combination   = Usually Avoid Combination  = Minimize Risk
 = No Action Needed   = No Interaction

Risperidone
  3 carbamazepine, 379
  4 clozapine, 630
  4 fluoxetine, 1112
  3 itraconazole, 1322
  4 maprotiline, 1448
  4 marijuana, 1453
  4 valproic acid, 1758

Ritalin
  see Methylphenidate

Ritonavir
  1 alfuzosin, 41
  3 budesonide, 301
  4 bupropion, 314
  3 buspirone, 323
  3 carbamazepine, 380
  2 cisapride, 551
  4 clarithromycin, 585
  2 colchicine, 656
  2 conivaptan, 673
  3 contraceptives, oral, 684
  3 desipramine, 777
  4 didanosine, 824
  3 digoxin, 853
  3 efavirenz, 943
  2 ergotamine, 973
  3 erythromycin, 992
  3 fentanyl, 1062
  4 fluconazole, 1085
  4 fluoxetine, 1112
  3 fluticasone, 1130
  3 indinavir, 1265
  3 ketoconazole, 1353
  4 loperamide, 1433
  3 maraviroc, 1449
  3 methadone, 1472
  3 midazolam, 1516
  3 olanzapine, 1589
  3 oxycodone, 1605
  2 pimozide, 1664
  3 quetiapine, 1709
  3 rifabutin, 1735
  3 rifampin, 1739
  3 saquinavir, 1758
  3 sildenafil, 1759
  2 simvastatin, 1779
  3 tadalafil, 1760
  4 telaprevir, 1760
  3 theophylline, 1761
  4 tipranavir, 1762
  4 trimethoprim/
      sulfamethoxazole,
      1762
  3 vardenafil, 1763
  3 vincristine, 1763
  4 zidovudine, 1764
  see also Tipranavir/
      Ritonavir

Rivastigmine
  3 atenolol, 247

Rizatriptan
  2 moclobemide, 1532
  3 propranolol, 1699

Robaxin
  see Methocarbamol

Robinul
  see Glycopyrrolate

Robitussin-DM
  see Dextromethorphan

Rocephin
  see Ceftriaxone

Rofecoxib
  3 enalapril, 951
  3 lisinopril, 1413
  3 lithium, 1764
  4 tizanidine, 1765
  4 warfarin, 1766

Roferon-A
  see Interferon Alfa-2a

Ropinirole
  3 ciprofloxacin, 537
  5 digoxin, 854

Ropivacaine
  3 ciprofloxacin, 538
  3 rifampin, 1739

Rosiglitazone
  3 ketoconazole, 1354
  4 nifedipine, 1573
  3 rifampin, 1740
  4 trimethoprim, 1766

Rosuvastatin
  4 cyclosporine, 745
  5 fenofibrate, 1058

Roxanol
  see Morphine

Roxithromycin
  3 cyclosporine, 745
  4 theophylline, 1767

Rozerem
  see Ramelteon

Rythmol
  see Propafenone

Sabril
  see Vigabatrin

Salmeterol
  3 ketoconazole, 1354

Sandimmune
  see Cyclosporine

Saquinavir
  3 efavirenz, 943
  4 fluconazole, 1086
  3 garlic, 1173
  3 grapefruit juice, 1215

Saquinavir *(cont.)*
  3 ketoconazole, 1355
  3 maraviroc, 1450
  3 midazolam, 1517
  3 nelfinavir, 1559
  3 omeprazole, 1593
  3 paclitaxel, 1610
  4 ranitidine, 1725
  3 rifabutin, 1736
  2 rifampin, 1740
  3 ritonavir, 1758
  3 sildenafil, 1768
  3 tipranavir, 1768

Saxagliptin
  3 diltiazem, 878
  3 ketoconazole, 1356
  3 rifampin, 1741

Secobarbital
  3 methoxyflurane, 1488

Seldane
  see Terfenadine

Selegiline
  3 contraceptives, oral, 685
  2 dextromethorphan, 789
  2 fluoxetine, 1113
  2 meperidine, 1462
  2 milnacipran, 1524
  3 moclobemide, 1533
  5 tacrine, 1769
  3 tyramine, 1770

Sensipar
  see Cinacalcet

Sensorcaine
  see Bupivacaine

Serax
  see Oxazepam

Serlect
  see Sertindole

Seromycin
  see Cycloserine

Seroquel
  see Quetiapine

Serpalan
  see Reserpine

Sertindole
  4 erythromycin, 992

Sertraline
  4 aripiprazole, 197
  4 bupropion, 314
  3 cisapride, 551
  4 clozapine, 631
  4 cyclosporine, 746
  4 diazepam, 805
  4 erythromycin, 993
  5 ethanol, 1026
  4 haloperidol, 1235

❶ = Avoid Combination **❷** = Usually Avoid Combination **❸** = Minimize Risk
4 = No Action Needed **5** = No Interaction

Sertraline *(cont.)*
4 lamotrigine, 1380
3 levothyroxine, 1399
3 linezolid, 1409
4 metoclopramide, 1497
5 olanzapine, 1589
3 oxycodone, 1606
4 phenytoin, 1650
1 pimozide, 1664
3 sumatriptan, 1770
3 tamoxifen, 1772
4 tolbutamide, 1773
3 tramadol, 1773
3 warfarin, 1774
4 zolpidem, 1775
Serzone
see Nefazodone
Sevelamer
3 levothyroxine, 1399
Siberian Ginseng
4 digoxin, 854
Sibutramine
2 dextromethorphan, 790
2 dihydroergotamine, 867
2 fluoxetine, 1113
2 lithium, 1424
2 meperidine, 1463
1 phenelzine, 1628
2 sumatriptan, 1775
2 tryptophan, 1776
Sildenafil
5 azithromycin, 277
3 cimetidine, 509
3 ciprofloxacin, 538
3 clarithromycin, 586
4 dihydrocodeine, 867
3 diltiazem, 879
3 erythromycin, 994
3 etravirine, 1037
3 fluvoxamine, 1142
3 grapefruit juice, 1216
3 indinavir, 1266
1 isosorbide mononitrate, 1308
3 ketoconazole, 1357
3 nelfinavir, 1559
3 ritonavir, 1759
3 saquinavir, 1768
4 simvastatin, 1777
2 telaprevir, 1777
5 tolbutamide, 1778
Silodosin
5 digoxin, 855
3 ketoconazole, 1357
Simethicone
4 warfarin, 1778
Simvastatin
2 amiodarone, 101

Simvastatin *(cont.)*
2 atazanavir, 243
3 carbamazepine, 381
3 cisapride, 552
2 clarithromycin, 586
3 colchicine, 657
2 conivaptan, 674
3 cyclosporine, 746
3 dronedarone, 922
3 efavirenz, 944
2 erythromycin, 995
3 fluconazole, 1087
4 glyburide, 1198
3 grapefruit juice, 1216
2 itraconazole, 1323
2 ketoconazole, 1358
2 nefazodone, 1555
2 nelfinavir, 1560
5 orlistat, 1601
3 phenytoin, 1651
3 posaconazole, 1672
3 ranolazine, 1730
2 rifampin, 1742
2 ritonavir, 1779
4 sildenafil, 1777
3 St. John's wort, 1780
3 tacrolimus, 1780
2 telithromycin, 1781
3 ticagrelor, 1782
5 tolbutamide, 1782
2 verapamil, 1783
4 warfarin, 1784
Sinequan
see Doxepin
Singulair
see Montelukast
Sintrom
see Acenocoumarol
Sirolimus
3 clarithromycin, 587
3 diltiazem, 880
3 dronedarone, 922
3 fluconazole, 1087
3 itraconazole, 1324
3 ketoconazole, 1359
4 micafungin, 1512
3 rifampin, 1784
2 voriconazole, 1785
Slo-Phyllin
see Theophylline
Sodium Bicarbonate
3 flecainide, 1071
3 lithium, 1424
3 methenamine, 1475
3 mexiletine, 1509
5 procainamide, 1685
3 quinidine, 1712
4 quinine, 1720

Sodium Chloride
3 lithium, 1425
Sodium Polystyrene Sulfonate Resin
3 antacids, 172
Solfoton
see Phenobarbital
Solifenacin
3 ketoconazole, 1359
Soma
see Carisoprodol
Somatostatin
3 methadone, 1473
3 morphine, 1539
Sonata
see Zaleplon
Soriatane
see Acitretin
Sotalol
3 amiodarone, 102
3 flecainide, 1072
4 telithromycin, 1814
2 ziprasidone, 1786
Sparfloxacin
4 cisapride, 553
3 sucralfate, 1787
2 ziprasidone, 1787
Sparine
see Promazine
Spiramycin
3 levodopa, 1389
Spironolactone
3 ammonium chloride, 126
4 aspirin, 224
3 candesartan, 1789
3 digoxin, 855
3 enalapril, 1790
4 lithium, 1425
1 mitotane, 1531
2 potassium, 1674
4 propoxyphene, 1695
4 warfarin, 1791
Sporanox
see Itraconazole
Sprycel
see Dasatinib
St. John's Wort
4 alprazolam, 64
4 amitriptyline, 117
3 contraceptives, oral, 686
2 cyclosporine, 747
3 digoxin, 856
3 duloxetine, 932
3 erlotinib, 979
3 exemestane, 1044

1 = Avoid Combination **2** = Usually Avoid Combination **3** = Minimize Risk

4 = No Action Needed **5** = No Interaction

St. John's Wort *(cont.)*
2 imatinib, 1251
1 indinavir, 1267
1 irinotecan, 1293
2 ixabepilone, 1331
2 maraviroc, 1450
3 methadone, 1474
3 midazolam, 1518
5 mycophenolate mofetil, 1792
3 nifedipine, 1573
3 omeprazole, 1593
5 pravastatin, 1676
2 rasagiline, 1792
3 simvastatin, 1780
2 tacrolimus, 1793
4 theophylline, 1793
3 warfarin, 1794
Starlix
see Nateglinide
Stavudine
5 didanosine, 824
4 food, 1157
Stelazine
see Trifluoperazine
Strattera
see Atomoxetine
Streptase
see Streptokinase
Streptokinase
4 heparin, 1238
Sublimaze
see Fentanyl
Succinylcholine
3 amphotericin B, 130
4 aprotinin, 189
3 cyclophosphamide, 703
4 diazepam, 806
3 digoxin, 857
2 echothiophate iodide, 936
4 lidocaine, 1406
4 lithium, 1426
3 magnesium, 1447
3 phenelzine, 1628
3 tacrine, 1795
Sucralfate
5 acetaminophen, 15
5 aspirin, 225
4 chlorpropamide, 445
5 cimetidine, 509
3 ciprofloxacin, 539
4 digoxin, 858
5 ibuprofen, 1247
3 ketoconazole, 1360
3 levothyroxine, 1400
3 moxifloxacin, 1542
3 norfloxacin, 1581

Sucralfate *(cont.)*
3 ofloxacin, 1586
3 phenytoin, 1652
5 procainamide, 1686
5 ranitidine, 1725
3 sparfloxacin, 1787
4 theophylline, 1796
3 trovafloxacin, 1796
3 warfarin, 1797
Sudafed
see Pseudoephedrine
Sufenta
see Sufentanil
Sufentanil
5 erythromycin, 995
Sular
see Nisoldipine
Sulfadiazine
3 methenamine, 1476
Sulfamethoxazole
4 fluconazole, 1088
2 para-aminobenzoic acid, 1612
see also Trimethoprim/ Sulfamethoxazole
Sulfamethoxypyridazine
4 oxacillin, 1603
Sulfaphenazole
3 phenytoin, 1652
Sulfasalazine
4 digoxin, 858
4 rifampin, 1742
3 talinolol, 1798
Sulfinpyrazone
3 aspirin, 225
4 probenecid, 1682
4 sulfisoxazole, 1798
3 tolbutamide, 1799
2 warfarin, 1799
Sulfisoxazole
4 sulfinpyrazone, 1798
4 thiopental, 1800
Sulindac
4 aspirin, 226
3 cyclosporine, 748
4 lithium, 1426
5 tolbutamide, 1801
2 warfarin, 1802
Sulphadimidine
3 cyclosporine, 749
Sulthiame
3 phenytoin, 1653
Sumatriptan
1 dihydroergotamine, 868
1 ergotamine, 974
3 fluoxetine, 1114
4 lithium, 1427

Sumatriptan *(cont.)*
1 methysergide, 1496
3 milnacipran, 1525
3 paroxetine, 1614
5 propranolol, 1699
3 sertraline, 1770
2 sibutramine, 1775
3 venlafaxine, 1803
Sumycin
see Tetracycline
Sunitinib
3 ketoconazole, 1361
3 rifampin, 1743
Suprane
see Desflurane
Suprax
see Cefixime
Surmontil
see Trimipramine
Sustiva
see Efavirenz
Sutent
see Sunitinib
Symmetrel
see Amantadine
Synalgos-DC
see Dihydrocodeine
Synercid
see Quinupristin/ Dalfopristin
Synthroid
see Levothyroxine

Tacrine
3 bethanechol, 284
3 cigarette smoking, 464
3 cimetidine, 510
5 diazepam, 807
4 digoxin, 859
3 enoxacin, 957
2 fluvoxamine, 1143
4 haloperidol, 1236
4 ibuprofen, 1247
3 levodopa, 1390
3 propranolol, 1700
5 quinidine, 1712
3 ramelteon, 1723
5 selegiline, 1769
3 succinylcholine, 1795
3 theophylline, 1805
3 trihexyphenidyl, 1805
5 warfarin, 1806
Tacrolimus
4 bromocriptine, 297
3 caspofungin, 398
3 clarithromycin, 588
3 clotrimazole, 622

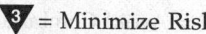

Tacrolimus *(cont.)*
3 diltiazem, 880
4 ergotamine, 974
3 erythromycin, 996
3 ethanol, 1027
3 fluconazole, 1089
3 itraconazole, 1324
3 ketoconazole, 1361
4 lansoprazole, 1381
4 metoclopramide, 1498
4 midazolam, 1519
3 nefazodone, 1555
3 nifedipine, 1574
4 omeprazole, 1594
3 phenytoin, 1654
3 posaconazole, 1807
3 rifampin, 1743
3 simvastatin, 1780
2 St. John's wort, 1793
4 tamoxifen, 1807
2 telaprevir, 1808
3 voriconazole, 1809
Tadalafil
3 bosentan, 290
3 doxazosin, 1809
3 ketoconazole, 1362
1 nitroglycerin, 1579
3 rifampin, 1744
3 ritonavir, 1760
4 tamsulosin, 1810
Tagamet
see Cimetidine
Talinolol
3 sulfasalazine, 1798
Talwin
see Pentazocine
Tambocor
see Flecainide
Tamoxifen
2 aminoglutethimide, 78
3 chloroquine, 424
3 cimetidine, 511
3 cinacalcet, 523
2 colchicine, 1811
3 diphenhydramine, 885
2 fluoxetine, 1115
3 haloperidol, 1236
3 imatinib, 1252
2 paroxetine, 1615
3 propoxyphene, 1695
2 quinidine, 1713
3 rifampin, 1745
3 sertraline, 1772
4 tacrolimus, 1807
3 terbinafine, 1815
Tamsulosin
4 atenolol, 248
3 cimetidine, 512

Tamsulosin *(cont.)*
5 digoxin, 859
4 enalapril, 952
4 erythromycin, 997
4 fluoxetine, 1117
4 ketoconazole, 1363
4 nifedipine, 1575
4 rifampin, 1745
4 tadalafil, 1810
5 theophylline, 1821
Tapentadol
3 almotriptan, 1811
3 clomipramine, 1812
3 fluoxetine, 1812
1 tranylcypromine, 1813
Tarceva
see Erlotinib
Taxol
see Paclitaxel
Tegison
see Etretinate
Tegretol
see Carbamazepine
Tekturna
see Aliskiren
Telaprevir
3 amlodipine, 122
2 atorvastatin, 261
2 colchicine, 658
2 cyclosporine, 750
3 digoxin, 860
3 ketoconazole, 1363
3 midazolam, 1519
2 rifampin, 1746
3 ritonavir, 1760
2 sildenafil, 1777
2 tacrolimus, 1808
Telithromycin
3 digoxin, 860
2 lovastatin, 1442
3 midazolam, 1520
3 oxycodone, 1607
2 simvastatin, 1781
4 sotalol, 1814
4 warfarin, 1814
Telmisartan
3 digoxin, 861
Temafloxacin
4 cimetidine, 513
4 warfarin, 1815
Temazepam
5 erythromycin, 997
4 itraconazole, 1325
Tenex
see Guanfacine
Tenidap
5 digoxin, 861

Teniposide
3 phenytoin, 1654
Tenofovir
4 atazanavir, 244
3 didanosine, 825
Tenormin
see Atenolol
Tenoxicam
4 aspirin, 227
Tensilon
see Edrophonium
Tenuate
see Diethylpropion
Tequin
see Gatifloxacin
Terbinafine
3 dextromethorphan, 790
5 digoxin, 862
5 midazolam, 1521
3 tamoxifen, 1815
5 triazolam, 1816
Terbutaline
3 furosemide, 1169
2 metoprolol, 1503
Terfenadine
5 azithromycin, 277
5 cimetidine, 513
2 clarithromycin, 589
5 dirithromycin, 888
1 erythromycin, 998
3 fluconazole, 1090
2 fluoxetine, 1117
1 fluvoxamine, 1143
3 grapefruit juice, 1217
1 itraconazole, 1326
1 ketoconazole, 1364
3 phenytoin, 1655
5 theophylline, 1816
2 troleandomycin, 1817
3 zafirlukast, 1818
Terramycin
see Oxytetracycline
Testosterone
4 fluconazole, 1091
Tetrabenazine
3 paroxetine, 1616
3 quinidine, 1714
1 reserpine, 1733
1 tranylcypromine, 1818
Tetracaine
3 propranolol, 1701
Tetracyclines
3 antacids, 173
2 bismuth, 288
3 colestipol, 667
3 contraceptives, oral, 687

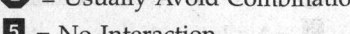

1 = Avoid Combination **2** = Usually Avoid Combination **3** = Minimize Risk

4 = No Action Needed **5** = No Interaction

Tetracyclines *(cont.)*
3 digoxin, 862
3 food, 1158
3 iron, 1299
4 lithium, 1428
2 methoxyflurane, 1489
3 penicillin G, 1623
4 theophylline, 1819
4 thiazides, 1820
3 zinc, 1820

Teveten
see Eprosartan

Thalidomide
5 contraceptives, oral,
688

Thalomid
see Thalidomide

Theo-24
see Theophylline

Theo-Dur
see Theophylline

Theolair
see Theophylline

Theophylline
3 adenosine, 31
3 allopurinol, 54
3 aminoglutethimide, 78
3 amiodarone, 103
5 azithromycin, 278
3 carbamazepine, 381
3 cigarette smoking, 465
3 cimetidine, 514
3 ciprofloxacin, 540
4 clarithromycin, 589
3 clinafloxacin, 594
4 contraceptives, oral,
688
4 dirithromycin, 889
4 disulfiram, 903
2 enoxacin, 958
4 ephedrine, 965
3 erythromycin, 998
2 febuxostat, 1049
5 fluconazole, 1091
2 fluvoxamine, 1144
4 furosemide, 1170
4 hydrocortisone, 1241
3 imipenem, 1253
4 influenza vaccine, 1280
3 interferon, 1289
3 isoniazid, 1304
4 ketoconazole, 1365
5 levofloxacin, 1392
3 lithium, 1428
4 methotrexate, 1485
2 mexiletine, 1510
3 moricizine, 1536
3 norfloxacin, 1582

Theophylline *(cont.)*
5 olanzapine, 1590
3 pefloxacin, 1623
3 pentoxifylline, 1625
3 phenobarbital, 1637
3 phenytoin, 1655
3 propafenone, 1692
2 propranolol, 1702
3 radioactive iodine, 1721
5 ranitidine, 1726
5 rifabutin, 1736
3 rifampin, 1746
3 ritonavir, 1761
4 roxithromycin, 1767
4 St. John's wort, 1793
4 sucralfate, 1796
3 tacrine, 1805
5 tamsulosin, 1821
5 terfenadine, 1816
4 tetracycline, 1819
3 thiabendazole, 1821
3 thyroid, 1822
3 ticlopidine, 1823
4 tocainide, 1823
2 troleandomycin, 1824
5 trovafloxacin, 1824
3 verapamil, 1825
4 vidarabine, 1826
3 zafirlukast, 1827

Thiabendazole
3 ramelteon, 1724
3 theophylline, 1821

Thiazides
3 calcium, 339
3 citalopram, 567
3 colestipol, 668
3 diazoxide, 810
4 indomethacin, 1275
3 insulin, 1287
3 methotrexate, 1486
3 paroxetine, 1617
4 propranolol, 1703
4 tetracycline, 1820
5 valacyclovir, 1827
4 warfarin, 1828

Thiopental
3 probenecid, 1682
4 sulfisoxazole, 1800

Thioridazine
1 amiodarone, 103
3 bromocriptine, 297
5 carbamazepine, 382
3 cigarette smoking, 466
3 cinacalcet, 523
4 codeine, 644
2 diphenhydramine, 886
2 disopyramide, 898
4 droperidol, 924
1 duloxetine, 933

Thioridazine *(cont.)*
2 fluoxetine, 1118
2 fluvoxamine, 1145
2 paroxetine, 1619
1 pimozide, 1665
2 procainamide, 1686
2 propafenone, 1693
4 quetiapine, 1709
1 quinidine, 1714
2 ziprasidone, 1829

Thiothixene
3 guanethidine, 1227

Thorazine
see Chlorpromazine

Thyroid
3 carbamazepine, 382
3 cholestyramine, 455
4 contraceptives, oral,
689
4 ketamine, 1335
4 lovastatin, 1443
3 phenytoin, 1656
3 theophylline, 1822
3 warfarin, 1830
see also Levothyroxine

Ticagrelor
4 digoxin, 863
3 diltiazem, 881
2 ketoconazole, 1365
3 rifampin, 1747
3 simvastatin, 1782

Ticlid
see Ticlopidine

Ticlopidine
4 antacids, 174
3 bupropion, 315
3 cyclosporine, 751
4 digoxin, 863
3 phenytoin, 1657
3 theophylline, 1823
4 warfarin, 1831

Tigecycline
4 warfarin, 1831

Tikosyn
see Dofetilide

Timolol
3 quinidine, 1715

Tindamax
see Tinidazole

Tinidazole
3 ethanol, 1027

Tipranavir
3 amprenavir, 137
4 antacids, 174
3 atorvastatin, 262
3 clarithromycin, 590
3 efavirenz, 945

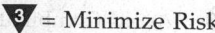

❶ = Avoid Combination ❷ = Usually Avoid Combination ❸ = Minimize Risk
④ = No Action Needed ⑤ = No Interaction

Tipranavir *(cont.)*
   3 ethinyl estradiol, 1033
   3 etravirine, 1038
   3 fluconazole, 1092
   3 lopinavir/ritonavir, 1435
   5 maraviroc, 1451
   3 rifabutin, 1737
   4 ritonavir, 1762
   3 saquinavir, 1768
   3 vitamin E, 1832
   3 zidovudine, 1832
Tizanidine
   3 cimetidine, 515
   2 ciprofloxacin, 541
   3 contraceptives, oral, 690
   3 ethanol, 1028
   2 fluvoxamine, 1146
   3 lisinopril, 1414
   3 mexiletine, 1511
   4 rofecoxib, 1765
Tobramycin
   3 carbenicillin, 389
   3 miconazole, 1512
Tocainide
   3 antacids, 175
   4 cimetidine, 516
   3 rifampin, 1748
   4 theophylline, 1823
Tofranil
   see Imipramine
Tolazamide
   3 doxepin, 913
Tolbutamide
   4 aprepitant, 188
   3 cimetidine, 516
   3 dicumarol, 816
   4 diltiazem, 882
   5 disulfiram, 904
   1 ethanol, 1028
   3 fluconazole, 1092
   4 fluvastatin, 1133
   3 halofenate, 1229
   3 ketoconazole, 1366
   3 methandrostenolone, 1475
   4 methyldopa, 1492
   4 omeprazole, 1594
   4 oxytetracycline, 1609
   2 phenylbutazone, 1642
   3 phenytoin, 1657
   3 rifampin, 1748
   4 sertraline, 1773
   5 sildenafil, 1778
   5 simvastatin, 1782
   3 sulfinpyrazone, 1799
   5 sulindac, 1801

Tolbutamide *(cont.)*
   3 trimethoprim/ sulfamethoxazole, 1833
Tolectin
   see Tolmetin
Tolinase
   see Tolazamide
Tolmetin
   4 aspirin, 227
   2 warfarin, 1834
Toloxatone
   3 tyramine, 1835
Tolterodine
   4 fluoxetine, 1119
   3 ketoconazole, 1367
   4 warfarin, 1836
Tolvaptan
   4 digoxin, 864
   4 grapefruit juice, 1218
   3 ketoconazole, 1368
   3 rifampin, 1749
Tonocard
   see Tocainide
Topamax
   see Topiramate
Topiramate
   3 contraceptives, oral, 690
   4 lithium, 1429
Toradol
   see Ketorolac
Tracleer
   see Bosentan
Tracrium
   see Atracurium
Tramadol
   3 amitriptyline, 117
   3 citalopram, 568
   3 duloxetine, 933
   3 fluoxetine, 1120
   3 mirtazapine, 1836
   4 morphine, 1540
   4 ondansetron, 1598
   3 paroxetine, 1620
   2 rasagiline, 1837
   3 sertraline, 1773
   2 tranylcypromine, 1837
   3 venlafaxine, 1838
Tranxene
   see Clorazepate
Tranylcypromine
   3 amobarbital, 127
   1 atomoxetine, 251
   4 chlorpromazine, 440
   1 dextroamphetamine, 782

Tranylcypromine *(cont.)*
   3 disulfiram, 904
   1 duloxetine, 934
   1 fluoxetine, 1121
   3 insulin, 1287
   1 linezolid, 1410
   1 milnacipran, 1525
   1 rasagiline, 1839
   1 tapentadol, 1813
   1 tetrabenazine, 1818
   2 tramadol, 1837
   1 tyramine, 1839
   1 venlafaxine, 1841
Trasylol
   see Aprotinin
Trazodone
   3 buspirone, 324
   3 chlorpromazine, 441
   4 fluoxetine, 1121
   4 tryptophan, 1841
   4 venlafaxine, 1842
   4 warfarin, 1842
Trental
   see Pentoxifylline
Triamterene
   3 amantadine, 69
   3 candesartan, 1843
   4 cimetidine, 518
   3 drospirenone, 927
   3 enalapril, 1844
   3 indomethacin, 1276
   2 potassium, 1675
   4 ranitidine, 1727
Triazolam
   5 azithromycin, 278
   3 clarithromycin, 591
   4 DHEA, 792
   3 diltiazem, 882
   3 erythromycin, 999
   2 fluconazole, 1093
   5 fluoxetine, 1122
   3 grapefruit juice, 1219
   3 isoniazid, 1305
   2 itraconazole, 1327
   3 ketoconazole, 1368
   3 modafinil, 1535
   3 rifampin, 1750
   5 terbinafine, 1816
   3 troleandomycin, 1845
Triclofos
   3 warfarin, 1845
Tricor
   see Fenofibrate
Trifluoperazine
   4 methyldopa, 1492
Trihexyphenidyl
   3 amantadine, 70
   4 levodopa, 1390

❶ = Avoid Combination ❷ = Usually Avoid Combination ❸ = Minimize Risk
❹ = No Action Needed ❺ = No Interaction

Trihexyphenidyl *(cont.)*
   3 tacrine, 1805
Trilafon
   see Perphenazine
Trileptal
   see Oxcarbazepine
Trimethoprim
   3 dapsone, 761
   4 digoxin, 864
   2 methotrexate, 1486
   3 phenytoin, 1658
   4 pindolol, 1668
   3 procainamide, 1687
   3 repaglinide, 1733
   4 rosiglitazone, 1766
   4 zidovudine, 1846
   see also Trimethoprim/
      Sulfamethoxazole
Trimethoprim/
   Sulfamethoxazole
   4 amantadine, 70
   4 cyclosporine, 751
   3 enalapril, 953
   4 glipizide, 1194
   3 glyburide, 1199
   4 lamivudine, 1378
   3 metronidazole, 1504
   4 rifampin, 1750
   4 ritonavir, 1762
   3 tolbutamide, 1833
   3 warfarin, 1847
Trimipramine
   4 venlafaxine, 1848
Troleandomycin
   3 alfentanil, 38
   3 carbamazepine, 383
   2 cisapride, 554
   3 clopidogrel, 1848
   3 fentanyl, 1063
   3 methylprednisolone,
      1495
   3 midazolam, 1521
   2 terfenadine, 1817
   2 theophylline, 1824
   3 triazolam, 1845
Trovafloxacin
   3 antacids, 175
   3 ferrous sulfate, 1064
   3 morphine, 1540
   4 omeprazole, 1595
   3 sucralfate, 1796
   5 theophylline, 1824
Trovan
   see Trovafloxacin
Tryptacin
   see Tryptophan
Tryptophan
   3 duloxetine, 934

Tryptophan *(cont.)*
   2 fluoxetine, 1122
   2 milnacipran, 1526
   2 sibutramine, 1776
   4 trazodone, 1841
Tubocurarine
   3 furosemide, 1170
   4 propranolol, 1703
   3 quinidine, 1716
Tylenol
   see Acetaminophen
Tyramine
   3 moclobemide, 1534
   3 selegiline, 1770
   3 toloxatone, 1835
   1 tranylcypromine, 1839

Uloric
   see Febuxostat
Ultram
   see Tramadol
Unipen
   see Nafcillin
Urea
   4 lithium, 1430
Ureaphil
   see Urea
Urecholine
   see Bethanechol
Urised
   see Methenamine
Urolene Blue
   see Methylene Blue

Valacyclovir
   5 thiazides, 1827
Valdecoxib
   3 lithium, 1850
Valium
   see Diazepam
Valproic Acid
   3 carbamazepine, 384
   3 chitosan, 408
   3 cholestyramine, 456
   3 cisplatin, 560
   3 clonazepam, 609
   3 clozapine, 631
   4 diazepam, 807
   3 ertapenem, 980
   3 erythromycin, 1000
   3 felbamate, 1052
   3 isoniazid, 1306
   3 lamotrigine, 1380
   3 meropenem, 1466
   3 nimodipine, 1577
   3 phenobarbital, 1638
   3 phenytoin, 1659

Valproic Acid *(cont.)*
   3 primidone, 1681
   5 quinidine, 1717
   4 risperidone, 1758
Valsartan
   4 aliskiren, 44
   2 atenolol, 249
Valtrex
   see Valacyclovir
Vancocin
   see Vancomycin
Vancomycin
   3 gentamicin, 1187
   3 indomethacin, 1277
   3 methotrexate, 1487
   4 vecuronium, 1850
Vantin
   see Cefpodoxime Proxetil
Vardenafil
   3 erythromycin, 1001
   3 indinavir, 1267
   3 ketoconazole, 1369
   1 nitroglycerin, 1580
   3 ritonavir, 1763
Vascor
   see Bepridil
Vasotec
   see Enalapril
Vecuronium
   4 vancomycin, 1850
   3 verapamil, 1851
Veetids
   see Penicillin V
Velban
   see Vinblastine
Venlafaxine
   5 aripiprazole, 197
   4 bupropion, 316
   3 desipramine, 777
   4 diphenhydramine, 887
   4 disulfiram, 905
   3 imipramine, 1259
   1 isocarboxazid, 1301
   3 ketoconazole, 1370
   3 linezolid, 1410
   3 lithium, 1430
   1 methylene blue, 1494
   4 metoclopramide, 1498
   3 milnacipran, 1526
   4 mirtazapine, 1529
   1 phenelzine, 1629
   3 sumatriptan, 1803
   3 tramadol, 1838
   1 tranylcypromine, 1841
   4 trazodone, 1842
   4 trimipramine, 1848
VePesid
   see Etoposide

1 = Avoid Combination   **2** = Usually Avoid Combination   **3** = Minimize Risk
4 = No Action Needed   **5** = No Interaction

Verapamil
4 aliskiren, 45
4 almotriptan, 57
3 antipyrine, 181
3 atorvastatin, 262
3 buspirone, 325
3 calcium, 340
2 carbamazepine, 385
4 ceftriaxone, 403
4 cigarette smoking, 1852
3 cimetidine, 518
3 clarithromycin, 591
3 clonazepam,
4 clonidine, 617
2 colchicine, 1852
4 colesevelam, 662
3 cyclosporine, 752
4 dantrolene, 759
3 diclofenac, 813
3 digoxin, 865
3 doxorubicin, 915
3 dronedarone, 923
3 eletriptan, 948
3 erythromycin, 1001
2 ethanol, 1029
4 etomidate, 1036
3 everolimus, 1040
4 fexofenadine, 1067
4 flecainide, 1072
4 grapefruit juice, 1220
3 imipramine, 1260
3 lithium, 1431
3 nebivolol, 1553
3 phenobarbital, 1639
2 pimozide, 1666
3 prazosin, 1679
3 propranolol, 1704
3 quinidine, 1717
3 ranolazine, 1731
3 rifampin, 1751
2 simvastatin, 1783
3 theophylline, 1825
1 tranylcypromine,
3 vecuronium, 1851

Vermox
see Mebendazole

Versed
see Midazolam

Vfend
see Voriconazole

Viagra
see Sildenafil

Vibramycin
see Doxycycline

Vidarabine
3 allopurinol, 55
4 theophylline, 1826

Videx
see Didanosine

Vigabatrin
5 contraceptives, oral,
691
3 phenytoin, 1660

Vinblastine
2 mitomycin, 1530

Vincristine
3 itraconazole, 1327
3 nifedipine, 1575
3 posaconazole, 1673
3 ritonavir, 1763
3 voriconazole, 1853

Vinorelbine
2 clarithromycin, 592
2 itraconazole, 1328

Vioxx
see Rofecoxib

Vira-A
see Vidarabine

Viracept
see Nelfinavir

Viramune
see Nevirapine

Viread
see Tenofovir

Vitamin A
3 acitretin, 26
5 mineral oil, 1527

Vitamin B$_6$
see Pyridoxine

Vitamin B$_{12}$
4 aminosalicylic acid, 82
4 neomycin, 1562

Vitamin C
1 amygdalin, 137
3 antacids, 176
5 choline salicylate, 458
4 ethanol, 1030
4 methenamine, 1477
3 warfarin, 1854

Vitamin E
3 iron, 1300
3 tipranavir, 1832
3 warfarin, 1855

Vitamin K
3 warfarin, 1855

Vivactil
see Protriptyline

Voltaren
see Diclofenac

Voriconazole
4 cimetidine, 519
3 cyclosporine, 753
3 diazepam, 808

Voriconazole (*cont.*)
5 digoxin, 866
3 efavirenz, 945
2 ergotamine, 975
3 ibuprofen, 1248
3 midazolam, 1522
3 nifedipine, 1576
3 omeprazole, 1596
3 oxycodone, 1607
3 phenytoin, 1661
2 pimozide, 1666
2 quinidine, 1718
5 ranitidine, 1728
3 rifabutin, 1737
2 rifampin, 1752
2 sirolimus, 1785
3 tacrolimus, 1809
3 vincristine, 1853
3 warfarin, 1856
3 zolpidem, 1857

Vumon
see Teniposide

Warfarin
3 acetaminophen, 15
5 alfuzosin, 41
3 allopurinol, 55
3 aminoglutethimide, 79
4 aminosalicylic acid, 82
3 amiodarone, 104
4 amitriptyline, 118
3 aprepitant, 189
2 aspirin, 228
5 atenolol, 249
2 azapropazone, 267
3 azathioprine, 275
5 azithromycin, 279
3 bezafibrate, 285
3 bosentan, 291
2 bromfenac, 294
5 bumetanide, 303
3 capecitabine, 342
3 carbamazepine, 386
4 celecoxib, 406
3 chitosan, 408
3 chloral hydrate, 410
5 chlordiazepoxide, 417
3 cholestyramine, 457
4 cigarette smoking, 466
2 cimetidine, 520
3 ciprofloxacin, 541
4 cisapride, 554
3 clarithromycin, 593
2 clofibrate, 598
3 colesevelam, 663
5 conivaptan, 674
2 contraceptives, oral,
692
4 cranberry juice, 693

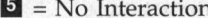

1 = Avoid Combination   **2** = Usually Avoid Combination   **3** = Minimize Risk
4 = No Action Needed   **5** = No Interaction

Warfarin *(cont.)*
3 cyclophosphamide, 703
4 cyclosporine, 753
2 danazol, 757
3 danshen, 758
2 dextrothyroxine, 791
5 diazepam, 808
4 diazoxide, 810
2 diclofenac, 814
4 dicloxacillin, 815
2 diflunisal, 827
4 diltiazem, 883
5 diphenhydramine, 888
4 disopyramide, 899
2 disulfiram, 905
5 dofetilide, 907
3 doxycycline, 918
3 erythromycin, 1002
4 ethacrynic acid, 1007
3 ethanol, 1031
2 etodolac, 1035
5 febuxostat, 1050
4 felbamate, 1052
5 felodipine, 1055
3 fenofibrate, 1058
2 fenoprofen, 1059
4 fish oil, 1068
3 fluconazole, 1094
3 fluorouracil, 1097
3 fluoxetine, 1123
5 flurazepam, 1127
3 fluvoxamine, 1147
3 furosemide, 1171
4 garlic, 1174
3 gemcitabine, 1178
2 gemfibrozil, 1184
4 ginger, 1188
2 *Ginkgo biloba*, 1189
3 ginseng, 1190
3 glucagon, 1196
2 glutethimide, 1196
3 glyburide, 1199
5 grapefruit juice, 1221
3 griseofulvin, 1222
3 heparin, 1238
2 ibuprofen, 1249
2 indomethacin, 1277
4 influenza vaccine, 1281
4 isoniazid, 1306
4 isotretinoin, 1308
3 itraconazole, 1329
3 ketoconazole, 1371
2 ketoprofen, 1375
4 levamisole, 1382
4 levofloxacin, 1392
3 lopinavir/ritonavir, 1436
3 lovastatin, 1444
2 meclofenamate, 1454

Warfarin *(cont.)*
2 mefenamic acid, 1455
3 mefloquine, 1457
3 menthol, 1458
5 meprobamate, 1463
3 mercaptopurine, 1466
3 mesalamine, 1467
2 metronidazole, 1505
3 miconazole, 1513
4 mineral oil, 1528
3 mitotane, 1531
5 moricizine, 1537
2 moxalactam, 1541
2 nabumetone, 1545
3 nafcillin, 1548
3 nalidixic acid, 1549
2 naproxen, 1550
3 neomycin, 1562
5 nitrazepam, 1578
3 norfloxacin, 1583
3 ofloxacin, 1587
4 omeprazole, 1596
4 orlistat, 1602
2 oxymetholone, 1608
3 paroxetine, 1621
4 penicillin G, 1624
4 phenformin, 1630
2 phenobarbital, 1640
1 phenylbutazone, 1644
3 phenytoin, 1662
2 piroxicam, 1669
5 pravastatin, 1676
4 prednisone, 1680
4 progestins, 1689
3 propafenone, 1694
3 propoxyphene, 1696
4 propranolol, 1705
3 propylthiouracil, 1706
5 psyllium, 1708
3 quilinggao, 1710
3 quinidine, 1719
5 ranitidine, 1728
3 reserpine, 1734
3 ribavirin, 1734
2 rifampin, 1753
4 rofecoxib, 1766
3 sertraline, 1774
4 simethicone, 1778
4 simvastatin, 1784
4 spironolactone, 1791
3 St. John's wort, 1794
3 sucralfate, 1797
2 sulfinpyrazone, 1799
2 sulindac, 1802
5 tacrine, 1806
4 telithromycin, 1814
4 temafloxacin, 1815
4 thiazides, 1828
3 thyroid, 1830

Warfarin *(cont.)*
4 ticlopidine, 1831
4 tigecycline, 1831
2 tolmetin, 1834
4 tolterodine, 1836
4 trazodone, 1842
3 triclofos, 1845
3 trimethoprim/ sulfamethoxazole, 1847
3 vitamin C, 1854
3 vitamin E, 1855
3 vitamin K, 1855
3 voriconazole, 1856
3 zafirlukast, 1858
Wellbutrin
  see Bupropion
Wine
  4 cisapride, 555
Wine, Red
  3 cyclosporine, 754
Wytensin
  see Guanabenz

Xanax
  see Alprazolam
Xenical
  see Orlistat
Xylocaine
  see Lidocaine

Zafirlukast
  3 aspirin, 230
  3 erythromycin, 1003
  3 terfenadine, 1818
  3 theophylline, 1827
  3 warfarin, 1858
Zagam
  see Sparfloxacin
Zalcitabine
  4 dapsone, 762
  5 foscarnet, 1161
Zaleplon
  3 rifampin, 1753
Zanaflex
  see Tizanidine
Zantac
  see Ranitidine
Zaroxolyn
  see Metolazone
Zecnil
  see Somatostatin
Zerit
  see Stavudine
Zetia
  see Ezetimibe

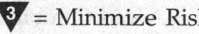

❶ = Avoid Combination **❷** = Usually Avoid Combination **▼❸** = Minimize Risk
❹ = No Action Needed **❺** = No Interaction

Zidovudine
4 acetaminophen, 17
4 acyclovir, 28
4 atovaquone, 263
5 azithromycin, 279
4 cimetidine, 521
4 clarithromycin, 594
5 dapsone, 762
4 didanosine, 826
4 fluconazole, 1095
3 food, 1159
5 foscarnet, 1161
1 ganciclovir, 1172
4 indinavir, 1268
3 interferon, 1290
5 itraconazole, 1330
4 methadone, 1474
5 naproxen, 1551
4 nelfinavir, 1561
4 oxazepam, 1604
4 phenytoin, 1663
3 probenecid, 1683
5 ranitidine, 1729
4 rifabutin, 1738
3 rifampin, 1754
4 ritonavir, 1764

Zidovudine *(cont.)*
3 tipranavir, 1832
4 trimethoprim, 1846
3 trimethoprim/
   sulfamethoxazole,
Zileuton
3 ramelteon, 1724
Zinc
3 ciprofloxacin, 542
3 tetracycline, 1820
Ziprasidone
3 carbamazepine, 387
2 dofetilide, 907
3 ketoconazole, 1371
2 moxifloxacin, 1543
2 pimozide, 1667
2 quinidine, 1719
2 sotalol, 1786
2 sparfloxacin, 1787
2 thioridazine, 1829
Zithromax
   see Azithromycin
Zocor
   see Simvastatin
Zofran
   see Ondansetron

Zolmitriptan
4 rifampin, 1755
Zoloft
   see Sertraline
Zolpidem
4 fluconazole, 1095
4 itraconazole, 1330
3 ketoconazole, 1372
4 paroxetine, 1622
3 rifampin, 1755
4 sertraline, 1775
3 voriconazole, 1857
Zomig
   see Zolmitriptan
Zopiclone
3 erythromycin, 1004
3 rifampin, 1756
Zovirax
   see Acyclovir
Zyloprim
   see Allopurinol
Zyprexa
   see Olanzapine
Zyvox
   see Linezolid

1 = Avoid Combination **2** = Usually Avoid Combination **3** = Minimize Risk
4 = No Action Needed **5** = No Interaction